**PART SEVEN  METABOLIC AND ELECTROLYTE DISORDERS, 816**

*Richard W. Nelson*
*Denise A. Elliott*

**54**  Disorders of Metabolism, 816
**55**  Electrolyte Imbalances, 828

**PART EIGHT  REPRODUCTIVE SYSTEM DISORDERS, 847**

*Cheri A. Johnson*

**56**  Disorders of the Estrous Cycle, 847
**57**  Disorders of the Vagina and Uterus, 870
**58**  Disorders of the Mammary Gland, 882
**59**  False Pregnancy, Disorders of Pregnancy, Parturition, and the Postpartum Period, 886
**60**  Disorders of Male Fertility, 905
**61**  Disorders of the Penis, Prepuce, and Testes, 918
**62**  Disorders of the Prostate Gland, 927
**63**  Genital Infections and Transmissible Venereal Tumor, 934
**64**  Artificial Insemination and Frozen Semen, 940

**PART NINE  NEUROMUSCULAR DISORDERS, 946**

*Susan M. Taylor*

**65**  The Neurologic Examination, 946
**66**  Diagnostic Tests for the Neuromuscular System, 961
**67**  Disorders of Locomotion, 974
**68**  Abnormalities of Mentation, Loss of Vision, and Pupillary Abnormalities, 983
**69**  Seizures, 991
**70**  Head Tilt, 1005
**71**  Encephalitis, Myelitis, and Meningitis, 1010
**72**  Disorders of the Spinal Cord, 1020
**73**  Disorders of Peripheral Nerves and the Neuromuscular Junction, 1049
**74**  Disorders of Muscle, 1062

**PART TEN  JOINT DISORDERS, 1071**

*Susan M. Taylor*

**75**  Clinical Manifestations of and Diagnostic Tests for Joint Disorders, 1071
**76**  Disorders of the Joints, 1079

**PART ELEVEN  ONCOLOGY, 1093**

*C. Guillermo Couto*

**77**  Cytology, 1093
**78**  Principles of Cancer Treatment, 1100
**79**  Practical Chemotherapy, 1103
**80**  Complications of Cancer Chemotherapy, 1108
**81**  Approach to the Patient with a Mass, 1117
**82**  Lymphoma in the Cat and Dog, 1122
**83**  Leukemias, 1133
**84**  Selected Neoplasms in Dogs and Cats, 1142

**PART TWELVE  HEMATOLOGY AND IMMUNOLOGY, 1156**

*C. Guillermo Couto*

**85**  Anemia, 1156
**86**  Erythrocytosis, 1170
**87**  Leukopenia and Leukocytosis, 1173
**88**  Combined Cytopenias and Leukoerythroblastosis, 1181
**89**  Disorders of Hemostasis, 1185
**90**  Lymphadenopathy and Splenomegaly, 1200
**91**  Hyperproteinemia, 1210
**92**  Immune-Mediated Diseases: Overview and Diagnosis, 1212
**93**  Immunosuppressive Drugs, 1216
**94**  Systemic Lupus Erythematosus, 1220
**95**  Fever of Undetermined Origin, 1222
**96**  Recurrent Infections, 1226

**PART THIRTEEN  INFECTIOUS DISEASES, 1229**

*Michael R. Lappin*

**97**  Laboratory Diagnosis of Infectious Diseases, 1229
**98**  Practical Antimicrobial Chemotherapy, 1240
**99**  Prevention of Infectious Diseases, 1250
**100**  Polysystemic Bacterial Diseases, 1259
**101**  Polysystemic Rickettsial Diseases, 1265
**102**  Polysystemic Viral Diseases, 1273
**103**  Polysystemic Mycotic Infections, 1287
**104**  Polysystemic Protozoal Infections, 1296
**105**  Zoonoses, 1307

# SMALL
# ANIMAL
# INTERNAL
# MEDICINE

# SMALL ANIMAL INTERNAL MEDICINE

## THIRD EDITION

**RICHARD W. NELSON,** DVM, DIPL. ACVIM
Professor, Department of Medicine and Epidemiology
School of Veterinary Medicine
University of California, Davis
Davis, California

**C. GUILLERMO COUTO,** DVM, DIPL. ACVIM
Professor, Department of Veterinary Clinical Sciences
College of Veterinary Medicine
Chief, Oncology/Hematology Service
Veterinary Teaching Hospital
The Ohio State University, Columbus, Ohio

*890 illustrations*

Mosby

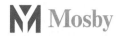

An Affiliate of Elsevier

11830 Westline Industrial Drive
St. Louis, Missouri 63146

---

NOTICE

Veterinary Medicine is an ever-changing field. Standard safety precautions must be followed, but as new research and clinical experience broaden our knowledge, changes in treatment and drug therapy may become necessary or appropriate. Readers are advised to check the most current product information provided by the manufacturer of each drug to be administered to verify the recommended dose, the method and duration of administration, and contraindications. It is the responsibility of the treating veterinarian, relying on experience and knowledge of the patient, to determine dosages and the best treatment for each individual patient. Neither the Publisher nor the editor assume any liability for any injury and/or damage to persons or property arising from this publication.

---

THIRD EDITION
Previous editions copyrighted 1992, 1998

**Library of Congress Cataloging-in-Publication Data**

Small animal internal medicine / [edited by] Richard W. Nelson, C. Guillermo Couto.—3rd ed.
    p.  cm.
    Includes bibliographical references and index.
    ISBN 0-323-01724-X
        1. Dogs—Diseases.  2. Cats—Diseases.  3. Veterinary internal medicine.  I. Nelson, Richard W. (Richard William), 1953-  II. Couto, C. Guillermo.

SF991.S5917   2003
636.7'0896—dc21                                           2003042106

*Senior Editor:* Elizabeth M. Fathman
*Managing Editor:* Teri Merchant
*Publishing Services Manager:* Linda McKinley
*Senior Project Manager:* Julie Eddy
*Designer:* Julia Dummitt
*Cover Art:* Kelli Bickman

Printed in China

Last digit is the print number:  9  8  7  6  5  4  3  2

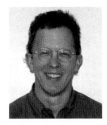

**RICHARD W. NELSON,** DVM, Dipl. ACVIM, Professor, Department of Medicine and Epidemiology, School of Veterinary Medicine, University of California, Davis. Dr. Nelson's interest lies in clinical endocrinology, with a special emphasis on disorders of the endocrine pancreas, thyroid gland, and adrenal gland. Dr. Nelson has authored numerous manuscripts and book chapters, has co-authored two textbooks, *Canine and Feline Endocrinology and Reproduction* with Dr. Ed Feldman and *Small Animal Internal Medicine* with Dr. Guillermo Couto, and has lectured extensively nationally and internationally. He was an Associate Editor for the *Journal of Veterinary Internal Medicine* and serves as a reviewer for several veterinary journals. Dr. Nelson is a co-founder and member of the Society for Comparative Endocrinology and a member of the European Society of Veterinary Endocrinology.

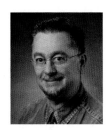

**C. GUILLERMO COUTO,** DVM, Dipl. ACVIM (Internal Medicine and Oncology), Professor, Department of Veterinary Clinical Sciences, College of Veterinary Medicine and Comprehensive Cancer Center, The Ohio State University. Dr. Couto earned his doctorate at Buenos Aires University, Argentina. Dr. Couto has been Editor-in-Chief of the *Journal of Veterinary Internal Medicine* and President of the Veterinary Cancer Society. He has received the Norden Distinguished Teaching Award, the OSU Clinical Teaching Award, and the BSAVA Bourgelat Award for outstanding contribution to small animal practice. Dr. Couto has published more than 250 articles and chapters in the areas of oncology, hematology, and immunology.

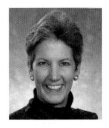

**SUSAN E. BUNCH,** DVM, PhD, Dipl. ACVIM, Professor of Medicine, Department of Clinical Sciences, College of Veterinary Medicine, North Carolina State University. Dr. Bunch is an internationally recognized veterinary internist with a special interest in hepatobiliary and pancreatic disorders of cats and dogs. Related to her interest in teaching simulator technology, she was awarded a Merck-AgVet Award for Teaching Creativity in 1997 and holds a U.S. patent for the Canine Abdominal Palpation Simulator. She has been invited to speak in the United States, Canada, Japan, and Western and Eastern Europe. She is a regular contributor to various journals and textbooks and is an invited reviewer for seven professional journals. Dr. Bunch has also been an active member of the ACVIM and, especially, of the Comparative Gastroenterology Society and Liver Study Group. She was named the NCVMA–Veterinary Teaching Hospital Clinician of the year in 1999.

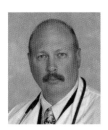

**GREGORY F. GRAUER,** DVM, MS, Dipl. ACVIM, Professor and Head of the Department of Clinical Sciences at the College of Veterinary Medicine, Kansas State University. Dr. Grauer received his DVM degree from Iowa State University in 1978 and completed his postgraduate training and MS degree at Colorado State University. He was a faculty member at the University of Wisconsin for 7 years and then returned to Colorado State University, where he served as Professor and Section Chief of Small Animal Medicine until 2000. Dr. Grauer has also served as President and Chairman of the Board of Regents of the American College of Veterinary Internal Medicine. His areas of clinical and research interest involve the small animal urinary system, specifically acute renal failure and proteinuric renal disease. He has authored more than 175 refereed scientific publications, abstracts, and book chapters and presented more than 750 hours of continuing education in the United States and abroad dealing with urinary tract disease in dogs and cats.

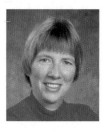

ELEANOR C. HAWKINS, DVM, Dipl. ACVIM (Internal Medicine), Professor, Department of Clinical Sciences, North Carolina State University College of Veterinary Medicine. Dr. Hawkins is an internationally recognized expert in respiratory diseases of the dog and cat. She is President-Elect of the specialty of Small Animal Internal Medicine of the American College of Veterinary Internal Medicine. She has served as a board member of the Comparative Respiratory Society (1991-1994). She has been invited to lecture in the United States, Europe, South America, and Japan. She is the author of many refereed publications and scientific proceedings. She has been a contributor or the respiratory editor for numerous well-known veterinary texts. Her areas of research include bronchoalveolar lavage as a diagnostic tool and canine chronic bronchitis.

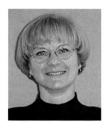

CHERI A. JOHNSON, DVM, MS, Dipl. ACVIM, Professor and Chief of Medicine, Department of Small Animal Clinical Sciences, College of Veterinary Medicine, Michigan State University. Dr. Johnson has been an invited speaker throughout North America and Europe. She has conducted research in areas relating to small animal internal medicine, particularly in reproduction and endocrinology. She has published numerous scientific articles and chapters and has served as an adhoc reviewer for several journals. Dr. Johnson has served on several committees in the ACVIM, including chairing the Credentials Committee. She is a member and past Secretary/Treasurer of the Society for Comparative Endocrinology. She is also a member of the AVMA and the Association for Women Veterinarians.

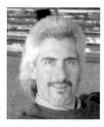

MICHAEL R. LAPPIN, DVM, PhD, Dipl. ACVIM, Professor of Small Animal Internal Medicine at the College of Veterinary Medicine and Biomedical Sciences at Colorado State University and Section Head of Small Animal Internal Medicine. After earning his DVM at Oklahoma State University in 1981, he completed a small animal internal medicine residency and earned his doctorate in parasitology at the University of Georgia. Dr. Lappin has studied feline infectious diseases and has authored more than 140 research papers and book chapters. Dr. Lappin is past Associate Editor for the *Journal of Veterinary Internal Medicine* and is serving on the editorial board of *Feline Medicine and Surgery* and *Compendium for Continuing Education for the Practicing Veterinarian*. Dr. Lappin has received the Beecham Research Award and the Norden Distinguished Teaching Award, and he is the Kenneth W. Smith Professor in Small Animal Clinical Veterinary Medicine at Colorado State University.

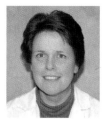

SUSAN M. TAYLOR, DVM, Dipl. ACVIM (Small Animal Internal Medicine), Professor and Chief of Small Animal Medicine, Department of Small Animal Clinical Sciences, Western College of Veterinary Medicine, University of Saskatchewan. Dr. Taylor has received several awards for teaching excellence, including the Norden Distinguished Teacher Award in 1992 and 1998. She has presented continuing education lectures throughout the United States, Canada, and Italy and has authored numerous refereed articles and book chapters. Dr. Taylor's current focus is on the investigation of medical and neurologic disorders of canine athletes. She has served on ACVIM's Certifying Examination Committee from 1992 to 1997 and is now a member of the Canadian Veterinary Medical Association, AAHA, the International Sled Dog Veterinary Medical Association (ISDVMA), and the American Canine Sports Medicine Association (ACSMA).

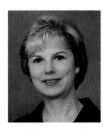 WENDY A. WARE, DVM, MS, Dipl. ACVIM (Cardiology), Professor, Departments of Veterinary Clinical Sciences and Biomedical Sciences, Iowa State University. Dr. Ware has served as Clinical Cardiologist in the Veterinary Teaching Hospital and as an educator for over 15 years. Her teaching skills in the areas of clinical cardiology and cardiovascular physiology are highly regarded. She has been invited to speak at many continuing education programs around the country and internationally. Dr. Ware has authored numerous journal articles and more than 35 book chapters. She has served as Associate Editor for Cardiology for the *Journal of Veterinary Internal Medicine* and has been a reviewer for several veterinary scientific journals. Dr. Ware is a member of the AVMA, ACVIM, and the American Heart Association Basic Sciences Council.

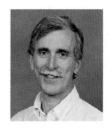 MICHAEL D. WILLARD, DVM, MS, Dipl. ACVIM, Professor, Department of Veterinary Small Animal Medicine and Surgery, Texas A&M University. Dr. Willard is an internationally recognized veterinary gastroenterologist and endoscopist. He has received the National SCAVMA teaching award for clinical teaching and the National Norden teaching award. A past President of the Comparative Gastroenterology Society and past Secretary of the specialty of Internal Medicine, his main interests are clinical gastroenterology and endoscopy (flexible and rigid), and he has published numerous papers on these topics. He has lectured on these subjects in North America, Europe, South America, Asia, and Australia.

**Denise A. Elliott, BVSc PhD, Dipl. ACVIM, ACVN**
Communications Manager, Waltham USA
Vernon, California

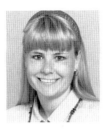

Dr. Elliott graduated from the University of Melbourne with a Bachelor in Veterinary Science with Honors in 1991. After completing an internship in small animal medicine and surgery at the University of Pennsylvania, Dr. Elliott moved to the University of California-Davis where she completed a residency in small animal medicine, a fellowship in renal medicine and hemodialysis, and a residency in small animal clinical nutrition. Dr. Elliott received board certification with the American College of Veterinary Internal Medicine in 1996 and with the American College of Veterinary Nutrition in 2001. The University of California-Davis awarded her a PhD in Nutrition in 2001 for her work on multifrequency bioelectrical impedance analysis in healthy cats and dogs. Dr. Elliott is currently the Communications Manager for Waltham USA, Inc.

*To Kay, Graciela, Beth Ann, Chris, Jason, and Kristen.*
*This project would not have been possible without their understanding,*
*encouragement, and patience.*

In the third edition of *Small Animal Internal Medicine,* we have retained our original goal of creating a practical text with a strong clinical slant that is useful for both practitioners and students. We have continued to limit authorship, with each author selected for clinical expertise in his or her respective field, to ensure as much consistency as possible within and among sections of the book. We have also continued to focus on the clinically relevant aspects of the most common internal medicine problems, presenting information in a concise, understandable, and logical format. An extensive use of tables, algorithms, cross-referencing within and among sections and a comprehensive index help make *Small Animal Internal Medicine* a quick, easy-to-use reference text.

## ORGANIZATION

*Small Animal Internal Medicine* contains 13 sections organized by organ systems (e.g., cardiology, respiratory); when multiple systems are involved, the sections are organized by discipline (e.g., oncology, infectious diseases). Each section, when possible, begins with a chapter on clinical signs and differential diagnoses and is followed by chapters on indications, techniques, and interpretation of diagnostic tests; general therapeutic principles; specific diseases; and, finally, a table listing recommended drug doses. Each section is extensively supported by tables, photographs, and illustrations, including many algorithms that address clinical presentations, differential diagnoses, diagnostic approaches, and treatment recommendations. Selected references and recommended readings are provided under the heading "Suggested Readings" at the end of each chapter, and specific studies are cited in the text by author name and year of publication and are included in the "Suggested Readings."

## FEATURES OF THE THIRD EDITION

We have retained all of the features that were popular in the first two editions and have added the following:

- Thorough revision and update of the content, with expanded coverage of hundreds of topics throughout the text

- Hundreds of new photographs, the majority of which are printed in full color
- Additional algorithms to aid readers in the decision-making process
- Extensive cross-referencing to other chapters and discussions, with a helpful "road map," as well as a reduction in redundancy
- Hundreds of functionally color-coded summary tables to draw the reader's eye to quickly accessible information, such as the following:

 Etiology

 Differential diagnoses

 Drugs (appearing within chapters)

 Drug formularies (appearing at the end of each section)

 Treatment

 General information (e.g., formulas, clinical pathology values, manufacturer information, breed predispositions)

A course management system (CMS) is available for this edition of *Small Animal Internal Medicine* to enhance faculty utility of the text. With the CMS, instructors who adopt this text for a course can use the accompanying course management website to post announcements, syllabi, assignments, additional course materials, quizzes and exams, password-protected grades, a course calendar, and more. You may also use the CMS to hold on-line discussions or to send e-mail to your students individually or as a group. To register for the CMS, go to http://evolve.elsevier.com/NelsonCouto/ and click "adopt."

# ACKNOWLEDGMENTS

We would like to extend our sincerest thanks to Susan, Greg, Eleanor, Cheri, Michael, Sue, Wendy, and Mike for the continued dedication and hard work to this project, as well as Linda Duncan, Liz Fathman, Teri Merchant, Julie Eddy, and many others at Mosby for their commitment and latitude in developing this text.

Finally, we are grateful to the many practitioners, faculty, and students worldwide who provided constructive comments on the first two editions, thereby making it possible to design an even stronger third edition. We believe the expanded content, features, and visual presentation will be positively received and will continue to make this text a valuable, user-friendly resource for all readers.

RICHARD W. NELSON
C. GUILLERMO COUTO

# CONTENTS

PART ONE  CARDIOVASCULAR SYSTEM
             DISORDERS, 1

*Wendy A. Ware*

**1  The Cardiovascular Examination, 1**
History and Clinical Signs, 1
Signs of Heart Disease and Heart
   Failure, 1
Physical Examination, 4
   *Mucous Membranes, 4*
   *Jugular Veins, 5*
   *Arterial Pulses, 6*
   *Precordium, 6*
   *Evaluation for Fluid Accumulation, 6*
   *Thoracic Auscultation, 6*
**2  Diagnostic Tests for the Cardiovascular
   System, 12**
Electrocardiography, 12
   *Benefits and Limitations, 12*
   *Normal ECG Waveforms, 12*
   *Lead Systems, 12*
   *Mean Electrical Axis, 13*
   *Chamber Enlargement and Bundle
      Branch Block Patterns, 15*
   *Sinus Rhythms, 15*
   *Ectopic Impulses, 16*
   *Conduction Disturbances, 23*
   *ST-T Abnormalities, 25*
   *ECG Manifestations of Drug Toxicities
      and Electrolyte Imbalances, 25*
   *Approach to ECG Interpretation, 26*
   *Common Artifacts, 29*
   *Ambulatory Electrocardiography, 29*
   *Other Methods of ECG Assessment, 29*
Thoracic Radiography, 32
   *Cardiomegaly, 32*
   *Cardiac Chamber Enlargement
      Patterns, 32*
   *Intrathoracic Blood Vessels, 34*
   *Patterns of Pulmonary Edema, 35*
Echocardiography (Cardiac
   Ultrasonography), 35
   *Benefits and Limitations, 35*
   *Basic Principles, 36*
   *Two-Dimensional Echocardiography, 36*

   *M-Mode Echocardiography, 38*
   *Contrast Echocardiography, 43*
   *Doppler Echocardiography, 44*
   *Transesophageal Echocardiography, 47*
Other Techniques, 47
**3  Management of Congestive Heart
   Failure, 51**
Pathophysiology of Heart Failure, 51
   *Neurohormonal Mechanisms, 52*
   *Renal Effects, 54*
   *Cardiac Responses, 54*
   *Other Effects of Chronic Heart Failure, 55*
Overview of Heart Failure Management, 55
   *General Causes of Heart Failure, 55*
   *Basic Principles of Treatment, 56*
Management of Chronic Heart Failure, 56
   *General Overview, 56*
   *Patient Monitoring, 58*
Treatment of Fulminant Congestive Heart
   Failure, 58
Dietary Management, 60
Diuretics, 62
   *Furosemide and Other Loop Diuretics, 62*
   *Spironolactone and Other Potassium-
      Sparing Diuretics, 64*
   *Thiazide Diuretics, 64*
Vasodilators, 64
   *Antiotensin-Converting Enzyme
      Inhibitors (ACEIs), 64*
   *Arteriolar and Other Mixed
      Vasodilators, 65*
   *Venodilators, 66*
Positive Inotropic Drugs, 66
   *Digitalis Glycosides, 66*
   *Sympathomimetic Agents
      (Catecholamines), 69*
   *Phosphodiesterase Inhibitors, 70*
Calcium Entry Blockers, 71
**4  Cardiac Rhythm Disturbances
   and Antiarrhythmic Therapy, 73**
General Considerations, 73
Common Heart Rhythm Abnormalities, 74
   *Irregular Tachyarrhythmias and Pulse
      Deficits, 75*
   *Rapid, Regular Rhythms, 83*
   *Bradyarrhythmias, 84*

Antiarrhythmic Drugs, 86
  *Class I Antiarrhythmic Drugs,* 87
  *Class II Antiarrhythmic Drugs:*
    *β-Adrenergic Blockers,* 91
  *Class III Antiarrhythmic Drugs,* 93
  *Class IV Antiarrhythmic Drugs: Calcium*
    *Entry Blockers,* 94
  *Anticholinergic Drugs,* 95
  *Sympathomimetic Drugs,* 96
  *Other Drugs,* 96

**5  Cardiopulmonary Resuscitation,** 98
General Considerations, 98
Signs of Impending Cardiopulmonary
  Arrest, 98
Approach to Cardiopulmonary
  Resuscitation, 99
  *Airway (A),* 99
  *Breathing (B),* 99
  *Circulation (C),* 100
  *Drugs (D),* 102
  *Electrocardiogram (E),* 104
  *Follow-Up (F),* 104

**6  Myocardial Diseases of the Dog,** 106
Dilated Cardiomyopathy, 106
  *Cardiomyopathy in Boxers*
    *and Doberman Pinschers,* 113
Hypertrophic Cardiomyopathy, 115
Arrhythmogenic Right Ventricular
  Cardiomyopathy, 116
Myocarditis, 116
  *Infective Myocarditis,* 116
  *Noninfective Myocarditis,* 118
  *Traumatic Myocarditis,* 118
Cardiogenic Shock, 118

**7  Myocardial Diseases of the Cat,** 122
Hypertrophic Cardiomyopathy, 122
  *Secondary Hypertrophic Myocardial*
    *Diseases,* 122
Restrictive Cardiomyopathy, 129
Dilated Cardiomyopathy, 130
Arrhythmogenic Right Ventricular
  Cardiomyopathy, 133
Myocarditis, 133
Arterial Thromboembolism, 134

**8  Acquired Valvular and Endocardial**
   **Diseases,** 139
Degenerative Mitral and Tricuspid Valve
  Disease, 139
  *Etiology, Pathology,*
    *and Pathophysiology,* 139
  *Complicating Factors,* 140

  *Epidemiology,* 141
  *Clinical Signs,* 141
  *Radiography,* 141
  *Electrocardiography,* 142
  *Echocardiography,* 142
  *Treatment and Prognosis,* 143
  *Patient Monitoring*
    *and Reevaluation,* 145
Infective Endocarditis, 145
  *Etiology,* 145
  *Pathophysiology,* 146
  *Clinical Features,* 146
  *Diagnosis,* 147
  *Treatment and Prognosis,* 149

**9  Common Congenital Cardiac**
   **Anomalies,** 151
General Considerations, 151
Extracardiac Arteriovenous Shunts, 153
  *Patent Ductus Arteriosus,* 153
Ventricular Outflow Obstructions, 155
  *Subaortic Stenosis,* 156
  *Pulmonic Stenosis,* 158
Intracardiac Shunts, 160
  *Ventricular Septal Defect,* 161
  *Atrial Septal Defect,* 162
Atrioventricular Valve Malformations, 162
  *Mitral Dysplasia,* 162
  *Tricuspid Dysplasia,* 162
Cardiac Anomalies Causing Cyanosis, 163
  *Tetralogy of Fallot,* 164
  *Pulmonary Hypertension with Shunt*
    *Reversal,* 164
Other Cardiovascular Anomalies, 166
  *Vascular Ring Anomalies,* 166
  *COR Triatriatum,* 166
  *Endocardial Fibroelastosis,* 167
  *Other Vascular Anomalies,* 167

**10  Heartworm Disease,** 169
Heartworm Life Cycle, 169
Pathophysiology, 169
Diagnostic Testing, 170
  *Serologic Tests,* 170
  *Detection of Microfilariae,* 171
Heartworm Disease in Dogs, 171
Heartworm Disease in Cats, 180

**11  Pericardial Diseases and Cardiac**
   **Tumors,** 185
General Considerations, 185
Pericardial Effusion, 185
  *Pericardiocentesis,* 191

Congenital Pericardial Disorders, 192
  *Peritoneopericardial Diaphragmatic*
    *Hernia,* 192
  *Other Pericardial Anomalies,* 192
Constrictive Pericardial Disease, 194
Cardiac Tumors, 194

**12** Systemic Arterial Hypertension, 198
General Considerations, 198
Blood Pressure Measurement, 200
Clinical Hypertension in Dogs
  and Cats, 201

PART TWO   RESPIRATORY SYSTEM
           DISORDERS, 210

*Eleanor C. Hawkins*

**13** Clinical Manifestations of Nasal
Disease, 210
General Considerations, 210
Nasal Discharge: Classification
  and Diagnostic Approach, 210
  *Classification and Etiology,* 210
  *Diagnostic Approach,* 211
Sneezing: Etiology and Diagnostic
  Approach, 215
  *Reverse Sneezing,* 215
Stertor, 216
Facial Deformity, 216

**14** Diagnostic Tests for the Nasal Cavity
and Paranasal Sinuses, 217
Nasal Radiography, 217
Computerized Tomography, 221
Rhinoscopy, 221
Nasal Biopsy: Indications
  and Techniques, 224
  *Nasal Swab,* 224
  *Nasal Flush,* 224
  *Pinch Biopsy,* 224
  *Core Biopsy,* 225
  *Turbinectomy,* 225
  *Complications,* 225
Nasal Cultures: Sample Collection
  and Interpretation, 226

**15** Disorders of the Nasal Cavity, 228
Feline Upper Respiratory Infection, 228
Nasopharyngeal Polyps, 232
Nasal Tumors, 233
Nasal Mycoses, 235
  *Cryptococcosis,* 235
  *Aspergillosis,* 235
Bacterial Rhinitis, 238

Nasal Parasites, 238
  *Nasal Mites,* 238
  *Nasal Capillariasis,* 238
Lymphoplasmacytic Rhinitis, 239
Allergic Rhinitis, 239

**16** Clinical Manifestations of Laryngeal
and Pharyngeal Disease, 241
Clinical Signs, 241
  *Larynx,* 241
  *Pharynx,* 241
Differential Diagnoses for Laryngeal Signs
  in Dogs and Cats, 242
Differential Diagnoses for Pharyngeal Signs
  in Dogs and Cats, 242

**17** Diagnostic Tests for the Larynx
and Pharynx, 243
Radiography and Ultrasonography, 243
Laryngoscopy and Pharyngoscopy, 243

**18** Disorders of the Larynx and Pharynx, 246
Laryngeal Paralysis, 246
Brachycephalic Airway Syndrome, 248
Obstructive Laryngitis, 249
Laryngeal Neoplasia, 249

**19** Clinical Manifestations of Lower
Respiratory Tract Disorders, 250
Clinical Signs, 250
  *Cough,* 250
  *Exercise Intolerance and Respiratory*
    *Distress,* 251
Diagnostic Approach to Dogs
  and Cats with Lower Respiratory
  Tract Disease, 252
  *Initial Diagnostic Evaluation,* 252
  *Further Diagnostic Evaluation,* 253

**20** Diagnostic Tests for the Lower Respiratory
Tract, 255
Thoracic Radiography, 255
  *General Principles,* 255
  *Trachea,* 256
  *Lungs,* 256
Angiography, 262
Ultrasonography, 262
Computed Tomography and Magnetic
  Resonance Imaging, 262
Nuclear Imaging, 262
Parasitologic Evaluation, 262
Serologic Tests for Pulmonary
  Pathogens, 264
Tracheal Wash, 264
Nonbronchoscopic Bronchoalveolar
  Lavage, 270

Transthoracic Lung Aspiration
and Biopsy, 274
Bronchoscopy, 276
Open-Chest Lung Biopsy
and Thoracoscopy, 281
Blood Gas Analysis, 281
Pulse Oximetry, 285

**21 Disorders of the Trachea and Bronchi, 287**
General Considerations, 287
Canine Infectious Tracheobronchitis, 287
Collapsing Trachea, 289
Feline Bronchitis, 291
Allergic Bronchitis, 295
Canine Chronic Bronchitis, 295
*Oslerus osleri*, 297

**22 Disorders of the Pulmonary Parenchyma, 299**
Viral Pneumonia, 299
Bacterial Pneumonia, 299
Toxoplasmosis, 302
Fungal Pneumonia, 302
Pulmonary Parasites, 302
*Capillaria aerophila*, 303
*Paragonimus kellicotti*, 303
*Aelurostrongylus abstrusus*, 303
Eosinophilic Lung Disease (Pulmonary
Infiltrates with Eosinophils
and Eosinophilic Pulmonary
Granulomatosis), 303
Miscellaneous Noninfectious Inflammatory
Lung Diseases, 304
Aspiration Pneumonia, 304
Pulmonary Neoplasia, 307
*Lymphomatoid Granulomatosis*, 309
Pulmonary Contusion, 309
Pulmonary Thromboembolism, 310
Pulmonary Edema, 312

**23 Clinical Manifestations of the Pleural
Cavity and Mediastinal Disease, 315**
General Considerations, 315
Pleural Effusion: Fluid Classification
and Diagnostic Approach, 315
*Transudates and Modified
Transudates*, 316
*Septic and Nonseptic Exudates*, 317
*Chylous Effusions*, 317
*Hemorrhagic Effusions*, 317
*Effusions due to Neoplasia*, 318
Pneumothorax, 318
Mediastinal Masses, 318
Pneumomediastinum, 319

**24 Diagnostic Tests for the Pleural Cavity
and Mediastinum, 320**
Radiography, 320
*Pleural Cavity*, 320
*Mediastinum*, 320
Ultrasonography, 322
Thoracocentesis, 322
Chest Tubes: Indications
and Placement, 323
Thoracoscopy and Thoracotomy, 326

**25 Disorders of the Pleural Cavity, 327**
Pyothorax, 327
Chylothorax, 330
Spontaneous Pneumothorax, 332
Neoplastic Effusion, 332

**26 Emergency Management of Respiratory
Distress, 333**
General Considerations, 333
Large Airway Disease, 333
*Extrathoracic (Upper) Airway
Obstruction*, 334
*Intrathoracic Large Airway
Obstruction*, 335
Pulmonary Parenchymal Disease, 335
Pleural Space Disease, 336

**27 Ancillary Therapy: Oxygen
Supplementation and Ventilation, 337**
Oxygen Supplementation, 337
*Oxygen Masks*, 337
*Oxygen Hoods*, 337
*Nasal Catheters*, 338
*Transtracheal Catheters*, 339
*Endotracheal Tubes*, 339
*Tracheal Tubes*, 339
*Oxygen Cages*, 340
Ventilatory Support, 340

## PART THREE    DIGESTIVE SYSTEM DISORDERS, 343

*Michael D. Willard*

**28 Clinical Manifestations of Gastrointestinal
Disorders, 343**
Dysphagia, Halitosis, and Drooling, 343
Distinguishing Regurgitation
from Vomiting, 345
Regurgitation, 346
Vomiting, 347
Hematemesis, 351
Diarrhea, 352

Hematochezia, 355
Melena, 356
Tenesmus, 356
Constipation, 357
Fecal Incontinence, 358
Weight Loss, 358
Anorexia, 360
Abdominal Effusion, 360
Acute Abdomen, 361
Abdominal Pain, 362
Abdominal Distention or Enlargement, 363

**29 Diagnostic Tests for the Alimentary Tract, 365**
Physical Examination, 365
Routine Laboratory Evaluation, 365
   *Complete Blood Count, 365*
   *Serum Biochemistry Profile, 366*
   *Urinalysis, 366*
Fecal Parasitic Evaluation, 366
Fecal Digestion Tests, 366
Miscellaneous Fecal Analyses, 367
Bacterial Fecal Culture, 367
Cytologic Evaluation of Feces, 368
Radiography of the Alimentary Tract, 368
Ultrasonography of the Alimentary Tract, 368
Imaging of the Oral Cavity, Pharynx, and Esophagus, 368
   *Indications, 368*
   *Indications for Imaging of the Esophagus, 369*
Imaging of the Stomach and Small Intestine, 371
   *Indications for Radiographic Imaging of the Abdomen without Contrast Media, 371*
   *Indications for Ultrasonography of the Stomach and Small Intestines, 374*
   *Indications for Contrast-Enhanced Gastrograms, 374*
   *Indications for Contrast-Enhanced Studies of the Small Intestine, 376*
   *Indications for Barium Contrast Enemas, 376*
Peritoneal Fluid Analysis, 377
Digestion and Absorption Tests, 378
Serum Concentrations of Vitamins, 378
Other Special Tests for Alimentary Tract Disease, 379
Endoscopy, 379

Biopsy Techniques and Submission, 384
   *Fine-Needle Aspiration Biopsy, 384*
   *Endoscopic Biopsy, 384*
   *Full-Thickness Biopsy, 385*

**30 General Therapeutic Principles, 387**
Fluid Therapy, 387
Dietary Management, 389
   *Special Nutritional Supplementation, 390*
   *Diets for Special Enteral Support, 395*
   *Parenteral Nutrition, 396*
Antiemetics, 396
Antacid Drugs, 397
Intestinal Protectants, 398
Digestive Enzyme Supplementation, 398
Motility Modifiers, 398
Antiinflammatory and Antisecretory Drugs, 399
Antibacterial Drugs, 401
Anthelmintic Drugs, 401
Enemas, Laxatives, and Cathartics, 402

**31 Disorders of the Oral Cavity, Pharynx, and Esophagus, 405**
Masses, Proliferations, and Inflammation of the Oropharynx, 405
   *Sialocele, 405*
   *Sialoadenitis/Sialoadenosis/Salivary Gland Necrosis, 405*
   *Neoplasms of the Oral Cavity in Dogs, 406*
   *Neoplasms of the Oral Cavity in Cats, 407*
   *Feline Eosinophilic Granuloma, 407*
   *Gingivitis/Peridontitis, 407*
   *Stomatitis, 408*
   *Feline Lymphocytic-Plasmacytic Gingivitis/Pharyngitis, 408*
Dysphagias, 409
   *Masticatory Muscle Myositis/Atrophic Myositis, 409*
   *Cricopharyngeal Achalasia/ Dysfunction, 409*
   *Pharyngeal Dysphagia, 409*
Esophageal Weakness/Megaesophagus, 410
   *Congenital Esophageal Weakness, 410*
   *Acquired Esophageal Weakness, 411*
   *Esophagitis, 412*
   *Hiatal Hernia, 412*
   *Dysautonomia, 412*
Esophageal Obstruction, 413
   *Vascular Ring Anomalies, 413*
   *Esophageal Foreign Objects, 414*
   *Esophageal Cicatrix, 414*
   *Esophageal Neoplasms, 415*

**32**  Disorders of the Stomach,  418
   Gastritis,  418
     *Acute Gastritis,*  418
     *Hemorrhagic Gastroenteritis,*  419
     *Chronic Gastritis,*  419
     *Helicobacter-Associated Disease,*  420
     *Physaloptera rara,*  420
     *Ollulanus tricuspis,*  421
   Gastric Outflow Obstruction/Gastric
    Statis,  421
     *Benign Muscular Pyloric Hypertrophy*
      *(Pyloric Stenosis),*  421
     *Gastric Antral Mucosal Hypertrophy,*  421
     *Gastric Foreign Objects,*  423
     *Gastric Dilation/Volvulus,*  424
     *Partial or Intermittent Gastric*
      *Volvulus,*  426
     *Idiopathic Gastric Hypomotility,*  427
     *Bilious Vomiting Syndrome,*  427
   Gastrointestinal Ulceration/Erosion,  427
   Infiltrative Gastric Diseases,  428
     *Neoplasms,*  428
     *Pythiosis,*  429
**33**  Disorders of the Intestinal Tract,  431
   Abbreviations Used in the Chapter,  432
   Acute Diarrhea,  432
     *Acute Enteritis,*  432
     *Dietary-Induced Diarrhea,*  433
   Infectious Diarrhea,  433
     *Canine Parvoviral Enteritis,*  433
     *Feline Parvoviral Enteritis,*  435
     *Canine Coronaviral Enteritis,*  436
     *Feline Coronaviral Enteritis,*  436
     *Feline Leukemia Virus–Associated*
      *Panleukopenia,*  436
     *Feline Immunodeficiency Virus–Associated*
      *Diarrhea,*  436
     *Salmon Poisoning,*  437
     *Campylobacteriosis,*  437
     *Salmonellosis,*  437
     *Clostridial Diseases,*  438
     *Miscellaneous Bacteria,*  439
     *Histoplasmosis,*  439
     *Protothecosis,*  440
   Alimentary Tract Parasites,  440
     *Whipworms,*  440
     *Roundworms,*  441
     *Hookworms,*  443
     *Tapeworms,*  443
     *Strongyloidiasis,*  444

     *Cryptosporidia,*  444
     *Giardiasis,*  445
     *Trichomoniasis,*  446
   Maldigestive Disease,  446
     *Exocrine Pancreatic Insufficiency,*  446
   Malabsorptive Diseases,  447
     *Canine Lymphocytic-Plasmacytic*
      *Enteritis,*  447
     *Canine Lymphocytic-Plasmacytic*
      *Colitis,*  448
     *Feline Lymphocytic-Plasmacytic*
      *Enteritis,*  448
     *Feline Lymphocytic-Plasmacytic*
      *Colitis,*  448
     *Canine Eosinophilic*
      *Gastroenterocolitis,*  448
     *Feline Eosinophilic Enteritis/*
      *Hypereosinophilic Syndrome,*  449
     *Granulomatous Enteritis/Gastritis,*  449
     *Immunoproliferative Enteropathy*
      *in Basenjis,*  449
     *Enteropathy in Sharpeis,*  450
     *Antibiotic Responsive Enteropathy,*  450
   Protein-Losing Enteropathy,  451
     *Causes of Protein-Losing Enteropathy,*  451
     *Intestinal Lymphangiectasia,*  451
     *Protein-Losing Enteropathy*
      *in Soft-Coated Wheaten Terriers,*  451
   Functional Intestinal Disease,  452
     *Irritable Bowel Syndrome,*  452
   Intestinal Obstruction,  452
     *Simple Intestinal Obstruction,*  452
     *Incarcerated Intestinal Obstruction,*  452
     *Mesenteric Torsion/Volvulus,*  453
     *Linear Foreign Objects,*  454
   Intussusception,  455
     *Ileocolic Intussusception,*  455
     *Jejunojejunal Intussusception,*  455
   Miscellaneous Intestinal Diseases,  456
     *Short Bowel Syndrome,*  456
   Neoplasms of the Small Intestine,  457
     *Alimentary Lymphoma,*  457
     *Intestinal Adenocarcinoma,*  457
     *Intestinal Leiomyoma/*
      *Leiomyosarcoma,*  458
   Inflammation of the Large Intestine,  458
     *Acute Colitis/Proctitis,*  458
     *Chronic Colitis,*  458
   Intussusception/Prolapse of the Large
    Intestine,  458
     *Cecocolic Intussusception,*  458
     *Rectal Prolapse,*  458

Neoplasms of the Large Intestine, 459
   *Adenocarcinoma,* 459
   *Rectal Polyps,* 459
Miscellaneous Large Intestinal
  Diseases, 460
   *Pythiosis,* 460
Perineal/Perianal Diseases, 460
   *Perineal Hernia,* 460
   *Perianal Fistulae,* 461
   *Anal Sacculitis,* 461
Perianal Neoplasms, 461
   *Anal Sac (Apocrine Gland)*
    *Adenocarcinoma,* 461
   *Perianal Gland Tumors,* 462
Constipation, 462
   *Pelvic Canal Obstruction due*
    *to Malaligned Healing of Old Pelvic*
    *Fractures,* 462
   *Benign Rectal Stricture,* 462
   *Dietary Indiscretion Leading*
    *to Constipation,* 463
   *Idiopathic Megacolon,* 463

**34** Disorders of the Peritoneum, 466
Inflammatory Diseases, 466
   *Septic Peritonitis,* 466
   *Sclerosing, Encapsulating Peritonitis,* 468
Hemoabdomen, 468
   *Abdominal Hemangiosarcoma,* 468
Miscellaneous Peritoneal Disorders, 469
   *Abdominal Carcinomatosis,* 469
   *Feline Infectious Peritonitis,* 469

PART FOUR   HEPATOBILIARY AND EXOCRINE
            PANCREATIC DISORDERS, 472

*Susan E. Bunch*

**35** Clinical Manifestations of Hepatobiliary
  Disease, 472
General Considerations, 472
Abdominal Enlargement, 472
   *Organomegaly,* 472
   *Abdominal Effusion,* 474
   *Abdominal Muscular Hypotonia,* 476
Jaundice, Bilirubinuria, and Change in
  Fecal Color, 476
Hepatic Encephalopathy, 479
Coagulopathies, 481
Polyuria and Polydipsia, 482

**36** Diagnostic Tests for the Hepatobiliary
  System, 483
Diagnostic Approach, 483
Diagnostic Tests, 485
   *Complete Blood Count,* 485
   *Tests to Assess Status of the Hepatobiliary*
    *System,* 486
   *Tests to Assess Function*
    *of the Hepatobiliary System,* 487
   *Urinalysis,* 490
   *Fecal Evaluation,* 491
   *Abdominocentesis/Fluid Analysis,* 491
   *Coagulation Tests,* 492
Diagnostic Imaging, 492
   *Survey Radiography,* 492
   *Ultrasonography,* 494
   *Scintigraphy,* 499
Liver Biopsy, 499

**37** Hepatobiliary Diseases in the Cat, 506
General Considerations, 506
Hepatic Lipidosis, 506
Inflammatory Hepatobiliary Disease, 513
Neoplasia, 517
Extrahepatic Bile Duct Obstruction, 518
Congenital Portosystemic Shunt, 520
Acute Toxic Hepatopathy, 521
Secondary Hepatobiliary Disease, 523

**38** Hepatobiliary Diseases in the Dog, 525
General Considerations, 525
Chronic Hepatitis, 525
   *Familial Chronic Hepatitis,* 526
   *Drug Administration,* 528
   *Infectious Agents,* 529
   *Idiopathic Chronic Hepatitis,* 530
Idiopathic Hepatic Fibrosis, 530
Congenital Portovascular Disorders
  with Normal Portal Pressure, 531
   *Congenital Portosystemic Shunt,* 531
   *Microvascular Dysplasia,* 533
Congenital Portovascular Disorders
  with High Portal Pressure, 533
   *Hepatoportal Fibrosis,* 534
   *Primary Portal Vein Hypoplasia,* 534
   *Idiopathic Noncirrhotic Portal*
    *Hypertension,* 534
   *Arterioportal Fistula,* 535
Treatment for Chronic Liver Disorders, 535
   *Prevention and Treatment of Copper*
    *Excess,* 535
   *Glucocorticoids,* 536
   *Azathioprine,* 537

*Antifibrotic Agents,* 537
*Dietary Modification,* 537
*Adjunctive Treatments,* 537
Acute Toxic Hepatopathy, 537
Biliary Tract Disorders, 538
Focal Hepatic Lesions, 541
*Abscesses,* 541
*Nodular Hyperplasia,* 542
Neoplasia, 542
Secondary Hepatic Disease, 542
*Pancreatitis,* 543
*Sepsis,* 543
*Miscellaneous Disorders,* 543

**39** **Treatment of Complications of Hepatic
Failure,** 546
General Considerations, 546
Hepatic Encephalopathy, 546
*Chronic Hepatic Encephalopathy,* 546
*Acute Hepatic Encephalopathy,* 547
*Massive Hepatic Necrosis,* 548
Ascites, 549
Coagulopathy/Gastrointestinal
Hemorrhage, 550
Sepsis, 551

**40** **The Exocrine Pancreas,** 552
General Considerations, 552
Acute Pancreatitis, 552
Feline Acute Pancreatitis—Comparative
Aspects, 560
Relapsing and Chronic Pancreatitis, 560
Exocrine Pancreatic Insufficiency, 560
Exocrine Pancreatic Neoplasia, 564

**PART FIVE   URINARY TRACT DISORDERS,** 568

*Gregory F. Grauer*

**41** **Clinical Manifestations of Urinary
Disorders,** 568
General Considerations, 568
*Pollakiuria and Dysuria-Stranguria,* 568
*Urethral Obstruction,* 568
*Urinary Tract Infection,* 568
*Transitional Cell Carcinoma,* 570
*Urolithiasis,* 570
*Feline Lower Urinary Tract
Inflammation,* 571
*Hematuria,* 572
Disorders of Micturition, 575
*Distended Bladder,* 576
*Small or Normal-Sized Bladder,* 576
*Geriatric Incontinence,* 577

*Polydipsia and Polyuria,* 577
Proteinuria, 579
Azotemia, 581
Renomegaly, 583

**42** **Diagnostic Tests for the Urinary
System,** 584
Renal Excretory Function, 584
*Glomerular Filtration Rate,* 584
*Fractional Clearance,* 585
Quantification of Proteinuria, 586
Plasma and Urine Osmolality, Water
Deprivation Test, and Response
to Exogenous Antidiuretic
Hormone, 587
Bladder and Urethral Function, 588
Bacterial Antibiotic Sensitivity Testing, 588
Diagnostic Imaging, 589
Cystoscopy, 596
Renal Biopsy, 598

**43** **Glomerulonephropathies,** 600
Etiology and Pathophysiology, 600
Clinical Features, 603
Diagnosis, 605
Treatment, 605
Prognosis, 607

**44** **Renal Failure,** 608
Acute Renal Failure, 608
*Etiology and Pathogenesis,* 608
*Clinical Features and Diagnosis,* 611
*Risk Factors for Renal Failure,* 611
*Monitoring Patients at Risk for ARF,* 613
*Treatment,* 613
Chronic Renal Failure, 615
*Etiology and Pathogenesis,* 615
*Clinical Features and Diagnosis,* 616
*Treatment,* 617

**45** **Urinary Tract Infections,** 624
Etiology and Pathogenesis, 624
Host Defense Mechanism, 625
Complicated Versus Uncomplicated
Urinary Tract Infections, 626
Relapses Versus Reinfections, 626
Clinical Features, 626
Treatment, 627

**46** **Canine Urolithiasis,** 631
Etiology and Pathogenesis, 631
Clinical Features and Diagnosis, 636
Treatment, 636
Reevaluation of the Patient
with Urolithiasis, 641

**47** Feline Lower Urinary Tract
Inflammation, 642
Etiology and Pathogenesis, 642
Clinical Features and Diagnosis, 645
Management, 645

**48** Disorders of Micturition, 650
Physiology of Micturition, 650
Etiology and Clinical Features of Disorders
of Micturition, 651
*Distended Bladder, 651*
*Small or Normal-Sized Bladder, 652*
*Geriatric Incontinence, 653*
Diagnosis, 653
*Initial Evaluation, 654*
*Pharmacologic Testing, 654*
Treatment, 655
*Lower Motor Neuron Disorders, 655*
*Upper Motor Neuron Disorders, 655*
*Reflex Dyssynergia, 655*
*Functional Urethral Obstruction, 655*
*Urethral Sphincter Mechanism*
*Incompetence, 656*
*Detrusor Hyperreflexia or Instability, 656*
*Congenial Disorders, 656*
*Anatomic Urethral Obstruction, 656*
Prognosis, 656

**PART SIX** ENDOCRINE DISORDERS, 660

*Richard W. Nelson*

**49** Disorders of the Hypothalamus
and Pituitary Gland, 660
Polyuria and Polydipsia, 660
Diabetes Insipidus, 661
Primary (Psychogenic) Polydipsia, 667
Endocrine Alopecia, 667
Growth Hormone-Responsive Dermatosis
in the Adult Dog, 670
Feline Acromegaly, 673
Pituitary Dwarfism, 677

**50** Disorders of the Parathyroid Gland, 681
Classification of Hyperparathyroidism, 681
Primary Hyperparathyroidism, 681
Primary Hypoparathyroidism, 686

**51** Disorders of the Thyroid Gland, 691
Hypothyroidism in Dogs, 691
Hypothyroidism in Cats, 709
Hyperthyroidism in Cats, 712
Canine Thyroid Neoplasia, 724

**52** Disorders of the Endocrine Pancreas, 729
Hyperglycemia, 729
Hypoglycemia, 729
Diabetes Mellitus in Dogs, 731
Diabetes Mellitus in Cats, 749
Diabetic Ketoacidosis, 762
Insulin-Secreting β-Cell Neoplasia, 769
Gastrinoma: Zollinger-Ellison
Syndrome, 775

**53** Disorders of the Adrenal Gland, 778
Hyperadrenocorticism in Dogs, 778
Hyperadrenocorticism in Cats, 798
Hypoadrenocorticism, 804
Pheochromocytoma, 809
Incidental Adrenal Mass, 812

**PART SEVEN** METABOLIC AND ELECTROLYTE
DISORDERS, 816

*Richard W. Nelson*
*Denise A. Elliott*

**54** Disorders of Metabolism, 816
*Denise A. Elliott*
Polyphagia with Weight Loss, 816
Obesity, 817
Hyperlipidemia, 822

**55** Electrolyte Imbalances, 828
*Richard W. Nelson*
Hypernatremia, 828
Hyponatremia, 830
Hyperkalemia, 832
Hypokalemia, 834
Hypercalcemia, 836
Hypocalcemia, 840
Hyperphosphatemia, 841
Hypophosphatemia, 842
Hypermagnesemia, 843
Hypomagnesemia, 843

**PART EIGHT** REPRODUCTIVE SYSTEM
DISORDERS, 847

*Cheri A. Johnson*

**56** Disorders of the Estrous Cycle, 847
Normal Estrous Cycle, 847
*The Bitch, 847*
*The Queen, 851*

Diagnostic Tests for the Female
  Reproductive Tract, 853
    *Vaginal Cytology, 853*
    *Vaginoscopy, 853*
    *Vaginal Bacterial Cultures, 854*
    *Virology, 854*
    *Assessment of Reproductive
      Hormones, 855*
    *Radiology and Ultrasonography, 858*
    *Karyotyping, 858*
    *Laparoscopy and Celiotomy, 858*
Female Infertility, 859
    *Failure to Cycle, 860*
    *Prolonged Interestrous Interval, 862*
    *Short Interestrous Interval, 862*
    *Abnormal Proestrus and Estrus, 863*
    *Prolonged Estrus, 863*
    *Short Estrus, 864*
    *Normal Cycles, 864*
Estrus Suppression and Population
  Control, 865
    *Megestrol Acetate, 866*
    *Androgens, 867*
    *GnRH Agonists, 867*
Ovarian Remnant Syndrome, 867
Estrus Induction, 868
    *The Queen, 868*
    *The Bitch, 868*
Induction of Ovulation, 869
    *The Queen, 869*
    *The Bitch, 869*

**57  Disorders of the Vagina and Uterus, 870**
Diagnostic Approach to Vulvar
  Discharge, 870
Hemorrhagic Vulvar Discharge, 870
Purulent Vulvar Discharge, 872
Mucoid Vulvar Discharge, 872
Uteroverdin and Cellular Debris, 872
Congenital Anomalies of the Vagina
  and Vulva, 872
Vaginitis, 874
Vaginal Hyperplasia and Prolapse, 875
Disorders of the Uterus, 877
Cystic Endometrial Hyperplasia
  and Pyometra, 877

**58  Disorders of the Mammary Gland, 882**
Mastitis, 882
Galactostasis, 882
Galactorrhea, 883
Feline Mammary Hyperplasia
  and Hypertrophy, 883
Mammary Neoplasia, 884

**59  False Pregnancy, Disorders of Pregnancy,
    Parturition, and the Postpartum
    Period, 886**
False Pregnancy, 886
Normal Events in Pregnancy
  and Parturition, 887
    *Fertilization and Implantation, 887*
    *Corpora Luteal Function and Serum
      Progesterone Concentrations, 888*
    *Litter Size, 888*
    *Confirmation of Pegnancy, 888*
    *Alterations in Bitch and Queen During
      Pregnancy, 890*
    *Gestation Length, 891*
    *Parturition, 891*
    *Predicting Labor, 891*
    *Stages of Labor, 891*
Dystocia, 892
Postpartum Disorders, 895
    *Agalactia, 895*
    *Puerperal Hypocalcemia (Puerperal
      Tetany, Eclampsia), 896*
    *Metritis, 896*
    *Subinvolution of Placental Sites, 897*
Abortifacients (Mismating), 898
    *Estrogens, 898*
    *Prostaglandins, 899*
    *Alternative Treatments, 899*
Fetal Resorption-Abortion-Stillbirth
  Complex, 900
Neonatal Morbidity and Mortality, 901
    *Environmental Factors, 901*
    *The Dam, 902*
    *The Neonate, 902*

**60  Disorders of Male Fertility, 905**
Normal Sexual Development
  and Behavior, 905
    *Testicular Descent, 905*
    *Puberty, 905*
    *Reproductive Physiology, 905*
    *Age-Related Effects, 906*
    *Breeding Behavior, 907*
Diagnostic Techniques to Assess
  Reproductive Function, 907
    *Semen Collection and Evaluation, 907*
    *Bacterial Culture of Semen, 911*
    *Radiography and Ultrasonography, 912*
    *Testicular Aspiration and Biopsy, 912*
    *Hormonal Evaluation, 912*
Diagnostic Approach to Infertility, 913
    *Physical Examination, 914*
    *Semen Evaluation, 914*

Oligozoospermia and Azoospermia, 915
Congenital Infertility, 916
Acquired Infertility, 916

**61** Disorders of the Penis, Prepuce, and Testes, 918
Acquired Penile Disorders, 918
*Penile Trauma,* 918
*Priapism,* 918
*Miscellaneous Acquired Disorders,* 919
Congenital Penile Disorders, 919
*Persistent Penile Frenulum,* 919
*Miscellaneous Congenital Disorders,* 919
Preputial Disorders, 920
*Balanoposthitis,* 920
*Phimosis,* 920
*Paraphimosis,* 920
Testicular Disorders, 921
*Orchitis and Epididymitis,* 921
*Cryptorchidism,* 922
*Testicular Torsion,* 923
*Testicular Neoplasia,* 924

**62** Disorders of the Prostate Gland, 927
Overview, 927
Benign Prostatic Hyperplasia, 928
Squamous Metaplasia of the Prostate, 930
Bacterial Prostatitis and Prostatic Abscess, 930
*Chronic Bacterial Prostatitis,* 931
Paraprostatic Cysts, 932
Prostatic Neoplasia, 932

**63** Genital Infections and Transmissible Venereal Tumor, 934
Genital Infection, 934
*Herpesvirus Infection,* 934
*Mycoplasma and Ureaplasma,* 935
*Brucella canis,* 936
Canine Transmissible Venereal Tumor, 938

**64** Artificial Insemination and Frozen Semen, 940
Principles, 940
Techniques, 941
Fresh Semen, 942
Frozen Semen, 942
Chilled Extended Semen, 943
Cat Semen, 943

## PART NINE  NEUROMUSCULAR DISORDERS, 946

*Susan M. Taylor*

**65** The Neurologic Examination, 946
Functional Anatomy of the Nervous System, 946

Screening Neurologic Examination, 948
*Diagnostic Approach,* 957
*Animal History,* 957
*Disease Onset and Progression,* 958

**66** Diagnostic Tests for the Neuromuscular System, 961
Hematology, 961
Serum Biochemistry Profile, 961
Urinalysis, 961
Radiography, 961
Cerebrospinal Fluid Analysis, 962
Contrast-Enhanced Radiography, 965
Electrodiagnostic Testing, 970
Biopsy of Muscle and Nerve, 972
Immunologic and Serologic Tests, 973

**67** Disorders of Locomotion, 974
Ataxia, 974
Paresis and Paralysis, 974
*Localizing Spinal Cord Lesions,* 975
*Generalized Lower Motor Neuron Paresis and Paralysis,* 976
*Episodic Weakness,* 976
Dysmetria and Hypermetria, 977
Involuntary Alterations in Muscle Tone, 980
*Dyskinesias,* 980
*Tremors,* 980
*Opisthotonos and Tetanus,* 980
*Myoclonus,* 981

**68** Abnormalities of Mentation, Loss of Vision, and Pupillary Abnormalities, 983
Mentation, 983
Head Trauma, 983
Loss of Vision and Pupillary Abnormalities, 984
*Optic Neuritis,* 985
*Optic Chiasm and Occipital Cortex,* 986
*Anisocoria,* 986
*Horner's Syndrome,* 987
*Protrusion of the Third Eyelid,* 989

**69** Seizures, 991
Overview and Diagnostic Approach, 991
Disorders Resulting in Seizures, 994
*Metabolic Disorders,* 994
*Toxins,* 994
*Congenital Malformations,* 994
*Degenerative Diseases,* 995
*Neoplasia,* 996
*Inflammatory Diseases,* 999
*Vascular Diseases,* 999
*Feline Ischemic Encephalopathy,* 999

*Trauma/Scar-Related Epilepsy,* 1000
*Thiamine Deficiency,* 1000
*Epilepsy,* 1000
Anticonvulsant Therapy, 1001
*Anticonvulsant Drugs,* 1001
*Alternative Therapies,* 1004
Emergency Therapy for Dogs and Cats
in Status Epilepticus, 1004

**70 Head Tilt,** 1005
General Considerations, 1005
Localization of the Lesion, 1005
Peripheral Vestibular Disease, 1006
Bilateral Peripheral Vestibular
Disease, 1009
Central Vestibular Disease, 1009
Congenital Nystagmus, 1009

**71 Encephalitis, Myelitis,
and Meningitis,** 1010
Synopsis of Clinical Features, 1010
Steroid-Responsive Suppurative
Meningitis, 1010
Meningeal Vasculitis, 1012
Granulomatous Meningoencephalitis, 1012
Pug Meningoencephalitis, 1013
Feline Polioencephalomyelitis, 1013
Feline Immunodeficiency Virus
Encephalopathy, 1014
Bacterial Meningitis and Myelitis, 1014
Canine Distemper Virus, 1015
Rabies, 1016
Feline Infectious Peritonitis, 1016
Toxoplasmosis, 1017
Neosporosis, 1017
Lyme Disease, 1018
Mycotic Infections, 1018
Rickettsial Diseases, 1018
Parasitic Meningitis, Myelitis,
and Encephalitis, 1018

**72 Disorders of the Spinal Cord,** 1020
General Considerations, 1020
Acute Spinal Cord Dysfunction, 1021
*Trauma,* 1021
*Hemorrhage/Infarction,* 1024
*Acute Intervertebral Disk Disease,* 1024
*Fibrocartilaginous Embolism,* 1030
Subacute Progressive Spinal Cord
Dysfunction, 1031
*Infectious Inflammatory Disease,* 1031
*Noninfectious Inflammatory
Disease,* 1031
*Diskospondylitis,* 1031

Chronic Progressive Spinal Cord
Dysfunction, 1034
*Neoplasia,* 1034
*Intraspinal Articular Cysts,* 1036
*Type II Intervertebral Disk Disease,* 1036
*Degenerative Myelopathy,* 1037
*Cauda Equina Syndrome,* 1038
*Cervical Vertebral Instability/
Malformation (Wobbler
Syndrome),* 1040
Progressive Spinal Cord Dysfunction
in Young Animals, 1043
*Neuronal Abiotrophies
and Degenerations,* 1043
*Metabolic Storage Diseases,* 1043
*Atlantoaxial Instability
and Luxation,* 1046
Congenital Spinal Cord Dysfunction:
Nonprogressive Signs, 1047
*Spina Bifida,* 1047
*Caudal Agenesis of Manx Cats,* 1047
*Spinal Dysraphism,* 1047
*Syringomyelia/Hydromyelia,* 1048

**73 Disorders of Peripheral Nerves
and the Neuromuscular Junction,** 1049
Focal Neuropathies, 1049
*Traumatic Neuropathies,* 1049
*Peripheral Nerve Tumors,* 1049
*Facial Nerve Paralysis,* 1051
*Trigeminal Nerve Paralysis,* 1053
Hyperchylomicronemia, 1054
Ischemic Neuromyopathy, 1054
Polyneuropathy, 1055
Acute Polyradiculoneuritis, 1056
Tick Paralysis, 1057
Botulism, 1058
Protozoal Polyradiculoneuritis, 1058
Dysautonomia, 1059
Myasthenia Gravis, 1059

**74 Disorders of Muscle,** 1062
Inflammatory Myopathies, 1062
*Masticatory Myositis,* 1062
*Canine Idiopathic Polymyositis,* 1063
*Feline Idiopathic Polymyositis,* 1064
*Dermatomyositis,* 1064
*Protozoal Myositis,* 1065
Metabolic Myopathies, 1065
*Glucocorticoid Excess,* 1065
*Hypothyroidism,* 1065
*Hypokalemic Polymyopathy,* 1065

Inherited Myopathies, 1066
    *Muscular Dystrophy,* 1066
    *Hereditary Labrador Retriever*
      *Myopathy,* 1067
    *Myotonia,* 1067
    *Miscellaneous,* 1068

## PART TEN   JOINT DISORDERS, 1071

*Susan M. Taylor*

**75**   **Clinical Manifestations of and Diagnostic Tests for Joint Disorders, 1071**
General Considerations, 1071
Clinical Manifestations, 1071
Diagnostic Tests, 1073
    *Clinical Pathology,* 1073
    *Radiography,* 1073
    *Synovial Fluid Collection*
      *and Analysis,* 1073
    *Synovial Fluid Culture,* 1076
    *Synovial Membrane Biopsy,* 1077
    *Immunologic and Serologic Tests,* 1077

**76**   **Disorders of the Joints, 1079**
Noninflammatory Joint Disease, 1079
    *Degenerative Joint Disease,* 1079
Infectious Inflammatory Joint
    Diseases, 1081
    *Septic (Bacterial) Arthritis,* 1081
    *Mycoplasma Polyarthritis,* 1083
    *Bacterial L Form-Associated*
      *Arthritis,* 1083
    *Rickettsial Polyarthritis,* 1084
    *Lyme Disease,* 1084
    *Fungal Arthritis,* 1084
    *Viral Arthritis,* 1085
Noninfectious Inflammatory Joint
    Diseases—Nonerosive, 1085
    *Systemic Lupus Erythematosus–Induced*
      *Polyarthritis,* 1085
    *Reactive Polyarthritis,* 1086
    *Idiopathic, Immune-Mediated,*
      *Nonerosive Polyarthritis,* 1086
    *Breed-Specific Polyarthritis*
      *Syndromes,* 1088
    *Lymphoplasmacytic Synovitis,* 1088
Noninfectious Inflammatory Joint
    Diseases—Erosive, 1089
    *Rheumatoid Arthritis,* 1089
    *Erosive Polyarthritis of Greyhounds,* 1091
    *Feline Chronic Progressive*
      *Polyarthritis,* 1091

## PART ELEVEN   ONCOLOGY, 1093

*C. Guillermo Couto*

**77**   **Cytology, 1093**
General Considerations, 1093
Fine-Needle Aspiration, 1093
Impression Smears, 1094
Staining of Cytologic Specimens, 1094
Interpretation of Cytologic
    Specimens, 1094
    *Normal Tissues,* 1094
    *Hyperplastic Processes,* 1094
    *Inflammatory Processes,* 1094
    *Malignant Cells,* 1095
    *Lymph Nodes,* 1098

**78**   **Principles of Cancer Treatment, 1100**
General Considerations, 1100
Patient-Related Factors, 1100
Owner-Related Factors, 1100
Treatment-Related Factors, 1101

**79**   **Practical Chemotherapy, 1103**
Cell and Tumor Kinetics, 1103
Basic Principles of Chemotherapy, 1103
Indications and Contraindications
    of Chemotherapy, 1105
Mechanism of Action of Anticancer
    Drugs, 1106
Types of Anticancer Drugs, 1106

**80**   **Complications of Cancer
Chemotherapy, 1108**
General Considerations, 1108
Hematologic Toxicity, 1108
Gastrointestinal Toxicity, 1111
Hypersensitivity Reactions, 1112
Dermatologic Toxicity, 1112
Pancreatitis, 1113
Cardiotoxicity, 1114
Urotoxicity, 1114
Hepatotoxicity, 1115
Neurotoxicity, 1115
Pulmonary Toxicity, 1115
Acute Tumor Lysis Syndrome, 1115

**81**   **Approach to the Patient with a Mass, 1117**
Approach to the Cat or Dog with a Solitary
    Mass, 1117
Approach to the Cat or Dog
    with a Metastatic Lesion, 1118
Approach to the Cat or Dog
    with a Mediastinal Mass, 1119

**82**   **Lymphoma in the Cat and Dog,** 1122
Etiology and Epidemiology, 1122
Clinical Features, 1122
Diagnosis, 1125
Treatment, 1126

**83**   **Leukemias,** 1133
Definitions and Classification, 1133
Leukemias in Dogs, 1133
*Acute Leukemias,* 1134
*Chronic Leukemias,* 1136
Leukemias in Cats, 1138
*Acute Leukemias,* 1138
*Chronic Leukemias,* 1139
Myelodysplastic Syndromes, 1140

**84**   **Selected Neoplasms in Dogs
and Cats,** 1142
Hemangiosarcoma in Dogs, 1142
Osteosarcoma in Dogs and Cats, 1144
Mast Cell Tumors in Dogs and Cats, 1146
*Mast Cell Tumors in Dogs,* 1146
*Mast Cell Tumors in Cats,* 1149
Oropharyngeal Neoplasms in Dogs
and Cats, 1149
*Oropharyngeal Neoplasms in Dogs,* 1150
*Oropharyngeal Neoplasms in Cats,* 1150
*Approach to Dogs and Cats with an
Oropharyngeal Mass,* 1150
Injection Site Sarcomas in Cats, 1151

**PART TWELVE**   **HEMATOLOGY
AND IMMUNOLOGY,** 1156

*C. Guillermo Couto*

**85**   **Anemia,** 1156
Definition, 1156
Clinical and Clinicopathologic
Evaluation, 1156
Principles of Management of the Anemic
Patient, 1160
Regenerative Anemias, 1160
*Blood Loss Anemia,* 1160
*Hemolytic Anemia,* 1160
Nonregenerative Anemias, 1164
*Anemia of Chronic Disease,* 1165
*Bone Marrow Disorders,* 1165
*Anemia of Renal Disease,* 1166
*Acute and Peracute Blood Loss
or Hemolysis (First 48 to
96 Hours),* 1167

*Semiregenerative Anemias,* 1167
*Iron Deficiency Anemia,* 1167
Principles of Transfusion Therapy, 1168
*Blood Groups,* 1168
*Crossmatching and Blood Typing,* 1168
*Blood Administration,* 1168
*Complications of Transfusion
Therapy,* 1169

**86**   **Erythrocytosis,** 1170
Definition and Classification, 1170
*Clinical and Clinicopathologic
Findings,* 1170
*Diagnosis and Treatment,* 1171

**87**   **Leukopenia and Leukocytosis,** 1173
General Considerations, 1173
Normal Leukocyte Morphology
and Physiology, 1173
Leukocyte Changes in Disease, 1174
*Neutropenia,* 1174
*Neutrophilia,* 1176
*Eosinopenia,* 1177
*Eosinophilia,* 1177
*Basopenia,* 1178
*Basophilia,* 1178
*Monocytopenia,* 1178
*Monocytosis,* 1178
*Lymphopenia,* 1179
*Lymphocytosis,* 1179

**88**   **Combined Cytopenias
and Leukoerythroblastosis,** 1181
Definitions and Classification, 1181

**89**   **Disorders of Hemostasis,** 1185
General Considerations, 1185
Normal Hemostasis, 1185
Clinical Manifestations of Spontaneous
Bleeding Disorders, 1186
Clinicopathologic Evaluation
of the Bleeding Patient, 1187
Management of the Bleeding Patient, 1189
Primary Hemostatic Defects, 1190
*Thrombocytopenia,* 1190
*Platelet Dysfunction,* 1192
Secondary Hemostatic Defects, 1194
*Congenital Clotting Factor
Deficiencies,* 1194
*Vitamin K Deficiency,* 1194
Mixed (Combined) Hemostatic
Defects, 1195
*Disseminated Intravascular
Coagulation,* 1195
Thrombosis, 1199

**90** Lymphadenopathy
and Splenomegaly, 1200
Applied Anatomy and Histology, 1200
Function, 1200
Lymphadenopathy, 1200
Splenomegaly, 1204
Approach to Patients
with Lymphadenopathy
or Splenomegaly, 1206
Management of Patients
with Lymphadenopathy
or Splenomegaly, 1208

**91** Hyperproteinemia, 1210

**92** Immune-Mediated Diseases: Overview
and Diagnosis, 1212
General Considerations, 1212
Immunology for the Clinician, 1212
Diagnostic Tests, 1213
*Direct Coombs' Test or Direct*
*Antiglobulin Test, 1213*
*Antinuclear Antibody Test, 1214*
*Direct Immunofluorescence*
*or Immunohistochemistry, 1214*
*Other Tests, 1214*

**93** Immunosuppressive Drugs, 1216
General Considerations, 1216
Corticosteroids, 1216
Cyclophosphamide, 1217
Azathioprine, 1217
Chlorambucil, 1218
Gold Salts, 1218
Cyclosporin A, 1218
Danazol, 1218

**94** Systemic Lupus Erythematosus, 1220
Etiology and Pathogenesis, 1220
*Clinical Features, 1220*
*Diagnosis, 1220*
*Treatment, 1221*

**95** Fever of Undetermined Origin, 1222
Fever, 1222
Fever of Undetermined Origin, 1222
*Disorders Associated with Fever*
*of Undetermined Origin, 1222*
*Diagnostic Approach to the Patient*
*with Fever of Undetermined*
*Origin, 1223*
*Treatment, 1224*

**96** Recurrent Infections, 1226
Classification and Clinical Features, 1226
*Diagnosis, 1227*
*Management, 1227*

**PART THIRTEEN** INFECTIOUS DISEASES, 1229

*Michael R. Lappin*

**97** Laboratory Diagnosis of Infectious
Diseases, 1229
Demonstration of the Organism, 1229
*Fecal Examination, 1229*
*Cytology, 1232*
*Tissue Techniques, 1235*
*Culture Techniques, 1235*
*Immunologic Techniques, 1236*
*Polymerase Chain Reaction, 1236*
*Animal Inoculation, 1237*
*Electron Microscopy, 1237*
Antibody Detection, 1237
*Serum, 1237*
*Body Fluids, 1238*

**98** Practical Antimicrobial
Chemotherapy, 1240
Anaerobic Infections, 1240
Bacteremia and Bacterial
Endocarditis, 1244
Skin and Soft Tissue Infections, 1245
Gastrointestinal Tract and Hepatic
Infections, 1245
Musculoskeletal Infections, 1246
Central Nervous System Infections, 1247
Respiratory Tract Infections, 1247
Urogenital Tract Infections, 1248

**99** Prevention of Infectious Diseases, 1250
Biosecurity Procedures for Small Animal
Hospitals, 1250
*General Biosecurity Guidelines, 1250*
*Patient Evaluation, 1251*
*Hospitalized Patients, 1251*
*Basic Disinfection Protocols, 1252*
Biosecurity Procedures for Clients, 1252
Vaccination Protocols, 1252
*Vaccine Types, 1252*
*Vaccine Selection, 1253*
*Vaccination Protocols for Cats, 1254*
*Vaccination Protocols for Dogs, 1256*

**100** Polysystemic Bacterial Diseases, 1259
Feline Plague, 1259
Leptospirosis, 1260
*Mycoplasma and Ureaplasma, 1262*

**101** Polysystemic Rickettsial Diseases, 1265
Rocky Mountain Spotted Fever, 1265
Canine Ehrlichiosis, 1267
Feline Ehrlichiosis, 1271
Other Rickettsial Infections, 1271

**102** **Polysystemic Viral Diseases,** 1273
Canine Distemper Virus, 1273
Feline Coronavirus, 1275
Feline Immunodeficiency Virus, 1278
Feline Leukemia Virus, 1281

**103** **Polysystemic Mycotic Infections,** 1287
Cryptococcosis, 1287
Blastomycosis, 1290
Histoplasmosis, 1291
Coccidioidomycosis, 1293

**104** **Polysystemic Protozoal Infections,** 1296
Feline Toxoplasmosis, 1296
Canine Toxoplasmosis, 1299
Neosporosis, 1299
Babesiosis, 1300
Cytauxzoonosis, 1301
Hepatozoonosis, 1302
Leishmaniasis, 1303
American Trypanosomiasis, 1304

**105** **Zoonoses,** 1307
Enteric Zoonoses, 1307
*Nematodes,* 1307
*Cestodes,* 1310
*Coccidians,* 1310
*Flagellates, Amoeba, and Ciliates,* 1311
*Bacteria,* 1312
Bite, Scratch, or Exudate Exposure
Zoonoses, 1312
*Bacteria,* 1312
*Fungi,* 1314
*Viruses,* 1315
Respiratory Tract and Ocular
Zoonoses, 1315
Genital and Urinary Tract Zoonoses, 1316

CHAPTER 1

# The Cardiovascular Examination

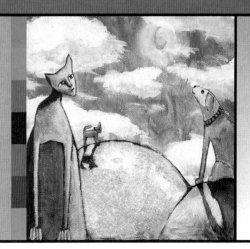

## CHAPTER OUTLINE

HISTORY AND CLINICAL SIGNS, 1
   Signs of heart disease and heart failure, 1
PHYSICAL EXAMINATION, 4
   Mucous membranes, 4
   Jugular veins, 5
   Arterial pulses, 6
   Precordium, 6
   Evaluation for fluid accumulation, 6
   Thoracic auscultation, 6

## HISTORY AND CLINICAL SIGNS

A thorough medical history provides valuable information and is an integral part of the cardiovascular evaluation. Examples of pertinent questions about the patient's medical history are listed in Table 1-1. This information may guide the choice of diagnostic tests by suggesting various cardiac or noncardiac diseases.

### SIGNS OF HEART DISEASE AND HEART FAILURE

Signs of heart disease may be present even if the animal is not in a state of heart failure. Objective signs of heart disease include cardiac murmurs, rhythm disturbances, jugular pulsations, and cardiac enlargement. Other clinical signs that can result from heart disease include syncope, excessively weak or strong arterial pulses, cough or respiratory difficulty, exercise intolerance, and cyanosis. Further evaluation using thoracic radiography, electrocardiography, echocardiography, and sometimes other tests is usually indicated when signs suggestive of cardiovascular disease are present.

The clinical signs of heart failure (Table 1-2) relate to high venous pressure behind the heart (congestive signs) or inadequate blood flow out of the heart (low output signs). Congestive signs secondary to right-sided heart failure stem from

systemic venous hypertension and its sequelae; congestion behind the left side of the heart results in pulmonary venous hypertension and edema. Chronic left-sided congestive heart failure may facilitate the development of right-sided heart failure if pulmonary arterial pressure rises secondary to pulmonary venous hypertension. Low output signs from right ventricular failure are similar to the low output signs of left ventricular failure because the left heart can pump only what it receives from the right heart. Biventricular failure develops in some animals. Heart failure is discussed further in Chapter 3 and within the context of specific diseases.

### Weakness and Syncope

Cardiac output often becomes inadequate in animals with heart disease or heart failure, especially in association with activity. Reduced exercise tolerance and tiring can result from impaired skeletal muscle perfusion during exercise and the vascular and metabolic changes that result over time. Episodes of exertional weakness or collapse can relate to these changes or to an acute decrease in cardiac output caused by arrhythmias (Table 1-3).

Syncope is an abrupt and transient loss of consciousness and postural tone caused by insufficient delivery of oxygen or glucose to the brain. As such, syncope is not a diagnosis itself but a sign of underlying disease. Various cardiac and noncardiac abnormalities can cause syncope as well as intermittent weakness (see Table 1-3). Syncope can be confused with episodes of intermittent weakness or seizures (Fig. 1-1). A careful description of the animal's behavior or activity before the collapse event, during the event itself, and after the collapse, as well as a drug history, helps the clinician differentiate among syncopal attacks, episodic weakness, and true seizures. Syncope is often associated with exertion or excitement. The actual event may be characterized by rear limb weakness or sudden collapse, lateral recumbency, stiffening of the forelimbs and opisthotonos, and micturition (Fig. 1-2). Vocalization is common; however, tonic/clonic motion, facial fits, and defecation are not. An aura (which often

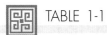 TABLE 1-1

**Important Historical Information**

Signalment (age, breed, gender)?
Vaccination status?
What is the diet? Have there been any recent changes in food or water consumption?
Where was the animal obtained?
Is the pet housed indoors or out?
How much time is spent outdoors? Supervised?
What activity level is normal? Does the animal tire easily now?
Has there been any coughing? When? Describe episodes.
Has there been any excessive or unexpected panting or heavy breathing?
Has there been any vomiting or gagging? Diarrhea?
Have there been any recent changes in urinary habits?
Have there been any episodes of fainting or weakness?
Do the tongue/mucous membranes always look pink, especially during exercise?
Have there been any recent changes in attitude or activity level?
Are medications being given for this problem? Which ones? How much? How often? Do they help?
Have medications been used in the past for this problem? Which ones? How much? Were they effective?

 TABLE 1-2

**Clinical Signs of Left- and Right-Sided Heart Failure**

| LOW OUTPUT SIGNS | CONGESTIVE SIGNS—LEFT SIDE | CONGESTIVE SIGNS—RIGHT SIDE |
| --- | --- | --- |
| Tiring | Pulmonary congestion and edema | Systemic venous congestion (high central venous pressure, |
| Exertional weakness | (resulting in cough, tachypnea, | jugular vein distention) |
| Syncope | dyspnea, orthopnea, pulmonary | Hepatic ± splenic congestion |
| Prerenal azotemia | crackles, tiring, hemoptysis, | Pleural effusion (resulting in dyspnea, orthopnea, cyanosis) |
| Cyanosis (from poor | cyanosis) | Ascites |
| cutaneous circulation) | Secondary right-sided heart failure | Small pericardial effusion |
| Cardiac arrhythmias | Cardiac arrhythmias | Subcutaneous edema |
| | | Cardiac arrhythmias |

 TABLE 1-3

**Causes of Syncope or Intermittent Weakness**

| CARDIAC CAUSES | PULMONARY CAUSES | METABOLIC AND HEMATOLOGIC CAUSES | NEUROLOGIC CAUSES |
| --- | --- | --- | --- |
| Bradyarrhythmias (e.g., second- or third-degree atrioventricular [AV] block, sinus arrest, sick sinus syndrome, atrial standstill) | Diseases causing hypoxemia | Hypoglycemia | Seizures |
| | Cough syncope | Hypoadrenocorticism | Neuromuscular disease |
| Tachyarrhythmias (e.g., paroxysmal atrial or ventricular tachycardia, reentrant supraventricular tachycardia, atrial fibrillation) | Pulmonary hypertension | Electrolyte imbalance (e.g., potassium, calcium) | Cerebrovascular accident |
| Congenital ventricular outflow obstruction (e.g., pulmonic stenosis, subaortic stenosis) | | Anemia | Narcolepsy, cataplexy |
| Acquired ventricular outflow obstruction (e.g., heartworm disease, hypertrophic obstructive cardiomyopathy, thrombus, tumor) | | Sudden hemorrhage | |
| Cyanotic heart disease (e.g., tetralogy of Fallot, "reversed" shunts) | | | |
| Impaired forward cardiac output (e.g., valvular insufficiency, dilated cardiomyopathy, myocardial infarction) | | | |
| Cardiac tamponade | | | |
| Constrictive pericarditis | | | |
| Cardiovascular drugs (e.g., diuretics, vasodilators) | | | |
| Vasodepressor reflexes | | | |

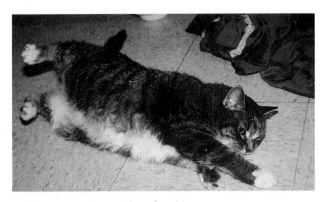

**FIG 1-1**
Cat experiencing syncope related to intermittent complete atrioventricular (AV) block with delayed onset of a ventricular escape rhythm. During these episodes the cat would appear dazed, then fall to the side and stiffen briefly. Within a few seconds she would regain consciousness and resume normal activity.

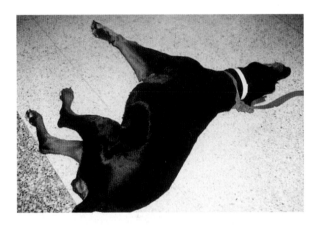

**FIG 1-2**
Syncope in a Doberman Pinscher with paroxysmal ventricular tachycardia. Note the extended head and neck with stiffened forelimbs. Just after this photograph was taken, involuntary micturition occurred, followed by return of consciousness and normal activity.

occurs before seizure activity), postictal dementia, and neurologic deficits are generally not seen in dogs and cats with cardiovascular syncope.

Testing to determine the cause of intermittent weakness or syncope usually includes an electrocardiogram (ECG) (obtained while resting, during exercise, and/or after exercise or a vagal maneuver), a complete blood count (CBC), serum biochemical analysis (including electrolytes and glucose), neurologic examination, thoracic radiographs, heartworm testing, and echocardiography. Other studies to rule out neuromuscular or neurologic disease may also be valuable. Intermittent cardiac arrhythmias not apparent on resting ECG may be uncovered by 24-hour ambulatory ECG (Holter monitor), event monitoring, or in-hospital continuous ECG monitoring.

**Cardiovascular causes of syncope.** Various arrhythmias, ventricular outflow obstructions, cyanotic congenital heart defects, and acquired diseases leading to poor cardiac output are the usual cardiac causes of syncope. Activation of vasodepressor reflexes and excessive dosages of cardiovascular drugs can also induce syncope (see Table 1-3). Causative arrhythmias are usually very fast or very slow and can occur with or without identifiable underlying organic heart disease. Ventricular outflow obstructions provoke syncope or sudden weakness if cardiac output becomes inadequate during exercise or if high systolic pressures activate ventricular mechanoreceptors, causing inappropriate reflex bradycardia and hypotension. Both dilated cardiomyopathy and severe mitral insufficiency can cause inadequate forward cardiac output, especially during exertion. Vasodilators and diuretics may induce syncope if given in excess. Syncope caused by abnormal peripheral vascular and/or neurologic reflex responses is not well defined in animals but is thought to occur occasionally. Postural hypotension, hyperventilation, and hypersensitivity of carotid sinus receptors could cause syncope by inappropriate peripheral vasodilation and bradycardia.

Fainting associated with a coughing fit (cough syncope; "cough-drop") occurs in some dogs with marked left atrial enlargement and bronchial compression, as well as in dogs with primary respiratory disease. Several mechanisms have been proposed, including an acute decrease in cardiac filling and output during the cough, peripheral vasodilation after the cough, and increased cerebrospinal fluid pressure with intracranial venous compression. Severe pulmonary diseases, anemia, certain metabolic abnormalities, and primary neurologic diseases can also cause collapse resembling cardiovascular syncope (see Table 1-3).

## Cough

Congestive heart failure in dogs is often manifested by coughing, tachypnea, and dyspnea. These signs also occur in association with the pulmonary vascular disease and pneumonitis of heartworm disease in both dogs and cats. Noncardiac conditions, including diseases of the upper and lower airways, pulmonary parenchyma (including noncardiogenic pulmonary edema), pulmonary vasculature, and pleural space, as well as certain nonrespiratory conditions, also can cause cough, tachypnea, and dyspnea. (Respiratory diseases are discussed in Chapters 19-23.) The cough accompanying left-sided heart failure in dogs is often soft and moist but sometimes sounds like gagging. In contrast, cough is an unusual sign of pulmonary edema in cats. Tachypnea progressing to dyspnea occurs in both species. Pleural and pericardial effusions occasionally are associated with coughing as well. Mainstem bronchus compression caused by severe left atrial enlargement can stimulate a cough (often described as dry or hacking) in dogs with chronic mitral insufficiency, even in the absence of pulmonary edema or congestion. A heartbase tumor or other mass that impinges on an airway can also mechanically stimulate coughing.

When respiratory signs are caused by heart disease, other evidence such as generalized cardiomegaly, left atrial enlargement, pulmonary venous congestion, lung infiltrates that resolve with diuretic therapy, and/or a positive heartworm test are usually present. Thorough physical examination, thoracic radiographs, an echocardiogram if possible, and an ECG facilitate differentiation of cardiac from noncardiac causes of cough and other respiratory signs.

## PHYSICAL EXAMINATION

Physical evaluation of the animal with suspected heart disease includes observation (e.g., attitude, posture, body condition, level of anxiety, respiratory pattern) and a general physical examination. The cardiovascular examination itself consists of evaluating the peripheral circulation (mucous membranes), systemic veins (especially the jugular veins), systemic arterial pulses (usually the femoral arteries), and the precordium (left and right chest wall over the heart); palpating or percussing for abnormal fluid accumulation (e.g., ascites, subcutaneous edema, pleural effusion); and auscultating the heart and lungs. Proficiency in the cardiovascular examination requires practice. But these skills are important for accurate patient assessment and monitoring.

Respiratory difficulty (dyspnea) usually causes the animal to appear anxious. Increased respiratory effort, flared nostrils, and often a rapid rate of breathing are evident (Fig. 1-3). Increased depth of respiration (hyperpnea) frequently results from hypoxemia, hypercarbia, or acidosis. Pulmonary edema (as well as other pulmonary infiltrates) increases lung stiffness; rapid and shallow breathing (tachypnea) results as an attempt to minimize the work of breathing. An increased resting respiratory rate is an early indicator of pulmonary edema in the absence of primary lung disease. Large-volume pleural effusion or other pleural space disease (e.g., pneumothorax) generally causes exaggerated respiratory motions as an effort to expand the collapsed lungs. It is important to note whether the respiratory difficulty is exaggerated during a particular phase of respiration. Prolonged, labored inspiration is usually associated with upper airway disorders (obstruction), whereas prolonged expiration occurs with lower airway obstruction or pulmonary infiltrative disease (including edema). Animals with severely compromised ventilation may refuse to lie down; they stand or sit with elbows abducted to allow maximal rib expansion, and they resist being positioned in lateral or dorsal recumbency (orthopnea). Cats with dyspnea often crouch in a sternal position with elbows abducted. Open-mouth breathing is usually a sign of severe respiratory distress in cats (Fig. 1-4). The increased respiratory rate associated with excitement, fever, fear, or pain can usually be differentiated from dyspnea by careful observation and physical examination.

### MUCOUS MEMBRANES

Mucous membrane color and capillary refill time (CRT) are used to estimate the adequacy of peripheral perfusion. Normally the oral membranes are assessed; however, caudal mucous membranes (prepuce or vagina) also can be evaluated. The color of the caudal membranes should be compared with

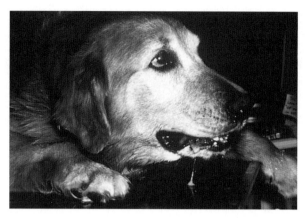

**FIG 1-3**
Dyspnea in an older male Golden Retriever with severe dilated cardiomyopathy and fulminant pulmonary edema. The dog was highly anxious, with rapid, labored respirations and hypersalivation. Shortly after the photograph was taken, he experienced respiratory arrest and was resuscitated. He lived another 9 months with therapy for heart failure.

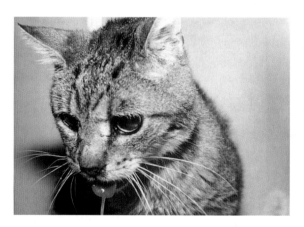

**FIG 1-4**
Severe dyspnea is manifested in this cat by open-mouth breathing, infrequent swallowing (drooling saliva), and reluctance to lie down. Note also the dilated pupils associated with heightened sympathetic tone.

that of the oral membranes in polycythemic cats and dogs regardless of whether a cardiac murmur is detected. If the oral membranes are pigmented, the ocular conjunctiva can be evaluated. The CRT is assessed by applying digital pressure to blanch the membrane; color should return within 2 seconds. Slower refill times occur from dehydration and other causes of decreased cardiac output because of high peripheral sympathetic tone and vasoconstriction. Pale mucous membranes result from anemia or peripheral vasoconstriction. However, the CRT is normal in anemic animals unless hypoperfusion is also present; the CRT can be difficult to assess in severely anemic animals because of the lack of color contrast (see Chapter 85). Table 1-4 outlines causes for abnormal mucous membrane color. Petechiae in the mucous membranes may be noticed in dogs and cats with platelet disorders (see Chapter 89). In addition, oral and ocular mucous

## TABLE 1-4
**Abnormal Mucous Membrane Color**

**Pale Mucous Membranes**

Anemia
Poor cardiac output/high sympathetic tone

**Injected, Brick-Red Membranes**

Polycythemia
Sepsis
Excitement
Other causes of peripheral vasodilation

**Cyanotic Mucous Membranes***

Pulmonary parenchymal disease
Airway obstruction
Pleural space disease
Pulmonary edema
Right-to-left shunting congenital cardiac defect
Hypoventilation
Shock
Cold exposure
Methemoglobinemia

**Differential Cyanosis**

Reversed patent ductus arteriosus (head and forelimbs
receive normally oxygenated blood, but caudal part of
body receives desaturated blood via the ductus, which
arises from the descending aorta)

**Icteric Mucous Membranes**

Hemolysis
Hepatobiliary disease
Biliary obstruction

*Because 5 g of desaturated hemoglobin per deciliter of blood is
necessary for visible cyanosis, anemic animals may not appear
cyanotic even with marked hypoxemia.

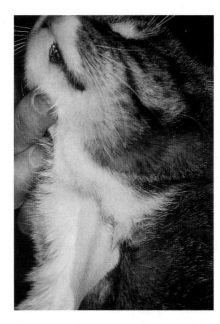

**FIG 1-5**
Prominent jugular vein distention is seen in this cat with signs
of right-sided congestive heart failure from dilated
cardiomyopathy.

## TABLE 1-5
**Causes of Jugular Vein Distention/Pulsation**

**Distention Alone**

Pericardial effusion/tamponade
Right atrial mass/inflow obstruction
Dilated cardiomyopathy
Cranial mediastinal mass
Jugular vein/cranial vena cava thrombosis

**Pulsation ± Distention**

Tricuspid insufficiency of any cause (degenerative,
cardiomyopathy, congenital)
Pulmonic stenosis
Heartworm disease
Pulmonary hypertension
Ventricular premature contractions
Complete (third-degree) heart block

membranes are often the sites where icterus (jaundice) is first detected. A yellowish cast to these membranes should prompt further evaluation for hemolysis (see Chapter 85) or hepatobiliary disease (see Chapter 35).

## JUGULAR VEINS

Systemic venous and right heart filling pressures are reflected at the jugular veins. These veins should not be distended when the animal is standing with its head in a normal position (jaw parallel to the floor). Persistent jugular vein distention occurs in association with right-sided congestive heart failure (because of high right heart filling pressure), external compression of the cranial vena cava, or jugular vein or cranial vena cava thrombosis (Fig. 1-5). Also abnormal are jugular pulsations extending higher than one third of the way up the neck from the thoracic inlet. Sometimes the carotid pulse wave is transmitted through adjacent soft tissues, mimicking a jugular pulse in thin or excited animals. To differentiate a true jugular pulse from carotid transmission, the jugular vein is occluded lightly below the area of

the visible pulse. If the pulse disappears, it is a true jugular pulsation; if the pulse continues, it is being transmitted from the carotid artery. Jugular pulse waves are related to atrial contraction and filling. Visible pulsations occur in animals with tricuspid insufficiency (after the first heart sound, during ventricular contraction), conditions causing a stiff and hypertrophied right ventricle (just before the first heart sound, during atrial contraction), or arrhythmias that cause the atria to contract against closed atrioventricular (AV) valves (so-called cannon *a* waves). Specific causes of jugular vein distention and/or pulsations are listed in Table 1-5. Impaired right ventricular filling, reduced pulmonary blood flow, or tricuspid regurgitation can cause a positive hepato-jugular reflux even in the absence of jugular distention or pulsations at rest. To test for this reflux, firm pressure is applied to the cranial abdomen while the animal stands quietly. This transiently increases venous return. Jugular distention that persists while abdominal pressure is applied constitutes a positive (abnormal) test; normal animals have little to no change in the jugular vein.

## ARTERIAL PULSES

The strength and regularity of the peripheral arterial pressure waves and the pulse rate are assessed by palpation of the femoral or other peripheral arteries. Subjective evaluation of pulse strength is based on the difference between the systolic and diastolic arterial pressures (pulse pressure). When the difference is wide, the pulse feels strong on palpation; abnormally strong pulses are termed *hyperkinetic.* When the pressure difference is small, the pulse feels weak *(hypokinetic).* If the rise to maximum systolic arterial pressure is prolonged, as in animals with severe subaortic stenosis, the pulse also feels weak *(pulsus parvus et tardus).* Both femoral pulses should be palpated and compared; absence of pulse or a weaker pulse on one side may be caused by thromboembolism. Femoral pulses can be difficult to palpate in cats, even when normal. Often an elusive pulse can be found by gently working a fingertip toward the cat's femur in the area of the femoral triangle, where the femoral artery enters the leg between the dorsomedial thigh muscles. Table 1-6 lists diseases that cause alteration of normal femoral pulse strength.

The femoral arterial pulse rate should be evaluated simultaneously with the direct heart rate, which is obtained by chest wall palpation or auscultation. Fewer femoral pulses than heartbeats constitute a pulse deficit. Various cardiac arrhythmias induce pulse deficits by causing the heart to beat before adequate ventricular filling has occurred. Consequently, minimal or even no blood is ejected for those beats, and a palpable pulse is absent. Other arterial pulse variations occur occasionally. Alternately weak then strong pulsations can result from severe myocardial failure *(pulsus alternans)* or from a normal heartbeat alternating with a premature beat (bigeminy), which causes reduced ventricular filling and ejection. An exaggerated decrease in systolic arterial pressure during inspiration occurs with cardiac tamponade; a weak arterial pulse strength *(pulsus paradoxus)* may be detected during inspiration in such a case.

## PRECORDIUM

The precordium is palpated by placing the palm and fingers of each hand on the corresponding side of the animal's chest wall over the heart. Normally the strongest impulse is felt during systole over the area of the left apex (located at approximately the left fifth intercostal space near the costochondral junction). Cardiomegaly or a space-occupying mass within the chest can shift the precordial impulse to an abnormal location. Decreased intensity of the precordial impulse can be caused by obesity, weak cardiac contractions, pericardial effusion, intrathoracic masses, pleural effusion, or pneumothorax. The precordial impulse should be stronger on the left chest wall than on the right. A stronger right precordial impulse can result from right ventricular hypertrophy or displacement of the heart into the right hemithorax by a mass lesion, lung atelectasis, or chest deformity. Very loud cardiac murmurs cause palpable vibrations on the chest wall known as a *precordial thrill.* This feels like a "buzzing" sensation on the hand. A precordial thrill is usually localized to the area of maximal intensity of the murmur.

## EVALUATION FOR FLUID ACCUMULATION

Right-sided congestive heart failure promotes abnormal fluid accumulation within body cavities (see Fig. 11-1) or, usually less noticeably, in the subcutis of dependent areas. Palpation and ballottement of the abdomen, palpation of dependent areas, and percussion of the chest in the standing animal are used to detect effusions and subcutaneous edema. Fluid accumulation secondary to right-sided heart failure is usually accompanied by abnormal jugular vein distention and/or pulsations, unless the animal's circulating blood volume has been decreased by diuretic use or other cause. Hepatomegaly and/or splenomegaly may also be noted in cats and dogs with right-sided heart failure.

## THORACIC AUSCULTATION

Thoracic auscultation is used to identify normal heart sounds, determine the presence or absence of abnormal sounds, assess heart rhythm and rate, and evaluate pulmonary sounds. Heart

 TABLE 1-6

**Abnormal Arterial Pulses**

| WEAK PULSES | STRONG PULSES | VERY STRONG, BOUNDING PULSES |
| --- | --- | --- |
| Dilated cardiomyopathy | Excitement | Patent ductus arteriosus |
| (Sub)aortic stenosis | Hypertrophic cardiopmyopathy (cats) | Fever/sepsis |
| Pulmonic stenosis | Hyperthyroidism | Severe aortic regurgitation |
| Shock | Fever/sepsis | |
| Dehydration | | |

sounds are created by turbulent blood flow and associated vibrations in adjacent tissue during the cardiac cycle. Although many of these sounds are too low in frequency and/or intensity to be audible, others can be heard with the stethoscope or even palpated. Heart sounds are classified as transient sounds (those of short duration) and cardiac murmurs (longer sounds occurring during a normally silent part of the cardiac cycle). Cardiac murmurs and transient sounds are described using general characteristics of sound: frequency (pitch), amplitude of vibrations (intensity/loudness), duration, and quality (timbre); the timbre is affected by the physical characteristics of the vibrating structures. Because many heart sounds are difficult to hear, cooperation of the animal and a quiet room are important during auscultation. If possible, the animal should be standing so that the heart is in its normal position. Panting in dogs is discouraged by holding the animal's mouth shut. Respiratory noise can be decreased further by placing a finger over one or both nostrils for a short time. Purring in cats may be stopped by holding a finger over one or both nostrils (Fig. 1-6), waving an alcohol-soaked cotton ball near the cat's nose, or turning on a water faucet near the animal. Various other artifacts can interfere with auscultation, including respiratory clicks, air movement sounds, shivering, muscle twitching, hair rubbing against the stethoscope (crackling sounds), gastrointestinal sounds, and extraneous room noises.

The traditional stethoscope has both a stiff, flat diaphragm and a bell on the chestpiece. The diaphragm, when applied firmly to the chest wall, allows better auscultation of higher frequency heart sounds than those of low frequency. The bell, applied lightly to the chest wall, facilitates auscultation of lower frequency sounds such as $S_3$ and $S_4$ (see gallop sounds below). Some stethoscopes have a single-sided chestpiece that is designed to function as a diaphragm when used with firm pressure and as a bell when used with light pressure. Ideally the stethoscope should have short double tubing and comfortable eartips. The binaural eartubes should be angled rostrally to align with the examiner's ear canals (Fig. 1-7).

Both sides of the chest should be carefully auscultated, with special attention paid to the valve areas (Fig. 1-8). The stethoscope is moved gradually to all areas of the chest. The examiner should concentrate on the various heart sounds, correlating them to the events of the cardiac cycle, and listen for any abnormal sounds in systole and diastole successively. The normal heart sounds ($S_1$ and $S_2$) are used as a framework for timing abnormal sounds. The point of maximal intensity (PMI) of any abnormal sounds should be located. The examiner should focus on cardiac auscultation separately from pulmonary auscultation because full assimilation of sounds from both systems simultaneously is unlikely. Pulmonary auscultation is described further in Chapter 19.

## Transient Heart Sounds

The heart sounds normally heard in dogs and cats are $S_1$ (associated with closure and tensing of the AV valves and associated structures at the onset of systole) and $S_2$ (associated with closure of the aortic and pulmonic valves following ejection). The diastolic sounds ($S_3$ and $S_4$) are not audible in normal dogs and cats. Fig. 1-9 correlates the hemodynamic events of the cardiac cycle with the ECG and timing of the heart sounds. It is important to understand these events and identify the timing of systole (between $S_1$ and $S_2$) and diastole (after $S_2$ until the next $S_1$) in the animal. The precordial impulse occurs just after $S_1$ (systole) and the arterial pulse between $S_1$ and $S_2$.

Sometimes the first ($S_1$) and/or second ($S_2$) heart sounds are altered in intensity. A loud $S_1$ may be heard in dogs and cats with a thin chest wall, high sympathetic tone, tachycardia, systemic arterial hypertension, or shortened PR intervals. A muffled $S_1$ can result from obesity, pericardial effusion, diaphragmatic hernia, dilated cardiomyopathy, hypovolemia/poor ventricular filling, or pleural effusion. A split or sloppy-sounding $S_1$ may be normal, especially in large dogs, or it may result from ventricular premature contractions or an intraventricular conduction delay. The intensity of the $S_2$ is

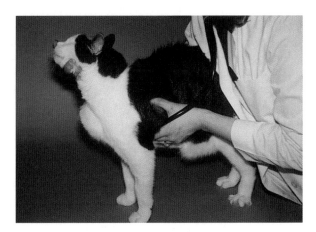

**FIG 1-6**
During cardiac auscultation, respiratory noise and purring can be decreased or eliminated by gently placing a finger over one or both nostrils for brief periods.

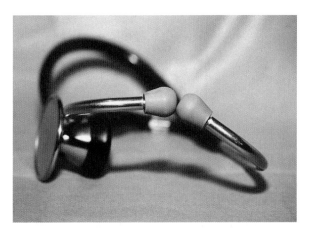

**FIG 1-7**
Note the angulation of the stethoscope's eartubes for optimal alignment with the clinician's ear canals (top of picture is rostral). The flat diaphragm of the chestpiece is facing left, and the concave bell is facing right.

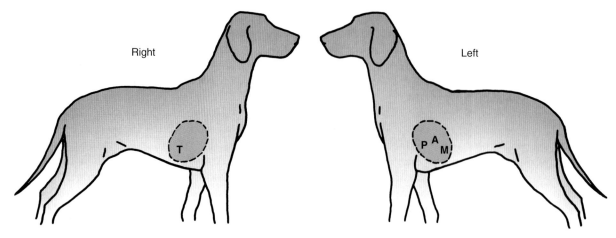

**FIG 1-8**
Approximate locations of various valve areas on the chest wall. *T,* Tricuspid; *P,* pulmonic; *A,* aortic; *M,* mitral.

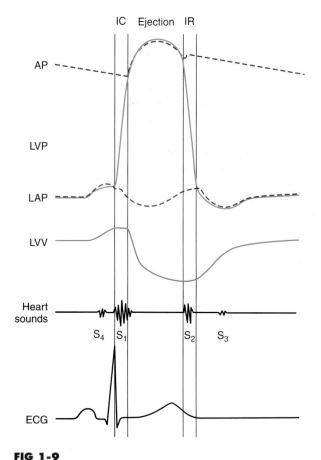

**FIG 1-9**
Cardiac cycle, depicting relationships among the great vessel, ventricular, and atrial pressures, ventricular volume, heart sounds, and electrical activation. *AP,* Aortic pressure; *ECG,* electrocardiogram; *IC,* isovolumic contraction; *IR,* isovolumic relaxation; *LVP,* left ventricular pressure; *LAP,* left atrial pressure; *LVV,* left ventricular volume.

increased by pulmonary hypertension, for example, from heartworm disease, a congenital shunt with Eisenmenger's physiology, or cor pulmonale. Normal physiologic splitting of $S_2$ can be heard in some dogs because of variation in stroke volume during the respiratory cycle. During inspiration, increased venous return to the right ventricle tends to delay closure of the pulmonic valve, and reduced filling of the left ventricle accelerates aortic closure. Pathologic splitting of $S_2$ can result from delayed ventricular activation or prolonged right ventricular ejection secondary to ventricular premature beats, right bundle branch block, a ventricular or atrial septal defect, or pulmonary hypertension. Cardiac arrhythmias often cause variation in the intensity (or even absence) of heart sounds.

**Gallop sounds.** The third ($S_3$) and fourth ($S_4$) heart sounds occur during diastole (see Figure 1-9) and are not normally audible in dogs and cats. When an $S_3$ or $S_4$ sound is heard, the heart may sound like a galloping horse, hence the term *gallop rhythm.* This term can be confusing because the presence or absence of an audible $S_3$ or $S_4$ has nothing to do with the heart's rhythm (i.e., the origin of cardiac activation and the intracardiac conduction process). Gallop sounds are usually heard best with the bell of the stethoscope (or by light pressure applied to a single-sided chestpiece) because they are of lower frequency than $S_1$ and $S_2$. At very fast heart rates, differentiation of $S_3$ from $S_4$ is difficult. If both sounds are present, they may be superimposed, which is called a *summation gallop.*

The $S_3$, also known as an $S_3$ *gallop* or *ventricular gallop,* is associated with low-frequency vibrations at the end of the rapid ventricular filling phase. An audible $S_3$ in the dog or cat usually indicates ventricular dilation with myocardial failure. The extra sound can be fairly loud or very subtle and is heard best over the cardiac apex. It may be the only auscultable abnormality in an animal with dilated cardiomyopathy. An $S_3$ gallop may also be audible in dogs with advanced valvular heart disease and congestive failure.

TABLE 1-7

**Grading of Heart Murmurs**

| GRADE | MURMUR |
|-------|--------|
| I | Very soft murmur; heard only in quiet surroundings after minutes of listening |
| II | Soft murmur but easily heard |
| III | Moderate-intensity murmur |
| IV | Loud murmur but not accompanied by a precordial thrill |
| V | Loud murmur with a palpable precordial thrill |
| VI | Very loud murmur that can be heard with the stethoscope off the chest wall; accompanied by a precordial thrill |

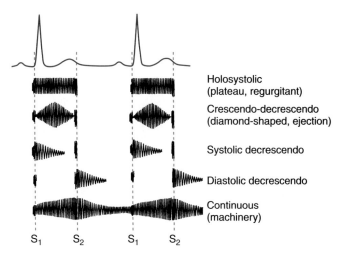

**FIG 1-10**
Murmur shapes and descriptions. The phonocardiographic shapes and timing of different murmurs are depicted and described.

The $S_4$ gallop, also called an *atrial* or *presystolic gallop,* is associated with low-frequency vibrations induced by blood flow into the ventricles during atrial contraction (just after the P wave of the ECG). An audible $S_4$ in the dog or cat is usually associated with increased ventricular stiffness and hypertrophy, as with hypertrophic cardiomyopathy or hyperthyroidism in cats. A transient $S_4$ gallop of unknown significance is sometimes heard in stressed or anemic cats.

**Other transient sounds.** Other brief abnormal sounds are sometimes audible. *Systolic clicks* are mid-to-late systolic sounds that are usually heard best over the mitral valve area. These sounds have been associated with degenerative valvular disease (endocardiosis), mitral valve prolapse, and congenital mitral dysplasia; a concurrent mitral insufficiency murmur may be present. In dogs with degenerative valvular disease, a mitral click may be the first abnormal sound noted, with a murmur developing over time. An early systolic, high-pitched ejection sound at the left base may occur in animals with valvular pulmonic stenosis or other diseases that cause dilation of a great artery. The sound is thought to arise from either the sudden checking of a fused pulmonic valve or the rapid filling of a dilated vessel during ejection. Rarely, restrictive pericardial disease causes an audible pericardial knock. This diastolic sound is caused by sudden checking of ventricular filling by the restrictive pericardium; its timing is similar to the $S_3$.

## Cardiac Murmurs

Cardiac murmurs are described by their timing within the cardiac cycle (systolic or diastolic, or portions thereof), intensity, PMI on the precordium, radiation over the chest wall, quality, and pitch. Systolic murmurs may occur in early (protosystolic), middle (mesosystolic), or late (telesystolic) systole or throughout systole (holosystolic). Diastolic murmurs generally occur in early diastole (protodiastolic) or throughout diastole (holodiastolic). Murmurs occurring at the very end of diastole are termed presystolic. The intensity of a murmur is arbitrarily graded on a I to VI scale (Table 1-7). The PMI is

usually indicated by the hemithorax (right or left) and intercostal space or valve area where it is located or by the terms *apex* or *base.* The areas to which the murmur radiates can be extensive, so the entire thorax, thoracic inlet, and carotid artery areas should be auscultated. The pitch and quality of a murmur relate to its frequency and subjective assessment. "Noisy" or "harsh" murmurs contain mixed frequencies. "Musical" murmurs are of essentially one frequency with its overtones.

A murmur is also described by its shape, as it appears on a phonocardiogram (graphic recording of cardiac sounds). Fig. 1-10 illustrates the shape and description of different murmurs. A plateau or regurgitant (holosystolic) murmur begins at about the time of $S_1$ and has a fairly uniform intensity throughout systole. Loud murmurs of this type may prevent distinction of $S_1$ and $S_2$ from the murmur. AV valve insufficiency and interventricular septal defects commonly cause this type of murmur because turbulent movement of blood occurs throughout ventricular systole. A crescendo-decrescendo or diamond-shaped murmur starts softly, builds intensity in midsystole, and then diminishes; $S_1$ and $S_2$ can usually be heard clearly before and after the murmur. This type is also called an *ejection murmur* because it occurs during blood ejection, usually because of ventricular outflow obstruction. A decrescendo murmur tapers from its initial intensity over time; it may occur in systole or diastole. Continuous (machinery) murmurs occur throughout systole and diastole.

**Systolic murmurs.** Systolic murmurs can be decrescendo, holosystolic (plateau shaped), or ejection (crescendo-decrescendo) in configuration. It can be difficult to differentiate these murmurs by auscultation alone, especially for the inexperienced listener. However, establishing that a murmur occurs in systole (rather than diastole), determining its PMI, and grading its intensity are the most important steps toward

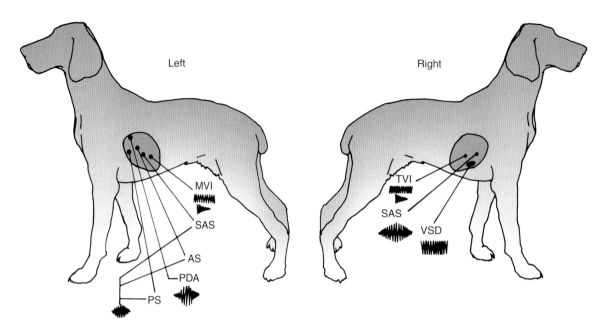

**FIG 1-11**
Location of murmurs. The usual PMI and the phonocardiographic shape of various congenital and acquired murmurs are depicted on the left chest wall **(A)** and the right chest wall **(B).** *AS,* Aortic (valvular) stenosis; *MVI,* mitral valve insufficiency; *PDA,* patent ductus arteriosus; *PS,* pulmonic stenosis; *SAS,* subaortic stenosis; *TVI,* tricuspid valve insufficiency; *VSD,* ventricular septal defect. (From Bonagura JD et al: Cardiovascular and pulmonary disorders. In Fenner W, editor: *Quick reference to veterinary medicine,* ed 2, Philadelphia, 1991, JB Lippincott.)

diagnosis. Fig. 1-11 indicates the typical location of various murmurs over different areas of the chest wall.

Functional murmurs tend to be heard best over the left base of the heart. They are usually of soft-to-moderate intensity and have a decrescendo (or crescendo-decrescendo) configuration. Functional murmurs may have no apparent cardiovascular cause (e.g., "innocent" puppy murmurs) or can result from an altered physiologic state (physiologic murmurs). Physiologic murmurs have been associated with anemia, fever, high sympathetic tone, hyperthyroidism, peripheral arteriovenous fistulae, hypoproteinemia, and athletic hearts.

The murmur of mitral insufficiency is heard best at the left apex in the area of the mitral valve. It radiates well dorsally and often to the left base and right chest wall. Mitral insufficiency characteristically causes a plateau or regurgitant murmur (holosystolic timing); however, in its early stages the murmur may be protosystolic, tapering to a decrescendo configuration. Occasionally this murmur has a musical or "whoop-like" quality.

Systolic ejection murmurs are most often heard at the left base and are caused by ventricular outflow obstruction, usually from a fixed narrowing (e.g., subaortic or pulmonic valve stenosis) or dynamic muscular obstruction. These murmurs become louder as cardiac output or contractile strength increases. The murmur of subaortic stenosis is heard well at the low left base and at the right base because the murmur radiates up the aortic arch, which curves toward the right. This

murmur also radiates up the carotid arteries and occasionally can be heard on the calvarium. The murmur of pulmonic stenosis is best heard high at the left base. Relative pulmonic stenosis occurs when flow through the valve is greatly increased even though the valve itself may be structurally normal (e.g., with a large left-to-right shunting atrial or ventricular septal defect).

Most murmurs heard on the right chest wall are holosystolic, plateau-shaped murmurs, with the exception of the murmur of subaortic stenosis as described earlier. The tricuspid insufficiency murmur is loudest at the right apex over the tricuspid valve. It may have a noticeably different pitch or quality from a concurrent mitral insufficiency murmur and often is accompanied by jugular pulsations. Ventricular septal defects also cause holosystolic murmurs. The PMI is usually at the right sternal border, reflecting the direction of the intracardiac shunt. A large ventricular septal defect may also cause the murmur of relative pulmonic stenosis.

**Diastolic murmurs.** Diastolic murmurs are uncommon in dogs and cats. Aortic insufficiency from bacterial endocarditis is the most common cause, although congenital malformation or degenerative aortic valve disease occasionally occurs. Clinically relevant pulmonic insufficiency is rare but would be more likely in the face of pulmonary hypertension. These diastolic murmurs begin at the time of $S_2$ and are heard best at the left base. They are decrescendo in configuration and extend a variable time into diastole, depending on the pressure difference between the associated great vessel and ventricle. Some aortic insufficiency murmurs have a musical quality.

**Continuous murmurs.** As implied by the name, continuous (machinery) murmurs occur throughout the cardiac cycle, indicating that a significant pressure gradient continuously exists between two connecting locations (vessels). There is no interruption of the murmur at the time of $S_2$; instead, the intensity is often greater at that time. The murmur becomes softer toward the end of diastole, and at slow heart rates it may even become inaudible. Patent ductus arteriosus (PDA) is by far the most common cause of a continuous murmur. The PDA murmur is loudest high at the left base above the pulmonic valve area; this murmur tends to radiate cranially, ventrally, and to the right. The systolic component is usually louder and heard well all over the chest, whereas the diastolic component is more localized to the left base in many cases. If only the cardiac apical area is auscultated, the diastolic component (and the correct diagnosis) may be missed.

Continuous murmurs can be confused with concurrent systolic ejection and diastolic decrescendo murmurs. But in these so-called *to-and-fro murmurs*, the ejection murmur component tapers in late systole, allowing the $S_2$ to be heard as a distinct sound. The most common cause of to-and-fro murmurs is the combination of subaortic stenosis with aortic insufficiency. Rarely, stenosis and insufficiency of the pulmonic valve cause this type of murmur.

## Suggested Readings

Davidow EB et al: Syncope: pathophysiology and differential diagnosis, *Compend Contin Educ* 23:608, 2001.

Goodwin JK: Pulse alterations. In Ettinger SJ et al, editors: *Textbook of veterinary internal medicine*, ed 5, Philadelphia, 2000, WB Saunders, p 174.

Hamlin RL: Normal cardiovascular physiology. In Fox PR et al, editors: *Canine and feline cardiology*, ed 2, New York, 1999, WB Saunders, p 25.

Perloff JK: Heart sounds and murmurs: physiological mechanisms. In Braunwald E, editor: *Heart disease: a textbook of cardiovascular medicine*, ed 4, Philadelphia, 1992, WB Saunders, p 43.

Ware WA: Abnormal heart sounds and heart murmurs. In Ettinger SJ et al, editors: *Textbook of veterinary internal medicine*, ed 5, Philadelphia, 2000, WB Saunders, p 170.

# CHAPTER 2

# Diagnostic Tests for the Cardiovascular System

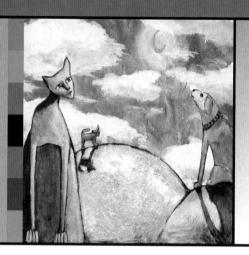

## CHAPTER OUTLINE

ELECTROCARDIOGRAPHY, 12
  Benefits and limitations, 12
  Normal ECG waveforms, 12
  Lead systems, 12
  Mean electrical axis, 13
  Chamber enlargement and bundle branch block
    patterns, 15
  Sinus rhythms, 15
  Ectopic impulses, 16
  Conduction disturbances, 23
  ST-T abnormalities, 25
  ECG manifestations of drug toxicities and electrolyte
    imbalances, 25
  Approach to ECG interpretation, 26
  Common artifacts, 29
  Ambulatory electrocardiography, 29
  Other methods of ECG assessment, 29
THORACIC RADIOGRAPHY, 32
  Cardiomegaly, 32
  Cardiac chamber enlargement patterns, 32
  Intrathoracic blood vessels, 34
  Patterns of pulmonary edema, 35
ECHOCARDIOGRAPHY (CARDIAC
ULTRASONOGRAPHY), 35
  Benefits and limitations, 35
  Basic principles, 36
  Two-dimensional echocardiography, 36
  M-mode echocardiography, 38
  Contrast echocardiography, 43
  Doppler echocardiography, 44
  Transesophageal echocardiography, 47
OTHER TECHNIQUES, 47

## ELECTROCARDIOGRAPHY

### BENEFITS AND LIMITATIONS

The electrocardiogram (ECG) provides a graphic representation of the electrical depolarization and repolarization processes of the cardiac muscle, as viewed from the body surface. The amplitude of these electrical potential differences is measured in millivolts (mV), and their duration is measured in seconds. The ECG provides information on heart rate, rhythm, and intracardiac conduction; it may also suggest the presence of specific chamber enlargement, myocardial disease, ischemia, pericardial disease, certain electrolyte imbalances, or some drug toxicities. However, the ECG alone cannot be used to make a diagnosis of congestive heart failure, assess the strength (or even presence) of cardiac contractions, or predict whether the animal will survive an anesthetic or surgical procedures.

### NORMAL ECG WAVEFORMS

The normal cardiac rhythm originates in the sinoatrial node and follows the cardiac conduction pathway outlined in Fig. 2-1. The ECG waveforms, P-QRS-T, are generated as the heart muscle is depolarized and then repolarized. Fig. 2-2 identifies the normal P-QRS-T waveforms, and Table 2-1 describes what each wave represents. The configuration of the QRS complex depends on the orientation of the lead being recorded. There can be some variation from animal to animal. The QRS complex as a whole represents electrical activation of ventricular muscle, regardless of whether individual Q, R, or S components (or variations thereof) are present or absent. The number of complexes (or beats) per minute is the heart rate.

### LEAD SYSTEMS

Various leads are used to evaluate the cardiac activation process. The orientation of a lead with respect to the heart is called the *lead axis*. Each lead has direction and polarity. A lead records the components of the depolarization and repolarization processes that are aligned with it. If the myocardial activation wave travels parallel to the lead, a relatively large

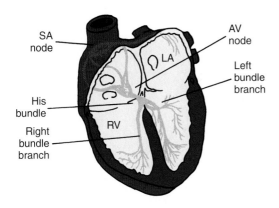

**FIG 2-1**
Schematic of cardiac conduction system. *AV,* Atrioventricular; *LA,* left atrium; *RV,* right ventricle; *SA,* sinoatrial. (Modified from Tilley LE: *Essentials of canine and feline electrocardiography,* ed 3, Philadelphia, 1992, Lea & Febiger.)

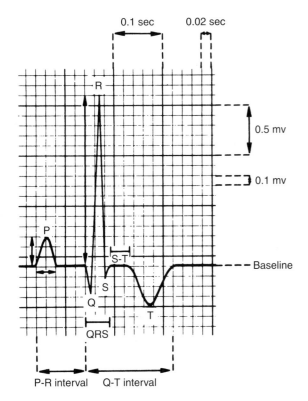

**FIG 2-2**
Normal canine P-QRS-T complex in lead II. Paper speed is 50 mm/sec; calibration is standard (1 cm = 1 mV). Time intervals (seconds) are measured from left to right; waveform amplitudes (millivolts) are measured as positive (upward) or negative (downward) motion from baseline. (From Tilley LE: *Essentials of canine and feline electrocardiography,* ed 3, Philadelphia, 1992, Lea & Febiger.)

deflection will be recorded. As the angle between the lead axis and the orientation of the activation wave increases toward 90 degrees, the ECG deflection for that lead becomes smaller; it becomes isoelectric when the activation wave is perpendicular to the lead axis. Each lead has a positive and a negative

 TABLE 2-1

**Normal Cardiac Waveforms**

| WAVEFORM | INTERPRETATION |
|---|---|
| P | Activation of atrial muscle; normally is positive in leads II and aV$_F$ |
| PQ interval | Time from onset of atrial muscle activation, through conduction over the atrioventricular (AV) node, bundle of His, and Purkinje fibers; also called PR interval |
| QRS complex | Activation of ventricular muscle; by definition, Q is the first negative deflection (if present), R is the first positive deflection, and S is the negative deflection after the R wave |
| J point | End of the QRS complex |
| ST segment | Represents the period between ventricular depolarization and repolarization (correlates with phase 2 of the action potential) |
| T wave | Ventricular muscle repolarization |
| QT interval | Total time of ventricular depolarization and repolarization |

pole or direction. A positive deflection will be recorded in a lead if the cardiac activation wave travels toward the positive pole (electrode) of that lead. If the wave of depolarization travels away from the positive pole, a negative deflection will be recorded in that ECG lead.

Both bipolar and unipolar ECG leads are used clinically. The standard bipolar leads record electrical potential differences between two electrodes on the body surface; the lead axis is oriented between these two points. The augmented unipolar leads employ a recording electrode (positive) on the body surface. The negative pole of the unipolar leads is formed by "Wilson's central terminal" (V), which is formed by the average from all other electrodes and is analogous to the center of the heart (or zero).

The standard limb lead system evaluates cardiac electrical activity in the frontal plane, which is the plane depicted by a ventrodorsal radiograph. In this plane, left-to-right and cranial-to-caudal currents are represented. Fig. 2-3 depicts the cardiac ventricles in the torso overlaid with the six standard frontal leads (hexaxial lead system). Unipolar chest (precordial) leads "view" the heart from the transverse plane (Fig. 2-4). The orthogonal lead system views the heart in three perpendicular planes. Table 2-2 outlines the common ECG lead systems.

## MEAN ELECTRICAL AXIS

The mean electrical axis (MEA) describes the average direction of the *ventricular* depolarization process in the frontal plane. It represents the summation of the various instantaneous vectors

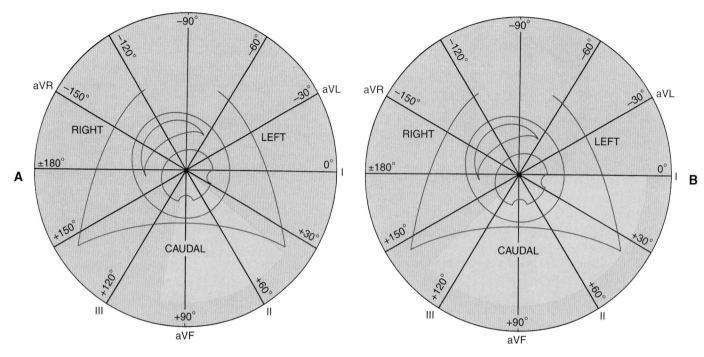

**FIG 2-3**

Frontal lead system: diagrams of six frontal leads over schematic of left and right ventricles within the thorax. Circular field is used for determining direction and magnitude of cardiac electrical activation. Each lead is labeled at its positive pole. Shaded area represents normal range for mean electrical axis. **A,** Dog. **B,** Cat.

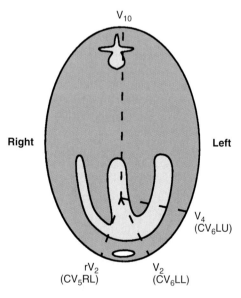

**FIG 2-4**

Commonly used chest leads seen from cross-sectional view. CV₅RL is located at right edge of sternum in fifth intercostal space (ICS); CV₆LL is near sternum at sixth ICS; CV₆LU is at costochondral junction at sixth ICS; and V₁₀ is located near seventh dorsal spinous process.

TABLE 2-2

### Small Animal ECG Lead Systems

| | |
|---|---|
| **Standard Bipolar Limb Leads** | |
| I | RA (−) compared with LA (+) |
| II | RA (−) compared with LL (+) |
| III | LA (−) compared with LL (+) |
| **Augmented Unipolar Limb Leads** | |
| $aV_R$ | RA (+) compared with average of LA and LL (−) |
| $aV_L$ | LA (+) compared with average of RA and LL (−) |
| $aV_F$ | LL (+) compared with average of RA and LA (−) |
| **Unipolar Chest Leads** | |
| $CV_6LL$ ($V_{2-3}$) | Sixth left ICS near sternum |
| $CV_6LU$ ($V_{4-6}$) | Sixth left ICS near costochondral junction |
| $V_{10}$ | Over dorsal spinous process of seventh thoracic vertebra |
| $CV_5RL$ ($rV_2$) | Fifth right ICS near sternum |
| **Orthogonal Leads** | |
| X | Lead I (right to left) in the frontal plane |
| Y | Lead $aV_F$ (cranial to caudal) in the midsagittal plane |
| Z | Lead $V_{10}$ (ventral to dorsal) in the transverse plane |

*RA,* Right arm; *LA,* left arm; *LL,* left leg; *ICS,* intercostal space.

that occur from the beginning until the end of ventricular muscle activation. Estimation of the MEA helps the clinician identify major intraventricular conduction disturbances and/or ventricular enlargement patterns that shift the average direction of ventricular activation. Because the MEA is determined in the frontal plane, only the six frontal leads are used. The MEA can be estimated by either of the following methods:

1. Find the lead (I, II, III, aV$_R$, aV$_L$, or aV$_F$) with the largest R wave (*Note:* the R wave is a positive deflection). The positive electrode of this lead is the approximate MEA orientation.
2. Find the lead (I, II, III, aV$_R$, aV$_L$, or aV$_F$) with the most isoelectric QRS (positive and negative deflections are about equal). Then identify the lead perpendicular to this lead on the hexaxial lead diagram (see Fig. 2-3). If the QRS in this perpendicular lead is mostly positive, the MEA is toward the positive pole of this lead. If the QRS in the perpendicular lead is mostly negative, the MEA is oriented toward the negative pole. If all leads appear isoelectric, the frontal axis is indeterminate. (See Fig. 2-3 for the normal MEA ranges for dogs and cats.)

## CHAMBER ENLARGEMENT AND BUNDLE BRANCH BLOCK PATTERNS

Changes in the ECG waveforms can suggest enlargement or conduction disturbance of a particular cardiac chamber, although enlargement is not consistently accompanied by these changes. Widening of the P wave has been associated with left atrial enlargement (p mitrale); sometimes the P wave is notched as well as wide. Right atrial enlargement may be manifested as a tall, spiked P wave (p pulmonale). With atrial enlargement the atrial repolarization (T$_a$ wave), which usually is obscured, may be evident as a baseline shift in the opposite direction of the P wave.

Because activation of the left ventricle is normally so dominant, right ventricular enlargement (dilation or hypertrophy) is usually pronounced if it is evident on the ECG. A right-axis deviation and an S wave in lead I are strong criteria for right ventricular enlargement (or right bundle branch block). Other ECG changes can usually be found as well. Three or more of the criteria listed in Table 2-3 are generally present when right ventricular enlargement exists.

Left ventricular dilation and eccentric hypertrophy (see p. 54) often cause increased R-wave voltages in the caudal leads (II and aV$_F$) and widening of the QRS. Left ventricular concentric hypertrophy (see Cardiac Responses section of Chapter 3) is inconsistently accompanied by a left-axis deviation. Conduction blocks in the major ventricular conduction pathways disturb the normal activation process and alter the QRS configuration. The region of ventricular muscle served by a diseased bundle branch is activated late and slowly, which causes QRS widening and orientation of the terminal QRS forces toward the area of delayed activation. Table 2-3 and Fig. 2-5 summarize ECG patterns seen in association with ventricular enlargement or conduction delay. Common clinical associations are listed in Table 2-4.

Small-voltage QRS complexes sometimes occur. Causes of reduced QRS amplitude include pleural or pericardial effusions, obesity, intrathoracic mass lesions, hypovolemia, and hypothyroidism. Small complexes are occasionally seen in dogs without identifiable abnormalities.

## SINUS RHYTHMS

Sinus rhythm is the normal cardiac rhythm, manifested by the P-QRS-T waveforms described previously. The P waves are positive in the caudal leads (II and aV$_F$), the PQ intervals are consistent, and the R to R intervals occur regularly, with less than 10% variation in timing. Normally the QRS complexes are narrow and upright in leads II and aV$_F$; however, if

 **TABLE 2-3**

**Ventricular Enlargement Patterns and Conduction Abnormalities**

**Normal**

Normal mean electrical axis
No S wave in lead I
Lead II R wave taller than that in lead I
Lead CV$_6$LL R wave larger than S wave

**Right Ventricular Enlargement**

Right-axis deviation
S wave present in lead I
S wave in V$_3$ (CV$_6$LL) deeper than R wave is tall or greater than 0.8 mV
Q-S (W shape) in V$_{10}$
Positive T wave in lead V$_{10}$ (except Chihuahua breed)
Deep S wave in leads II, III, and aV$_F$

**Right Bundle Branch Block (RBBB)**

Same as right ventricular enlargement with the end of the QRS prolonged (wide, sloppy S wave)

**Left Ventricular Hypertrophy**

Left-axis deviation
R wave in lead I taller than R wave in leads II or aV$_F$
No S wave in lead I

**Left Anterior Fascicular Block (LAFB)**

Same as left ventricular hypertrophy, possibly with wider QRS

**Left Ventricular Dilation**

Normal frontal axis
Taller than normal R wave in leads II, aV$_F$, CV$_6$LL
Widened QRS; slurring and displacement of ST segment and T-wave enlargement may also occur

**Left Bundle Branch Block (LBBB)**

Normal frontal axis
Very wide and sloppy QRS
Small Q wave may be present in leads II, III, and aV$_F$ (incomplete LBBB)

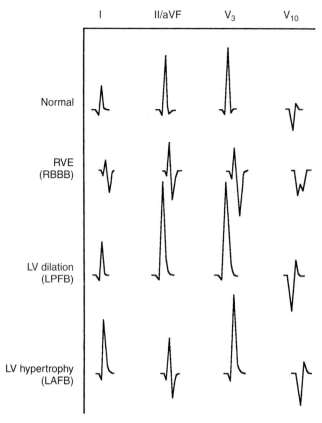

**FIG 2-5**
Schematic of common ventricular enlargement patterns and conduction abnormalities. ECG leads are listed across top. *LAFB,* Left anterior fascicular block; *LPFB,* left posterior fascicular block; *LV,* left ventricular; *RVE,* right ventricular enlargement; *RBBB,* right bundle branch block.

 TABLE 2-4

**Clinical Associations of ECG Enlargement Patterns**

**Left Atrial Enlargement**

Mitral insufficiency (acquired or congenital)
Cardiomyopathies
Patent ductus arteriosus
Subaortic stenosis
Ventricular septal defect

**Right Atrial Enlargement**

Tricuspid insufficiency (acquired or congenital)
Chronic respiratory disease
Interatrial septal defect
Pulmonic stenosis

**Left Ventricular Enlargement (Dilation)**

Mitral insufficiency
Dilated cardiomyopathy
Aortic insufficiency
Patent ductus arteriosus
Ventricular septal defect
Subaortic stenosis

**Left Ventricular Enlargement (Hypertrophy)**

Hypertrophic cardiomyopathy
Subaortic stenosis

**Right Ventricular Enlargement**

Pulmonic stenosis
Tetralogy of Fallot
Tricuspid insufficiency (acquired or congenital)
Severe heartworm disease
Pulmonary hypertension (of any cause)

an intraventricular conduction disturbance or ventricular enlargement pattern is present, they may be wide and abnormally shaped. Sinus arrhythmia is characterized by a cyclic slowing and speeding of the sinus rate; it is usually associated with respiration. The sinus rate tends to increase on inspiration and decrease with expiration as a result of fluctuations in vagal tone. There may also be a cyclic change in P-wave configuration ("wandering pacemaker"), with the P waves becoming taller and spiked during inspiration and flatter in expiration. Sinus arrhythmia is a common and normal rhythm variation in dogs. It also occurs in resting cats, but it is not often seen clinically. Pronounced sinus arrhythmia occurs in some animals with chronic pulmonary disease. Reflex fluctuations in vagal tone during the respiratory cycle can be accentuated by intrapleural, intrapulmonary, and/or intravascular changes accompanying lung disease.

Table 2-5 lists normal heart rate ranges for sinus rhythms in dogs and cats. The term *bradyarrhythmia* describes a heart rhythm that is slow, without identifying its site of origin. Conversely, a *tachyarrhythmia* is a heart rhythm with a faster rate than normal. Both sinus bradycardia and sinus tachycardia are rhythms that originate in the sinus node and are conducted normally; however, the rate of sinus bradycardia is slower than normal for the species, whereas that of sinus tachycardia is faster than normal. Some causes of sinus bradycardia and tachycardia are listed in Table 2-6.

Sinus arrest is a cessation of sinus activity lasting at least twice as long as the animal's longest expected RR interval. The resulting pause is interrupted by either an escape beat or resumption of sinus activity. Long pauses can cause fainting or weakness. Sinus arrest cannot be differentiated with certainty from sinoatrial (SA) block by the surface ECG. Fig. 2-6 illustrates various sinus rhythms.

## ECTOPIC IMPULSES

Impulses originating elsewhere than the sinus node (ectopic impulses) are abnormal and create an arrhythmia (dysrhythmia). Ectopic impulses are described on the basis of their general site of origin (atrial, junctional, supraventricular, ventricular) and their timing (Fig. 2-7). Timing refers to whether

TABLE 2-5

Normal ECG Reference Ranges for Dogs and Cats

| DOGS | CATS |
|---|---|
| **Heart Rate** | |
| 70 to 160 beats/min (adults)* to 220 beats/min (puppies) | 120 to 240 beats/min |
| **Mean Electrical Axis (Frontal Plane)** | |
| +40 to +100 degrees | 0 to +160 degrees |
| **Measurements (Lead II)** | |
| **P-wave duration (maximum)** | |
| 0.04 set (0.05 sec, giant breeds) | 0.035 to 0.04 sec |
| **P-wave height (maximum)** | |
| 0.4 mV | 0.2 mV |
| **PR interval** | |
| 0.06 to 0.13 sec | 0.05 to 0.09 sec |
| **QRS complex duration (maximum)** | |
| 0.05 sec (small breeds) | 0.04 sec |
| 0.06 sec (large breeds) | |
| **R-wave height (maximum)** | |
| 2.5 mV (small breeds) | 0.9 mV; QRS total in any lead <1.2 mV |
| 3 mV (large breeds)† | |
| **ST segment deviation** | |
| <0.2 mV depression | No marked deviation |
| <0.15 mV elevation | |
| **T wave** | |
| Normally <25% of R-wave height; can be positive, negative, or biphasic | Maximum 0.3 mV; can be positive (most common), negative, or biphasic |
| **QT interval duration** | |
| 0.15 to 0.25 (to 0.27) sec; varies inversely with heart rate | 0.12 to 0.18 (range 0.07 to 0.2) sec; varies inversely with heart rate |
| **Chest Leads** | |
| $CV_5RL$ ($rV_2$): positive T wave | R wave 1.0 mV maximum in chest leads |
| $CV_6LL$ ($V_2$): S wave 0.8 mV maximum; R wave 2.5 mV maximum† | |
| $CV_6LU$ ($V_4$): S wave 0.7 mV maximum; R wave 3 mV maximum† | |
| $V_{10}$: negative QRS; negative T wave (except Chihuahua) | $V_{10}$: R/Q <1.0; negative T wave |

Each small box on the ECG paper grid is 0.02 second wide at 50 mm/sec paper speed, 0.04 second wide at 25 mm/sec, and 0.1 mV high at a calibration of 1 cm = 1 mV.
*Range may extend lower for large breeds and higher for toy breeds.
†May be greater in young (under 2 years), thin, deep-chested dogs.

TABLE 2-6

Causes of Sinus Bradycardia and Sinus Tachycardia

| Sinus Bradycardia | Sinus Tachycardia |
|---|---|
| Hypothermia | Hyperthermia/fever |
| Hypothyroidism | Hyperthyroidism |
| Cardiac arrest (before or after) | Anemia/hypoxia |
| Drugs (e.g., tranquilizers, anesthetics, β-blockers, calcium entry blockers, digitalis) | Heart failure |
| Increased intracranial pressure | Shock |
| Brainstem lesions | Hypotension |
| Severe metabolic disease (e.g., uremia) | Sepsis |
| Ocular pressure | Anxiety/fear |
| Carotid sinus pressure | Excitement |
| Other causes of high vagal tone | Exercise |
| Sinus node disease | Pain |
| Normal variation (athletic dog) | Drugs (anticholinergics, sympathomimetics) |
| | Toxicities (e.g., chocolate, hexachlorophene) |
| | Electric shock |
| | Other causes of high sympathetic tone |

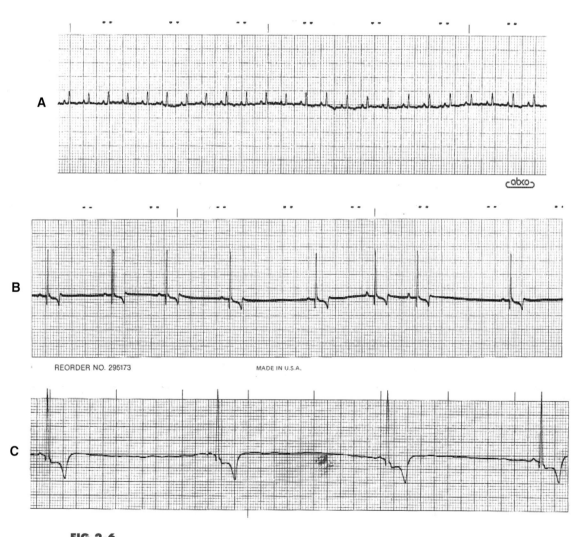

**FIG 2-6**
Sinus rhythms. **A,** Sinus rhythm in normal cat (lead II, 25 mm/sec). **B,** Sinus arrhythmia with wandering pacemaker in a dog. Note gradual variation in P-wave height associated with respiratory changes in heart rate; this variation is normal in the dog (lead aV_F, 25 mm/sec). **C,** Sinus bradycardia (lead II, 25 mm/sec, dog).

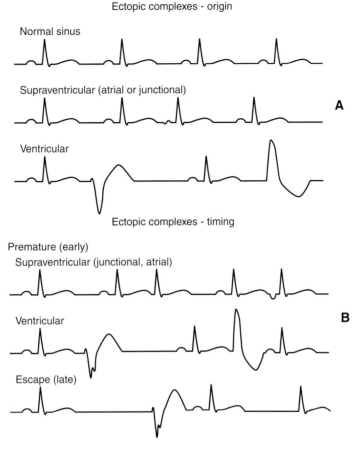

**FIG 2-7**
Diagrams illustrating the appearance of ectopic complexes. Abnormal impulses can originate **(A)** above the AV node (supraventricular) or from within the ventricles (ventricular). Supraventricular ectopic complexes have a normal-appearing QRS. An abnormal P wave usually precedes a complex originating in atrial tissue; no P wave (or a retrograde P wave in the ST segment [not shown]) is common with an impulse originating from the AV junction. Ventricular-origin QRS complexes have a different configuration from the normal sinus QRS. The timing **(B)** of ectopic complexes refers to whether they appear before the next expected sinus complex (premature or early) or after a longer than expected pause (escape or late).

the impulse occurs earlier than the next expected sinus impulse (premature) or after a longer pause (late or escape). Escape complexes represent activation of a subsidiary pacemaker and function as a rescue mechanism for the heart. Premature ectopic impulses (complexes) occur singly or in multiples; groups of three or more comprise an episode of tachycardia. Episodes of tachycardia can be brief (paroxysmal tachycardia) or quite prolonged (sustained tachycardia). When one premature complex follows each normal QRS, a bigeminal pattern exists; the origin of the premature complexes determines whether the rhythm is described as atrial or ventricular bigeminy. Fig. 2-8 shows examples of supraventricular and ventricular complexes.

## Supraventricular Premature Complexes

Supraventricular premature complexes are impulses that originate above the atrioventricular (AV) node, either in the atria or the AV junctional area. Because they are conducted

into and through the ventricles via the normal conduction pathway, their QRS configuration is normal (unless an intraventricular conduction disturbance is also present). Premature complexes arising within the atria are usually preceded by an abnormal P wave (positive, negative, or biphasic configuration) called a *P′ wave.* If an ectopic P′ wave occurs before the AV node has completely repolarized, the impulse may not be conducted into the ventricles (an example of physiologic AV block). In some cases, the premature impulse is conducted slowly (prolonged P′Q interval) or with a bundle branch block pattern. Junctional complexes are usually not preceded by a P′ wave, although retrograde conduction of the impulse back through the atria may occur, which causes a negative P′ wave to follow, be superimposed on, or even precede the resulting QRS complex. If the origin of the ectopic complex(es) is unclear, the more general term *supraventricular premature complex* (or *supraventricular tachycardia*) is used. Clinically it is more important to distinguish whether

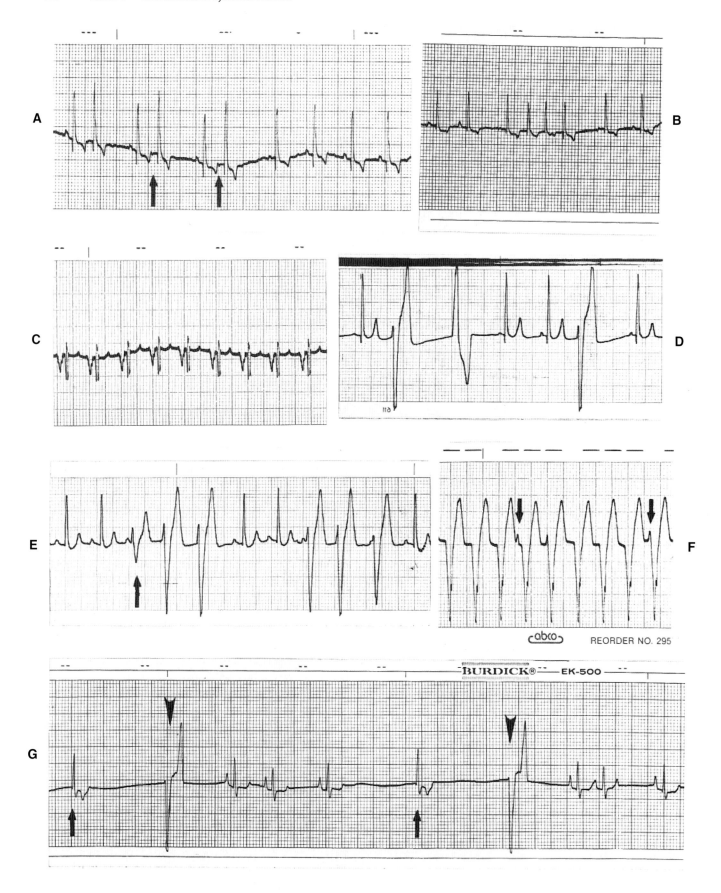

**FIG 2-8**
Ectopic complexes and rhythms. **A,** Atrial premature complexes in an old Cocker Spaniel with mitral insufficiency. Note small negative P waves *(arrows)* preceding early complexes. Slight increase in QRS size is thought to be related to minor intraventricular conduction delay with prematurity (lead III, 25 mm/sec). **B,** Short paroxysm of atrial tachycardia (lead II, 25 mm/sec, dog). **C,** Sustained atrial tachycardia in Irish Setter with mitral stenosis. Note negative, abnormal P waves (lead II, 25 mm/sec). **D,** Multiform ventricular premature complexes (lead II, 25 mm/sec, dog). **E,** Intermittent paroxysms of ventricular tachycardia demonstrating fusion complex *(arrow)* (lead II, 25 mm/sec, dog). **F,** Sustained ventricular tachycardia with several nonconducted P waves *(arrows)* superimposed (lead $aV_F$, 25 mm/sec, dog). **G,** Sinus arrhythmia with periods of sinus arrest interrupted by junctional *(arrows)* and ventricular *(arrowheads)* escape complexes (lead II, 25 mm/sec, dog). Differentiation of escape and premature complexes is crucial.

---

an arrhythmia originates from above the AV node (supraventricular) or below it (ventricular) rather than determine the more specific localization. Supraventricular premature complexes usually depolarize the sinus node as well, resetting the sinus rhythm and creating a "noncompensatory pause" (i.e., the interval between the sinus complexes preceding and following the premature complex is less than that of three consecutive sinus complexes).

### Supraventricular Tachycardia

Atrial tachycardia is caused by rapid discharge of an abnormal atrial focus or by atrial reentry (repetitive activation caused by conduction of the electrical impulse around an abnormal circuit within the atria). In the dog, the atrial activation rate per minute is usually between 260 and 380. The P' waves are often hidden in the QRS-T complexes. Atrial tachycardia can be paroxysmal or sustained. It is usually a regular rhythm unless the rate is too fast for the AV node to conduct every impulse, in which case physiologic AV block and irregular ventricular activation result. A consistent ratio of atrial impulses to ventricular activation (e.g., 2:1 or 3:1 AV conduction) preserves the regularity of this arrhythmia. Sometimes the impulses traverse the AV node but are delayed within the ventricular conduction system, causing a bundle branch block pattern on the ECG; differentiation from ventricular tachycardia may be difficult in these cases.

Supraventricular tachycardia often involves a reentrant loop using the AV node (either within the AV node or using an accessory pathway). A premature supraventricular or ventricular impulse can initiate this arrhythmia. During episodes of reentrant supraventricular tachycardia in animals with ventricular preexcitation (see p. 25), the PR interval usually normalizes or is prolonged, with retrograde P' waves. The QRS complexes are of normal configuration unless a simultaneous intraventricular conduction disturbance is present.

### Atrial Flutter

Atrial flutter is caused by a very rapid (usually greater than 400 impulses/min) wave of electrical activation regularly cycling through the atria. The ventricular response may be irregular or regular, depending on the pattern of AV conduction. The ECG baseline consists of "sawtooth" flutter waves that represent the fast, recurrent atrial activation. Atrial flutter is not a stable rhythm; it often degenerates into atrial fibrillation or may convert back to sinus rhythm.

### Atrial Fibrillation

Atrial fibrillation is a common arrhythmia characterized by many small reentrant circuits throughout the atrial tissue, which cause the overall electrical activation pattern of the atria to be rapid and chaotic. There are no P waves on the ECG because there is no uniform atrial depolarization wave. Rather, the baseline usually shows irregular undulations (fibrillation waves). Because there is no organized electrical activity, meaningful atrial contraction is absent. The AV node, being constantly bombarded with these chaotic electrical impulses, conducts as many as it can to the ventricles. Therefore the (ventricular) heart rate is determined by AV conduction velocity and recovery time. Atrial fibrillation causes an irregular heart rhythm that is usually quite rapid (Fig. 2-9). Most often the QRS complexes are normal in configuration because the normal intraventricular conduction pathway is used. Minor variation in the height of the QRS complexes is common, however, and intermittent or sustained bundle branch blocks can occur. Atrial fibrillation tends to be a consequence of severe atrial disease and enlargement in dogs and cats; it is usually preceded by intermittent atrial tachyarrhythmias and perhaps atrial flutter. However, atrial fibrillation sometimes occurs spontaneously in giant breed dogs without evidence of underlying heart disease. The heart rate is generally normal in these dogs.

### Ventricular Premature Complexes

Ventricular premature complexes (VPCs or PVCs) originate below the AV node and cannot access the normal ventricular conduction pathway. Therefore their QRS configuration is abnormal compared to the animal's sinus complexes. Ventricular ectopic complexes are usually wider than the normal complexes because of the slower intramuscular conduction. Because VPCs usually are not conducted backward through

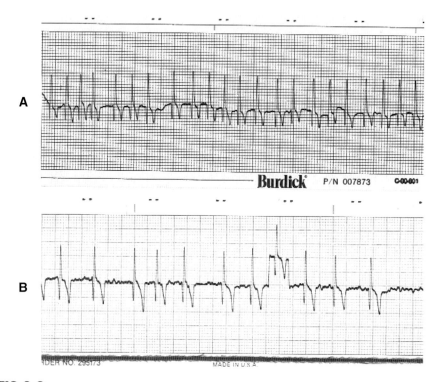

**FIG 2-9**
Atrial fibrillation. **A,** Uncontrolled atrial fibrillation (heart rate 220 beats/min) in a Doberman Pinscher with dilated cardiomyopathy (lead II, 25 mm/sec). **B,** Slower ventricular response rate after therapy in a different Doberman Pinscher with dilated cardiomyopathy showing baseline fibrillation waves. Note lack of P waves and irregular RR intervals. Eighth complex from left superimposed on calibration mark (lead II, 25 mm/sec).

the AV node into the atria, the sinus rate continues undisturbed; thus the VPC is followed by a "compensatory pause" in the sinus rhythm. When the configuration of multiple VPCs or ventricular tachycardia is consistent in an animal, the complexes are described as being uniform, unifocal, or monomorphic. When the VPCs occurring in an individual have differing configurations, they are said to be multiform or polymorphic. Increased electrical instability is thought to accompany multiform VPCs or tachycardia.

### Ventricular Tachycardia

Ventricular tachycardia is a series of VPCs (usually greater than 100 beats/min). The RR interval is most often regular, although some variation can occur. Nonconducted sinus P waves may be superimposed on or between the ventricular complexes, but they are unrelated to the VPCs because the AV node and/or ventricles are in the refractory period (physiologic AV dissociation). The term *capture beat* refers to the successful conduction of a sinus P wave into the ventricles uninterrupted by another VPC (i.e., the sinus node has "recaptured" the ventricles). If the normal ventricular activation sequence is interrupted by another VPC, a "fusion" complex can result. The configuration of a fusion complex represents a melding of the normal QRS and that of the VPC (see Fig. 2-8, *E*). Fusion complexes are often observed at the

onset or end of a paroxysm of ventricular tachycardia; they are preceded by a P wave and shortened PR interval. Identification of P waves (whether conducted or not) or fusion complexes helps to differentiate ventricular tachycardia from supraventricular tachycardia with abnormal intraventricular conduction.

### Accelerated Ventricular Rhythm

Also called *idioventricular tachycardia,* accelerated ventricular rhythm is an enhanced ventricular rhythm with a rate of about 60 to 100 beats/min in the dog (perhaps somewhat faster in the cat). Because the rate is slower than true ventricular tachycardia, it is usually a less serious rhythm disturbance. An accelerated ventricular rhythm may appear intermittently with sinus arrhythmia, as the sinus rate decreases; the ventricular rhythm is often suppressed as the sinus rate increases. This is observed commonly in dogs recovering from motor vehicle trauma. Clinically this rhythm disturbance may have no deleterious effects, although it could progress to ventricular tachycardia. Deterioration of the patient's condition would make this more likely.

### Ventricular Fibrillation

Ventricular fibrillation is a lethal rhythm characterized by multiple reentrant circuits causing chaotic electrical activity

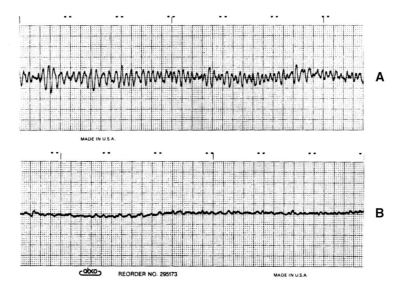

**FIG 2-10**
Ventricular fibrillation. Note chaotic baseline motion and absence of organized waveforms.
**A,** Coarse fibrillation. **B,** Fine fibrillation (lead II, 25 mm/sec, dog).

in the ventricles; the ECG consists of an irregularly undulating baseline (Fig. 2-10). Like the atria during atrial fibrillation, the ventricles have no coordinated mechanical activity in the presence of uncoordinated electrical activation and cannot function as a pump. Ventricular flutter, appearing as rapid sine-wave activity on the ECG, may precede fibrillation. Ventricular fibrillation may be "coarse," with larger ECG oscillations, or "fine." Ventricular asystole is the absence of ventricular electrical (and mechanical) activity.

### Escape Complexes

Escape complexes and escape rhythms constitute a protective mechanism. An escape complex occurs after a pause in the dominant (usually sinus) rhythm. If the dominant rhythm does not resume, the escape focus continues to discharge at its own intrinsic rate; escape rhythms are usually regular. Escape complexes originate from automatic cells in the atria, the AV junction, or the ventricles (see Fig. 2-8, *G*). Ventricular escape rhythms (idioventricular rhythms) usually occur at a rate less than 40 to 50 beats/min in the dog and 100 beats/min in the cat, although ventricular escape rates in both species can be higher. Junctional escape rhythms usually range from 40 to 60 beats/min in the dog, with a faster rate expected in the cat. It is important to differentiate escape from premature complexes because escape activity should *never* be suppressed with antiarrhythmic drugs.

### CONDUCTION DISTURBANCES

Abnormalities of impulse conduction within the atrium may arise at several sites. In *sinoatrial block,* impulse transmission from the SA node to the atrial muscle is prevented; this occurrence cannot reliably be differentiated from sinus arrest on the ECG, although with SA block the interval between P

waves is a multiple of the normal P to P interval. An atrial, junctional, or ventricular escape rhythm should take over after prolonged sinus arrest or block. In *atrial standstill,* diseased atrial muscle prevents normal electrical and mechanical function, regardless of sinus node activity; this situation results in the absence of P waves and a junctional or ventricular escape rhythm. Hyperkalemia interferes with normal atrial function and can mimic atrial standstill.

### Conduction Disturbances within the AV Node

Abnormalities of AV conduction can be caused by excessive vagal tone, drugs (e.g., digoxin, xylazine, verapamil, and anesthetic agents), and organic disease of the AV node and/or intraventricular conduction system. Three categories of AV conduction disturbances are commonly described (Fig. 2-11). *First-degree AV block* occurs when conduction from the atria into the ventricles is prolonged, although all impulses are conducted. *Second-degree AV block* is characterized by intermittent AV conduction; some P waves are not followed by a QRS complex. When many P waves are not conducted, the patient has high-grade second-degree heart block. There are two subtypes of second-degree AV block. Mobitz type I (Wenckebach) is characterized by progressive prolongation of the PR interval until a nonconducted P wave occurs; it is frequently associated with disorders within the AV node itself and/or high vagal tone. Mobitz type II is characterized by uniform PR intervals preceding the blocked impulse and is thought to be more often associated with disease lower in the AV conduction system (e.g., bundle of His or major bundle branches). An alternate classification of second-degree AV block based on QRS configuration has been described. Patients with type A second-degree block have a normal, narrow

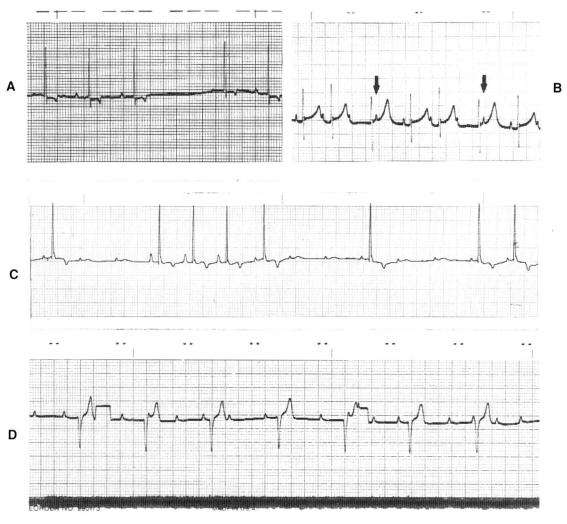

**FIG 2-11**

AV conduction abnormalities. **A,** First-degree AV block in a dog with digoxin toxicity (lead aVF, 25 mm/sec). **B,** Second-degree AV block (Wenckebach) in an old cat under anesthesia. Note gradually prolonged PR interval with failed conduction of third (and seventh) P wave(s) followed by an escape complex. The fourth and eighth P waves *(arrows)* are not conducted because the ventricles are refractory (lead II, 25 mm/sec). **C,** Second-degree AV block in a comatose old dog with brainstem signs and seizures. Note the changing configuration of the P waves (wandering pacemaker) (lead II, 25 mm/sec). **D,** Complete (third-degree) heart block in a Poodle. There is underlying sinus arrhythmia, but no P waves are conducted; a slow ventricular escape rhythm has resulted. Two calibration marks (half-standard, 0.5 cm = 1 mV) are seen (lead II, 25 mm/sec).

QRS configuration; those with type B second-degree block have a wide or abnormal QRS configuration, which suggests diffuse disease lower in the ventricular conduction system. Mobitz type I AV block usually is type A, whereas Mobitz type II frequently is type B. Supraventricular or ventricular escape complexes are common during long pauses in ventricular activation. *Third-degree* or *complete AV block* is present when no sinus (or supraventricular) impulses are conducted into the ventricles. Often a regular sinus rhythm or sinus arrhythmia is evident; however, the P waves are not related to the QRS complexes, which result from a (usually) regular ventricular escape rhythm.

## Intraventricular Conduction Disturbances

Slowed or blocked impulse transmission within any of the major bundle branches causes an intraventricular conduction disturbance. The right bundle branch or the left anterior or posterior fascicles of the left bundle branch can be affected singly or in combination. A block in all three major branches results in third-degree (complete) heart block. Activation of the myocardium served by the blocked pathway occurs relatively slowly, from myocyte to myocyte, therefore the QRS complexes appear wide and abnormal (see Fig. 2-5). Right bundle branch block (RBBB) is sometimes identified in otherwise normal dogs and cats, although it can result from dis-

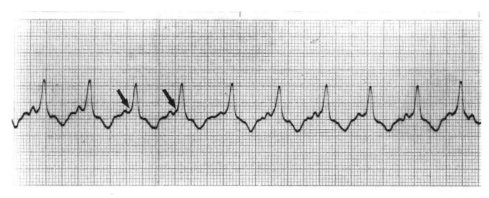

**FIG 2-12**
Ventricular preexcitation in a cat. Note slowed QRS upstroke (delta wave; *arrows*) immediately following each P wave (lead II, 50 mm/sec, 1 cm = 1 mV).

ease or distention of the right ventricle. Left bundle branch block (LBBB) is usually related to clinically relevant underlying disease of the left ventricle. The left anterior fascicular block (LAFB) pattern is common in cats with hypertrophic cardiomyopathy.

### Ventricular Preexcitation

Early activation (preexcitation) of part of the ventricular myocardium can occur when there is an accessory conduction pathway that bypasses the normal slow-conducting AV nodal pathway. Several types of preexcitation and accessory pathways have been described; most cause a shortened PR interval. Wolff-Parkinson-White (WPW) preexcitation is also characterized by early widening and slurring of the QRS by a so-called delta wave (Fig. 2-12). This pattern occurs because the accessory pathway (Kent's bundle) lies outside the AV node (extranodal) and allows early depolarization (represented by the delta wave) of a part of the ventricle distant to where normal ventricular activation begins. Other accessory pathways connect the atria or dorsal areas of the AV node directly to the bundle of His. These cause a short PR interval without early QRS widening. Preexcitation can be intermittent or concealed (not evident on ECG). The danger with preexcitation is that a reentrant supraventricular tachycardia can occur using the accessory pathway and AV node (also called AV reciprocating tachycardia). Usually the tachycardia impulses travel into the ventricles via the AV node (antegrade or orthodromic conduction) and then back to the atria via the accessory pathway, but sometimes the direction is reversed. Rapid AV reciprocating tachycardia can cause weakness, syncope, congestive heart failure, and death. The presence of the WPW pattern on ECG in conjunction with reentrant supraventricular tachycardia that causes clinical signs characterizes the WPW syndrome.

### ST-T ABNORMALITIES

The ST segment extends from the end of the QRS complex (also called the J point) to the onset of the T wave. In dogs and cats this segment tends to slope into the following T wave, therefore clear demarcation is uncommon. Abnormal elevation ($>0.15$ mV in dogs or 0.1 mV in cats) or depression ($>0.2$ mV in dogs or $>0.1$ mV in cats) of the J point and ST segment in leads I, II, or $aV_F$ may be significant and can be caused by ischemia or other causes of myocardial injury. Atrial enlargement or tachycardia can cause pseudodepression of the ST segment because of prominent $T_a$ waves. Other secondary causes of ST segment deviation include ventricular hypertrophy, slowed conduction, and some drugs (e.g., digoxin). Table 2-7 lists common causes of ST segment abnormalities. The T wave represents ventricular muscle repolarization; it may be positive, negative, or biphasic in normal cats and dogs. Changes in size, shape, or polarity from previous recordings in a given animal are probably clinically important. Abnormalities of the T wave can be primary (i.e., not related to the depolarization process) or secondary (i.e., related to abnormalities of ventricular depolarization). Secondary ST-T changes tend to be in the opposite direction of the main QRS deflection. Table 2-7 lists some causes of ST-T abnormalities.

### QT Interval

The QT interval represents the total time of ventricular activation and repolarization. This interval varies inversely with average heart rate; faster rates have a shorter QT interval. Autonomic nervous tone, various drugs, and electrolyte disorders influence the duration of the QT interval (see Table 2-7). In an attempt to more clearly define the QT interval–heart rate relationship, prediction equations for the expected QT duration have been derived for normal dogs and cats (see Suggested Readings). Inappropriate prolongation of the QT interval may facilitate development of serious reentrant arrhythmias when underlying nonuniformity in ventricular repolarization exists.

### ECG MANIFESTATIONS OF DRUG TOXICITIES AND ELECTROLYTE IMBALANCES

Digoxin, antiarrhythmic agents, and anesthetic drugs often alter heart rhythm and/or conduction either by their direct electrophysiologic effects or by affecting autonomic tone. Table 2-8 summarizes common ECG manifestations of these drug effects.

## TABLE 2-7

### Causes of ST Segment, T Wave, and QT Abnormalities

**Depression of J Point/ST Segment
(>0.2 mV in caudal leads)**

Myocardial ischemia
Myocardial infarction/injury (subendocardial)
Hyperkalemia or hypokalemia
Cardiac trauma
Secondary change (ventricular hypertrophy, conduction
   disturbance, ventricular premature complexes [VPCs])
Digitalis ("sagging" appearance)
Pseudodepressian (prominent Ta)

**Elevation of the J Point/ST Segment
(>0.15 mV in Caudal Leads)**

Pericarditis
Left ventricular epicardial injury
Myocardial infarction (transmural)
Myocardial hypoxia
Secondary change (ventricular hypertrophy, conduction
   disturbance, VPCs)
Digoxin toxicity

**Prolongation of QT Interval**

Hypocalcemia
Hypokalemia
Quinidine toxicity
Ethylene glycol poisoning
Secondary to prolonged QRS
Hypothermia
Central nervous system abnormalities

**Shortening of QT Interval**

Hypercalcemia
Hyperkalemia
Digitalis toxicity

**Large T Waves**

Myocardial hypoxia
Ventricular enlargement
Intraventricular conduction abnormalities
Hyperkalemia
Metabolic or respiratory diseases and cardiac
   drug toxicities
Normal variation

**Tented T Waves**

Hyperkalemia

---

Abnormalities of potassium homeostasis have marked and complex influences on cardiac electrophysiology and, consequently, on the ECG. Hypokalemia may increase spontaneous automaticity of cardiac cells, as well as nonuniformly slow repolarization and conduction; these effects predispose to both supraventricular and ventricular arrhythmias. Hypokalemia can cause progressive ST segment depression, reduced T-wave amplitude, and QT interval prolongation. Severe hypokalemia can also increase QRS and P-wave amplitudes and durations. In addition, hypokalemia exacerbates digoxin toxicity and reduces the effectiveness of class I antiarrhythmic agents (see Chapter 4). Hypernatremia and alkalosis worsen the effects of hypokalemia on the heart.

Moderate hyperkalemia actually has an antiarrhythmic effect by reducing automaticity and enhancing uniformity and speed of repolarization. However, rapid or severe increases in serum potassium concentration are arrhythmogenic primarily because they slow conduction velocity and shorten the refractory period. Fig. 2-13 describes the progression of ECG changes as the serum potassium concentration rises. The sinus node is relatively resistant to the effects of hyperkalemia and continues to function, although its rate often decreases. Despite the progressive unresponsiveness of atrial muscle, specialized fibers transmit sinus impulses to the ventricles, resulting in a sinoventricular rhythm. The characteristic "tented" T-wave appearance may be more apparent in some leads than in others. Fig. 2-14 illustrates the ECG effects of severe hyperkalemia and the response to therapy in a dog with Addison's disease. Hypocalcemia, hyponatremia, and acidosis accentuate the ECG changes caused by hyperkalemia, whereas hypercalcemia and hypernatremia tend to counteract them. Therapy for severe hyperkalemia is discussed on p. 832.

Marked ECG changes caused by other electrolyte disturbances are infrequent. Severe hypercalcemia or hypocalcemia could have noticeable effects (see Table 2-8), but this is rarely seen clinically. Hypomagnesemia has no reported effects on the ECG, but it can predispose to digoxin toxicity and exaggerate the effects of hypocalcemia.

## APPROACH TO ECG INTERPRETATION

For standard ECG recording, the animal should be placed on a nonconducting pad in right lateral recumbency. The proximal limbs should be parallel to each other and perpendicular to the torso. Other body positions may cause changes in recorded waveform amplitudes and affect the calculated MEA. However, if the only information needed is the heart rate and rhythm, the standard recording position is not essential. Front limb electrodes are placed at the elbows or slightly below, not touching the chest wall or each other. Rear limb electrodes are placed at the stifles or hocks. When alligator clip or plate electrodes are used, copious ECG paste or (less ideally) alcohol should be applied to ensure good contact. Communication between two electrodes via a bridge of paste or alcohol or by physical contact should be avoided. The animal is gently held in position to minimize movement artifacts. A better quality tracing is obtained when the animal is relaxed and quiet. Holding the mouth shut to discourage panting or placing a hand on the chest of a trembling animal may be helpful.

A good ECG recording has minimal artifact from patient movement, no electrical interference, and a clean baseline. The ECG complexes should be centered and totally contained within the paper gridwork so that neither the top nor bottom of the QRS complex is clipped off. If the complexes are too

TABLE 2-8

ECG Changes Associated With Selected Drug Toxicities and Electrolyte Imbalances

**Hyperkalemia (see Figs. 2-13, 2-14)**

Large, spiked (± tented) T waves
QT interval abbreviation
Flat or absent P waves
Widened QRS
ST segment depression

**Hypokalemia**

ST segment depression
Small, biphasic T waves
QT interval prolongation
Tachyarrhythmias

**Hypercalcemia**

Few effects
Abbreviated QT interval
Prolonged conduction
Tachyarrhythmias

**Hypocalcemia**

Prolonged QT interval
Tachyarrhythmias

**Digoxin**

PR prolongation
Second- (or third-) degree atrioventricular (AV) block
Sinus bradycardia or arrest
Accelerated junctional rhythm
Ventricular premature complexes
Ventricular tachycardia
Paroxysmal atrial tachycardia with block
Atrial fibrillation with slow ventricular rate

**Quinidine/Procainamide**

Atropine-like effects
QT prolongation
AV blocks
Ventricular tachyarrhythmias
QRS widening
Sinus arrest

**Lidocaine**

AV block
Ventricular tachycardia
Sinus arrest

**Barbiturate/Thiobarbiturates**

Ventricular bigeminy

**Halothane/methoxyflurane**

Sinus bradycardia
Ventricular arrhythmias (increased sensitivity to catecholamines, especially halothane)

**Xylazine**

Sinus bradycardia
Sinus arrest/sinoatrial block
AV block
Ventricular tachyarrhythmias (especially with halothane, epinephrine)

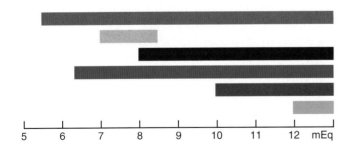

| 5 | 6 | 7 | 8 | 9 | 10 | 11 | 12 | mEq |

↑ Rate of repolarization → Peaked, tented T wave
    Shortened Q-T interval

Slowed conduction in atria → Flattened P wave

Conduction through atria fails → P wave disappears;
    sinus node continues → "Sinoventricular" rhythm

Progressive slowing of intraventricular conduction →
    QRS widens

Activation of ectopic pacemakers → Irregular ventricular
    rhythm

Ventricular fibrillation or asystole

**FIG 2-13**
Progressive ECG changes that develop with worsening hyper-kalemia (scale represents serum K⁺ concentration in mEq/L). Although ECG changes correlate poorly with serum K⁺ concentration, they accurately reflect cardiac electrophysiologic changes.

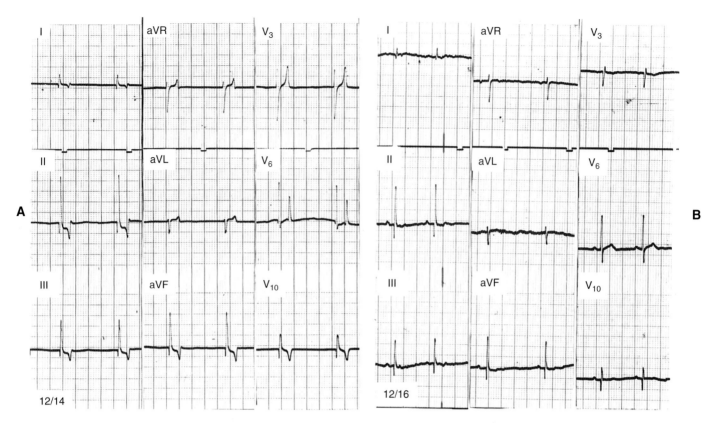

**FIG 2-14**

ECGs recorded in a female Poodle with Addison's disease at presentation (**A,** K$^+$ = 10.2; Na$^+$ = 132 mEq/L) and 2 days later after treatment (**B,** K$^+$ = 3.5; Na$^+$ = 144 mEq/L). Note absence of P waves, accentuated and tented T waves (especially in chest leads), shortened QT interval, and slightly widened QRS complexes in **A** compared to **B** (leads as marked, 25 mm/sec, 1 cm = 1 mV).

large to fit entirely within the grid, the calibration should be changed from standard (1 cm = 1 mV) to ½ standard (0.5 cm = 1 mV). To measure waveform amplitude, the calibration used during the recording must be known. A calibration square wave (1 mV amplitude) can be inscribed manually during the recording if this is not done automatically. The paper speed and lead(s) recorded also must be evident for interpretation.

A consistent approach to ECG interpretation is recommended. After the paper speed, lead(s) used, and calibration have been identified, the heart rate, heart rhythm, and MEA are determined. Finally, individual waveforms are measured. The heart rate can be calculated by counting the number of complexes in 3 or 6 seconds and then multiplying by 20 or 10, respectively. Some ECG machines inscribe 1-second marks on the paper during recording. Some one-channel recorders use paper with small vertical hash marks at the top margin that can be used to calculate time elapsed (e.g., at 25 mm/sec there are 3 seconds between two marks; at 50 mm/sec, 1.5 seconds). If the heart rhythm is regular, 3000 divided by the number of small boxes (at a paper speed of 50 mm/sec) between successive RR intervals equals the ap-

proximate heart rate. Because variations in heart rate are so common (in dogs especially), calculating an estimated heart rate over several seconds is usually more accurate and practical than calculating an instantaneous heart rate.

Heart rhythm is evaluated by scanning the ECG for irregularities and identifying individual waveforms. The presence and pattern of P waves and QRS-T complexes are determined first. The relationship between the P waves and QRS-Ts is then evaluated. Calipers are often useful for assessing the regularity and interrelationships of the waveforms. Estimation of the MEA is described on p. 15.

Waveforms and intervals are usually measured using lead II. Amplitudes are recorded in millivolts and durations in seconds. Only one thickness of the inscribed pen line should be included for each measurement. At a paper speed of 25 mm/sec, each small (1-mm) box on the ECG gridwork is 0.04 seconds in duration from left to right. At a paper speed of 50 mm/sec, each small box equals 0.02 seconds. At standard calibration, a deflection of the pen up or down 10 small boxes (1 cm) equals 1 mV. Table 2-5 contains normal ECG reference ranges for cats and dogs. Although these values are representative of most normal animals, complex measurements for some subpopulations can fall outside these ranges. For example, endurance-trained sled dogs typically have ECG measurements that exceed the "normal" range for non-sled dogs, which probably reflects the effects of training on heart size. However, such changes in nontrained dogs could suggest pathologic cardiac enlargement. Manual frequency filters are available on many ECG machines. Activating the frequency filter can markedly attenuate the recorded voltages of some waveforms, although baseline artifact is reduced. The effects of filtering on QRS amplitude may complicate the assessment for ECG chamber enlargement criteria.

## COMMON ARTIFACTS

Fig. 2-15 illustrates some common ECG artifacts. Electrical interference can be minimized or eliminated by properly grounding the ECG machine; turning off other electrical equipment or lights on the same circuit or having a different person restrain the animal may also help. Artifacts are sometimes confused with arrhythmias; however, artifacts do not disturb the underlying cardiac rhythm. Ectopic complexes often disrupt the underlying rhythm and are followed by a T wave. Careful examination for these characteristics usually allows differentiation between intermittent artifacts and arrhythmias.

## AMBULATORY ELECTROCARDIOGRAPHY

### Holter Monitoring

Holter monitoring allows the continuous recording of cardiac electrical activity during normal daily activities (except swimming), strenuous exercise, and sleep. This technique is useful for detecting and quantifying intermittent cardiac arrhythmias and therefore can help identify cardiac causes of syncope and episodic weakness. Holter monitoring is also used to assess the efficacy of antiarrhythmic drug therapy and to screen for arrhythmias associated with cardiomyopathy or other diseases. The Holter monitor consists of a small, battery-powered tape recorder that is worn by the patient, typically for 24 hours (Figs. 2-16 and 2-17). Two or three ECG channels are recorded from modified chest leads using adhesive patch electrodes. During the recording period, the animal's activities are noted in a patient diary for later correlation with simultaneous ECG events. An event button on the Holter recorder can be pressed to mark the tape if syncope or some other episode is witnessed.

The signals recorded on tape are converted to digital format and analyzed using computer algorithms that classify the recorded complexes. Because fully automated computer analysis can result in significant misclassification of QRS complexes and artifacts from dog and cat recordings, interaction and editing by a trained Holter technician experienced with veterinary recordings is important for accurate analysis. A summary report and selected portions of the recording are enlarged and printed for examination by the clinician. In addition, a full disclosure printout of the entire recording should be visually scanned and compared with the selected ECG strips as well as to the times of clinical signs and/or activities noted in the patient diary (see Suggested Readings for more information). A Holter monitor, hook-up supplies, and tape analysis can be obtained from some commercial human Holter scanning services (e.g., LabCorp, Burlington, NC; 800-289-4358). Holter monitoring is also available at many university veterinary teaching hospitals and cardiology referral practices (also Veterinary Imaging Assoc., Hopatcong, NJ; 800-773-7944).

Wide variation in heart rate is seen throughout the day in normal animals. In dogs, maximum heart rates of up to 300 beats/min have been recorded in association with excitement or activity. Episodes of bradycardia (50 beats/min or less) are common, especially during quiet periods and sleep; heart rates as low as 17 beats/min have been recorded (Hall and colleagues, 1991). Sinus arrhythmia, sinus pauses (sometimes for longer than 5 seconds), and occasional second-degree AV block are apparently common in dogs, especially at times when the mean heart rate is lower. In normal cats, heart rates also vary widely over 24 hours, ranging from 68 to 294 beats/min in one study (Ware, 1999). Although regular sinus rhythm predominates in normal cats, sinus arrhythmia is evident at slower heart rates. Ventricular premature complexes occur only sporadically in normal dogs and cats; their prevalence likely increases only slightly with age.

### Event Recording

Cardiac event recorders are smaller than typical Holter units and contain a microprocessor with memory loop that can store a brief period of a single modified chest lead ECG. The event recorder can be worn for periods of a week or so, but it cannot store prolonged, continuous ECG activity. Event recorders are used most often to determine if episodic weakness or syncope is caused by a cardiac arrhythmia. When an episode is observed, the owner activates the recorder, which then stores the ECG from a predetermined time frame (e.g., from 30 seconds before activation to 30 seconds after) for later retrieval and analysis.

## OTHER METHODS OF ECG ASSESSMENT

### Heart Rate Variability (HRV)

The amount of variation in time between consecutive heartbeats is influenced by phasic fluctuations in vagal and sympathetic tone. These occur during the respiratory cycle and also during slower periodic oscillations of arterial blood pressure. Heart rate variability refers to the fluctuation of beat-to-beat time intervals around their mean value. HRV is influenced by baroreceptor function as well as by the respiratory cycle and sympathetic/parasympathetic balance. The degree of HRV decreases in association with severe myocardial dysfunction and heart failure, as well as with other causes of increased sympathetic tone. In people with cardiomyopathy and/or coronary artery disease, reduced HRV can indicate an increased risk for sudden death. The potential clinical usefulness of HRV as an indicator of autonomic function, and possibly of prognosis, for veterinary patients is being explored (see Suggested Readings). However, numerous technical limitations and challenges exist.

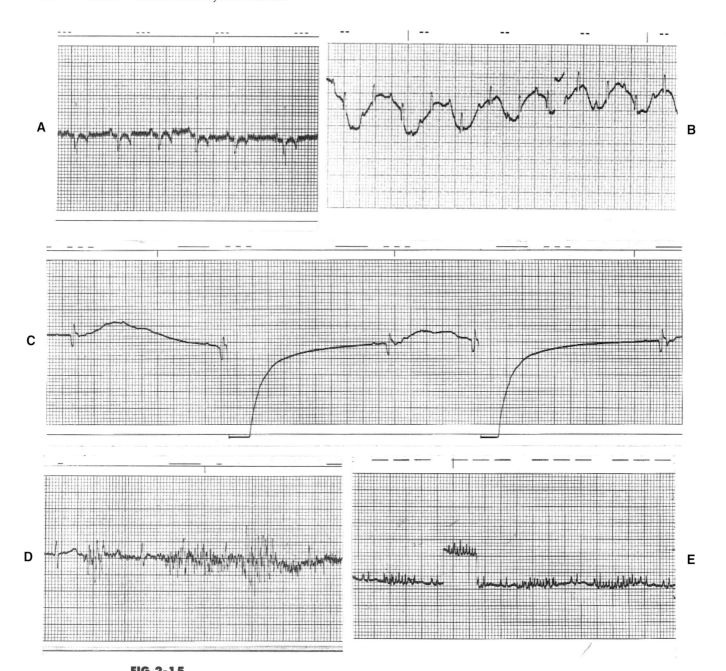

**FIG 2-15**
Common ECG artifacts. **A,** 60 Hz electrical interference (lead III, 25 mm/sec, dog).
**B,** Baseline movement caused by panting (lead II, 25 mm/sec, dog). **C,** Respiratory motion
artifact (lead V₃, 50 mm/sec, dog). **D,** Severe muscle tremor artifact (lead V₃, 50 mm/sec,
cat). **E,** Intermittent, rapid baseline spikes caused by purring in a cat; a calibration mark is
seen just left of the center of the strip (lead aV_F, 25 mm/sec).

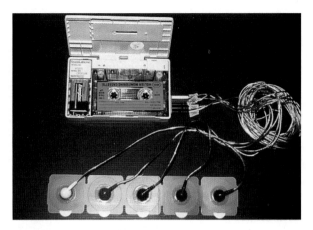

**FIG 2-16**
Holter monitor with cassette recording tape and battery inside. Five lead wires (for two leads plus ground) are attached to pre-gelled electrode pads for placement on the patient's chest. The entire assembly weighs less than a pound.

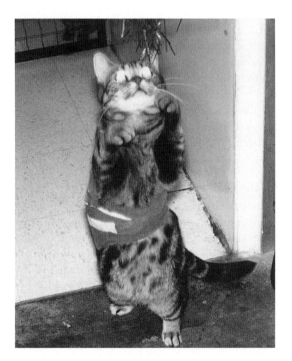

**FIG 2-17**
Holter monitor attached to a cat with mild hypertrophic cardiomyopathy. This cat tolerated wearing the monitor quite well and is seen here jumping after a toy. Most dogs and some cats appear relatively undisturbed by the presence of the monitor.

The variation in instantaneous heart rate (R-to-R intervals) can be evaluated as a function of time (time-domain analysis) as well as in terms of the frequency and amplitude of its summed oscillatory components (frequency-domain analysis). The time frame for HRV analysis can be relatively short (several minutes) or extended over longer periods (e.g., 24-hour Holter recordings). Time-domain indices include the standard deviation of normal beat R-to-R intervals (SDNN), which reflects low-frequency (longer-term) variation in heart rate, and the percentage of consecutive normal R-to-R intervals that vary by more than 50 msec (pNN50), which reflects high-frequency (short-term; respiratory) variation in heart rate. Other time-domain indices are also used.

Frequency-domain analysis allows assessment of the balance between sympathetic and vagal modulation of the cardiovascular system. It may differentiate sympathetic and parasympathetic influences better than time-domain indices. Fast Fourier transformation (or an alternative method) is used to analyze consecutive R-R intervals over a period of time to detect the number, frequency, and amplitude of oscillatory components; this is known as power spectral analysis. A high-frequency spectral component is a marker of vagal changes and is associated with respiratory-influenced change in HRV. A low-frequency component represents the rhythm corresponding to slow vasomotor waves that influence HRV as well as variability in arterial blood pressure. The low-frequency component is mainly a marker of sympathetic modulation, although there is some vagal effect. Power spectral analysis also reveals some very-low-frequency components of unclear significance. There are parallels between time- and frequency-domain indices: SDNN (and others) reflects low-frequency variability in heart rate and correlates with total power; pNN50 (and others) reflects high-frequency (vagal) influences on HRV.

## Signal-Averaged Electrocardiography (SAECG)

Digital signal averaging of the ECG provides a means of enhancing ECG signal resolution by discarding random components (noise). The process allows detection of small-voltage potentials that may occur at the end of the QRS complex and into the early ST segment. These so-called ventricular late potentials are found in patients with injured myocardium; they indicate the presence of conditions that predispose to reentrant ventricular tachyarrhythmias. The presence of late potentials can be useful in identifying patients at high risk of ventricular tachycardia and sudden death. This technique is available at some veterinary teaching hospitals. Both time- and frequency-domain analyses can be done to detect late potentials. Time-domain indices include the QRS complex duration (HFQRS), duration of the terminal portion of the filtered QRS complex below 40 $\mu$V (LAS$_{40}$), and the root mean square (RMS) voltages of various time durations at the end of the QRS complex. Fast Fourier transformation can be used to assess frequency components within the QRS and to derive maps relating power, frequency, and also time (spectrotemporal mapping). The presence of late potentials on SAECG has been identified in some Dobermans with ventricular tachycardia and significant ventricular dysfunction, but the sensitivity for predicting the risk of ventricular tachycardia is unclear (Calvert and colleagues, 1998a).

## THORACIC RADIOGRAPHY

Chest radiographs are important in the assessment of dogs and cats with heart disease. At least two radiographic views should be evaluated: lateral and dorsoventral (DV) or ventrodorsal (VD). High kilovoltage peak (kVp) and low milliamperes (mAs) radiographic technique is recommended for better resolution among soft tissue structures. The films should be examined systematically, beginning with assessment of technique, patient positioning, presence of artifacts, and phase of respiration during exposure. Exposure is ideally made at the time of peak inspiration. On expiration, the lungs appear denser, the heart is relatively larger, the diaphragm may overlap the caudal heart border, and pulmonary vessels are poorly delineated. Use of exposure times short enough to minimize respiratory motion and proper, straight (not obliquely tilted) patient positioning are important for accurate interpretation of cardiac shape and size, and pulmonary parenchyma. On lateral view, the ribs should be aligned with each other dorsally. On DV or VD views, the sternum, vertebral bodies, and dorsal spinous processes should be superimposed. The views chosen should be used consistently because slight changes in the appearance of the cardiac shadow occur with different positions. For example, the heart tends to look more elongated on the VD compared with the DV view. In general, better definition of the hilar area and caudal pulmonary arteries is obtained using the DV view.

Chest conformation should be considered when evaluating cardiac size and shape in dogs because normal cardiac appearance may vary from breed to breed. The cardiac shadow in dogs with round or barrel-shaped chests has greater sternal contact on lateral view and an oval shape on DV or VD view. In contrast, the heart has an upright, elongated appearance on lateral view and a small, almost circular shape on DV or VD view in narrow- and deep-chested dogs. Because of variations in chest conformation and the influences of respiration, cardiac cycle, and positioning on the apparent size of the cardiac shadow, mild cardiomegaly may be difficult to identify. Also, excess pericardial fat may mimic the appearance of cardiomegaly. The cardiac shadow in puppies normally appears slightly large relative to thoracic size compared to adult dogs.

Good correlation exists between body length and heart size regardless of chest conformation. Because of this relationship, the vertebral heart score (VHS) can be used to determine the presence and quantify the degree of cardiomegaly in dogs and cats. Measurements for the VHS are obtained using the lateral view (Fig. 2-18) in dogs, although the technique also has been described using the DV view. The cardiac long axis is measured from the ventral border of the left mainstem bronchus to the most ventral aspect of the cardiac apex. This same distance is compared to the thoracic spine beginning at the cranial edge of T4; length is estimated to the nearest 0.1 vertebra. The maximum perpendicular short axis is measured in the central third of the heart shadow; the short axis is also measured in number of vertebrae (to the nearest 0.1) beginning with T4. The two measurements are added to yield the VHS. A VHS of 8.5 to 10.5 vertebrae is considered normal for most breeds. Some variation may exist among breeds; an upper limit of 11 vertebrae may be normal in dogs with a short thorax (e.g., Miniature Schnauzer), whereas an upper limit of 9.5 vertebrae may be normal in dogs with a long thorax (e.g., Dachshund). The VHS in normal puppies falls within the reference range for adult dogs (Sleeper and colleague, 2001).

The cardiac silhouette on lateral view in cats is aligned more parallel to the sternum than in dogs; this parallel positioning may be accentuated in old cats. Radiographic positioning can significantly influence the relative size, shape, and position of the heart because the feline thorax is so flexible. Nevertheless, measurement of VHS is also useful in cats. The range of VHS derived from lateral radiographs in cats was reported as 6.7 to 8.1 vertebrae, with a mean of 7.5 vertebrae (Litster and colleague, 2000). The mean short axis cardiac dimension taken from DV or VD view, compared with the thoracic spine beginning at T4 on lateral view, was 3.4 to 3.5 vertebrae. An upper limit of normal of 4 vertebrae was identified. In kittens, as in puppies, the relative size of the heart compared to the thorax is larger than in adults because of smaller lung volume.

An abnormally small heart shadow results from reduced venous return, for example, from shock or hypovolemia. The apex appears more pointed and may be elevated from the sternum. Radiographic suggestion of abnormal cardiac size or shape should be considered within the context of the physical examination and other test findings.

### CARDIOMEGALY

Generalized enlargement of the heart shadow on plain thoracic radiographs may indicate true cardiomegaly or distention of the surrounding pericardial sac. When the heart itself is enlarged, the contours of different chambers are usually still evident, although massive right ventricular and atrial dilation can make the heart appear very round. Filling of the pericardial sac with fluid, fat, or viscera tends to obliterate these contours and create a globoid heart shadow. Table 2-9 provides common differential diagnoses for cardiac enlargement patterns. Radiographic patterns of specific chamber enlargement are discussed below.

### CARDIAC CHAMBER ENLARGEMENT PATTERNS

Rarely is there isolated enlargement of one cardiac chamber. Most diseases that cause dilation or hypertrophy of the heart affect two or more chambers. For example, mitral insufficiency leads to both left ventricular and left atrial enlargement; pulmonic stenosis causes right ventricular enlargement, a main pulmonary artery bulge and, often, right atrial dilation. Nevertheless, enlargement of specific chambers and great vessels is described individually. Fig. 2-19 illustrates various patterns of chamber enlargement.

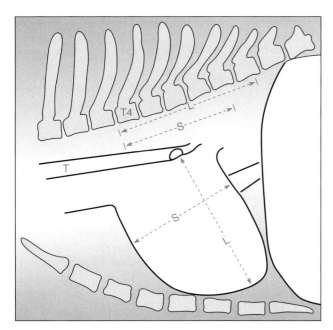

**FIG 2-18**
Diagram illustrating the vertebral heart score (VHS) measurement method using the lateral chest radiograph. The long-axis *(L)* and short-axis *(S)* heart dimensions are transposed onto the vertebral column and recorded as the number of vertebrae, beginning with the cranial edge of T4. These values are added to obtain the VHS. In this example, L = 5.8 v and S = 4.6 v, therefore VHS = 10.4 v. *T,* Trachea. (Modified from Buchanan JW et al: Vertebral scale system to measure canine heart size in radiographs, *J Am Vet Med Assoc* 206:194, 1995.)

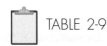 TABLE 2-9

**Common Differential Diagnoses for Radiographic Signs of Cardiomegaly**

**Generalized Enlargement of the Cardiac Shadow**

Dilated cardiomyopathy
Mitral and tricuspid insufficiency
Pericardial effusion
Pericardioperitoneal diaphragmatic hernia
Tricuspid dysplasia
Ventricular septal defect
Patent ductus arteriosus

**Left Atrial Enlargement**

Early mitral insufficiency
Hypertrophic cardiomyopathy
Early dilated cardiomyopathy (especially Doberman Pinschers)
(Sub)aortic stenosis

**Left Atrial and Ventricular Enlargement**

Dilated cardiomyopathy
Hypertrophic cardiomyopathy

**Left Atrial and Ventricular Enlargement—cont'd**

Mitral insufficiency (acquired or congenital)
Aortic insufficiency
Ventricular septal defect
Patent ductus arterious
(Sub)aortic stenosis

**Right Atrial and Ventricular Enlargement**

Advanced heartworm disease
Chronic, severe pulmonary disease
Tricuspid insufficiency (acquired or congenital)
Pulmonic stenosis
Tetralogy of Fallot
Atrial septal defect
Reversed shunting congenital defects (pulmonary hypertension)

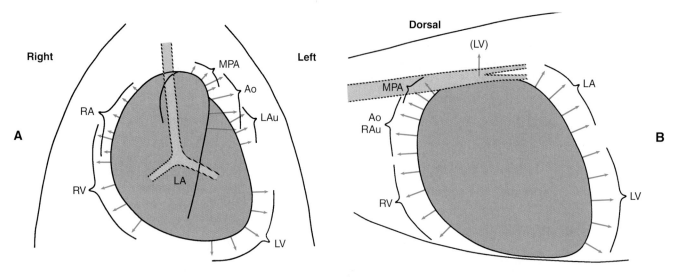

**FIG 2-19**
Common radiographic enlargement patterns. Diagrams indicating direction of enlargement of cardiac chambers and great vessels in the dorsoventral **(A)** and lateral **(B)** views. *Ao,* Aorta (descending); *LA,* left atrium; *LAu,* left auricle; *LV,* left ventricle; *MPA,* main pulmonary artery; *RA,* right atrium; *RAu,* right auricle; *RV,* right ventricle. (Modified from Bonagura JD et al: Cardiovascular and pulmonary disorders. In Fenner W, editor: *Quick reference to veterinary medicine,* ed 3, Philadelphia, 2000, JB Lippincott.)

## Left Atrium

The left atrium is the most dorsocaudal chamber of the heart, although its auricular appendage extends to the left and craniad. An enlarged left atrium bulges dorsally and caudally on lateral view. There is elevation of the left and possibly right mainstem bronchi; compression of the left mainstem bronchus occurs with severe left atrial enlargement (especially on expiration). In cats the caudal heart border is normally quite straight on lateral view; left atrial enlargement causes subtle to marked convexity of the dorsocaudal heart border, with elevation of the mainstem bronchi. On DV or VD view, the mainstem bronchi are pushed laterally and curve slightly around a markedly enlarged left atrium (sometimes referred to as the "bow-legged cowboy sign"). A bulge in the 2- to 3-o'clock position of the cardiac silhouette is common in cats and dogs with concurrent left auricular enlargement. Massive left atrial enlargement sometimes appears as a large, rounded, soft tissue opacity superimposed over the central to caudal cardiac silhouette on DV (VD) view. The size of the left atrium is a function not only of the pressure or volume load imposed on it, but also of the length of time the overload has been present. For example, mitral regurgitation of slowly increasing severity may cause massive left atrial enlargement without pulmonary edema if the chamber has had time to dilate at relatively low pressures. Conversely, rupture of chordae tendineae causes acute valvular regurgitation; there can be pulmonary edema with little radiographic evidence of left atrial enlargement because atrial pressure rises quickly.

## Left Ventricle

Left ventricular enlargement is manifested on lateral view by an elevation of the carina and caudal vena cava. The caudal heart border becomes convex. On DV or VD view, there is rounding and enlargement in the 2- to 5-o'clock position.

## Right Atrium

Right atrial enlargement causes a bulge of the cranial heart border and widening of the cardiac silhouette on lateral view. Tracheal elevation may occur over the cranial portion of the heart shadow. Bulging of the cardiac shadow on DV or VD view occurs in the 9- to 11-o'clock position. Because the right atrium is largely superimposed on the right ventricle, differentiation from right ventricular enlargement is difficult; however, concurrent enlargement of both chambers is common.

## Right Ventricle

Right ventricular enlargement (dilation or hypertrophy) usually causes increased convexity of the cranioventral heart border and elevation of the trachea over the cranial heart border on lateral view. With severe right ventricular enlargement and relatively normal left heart size, the apex is elevated from the sternum. The carina and caudal vena cava are also elevated. The heart on DV or VD view tends to take on a reverse-D configuration if left-sided enlargement is absent; the apex may be shifted leftward, and the right heart border bulges to the right.

## INTRATHORACIC BLOOD VESSELS

The aorta and main pulmonary artery tend to dilate in response to chronic arterial hypertension or increased turbulence (poststenotic dilation). Subaortic stenosis causes dilation of the ascending aorta. Because of its location within the mediastinum, dilation here is not easily detected, although widening and increased opacity of the dorsocranial heart shadow may be observed. Patent ductus arteriosus (PDA) causes a localized dilation in the descending aorta just caudal to the arch, which is where the ductus exits; this "ductus bump" is seen on DV or VD view. Severe dilation of the main pulmonary trunk can be seen as a bulge superimposed over the trachea on lateral radiograph. On DV view in the dog, main pulmonary trunk enlargement causes a bulge in the 1- to 2-o'clock position; pulmonic stenosis or pulmonary hypertension are the usual causes. In the cat, the main pulmonary trunk is slightly more medial and is usually obscured within the mediastinum.

The width of the caudal vena cava (CaVC) is approximately that of the descending thoracic aorta, although its size changes with respiration. The CaVC is pushed dorsally with enlargement of either ventricle. Persistent widening of the CaVC could indicate right ventricular failure, cardiac tamponade, pericardial constriction, or other obstruction to right heart inflow; a thin vena cava might indicate hypovolemia, poor venous return, or pulmonary overinflation. Lehmkuhl and colleagues (1997) compared the CaVC diameter with other thoracic structures. Dogs with right heart disease and abnormal caudal caval distension are expected to have the following comparative findings: CaVC/aortic diameter (at the same intercostal space as CaVC measurement) >1.5; CaVC/ length of the thoracic vertebra directly above the tracheal bifurcation >1.3; and CaVC/width of right fourth rib (just ventral to the spine) >3.5.

The size and appearance of the pulmonary vasculature should be closely evaluated. Pulmonary arteries are located dorsal and lateral to their accompanying veins and bronchi. Several patterns occur: overcirculation, undercirculation, prominent pulmonary arteries, and prominent pulmonary veins. An overcirculation pattern occurs when the lungs are hyperperfused, as in left-to-right shunts, overhydration, and other hyperdynamic states. Pulmonary arteries and veins are both prominent; the increased perfusion also gives a generally hazy appearance to the lungs.

Pulmonary undercirculation is characterized by narrowed pulmonary arteries and veins, along with an increased lucency of the lung fields. Severe dehydration, hypovolemia, obstruction to right ventricular inflow, right-sided congestive heart failure, and tetralogy of Fallot can cause this pattern. Some animals with pulmonic stenosis appear to have pulmonary undercirculation. Overinflation of the lungs or overexposure of radiographs also minimizes the appearance of pulmonary vessels.

Pulmonary arteries larger than their accompanying veins indicate pulmonary arterial hypertension; heartworm disease is a common cause (see Chapter 10). The pulmonary arteries become dilated, tortuous, and blunted, and visualization of the terminal portions is lost. On lateral view, the cranial lobar artery near the base of the heart is normally no wider than the proximal one third of the third or fourth rib. The DV view is best for evaluating the caudal pulmonary arteries in both cats and dogs. The caudal pulmonary arteries should be no wider than the ninth rib at their point of intersection. Heartworm disease often causes patchy to diffuse interstitial pulmonary infiltrates.

Prominent pulmonary veins are a sign of pulmonary venous congestion, usually from left-sided congestive heart failure. On lateral view, the cranial lobar veins are larger and denser than their accompanying arteries and may sag ventrally. Dilated, tortuous pulmonary veins may be seen entering the dorsocaudal aspect of the enlarged left atrium in dogs and cats with chronic pulmonary venous hypertension. However, pulmonary venous dilation is not always visualized in patients with left-sided heart failure. In cats with acute cardiogenic pulmonary edema, enlargement of both pulmonary veins and arteries can be seen.

## PATTERNS OF PULMONARY EDEMA

Pulmonary interstitial fluid accumulation causes the pulmonary parenchyma to appear hazy; pulmonary vessels become ill defined, and bronchial walls thicken. As pulmonary edema worsens, areas of fluffy or mottled fluid opacity progressively become more confluent. Alveolar edema causes greater opacity in the lung fields and obscures vessels and outer bronchial walls. The air-filled bronchi appear as lucent, branching lines surrounded by fluid density (air bronchograms). Interstitial and alveolar patterns of pulmonary infiltration can be caused by many pulmonary diseases as well as by cardiogenic edema (see p. 255). The distribution of these pulmonary infiltrates is important, especially in dogs. Cardiogenic pulmonary edema in dogs is generally located in dorsal and perihilar areas and is often bilaterally symmetric. In contrast, the distribution of cardiogenic edema in cats is usually uneven and patchy; the edema is either distributed throughout the lung fields or concentrated in the middle zones. Radiographic technique as well as the phase of respiration influence the apparent severity of interstitial infiltrates.

## *ECHOCARDIOGRAPHY (CARDIAC ULTRASONOGRAPHY)*

### BENEFITS AND LIMITATIONS

Echocardiography is an important noninvasive tool for imaging the heart and surrounding structures. It is used to evaluate cardiac chamber size, wall thickness, wall motion, valve configuration and motion, and the proximal great vessels. With ultrasound, anatomic relationships can be determined and information on cardiac function can be derived. Echocardiography is a sensitive method for pericardial and pleural fluid detection. It also can permit identification of mass lesions within and adjacent to the heart. Echocardiographic examination can usually be performed with minimal or no chemical restraint.

Echocardiography, like other diagnostic modalities, is most useful within the context of a thorough history, cardiovascular examination, and other appropriate tests. Technical expertise is essential to adequately perform and interpret the echocardiographic examination. The importance of the echocardiographer's skill and understanding of normal and abnormal cardiovascular anatomy and physiology cannot be overemphasized. The ultrasound equipment used, as well as individual patient characteristics, also affects the quality of images obtained. Sound waves do not travel well though bone (e.g., ribs) or air (lungs); these structures may preclude good visualization of the entire heart.

## BASIC PRINCIPLES

Diagnostic ultrasonography uses pulsed, high-frequency sound waves that are reflected from body tissue interfaces. Ultrasound can be aimed in a specific direction and obeys the laws of geometric optics with regard to reflection, transmission, and refraction. When an ultrasonic wave meets an interface of differing biologic tissues, the wave is reflected, refracted, and absorbed. Only the reflected part can be received and processed by the transducer, which acts as a receiver more than 99% of the time. Echocardiographic images are displayed on an oscilloscope screen and can be recorded digitally or on videotape, paper, and/or special radiographic film.

Because sound waves are propagated to the surrounding medium at a characteristic speed, the thickness, size, and location of various soft tissue structures in relation to the origin of the ultrasound beam can be determined at any point in time. The intensity of the ultrasound beam decreases as it travels away from the transducer because of beam divergence, absorption, scatter, and reflection of wave energy at tissue interfaces; these factors influence the intensity of the returning echoes. Stronger echoes are returned when the beam is perpendicular to the imaged structure. In addition, the greater the mismatch in acoustic impedance (which is related to tissue density) between two adjacent tissues, the more reflective their boundary and the stronger the resulting echoes. Very reflective interfaces such as bone/tissue or air/tissue prevent the imaging of weaker echoes from deeper, soft tissue interfaces.

Higher frequency ultrasound waves have a longer near field and less divergence in the far field; they permit better resolution of small structures. However, because more energy is absorbed and scattered by the soft tissues, higher frequencies have less penetrating ability. Conversely, a transducer that produces lower frequency ultrasound provides greater depth of penetration but less-well-defined images. Frequencies generally used for small animal echocardiography range from 3.5 MHz for large dogs to 7.5 MHz for cats and small dogs. A megahertz (MHz) represents 1,000,000 cycles/sec.

Certain descriptive terms are used in ultrasonography. Tissues that strongly reflect ultrasound are *hyperechoic*, or of great echogenicity. Poorly reflecting tissues are *hypoechoic*, whereas fluid, which does not reflect sound, is *anechoic* or *sonolucent*. Tissue behind an area of sonolucency appears hyperechoic because of *acoustic enhancement*. On the other hand, through-transmission of the ultrasound beam is blocked by a strongly hyperechoic object (such as a rib), and an *acoustic shadow* (where no image appears) is cast behind the object.

Three types of echocardiography are used clinically: M-mode, two-dimensional (2-D, real-time), and Doppler. Each has important applications, which are described briefly below. For most echocardiographic examinations, the hair over the transducer placement site is shaved to improve skin con-

tact and image clarity. Coupling gel is applied to produce air-free contact between skin and transducer. The transducer is placed over the area of the precordial impulse (or other appropriate site), and its position is adjusted to find a good "acoustic window" that allows clear visualization of the heart. The right and left parasternal transducer positions are used most often. Minor adjustment of the animal's forelimb or torso position may be required to obtain a good acoustic window. Once the heart has been located, the transducer is angled or rotated and the echocardiograph's controls are adjusted as necessary to optimize the image. For 2-D and M-mode echocardiography, optimal visualization generally is achieved when the ultrasound beam is perpendicular to the cardiac structures and endocardial surfaces being imaged. The ultrasound machine has various controls for factors such as beam strength, focus, and postprocessing that can be adjusted to optimize image quality. Image artifacts are common and can mimic a cardiac abnormality. However, if a suspected lesion can be visualized in more than one imaging plane, it is likely to be real.

The basic echocardiographic examination includes carefully obtained M-mode measurements and all standard 2-D imaging planes from both sides of the chest, as well as any other views needed to further evaluate specific lesions. Doppler evaluation, if available, provides important additional information and is described further below. The entire examination can be quite time-consuming. Light tranquilization is helpful if the animal does not lie quietly. Buprenorphine (0.0075 to 0.01 mg/kg IV) with acepromazine (0.03 mg/kg IV) usually works well for dogs. Butorphanol (0.2 mg/kg IM) with acepromazine (0.1 mg/kg IM) is adequate for many cats, although some require more intense sedation. Acepromazine (0.1 mg/kg IM) followed in 15 minutes by ketamine (2 mg/kg IV) can be used in cats, but this regimen can increase the heart rate undesirably.

## TWO-DIMENSIONAL ECHOCARDIOGRAPHY

A plane of tissue (both depth and width) can be evaluated with 2-D echocardiography, which makes the resulting image "slices" more intuitively recognizable. Anatomic changes resulting from various diseases or congenital defects can be seen, although actual blood flow is not usually visualized with 2-D or M-mode imaging alone.

### Common 2-D Echocardiographic Views

A variety of planes can be imaged from several chest wall locations. Most standard views are obtained from either the right or left parasternal positions (directly over the heart and close to the sternum). Images are occasionally obtained from subxiphoid (subcostal) or thoracic inlet (suprasternal) positions. The animal is gently restrained in lateral recumbency for the examination; better quality images are usually obtained when the heart is imaged from the recumbent side. For this, the animal is placed on a table or platform with an edge cutout, which allows the echocardiographer to position and manipulate the transducer from the animal's dependent side. Some animals can be adequately imaged while standing. The orientation, relative size, and wall thickness of the cardiac chambers; all valves and related structures; and the great vessels are systematically examined. Any suspected abnormality is scanned in multiple planes to further verify and delineate it.

Long-axis views are obtained with the imaging plane parallel to the long axis of the heart, whereas short-axis views are perpendicular to this plane. Images are described by the location of the transducer and the imaging plane used (e.g., right parasternal short-axis view, left cranial parasternal long-axis view). Figs. 2-20 to 2-25 illustrate standard 2-D imaging

planes and display formats. Two-dimensional imaging allows an overall assessment of cardiac chamber size and wall thickness. The right ventricular wall is usually about one third the thickness of the left ventricular free wall and should be no more than one half its thickness. The size of the right atrial and ventricular chambers is subjectively compared to that of the left atrium and ventricle; the left apical four-chamber view is useful for this.

Left ventricular internal dimensions and wall thickness are usually obtained using M-mode imaging, but appropriately timed 2-D frames can also be used. There are also several methods that can be used to estimate left ventricular volume

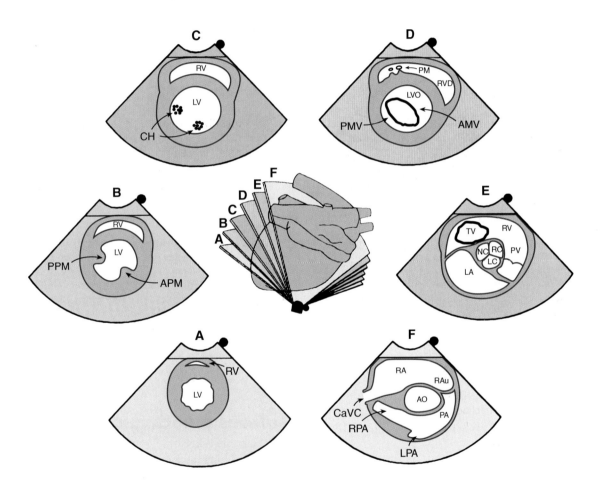

**FIG 2-20**
Two-dimensional short-axis echocardiographic views from the right parasternal position. The center diagram indicates the orientation of the ultrasound beam used to image cardiac structures at the six levels shown. Several of these positions guide M-mode beam placement as well as Doppler evaluation of tricuspid and pulmonary flows. Corresponding echo images are shown clockwise from the bottom. **A,** Apex. **B,** Papillary muscle. **C,** Chordae tendineae. **D,** Mitral valve. **E,** Aortic valve. **F,** Pulmonary artery. *AMV,* Anterior (septal) mitral valve cusp; *AO,* aorta; *APM,* anterior papillary muscle; *CaVC,* caudal vena cava; *CH,* chordae tendineae; *LA,* left atrium; *LPA,* left pulmonary artery; *LV,* left ventricle; *LVO,* left ventricular outflow tract; *PA,* pulmonary artery; *PM,* papillary muscle; *PMV,* posterior mitral valve cusp; *PPM,* posterior papillary muscle; *PV,* pulmonary valve; *RA,* right atrium; *RAu,* right auricle; *RC, LC, NC,* right, left, and noncoronary cusps of aortic valve; *RPA,* right pulmonary artery; *RV,* right ventricle; *RVO,* right ventricular outflow tract; *TV,* tricuspid valve. (From Thomas WP et al: Recommendations for standards in transthoracic 2-dimensional echocardiography in the dog and cat, *J Vet Intern Med* 7:247, 1993.)

Long-axis 4-chamber view

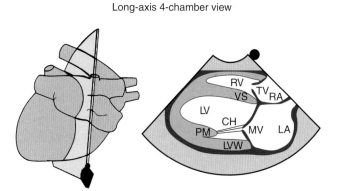

4-chamber (inflow) view

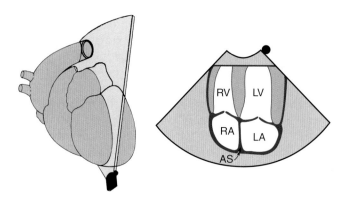

Long-axis LV outflow view

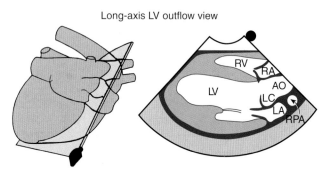

5-chamber (LV outflow) view

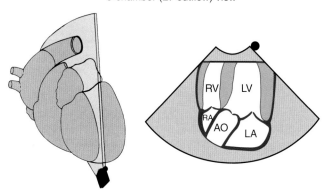

**FIG 2-21**
Two-dimensional long-axis echocardiographic views from right parasternal position. Each diagram on the left indicates the location of the ultrasound beam as it transects the heart from the right side, resulting in the corresponding echo image on the right. Long-axis four-chamber (left ventricular inflow) view is above. Long-axis view of the left ventricular outflow region is below. *AO,* Aorta; *CH,* chordae tendineae; *LA,* left atrium; *LC,* left coronary cusp of aortic valve; *LV,* left ventricle; *LVW,* left ventricular wall; *MV,* mitral valve; *PM,* papillary muscle; *RA,* right atrium; *RPA,* right pulmonary artery; *RV,* right ventricle; *TV,* tricuspid valve; *VS,* interventricular septum. (From Thomas WP et al: Recommendations for standards in transthoracic 2-dimensional echocardiography in the dog and cat, *J Vet Intern Med 7*:247, 1993.)

**FIG 2-22**
Left caudal (apical) parasternal position. Four-chamber view optimized for ventricular inflow is above. Five-chamber view optimized for left ventricular outflow is below. These views provide good Doppler velocity signals from mitral and aortic valve regions. *AO,* Aorta; *AS,* interatrial septum; *LA,* left atrium; *LV,* left ventricle; *RA,* right atrium; *RV,* right ventricle. (From Thomas WP et al: Recommendations for standards in transthoracic 2-dimensional echocardiography in the dog and cat, *J Vet Intern Med 7*:247, 1993.)

and wall mass. Left atrial size is better assessed using 2-D rather than M-mode. Several methods for measuring left atrial size have been described. One is to measure the cranial-caudal diameter (top to bottom on the screen) at end-systole using a right parasternal long axis four-chamber view. For cats, this left atrial dimension normally is less than 16 mm; a diameter exceeding 19 mm is thought to indicate greater risk for thromboembolism (Bonagura, 2001). In dogs, however, there is greater variation related to body size. Instead, the left atrial dimension can be compared to the 2-D aortic root diameter measured across the sinuses of Valsalva; normally this left atrial diameter/aortic root ratio is 1.7 to 1.9 (Bonagura, 2001).

## M-MODE ECHOCARDIOGRAPHY

The M-mode echocardiogram provides a one-dimensional view (depth) into the heart. M-mode images represent echoes from various tissue interfaces along the axis of the beam (displayed vertically on the screen). These echoes, which move during the cardiac cycle, are displayed against time (on the horizontal axis). Thus the "wavy" lines seen on these recordings correspond to the positions of particular structures in relation to the transducer as well as to each other at any point in time. Most machines allow for more accurate placement of the M-mode beam using a movable cursor line superimposed on a 2-D (real-time) image. The M-mode image usually provides cleaner resolution of cardiac borders than a 2-D image because of its high sampling rate. Measurements of cardiac dimensions and motion throughout the cardiac cycle are often more accurately obtained from M-mode tracings, especially when coupled with a simultaneously recorded

Long-axis 2-chamber view

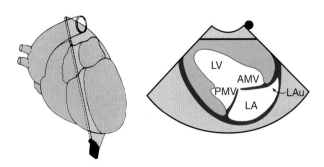

Long-axis LV outflow view

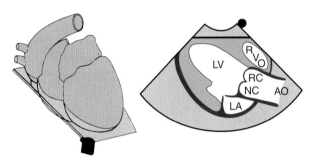

**FIG 2-23**
Left caudal (apical) parasternal 2-dimensional views optimized for left ventricular inflow and left auricle *(above)* and left ventricular outflow *(below)*. AMV, Anterior (septal) mitral valve cusp; AO, aorta; LA, left atrium; LAu, left auricle; LV, left ventricle; PMV, posterior mitral valve cusp; RC, NC, right and noncoronary cusps of aortic valve; RVO, right ventricular outflow tract. (From Thomas WP et al: Recommendations for standards in transthoracic 2-dimensional echocardiography in the dog and cat, *J Vet Intern Med* 7:247, 1993.)

Short-axis view

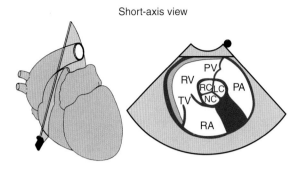

**FIG 2-24**
Left cranial parasternal short-axis view optimized for right ventricular inflow and outflow. This view is useful for Doppler interrogation of tricuspid and pulmonary artery flows. *PA,* Pulmonary artery; *PV,* pulmonary valve; *RA,* right atrium; *RC, LC, NC,* right, left, and noncoronary cusps of aortic valve; *RV,* right ventricle; *TV,* tricuspid valve. (From Thomas WP et al: Recommendations for standards in transthoracic 2-dimensional echocardiography in the dog and cat, *J Vet Intern Med* 7:247, 1993.)

ECG (or phonocardiogram). Difficulty achieving consistent and accurate beam placement for standard measurements and calculations can be a limitation. Beam placement guided by 2-D imaging lessens this problem.

## M-Mode Views

Standard M-mode views are obtained from the right parasternal transducer position. The M-mode cursor is positioned with 2-D guidance using the right parasternal short-axis view. Precise positioning of the ultrasound beam within the heart and clear endocardial surface images are essential for accurate M-mode measurements and calculations. For example, papillary muscles within the left ventricle must be avoided when measuring free-wall thickness. Fig. 2-26 illustrates standard M-mode views.

## Common Measurements and Normal Values

The standard dimensions measured with M-mode and the time in the cardiac cycle at which they are taken are also indicated in Fig. 2-26. Measurements are made using the lead-

ing edge technique when possible (i.e., from the edge closest to the transducer [leading edge] of one side of the dimension to the leading edge of the other). In this way, only one endocardial surface is included in the measurement. The systolic and diastolic thickness of the left ventricular wall and interventricular septum, as well as left ventricular chamber dimensions, should be determined at the level of the chordae tendineae, not at the apex or mitral valve level. It is often difficult to measure right ventricular structures. Calculation of indices to estimate myocardial function (e.g., fractional shortening) is done using these measurements (Fig. 2-27). Measurements may also be taken from the 2-D echocardiogram if the images are of high resolution and frames from the appropriate times in the cardiac cycle are used. Chamber volume and ejection fraction can be calculated, but both contain inaccuracies created by the geometric assumptions that must be made from one-dimensional measurement alone. Greater reliability is obtained by using the modified Simpsons' method, with accurate left ventricular area and length measurements (see Suggested Readings for further information).

Diastolic measurements are made at the onset of the QRS complex of a simultaneously recorded ECG. Systolic measurements of the left ventricle are made from the point of peak downward motion of the septum to the leading edge of the left ventricular free-wall endocardium at the same instant. The septum and left ventricular wall normally move toward each other in systole, although their peak movement may not coincide if electrical activation is not simultaneous. Paradoxic septal motion, in which the septum seems to move away from the left ventricular wall and toward the transducer in systole, occurs in some cases of right ventricular volume and/or pressure overload. This abnormal septal motion can also be visualized on 2-D images; it precludes accurate assessment of left ventricular function using fractional shortening.

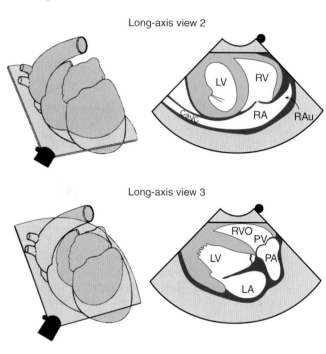

**FIG 2-25**

Left cranial parasternal long-axis views optimized for aortic root *(above)*, right atrium and auricle *(middle)*, and right ventricular outflow and main pulmonary artery *(below)*. These views are used to evaluate the heart base and can provide good Doppler signals for tricuspid and pulmonary flows. *AO,* Aorta; *CaVC,* caudal vena cava; *LA,* left atrium; *LV,* left ventricle; *PA,* pulmonary artery; *PV,* pulmonary valve; *RA,* right atrium; *RAu,* right auricle; *RC, NC,* right and noncoronary cusps of aortic valve; *RV,* right ventricle; *RVO,* right ventricular outflow tract. (From Thomas WP et al: Recommendations for standards in transthoracic 2-dimensional echocardiography in the dog and cat, *J Vet Intern Med* 7:247, 1993.)

The fractional shortening (FS; % Δ D) is the index used most often to estimate left ventricular function. Fractional shortening is the percent change in left ventricular dimension from diastole to systole. This index of contractility, like others taken during cardiac ejection, has the significant limitation of being dependent on ventricular loading conditions. For example, reduced left ventricular afterload (as occurs from mitral insufficiency, ventricular septal defect, or peripheral vasodilation) facilitates ejection of blood and allows greater fractional shortening, although intrinsic myocardial contractility is not increased. Hence the apparent hypercontractility (exaggerated fractional shortening) in patients with severe mitral regurgitation and normal myocardial function. The use of the calculated end-systolic volume index has been suggested as a more accurate way to assess myocardial contractility in the presence of mitral regurgitation. This index compares ventricular size after ejection to body size rather than to the volume-overloaded end-diastolic ventricular size.

Mitral valve motion is also evaluated on the M-mode scan. The anterior (septal) leaflet is most prominent and has an M configuration. The posterior (parietal) leaflet is smaller and more difficult to image; its motion mirrors the anterior leaflet, appearing as a W. The motion pattern of the tricuspid

valve is similar. The mitral valve motion pattern is identified by letters (see Fig. 2-26). Point *D* occurs at the time of early diastole when the valve first opens, and point *E* occurs at maximal opening of the valve during the rapid ventricular filling phase. An indication of the velocity of blood flow through the mitral valve at this time is provided by the slope from points *D* to *E*. Point *F* represents the end of rapid ventricular filling when the valve drifts into a more closed position. Atrial contraction causes the valve to open again to point *A*. Normally the valve excursion is greater at point *E;* sometimes a more prominent *A* point occurs because of higher left atrial systolic pressure from increased left ventricular stiffness. Point *C* occurs with closure of the mitral valve during the onset of ventricular systole. Inconsistently, high left ventricular end-diastolic pressure causes a *B* "shoulder" or "bump," which interrupts the normally straight *A*-to-*C* line. In normal animals, the *E* point of the mitral valve lies close to the interventricular septum. Poor myocardial contractility is the most common cause of an increased *E* point-to-septal separation. In animals with left ventricular outflow obstruction, the anterior mitral leaflet can be sucked toward the septum during ejection. This is called systolic anterior motion (SAM), and it causes the normally straight

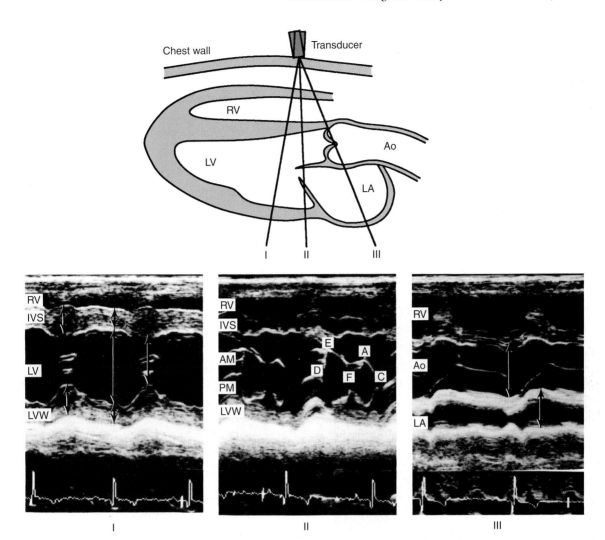

## FIG 2-26

Common M-mode views. The top diagram indicates the approximate orientation of the one-dimensional ultrasound beam through the heart to achieve the corresponding M-mode images below. A lead II ECG is recorded below the echo images and is used for timing. End diastole occurs at the onset of the QRS complex; end systole is at the time of the smallest dimension between the interventricular septum and posterior left ventricular wall. In panel I, at the level of the chordae tendineae, the internal dimensions of the left ventricle are measured from the leading (anterior) edge of the left endocardial wall of the septum to the leading edge (luminal surface) of the posterior left ventricular wall *(arrows)*. The thickness of the septum is measured from the right endocardial surface of the septum to the leading edge of the left endocardial septal wall at end diastole and end systole; the posterior left ventricular wall is measured at the same times from the endocardial surface to (but not including) the leading edge of the epicardial echo *(arrows)*. Panel II, at the mitral valve level, illustrates the appearance of the anterior and posterior mitral leaflets. The motion of the anterior leaflet is described by the letters shown. Diastolic opening of the valve occurs at point *D* and systolic closing occurs at point *C* (see text for more information). In panel III, aortic root diameter at the level at which valve cusps are seen is measured from the leading (anterior) edge of the anterior aortic wall to the leading edge of the posterior wall and timed with the onset of the QRS complex *(arrow)*. The left atrium (auricle) is measured from the leading edge of the posterior aortic wall to the leading edge of the atrial wall at the time of peak anterior aortic movement *(arrow)*. *AM,* Anterior leaflet of mitral valve; *Ao,* aorta; *IVS,* interventricular septum; *LA,* left atrium; *LV,* left ventricular lumen; *LVW,* left ventricular posterior wall; *PM,* posterior leaflet of mitral valve; *RV,* right ventricular lumen.

$$FS = \frac{LVID_d - LVID_s}{LVID_d} \times 100$$

**FIG 2-27**
Echocardiographic indices commonly used to assess myocardial function. *BSA,* Body surface area (m²); *ESVI,* end-systolic volume index (ml/m²); *FS,* fractional shortening (%); *LVET,* left ventricular ejection time(s); *LVID_d,* left ventricular internal dimension at end diastole (cm); *LVID_s,* left ventricular internal dimension at end systole (cm); *VCF,* mean velocity of circumferential shortening (circumferences/sec).

$$ESVI^* = \frac{LVID_s^3 \times \dfrac{7}{(2.4 + LVID_s)}}{BSA}$$

Estimated degree of myocardial failure:

Mild: 30-60 ml/m²
Moderate: 60-90 ml/m²
Severe: >90 ml/m²
Normal: <30 ml/m²

$$VCF = \frac{LVID_d - LVID_s}{LVID_d \times LVET}$$

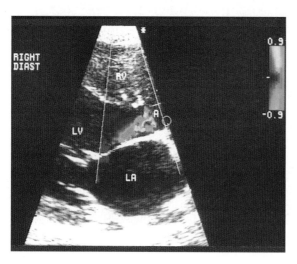

**FIG 2-28**
Color flow Doppler image of an aortic regurgitation jet angled toward and along the anterior leaflet of the mitral valve in a young English Toy Spaniel with a ventricular septal defect. The regurgitant jet causes the mitral leaflet to flutter in diastole, as seen in Fig. 2-29. Imaged from the right parasternal long axis position. *A,* Aorta; *LA,* left atrium; *LV,* left ventricle; *RV,* right ventricle.

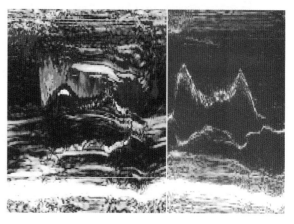

**FIG 2-29**
Color M-mode and standard M-mode images of the mitral valve of an English Toy Spaniel with a ventricular septal defect and aortic regurgitation. The turbulence from aortic regurgitation is seen as the yellow/green/blue color along the anterior leaflet in the left ventricular outflow region. The black and white image shows fluttering of the anterior mitral leaflet, which appears wide and "fuzzy" compared to the thin, discrete posterior leaflet image.

mitral echoes (between points *C* and *D*) to bend toward the septum during systole (see Fig. 7-3). Diastolic flutter of the anterior mitral leaflet can sometimes be seen when an aortic insufficiency jet causes the leaflet to vibrate (Figs. 2-28 and 2-29).

The diameters of the aortic root and left atrium are also commonly measured with M-mode imaging. The walls of the aortic root appear as two parallel lines shifting upward in systole. During diastole, one or two aortic valve cusps may be seen as a straight line parallel to and centered between the aortic wall echoes. At the onset of ejection, the cusps quickly separate to opposite sides of the aortic root and then come together again at the end of ejection. The shape of these echoes (two cusps) has been described as a train of boxcars or little rectangular boxes attached together by a string. The diameter of the aorta is determined at end-diastole. The amplitude of posterior-to-anterior motion of the aortic root is often decreased in animals with poor cardiac output. The left atrial dimension is taken at maximal systolic excursion. In normal cats and dogs, the ratio of left atrial to aortic root diameters is about 1:1. However, this is an imprecise measure of left atrial size, because (especially in dogs) the part of the left atrium imaged on this M-mode view is usually the area between the body of the left atrium and the left auricle. This

TABLE 2-10

**Approximate Echocardiographic Measurements for Dogs***

| | WEIGHT (kg) | | | | | | | | | | |
|---|---|---|---|---|---|---|---|---|---|---|---|
| | **3** | **5** | **7** | **10** | **15** | **20** | **25** | **30** | **35** | **40** | **50** |
| LVID$_d$ (mm) | 24.6† | 27.4 | 30.0 | 32.7 | 37.1 | 41.4 | 44.8 | 48.3 | 51.7 | 54.8 | 60.7 |
| | (6.2) | (5.2) | (4.5) | (3.5) | (2.4) | (2.2) | (2.9) | (3.9) | (5.0) | (6.1) | (8.3) |
| LVID$_s$ (mm) | 13.6 | 16.0 | 17.9 | 20.6 | 24.3 | 28.0 | 31.0 | 33.9 | 36.9 | 39.6 | 44.6 |
| | (5.5) | (4.7) | (4.0) | (3.1) | (2.1) | (2.0) | (2.5) | (3.4) | (4.5) | (5.4) | (7.4) |
| LVW$_d$ (mm) | 5.0 | 5.4 | 5.7 | 6.2 | 6.8 | 7.4 | 7.9 | 8.4 | 8.9 | 9.3 | 10.2 |
| | (2.1) | (1.7) | (1.5) | (1.2) | (0.8) | (0.7) | (1.0) | (1.3) | (1.7) | (2.0) | (2.8) |
| LVW$_s$ (mm) | 7.2 | 7.9 | 8.4 | 9.2 | 10.2 | 11.3 | 12.1 | 13.0 | 13.8 | 14.5 | 16.0 |
| | (1.7) | (1.6) | (1.4) | (1.3) | (1.1) | (1.1) | (1.2) | (1.3) | (1.5) | (1.7) | (2.2) |
| IVS$_d$ (mm) | 5.8 | 6.2 | 6.5 | 7.0 | 7.6 | 8.2 | 8.7 | 9.2 | 9.7 | 10.2 | 11.0 |
| | (2.1) | (1.7) | (1.5) | (1.2) | (0.8) | (0.7) | (0.9) | (1.3) | (1.7) | (2.0) | (2.7) |
| IVS$_s$ (mm) | 9.8 | 10.2 | 10.4 | 10.9 | 11.5 | 12.3 | 13.0 | 13.9 | 14.6 | 15.4 | — |
| | (2.6) | (2.2) | (2.0) | (1.7) | (1.2) | (1.1) | (1.5) | (2.3) | (2.6) | (3.5) | |
| LA‡ (mm) | 12.7 | 14.0 | 15.0 | 16.3 | 18.3 | 20.2 | 21.8 | 23.3 | 24.8 | 26.2 | 28.8 |
| | (5.3) | (4.5) | (3.8) | (3.0) | (2.0) | (1.9) | (2.4) | (3.3) | (4.3) | (5.2) | (7.1) |
| Ao (mm) | 13.8 | 15.3 | 16.4 | 18.1 | 20.4 | 22.8 | 24.6 | 26.4 | 28.3 | 30.0 | 33.1 |
| | (3.6) | (3.0) | (2.6) | (2.0) | (1.4) | (1.3) | (1.6) | (2.2) | (2.9) | (3.5) | (4.8) |

From Bonagura JD et al: Echocardiography: principles of interpretation, *Vet Clin North Am* 15:1177, 1985. (See Suggested Readings for additional references.)
Some athletic normal dogs have a slightly lower FS (20% to 25%); normal Dobermans also may have FS values below the usual normal range. *LVID$_d$*, Left ventricular internal diameter at end diastole; *LVID$_s$*, left ventricular internal diameter at end systole; *LVW$_d$*, left ventricular wall at end diastole; *LVW$_s$*, left ventricular wall at end systole; *IVS$_d$*, interventricular septum at end diastole; *IVS$_s$*, interventricular septum at end systole; *LA*, left atrium (systole); *Ao*, aortic root; *FS*, fractional shortening; *EPSS*, mitral E-point septal separation.
*These are approximate guidelines only; normal dogs may be above or below these values, especially those near the outer range of body weight.
†Mean value given; ± standard deviation in parentheses below.
‡M-mode cursor position for LA measurement is often variable among animals; usually the maximal LA dimension is not represented by this dimension (see text for more information).

measurement therefore usually does not represent maximal atrial size. In cats the M-mode beam is more likely to cross the body of the left atrium, but its orientation can be inconsistent. Echo beam placement may be difficult in some animals, and the pulmonary artery can be inadvertently imaged instead.

Systolic time intervals (STIs) have been used sporadically for estimation of cardiac function, although they also are influenced by cardiac filling and afterload. These intervals can be calculated if the opening and closing of the aortic valve are clearly seen with M-mode imaging and a simultaneous ECG is recorded for timing. The STIs are left ventricular ejection time (duration of time the aortic valve is open), preejection period (time from the onset of the QRS to aortic valve opening), and total electromechanical systole (left ventricular ejection time plus preejection period).

Several reports of normal reference ranges for echocardiographic measurements in dogs and cats have been published, most derived from relatively small numbers of animals. The reported values vary from study to study. Values for dogs are greatly affected by body size, and breed differ-

ences have been reported as well. Endurance training also affects measured parameters, reflecting the increased cardiac mass and volume associated with frequent and sustained strenuous exercise. Although guidelines for commonly used echocardiographic measurements are given in Tables 2-10 and 2-11, these values should be regarded as only approximate. The Suggested Readings list also includes reports of reference values for various dog breeds and cats.

## CONTRAST ECHOCARDIOGRAPHY

Contrast echocardiography, or "bubble study," is a technique in which a substance containing "microbubbles" is rapidly injected either into a peripheral vein or selectively into the heart. The passage of these microbubbles into the ultrasound beam generates many tiny echoes that temporarily opacify the blood pool being imaged. The microbubbles look like bright sparkles that move with the blood flow. Agitated saline solution, a mixture of saline and the patient's blood, and other substances can be used as echo-contrast material. Injection into a peripheral vein opacifies the right heart chambers; bubbles seen in the left heart or aorta indicate a

TABLE 2-11

Echocardiographic Measurement Guidelines for Cats*

| LVIDd† (mm) | LVIDs (mm) | LVWd (mm) | LVWs (mm) | IVSd (mm) | IVSs (mm) | LA‡ (mm) | Ao (mm) | FS§ (%) | EPSS‖ (mm) |
|---|---|---|---|---|---|---|---|---|---|
| 12-18 | 5-10 | ≤5.5 | ≤9 | ≤5.5 | ≤9 | 8-13 | 8-11 | 35-65 | ≤4 |

*LVID*d, Left ventricular internal diameter at end diastole; *LVID*s, left ventricular internal diameter at end systole; *LVW*d, left ventricular wall at end diastole; *LVW*s, left ventricular wall at end systole; *IVS*d, interventricular septum at end diastole; *IVS*s, interventricular septum at end systole; *LA*, left atrium (systole); *Ao*, aortic root; *FS*, fractional shortening; *EPSS*, mitral E-point septal separation.
*These values are based on the author's experience and compilation of published studies. (See Suggested Readings for additional references.)
†Ketamine increases heart rate and decreases LVIDd.
‡M-mode cursor position for LA measurement varies among animals; the maximal LA dimension is better assessed with 2-D imaging and is normally <16 mm.
§FS 25% to 40% is usual normal range for all body weights.
‖EPSS ≤5 to 6 mm.

right-to-left shunt. Saline microbubbles do not pass through the pulmonary capillaries (although some commercially available echo-contrast agents do), therefore echo-contrast injection via selective left-sided heart catheterization is required to visualize intracardiac left-to-right shunts or mitral regurgitation. Doppler echocardiography is now generally used instead of echo-contrast injections.

## DOPPLER ECHOCARDIOGRAPHY

Doppler echocardiography detects blood flow direction and velocity. The most important clinical applications relate to finding abnormal flow direction or turbulence and increased flow velocity. The Doppler modality is based on the detection of frequency shifts between the emitted ultrasound energy and echoes reflected from moving blood cells (the Doppler shift).* Echoes returning from cells moving away from the transducer are of lower frequency, whereas those from cells moving toward the transducer cause are of higher frequency. The higher the velocity of the cells, the greater the frequency shift. Optimal blood flow profiles and calculation of maximal blood flow velocity are possible when the ultrasound beam is aligned parallel to the flow. The parallel beam alignment necessary for accurate Doppler imaging is in contrast to the perpendicular beam orientation needed for optimal M-mode and 2-D imaging. With Doppler imaging, the calculated blood flow velocity diminishes as the ultrasound beam's angle of incidence and the direction of blood flow diverge from 0 degrees, because the calculated flow velocity is inversely related to the cosine of this angle (cosine 0 degrees = 1). As long as the angle between the ultrasound beam and the path of blood flow is less than 20 degrees, maximal flow velocity can be estimated with reasonable accuracy. As this angle of incidence increases, the calculated velocity decreases. At an angle of 90 degrees, the calculated velocity is 0 (cosine 90 degrees = 0), therefore no flow signal is recorded when the ultrasound beam is perpendicular to blood flow. Flow signals are usually displayed with time on the *x* axis and velocity (scaled in m/sec) on the *y* axis. A zero baseline demarcates flow away from (below baseline) or toward (above baseline) the transducer. Higher velocities are displayed farther from baseline. Other flow characteristics (e.g., turbulence) also affect the Doppler spectral display.

Characteristic blood flow patterns are obtained from the different valve areas. Flow across both AV valves has a similar pattern; likewise, flow patterns across the semilunar valve areas are similar. Normal diastolic flow across the mitral valve (Fig. 2-30) and tricuspid valve consists of an initial higher velocity signal during the rapid ventricular filling phase (E wave), which is followed by a smaller velocity signal associated with atrial contraction (A wave). Breed, age, and body weight appear to have little influence on normal Doppler measurements. Peak velocities are normally higher across the mitral (peak E usually less than or equal to 0.9 to 1.0 m/sec; peak A usually less than or equal to 0.6 to 0.7 m/sec) compared to the tricuspid valve (peak E usually ≤ to 0.8 to 0.9 m/sec; peak A usually ≤ 0.5 to 0.6 m/sec). Flow across the pulmonary and aortic valves (Fig. 2-31) accelerates rapidly during ejection, with more gradual deceleration. The peak systolic pulmonary velocity is less than or equal to 1.4 to 1.5 m/sec in most normal dogs, and the peak aortic velocity is usually less than or equal to 1.6 to 1.7 m/sec. Some normal dogs may have peak aortic velocities slightly above 2 m/sec related to increased stroke volume or high sympathetic tone, especially if unsedated. Ventricular outflow obstruction causes more rapid flow acceleration, increased peak velocities, and turbulence. In general, aortic velocities over 2.1 or 2.2 m/sec are suggestive of outflow obstruction. However, between 1.7 and around 2.2 m/sec lies a "grey zone" in which very mild left ventricular outflow obstruction (e.g., some cases of subaortic stenosis) cannot be differentiated with certainty from normal but vigorous left ventricular ejection direction.

---

*$V = C\dfrac{\pm\Delta f}{2f_0\cos\theta}$

*V*, Calculated blood flow velocity (m/sec); *C*, speed of sound in soft tissue (1540 m/sec); ± Δ*f*, Doppler frequency shift; $f_0$, transmitted frequency; θ, intercept angle (between ultrasound beam and blood flow).

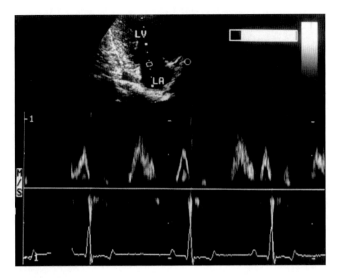

**FIG 2-30**
Normal mitral valve inflow recorded with pulsed-wave (PW) Doppler imaging from left caudal parasternal position in a dog. The flow signal (above baseline) following the QRS-T of the ECG represents early diastolic flow into the ventricle; the second, smaller peak after the P wave represents inflow from atrial contraction. Velocity scale in meters per second is on the left. *LA,* Left atrium; *LV,* left ventricle.

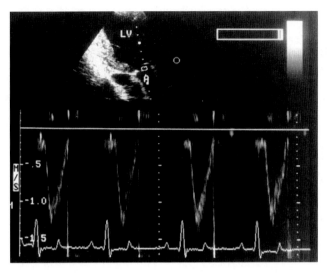

**FIG 2-31**
Normal aortic outflow recorded with pulsed-wave (PW) Doppler imaging from left caudal parasternal position in a dog. Note rapid blood acceleration (below baseline) into the aorta with a peak velocity of about 1.35 m/sec. Velocity scale in meters per second is on the left. *A,* Aorta; *LV,* left ventricle.

Because blood flow patterns and velocity can be evaluated with Doppler imaging, detection and quantification of valvular insufficiency, obstructive lesions, and cardiac shunts are possible. Cardiac output and other indicators of systolic and diastolic function can be assessed (see Suggested Readings). Doppler-derived diastolic function indices include the isovolumic relaxation time, mitral valve peak E velocity/peak A velocity (E/A) ratio, and others. Numerous factors can complicate the accurate evaluation of diastolic function.

Several types of Doppler echocardiography are used clinically: pulsed wave (PW), continuous wave (CW), and color flow mapping. PW Doppler uses short bursts of ultrasound to analyze echoes returning from a specified area distant to the transducer (designated the sample volume). The advantage of PW Doppler imaging is that blood flow velocity, direction, and spectral characteristics can be calculated from a specific location in the heart or blood vessel. The main disadvantage is that the maximum velocity that can be measured is limited because the pulse repetition frequency is limited. This relates to the time required to receive and process echoes returning from the selected location. The maximum measurable velocity (called the Nyquist limit) is influenced by the transmitted frequency and the distance of the sample volume from the transducer. Lower frequency transducers and closer sample volume placement increase the Nyquist limit. If blood flow velocity is higher than the Nyquist limit, "aliasing," or velocity ambiguity, occurs. This is displayed as a band of velocity signals extending above and below ("wrapped around") the baseline, so that neither velocity nor direction is measurable (Fig. 2-32).

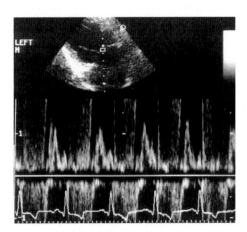

**FIG 2-32**
Mitral diastolic inflow and systolic regurgitant flow in a dog with degenerative mitral valve disease recorded with PW Doppler imaging from left caudal parasternal position. The direction of mitral regurgitant flow is away from the transducer (below baseline); however, this direction cannot be discerned with pulsed-wave imaging because the flow velocity is too high. The signal is instead "wrapped around" the baseline (aliased).

CW Doppler imaging uses dual crystals so that ultrasound can be continuously and simultaneously transmitted and received. Theoretically there is no maximum velocity limit with this modality, therefore high-velocity flows can be measured (Fig. 2-33). The disadvantage of CW Doppler imaging is that sampling of blood flow velocity and direction occurs all along

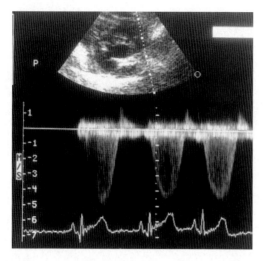

**FIG 2-33**
Continuous-wave (CW) Doppler recording of high-velocity pulmonary outflow in a dog with pulmonic stenosis imaged from the right parasternal short-axis position. Estimated systolic pressure gradient across the pulmonary valve is about 100 mm Hg based on a peak velocity of 5 m/sec. Peak velocity varies slightly with changes in ventricular filling. Velocity scale in meters per second is on the left.

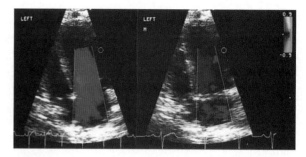

**FIG 2-34**
Color flow Doppler images from left caudal parasternal position. Left panel indicates diastolic flow moving toward the transducer into the ventricle (coded red). Right panel, in systole, shows mitral valve closed and blue-coded flow moving away, in left ventricular outflow tract. Imaged from the left caudal parasternal position.

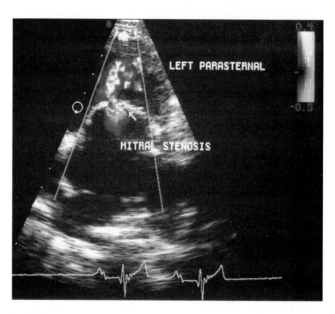

**FIG 2-35**
Example of color flow aliasing in a dog with mitral valve stenosis. Diastolic flow toward the narrowed mitral orifice *(arrow)* accelerates beyond the Nyquist limit, causing red-coded flow (blood moving toward transducer) to alias to blue, then again to red, and once more to blue. Turbulent flow, indicated by shades of yellow and green, is seen within the left ventricle at the top of the 2-D image.

the ultrasound beam, not in a specified area (so-called range ambiguity).

Color flow mapping is a form of PW Doppler echocardiography that combines the M-mode or 2-D modality with blood flow imaging. However, instead of one sample volume along one scan line, many are analyzed along multiple scan lines. The mean frequency shift obtained from the multiple sample volumes is color coded for direction and velocity. Several types of mapping are usually available. Most systems code blood flow toward the transducer as red and flow away from the transducer as blue (Fig. 2-34). Differences in relative velocity of flow can be accentuated, and the presence of multiple velocities and directions of flow (turbulence) can be indicated by different display maps that use variations in brightness and color. Aliasing occurs often, even with normal blood flows; it is displayed as a reversal of color (e.g., red shifting to blue [Fig. 2-35]). Multiple velocities and directions of flow in an area are indicated using a variance map, which adds shades of yellow or green to the red/blue display (Figs. 2-36 and 2-37).

The instantaneous pressure gradient across a stenotic or regurgitant valve area is estimated using the maximum measured velocity of the flow jet. CW Doppler is used if aliasing occurs with PW Doppler. Parallel Doppler beam alignment is essential to measure maximum velocity. A modification of the Bernoulli equation is used:

$$\text{Pressure gradient} = 4(\text{maximum velocity})^2$$

Other factors involved in this relationship are usually of little clinical consequence and are generally ignored, although they could be influential in some types of flow obstruction.

Doppler estimation of pressure gradients is used in combination with M-mode and 2-D imaging to assess the severity of congenital or acquired outflow obstructions. The maximum velocity of a regurgitant jet also can be used to estimate the peak pressure gradient across the regurgitant valve. For example, the peak velocity of a tricuspid regurgitation jet can be used to estimate pulmonary artery pressure in the absence of pulmonic stenosis. The calculated systolic pressure gradient plus the central venous pressure equals the peak right ventricular systolic pressure, which approximates the pulmonary artery pressure.

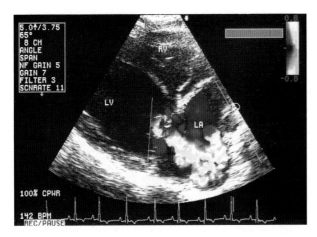

**FIG 2-36**
Systolic frame showing turbulent flow (indicated using a variance map of yellow and green) backward into an enlarged left atrium in a dog with mitral regurgitation. The regurgitant jet extends to the dorsal aspect of the left atrium. Imaged from the right parasternal long axis, four-chamber view. *LA,* Left atrium; *LV,* left ventricle; *RV,* right ventricle.

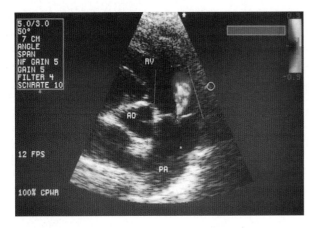

**FIG 2-37**
Color flow Doppler image of pulmonic regurgitation in a terrier with pulmonary hypertension and secondary distension of the right ventricular outflow region and main pulmonary artery. Diastolic frame taken from a right parasternal short-axis view. *Ao,* Aorta; *PA,* pulmonary artery; *RV,* right ventricle.

Semiquantification of valve regurgitation by determining the size and shape of the regurgitant jet is sometimes done, especially with color flow Doppler. Although technical and hemodynamic factors confound the accuracy of such assessment, wide and long regurgitant jets are generally associated with more severe regurgitation than narrow jets. Other methods have been described as well. Measurement of maximum regurgitant jet velocity is not an indicator of the severity of regurgitation, especially mitral regurgitation. Changes in chamber size provide a better indication of severity with chronic regurgitation.

The quantification of abnormal blood flow and calculation of cardiac output are subject to numerous sources of er-

ror, although these values are sometimes clinically useful. There is increasing interest in the use of Doppler-derived indices of diastolic function to evaluate patients with cardiac disease. Further information about these methods can be found elsewhere (see Suggested Readings). Adequate Doppler examinations are often very time-consuming. They are technically demanding and require a good understanding of cardiac anatomy and hemodynamic principles.

## TRANSESOPHAGEAL ECHOCARDIOGRAPHY

Cardiac structures can be imaged through the esophageal wall with specialized transducers mounted on a flexible, steerable endoscope tip. Transesophageal echocardiography (TEE) can provide clearer images of some cardiac structures (especially those at or above the AV junction) compared to transthoracic echocardiography because chest wall and lung interference is avoided. The need for heavy sedation or general anesthesia, the expense of the endoscopic transducers, and the potential complications of the endoscopy procedure are the main disadvantages of TEE.

## OTHER TECHNIQUES

### Angiocardiography

Nonselective angiocardiography can be useful for diagnosing several acquired and congenital diseases, including cardiomyopathy and heartworm disease in cats, severe pulmonic or aortic or subaortic stenosis, PDA, and tetralogy of Fallot. Intracardiac septal defects and valvular regurgitation cannot usually be identified. The quality of such studies is higher with rapid injection of radiopaque dye via a large-bore catheter and small patient size. In most cases, echocardiography can provide similar information more safely than nonselective angiocardiography. However, evaluation of the pulmonary vasculature is better accomplished using nonselective angiocardiography.

Selective angiocardiography is performed by placing cardiac catheters into specific areas of the heart or great vessels. Injection of contrast material is generally preceded by the measurement of pressures and oxygen saturations. This technique allows identification of anatomic abnormalities and the path of blood flow. Doppler echocardiography now is used more commonly; it usually provides comparable information noninvasively with less expense, time, and risk involved.

### Cardiac Catheterization

Cardiac catheterization entails the placement of specialized catheters selectively into different areas of the heart and vasculature via the jugular vein, carotid artery, or femoral vessels. Measurement of pressures, cardiac output, and blood oxygen concentrations can thus be obtained from specific areas. Identification and quantification of congenital and certain acquired cardiac abnormalities are possible using these procedures along with selective angiocardiography. Cardiac catheterization is still considered the gold standard for estimating the severity of cardiac defects, although the advantages of Doppler echocardiography often outweigh those of cardiac catheterization, especially in view of the good correlation between certain Doppler- and catheterization-derived measurements. Cardiac catheterization is necessary for balloon valvuloplasty and other interventional procedures.

**Pulmonary capillary wedge pressure.** Pulmonary capillary wedge pressure (PCWP) monitoring is sometimes performed in dogs with heart failure because the PCWP provides an estimate of left heart filling pressure (in the absence of left ventricular inflow obstruction). The PCWP is obtained by passing an end-hole, balloon-tipped (Swan-Ganz) catheter through the right side of the heart and into the main pulmonary artery. The balloon is inflated, and the catheter is allowed to become "wedged" in a smaller pulmonary artery, effectively occluding flow. The pressure measured at the catheter tip reflects pulmonary capillary pressure, which is essentially equivalent to left atrial pressure. This invasive technique allows differentiation of cardiogenic from noncardiogenic pulmonary edema and provides a means of monitoring the effectiveness of heart failure therapy. However, its use requires meticulous, aseptic catheter placement and maintenance, as well as continuous patient monitoring.

### Central Venous Pressure Measurement

Central venous pressure (CVP) is influenced by intravascular volume, venous compliance, and cardiac function. Its measurement can help the clinician differentiate high right heart filling pressure (e.g., from right heart failure or pericardial disease) from other causes of pleural or peritoneal effusion. However, pleural effusion of sufficient volume increases intrapleural pressure to the point where cardiac filling is impaired; this can raise CVP in the absence of cardiac disease. CVP therefore should be measured after thoracocentesis in patients with moderate-to-large pleural effusions. CVP is sometimes used to monitor critical patients receiving large-volume fluid infusions. However, CVP is not an accurate reflection of left heart filling pressure and therefore should not be relied on to monitor treatment of cardiogenic pulmonary edema. CVP in normal dogs and cats usually ranges from 0 to 8 (up to 10) cm $H_2O$; fluctuations that parallel intrapleural pressure changes occur during respiration.

CVP is measured by aseptically placing a large-bore jugular catheter that extends into or close to the right atrium and connecting it via extension tubing and a three-way stopcock to the patient's fluid administration set. A water manometer is attached to the stopcock and positioned vertically, with the stopcock (representing 0 cm $H_2O$) located at the same horizontal level as the patient's right atrium. The stopcock is turned off to the animal, allowing the manometer to fill with crystalloid fluid; then the stopcock is turned off to the fluid reservoir to allow equilibration of the fluid column in the manometer with the animal's CVP. Repeated measurements are more consistent when taken with the animal and manometer in the same position and during the expiratory phase of respiration. Small fluctuations in the manometer's fluid meniscus occur with the heartbeat, and slightly larger movement is associated with respiration. A marked change in the height of the fluid column associated with the heartbeat suggests either severe tricuspid insufficiency or that the catheter tip is within the right ventricle.

### Biochemical Markers of Myocardial Injury

Cardiac troponins are regulatory proteins associated with the thin contractile filaments. Most are structurally bound, with only a small percentage free in the myocardial cytoplasm. Circulating concentrations of cardiac troponin I (cTnI) and cardiac troponin T (cTnT) increase within several hours after acute myocardial injury or necrosis. cTnI has greater sensitivity in detecting myocardial injury than myocardial-bound creatine kinase (CK-MB) and other biochemical markers of muscle damage. In dogs the CK-MB isoform comprises only a minority of total cardiac CK, and it is also present in noncardiac tissues. cTnI is also a more sensitive and specific marker of cardiac cell necrosis in people than cTnT; cTnI is specific to the heart, whereas cTnT can increase with some noncardiac conditions. The structure of cardiac troponins is highly conserved across species, therefore human assays can be used for dogs and cats. Newer assays using monoclonal antibody to cTnI do not show cross-reactivity with skeletal muscle; assays for cTnT have only minor cross-reactivity. The normal plasma concentration of cTnI in dogs has been estimated at less than 0.04 ng/ml (Sleeper and colleague, 2001b), and preliminary work suggested that plasma concentrations greater than 0.07 ng/ml indicate cardiac pathology in dogs. Concentrations greater than 0.11 to 0.16 ng/ml appear abnormal in cats (Sleeper and colleague, 2001b). However, others have suggested that the normal concentrations for both dogs and cats are cTnI less than 0.5 ng/ml and cTnT less than 0.1 ng/ml (Schober and colleagues, 2001c). In people the threshold for separating significant from nonsignificant myocyte injury is 2 ng/ml for cTnI, and 0.1 ng/ml for cTnT (Schober and colleagues, 2001c). Elevated cardiac troponin concentrations have been measured in more than half of studied animals with blunt chest trauma, dogs with dilated cardiomyopathy, cats with hypertrophic cardiomyopathy (HCM), dogs with gastric dilation–volvulus and cardiac arrhythmias, and a few other conditions (Schober and colleagues, 2001c). Measured concentrations of cTnI were higher in HCM cats with congestive failure, especially thromboembolism (Herndon and colleagues, 2002).

### Endomyocardial Biopsy

Small samples of endocardium and adjacent myocardium can be obtained using a special bioptome passed into the right ventricle via a jugular vein. Routine histopathology and other techniques to evaluate myocardial metabolic abnormalities can be performed on the biopsy samples. This technique is most often used for myocardial disease research and is not commonly used in clinical veterinary cardiology.

### Nuclear Cardiology

Radionuclide methods of evaluating cardiac function are available at some veterinary referral centers. These techniques can provide noninvasive assessment of cardiac output, ejection fraction, and other measures of cardiac performance, as well as of myocardial blood flow and metabolism.

## Pneumopericardiography

Pneumopericardiography may be helpful in delineating the cause of pericardial effusions, especially if echocardiography is unavailable. This technique and pericardiocentesis are described in Chapter 11.

## Suggested Readings

ELECTROCARDIOGRAPHY

Bright JM et al: Clinical usefulness of cardiac event recording in dogs and cats examined because of syncope, episodic collapse, or intermittent weakness: 60 cases (1997-1999), *J Am Vet Med Assoc* 216:1110, 2000.

Calvert CA: High-resolution electrocardiography, *Vet Clin North Am Small Anim Pract* 28:1429, 1998.

Calvert CA et al: Possible late potentials in 4 dogs with sustained ventricular tachycardia, *J Vet Intern Med* 12:96, 1998a.

Calvert CA et al: Signal-averaged electrocardiograms in normal Doberman Pinschers, *J Vet Intern Med* 12:355, 1998b.

Calvert CA et al: Correlations among time and frequency measures of heart rate variability recorded by use of a Holter monitor in overtly healthy Doberman Pinschers with and without echocardiographic evidence of dilated cardiomyopathy, *Am J Vet Res* 62:1787, 2001a.

Calvert CA et al: Effect of severity of myocardial failure on heart rate variability in Doberman Pinschers with and without echocardiographic evidence of dilated cardiomyopathy, *J Am Vet Med Assoc* 219:1076, 2001b.

Calvert CA et al: Evaluation of stability over time for measures of heart-rate variability in overtly healthy Doberman Pinschers, *Am J Vet Res* 63:53, 2002.

Constable PD et al: Effects of endurance training on standard and signal-averaged electrocardiograms of sled dogs, *Am J Vet Res* 61:582, 2000.

Cote E et al: Event-based cardiac monitoring in small animal practice, *Compend Contin Educ* 21:1025, 1999.

Fox PR et al: Analysis of continuous ECG (Holter) monitoring in normal cats and cardiomyopathic cats in congestive heart failure, *J Vet Intern Med* 12:199, 1998 (abstract).

Goodwin JK: Holter monitoring and cardiac event recording, *Vet Clin North Am Small Anim Pract* 28:1391, 1998.

Haggstrom J et al: Heart rate variability in relation to severity of mitral regurgitation in Cavalier King Charles Spaniels, *J Small Anim Pract* 37:69, 1996.

Hall LW et al: Ambulatory electrocardiography in dogs, *Vet Rec* 129:213, 1991.

Hinchcliff KW et al: Electrocardiographic characteristics of endurance-trained Alaskan sled dogs, *J Am Vet Med Assoc* 211:1138, 1997.

Meurs KM et al: Use of ambulatory electrocardiography for detection of ventricular premature complexes in healthy dogs, *J Am Vet Med Assoc* 218:1291, 2001.

Miller RH et al: Retrospective analysis of the clinical utility of ambulatory electrocardiographic (Holter) recordings in syncopal dog: 44 cases (1991-1995), *J Vet Intern Med* 13:111, 1999.

Moise NS et al: Twenty-four hour ambulatory electrocardiography (Holter monitoring). In Bonagura JD, editor: *Kirk's current veterinary therapy XII,* Philadelphia, 1995, WB Saunders, p 792.

Nakayama H et al: Correlation of cardiac enlargement as assessed by vertebral heart size and echocardiographic and electrocardiographic findings in dogs with evolving cardiomegaly due to rapid ventricular pacing, *J Vet Intern Med* 15:217, 2001.

Oguchi Y et al: Duration of QT interval in clinically normal dogs, *Am J Vet Res* 54:2145, 1993.

Rishniw M et al: Effect of body position on the 6-lead ECG of dogs, *J Vet Intern Med* 16:69, 2002.

Tilley LP: *Essentials of canine and feline electrocardiography,* ed 3, Philadelphia, 1992, Lea & Febiger.

Ulloa HM et al: Arrhythmia prevalence during ambulatory electrocardiographic monitoring of Beagles, *Am J Vet Res* 56:275, 1995.

Ware WA: Practical use of Holter monitoring. *Compend Contin Educ* 20:1, 1998.

Ware WA: Twenty-four hour ambulatory electrocardiography in normal cats. *J Vet Intern Med* 13:175, 1999.

Ware WA et al: Duration of the QT interval in healthy cats. *Am J Vet Res* 60:1426, 1999.


RADIOGRAPHY

Buchanan JW et al: Vertebral scale system to measure canine heart size in radiographs, *J Am Vet Med Assoc* 206:194, 1995.

Farrow CS et al: *Radiology of the cat,* St Louis, 1994, Mosby.

Lehmkuhl LB et al: Radiographic evaluation of caudal vena cava size in dogs, *Vet Radiol Ultrasound* 38:94, 1997.

Litster AL et al: Vertebral scale system to measure heart size in radiographs of cats, *J Am Vet Med Assoc* 216:210, 2000.

Moon ML et al: Age-related changes in the feline cardiac silhouette, *Vet Radiol Ultrasound* 34:315, 1993.

Sleeper MM et al: Vertebral scale system to measure heart size in growing puppies, *J Am Vet Med Assoc* 219:57, 2001a.


ECHOCARDIOGRAPHY

Atkins CE et al: Systolic time intervals and their derivatives for evaluation of cardiac function, *J Vet Intern Med* 6:55, 1992.

Bonagura JD et al: Echocardiography: principles of interpretation, *Vet Clin North Am* 15:1177, 1985.

Bonagura JD et al: Doppler echocardiography. I. Pulsed and continuous wave studies, *Vet Clin North Am Small Anim Pract* 28:1325, 1998a.

Bonagura JD et al: Doppler echocardiography. II. Color Doppler imaging, *Vet Clin North Am Small Anim Pract* 28:1361, 1998b.

Bonagura JD et al: Echocardiography. In Ettinger SJ et al, editors: *Textbook of veterinary internal medicine,* ed 5, Philadelphia, 2000, WB Saunders, p 834.

Bonagura JD: Echocardiography case studies. In *Proceedings of the 19th ACVIM Forum,* 2001, Denver, p 133.

Brown DJ et al: Use of pulsed-wave Doppler echocardiography to determine aortic and pulmonary velocity and flow variables in clinically normal dogs, *Am J Vet Res* 52:543, 1991.

Crippa L et al: Echocardiographic parameters and indices in the normal Beagle dog, *Lab Anim* 26:190, 1992.

Darke PGG et al: Transducer orientation for Doppler echocardiography in dogs, *J Small Anim Pract* 34:2, 1993.

DeMadron E et al: Two-dimensional echocardiography in the normal cat, *Vet Radiol* 26:149, 1985.

Fox PR et al: Echocardiographic reference values in healthy cats sedated with ketamine HCl, *Am J Vet Res* 46:1479, 1985.

Gooding JP et al: Echocardiographic assessment of left ventricular dimensions in clinically normal English Cocker Spaniels. *Am J Vet Res* 47:296, 1986.

Herrtage ME: Echocardiographic measurements in the normal Boxer. *Proceedings of the 4th European Society of Veterinary Internal Medicine Congress,* Brussels, Belgium, 1994, p 172 (abstract).

Jacobs G et al: M-mode echocardiographic measurements in non-anesthetized healthy cats: effects of body weight, heart rate, and other variables, *Am J Vet Res* 46:1705, 1985.

Jacobs G et al: Influence of alterations in heart rate on echocardiographic measurements in the dog, *Am J Vet Res* 49:548, 1988.

Lonsdale RA et al: Echocardiographic parameters in training compared with nontraining Greyhounds, *Vet Radiol Ultrasound* 39:325, 1998.

Loyer C et al: Biplane transesophageal echocardiography in the dog: technique, anatomy and imaging planes, *Vet Radiol Ultrasound* 36:212, 1995.

Luis Fuentes V et al: Diastology: theory and practice II. In *Proceedings of the 19th ACVIM Forum,* 2001, Denver, p 142.

McEntee K et al: Doppler echocardiographic study of left and right ventricular function during dobutamine stress testing in conscious healthy dogs, *Am J Vet Res* 60:865, 1999.

Minors SL et al: Resting and dobutamine stress echocardiographic factors associated with the development of occult dilated cardiomyopathy in healthy Doberman Pinscher dogs, *J Vet Intern Med* 12:369, 1998.

Moise NS et al: Echocardiography, electrocardiography, and radiography of cats with dilatation cardiomyopathy, hypertrophic cardiomyopathy, and hyperthyroidism, *Am J Vet Res* 47:1476, 1986.

Moise NS et al: Echocardiography and Doppler imaging. In Fox PR et al, editors: *Textbook of canine and feline cardiology,* ed 2, Philadelphia, 1999, WB Saunders, p 130.

Morrison SA et al: Effect of breed and body weight on echocardiographic values in four breeds of dogs of differing somatotype, *J Vet Intern Med* 6:220, 1992.

Nakayama T et al: Prevalence of valvular regurgitation in normal Beagle dogs detected by color Doppler echocardiography, *J Vet Med Sci* 56:973, 1994.

O'Grady MR et al: Outcome of 103 asymptomatic Doberman Pinschers: incidence of dilated cardiomyopathy in a longitudinal study, *J Vet Intern Med* 9:199, 1995 (abstract).

Page A et al: Echocardiographic values in the Greyhound, *Aust Vet J* 70:361, 1993.

Pipers FS et al: Echocardiography in the domestic cat, *Am J Vet Res* 40:882, 1979.

Rishniw M et al: Evaluation of four 2-dimensional echocardiographic methods of assessing left atrial size in dogs, *J Vet Intern Med* 14:429, 2000.

Schober KE et al: Effects of age, body weight, and heart rate on transmitral and pulmonary venous flow in clinically normal dogs, *Am J Vet Res* 62:1447, 2001a.

Schober KE et al: Diastology: theory and practice I. In *Proceedings of the 19th ACVIM Forum,* 2001b, Denver, p 139.

Sisson DD et al: Changes in linear dimensions of the heart, relative body weight as measured by M-mode echocardiography in growing dogs, *Am J Vet Res* 52:1591, 1991.

Snyder PS et al: A comparison of echocardiographic indices of the non-racing, healthy Greyhound to reference values from other breeds, *Vet Radiol Ultrasound* 36:387, 1995.

Stepien RL et al: Effect of endurance training on cardiac morphology in Alaskan sled dogs, *J Appl Physiol* 85:1368, 1998.

Thomas WP et al: Recommendations for standards in transthoracic two-dimensional echocardiography in the dog and cat, *J Vet Intern Med* 7:247, 1993.

Vollmar AC: Echocardiographic measurements in the Irish Wolfhound: reference values for the breed, *J Am Anim Hosp Assoc* 35:271, 1999.

Vollmar AC et al: Clinical echocardiographic and ECG findings in 232 sequentially examined Irish Wolfhounds, *J Vet Intern Med* 15:279, 2001 (abstract).

Yuill CD et al: Doppler-derived velocity of blood flow across cardiac valves in the normal dog, *Can J Vet Res* 55:185, 1991.

**OTHER TECHNIQUES**

Gookin JL et al: Evaluation of the effect of pleural effusion on central venous pressure in cats, *J Vet Intern Med* 13:561, 1999.

Herndon WE et al: Cardiac troponin I in feline hypertrophic cardiomyopathy. *J Vet Intern Med* 16:558, 2002.

Lobetti R et al: Cardiac troponins in canine babesiosis, *J Vet Intern Med* 16:63, 2002.

Oakley RE et al: Experimental evaluation of central venous pressure monitoring in the dog, *J Am Anim Hosp Assoc* 33:77, 1997.

Schober KE et al: Circulating cardiac troponins in small animals. In *Proceedings of the 19th ACVIM Forum,* 2001c, Denver, p 91.

Sleeper MM et al: Cardiac troponin I in the normal dog and cat, *J Vet Intern Med* 15:501, 2001b.

# CHAPTER 3

# Management of Congestive Heart Failure

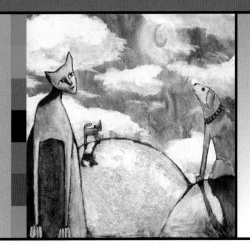

## CHAPTER OUTLINE

PATHOPHYSIOLOGY OF HEART FAILURE, 51
   Neurohormonal mechanisms, 52
   Renal effects, 54
   Cardiac responses, 54
   Other effects of chronic heart failure, 55
OVERVIEW OF HEART FAILURE MANAGEMENT, 55
   General causes of heart failure, 55
   Basic principles of treatment, 56
MANAGEMENT OF CHRONIC HEART FAILURE, 56
   General overview, 56
   Patient monitoring, 58
TREATMENT OF FULMINANT CONGESTIVE HEART
FAILURE, 58
DIETARY MANAGEMENT, 60
DIURETICS, 62
   Furosemide and other loop diuretics, 62
   Spironolactone and other potassium-sparing diuretics, 64
   Thiazide diuretics, 64
VASODILATORS, 64
   Angiotensin-converting enzyme inhibitors (ACEIs), 64
   Arteriolar and other mixed vasodilators, 65
   Venodilators, 66
POSITIVE INOTROPIC DRUGS, 66
   Digitalis glycosides, 66
   Sympathomimetic agents (catecholamines), 69
   Phosphodiesterase inhibitors, 70
CALCIUM ENTRY BLOCKERS, 71

## PATHOPHYSIOLOGY OF HEART FAILURE

Clinical heart failure occurs when the heart is either unable to adequately deliver blood for the body's metabolic demands or when it can do so only with elevated filling pressures. Heart failure is not a specific diagnosis, but a syndrome caused by one or more underlying processes. Poor myocardial contractility (systolic dysfunction), as a primary cause, can initiate the cascade of neurohormonal and other responses that result in clinical heart failure. However, other causes of chronic cardiac stress or injury can underlie the development of circulatory congestion and secondarily lead to myocardial systolic (and/or diastolic) dysfunction.

Chronic heart failure cannot be framed simply and only in terms of a "bad pump" that needs positive inotropic stimulation and a diuretic, although this therapeutic approach may be transiently necessary in some cases of acute, decompensated myocardial failure. The pathophysiology of the failing heart is much more complex and involves a number of structural and functional changes within cardiac and vascular cells, as well as within the extracellular matrix. The syndrome of heart failure can be viewed in terms of progressive ventricular remodeling that develops secondary to a cardiac injury or stress such as valvular disease, genetic mutations, acute inflammation, ischemia, increased systolic pressure load, and other causes.

Ventricular remodeling refers to the changes in myocardial size and shape that occur in response to various mechanical, biochemical, and molecular signals induced by the underlying injury or stress. It includes myocardial cell hypertrophy, cardiac cell dropout or self-destruction (apoptosis), excessive interstitial matrix formation, and dissolution of collagen struts that bind individual myocytes together. The dissolution of collagen struts, which results from effects of myocardial collagenases or matrix metalloproteinases, can cause dilation or distortion of the ventricle from myocyte slippage.

Stimuli for remodeling include mechanical forces (e.g., increased wall stress from volume or pressure overload) and various neurohormones (e.g., angiotensin II, norepinephrine, endothelin, aldosterone) and cytokines (e.g., tumor necrosis factor [TNF]-$\alpha$). Contributing biochemical abnormalities of oxidative phosphorylation, high-energy phosphate metabolism, calcium ion movements, contractile proteins, protein synthesis, and catecholamine metabolism have been variably identified in different models of heart failure and in clinical patients. Myocyte hypertrophy and reactive fibrosis increase total cardiac mass by eccentric and, in some cases, concentric patterns of hypertrophy (see p. 54). Ventricular hypertrophy can increase chamber stiffness, impair relaxation, and increase filling pressures; these abnormalities of diastolic function can promote and contribute to systolic failure. Interstitial matrix growth, apoptosis, and myocyte slippage also can contribute to progressive changes in ventricular size, shape, and stiffness that lead to failure. Ventricular remodeling also promotes the development of arrhythmias.

The mechanism of progression from ventricular hypertrophy to reduced pump function and overt failure is not well understood. The initiating stimulus underlying chronic cardiac remodeling may occur years before clinical evidence of heart failure appears. As far as possible, the underlying cause should be defined, because in some cases it can be treated or reversed.

## NEUROHORMONAL MECHANISMS

Neurohormonal responses that contribute to cardiac remodeling also have more far-reaching effects. In general, the clinical syndromes of congestive heart failure result from chronic,

overexuberant activation of several neurohormonal "compensatory" mechanisms. Although these mechanisms support the circulation in the face of acute hypotension and hypovolemia, chronic activation accelerates further deterioration of cardiac function. Major neurohormonal changes in heart failure include increases in sympathetic nervous tone, attenuated vagal tone, activation of the renin-angiotensin-aldosterone system, and release of antidiuretic hormone (vasopressin). These neurohormonal systems work independently and together to increase vascular volume (by sodium and water retention and increased thirst) and vascular tone (Fig. 3-1). Excessive volume retention results in edema and effusions. Prolonged systemic vasoconstriction increases the workload on the heart, can reduce forward cardiac output, and may ex-

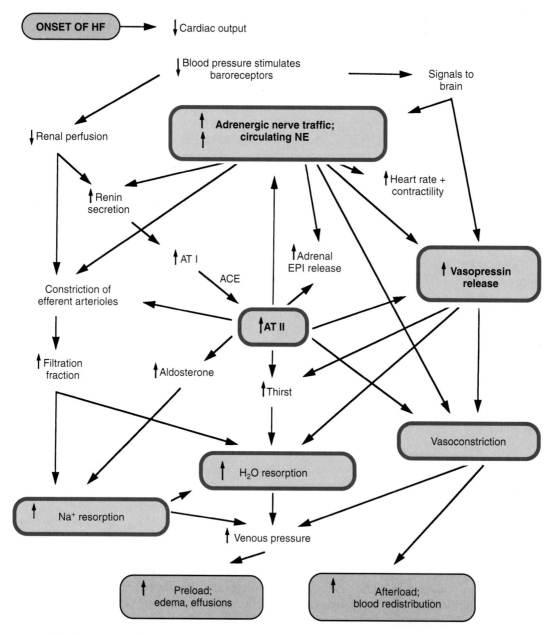

**FIG 3-1**

Neurohormonal compensatory mechanisms and their major effects in heart failure. *ACE,* Angiotensin-converting enzyme; *AT,* angiotensin; *EPI,* epinephrine; *HF,* heart failure; *NE,* norepinephrine.

acerbate valvular regurgitation. The extent to which they are activated varies with the severity and etiology of heart failure. In general, however, as failure worsens, neurohormonal activation increases, and the degree of neurohormonal activation appears to be related to mortality as well as morbidity.

The immediate circulatory benefits of sympathetic stimulation (e.g., increased contractility, heart rate, and venous return) are detrimental over time by increasing afterload stress and myocardial oxygen requirements, contributing to myocardial remodeling and cellular damage, and enhancing the potential for cardiac arrhythmias. Normal feedback regulation of sympathetic nervous and hormonal systems depends on arterial and atrial baroreceptor function. Baroreceptor responsiveness becomes attenuated in chronic heart failure, which contributes to sustained sympathetic and hormonal activation and reduced inhibitory vagal effects. However, baroreceptor dysfunction can improve with reversal of heart failure, increased myocardial contractility, decreased cardiac loading conditions, or inhibition of angiotensin II (which directly attenuates baroreceptor sensitivity). Digoxin has a positive effect on baroreceptor sensitivity, which may be its main therapeutic benefit.

The renin-angiotensin system (Fig. 3-2) has many important effects. Renin release from the renal juxtaglomerular apparatus is promoted by low renal artery perfusion pressure, renal β-adrenergic receptor stimulation, and reduced sodium delivery to the macula densa of the distal renal tubule. Stringent dietary salt restriction and diuretic or vasodilator therapy can promote renin release. Renin facilitates conversion of the precursor peptide angiotensinogen to angiotensin I (an inactive form). Angiotensin-converting enzyme (ACE), found in the lungs and elsewhere, converts angiotensin I to the active angiotensin II and is involved in the degradation of certain vasodilator kinins. Other pathways also generate angiotensin II.

The effects of angiotensin II are far-reaching and potent; major effects include direct vasoconstriction and stimulation of aldosterone release from the adrenal cortex. Aldosterone promotes sodium and chloride reabsorption, as well as potassium and hydrogen ion secretion in the renal collecting tubules; the concurrent water reabsorption augments vascular volume. Additional effects of angiotensin II include enhancement of thirst and salt appetite, facilitation of neuronal norepinephrine synthesis and release, blockade of neuronal norepinephrine reuptake, stimulation of antidiuretic hormone (vasopressin) release, and increased adrenal epinephrine secretion. Pharmacologic inhibition of ACE, therefore, can reduce neurohormonal activation and promote vasodilation and diuresis. Local production of angiotensin II also occurs in the heart, blood vessels, adrenal glands, and other tissues. Local activity affects cardiovascular structure and function by enhancing sympathetic effects and promoting remodeling.

Antidiuretic hormone (vasopressin) is released from the posterior pituitary gland. This hormone directly causes vasoconstriction and also promotes free water reabsorption in the distal nephrons. Although increased plasma osmolality or reduced blood volume are the normal stimuli for antidiuretic

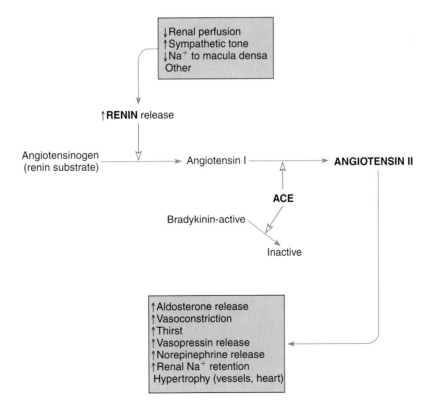

**FIG 3-2**
Summary of the renin-angiotensin mechanism in heart failure. *ACE,* Angiotensin-converting enzyme. (From Ware WA: Drugs acting on the cardiovascular system. In Ahrens FA, editor: *National veterinary medical series: pharmacology,* Baltimore, 1996, Williams & Wilkins.)

hormone release, reduced effective circulating volume and other nonosmotic stimuli cause continued release of antidiuretic hormone in patients with heart failure. The continued release of antidiuretic hormone contributes to the dilutional hyponatremia sometimes found in patients with heart failure.

Increased circulating concentrations of other substances that play a role in abnormal myocardial hypertrophy and/or fibrosis, including cytokines (e.g., TNF-$\alpha$) and endothelins, have also been detected in patients with severe heart failure.

Some endogenous mechanisms oppose the vasoconstrictor responses. Normally, a balance between vasodilator and vasoconstrictor effects maintains circulatory homeostasis as well as renal solute excretion. As heart failure progresses, the influence of the vasoconstrictor mechanisms predominates despite increased activation of vasodilator mechanisms.

Natriuretic peptides are made and released from the heart; they play an important role in regulation of blood volume and pressure. Several natriuretic peptides have been identified. Atrial natriuretic peptide (ANP) is synthesized by atrial myocytes as a prohormone, which is cleaved to the active peptide after release is stimulated by mechanical stretch of the atrial wall. Brain natriuretic peptide (BNP) is also synthesized in the heart, but it is produced mainly by the ventricles in response to myocardial dysfunction or ischemia. Natriuretic peptides cause diuresis, natriuresis, and peripheral vasodilation. They act to antagonize the effects of the renin-angiotensin system and can also alter vascular permeability and inhibit growth of smooth muscle cells. Natriuretic peptides are degraded by neutral endopeptidases. Circulating concentrations of ANP and BNP increase in patients with heart failure. This increase has been correlated with pulmonary capillary wedge pressure and severity of heart failure in dogs as well as people. Reduced renal responsiveness to ANP may occur with persistently high circulating concentrations of natriuretic peptides. In people, plasma BNP is considered a sensitive and specific marker for chronic left ventricular dysfunction, and increased concentrations are negatively correlated with prognosis.

Intrarenal vasodilator prostaglandins also oppose the action of angiotensin II on the renal vasculature. The use of prostaglandin synthesis inhibitors in dogs or cats with severe heart failure may increase arteriolar resistance, reduce glomerular filtration, and enhance sodium retention.

## RENAL EFFECTS

Renal efferent glomerular arteriolar constriction, mediated by sympathetic stimulation and angiotensin II, helps maintain glomerular filtration in the face of reduced cardiac output and renal blood flow. Higher oncotic and lower hydrostatic pressures develop in the peritubular capillaries, enhancing the reabsorption of tubular fluid and sodium. Angiotensin II–mediated aldosterone release further promotes sodium and water retention. Continued activation of these mechanisms leads to clinical edema and effusions.

Afferent arteriolar vasodilation mediated by endogenous prostaglandins and natriuretic peptides can partially offset the effects of efferent vasoconstriction, but progressive impairment of renal blood flow leads to renal insufficiency. Diuretics not only can magnify azotemia and electrolyte loss, they also can further reduce cardiac output and activate the neurohormonal mechanisms.

## CARDIAC RESPONSES

Increased ventricular filling (preload) causes greater contraction force and blood ejection. This response, known as *the Frank-Starling mechanism,* allows beat-to-beat adjustments that balance the output of the two ventricles and increase overall cardiac output in response to acute increases in hemodynamic load. Acute increases in cardiac load result from development or rapid worsening of valvular insufficiency, arterial hypertension, or outflow obstructions. The Frank-Starling effect helps normalize cardiac output under conditions of increased pressure and/or volume loading. However, these conditions also increase ventricular wall stress and oxygen consumption.

Ventricular wall stress is directly related to ventricular pressure and internal dimensions, but inversely related to wall thickness (Laplace's law). Myocardial hypertrophy can reduce wall stress, and different patterns of hypertrophy develop, depending on the underlying cardiac disease. Ventricular systolic pressure loads mainly cause "concentric" hypertrophy; myocardial fibers and ventricular walls thicken as contractile units are added in parallel. Volume loads cause "eccentric" hypertrophy; myocardial fiber elongation and chamber dilation occur as new sarcomeres are laid down in series. Compensatory hypertrophy lessens the importance of the Frank-Starling mechanism in stable, chronic heart failure.

Cardiac hypertrophy and remodeling begin long before heart failure becomes manifest. Clinical heart failure can also be considered the state of decompensated hypertrophy, in which ventricular function progressively deteriorates as contractility and relaxation become more abnormal. Abnormal pressure and volume loads both impair cardiac performance over time, although volume loads are better tolerated because myocardial oxygen demand is not as severe. Eventually, though, decompensation and myocardial failure develop. In contrast, initial cardiac pressure and volume loads are normal in patients with primary myocardial diseases; however, intrinsic defects of the heart muscle lead to the hypertrophy and dilation observed.

Continued exposure to increased sympathetic stimulation causes reduced cardiac sensitivity to catecholamines. Desensitization or down-regulation (reduced number) of myocardial $\beta_1$-receptors may represent a protective mechanism against the cardiotoxic and arrhythmogenic effects of catecholamines. The ability of the failing heart to produce cyclic adenosine monophosphate (cAMP)—and therefore its responsiveness to drugs that act by this mechanism (e.g., dobutamine, dopamine, amrinone)—is diminished. $\beta$-Blocking agents can reverse $\beta_1$-receptor down-regulation, but they may worsen heart failure.

Also present in the heart are $\beta_2$- and $\alpha_1$-receptors, which are not down-regulated and are thought to contribute to myocardial remodeling and arrhythmogenesis. In addition, $\beta_3$-receptors, which mediate a negative inotropic effect, may contribute to deterioration of myocardial function.

## OTHER EFFECTS OF CHRONIC HEART FAILURE

Reduced exercise capacity occurs in association with heart failure. Poor diastolic filling and inadequate forward output, as well as pulmonary edema or pleural effusion, interfere with exercise ability. However, peripheral abnormalities also play an important role. Impaired exercise-induced vasodilation contributes to inadequate skeletal muscle perfusion and fatigue. Excessive peripheral sympathetic tone, angiotensin II (both circulating and locally produced), and vasopressin can contribute to impaired skeletal muscle vasodilatory capacity with chronic heart failure. Increased vascular wall sodium content and interstitial fluid pressure cause stiffening and compression of vessels. Other mechanisms can include impaired endothelium-dependent relaxation, increased endothelin levels, and vascular wall changes induced by the growth factor effects of various neurohormonal vasoconstrictors. The improvement in exercise capacity shown in people and some dogs after chronic ACE inhibitor therapy suggests that the renin-angiotensin system plays an important role.

## OVERVIEW OF HEART FAILURE MANAGEMENT

### GENERAL CAUSES OF HEART FAILURE

The causes of heart failure are quite diverse, and it is useful to think of them in terms of general pathophysiologic groups. These groups are *myocardial failure, pressure overload, volume overload,* and *reduced ventricular compliance* (impaired filling). The major underlying abnormality for most cases of heart failure falls into one of these pathophysiologic groups, although other pathophysiologic abnormalities often are also present. In advanced failure, abnormalities of both systolic and diastolic function are common. Heart failure can result from persistent cardiac arrhythmias as well.

Myocardial failure is characterized by poor ventricular contractile function; valvular insufficiency may or may not be present. Diseases that cause a volume or flow overload to the heart usually involve a primary "plumbing" problem (e.g., a leaky valve or abnormal systemic-to-pulmonary connection). Cardiac pump function is often maintained near normal for a prolonged time, but myocardial contractility does eventually deteriorate. Pressure overload results when the ventricle must generate higher than normal systolic pressure to eject blood. Concentric hypertrophy increases ventricular wall thickness and stiffness and predisposes to ischemia. Excessive pressure loads eventually cause myocardial contractility to decline.

Diseases that restrict ventricular filling cause abnormal diastolic function. Contractile ability is usually normal initially, but inadequate filling causes congestion behind one or both ventricles and may diminish cardiac output. Therapy for these cases centers on enhancing ventricular filling. Examples of common diseases are grouped in Table 3-1 according to main initiating pathophysiology and typical clinical presentation (e.g., primarily left- or right-sided heart failure). (See discussions in other chapters for more information about individual diseases.)

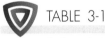 TABLE 3-1

Causes of Chronic Heart Failure (CHF)

| LEFT-SIDED CHF | EITHER | RIGHT-SIDED CHF |
|---|---|---|
| **Myocardial Failure** | | |
| Drug toxicities (e.g., doxorubicin) | Idiopathic dilated cardiomyopathy | |
| Myocardial ischemia/infarction | Infective myocarditis | |
| **Volume-Flow Overload** | | |
| Mitral endocardiosis | Chronic anemia | Tricuspid endocardiosis |
| Mitral/aortic endocarditis | Thyrotoxicosis | Tricuspid endocarditis |
| Ventricular septal defect | | Tricuspid dysplasia |
| Patent ductus arteriosus | | |
| Mitral dysplasia | | |
| **Pressure Overload** | | |
| (Sub)aortic stenosis | | Pulmonic stenosis |
| Systemic hypertension | | Heartworm disease/pulmonary hypertension |
| **Restriction to Ventricular Filling** | | |
| Hypertrophic cardiomyopathy | | Cardiac tamponade |
| Restrictive cardiomypathy | | Constrictive pericardial disease |

## TABLE 3-2

**Therapeutic Goals According to Pathophysiologic Group of Heart Failure**

| PATHOPHYSIOLOGIC GROUP | GOALS |
| --- | --- |
| Myocardial failure | Improve cardiac output (angiotensin-converting enzyme inhibitor [ACEI], digoxin, other positive inotropic drugs or vasodilators).<br>Control edema and effusions (diuretics, vasodilators, diet).<br>Improve myocardial function? (ACEI, digoxin, spironolactone?, other?)<br>Reduce cardiac workload (rest, vasodilators).<br>Control arrhythmias and avoid complications.<br>Specific therapy if possible. |
| Volume-flow overload | Control edema and effusions (diuretics, ACEI or other vasodilators, diet).<br>Reduce valvular regurgitation if present (ACEI or arteriolar vasodilators).<br>Improve forward cardiac output (ACEI, other arteriolar vasodilators, digoxin).<br>Reduce cardiac workload (rest, diuretics, vasodilators).<br>Control arrhythmias and avoid complications.<br>Specific therapy if possible. |
| Pressure overload | Relieve stenosis or reduce arterial hypertension if possible.<br>Reduce cardiac workload (rest, diuretic; depending on etiology: β-blocker, ACEI, other antihypertensives).<br>Control edema or effusions (diuretic, diet; depending on etiology: ACEI, other vasodilators).<br>Support cardiac function (± digoxin).<br>Control arrhythmias and avoid complications. |
| Restricted ventricular filling— pericardial disease | Drain pericardial fluid.<br>Remove pericardium if necessary.<br>Treat underlying disease if possible. |
| Restricted ventricular filling— hypertrophic cardiomyopathy | Enhance cardiac filling/slow heart rate (β-blocker or diltiazem).<br>Reduce edema and effusions (diuretics, diet, ± ACEI).<br>Reduce cardiac workload and stress (rest).<br>Control arrhythmias and avoid complications (including thromboembolism).<br>Seek/treat possible underlying disease (e.g., feline hyperthyroidism). |

## BASIC PRINCIPLES OF TREATMENT

Most current treatment strategies for heart failure are aimed at modifying either the results of neurohormonal activation (i.e., sodium and water retention) or the activation process itself (e.g., angiotensin-converting enzyme inhibition). In most cases, therapy centers on controlling edema and effusions, improving cardiac output, reducing cardiac workload, supporting myocardial function, and managing concurrent arrhythmias. The approach to these goals varies somewhat with different diseases, most notably those causing restriction to ventricular filling. Table 3-2 provides an overview of these principles.

The signs of heart failure were listed in Table 1-2. The clinical severity of heart failure is sometimes described according to a modified New York Heart Association classification scheme. This system groups patients into four functional classes based on subjective evaluation of the clinical condition, without consideration of etiology or myocardial function (Table 3-3). This classification can be helpful conceptually and for categorizing study patients. However, to best individualize therapy, it is important to determine the etiology as well as the severity of heart failure. Forrester's classification is another method of grouping heart failure patients (Table 3-3). Dogs with chronic mitral regurgitation often fall into group II; severe dilated cardiomyopathy is the most common diagnosis in group IV. Diseases that cause group III characteristics are rare in dogs and cats. Regardless of the clinical classification scheme, identification of the underlying disease and pathophysiology is important for guiding therapy.

## MANAGEMENT OF CHRONIC HEART FAILURE

### GENERAL OVERVIEW

A brief summary of current approaches to chronic heart failure therapy is presented here. More specific therapeutic guidelines are found in the chapters on different diseases and in the discussion of medications that follows in this chapter. As heart disease progresses, therapy is tailored to the individual animal's needs by adjusting dosages, adding or substituting drugs, and modifying lifestyle or diet. Exercise and dietary salt restriction help reduce cardiac workload regardless of

TABLE 3-3

Classification Systems for Heart Failure Severity

| CLASSIFICATION | DEGREE OF SEVERITY |
|---|---|
| **New York Heart Association Functional Classification** | |
| I | Heart disease present but no evidence of heart failure or exercise intolerance; cardiomegaly minimal to absent |
| II | Signs of heart disease with evidence of exercise intolerance; radiographic cardiomegaly present |
| III | Signs of heart failure with normal activity or at night (e.g., cough, orthopnea); radiographic signs of significant cardiomegaly and pulmonary edema or pleural/abdominal effusion |
| IV | Severe heart failure with clinical signs at rest or with minimal activity; marked radiographic signs of congestive heart failure (CHF) and cardiomegaly |
| **Forrester's Classification (Group)** | |
| I | Normal cardiac output and pulmonary venous pressures |
| II | Pulmonary congestion but normal cardiac output |
| III | Low cardiac output and peripheral hypoperfusion with no pulmonary congestion |
| IV | Low cardiac output with pulmonary congestion |

heart failure etiology. Nutritional issues in the management of chronic heart failure are discussed below. The evolving perspective on chronic heart failure management is based on blocking excessive neurohormonal activation and preventing progression of myocardial remodeling and dysfunction, using diuretics to control signs of congestion. Future strategies may also involve drugs that block cytokines, antagonize endothelins, and enhance atrial peptides, as well as other strategies to block the effects of neurohormonal activation.

*Diuretic* therapy is indicated for controlling cardiogenic pulmonary edema and effusions. However, pleural effusion and large-volume ascites should first be drained to facilitate respiration. Likewise, pericardial effusion that compromises cardiac filling must be drained. Although aggressive furosemide treatment is indicated for acute, fulminant pulmonary edema, the smallest effective doses are used for chronic heart failure therapy. Furosemide (or other diuretic) alone is not recommended as the sole treatment for chronic heart failure, because it can exacerbate neurohormonal activation and reduce renal function.

*ACE inhibitors (ACEIs)* have become the cornerstone of therapy for most causes of chronic heart failure, especially myocardial contractile dysfunction and chronic valvular insufficiency. ACEIs have only modest diuretic and vasodilatory effects; their main benefits arise from opposing the effects of neurohormonal activation and abnormal cardiovascular remodeling changes. ACEIs improve the clinical status and survival in dogs with dilated cardiomyopathy and chronic mitral regurgitation (Ettinger and colleagues, 1998) and probably other causes of heart failure as well.

*Digoxin* is usually indicated for patients with myocardial failure or supraventricular tachyarrhythmias (except cats with hypertrophic cardiomyopathy); it is also often added to the therapy of advanced mitral regurgitation in dogs. Digoxin ap-

pears to have a neutral effect on mortality in people with heart failure. Its ability to sensitize baroreceptors and thereby modulate neurohormonal activation and its modest positive inotropic effect are probably digoxin's most important attributes. Because the drug is potentially toxic, low doses are used and serum concentrations are monitored; serum concentrations in the low to middle "therapeutic" range are desired (see p. 68).

Chronic heart failure that becomes refractory to initial furosemide and ACEI therapy, with or without digoxin, is usually handled by intensifying the dose of furosemide and/or ACEI (for dosages, see Table 3-6). When dosages approach the maximum recommended levels, another diuretic or vasodilator can be cautiously added. Spironolactone is recommended as the first agent for this because of its action as an aldosterone antagonist. Not only can insufficient suppression of aldosterone develop despite ACE inhibition (so-called aldosterone escape), now it is known that aldosterone can also promote collagen synthesis and contribute to abnormal cardiac remodeling. In people with myocardial dysfunction, the addition of spironolactone to standard therapy reduces mortality. Thus, the benefits of spironolactone are thought to extend beyond its effect to promote additional diuresis, and the addition of spironolactone earlier in the course of therapy may be advantageous.

Further intensification of therapy for dogs with chronic heart failure from mitral regurgitation or dilated cardiomyopathy also can be achieved by using low doses of another vasodilator to further reduce afterload (e.g., amlodipine [p. 64] or hydralazine; see Table 3-6). Blood pressure should be monitored in these cases. However, an arteriolar vasodilator is not recommended for cats with hypertrophic cardiomyopathy or dogs with fixed ventricular outflow obstruction (e.g., subaortic stenosis). Some animals benefit from the addition of a thiazide diuretic as failure becomes more refractory.

Chronic heart failure is associated with skeletal muscle changes that lead to fatigue and dyspnea. Exercise restriction is usually recommended in the face of decompensated heart failure. Furthermore, strenuous exercise can provoke dyspnea and potentially serious cardiac arrhythmias. However, physical training can improve cardiopulmonary function and quality of life in patients with chronic heart failure. This is partly mediated by improvement in vascular endothelial function and restoration of flow-dependent vasodilation. It is difficult to know how much exercise is beneficial rather than detrimental to an individual. In general, regular (not sporadic) mild to moderate activity is encouraged, as long as signs of excessive respiratory effort do not develop. Strenuous bursts of activity should be avoided.

Chronic therapy with certain β-blockers reduces mortality and improves cardiac function in people with myocardial failure; however, not all β-blockers are effective for this. Furthermore, some patients experience possibly fatal clinical deterioration and worsening failure before any chronic benefits are seen. Agents that have been effective in human clinical trials are either second-generation (metoprolol) or third-generation (carvedilol) β-blockers (see p. 91 in Chapter 4). Carvedilol blocks $\beta_1$-, $\beta_2$-, and $\alpha_1$-receptors; it appears to have greater benefits than the selective $\beta_1$ agent, metoprolol. Whether veterinary patients will consistently achieve the improved myocardial function and survival seen in people after chronic (at least 3 to 6 months) therapy is not known. Caution is warranted in all patients with myocardial failure, especially those with clinical signs of congestion. Carvedilol or metoprolol could be considered for stable, compensated patients only. Very low doses should be used initially and titrated upward every 2 to 3 weeks as tolerated. Results of veterinary clinical studies are needed before more definitive guidelines can be established.

## PATIENT MONITORING

Periodic reevaluation of animals with chronic heart failure is important, because underlying disease progression and complications can develop. Medications and dosage should be reviewed with the owner at each visit. Any problems with drug administration, adverse effects, or signs of toxicity should be ascertained. The animal's response to the medications, diet and appetite, and activity level, as well as any other concerns, should also be discussed. Client education is important when managing chronic heart failure. A good understanding of the pet's underlying disease, the signs of heart failure, and the purpose and potential adverse effects of each medication make early identification of complications more likely. Monitoring of the pet's respiratory and heart rates during sleep or while it is resting at home is also helpful. The normal resting respiratory rate for most animals in their home environment is 30 or fewer breaths per minute. Pulmonary edema increases lung stiffness and induces faster, shallower respirations; a persistent increase in the resting respiratory rate is often an early sign of worsening heart failure. Likewise, a persistent increase in the resting heart rate accompanies the heightened sympathetic tone of decompensating failure.

A thorough physical examination, with emphasis on the cardiovascular system (see Chapter 1), is important at each evaluation. Depending on the patient's status, clinical tests might include a resting electrocardiogram (ECG) or ambulatory monitoring, thoracic radiographs, serum biochemistry analyses, an echocardiogram, serum digoxin concentration, and other tests. Periodic measurement of serum electrolyte and creatinine or blood urea nitrogen (BUN) concentrations is recommended. Electrolyte imbalance (especially hypokalemia or hyperkalemia, hypomagnesemia, and sometimes hyponatremia) can occur from the use of diuretics, ACEIs, and salt restriction. Prolonged anorexia can contribute to hypokalemia. However, potassium supplementation should not be used without documenting hypokalemia, especially when ACEIs and spironolactone are prescribed. The serum magnesium concentration does not accurately reflect total body stores; however, supplementation may be especially beneficial in animals that develop ventricular arrhythmias while receiving furosemide and digoxin.

Many factors can exacerbate the signs of heart failure, including physical exertion, infection, anemia, exogenous fluid administration (excess volume or sodium load), high-salt diet or dietary indiscretion, erratic administration of medication, inappropriate medication dosage for the level of disease, development of cardiac arrhythmias, environmental stress (e.g., heat, humidity, cold, smoke), development or worsening of concurrent extracardiac disease, and progression of underlying heart disease (e.g., ruptured chordae tendineae, left atrial tear, or secondary right heart failure). Repeated episodes of acute, decompensated congestive heart failure that may require hospitalization and intensive diuresis are relatively common in patients with chronic progressive heart failure.

## TREATMENT OF FULMINANT CONGESTIVE HEART FAILURE

Fulminant congestive heart failure is characterized by severe cardiogenic pulmonary edema, with or without pleural and/or abdominal effusions or poor cardiac output. Therapy is designed to rapidly reduce pulmonary edema, improve oxygenation, and optimize cardiac output (Table 3-4). Thoracocentesis should be performed expediently if marked pleural effusion exists. Animals with severe congestive heart failure are greatly stressed, therefore physical activity must be maximally curtailed to reduce total oxygen consumption; cage confinement is preferred. When transported, the animal should be placed on a cart or carried. Unnecessary handling of the patient and administration of oral medications are avoided when possible. Supplemental oxygen administered by face mask, nasal catheter, endotracheal tube, or oxygen cage is beneficial. Whatever means is chosen, patient struggling is to be avoided. An oxygen cage with temperature and humidity controls is preferred, and a setting of 65° F is recommended for normothermic animals. An oxygen flow of 6 to 10 L/min is usually adequate; initially concentrations of 50% to 100% oxygen may be needed. Extremely severe cases may respond to endotracheal or tracheotomy tube placement

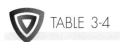

## TABLE 3-4

**Therapy of Fulminant Congestive Heart Failure**

Avoid stress!
Provide cage rest
Enhance oxygenation:
  Check airway patency
  Give supplemental oxygen (avoid >50% for >24 hours)
  If frothing is evident, suction airways
  Intubate and mechanically ventilate if needed
  Perform thoracocentesis if pleural effusion suspected
Remove alveolar fluid:
  Initiate diuresis:
    Furosemide (dogs: 2-5 mg/kg IV or IM, q1-4h until
      respiratory rate decreases, then q6-12h; cats:
      1-2 mg/kg IV or IM, q1-4h until respiratory rate
      decreases, then q6-12h)
  Redistribute blood volume:
    Vasodilators (2% nitroglycerin ointment—dogs:
      ½-1½ inch cutaneously q6h; cats: ¼-½ inch
      cutaneously q6h; or sodium nitroprusside—
      0.5-1 µg/kg/min CRI, titrate upward as needed)
    Morphine (dogs only: 0.05-0.1 mg/kg IV boluses
      q2-3 min to effect, or 0.1-0.5 mg/kg single IM
      or SC dose)
    ± Phlebotomy (6-10 ml/kg)
Reduce bronchoconstriction:
  Aminophylline (dogs: 6-10 mg/kg slow IV, IM, SC, PO
    q6-8h; cats: 4-8 mg/kg IM, SC, PO q8-12h) or
    similar drug
Minimize anxiety:
  Morphine (dogs: dose above)
  Acepromazine (cats: 0.05-0.2 mg/kg SC) or
  Diazepam (cats: 2-5 mg IV; dogs: 5-10 mg IV)
Reduce afterload:
  Enalapril (0.5 mg/kg PO q12-24h) or other ACEI—
    avoid nitroprusside—or
  Hydralazine (dogs: 0.5-1 mg/kg PO repeated in 2-4h,
    then q12h; see text)—avoid nitroprusside—or
  Amlodipine (dogs: 0.1-0.3 mg/kg PO q12-24h;
    see text)
Increase contractility (if myocardial failure present):
  Digoxin (see Table 3-8)
  Dobutamine (1-10 µg/kg/min CRI; start low) or
  Dopamine (dogs: 1-10 µg/kg/min CRI; cats: 1-5
    µg/kg/min CRI; start low)
  Amrinone (1-3 mg/kg IV; 10-100 µg/kg/min CRI)
Monitor and manage abnormalities as possible:
  Respiratory rate, heart rate and rhythm, pulse strength,
    body weight, urine output, hydration, attitude, serum
    biochemistry and blood gas analyses, arterial and
    pulmonary capillary wedge pressures

*ACEI,* Angiotensin-converting enzyme inhibitor; *CRI,* constant rate infusion.

can adversely affect hemodynamics, and chronic high oxygen concentrations (>70%) can injure lung tissue. Continuous monitoring is essential for intubated animals.

Rapid diuresis can be achieved with furosemide administered intravenously. Some patients are unresponsive to traditional doses (1 to 2 mg/kg) but do respond to higher initial doses or to cumulative doses administered at frequent intervals (see Table 3-4). Once diuresis has begun and respiration improves, the dosage is reduced to prevent excessive volume contraction or electrolyte depletion. Aminophylline, given by slow intravenous administration or intramuscular injection, has mild diuretic and positive inotropic actions and a bronchodilating effect; it also decreases fatigue of respiratory muscles. Adverse effects include increased sympathomimetic activity and arrhythmias. Oral therapy can be used when respiration improves because gastrointestinal (GI) absorption is rapid.

Tranquilizers (morphine for dogs, low doses of acepromazine for cats) can reduce anxiety (see Table 3-4). Other beneficial effects of morphine include slower, deeper breathing from respiratory center depression and redistribution of blood away from the lungs via splanchnic vasodilation. Because morphine can increase intracranial pressure, it is contraindicated in dogs with neurogenic edema. Morphine is contraindicated in cats.

Vasodilating drugs can reduce pulmonary edema by increasing systemic venous capacitance, lowering pulmonary venous pressure, and reducing systemic arterial resistance. Hydralazine, a pure arteriolar dilator, is used for treating refractory pulmonary edema caused by mitral regurgitation (and sometimes dilated cardiomyopathy). It effectively reduces regurgitant fraction and lowers left atrial pressure. An initial dose of 0.75 to 1 mg/kg is given orally, followed by repeated doses every 2 to 3 hours until the systolic blood pressure is between 90 and 110 mm Hg or clinical improvement is obvious. If blood pressure cannot be monitored, an initial dose of 1 mg/kg is repeated in 2 to 4 hours if sufficient clinical improvement has not been observed. The addition of 2% nitroglycerin ointment may provide beneficial venodilating effects.

An alternative therapy to nitroglycerine/hydralazine is the infusion of sodium nitroprusside, beginning at 0.5 to 1 µg/kg/min and titrating upward as needed; but, blood pressure must be closely monitored. The dose is titrated to maintain a systolic blood pressure of 90 to 100 mm Hg. The infusion is usually continued for 12 to 24 hours. Another choice for vasodilation is an ACEI or amlodipine, with or without nitroglycerin ointment. The onset of action is slower and the effects are less pronounced, but this regimen can still be helpful.

Positive inotropic therapy (see p. 66) is indicated for patients with heart failure caused by poor myocardial contractility (dilated cardiomyopathy [DCM]), but it must be administered cautiously. IV dobutamine is usually preferred over dopamine because it has less effect on the heart rate and afterload. Amrinone or milrinone can also be used acutely by IV infusion. Catecholamines can increase pulmonary and systemic vascular resistance, potentially exacerbating interstitial fluid accumulation; they also can cause arrhythmias.

and mechanical ventilation with positive end-expiratory pressure (PEEP), continuous positive airway pressure (CPAP), or high-frequency jet ventilation. PEEP ventilation helps clear small airways and expand alveoli and may force alveolar fluid back into the interstitium. However, positive airway pressures

Digoxin is usually not administered IV, except for some supraventricular tachyarrhythmias. Furthermore, the acidosis and hypoxemia associated with severe pulmonary edema can increase myocardial sensitivity to digitalis-induced arrhythmias; thus, monitoring of electrolyte and acid-base balance is important.

For cats with hypertrophic cardiomyopathy, diuretic and oxygen therapy are given as outlined above. Diltiazem or a $\beta_1$-blocker is used once severe dyspnea has abated; or, IV administration (esmolol or diltiazem) could be considered. Moderate-to-large pleural effusions should be drained. Arteriolar vasodilators could be detrimental if left ventricular outflow obstruction exists (see Chapter 7).

Other approaches that have been used in patients with acute cardiogenic edema include phlebotomy of up to 25% of total blood volume and rotating limb tourniquets (probably not very effective in animals). Environmental stressors such as excess heat and humidity or extreme cold should be avoided. Once diuresis has begun and respiratory signs begin to abate, low-sodium water is offered by mouth. Very conservative parenteral fluid therapy (e.g., 15 to 30 ml/kg/day) may be required in very ill or anorectic animals; a 5% dextrose in water solution or a low-sodium fluid should be used. Arterial blood pressure monitoring and serial serum creatinine or BUN and electrolyte concentration measurement are advised to avoid excessive diuresis and hypotension.

## DIETARY MANAGEMENT

Heart failure causes impaired ability to excrete sodium and water loads. Therefore dietary salt restriction is recommended to help control fluid accumulation and to reduce necessary drug therapy. The degree of sodium restriction recommended generally depends on the severity of the heart failure. Chloride restriction also appears to be important. Before signs of heart failure develop, merely avoiding high-salt table scraps or treats may be sufficient, although a diet somewhat reduced in sodium is often recommended. Foods that are high in salt include processed meats, liver and kidney, canned fish, cheese, margarine or butter, canned vegetables, breads, potato chips, pretzels and other "munchies," and dog treats such as rawhide and biscuits.

Moderate salt restriction is advised when clinical heart failure develops. This represents a sodium intake of about 30 mg/kg/day (about 0.06% sodium for canned food, or 210 to 240 mg/100 g of dry food). Diets designed for geriatric animals or renal disease usually provide this level of salt (Table 3-5). Further sodium restriction is found in prescription cardiac diets (e.g., 13 mg of sodium per kilogram of body weight per day, or about 90 to 100 mg of sodium per 100 g of dry food, or 0.025% sodium in a canned food), which can be helpful in patients with advanced heart failure. Severe sodium restriction (e.g., 7 mg/kg/day) can exacerbate neurohormonal activation and contribute to hyponatremia. Recipes for homemade low-salt diets are available.* However, providing a balanced vitamin and mineral content may be difficult. Supplementation of homemade diets with brewer's yeast (1 g/kg body weight/day) or a B-complex vitamin preparation helps offset loss of these vitamins through diuresis. Some drinking water contains considerable sodium. Nonsoftened water or, where the public water supply contains more than 150 ppm of sodium, distilled water can be recommended to further reduce salt intake.

A well-balanced diet and an adequate caloric and protein intake are important. However, inappetence is common in dogs and cats with heart failure. Warming the food to enhance its flavor, adding small amounts of very palatable "human" foods (e.g., unsalted meats or gravy, low-sodium soup), using a salt substitute (potassium chloride [KCl]) or garlic powder, handfeeding, and providing small quantities of the diet several times a day may help when appetite is poor. If a change in diet is indicated, gradually switching improves acceptance (e.g., mixing the new with the old diet in a 1:3 ratio for several days, then 1:1 for several days, then 3:1, and finally the new diet alone). Malaise, increased respiratory effort, and adverse effects of medication all can contribute to poor appetite. Yet more calories may be needed because of increased cardiopulmonary energy consumption and/or stress. Meanwhile, poor splanchnic perfusion, bowel and pancreatic edema, and secondary intestinal lymphangiectasia may reduce nutrient absorption and promote protein loss. Hypoalbuminemia and reduced immune function may develop. These factors and concurrent renal or hepatic dysfunction may alter the pharmacokinetics of certain drugs as well.

Cardiac cachexia refers to the syndrome of muscle wasting and fat loss associated with some cases of chronic congestive heart failure. Loss of muscle over the spine and gluteal region is usually noted first. Weakness and fatigue are seen with loss of lean body mass; cardiac mass also can be affected. In people, cardiac cachexia also has been associated with reduced immune function, and it is a predictor of poor survival. Multiple factors are involved in the pathogenesis of cardiac cachexia, including the cytokines, TNF-$\alpha$, and interleukin-1 (IL-1). These substances suppress appetite and cause hypercatabolism. Dietary supplementation with fish oils, which are high in *n*-3 fatty acids (eicosapentaenoic [EPA] and docosahexaenoic [DHA] acids), can reduce cytokine production. They also may improve endothelial function and have other beneficial effects. Freeman and colleagues (1998) found improvements in cachexia and lower IL-1 levels in dogs with DCM using approximately 27 mg/kg/day EPA and 18 mg/kg/day DHA. A decreased IL-1 concentration correlated with length of survival in these patients, although there was no effect of fish oil on overall mortality.

---

*For recipes see Hand MS et al, editors: *Small animal clinical nutrition IV*, Topeka, Kan, 1997, Mark Morris Institute; and Wills JM et al, editors: *The Waltham book of clinical nutrition of the dog & cat*, Tarrytown, NY, 1994, Pergamon/Elsevier Science.

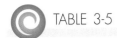

TABLE 3-5

Commercial Reduced-Sodium Diets*

| | PROTEIN | FAT | SODIUM | CHLORIDE | POTASSIUM | MAGNESIUM | PHOSPHORUS |
|---|---|---|---|---|---|---|---|
| **Canned Canine Products** | | | | | | | |
| Hill's Prescription Diet Canine h/d | 17.3 | 28.8 | 0.10 | 0.35 | 0.83 | 0.13 | 0.47 |
| Hill's Prescription Diet Canine k/d | 14.8 | 27.3 | 0.21 | 0.25 | 0.30 | 0.13 | 0.11 |
| Hill's HealthBlend Canine Geriatric | 17.4 | 14.0 | 0.15 | 0.59 | 0.63 | 0.09 | 0.41 |
| Hill's Prescription Diet Canine w/d | 16.2 | 12.1 | 0.26 | 0.78 | 0.60 | 0.08 | 0.42 |
| Purina CNM Canine CV-Formula | 17.8 | 31.9 | 0.12 | 1.27 | 1.21 | 0.06 | 0.40 |
| Purina CNM Canine NF-Formula | 16.6 | 25.3 | 0.23 | 0.49 | 0.33 | 0.07 | 0.26 |
| Select Care Canine Modified Formula | 16.8 | 21.8 | 0.24 | NA | 0.96 | 0.07 | 0.35 |
| Waltham Low Sodium | 26.3 | 38.0 | 0.10 | NA | 1.50 | 0.10 | 0.67 |
| Leo Specific Cardil CHW | 17.7 | 21.3 | 0.11 | NA | 1.31 | 0.07 | 0.57 |
| **Dry Canine Products** | | | | | | | |
| Hill's Prescription Diet Canine h/d | 17.2 | 20.9 | 0.07 | 0.35 | 0.72 | 0.11 | 0.62 |
| Hill's Prescription Diet Canine k/d | 14.6 | 19.5 | 0.21 | 0.38 | 0.32 | 0.06 | 0.29 |
| Hill's HealthBlend Canine Geriatric | 17.7 | 10.0 | 0.15 | 0.52 | 0.60 | 0.10 | 0.51 |
| Hill's Prescription Diet Canine w/d | 16.7 | 6.9 | 0.21 | 0.50 | 0.60 | 0.12 | 0.51 |
| Purina CNM Canine NF-Formula | 14.9 | 16.4 | 0.23 | 0.40 | 0.36 | 0.08 | 0.27 |
| Select Care Canine Modified Formula | 14.4 | 19.7 | 0.28 | NA | 0.88 | 0.09 | 0.34 |
| MediCal Cardio | 18.6 | 17.2 | 0.17 | NA | 1.04 | 0.10 | 0.60 |
| **Canned Feline Products** | | | | | | | |
| Hill's Prescription Diet Feline h/d | 43.6 | 27.0 | 0.24 | 0.75 | 0.90 | 0.06 | 0.73 |
| Hill's Prescription Diet Feline k/d | 29.3 | 41.1 | 0.26 | 0.27 | 1.00 | 0.04 | 0.57 |
| Hill's HealthBlend Feline Adult | 41.1 | 22.3 | 0.24 | 0.70 | 0.79 | 0.06 | 0.65 |
| Hill's HealthBlend Feline Geriatric | 40.9 | 20.5 | 0.33 | 0.67 | 0.88 | 0.10 | 0.61 |
| Purina CNM Feline CV-Formula | 42.5 | 26.8 | 0.20 | 1.09 | 1.33 | 0.07 | 0.92 |
| Select Care Feline Modified Formula | 35.0 | 53.0 | 0.23 | NA | 1.07 | 0.06 | 0.49 |
| Leo Specific FHW | 44.3 | 26.7 | 0.14 | NA | 1.31 | 0.11 | 0.71 |
| **Dry Feline Products** | | | | | | | |
| Hill's Prescription Diet Feline k/d | 28.1 | 27.4 | 0.28 | 0.50 | 0.89 | 0.05 | 0.57 |
| Hill's HealthBlend Feline Adult | 32.7 | 20.2 | 0.23 | 0.62 | 0.65 | 0.07 | 0.70 |
| Hill's HealthBlend Feline Geriatric | 33.2 | 18.6 | 0.33 | 0.89 | 0.79 | 0.07 | 0.68 |
| Purina CNM Feline NF-Formula | 28.8 | 11.8 | 0.18 | 0.60 | 0.82 | 0.09 | 0.38 |
| Select Care Feline Modified Formula | 28.3 | 22.1 | 0.27 | NA | 0.92 | 0.07 | 0.52 |

From Roudebush P et al: Cardiovascular disease. In Hand MS et al, editors: *Small animal clinical nutrition IV*, Topeka, Kan, 1997, Mark Morris Institute.
*NA*, Informed not published by manufacturer.
*Expressed as % dry matter; manufacturer's published values.

Obesity, on the other hand, increases metabolic demands on the heart and expands blood volume. Increased cardiac filling, stimulation of hypertrophy, increased venous pressures, and predisposition to arrhythmias may result. Intrinsic myocardial changes that decrease contractility also can occur in association with obesity. Mechanical interference with respiration promotes hypoventilation; this can contribute to cor pulmonale and complicate preexisting heart disease. A reducing diet is indicated for grossly overweight pets with heart disease.

Supplementation of specific nutrients is important in some cases. Taurine is an essential nutrient for cats. Prolonged deficiency causes myocardial failure as well as other abnormalities (see the section on feline dilated cardiomyopathy,

## TABLE 3-6

### Dosage of Diuretics and Vasodilators

| DRUG | DOG | CAT |
|---|---|---|
| **Diuretics** | | |
| Furosemide | 1-3 mg/kg q8-24h chronic PO; or 2-5 mg/kg q4-6h IV, IM, SC | 1-2 mg/kg q12h up to 4 mg/kg q8-12h, IV, IM, SC, PO |
| Spironolactone | 2 mg/kg q12h PO | 1-2 mg/kg q12h PO |
| Chlorothiazide | 20-40 mg/kg q12h PO | Same |
| Hydrochlorothiazide | 2-4 mg/kg q12h PO | 1-2 mg/kg q12h PO |
| Triamterene | 2 (to 4) mg/kg/day PO | — |
| **ACEI and other Vasodilators** | | |
| Enalapril | 0.5 mg/kg q24(to 12)h PO | 0.25-0.5 mg/kg q24(to 12)h |
| Captopril | 0.5-2 mg/kg q8-12h PO (low initial dose) | 0.5-1.25 mg/kg q12-24h |
| Benazepril | 0.25-0.5 mg/kg q24h PO | Same |
| Lisinopril | 0.5 mg/kg q24h PO | 0.25-0.5 mg/kg q24h PO |
| Fosinopril | 0.25-0.5 mg/kg q24h PO | — |
| Hydralazine | 0.5-2 mg/kg q12h PO (to 1 mg/kg initial) | 2.5 (up to 10) mg/cat q12h PO |
| Amlodipine | (0.05 to) 0.1-0.3 (to 0.5) mg/kg q(12 to)24h PO | 0.625 mg/cat q24(to 12)h PO |
| Prazosin | Small dogs (<5 kg): Do not use<br>Medium dogs: 1 mg q8-12h PO<br>Large dogs: 2 mg q8h PO | |
| Sodium nitroprusside | 0.5-1 µg/kg/min constant rate infusion (CRI) (initial), to 5-15 µg/kg/min CRI | Same |
| Nitroglycerine ointment | ½-1½ inch q4-6h cutaneously | ¼-½ inch q4-6h cutaneously |
| Isosorbide dinitrate | 0.5-2 mg/kg q8h PO | — |

*CRI,* Constant rate infusion.

p. 130). Reformulation of most commercial and prescription cat foods has significantly reduced the prevalence of taurine-responsive dilated cardiomyopathy in cats. However, some diets may still be deficient. Taurine-deficient cats are given oral supplements of taurine (250 to 500 mg) twice daily. Some dogs with dilated cardiomyopathy appear deficient in taurine and/or L-carnitine (see the section on canine myocardial disease in Chapter 6). Dogs fed protein-restricted diets can become taurine deficient, and some develop evidence of dilated cardiomyopathy (Sanderson and colleagues, 2001). Oral supplementation with 1 to 2 g of L-carnitine (or 50 to 100 mg/kg) two or three times daily and 500 mg taurine twice daily has been recommended for dogs with these deficiencies.

The role of antioxidants and other dietary supplements is unclear. There is increasing evidence of oxidative stress in patients with myocardial failure, and free-radical damage probably plays a role in the pathogenesis of myocardial dysfunction. Cytokines such as TNF-α, which increase in the circulation in heart failure, can promote oxidative stress. In people, vitamin C supplementation has a beneficial effect on endothelial function, cardiac morbidity, and mortality. There is controversy as to whether coenzyme Q-10 provides any measurable benefit. A recent review concluded that there was no beneficial effect in human heart failure patients (Khatta and colleagues, 2000). Others have suggested that coenzyme Q-10 may have some use as an adjuvant therapy. The poten-

tial benefit of other antioxidant supplements in dogs and cats with heart failure is likewise unclear.

## DIURETICS

Diuretics remain fundamental to the management of congestive heart failure because of their ability to decrease venous congestion and fluid accumulation (Tables 3-6 and 3-7). Agents that interfere with ion transport in the loop of Henle have potent ability to promote both salt and water loss. Diuretics of other classes such as thiazides and potassium-sparing agents are sometimes combined with furosemide for chronic heart failure therapy. However, given in excess, diuretics promote excessive volume contraction and activate the renin-angiotensin-aldosterone cascade. Diuretics also can exacerbate preexisting dehydration or azotemia. So, the indication for their use in such animals should be clearly established, and the lowest effective dose should be used.

### FUROSEMIDE AND OTHER LOOP DIURETICS

Furosemide is the loop or "high-ceiling" diuretic used most widely for cats and dogs with heart failure (see Tables 3-6 and 3-7). Bumetanide and ethacrynic acid are others. These potent agents act on the ascending limb of the loop of Henle to

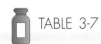 TABLE 3-7

**Diuretics and Vasodilators, Commercial Preparations**

| DRUG | PREPARATIONS | BRAND/MANUFACTURER |
|---|---|---|
| **Diuretics** | | |
| Furosemide | *Veterinary:* 12.5 and 50 mg tablets<br>50 mg/ml injectable solution<br>10 mg/ml oral syrup | Lasix (Intervet, Kansas City, Mo); generics |
| | *Human:* 20, 40, and 80 mg tablets<br>10 mg/ml and 40 mg/5 ml oral solutions<br>10 mg/ml injectable solution | Lasix (Aventis, Bridgewater, N.J.); generics |
| Spironolactone | 25, 50, and 100 mg tablets | Aldactone (Searle, Chicago, Ill); generics |
| Chlorothiazide | 250 and 500 mg tablets<br>250 mg/5 ml oral suspension | Diuril (Merck, West Point, Pa); generics |
| Hydrochlorothiazide | 25, 50, and 100 mg tablets<br>100 mg/ml and 50 mg/5 ml solutions | Hydrodiuril (Merck, West Point, Pa); generics |
| Triamterene | 50 and 100 mg capsules | Dyrenium (GlaxoSmithKline, Pa); generics |
| **Vasodilators** | | |
| Enalapril | *Veterinary:* 1, 2.5, 5, 10, and 20 mg tablets<br>*Human:* 2.5, 5, 10, and 20 mg tablets<br>1.25 mg/ml enalaprilat IV injectable solution | Enacard (Merial, Rahway, N.J.)<br>Vasotec (Merck, West Point, Pa); generic<br>Vasotec IV (Merck, West Point, Pa) |
| Captopril | 12.5, 25, 50, and 100 mg tablets | Capoten (Bristol-Meyers Squibb, Princeton, N.J.); generics |
| Benazepril | 5, 10, 20, and 40 mg tablets | Lotensin (Novartis, Summit, N.J.) |
| Lisinopril | 2.5, 5, 10, 20, and 40 mg tablets | Prinivil (Merck, West Point, Pa); Zestril (AstraZeneca, Wilmington, Del) |
| Fosinopril | 10, 20, and 40 mg tablets | Monopril (Bristol-Myers Squibb, New York, N.Y.) |
| Hydralazine | 10, 25, 50, and 100 mg tablets | Apresoline (Novartis, Summit, N.J.); generics |
| Amlodipine | 2.5, 5, and 10 mg tablets | Norvasc (Pfizer, New York, N.Y.) |
| Prazosin | 1, 2, and 5 mg capsules | Minipress (Pfizer, New York, N.Y.) |
| Sodium nitroprusside | 50 mg vials, powder for injection | Nitropress (Abbott, Abbott Park, Ill); generics |
| Nitroglycerine | 2% ointment | Nitrobid (Hoechst Marion Roussel, Kansas City, Mo); Nitrol (Savage, Melville, N.Y.); generics |
| Isorbide dinitrate | 5, 10, 20, and 30 mg tablets | Isordil Titradose (Wyeth-Ayerst, Philadelphia, Pa); generics |

inhibit active $Cl^-$, $K^+$, and $Na^+$ cotransport, thereby promoting excretion of these electrolytes; $Ca^{++}$ and $Mg^{++}$ are also lost in the urine. Loop diuretics can increase systemic venous capacitance, possibly by mediating renal prostaglandin release. Furosemide (and ethacrynic acid) may also promote salt loss by increasing total renal blood flow and by preferentially enhancing renal cortical flow. The loop diuretics are well absorbed when given orally. Bumetanide is 40 to 50 times more potent than furosemide.

Diuresis begins within 5 minutes after IV furosemide administration; the effect peaks in about 30 minutes and lasts for approximately 2 hours. After oral administration, diuresis occurs within 1 hour, peaks between 1 to 2 hours, and may last for 6 hours. Furosemide is highly protein-bound; about 80% is actively secreted unchanged in the proximal renal tubules, with the remainder excreted as glucuronide.

The dosage of furosemide varies, depending on the clinical situation (see Table 3-6). The respiratory pattern, hydration status, body weight, exercise tolerance, renal function, and serum electrolyte concentrations are used to monitor the response to furosemide (and other diuretic) therapy. According to the manufacturer, a slight yellowish discoloration of the parenteral solution before the expiration date does not affect the drug's efficacy.

Adverse effects are usually related to excessive fluid and/or electrolyte losses. Cats are more sensitive than dogs, therefore lower doses are used. Although hypokalemia is the most common electrolyte disturbance, it is unusual in dogs that are not anorexic. Hyponatremia develops in some patients with severe congestive heart failure and results from an inability to excrete free water (dilutional hyponatremia) rather than a total body sodium deficit. Rapid IV administration of furosemide (and ethacrynic acid) or concurrent ototoxic drug use (e.g., aminoglycosides) has been associated with hearing loss in people. Transient thrombocytopenia and granulocytopenia also have been reported occasionally in people.

## SPIRONOLACTONE AND OTHER POTASSIUM-SPARING DIURETICS

Spironolactone, triamterene, and amiloride generally have mild diuretic effects but can augment therapy for chronic refractory heart failure when furosemide and an ACEI alone are insufficient to control fluid accumulation (see Tables 3-6 and 3-7). They reduce the renal potassium wasting of furosemide and other diuretics.

Spironolactone is a competitive antagonist of aldosterone. It promotes $Na^+$ loss and $K^+$ retention in the distal renal tubule; its effects are more pronounced with high circulating aldosterone concentrations. The drug's onset of action is slow; peak diuresis occurs within 2 to 3 days. Its antialdosterone effects are also thought to be important locally within the heart (see above, p. 57).

Triamterene and amiloride inhibit $Na^+$ reabsorption in the distal tubule, which decreases $K^+$ secretion independent of aldosterone's effects. Triamterene's effect begins within 2 hours of administration, peaks at 6 to 8 hours, and lasts 12 to 16 hours.

The potassium-sparing diuretics must be used cautiously in patients receiving an ACEI or potassium supplement. Potassium-sparing diuretics are absolutely contraindicated in patients with hyperkalemia. Adverse effects relate to excess $K^+$ retention and gastrointestinal disturbances. Spironolactone may reduce the clearance of digoxin.

## THIAZIDE DIURETICS

Thiazide diuretics decrease sodium and chloride absorption and increase calcium absorption in the early part of the distal tubules. Excretion of $Na^+$, $Cl^-$, $K^+$, and $Mg^{++}$ results, with mild to moderate diuresis (see Tables 3-6 and 3-7). The thiazides decrease renal blood flow and should not be used in azotemic animals.

Chlorothiazide's effects begin within 1 hour, peak at 4 hours, and last 6 to 12 hours. The action of hydrochlorothiazide begins within 2 hours, peaks at 4 hours, and lasts about 12 hours. Adverse effects are uncommon in nonazotemic animals; however, hypokalemia or other electrolyte disturbances and dehydration can occur with excessive use or in patients with anorexia. Thiazides can cause hyperglycemia in diabetic or prediabetic animals by inhibiting conversion of proinsulin to insulin.

## VASODILATORS

Vasodilator therapy improves cardiac output and reduces edema and effusions associated with heart failure (see Tables 3-6 and 3-7). In most cases ACEIs are the agents of first choice because they have important effects in addition to vasodilation. Vasodilators can affect arterioles, venous capacitance vessels, or both ("balanced" vasodilators). Arteriolar dilators relax arteriolar smooth muscle and thus reduce systemic vascular resistance and afterload on the heart. This facilitates ejection of blood. Agents that diminish arteriolar resistance are also used in the treatment of hypertension. In patients with mitral regurgitation, arteriolar dilators decrease the systolic pressure gradient across the mitral valve, reduce regurgitant flow, and enhance forward flow into the aorta. Reduced regurgitant flow can diminish left atrial pressure and pulmonary congestion. Left atrial size may also be decreased.

Arteriolar or mixed vasodilator therapy is generally begun with a low dose to avoid hypotension and reflex tachycardia. A reduction in concurrent diuretic dosage may be advisable. Monitoring for signs of hypotension is especially important after initiating treatment. Sequential arterial blood pressure measurement is preferred. Clinical signs of drug-induced hypotension include weakness, lethargy, tachycardia, and poor peripheral perfusion. The vasodilator dosage can be titrated upward if necessary; monitoring for hypotension accompanies each increase in dose. A mean arterial pressure of 70 to 80 mm Hg or a venous $P_{O_2}$ of greater than 30 mm Hg (from a free-flowing jugular vein) is the suggested therapeutic endpoint for dosage titration. Systolic pressures of less than 90 to 100 mm Hg should be avoided.

Venodilators relax systemic veins, increase venous capacitance, decrease cardiac filling pressures (preload), and reduce pulmonary congestion. The goals of venodilator therapy are to maintain the central venous pressure at 5 to 10 cm $H_2O$ and the pulmonary capillary wedge pressure at 12 to 18 mm Hg.

## ANGIOTENSIN-CONVERTING ENZYME INHIBITORS (ACEIs)

Angiotensin II promotes volume retention and vasoconstriction in several ways (see Figs. 3-1 and 3-2). By blocking the formation of angiotensin II, ACEIs allow arteriolar and venous vasodilation and reduced $Na^+$ and water retention (via decreased circulating aldosterone). The vasodilating effects of ACEIs may be enhanced by vasodilator kinins normally degraded by ACE. A local vasodilating effect may occur through inhibition of ACE found within vascular walls even in the absence of high circulating renin levels. Local ACE inhibition is also beneficial by modulating vascular smooth muscle and myocardial remodeling.

Because of their multiple effects in moderating excess neurohormonal responses, ACEIs have considerable advantages over hydralazine and other arteriolar dilators (see Tables 3-6 and 3-7). The addition of an ACEI to diuretic and digoxin therapy leads to sustained clinical improvement and lower mortality rates in people and dogs with heart failure from myocardial disease or volume overload. ACEIs also appear to delay the onset of clinical heart failure from myocardial dysfunction. ACEIs reduce cardiac filling pressures and improve clinical heart failure. A measurable reduction in the heart rate, decreased peripheral vascular resistance, and improved cardiac output have been variably reported. The secondary inhibition of aldosterone release helps reduce edema/effusions, as well as aldosterone's direct adverse effects on the heart. ACEIs reduce ventricular arrhythmias and the rate of sudden death in people (and probably animals) with heart failure, likely because angiotensin II–induced facilitation of norepinephrine and epinephrine release is inhibited. ACEIs have been variably effective in treating dogs with hypertension.

Adverse effects of ACEIs include hypotension, GI upset, renal function deterioration, and hyperkalemia (especially when the drugs are used with a potassium-sparing diuretic or potassium supplement). Angiotensin II is important in mediating renal efferent arteriolar constriction, which maintains glomerular filtration when renal blood flow decreases. As long as cardiac output and renal perfusion improve with therapy, renal function is usually maintained. Poor glomerular filtration is more likely to result with overdiuresis, excess vasodilation, or severe myocardial dysfunction. Reducing the diuretic dosage may restore renal function. If not, the ACEI dosage is reduced or sometimes discontinued. Hypotension can usually be avoided with low initial doses. Other adverse effects reported in people include rash, pruritus, impairment of taste, proteinuria, cough, and neutropenia. The mechanism of ACEI-induced cough in people is unclear but may involve inhibition of endogenous bradykinin degradation or may be associated with increased nitric oxide generation. Nitric oxide has an inflammatory effect on bronchial epithelial cells; a preliminary study in people found that iron supplementation (ferrous sulfate) improved ACEI-induced cough, possibly by reducing nitric oxide generation or associated cell damage (Lee and colleagues, 2001). The ACEI fosinopril appears to have less of a propensity to induce coughing.

### Enalapril

Enalapril is absorbed well when taken orally; administration with food does not reduce its bioavailability (see Tables 3-6 and 3-7). It is hydrolyzed in the liver to enalaprilat, its most active form. Peak ACE-inhibiting activity occurs within 4 to 6 hours in dogs. The duration of action is 12 to 14 hours, and effects are minimal by 24 hours at the recommended once-daily dose. Enalapril is generally administered once daily, although some dogs respond better when dosed every 12 hours. In cats, maximal activity occurs within 2 to 4 hours after an oral dose of either 0.25 or 0.5 mg/kg; some ACE inhibition (50% of control) persists for 2 to 3 days. Enalapril and its active metabolite are excreted in the urine. Renal failure and severe congestive heart failure prolong its half-life; therefore reduced doses should be used in such patients. Severe liver dysfunction interferes with the conversion of the prodrug to the active enalaprilat; lisinopril or captopril should be considered in such patients instead. Injectable enalaprilat is also available but there is little veterinary experience with it; this form is not well absorbed orally. Enalapril maleate is available in both veterinary and human preparations.

### Captopril

Captopril was the first ACEI to be used clinically (see Tables 3-6 and 3-7). In contrast to enalapril and others, captopril contains a sulfhydryl group; disulfide metabolites can act as free-radical scavengers. This might have beneficial effects for the treatment of some heart diseases, although the clinical significance is presently unclear. However, captopril was less effective than several other ACEIs in reducing ACE activity in a normal dog study (Hamlin and colleagues, 1998). Captopril is well absorbed when taken orally (75% bioavailable);

however, food reduces its bioavailability by 30% to 40%. The drug is about 40% protein-bound. In dogs, hemodynamic effects appear within 1 hour, peak in 1 to 2 hours, and last less than 4 hours, therefore it is administered to dogs two or three times daily. The drug has also been used in cats one or two times daily. Captopril is excreted in the urine.

### Benazepril

Benazepril, like enalapril, is a prodrug that is metabolized to its active form, benazeprilat. Only about 40% is absorbed when the drug is administered orally, but feeding does not affect absorption. After oral administration, peak ACE inhibition occurs within 2 hours in dogs and cats; its effect can last longer than 24 hours (see Tables 3-6 and 3-7). In cats, dosages of 0.25 to 0.5 mg/kg resulted in 100% inhibition of ACE, which was maintained at over 90% at 24 hours and tapered off to about 80% by 36 hours. Benazepril has an initial half-life of 2.4 hours and a terminal half-life of about 29 hours in cats. Repeated doses produce moderate increases in the drug plasma concentration. Benazepril is eliminated equally in urine and bile in dogs, an advantage for animals with renal disease. In cats, about 85% of the drug is excreted in the feces and only 15% in the urine. The drug appears to be well tolerated.

### Lisinopril

Lisinopril is a lysine analog of enalaprilat with direct ACE-inhibiting effects. It is 25% to 50% bioavailable, and absorption is not affected by feeding. The time to peak effect is 6 to 8 hours. The duration of ACE inhibition appears long, but more specific information in animals is lacking. Once-daily administration has been tried, with apparent effectiveness (see Tables 3-6 and 3-7).

### Fosinopril

Fosinopril is structurally different in that it contains a phosphinic acid radical (rather than sulfhydryl or carboxyl) (see Tables 3-6 and 3-7). It may be retained longer in myocytes. Fosinopril is also a prodrug, which is converted to the active fosinoprilat in the GI mucosa and liver. Elimination occurs equally between the kidneys and the liver; compensatory increases in one pathway occur with impairment of the other. The duration of action is well over 24 hours in people. Fosinopril may cause falsely low serum digoxin measurements using RIA assays but does not affect tests using EIA methodology.

## ARTERIOLAR AND OTHER MIXED VASODILATORS

### Hydralazine

Hydralazine directly relaxes arteriolar smooth muscle when the vascular endothelium is intact, but it has little effect on the venous system (see Tables 3-6 and 3-7). The drug reduces arterial blood pressure, improves pulmonary edema, and increases jugular venous oxygen tension (presumably from increased cardiac output) in dogs with mitral insufficiency and heart failure. The most common indication for hydralazine is acute, severe congestive heart failure from mitral regurgitation.

Hydralazine has been associated with significant reflex tachycardia in some animals, and the dosage should be reduced if this occurs. Hydralazine can contribute to the enhanced neurohormonal response in heart failure, which makes it less desirable than the ACEIs for chronic use. However, it can be useful for animals that cannot tolerate an ACEI.

Administration of hydralazine with food reduces bioavailability by over 60%. There is extensive first-pass hepatic metabolism of this drug. However, in dogs, increased doses saturate this mechanism and increase bioavailability. The general precautions for initiating and titrating therapy are the same as those previously outlined for all vasodilators.

Hypotension is the most common adverse effect of hydralazine therapy. Gastrointestinal upset also can occur, which may require drug discontinuation. High dosages have been associated with a lupuslike syndrome in people, although this has not been reported in animals.

### Prazosin

Prazosin selectively blocks $\alpha_1$-receptors in both arterial and venous walls. Initial hemodynamic improvement may be followed by drug tolerance over time. For this reason, the drug is rarely used; the capsule sizes available are inconvenient as well. Controlled clinical studies in dogs are lacking. Hypotension is the most common adverse effect, especially after the first dose. Tachycardia should occur less frequently than with hydralazine because presynaptic $\alpha_2$-receptors, important in the feedback control of norepinephrine release, are not blocked.

### Sodium Nitroprusside

Sodium nitroprusside is a nitrate that acts directly on vascular smooth muscle and causes potent arteriolar and venous dilation (see Tables 3-6 and 3-7). Sodium nitroprusside is given by intravenous infusion because of its short duration of action; its major indication is fulminant congestive heart failure (see Tables 3-6 and 3-7). However, it should be used only when hemodynamic monitoring is available because of the potential for severe hypotension. The dose is titrated to maintain the mean arterial pressure above 70 mm Hg. The manufacturer's instructions for reconstitution and dilution of the drug should be followed. Solutions that are discolored or that contain particulate matter should not be used. Tolerance develops rapidly, further necessitating careful monitoring and dosage adjustment. Profound hypotension is the major adverse effect. Cyanide toxicity can result from excessive or prolonged use.

## VENODILATORS

### Nitroglycerine and Isosorbide Dinitrate

Nitroglycerine and other nitrates that are administered orally or transcutaneously act mainly on venous smooth muscle, thereby increasing venous capacitance and reducing cardiac filling pressures. The major indication for these agents is acute cardiogenic pulmonary edema (see Tables 3-6 and 3-7). Because of extensive first-pass hepatic metabolism after oral adminis-

tration, the transcutaneous route is used most often in animals; the drug is also well absorbed sublingually. Nitroglycerin ointment (2%) is usually applied to the skin of the groin, axillary area, or ear pinna. Dosage and absorption vary, but a lower dose is used initially in small dogs and in cats. Application papers or gloves should be used so that the person administering the drug avoids skin contact. Self-adhesive, sustained-release preparations may be useful, but they have not been systematically evaluated in small animals. Transdermal patches (5 mg) applied for 12 hr/day have been used with anecdotal success in large dogs. In some cases nitroglycerin ointment or isosorbide dinitrate is used chronically in combination with hydralazine, especially if an ACEI is not tolerated. The efficacy of oral nitrates is in question, even with adequate drug absorption (Adin and colleagues, 2001).

Hypotension can result from excessive or inappropriate use of nitrates. Large doses and frequent application or long-acting formulations are most likely to be associated with drug tolerance.

## POSITIVE INOTROPIC DRUGS

### DIGITALIS GLYCOSIDES
#### Digoxin

Digoxin is the digitalis glycoside used almost exclusively for heart failure in small animals (Tables 3-8 and 3-9); although digitoxin is still available, it is rarely used. Clinical benefits of digoxin may arise from a modest positive inotropic effect or suppression of supraventricular arrhythmias, but direct sensitization of arterial baroreceptors is probably most important in heart failure. Digoxin is indicated in heart failure caused by myocardial dysfunction, chronic mitral insufficiency, and other chronic volume or pressure overloads. Digoxin is usually contraindicated in patients with hypertrophic cardiomyopathy, especially those with ventricular outflow obstruction. Digoxin is not useful for pericardial diseases and, in view of its potential toxicity, should not be used in such cases. Digoxin is only moderately effective in slowing the ventricular response rate to atrial fibrillation and does not cause conversion to sinus rhythm. It is usually contraindicated when sinus or atrioventricular (AV) node disease is present. In most patients with serious ventricular arrhythmias, digoxin is relatively contraindicated because it may exacerbate such arrhythmias.

The digitalis glycosides are relatively weak positive inotropic agents. They increase the $Ca^{++}$ available to contractile proteins by competitively binding and inhibiting the $Na^+$, $K^+$-ATPase pump at the myocardial cell membrane. Intracellular $Na^+$ accumulation promotes $Ca^{++}$ entry via the sodium-calcium exchange. However, in diseased myocardial cells, diastolic sequestration and systolic release of $Ca^{++}$ may be impaired. Digitalis glycosides may be ineffective inotropic agents in these cells and could predispose to cellular $Ca^{++}$ overload and electrical instability.

The antiarrhythmic effects of the digitalis glycosides are mediated primarily via increased parasympathetic tone to the sinus and AV nodes and the atria. There are also some direct

## TABLE 3-8

Dosage of Positive Inotropic Drugs

| DRUG | DOG | CAT |
|------|-----|-----|
| Digoxin | PO: dogs <22 kg, 0.011 mg/kg q12h; dogs >22 kg, 0.22 mg/m$^2$ q12h *or* 0.005 mg/kg q12h<br>Decrease by 10% for elixir. Maximum: 0.5 mg/day or 0.375 mg/day for Dobermans<br>IV loading: 0.01-0.02 mg/kg—give ¼ of this total dose in slow boluses over 2-4 hr to effect | PO: 0.007 mg/kg q48h<br>IV loading: 0.005 mg/kg—give ½ of total, then 1-2 hr later give ¼ dose bolus(es) if needed |
| Digitoxin | 0.02-0.03 mg/kg q8h (small dogs) to q12h (large dogs) | Do not use |
| Dopamine | For CHF—1-10 μg/kg/min CRI; for shock—5-15 μg/kg/min CRI (40 mg of dopamine into 500 ml of fluid provides 80 μg/ml; infusion at 0.75 ml/kg/hr provides 1 μg dopamine/kg/min) | 1-5 μg/kg/min CRI |
| Dobutamine | 1-10 μg/kg/min CRI (250 mg of dobutamine into 500 ml of fluid yields 500 μg/ml; infusion at 0.6 ml/kg/hr provides 5 μg dobutamine/kg/min) | Same |
| Amrinone | 1-3 mg/kg initial bolus IV; 10-100 μg/kg/min CRI | Same? |
| Milrinone | 50 μg/kg IV over 10 minutes initially; 0.375-0.75 μg/kg/min CRI (human dose) | Same? |

*CHF,* Congestive heart failure; *CRI,* constant rate infusion.

## TABLE 3-9

Positive Inotropic Drugs, Commercial Preparations

| DRUG | PREPARATIONS | BRAND/MANUFACTURER |
|------|--------------|--------------------|
| Digoxin | *Veterinary:* 0.15 mg/ml elixir<br>0.05 mg/ml elixir<br>*Human:* 0.125, 0.25, and 0.5 mg tablets<br>0.05 mg/ml pediatric elixir<br>0.25 mg/ml and 0.1 mg/ml injectable | Cardoxin (EVSCO, Buena, N.J.)<br>Cardoxin LS (EVSCO)<br>Lanoxin (GlaxoSmithKline, Research Triangle Park, N.C.) |
| Digitoxin | 0.05 and 0.1 mg tablets | Crystodigin (Eli Lilly, Indianapolis, Ind) |
| Dopamine | 40, 80, or 160 mg/ml injectable solution | Intropin (Faulding, Elizabeth, N.J.); generics |
| Dobutamine | 12.5 mg/ml injectable solution, 20 ml vials | Dobutrex (Eli Lilly, Indianapolis, Ind); generics |
| Amrinone | 5 mg/ml injectable solution | Inocor (Sanofi, New York, N.Y.) |
| Milrinone | 1 mg/ml injectable solution<br>Premixed 200 μg/ml in D5W | Primacor (Sanofi, New York, N.Y.) |

effects that further prolong conduction time and the refractory period of the AV node. Slowing of the sinus rate, a reduced ventricular response rate to atrial fibrillation and flutter, and suppression of atrial premature depolarizations result. Although ventricular arrhythmias might be suppressed (probably via enhanced vagal tone), the potential arrhythmogenic effects of these drugs should be considered, especially in the setting of heart failure.

When taken by mouth, digoxin is well absorbed and undergoes minimal hepatic metabolism. Absorption is approximately 60% for the tablet form and 75% for the elixir. Bioavailability is reduced by kaolin-pectin compounds, antacids, the presence of food, and malabsorption syndromes. About 27% of the drug in serum is protein-bound; the serum half-life in dogs ranges from 23 to 39 hours. Therapeutic serum concentrations are achieved within 2 to 4½ days with dosing every 12 hours.

In cats, the reported serum half-life of digoxin ranges widely, from about 25 to longer than 78 hours; chronic oral administration increases the half-life. The alcohol-based elixir, which is poorly palatable, results in serum concentrations approximately 50% higher than the tablet form. Administration of the tablets with food has resulted in serum concentrations about 50% lower than in the fasted state in this species. The pharmacokinetics in cats with heart failure is similar to that in control cats receiving aspirin, furosemide, and a low-salt diet, although much intercat variation is present. Digoxin treatment every 48 hours in these cats produces effective serum concentrations, with steady state achieved in about 10 days. A dose of 0.007 mg/kg every 48 hours is recommended; approximately 50% of patients become toxic at a dose of 0.01 mg/kg every 48 hours. Serum concentrations can be measured 8 hours postdosing once steady state has been reached (after about 10 days).

Oral maintenance doses of digoxin are used to initiate therapy in most cases because loading doses often result in toxic serum concentrations. When more rapid achievement of therapeutic serum concentrations is deemed critical (e.g., for supraventricular tachyarrhythmia), the drug can be given at twice the PO maintenance dose for 1 to 2 doses or intravenously with caution. Intravenous digoxin must be given slowly (over at least 15 minutes) because rapid injection causes peripheral vasoconstriction. Usually the calculated dose is divided, and boluses of one fourth the dose are given slowly over several hours (see Table 3-8). However, alternate IV therapy for supraventricular tachycardia is usually more effective (see Chapter 4). Other intravenous positive inotropic drugs (see below) are safer and more effective than digoxin for immediate support of myocardial contractility.

Elimination of digoxin is primarily by glomerular filtration and renal secretion in dogs, although approximately 15% is metabolized by the liver. Renal and hepatic elimination are equally important in cats. A prolonged sulfobromophthalein (SBP) retention of over 5% at 30 minutes has been associated with digoxin toxicity in cats. The serum digoxin concentration (and risk of toxicity) increases in patients with renal failure because of reduced clearance and volume of distribution. There appears to be no correlation between the degree of azotemia and the serum digoxin concentration in dogs, which makes extrapolations from human formulas for calculating drug dosage in renal failure unusable in this species. Lower doses and close monitoring of serum digoxin concentration are recommended in animals with renal disease. Use of digitoxin rather than digoxin in dogs with renal failure might be feasible; however, digitoxin should not be used in cats because of its extended half-life.

Brand name digoxin is generally recommended over generic formulations (dosing is outlined in Table 3-8). The dosage in dogs weighing over 22 kg is sometimes based on body surface area rather than on body weight. There is only a weak correlation between digoxin dose and serum concentration in dogs with heart failure, indicating that other factors influence the serum concentrations of this drug. Because much of the drug is bound to skeletal muscle, animals with reduced muscle mass or cachexia and those with compromised renal function can easily become toxic at the usual calculated doses. Because digoxin has poor lipid solubility, the dose should be based on the calculated lean body weight; this consideration is especially important in obese animals. Management of digoxin toxicity is outlined on p. 69. Conservative dosing and measurement of serum digoxin concentra-

tions help prevent toxicity. Measurement of the serum concentration is recommended at 7 to 10 days after initiation of therapy (or dosage change). Samples are drawn 8 to 10 hours after the previous dose. Many veterinary and most human hospital laboratories can provide this service. The therapeutic serum concentration range is 1 to 2 (or 2.4) ng/ml. If the serum concentration is less than 0.8 ng/ml, the digoxin dose can be increased by up to 30% and the serum concentration measured the following week. However, a serum concentration in the middle to low therapeutic range is probably safer. People with high-normal serum digoxin concentrations are at greater risk of sudden death. If serum concentrations cannot be measured and toxicity is suspected, the drug should be discontinued for 1 to 2 days and then reinstituted at half the original dose.

Certain drugs affect serum digoxin concentrations when administered concurrently. Quinidine increases serum digoxin concentrations by displacing the drug from skeletal muscle binding sites and reducing its renal clearance. This drug combination therefore is not recommended; however, if both must be used, the digoxin dose is reduced by 50% initially and guided by serum concentration measurement. Other drugs known to increase the serum digoxin concentration are verapamil and amiodarone. Diltiazem, prazosin, spironolactone, and triamterene may increase the serum digoxin concentration. Hypokalemia especially, as well as other electrolyte and thyroid disturbances, can potentiate digoxin toxicity (see p. 69). Drugs affecting hepatic microsomal enzymes may also affect digoxin metabolism.

## Digitoxin

Digitoxin is well absorbed orally, is approximately 90% protein-bound in serum, and is lipid soluble. Its half-life in dogs is 8 to 12 hours. Digitoxin is cleared by the liver, although it appears to be tolerated in the presence of liver disease. Digitoxin has an extremely long half-life (over 100 hours) in the cat and is not used in this species. The drug has been given to large dogs twice daily and to small dogs three times daily to achieve a similar dosage per body surface area. Quinidine does not increase serum concentrations of digitoxin. The serum digitoxin concentration is measured 6 to 8 hours postdose; the therapeutic serum concentration is 15 to 35 ng/ml.

## Digitalis Toxicity

Myocardial toxicity from digitalis glycosides can cause almost any cardiac rhythm disturbance, including ventricular tachyarrhythmias, supraventricular premature complexes and tachycardia, sinus arrest, Mobitz type I second-degree AV block, and junctional rhythms. Myocardial toxicity can occur before any other signs and can lead to collapse and death, especially in animals with myocardial failure. Therefore the appearance of PR interval prolongation or signs of gastrointestinal toxicity should not be used to guide progressive dosing of digitalis. Rather, measurement of therapeutic serum concentrations and clinical improvement should guide therapy. Loading doses are not advised in the presence of myocardial failure. Digitalis can aggravate the cellular calcium overloading and electrical instability common in failing myocardial cells. It can stimulate spontaneous automaticity of myocardial cells by inducing and potentiating late afterdepolarizations; cellular stretch, calcium overloading, and hypokalemia enhance this effect. Toxic concentrations of digitalis also enhance automaticity by increasing sympathetic tone to the heart. Furthermore, the parasympathetic effects of slowed conduction and altered refractory period facilitate the development of reentrant arrhythmias. Digitalis intoxication should be suspected in patients taking the drug if ventricular arrhythmias and/or tachyarrhythmias with impaired conduction appear.

Gastrointestinal toxicity may develop before signs of myocardial toxicity. Signs include anorexia, depression, vomiting, borborygmus, and diarrhea. Some of these gastrointestinal signs result from the direct effects of digitalis on chemoreceptors in the area postrema of the medulla.

Hypokalemia predisposes to myocardial toxicity by leaving more available binding sites on membrane $Na^+$, $K^+$-ATPase for digitalis; conversely, hyperkalemia displaces digitalis from those binding sites. Hypercalcemia and hypernatremia potentiate both the inotropic and toxic effects of the drug.

Abnormal thyroid hormone concentrations can influence the response to digoxin. Hyperthyroidism may potentiate the myocardial effects of the drug. Hypothyroidism prolongs the half-life of digoxin in people but had no pharmacokinetic effect in one study using dogs. Hypoxia sensitizes the myocardium to the toxic effects of digitalis. Some drugs cause increased serum concentrations of various digitalis glycosides (see p. 68). In addition, alteration of hepatic and renal function may affect the clearance of these drugs.

Therapy for digitalis toxicity depends on its manifestations. Gastrointestinal signs usually respond to drug withdrawal and correction of fluid or electrolyte disturbances. AV conduction abnormalities also resolve after drug withdrawal, although sometimes anticholinergic therapy is needed. However, digitalis-induced ventricular tachycardia and frequent ventricular premature complexes should be treated vigorously. Lidocaine, the drug of choice, reduces sympathetic nervous tone and can suppress arrhythmias caused by reentry and late afterdepolarizations, but it has little effect on the sinus rate or AV nodal conduction. The second drug of choice in the dog is phenytoin (diphenylhydantoin), which has effects similar to those of lidocaine. Intravenous administration of phenytoin must be slow to avoid hypotension and myocardial depression caused by the propylene glycol vehicle. Phenytoin has occasionally been used orally to treat or prevent ventricular tachyarrhythmias caused by digitalis.

Other measures can also be beneficial for digitalis toxicity. Intravenous potassium supplementation is given if the serum potassium concentration is less than 4 mEq/L. Magnesium supplementation may also be effective in suppressing arrhythmias; magnesium sulfate has been used at 25 to 40 mg/kg slow IV bolus, followed by infusion of the same dose over 12 to 24 hours. Fluid therapy is indicated to correct dehydration and maximize renal function. In some cases, propranolol helps control ventricular tachyarrhythmias, but it is not used if AV conduction block is present. Quinidine should not be used because it increases the serum concentration of digitalis. Oral administration of the steroid-binding resin cholestyramine is useful only very soon after accidental overdose of digoxin because this drug undergoes minimal enterohepatic circulation. Much greater enterohepatic circulation occurs with digitoxin, which allows for increased binding to cholestyramine within the gut. A preparation of digoxin-specific antigen–binding fragments (digoxin-immune Fab) derived from ovine antidigoxin antibodies (Digibind, Burroughs-Wellcome, Research Triangle Park, N.C.) has occasionally been used for digoxin and digitoxin overdose. The Fab fragment binds with antigenic determinants on the digoxin molecule, preventing and reversing the pharmacologic and toxic effects of digoxin. The Fab fragment–digoxin complex is subsequently excreted by the kidneys. Each 38 mg vial binds about 0.6 mg of digoxin. The recommended human dose is:

$$\text{Number of vials needed} = \frac{(\text{Serum digoxin concentration [ng/ml]} \times \text{Body weight [kg]})}{100}$$

A modified formula taking into account the volume of distribution of digoxin in the dog (Senior and colleagues, 1991):

$$\text{Number of vials needed} = \frac{\text{Body load of digoxin (mg)}}{0.6 \text{ mg of digoxin}}$$

$$\text{Body load of digoxin} = \frac{(\text{Serum digoxin concentration [ng/ml]} \times 14 \text{ L/kg} \times \text{Body weight [kg]})}{1000}$$

## SYMPATHOMIMETIC AGENTS (CATECHOLAMINES)

Sympathomimetic agents act by binding to cardiac $\beta_1$-adrenergic receptors and activating adenylate cyclase, which increases the production of cAMP (see Tables 3-8 and 3-9). In turn, cAMP stimulates a protein kinase system that, by phosphorylation of certain membrane proteins, leads to increased calcium influx. Increased calcium availability during systole allows a stronger contraction. Because of their short half-life (less than 2 minutes) and extensive hepatic metabolism of the catecholamines used clinically, they are administered by constant IV infusion. Their long-term use is limited also by the development of $\beta_1$-receptor down-regulation. In general, these drugs are used for less than 3 days. Catecholamines also variably stimulate $\beta_2$- and $\alpha$-adrenergic receptors.

### Dopamine

Dopamine has less vasoconstrictor and chronotropic effects than norepinephrine, of which it is the precursor. At low doses (less than 2 to 5 $\mu$g/kg/min IV infusion), it stimulates vasodilator dopaminergic receptors in the renal, mesenteric, coronary, and cerebral circulations; it also stimulates $\beta$- and $\alpha$-receptors, especially at higher doses. Peripheral vasoconstriction occurs at 10 to 15 $\mu$g/kg/min and can help maintain blood pressure after cardiac arrest or in cardiogenic shock. At these higher dosages the heart rate, myocardial oxygen demand, and the risk of inducing ventricular arrhythmias also increase. Low-to-moderate doses are useful for increasing contractility and cardiac output in patients with acute myocardial failure. An initial IV dose of 1 µg/kg/min can be titrated upward to obtain the desired clinical effect. The infusion rate should be decreased if sinus tachycardia or other tachyarrhythmias develop. Dopamine is available as an injectable solution of several concentrations that is diluted in saline solution, 5% dextrose in water, or lactated Ringer's solution. For example, dilution of 40 mg of dopamine into 500 ml of fluid yields a solution of 80 µg/ml; a volume of 0.75 ml/kg/hr provides 1 µg/kg/min (also see Table 4-7 for constant rate infusion [CRI] calculation). The manufacturer's preparation and storage information should be reviewed. By increasing renal blood flow, dopamine may enhance the renal clearance of other drugs.

### Dobutamine

A synthetic analog of dopamine, dobutamine is used for short-term inotropic support in animals with severe myocardial failure. It stimulates $\beta_1$-receptors but has only weak action on $\beta_2$- and $\alpha$-receptors; it does not stimulate dopaminergic receptors. The drug increases contractility with minimal effects on heart rate and blood pressure at lower infusion rates (3 to 7 µg/kg/min). Although less arrhythmogenic than other catecholamines, at higher rates (10 to 20 µg/kg/min) it may precipitate supraventricular and ventricular arrhythmias. The initial infusion rate should be low and can be gradually increased over hours to achieve greater inotropic effect; the heart rate and rhythm should be closely monitored. Dilution of 250 mg dobutamine into 500 ml of fluid yields 500 µg of dobutamine per milliliter. An infusion rate of 0.6 ml/kg/hr provides 5 µg/kg/min (also see Table 4-7 for CRI calculation). Cats are more sensitive to dobutamine than dogs and may exhibit seizures or other adverse effects at relatively low doses.

### Epinephrine

Epinephrine has strong stimulating effects on $\alpha$- and $\beta$-receptors and causes increased blood pressure, heart rate, and contractility. It is very arrhythmogenic, which, combined with its effects on blood pressure and heart rate, makes it unsuitable for inotropic support in patients with heart failure. However, epinephrine is the drug of choice for resuscitation after cardiac arrest (see Table 5-1).

### Other Catecholamines

Isoproterenol stimulates $\beta$-receptors, thereby increasing heart rate, contractility, and cardiac output. This drug decreases blood pressure and is quite arrhythmogenic. It should not be used in patients with heart failure, and it is contraindicated for cardiac arrest because of its hypotensive effects. Isoproterenol has been used for symptomatic AV block refractory to atropine (see p. 86).

Norepinephrine, methoxamine, and others (see Table 5-1) are strong stimulators of $\alpha$-adrenergic receptors that increase contractility but also increase blood pressure. These potent $\alpha$-agonists are sometimes used as pressor agents; they are not indicated for treatment of heart failure.

## PHOSPHODIESTERASE INHIBITORS

Bipyridine compounds such as amrinone and milrinone inhibit phosphodiesterase III, an intracellular enzyme that degrades cAMP (see Tables 3-8 and 3-9). Increased myocardial cAMP leads to greater $Ca^{++}$ influx and greater contractility. These drugs cause vasodilation because increased cAMP reduces $Ca^{++}$ uptake and promotes relaxation in vascular smooth muscle. Much of the clinical benefit of these agents may come from the vasodilating effects. Higher doses can cause hypotension, tachycardia, and GI signs. Improvements in contractility of 40% to 200% have been reported in dogs with experimentally induced myocardial failure.

### Amrinone

Amrinone's effects are short-lived (less than 30 minutes) after IV injection in normal dogs, therefore constant infusions are required for sustained effect. Peak effects occur after 45 minutes of constant infusion in dogs. Amrinone has a relatively wide margin of safety in people, although it may exacerbate ventricular arrhythmias. The drug is used only for short-term inotropic support in dogs and cats with myocardial failure. An initial slow intravenous bolus is followed by a constant infusion (see Table 3-8). One half the original bolus dose can be repeated after 20 to 30 minutes.

### Milrinone

Milrinone is much more potent (10 to 30 times) than amrinone. During clinical investigations it was shown to be an effective inotropic agent in normal dogs and in dogs with heart failure, but it is not available in oral form. An intravenous form is marketed for acute use in people. It appears to be a relatively safe drug, but it exacerbates ventricular tachyarrhythmias in some animals. Milrinone was associated with decreased long-term survival in human trials. Higher doses increase the heart rate. Peak effects occur within 30 minutes of initiating constant infusion. Milrinone's effects last less than 30 minutes after intravenous bolus. Oral administration (0.5 to 1 mg/kg) in dogs with myocardial failure resulted in clinical, hemodynamic, and echocardiographic improvement during clinical trials. However, there is little veterinary experience with IV milrinone.

### Pimobendan

Pimobendan is a different phosphodiesterase inhibitor that causes arterial dilation and venodilation, as well as positive inotropic effects. It also has a calcium-sensitizing effect on the myocardium. This drug may additionally have favorable effects on myocardial oxygen requirements and diastolic function. The drug is available for oral administration in Europe and appears to cause marked clinical improvement in some dogs with myocardial failure. Clinical veterinary trials are ongoing.

## CALCIUM ENTRY BLOCKERS

Calcium entry blockers as a group can cause coronary and systemic vasodilation, enhanced myocardial relaxation, and reduced cardiac contractility. Some of these agents have antiarrhythmic effects by their action on the slow inward $Ca^{++}$ current. As such, they comprise the class IV antiarrhythmic drugs and are discussed further on p. 94. The calcium entry blockers are potentially useful for treating hypertrophic cardiomyopathy, hypertension, and myocardial ischemia. Diltiazem is the calcium entry blocker used most for feline hypertrophic cardiomyopathy (see Table 4-5). Amlodipine is also used in chronic heart failure as an adjunctive vasodilator (see Table 3-6). It has been used for this purpose in people without increasing cardiovascular mortality.

### Suggested Readings

PATHOPHYSIOLOGY OF HEART FAILURE

Asano K et al: Plasma atrial and brain natriuretic peptide levels in dogs with congestive heart failure, *J Vet Med Sci* 61:523, 1999.

Biondo AW et al: Genomic sequence and cardiac expression of atrial natriuretic peptide in cats, *Am J Vet Res* 63:236, 2002.

Burger AJ et al: Activity of the neurohormonal system and its relationship to autonomic abnormalities in decompensated heart failure, *J Card Fail* 7:122, 2001.

Constable P et al: Clinical assessment of left ventricular relaxation, *J Vet Intern Med* 13:5, 1999.

Francis GS: Pathophysiology of chronic heart failure, *Am J Med* 110:37S, 2001.

Haggstrom J et al: Effects of naturally acquired decompensated mitral valve regurgitation on the renin-angiotensin-aldosterone system and atrial natriuretic peptide concentration in dogs, *Am J Vet Res* 58:77, 1997.

Kramer GA et al: Plasma taurine concentrations in normal dogs and in dogs with heart disease, *J Vet Intern Med* 9:253, 1995.

Meredith IT et al: Cardiac sympathetic nervous activity in congestive heart failure, *Circulation* 88:136, 1993.

Pedersen HD et al: Activation of the renin-angiotensin system in dogs with asymptomatic and mildly symptomatic mitral valvular insufficiency, *J Vet Intern Med* 9:328, 1995.

Sanderson SL et al: Effects of dietary fat and L-carnitine on plasma and whole blood taurine concentrations and cardiac function in healthy dogs fed protein-restricted diets, *Am J Vet Res* 62:1616, 2001.

Turk JR: Physiologic and pathophysiologic effects of natriuretic peptides and their implication in cardiopulmonary disease, *J Am Vet Med Assoc* 216:1970, 2000.

Weber KT: Aldosterone in congestive heart failure, *N Engl J Med* 345:1689, 2001.

THERAPY OF HEART FAILURE

Adin DB et al: Efficacy of a single oral dose of isosorbide 5-mononitrate in normal dogs and in dogs with congestive heart failure, *J Vet Intern Med* 15:105, 2001.

Atkins CE et al: Effect of aspirin, furosemide, and commercial low-salt diet on digoxin pharmacokinetic properties in clinically normal cats, *J Am Vet Med Assoc* 193:1264, 1988.

Atkins CE et al: Effects of compensated heart failure on digoxin pharmacokinetics in cats, *J Am Vet Med Assoc* 195:945, 1989.

Bristow MR: β-Adrenergic receptor blockade in chronic heart failure, *Circulation* 101:558, 2000.

COVE Study Group: Controlled clinical evaluation of enalapril in dogs with heart failure: results of the Cooperative Veterinary Study Group, *J Vet Intern Med* 9:243, 1995.

Davidson G: Enalapril maleate, *Compend Contin Educ Small Anim Pract* 21:1118, 1999.

Ettinger SJ et al: Effects of enalapril maleate on survival of dogs with naturally acquired heart failure, *J Am Vet Med Assoc* 213:1573, 1998.

Freeman LM et al: Nutritional alterations and the effect of fish oil supplementation in dogs with heart failure, *J Vet Intern Med* 12:440, 1998.

Garg R et al: The effects of digoxin on mortality and morbidity in patients with heart failure, *N Engl J Med* 336:525, 1997.

Hamlin RL: Carvedilol. *Proceedings of the 19th ACVIM Forum,* Denver, 2001, p 104.

Hamlin RL et al: Effects of enalapril on exercise tolerance and longevity in dogs with heart failure produced by iatrogenic mitral regurgitation, *J Vet Intern Med* 10:85, 1996.

Hamlin RL et al: Comparison of some pharmacokinetic parameters of 5 angiotensin-converting enzyme inhibitors in normal Beagles, *J Vet Intern Med* 12:93, 1998.

Hoffman RL et al: Vitamin C inhibits endothelial cell apoptosis in congestive heart failure, *Circulation* 104:2182, 2001.

Hornig B et al: Physical training improves endothelial function in patients with chronic heart failure, *Circulation* 93:210, 1996.

IMPROVE Study Group: Acute and short-term hemodynamic, echocardiographic, and clinical effects of enalapril maleate in dogs with naturally acquired heart failure: results of the Invasive Multicenter Prospective Veterinary Evaluation of Enalapril study, *J Vet Intern Med* 9:234, 1995.

Keister DM et al: Milrinone: a clinical trial in 29 dogs with moderate-to-severe congestive heart failure, *J Vet Intern Med* 4:79, 1990.

Khatta M et al: The effect of coenzyme Q10 in patients with congestive heart failure, *Ann Intern Med* 132:636, 2000.

King JN et al: Pharmacokinetics of the active metabolite of benazepril, benazeprilat, and inhibition of plasma angiotensin-converting enzyme activity after single and repeated administration to dogs, *Am J Vet Res* 56:1620, 1995.

King JN et al: Pharmacokinetics of benazepril and inhibition of plasma ACE activity in cats, *J Vet Intern Med* 10:163, 1996 (abstract).

Kittleson MD et al: The acute hemodynamic effects of milrinone in dogs with severe idiopathic myocardial failure, *J Vet Intern Med* 1:121, 1987.

Kvart C et al: Efficacy of enalapril for prevention of congestive heart failure in dogs with myxomatous valve disease and asymptomatic mitral regurgitation, *J Vet Intern Med* 16:80, 2002.

Lee SC et al: Iron supplementation inhibits cough associated with ACE inhibitors, *Hypertension* 38:166, 2001.

Lefebvre HP et al: Effects of renal impairment on the disposition of orally administered enalapril, benazepril and their active metabolites, *J Vet Intern Med* 13:21, 1999.

Lovern CS et al: Additive effects of a sodium chloride restricted diet and furosemide administration in healthy dogs, *Am J Vet Res* 62:1793, 2001.

Packer M: Current role of β-adrenergic blockers in the management of chronic heart failure, *Am J Med* 110:81S, 2001.

Parameswaran N et al: Increased splenic capacity in response to transdermal application of nitroglycerine in the dog, *J Vet Intern Med* 13:44, 1999.

Pion PD et al: The effectiveness of taurine and levocarnitine in dogs with heart disease, *Vet Clin North Am Small Anim Pract* 28:1495, 1998.

Pouchelon JL et al: Treatment of heart failure in dogs with benazepril: results of European double blind placebo controlled study, *J Vet Intern Med* 10:163, 1996 (abstract).

Roudebush P et al: The effect of combined therapy with captopril, furosemide, and a sodium-restricted diet on serum electrolyte levels and renal function in normal dogs and dogs with congestive heart failure, *J Vet Intern Med* 8:337, 1994.

Rush JE et al: Clinical, echocardiographic and neurohormonal effects of a sodium-restricted diet in dogs with heart failure, *J Vet Intern Med* 14:512, 2000.

Sanders N et al: Effects of enalapril on healthy cats, *J Vet Intern Med* 6:139, 1992 (abstract).

Senior DF et al: Treatment of acute digoxin toxicosis with digoxin immune Fab (ovine), *J Vet Intern Med* 5:302, 1991.

Snyder PS et al: Digoxin pharmacokinetics in dogs with experimental hypothyroidism, *J Vet Intern Med* 7:137, 1993 (abstract).

Straeter-Knowlen IM et al: ACE inhibitors in HF restore canine pulmonary endothelial function and ANGII vasoconstriction, *Am Physiol Soc* 277:H1924, 1999.

Ward DM et al: Treatment of severe chronic digoxin toxicosis in a dog with cardiac disease using ovine digoxin-specific immunoglobulin G Fab fragments, *J Am Vet Med Assoc* 215:1808, 1999.

# CHAPTER 4

## Cardiac Rhythm Disturbances and Antiarrhythmic Therapy

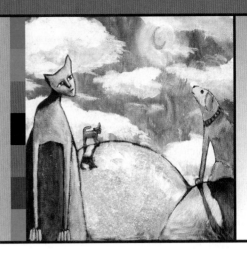

### CHAPTER OUTLINE

GENERAL CONSIDERATIONS, 73
COMMON HEART RHYTHM ABNORMALITIES, 74
    Irregular tachyarrhythmias and pulse deficits, 75
    Rapid, regular rhythms, 83
    Bradyarrhythmias, 84
ANTIARRHYTHMIC DRUGS, 86
    Class I antiarrhythmic drugs, 87
    Class II antiarrhythmic drugs: β-adrenergic blockers, 91
    Class III antiarrhythmic drugs, 93
    Class IV antiarrhythmic drugs: calcium entry
      blockers, 94
    Anticholinergic drugs, 95
    Sympathomimetic drugs, 96
    Other drugs, 96

## GENERAL CONSIDERATIONS

Cardiac arrhythmias occur for many reasons. Although some arrhythmias are of no clinical consequence, others cause serious hemodynamic compromise and sudden death, especially in animals with underlying heart disease. In order to make the best therapeutic decisions, it is important not only to make an accurate ECG diagnosis, but also to consider the arrhythmia's clinical context. It is well known that the risk of death associated with ventricular tachyarrhythmias in people is higher when myocardial function is impaired. Dogs with cardiomyopathy also have increased risk for sudden death, especially Doberman Pinschers and Boxers. An inherited disorder predisposing to sudden death has also been identified in young German Shepherds. On the other hand, in previously healthy animals, the ventricular ectopy common after thoracic trauma (see p. 118) generally resolves without therapy. Occasional ventricular premature complexes have also been identified in healthy animals. However, arrhythmias that compromise cardiac output and coronary perfusion can promote myocardial ischemia, deterioration of cardiac pump function, and sometimes sudden death. These arrhythmias tend to be either very rapid (e.g., sustained ventricular or supraventricular tachyar-

rhythmias) or very slow (e.g., advanced AV block with a slow or unstable ventricular escape rhythm). Sometimes, however, a lethal arrhythmia such as ventricular fibrillation may occur without antecedent sustained arrhythmia. Rapid, sustained tachycardia of either supraventricular or ventricular origin reduces cardiac output acutely and eventually leads to myocardial dysfunction and congestive heart failure.

Multiple factors underlie the development of cardiac rhythm disturbances. Abnormalities of conduction or automaticity caused by cardiac structural or physiologic remodeling can predispose to arrhythmias, even in the absence of overt cardiac disease. Genetic factors and environmental stresses contribute to this. However, to provoke and sustain a rhythm disturbance, additional triggering (e.g., premature stimulus or abrupt change in heart rate) and/or modulating factors (e.g., changes in autonomic tone, circulating catecholamines, ischemia, or electrolyte disturbances) are thought to be necessary. For example, episodes of anger or aggressive behavior have been linked to increased susceptibility to ischemic arrhythmias and sudden arrhythmic death in both dogs and people. Increasing attention also is being focused on the relation between various stresses that lead to remodeling of heart tissue and the development of arrhythmias. Such remodeling can involve myocyte hypertrophy, changes in the structure or function of ion channels, tissue fibrosis, or the activity of the autonomic nervous system.

Although some remodeling changes act as beneficial compensatory mechanisms in the short term, they can have harmful and arrhythmogenic long-term effects. If the underlying arrhythmogenic modulators that cause cardiac structural and functional remodeling can be controlled, arrhythmias should be lessened. Such modulators include catecholamines, free radicals, angiotensin II, ACE, cytokines, and nitric oxide. The increased survival in human heart failure patients whose therapy includes ACE inhibitors (ACEI), spironolactone, and/or some β-blockers supports this approach. There is similar evidence for ACEI in dogs with dilated cardiomyopathy (DCM), and there is reason to suspect that the other therapies would be beneficial as well.

If antiarrhythmic drug therapy is contemplated, its goals should be defined. An immediate goal is to restore hemodynamic stability. Although the ideal goals include conversion to sinus rhythm, correction of the underlying cause, and prevention of further arrhythmia and sudden death, suppression of all abnormal beats is generally not a realistic goal. Successful therapy may imply sufficient reduction in frequency (e.g. by ≥70% to 80%) or repetitive rate of ectopic beats to promote normal hemodynamics and eliminate clinical signs. However, even with apparently complete conversion to sinus rhythm, the risk of sudden death from a lethal arrhythmia may remain.

Various arrhythmias and their ECG characteristics are described in Chapter 2. A general approach to managing cardiac rhythm disturbances is provided here, recognizing that much remains to be learned about effective arrhythmia management and the prevention of sudden death.

1. Record and interpret an ECG (Table 4-1); identify and define any arrhythmia. An extended ECG recording period may be needed (e.g., Holter monitor or prolonged in-hospital monitoring).
2. Evaluate the whole patient, including the history, physical examination findings, and clinical/laboratory test results.

Are signs of hemodynamic impairment evident (e.g., episodic weakness, syncope, signs of congestive heart failure)? Are other signs of cardiac disease present (e.g., heart murmur, cardiomegaly)? Are there additional abnormalities (e.g., fever, abnormal blood chemistry values, respiratory or other extracardiac disease, trauma)? Is the animal receiving any medications? Correct what can be corrected.

3. Decide whether to use antiarrhythmic drug therapy. Consider the signalment, history, clinical signs, and underlying disease, as well as the potential benefits/risks of the drug(s) being contemplated.
4. If an antiarrhythmic drug is to be used, define the goals of therapy for this patient.
5. Initiate treatment and determine drug effectiveness. Adjust dose or try alternate agents if needed.
6. Monitor patient status. Assess arrhythmia control (consider repeated Holter monitoring), manage underlying disease(s), and watch for adverse drug effects and other complications.

## COMMON HEART RHYTHM ABNORMALITIES

Table 4-2 lists common arrhythmias according to a clinical description of the heartbeat. Cardiac arrhythmias in a given animal often occur inconsistently and are influenced by drug therapy, prevailing autonomic tone, baroreceptor reflexes, and variations in heart rate. Treatment decisions are based on

 TABLE 4-1

**Guide for ECG Interpretation**

1. Determine the heart rate. Is it too fast, too slow, or normal?
2. Is the rhythm regular or irregular?
3. Is sinus rhythm present (with or without other abnormalities), or are there no consistent P-QRS-T relationships?
4. Are all P waves followed by a QRS and all QRS complexes preceded by a P wave?
5. If premature (early) complexes are present, do they look the same as sinus QRS complexes (implying atrial or junctional [supraventricular] origin), or are they wide and of different configuration than sinus complexes (implying a ventricular origin or possibly abnormal ventricular conduction of a supraventricular complex)?
6. Are premature QRS complexes preceded by an abnormal P wave (suggesting atrial origin)?
7. Are there baseline undulations instead of clear and consistent P waves, with a rapid, irregular QRS occurrence (compatible with atrial fibrillation)?
8. Are there long pauses in the underlying rhythm before an abnormal complex occurs (escape beat)?
9. Is an intermittent AV conduction disturbance present?
10. Is there no consistent relation between P waves and QRS complexes, with a slow and regular QRS occurrence (implying complete AV block with escape rhythm)?
11. For sinus and supraventricular complexes, is the frontal axis normal?
12. Are all measurements and waveform durations within normal limits?

Please refer to Chapter 2 for more specific information.

 TABLE 4-2

**Differential Diagnoses for Common Heart Rate and Rhythm Disturbances**

**Slow, Irregular Rhythms**

Sinus bradyarrhythmia
Sinus arrest
Sick sinus syndrome
High-grade second-degree AV block

**Slow, Regular Rhythms**

Sinus bradycardia
Complete AV block with ventricular escape rhythm
Atrial standstill with ventricular escape rhythm

**Fast, Irregular Rhythms**

Atrial or supraventricular premature contractions
Paroxysmal atrial or supraventricular tachycardia
Atrial flutter or fibrillation
Ventricular premature contractions
Paroxysmal ventricular tachycardia

**Fast, Regular Rhythms**

Sinus tachycardia
Sustained supraventricular tachycardia
Sustained ventricular tachycardia

consideration of the origin (supraventricular or ventricular), timing (premature or escape), and severity of the rhythm disturbance, as well as the clinical context. Correct ECG interpretation is obviously important. Although a routine (resting) ECG documents arrhythmias present during the recording period, it provides only a glimpse of the cardiac rhythms occurring over the course of a day. Because arrhythmias can have marked variation in frequency and severity over time, potentially critical arrhythmias can easily be missed. For this reason, Holter monitoring or other forms of extended ECG acquisition are useful in assessing the severity and frequency of arrhythmias and for monitoring treatment efficacy. Some rhythm abnormalities do not require therapy, whereas others demand immediate, aggressive treatment. Close patient monitoring is especially important in animals with more serious arrhythmias.

## IRREGULAR TACHYARRHYTHMIAS AND PULSE DEFICITS

Irregular heart rhythms are common, and the ECG is important for differentiating abnormal rhythms as well as sinus arrhythmia. Pulse deficits and an irregular, weak pulse with heart sounds of varying intensity and regularity may be detected during physical examination. A pulse deficit occurs when cardiac contraction does not cause a palpable pulse; early contractions interrupt ventricular filling and reduce the resulting stroke volume. Ventricular filling may be so inadequate that there is no semilunar valve opening and ejection for that cycle (Fig. 4-1). Rapid atrial fibrillation and premature contractions of any origin often cause pulse deficits. Ventricular premature complexes (VPCs) can cause audible splitting of the heart sounds because of asynchronous ventricular activation. Ventricular and supraventricular tachycardias and atrial fibrillation cause more severe hemodynamic compromise than isolated premature contractions do. Sustained, rapid arrhythmias lead to decreases in cardiac output, arterial blood pressure, and coronary perfusion; eventually, congestive and/or low-output heart failure can result. Signs of poor cardiac output and hypotension include weakness, depression, pallor, capillary refill time prolongation, exercise intolerance, syncope, dyspnea, prerenal azotemia, worsening rhythm disturbances and, sometimes, altered mentation, seizure activity, and sudden death.

### Premature Contractions and Paroxysmal Tachycardias

Frequent premature contractions and paroxysmal tachycardias can compromise ventricular filling, especially if underlying heart disease exists. Supraventricular tachyarrhythmias can result from various mechanisms, including reentry involving

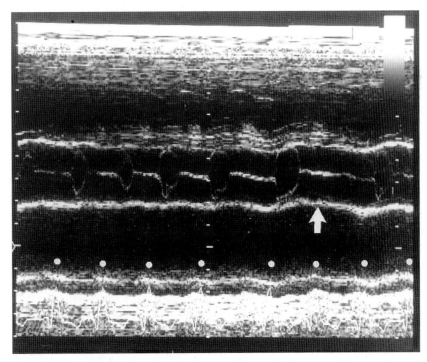

**FIG 4-1**
M-mode echocardiogram at the aortic root level in a Doberman Pinscher with atrial fibrillation and dilated cardiomyopathy. Pulse deficits and variable-intensity pulses occurred secondary to the variable (or absent) aortic valve opening caused by the arrhythmia and illustrated in this echocardiogram. The motion of two aortic valve leaflets is seen within the parallel aortic root echoes. Most cycles are associated with variable and poor stroke volume and with abbreviated aortic valve opening, but there is no opening at all after the sixth QRS complex from the left *(arrow)*. R waves are indicated by white dots.

## TABLE 4-3

Factors Predisposing to Arrhythmias

| | |
|---|---|
| **Atrial Arrhythmias**<br>***Cardiac*** | **Ventricular Arrhythmias—cont'd**<br>***Cardiac—cont'd*** |

**Atrial Arrhythmias**
***Cardiac***

Mitral or tricuspid insufficiency
Dilated cardiomyopathy
Hypertrophic cardiomyopathy
Restrictive cardiomyopathy
Cardiac neoplasia
Congenital malformation
Accessory AV nodal bypass tract(s)
Myocardial fibrosis
High sympathetic tone
Digitalis glycosides
Other drugs (anesthetic agents, bronchodilators)
Ischemia
Intraatrial catheter placement

***Extracardiac***

Catecholamines
Electrolyte imbalances
Acidosis/alkalosis
Hypoxia
Thyrotoxicosis
Severe anemia
Electric shock
Thoracic surgery

**Ventricular Arrhythmias**
***Cardiac***

Congestive heart failure
Cardiomyopathy (especially Doberman Pinschers and Boxers)
Myocarditis
Pericarditis
Degenerative valvular disease with myocardial fibrosis
Ischemia

**Ventricular Arrhythmias—cont'd**
***Cardiac—cont'd***

Trauma
Cardiac neoplasia
Heartworm disease
Congenital heart disease
Ventricular dilation
Mechanical stimulation (intracardiac catheter, pacing wire)
Drugs (digitalis, sympathomimetics, anesthetics, tranquilizers, anticholinergics, antiarrhythmics)

***Extracardiac***

Hypoxia
Electrolyte imbalances (especially $K^+$)
Acidosis/alkalosis
Thyrotoxicosis
Hypothermia
Fever
Sepsis/toxemia
Trauma (thoracic or abdominal)
Gastric dilation/volvulus
Splenic mass or splenectomy
Hemangiosarcoma
Pulmonary disease
Uremia
Pancreatitis
Pheochromocytoma
Other endocrine diseases (diabetes mellitus, Addison's disease, hypothyroidism)
High sympathetic tone (pain, anxiety, fever)
Central nervous system disease (increases in sympathetic or vagal stimulation)
Electric shock

---

the AV node, accessory pathways, or SA node, as well as ectopic foci within atrial or junctional tissue. Many are associated with atrial enlargement. Common underlying heart diseases include chronic mitral or tricuspid valve degeneration with regurgitation, dilated cardiomyopathy, congenital malformations, and cardiac neoplasia. Other factors also may predispose to atrial tachyarrhythmias (Table 4-3).

Ventricular premature contractions are associated with disorders that affect cardiac tissue directly or indirectly through neurohormonal effects (see Table 4-3). For instance, central nervous system disease can produce abnormal neural effects on the heart and cause ventricular or supraventricular arrhythmias (brain-heart syndrome). Adverse hemodynamic effects may be clinically insignificant when VPCs are infrequent or underlying cardiac function is normal. However, hemodynamic impairment can be severe in dogs or cats with underlying heart disease, rapid ventricular rates, or myocardial depression stemming from a systemic disease. Correct-

ing underlying hypoxia, electrolyte or acid-base imbalances, or abnormal hormone concentrations (e.g., thyroid) or discontinuing certain drugs may be important for arrhythmia control.

**Treatment of supraventricular premature contractions and tachycardia.** Occasional premature beats do not require specific therapy. If possible, factors that predispose to these arrhythmias should be minimized (e.g., discontinue or reduce dosage of suspect drugs, manage heart failure if present, and correct metabolic abnormalities). Digoxin (see Table 3-8) is usually the initial PO drug of choice for treating frequent atrial premature contractions or paroxysmal atrial tachycardia in dogs with heart failure and cats with dilated cardiomyopathy (Fig. 4-2). A β-blocker or the calcium entry blocker diltiazem (Table 4-4) may be added to the regimen if the arrhythmia is not controlled with digoxin plus an ACEI and furosemide for heart failure. Cats with hypertrophic cardiomyopathy or hyperthyroidism are usually

**SUPRAVENTRICULAR TACHYARRHYTHMIAS**

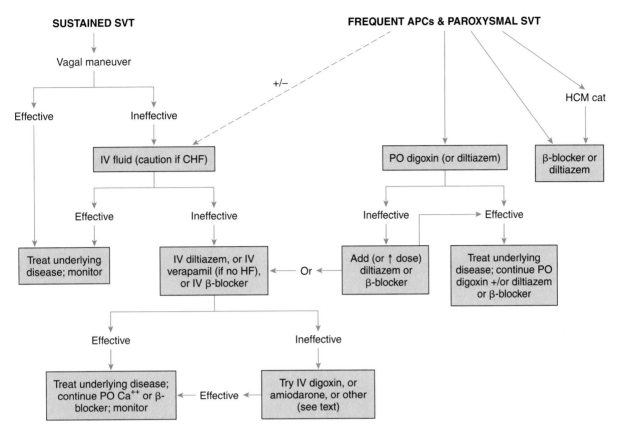

**FIG 4-2**

A therapeutic approach to supraventricular tachyarrhythmias. See Table 4-5 for drug doses and text for more information. *APCs,* Atrial premature contractions; *CHF,* congestive heart failure; *HCM,* hypertrophic cardiomyopathy; *HF,* heart failure or significant underlying cardiac disease; *SVT,* supraventricular tachycardia.

given a β-adrenergic blocker such as atenolol or propranolol, although diltiazem is an alternative (Table 4-5).

More aggressive initial therapy is warranted for patients with rapid and persistent supraventricular tachyarrhythmias, especially in the face of hemodynamic impairment. The calcium channel blocker diltiazem (IV or PO loading) is preferred because of its lesser negative inotropic effects. Verapamil (IV) can be very effective against supraventricular tachycardias but is not recommended for dogs with myocardial dysfunction or heart failure because of its greater negative inotropic effects. A β-blocker given slowly IV (propranolol, esmolol) is an alternative therapy, but it also has negative inotropic effects in animals with high underlying sympathetic tone. IV digoxin also can be used, but it has been less effective than the calcium channel blockers. Digoxin has a slower onset of action, and although it increases vagal tone, its IV administration can also increase central sympathetic output. Once the rhythm has been better controlled, maintenance doses of PO digoxin and/or diltiazem or a β-blocker are options for chronic therapy. Amiodarone could be an alternative agent in cases refractory to conventional drugs.

Paroxysmal AV reciprocating tachycardia, which is a reentrant tachycardia involving an accessory pathway and the AV node (see p. 21) is interrupted by slowing conduction or prolonging the refractory period of either or both tissues. β-Blockers and diltiazem slow AV conduction and increase refractoriness. Digoxin slows AV conduction but has variable effects on the accessory pathway; its use tends to be avoided in people with preexcitation syndromes. Procainamide and quinidine (see Table 4-5) may prevent AV reciprocating tachycardia because they lengthen the refractory period of the accessory pathway. High-dose procainamide, with or without a β-blocker or diltiazem, has been successful in preventing the recurrence of tachycardia in some cases. Class IC and class III antiarrhythmic agents are also used in people with ventricular preexcitation, but experience in dogs is limited (see Table 4-4). Intracardiac electrophysiologic mapping and radiofrequency catheter ablation of accessory pathways has been successful in abolishing refractory supraventricular tachycardia associated with preexcitation in dogs (Wright and colleagues, 1999). Although of limited availability, this technique provides a therapeutic alternative for dogs with nonresponsive tachycardias and tachycardia-induced congestive heart failure.

TABLE 4-4

Classes and Effects of Antiarrhythmic Drugs

| CLASS | DRUG | MECHANISM AND ECG EFFECTS |
|---|---|---|
| I | | Decreases fast inward $Na^+$ current; membrane-stabilizing effects (decreased conductivity, excitability, and automaticity) |
| IA | Quinidine<br>Procainamide<br>Disopyramide | Moderately decreases conductivity, increases action potential duration; can prolong QRS complex and Q-T interval |
| IB | Lidocaine<br>Mexiletine<br>Tocainide<br>Phenytoin | Little change in conductivity, decreases action potential duration; QRS complex and Q-T interval unchanged |
| IC | Flecainide<br>Encainide<br>Propafenone | Markedly decreases conductivity without changing action potential duration |
| II | Propranolol<br>Atenolol<br>Esmolol<br>Metoprolol<br>Carvedilol<br>Others | β-Adrenergic blockade—reduces effects of sympathetic stimulation (no direct myocardial effects at clinical doses) |
| III | Sotalol<br>Amiodarone<br>Bretylium<br>Ibutilide<br>Dofetilide<br>Others | Selectively prolongs action potential duration and refractory period; antiadrenergic effects; Q-T interval prolonged |
| IV | Verapamil<br>Diltiazem<br>Others | Decreases slow inward $Ca^{++}$ current (greatest effects on sinoatrial and AV nodes) |

**Other Antiarrhythmic Agents**

| | | |
|---|---|---|
| | Digoxin | Antiarrhythmic action results mainly from indirect autonomic effects (especially increased vagal tone) |
| | Atropine | Anticholinergic agents oppose vagal effects on SA and AV nodes (glycopyrrolate and other drugs also have this effect) |
| | Adenosine | Briefly opens $K^+$ channels and indirectly slows $Ca^{++}$ current (strongest effects on sinoatrial and AV nodes); can transiently block AV conduction |

**Acute treatment of VPCs and ventricular tachycardia.** There is controversy over whether, when, and how to treat ventricular tachyarrhythmias. Antiarrhythmic drugs can have serious adverse effects, can provoke additional arrhythmias (proarrhythmic effects), and may not be efficacious. Several factors influence the decision on whether to use an antiarrhythmic drug. These include the nature of the animal's underlying disease, the perceived severity of the arrhythmia, and whether hemodynamic compromise is evident. Because diseases such as dilated cardiomyopathy, "Boxer cardiomyopathy," hypertrophic cardiomyopathy, and subaortic stenosis, among others, are frequently associated with sudden death from arrhythmias, ventricular antiarrhythmic therapy would appear most urgent in animals with these diseases. However, it is difficult to accurately assess the apparent efficacy of a particular therapy. Furthermore, it is not known whether such therapy actually prolongs survival. Pretreatment and posttreatment 24- to 48-hour ambulatory ECG recordings showing at least a 70% to 80% reduction in arrhythmia frequency provide the best indicator of drug arrhythmia-suppression efficacy. Intermittent ECG recordings cannot truly differentiate between drug effect (or lack thereof) and the spontaneous, marked variability of arrhythmia frequency that occurs in any individual. However, in-hospital ECG recordings of 15 seconds to several minutes in duration are often the most practical attempt to monitor arrhythmias. The following guidelines are offered with these issues and limitations in mind.

Occasional VPCs in an otherwise asymptomatic animal are usually not treated. Moderately frequent (e.g., 20 to 40/min), single VPCs of uniform configuration may not require antiar-

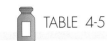

TABLE 4-5

Dosage of Antiarrhythmic Drugs

| AGENT | DOSAGE |
|---|---|
| **Class I** | |
| Lidocaine | Dog: Initial boluses of 2 mg/kg slowly IV, up to 8 mg/kg; or rapid IV infusion at 0.8 mg/kg/min; if effective, then 25 to 80 μg/kg/min CRI (see Table 4-7); can also be used intratracheally for CPR<br>Cat: Initial bolus of 0.25 to 0.5 mg/kg slowly IV; can repeat at a dose of 0.15 to 0.25 mg/kg in 5 to 20 min; if effective, 10 to 20 μg/kg/min CRI |
| Procainamide | Dog: 6 to 10 (up to 20) mg/kg IV over 5 to 10 min; 10 to 50 μg/kg/min CRI; 6 to 20 (up to 30) mg/kg q4-6h IM; 10 to 25 mg/kg q6h PO (sustained release: q6-8h)<br>Cat: 1 to 2 mg/kg slowly IV; 10 to 20 μg/kg/min CRI; 7.5 to 20 mg/kg q(6 to)8h IM or PO |
| Quinidine | Dog: 6 to 20 mg/kg q6h IM (loading dose, 14 to 20 mg/kg); 6 to 16 mg/kg q6h PO; sustained action preparations, 8 to 20 mg/kg q8h PO<br>Cat: 6 to 16 mg/kg q8h IM or PO |
| Tocainide | Dog: 10 to 20 (to 25) mg/kg q8h PO<br>Cat: — |
| Mexiletine | Dog: 4 to 10 mg/kg q8h PO<br>Cat: — |
| Phenytoin | Dog: 10 mg/kg slowly IV; 30 to 50 mg/kg q8h PO<br>Cat: Do not use |
| **Class II** | |
| Propranolol | Dog: 0.02 mg/kg initial bolus slowly IV (up to maximum of 0.1 mg/kg); initial dose, 0.1 to 0.2 mg/kg q8h PO, up to 1 mg/kg q8h<br>Cat: Same IV instructions; 2.5 up to 10 mg/cat q8-12h PO |
| Atenolol | Dog: 0.2 to 1 mg/kg q12-24h PO<br>Cat: 6.25 to 12.5 mg/cat q(12 to)24h PO |
| Esmolol | Dog: 200 to 500 μg/kg IV over 1 min (loading dose), followed by infusion of 25 to 200 μg/kg/min<br>Cat: Same |
| Metoprolol | Dog: initial dose, 0.2 mg/kg q8h PO, up to 1 mg/kg q8h<br>Cat: — |
| Nadolol | Dog: initial dose, 0.2 mg/kg q8-12h PO, up to 1 mg/kg q8-12h<br>Cat: — |
| **Class III** | |
| Sotalol | Dog: 1 to 3.5 mg/kg q12h PO<br>Cat: — |
| Amiodarone | Dog: 10 mg/kg q12h PO for 7 days, then 8 mg/kg q24h PO (higher doses have been used); 3 to 5 mg/kg slowly IV (can repeat but do not give more than 10 mg/kg in 1 hour)<br>Cat: — |
| Bretylium | Dog: 2 to 6 mg/kg IV; can repeat in 1 to 2 hr (humans)<br>Cat: — |
| **Class IV** | |
| Diltiazem | Dog: Initial dose, 0.5 mg/kg q8h PO up to 2 mg/kg; for atrial tachycardia, 0.15 to 0.25 mg/kg over 2 to 3 min IV (can repeat q15min until conversion or maximum dose of 0.75 mg/kg), or 0.5 mg/kg PO followed by 0.25 mg/kg PO q1h to a total of 1.5 (to 2) mg/kg or conversion<br>Cat: Same?; for hypertrophic cardiomyopathy, 1 to 2.5 mg/kg q8h; sustained-release preparations Cardizem-CD, 10 mg/kg/day (45 mg/cat is about 105 mg of Cardizem-CD, or the amount that fits into the small end of a No. 4 gelatin capsule); Dilacor XR, 30 mg/cat/day (one half of a 60-mg tablet contained within the 240-mg gelatin capsule) |
| Verapamil | Dog: Initial dose, 0.05 mg/kg slowly IV, can repeat q5min up to a total of 0.15 (to 0.2) mg/kg; 0.5 to 2 mg/kg q8h PO<br>Cat: Initial dose, 0.025 mg/kg slowly IV, can repeat q5min up to a total of 0.15 (to 0.2) mg/kg; 0.5 to 1 mg/kg q8h PO |

*CRI,* Constant rate infusion; *CPR,* cardiopulmonary resuscitation; —, effective dosage not known.

*Continued*

TABLE 4-5

Dosage of Antiarrhythmic Drugs—cont'd

| AGENT | DOSAGE |
|---|---|
| **Anticholinergic** | |
| Atropine | Dog: 0.02 to 0.04 mg/kg IV, IM, SC; can also be given intratracheally for CPR<br>Cat: Same |
| Glycopyrrolate | Dog: 0.005 to 0.01 mg/kg IV or IM; 0.01 to 0.02 mg/kg SC<br>Cat: Same |
| Propantheline Br | Dog: 3.73 to 7.5 mg q8-12h PO<br>Cat: — |
| **Sympathomimetic** | |
| Isoproterenol | Dog: 0.045 to 0.09 μg/kg/min CRI<br>Cat: Same |
| Terbutaline | Dog: 2.5 to 5 mg/dog q8-12h PO<br>Cat: 1.25 mg/cat q12h PO |
| **Other Agents** | |
| Digoxin | See Table 3-8 |
| Adenosine | Dog: Up to 12 mg as rapid IV bolus<br>Cat: — |

rhythmic drug treatment either, especially if underlying heart function is normal. Traditionally, the guidelines for instituting ventricular antiarrhythmic therapy have been based on frequency, prematurity, and variability of the QRS configuration of the arrhythmia. These have included frequent VPCs (e.g., more than about 30/min), paroxysmal or sustained ventricular tachycardia (e.g., at rates over 130 beats/min), multiform VPCs, or close coupling of the VPCs to preceding complexes (R-on-T phenomenon). However, clear evidence supporting these guidelines as predictive of greater risk of sudden death in all patients is lacking. Therefore consideration of underlying heart disease and whether signs of hypotension are related to the arrhythmia is thought to be of greater importance. Animals thought to be hemodynamically unstable or that have a disease associated with sudden cardiac death (i.e., from arrhythmias) should be treated earlier and more aggressively.

Lidocaine, administered IV, is usually the first-choice drug for controlling serious ventricular tachyarrhythmias in hospitalized dogs. It is effective against arrhythmias of multiple underlying mechanisms, and it has minimal adverse hemodynamic effects. Because IV boluses last only about 10 to 15 minutes, a constant rate infusion (CRI) is warranted if the drug is effective. Small supplemental IV boluses can be given in addition to a CRI to maintain therapeutic drug concentrations until a steady state is achieved. IV infusions can be continued for several days if needed.

If lidocaine is ineffective, procainamide (given IV, IM, or PO) or quinidine (given IM or PO) is often tried next (see Table 4-5 and Fig. 4-3). The effects of a single IM or PO loading dose of either drug should occur within 2 hours. If this is

effective, lower doses can be given every 4 to 6 hours IM or PO. If it is ineffective, the dose can be increased or another antiarrhythmic drug can be chosen. Quinidine is generally not given IV because of its hypotensive effects. If the arrhythmia has not been controlled, a β-blocker can be added. Alternative approaches include use of mexiletine HCl or sotalol HCl, PO. Amiodarone HCl, given IV, has been effective in people for both ventricular and supraventricular tachyarrhythmias. Veterinary experience with this drug is still limited, but early anecdotal evidence is encouraging. Experimentally, 3 to 5 mg/kg slowly IV has been effective in dogs (Awaji and colleagues, 1995).

Cats with frequent ventricular tachyarrhythmias are usually given a β-blocker first. Alternatively, very low doses of lidocaine can be administered (see Table 4-5). Procainamide may also be used.

Digoxin is not used for treating ventricular tachyarrhythmias specifically, although it may be a component of therapy for concurrent heart failure or supraventricular arrhythmias. Because digoxin can predispose to the development of ventricular arrhythmias, simultaneous use of another antiarrhythmic drug may also be necessary and should precede administration of digoxin if frequent or repetitive VPCs are present. Phenytoin is used in dogs only for the management of digitalis-induced ventricular arrhythmias refractory to lidocaine.

If the ventricular tachyarrhythmia appears refractory to initial treatment attempts, one or more of the following considerations may be helpful:

1. Reevaluate the ECGs—could the rhythm have been incorrectly diagnosed initially? For example, supraventricular

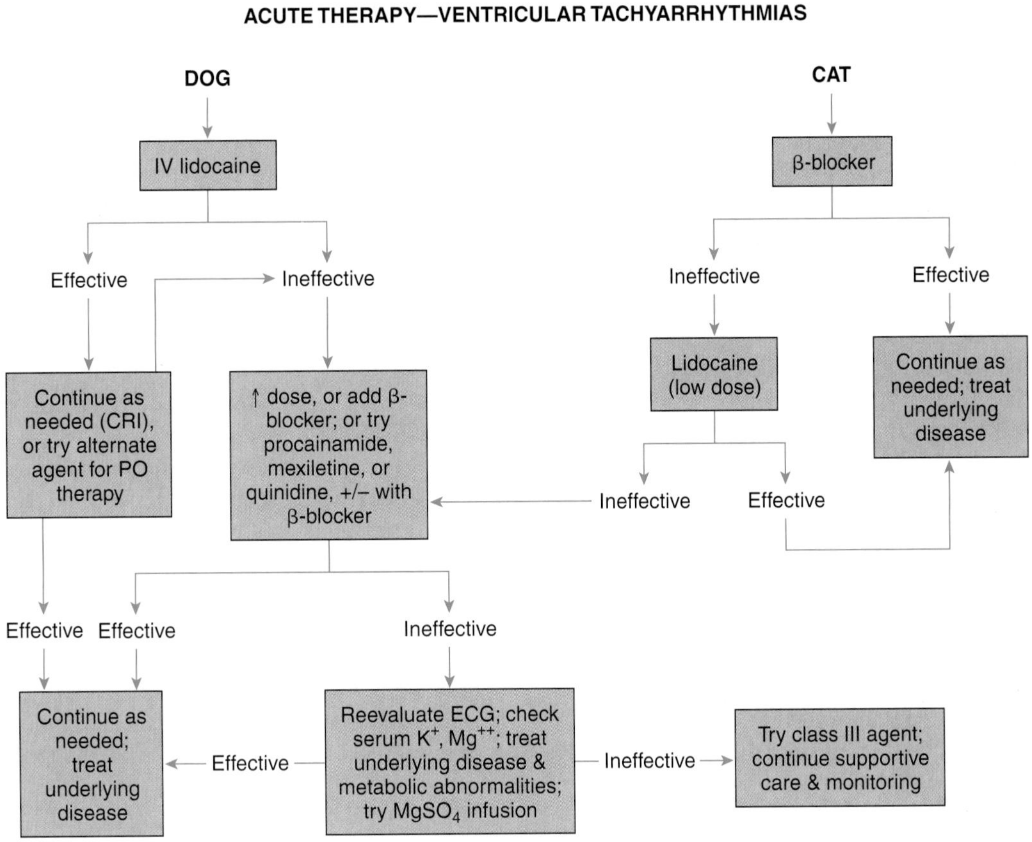

## ACUTE THERAPY—VENTRICULAR TACHYARRHYTHMIAS

**FIG 4-3**
An approach to acute therapy for ventricular tachyarrhythmias. See Table 4-5 for drug doses and text for more information. *CRI,* Constant rate infusion; *ECG,* electrocardiogram.

tachycardia with an intraventricular conduction disturbance can mimic ventricular tachycardia.

2. Reevaluate the serum potassium (and magnesium) concentration. Hypokalemia reduces the efficacy of class I antiarrhythmic drugs (e.g., lidocaine, procainamide, quinidine) and can predispose to the development of arrhythmias. If the serum potassium concentration is lower than 3 mEq/L, potassium chloride (KCl) can be infused at a rate of 0.5 mEq/kg/hr; if it is 3 to 3.5 mEq/L, KCl can be infused at a rate of 0.25 mEq/kg/hr. Aim for a serum potassium concentration in the high-normal range. If the serum magnesium concentration is less than 1.0 mg/dl, magnesium sulfate or magnesium chloride, diluted in 5% dextrose in water, can be administered at 0.75 to 1.0 mEq/kg/day by CRI.

3. Increase the dose of the conventional antiarrhythmic drug having the greatest effect.

4. Administer a β-blocker in conjunction with a class I drug (e.g., propranolol, esmolol, or atenolol with procainamide), or a class IA drug with a IB drug (e.g., procainamide with lidocaine or mexiletine), or try sotalol.

5. Consider the possibility that the drug therapy is exacerbating the rhythm disturbance (a proarrhythmic effect). Polymorphous ventricular tachycardia *(torsades de pointes)*

has been associated with quinidine, procainamide, and other drug toxicities.

6. Magnesium sulfate may be effective in animals with ventricular tachyarrhythmias associated with digoxin toxicity or with suspected polymorphous ventricular tachycardia *(torsades de pointes).* A slowly administered IV bolus of 25 to 40 mg/kg, diluted in 5% dextrose in water, followed by an infusion of the same dose over 12 to 24 hours, has been suggested. Because magnesium sulfate contains 8.13 mEq of magnesium per gram, a similar magnesium dose is provided by calculating 0.15 to 0.3 mEq/kg.

7. If the animal is tolerating the arrhythmia well, continue supportive care and close cardiovascular monitoring alone or with the most effective antiarrhythmic drug.

8. Try IV amiodarone, bretylium, or a newer or investigational antiarrhythmic agent if available. Alternatively, direct current (DC) cardioversion or ventricular pacing may be available at a referral center.

**Chronic oral therapy of ventricular tachyarrhythmias.** Traditionally, long-term oral therapy has consisted of the so-called class I antiarrhythmic drugs, sometimes in combination with a β-blocker. Although these agents may effectively suppress ventricular arrhythmias, they are unlikely to reduce the risk of sudden death. The Class IB drugs (lidocaine and mexiletine) experimentally have more ability to raise the fibrillation threshold than the class IA agents (procainamide and quinidine). Mexiletine has been used effectively against ventricular tachyarrhythmias and has been associated with fewer adverse effects than tocainide (see Suggested Readings). Uncontrolled observations in dogs suggest that mexiletine may be more effective than procainamide or quinidine. The combination of mexiletine with quinidine has been effective in some patients with arrhythmias refractory to either agent alone.

Although the class IB agent tocainide may effectively control ventricular tachyarrhythmias, its use has declined because of the incidence of adverse effects associated with chronic administration. Sustained-release procainamide has suppressed ventricular ectopia in some cases, but there are concerns about long-term efficacy, lack of protection from sudden death, and adverse effects, including gastrointestinal disturbances, lethargy, and proarrhythmia. Quinidine is a less desirable agent because of its frequent adverse effects and its interference with digoxin pharmacokinetics. Because there is questionable protection from ventricular fibrillation, even with effective suppression of ventricular ectopia, and considering the proarrhythmia risk of the class I agents (especially classes IA and IC), reliance on these drugs must be questioned.

Class III agents appear to have much greater antifibrillatory effects than the class I drugs. In people, use of the traditional class I drugs has been largely replaced by use of class III agents (especially amiodarone) or invasive techniques (catheter ablation or implantable cardioverter-defibrillators). People with underlying heart disease and arrhythmias have also benefited from the use of β-blockers and ACE inhibitors, as well as other therapies.

β-Blockers (e.g., atenolol, propranolol) can be useful for both ventricular and supraventricular arrhythmias that are provoked by sympathetic stimulation or catecholamines. In people and experimentally in dogs with myocardial ischemia or infarction, β-blockers have conferred protection against ventricular fibrillation. However, β-blockers alone do not appear to be very effective in suppressing ventricular ectopia in Dobermans with cardiomyopathy (Calvert and colleague, 2000). They are often used in combination with a class I agent (e.g., procainamide or mexiletine), although their negative inotropic effect demands caution when used in animals with myocardial failure.

Sotalol is a nonselective β-blocker with class III effects that has been used with apparent success in Boxers and Dobermans with cardiomyopathy. Anecdotally it seems to reduce the occurrence of sudden death, but evidence-based studies are awaited. Some dogs with dilated cardiomyopathy have experienced worsening myocardial function while on sotalol (Calvert and colleague, 2000). Amiodarone appears to be a promising alternative, although there are concerns about its prolonged half-life and an array of potential adverse effects. However, amiodarone may have lesser proarrhythmic effects and may confer greater antifibrillatory protection than other agents.

In summary, drugs currently used for the chronic management of ventricular tachyarrhythmias in dogs include the following:

- Sustained-release procainamide or mexiletine (or possibly tocainide);
- Sustained-release procainamide or mexiletine combined with atenolol or propranolol;
- Sotalol; or
- Amiodarone

The last three options are favored because they likely provide a greater antifibrillatory effect.

Frequent reevaluation is important for animals on long-term antiarrhythmic therapy for any rhythm disturbance. Clients can be shown how to use a stethoscope or palpate the chest wall to count the number of "skipped" beats per minute at home; this may yield an approximation of the frequency of arrhythmic events (either single or paroxysms). However, continuous 24- to 48-hour ambulatory ECG recordings are more accurate. The decision to continue or discontinue successful antiarrhythmic therapy is also based on consideration of the clinical situation and any underlying cardiac disease.

## Atrial Fibrillation

In cats and dogs, atrial fibrillation most often occurs when marked atrial enlargement is present. Atrial fibrillation is a serious arrhythmia, especially when the ventricular response rate is high. Predisposing conditions include dilated cardiomyopathy, chronic degenerative AV valve disease, congenital malformations that cause atrial enlargement, and hypertrophic or restrictive cardiomyopathy in cats. Clinical heart failure is common in these animals. Uncontrolled atrial fibrillation is characterized by an irregular and rapid ventricular response rate. Little time is available for ventricular filling, which compromises stroke volume. Furthermore, the contribution of atrial contraction to ventricular filling (the "atrial kick"), which is especially important at faster heart rates, is lost. Consequently, cardiac output tends to decrease considerably when atrial fibrillation develops; poor myocardial function exacerbates this.

Long-lasting conversion to sinus rhythm is rare when clinically significant underlying cardiac disease exists, even after successful electrical cardioversion. Therefore treatment is directed at reducing the ventricular response rate by slowing AV conduction (Fig. 4-4). A slower heart rate allows more time for ventricular filling and lessens the relative importance of atrial contraction. An in-hospital heart rate of less than 150 (or 180 in cats) beats/min is desirable. The pet's resting heart rate at home is a better indicator of drug effectiveness; many owners can monitor this. Heart rates of 70 to 120 beats/min in dogs and 80 to 140 beats/min in cats are acceptable, especially if the animal's activity level is good. The initial drug of choice for most dogs with atrial fibrillation is digoxin PO (see Table 3-8). If the heart rate exceeds

**ATRIAL FIBRILLATION**

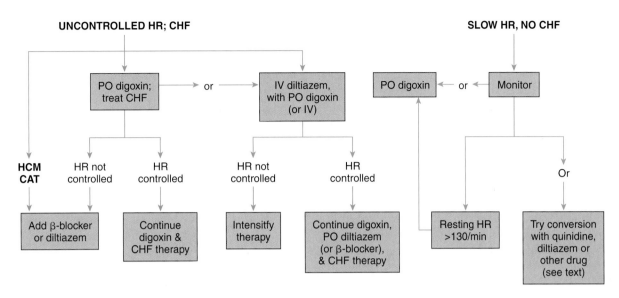

**FIG 4-4**
A therapeutic approach to atrial fibrillation. See Table 4-5 for drug doses and text for more information. *CHF,* Congestive heart failure; *HCM,* hypertrophic cardiomyopathy; *HR,* heart rate.

200 to 220 beats/min at rest, twice the eventual PO maintenance dosage can be given for 1 (to 2) days. For a more immediate decrease in heart rate, IV diltiazem should have less negative inotropic effect than an IV β-blocker or verapamil. When dobutamine or dopamine infusion is used to support myocardial function (see p. 69 and Table 3-8), IV diltiazem or an IV loading dose of digoxin can be used, but a β-blocker should be avoided.

Digoxin alone does not adequately reduce the heart rate in many animals. For chronic therapy, either a β-blocker or diltiazem can be added and titrated upward as needed to further slow AV conduction and the ventricular rate (see pp. 91 and 94 and Table 4-5). Because of their potential myocardial depressive effects, these drugs are usually added 1 to 2 days after PO digoxin institution in most dogs and in cats with dilated cardiomyopathy. An occasional dog will revert to sinus rhythm in response to diltiazem therapy. Digoxin is not used in cats with hypertrophic cardiomyopathy that develop atrial fibrillation; a β-blocker or diltiazem is used instead. Experimentally, in normal dogs with artificially induced atrial fibrillation, an acute PO dose of diltiazem at 5 mg/kg reduced the ventricular response rate to a heart rate similar to the baseline sinus rhythm rate (Miyamoto and colleagues, 2001). Whether such high doses can be safely used in dogs with underlying cardiac disease is not known, and caution is warranted.

Atrial fibrillation sometimes develops in large- or giant-breed dogs without cardiomegaly or other evidence of heart disease. This can occur in association with trauma or surgery, but atrial fibrillation with a slow ventricular response rate may also be an incidental finding in such a dog. Acute atrial fibrillation without signs of heart disease or failure may convert to sinus rhythm either spontaneously or in response to PO or IM quinidine therapy (see Table 4-5). The drug is discontinued after sinus rhythm has been achieved. Alternatively, diltiazem, given PO for 3 days, may be effective. Dogs that do not convert to sinus rhythm are either given digoxin (preferred) or monitored periodically without therapy if the ventricular rate is consistently low at rest.

Other drugs are being used in people to suppress atrial fibrillation but little veterinary experience exists. Ibutilide, amiodarone, sotalol, and dofetilide are class III antiarrhythmic drugs that have had some success in converting atrial fibrillation to sinus rhythm and preventing recurrence. Success is more likely in patients with normal left atrial size and recent onset atrial fibrillation. Propafenone (class IC) has also been used.

## RAPID, REGULAR RHYTHMS

### Sinus Tachycardia

High sympathetic tone or drug-induced vagal blockade causes sinus tachycardia. Underlying causes include anxiety, pain, fever, thyrotoxicosis, heart failure, hypotension, shock, the ingestion of stimulants or toxins (e.g., chocolate, caffeine), and drugs (e.g., catecholamines, anticholinergics, theophylline, and related agents). The heart rate in dogs and cats with sinus tachycardia is usually less than 300 beats/min, although it can be higher in those with thyrotoxicosis or those that have ingested exogenous stimulants or drugs (particularly cats). Alleviation of the underlying cause and the IV administration of fluids to reverse hypotension (in animals without edema) should cause the sympathetic tone and sinus rate to decrease.

## Sustained Supraventricular Tachycardia

Differentiation of sustained supraventricular tachycardia (SVT) from sinus tachycardia is sometimes difficult. The heart rate with SVT is often over 300 beats/min, but it is rare for the sinus rate to be this rapid. SVTs, like sinus tachycardias, usually have a normal QRS configuration (narrow and upright in lead II). However, if an intraventricular conduction disturbance is present, SVT may look like ventricular tachycardia.

The initial approach to SVT includes performing a *vagal maneuver.* This can help the clinician differentiate among tachycardias caused by an ectopic automatic focus, those dependent on a reentrant circuit involving the AV node, or excessive rapid sinus node activation. The vagal maneuver may transiently slow or intermittently block AV conduction, exposing abnormal atrial P' waves and allow an ectopic atrial focus to be identified. Vagal maneuvers can terminate reentrant supraventricular tachycardias involving the AV node by interrupting the reentrant circuit. The maneuver tends to temporarily slow the rate of sinus tachycardia. Vagal maneuvers are performed by massaging the area over the carotid sinuses (below the mandible in the jugular furrows) or by applying firm, bilateral ocular pressure for 15 to 20 seconds. The vagal maneuver can be potentiated in dogs by administering morphine sulfate (0.2 mg/kg IM; various manufacturers) or edrophonium chloride (1 to 4 mg IV [Tensilon, ICN Pharm, Costa Mesa, Calif; Enlon, Baxter, New Providence, N.J.]; atropine and an endotracheal tube should be readily available). β-Blockers, calcium entry blockers, digoxin, and other agents may also increase the effectiveness of vagal maneuvers.

If the vagal maneuver does not terminate SVT, drug therapy is used as described for rapid paroxysmal SVT (see p. 77, Table 4-5, and Fig. 4-2). Concurrently, IV fluids are administered to maintain blood pressure and enhance endogenous vagal tone. However, patients with known or suspected heart failure should receive a small volume slowly, if at all. Further cardiac diagnostic tests are indicated once conversion has been achieved or the ventricular rate has decreased to fewer than 200 beats/min. Adenosine has been used in people for terminating supraventricular tachycardias, but this has generally been ineffective in dogs. Refractory SVT might respond to sotalol, amiodarone, or a class IA or IC drug.

Reentrant supraventricular tachycardia involving an accessory pathway and the AV node occurs in cats and dogs with ventricular preexcitation. When vagal maneuvers fail to interrupt the tachycardia, IV diltiazem or verapamil is tried (although IV verapamil is not used in the setting of preexisting atrial fibrillation). Another alternative is procainamide, administered slowly IV (see Table 4-5). Vagal maneuvers can be repeated after these drugs are given. If these approaches are unsuccessful, an IV β-blocker or amiodarone may help. Chronic therapy to prevent recurrent AV reciprocating tachycardia was discussed earlier (p. 77).

## Sustained Ventricular Tachycardia

Sustained ventricular tachycardia is treated aggressively because marked decreases in arterial blood pressure can result, especially at faster rates. IV lidocaine is usually the first-choice antiarrhythmic agent in dogs because of its minimal adverse hemodynamic effects (see Table 4-5). Other therapeutic options for ventricular tachycardia are outlined in Fig. 4-3 and discussed on p. 80. Direct current cardioversion can be attempted if equipment is available, but ECG-synchronized equipment and anesthesia or sedation are required.

A β-blocker is usually considered the drug of first choice for ventricular tachycardia in cats. Lidocaine in small doses can be used instead (see Table 4-5). However, cats, especially if not anesthetized, are quite sensitive to its neurotoxic effects. Procainamide and quinidine have also been used in this species.

Close ECG monitoring and further diagnostic testing should follow initial therapy. Total suppression of persistent ventricular tachyarrhythmias is not expected. Consideration of the animal's clinical status and underlying disease, how well the drug has suppressed the arrhythmia, and the drug dosage (e.g., can it be increased?) influence the decision whether to continue or discontinue current treatment or to use a different drug. The patient's clinical status and the results of diagnostic testing also guide decisions about chronic PO therapy (see p. 81).

## BRADYARRHYTHMIAS

### Sinus Bradycardia

Slow sinus rhythm (or arrhythmia) can be a normal finding, especially in athletic dogs. Sinus bradycardia has also been associated with the administration of various drugs (e.g., xylazine, thorazine tranquilizers, anesthetic agents, digoxin, calcium entry blockers, β-blockers, parasympathomimetic drugs), trauma or diseases of the central nervous system, organic disease of the sinus node, hypothermia, hyperkalemia, and hypothyroidism, among other disorders. Conditions that increase vagal tone (e.g., respiratory or gastrointestinal tract disease or a mass involving the vagosympathetic trunk) may induce sinus bradycardia. Chronic pulmonary disease often is associated with pronounced respiratory sinus arrhythmia.

In most cases of sinus bradycardia, the heart rate increases in response to exercise or atropine administration, and no clinical signs are associated with the slow heart rate. Symptomatic dogs usually have a heart rate slower than 50 beats/min and/or pronounced underlying disease. Because sinus bradycardia and sinus bradyarrhythmia are extremely rare in cats, a search for underlying cardiac or systemic disease (e.g., hyperkalemia) is warranted in any cat with a slow heart rate.

When sinus bradycardia is associated with signs of weakness, exercise intolerance, syncope, or worsening underlying disease, an anticholinergic (or adrenergic) agent is given (Fig. 4-5; see Tables 3-8 and 4-5). If sinus bradycardia is the result of a drug effect, discontinuation, dosage reduction, or other therapy should be used as appropriate (e.g., reversal of anesthesia, calcium salts for calcium entry blocker overdose, dopamine or atropine for β-blocker toxicity). If there is inadequate acceleration of the heart rate after medical therapy, temporary or permanent pacing is indicated (see Suggested Readings).

## Sick Sinus Syndrome

Erratic sinoatrial function, resulting in clinical signs of episodic weakness, syncope, and Stokes-Adams seizures, characterizes the sick sinus syndrome. Older female Miniature Schnauzers are most often affected, but the syndrome is also seen in Dachshunds, Pugs, and mixed-breed dogs. Sick sinus syndrome is extremely rare in cats. Affected dogs have episodes of marked sinus bradycardia with sinus arrest (or sinoatrial block). Abnormalities of the AV conduction system may coexist, causing the activity of subsidiary pacemakers to be depressed and resulting in prolonged periods of asystole. Some affected dogs also have various paroxysmal supraventricular tachyarrhythmias, prompting the name bradycardia-tachycardia syndrome (Fig. 4-6). Premature complexes may be followed by long pauses before sinus node activity resumes, indicating a prolonged sinus node recovery time. Intermittent periods of accelerated junctional rhythms and variable junctional or ventricular escape rhythms may also occur.

Clinical signs can result from bradycardia and sinus arrest, paroxysmal tachycardia, or both. Signs can mimic seizures stemming from neurologic or metabolic disorders. Concurrent degenerative AV valve disease is also often present. Some dogs have evidence of congestive heart failure, usually secondary to AV valve regurgitation, although the arrhythmias may be a complicating factor.

The ECG abnormalities are frequently pronounced in dogs with long-standing sick sinus syndrome. Nevertheless, some dogs have one or more normal resting ECGs. Establishment of a definitive diagnosis is aided by 24-hour ambulatory or prolonged visual ECG monitoring. An atropine challenge test is done in dogs with persistent bradycardia (see p. 96). The normal response is an increase in the heart rate of 150% or to over 130 to 150 beats/min. Dogs with sick sinus syndrome generally have a subnormal response.

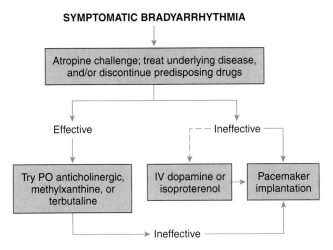

**SYMPTOMATIC BRADYARRHYTHMIA**

Atropine challenge; treat underlying disease, and/or discontinue predisposing drugs

Effective — Ineffective

Try PO anticholinergic, methylxanthine, or terbutaline

IV dopamine or isoproterenol

Pacemaker implantation

Ineffective

**FIG 4-5**
A therapeutic approach to symptomatic bradyarrhythmias. See Tables 3-8 and 4-5 and text for more information.

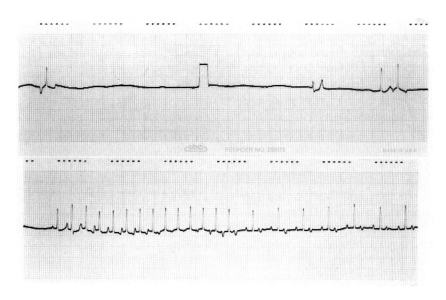

**FIG 4-6**
Continuous electrocardiogram from an 11-year-old female Miniature Schnauzer with sick sinus syndrome, illustrating a combination of bradycardia and tachycardia. The top portion shows persistent sinus arrest with three different escape complexes, followed by an atrial premature complex. There is a 1 mV calibration mark in the middle of the top strip. The bradycardia is interrupted by a run of atrial tachycardia at a rate of 250 beats/min, with 1:1 atrioventricular conduction initially; however, starting in the middle of the bottom strip, every other P' wave is blocked (2:1 atrioventricular conduction).

Therapy with an anticholinergic agent, methylxanthine bronchodilator, or terbutaline given PO may temporarily help animals that have a positive response to atropine challenge (see Fig. 4-5; Table 4-5); however, such therapy is often unrewarding. Anticholinergic or sympathomimetic drugs used to accelerate the sinus rate can also exacerbate any tachyarrhythmias that may already exist. Conversely, drugs used to suppress these supraventricular tachyarrhythmias can magnify the bradycardia, although digoxin or diltiazem is helpful in some dogs if used cautiously. Sick sinus syndrome with frequent or severe clinical signs is best managed by permanent artificial pacing. The Suggested Readings list includes sources of further details on pacing. Dogs that remain symptomatic because of paroxysmal supraventricular tachyarrhythmias can safely be given appropriate antiarrhythmic therapy once a normally functioning pacemaker is in place.

### Atrial Standstill

Persistent atrial standstill is a rhythm disturbance characterized by lack of effective atrial electrical activity (i.e., no P waves and a flat baseline) in which a junctional or ventricular escape rhythm controls the heart. This bradyarrhythmia is rare in dogs and extremely rare in cats; most cases have occurred in English Springer Spaniels with muscular dystrophy of the fascioscapulohumeral type, although infiltrative and inflammatory diseases of the atrial myocardium can also result in atrial standstill. Because organic disease of the atrial myocardium may also involve the ventricular myocardium, persistent atrial standstill may be a harbinger of a serious and progressive cardiac disorder.

Medical treatment for persistent atrial standstill is rarely rewarding; however, an anticholinergic drug or an infusion of dopamine or isoproterenol can sometimes temporarily accelerate the escape rhythm (see Fig. 4-5; Tables 3-8 and 4-5). If ventricular tachyarrhythmias result from this treatment, the drug should be discontinued or the dose reduced. Terbutaline PO may also have some beneficial effect. Antiarrhythmic agents are contraindicated in these animals because they may suppress the escape focus as well as the tachyarrhythmia. Permanent pacemaker implantation is the treatment of choice, although the prognosis is poor in dogs with concurrent ventricular myocardial dysfunction.

An apparent lack of atrial electrical and mechanical activity can be seen transiently ("silent atrium") in cats and dogs with hyperkalemia; as the serum potassium concentration returns to normal, sinus node activity (and P waves) become evident. The treatment of hyperkalemia is discussed on p. 832.

### Second- and Third-Degree AV Blocks

Second-degree, or intermittent, AV block usually causes an irregular heartbeat. In contrast, the ventricular escape rhythm that occurs with a third-degree, or complete, AV block is regular, although premature contractions or shifts in the escape focus may cause some irregularities. AV conduction disturbances may result from therapy with certain drugs (e.g., $\alpha_2$-agonists, opioids, digoxin), high vagal tone, or organic disease of the AV node. Diseases that have been associated with AV conduction disturbances include bacterial endocarditis

(of the aortic valve), hypertrophic cardiomyopathy, infiltrative myocardial disease, and myocarditis. Idiopathic heart block may occur in middle-aged to older dogs; congenital third-degree heart block has also been seen in dogs. Symptomatic heart block is less common in cats, but evidence of any AV conduction disturbance should prompt further diagnostic evaluation. Most cases have been associated with hypertrophic cardiomyopathy. Heart block is occasionally found in old cats without detectable organic heart disease.

Type I second-degree AV block and first-degree AV block are frequently associated with high vagal tone or drug effects in dogs. These animals are often asymptomatic; exercise or injection of an anticholinergic drug (atropine or glycopyrrolate) usually abolishes the conduction disturbance. High-grade (many blocked P waves) second-degree AV block and complete heart block usually cause lethargy, exercise intolerance, weakness, syncope, and other signs of low cardiac output. These signs become severe when the heart rate is consistently less than 40 beats/min. Congestive heart failure develops secondary to chronic bradycardia in some dogs, especially if other cardiac disease is present.

An atropine challenge test (p. 96) is used to determine the degree of vagal influence on the AV block. Long-term PO anticholinergic therapy (e.g., propantheline bromide) can be attempted in symptomatic animals that are atropine-responsive (see Fig. 4-5; Table 4-5). Atropine or subsequent PO anticholinergic therapy is often ineffective, however; therefore artificial pacing is usually indicated. An emergency infusion of dopamine (see Table 3-8) or isoproterenol (see Table 4-5) may increase the ventricular escape rate in animals with high-grade second- or third-degree block, although ventricular tachyarrhythmias may also be provoked. Isoproterenol PO is usually ineffective. A thorough cardiac workup is indicated before permanent artificial pacemaker implantation because some underlying diseases (e.g., myocardial disease, endocarditis) are associated with a poor prognosis, even after pacing. Temporary transvenous pacing is sometimes used for 1 to 2 days to assess the animal's response to a normal heart rate before permanent pacemaker surgery is performed.

## ANTIARRHYTHMIC DRUGS

Drugs used to suppress arrhythmias have been grouped according to their electrophysiologic effects on cardiac cells (Vaughan-Williams classification; Table 4-4), although the clinical usefulness of this classification is rapidly fading. Class I agents tend to slow conduction and decrease automaticity and excitability by means of their membrane-stabilizing effects; the "traditional" ventricular antiarrhythmic drugs belong to this class. Class II drugs include the β-adrenergic antagonists, which act by inhibiting the effects of catecholamines on the heart. Class III drugs prolong the effective refractory period of cardiac action potentials without decreasing conduction velocity; they may be most effective in suppressing reentrant arrhythmias or in preventing ventricular fibrillation. Class IV drugs are the calcium entry blockers; ventricular arrhythmias are usually not responsive to these agents. Dosages of antiarrhythmic drugs are given in Table 4-5, and various preparations and manufacturers are listed in Table 4-6.

## CLASS I ANTIARRHYTHMIC DRUGS

Class I drugs block membrane sodium channels and depress the action potential upstroke (phase 0). They have been sub-classified according to differences in other electrophysiologic characteristics. These differences (see Table 4-4) may influence their efficacy in the treatment of particular arrhythmias. Most of these agents depend on the extracellular potassium concentration for their effects.

### Lidocaine

Lidocaine is usually the intravenous ventricular antiarrhythmic agent of first choice in dogs, but it is generally ineffective in the management of supraventricular arrhythmias. It has little effect on the sinus rate, AV conduction rate, and refractoriness. The electrophysiologic effects of lidocaine are extremely dependent on the extracellular potassium concentration; hypokalemia may render the drug ineffective, whereas hyperkalemia intensifies its depressant effects on cardiac membranes. Lidocaine suppresses automaticity in both normal Purkinje fibers and diseased myocardial tissue, slows conduction, and reduces the supernormal period (during which the cell can be reexcited before complete repolarization occurs). It has greater effects on diseased and hypoxic cardiac

 TABLE 4-6

Commercial Preparations of Antiarrhythmic Drugs

| DRUG | PREPARATIONS | MANUFACTURERS |
|---|---|---|
| **Class I** | | |
| Lidocaine | 20 mg/ml (2%) injectable solution | Xylocaine (AstraZeneca, Wilmington, Del); generics |
| Procainamide | 250, 375, and 500 mg tablets and capsules; 100 and 500 mg/ml injectable solution | Pronestyl (Bristol-Myers Squibb, Princeton, N.J.); generics |
| Procainamide, SR | 250, 500, 750, and 1000 mg tablets | Procan SR (Parke-Davis, Morris Plains, N.J.); Pronestyl SR (Bristol-Myers Squibb); Procanbid (Monarch, Bristol, Tenn); generics |
| Quinidine sulfate | 200 and 300 mg tablets | Various generics |
| Quinidine sulfate, SR | 300 mg tablets | Quinidex Extentabs (A.H. Robins, Richmond, Va) |
| Quinidine gluconate, SR | 324 mg tablets | Quinaglute Dura-Tabs (Berlex Laboratories, Wayne, NJ); generics (Eli Lilly, Indianapolis, Ind) |
| | 80 mg/ml injectable solution | |
| Quinidine polygalacturonate | 275 mg tablets (equivalent to 200 mg of quinidine sulfate) | Cardioquin (Purdue Frederick, Norwalk, Conn) |
| Tocainide | 400 and 600 mg tablets | Tonocard (AstraZeneca, Wilmington, Del) |
| Mexiletine | 150, 200, and 250 mg capsules | Mexitil (Boehringer Ingelheim Pharmaceuticals, Ridgefield, Conn); generics |
| Phenytoin | 50 mg/ml injectable solution | Dilantin (Parke-Davis, Morris Plains, N.J.); generics |
| **Class II** | | |
| Propranolol | 10, 20, 40, 60, 80 mg tablets; 1 mg/ml injectable solution 4 and 8 mg/ml oral solutions; also Inderal LA sustained-release capsules | Inderal (Wyeth-Ayerst, Philadelphia, Pa); (Roxane, Columbus, Ohio); other generics |
| Atenolol | 25, 50, and 100 mg tablets 5 mg/10 ml injectable solution | Tenormin (AstraZeneca, Wilmington, Del); generics |
| Esmolol | 10 and 250 mg/ml injectable solutions | Brevibloc (Baxter Anesthesia, New Providence, N.J.) |
| Metoprolol tartrate | 50 and 100 mg tablets; 5 mg/5 ml injectable | Generics |
| **Class III** | | |
| Amiodarone | 200 and 400 mg tablets; 50 mg/ml injectable solution | Cordarone (Wyeth-Ayerst, Philadelphia, Pa); Pacerone (Upsher-Smith, Minneapolis, Minn); generic |
| Sotalol | 80, 160, and 240 mg tablets | Betapace (Berlex, Wayne, N.J.); generics |
| Bretylium tosylate | 50 mg/ml injectable solution | Generics |

*SR,* Sustained release.

*Continued*

TABLE 4-6

Commercial Preparations of Antiarrhythmic Drugs—cont'd

| DRUG | PREPARATIONS | MANUFACTURERS |
|---|---|---|
| **Class IV** | | |
| Diltiazem | 30, 60, 90, and 120 mg tablets; 5 mg/ml injectable solution | Generics |
| Diltiazem, SR | 120, 180, 240, and 300 mg capsules | Cardizem-CD (Biovail Pharm, Morrisville, N.C.); Cartia XT (Andrx Pharm, Jackson, Miss) |
| | 120, 180, and 240 mg capsules | Dilacor XR (Watson Pharm, Corona, Calif); Diltia XT (Andrx Pharm, Jackson, Miss) |
| Verapamil | 40, 80, and 120 mg tablets; 5 mg/2 ml injectable solution | Calan (Pharmacia, Peapack, N.J.); Isoptin (Abbott, Abbott Park, Ill); generics |
| **Anticholinergic** | | |
| Atropine sulfate USP | Various concentrations for injection; 0.4 mg tablets | Generics |
| Glycopyrrolate | *Veterinary:* 0.2 mg/ml injectable solution | Robinul-V (Fort Dodge Laboratories, Fort Dodge, Iowa) |
| | *Human:* 1 and 2 mg tablets; 0.2-mg/ml injectable solution | Robinul (A.H. Robins, Richmond, Va; Baxter Anesthesia, New Providence, N.J.) |
| Propantheline bromide | 15 mg tablets | Generics |
| **Sympathomimetic** | | |
| Isoproterenol | 0.2 mg/ml injectable solution | Generics |
| Terbutaline | 2.5 and 5 mg tablets | Brethine (Novartis, Summit, N.J.) |
| **Other Agents** | | |
| Digoxin | See Table 3-9 | |
| Adenosine | 3 mg/ml injectable solution | Adenocard (Fujisawa USA, Deerfield, Ill) |

cells and at faster stimulation rates. If given slowly IV, lidocaine produces little or no depression of contractility at therapeutic doses. This makes it the drug of choice in dogs with heart failure; the lidocaine congeners tocainide and mexiletine similarly produce minimal negative inotropic and hypotensive effects. Lidocaine should be used carefully to avert the hypotension associated with toxic concentrations. The drug is contraindicated in dogs with complete heart block and should be used only cautiously in animals with sinus bradycardia, sick sinus syndrome, and first- or second-degree AV block.

Lidocaine undergoes rapid hepatic metabolism; some of the drug's metabolites may contribute to its antiarrhythmic and toxic effects. Lidocaine is not effective PO because of its almost complete first-pass hepatic elimination; it should be administered IV, usually as slow boluses followed by a constant rate infusion (CRI) (see Tables 4-5 and 4-7). The half-life after IV injection is about 90 minutes in the dog; CRI without a loading dose results in steady state concentrations in 4 to 6 hours. An initial bolus of 2 mg/kg is used in dogs and can be repeated two to three times if necessary. Lower doses should be used in cats to avoid toxicity (loading dose of 0.25 to 0.5 mg/kg). Therapeutic plasma concentrations are thought to range from 1.5 to 6 μg/ml in dogs. Only lidocaine without epinephrine should be used for antiarrhythmic therapy.

The most common toxic effect of lidocaine is central nervous system excitation. Signs include agitation, disorientation, muscle twitches, nystagmus, and generalized seizures. Nausea can also occur. Worsening of arrhythmias (a proarrhythmic effect) is seen occasionally, as it is with any drug having cardiac electrophysiologic effects. Cats are particularly sensitive to the drug's toxic effects and may undergo respiratory arrest along with seizures. In the event of toxicity, lidocaine should be discontinued until the toxicity signs disappear; a lower infusion rate may then be instituted. Diazepam (0.25 to 0.5 mg/kg IV) is used to control lidocaine-induced seizures. There are anecdotal reports of respiratory depression and arrest after the administration of lidocaine in unconscious dogs and cats. Propranolol, cimetidine, and other drugs that decrease liver blood flow slow the metabolism of lidocaine and predispose to the development of toxicity. Animals with heart failure may also

TABLE 4-7

## Formulas to Calculate Constant-Rate Infusion

### Method 1

(Allows for "fine-tuning" fluid as well as drug administration rate)

Determine desired drug infusion rate:

μg/kg/min × kg body weight = μg/min     (A)

Determine desired fluid infusion rate:

ml/hour ÷ 60 = ml/min     (B)

(A) ÷ (B) = μg/min ÷ ml/min = μg drug/ml of fluid

Convert from μg to mg of drug needed (1 μg = 0.001 mg)

mg drug/ml fluid × ml of fluid in bag (or bottle or burette) = mg of drug to add to fluid bag

### Method 2

(For total dose over a 6-hour period, must also calculate fluid volume and administration rate)

*Total* dose in mg to infuse over a 6-hour period = Body weight (kg) × Dose (μg/kg/min) × 0.36

### Method 3 (for Lidocaine)

(Faster but less helpful if fluid rate is important or fine drug-dosage adjustments are needed)

For CRI of 44 μg/kg/min of lidocaine, add 25 ml of 2% lidocaine to 250 ml of D5W

Infuse at 0.25 ml/25 lb of body weight/min

---

have reduced hepatic blood flow and may require a lower dosage of the drug.

## Procainamide

Procainamide is similar to quinidine in its electrophysiologic effects (see Table 4-4), although some arrhythmias may respond better to one or the other of these drugs. Procainamide has both direct and indirect (vagolytic) effects; it is indicated for the treatment of premature ventricular (and sometimes atrial) depolarizations and tachycardias. It is less effective than quinidine in the management of atrial arrhythmias and is usually not effective in converting chronic atrial flutter-fibrillation to sinus rhythm. Procainamide should be used only with great caution in animals with sinus bradycardia, sick sinus syndrome, AV blocks, intraventricular conduction disturbances, or hypotensive states. As with all ventricular antiarrhythmic agents, its use is contraindicated in animals with complete heart block.

Procainamide is well absorbed PO in the dog but has a half-life of only 2.5 to 4 hours. The sustained-release preparation has a slightly longer half-life of 3 to 6 hours. The drug undergoes hepatic metabolism and renal excretion in proportion to the creatinine clearance. The metabolite N-acetylprocainamide is not present to any significant degree in dogs and cats. PO and IM administration of this drug are not associated with marked hemodynamic effects; however, rapid IV injection can cause hypotension and cardiac depression, although to a much lesser degree than quinidine administered IV. CRI may be used if the arrhythmia responds to an IV bolus; a steady state is reached in 12 to 22 hours. General dosage recommendations are given in Table 4-5. Therapeutic plasma concentrations are thought to be 4 to 10 μg/ml.

The toxic effects of procainamide are similar to those of quinidine (see later discussion) but are usually milder. Gastrointestinal upset and prolongation of the QRS or QT intervals may occur. Procainamide can enhance the ventricular response rate to atrial fibrillation if used without digoxin or a β-blocker or calcium entry blocker. More serious toxic effects include hypotension, depressed AV conduction (sometimes causing second- or third-degree heart block), and proarrhythmia. Proarrhythmia can cause syncope or ventricular fibrillation. IV fluids, catecholamines, or calcium-containing solutions can be used to treat hypotension. Gastrointestinal signs associated with PO therapy may respond to dosage reduction; they appear to be less frequent than those associated with quinidine. High-dose PO procainamide therapy in people has been associated with a reversible lupus-like syndrome characterized by neutropenia, fever, depression, and hepatomegaly, but this has not been documented in dogs. Long-term use can cause brown discoloration of the haircoat in black Dobermans.

## Quinidine

Quinidine (see Table 4-5) has been used for the treatment of ventricular and, occasionally, supraventricular tachyarrhythmias. In large dogs with atrial fibrillation of recent onset but with normal ventricular function, quinidine may cause conversion to sinus rhythm. The drug is contraindicated in animals with sinus bradycardia, sick sinus syndrome, high-grade second-degree AV block, or complete heart block. Quinidine should be used only cautiously in animals with heart failure or hyperkalemia.

Depression of automaticity and conduction velocity and prolongation of the effective refractory period are characteristic electrophysiologic effects of this drug. Corresponding dose-dependent ECG changes (e.g., PR, QRS, and QT prolongation) result from direct electrophysiologic and vagolytic effects. At low doses, quinidine's vagolytic effects may cause the sinus rate or the ventricular response rate to atrial fibrillation to increase by antagonizing the direct effects of the drug. As with other class I agents, hypokalemia reduces the antiarrhythmic effectiveness of quinidine.

The drug is well absorbed PO but is has fallen out of favor for chronic oral therapy. Quinidine's extensive hepatic metabolism is not greatly dependent on liver blood flow, and it is unclear whether severe heart failure or liver disease significantly alters drug metabolism. Quinidine has a half-life of about 6 hours in dogs but only 2 hours in cats. Because it is highly protein-bound, severe hypoalbuminemia can predispose to the development of toxicity. Cimetidine, by slowing the drug's elimination, may also predispose to the development of toxicity. Quinidine can precipitate digoxin toxicity if the two drugs are used simultaneously because it displaces digoxin from skeletal muscle binding sites and decreases the renal clearance of digoxin. Anticonvulsants and other drugs that induce hepatic microsomal enzymes can speed the metabolism of quinidine and necessitate an increased dosage.

IV administration is not recommended because of quinidine's propensity to cause vasodilation (by means of nonspecific α-adrenergic receptor blockade), cardiac depression, and hypotension. Use of the PO and IM routes is usually not associated with adverse hemodynamic effects, but close monitoring is warranted initially, especially in animals with underlying cardiac disease. Blood concentrations in the human therapeutic range (2.5 to 5 μg/ml) are usually reached within 12 to 24 hours after PO and IM administration.

Slow-release sulfate, gluconate, and polygalacturonate salts of quinidine prolong the drug's absorption and elimination. Administration of these products every 8 hours is probably adequate for dogs, whereas standard quinidine sulfate should be given every 6 hours. Approximate concentrations of active drug are 83% for quinidine sulfate, 62% for quinidine gluconate, and 80% for quinidine galacturonate. The sulfate salt is more rapidly absorbed than the gluconate. A peak effect is usually achieved 1 to 2 hours after PO administration.

Quinidine toxicity occurs as an extension of the drug's electrophysiologic and hemodynamic actions. The PR interval and QRS duration lengthen as the plasma concentration increases. The development of marked QT prolongation, right bundle branch block, or QRS widening exceeding 25% of the pretreatment value suggests drug toxicity. Various conduction blocks as well as ventricular tachyarrhythmias can result from high blood concentrations of this drug. *Torsades de pointes* (a form of ventricular tachycardia in which the electrical axis appears to rotate) or ventricular fibrillation can develop as a result of increased temporal dispersion of myocardial refractoriness, which is implied by marked QT prolongation. Transient episodes of these serious arrhythmias have been implicated as a cause of syncopal attacks in people receiving quinidine. Lethargy, weakness, and congestive heart failure can result from the negative inotropic and vasodilatory effects of the drug and subsequent hypotension. Cardiotoxicity and hypotension may be partially reversed by administering sodium bicarbonate (1 mEq/kg IV), which temporarily decreases serum potassium concentrations, enhances quinidine's binding to albumin, and reduces its cardiac electrophysiologic effects. Gastrointestinal signs (nausea, vomiting, and diarrhea) are common in animals receiving quinidine PO. Thrombocytopenia, which is reversible after quinidine discontinuation, has occurred in people and possibly in dogs and cats. As noted earlier, quinidine increases serum digoxin concentrations.

## Mexiletine

Mexiletine is similar to lidocaine in its electrophysiologic, hemodynamic, toxic, and antiarrhythmic properties. It has been effective in terminating or controlling ventricular tachyarrhythmias in dogs. The combination of a β-blocker (or procainamide or quinidine) with mexiletine may be more efficacious and associated with fewer adverse effects in some animals than mexiletine alone. The drug is easily absorbed when administered PO, but antacids, cimetidine, and narcotic analgesics reportedly slow its absorption in people. Mexiletine undergoes hepatic metabolism (influenced by liver blood flow) and some renal excretion (which is slower if the urine is alkaline). Hepatic microsomal enzyme inducers may accelerate its clearance. The half-life in dogs is 4.5 to 7 hours (depending to some degree on the urine pH). Approximately 70% of the drug is protein-bound. The therapeutic serum concentration is thought to range from 0.5 to 2.0 μg/ml (as in people). Information on the effects of this drug in cats is not available. Adverse effects have included vomiting, anorexia, tremor, and disorientation. Overall, mexiletine appears to produce fewer adverse effects than tocainide (see below).

## Tocainide

Tocainide has been effective in controlling various ventricular tachyarrhythmias, but is less favored for chronic PO therapy. It is similar to lidocaine in its electrophysiologic, hemodynamic, and toxic properties but is administered PO. Tocainide is well absorbed by this route and does not undergo extensive first-pass metabolism. The plasma concentration peaks about 2 hours after administration in dogs. Effective serum concentrations can be maintained for 6 to 8 hours after three doses. A "loading" dose can be achieved by administering two doses 2 hours apart, with a third dose given 6 hours later; this is not recommended for dogs concurrently receiving lidocaine, however. Effective plasma concentrations in dogs are reportedly 6 μg/ml 8 hours after administration (trough) and 10 μg/ml 2 hours after administration (peak). There does not appear to be a close correlation between the dose and plasma concentration in dogs. Plasma concentrations of greater than 12 μg/ml may cause neurotoxicity. Furthermore, toxicity signs can occur in the presence of "therapeutic" plasma concentrations. The drug is eliminated by both renal and hepatic routes. Because its clearance is not significantly influenced by changes in liver blood flow, drugs such as propranolol and cimetidine are not expected to slow its elimination. Gastrointestinal adverse effects (anorexia and vomiting) seem to be common; occasional neurotoxic signs such as ataxia, disorientation, and twitching have been observed. The administration of tocainide for more than 3 months has been associated with serious ocular and renal toxicity in some dogs (see Suggested Readings).

## Phenytoin

Phenytoin has electrophysiologic effects similar to those of lidocaine. However, it also has some slow–calcium channel inhibitory and central nervous system effects that may contribute to its effectiveness against digitalis-induced arrhythmias. It is currently used only for the therapy of digitalis-induced ventricular arrhythmias that are not responsive to lidocaine in dogs. The contraindications to its use are the same as those for lidocaine. Rapid IV injection should be avoided because the propylene glycol vehicle can depress myocardial contractility and cause vasodilation, hypotension, and respiratory arrest and can exacerbate arrhythmias. Slow IV infusion and PO administration do not cause relevant hemodynamic disturbances; however, the oral bioavailability of phenytoin is poor.

The half-life of phenytoin is only about 3 hours in the dog. The drug is metabolized in the liver, and it may speed up its own elimination by stimulating hepatic microsomal enzymes. The co-administration of cimetidine, chloramphenicol, or other drugs that inhibit the activity of microsomal enzymes can result in toxic serum concentrations of phenytoin. The IV administration of phenytoin has been associated with the development of bradycardia, AV blocks, ventricular tachycardia, and cardiac arrest. Other manifestations of phenytoin toxicity include central nervous system signs (depression, nystagmus, disorientation, and ataxia); blood dyscrasias have been associated with long-term use in people. The drug is not recommended for use in cats because it has a half-life of more than 24 hours in this species and even low doses produce toxic serum concentrations.

## Other Class I Agents

Disopyramide is similar to quinidine and procainamide electrophysiologically. It has a very short half-life in the dog (less than 2 hours) as well as marked depressive effects on the canine myocardium. These factors make the drug undesirable for clinical use.

Flecainide (Tambocor, 3M Pharm, Northridge, Calif; and generic) and propafenone (Rythmol, Abbott Labs, Abbott Park, Ill; and generic), which are class IC agents, characteristically produce a marked reduction in the cardiac conduction velocity but have little effect on sinus rate or refractoriness. However, high doses lead to a depression of automaticity in the sinus node and specialized conducting tissues. Vasodilation and myocardial depression can result in severe hypotension after IV injection, especially in animals with underlying cardiac disease. Proarrhythmia is a serious potential adverse effect of these agents. Bradycardia, intraventricular conduction disturbance, and consistent (although transient) hypotension, as well as nausea, vomiting, and anorexia, have occurred in dogs. Flecainide (and encainide) have been associated with increased mortality in people. Thus these agents should be used only with great caution and for the treatment of life-threatening ventricular arrhythmias refractory to other therapy.

## CLASS II ANTIARRHYTHMIC DRUGS: β-ADRENERGIC BLOCKERS

The β-blockers act by blocking catecholamine effects and reducing myocardial $O_2$ demand. β-Adrenergic receptors have been classified into subtypes. $\beta_1$-Receptors are primarily located in the myocardium and mediate increases in contractility, heart rate, AV conduction velocity, and automaticity in specialized fibers. $\beta_2$-Receptors mediate bronchodilation and vasodilation, as well as renin and insulin release. There are also some $\beta_2$-receptors in the heart. Some drugs that block β-receptors are "nonselective" in that they inhibit catecholamine binding to both $\beta_1$- and $\beta_2$-adrenergic receptors; others are more selective and antagonize primarily one or the other receptor subtype (Table 4-8). The first-generation β-blockers (e.g., propranolol) have nonselective β-blocking effects. Second-generation agents (e.g., atenolol, metoprolol) are relatively $\beta_1$ selective. The third-generation β-blockers affect both $\beta_1$- and $\beta_2$-receptors but also antagonize $\alpha_1$-receptors and may have other effects. A few β-blockers have some degree of intrinsic sympathomimetic activity.

 TABLE 4-8

Characteristics of Selected β-Blockers

| DRUG | ADRENERGIC RECEPTOR SELECTIVITY | LIPID SOLUBILITY | MAIN ROUTE OF ELIMINATION | AVAILABLE AS |
|---|---|---|---|---|
| Atenolol | $\beta_1$ | 0 | RE | Tenormin (AstraZeneca), generic |
| Carvedilol | $\beta_1$, $\beta_2$, $\alpha_1$ | + | HM | Coreg (GlaxoSmithKline) |
| Esmolol | $\beta_1$ | 0 | BE | Brevibloc (Baxter Anesthesia) |
| Labetalol | $\beta_1$, $\beta_2$, $\alpha_1$ | ++ | HM | Normodyne (Schering), Trandate (Promethius) |
| Metoprolol | $\beta_1$ | ++ | HM | Lopressor (Novartis), generic |
| Nadolol | $\beta_1$, $\beta_2$ | 0 | RE | Corgard (Monarch), generic |
| Pindolol* | $\beta_1$, $\beta_2$ | ++ | B | Visken (Novartis), generic |
| Propranolol | $\beta_1$, $\beta_2$ | ++ | HM | Inderal (Wyeth-Ayerst), generic |
| Sotalol† | $\beta_1$, $\beta_2$ | 0 | RE | Betapace (Berlex) |
| Timolol | $\beta_1$, $\beta_2$ | 0 | RE | Blocadren (Merck), generic |

*Has intrinsic sympathomimetic activity.
†Also has class III antiarrhythmic activity.
*RE*, Renal excretion; *BE*, blood esterases; *HM*, hepatic metabolism; *B*, both renal excretion and hepatic metabolism are important.

β-Receptor blockers are used in the treatment of hypertrophic cardiomyopathy, certain congenital and acquired ventricular outflow obstructions, systemic hypertension, hyperthyroid heart disease, supraventricular and ventricular tachyarrhythmias (especially those caused by enhanced sympathetic tone), and other diseases or toxicities that cause excessive sympathetic stimulation. Studies in people with stable heart failure have shown that long-term therapy with certain β-blockers improves cardiac function and prolongs survival in patients who tolerate the drug (see p. 93). These drugs slow the heart rate (thereby increasing ventricular filling time), reduce myocardial oxygen demand, and increase AV conduction time and refractoriness. A β-blocker is often used in conjunction with digoxin to slow the ventricular response rate to atrial fibrillation. A β-blocker such as propranolol or atenolol is considered the first-line antiarrhythmic agent in cats with supraventricular or ventricular tachyarrhythmias.

The clinical antiarrhythmic effect of class II drugs is thought to be caused solely by $\beta_1$-receptor blockade rather than by direct electrophysiologic mechanisms. In normal animals, β-receptor blockers have little negative inotropic effect. However, animals with severe underlying myocardial disease may be dependent on increased sympathetic drive to maintain cardiac output. Therefore these drugs must be used cautiously because marked depression of cardiac contractility, conduction, or heart rate could result. β-Blockers are generally contraindicated in patients with sinus bradycardia, sick sinus syndrome, high-grade AV block, or severe congestive heart failure and in animals also receiving a calcium entry blocker. Drugs that antagonize both $\beta_1$- and $\beta_2$-adrenergic receptors (nonselective β-blockers) may increase peripheral vascular resistance (resulting from unopposed α effects) and cause bronchoconstriction. β-Blockers may also prevent the appearance of early signs of acute hypoglycemia in diabetics (e.g., tachycardia and blood pressure changes), and they also reduce the release of insulin in response to hyperglycemia.

β-Blockers enhance the depression of AV conduction produced by digitalis, class I antiarrhythmic drugs, and calcium entry blockers. The simultaneous use of a β-blocker and a calcium entry blocker is not recommended because it can lead to marked decreases in heart rate and myocardial contractility. Because of the possibility of β-receptor up-regulation (increased number or affinity of receptors) during long-term β-blockade, abrupt discontinuation of therapy could result in serious cardiac arrhythmias.

### Propranolol

Propranolol is a nonselective β-blocker that has been widely used in dogs and cats, although other β-blockers are used often now. The combination of propranolol with a class I agent often produces better ventricular tachyarrhythmia suppression than either agent alone. Propranolol has been used successfully to reduce arterial pressure in some hypertensive dogs, especially in conjunction with a low-sodium diet. Propranolol (or any β-blocker) should be used only cautiously in animals with heart failure; prior digitalization is advised if myocardial failure is present. It is suggested that propranolol therapy be delayed until after pulmonary edema resolves because of the potential for bronchoconstriction from $\beta_2$-receptor antagonism. The $\beta_2$-receptor blocking effects of propranolol also make it relatively contraindicated in patients with asthma or chronic small airway disease.

Propranolol has a relatively low bioavailability when given PO because of extensive first-pass hepatic metabolism; however, long-term administration and higher doses cause hepatic enzyme saturation and increase bioavailability. Propranolol decreases hepatic blood flow, thereby prolonging its own elimination and that of other drugs dependent on liver blood flow for their metabolism (e.g., lidocaine). Feeding delays the rate of PO absorption and increases the clearance of an IV dose (by increasing hepatic blood flow). The half-life of propranolol in the dog is only about 1.5 hours (0.5 to 4.2 hours in cats), but active metabolites exist. Dosing every 8 hours appears to be adequate in both dogs and cats. Because the effects of this drug (and other β-blockers) depend on the level of sympathetic activation, individual patient response is quite variable. Therefore initial dosages should be low and titrated upward as needed, according to the animal's response (see Table 4-5). The IV form is used mainly in the treatment of refractory ventricular tachycardia (in conjunction with a class I drug) and in the emergency management of atrial or junctional tachycardia.

Toxicity of propranolol is usually related to excessive β-blockade stemming from overzealous use. However, some animals are unable to tolerate even small doses, and the importance of careful dosage titration from an initial low dose cannot be overemphasized for this and all β-blockers. Bradycardia, heart failure, hypotension, bronchospasm, and hypoglycemia can occur. Infusion of a catecholamine (e.g., dopamine or dobutamine) will help reverse these effects. Propranolol and other lipophilic β-blockers can cause a depressed attitude and disorientation as a result of central nervous system effects.

### Atenolol

Atenolol is a selective $\beta_1$-blocker that is now used more often than propranolol in dogs and cats with clinical heart disease to slow sinus rate and AV conduction and to suppress ventricular premature depolarizations. The half-life of atenolol is slightly over 3 hours in dogs and about 3.5 hours in cats. Its oral bioavailability in both species is 90%. Atenolol is excreted in the urine; renal impairment delays clearance. Its β-blocking effects are evident for 12 hours but are gone by 24 hours in normal animals. This hydrophilic drug does not readily cross the blood-brain barrier, therefore adverse central nervous system effects are unlikely. However, weakness or exacerbation of heart failure can be observed, as with other β-blockers.

### Other β-Blockers

Many β-blocking drugs are available. Their basic effects are similar, although their relative selectivity for $\beta_1$- as opposed to both $\beta_1$- and $\beta_2$-receptors, as well as their pharmacologic characteristics, vary. Some of these drugs are listed in Tables 4-5,

4-6, and 4-8. Esmolol has $\beta_1$-receptor selectivity and a very short half-life (less than 10 minutes). Although expensive, this drug has been used for the short-term treatment of tachyarrhythmias and feline hypertrophic obstructive cardiomyopathy.

Certain $\beta$-blockers have proved useful in the treatment of chronic, stable myocardial failure by reducing the cardiotoxic effects of excess sympathetic stimulation, improving cardiac function, promoting upregulation of cardiac $\beta$-receptors, and increasing survival time. The third-generation $\beta$-blocker carvedilol and the second-generation agent metoprolol have effectiveness in this regard. Nonselective (first-generation) agents such as propranolol and some later-generation agents do not appear to confer these survival benefits. Agents with intrinsic sympathomimetic activity appear to have deleterious effects.

Carvedilol blocks $\beta_1$-, $\beta_2$-, and $\alpha_1$-receptors but is without intrinsic sympathomimetic activity. It also acts as an oxygen free-radical scavenger, is thought to block certain $Ca^{++}$ channels, and also promotes vasodilation by affecting either nitric oxide or prostaglandin mechanisms. Carvedilol is metabolized in the liver; excretion is mainly biliary, with a minor renal contribution. The drug's vasodilatory effects may offset negative inotropic effects of $\beta$-blockade, although in chronic human studies, improvements in left ventricular function occurred without a change in systemic vascular resistance. It appears that carvedilol may be superior to metoprolol for chronic heart failure therapy in people. Veterinary studies are in progress to evaluate whether similar improvements in morbidity and mortality occur in dogs with stable dilated cardiomyopathy that are given chronic low-dose carvedilol therapy. Caution is warranted, because any $\beta$-blocker can provoke clinical decompensation in patients dependent on high sympathetic tone to maintain cardiac output. Furthermore, the beneficial effects seen in people only become evident after several months of therapy. There is also some preliminary evidence in people that carvedilol may have a protective effect against doxorubicin-induced cardiotoxicity.

## CLASS III ANTIARRHYTHMIC DRUGS

Prolongation of cardiac action potential duration and effective refractory period without decreasing conduction velocity are the common features of class III drugs (see Tables 4-4 to 4-6). They are useful for the treatment of refractory ventricular arrhythmias, especially those caused by reentry. These drugs have antifibrillatory effects as well. Currently available agents share some characteristics of other antiarrhythmic drug classes in addition to their class III effects.

### Sotalol

Sotalol is a nonselective $\beta$-blocker that has class III effects. It prolongs the refractory period by selectively blocking the rapid component of $K^+$ channels responsible for repolarization (delayed rectifier current). The bioavailability of sotalol in people is almost 100%, with peak plasma concentrations reached within 2 to 3 hours, and a half-life of 7 to 15 hours. It is eliminated unchanged by the kidneys, and renal dysfunction prolongs elimination. Sotalol's $\beta$-blocking effects

last longer than its plasma half-life. The drug has minimal hemodynamic effects other than a slowing of sinus rate in normal people. Sotalol can cause proarrhythmia (as can all antiarrhythmic agents), including *torsades de pointes*. It appears that dogs require much higher doses than people to manifest the class III effects. Doses that have been used clinically in dogs may be producing primarily $\beta$-blocking effects. On the other hand, the high incidence of proarrhythmia (especially *torsades de pointes*), which is of concern in people taking sotalol, has not been reported clinically in dogs. Experimentally, in hypokalemic dogs, co-administration of the class IB agent mexiletine reduced this proarrhythmic potential.

Sotalol may worsen heart failure when serious myocardial disease is present. Although there is experimental evidence that sotalol has less of a negative inotropic effect than propranolol and may even have a mild positive inotropic effect related to its ability to prolong action potential duration, it has been associated with clinical deterioration in dogs with moderately to markedly reduced myocardial contractility. Sotalol has been used successfully in large-breed dogs with persistent ventricular tachyarrhythmias and good myocardial function. Other adverse effects of sotalol have included hypotension, depression, nausea, vomiting, diarrhea, and bradycardia.

### Amiodarone

Amiodarone is thought to produce its antiarrhythmic effects by prolonging the action potential duration and effective refractory period in both atrial and ventricular tissues. Although considered a class III agent, it shares properties with all three other antiarrhythmic drug classes. Amiodarone is an iodinated compound that also has noncompetitive $\alpha_1$- and $\beta$-blocking effects, as well as calcium channel blocking effects. The $\beta$-blocking effects occur soon after administration, but maximal class III effects (and prolongation of the action potential duration and QT interval) are not achieved for weeks with chronic administration. Amiodarone's $Ca^{++}$ blocking effects may inhibit triggered arrhythmias by reducing afterdepolarizations. Therapeutic doses slow the sinus rate, decrease AV conduction velocity, and minimally depress myocardial contractility and blood pressure. Indications for amiodarone in people include refractory tachyarrhythmias of both atrial and ventricular origin, especially reentrant arrhythmias using an accessory pathway. Intravenous amiodarone has been used in people with atrial fibrillation or ventricular tachycardia, and during cardiopulmonary resuscitation from recurrent ventricular tachycardia or fibrillation. There is still relatively limited veterinary experience with amiodarone, although it appears to be a promising drug for dogs. It has been used PO most often, although an IV form is available. The IV form is not labeled for human pediatric patients and has caused a potentially fatal "gasping syndrome" in neonates. However, doses of 1 mg/kg given over 5 to 10 minutes and repeated up to a total initial dose of 5 mg/kg over 25 to 50 minutes, or continuous infusion of 10 to 15 mg/kg/day, has been used successfully in children (Perry and colleagues, 1996) and could be tried in dogs.

Amiodarone's pharmacokinetics are complex, with a prolonged time to steady state, concentration in myocardial and other tissues, and accumulation of an active metabolite (desethylamiodarone) with chronic PO use. The human therapeutic serum concentration range of 1 to 2.5 μg/ml is thought to apply to dogs also. Electrophysiologic effects occur in dogs at these concentrations. Amiodarone may have a lesser proarrhythmic effect than other agents and may reduce the risk of sudden death because of uniform effects on repolarization throughout the ventricles. Experimentally in dogs, chronic amiodarone treatment moderately prolonged QT interval without affecting dispersion of repolarization (Merot and colleagues, 1999). Another study in normal dogs given PO amiodarone (25 mg/kg q12h × 4 weeks, then 25 mg/kg q24h × 2 weeks) found QT and myocardial action potential duration prolongation, as well as suppression of Purkinje fiber automaticity. Plasma drug concentrations within the therapeutic range for humans were reported in this study (Bicer and colleagues, 2001). IV amiodarone administered to normal dogs did not decrease myocardial contractility ($dP/dt_{max}$) until cumulative doses of 12.5 and 15 mg/kg were reached (given in 2.5 mg/kg increments q15min) (Bicer and colleagues, 2000). However, the potential for more profound cardiac depression and hypotension with IV amiodarone is of concern in dogs with myocardial disease.

Long-term therapy in people is associated with numerous and potentially severe adverse effects, including corneal microdeposits, abnormalities in thyroid function, liver disease, pneumonitis and pulmonary fibrosis, photosensitivity, bluish skin discoloration, and peripheral neuropathy. Gastrointestinal upset, hepatic dysfunction, and positive Coombs' test have been reported in dogs receiving PO amiodarone. Amiodarone reduces the clearance and increases the serum concentration of digoxin and diltiazem.

## Bretylium Tosylate

The antiarrhythmic effects of bretylium also are related to prolongation of action potential duration and effective refractory period in ventricular muscle and Purkinje fibers. The drug also increases the ventricular fibrillation threshold. Bretylium causes an initial release of catecholamines from sympathetic nerve terminals, followed by a longer period during which norepinephrine release is inhibited. The transient increase followed by the prolonged decrease in sinus rate, AV conduction velocity, vascular resistance, and arterial blood pressure seen after IV drug administration is attributed to this. Bretylium is eliminated through the kidneys, so renal disease reduces drug clearance. Bretylium's half-life in dogs is about 10.4 hours. Extremely poor absorption PO limits its use to the IM or IV routes. Tissue concentrations rise slowly to peak within 1.5 to 6 hours after administration and are more closely related to the antifibrillatory effects of the drug than plasma concentrations.

Bretylium is potentially indicated for the treatment of life-threatening ventricular arrhythmias that are nonresponsive to conventional therapy and for animals at risk for ventricular fibrillation. It is not indicated as initial therapy for ventricular arrhythmias. Although early studies suggested that the drug might convert ventricular fibrillation to sinus rhythm, later studies of electrically induced fibrillation in dogs did not support this. It is thought that the antifibrillatory effects of bretylium may be delayed 4 to 6 hours after administration. For this reason, clinical usefulness might be realized by giving it early to high-risk animals (e.g., prior to surgical procedures in dogs with serious underlying cardiac disease), but in conjunction with other antiarrhythmic drugs. However, further clinical study is needed.

Adverse effects of bretylium after rapid IV injection include ataxia, nausea, and vomiting. Significant hypotension is uncommon and responds to fluid administration. Extreme bradycardia or hypotension is a contraindication to its use. There appear to be no drug interactions of importance. Aggravation of arrhythmias and tachycardia (early) can occur.

## Other Class III Agents

Ibutilide fumarate (Corvert, Pharmacia & Upjohn, Kalamazoo, Mich) is somewhat effective for converting recent onset atrial fibrillation in people, but there is little veterinary experience with this drug. In experimental rapid pacing–induced cardiomyopathy in dogs, ibutilide caused increased dispersion of ventricular repolarization and episodes of *torsades de pointes* (Hsieh and colleagues, 2000). Dofetilide (Tikosyn, Pfizer, New York, N.Y.) is another drug that selectively blocks the rapid component of the $K^+$ current responsible for repolarization. It is approved in people for the conversion of atrial fibrillation and subsequent maintenance of sinus rhythm. Its efficacy for this appears comparable to other class III drugs, but it does not have a negative inotropic effect and appears safer in the presence of left ventricular dysfunction. Other class III agents are also being investigated.

## CLASS IV ANTIARRHYTHMIC DRUGS: CALCIUM ENTRY BLOCKERS

The calcium entry blockers are a diverse group of drugs that have the common property of decreasing cellular $Ca^{++}$ influx by blocking transmembrane L-type calcium channels (see Tables 4-4 to 4-6). Calcium is important to the electrical and mechanical functions of the heart and vasculature. Calcium entry blockers as a group can cause coronary and systemic vasodilation, enhance myocardial relaxation, and reduce cardiac contractility. Some calcium entry blockers have antiarrhythmic effects, especially on tissues dependent on the slow inward $Ca^{++}$ current, such as the sinus and AV nodes. Other conditions for which calcium entry blockers are potentially useful include hypertrophic cardiomyopathy, myocardial ischemia, and hypertension.

## Diltiazem

Diltiazem is a benzothiazepine calcium channel blocker. It slows AV conduction, causes potent coronary and mild peripheral vasodilation, and has a lesser negative inotropic effect than the prototypical calcium entry blocker, verapamil. Diltiazem is often combined with digoxin to further slow the ventricular response rate to atrial fibrillation in dogs. It is indicated for the treatment of other supraventricular tachyarrhythmias as well. Diltiazem is often used in cats with hypertrophic cardiomyopathy, where its beneficial effects can include enhancement of myocardial relaxation and perfusion, as well as mild reductions in heart rate, contractility, and myocardial oxygen demand (see Chapter 7). Chronic diltiazem therapy may possibly be associated with a decrease in left ventricular wall and septal thickness in cats with hypertrophic cardiomyopathy.

Peak effects are seen within 2 hours after PO dosing, and the effects last at least 6 hours. The half-life of diltiazem in the dog is just over 2 hours; this may be prolonged with chronic PO treatment because of its enterohepatic circulation. Peak plasma concentrations occur 30 to 60 minutes after PO dosing. In cats, peak plasma concentrations of diltiazem are reached in 30 minutes and remain in the therapeutic range (50 to 300 µg/ml) for 8 hours. Potentially active metabolites exist; very little of the parent drug is excreted unchanged in the urine. Drugs that inhibit hepatic enzyme systems (e.g., cimetidine) decrease diltiazem's metabolism. Also, propranolol and diltiazem reduce each other's clearance when used simultaneously. Initial dosages should be low, with the dosage increased as needed to effect or to the maximal recommended dose (see Table 4-5). The sustained-release preparation, Cardizem-CD, has been evaluated in cats at a dosage of 10 mg/kg daily. Peak plasma concentrations are reached in 6 hours, and therapeutic concentrations are maintained for 24 hours. A dose of 45 mg per cat once a day is approximately equal to 105 mg of Cardizem-CD (or the amount that fits into the small end of a No. 4 gelatin capsule; a 300-mg capsule provides about 6.5 doses). Dilacor XR (now available as Diltia XT) is another sustained-release diltiazem preparation that has four tablets contained within a 240-mg gelatin capsule. Each of these internal tablets has 60 mg of diltiazem; one-half tablet (30 mg) per cat can be administered once daily.

Adverse effects are uncommon at therapeutic doses, although anorexia, nausea, and bradycardia may occur. Rarely, other gastrointestinal, cardiac, and neurologic adverse effects have occurred in people and cats. High liver enzyme activities in association with anorexia have sporadically occurred in cats. Some cats have become aggressive or shown other personality change when treated with diltiazem. As with other calcium entry blockers, an overdose or an exaggerated response is treated with supportive care: atropine (see Table 4-5) for bradycardia or AV blocks; dopamine or dobutamine (see Table 3-8) and furosemide (see Table 3-6) for heart failure; and dopamine or IV calcium salts for hypotension.

## Verapamil

Verapamil, a phenylalkylamine, has the most potent cardiac effects of the clinically used calcium entry blockers. It causes dose-related slowing of the sinus rate and AV conduction. The drug increases the refractory period of nodal tissues and thus is effective in abolishing reentrant supraventricular tachycardia and slowing the ventricular response rate in atrial fibrillation. Verapamil has important negative inotropic and some vasodilatory effects that can cause serious decompensation, hypotension, and even death in the presence of underlying myocardial disease. Because of this, verapamil is not recommended for use in animals with heart failure. Verapamil is often effective against supraventricular and atrial

tachycardias in animals that do not have heart failure. An initially low dose (see Table 4-5) is given very slowly IV; this can be repeated at 5 (or more)–minute intervals if no adverse effects have occurred and the arrhythmia persists. Blood pressure monitoring is advisable when using the IV route because of the potential for hypotension. Contraindications to verapamil use include congestive heart failure, sick sinus syndrome, AV conduction disturbances, digitalis toxicity, and preexisting β-blocker therapy. The concurrent use of verapamil and a β-blocking drug can cause a sudden decrease in the sinus rate or complete heart block.

The half-life of verapamil in the dog is about 2.5 hours. It is poorly absorbed and undergoes first-pass hepatic metabolism, resulting in low bioavailability of the PO form. The pharmacokinetics in cats are similar to those in dogs. The toxic effects of verapamil include sinus bradycardia, AV block, hypotension, reduced myocardial contractility, and cardiogenic shock. The negative inotropic effects of verapamil may be reversed by the IV administration of calcium salts, sympathomimetic drugs, or amrinone (see Table 3-8). Atropine may also be required to treat bradycardia or conduction blocks precipitated by verapamil. Verapamil reduces the renal clearance of digoxin, thereby raising its serum concentration.

### Other Calcium Entry Blockers

There are several other drugs available that have calcium channel blocking activity. Most (dihydropyridine group) are used as antihypertensives in people; some, such as amlodipine and felodipine, are used in chronic heart failure therapy. Amlodipine is recommended as the first-line antihypertensive agent in cats and is also used in some hypertensive dogs (see Chapter 12). It is being incorporated into the therapy of chronic refractory heart failure for some dogs, beginning at lower doses (e.g. 0.05 to 0.1 mg/kg q24 or 12h; see Table 3-6). Amlodipine besylate is a long-acting dihydropyridine calcium entry blocker, with a plasma half-life of about 30 hours in dogs, and maximal effects that occur 4 to 7 days after initiating therapy. Oral bioavailability is high (88% in dogs), and peak plasma concentrations are reached 3 to 8 hours after administration; plasma concentrations increase with chronic therapy. The drug undergoes hepatic metabolism, but there is not extensive first-pass elimination; caution is warranted in animals with poor liver function. Excretion is through the urine and feces. Pharmacokinetic data for cats are unavailable, but amlodipine's effects on blood pressure are thought to last at least 24 hours in that species. Amlodipine generally does not have significant effects on the serum creatinine concentration or body weight in cats with chronic renal failure. Nifedipine, also a potent vasodilator, has no relevant effect on AV conduction and is not useful as an antiarrhythmic agent.

## ANTICHOLINERGIC DRUGS

### Atropine and Glycopyrrolate

Anticholinergic drugs can increase sinus node rate and AV conduction in the presence of excessive vagal tone (see Tables 4-5 and 4-6). Atropine is a competitive muscarinic receptor antagonist. Parenteral atropine or glycopyrrolate is indicated for bradycardia or AV block induced by anesthesia, central nervous system lesions, and certain other diseases or toxicities. Unlike atropine, glycopyrrolate does not have centrally mediated effects and its effects are longer lasting than those of atropine.

An **atropine challenge** test is used to determine the degree of vagal influence on sinus and/or AV nodal function. Atropine given by any parenteral route can transiently exacerbate vagally mediated AV block when the atrial rate increases faster than AV conduction can respond. However, IV administration (0.02 mg/kg) has been shown to cause the fastest and most consistent onset and resolution of the exacerbated block, as well as the most rapid postbradycardia heart rates, compared with the IM and SC routes. It is thought that atropine challenge test results are most consistent using IV administration of (0.02 to) 0.04 mg/kg, followed by ECG recording in 5 to 10 minutes. If the heart rate has not increased by at least 150%, the ECG should be repeated at 15 to 20 minutes after the atropine injection, because the AV nodal vagomimetic effect may last longer than 5 minutes in some dogs. The normal sinus node response is an increase in rate to 150 to 160 beats/min (or over 135 beats/min). Evaluation of heart rate variability after different atropine doses in an experimental study indicated that 0.04 mg/kg did, but 0.02 mg/kg did not, completely abolish parasympathetic tone (Rishniw and colleagues, 1999). In animals with organic AV nodal disease, AV block may remain unchanged or worsen after anticholinergic injection.

### Oral Anticholinergic Drugs

Some animals that respond to parenteral atropine or glycopyrrolate will also respond to PO anticholinergics, at least transiently. Oral therapy may relieve the clinical signs in these animals (see Table 4-5). However, animals with symptomatic bradyarrhythmias usually require permanent pacemaker implantation to effectively control the heart rate. Propantheline bromide has been used commonly, but other oral anticholinergic agents are also available.

Vagolytic drugs may aggravate paroxysmal supraventricular tachyarrhythmias (as occur in the sick sinus syndrome) and should not be used as chronic therapy in animals with them. Other adverse effects of anticholinergic therapy include vomiting, dry mouth, constipation, keratoconjunctivitis sicca, and drying of respiratory secretions.

### SYMPATHOMIMETIC DRUGS

Isoproterenol is a $\beta$-receptor agonist that has been used in the treatment of symptomatic AV block or bradycardia refractory to atropine (see earlier discussion and Tables 4-5 and 4-6), although electrical pacing is safer and more effective. Because of its affinity for $\beta_2$-receptors, it can cause hypotension, and it is not used for treating either heart failure or cardiac arrest. Isoproterenol can be arrhythmogenic, as can other catecholamines. The lowest effective dose (see Table 4-5) should be used and the animal monitored closely for the development of arrhythmias. Administration PO is not effective because

of marked first-pass hepatic metabolism. Terbutaline PO, a $\beta_2$-receptor agonist, may have a mild stimulatory effect on the heart rate. The methylxanthine bronchodilators (aminophylline and theophylline) have increased the heart rate in some dogs with sick sinus syndrome when used at higher doses.

### OTHER DRUGS

Adenosine is an endogenous nucleoside that has been used for the acute termination of supraventricular tachycardias in people. Veterinary experience with adenosine has been limited and not encouraging. Adenosine binds with $\alpha_1$-receptors on the cardiac cell surface and activates potassium channels in the same manner as acetylcholine to shorten action potential duration and to hyperpolarize the membrane. It also indirectly antagonizes catecholamine effects in the sinus node. Other effects include transient sinus node exit block, AV blocks, and a secondary reflex tachycardia. Adenosine is rapidly degraded by enzyme systems in vascular endothelium and blood cells. The elimination half-life in people is 1 to 6 seconds, therefore most of the drug's effects are produced by its first passage through the circulation. Adenosine must be administered rapidly IV, preferably into a central vein. Doses of 6 to 12 mg are used in people. Transient sinus rate slowing or AV block occurs. Methylxanthine bronchodilators block the effects of adenosine.

### Suggested Readings

Arrhythmias and Antiarrhythmic Drugs

Awaji T et al: Acute antiarrhythmic effects of intravenously administered amiodarone on canine ventricular arrhythmias, *J Cardiovasc Pharmacol* 26:869, 1995.

Baty CJ et al: Torsades de pointes–like polymorphic ventricular tachycardia in a dog, *J Vet Intern Med* 8:439, 1994.

Bicer S et al: Hemodynamic and electrocardiographic effects of graded doses of amiodarone in healthy dogs anesthetized with morphine/$\alpha$ chloralose, *J Vet Intern Med* 14:90, 2000.

Bicer S et al: Effects of chronic oral amiodarone on left ventricular pressure, electrocardiograms, and action potentials from myocardium in vivo and from Purkinje fibers in vitro, *Vet Therap* 2:325, 2001.

Bonagura JD et al: Acute effects of esmolol on left ventricular outflow tract obstruction in cats with hypertrophic cardiomyopathy: a Doppler echocardiographic study, *J Vet Intern Med* 5:123, 1991 (abstract).

Calvert CA et al: Efficacy and toxicity of tocainide for the treatment of ventricular tachyarrhythmias in Doberman Pinschers with occult cardiomyopathy, *J Vet Intern Med* 10:235, 1996.

Calvert CA et al: CVT update: Doberman Pinscher occult cardiomyopathy. In Bonagura JD, editor: *Kirk's current veterinary therapy XIII*, Philadelphia, 2000, WB Saunders, p 756.

Calvert CA et al: Positive Coombs' test results in two dogs treated with amiodarone, *J Am Vet Med Assoc* 216:1933, 2000.

Chezalviel-Guilbert F et al: Mexiletine antagonizes the effects of sotalol on QT interval duration and its proarrhythmic effects in a canine model of torsades de pointes, *J Am Coll Cardiol* 26:787, 1995.

Cooke KL et al: Calcium channel blockers in veterinary medicine, *J Vet Intern Med* 12:123, 1998.

Hsieh MH et al: Proarrhythmic effects of ibutilide in a canine model of pacing induced cardiomyopathy, *Pacing Clin Electrophysiol* 23:149, 2000.

Jacobs G et al: Hepatopathy in 4 dogs treated with amiodarone, *J Vet Intern Med* 14:96, 2000.

Johnson LM et al: Pharmacokinetic and pharmacodynamic properties of conventional and CD-formulated diltiazem in cats, *J Vet Intern Med* 10:316, 1996.

Lunney J et al: Mexiletine administration for management of ventricular arrhythmia in 22 dogs, *J Am Anim Hosp Assoc* 27:597, 1991.

Merot J et al: Effects of chronic treatment by amiodarone on transmural heterogeneity of canine ventricular repolarization in vivo: interactions with acute sotalol, *Cardiovasc Res* 44:303, 1999.

Miyamoto M et al: Cardiovascular effects of intravenous diltiazem in dogs with iatrogenic atrial fibrillation, *J Vet Intern Med* 14:445, 2000.

Miyamoto M et al: Acute cardiovascular effects of diltiazem in anesthetized dogs with induced atrial fibrillation, *J Vet Intern Med* 15:559, 2001.

Moise NS et al: Diagnosis of inherited ventricular tachycardia in German Shepherd dogs, *J Am Vet Med Assoc* 210:403, 1997.

Moise NS: Diagnosis and management of canine arrhythmias. In Fox PR et al, editors: *Textbook of canine and feline cardiology,* ed 2, 1999, Philadelphia, WB Saunders, p 331.

Perry JC et al: Pediatric use of intravenous amiodarone: efficacy and safety in critically ill patients from a multicenter protocol, *J Am Coll Cardiol* 27:1246, 1996.

Pinson DM: Myocardial necrosis and sudden death after an episode of aggressive behavior in a dog, *J Am Vet Med Assoc* 211:1371, 1997.

Poole JE et al: Sudden cardiac death. In Zipes DP et al, editors: *Cardiac electrophysiology, from cell to bedside,* ed 3, Philadelphia, 2000, WB Saunders, p 615.

Quiñones M et al: Pharmacokinetics of atenolol in clinically normal cats, *Am J Vet Res* 57:1050, 1996.

Restivo M et al: Efficacy of azimilide and dofetilide in the dog right atrial enlargement model of atrial flutter, *J Cardiovasc Electrophysiol* 12:1018, 2001.

Rishniw M et al: Characterization of chronotropic and dysrhythmogenic effects of atropine in dogs with bradycardia, *Am J Vet Res* 57:337, 1996.

Rishniw M et al: Characterization of parasympatholytic chronotropic responses following intravenous administration of atropine to clinically normal dogs, *Am J Vet Res* 60:1000, 1999.

Sawangkoon S et al: Acute cardiovascular effects and pharmacokinetics of carvedilol in healthy dogs, *Am J Vet Res* 61:57, 2000.

Schiffer SP: Evidence linking behavior states with cardiac vulnerability, *J Am Vet Med Assoc* 212:488, 1998 (letter).

Seidler RW et al: Influence of sotalol on the time constant of isovolumic left ventricular relaxation in anesthetized dogs, *Am J Vet Res* 60:717, 1999.

Sicilian Gambit members: New approaches to antiarrhythmic therapy, Part I. *Circulation* 104:2865, 2001.

Sicilian Gambit members: New approaches to antiarrhythmic therapy, Part II. Circulation 104:2990, 2001.

Sicouri S et al: Chronic amiodarone reduces transmural dispersion of repolarization in the canine heart, *J Cardiovasc Electrophysiol* 8:1269, 1997.

Stambler BS et al: Efficacy and safety of repeated intravenous doses of ibutilide for rapid conversion of atrial flutter or fibrillation, *Circulation* 94:1613, 1996.

Wright KN et al: Radiofrequency catheter ablation of atrioventricular accessory pathways in 3 dogs with subsequent resolution of tachycardia-induced cardiomyopathy, *J Vet Intern Med* 13:361, 1999.

Wright KN: Assessment and treatment of supraventricular tachyarrhythmias. In Bonagura JD, editor: *Kirk's current veterinary therapy XIII,* Philadelphia, 2000, WB Saunders, p 726.

CARDIAC PACING

Darke PGG: Update: transvenous pacing. In Kirk RW et al, editors: *Current veterinary therapy XI,* Philadelphia, 1992, WB Saunders, p 708.

Flanders JA et al: Introduction of an endocardial pacing lead through the costocervical vein in six dogs, *J Am Vet Med Assoc* 215:46, 1999.

Moise NS: Pacemaker therapy. In Fox PR et al, editors: *Textbook of canine and feline cardiology,* ed 2, 1999, Philadelphia, WB Saunders, p 400.

Oyama MA et al: Practices and outcomes of artificial cardiac pacing in 154 dogs, *J Vet Intern Med* 15:229, 2001.

Sisson D et al: Permanent transvenous pacemaker implantation in forty dogs, *J Vet Intern Med* 5:322, 1991.

Snyder PS et al: Syncope in three dogs with cardiac pacemakers, *J Am Anim Hosp Assoc* 27:611, 1991.

# CHAPTER 5

# Cardiopulmonary Resuscitation

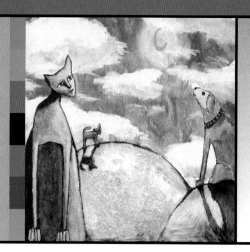

## CHAPTER OUTLINE

GENERAL CONSIDERATIONS, 98
SIGNS OF IMPENDING CARDIOPULMONARY
ARREST, 98
APPROACH TO CARDIOPULMONARY
RESUSCITATION, 99
    Airway (A), 99
    Breathing (B), 99
    Circulation (C), 100
    Drugs (D), 102
    Electrocardiogram (E), 104
    Follow-up (F), 104

## GENERAL CONSIDERATIONS

Respiratory arrest is characterized by apnea but continued heartbeats. If not reversed, it soon leads to a lethal cardiac rhythm and cardiopulmonary arrest. Cardiac pump activity and blood circulation cease with ventricular fibrillation, ventricular asystole, or electromechanical dissociation (EMD). Conditions leading to the development of these lethal arrhythmias include extreme bradycardia, tachyarrhythmias, hypotension, advanced shock, trauma, and causes of respiratory arrest, such as anesthetics or other drugs, severe pulmonary or central nervous system disease, suffocation, and airway obstruction. Because of the potential for EMD in animals with severe cardiopulmonary disease and arrest, it is important to verify the presence of heartbeats and pulses, even if the electrocardiogram (ECG) appears reasonably normal.

Ventricular fibrillation is the most common lethal arrhythmia in dogs and people; EMD appears to be the most common in cats. Because a critical myocardial mass is necessary to sustain ventricular fibrillation, the small size of the feline heart may preclude sustained fibrillation and allow sinus rhythm to resume spontaneously. In cats and young dogs, primary respiratory arrest often occurs first and progresses to cardiac arrest. The rapid institution of assisted ventilation with oxygen may avert cardiac arrest, especially if there is no

serious underlying disease. Cardiopulmonary arrest appears to be more common than respiratory arrest alone in dogs over 4 years of age. A much higher percentage of both dogs and cats are successfully resuscitated from respiratory arrest than from cardiopulmonary arrest. The severity of any underlying disease, as well as the rapidity with which resuscitative efforts are begun, greatly influence the outcome.

Reported survival rates for dogs and cats undergoing cardiopulmonary resuscitation (CPR) vary and are difficult to compare because of differences in the definition of survival and the techniques used. The percentage of animals with cardiopulmonary arrest that temporarily regain spontaneous circulation after CPR appears to be less than 25%. Less than 5% of dogs and only 9% of cats are discharged from the hospital alive after experiencing cardiopulmonary arrest. Arrest secondary to drug and anesthetic reactions is associated with a better long-term outcome than that secondary to a serious underlying disease. The decision to begin or continue CPR should be based on the potential reversibility of the animal's underlying problems as well as the owner's wishes.

## SIGNS OF IMPENDING CARDIOPULMONARY ARREST

Early recognition of the signs of cardiopulmonary deterioration may help in the prevention of cardiac arrest or at least allow a more rapid response when it occurs. Signs of impending arrest include slowing of the heart or respiratory rate, gasping or irregular respirations, deteriorating consciousness, progressive T-wave enlargement on the ECG (suggesting myocardial hypoxia), ST segment changes, and cardiac arrhythmias. The appearance of any of these signs should prompt appropriate action, such as providing supplemental oxygen, placing an intravenous (IV) line, locating a suitable endotracheal tube, monitoring the ECG, administering any appropriate drugs to manage arrhythmias, increasing the ventilation of anesthetized animals and discontinuing inhaled anesthetics, and gathering the equipment and drugs needed should arrest occur.

Animals in respiratory arrest, with or without concurrent cardiac arrest, may exhibit agonal gasps or show no respiratory motion. They quickly become unconscious, their mucous membranes become pale gray or cyanotic, pupils dilate, and muscular tone is lost. Palpable pulse and heartbeat disappear when systolic pressures decrease below 50 to 60 mm Hg; bleeding from surgical sites or wounds also may stop. Immediate and effective CPR is imperative.

## APPROACH TO CARDIOPULMONARY RESUSCITATION

Successful cardiac resuscitation begins with advanced planning. Guidelines and drug doses for CPR should be posted for easy reference (Table 5-1; Fig. 5-1). Both lay and professional staff should be familiar with the procedures and equipment used for resuscitation, and emergency equipment should be readily accessible so that a coordinated and efficient "team effort" can be mounted. Most hospitals maintain a "crash cart" of the drugs and supplies likely to be needed for CPR.

The immediate goal of CPR is to restore ventilation and effective circulation to the heart and brain. Further goals are to restore normal heart rhythm and output and to correct tissue hypoxia and acidosis. The drugs commonly used in CPR and their dosages are listed in Table 5-1. The components of CPR—A (airway), B (breathing), C (circulation), D (drugs), E (ECG), and F (follow-up)—are discussed in the following paragraphs. This approach to resuscitation is outlined in Fig. 5-1.

## AIRWAY (A)

Establishing a patent airway is critical to ensuring effective resuscitation. A properly placed and secured cuffed endotracheal tube should be used. Suction is used to remove any mucus, fluid, or vomitus from the pharynx and trachea. Tracheostomy may be necessary in some animals.

## BREATHING (B)

Intermittent positive-pressure ventilation can be accomplished using the reservoir bag on an anesthetic machine, a self-inflating resuscitation bag (e.g., Ambu bag), or a mouth-to-tube technique. Use of 100% oxygen has been recommended. However, there is concern that prolonged use of 100% $O_2$ contributes to oxidative stress and delayed brain injury after reperfusion. Use of room air may reduce oxidation of brain lipids and improve neurological outcome. Two long breaths (1 to 1.5 seconds in duration) should be given initially; artificial ventilation is begun if the animal does not spontaneously start to breathe. Various ventilation rates have been used; a rate of 20 (large dogs) to 24 (small dogs and possibly higher in cats) breaths/min appears to be more effective than the previously recommended 12 to 15 breaths/min. Sufficient volume is given to approximate normal chest expansion. Peak airway pressure should generally not exceed 20 cm $H_2O$ in order to avoid pulmonary injury and pneumothorax. Short-term artificial ventilation alone may resuscitate an animal with respiratory arrest.

Cardiac massage is begun if arterial pulses are not palpable. Simultaneous ventilation with every second to third chest compression can enhance forward flow by intermittently generating higher intrathoracic pressure; however, it may impede

### TABLE 5-1

Drug Dosages for CPR in Dogs and Cats

| DRUG | DOSAGE |
| --- | --- |
| Epinephrine | (0.1 to) 0.2 mg/kg IV or 0.4 mg/kg IT (diluted with 2-5 ml of sterile water or saline) q(3 to) 5min as needed; also can use IO. (Previously recommended: 0.1 to 0.5 mg/10 kg) 1:1000 = 1 mg/ml |
| Methoxamine | 0.1 to 0.2 mg/kg IV; can use IT |
| Metaraminol | 0.1 to 0.2 mg/kg IV |
| Mephentermine | 0.1 to 0.5 mg/kg IV |
| Phenylephrine | 0.01 to 0.1 mg/kg IV |
| Norepinephrine | 0.01 to 0.1 mg/average dog |
| Dopamine | Dogs: 5 to 15 μg/kg/min; cats: 1 to 5 μg/kg/min CRI; can use IO |
| Sodium bicarbonate | 0.5 to 1 mEq/kg initial dose; up to 8 mEq/kg if prolonged arrest and/or CPR. Do *not* give IT; can use IO |
| Calcium chloride (10%) | 0.1 to 0.26 ml/kg IV (or 1.5 to 2 ml/dog) |
| Calcium gluconate (10%) | 0.1 to 0.3 ml/kg IV; can use IO |
| Dexamethasone SP | 4 mg/kg IV; can use IO |
| Atropine | 0.04 mg/kg IV, IM, IT, IO |
| Lidocaine | Dogs: 2 mg/kg, up to 8 mg/kg IV; cats: 0.25 to 0.5 mg/kg slowly IV; see Table 4-5, p.79; can use IT or IO |
| Bretylium tosylate | 10 mg/kg IV |

*IT,* Intratracheally; *IO,* intraosseously; *CRI,* constant rate infusion; see p. 89.

AIRWAY -          Clear airway; intubate trachea.

BREATHE -         Give 2 deep breaths; check for spontaneous respirations, if absent begin artificial
                  ventilation (20-30/min) with 100% $O_2$ (see text).

CIRCULATION -     Check for pulse, if absent begin external chest compressions (at least 80/min—see
                  text). If 1 rescuer, give 2 breaths every 15 compressions.

           Additional measures:
             Attach ECG monitor
             IV fluids (10-20 ml/kg, more if hypovolemic)
             Wrap abdomen or compress abdomen alternately with chest
             Simultaneous ventilation with every second to third chest compression
           Assess effectiveness:
             Palpable artificial pulse?
             Return of mucous membrane color?
             Return of spontaneous circulation?
           Modify CPR technique or fluid administration rate if needed.

           If external cardiac massage is ineffective after 2-3 min, consider
             internal cardiac massage (see text).

DRUGS -           Continue IV fluids; use ECG to guide cardiac drug administration (below); if no ECG
                  available:

           No heartbeat:                    Bradycardia:
           give epinephrine*                give atropine†

           If prolonged CPR or unwitnessed arrest, give Na bicarbonate (0.5-1.0 mEq/kg IV),
             repeat after each 10-15 min of CPR or dose based on central venous blood gas
             assessments.
           Consider use of pressor agent if fluids and CPR give inadequate blood pressure.

**FIG 5-1**
Guidelines for cardiopulmonary resuscitation once breathlessness and pulselessness have
been determined.                                                         *Continued*

coronary blood flow by increasing right atrial as well as aortic pressure.

## CIRCULATION (C)

### External Cardiac Massage

External (closed-chest) cardiac massage is begun as soon as cardiac arrest is recognized, unless the animal has a condition known to make it ineffective (see later discussion). In all but the smallest animals, forward arterial blood flow is produced mainly by fluctuations in intrathoracic pressure (causing compression of all intrathoracic structures) that are generated during external cardiac massage rather than by direct compression of the heart itself. Many studies have been conducted in an attempt to determine the optimal method of artificial circulation. Although there is still controversy over this, the following is generally agreed upon. External massage is often effective for small or medium dogs and cats, but it is unlikely to generate adequate cardiac output and coronary or brain perfusion in dogs weighing more than 10 to 15 kg. If external massage is judged ineffective after 5 minutes of application, open-chest massage should be tried.

Small dogs (weight of less than 15 kg) and cats should be placed in lateral recumbency for cardiac massage; the chest is compressed with one hand placed on either side of the chest over the heart (fourth to fifth intercostal space). In very small dogs and cats, it may be possible to perform effective mas-

sage using one hand by placing the thumb on one side of the chest and the fingers on the other. Large (weight of more than 15 to 20 kg) dogs are placed in dorsal recumbency after tracheal intubation, because greater intrathoracic pressures can be generated in this position. A "V" table or sandbags placed along the dog's sides help keep the animal from rotating into a lateral position. For dogs in dorsal recumbency, the chest is compressed over the caudal third of the sternum.

The chest should be abruptly compressed 100 to 120 times per minute in small dogs and cats and 80 to 100 times per minute in large dogs. The compression and relaxation phases should take the same amount of time (50% duty cycle) to optimize the blood flow produced by thoracic pressure changes. It is recommended that the chest wall be displaced by 30% with each compression. If only one rescuer is present, a cardiac compression rate of 80 to 100 per minute is used and two breaths are given after every 15 chest compressions.

Abdominal pressure, applied either manually by an assistant or with a compression bandage, may prevent paroxysmal diaphragmatic motion during the chest compressions and reduce the size of the perfused vasculature. Wrapping the pelvic limbs may further improve blood pressure. Abruptly compressing the abdomen in-between chest compressions may significantly increase coronary and cerebral blood flow. A third rescuer is needed for this maneuver, however. Simultaneous chest and abdominal compression is not recommended because of the risk for liver injury and hemorrhage.

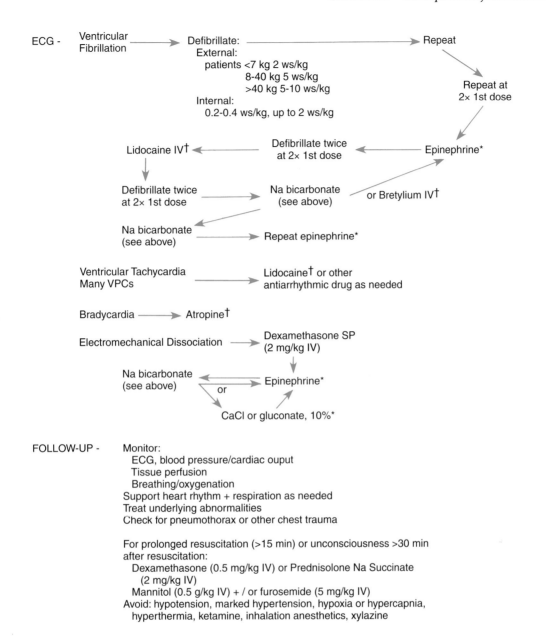

ECG -   Ventricular → Defibrillate: ──────────────────→ Repeat
        Fibrillation    External:
                          patients <7 kg 2 ws/kg
                          8-40 kg 5 ws/kg
                          >40 kg 5-10 ws/kg
                        Internal:
                          0.2-0.4 ws/kg, up to 2 ws/kg

                                                              Repeat at
                                                              2× 1st dose

Lidocaine IV† ←── Defibrillate twice          Epinephrine*
                  at 2× 1st dose

Defibrillate twice ──→ Na bicarbonate    or Bretylium IV†
at 2× 1st dose          (see above)

Na bicarbonate ──────→ Repeat epinephrine*
(see above)

Ventricular Tachycardia ──────→ Lidocaine† or other
Many VPCs                        antiarrhythmic drug as needed

Bradycardia ──→ Atropine†

Electromechanical Dissociation ──→ Dexamethasone SP
                                   (2 mg/kg IV)

Na bicarbonate ←──  ──→ Epinephrine*
(see above)      or
                 CaCl or gluconate, 10%*

FOLLOW-UP -   Monitor:
                ECG, blood pressure/cardiac ouput
                Tissue perfusion
                Breathing/oxygenation
              Support heart rhythm + respiration as needed
              Treat underlying abnormalities
              Check for pneumothorax or other chest trauma

              For prolonged resuscitation (>15 min) or unconsciousness >30 min
              after resuscitation:
                Dexamethasone (0.5 mg/kg IV) or Prednisolone Na Succinate
                  (2 mg/kg IV)
                Mannitol (0.5 g/kg IV) + / or furosemide (5 mg/kg IV)
              Avoid: hypotension, marked hypertension, hypoxia or hypercapnia,
                hyperthermia, ketamine, inhalation anesthetics, xylazine

* See Table 5-1 for dosage information.
† See Tables 4-6 and 5-1 for dosage information.

**FIG 5-1, cont'd**
For legend see opposite page.

Successful external massage and positive-pressure ventilation should result in detectable arterial pulses and improved mucous membrane color. A reduction in pupillary size may be seen; however, because drugs used in CPR may affect pupillary size, and hypoxic injury to the retina may cause nonresponsive pupils, this finding does not necessarily indicate ineffective CPR.

If the desired effects are not seen within 1 to 2 minutes, the CPR technique should be modified. More or less compressive force, abdominal or pelvic limb binding, a change in the position of the animal, an adjustment of the hand position on the animal's chest, a longer compression phase, or a change in the rate of compressions are some measures that can be tried. Use of a pressor agent and an increase in the rate of IV fluid administration may help by improving venous return. Complications associated with external cardiac massage include fractured ribs, pulmonary or other intrathoracic tissue injury, and pneumothorax.

## Internal Cardiac Massage

Direct cardiac massage is more effective than closed-chest massage. It is indicated if external massage has proved ineffective after about 5 minutes; if the animal is a large or barrel-chested dog; if fractured ribs or other chest wall trauma is evident; or if pneumothorax, pulmonary contusion, pleural effusion, pericardial effusion, diaphragmatic hernia, or hypovolemia is suspected. Open-chest massage permits the evaluation of venous return and lung inflation, as well as the detection of ventricular fibrillation and spontaneous contractions. However, the effectiveness of internal cardiac massage is reduced if it is delayed. The decision to perform internal cardiac massage may also be influenced by the nature of the animal's underlying condition and the owner's wishes.

The left fifth or sixth intercostal space is used for the emergency thoracotomy. It is advantageous to clip a strip of hair directly over the incision site and swab the skin quickly with alcohol or other disinfectant; however, no more than a few seconds should be allowed for this. The incision down to the pleura should be accomplished rapidly but carefully to avoid cutting an intercostal vessel just caudal to the rib and the internal thoracic artery lateral to the sternum. The pleural space is entered bluntly while the animal is exhaling so that the lungs are not cut. The opening in the pleural space is then enlarged with scissors, and a self-retaining retractor is used to spread the ribs so that the heart can be grasped. Pericardiotomy allows maximal diastolic filling and prevents the development of cardiac tamponade should blood or a transudate accumulate, but it may not be necessary in all cases.

Direct cardiac massage is performed by compressing the heart between two fingers (small heart), between the palm and flat portion of the fingers of one hand (mid-sized heart), or between the palm and the opposite chest wall or both hands (large heart). The rescuer must be careful to not traumatize or perforate the heart nor rotate it so that filling is compromised. Enough compressive force is applied to empty the ventricles (from apex to base), allowing time for the ventricle to fill before the next compression. The descending aorta can be compressed with a finger of the opposite hand or a vascular clamp to maximize blood flow to the heart and brain. If this technique is used, aortic compression should be maintained for the duration of resuscitation until stable, spontaneous cardiac activity is restored; aortic compression should be removed gradually over 10 to 20 minutes.

If cardiac massage is successful, the chest is then thoroughly lavaged with sterile isotonic solution and the skin edges cleaned and disinfected before the incision is closed. If the pericardium was incised, it should be left open. The chest should be carefully evacuated of air. Broad-spectrum antibiotic therapy is indicated.

## Defibrillation

Ventricular fibrillation is treated by electrical defibrillation using DC current and is most effective early in the arrest. It involves the passage of a brief high-energy electrical charge through the myocardium in an attempt to depolarize the entire heart, thus allowing a normal rhythm to be reestablished. Lower energy levels are used initially, but if these are unsuccessful, repeated shocks are given at progressively higher energy levels and/or paired in rapid succession. Generally the longer the animal has been in ventricular fibrillation, the higher the energy required to accomplish defibrillation and

the lower the chance for successful defibrillation. Excessive energy levels can cause cardiac injury. If the ECG shows fine ventricular fibrillation waves, the heart tends to be much less responsive to electrical defibrillation. Epinephrine may be administered to coarsen the waves and increase the chance of successful defibrillation, but it has also been shown to promote deterioration of left ventricular function during fibrillation.

For external defibrillation, paddles are placed firmly on either side of the chest over the heart so that the charge passes through as much myocardium as possible. Good skin contact with the entire face of the paddle is important to maximize distribution of the shock and defibrillation efficiency and to minimize tissue damage. Contact paste is used to enhance conduction of the electrical current to the body; commercial ECG gels, pHisoHex soap, or K-Y Jelly and salt can also be used. Care should be taken to ensure that the paddles do not touch each other and that the contact paste (or other conductive material) on the skin does not form a connection between the two paddles. Alcohol should not be used to enhance skin-paddle contact because it is flammable. The recommended initial energy settings are based on animal size: 2 watt-sec/kg for animals weighing less than 7 kg, 5 watt-sec/kg for dogs weighing 8 to 40 kg, and 5 to 10 watt-sec/kg for very large dogs. Before the defibrillator is discharged, all personnel should be clear of the animal, ECG machine, anesthesia machine, table, and defibrillator. If defibrillation does not occur, CPR is continued while preparations are made for another try at a higher power setting.

Internal defibrillation is accomplished with sterile, internal paddles that may be covered with saline-soaked gauze sponges. The paddles are placed on opposite sides of the heart so that their entire surface makes contact with the heart and the current flows across as much myocardium as possible. Recommended energy settings for internal defibrillation are 0.2 to 0.4 watt-sec/kg (up to 2 watt-sec/kg).

Chemical defibrillators such as ionic choline cocktails (acetylcholine, potassium chloride, and calcium salts) or bretylium tosylate have had little to no effectiveness. A sharp precordial thump may occasionally convert ventricular fibrillation or tachycardia to sinus rhythm, but it can also precipitate fibrillation during ventricular tachycardia. In people, IV amiodarone in conjunction with defibrillation has been used with some success in the management of refractory, recurrent ventricular tachycardia and fibrillation. Bretylium and amiodarone may prevent recurrent ventricular fibrillation by raising the fibrillation threshold (see Chapter 4). If hypomagnesemia is suspected, IV infusion of 0.15 to 0.3 mEq/kg of MgCl or MgSO$_4$ over a few minutes might be helpful.

## DRUGS (D)

Drugs administered during CPR are best given through a central vein. However, this route is not always available. Alternate routes (in order of preference) include the intratracheal, intraosseous, peripheral venous, and intralingual routes. Intracardiac injections are best avoided unless they are done under direct visualization and while the ascending aorta is compressed. "Blind" intracardiac injections can result in coronary vessel laceration and lead to myocardial infarction or cardiac tamponade. Furthermore, CPR must be stopped during the injection, and intramyocardial injection may precipitate resistant ventricular fibrillation. Intratracheal administration can be accomplished using a long, flexible catheter inserted into the endotracheal tube. The IV dose of the drug in this instance is doubled and diluted with 2 to 5 ml of sterile water or saline. Sodium bicarbonate should not be administered by this route (see p. 104). The intraosseous route has received increased interest lately; it can be used for fluid replacement, as well as drug administration, because the intramedullary space is closely connected with the vascular system. A bone marrow needle (or spinal needle in small animals) can be inserted into the proximal tibia, trochanteric fossa of the femur, or another site to gain access to the intramedullary space. Intralingual injections are made under the dorsal mucosal surface.

## Support of Circulation

Epinephrine is usually indicated in the management of cardiac arrest because of its cardiostimulatory and pressor effects. The vasoconstriction induced by the $\alpha$-adrenergic effects of epinephrine helps maintain blood pressure and improve venous return. Its $\beta$-adrenergic effects cause heart rate, contractility, and automaticity to increase. The $\alpha$-agonist effects are thought more important than the $\beta$-agonist effects, which can worsen myocardial ischemia. Epinephrine HCl is available in 1-mg/ml ampules at a 1:1000 dilution (Adrenaline Chloride; Monarch, Bristol, Tenn; generic). The central venous route is the preferred route of administration, although intratracheal administration has also been advocated. When administered by the intratracheal route, dilution of epinephrine in a small volume (e.g., 2 ml) of distilled water has resulted in higher plasma concentrations and blood pressure compared to the same dose diluted in saline (Naganobu and colleagues, 2000). However, there is some controversy as to whether intratracheal administration is likely to reduce blood pressure because of $\beta$-receptor–mediated vasodilation. The effectiveness of peripheral IV (and probably intratracheal) administration is limited by the effectiveness of artificial circulation. The effectiveness of intranasal administration of 14 mg of epinephrine per nostril compared favorably with that of IV administration of 0.015 mg/kg of the catecholamine in one study (Bleske and colleagues, 1992). It may also be given by intralingual or intraosseous injection. Intracardiac injections can cause significant cardiac and pulmonary damage, including direct myocardial injury, cardiac tamponade, coronary laceration, pneumothorax, and lung laceration. The intramyocardial delivery of epinephrine also can induce refractory ventricular fibrillation. It is currently recommended that undiluted (1:1000) epinephrine be administered every (3 to) 5 minutes as needed (see Table 5-1). However, the hemodynamic effects of high-dose epinephrine ($\geq$0.1 mg/kg) during CPR appear to last longer than 5 minutes, therefore longer intervals between injections could be used (Bar-Joseph and colleagues, 2000). Epinephrine diluted to 1:10,000 can be used in very small animals.

Dopamine (see p. 67, Table 3-8) is another catecholamine that has been used successfully to stimulate the heart during cardiac arrest. However, both dopamine and epinephrine can induce arrhythmias, including ventricular fibrillation. Catecholamine-induced arrhythmias are facilitated in the presence of hypoxia, acidosis, the use of halothane or other anesthetics, and myocardial trauma. Dobutamine has been shown to not be effective in the initial treatment of cardiac arrest. Agents that stimulate $\alpha$-receptors only may be as effective as epinephrine in treating cardiac arrest because of their ability to cause vasoconstriction and to increase blood pressure and circulating volume; norepinephrine, methoxamine, metaraminol, and phenylephrine are potent $\alpha$-agonists. Norepinephrine is available in 4-ml (1-mg/ml) ampules (Levophed; Sanofi Winthrop, New York, N.Y.); methoxamine is available in 20-mg/ml ampules (Vasoxyl; Glaxo Wellcome, Research Triangle Park, N.C.). Metaraminol bitartrate (Aramine; Merck, West Point, Pa) and phenylephrine HCl injection (generic) are both available as 10-mg/ml solutions for injection. Isoproterenol should not be used to treat cardiac arrest because it causes peripheral vasodilation through its $\beta$-agonist effects. Drugs that block $\alpha$-receptors, such as phenothiazine tranquilizers, also cause vasodilation and should not be used. Bradycardia may respond to atropine, glycopyrrolate, or dopamine (see Table 5-1). Atropine can be given through an endotracheal tube, but endobronchial administration via a flexible catheter wedged into a peripheral bronchus is associated with higher plasma concentrations, longer half-life, and greater increases in heart rate (Paret and colleagues, 1999).

Rapid vasodilation occurs during cardiac arrest as a result of tissue anoxia. Successful resuscitation may require both intravascular fluid administration and pressor agents to restore effective circulating blood volume and venous return. However, the use of large loading doses of IV fluids (e.g., 40 to 80 ml/kg for dogs and 20 to 40 ml/kg for cats) may predispose to the development of pulmonary edema in some animals. Furthermore, fluid loading during cardiac arrest impedes coronary perfusion by disproportionately raising right atrial pressure more than aortic diastolic pressure; coronary perfusion is dependent on the difference between aortic and right atrial pressures, especially during diastole. Therefore the use of initial fluid doses of only 10 to 20 ml/kg has been suggested for animals that show an incomplete vasoconstrictor response to epinephrine (or an $\alpha$-adrenergic agent) or that have hypovolemia. If CPR is successful, the fluid rate should then be adjusted to maintain organ perfusion. In some situations, whole blood, plasma, colloid blood expanders, or hypertonic saline solutions, in conjunction with crystalloid solutions, are indicated to maintain vascular volume and pressure.

It is generally not recommended that calcium chloride be administered during CPR. This is because large amounts of free calcium can accumulate in ischemic cells, which leads to cellular dysfunction and death. There appears to be no increase in the success of resuscitation with the use of calcium salts. Ventricular arrhythmias, myocardial tetany and hyperpolarization, and postanoxic tissue damage are among the adverse effects of calcium administered in the treatment of cardiac arrest. However, there are several situations in which calcium is indicated for the management of cardiac arrest: severe hyperkalemia (effects on excitable tissues are lessened by calcium), hypocalcemia, and an overdose of calcium entry blocking drugs. The use of calcium salts for the management of EMD is controversial.

### Minimize Acidosis

Both metabolic and respiratory acidosis develop after cardiac arrest. This is because anaerobic metabolism during periods of hypoxia generates lactic acid, and respiratory arrest leads to the accumulation of carbon dioxide. Acidosis can in turn worsen cardiac arrest in several ways. It decreases cardiac automaticity, myocardial contractility, and responsiveness to catecholamines; it lowers the ventricular fibrillation threshold; and it increases pulmonary vascular resistance. Inadequate ventilation is a major factor in the development of refractory acidosis.

Immediate and effective artificial ventilation and cardiac massage should prevent the development of serious acidosis, making sodium bicarbonate therapy unnecessary. In contrast, if its institution is delayed or CPR is prolonged, it may be necessary to administer large doses of bicarbonate to reverse the resultant acidosis. Unfortunately, it is difficult to know exactly when and how much bicarbonate to give. An overdose can be detrimental by causing metabolic alkalosis, hyperosmolality, an increased $PaCO_2$, leftward displacement of the oxyhemoglobin dissociation curve (diminishing oxygen release to the tissues), an acute decrease in the serum $K^+$ concentration (resulting from an intracellular shift), cerebrospinal fluid acidosis (resulting from the rapid diffusion of newly generated carbon dioxide), and a possible inactivation of catecholamines. An arterial pH greater than 7.55 during CPR has been associated with decreased survival.

Sodium bicarbonate may be helpful if cardiac arrest is not immediately recognized, if effective CPR is otherwise delayed for more than 2 minutes, or if preexistent metabolic acidosis is suspected. Initial doses of 0.5 to 1 mEq/kg are usually given. Sometimes total doses of up to 8 mEq/kg are needed. If results of blood gas analysis are available, they can be used to guide bicarbonate therapy; central (or large) venous rather than arterial samples should be used to assess tissue perfusion adequacy and guide bicarbonate therapy. Bicarbonate is given if the pH is less than 7.20. If blood gases cannot be measured, 0.5 mEq/kg of bicarbonate is given every 10 minutes up to two times, after the initial 15 to 20 minutes of CPR. Adequate ventilation is necessary to eliminate the carbon dioxide generated. Sodium bicarbonate should not be combined with (or given in the same IV line as) solutions containing calcium salts or catecholamines, because it precipitates the former and inactivates the latter. Sodium bicarbonate should also not be administered by the intratracheal route, because it inactivates surfactant and causes lung atelectasis. Arterial blood gas analysis is useful to assess blood oxygenation during CPR, although results do not accurately reflect acid-base status.

### Stabilize Heart Rhythm

Animals in which cardiac arrest appears imminent may respond to antiarrhythmic therapy and other supportive care.

Atropine or glycopyrrolate should be used for the control of bradycardia. Frequent ventricular premature contractions or ventricular tachycardia may be suppressed by lidocaine or other antiarrhythmic agents (see p. 80).

An ECG-based diagnosis of the heart rhythm is important for choosing appropriate therapy throughout CPR (see following paragraph). After successful resuscitation, antiarrhythmic or anticholinergic agents may be useful to normalize the heart rhythm and prevent recurrence of arrest. Continued attention to blood pressure, venous return, oxygenation, and acid-base balance is important.

### ELECTROCARDIOGRAM (E)

As soon as possible after cardiac arrest is detected, an ECG monitor should be attached to the animal. Accurate diagnosis of the cardiac rhythm facilitates successful CPR. Ventricular fibrillation, ventricular asystole, and EMD all sound the same through the stethoscope (i.e., no heartbeat), but their therapy differs somewhat. Extreme bradycardia or a weakly beating heart may also be difficult to discern using auscultation. Ventricular fibrillation should be treated with electrical defibrillation as soon as possible. Ventricular asystole may respond to repeated doses of epinephrine; the spontaneous electrical activity that develops is often ventricular fibrillation, which is treated as described on p. 102. Successful treatment of EMD is difficult. In animals with EMD the ECG may be normal or at least show organized electrical activity, yet the ventricles do not contract effectively. Epinephrine and the potent $\alpha$-agonist methoxamine (see Table 5-1) have each been advocated for the treatment of EMD, as has calcium chloride. Atropine, in addition to epinephrine, may also have a role in the therapy of asystole and EMD. However, the most effective approach is not clear at this time. The opiate antagonist naloxone HCl (Narcan; Endo Labs, Chadds Ford, Pa; generic; 0.03 mg/kg IV or IT) may be helpful against the myocardial depressant effects of endogenous opiates by increasing myocardial responsiveness to catecholamines.

### FOLLOW-UP (F)

If CPR is successful, the animal should be monitored closely because of the high prevalence of recurrent cardiac arrest. Specific recommendations for care after resuscitation have not been firmly established. However, general supportive measures include maintenance of the $PaCO_2$ at about 25 mm Hg and the diastolic blood pressure at greater than 60 mm Hg; the provision of supplemental oxygen and an adequate circulating volume; and normalization of acid-base, electrolyte, or other metabolic disturbances. An infusion of dopamine or dobutamine may help offset the depressed ventricular function that frequently occurs after cardiac arrest. Continuous ECG monitoring is advisable. IV fluids are usually indicated to prevent hypovolemia and optimally perfuse previously ischemic tissue capillary beds. The rate of administration is guided by the animal's hemodynamic state and urine output. Some animals require continued ventilatory support after resuscitation. Artificial hyperventilation may be helpful in decreasing intracranial pressure. It is important to manage cardiac arrhythmias and frequently assess hemodynamic state by checking mucous membrane color and perfusion, heart rate, femoral pulse quality, and, if possible, arterial blood pressure. A constant infusion of lidocaine may prevent the recurrence of ventricular arrhythmias or fibrillation. The lungs and heart should be auscultated periodically.

Underlying abnormalities that may have led to the arrest should also be dealt with, and these could include acid-base or electrolyte disturbances, hypoxia, sepsis, toxicity, neurologic disease, anesthesia, hypovolemia, advanced metabolic disorders, or primary lung or cardiac disease. Thoracic radiographs should be obtained after CPR to detect pulmonary contusions or edema, rib fractures, pneumothorax, or pleural effusion that may have resulted from resuscitation. A complete blood count, serum biochemical profile, and urinalysis may also be helpful.

Brain injury resulting from cardiac arrest and resuscitation arises as a result of a complex interaction of factors, which include neuronal calcium overloading and postresuscitative decreases in cerebral blood flow. Calcium antagonists, iron chelators, free-radical scavengers, antiprostaglandins, dimethylsulfoxide, and other therapies have been found in experiments to be variably helpful in minimizing postresuscitation neurologic damage. Deferoxamine mesylate (Desferal; Novartis, East Hanover, N.J.) is an iron chelator that has been advocated for postresuscitation reperfusion injury. Doses of 10 mg/kg IV or IM, repeated in 2 hours, then every 8 hours for 24 hours, have been used. Other experiments involving the use of mild hypothermia (to about 93° F or 34° C), the promotion of cerebral blood flow by inducing mild hypertension and hemodilution, and the maintenance of normocapnia have resulted in normal neurologic function or milder deficits. Hyperventilation to maintain a high level of respiratory alkalosis during recirculation also has been found in experiments to result in less histologic neuronal degeneration. Cerebral edema should be assumed to exist if consciousness is not improving by 15 to 30 minutes after successful CPR or if CPR has been performed for more than 15 minutes. Corticosteroids, mannitol, and furosemide have been used in an attempt to reduce postresuscitative cerebral edema. However, there may be no benefit from steroids, either in terms of survival or neurologic recovery.

## Suggested Readings

Bar-Joseph G et al: Response to repeated equal doses of epinephrine during cardiopulmonary resuscitation in dogs, *Ann Emerg Med* 35:3, 2000.

Bleske BE et al: Comparison of intravenous and intranasal administration of epinephrine during CPR in a canine model, *Ann Emerg Med* 21:1125, 1992.

Eisenberg MS et al: Cardiac resuscitation, *N Engl J Med* 344:1304, 2001.

Feneley MP et al: Influence of compression rate on initial success of resuscitation and 24-hour survival after prolonged manual cardiopulmonary resuscitation in dogs, *Circulation* 77:240, 1988.

Haskins SC: Internal cardiac compression, *J Am Vet Med Assoc* 200:1945, 1992.

Henik RA et al: Effects of body position and ventilation/compression ratios during cardiopulmonary resuscitation in cats, *Am J Vet Res* 48:1603, 1987.

Henik RA et al: Cardiopulmonary resuscitation in cats, *Semin Vet Med Surg (Small Anim)* 3:185, 1988.

Henik RA: Basic life support and external cardiac compression in dogs and cats, *J Am Vet Med Assoc* 200:1925, 1992.

Jastremski M et al: Glucocorticoid treatment does not improve neurological recovery following cardiac arrest, *J Am Med Assoc* 262:3427, 1989.

Kass PH et al: Survival following cardiopulmonary resuscitation in dogs and cats, *Vet Emerg Crit Care* 2:57, 1992.

Liu Y et al: Normoxic ventilation after cardiac arrest reduces oxidation of brain lipids and improves neurological outcome, *Stroke* 29:1679, 1998.

Marks SL: Cardiopulmonary resuscitation and oxygen therapy, *Vet Clin North Am Small Anim Pract* 29:959, 1999.

Naganobu K et al: A comparison of distilled water and normal saline as diluents for endobronchial administration of epinephrine in the dog, *Anesth Analg* 91:317, 2000.

Paret G et al: Atropine pharmacokinetics and pharmacodynamics following endotracheal versus endobronchial administration in dogs, *Resuscitation* 41:57, 1999.

Safar P et al: Improved cerebral resuscitation from cardiac arrest in dogs with mild hypothermia plus blood flow promotion, *Stroke* 27:105, 1996.

Vaknin Z et al: Is endotracheal adrenaline deleterious because of the β adrenergic effect? *Anesth Analg* 92:1408, 2001.

Wingfield WE et al: Respiratory and cardiopulmonary arrest in dogs and cats: 265 cases (1986-1991), *J Am Vet Med Assoc* 200:1993, 1992.

# CHAPTER 6

# Myocardial Diseases of the Dog

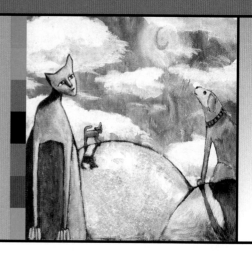

## CHAPTER OUTLINE

DILATED CARDIOMYOPATHY, 106
    Cardiomyopathy in Boxers and Doberman
      Pinschers, 113
HYPERTROPHIC CARDIOMYOPATHY, 115
ARRHYTHMOGENIC RIGHT VENTRICULAR
CARDIOMYOPATHY, 116
MYOCARDITIS, 116
    Infective myocarditis, 116
    Noninfective myocarditis, 118
    Traumatic myocarditis, 118
CARDIOGENIC SHOCK, 118

Myocardial diseases resulting in poor contractile function and cardiac chamber enlargement are an important cause of heart failure in dogs. Most clinically recognized cases are considered idiopathic dilated cardiomyopathy (DCM) and affect the larger breeds of dog, although Cocker Spaniels are commonly affected as well. Secondary and infective myocardial diseases (pp. 106 and 116) are documented less frequently and do not show particular breed predispositions. Hypertrophic cardiomyopathy (HCM) and arrhythmogenic right ventricular cardiomyopathy (ARVC) are uncommon in dogs. The pathophysiology and therapeutic principles of HCM in dogs are similar to those of HCM in cats, which is discussed more fully in Chapter 7.

## DILATED CARDIOMYOPATHY

### Etiology

Dilated cardiomyopathy is characterized by poor myocardial contractility, with or without arrhythmias. Most cases of DCM in dogs are primary or idiopathic. Up to 50% of DCM cases in people are thought to be familial; abnormalities of various cytoskeletal proteins and a sarcomeric protein have been found in different kindreds. Genetic factors are also thought to play a role in dogs, especially in breeds that have a high incidence or a familial occurrence of the disease, such as Doberman Pinschers, Boxers, and Cocker Spaniels. Pedigree analysis of a group of Great Danes with DCM suggested inheritance as an X-linked recessive trait (Meurs and colleagues, 2001). An autosomal dominant inheritance pattern has been found in Boxers with ventricular arrhythmias (Meurs and colleagues, 1998). A rapidly fatal familial DCM affecting very young Portuguese Water dogs is thought to have an autosomal recessive inheritance pattern (Dambach and colleagues, 1999). DCM as an entity probably represents the end-stage of different pathologic processes or metabolic defects involving myocardial cells or the intercellular matrix, rather than a single disease. Idiopathic DCM has also been associated with prior viral infections in people. However, based on polymerase chain reaction (PCR) analysis of myocardial samples from a small number of dogs with DCM, viral agents do not seem to be commonly associated with DCM in this species (Maxson and colleagues, 2001).

**Secondary myocardial diseases.** Poor myocardial function can result from a variety of identifiable insults and nutritional deficiencies. Myocardial infections (see p. 116), inflammation, trauma (see p. 118), ischemia, neoplastic infiltrations, and metabolic abnormalities can impair normal contractile function. Hyperthermia, irradiation, electric shock, and other insults can also damage the myocardium. Some substances are known cardiac toxins.

The antineoplastic drug doxorubicin induces both acute and chronic cardiotoxicity. Histamine, secondary catecholamine release, and free-radical production appear to be involved in the pathogenesis of this myocardial damage, which leads to decreased cardiac output, arrhythmias, and degeneration of myocytes. Doxorubicin-induced cardiotoxicity is directly related to the peak serum concentration of the drug. The risk is reduced if prolonged infusion times or a low-dose weekly schedule are used, although it is unclear if the latter also results in a reduced tumoricidal effect. Progressive myocardial damage and fibrosis have developed in association with cumulative doses of greater than 160 mg/m$^2$ and sometimes as low as 100 mg/m$^2$; however, clinical cardiotoxicity is uncommon in dogs with normal pretreatment cardiac function until the cumulative dose exceeds 240 mg/m$^2$. It is difficult to predict whether clinical cardiotoxicity will occur, and electrocardiographic (ECG) changes do not necessarily precede clinical heart failure. Measurement of circulating cardiac troponin concentrations may become useful in monitoring dogs for doxorubicin-induced myocardial injury, but more work is needed to clarify this. Breeds in which there is a higher prevalence of idiopathic DCM and dogs with underlying cardiac abnormalities are thought to be at greater risk for doxorubicin-induced cardiotoxicity. Clinical features of this cardiomyopathy are similar to those of idiopathic DCM. Other cardiotoxic effects of doxorubicin include infranodal atrioventricular (AV) and bundle branch blocks, and ventricular and supraventricular tachyarrhythmias.

Ethyl alcohol, especially if given intravenously (IV) for the treatment of ethylene glycol intoxication, can cause severe myocardial depression and death; the slow administration of a diluted (20% or less) solution is therefore advised. Other cardiac toxins include plant toxins (e.g., *Taxus,* foxglove, black locust, buttercups, lily of the valley, gossypol), cocaine, anesthetic drugs, cobalt, catecholamines, and ionophores such as monensin.

In some dogs, DCM has been associated with L-carnitine–linked defects in myocardial metabolism. One or more underlying genetic or acquired metabolic defects, rather than simple L-carnitine deficiency, are suspected. L-Carnitine is an essential component of the mitochondrial membrane transport system for fatty acids, which are the heart's most important energy source. It also transports potentially toxic metabolites out of the mitochondria in the form of carnitine esters. The excess production of such metabolites can result in L-carnitine depletion. L-Carnitine is mainly present in foods of animal origin, and DCM has developed in some dogs fed strict vegetarian diets. There may be an association between DCM and carnitine deficiency in some families of Boxers, Doberman Pinschers, Great Danes, Irish Wolfhounds, Newfoundlands, and Cocker Spaniels. Unfortunately, the plasma carnitine concentration is not a sensitive indicator of myocardial carnitine deficiency, although it is specific. Most dogs with myocardial carnitine deficiency diagnosed on the basis of findings from endomyocardial biopsy have had normal or high plasma carnitine concentrations. Furthermore, the response to oral carnitine supplementation is inconsistent. Subjective improvement can occur, but few dogs have echocardiographic evidence of improved function. L-Carnitine supplementation does not suppress preexisting arrhythmias or prevent sudden death.

Low plasma taurine, and sometimes carnitine concentrations have been found in American Cocker Spaniels with DCM. Oral supplementation of these amino acids has improved left ventricular size and function and reduced the need for heart failure medications in this breed (Kittleson and colleagues, 1997). How taurine deficiency might contribute to the pathogenesis of DCM is not known. Other dogs with DCM, including some Golden Retrievers, Labrador Retrievers, Saint Bernards, and other breeds also have had low plasma taurine concentrations. However, the role of taurine supplementation is unclear. In a retrospective study, Freeman

and colleagues (2001) found that dietary levels of taurine in taurine-deficient dogs were no different from those of dogs with DCM and a normal blood taurine concentration. Although the taurine-deficient dogs showed some echocardiographic improvement after supplementation, survival time was not clearly longer.

Acute myocardial infarction from coronary embolization occurs uncommonly. Most cases have underlying disease associated with a tendency for embolus and/or thrombus formation, such as bacterial endocarditis, neoplasia, severe renal disease, immune-mediated hemolytic anemia, acute pancreatitis, DIC, and/or corticosteroid use. Although atherosclerosis of major coronary arteries is rare in dogs, it can accompany severe hypothyroidism and lead to acute myocardial infarction. The abrupt onset of arrhythmias, pulmonary edema, marked ST segment changes on the ECG, and regional or widespread myocardial dysfunction evident on an echocardiogram would be likely with acute obstruction of a major coronary artery. In contrast, nonatherosclerotic narrowing of small coronary arteries may be more clinically important than previously appreciated. Hyalinization of small coronary vessels and intramural myocardial infarctions have been described in association with chronic degenerative AV valve disease, but these also occur in older dogs without endocardiosis. Fibromuscular arteriosclerosis of small coronary vessels has also been described. These changes in the walls of the small coronary arteries cause luminal narrowing and can impair resting coronary blood flow as well as vasodilatory responses. Small myocardial infarctions and secondary fibrosis can lead to deterioration of myocardial function and a variety of tachyarrhythmias, as well as conduction disturbances. A retrospective study of dogs with histopathologically confirmed intramural coronary arteriosclerosis, with or without evidence of multiple chronic or acute infarctions, found that almost half of the cases died from congestive heart failure (Falk and colleague, 2000). An additional 20% of cases died suddenly; most of these had hyaline arteriosclerosis but not degenerative valve disease. Another 15% of cases died during or after general anesthesia. Of the cases that had an echocardiogram, most had a moderate decrease in contractility. Surprisingly, the majority of dogs in this study were of larger breeds; Cocker Spaniels and Cavalier King Charles Spaniels were the most common small breeds.

To what extent myocardial injury may be induced by free radicals is not clear. Evidence for increased oxidative stress has been found in dogs as well as people with congestive heart failure and myocardial failure; a negative correlation between disease severity and plasma vitamin E concentration has been noted in dogs with DCM (Freeman and colleagues, 1999). Reduced myocardial function has been associated with diseases such as hypothyroidism, pheochromocytoma, and diabetes mellitus, but it is unusual for clinical heart failure to occur in dogs secondary to these conditions alone. Excessive sympathetic stimulation stemming from brain or spinal cord injury results in myocardial hemorrhage, necrosis, and arrhythmias (brain-heart syndrome). Muscular dystrophy of the fasciohumeral type (reported in Springer Spaniels) can result in atrial standstill and heart failure. Canine X-linked (Duchenne's) muscular dystrophy in Golden Retrievers and other breeds also has been associated with myocardial fibrosis and mineralization. Rarely, nonneoplastic (e.g., glycogen storage disease) and neoplastic (metastatic and primary) infiltrative myocardial diseases interfere with normal myocardial function. Immunologic mechanisms may also play an important role in the pathogenesis of myocardial dysfunction in some dogs with myocarditis.

Rapid, incessant tachycardia leads to progressive myocardial dysfunction, activation of neurohormonal compensatory mechanisms, and congestive heart failure. This is known as tachycardia-induced cardiomyopathy (TICM). The myocardial failure is sometimes reversible if the heart rate can be normalized. TICM has been described in several dogs with AV nodal reciprocating tachycardias associated with accessory conduction pathways bypassing the AV node (e.g., Wolff-Parkinson-White syndrome; see p. 21). Rapid artificial pacing (e.g., >200 beats/min) is a common model for inducing experimental myocardial failure that simulates DCM.

## Pathophysiology of Dilated Cardiomyopathy

The major functional defect in DCM is decreased ventricular contractility (systolic dysfunction). Progressive cardiac chamber dilation occurs as a result of worsening systolic pump function and cardiac output (see Fig. 7-6, p. 131). Poor cardiac output can cause weakness, syncope, and cardiogenic shock. Increased diastolic stiffness is also thought to contribute to the development of higher end-diastolic pressures, venous congestion, and ultimately congestive heart failure. Cardiac enlargement and papillary muscle dysfunction often cause poor systolic apposition of mitral and tricuspid leaflets resulting in valve insufficiency. Most dogs with DCM do not have severe degenerative AV valve disease (endocardiosis), although some have mild to moderate valve changes that can exacerbate the mitral and/or tricuspid valve regurgitation. DCM probably develops slowly, although the onset of clinical signs may appear acute. For example, left ventricular dysfunction reportedly declines gradually in Dobermans over 2 to 3 years before signs of heart failure and final deterioration occur.

As cardiac output decreases, sympathetic, hormonal, and renal compensatory mechanisms become activated. These mechanisms increase heart rate, peripheral vascular resistance, and volume retention (see Chapter 3). Chronic neurohormonal activation is thought to contribute to progressive myocardial damage as well as the syndrome of congestive heart failure. Coronary perfusion can be compromised by poor forward blood flow and increased ventricular diastolic pressure; myocardial ischemia further impairs myocardial function and predisposes to the development of arrhythmias. Atrial arrhythmias, especially atrial tachycardia and atrial fibrillation, commonly develop in association with atrial enlargement. Because atrial contraction contributes significantly to ventricular filling, especially at faster heart rates, the loss of the "atrial kick" secondary to atrial fibrillation can markedly reduce cardiac output and cause acute clinical de-

compensation. The tachycardia associated with atrial fibrillation probably also accelerates disease progression. Signs of low-output heart failure and right- or left-sided congestive failure (see Chapters 1 and 3) are common in dogs with DCM. Ventricular tachyarrhythmias also occur frequently and can cause sudden death.

## Pathology

It is typical to see dilation of all cardiac chambers in dogs with DCM, although left atrial and ventricular enlargement may predominate. The ventricular wall thickness appears decreased compared with the lumen size. Papillary muscles often look flattened and atrophic; endocardial thickening may be noted. The AV valves generally have only mild to moderate, if any, degenerative changes. Histopathologic findings include scattered areas of myocardial necrosis, degeneration, and fibrosis, especially in the left ventricle. The presence of narrowed (attenuated) myocardial cells with a wavy appearance is reported to be a common finding (Tidholm and colleagues, 1998). Such abnormal cells have also been noted in some Newfoundlands thought to be predisposed to DCM but without any clinical or echocardiographic evidence of the disease (Tidholm and colleagues, 2000). Inflammatory cell infiltrates and myocardial hypertrophy are inconsistent features.

## Clinical Features

Idiopathic DCM is most common in large and giant breeds of dogs, including Great Danes, Doberman Pinschers, Saint Bernards, Scottish Deerhounds, Irish Wolfhounds, Boxers, Newfoundlands, Afghan Hounds, and Dalmatians. Among smaller breeds, English and American Cocker Spaniels, English Bulldogs, and others are affected, but the disease is rare in dogs weighing less than 12 kg. The prevalence of DCM increases with age, although most dogs presenting with heart failure are 4 to 10 years old. Most reports indicate that more male than female dogs are affected. Others suggest no gender predilection in Boxers and Doberman Pinschers once dogs with occult disease are included in the analysis. The nature of the cardiomyopathy in Boxers and Dobermans appears to be somewhat different from that in other large and giant breeds (see p. 113).

## Clinical Findings

Clinical signs may develop rapidly, especially in sedentary dogs in which ordinarily early signs may not be noticed until the disease is advanced. Presenting complaints include any or all of the following: weakness, lethargy, tachypnea or dyspnea, exercise intolerance, cough (sometimes described as "gagging"), anorexia, abdominal distention (ascites), and syncope (see Fig. 1-2, p. 3). Loss of muscle mass (cardiac cachexia), accentuated along the dorsal midline, may be severe. Conversely, subclinical DCM is now being recognized more frequently, especially through the use of echocardiography. Some giant-breed dogs with mild-to-moderate left ventricular dysfunction are relatively asymptomatic, even in the presence of atrial fibrillation.

Physical examination findings vary with the degree of cardiac decompensation. Poor cardiac output with high sympathetic tone and peripheral vasoconstriction causes pale mucous membranes and a prolonged capillary refill time. The femoral arterial pulse and precordial impulse are often weak and rapid; cardiac tachyarrhythmias usually cause pulse deficits (see Fig. 4-1, p. 75). Signs of left- and/or right-sided congestive heart failure, such as tachypnea, increased breath sounds, pulmonary crackles, jugular venous distention or pulsations, pleural effusion or ascites, and/or hepatosplenomegaly, are usually present. Heart sounds can be muffled secondary to pleural effusion or poor cardiac contractile strength. An audible third heart sound (S₃ gallop) is a classic finding, although it may be obscured by an irregular heart rhythm. Uncontrolled atrial fibrillation and frequent ventricular premature contractions (VPCs) cause a rapid and irregular heartbeat, with frequent pulse deficits and variable pulse strength. Systolic murmurs of mitral or tricuspid regurgitation that are soft to moderate in intensity are common.

## Radiography

Generalized cardiomegaly is usually evident, although left heart enlargement may predominate (Fig. 6-1). Cardiomegaly may be severe enough to mimic the globoid cardiac silhouette typical of large pericardial effusions. In contrast, Doberman Pinschers and some Boxers appear to have mainly left atrial enlargement without marked cardiomegaly. The stage of disease, chest conformation, and hydration status influence these radiographic findings. Distended pulmonary veins and pulmonary interstitial or alveolar opacities, especially in the hilar and dorsocaudal regions, indicate the presence of left heart failure and pulmonary edema. Some dogs have an asymmetric or widespread distribution of pulmonary edema infiltrates. Pleural effusion, distention of the caudal vena cava, hepatomegaly, and ascites usually accompany right-sided heart failure.

## Electrocardiography

The ECG findings in dogs with DCM are quite variable. The QRS complexes may be tall (consistent with left ventricular dilation), normal in size, or smaller than usual. Myocardial disease can produce a widened QRS complex with a sloppy R-wave descent and a slurred ST segment. Sometimes a bundle branch block pattern or other intraventricular conduction disturbance is present. The P waves in dogs with sinus rhythm are frequently widened and notched, suggesting left atrial enlargement. Premature atrial complexes, paroxysmal atrial tachycardia, or atrial fibrillation commonly occur (see p. 22 and Fig. 2-9), especially in Great Danes and other giant breeds. Uniform or multiform VPCs and paroxysmal ventricular tachycardia can coexist with sinus rhythm or atrial fibrillation.

## Echocardiography

Echocardiography is the best means of assessing cardiac chamber dimensions and myocardial function and for differentiating pericardial effusion or chronic valvular insufficiency from DCM. Dilated cardiac chambers and poor systolic ventricular wall and septal motion are characteristic findings in DCM. All chambers are usually affected, but right atrial and ventricular dimensions may appear normal, especially in Dobermans and Boxers. Left ventricular systolic dimension is increased, and fractional shortening is decreased (Fig. 6-2). Other common features are a wide mitral valve E point–septal separation and reduced aortic root motion. Left ventricular free-wall and septal thicknesses are normal to decreased. Mild to moderate AV valve regurgitation may be seen with Doppler echocardiography (Fig. 6-3). Dobutamine stress testing may provide insight as to the presence of early myocardial dysfunction in dogs thought to be at risk for DCM, but further research is needed to define the clinical applicability and optimal dosage for this more clearly.

## Clinical Pathology

Prerenal azotemia resulting from poor renal perfusion or mildly increased liver enzyme activities secondary to passive hepatic congestion may be present in dogs with DCM. Severe heart failure can be associated with hypoproteinemia and dilutional hyponatremia. Clinicopathologic findings are noncontributory in many cases. Hypothyroidism with associated hypercholesterolemia occurs in some dogs with DCM. However, because dogs with DCM can have decreased serum thyroid hormone concentrations without hypothyroidism (sick euthyroid), TSH stimulation or free T₄ determination may be useful. A recent small study documented increased plasma renin activity, aldosterone concentrations, urine aldosterone/creatinine ratio, and atrial natriuretic peptide (ANP) precursor concentrations in DCM dogs with clinical heart failure, but not in those without clinical signs or normal dogs (Tidholm and colleagues, 2001). Serum cardiac troponin (cTnT or cTnI) concentration elevations occur in some dogs with DCM as well as other causes of myocyte injury (Schober and colleagues, 2001; DeFrancesco and colleagues, 2002). In people with DCM, persistently elevated cTnT has been associated with poor survival. Further work is needed to assess the clinical usefulness of measuring circulating cardiac troponin concentrations in animals.

## Treatment

Therapy is aimed at controlling the signs of congestive heart failure, optimizing cardiac output, managing arrhythmias, improving the animal's quality of life, and prolonging survival, if possible. Digoxin, an angiotensin-converting enzyme inhibitor (ACEI), and furosemide form the core treatment for most dogs (Table 6-1). A stronger inotropic agent and other therapy may be needed for dogs with fulminant heart failure. Antiarrhythmic agents and other drugs are used on an individual-need basis. Exercise and dietary salt restriction can help decrease cardiac workload and water retention. Client education regarding the disease process, therapeutic goals, and medications is important for a realistic appreciation of the pet's physical limitations and possible future complications.

Most dogs with DCM have some degree of congestive heart failure when first examined; the severity of the failure generally determines the aggressiveness of therapy. Because

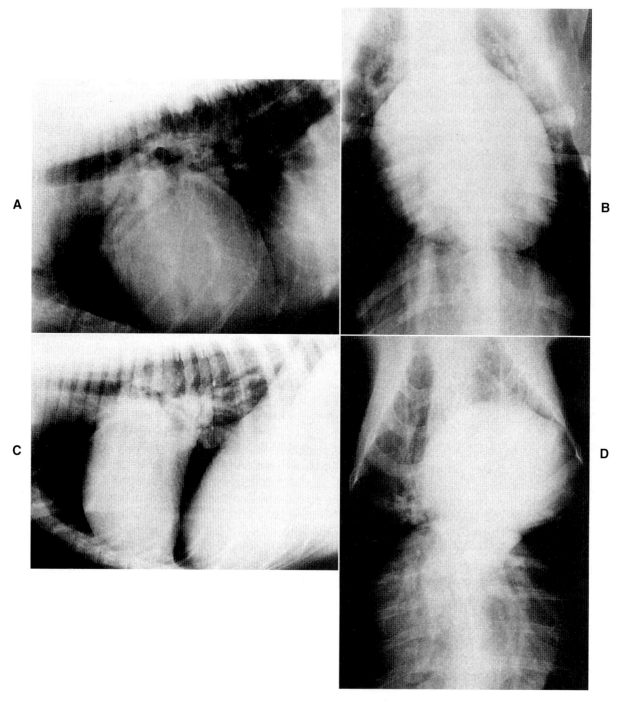

**FIG 6-1**
Radiographic examples of dilated cardiomyopathy in dogs. Lateral **(A)** and dorsoventral **(B)** views showing generalized cardiomegaly and hilar interstitial pulmonary infiltrates of edema in a male Great Dane. Lateral **(C)** and dorsoventral **(D)** views of a female Doberman Pinscher depicting the prominent left atrial and relatively moderate ventricular enlargements commonly found in affected dogs of this breed.

clinical status can deteriorate rapidly, it is important to frequently evaluate the patient's respiratory rate and character, lung sounds, pulse quality, heart rate and rhythm, peripheral perfusion, rectal temperature, hydration status, body weight, renal function, mentation, and blood pressure (if possible). Cardiogenic shock can result from the abysmal ventricular

contractility present in dogs with severe DCM, especially after excessive diuresis and vasodilation.

In critical cases, IV or intramuscular (IM) furosemide (see Table 3-6, p. 62), 2% nitroglycerin ointment, or sodium nitroprusside infusion (see Table 3-6), aminophylline (4 to 8 mg/kg IM), oxygen therapy (40% to 50%), and cage rest

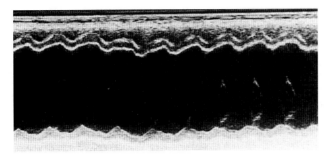

**FIG 6-2**
M-mode echocardiogram from a dog with dilated cardiomyopathy at the chordal (left side of figure) and mitral valve (right side of figure) levels. Note attenuated wall motion (fractional shortening = 18%) and the wide mitral valve E point–septal separation (28 mm).

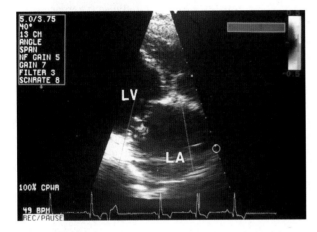

**FIG 6-3**
Mild mitral regurgitation is indicated by a relatively small area of disturbed flow in this systolic frame from a Doberman Pinscher with dilated cardiomyopathy. Note also the left atrial and ventricular dilation as well as a premature ventricular complex on the ECG. Right parasternal long axis view, optimized for the left ventricular inflow tract. *LA,* Left atrium; *LV,* left ventricle.

with or without morphine (0.2 to 0.3 mg/kg subcutaneously [SC] or IM) are used initially to help stabilize the animal's condition and allow baseline diagnostic testing. Thoracocentesis is indicated if pleural effusion is suspected or identified. Table 3-4 (p. 59) provides a guide for the therapy of acute congestive heart failure.

**Inotropic support.** Therapy for dogs with DCM includes inotropic support, usually in the form of digoxin, given orally (PO). Digoxin has only mild to moderate inotropic effects, but it has neurohormonal modulating effects and helps slow the ventricular response rate to atrial fibrillation (see Chapter 3). Stronger inotropic support for dogs with extremely poor contractility, cardiogenic shock, or fulminant congestive heart failure can be temporarily provided by IV infusion of dobutamine or dopamine administered for 2 (to 3) days and/or amrinone or milrinone (see Table 3-8, p. 67).

 TABLE 6-1

**Treatment Outline for Dogs with Dilated Cardiomyopathy**

| THERAPY | DRUG |
|---|---|
| **Initial Therapy of Acute Failure** | |
| Diuretic | Furosemide |
| Inotropic support | Digoxin |
| | ± Dobutamine or dopamine |
| | ± Amrinone (or milrinone) |
| ACEI | Enalapril or other |
| *and/or* | |
| Other vasodilator | ± Nitroprusside or hydralazine-nitroglycerin, or amlodipine |
| Oxygen | — |
| Bronchodilator | ± Theophylline or aminophylline |
| Cage confinement | — |
| Other therapy | ± Morphine |
| | ± Fluids |
| Antiarrhythmic drugs as needed (see Chapter 4 and Table 4-5) | |
| **Chronic Therapy** | |
| Diuretic | Furosemide and spironolactone |
| Inotropic support | Digoxin |
| ACEI | Enalapril or other |
| ± Other vasodilator | Amlodipine or hydralazine (± nitrate) |
| Exercise restriction | — |
| Sodium restriction | — |
| Other therapy | ± Trial of L-carnitine, taurine, other (see text) |
| Antiarrhythmic drugs as needed (see Chapter 4 and Table 4-5) | |
| **Therapy for Atrial Fibrillation if Inadequate Heart Rate Control with Digoxin** | |
| β-Blocker | Atenolol, propranolol, or other |
| *or* | |
| Calcium entry blocker | Diltiazem |

See Tables 3-4 (p. 59), 3-6 (p. 62), 3-8 (p. 67), and 4-5 (p. 79) for dosages and Chapters 3 and 4 for further information.
*ACEI,* Angiotensin-converting enzyme inhibitor.

However, the long-term use of strong positive inotropic drugs is thought to have detrimental effects on the myocardium. During infusion of these drugs, the animal must be closely observed for worsening tachycardia or arrhythmias (especially VPCs). If arrhythmias develop, the drug is discontinued or infused at up to half the original rate. In the presence of atrial fibrillation, catecholamine infusion can be detrimental because it can facilitate AV conduction and increase the ventricular response rate. If dopamine or dobutamine is thought necessary for such a case, digoxin should be given first, either PO or through the cautious use of IV loading doses (see Table 3-8). Rapid PO or cautious IV diltiazem is an alternative to IV digoxin. The phosphodiesterase inhibitors amrinone and milrinone (see Table 3-8 and p. 70) have been helpful for the short-term stabilization of some dogs and can be used concurrently with digoxin and a catecholamine.

Digoxin therapy is usually initiated with maintenance doses given PO (see p. 66). Toxicity appears to develop in some dogs, especially Dobermans, at relatively low dosages. A total maximum daily dose of 0.5 mg is generally used for large and giant-breed dogs, except for Dobermans, which are given a total maximum dose of 0.25 mg to 0.375 mg/day. It is recommended that the serum digoxin concentration be measured 7 to 10 days after digoxin therapy is initiated or the dose is changed (see p. 66).

Digoxin is also used to suppress supraventricular tachyarrhythmias and to slow the ventricular response rate in animals with atrial fibrillation. Dogs with atrial fibrillation and a ventricular rate exceeding 200 beats/min can be cautiously given digoxin IV (see Table 3-8) or twice the PO maintenance dose on the first day to more rapidly achieve effective blood concentrations. However, the use of IV or rapid oral diltiazem is probably safer (see Table 4-5, p. 80). The serum electrolyte and creatinine or blood urea nitrogen (BUN) concentrations should be monitored, because hypokalemia and azotemia predispose to the development of digoxin toxicity. If digoxin alone has not significantly reduced the heart rate after 36 to 48 hours, a β-blocker or diltiazem can be added (see Table 4-5, p. 80). Because these agents can have negative inotropic effects, a low initial dose and gradual dosage titration to effect or a maximum recommended level is advised. Heart rate control in dogs with atrial fibrillation is very important. A maximum ventricular rate of 140 to150 beats/min in the hospital (i.e., stressful) setting is the recommended target; lower heart rates (e.g., ~100 beats/min or less) are expected at home. Because accurate counting of heart rate by auscultation or chest palpation in dogs with atrial fibrillation is difficult, an ECG recording is recommended. Femoral pulses should not be used to assess heart rate in the presence of atrial fibrillation.

The ECG should also be monitored for the appearance of ventricular arrhythmias, which can be worsened by digitalis glycosides. If frequent or repetitive VPCs are present initially, digoxin should be used only at low doses or withheld until the VPCs are controlled with antiarrhythmic therapy (see Chapter 4). Quinidine should be avoided because it can lead to increased serum digoxin concentrations, among other concerns.

**Diuretics.** Furosemide is the most commonly used diuretic (see Table 3-6 and p. 62). High doses (i.e., 3 to 5 mg/kg or even 8 mg/kg) can be given parenterally initially if needed. For long-term therapy, the lowest effective dose given PO at consistent time intervals is best. The dose and frequency of administration can be increased as necessary. Hypokalemia and alkalosis appear to be uncommon sequelae unless anorexia or vomiting occurs. Potassium supplements may be given if hypokalemia is documented, but they must be used cautiously if an ACEI and/or spironolactone (see Table 3-6) is also being administered. Hyperkalemia can occur if a potassium-sparing diuretic or potassium supplements are used in conjunction with an ACEI or if renal disease is present. Spironolactone is an aldosterone-receptor antagonist that, in combination with ACEIs and loop diuretics, has reduced mortality in people with moderate to severe heart failure. Increased plasma concentrations of aldosterone develop as a component of neurohormonal activation in patients with heart failure. Aldosterone is known to promote cardiac fibrosis and abnormal vascular remodeling and as such contributes to the progression of cardiac disease. Therefore, in addition to the ACEI, furosemide, and digoxin used for chronic therapy of DCM, the simultaneous use of spironolactone is gaining favor.

**Vasodilators.** An ACEI should be used in the treatment of DCM. Angiotensin-converting enzyme inhibition can attenuate progressive ventricular dilation and secondary mitral regurgitation. ACEIs have a positive effect on survival in both people and dogs with myocardial failure. These drugs minimize clinical signs and increase exercise tolerance. Enalapril has been the most extensively studied ACEIs in dogs, but other ACEIs probably have similar effects. Therapy with an ACEI is also thought to be beneficial for dogs with subclinical myocardial dysfunction. The pure arteriolar dilator hydralazine can also improve cardiac output and exercise tolerance, as well as help reduce congestion; however, it can precipitate hypotension and reflex tachycardia and tends to augment the neurohormonal activation of heart failure. Hydralazine can be used in combination with a nitrate in dogs that do not tolerate an ACEI. Hydralazine or amlodipine (see Table 3-6) could also be useful as adjunct therapy for dogs with refractory heart failure, although it is necessary to carefully monitor arterial blood pressure in such animals.

Any vasodilator must be used judiciously in dogs with a low cardiac reserve because of the increased potential for hypotension. Therapy is initiated at a low dose; if this is well tolerated, the next dose is increased to a low maintenance level. The animal should be evaluated for several hours after each incremental dose, ideally by blood pressure measurement. Signs of worsening tachycardia, weakened pulses, or lethargy also can indicate the presence of hypotension. The jugular venous $P_{O_2}$ can be used to estimate directional changes in cardiac output; a venous $P_{O_2}$ greater than 30 mm Hg is desirable. The vasodilator dosage is carefully increased if necessary.

**Fluid therapy.** Fluid administration (either SC or IV) may be needed in some dogs, especially after aggressive diuretic therapy. High cardiac filling pressures are often necessary to maintain cardiac output in these dogs. Although venous congestion and edema may be alleviated by diuresis, the resulting reduction in filling pressure (preload) may cause inadequate cardiac output and hypotension. 5% dextrose in water with potassium chloride added (12 mEq/500 ml), or 0.45% sodium chloride and 2.5% dextrose with potassium chloride added, can be administered at conservative rates, such as 20 to 40 ml/kg/day. Careful monitoring is essential, however, because overhydration and pulmonary edema may develop rapidly.

**Bronchodilators.** Bronchodilator therapy may be beneficial in some dogs with severe, acute pulmonary edema and bronchoconstriction. Aminophylline also has transient diuretic properties and a mild positive inotropic effect. It can be given IV or IM (4 to 8 mg/kg), or PO (6 to 10 mg/kg) every 8 hours. Long-term bronchodilator administration is not recommended.

**Monitoring.** Many dogs can be maintained fairly well with digoxin, furosemide, an ACEI, a low- to moderate-sodium diet, exercise restriction, and, if atrial fibrillation is present, a β-blocker or diltiazem. Owner education regarding the purpose, dosage, and adverse effects of each drug used is also important. Clients should be instructed to monitor the dog's resting respiratory and heart rates at home. Periodic reevaluation of the patient is important, but the time frame for this depends on the animal's status. Visits once or twice a week may be needed initially. Serum electrolyte and creatinine (or BUN) concentrations, an ECG, pulmonary status, serum digoxin concentration, body weight, and other appropriate factors can be evaluated and the treatment adjusted as needed.

**Other therapy.** Oral L-carnitine supplementation may improve survival in dogs with low myocardial carnitine concentrations. Doses of 50 to 200 mg/kg every 8 hours or 1 g (Cocker Spaniels) to 2 g (large/giant breeds) every 8 to 12 hours have been used for this purpose. However, although a small percentage of dogs have shown marked clinical improvement in response to such treatment, it is doubtful that the use of high doses of L-carnitine in the absence of myocardial carnitine deficiency will prove beneficial. Nevertheless, because serious adverse effects of carnitine supplementation have not been reported, a 3- to 6-month trial of the therapy is reasonable, given the guarded prognosis for this disease. However, the cost of carnitine supplementation is not insignificant. Dogs treated with carnitine supplementation may give off a peculiar odor. Dogs that respond exhibit improved activity within 1 to 4 weeks; echocardiographic improvement appears in some dogs after 2 to 3 months of supplementation. However, a response plateau is reached in 6 to 8 months; the animal seems well but still has a subnormal echocardiographic shortening fraction and usually requires medication.

It may be helpful to measure the plasma taurine concentration in some dogs; this test is offered by most diagnostic laboratories. Supplemental taurine therapy (500 mg PO q8h) can be given to dogs with plasma concentrations of less than 25 nmol/ml. In the absence of plasma measurement, empirical taurine and carnitine supplementation may be beneficial in American Cocker Spaniels with DCM. At this time, the use of other nutritional supplement is controversial. There is preliminary evidence that supplementation of omega-3 fatty acids in the form of fish oil capsules may help reduce the production of cytokines associated with the development of cardiac cachexia (e.g., tumor necrosis factor). Oxygen free-radical damage can also contribute to myocardial dysfunction. There is experimental evidence in other species that antioxidant vitamins can reduce oxidative stress and possibly attenuate associated myocardial and endothelial dysfunction. Whether supplementation with vitamin C or other antioxidant vitamins would have a measurable benefit in canine DCM remains to be seen.

Long-term, low-dose β-blocker therapy with carvedilol or metoprolol may be beneficial over time if the dog can tolerate the drug. It is emphasized that this approach is only for dogs with chronic, stable DCM. β-Blockers acutely can worsen myocardial function and cause clinical deterioration. Definitive recommendations await the results of further study and clinical experience in dogs (see Chapter 4, p. 93).

Pimobendan (Vetmedin, Boehringer Ingelheim) is a phosphodiesterase III inhibitor that sensitizes the contractile proteins to intracellular $Ca^{++}$, thus increasing contractile strength. This drug also has vasodilatory effects, which contribute to its ability to improve cardiac function. Pimobendan is not yet available in the United States but is being used in Europe and elsewhere. Many dogs appear to experience marked clinical improvement when this agent is added to conventional therapy. Several controlled clinical trials are ongoing in dogs with heart failure from DCM as well as chronic mitral regurgitation. It is not clear whether pimobendan increases the frequency of ventricular ectopy and sudden death, as has occurred with other phosphodiesterase inhibitors.

Dynamic cardiomyoplasty has been described for the treatment of DCM. This procedure involves the surgical transposition of the latissimus dorsi muscle into the thoracic cavity, where it is wrapped around the failing ventricles. A myostimulator is implanted to activate the muscle synchronously with the heart, and the skeletal muscle undergoes a period of adaptation to repetitive stimulation. Although the results in some dogs have been encouraging, this is unlikely to be a widely used treatment. Other surgical techniques, such as plication or partial excision of the LV free wall in order to reduce ventricular dimension and wall stress, have been described, but their clinical usefulness in dogs is unknown. Partial left ventriculectomy (Batista procedure) in people has been associated with short-term improvement followed by some worsening.

## Prognosis

The prognosis for dogs with DCM is generally guarded to poor. Most dogs do not survive longer than 3 months following the clinical manifestations of heart failure, although approximately 25% to 40% of affected dogs live longer than 6 months if the initial response to therapy is good. The probability of survival for 2 years is estimated at 7.5% to 28%. Overall, pleural effusion and possibly ascites and pulmonary edema appear to be independent indicators of poorer prognosis. Sudden death can occur even in the occult stage, before heart failure is apparent. Doberman Pinschers have especially poor survival times. In each case, however, it is reasonable to assess the animal's response to initial treatment before pronouncing an unequivocally dismal prognosis.

## CARDIOMYOPATHY IN BOXERS AND DOBERMAN PINSCHERS

### Boxers

The prevalence of ventricular arrhythmias and syncope is high in Boxers with cardiomyopathy. Clinical features vary, and three disease categories have been described. The first consists of asymptomatic dogs that have ventricular tachyarrhythmia.

The second consists of dogs that have normal heart size and LV function, but also signs of syncope and weakness resulting from paroxysmal or sustained ventricular tachycardia. The third group, which seems less prevalent, is comprised of Boxers with poor myocardial function and congestive failure, as well as ventricular arrhythmias. Histologic changes in the myocardium are more extensive than those in dogs of other breeds with cardiomyopathy and include atrophy of myofibers, fibrosis, and fatty infiltration. These changes resemble those of arrhythmogenic right ventricular cardiomyopathy in people. Focal areas of myocytolysis, necrosis, hemorrhage, and mononuclear cell infiltration are also common.

Clinical signs can appear at any age, although the mean age is reported to be 8.5 years (range of less than 1 to 15 years). A genetic basis is believed to exist because the disease is more prevalent in some bloodlines. The most consistent clinical finding is a cardiac arrhythmia. When congestive failure occurs, left-sided signs are more common than ascites or other signs of right-sided heart failure; many Boxers also develop a mitral insufficiency murmur.

The radiographic findings are variable; many Boxers have no visible abnormalities. Those with congestive signs generally show evidence of cardiomegaly and pulmonary edema. The ECG usually documents an underlying sinus rhythm. Atrial fibrillation is less common; supraventricular tachycardia, conduction abnormalities, and evidence of chamber enlargement sometimes occur. The characteristic finding is ventricular ectopy; VPCs occur singly, in pairs, in short runs, or as sustained ventricular tachycardia. Most ectopic ventricular complexes appear upright in leads II and aV$_F$; some Boxers have multiform VPCs. Twenty-four-hour Holter monitoring is often recommended as a screening test for Boxer cardiomyopathy, as well as as a means of evaluating the efficacy of antiarrhythmic drug therapy. Frequent VPCs and/or complex ventricular arrhythmias are characteristic findings in affected dogs. However, an absolute number of VPCs per 24 hours that might separate normal from abnormal dogs is not (and may never be) clear. An arbitrary cutoff of 50 VPCs per 24 hours is sometimes used. However, there can be enormous variability in the number of VPCs between repeated Holter recordings in the same dog. Very frequent VPCs or episodes of ventricular tachycardia are thought to signal increased risk for syncope and sudden death. Echocardiographic findings also vary, from normal cardiac size and function to chamber dilation with poor fractional shortening. Congestive heart failure may develop later in dogs with mild echocardiographic changes and those with syncope or weakness.

Therapy for symptomatic Boxers with normal heart size and LV function is usually limited to antiarrhythmic drugs. The best regimen(s) and when to institute therapy are still not clear. Antiarrhythmic drug therapy that is apparently successful in reducing the number of VPCs, based on Holter recording, may still not prevent sudden death. The focus now is on drugs or drug combinations that also increase the ventricular fibrillation threshold, with the hope that not only will arrhythmia frequency and severity be decreased, but also that the risk for sudden death from ventricular fibrillation might be reduced. Recently, sotalol, procainamide with atenolol, amiodarone, or mexiletine with atenolol have been advocated (see Chapter 4). The class III agents (sotalol, amiodarone) are gaining favor. Suppression of persistent supraventricular tachyarrhythmias is sometimes necessary. Therapy for congestive failure is similar to that described for dogs with DCM; however, digoxin is used sparingly or not at all if frequent ventricular tachyarrhythmias are present.

The prognosis for affected Boxers is guarded to poor. If heart failure is present, the animal usually dies within 6 months. Asymptomatic dogs may have a more optimistic future, but the likelihood of developing serious refractory arrhythmias and congestive heart failure is high. Many Boxers with cardiomyopathy die suddenly, presumably from VPCs leading to ventricular fibrillation. The ventricular arrhythmias can be refractory to antiarrhythmic therapy. Furthermore, the ability of antiarrhythmic drugs to prolong life even if most arrhythmias are suppressed is unknown. Myocardial carnitine deficiency has been documented in some Boxers with DCM and heart failure; some of these dogs responded to PO L-carnitine supplementation.

## Doberman Pinschers

This breed appears to have the highest prevalence of DCM. A genetic basis is believed to exist, but the inheritance pattern is not clear. Impaired intracellular energy homeostasis, leading to decreased myocardial ATP concentrations, has been documented by myocardial biochemical studies conducted in Dobermans with DCM. Subclinical (occult) disease has been estimated to be present in as many as 44% of asymptomatic adult Dobermans. The disease is thought to evolve over a period of years before clinical signs become evident. Males generally become symptomatic at an earlier age than females. Sudden death before the onset of congestive heart failure is common. Ventricular tachyarrhythmias occur frequently in Dobermans with cardiomyopathy. Serial Holter recordings have documented the appearance of VPCs months to more than a year before early echocardiographic abnormalities are noted. Once left ventricular function begins to deteriorate, the frequency of tachyarrhythmias increases. Histopathologic findings include myocardial fibrosis, fatty infiltration, and myocyte degeneration.

The disease is clinically similar to idiopathic DCM in other large-breed dogs; however, the combination of ventricular tachyarrhythmias and severely compromised left ventricular contractility is highly prevalent in Dobermans. The history often includes episodic weakness or syncope. Sudden death from ventricular tachycardia-fibrillation is common. Some Dobermans exhibit syncope resulting from bradycardia associated with excitement or exertion rather than from ventricular tachycardia. Fulminant pulmonary edema often appears acutely, and cardiogenic shock can result from poor cardiac output and congestive failure.

Radiographically the heart may not appear greatly enlarged, with the exception of the left atrium (see Fig. 6-1, *C* and *D*). Severe and diffuse infiltrates of pulmonary edema occur in dogs with congestive heart failure. The ECG often documents an underlying sinus rhythm, although atrial fibrillation is relatively common. Paroxysmal or sustained ventricular tachycardia, fusion complexes, and multiform VPCs also are frequent findings, and the QRS complexes often appear wide and sloppy. Twenty-four–hour Holter monitoring usually documents frequent ventricular ectopy. Dobermans with fulminant congestive failure typically have prominent left ventricular dilation and extremely low fractional shortening (often less than 10%) on echocardiogram. Therapy is the same as that described for DCM in large and giant-breed dogs (see Table 6-1), with antiarrhythmic therapy frequently indicated as for Boxers (see Chapter 4).

The prognosis for most of these dogs is guarded to grave, depending on the severity of heart failure and response to initial therapy. Sudden death occurs in about 20% to 40% of affected Dobermans, often before the onset of clinical congestive heart failure. Although ventricular tachyarrhythmias are thought to precipitate cardiac arrest most commonly, bradyarrhythmias may be involved in some dogs. Mild DCM is diagnosed in some Dobermans before clinical signs appear. These dogs do well for a time, although their condition usually deteriorates within 6 to 12 months. Dogs in overt congestive failure when first seen generally do not live long (reported median survival of less than 7 weeks). The prognosis is worse if atrial fibrillation is present in dogs with congestive failure. Most symptomatic dogs are between 5 and 10 years old at the time of death.

Early diagnosis may help prolong life; further cardiac evaluation is indicated for dogs with a history of reduced exercise tolerance, weakness or syncope, or in those in which an arrhythmia, murmur, or gallop sound is detected. Owners and breeders are also increasingly requesting screening for subclinical disease. Ambulatory (Holter) ECG monitoring for 24 to 48 hours and echocardiography are most useful for this. The finding of over 50 VPCs per 24 hours or any couplets or triplets is thought to be predictive of future DCM (Calvert and colleagues, 2000). However, many dogs with fewer than 50 VPCs per 24 hours on initial evaluation also have developed cardiomyopathy several years later. Analysis of heart rate variability (HRV) has not been helpful in differentiating mildly or moderately affected dogs from normal ones or in predicting sudden death (Calvert and colleague, 2001). The technique of signal-averaged electrocardiography (SAECG) may be useful if available. The SAECG is abnormal in some but not all Dobermans with occult DCM that die suddenly (Calvert and colleagues, 1998). However, detection of ventricular late potentials with this test appears to be a clear indicator of increased risk for sudden death.

Echocardiographic abnormalities may be absent early in the disease. It is important to note that apparently healthy Dobermans often have reduced myocardial function compared to what is considered normal for other breeds. Based on studies of over 100 Dobermans, O'Grady and colleagues (1995) identified the following echocardiographic criteria as predictors of high risk for overt DCM within 2 to 3 years in asymptomatic dogs: left ventricular internal diameter in diastole (LVID$_d$) over 46 mm; left ventricular internal diameter in systole (LVID$_s$) over 38 mm, or VPCs during initial examination. Calvert and colleagues (1997) also reported criteria for identifying occult

DCM in clinically normal Dobermans: LVID$_d$ over 45 mm for dogs under 38 kg body weight or over 49 mm for dogs over 37 kg; fractional shortening of less than 25%, and/or mitral valve E point–septal separation over 8 mm.

# HYPERTROPHIC CARDIOMYOPATHY

Hypertrophic cardiomyopathy is uncommon in dogs, in contrast to cats. Although its cause is unknown, a genetic basis is suspected. It may be that several disease processes produce similar ventricular changes. The abnormal and marked myocardial hypertrophy typical of this disease increases the stiffness of the ventricle and causes diastolic dysfunction. The hypertrophy is usually symmetric, but regional variation in wall or septal thickness can occur. Severe ventricular hypertrophy is likely to cause compromised coronary perfusion and myocardial ischemia, which exacerbate arrhythmias and worsen ventricular relaxation and filling. These abnormalities are magnified as the heart rate increases; high ventricular filling pressures predispose to the development of left-sided congestive failure. Besides diastolic dysfunction, dynamic systolic left ventricular outflow obstruction occurs in some dogs. Malposition of the mitral apparatus may contribute to systolic anterior mitral valve motion and outflow tract obstruction as well as to mitral regurgitation. In some dogs, asymmetric septal hypertrophy also contributes to outflow obstruction. Left ventricular outflow obstruction increases ventricular wall stress and myocardial oxygen requirement; it also impairs coronary blood flow and worsens ischemia. These abnormalities become more pronounced as the heart rate increases.

## Clinical Features

HCM is most commonly diagnosed in young to middle-aged, large-breed dogs, although there is a wide age distribution, and dogs of various breeds are affected. There may be a higher incidence of HCM in males. Clinical signs of heart failure, episodic weakness, and/or syncope occur in some dogs; however, sudden death can occur before other cardiac signs develop. Ventricular arrhythmias secondary to myocardial ischemia are thought to cause the low-output signs and sudden death. A systolic murmur of left ventricular outflow tract obstruction or mitral insufficiency may be heard on auscultation. The systolic ejection murmur of ventricular outflow obstruction is accentuated when ventricular contractility is increased (e.g., by exercise or in the heartbeats after VPCs) or when systemic arterial pressure is decreased (by a vasodilator). An atrial gallop sound (S$_4$) may be heard in some affected dogs.

## Diagnosis

Echocardiography is the best diagnostic tool in dogs with HCM. An abnormally thick left ventricle, with or without narrowing of the left ventricular outflow tract area or asymmetric septal hypertrophy, and left atrial enlargement are characteristic findings. Mitral regurgitation may be evident on Doppler studies. Severe outflow obstruction causes systolic anterior motion of the mitral valve and partial systolic aortic valve closure. Other causes of left ventricular hypertrophy include congenital subaortic stenosis, hypertensive renal disease, thyrotoxicosis, and pheochromocytoma. Thoracic radiographs may show normal findings or left atrial and ventricular enlargement, with or without pulmonary congestion or edema. Ventricular tachyarrhythmias and conduction abnormalities, including complete heart block, first-degree AV block, and fascicular blocks, appear to be common ECG findings. Criteria for left ventricular enlargement are variably present.

### Treatment

The goals of treatment for HCM are to enhance myocardial relaxation and ventricular filling, control pulmonary edema, and suppress arrhythmias. A β-blocker (see p. 91) or calcium entry blocker (see p. 94) may lower the heart rate, prolong the ventricular filling time, and reduce ventricular contractility and the myocardial oxygen requirement. β-Blockers may also increase the threshold for arrhythmias induced by heightened sympathetic activity, whereas calcium entry blockers facilitate the myocardial relaxation process. The β-blockers and verapamil reduce and may eliminate dynamic outflow obstruction because of their negative inotropic effects. Diltiazem has a lesser inotropic effect and would be less useful against dynamic outflow obstruction, especially in view of its vasodilating effects. The β-blocker and calcium entry blocker drugs can also worsen AV conduction abnormalities and thus may be relatively contraindicated in certain animals. Diuretics are indicated if congestive signs are present. Digoxin should not be used because it may increase myocardial oxygen requirements, worsen outflow obstruction, and predispose to the development of ventricular arrhythmias. Marked exercise restriction is advised in dogs with HCM.

## ARRHYTHMOGENIC RIGHT VENTRICULAR CARDIOMYOPATHY

A rare form of cardiomyopathy limited mainly to the right ventricle has been observed in dogs. It appears to be similar to the right ventricular cardiomyopathy described in people and cats (see p. 133). Pathologic changes are characterized by widespread replacement of the right ventricular myocardium by fibrous and fatty tissue. A possible differential diagnosis in certain geographic areas could be trypanosomiasis. Clinical manifestations are largely related to right-sided congestive heart failure with marked right heart dilation and severe ventricular tachyarrhythmias. Sudden death is a common outcome in people with the disease.

## MYOCARDITIS

### INFECTIVE MYOCARDITIS
### Etiology and Clinical Features

A wide variety of agents can affect the myocardium, although disease manifestations in other organ systems may overshadow the cardiac involvement. The heart can be injured by direct invasion of the infective agent, by toxins it elaborates, or by the host's immune response. Noninfective causes of myocarditis include cardiotoxic drugs and drug hypersensitivity reactions. Myocarditis can cause persistent cardiac arrhythmias and progressively impair myocardial function. Cardiotropic viruses may play an important role in the pathogenesis of myocarditis and cardiomyopathy in several species. In people an association between acute (viral) myocarditis and subsequent DCM has long been recognized. Using PCR techniques, viral genetic material (e.g., enterovirus, adenovirus, parvovirus, and other viruses) has been amplified inconsistently from myocardial samples from people with DCM as well as myocarditis. However, similar evidence from dogs is weak. Links between the host animal's immune system, genetic factors, and the development, severity, and consequences of myocarditis have also been identified.

**Viral myocarditis.** Lymphocytic myocarditis has been associated with acute viral infections in experimental animals and in people. A syndrome of parvoviral myocarditis became widely recognized in the late 1970s and early 1980s. It was characterized by a peracute necrotizing myocarditis that occurred mostly in 4- to 8-week-old puppies unprotected by maternal antibodies, and it resulted in the sudden death (with or without signs of acute respiratory distress) of these apparently healthy pups. Necropsy findings included cardiac dilation with pale streaks in the myocardium, gross evidence of congestive failure, large basophilic or amorphophilic intranuclear inclusion bodies, myocyte degeneration, and focal mononuclear cell infiltrates. This syndrome is uncommon today, probably as a result of maternal antibody production in response to virus exposure and vaccination. However, parvovirus can also cause a form of DCM in young dogs that survive neonatal infection. Viral genetic material has been identified in some canine ventricular myocardial samples in the absence of classic intranuclear inclusion bodies. There may be a relation between persistent viral infection and subsequent dilated cardiomyopathy, although the relative clinical importance of this is unclear at present. Experimentally, canine distemper virus has been observed to cause myocarditis in young puppies, but multisystemic signs usually predominate. Histologic changes in the myocardium are mild compared with those in the classic form of parvovirus myocarditis. Experimentally induced herpesvirus infection of pups during gestation has also been observed to cause necrotizing myocarditis with intranuclear inclusion bodies leading to fetal or perinatal death.

**Bacterial myocarditis.** Bacteremia and bacterial endocarditis or pericarditis can cause focal or multifocal suppurative myocardial inflammation or abscess formation. Localized infections elsewhere in the body may be the source of the organisms. Clinical signs include malaise, weight loss, and, inconsistently, fever. Arrhythmias and cardiac conduction abnormalities are common, but murmurs are rare unless concurrent valvular endocarditis or another underlying cardiac defect is present. Serial bacterial (or fungal) blood cultures may allow identification of the organism (see p. 1235). *Bartonella vinsonii* subspecies recently have been associated with cardiac arrhythmias, myocarditis, and endocarditis in dogs (Breitschwerdt and colleagues, 1999).

**Lyme disease.** Lyme carditis is recognized more frequently in animals in certain geographic areas, especially the northeastern, western coastal, and north central United States. The spirochete *Borrelia burgdorferi* is transmitted to dogs by ticks (especially *Ixodes dammini*) and possibly other biting insects. High-grade AV block is a manifestation of Lyme carditis in people; third-degree (complete) and high-grade second-degree heart block have been identified in dogs with Lyme disease. Syncope, congestive heart failure, impaired myocardial contractility, and ventricular arrhythmias have also been identified in affected dogs. The pathologic findings of myocarditis with infiltrates of plasma cells, macrophages, neutrophils, and lymphocytes, in conjunction with areas of myocardial necrosis, are similar to those seen in human Lyme carditis. However, it appears that appropriate antimicrobial therapy may not routinely result in the resolution of AV conduction disturbances in dogs, as it does in people. A presumptive diagnosis is made on the basis of the finding of positive (or increasing) serum titers and concurrent signs of myocarditis, with or without other systemic signs. The findings from endomyocardial biopsy, if available, may be helpful in confirming the diagnosis. Treatment with an appropriate antibiotic should be instituted pending diagnostic test results (see p. 1240). Cardiac drugs are used as needed.

**Protozoal myocarditis.** The protozoal organisms *Trypanosoma cruzi, Toxoplasma gondii, Neosporum caninum, Babesia canis,* and *Hepatozoon canis* can affect the myocardium. Trypanosomiasis (Chagas' disease) is an important cause of myocarditis in people in Central and South America. In the United States it has occurred mainly in young dogs in Texas, Louisiana, Oklahoma, Virginia, and other southern states, but the possibility for human infection should be recognized. The organism is carried by bloodsucking insects of the family Reduviidae and is enzootic in wild animals of the region. Amastigotes of *T. cruzi* cause myocarditis with a mononuclear cell infiltrate and disruption and necrosis of myocardial fibers. Acute, latent, and chronic phases of Chagas' myocarditis have been described. Lethargy, depression, and other systemic signs, as well as various tachyarrhythmias, AV conduction defects, and sudden death, have been observed in dogs with acute trypanosomiasis, although clinical signs are sometimes subtle. The disease is diagnosed in the acute stage by the finding of trypomastigotes in thick peripheral blood smears; the organism can be isolated in cell culture or by inoculation into mice. Animals that survive the acute phase enter a latent phase of variable duration in which the parasitemia is resolved and antibodies against the organism develop. Chronic Chagas' disease is characterized by progressive, right-sided or generalized cardiomegaly and arrhythmias. Ventricular tachyarrhythmias may be most notable, but supraventricular tachyarrhythmias can occur. Right bundle branch block and AV conduction disturbances are also reported. Ventricular dilation and reduced myocardial function are usually evident on echocardiograms, and clinical signs of biventricular failure are common. Findings from serologic testing may provide the basis for an antemortem diagnosis in chronic cases. Therapy in the acute stage is aimed at eliminating the organism and minimizing myocardial inflammation; several treatments have been tried with variable success (see p. 1304). The therapy for chronic Chagas' disease is directed at supporting myocardial function, controlling congestive signs, and suppressing arrhythmias.

Toxoplasmosis and neosporiosis occasionally cause clinical myocarditis as part of a generalized systemic process, especially in the immunocompromised animal. After the initial infection, the organism becomes encysted in the heart and various other body tissues. With rupture of these cysts, expelled bradyzoites induce hypersensitivity reactions and tissue necrosis. Often other systemic signs predominate over signs of myocarditis. Immunosuppressed dogs with chronic toxoplasmosis (or neosporiosis) may be at risk for active disease, including clinically relevant myocarditis, pneumonia, chorioretinitis, and encephalitis (see p. 1299). Therapy with appropriate antiprotozoal agents may be successful.

Babesiosis has sometimes been associated with cardiac lesions in dogs, including myocardial hemorrhage, inflammation, and necrosis. Pericardial effusion and variable ECG changes are also noted in some cases. A correlation between plasma cardiac troponin I (cTnI) concentration (a biochemical marker of myocardial injury) and clinical severity, survival, and cardiac histologic changes has been reported in dogs with babesiosis (Lobetti and colleagues, 2002). Myocardial involvement with *H. canis* during part of its life cycle has been found in dogs along the Texas coast. Infection results from ingestion of the organism's definitive host, the brown dog tick (*Rhipicephalus sanguineus*). Reported clinical signs include stiffness, anorexia, fever, neutrophilia, and periosteal new bone reaction (see p. 1302).

**Miscellaneous causes.** In rare instances, fungi (*Aspergillus, Cryptococcus, Coccidioides, Histoplasma, Paecilomyces*), rickettsiae (*Rickettsia rickettsii, Ehrlichia canis, Bartonella elizabethae*), algaelike organisms (*Prototheca*), and nematode larval migration (*Toxocara* sp.) cause myocarditis. Affected animals are usually immunosuppressed and have systemic signs of disease. Rocky Mountain spotted fever (*R. rickettsii*) occasionally causes fatal ventricular arrhythmias, along with necrotizing vasculitis, myocardial thrombosis, and ischemia (see p. 1265). *Angiostrongylus vasorum* infection in association with immune-mediated thrombocytopenia has rarely caused myocarditis, thrombosing arteritis, and sudden death (Gould and colleague, 1999).

## Diagnosis

The classic clinical presentation of acute myocarditis involves the unexplained onset of arrhythmias or heart failure after a recent episode of infectious disease. Yet even in this setting, the diagnosis may be equivocal because there are no clinical or clinicopathologic findings specific for myocarditis. A complete blood count, serum biochemical profile including determination of creatine kinase activity, thoracic and abdominal radiographs, and urinalysis are usually obtained as part of a broad database. The utility of circulating cardiac troponin concentrations to detect myocardial injury is expected to grow as more veterinary experience is gained. There may be nonspecific ECG changes (e.g., ST segment shifts, T-wave or QRS voltage changes, AV conduction abnormalities) or echocardiographic signs of poor regional or global wall motion, altered myocardial echogenicity, or pericardial effusion. In dogs with persistent fever, serial bacterial (or fungal) blood cultures may be rewarding. Serologic screening for known infectious causes may or may not be helpful. The lack of a consistent clinical presentation and effective noninvasive tests contributes to the difficulty of establishing a definitive diagnosis; the diagnostic criteria for myocarditis are histologic and include the finding of inflammatory infiltrates with myocyte degeneration and necrosis. Endomyocardial biopsy specimens are currently the only means of obtaining a definitive antemortem diagnosis, but the findings may not be diagnostic if the lesions are focal.

### Treatment

Therapy for suspected myocarditis is largely supportive unless a specific etiology can be identified and treated. This includes strict rest, antiarrhythmic therapy as needed (see Chapter 4), an ACEI with or without digoxin for reduced myocardial function, a diuretic for signs of congestion or edema, and other support as needed (see Chapter 3). Corticosteroids have not been proved to be clinically beneficial in dogs with myocarditis, and considering the possible infective cause, they are not recommended as nonspecific therapy.

## NONINFECTIVE MYOCARDITIS

Myocardial inflammation can result from the effects of drugs, toxins, or immunologic responses. Although there is little clinical documentation for many of these in dogs, a large number of potential causes have been identified in people. Besides the well-known toxic effects of doxorubicin and catecholamines, other potential causes of noninfective myocarditis include heavy metals (e.g., arsenic, lead, mercury), antineoplastic drugs (cyclophosphamide, 5-fluorouracil, interleukin-2, alpha-interferon), other drugs (e.g., thyroid hormone, cocaine, amphetamines, lithium), and toxins (wasp or scorpion stings, snake venom, spider bites). Immune-mediated diseases and pheochromocytoma can cause myocarditis as well. Hypersensitivity reactions to many antiinfective agents and other drugs have also been identified as causing myocarditis in people. Drug-related myocarditis is usually characterized by eosinophilic as well as lymphocytic infiltrates.

## TRAUMATIC MYOCARDITIS

Nonpenetrating or blunt trauma to the chest and heart is more common than penetrating wounds in dogs and cats. Posttraumatic cardiac arrhythmias are frequently observed in such animals, especially in dogs. Cardiac damage can result from impact against the chest wall, compression, or acceleration-deceleration forces. Other mechanisms of myocardial injury and arrhythmogenesis might include an autonomic imbalance, ischemia, reperfusion injury, or electrolyte and acid-base disturbances. Chest radiographs, serum biochemistries, and ECG are recommended components in the assessment of these cases. Echocardiography may be indicated to define

preexisting heart disease or unexpected cardiovascular findings, but it has not been a sensitive test for identifying small areas of myocardial injury. Measurement of serum cardiac troponin concentrations may become more widely used in the near future to assess myocardial injury.

Arrhythmias usually appear within 24 to 48 hours after trauma, although they can be missed on intermittent ECG recordings. VPCs, ventricular tachycardia, and accelerated idioventricular rhythms (with rates of 60 to 100 beats/min or slightly faster) are more common than supraventricular tachyarrhythmias or bradyarrhythmias in this setting. Accelerated idioventricular rhythms usually are manifested only when the sinus rate slows or pauses; they are benign in most dogs with normal underlying heart function and disappear with time (generally within a week or so). Antiarrhythmic therapy for such ventricular ectopic beats is usually unnecessary. The animal and ECG should be closely monitored, however. If more serious arrhythmias (e.g., faster rate or multiform configuration) or hemodynamic deterioration develops, antiarrhythmic therapy may be indicated (see p. 78, Chapter 4).

Traumatic avulsion of AV valve papillary muscles, septal perforation, and rupture of the heart or pericardium have also been reported. Acute low-output failure and shock, as well as arrhythmias, can develop quickly in such animals. Traumatic papillary muscle avulsion causes acute volume overload and the rapid onset of congestive failure.

## CARDIOGENIC SHOCK

### Etiology

Shock stemming from any cause results in acute, severe circulatory failure. The delivery of oxygen and nutrients to vital organs and the removal of accumulated metabolites are inadequate as a result, and progressive and eventually fatal derangement of physiologic processes ensues. Cardiogenic shock results from profound impairment of cardiac pumping ability. The causes are diverse and include myocardial contractility failure, acute disruption of valvular structures with severe blood regurgitation, sustained severe bradyarrhythmias or tachyarrhythmias, an intracardiac obstruction to blood flow, and an overdose of hypotensive or negative inotropic drugs, especially in the face of preexisting cardiac disease (Table 6-2). Extracardiac obstruction to blood flow resulting from cardiac tamponade, pulmonary hypertension, or massive pulmonary embolism can also severely reduce forward cardiac output. Acute myocardial infarction, although a frequent cause of cardiogenic shock in people, is uncommon in dogs and cats. Severe DCM is probably the most common cause of cardiogenic shock in dogs (and cats).

### Clinical Features

Signs of cardiogenic shock are related to low cardiac output and arterial hypotension, as well as to the compensatory neurohumoral responses activated to increase vascular volume and maintain blood pressure. These responses include heightened sympathetic tone, the adrenal medullary release of cat-

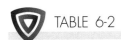 TABLE 6-2

## Causes of Cardiogenic Shock

**Myopathic**

Dilated cardiomyopathy
Myocarditis
Myocardial infarction

**Valvular**

Rupture of chordae tendineae
Papillary muscle avulsion
Acute aortic regurgitation

**Intracardiac Obstruction**

Intracardiac tumor
Hypertrophic obstructive cardiomyopathy
Aortic stenosis

**Arrhythmias**

Sustained ventricular tachycardia
Sustained atrial or supraventricular tachycardia
Uncontrolled atrial fibrillation or flutter
Complete heart block or atrial standstill with slow escape
   rhythm
Severe sinus bradycardia

**Drug Overdose**

Vasodilators
β-Adrenergic blockers
Calcium entry blockers

**Extracardiac Obstruction**

Cardiac tamponade
Heartworm disease
Massive pulmonary thromboembolism
Other causes of pulmonary hypertension

echolamines, and the elaboration of angiotensin, vasopressin, aldosterone, cortisol, and other hormones. Tachycardia (unless shock is caused by a bradyarrhythmia), weak arterial pulses, pallor, a prolonged capillary refill time, peripheral cyanosis, hyperventilation, oliguria, and depression are common manifestations. In addition, cardiac arrhythmias, a murmur or gallop sound, decreased-intensity heart sounds, acute pulmonary edema, and systemic venous distention (with right heart failure or cardiac tamponade) can occur.

## Treatment

Therapy is aimed at restoring organ perfusion to provide adequate tissue oxygenation. Therefore support of arterial blood pressure, forward cardiac output, and vascular volume is crucial. The basic pathophysiologic abnormality must be identified in order for optimal treatment to be implemented. Specific measures to control the underlying disease may be possible. Inotropic support in combination with diuresis, vasodilation, fluids, and other supportive measures is indicated

for the management of DCM (see Table 6-1). In contrast, pericardiocentesis is necessary for the treatment of cardiac tamponade. It is also important to control arrhythmias. Cardiogenic shock resulting from overdose of a vasodilator drug may respond to an infusion of fluids and dopamine, or another pressor agent. Overdose of a β-adrenergic blocker, resulting in bradycardia and poor contractility, may also respond to an infusion of dopamine or dobutamine. Supplemental calcium is indicated for an overdose of a calcium entry blocker.

Early recognition of the complications of shock increases the chance of successful treatment. Acute renal failure is a major sequela of prolonged hypotension and renal hypoperfusion. Dopamine, infused at low doses, promotes renal vasodilation through the stimulation of dopaminergic receptors; however, at higher doses it can stimulate peripheral α-adrenergic receptors and cause vasoconstriction (see Table 3-8). Fluid replacement therapy is important but must be administered cautiously to animals in heart failure.

Severe metabolic acidosis resulting from anaerobic tissue metabolism can occur in animals in shock. Bicarbonate therapy is ideally guided by venous blood gas values. If these are unavailable, the total carbon dioxide concentration can be used to estimate acid-base status, as long as pulmonary function is relatively normal. In the absence of these measurements, a clinical estimation of the adequacy of peripheral perfusion can help guide bicarbonate therapy. Mild, moderate, and severe impairment of perfusion has been empirically treated with IV sodium bicarbonate given at doses of 1, 3, and 5 mEq/kg, respectively. Complications of rapid or excessive bicarbonate administration include alkalosis, hypotension, paradoxical cerebrospinal fluid acidosis, cerebral edema, hypercapnia, and vomiting.

Supplemental oxygen therapy is indicated for animals with pulmonary edema; likewise, thoracocentesis should be performed if pleural effusion is present. Assisted ventilation, with positive end-expiratory pressure, may be of benefit in animals with severe edema or other pulmonary complications (see p. 340).

Frequent assessment of the patient is important, as with any critical condition. Indirect or direct measurement of arterial blood pressure is indicated. A mean arterial pressure consistently greater than 60 mm Hg or a systolic pressure greater than 80 mm Hg is desired. Indirect measures of organ perfusion, such as the capillary refill time, mucous membrane color, urine output, toe-web temperature, and mentation, are also helpful. The reversal of severe peripheral vasoconstriction combined with strong femoral pulses often indicates that therapy has been effective. However, because of the profound vasoconstrictive response that occurs in shock, arterial blood pressure and femoral pulse strength are not always associated with adequate tissue perfusion or volume replacement.

The central venous pressure (CVP) does not adequately reflect the status of the circulating blood volume or left heart filling pressures in animals in cardiogenic shock. Reduced right heart function and obstruction to cardiac filling or output elevate the CVP, independent of left heart filling or output. Thus CVP is likely to be misleading if used to guide fluid therapy. The placement of a Swan-Ganz catheter into the pulmonary artery allows measurement of pulmonary arterial and pulmonary capillary wedge pressures and also provides access to mixed venous blood samples. The pulmonary wedge pressure reflects the left atrial (and therefore left ventricular) filling pressure in the absence of significant pulmonary vascular disease or obstruction to left ventricular inflow. Maintaining this pressure in the high-normal range (10 to 15 mm Hg) is desirable. Although use of the pulmonary capillary wedge pressures to guide fluid therapy is helpful, the placement and care of an indwelling pulmonary artery catheter requires meticulous attention to asepsis and close monitoring.

Electrolyte balance and renal function should also be monitored. A serum potassium concentration maintained in the mid- to high-normal range is especially important in animals with arrhythmias. Aggressive antimicrobial therapy is also indicated in animals in cardiogenic shock associated with bacterial endocarditis or sepsis. Glucocorticoids are unlikely to be of benefit in dogs or cats in cardiogenic shock.

## Suggested Readings

NONINFECTIVE MYOCARDIAL DISEASE

Bright JM et al: Isolated right ventricular cardiomyopathy in a dog, *J Am Vet Med Assoc* 207:64, 1995.

Calvert CA et al: Bradycardia-associated episodic weakness, syncope, and aborted sudden death in cardiomyopathic Doberman Pinschers, *J Vet Intern Med* 10:88, 1996.

Calvert CA et al: Clinical and pathological findings in Doberman Pinschers with occult cardiomyopathy that died suddenly or developed congestive heart failure: 54 cases (1984-1991), *J Am Vet Med Assoc* 210:505, 1997.

Calvert CA et al: Signalment, survival, and prognostic factors in Doberman Pinschers with end-stage cardiomyopathy, *J Vet Intern Med* 11:323, 1997.

Calvert CA et al: Thyroid-stimulating hormone stimulation tests in cardiomyopathic Doberman Pinschers: a retrospective study, *J Vet Intern Med* 12:343, 1998.

Calvert CA et al: Doberman Pinscher occult cardiomyopathy. In Bonagura JD, editor: *Kirk's current veterinary therapy XIII*, Philadelphia, 2000, WB Saunders, p 756.

Calvert CA et al: Results of ambulatory electrocardiography in overtly healthy Doberman Pinschers with echocardiographic abnormalities, *J Am Vet Med Assoc* 217:1328, 2000.

Calvert CA et al: Effect of severity of myocardial failure on heart rate variability in Doberman Pinschers with and without echocardiographic evidence of dilated cardiomyopathy, *J Am Vet Med Assoc* 219:1084, 2001.

Carroll MC et al: Carnitine: a review, *Compend Contin Educ* 23:45, 2001.

Dambach DM et al: Familial dilated cardiomyopathy of young Portuguese water dogs, *J Vet Intern Med* 13:65, 1999.

De Andrade JN et al: Reduction of diameter of the left ventricle of dogs by plication of the left ventricular free wall, *Am J Vet Res* 62:297, 2001.

DeFrancesco TC et al: Prospective clinical evaluation of serum cardiac troponin T in dogs admitted to a veterinary teaching hospital, *J Vet Intern Med* 16:553, 2002.

Driehuys S et al: Myocardial infarction in dogs and cats: 37 cases (1985-1994), *J Am Vet Med Assoc* 213:1444, 1998.

Falk T et al: Ischaemic heart disease in the dog: a review of 65 cases, *J Small Anim Pract* 41:97, 2000.

Freeman LM et al: Idiopathic dilated cardiomyopathy in Dalmatians: nine cases (1990-1995), *J Am Vet Med Assoc* 209:1592, 1996.

Freeman LM et al: Assessment of degree of oxidative stress and antioxidant concentration in dogs with idiopathic dilated cardiomyopathy, *J Am Vet Med Assoc* 215:644, 1999.

Freeman LM et al: Relationship between circulating and dietary taurine concentration in dogs with dilated cardiomyopathy, *Vet Therapeutics* 2:370, 2001.

Keene BW: Carnitine supplementation: what have we learned? *Proceedings of the 18th ACVIM Forum*, Seattle, 2000, p 105.

Kittleson MD et al: Results of the multicenter spaniel trial (MUST): taurine- and carnitine-responsive dilated cardiomyopathy in American Cocker Spaniels with decreased plasma taurine concentration, *J Vet Intern Med* 11:204, 1997.

Kramer GA et al: Plasma taurine concentrations in normal dogs and in dogs with heart disease, *J Vet Intern Med* 9:253, 1995.

Mauldin GE et al: Doxorubicin-induced cardiotoxicosis: clinical features in 23 dogs, *J Vet Intern Med* 6:82, 1992.

Maxson TR et al: Polymerase chain reaction analysis for viruses in paraffin-embedded myocardium from dogs with dilated cardiomyopathy or myocarditis, *Am J Vet Res* 62:130, 2001.

Meurs KM et al: Familial ventricular arrhythmias in Boxers, *J Vet Intern Med* 13:437, 1999.

Meurs KM et al: Clinical features of dilated cardiomyopathy in Great Danes and results of a pedigree analysis: 17 cases (1990-2000), *J Am Vet Med Assoc* 218:729, 2001.

McEntee K et al: Usefulness of dobutamine stress tests for detection of cardiac abnormalities in dogs with experimentally induced early left ventricular dysfunction, *Am J Vet Res* 62:448, 2001.

Minors SL et al: Resting and dobutamine stress echocardiographic factors associated with the development of occult dilated cardiomyopathy in healthy Doberman Pinscher dogs, *J Vet Intern Med* 12:369, 1998.

Monnet E et al: Idiopathic dilated cardiomyopathy in dogs: survival and prognostic indicators, *J Vet Intern Med* 9:12, 1995.

O'Brien PJ: Deficiencies of myocardial troponin-T and creatine kinase MB isoenzyme in dogs with idiopathic dilated cardiomyopathy, *Am J Vet Res* 58:11, 1997.

O'Grady MR et al: Outcome of 103 asymptomatic Doberman Pinschers: incidence of dilated cardiomyopathy in a longitudinal study, *Proceedings of the 13th ACVIM Forum*, Lake Buena Vista, Fla, 1995, p 1014 (abstract).

Orton EC et al: Dynamic cardiomyoplasty for treatment of idiopathic dilatative cardiomyopathy in a dog, *J Am Vet Med Assoc* 205:1415, 1994.

Panciera DL: An echocardiographic and electrocardiographic study of cardiovascular function in hypothyroid dogs, *J Am Vet Med Assoc* 205:996, 1994.

Schober KE et al: Circulating cardiac troponins in small animals, *Proceedings of the 19th ACVIM Scientific Forum*, Denver, 2001, p 91.

Sisson DD et al: Primary myocardial diseases in the dog. In Ettinger SJ et al, editors: *Textbook of veterinary internal medicine*, ed 5, WB Saunders, Philadelphia, 2000, p 874.

Sleeper MM et al: Cardiac troponin I in the normal dog and cat, *J Vet Intern Med* 15:501, 2001.

Sleeper MM et al: Dilated cardiomyopathy in juvenile Portuguese water dogs, *J Vet Intern Med* 16:52, 2002.

Tidholm A et al: Dilated cardiomyopathy in the Newfoundland: a study of 37 cases (1983-1994), *J Am Anim Hosp Assoc* 32:465, 1996.

Tidholm A et al: Survival and prognostic factors in 189 dogs with dilated cardiomyopathy, *J Am Anim Hosp Assoc* 33:364, 1997.

Tidholm A et al: Prevalence of attenuated wavy fibers in myocardium of dogs with dilated cardiomyopathy, *J Am Vet Med Assoc* 212:1732, 1998.

Tidholm A et al: Detection of attenuated wavy fibers in the myocardium of Newfoundlands without clinical or echocardiographic evidence of heart disease, *Am J Vet Res* 61:238, 2000.

Tidholm A et al: Effects of dilated cardiomyopathy on the renin-angiotensin-aldosterone system, atrial natriuretic peptide activity, and thyroid hormone concentrations in dogs, *Am J Vet Res* 62:961, 2001.

Vollmar AC: The prevalence of cardiomyopathy in the Irish Wolfhound: a clinical study of 500 dogs, *J Am Anim Hosp* 36:126, 2000.

Weber KT: Aldosterone in congestive heart failure, *N Engl J Med* 345:1689, 2001.

Wright KN et al: Radiofrequency catheter ablation of atrioventricular accessory pathways in 3 dogs with subsequent resolution of tachycardia-induced cardiomyopathy, *J Vet Intern Med* 13:361, 1999.

MYOCARDITIS

Barber JS et al: Clinical aspects of 27 cases of neosporosis in dogs, *Vet Rec* 139:439, 1996.

Barr SC et al: Electrocardiographic and echocardiographic features of trypanosomiasis in dogs inoculated with North American *Trypanosoma cruzi* isolates, *Am J Vet Res* 53:521, 1992.

Barr SC et al: *Trypanosoma cruzi* infection in Walker hounds from Virginia, *Am J Vet Res* 56:1037, 1995.

Bradley KK et al: Prevalence of American trypanosomiasis (Chagas' disease) among dogs in Oklahoma, *J Am Vet Med Assoc* 217:1853, 2000.

Breitschwerdt EB et al: *Bartonella vinsonii* subsp. *berkhoffii* and related members of the alpha subdivision of the Proteobacteria in dogs with cardiac arrhythmias, endocarditis, or myocarditis, *J Clin Microbiol* 37:3618, 1999.

Gould SM et al: Immune-mediated thrombocytopenia associated with *Angiostrongylus vasorum* infection in a dog, *J Small Anim Pract* 40:227, 1999.

Keene BW: Evidence for the role of myocarditis in the pathophysiology of dilated cardiomyopathy. *Proceedings of the 11th ACVIM Forum*, Washington, DC, 1993, p 565.

Lobetti R et al: Cardiac troponins in canine babesiosis, *J Vet Intern Med* 16:63, 2002.

Meurs KM et al: Aberrant migration of *Toxocara* larvae as a cause of myocarditis in the dog, *J Am Anim Hosp Assoc* 30:580, 1994.

Meurs KM et al: Chronic *Trypanosoma cruzi* infection in dogs: 11 cases (1987-1996), *J Am Vet Med Assoc* 213:497, 1998.

Pisani B et al: Inflammatory myocardial diseases and cardiomyopathies, *Am J Med* 102:459, 1997.

Snyder PS et al: Electrocardiographic findings in dogs with motor vehicle–related trauma, *J Am Anim Hosp Assoc* 37:55, 2001.

# CHAPTER 7

# Myocardial Diseases
## of the Cat

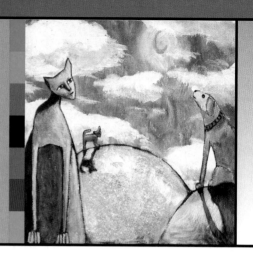

## CHAPTER OUTLINE

HYPERTROPHIC CARDIOMYOPATHY, 122
   Secondary hypertrophic myocardial diseases, 122
RESTRICTIVE CARDIOMYOPATHY, 129
DILATED CARDIOMYOPATHY, 130
ARRHYTHMOGENIC RIGHT VENTRICULAR
CARDIOMYOPATHY, 133
MYOCARDITIS, 133
ARTERIAL THROMBOEMBOLISM, 134

Myocardial diseases that affect cats encompass a diverse collection of idiopathic and secondary diseases affecting the myocardium. The spectrum of anatomic and pathophysiologic characteristics of these diseases is wide. Disease characterized by myocardial hypertrophy is most often seen clinically in cats and is discussed at length in this chapter; myocardial disease with restrictive pathophysiology is also common. Classic dilated cardiomyopathy is now rarely seen clinically in cats; characteristic features of this disease are discussed more fully in Chapter 6. The myocardial disease of some cats does not fit neatly into the categories of hypertrophic, dilated, or restrictive cardiomyopathy; rather, it is considered "indeterminate" or unclassified myocardial disease. Systemic thromboembolism remains a troubling complication in cats with myocardial disease.

## HYPERTROPHIC CARDIOMYOPATHY

### Etiology

The cause of primary or idiopathic hypertrophic cardiomyopathy (HCM) in cats is unknown, but a genetic basis is thought to underlie some cases. Disease prevalence appears to be high in several breeds, such as Maine Coon, Persian, Ragdoll, and American Shorthair. There are also reports of HCM in littermates and other closely related domestic short-hair cats. An autosomal dominant inheritance pattern that is similar to the most common inheritance pattern seen in people

has been found in the families studied (Meurs and colleagues, 1997). Most cases of HCM in people are familial, and a large number of specific abnormalities in nine genes coding for myocardial proteins have been identified in different kindreds. A reduction in the sarcomeric protein myomesin has been found in a group of affected Maine Coon cats (Meurs and colleagues, 2001), although several common human gene mutations have not yet similarly been found in cats with HCM. In addition to mutations of genes that encode for myocardial contractile or regulatory proteins, postulated causes of the disease include an increased myocardial sensitivity to or excessive production of catecholamines; an abnormal hypertrophic response to myocardial ischemia, fibrosis, or trophic factors; a primary collagen abnormality; or abnormalities of the myocardial calcium-handling process. Myocardial hypertrophy with foci of mineralization but infrequent congestive failure has been described in association with hypertrophic feline muscular dystrophy, an X-linked recessive dystrophin deficiency similar to Duchenne's muscular dystrophy in people. Some cats with HCM have high serum growth hormone concentrations. Whether viral myocarditis has a role in the pathogenesis of feline cardiomyopathy is not clear. In one study of formalin-fixed cardiomyopathic feline hearts, 55% of HCM samples showed evidence of myocarditis; panleukopenia virus DNA was documented in some (Meurs and colleagues, 2000).

### SECONDARY HYPERTROPHIC MYOCARDIAL DISEASES

Myocardial hypertrophy develops as a compensatory response to certain identifiable stresses or disease; marked left ventricular wall and septal thickening and clinical heart failure can occur in some cats. Such cases are not considered idiopathic HCM. Secondary causes should be ruled out if left ventricular hypertrophy is identified.

Testing for hyperthyroidism is indicated in cats 6 years of age or older with myocardial hypertrophy (see p. 712). Hyperthyroidism alters cardiovascular function by its direct effects on the myocardium and through the effects of the interaction of heightened sympathetic nervous system activity and excess thyroid hormone on the heart and peripheral circulation. Cardiac effects of thyroid hormone include myocardial hypertrophy and enhanced heart rate and contractility. The metabolic acceleration accompanying hyperthyroidism creates a hyperdynamic circulatory state characterized by increased cardiac output, oxygen demand, blood volume, and heart rate. Systemic hypertension can result and further stimulate myocardial hypertrophy. Clinical cardiovascular signs often include a systolic murmur, hyperdynamic precordial and arterial impulses, tachycardia and arrhythmias, and evidence of left ventricular enlargement or hypertrophy seen on electrocardiogram (ECG), thoracic radiographs, or echocardiogram. Signs of congestive heart failure develop in approximately 15% of hyperthyroid cats; most have normal to high fractional shortening, but a few have poor contractile function. Specific therapy, in addition to the antithyroid treatment, may be necessary to manage the cardiac complications of hyperthyroidism. β-Blockers can temporarily control many of the adverse cardiac effects of excess thyroid hormone, especially tachyarrhythmias. Diltiazem is an alternative therapy. Treatment for congestive failure is the same as that described later for HCM. The rare hypodynamic (dilated) cardiac failure is treated in the same way as dilated cardiomyopathy. β-Blocker or other cardiac therapy is not a substitute for antithyroid treatment, however.

Left ventricular concentric hypertrophy is the expected response to increased ventricular systolic pressure (afterload). Systemic arterial hypertension (see Chapter 12) increases afterload because of high arterial pressure and resistance. Increased resistance to ventricular outflow also occurs in the presence of a fixed (e.g., congenital subaortic stenosis) or dynamic left ventricular outflow tract obstruction. The latter occurs in some cats with idiopathic HCM and is described later.

Cardiac hypertrophy also develops in cats with hypersomatotropism (acromegaly) as a result of growth hormone's trophic effects on the heart; congestive heart failure ensues in some of these cats. Increased myocardial thickness occasionally results from infiltrative myocardial disease, most notably from lymphoma.

## Pathophysiology

The extent and distribution of hypertrophy among cats with HCM is variable. However, this myocardial thickening leads to diastolic dysfunction from increased ventricular stiffness and the development of relaxation abnormalities. Fibrosis and disorganized myocardial cell structure also contribute to the development of abnormal ventricular stiffness. Left ventricular filling is impaired and higher diastolic pressures are required when ventricular distensibility is reduced. Furthermore, early active myocardial relaxation may be slowed and incomplete, especially in the presence of myocardial ischemia. Because progressively higher filling pressures are required as the left ventricle becomes stiffer, left atrial and ventricular end-diastolic pressures rise and pulmonary congestion and edema can result. The atrium enlarges, sometimes markedly, but the left ventricular volume remains normal or decreased.

A reduced ventricular volume results in a lower stroke volume and may contribute to the activation of the renin-angiotensin and sympathetic nervous systems. Geometric changes of the left ventricle and papillary muscles or abnormal (anterior) systolic motion of the mitral valve may prevent normal valve closure. The resulting mitral regurgitation exacerbates the increased left atrial volume and pressure. Higher heart rates further interfere with left ventricular filling, exacerbate myocardial ischemia, and promote pulmonary venous congestion and edema by shortening the diastolic filling period. Contractility, or systolic function, is usually normal in affected cats. However, some cats experience progression to ventricular systolic failure and dilation.

Some cats also have dynamic left ventricular outflow obstruction during systole (i.e., functional subaortic stenosis or hypertrophic obstructive cardiomyopathy). Excessive and asymmetric hypertrophy of the basilar interventricular septum may be evident on echocardiograms or at necropsy. Systolic outflow obstruction increases left ventricular pressure, wall stress, and myocardial oxygen demand and promotes myocardial ischemia. Mitral regurgitation is exacerbated by forces tending to pull the anterior leaflet toward the interventricular septum during ejection (mitral systolic anterior motion; see Fig. 7-3). An audible ejection murmur is common in cats with outflow obstruction.

Several factors probably contribute to the development of myocardial ischemia in cats with HCM. These include a myocardial capillary density inadequate for the degree of hypertrophy, narrowing of intramural coronary arteries, increased left ventricular filling pressure, and decreased coronary artery perfusion pressure. Ischemia impairs early, active ventricular relaxation, which further increases the ventricular filling pressure and chronically leads to myocardial fibrosis. It is also thought to predispose to the development of lethal arrhythmias and possibly thoracic pain. Diastolic dysfunction and ischemia are exacerbated by increases in heart rate.

Pulmonary venous congestion and edema frequently result from increased left atrial pressure; some cats with HCM also have pleural effusion. A modified transudate is more common, although the effusion may be (or become) chylous. Increased pulmonary venous and capillary pressures are thought to cause pulmonary vasoconstriction, increased pulmonary arterial pressure, and secondary right-sided heart failure. Accumulation of pleural effusion may also be promoted if pleural venous drainage into the pulmonary veins occurs in cats, as it does in people.

Thrombi may form within the dilated left atrium or other areas of the heart; systemic thromboembolism results if portions are dislodged into the circulation. Moderate-to-severe left atrial enlargement and secondary blood stasis are considered risk factors for thromboembolism. This complication is discussed later (see p. 134).

## Pathology

Postmortem findings in cats with HCM consist of left ventricular free-wall and interventricular septal hypertrophy. The hypertrophy is symmetric in many cats, but some have asymmetric septal thickening, and a few have hypertrophy limited to the free wall or papillary muscles. The degree of left atrial enlargement varies from mild to massive. A thrombus is sometimes found within the left atrium or attached to a ventricular wall. The left ventricular lumen usually appears small. Focal or diffuse areas of fibrosis within the endocardium, conduction system, or myocardium and narrowing of small intramural coronary arteries may also be noted. Areas of myocardial infarction may be present. Myocardial fiber disarray, common in people with HCM, is also found in some cats. Evidence of congestive heart failure or systemic thromboembolism may also be present.

## Clinical Features

HCM has historically been most common in middle-aged male cats, but clinical signs can occur at ages ranging from several months to geriatric. Cats with milder disease may be asymptomatic for years. Symptomatic cats are most often presented for respiratory signs of variable severity or acute signs of thromboembolism (see p. 134). Respiratory signs include tachypnea, panting associated with activity, dyspnea, or, rarely, coughing (which can be misinterpreted as vomiting). Disease onset may seem acute in sedentary cats, even though pathologic changes have developed gradually. Occasionally lethargy or anorexia is the only evidence of disease. Some cats have syncope or sudden death in the absence of other signs. Stresses such as anesthesia, surgery, fluid administration, systemic illnesses (e.g., fever or anemia), and even boarding can precipitate heart failure in an otherwise compensated cat. Asymptomatic disease is sometimes discovered by detecting a murmur or gallop sound on auscultation.

Systolic murmurs indicative of either mitral regurgitation or left ventricular outflow tract obstruction are common. However, some cats do not have an audible murmur, even with marked ventricular hypertrophy. A diastolic gallop sound (usually $S_4$) may be heard, especially if heart failure is evident or imminent. Cardiac arrhythmias are relatively common. Femoral pulses are usually strong, unless distal aortic thromboembolism has occurred. A vigorous precordial impulse is often palpable. Prominent lung sounds, pulmonary crackles, and sometimes cyanosis accompany severe pulmonary edema; pleural effusion usually attenuates ventral pulmonary sounds. However, the physical examination findings can be normal.

## Radiography

Radiographic features of HCM include a prominent left atrium and variable left ventricular enlargement (Fig. 7-1). The classic valentine-shaped appearance of the heart on dorsoventral or ventrodorsal views is not always present, although usually the point of the left ventricular apex is maintained. The cardiac silhouette appears normal in most cats with mild HCM. Enlarged and tortuous pulmonary veins may be seen in the presence of chronically high left atrial and pulmonary venous pressures. Variable degrees of patchy interstitial or alveolar pulmonary edema develop in the setting of left-sided heart failure. The radiographic distribution of pulmonary edema is variable; a diffuse or focal distribution throughout the lung fields is common, in contrast to the perihilar distribution characteristic of cardiogenic pulmonary edema seen in dogs. The finding of pleural effusion suggests biventricular failure; hepatomegaly may also be noted in the setting of right-sided failure.

## Electrocardiography

Many cats (up to 70%) with HCM have ECG abnormalities. These commonly include criteria for left atrial and ventricular enlargement, ventricular and/or (less often) supraventricular tachyarrhythmias, or a left anterior fascicular block pattern. Occasionally an atrioventricular (AV) conduction delay, complete AV block, or sinus bradycardia is found.

## Echocardiography

Echocardiography is the best means of diagnosis (see Chapter 2). It allows the differentiation of HCM from other myocardial disorders, including the now uncommon dilated cardiomyopathy. Two-dimensional echocardiography demonstrates the extent of hypertrophy and its distribution within the ventricular wall, septum, and papillary muscles. Nonselective angiocardiography is an alternative means of diagnosis, but it poses a greater risk to the cat.

Because the distribution of hypertrophy is variable, the entire ventricle should be carefully scanned. Widespread thickening is common, and the hypertrophy is often asymmetrically distributed among various LV wall, septal, and papillary muscle locations. Focal areas of hypertrophy also occur. Use of two-dimensional–guided M-mode is important to ensure proper beam position. Standard M-mode views and measurements are obtained, but thickened areas outside these standard positions should also be measured (Fig. 7-2). The diagnosis may be questionable in cats with mild or only focal thickening. I consider 5 mm the upper limit of normal for diastolic left ventricular wall and septal thicknesses. Cats with severe HCM have diastolic left ventricular wall or septal thicknesses of 8 mm or more, although the degree of hypertrophy is not necessarily correlated with the severity of clinical signs. Papillary muscle hypertrophy can be marked, and systolic left ventricular cavity obliteration is observed in some cats. Increased echogenicity (brightness) of papillary muscles and subendocardial areas is thought to be a marker for chronic myocardial ischemia with resulting fibrosis. Left ventricular fractional shortening (FS) is generally normal to increased. However, some cats have mild-to-moderate LV dilation and reduced contractility (FS ~23% to 29%; normal FS is 35% to 65%). Right ventricular enlargement and pericardial or pleural effusion are occasionally detected.

Cats with dynamic left ventricular outflow tract obstruction also often have systolic anterior motion of the mitral valve (Fig. 7-3) or premature closure of the aortic valve leaflets on M-mode scans. Doppler modalities can demonstrate mitral regurgitation and left ventricular outflow turbulence

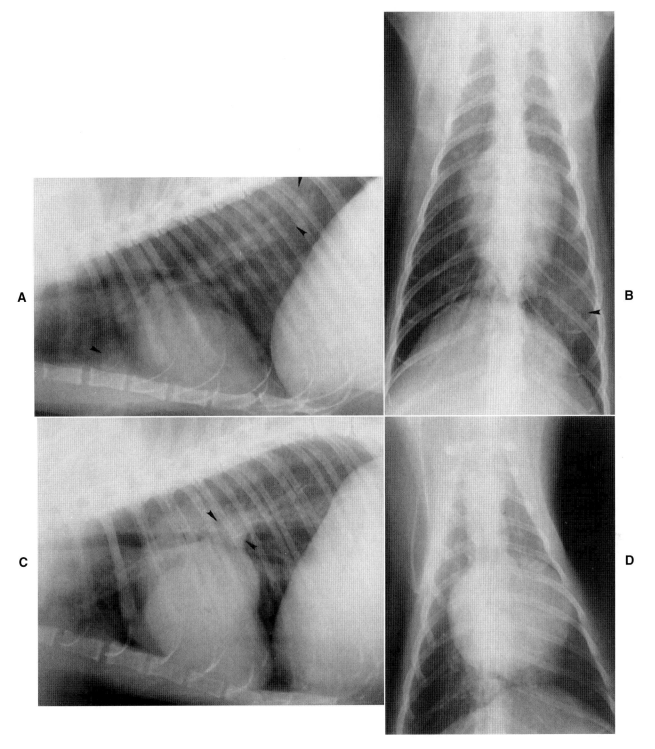

**FIG 7-1**
Radiographic examples of feline hypertrophic cardiomyopathy. Lateral **(A)** and dorsoventral **(B)** views showing atrial and mild ventricular enlargement along with patchy interstitial pulmonary edema *(arrowheads)* in a male Domestic Shorthair cat with left-sided congestive heart failure. Lateral **(C)** and dorsoventral **(D)** views of a male Siamese cat with marked atrial enlargement, dilated pulmonary veins *(arrowheads* in C), and atrial fibrillation.

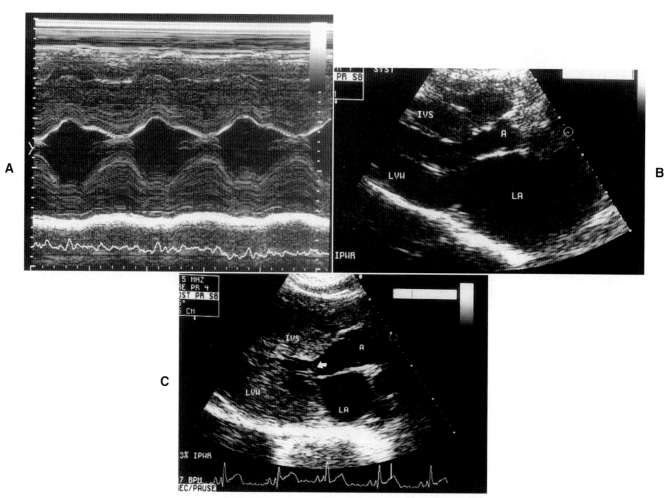

**FIG 7-2**

Echocardiographic examples of feline hypertrophic cardiomyopathy. M-mode image **(A)** at the left ventricular level from a 7-year-old male domestic shorthair cat that also had a marked left ventricular outflow tract obstruction. The left ventricular diastolic free-wall thickness is 7 mm; the septal thickness is more than 8 mm. Two-dimensional right parasternal long-axis views optimized for the left ventricular outflow tract and obtained during systole in a 6-year-old male Domestic Shorthair cat **(B)** and a 1-year-old male Persian cat **(C)**. In **B,** note the markedly enlarged left atrium but moderate degree of ventricular hypertrophy. This cat had no evidence of outflow tract obstruction. In **C,** note the systolic obliteration of the apical portion of the left ventricle resulting from severe hypertrophy. In this cat with hypertrophic obstructive cardiomyopathy, echoes from the anterior mitral leaflet are seen within the left ventricular outflow tract *(arrow)* because of the abnormal systolic anterior motion (SAM) of the mitral valve. *A,* Aorta; *IVS,* interventricular septum; *LA,* left atrium; *LVW,* left ventricular free wall.

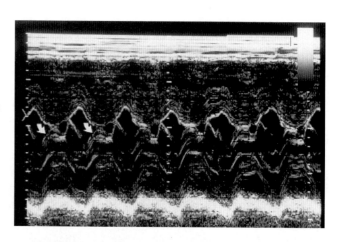

**FIG 7-3**

M-mode echocardiogram taken at the mitral valve level from the same cat as in Fig. 7-2, *C.* Note the systolic anterior (toward the septum) motion of the anterior mitral leaflet *(arrows).*

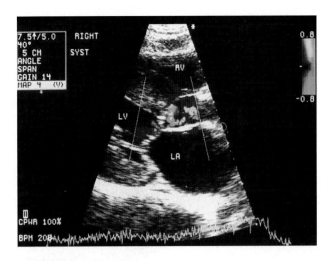

**FIG 7-4**
Color flow Doppler image taken in systole from a cat with hypertrophic obstructive cardiomyopathy. Note the turbulent flow just above where the thickened interventricular septum protrudes into the left ventricular outflow tract. Hypertrophy of the left ventricular free wall and left atrial enlargement are also seen. Right parasternal long-axis view; *A,* aorta; *LA,* left atrium; *LV,* left ventricle; *RV,* right ventricle.

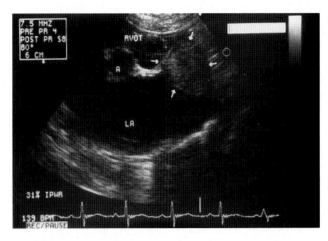

**FIG 7-5**
Echocardiogram obtained from the right parasternal short-axis position at the aortic–left atrial level in an old male Domestic Shorthair cat with restrictive cardiomyopathy. Note the massive left atrial enlargement and thrombus *(arrows)* within the auricle. *A,* Aorta; *LA,* left atrium; *RVOT,* right ventricular outflow tract.

(Fig. 7-4), although optimal alignment with the maximal velocity outflow jet is often difficult and it is easy to underestimate the systolic gradient. Doppler-derived estimates of diastolic function, such as isovolumic relaxation time and mitral inflow velocity pattern, are sometimes employed, but these can be difficult to reliably obtain and interpret. Pulsed wave Doppler tissue imaging of the mitral annulus and M-mode–derived global left atrial shortening fraction have also been described in the evaluation of LV diastolic function, although their clinical utility remains to be clarified (Gavaghan and colleagues, 1999; Strickland, 2001).

Left atrial enlargement may be mild to marked. Spontaneous contrast (swirling, smoky echoes) is visible within the enlarged left atrium of some cats. This is thought to result from blood stasis with cellular aggregations and to be a harbinger of thromboembolism. A thrombus is occasionally visualized within the left atrium, usually in the auricle (Fig. 7-5).

Other causes of myocardial hypertrophy (see p. 122) should be excluded before a diagnosis of idiopathic HCM is made. Myocardial thickening can also result from infiltrative disease. Variation in myocardial echogenicity or wall irregularities may be noted in such cases. Excess moderator bands appear as bright, linear echoes within the left ventricular cavity.

## Treatment

The main goals of therapy are to facilitate ventricular filling, relieve congestion, control arrhythmias, minimize ischemia, and prevent thromboembolism (Table 7-1). Ventricular filling is improved by slowing the heart rate and enhancing relaxation. Stress and activity level should be minimized toward this end. Diltiazem or a β-blocker (see Chapter 4 and Table 4-5) is the foundation of long-term oral therapy. The decision to use one particular drug over another may be influenced by the specific abnormalities in the individual case or the response to medication.

There is debate about whether (and how) asymptomatic cats with HCM should be treated. It is unclear whether disease progression can be slowed or survival prolonged by the institution of drug therapy before the onset of clinical signs. Nevertheless, some cats show an increased activity level or improved "attitude" after they start to receive diltiazem or a β-blocker on the basis of echocardiographic or ECG abnormalities, even when the owners had not previously noted a problem.

The β-adrenergic blockers can produce greater decreases in heart rate than diltiazem. They are also useful in controlling tachyarrhythmias and reducing systolic outflow obstruction and myocardial oxygen demand through their negative inotropic effect. These effects can be especially important in cats with severe outflow obstruction, paroxysmal arrhythmias, or myocardial infarction. I favor atenolol (6.25 to 12.5 mg/cat q24[to 12]h) over diltiazem for cats with these disease features. The reduction in heart rate and decrease in myocardial ischemia that results from β-blocker therapy may also indirectly alleviate left ventricular diastolic stiffness and enhance filling. However, there is no direct enhancement of relaxation, and β-blockers may even slow the relaxation process. If propranolol is used in the presence of congestive heart failure, its administration is usually delayed until after pulmonary edema is largely resolved. Because propranolol is a nonselective β-blocker, an adverse effect can be bronchoconstriction stemming from antagonism of airway $\beta_2$-receptors. This is not such a concern with the more $\beta_1$-receptor–selective agents (e.g., atenolol). Yet the advantages of slowing sinus tachycardia and minimizing ventricular arrhythmias may outweigh the risk

TABLE 7-1

**Outline of Therapy for Hypertrophic Cardiomyopathy**

| THERAPY | DRUG |
|---|---|
| **Initial Therapy of Acute Failure** | |
| Diuretic | Furosemide |
| Oxygen | — |
| Vasodilator | Nitroglycerin, possibly ACEI |
| Bronchodilator | Aminophylline or theophylline |
| Cage confinement | |
| Calcium entry blocker | Diltiazem |
| *or* | |
| β-Blocker | Atenolol, propranolol (avoid with pulmonary edema or thrombo-embolism), or esmolol |
| ± Anticoagulants | Aspirin |
| | Heparin |
| | ± Others (see text) |
| Other therapy | ± Acepromazine |
| | ± Fluids |
| Antiarrhythmic drugs | β-Blocker (or diltiazem) |
| | ± Lidocaine |
| | ± Procainamide |
| **Chronic Therapy** | |
| Diuretics (±) | Furosemide |
| | ± Other |
| Calcium entry blocker | Diltiazem |
| *or* | |
| β-Blocker | Atenolol or propranolol |
| ± Anticoagulants | Aspirin, warfarin, (LMWH) |
| Exercise restriction | — |
| Sodium restriction | — |
| Antiarrhythmic (±) | β-Blocker or other |

See text, Tables 3-4, 3-6, and 4-5 for dosages, and Chapters 3 and 4 for further information.
*ACEI,* Angiotensin-converting enzyme inhibitor; *LMWH,* low molecular weight heparin.

of bronchospasm, even with propranolol. Some cats do not tolerate propranolol well (e.g., lethargy, depressed appetite). In these cases, atenolol or another β-blocker may be better tolerated instead, or diltiazem could be used.

Diltiazem (1.75 to 2.5 mg/kg or 7.5 mg/cat PO q8h) is well tolerated and effective in many cases. It promotes coronary vasodilation and enhances ventricular relaxation. The drug causes mild decreases in heart rate and contractility; it may also decrease systolic outflow gradients if peripheral vasodilation does not enhance ventricular shortening. It is generally less effective than the β-blockers in decreasing heart rate. Longer-acting diltiazem products are more convenient for chronic use. Dilacor XR (Watson Pharma, Corona, Calif) is dosed at ½ of an internal (60 mg) tablet from the 240 mg capsule size q24 (to 12) h; an alternative is Cardizem CD (Biovail Pharm., Morrisville, N.C.) dosed at 10 mg/kg q24h, which must be compounded. Calcium entry blockers that have pri-

marily vasodilatory effects (e.g., nifedipine, nicardipine) can cause reflex tachycardia and worsen systolic outflow gradients; therefore they are not used for cats with HCM. Verapamil has a greater negative inotropic effect than diltiazem and thus should be better for reducing ventricular outflow obstruction. However, it is not recommended because of its variable bioavailability and risk of toxicity in cats.

Pulmonary edema is treated with furosemide; cats with severe respiratory distress are usually given the drug intramuscularly (IM) (2 mg/kg, q1-4h; see Table 3-6), because intravenous (IV) injection can be excessively stressful. If pleural effusion is suspected, thoracocentesis is performed expediently, with the cat restrained gently in sternal position. Nitroglycerin ointment is often applied (q4-6h; see Table 3-6), although no studies of its efficacy in this situation have been done. Once initial medications have been given, the cat should be allowed to rest, preferably while receiving supplemental oxygen. The respiratory rate is noted initially, then every 30 minutes or so without disturbing the cat. Catheter placement, blood sampling, radiographs, and other tests and therapies should be delayed until the cat's condition is more stable. Airway suctioning and mechanical ventilation with positive end-expiratory pressure can be considered in extreme cases. The bronchodilating and mild diuretic effects of aminophylline (5 mg/kg q12h, IM, IV) may be helpful in cats with severe pulmonary edema, as long as the drug does not increase the heart rate. Acepromazine has been used to reduce anxiety and promote the peripheral redistribution of blood by its β-adrenergic–blocking effects (0.05 to 0.2 mg/kg subcutaneously [SC]), but preexisting hypothermia can be exacerbated by peripheral vasodilation. Morphine should not be used in cats. When respiratory distress has been alleviated, furosemide (~1 mg/kg) can be continued q8-12h; diuretic therapy is guided by the animal's respiratory rate and effort. Once pulmonary edema has been controlled, furosemide is gradually reduced to the lowest dose and longest dosing interval at which it is effective, and given orally (PO). Usually this is started at 6.25 mg/cat q12-24h and slowly reduced over days to weeks, depending on the cat's response. Some cats do well with dosing a couple times per week, whereas others require it several times per day. Complications of excessive diuresis include azotemia, anorexia, electrolyte disturbances, and suboptimal left ventricular filling pressure. Cautious fluid administration may be needed in some cats after excessive diuresis (e.g., 15 to 20 ml/kg/day of half-strength saline, 5% dextrose in water, or other low-sodium fluid). Some cats that have had an episode of congestive failure but are responding well to long-term therapy with diltiazem or a β-blocker can be weaned off furosemide therapy, but close monitoring for the recurrence of pulmonary edema is necessary.

There is evidence that enalapril (and other angiotensin-converting enzyme inhibitors [ACEIs]) may be beneficial in modulating neurohormonal activation, especially in cats with refractory heart failure. Inhibition of the renin-angiotensin system may mitigate angiotensin II–mediated ventricular hypertrophy (remodeling). There is preliminary evidence that suggests that ACEIs might reduce left atrial size and ventricular/

septal wall thickness in some cats. Enalapril is the ACEI used most commonly in cats, although others are available (see Chapter 3 and Table 3-6). An additional theoretical rationale for ACEI use is based on the improved survival in people after myocardial infarction. However, further study in cats with HCM is needed to determine if there is enhanced survival with ACEIs.

Occasionally a β-blocker is added to diltiazem therapy (or vice versa) in cats whose failure is hard to control or to further reduce heart rate in cats with atrial fibrillation. However, care must be taken to prevent bradycardia or hypotension in animals receiving this combination.

Certain drugs are generally contraindicated in cats with HCM. These include digoxin and other positive inotropic agents, because they increase the myocardial oxygen demand and can worsen dynamic outflow tract obstruction. Any drug that accelerates the heart rate is potentially detrimental, because tachycardia decreases filling time and predisposes to the development of myocardial ischemia. Arterial vasodilators can cause hypotension and reflex tachycardia, because cats with HCM have little preload reserve. Hypotension can also exacerbate dynamic outflow obstruction. The ACEIs also have this potential; however, their vasodilating effects are usually mild.

Refractory pulmonary edema or pleural effusion is difficult to manage. Moderate-to-large pleural effusions should be treated by thoracocentesis. Various therapeutic strategies may also be useful, including increasing doses of furosemide (up to 4 mg/kg q8h), adding an ACEI, maximizing the dose of diltiazem or β-blocker, or adding another diuretic, such as spironolactone, with or without hydrochlorothiazide (see Table 3-6). Frequent monitoring for the development of azotemia or electrolyte disturbances is warranted. Digoxin can also be considered for the treatment of refractory right-sided heart failure in the absence of outflow obstruction. The progressive development of LV dilation and myocardial systolic failure is difficult to manage successfully. An ACEI, digoxin, and cautious β-blocker therapy along with diuretics is suggested. The blood taurine concentration should be measured and oral supplementation initiated if needed (see Dilated Cardiomyopathy, below).

Long-term therapy usually also includes a drug to decrease the likelihood of thromboembolism, such as aspirin (25 mg/kg PO every 3 days) or warfarin (see p. 136, below). Exercise and dietary sodium restrictions, if possible, are also recommended.

## Complications

A major complication of hypertrophic and other forms of cardiomyopathy in cats is arterial thromboembolism (discussed later, see p. 134). Atrial fibrillation and other tachyarrhythmias further impair diastolic filling and exacerbate venous congestion; the loss of the atrial "kick" and the rapid heart rate associated with atrial fibrillation are especially detrimental. Ventricular tachycardia or other arrhythmias may lead to syncope or sudden death. Refractory biventricular failure is another serious complication that may develop.

## Prognosis

The prognosis for cats with HCM is quite variable and depends on several factors. These include the response to therapy and whether thromboembolic events occur, the disease progresses, and/or arrhythmias develop. Asymptomatic cats with only mild-to-moderate left ventricular hypertrophy and atrial enlargement often live well for several years. However, cats with more severe hypertrophy and left atrial enlargement appear to be at greater risk for heart failure, thromboembolism, and sudden death. A recent study identified left atrial size and age as parameters negatively correlated with survival on multivariate analysis (Rush and colleagues, 2002). Cats with congestive failure may live for several days to several years, but the median survival time is probably 1 to 2 years. The prognosis is worse if there is atrial fibrillation or refractory right-sided heart failure. The prognosis is generally guarded for cats presented with thromboembolism and congestive failure (median survival of 2 to 6 months), although some do well if congestive signs can be controlled and infarction of vital organs has not occurred. Recurrence of thromboembolism is common.

## *RESTRICTIVE CARDIOMYOPATHY*

### Etiology and Pathophysiology

Restrictive cardiomyopathy (RCM) is associated with extensive endocardial, subendocardial, or myocardial fibrosis. The etiology is not clear but probably is multifactorial. The disease may be a sequela of endomyocarditis or represent the end-stage of myocardial failure and infarction stemming from HCM. Severe perivascular and interstitial fibrosis and intramural coronary artery narrowing have been reported as typical histologic findings. Occasionally, secondary RCM results from neoplastic (e.g., lymphoma) or other infiltrative or infectious diseases.

The major pathophysiologic abnormality is impaired diastolic filling secondary to left ventricular and/or endocardial fibrosis. Most affected cats have normal to mildly reduced contractility, but this may progress with time as more functional myocardium is lost. In some cats regional left ventricular dysfunction occurs, which decreases overall systolic function; however, these cases are perhaps better categorized as unclassified rather than restrictive. Mitral regurgitation may be present but is usually mild. The massive left atrial enlargement often seen is mainly caused by increased left ventricular wall stiffness from the fibrosis. Arrhythmias, ventricular dilation, and myocardial ischemia or infarction also contribute to the development of diastolic dysfunction. Chronic elevation of left heart filling pressures in combination with compensatory neurohormonal activation leads to left-sided or biventricular failure.

A prominent pathologic feature is marked atrial enlargement and hypertrophy. The left ventricle shows variable dilation, with or without hypertrophy, which can be regional. Endomyocardial fibrosis may be focal or widespread, with extensive scarring that deforms the ventricle. The mitral valve apparatus and papillary muscles may be distorted and fused to surrounding structures. Thrombi are commonly found within the left atrium, left ventricle, or systemic vasculature. Histopathologic changes include endocardial and myocardial fibrosis, intramural coronary arteriosclerosis, hypertrophied myocytes, areas of myocardial degeneration and necrosis, and sometimes endomyocardial cellular infiltrates. Excess moderator bands (branching, fibrous bands extending along or between the left ventricular wall and septum) are found in some cats, but their role in the development of myocardial disease and congestive heart failure is unclear. They may represent a congenital anomaly, because they have been identified in young kittens as well as old cats.

## Clinical Features and Diagnosis

RCM appears most often in middle-aged or older cats. The clinical signs are variable but usually reflect the presence of left- or right-sided congestive heart failure, or both. Signs are often precipitated by stress or concurrent disease that increases demands on the cardiovascular system and are likely to develop or worsen suddenly. Thromboembolic events are common. Inactivity, poor appetite, vomiting, and weight loss may be part of the cat's recent history. Sometimes asymptomatic disease is discovered by the finding of auscultation abnormalities or radiographic evidence of cardiomegaly.

Common physical examination findings in cats with RCM can include a systolic murmur of mitral or tricuspid regurgitation, a gallop sound, or arrhythmias. Abnormal pulmonary sounds may accompany pulmonary edema or a pleural effusion. Femoral arterial pulses are normal or slightly weak. Jugular vein distention and pulsation are associated with right-sided heart failure. Signs of distal aortic (or other) thromboembolism may be the reason for presentation.

Diagnostic test results are often similar to those in cats with HCM. Radiographs show left atrial enlargement, which can be massive, and left ventricular or generalized heart enlargement (see Fig. 7-1, *C* and *D*). Pericardial effusion exacerbates the cardiomegaly. Dilated, tortuous proximal pulmonary veins may be noted; infiltrates of pulmonary edema or a pleural effusion, and sometimes hepatomegaly, are seen in cats with heart failure. The ECG is often abnormal; wide QRS complexes, tall R waves, evidence of intraventricular conduction disturbances, wide P waves, and atrial tachyarrhythmias or fibrillation are common.

Echocardiographic features include marked left (and sometimes right) atrial enlargement, variable left ventricular free-wall and septal thickening, and often normal to somewhat depressed wall motion (fractional shortening usually exceeding 25%). Hyperechoic areas of fibrosis may appear within the LV wall and/or endocardial areas. Endocardial scarring can be extensive and bridge to the septum, thus constricting portions of the ventricular lumen. Extraneous intraluminal echoes representing excess moderator bands are occasionally seen. Right ventricular dilation is frequently identified. Sometimes an intracardiac thrombus is found, usually in the left auricle or atrium but occasionally in the left ventricle (see Fig. 7-4). Doppler evaluation may show mild mitral or tricuspid regurgitation. Nonselective angiocardiog-

raphy will reveal the same anatomic findings and highlight the distended and tortuous pulmonary veins. Some cats have marked regional wall dysfunction, especially of the left ventricular free wall, which depresses fractional shortening, along with mild left ventricular dilation. These may represent cases of myocardial infarction or unclassified cardiomyopathy rather than RCM.

The clinicopathologic findings are nonspecific. Pleural effusions usually consist of modified transudate or chyle. The plasma taurine concentration is low in some affected cats and should be measured if decreased contractility is identified.

## Treatment and Prognosis

Therapy for acute heart failure is the same as that described for cats with HCM (p. 128) and involves the use of furosemide, oxygen, nitroglycerin, and thoracocentesis for the treatment of pleural effusion. Treatment for thromboembolism is outlined later (p. 134). Long-term therapy for heart failure includes furosemide, as needed; the resting respiratory rate, activity level, and radiographic findings are used to monitor efficacy. Enalapril is also used, starting with very low doses and increasing to the usual maintenance dose of 0.25 to 0.5 mg/kg/day. Twice-daily administration can be helpful in refractory cases. Ideally, blood pressure should be monitored when initiating or adjusting ACEI therapy. Creatinine or the blood urea nitrogen and electrolyte concentrations should be measured periodically. The doses of furosemide or enalapril, or both, should be reduced if hypotension or azotemia occurs. A β-blocker is usually used for tachyarrhythmias or if myocardial infarction is suspected. Alternatively, diltiazem can also be used, although its value in the face of significant fibrosis is controversial. Cats with refractory failure or reduced systolic function are also given digoxin (see Table 3-8). Prophylaxis against thromboembolism using aspirin or warfarin is recommended (see p. 136), and a low-sodium diet is fed, if accepted.

Refractory heart failure with pleural effusion is difficult to manage. Besides repeated thoracocenteses, enalapril or furosemide dosages can be increased cautiously; hydrochlorothiazide and spironolactone (2 to 3 mg/kg of the combination daily), or nitroglycerin ointment, can be added to the regimen.

The overall prognosis for cats with heart failure from RCM is guarded to poor, although occasional cats live well for more than a year after diagnosis. The time course of subclinical RCM is unknown. Thromboembolism and refractory pleural effusion commonly occur.

## DILATED CARDIOMYOPATHY

### Etiology

In the late 1980s taurine deficiency was discovered to be a major cause of dilated cardiomyopathy (DCM) in cats. The taurine content of commercial feline diets has since been increased, and clinical DCM is now uncommon in cats. Because DCM does not develop in all cats fed taurine-deficient diets, factors other than a simple deficiency of this essential amino acid are thought to be involved and include genetic factors and a possible link with potassium depletion. Despite the presence of low plasma taurine concentrations in most cats with DCM, there may actually be no significant difference in the myocardial taurine concentrations in these cats compared with those in cats with other forms of heart disease. Since the link between taurine deficiency and DCM was discovered, the incidence of feline DCM has markedly decreased. The relatively few cases identified now usually are not taurine deficient and may be the end-stage of another myocardial metabolic abnormality, toxicity, or infection.

**Secondary dilated myocardial disease.** Doxorubicin causes characteristic myocardial histologic lesions in cats as well as dogs; however, this species appears fairly resistant to clinical dilated myocardial failure. Some cats show echocardiographic changes consistent with DCM after receiving cumulative doses of 170 to 240 mg/m$^2$.

## Pathophysiology

The pathophysiologic features of DCM in cats are similar to those in dogs (see p. 108). The hallmark is poor myocardial contractility (Fig. 7-6). Usually all cardiac chambers become

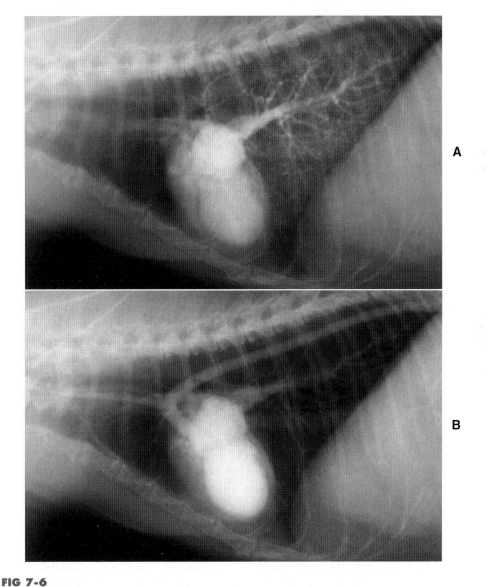

**FIG 7-6**
Nonselective angiogram from a 13-year-old female Siamese cat with dilated cardiomyopathy. A bolus of radiographic contrast material was injected into the jugular vein. **A,** Three seconds after injection some dye remains in the right ventricle and pulmonary vasculature. Dilated pulmonary veins are seen entering the left atrium. Note the dilated left atrium and ventricle. **B,** Thirteen seconds after the injection the left heart and pulmonary veins are still opacified, illustrating the poor cardiac contractility and extremely slow circulation time. The thin left ventricular caudal wall and papillary muscles are better seen in this frame.

dilated; AV valve insufficiency occurs secondary to chamber enlargement and papillary muscle atrophy. As cardiac output decreases, compensatory neurohormonal mechanisms are activated, leading to an increased cardiac volume and clinical manifestations of left- or right-sided congestive heart failure, or both. Arrhythmias and pleural effusion are common in cats with DCM.

## Clinical Features and Diagnosis

DCM historically has occurred in cats of all ages, with no breed or gender predilection. Clinical signs are frequently vague and include the acute onset of anorexia, lethargy, or dyspnea, or a combination of these. Subtle evidence of poor ventricular function is found in conjunction with signs of respiratory compromise. Increased respiratory effort, depression, dehydration, and hypothermia are frequent findings. Jugular venous distention, an attenuated precordial impulse, weak femoral pulses, a gallop sound (usually $S_3$), and a left or right apical systolic murmur (of mitral or tricuspid regurgitation) are common. Bradycardia and arrhythmias are frequent, although many cats have a normal sinus rhythm. Increased lung sounds and pulmonary crackles can be auscultated in some cats, or pleural effusion may muffle ventral lung sounds. There may also be clinical signs of arterial thromboembolism (see p. 134).

Generalized cardiomegaly with rounding of the cardiac apex is a common radiographic finding. Pleural effusion is common and tends to obscure the heart shadow and coexisting evidence of pulmonary edema or venous congestion. Hepatomegaly and occasionally ascites may be detected. A left ventricular enlargement pattern, AV conduction disturbances, and arrhythmias are frequent ECG findings.

Definitive diagnosis is best made on the basis of the echocardiographic findings. These are analogous to those in dogs with DCM (see p. 109). A thrombus may be identified within the left atrium. Nonselective angiocardiography is a more risky alternative to echocardiography, as it is for the diagnostic evaluation of other cardiomyopathies. Characteristic angiographic features include generalized chamber enlargement, atrophied papillary muscles, a decreased aortic diameter, and a slow circulation time (see Fig. 7-5). Complications of the procedure, especially in cats with poor myocardial function or decompensated heart failure, include vomiting and aspiration, arrhythmias, and cardiac arrest.

The pleural effusion in cats with DCM is usually a modified transudate, although true chylous effusions occur. Prerenal azotemia, mild increases in liver enzyme activities, and a stress leukogram are other common clinicopathologic findings. High serum muscle enzyme activities, an abnormal blood clotting profile, and disseminated intravascular coagulation (DIC) can occur in association with thromboembolism.

Plasma taurine quantification is offered by several commercial laboratories. In the event this is desired, specific instructions should be obtained from the laboratory regarding sample collection and mailing. Plasma taurine concentrations are influenced by the amount of taurine in the diet, the type of diet, and the time of sampling sin relation to eating; however, a plasma taurine concentration of 20 nmol/ml or less in

a cat with DCM is considered diagnostic for taurine deficiency. Non-anorexic cats with a plasma taurine concentration of less than 60 nmol/ml probably should receive taurine supplementation or have their diet changed. Results are more consistent if whole blood samples rather than plasma samples are used for taurine determinations. Normal whole blood taurine concentrations are over 200 nmol/ml.

## Treatment and Prognosis

The goals of treatment are to increase cardiac output and improve pulmonary function, as for dogs with DCM. Pleural fluid is removed by thoracocentesis. In acute failure, furosemide is given to promote diuresis, as described earlier for HCM. However, diuresis that is too aggressive can significantly reduce cardiac output in these cases with poor systolic function. Supplemental $O_2$ may be needed. The venodilator nitroglycerin may be helpful in cats with severe pulmonary edema. Vasodilators (e.g., hydralazine, an ACEI, or amlodipine) may help maximize cardiac output, although with the risk of hypotension (see Table 3-6). Blood pressure, hydration, renal function, electrolyte balance, and peripheral perfusion should be monitored closely. Hypothermia is common in cats with decompensated DCM, therefore external warming should be provided as needed. Once pulmonary edema has been controlled, furosemide is tapered to the lowest effective PO dosage.

Positive inotropic support is indicated. Dobutamine or dopamine (see p. 69 and Table 3-8) administered by constant rate infusion can be used for critical cases. Adverse effects of dobutamine can include seizures or tachycardia; if they occur, the infusion rate should be decreased by 50% or the drug discontinued. The adverse effects of dopamine usually occur at higher doses; they include tachycardia and increased peripheral vascular resistance resulting from the α-adrenergic effects of the drug. Dopaminergic effects may cause renal blood flow to increase at low infusion rates. Amrinone (see p. 70) is a positive inotropic agent with peripheral vasodilating properties, although the dose for cats is not well established (see Table 3-8). Digoxin PO (see p. 66 and Table 3-8) is the positive inotropic drug of choice for maintenance therapy. Digoxin tablets are usually used, because many cats dislike the taste of digoxin elixir. Toxicity can easily occur, especially if other drugs are being used concurrently, therefore periodic evaluation of serum digoxin concentration is recommended (see p. 66).

Furosemide and vasodilating agents can reduce cardiac filling and predispose to the development of cardiogenic shock in cats with DCM. Half-strength saline solution with 2.5% dextrose or other low-sodium fluids can be given IV at 15 to 35 ml/kg/day in several divided doses or by constant rate infusion; potassium supplementation may be needed. Fluid can be administered SC if necessary, although the absorption of the fluids from the extravascular space may be impaired.

Chronic therapy for DCM in cats that survive acute heart failure includes oral furosemide, an ACEI, digoxin, aspirin (or warfarin), and (if taurine deficient) taurine supplementation or a high-taurine diet. Taurine supplementation, at a dosage of 250 to 500 mg PO q12h, should be instituted as soon as possible in cats with low or unmeasured plasma taurine concentrations. Taurine is available in 500-mg capsules from health food stores. Because clinical improvement generally does not begin until after 1 to 2 weeks of taurine supplementation, supportive cardiac care is vital. Aspirin or warfarin therapy is usually instituted to reduce the risk of thromboembolism.

Echocardiographic evidence of improved systolic function is seen in most taurine-deficient cats within 6 weeks of initiation of taurine supplementation. Drug therapy may become unnecessary in some cats after 6 to 12 weeks, although it is advised that the resolution of pleural effusion and pulmonary edema be confirmed radiographically before weaning the cat from medications. When echocardiographic measures of systolic function are at or near normal, the amount of taurine supplementation can be decreased and therapy eventually discontinued, as long as the cat eats a diet known to support adequate plasma taurine concentrations (e.g., most name-brand commercial foods). Dry diets with 1000 to 1200 mg of taurine per kilogram of dry weight and canned diets with 2000 to 2500 mg of taurine per kilogram of dry weight are thought to maintain normal plasma taurine concentrations in adult cats. Reevaluation of the plasma taurine concentration 2 to 4 weeks after supplement discontinuation is also advised.

Taurine-deficient cats that survive a month after initial diagnosis often can be weaned from all or most medications, except for taurine. These cats appear to have about a 50% chance for 1-year survival. The prognosis for cats not supplemented with taurine or those that are do not respond to taurine is guarded to poor. Thromboembolism in a cat with DCM is a grave sign. Supportive therapy for cats with thromboembolism is described on p. 134.

## ARRHYTHMOGENIC RIGHT VENTRICULAR CARDIOMYOPATHY

An idiopathic cardiomyopathy mainly involving the right ventricle (RV), which is similar to the uncommon arrhythmogenic right ventricular cardiomyopathy in people, also occurs in cats (Fox and colleagues, 2000). Moderate-to-severe dilation of the RV chamber, with either focal or diffuse RV wall thinning, is characteristic. A RV wall aneurysm is also common. Right, and less often left, atrial dilation may occur. Histologic findings include myocardial atrophy with fatty and/or fibrous replacement tissue, focal myocarditis, and evidence of apoptosis. These are most prominent in the RV wall. Fibrous tissue or fatty infiltration is sometimes found in the LV and atrial walls.

The clinical presentation is usually that of right-sided congestive failure, with labored respirations, jugular venous distension, ascites or hepatosplenomegaly, and occasionally syncope. Presenting signs can also be lethargy and inappetence without overt heart failure.

Thoracic radiography demonstrates right heart and sometimes left atrial enlargement. Pleural effusion is common; ascites, caudal vena caval distension, and evidence for pericardial effusion may also be noted. Various arrhythmias have been documented on ECG in affected cats, including ventricular premature complexes (VPCs), ventricular tachycardia, atrial fibrillation, and supraventricular tachyarrhythmias. A right bundle branch block pattern appears to be common; some cats have had first-degree AV block. Echocardiography shows severe right atrial and RV enlargement. Other echo findings can include abnormal muscular trabeculation, aneurysmal dilation, areas of dyskinesis, and paradoxical septal motion. Tricuspid regurgitation appears to be a consistent finding on Doppler examination.

The prognosis is guarded once signs of heart failure appear. Recommended therapy includes diuretics as necessary, digoxin, and an ACEI. Additional therapy for specific arrhythmias may be needed (see Chapter 4). In people with similar disease, both supraventricular and ventricular tachyarrhythmias are a prominent feature and sudden death is common.

## MYOCARDITIS

Inflammation of the myocardium and adjacent structures also occurs in cats (see also p. 116). Histologic evidence of myocarditis was identified in myocardial samples from 58% of cardiomyopathic cats but none from control cats in one study. Using polymerase chain reaction (PCR) techniques, panleukopenia viral DNA was amplified in almost one third of the cases (Meurs and colleagues, 2000). However, the possible role of viral myocarditis in the pathogenesis of cardiomyopathy needs further clarification. Congestive heart failure or fatal arrhythmias may result from severe, widespread myocarditis. Cats with focal myocardial inflammation may remain asymptomatic. Acute and chronic cases of suspected viral myocarditis have been described. Although a viral cause is rarely documented, feline coronavirus has been shown to cause pericarditis-epicarditis. Endomyocarditis found during histopathologic examination has occurred mostly in young cats. Acute death, with or without signs of pulmonary edema lasting 1 to 2 days, is the most common presentation. Histopathologic characteristics of acute endomyocarditis include focal or diffuse lymphocytic, plasmacytic, and histiocytic infiltrates with a few neutrophils. Degenerative and lytic changes are seen in adjacent myocytes. Chronic endomyocarditis has been associated with a minimal inflammatory response but much myocardial degeneration and fibrosis. It is speculated that RCM represents the end stage of nonfatal endomyocarditis. Therapy involves the management of congestive signs and arrhythmias and other supportive care.

Bacterial myocarditis may result from sepsis or from bacterial endocarditis or pericarditis, as it does in dogs. Subclinical lymphoplasmacytic myocarditis has been found in cats with experimental *Bartonella* infections, but it is unclear whether natural infections have any role in the development of cardiomyopathy. Myocarditis caused by *Toxoplasma gondii* also occurs occasionally, usually in immunosuppressed cats as part of a generalized disease process. Traumatic myocarditis is infrequently recognized in cats.

## ARTERIAL THROMBOEMBOLISM

Thromboembolism can occur with any form of feline cardiomyopathy. Thrombosis and embolization result from circulatory stasis, altered blood coagulability, local tissue or blood vessel injury, or a combination of these. Poor intracardiac blood flow, especially within the left atrium, may result in blood stasis and clot formation. Hypercoagulability has been demonstrated in cats with thromboembolic disease, in which platelets are known to be quite reactive. Disseminated intravascular coagulation also may develop in cats with thromboembolism. Changes in cardiac endothelial surfaces secondary to the cardiomyopathy could induce platelet adhesion, leading to activation of the coagulation cascade.

The most common site of embolization is the distal aortic trifurcation ("saddle thrombus"), noted in more than 90% of cats with thromboembolic disease. Thromboemboli can also lodge within a brachial artery, various organs, and the heart itself. Small, "silent" emboli may occur as well. Vasoactive substances that impair the development of collateral circulation are released after thromboembolization. Experimental ligation of the distal aorta does not result in the clinical syndrome seen in cats with thromboembolic disease, however. Instead, an ischemic neuromyopathy results from the thromboembolus and the resulting impaired collateral circulation. Nerve conduction failure, ischemic damage to nerve sheaths, and wallerian-type degeneration cause peripheral nerve dysfunction; pathologic changes also occur in the associated muscle tissue.

### Clinical Features and Diagnosis

Middle-aged male cats appear to be at highest risk for thromboembolism. The clinical signs occur acutely and are usually dramatic. Often there is no history of cardiac disease. The clinical findings depend on the area embolized as well as the extent and duration of arterial blockage. For example, acute distal aortic embolization is manifested by paresis in the hindlimbs. The femoral pulses are absent, the limbs cool, the nailbeds cyanotic, and the affected muscles become firm and painful. The cranial tibial and gastrocnemius muscles are most affected. The cat is usually able to flex and extend the hips but drags the lower legs (Fig. 7-7); sensation to the lower legs is poor. One side may show greater neurologic deficits than the other; occasionally only distal embolization of one limb occurs, resulting in paresis of the lower limb alone. Embolization of a (usually the right) brachial artery causes forelimb monoparesis; intermittent claudication occurs occasionally. Thromboembolism of the renal, mesenteric, or pulmonary arterial circulation may result in failure of these organs and death. Emboli lodging in the CNS can cause seizures and various neurologic deficits.

Respiratory distress, a cardiac murmur, or an arrhythmia is often noted at presentation. Common clinical findings asso-

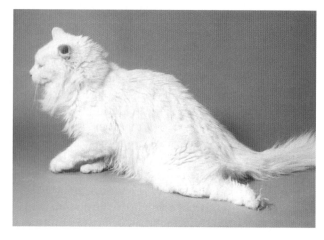

**FIG 7-7**
Cat with thromboembolism to the distal aorta. The left rear limb was dragged behind as the cat tried to walk; there was slightly better function in the right rear.

ciated with thromboembolism are summarized in Table 7-2. Azotemia is common and may result from dehydration, poor cardiac output related to the cardiomyopathy, embolization of the renal arteries, or a combination of these. Skeletal muscle damage and necrosis are accompanied by elevations of alanine aminotransferase and aspartate aminotransferase activities, beginning within 12 hours of the thromboembolic event and peaking by 36 hours. Widespread muscle injury causes lactate dehydrogenase and creatine kinase activities to be increased soon after the event; elevations in these enzyme activities may persist for weeks. Metabolic acidosis, disseminated intravascular coagulation, and hyperkalemia may also be present secondary to ischemic muscle damage and reperfusion. Stress hyperglycemia is also common.

Echocardiography delineates the type of myocardial disease and may reveal the presence of an intracardiac thrombus (see Fig. 7-5). Most cats have prominent left atrial enlargement. If echocardiography is unavailable, nonselective angiocardiography can be done to define the nature of the cardiac disease and allow the anatomic location and extent of the embolus to be determined; however, angiocardiography should be delayed until the animal's condition has been stabilized. The finding of no palpable femoral pulses, in conjunction with other physical examination, auscultatory, and plain thoracic radiographic findings, is often diagnostic. However, a cardiac murmur, gallop sound, or arrhythmia is an inconsistent finding, and a minority of affected cats have no radiographic evidence of cardiomegaly (Harpster and colleague, 1995). Other causes of acute posterior paresis to be considered include intervertebral disc disease, spinal neoplasia (e.g., lymphoma), trauma, fibrocartilaginous infarction, diabetic neuropathy, and possibly, myasthenia gravis.

### Treatment and Prognosis

The goals of treatment are to manage concurrent congestive heart failure and arrhythmias (if present), prevent extension of the embolus and formation of additional thrombi, pro-

## TABLE 7-2

Common Clinical Findings in Cats with
Thromboembolism

### Acute Limb Paresis

Posterior paresis
Monoparesis
± Intermittent claudication

### Characteristics of Affected Limb(s)

Painful
Cool distal limbs
Pale footpads
Cyanotic nailbeds
Absent arterial pulse
Contracture of affected muscles (especially gastrocnemius
    and cranial tibial)

### Signs of Congestive Heart Failure

Tachypnea/dyspnea
Anorexia
Lethargy/weakness
Systolic murmur
Gallop sounds
Arrhythmias
Pulmonary edema
Cardiomegaly
Effusions

### Vocalization (Pain and Distress)

### Hypothermia

### Hematologic and Biochemical Abnormalities

Azotemia
Increased alanine aminotransferase activity
Increased aspartate aminotransferase activity
Increased lactate dehydrogenase activity
Increased creatine kinase activity
Hyperglycemia
Lymphopenia
Disseminated intravascular coagulation (see Chapter 89,
    Disorders of Hemostasis)

mote collateral circulation, and provide supportive care. The treatment of heart failure is outlined in preceding paragraphs and in Table 7-1 (HCM). Digoxin is generally not used unless DCM has been identified. Propranolol is also avoided because its β-blocking effects may leave vascular α-adrenergic receptors unopposed and contribute to peripheral vasoconstriction. In addition, propranolol has no antithrombotic effects at clinical doses.

The therapy for the thromboembolism is somewhat controversial, and there is no proven best treatment. At a minimum, supportive care should be given to allow time for the establishment of collateral circulation (2 to 5 days). The conditions of some cats improve with or despite specific therapy. An analgesic is recommended because this is a painful condition. Butorphanol (0.15 to 0.5 mg/kg IM into the cranial lum-

bar area or SC q1-3h), has been recommended, especially for the first 24 to 36 hours after the embolic event. Low-dose morphine (0.1 to 0.3 mg/kg q3-6h IM, SC) could be considered, but occasional cats experience dysphoria. A fentanyl patch (25 μg/hour size, Duragesic, Janssen Pharm. Titusville, N.J.), applied to a shaved area of skin, could be used to help alleviate pain for up to 3 days. However, because it takes about 12 hours to become effective, another analgesic is used simultaneously during this initial period. Respiratory depression and reduced GI motility are potential side effects. Acepromazine has been advocated for its α-adrenergic receptor–blocking effects (0.05 to 0.3 mg/kg SC q8h). However, because it has not been documented to improve collateral flow and because it (as well as other vasodilators, such as hydralazine) could worsen cardiac function by causing hypotension or exacerbating a preexisting outflow tract obstruction, it is not recommended.

Sodium heparin (initial dose of 200 IU/kg IV, then 150 to 200 IU/kg SC q6-8h) is often administered for 2 to 4 days in an attempt to prevent further thrombus formation, although its efficacy is unclear. Heparin is a cofactor for antithrombin III. The antithrombin III–heparin complex neutralizes factors IX, X, XI, XII, and thrombin (factor II), thereby preventing further coagulation. Heparin does not affect existing thromboemboli. SC doses are adjusted to prolong the cat's thromboplastin time or activated coagulation time from 1.5 to 2.5 times the pretreatment level (see p. 1199). The coagulation test should be monitored daily. As expected, bleeding can be a major complication of therapy. If this occurs, protamine sulfate may be given, but care must be taken because an overdose of protamine can paradoxically cause irreversible hemorrhage. Dosage guidelines for protamine sulfate are as follows: 1 mg/100 U of heparin is given if the heparin was given within the previous 60 minutes; 0.5 mg/100 U of heparin is given if the heparin was given more than 1 but less than 2 hours earlier; and 0.25 mg/100 U of heparin is given if more than 2 hours have elapsed since heparin was administered.

Low molecular weight heparins (LMWH) may be a safer alternative to unfractionated heparin, but more clinical experience is needed before definitive recommendations can be made. Low molecular weight heparins are derived by chemical or enzymatic depolymerization of heparin, which yields mixtures of smaller polymers (2000 to 15,000 kDa). The LMWH have greater anti-Xa:anti-IIa ratios compared to unfractionated heparin. They have fewer side effects, appear not to be inactivated by platelet factor 4, have less plasma protein binding, and little to no heparin-induced platelet activation compared with unfractionated heparin. The LMWH have differences in biologic and clinical effects and are not interchangeable. They are being used in people for venous thromboembolic and acute coronary diseases. Determining the level of anticoagulation can be difficult, because there are minimal changes in coagulation test results. Several LMWH are commercially available. Initial veterinary experience in cats has been variable but appears promising. Doses based on recommendations in humans have been used for enoxaparin (Lovenox, Aventis Pharm., Bridgewater, NJ; 1 mg/kg q12[to

24]h, SC ) and dalteparin (Fragmin, Pharmacia Upjohn, Peapack, N.J.; 100 U/kg q24h SC ), but the optimum dosage and administration frequency for cats are not yet known.

More aggressive thrombolytic therapy has proved problematic, even if instituted within 8 hours of the thromboembolic event and closely monitored. Streptokinase (Streptase; AstraZenica, Wilmington, Del) is a nonspecific plasminogen activator that leads to the degradation of fibrin in thrombi and clot lysis but also potentially leads to systemic fibrinolysis, coagulopathy, and bleeding. The reported protocol is 90,000 IU/cat of streptokinase infused IV within 30 minutes, then 45,000 IU/hr is given for 3 to 8 hours. However, the mortality in these cats is very high. It is unclear if lower doses would be effective with fewer complications. Acute hyperkalemia (secondary to thrombolysis and reperfusion), metabolic acidosis, bleeding, and other complications are thought to be responsible for causing death. Streptokinase therapy should not even be considered if heparin has already been administered (because of the risk for excess hemorrhage), if the cat is anuric, or if the serum potassium concentration and the ECG cannot be monitored continuously. Tissue plasminogen activator (TPA) (Activase, Genentech, San Francisco, Calif; Retavase, Centocor, Malvern, Pa) has a higher specificity of action against fibrin within thrombi, with a low affinity for circulating plasminogen. A dose of 0.25 to 1 mg/kg/hr up to a total of 1 to 10 mg/kg IV has been used. However, this also has yielded disappointing results in the few cats evaluated. Although evidence of reperfusion was found, the mortality rate during therapy was high. The cause of death in most cats was related to reperfusion (hyperkalemia, metabolic acidosis), although congestive heart failure and arrhythmias were also involved.

Other supportive therapy includes general nursing care, correcting hypothermia, treating dehydration, and monitoring renal function and serum electrolyte concentrations daily. Continuous ECG monitoring during the first several days can help in detecting the development of acute hyperkalemia. Nutritional support and/or loosely bandaging the affected limb(s) to prevent self-mutilation may be needed in some cats. Surgical removal of the clot is not advised (except, perhaps, for a suprarenal thrombus). The surgical risk is high in most cases because of the presence of decompensated heart failure, arrhythmias, disseminated intravascular coagulation, and hypothermia. Furthermore, significant neuromuscular ischemic injury has probably already occurred by the time surgery is performed, thus further reducing the likelihood for a good outcome. Clot removal using an embolectomy catheter has not been very effective in cats either.

If concurrent congestive heart failure can be controlled and other complications avoided, function should begin to return in the affected limbs within 7 to 14 days. Some cats become clinically normal within 1 to 2 months, although residual deficits may persist for a variable length of time. Permanent limb atrophy and/or deformity may develop; amputation may occasionally be necessary. In general, the prognosis is guarded. About two thirds of affected cats die or are euthanized soon after the thromboembolic event. Some cats survive well for

more than a year, although repeated events are common and worsen the long-term prognosis. Significant embolization of the kidneys, intestines, or other organs carries a grave prognosis. Other poor prognostic signs include refractory heart failure or arrhythmias, progressive hyperkalemia or azotemia, progressive limb injury (continued muscle contracture after 2 to 3 days, necrosis), persistent hypothermia, severe left atrial enlargement, presence of intracardiac thrombi or spontaneous contrast ("swirling smoke") on echocardiogram, disseminated intravascular coagulation, and previous thromboembolism.

## Prevention of Thromboembolism

No current therapeutic strategy has been found to consistently prevent thromboembolism. The risk of thromboembolism is thought to be greater in cats with marked left atrial enlargement, echocardiographic evidence of intracardiac spontaneous contrast or visible intracardiac thrombi, and in those with a prior thromboembolic event.

Aspirin has been observed to inhibit platelet aggregation and improve collateral circulation in experimental aortic thrombosis at a dose of 10 to 25 mg/kg (1.25 grains/cat) administered once every (2 to) 3 days PO. The drug acts by irreversibly inhibiting the enzyme cyclooxygenase, thereby reducing thromboxane $A_2$ synthesis and subsequent platelet aggregation, serotonin release, and vasoconstriction. However, the optimal dose of aspirin that can inhibit thromboxane $A_2$ production but minimally affect prostacyclin synthesis by the vascular endothelium has not yet been established. Prostacyclin causes vasodilation and inhibits platelet aggregation. Although aspirin has been used widely with generally little risk, it does not consistently prevent initial or recurrent thromboembolism. Nevertheless, aspirin is still often recommended for cats with at least moderate left atrial enlargement, especially if the closer monitoring needed for warfarin is deemed problematic. Vomiting and inappetence, requiring drug discontinuation, can be side effects in some cats. The aspirin-Maalox combination (Ascriptin) may be helpful. More aggressive preventative therapy (e.g., warfarin, LMWH) is thought prudent in cats that have survived an episode of thromboembolism. Diltiazem given at clinical doses does not appear to have significant platelet-inhibiting effects.

Long-term therapy with warfarin (Coumadin, DuPont, Wilmington, Del; generics) has been advocated for cats that survive an acute thromboembolic event or are otherwise presumed to be at high risk for thromboembolism. It may afford better protection than aspirin, but thromboembolism can still recur. Furthermore, warfarin has a greater potential for causing serious adverse effects, even in cats that are closely monitored. Warfarin works by inhibiting the formation of vitamin K–dependent clotting factors (II, VII, IX, and X) as well as the anticoagulant proteins C and S. In people, a transient hypercoagulable state occurs after the initiation of therapy until the levels of clotting factors decrease. Studies regarding this phenomenon in animals are not available, but heparin is usually given for the first 2 to 5 days of warfarin therapy. The pharmacokinetics of warfarin in cats are not well documented; in people, the bioavailability varies with different drug preparations and elimination is mainly by hepatic metabolism. Many drug interactions with warfarin are observed in people.

Monitoring of the patient is very important because of the potentially wide variability in dose response and the risk of bleeding. It is prudent to hospitalize the patient during the initiation of warfarin therapy. A baseline coagulation profile and platelet count should be obtained. Aspirin, if previously being given, should be discontinued. The usual initial dose is 0.1 mg/kg/day PO (or a quarter to half of a 1-mg warfarin tablet), although a quarter of a tablet q48h may be sufficient in some cats. Heparin (100 IU/kg SC q8h) is administered for 3 to 4 days if not already being used for a prior thromboembolic event. It is preferable to keep the medication administration and blood sampling times consistent. The prothrombin time (PT) is evaluated daily (several hours after warfarin dosing) for 5 to 6 days initially. The PT can then be evaluated at progressively increasing time intervals (e.g., twice a week, then once a week, then every month to 2 months) as long as the cat's condition appears stable. Use of the same brand of warfarin may provide more consistent results. Clinical signs of bleeding may be weakness, lethargy, or pallor rather than overt hemorrhage.

The initial warfarin dose is adjusted to maintain a desirable PT. Variable recommendations for this exist; a PT value from 1.3 to 2 times the baseline value at 8 to 10 hours after dosing may be used. A more precise method is the standardized PT represented by the international normalization ratio (INR). This method has been recommended to eliminate the problems posed by variations in commercial PT assays. The INR is calculated by dividing the animal's PT by the control PT and raising the quotient to the power of the international sensitivity index (ISI) of the thromboplastin used in the assay, or INR = (animal PT/control PT)$^{ISI}$. The ISI is provided with each batch of thromboplastin manufactured. Extrapolation from data in people would indicate that an INR of 2 to 3 is as effective as higher values, with less chance for bleeding. However, it may be difficult to achieve fine dose adjustments in cats because of the size of commercial drug tablets.

If the PT or INR is excessively increased, warfarin should be discontinued and vitamin $K_1$ administered (1 to 2 mg/kg/day PO or SC). If the PT is still prolonged after 3 days, vitamin $K_1$ treatment is continued until the PT is normal and the packed cell volume is stable. Some cats with severe bleeding need fresh frozen plasma, packed red blood cells, or whole fresh blood transfusions. Warfarin treatment can be resumed at half the original dose, along with heparin, which is given for several days.

The combination of aspirin and warfarin has been used in some cats judged to be at very high risk for thromboembolism. However, preliminary experience indicates that the combination is no more effective than either alone in preventing recurrent thromboembolism. Low molecular weight heparin is another option for chronic therapy, although it must be given by injection (see p. 135). The overall efficacy and the optimal dose and administration schedule for the different products available are not known.

Hyperhomocysteinemia has been found in some cats with aortic thromboembolism but not others; some cats with thromboembolism have decreased plasma arginine and vitamins $B_6$ and $B_{12}$ (Hohenhaus and colleagues, 1999; McMichael and colleagues, 2000). Hyperhomocysteinemia and reduced plasma vitamin B concentrations are risk factors for thromboembolism in people. It is not known whether B vitamin or arginine supplementation would be helpful in improving endothelial function and/or inhibiting platelet aggregation and so reduce the risk of thromboembolism in cats with cardiomyopathy.

## Suggested Readings

**MYOCARDIAL DISEASES**

Baty CJ et al: Natural history of hypertrophic cardiomyopathy and aortic thromboembolism in a family of domestic shorthair cats, *J Vet Intern Med* 15:595, 2001.

Bonagura JD et al: Acute effects of esmolol on left ventricular outflow tract obstruction in cats with hypertrophic cardiomyopathy: a Doppler-echocardiographic study, *J Vet Intern Med* 5:123, 1991 (abstract).

Bright JM et al: Evaluation of the calcium channel–blocking agents diltiazem and verapamil for treatment of feline hypertrophic cardiomyopathy, *J Vet Intern Med* 5:272, 1991.

Bright JM et al: Pulsed Doppler assessment of left ventricular diastolic function in normal and cardiomyopathic cats, *J Am Anim Hosp Assoc* 35:285, 1999.

Dow SW et al: Taurine depletion and cardiovascular disease in adult cats fed a potassium-depleted acidified diet, *Am J Vet Res* 53:402, 1992.

Fox PR: Feline cardiopathy. I. Hypertrophic cardiomyopathy, *Proceedings of the 19th ACVIM Forum,* Denver, 2001, p 145.

Fox PR et al: Echocardiographic assessment of spontaneously occurring feline hypertrophic cardiomyopathy: an animal model of human disease, *Circulation* 92:2645, 1995.

Fox PR et al: Spontaneously occurring arrhythmogenic right ventricular cardiomyopathy in the domestic cat: a new animal model similar to the human disease, *Circulation* 102:1863, 2000.

Gaschen L et al: Cardiomyopathy in dystrophin-deficient hypertrophic feline muscular dystrophy, *J Vet Intern Med* 13:346, 1999.

Gavaghan BJ et al: Quantification of left ventricular diastolic wall motion by Doppler tissue imaging in healthy cats and cats with cardiomyopathy, *Am J Vet Res* 60:1478, 1999.

Jacobs G et al: Cardiovascular complications of feline hyperthyroidism. In Bonagura JD et al, editors: *Kirk's current veterinary therapy XI,* Philadelphia, 1992, WB Saunders, p 756.

Johnson LM et al: Pharmacokinetic and pharmacodynamic properties of conventional and CD-formulated diltiazem in cats, *J Vet Intern Med* 10:316, 1996.

Kittleson MD et al: Familial hypertrophic cardiomyopathy in Maine Coon cats: an animal model of human disease, *Circulation* 99:3172, 1999.

Kraus MS et al: Hypertrophic cardiomyopathy in a litter of five mixed-breed cats, *J Am Anim Hosp Assoc* 35:293, 1999.

Lawler DF et al: Evidence for genetic involvement in feline dilated cardiomyopathy, *J Vet Intern Med* 7:383, 1993.

Liu SK et al: Myocarditis in the dog and cat. In Bonagura JD, editor: *Kirk's current veterinary therapy XII,* Philadelphia, 1995, WB Saunders, p 842.

Meurs KM et al: Familial systolic anterior motion of the mitral valve and/or hypertrophic cardiomyopathy is apparently inherited as an autosomal dominant trait in a family of American shorthair cats, *J Vet Intern Med* 11:138, 1997 (abstract).

Meurs KM et al: Molecular screening by polymerase chain reaction detects panleukopenia virus DNA in formalin-fixed hearts from cats with idiopathic cardiomyopathy and myocarditis, *Cardiovasc Pathol* 9:119, 2000.

Meurs KM et al: Myomesin, a sarcomeric protein, is reduced in Maine Coon cats with familial hypertrophic cardiomyopathy, *J Vet Intern Med* 15:281, 2001.

Novotny MJ et al: Echocardiographic evidence for myocardial failure induced by taurine deficiency in domestic cats, *Can J Vet Res* 58:6, 1994.

O'Keefe DA et al: Systemic toxicity associated with doxorubicin administration in cats, *J Vet Intern Med* 7:309, 1993.

Peterson EN et al: Heterogeneity of hypertrophy in feline hypertrophic heart disease, *J Vet Intern Med* 7:183, 1993.

Peterson ME et al: Acromegaly in 14 cats, *J Vet Intern Med* 4:192, 1990.

Pion PD et al: Response of cats with dilated cardiomyopathy to taurine supplementation, *J Am Vet Med Assoc* 201:275, 1992.

Rush JE et al: The use of enalapril in the treatment of feline hypertrophic cardiomyopathy, *J Am Anim Hosp Assoc* 34:38, 1998.

Rush JE et al: Population and survival characteristics of cats with hypertrophic cardiomyopathy: 260 cases (1990-1999), *J Am Vet Med Assoc* 220:202, 2002.

Stalis IH et al: Feline endomyocarditis and left ventricular endocardial fibrosis, *Vet Pathol* 32:122, 1995.

Strickland KN: Left atrial global shortening fraction in cats with cardiomyopathy, *Proceedings of the 19th ACVIM Forum,* Denver, 2001, p 86.

THROMBOEMBOLISM

Harpster NK et al: Warfarin therapy of the cat at risk of thromboembolism. In Bonagura JD, editor: *Kirk's current veterinary therapy XII,* Philadelphia, 1995, WB Saunders, p 868.

Hohenhaus AE et al: Evaluation of plasma homocysteine and B vitamin concentrations in cardiomyopathic cats with congestive heart failure and arterial thromboembolism, *Proceedings, 1999 Purina Nutrition Forum,* p 89 (abstract), St Louis.

Laste NJ et al: A retrospective study of 100 cases of feline distal aortic thromboembolism: 1977-1993, *J Am Anim Hosp Assoc* 31:492, 1995.

McMichael MA et al: Plasma homocysteine, B vitamins, and amino acid concentrations in cats with cardiomyopathy and arterial thromboembolism, *J Vet Intern Med* 14:507, 2000.

Pion PD et al: Therapy for feline aortic thromboembolism. In Kirk RW, editor: *Current veterinary therapy X,* Philadelphia, 1989, WB Saunders, p 295.

Welles EG et al: Platelet function and antithrombin, plasminogen, and fibrinolytic activities in cats with heart disease, *Am J Vet Res* 55:619, 1994.

# CHAPTER 8

## Acquired Valvular and Endocardial Diseases

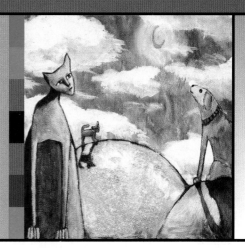

### CHAPTER OUTLINE

DEGENERATIVE MITRAL AND TRICUSPID VALVE
DISEASE, 139
INFECTIVE ENDOCARDITIS, 145

## DEGENERATIVE MITRAL AND TRICUSPID VALVE DISEASE

Chronic degenerative atrioventricular (AV) valvular disease is the most common cause of heart failure in the dog. Other terms for the condition include *endocardiosis, mucoid* or *myxomatous valvular degeneration,* and *chronic valvular fibrosis.* Clinically important degenerative valve lesions are extremely rare in cats. Hence this discussion pertains only to chronic valvular disease in dogs. Degenerative lesions most often involve the mitral valve; however, both AV valves are affected in many dogs. Isolated degenerative disease of the tricuspid valve is uncommon; degenerative disease of the aortic or pulmonic valve is rare.

### ETIOLOGY, PATHOLOGY, AND PATHOPHYSIOLOGY

The etiology of endocardiosis is unknown, but a hereditary basis is likely. Multiple factors involving collagen degeneration, valve leaflet stress, and possibly endothelial function are thought to be involved. Mitral valve prolapse may be important in the pathogenesis of the disease, at least in some breeds. A high prevalence of mitral prolapse is seen in clinically normal dogs of some predisposed breeds, and further, the degree of prolapse may be associated with severity of the disease (Pedersen, 1999b).

Pathologic changes in the valves of affected dogs develop gradually with age. Early lesions consist of small nodules on the free margins of the valve; these become larger, coalescing plaques that distort the valve. The affected valve leaflets become thickened. They may enlarge, and redundant tissue between chordal attachments often bulges (prolapses) like a parachute or balloon toward the atrium. The valve gradually begins to leak because the edges do not coapt properly. In ad-

vanced cases, grossly deformed, thickened, and possibly shrunken leaflets occur. The chordae tendineae are also affected, becoming thickened and weak. As the lesions progress, the valve insufficiency becomes clinically evident. The histologic changes have been described as "myxomatous degeneration." Collagen within the affected leaflets degenerates and may disintegrate, whereas acid mucopolysaccharides and other substances accumulate within the layers of the leaflets. This results in the nodular thickening, deformity, and weakening of the valve and its chordae tendineae. The valve lesions in dogs with degenerative valvular disease are similar to those found in the mitral valve prolapse syndrome of humans.

Valve regurgitation leads to dilation of the adjacent atrium, valve annulus, and ventricle. Atrial jet lesions, endocardial fibrosis, and partial or even full-thickness atrial tears can form. Chronic valvular disease is also associated with intramural coronary arteriosclerosis, microscopic intramural myocardial infarctions, and focal myocardial fibrosis. The extent to which these changes cause clinical myocardial dysfunction is not clear; however, impaired myocardial contractility is observed late in the disease. Geriatric dogs without valvular disease also have similar vascular lesions.

The pathophysiologic changes relate to volume overloading on the affected side of the heart after the valve or valves become incompetent. Regurgitation usually develops slowly over months to years, and mean left atrial (LA) pressure remains fairly low unless the regurgitant volume suddenly increases greatly (e.g., ruptured chordae). With advancing valve degeneration, a progressively larger volume of blood moves ineffectually back and forth between the ventricle and atrium, diminishing the forward flow to the aorta. Compensatory mechanisms augment blood volume to meet the circulatory needs of the body (see Chapter 3). These include increased sympathetic neural activity, attenuated vagal tone, and renin-angiotensin-aldosterone system (RAAS) activation. Release of atrial natriuretic peptide (ANP) may help to counter the effects of RAAS activation in earlier stages of the disease. Higher ANP concentrations are associated with marked LA enlargement and severity of congestive failure. The affected ventricle and atrium dilate to accept the growing regurgitant volume and the required forward stroke volume; eccentric

**139**

myocardial hypertrophy develops in the attempt to normalize the resulting increase in wall stress.

These compensatory changes in heart size and blood volume allow most dogs to remain asymptomatic for a prolonged period. Massive LA enlargement may develop before any signs of heart failure appear, and some dogs never show clinical signs of heart failure. The rate at which the regurgitation worsens, as well as the degree of atrial distensibility and ventricular contractility, influences how well the animal tolerates the disease.

The ability of the compensatory mechanisms to maintain homeostasis is eventually exceeded in many dogs, leading to a rise in atrial pressures with or without a decrease in forward cardiac output. Gradual increases in atrial, pulmonary venous, and capillary hydrostatic pressures stimulate compensatory increases in pulmonary lymphatic flow. Overt pulmonary edema develops when the capacity of the pulmonary lymphatic system is exceeded. Impaired pulmonary vasomotor function has also been associated with pulmonary congestion (Straeter-Knowlen and colleagues, 1999). In some dogs, tricuspid insufficiency is severe enough to cause signs of right-sided congestive heart failure. Increased pulmonary vascular pressures secondary to chronic left-sided heart failure may also contribute to the development of right-sided heart failure. Compensatory neurohormonal responses further cause the blood volume to expand and vascular tone to increase, exacerbating congestion and valve insufficiency.

Ventricular function appears to be maintained fairly well in many dogs until late in the disease, even though severe congestive heart failure may occur. Nevertheless, chronic volume overload eventually reduces myocyte contractility, although heightened sympathetic activity can mask this. There is evidence that oxygen free radicals may be involved in the depression of contractility associated with chronic volume overload (Prasad and colleagues, 1996). Chronic β-blockade improves myocyte contractility experimentally (Tsutsui and colleagues, 1994). Reduced contractility exacerbates ventricular dilation and valve regurgitation and therefore may worsen congestive failure. In the clinic, it is difficult to assess myocardial contractility in dogs with mitral regurgitation; ejection phase indices (e.g., echocardiographic fractional shortening, mean velocity of circumferential fiber shortening, ejection fraction) overestimate contractility because the regurgitation of blood into the low-pressure atrium facilitates ventricular wall shortening by reducing afterload. Isovolumetric indices (e.g., the maximum rate of increase in left ventricular pressure) are not valid because there is no isovolumetric contraction (regurgitation begins early in systole). The end-systolic stress (or pressure)–end-systolic volume indices are better, although not ideal, for gauging contractility but are not usually assessed in veterinary patients. The echocardiographic estimation of the end-systolic volume index may be useful (see p. 35). Using this index, it appears that myocardial function is normal to mildly depressed in most dogs with chronic mitral degeneration.

## COMPLICATING FACTORS

Although endocardiosis usually progresses slowly, certain complicating events can cause the acute onset of clinical signs in dogs with previously compensated disease (Table 8-1). For example, tachyarrhythmias may be severe enough to cause decompensated congestive failure, syncope, or both. Frequent atrial premature contractions, paroxysmal atrial tachycardia, or atrial fibrillation can reduce ventricular filling time and cardiac output, increase myocardial oxygen needs, and worsen pulmonary congestion and edema. Ventricular tachyarrhythmias also occur but are less common.

Rupture of diseased chordae tendineae suddenly increases the regurgitant volume and can precipitate fulminant pulmonary edema within hours in previously compensated or even asymptomatic dogs. Low cardiac output signs may also be noted. Sometimes, ruptured chordae are an incidental finding (on an echocardiogram or at necropsy), especially if second- or third-order chordae are involved.

Massive LA enlargement itself can compress the left mainstem bronchus and stimulate persistent coughing, even in the

 TABLE 8-1

**Potential Complications of Chronic Atrioventricular Valve Disease**

**Causes of Acutely Worsened Pulmonary Edema**

Arrhythmias
  Frequent atrial premature complexes
  Paroxysmal atrial/supraventricular tachycardia
  Atrial fibrillation
  Frequent ventricular tachyarrhythmias
  Rule out drug toxicity (e.g., digoxin)
Ruptured chordae tendineae
Iatrogenic volume overload
  Excessive volumes of IV fluids or blood
  High-sodium fluids
Erratic or improper medication administration
Insufficient medication for stage of disease
Increased cardiac workload
  Physical exertion
  Anemia
  Infections/sepsis
  Hypertension
  Disease of other organ systems (e.g., pulmonary, renal, liver, endocrine)
  Hot, humid environment
  Excessively cold environment
  Other environmental stresses
High sodium intake
Myocardial degeneration and poor contractility

**Causes of Reduced Cardiac Output or Weakness**

Arrhythmias (see above)
Ruptured chordae tendineae
Cough syncope
Left atrial tear
  Intrapericardial bleeding
  Cardiac tamponade
Increased cardiac workload (see above)
Secondary right-sided heart failure
Myocardial degeneration and poor contractility

absence of congestive heart failure. Further, when the left (or right) atrium is stretched beyond its elastic limit, partial- or full-thickness tears occur. Atrial wall rupture usually causes acute cardiac tamponade; there appears to be a higher prevalence of this complication in male Miniature Poodles, Cocker Spaniels, and Dachshunds. In most of these cases, severe valve disease, marked atrial enlargement, atrial jet lesions, and often, ruptured first-order chordae tendineae are present.

## EPIDEMIOLOGY

The prevalence and severity of chronic, degenerative AV valve disease increase with age. Clinical evidence of the condition is found most commonly in middle-age and older small to midsize breeds. More than 30% of small-breed dogs older than 10 years are affected. A higher prevalence has been noted in Poodles, Miniature Schnauzers, Chihuahuas, Fox Terriers, Cocker Spaniels, and Boston Terriers. An especially high incidence and an early onset of degenerative mitral valve disease have been noted in Cavalier King Charles Spaniels; more than 50% of these dogs older than 4 years have characteristic murmurs. In this breed, the inheritance is thought to be polygenic, with gender and age influencing expression. The overall prevalence of mitral regurgitation murmurs and degenerative valve disease is similar in males and females; but males have faster progression, greater severity, and a higher prevalence of congestive failure than females. Many times the accompanying cardiac murmur of mitral (or tricuspid) insufficiency is an incidental finding, and it may take years before a dog with a murmur resulting from degenerative mitral or tricuspid disease becomes symptomatic.

## CLINICAL SIGNS

Degenerative AV valve disease may cause no clinical signs for years, and some dogs never develop signs of heart failure. In those that do, the signs usually relate to decreased exercise tolerance and manifestations of pulmonary congestion and edema. Diminished exercise capacity and cough or tachypnea with exertion are common initial owner complaints. As pulmonary congestion and interstitial edema worsen, the resting respiratory rate also increases. Coughing occurs at night and early morning, as well as with activity. Severe edema results in obvious respiratory distress, often with a moist cough. Signs of severe pulmonary edema can develop gradually or acutely. Intermittent episodes of symptomatic pulmonary edema interspersed with periods of compensated heart failure occurring over months to years are also common.

Episodes of transient weakness or acute collapse (syncope) may occur secondary to arrhythmias, coughing, or an atrial tear. Signs of tricuspid regurgitation, often overshadowed by those of mitral disease, include ascites, respiratory distress resulting from pleural effusion, and, rarely, peripheral tissue edema. Gastrointestinal signs may accompany splanchnic congestion.

Mitral regurgitation is generally accompanied by a holosystolic murmur best heard in the area of the left apex (left fourth to sixth intercostal space). However, mild regurgitation may cause a murmur heard only in early systole (protosystolic) or may be inaudible. The murmur may radiate in any direction. Exercise and excitement often increase the intensity of soft mitral regurgitation murmurs. Louder murmurs have been associated with more advanced disease; but it is important to remember that the murmur can be soft or even inaudible in dogs with massive regurgitation and severe heart failure. Occasionally the murmur will sound like a musical tone or whoop. Some dogs have an audible mid- to late-systolic click, with or without a murmur. An $S_3$ gallop may be audible at the left apex in dogs with advanced disease. Tricuspid regurgitation causes a murmur similar to that of mitral regurgitation, but it is best heard at the right apex. The radiation of a mitral murmur to the right chest wall may mimic or mask a tricuspid murmur. Jugular vein pulsations, a precordial thrill over the right apex, and a different quality to the murmur heard over the tricuspid region help in identifying tricuspid insufficiency.

Pulmonary sounds can be normal or abnormal. Normal breath sounds are heard in the absence of congestive heart failure or in dogs with mild pulmonary edema. Accentuated, harsh breath sounds and end-inspiratory crackles (especially in ventral lung fields) develop as the edema worsens. Fulminant pulmonary edema causes widespread inspiratory as well as expiratory crackles and wheezes. Some dogs with chronic mitral regurgitation have abnormal lung sounds associated with underlying pulmonary or airway disease, rather than with heart failure. Dogs with congestive heart failure tend to have sinus tachycardia, whereas those with chronic pulmonary disease frequently have marked sinus arrhythmia and a normal heart rate. Pleural effusion causes diminished pulmonary sounds ventrally.

Other physical examination findings may be normal or noncontributory. Peripheral capillary perfusion and arterial pulse strength are usually good, although pulse deficits accompany some tachyarrhythmias. A palpable precordial thrill accompanies loud (grade V to VI) murmurs. Jugular vein distention and pulsations are not expected in the presence of mitral regurgitation alone. In animals with tricuspid regurgitation, jugular pulsations occur during ventricular systole and tend to be more evident after exercise or with excitement. Distention of the vein results from elevated right side of the heart filling pressures. Jugular pulsations and distention are more evident during the application of cranial abdominal compression (positive hepatojugular reflux). Abdominal signs of right-sided heart failure (e.g., hepatomegaly, ascites) may also be noted.

## RADIOGRAPHY

Thoracic radiographs typically show some degree of LA and ventricular enlargement (see p. 32), which progresses over months to years (Fig. 8-1). Elevation of the left and sometimes right mainstem bronchi, with compression of the left mainstem bronchus, occurs in dogs with severe LA enlargement. Fluoroscopy may show dynamic main bronchus collapse that is associated with coughing or even quiet breathing in such animals. Extreme dilation of the left atrium can develop over time, even in the absence of clinical heart failure. Variable right-sided heart enlargement occurs in animals with chronic tricuspid regurgitation, but this may be masked by

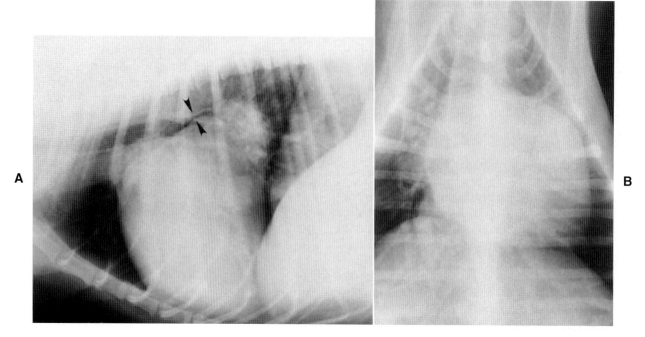

**FIG 8-1**
**A,** Lateral and, **B,** dorsoventral radiographs from a Poodle with advanced mitral valve insufficiency. Note marked left ventricular and atrial enlargement and narrowing of left mainstem bronchus *(arrowheads in* **A**).

left-sided heart and pulmonary changes resulting from concurrent mitral disease.

Pulmonary venous congestion and interstitial edema occur with the onset of left-sided congestive failure; progressive interstitial and alveolar pulmonary edema may follow. The radiographic distribution pattern of cardiogenic pulmonary edema in dogs is classically hilar, dorsocaudal, and bilaterally symmetric. However, an asymmetric distribution is seen in some dogs. The presence and severity of pulmonary edema do not necessarily correlate with the degree of cardiomegaly. Acute, severe mitral regurgitation (e.g., with rupture of the chordae tendineae) can cause cardiogenic edema with minimal LA enlargement, whereas slowly developing regurgitation can produce massive LA enlargement with no evidence of congestive failure. Early signs of right-sided heart failure include caudal vena caval distention, pleural fissure lines, and hepatomegaly. Overt pleural effusion and ascites occur with advanced failure.

## ELECTROCARDIOGRAPHY

The electrocardiogram (ECG) may indicate the presence of left atrial or biatrial enlargement and left ventricular dilation (see p. 15), although the tracing is often normal. Typical characteristics of right ventricular enlargement occasionally are seen in dogs with severe tricuspid regurgitation. Arrhythmias are common in dogs with advanced disease, especially sinus tachycardia, supraventricular premature complexes, paroxysmal or sustained supraventricular tachycardias, ventricular premature complexes, and atrial fibrillation. These arrhythmias may be associated with decompensated congestive failure, weakness, or syncope.

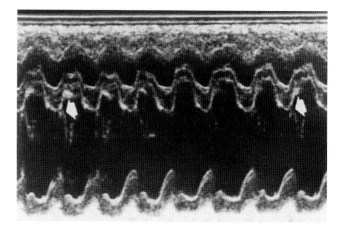

**FIG 8-2**
Sample M-mode echocardiogram from male Maltese with advanced mitral valve insufficiency and left-sided heart failure. Note accentuated septal and left ventricular posterior wall motion (fractional shortening = 50%) and lack of mitral valve E point–septal separation *(arrows)*.

## ECHOCARDIOGRAPHY

The atrial and ventricular chamber dilation secondary to chronic AV valve insufficiency is evident on echocardiograms. Depending on the degree of volume overload, this enlargement can be severe. In the presence of mitral regurgitation, left ventricular wall and septal motion is accentuated when contractility is normal (Fig. 8-2); little to no E point–septal separation and a high fractional shortening are seen. The diastolic ventricular dimension is increased, but the systolic di-

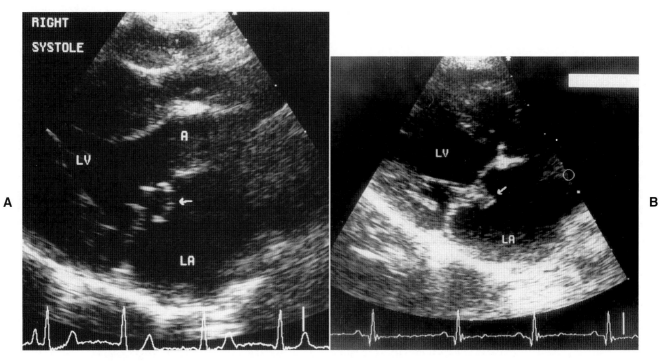

**FIG 8-3**
Echocardiograms showing abnormal systolic mitral valve motion secondary to degenerative mitral valve disease. **A,** Ballooning area *(arrow)* of mitral prolapse seen in a 14-year-old male Poodle. **B,** Chordae tendineae rupture allows the tip of this thickened mitral leaflet to flail into the left atrium in this 13-year-old male Lhasa Apso. *A,* Aorta; *LA,* left atrium; *LV,* left ventricle.

mension is normal until the myocardium itself begins to fail. The end-systolic volume index may be helpful for assessing myocardial function. The ventricular wall thickness is typically normal. Right ventricular and atrial enlargement is seen in dogs with severe tricuspid disease, in which volume overload of the right ventricle possibly causes paradoxic septal motion. Pericardial fluid is evident after an LA tear occurs.

The affected valve cusps are thicker than normal and may appear knobby. Exaggerated motion and thick mitral echoes are commonly seen on M-mode examinations. Valve thickening is usually most evident on the anterior leaflet. Smooth thickening is characteristic of degenerative disease (endocardiosis), whereas bacterial endocarditis tends to cause the formation of rough and irregular vegetative valve lesions. In actuality, however, it is often impossible to differentiate between degenerative and infective thickening. Systolic prolapse or ballooning of a portion of one or both valve leaflets into the atrium is common in dogs with degenerative AV valve disease (Fig. 8-3, *A*). Sometimes a ruptured chorda tendinea or leaflet tip flails into the atrium during systole (Fig. 8-3, *B*). The direction and extent of disturbed flow in the atrium can be seen with color-flow Doppler (see Fig. 2-36). Spectral Doppler interrogation of the high-velocity regurgitant jet allows estimation of the systolic pressure gradient between the affected atrium and ventricle.

Clinical laboratory data may be normal or may reflect changes compatible with congestive heart failure or concurrent extracardiac disease. Other diseases that may be confused

with symptomatic degenerative mitral or tricuspid valve disease include tracheal collapse, chronic bronchitis, bronchiectasis, pulmonary fibrosis, pulmonary neoplasia, pneumonia, pharyngitis, heartworm disease, dilated cardiomyopathy, and bacterial endocarditis. The cough caused by major airway collapse often is described as "honking."

## TREATMENT AND PROGNOSIS

Although surgical procedures such as mitral annuloplasty, other valve repair techniques, and mitral valve replacement are available at some referral centers, most cases are treated medically. The main goals of medical therapy are to control signs of congestive heart failure, enhance forward blood flow, reduce the regurgitant volume, and modulate the excessive neurohormonal activation that contributes to the disease process (see Table 3-2). Drugs that decrease left ventricular size (e.g., diuretics, vasodilators, positive inotropic agents) may reduce the regurgitant volume by decreasing mitral annulus size. Arteriolar vasodilators enhance forward cardiac output and reduce regurgitant volume by decreasing systemic arteriolar resistance. Clinical compensation can be maintained for months to years with appropriate therapy in many dogs with advanced mitral regurgitation (with or without tricuspid regurgitation), although frequent reevaluation and medication adjustment become necessary as the disease progresses. Although congestive signs appear gradually in some dogs, severe pulmonary edema or episodes of syncope develop rapidly in others. Many dogs receiving long-term therapy for heart failure have intermittent episodes of decompensation that can be successfully managed. Therapy must be tailored to the individual dog and guided by its clinical status, the nature of complicating factors, and the animal's medication history. Categorizing animals into a "functional class" of heart failure (see p. 57) may be helpful conceptually; however, the clinical progression of disease in an individual dog does not necessarily follow an orderly sequence.

**Asymptomatic AV valve regurgitation.** Dogs that are asymptomatic (functional class I) do not require drug therapy. Convincing evidence of the benefit of angiotensin-converting enzyme inhibitor (ACEI) therapy in asymptomatic dogs is presently lacking. Owner education is important so that he or she is alert to the early signs of heart failure. During this preclinical stage it is wise to pursue weight reduction for obese dogs, to advise moderate exercise restriction, and to delete high-salt foods from the dog's diet. A diet moderately restricted in sodium chloride may be helpful (see Table 3-5).

**Mild to moderate congestive heart failure.** Dogs with clinical signs that occur in response to exercise or activity (functional classes II and III) are treated with several modalities. The severity of the heart failure and the nature of any complicating factors influence the aggressiveness of therapy. Moderate dietary salt restriction (e.g., diets formulated for dogs with kidney disease or for geriatric dogs; see Table 3-5) is recommended initially. Further salt restriction is achieved using diets formulated for patients with heart failure (see Table 3-5).

An ACEI is generally prescribed for dogs with early signs of failure (see Chapter 3). Although ACEIs are not pure arteriolar vasodilating agents, their overall ability to modulate the neurohormonal response to heart failure is advantageous for long-term use (see p. 64). Long-term enalapril (or other ACEI) therapy may improve exercise tolerance, cough, and respiratory effort, although the issue of enhanced survival is unclear. In dogs with respiratory signs that could be caused by either heart failure or a noncardiac cause, an initial therapeutic trial of furosemide (e.g., 1 to 2 mg/kg PO q8-12h) is indicated. Cardiogenic pulmonary edema usually responds rapidly.

Dogs with radiographic evidence of pulmonary edema and/or more severe clinical signs are also treated with furosemide (see Table 3-6). Higher and more frequent doses are administered for the treatment of more severe edema. When signs of failure are controlled, the dose and frequency of administration are reduced to the lowest effective levels for long-term therapy. The use of furosemide alone (e.g., without an ACEI or digoxin) for the long-term treatment of heart failure is not recommended.

Digoxin therapy is advocated for the chronic treatment of failure resulting from advanced AV valve regurgitation. Its effects on baroreceptors may be of greater benefit than any positive inotropic effects (see Chapter 3). Digoxin is usually added after ACEI and furosemide therapy has been initiated, especially if there is marked left ventricular enlargement. Other indications for digoxin include frequent atrial premature beats or tachycardia, atrial fibrillation, and recurrent episodes of

pulmonary edema despite furosemide and ACEI treatment. Conservative doses (see Table 3-8) are given, and serum concentrations are measured to prevent toxicity (see p. 66).

Exercise restriction is enforced until signs of failure abate. However, mild-to-moderate regular activity can be beneficial during chronic, compensated disease. Strenuous exercise is best avoided. Dogs with persistent cough caused by mechanical compression of their mainstem bronchi may require antitussive therapy (see p. 288). See Management of Chronic Heart Failure in Chapter 3 for more information.

**Severe congestive heart failure.** Dogs with severe pulmonary edema and shortness of breath at rest (functional class IV) constitute true emergencies (see Table 3-4). Aggressive treatment but gentle handling is crucial, because any added stress can lead to death. Cage rest, supplemental oxygen therapy, high-dose (e.g., 2 to 4 mg/kg q1-4h initially) parenteral furosemide therapy, and vasodilator therapy are indicated (see Table 3-6). Hydralazine is recommended for acute therapy because of its direct and rapid vasodilating effect on arterioles, which increases forward flow and decreases regurgitation. A reduced dose is used in animals already receiving an ACEI (see p. 65). Topical nitroglycerin can also be used in an attempt to reduce pulmonary venous pressure by direct venodilation. Intravenous (IV) nitroprusside can be used instead of other vasodilators because it produces arteriolar and venous dilation; however, blood pressure must be closely monitored to prevent hypotension.

Digoxin therapy (see Table 3-8) can be initiated (or continued if previously prescribed) once the acute dyspnea subsides. Paroxysmal atrial tachycardia or atrial fibrillation may respond to digoxin. Although it takes several days for a therapeutic blood concentration to be reached with oral maintenance doses, IV digitalization is generally avoided unless the arrhythmia appears to be life-threatening. Diltiazem or a β-blocker (see Table 4-5) can be used instead of or in addition to digoxin for the control of supraventricular tachyarrhythmias (see Chapter 4). Myocardial function is usually adequate in these dogs; however, if poor contractility is documented, other more potent inotropic agents (e.g., dobutamine, dopamine, amrinone) can be given IV (see Table 3-8) or pimobendan used, if available.

Mild sedation can be useful to reduce anxiety (e.g., morphine; see p. 58 and Table 3-4). Minimal handling of the animal also helps reduce stress. Thoracic radiographs and other diagnostic procedures are postponed until the dog's respiratory condition is more stable. Bronchodilators (e.g., theophylline, aminophylline) have been used because of possible bronchospasm induced by severe pulmonary edema (see p. 58); although the efficacy of this is unclear, these agents may help support respiratory muscle function. In dogs with moderate- to large-volume pleural effusion, thoracocentesis is indicated to improve pulmonary function. Ascites severe enough to impede respiration should also be drained. Occasionally therapy for ventricular tachyarrhythmias is warranted. It is important, as always, to watch for drug toxicities and adverse effects (e.g., azotemia, electrolyte abnormalities, arrhythmias).

After the animal's condition is stabilized, medications are adjusted over several days to weeks to determine the best regimen for long-term treatment. Furosemide is titrated to the lowest dose (and longest interval) that controls signs of congestive heart failure. Changing to an ACEI for ongoing therapy is recommended if hydralazine or nitroprusside was the vasodilator used initially. As the effects of previously administered hydralazine wane, the first enalapril (or other ACEI) dose given should be one-half the usual dose (i.e., 0.25 mg/ kg). Because nitroprusside has such a short half-life, enalapril administration can begin at the standard dose if this vasodilator was used for acute therapy.

**Chronic refractory congestive heart failure.** When congestive heart failure becomes decompensated, therapy is intensified or modified as needed for the individual dog. The following suggestions for modifying therapy are listed in approximate order of use. Some dogs respond to an increased dose of furosemide and rest for a few days and then can be returned to their previous or a slightly higher dose. Increasing the frequency of ACEI administration (e.g., enalapril from once to twice daily) can be effective. Digoxin can be added if it is not already being used; the dose of digoxin is not titrated upward unless subtherapeutic serum concentrations are documented (see Chapter 3). Dietary sodium restriction can be intensified. If the ACEI and furosemide doses are already maximal, low-dose hydralazine (e.g., 0.25 to 0.5 mg/kg PO q12h) or amlodipine (e.g., 0.05 to 0.2 mg/kg PO q24h) can be added, but blood pressure should be monitored. Another diuretic with a different mechanism of action, such as spironolactone (1 to 2 mg/kg PO q12-24h) or the spironolactone/hydrochlorothiazide combination product (1 to 2 mg/kg of the combination 25 mg/25 mg product), may reduce the severity of chronic refractory pulmonary edema or effusions. Continued monitoring, especially of renal function and serum electrolyte concentrations, is important. Intermittent tachyarrhythmias can cause decompensated congestive failure as well as episodes of transient weakness or syncope. Cough-induced syncope, atrial rupture, or other causes of reduced cardiac output may also occur. Despite the periodic recurrence of signs of congestive heart failure, many dogs with chronic AV valve regurgitation can enjoy a good quality of life for several years after the signs of failure first appear.

## PATIENT MONITORING AND REEVALUATION

Client education regarding the disease process, the clinical signs of failure, and the drugs used to control them is essential for long-term therapy to be successful. As the disease progresses, medication readjustment (i.e., different dosages of currently used drugs and/or additional drugs) is usually required. Common potential complications of chronic degenerative AV valve disease that can lead to decompensation are listed in Table 8-1. At-home monitoring by the owner is important, especially because decompensation often occurs unexpectedly. Respiratory and heart rates can be noted when the dog is quietly resting or sleeping; a persistent increase in either can signal the existence of early decompensation.

It is recommended that asymptomatic dogs not receiving cardiac medication be reevaluated at least yearly in the context of a routine preventive health program. The timing of reevaluations in dogs receiving heart failure medications depends on the stability of the animal's condition and the nature of any complicating factors. Dogs with recently diagnosed or decompensated heart failure should be checked more frequently (several days to 1 week or so) until their condition is stable. Those with chronic heart failure that appears well controlled can be reevaluated less frequently, usually several times per year. The medication supply, administration compliance, drugs and doses being given, and diet should be reviewed with the owner at each visit.

A general physical examination as well as a careful cardiovascular examination is done at the time of reevaluation. An ECG is indicated if an arrhythmia or unexpectedly low or high heart rate is auscultated. When an arrhythmia is suspected but not documented on routine ECG, ambulatory electrocardiography (e.g., 24-hour Holter monitoring) can be helpful. The respiratory rate and pattern are also noted, and thoracic radiographs are warranted if abnormal pulmonary sounds are heard or if the owner reports coughing, other respiratory signs, or an increased resting respiratory rate. Other causes of cough should be considered if neither pulmonary edema nor venous congestion is seen radiographically and if the resting respiratory rate has not increased. Left mainstem bronchus compression by the enlarged left atrium can stimulate a dry cough. Cough suppressants are helpful for this but should only be prescribed after other causes of cough are ruled out. Echocardiography may show evidence of chordal rupture, progressive cardiomegaly, or worsened myocardial function. Frequent monitoring of serum electrolyte concentrations and renal function is important. Other routine blood and urine tests should be done periodically also. Dogs receiving digoxin should have serum concentration measured 7 to 10 days after the initiation of treatment or a dosage change. Additional measurements are recommended if signs consistent with toxicity appear or if renal disease or electrolyte imbalance (hypokalemia) is suspected.

The prognosis in dogs with degenerative valve disease that has become symptomatic is quite variable. With appropriate therapy and attentive management of complications, some dogs live well for more than 4 years after the signs of heart failure first appear. Some dogs die during an initial episode of fulminant pulmonary edema. Survival for most symptomatic dogs ranges from several months to a few years.

## *INFECTIVE ENDOCARDITIS*

### ETIOLOGY

Endocarditis is an infection involving the cardiac valves or endocardial tissues. Although it can occur in any species, it is more common in dogs than in cats. Bacteremia, either persistent or transient, is necessary for an endocardial infection to occur. Recurrent bacteremia can result from infections of the skin, mouth, urinary tract, prostate, lungs, or other organs. Dentistry procedures are known to cause a transient bacteremia. Other procedures are presumed to cause transient bacteremia in some cases (e.g., endoscopy, urethral catheterization, anal surgery, and other "dirty" procedures). The chance of a cardiac infection becoming established is increased in the presence of highly virulent organisms or a heavy bacterial load. The endocardial surface of the valve is infected directly from the blood flowing past it. Previously normal valves may be invaded by virulent bacteria, causing acute bacterial endocarditis. Subacute bacterial endocarditis is thought to result from infection of previously damaged or diseased valves after a persistent bacteremia. Such damage can result from mechanical trauma (e.g., jet lesions resulting from turbulent blood flow or endocardial injury from a vascular catheter extending into the heart). Myxomatous degeneration of the mitral valve has not been associated with a higher risk for infective endocarditis. The lesions of endocarditis are typically located downstream from the disturbed blood flow; common sites include the ventricular side of an aortic valve in the presence of subaortic stenosis, the right ventricular side of a ventricular septal defect, and the atrial surface of a regurgitant mitral valve. Bacterial clumping caused by the action of an agglutinating antibody may facilitate attachment to the valves. Alternatively, chronic stress and mechanical trauma can predispose to the development of nonbacterial thrombotic endocarditis, a sterile accumulation of platelets and fibrin on the valve surface. Nonseptic emboli may break off from such vegetations and cause infarctions elsewhere. Bacteremia can also cause a secondary infective endocarditis at these sites.

Organisms identified in dogs and cats with endocarditis have most often been *Streptococcus* sp., *Staphylococcus* sp., or *Escherichia coli*. Additional organisms isolated from infected valves have included *Corynebacterium (Arcanobacterium)* sp., *Pasteurella* sp., *Pseudomonas aeruginosa*, *Erysipelothrix rhusiopathiae*, and others. *E. rhusiopathiae* isolates from dogs with endocarditis have also been identified as *E. tonsillaris*. *Bartonella vinsonii* subsp. *berkhoffii* has also been identified in dogs with endocarditis. Culture-negative endocarditis may be caused by fastidious organisms.

## PATHOPHYSIOLOGY

The mitral and aortic valves are the ones most commonly infected in dogs and cats. Microbial colonization results in ulceration of the valve endothelium; exposure of subendothelial collagen in turn stimulates platelet aggregation and activation of the coagulation cascade, leading to the formation of vegetations. Vegetations consist mainly of aggregated platelets, fibrin, blood cells, and bacteria. Newer vegetations are friable. With time, the lesions become fibrous and may calcify. As additional fibrin is deposited over bacterial colonies, they become protected from normal host defenses as well as many antibiotics. Although vegetations usually involve the valve leaflets, lesions may extend to the chordae tendineae, sinuses of Valsalva, mural endocardium, or adjacent myocardium. Vegetations cause valve deformity, including perforations or tearing of the leaflet or leaflets, and result in valve

insufficiency. Rarely, large vegetations may cause the valve to become stenotic.

Congestive heart failure commonly results from valve insufficiency and the resulting volume overload. Because the mitral and aortic valves are usually affected, pulmonary congestion and edema resulting from left-sided heart failure are expected. Clinical heart failure develops rapidly in association with severe valve destruction, rupture of chordae tendineae, and multiple valve involvement or when other predisposing factors are present. Cardiac function is also compromised by myocardial injury, such as that resulting from coronary arterial embolization with myocardial infarction and abscess formation or from direct extension of the infection into the myocardium. Reduced contractility and atrial or ventricular tachyarrhythmias often result. Aortic valve endocarditis may extend into the AV node and cause partial or complete AV block. Arrhythmias may cause weakness, syncope, and sudden death or contribute to the development of congestive heart failure.

Fragments of vegetative lesions often break loose. Embolization of other body sites causes infarction or metastatic infection, which results in diverse clinical signs. Larger and more mobile vegetations (as assessed by echocardiography) are associated with a higher incidence of embolic events in people, although other factors can also be important (DiSalvo and colleagues, 2001). Emboli may be septic or bland (containing no infectious organisms). Septic arthritis, diskospondylitis, urinary tract infections, and renal and splenic infarctions are common in affected animals. Local abscess formation resulting from septic thromboemboli contributes to the recurrence of bacteremia and fever. Hypertrophic osteopathy has also been associated with bacterial endocarditis. Circulating immune complexes contribute to the disease syndrome. Sterile polyarthritis, glomerulonephritis, and other immune-mediated organ damage are common. Rheumatoid factor and antinuclear antibody test results may be positive.

## CLINICAL FEATURES

The prevalence of bacterial endocarditis is relatively low in dogs and even lower in cats. Male dogs are affected more commonly than females, and the prevalence of endocarditis increases with age. There are conflicting reports as to whether German Shepherd and other large-breed dogs are at greater risk. Subaortic stenosis is a known risk factor for aortic valve endocarditis. Immunocompromised animals may also be at greater risk for endocarditis, but this has not been substantiated.

The clinical signs are quite variable. Cardiac signs (e.g., those resulting from left-sided congestion or arrhythmias) may be the reason for presentation; however, the cardiac signs may be overshadowed by systemic signs resulting from infarction, infection, or immune-mediated damage or a combination of these. Nonspecific signs of lethargy, weight loss, inappetence, recurrent fever, and weakness may be the predominant abnormalities. It is important to maintain an index of suspicion for this disease, which has been nicknamed "the great imitator." Many affected animals have evidence of past or concurrent infections, although often a clear history of predisposing factors is absent. It is important to recognize that infective endocarditis often mimics immune-mediated disease. Dogs with endocarditis are commonly evaluated for a "fever of unknown origin" (see Chapter 95). Some of the consequences of infective endocarditis are outlined in Table 8-2.

Signs of heart failure occurring in an unexpected clinical setting or in an animal with a murmur of recent onset could indicate the existence of infected valve damage, especially if other suggestive signs are present. However, such a murmur could be caused by noninfective acquired disease (e.g., degenerative valve disease, cardiomyopathy), previously undiagnosed congenital disease, or physiologic alterations (e.g., fever, anemia). Conversely, endocarditis may develop in an animal with a known murmur resulting from another cardiac disease. Although a change in murmur quality or intensity over a short time may indicate active valve damage, physiologic causes of murmur variation are common. The onset of a diastolic murmur at the base of the left side of the heart is suspicious for aortic valve endocarditis, especially if fever or other signs are present.

## DIAGNOSIS

It is difficult to make a definitive ante-mortem diagnosis. A presumptive diagnosis of infective endocarditis is made on the basis of positive findings in two or more blood cultures, in addition to either echocardiographic evidence of vegetations or valve destruction or the documented recent appearance of a regurgitant murmur. Endocarditis is likely even when blood culture results are negative or intermittently positive if there is echocardiographic evidence of vegetations or

### TABLE 8-2

**Potential Sequelae of Infective Endocarditis**

**Heart**

Valve insufficiency or stenosis
  Murmur
  Congestive heart failure
Coronary embolization (aortic valve*)
  Myocardial infarction
  Myocardial abscess
  Myocarditis
  Decreased contractility (segmental or global)
  Arrhythmias
Myocarditis (direct invasion by microorganisms)
  Arrhythmias
  Atrioventricular conduction abnormalities (aortic valve*)
  Decreased contractility
Pericarditis (direct invasion by microorganisms)
  Pericardial effusion
  Cardiac tamponade (?)

**Kidney**

Infarction
  Reduced renal function
Abscess formation and pyelonephritis
  Reduced renal function
  Urinary tract infection
  Renal pain
Glomerulonephritis (immune mediated)
  Proteinuria
  Reduced renal function

**Musculoskeletal**

Septic arthritis
  Joint swelling and pain
  Lameness
Immune-mediated polyarthritis
  Shifting leg lameness
  Joint swelling and pain

**Musculoskeletal—cont'd**

Septic osteomyelitis
  Bone pain
  Lameness
Myositis
  Muscle pain

**Brain and Meninges**

Abscesses
  Associated neurologic signs
Encephalitis and meningitis
  Associated neurologic signs

**Vascular System in General**

Vasculitis
  Thrombosis
  Petechiae and small hemorrhages (e.g., eye, skin)
Obstruction
  Ischemia of tissues served, with associated signs

**Lung**

Pulmonary emboli (tricuspid or pulmonic valves, rare*)
Pneumonia (tricuspid or pulmonic valves, rare*)

**Nonspecific**

Sepsis
Fever
Anorexia
Malaise and depression
Shaking
Vague pain
Inflammatory leukogram
Mild anemia
± Positive antinuclear antibody test
± Positive blood cultures

*Diseased valve most commonly associated with abnormality.

## TABLE 8-3

Criteria for Diagnosis of Infective Endocarditis

**Definite Endocarditis by Pathologic Criteria**

Pathologic (post-mortem) lesions of active endocarditis with evidence of microorganisms in vegetation (or embolus) or intracardiac abscess

**Definite Endocarditis by Clinical Criteria**

Two major criteria (below), or
One major and three minor criteria, or
Five minor criteria

**Possible Endocarditis**

Findings consistent with infective endocarditis that fall short of "definite" but not "rejected"

**Rejected Diagnosis of Endocarditis**

Firm alternative diagnosis for clinical manifestations
Resolution of manifestations of infective endocarditis with 4 or fewer days of antibiotic therapy
No pathologic evidence of infective endocarditis at surgery or necropsy after 4 or fewer days of antibiotic therapy

**Major Criteria**

Positive blood cultures
- Typical microorganism for infective endocarditis from two separate blood cultures

**Major Criteria—cont'd**

- Persistently positive blood cultures for organism consistent with endocarditis (samples drawn >12 hr apart or three or more cultures drawn at least 1 hr apart)

Evidence of endocardial involvement
- Positive echocardiogram for infective endocarditis (oscillating mass on heart valve or supportive structure or in path of regurgitant jet; or evidence of cardiac abscess)
- New valvular regurgitation (increase or change in preexisting murmur not sufficient evidence)

**Minor Criteria**

Predisposing heart condition (see p. 146)
Fever
Vascular phenomena: major arterial emboli, septic infarcts
Immunologic phenomena: glomerulonephritis, positive antinuclear antibody or rheumatoid factor tests
Microbiologic evidence: positive blood culture not meeting major criteria above
Echocardiogram consistent with infective endocarditis but not meeting major criteria above
(Rare in dogs and cats: repeated nonsterile IV drug administration)

Modified from Duke Criteria for Endocarditis. In Durack DT et al: New criteria for diagnosis of infective endocarditis: utilization of specific echocardiographic findings, *Am J Med* 96:200, 1994.

valve destruction along with a combination of other criteria (Table 8-3). A new diastolic murmur, hyperkinetic pulses, and fever are strongly suggestive of aortic valve endocarditis. Table 8-3 is an adaptation of the Duke criteria for the diagnosis of infective endocarditis used in people.

Several samples of at least 10 ml of blood should be aseptically collected over a 24-hour period for bacterial blood culture, with more than 1 hour elapsing between collections. Different venipuncture sites should be used for each sample. Larger sample volumes (e.g., 20 to 30 ml) increase culture sensitivity. Both aerobic and anaerobic cultures have been recommended, although the value of routine anaerobic culture is questionable. Prolonged incubation (3 weeks) is recommended, because some bacteria are slow-growing. Although blood culture results are positive in many dogs with this disease, negative results do not necessarily rule out infective endocarditis. Results can be negative in the setting of chronic endocarditis, recent antibiotic therapy, intermittent bacteremia, and infection with fastidious or slow-growing organisms, as well as noninfective endocarditis. Serologic and polymerase chain reaction (PCR) testing, as well as culture, is also commercially available for *Bartonella* sp.

Echocardiography is especially supportive if oscillating vegetative lesions and abnormal valve motion can be identified (Fig. 8-4). The visualization of lesions depends on their size and location as well as the resolution capabilities of the ultra-

sound equipment. False-negative and false-positive findings of "lesions" can occur; cautious interpretation of the findings is therefore important. Early lesions consist of mild valve thickening and/or enhanced echogenicity. Vegetative lesions appear as irregular, dense masses. As valve destruction progresses, ruptured chordae, flail leaflet tips, or other abnormal valve motion can be seen. Differentiation of mitral vegetations from degenerative thickening may be impossible. However, classically, vegetative endocarditis has a rough, ragged appearance, whereas degenerative disease is associated with smooth valvular thickenings. Poor or marginal-quality images or the use of lower-frequency transducers may prevent the identification of some vegetations because of suboptimal resolution. Cardiac sequelae of valve dysfunction can be identified. These include chamber enlargement resulting from volume overload and flail or otherwise abnormal valve leaflet motion. Aortic insufficiency may cause a high-frequency flutter of the anterior mitral valve leaflet during diastole as the regurgitant jet hits this leaflet. Aortic valve regurgitation appears as a diastolic "flame" of color extending from the valve on color-flow Doppler studies (Fig. 8-5). Echocardiography may also identify myocardial dysfunction and arrhythmias.

The ECG may be normal or document premature beats, tachycardias, conduction disturbances, or evidence of myocardial ischemia. Radiographic findings may be unremarkable or show evidence of left-sided heart failure. Cardio-

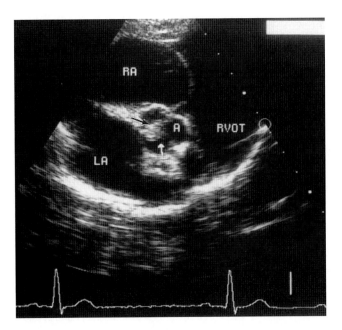

**FIG 8-4**
Right parasternal short-axis echocardiogram at the aortic–left atrial level in a 2-year-old male Vizsla with congenital subaortic stenosis and pulmonic stenosis. Note the aortic valve vegetation *(arrows)* caused by endocarditis. *A,* Aorta; *LA,* left atrium; *RA,* right atrium; *RVOT,* right ventricular outflow tract.

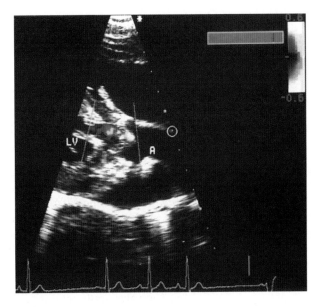

**FIG 8-5**
Right parasternal long axis, color-flow Doppler image taken during diastole from the same dog as in Fig. 8-4. The flamelike jet of aortic regurgitation extends from the closed aortic valve into the left ventricular outflow tract. *A,* Aorta; *LV,* left ventricle.

megaly is minimal early in the disease but progresses over time as a result of valve insufficiency. Radiographs may show other organ involvement (e.g., diskospondylitis).

Clinical laboratory findings usually reflect the presence of an inflammatory process, and biochemical abnormalities can

be variable. Neutrophilia with a left shift is typical of acute endocarditis, whereas mature neutrophilia with or without monocytosis usually develops in the presence of chronic disease. Nonregenerative anemia has been associated with about one half of the cases in dogs. Azotemia, hyperglobulinemia, hematuria, pyuria, and proteinuria are common as well. The antinuclear antibody test result may be positive in dogs with subacute or chronic bacterial endocarditis.

## TREATMENT AND PROGNOSIS

Aggressive therapy with bactericidal antibiotics capable of penetrating fibrin and supportive care are indicated for animals with infective endocarditis. Antimicrobials must reach bacteria deep within the vegetative lesions to be effective. Drug choice is ideally guided by culture results and results of in vitro susceptibility tests, but because a delay in treatment while such results are awaited can be harmful, broad-spectrum combination therapy is usually begun immediately after blood culture samples have been obtained. Therapy can be altered, if necessary, when culture results are available; however, animals with negative culture results should continue to be given a broad-spectrum regimen. An initial combination of a cephalosporin, penicillin, or a synthetic penicillin derivative (e.g., ampicillin) with an aminoglycoside (gentamicin or amikacin) or a fluoroquinolone (e.g., enrofloxacin) is commonly used and should be effective against the organisms most often associated with infective endocarditis (for doses, see p. 1244). Antibiotics are administered IV (or at least intramuscularly) for the first week or longer to obtain higher and more predictable blood concentrations. Orally administered therapy is often used thereafter for the sake of practicality, although parenteral administration is probably better. Antimicrobial therapy is continued for at least 4 weeks, although therapy for 6 (to 8) weeks is often recommended. However, aminoglycosides are discontinued after 2 (to 3) weeks or sooner if renal toxicity develops. Close monitoring of the urine sediment is indicated to detect early aminoglycoside nephrotoxicity (see p. 611).

Supportive care includes treatment of congestive heart failure (see Chapter 3) and arrhythmias (see Chapter 4) when present, as well as complications related to the primary source of infection, embolic events, or immune responses. Attention to hydration status, nutritional support, and general nursing care is also important. Corticosteroids are contraindicated. It is unclear whether the use of aspirin to inhibit platelet aggregation and growth of vegetative lesions is of benefit in reducing the incidence of embolic events. The potential adverse effects of aspirin must be considered.

Long-term prognosis is generally guarded to poor. Evidence of vegetations and volume overload seen on echocardiograms points toward a poor prognosis. Occasionally, aggressive therapy is successful if valve dysfunction is not severe and large vegetations are not present. Congestive heart failure is the most common cause of death, although sepsis, systemic embolization, arrhythmias, or renal failure may be the cause. Aortic valve involvement and gram-negative organisms are factors that independently appear to worsen the prognosis.

The use of prophylactic antibiotics is controversial. Experience in people indicates that most cases of infective endocarditis are not preventable; the risk of endocarditis involved with a specific (e.g. dental) procedure is very low compared with the cumulative risk associated with normal daily activities. However, in view of the increased incidence of endocarditis with certain cardiovascular malformations, antimicrobial prophylaxis is recommended for animals with the following defects before dental or other "dirty" procedures (e.g., involving the oral cavity or intestinal or urogenital systems). Subaortic stenosis is a well-recognized predisposing lesion; endocarditis has also been associated with ventricular septal defect, patent ductus arteriosus, and cyanotic congenital heart disease. Antimicrobial prophylaxis should be given to animals with an implanted pacemaker or with a history of endocarditis and should be considered in immunocompromised animals as well. Recommendations extrapolated from human medicine have included the administration of high-dose ampicillin or amoxicillin (with or without an aminoglycoside, depending on the procedure) 1 hour before and 6 hours following the procedure. The American Heart Association has recently dropped the recommendation for a second dose after the procedure in people.

## Suggested Readings

### Degenerative AV Valve Disease

Beardow AW et al: Chronic mitral valve disease in Cavalier King Charles Spaniels: 95 cases (1987-1991), *J Am Vet Med Assoc* 203:1023, 1993.

Buchanan JW: Causes and prevalence of cardiovascular disease. In Kirk RW et al, editors: *Current veterinary therapy XI,* Philadelphia, 1992, WB Saunders.

Buchanan JW et al: Circumferential suture of the mitral annulus for correction of mitral regurgitation in dogs, *Vet Surg* 27:182, 1998.

Davila-Roman VG et al: Myocardial contractile state in dogs with chronic mitral regurgitation: echocardiographic approach to the peak systolic pressure/end systolic area relationship, *Am Heart J* 126:155, 1993.

Haggstrom J et al: Chronic valvular disease in the Cavalier King Charles Spaniel in Sweden, *Vet Rec* 131:549, 1992.

Haggstrom J et al: Heart sounds and murmurs: changes related to severity of chronic valvular disease in the Cavalier King Charles Spaniel, *J Vet Intern Med* 9:75, 1995.

Haggstrom J et al: Effects of naturally acquired decompensated mitral valve regurgitation on the renin-angiotensin-aldosterone system and atrial natriuretic peptide concentration in dogs, *Am J Vet Res* 58:77, 1997.

Hamlin RL et al: Effects of enalapril on exercise tolerance and longevity in dogs with heart failure produced by iatrogenic mitral regurgitation, *J Vet Intern Med* 10:85, 1996.

Jacobs GJ et al: Echocardiographic detection of flail left atrioventricular valve cusp from ruptured chordae tendineae in 4 dogs, *J Vet Intern Med* 9:341, 1995.

Kitagawa H et al: Efficacy of monotherapy with benazepril, an angiotensin converting enzyme inhibitor, in dogs with naturally acquired chronic mitral insufficiency, *J Vet Med Sci* 59:513, 1997.

Kittleson MD et al: Myocardial function in small dogs with chronic mitral regurgitation and severe congestive heart failure, *J Am Vet Med Assoc* 184:455, 1984.

Mow T et al: Increased endothelin-receptor density in myxomatous canine mitral leaflets, *J Cardiovasc Pharmacol* 34:254, 1999.

Orton EC: Surgical treatment of valvular disease. In *Proceedings of the 19th ACVIM Forum,* Denver, 2001, p 156.

Pedersen HD et al: Auscultation in mild mitral regurgitation in dogs: observer variation, effects of physical maneuvers, and agreement with color Doppler echocardiography and phonocardiography, *J Vet Intern Med* 13:56, 1999a.

Pedersen HD et al: Echocardiographic mitral prolapse in Cavalier King Charles spaniels: epidemiology and prognostic significance for regurgitation, *Vet Rec* 144:315, 1999b.

Prasad K et al: Oxidative stress as a mechanism of cardiac failure in chronic volume overload in canine model, *J Mol Cell Cardiol* 28:375, 1996.

Sisson D: Acquired valvular heart disease in dogs and cats. In Bonagura JD, editor: *Contemporary issues in small animal practice. Cardiology,* New York, 1987, Churchill Livingstone, p 59.

Straeter-Knowlen IM et al: ACE inhibitors in heart failure restore canine pulmonary endothelial function and ANG II vasoconstriction, *Am J Physiol* 277:H1924, 1999.

Swenson L et al: Relationship between parental cardiac status in Cavalier King Charles Spaniels and prevalence and severity of chronic valvular disease in offspring, *J Am Vet Med Assoc* 208:2009, 1996.

Tsutsui H et al: Effects of chronic beta-adrenergic blockade on the left ventricular and cardiocyte abnormalities of chronic canine mitral regurgitation, *J Clin Invest* 93:2639, 1994.

### Infective Endocarditis

Breitschwerdt EB et al: Endocarditis in a dog due to infection with a novel *Bartonella* subspecies, *J Clin Microbiol* 33:154, 1995.

Calvert CA et al: Cardiovascular infections in dogs: epizootiology, clinical manifestations and prognosis, *J Am Vet Med Assoc* 187:612, 1985.

DiSalvo G et al: Echocardiography predicts embolic events in infective endocarditis, *J Am Coll Cardiol* 37:1069, 2001.

Durack DT et al: New criteria for diagnosis of infective endocarditis: utilization of specific echocardiographic findings, *Am J Med* 96:200, 1994.

Elwood CM et al: Clinical and echocardiographic findings in 10 dogs with vegetative bacterial endocarditis, *J Small Anim Practice* 34:420, 1993.

Miller MW et al: Infectious endocarditis. In Fox P et al, editors: *Textbook of canine and feline cardiology,* ed 2, Philadelphia, 1999, WB Saunders, p 567.

Sisson D et al: Endocarditis of the aortic valve, *J Am Vet Med Assoc* 184:570, 1984.

Sisson D: Bacterial endocarditis. In *Proceedings of the 18th Annual Waltham/OSU Symposium,* Vernon, Calif, 1994, Waltham USA.

Takahashi T et al: *Erysipelothrix tonsillarum* isolated from dogs with endocarditis in Belgium, *Res Vet Sci* 54:264, 1993.

# Common Congenital Cardiac Anomalies

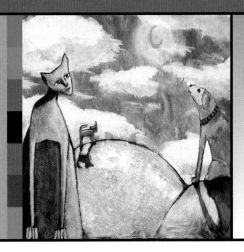

## CHAPTER OUTLINE

GENERAL CONSIDERATIONS, 151
EXTRACARDIAC ARTERIOVENOUS SHUNTS, 153
    Patent ductus arteriosus, 153
VENTRICULAR OUTFLOW OBSTRUCTIONS, 155
    Subaortic stenosis, 156
    Pulmonic stenosis, 158
INTRACARDIAC SHUNTS, 160
    Ventricular septal defect, 161
    Atrial septal defect, 162
ATRIOVENTRICULAR VALVE MALFORMATIONS, 162
    Mitral dysplasia, 162
    Tricuspid dysplasia, 162
CARDIAC ANOMALIES CAUSING CYANOSIS, 163
    Tetralogy of Fallot, 164
    Pulmonary hypertension with shunt reversal, 164
OTHER CARDIOVASCULAR ANOMALIES, 166
    Vascular ring anomalies, 166
    COR triatriatum, 166
    Endocardial fibroelastosis, 167
    Other vascular anomalies, 167

## GENERAL CONSIDERATIONS

The congenital cardiac anomalies most often encountered in dogs and cats are described in this chapter. Other defects and malformations have been reported sporadically. Most congenital lesions are accompanied by an audible murmur, although some serious malformations are not. A murmur, especially if it is loud, in a young puppy or kitten may be an indication of congenital disease (Fig. 9-1). Conversely, clinically insignificant "innocent" murmurs are relatively common in young animals. Innocent murmurs are usually soft systolic ejection–type murmurs heard best at the left heart base; their intensity may vary with heart rate or body position. These murmurs tend to get softer and usually disappear by about 4 months of age. Murmurs associated with congenital disease usually persist and may get louder with time, although this is not always the case. Careful examination and auscultation of the young patient are important, not only in animals intended for breeding, but also in working dogs and pets. Periodic auscultation to check for the persistence of a murmur is advisable as the animal grows, even if no other clinical signs exist. Further diagnostic tests are indicated in animals that manifest other signs or in valuable animals. Adult dogs and cats with a previously undiagnosed congenital defect may or may not be found to have clinical signs of their disease at the time of presentation.

Identification of the specific defect is only part of the evaluation process, because congenital malformations vary widely in severity. A veterinary cardiologist or practitioner with advanced cardiology training can provide a definitive diagnosis, estimate the severity, identify likely sequelae, and make suggestions for medical management. Surgical repair or palliation, balloon valvuloplasty, or other interventional techniques can be discussed in selected cases. Initial noninvasive testing usually includes thoracic radiographs, an electrocardiogram (ECG), and echocardiographic studies (M-mode, 2-dimensional [2-D], and Doppler). A packed cell volume (PCV) is useful if right-to-left shunting is a consideration. Cardiac catheterization with selective angiocardiography may also be needed to define congenital structural abnormalities and their severity or in preparation for an interventional procedure.

Patent ductus arteriosus (PDA) and subaortic stenosis (SAS) have been identified in different surveys as the most common congenital cardiovascular anomaly in the dog; pulmonic stenosis (PS) is also quite common. Persistent right aortic arch (a vascular ring anomaly), ventricular septal defect (VSD), malformations (dysplasia) of the atrioventricular (AV) valves, atrial septal defect (ASD), and tetralogy of Fallot (T of F) occur less frequently but are not rare. An endocardial cushion defect consists of all or some of the following: a high VSD, a low ASD, and malformations of one or both AV valves. The most common malformations in cats are AV valve dysplasias, atrial or ventricular septal defects (which may occur as part of an endocardial cushion defect), and endocardial fibroelastosis (mainly in Burmese and Siamese cats). Other lesions in cats include SAS, PDA, T of F, and PS. Congenital malformations are more prevalent in male than female cats. Congenital malformations in both

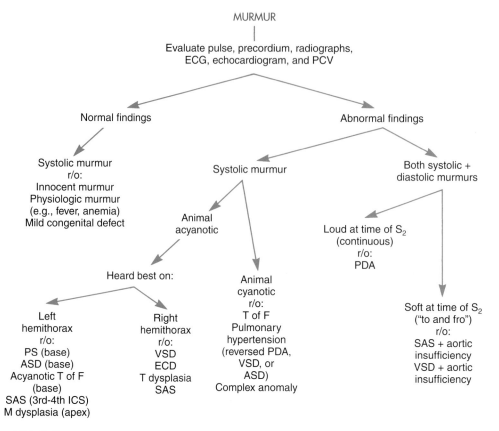

**FIG 9-1**
Flow chart for differentiating murmurs in puppies and kittens. *ASD,* Atrial septal defect; *ECD,* endocardial cushion defect; *ECG,* electrocardiogram; *ICS,* intercostal space; *M,* mitral valve; *PCV,* packed cell volume; *PDA,* patent ductus arteriosus; *r/o,* rule out; *SAS,* subaortic stenosis; *T,* tricuspid valve; *T of F,* tetralogy of Fallot; *VSD,* ventricular septal defect.

 TABLE 9-1

### Breed Predispositions for Congenital Heart Disease

| DISEASE | BREED |
|---|---|
| Patent ductus arteriosus | Maltese, Pomeranian, Shetland Sheepdog, English Springer Spaniel, Keeshond, Bichon Frise, Toy and Miniature Poodles, Yorkshire Terrier, Collie, Cocker Spaniel, German Shepherd Dog; Chihuahua, Kerry Blue Terrier, Labrador Retriever, Newfoundland; female > male |
| Subaortic stenosis | Newfoundland, Golden Retriever, Rottweiler, Boxer, German Shepherd Dog, English Bulldog, Great Dane, German Short-Haired Pointer, Bouvier des Flandres, Samoyed(?) |
| Pulmonic stenosis | English Bulldog (male > female), Mastiff, Samoyed, Miniature Schnauzer, West Highland White Terrier, Cocker Spaniel, Beagle, Airedale Terrier, Boykin Spaniel, Chihuahua, Scottish Terrier, Boxer, Fox Terrier(?) |
| Ventricular septal defect | English Bulldog, English Springer Spaniel, Keeshond; cats |
| Atrial septal defect | Samoyed, Doberman Pinscher, Boxer |
| Tricuspid dysplasia | Labrador Retriever, German Shepherd Dog, Boxer, Weimaraner, Great Dane, Old English Sheepdog, Golden Retriever; other large breeds; (male > female?) |
| Mitral dysplasia | Bull Terrier, German Shepherd Dog, Great Dane, Golden Retriever, Newfoundland, Mastiff, Rottweiler(?); cats; (male > female?) |
| Tetralogy of Fallot | Keeshond, English Bulldog |
| Persistent right aortic arch | German Shepherd Dog, Great Dane, Irish Setter |

species can occur as isolated defects, which is most often the case, or in various combinations.

The prevalence of congenital defects is higher in purebred animals than in mixed-breed animals. In some studies, a polygenic inheritance pattern has been suggested, although there is more recent focus on a single major gene effect influenced by other modifying genes. The recognized predispositions of particular breeds to certain congenital defects are listed in Table 9-1, though other breeds of animals and mixed-breed animals can have any of these defects as well.

## EXTRACARDIAC ARTERIOVENOUS SHUNTS

The most common congenital arteriovenous shunt is the PDA. Rarely, similar hemodynamic and clinical abnormalities are caused by an aorticopulmonary window (a communication between the ascending aorta and pulmonary artery) or some other functionally similar communication in the hilar region.

## PATENT DUCTUS ARTERIOSUS

### Etiology and Pathophysiology

Functional closure of the ductus arteriosus normally occurs within hours after birth and is followed by structural changes, occurring over several months, that cause permanent closure. The ductal wall in animals with an inherited PDA is histologically abnormal and unable to constrict. The size of the patent ductus may depend on the number, or "dose," of associated genes. When the ductus fails to close, blood shunts through it from the descending aorta into the pulmonary artery. Shunting occurs during both systole and diastole, because aortic pressure normally is higher than pulmonic pressure throughout the cardiac cycle. This left-to-right shunt causes a volume overload of the pulmonary circulation, left atrium, and left ventricle. The shunt volume is directly related to the pressure difference (gradient) between the two circulations and the diameter of the ductus.

Hyperkinetic arterial pulses are characteristic of PDA. Blood runoff from the aorta into the pulmonary system allows diastolic aortic pressure to decrease below normal. A palpably stronger arterial pulse results from the widened pulse pressure (systolic minus diastolic pressure) (Fig. 9-2).

Compensatory mechanisms (e.g., increased heart rate, volume retention) maintain blood flow to the body. However, a great hemodynamic burden is imposed on the left ventricle, especially by a large ductus, because the increased volume is pumped into the relatively high-pressure aorta. Left ventricular and mitral annulus dilation in turn cause mitral regurgitation and further volume overload. Excess fluid retention, declining myocardial contractility stemming from the chronic volume overload, and arrhythmias contribute to the development of congestive heart failure.

Occasionally the excess pulmonary blood flow leads to pulmonary vascular changes, increased resistance, and pulmonary hypertension (see p. 164). If the pulmonary pressure rises to equal the aortic pressure, very little blood shunting occurs. If the pulmonary artery pressure exceeds the aortic pressure, reverse shunting (right-to-left flow) occurs. Reversed shunt was noted in 15% of dogs with inherited PDA (Buchanan, 1994). Female Cocker Spaniels may be at increased risk for reversed PDA.

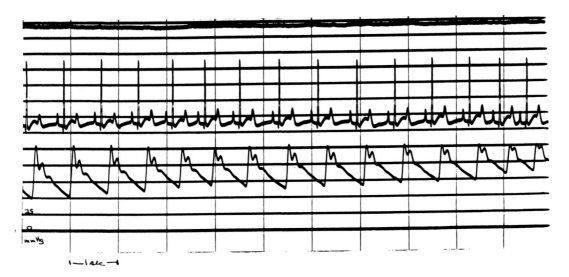

**FIG 9-2**
Continuous femoral artery pressure recording during surgical ligation of a patent ductus arteriosus in a Poodle. The wide pulse pressure (left side of trace) narrows as the ductus is closed (right side of trace). Diastolic arterial pressure rises because blood runoff into the pulmonary artery is curtailed. (Courtesy Dr. Dean Riedesel.)

## TABLE 9-2

### Radiographic Findings in Common Congenital Heart Defects

| DEFECT | HEART | PULMONARY VESSELS | OTHER |
|---|---|---|---|
| PDA | LAE, LVE; L auricular bulge; ± increased cardiac width | Overcirculated | Bulge in descending aorta + pulmonary trunk; ± pulmonary edema |
| SAS | ± LAE, LVE | Normal | Wide cranial waist (ascending aorta dilation) |
| PS | RAE, RVE; reverse D | Normal to undercirculated | Pulmonary trunk bulge |
| VSD | LAE, LVE; ± RVE | Overcirculated | ± Pulmonary edema; ± pulmonary trunk bulge (large shunts) |
| ASD | RAE, RVE | ± Overcirculated | ± Pulmonary trunk bulge |
| T dys. | RAE, RVE; ± globoid shape | Normal | Caudal cava dilation; ± pleural effusion, ascites, hepatomegaly |
| M dys. | LAE, LVE | ± Venous hypertension | ± Pulmonary edema |
| T of F | RVE, RAE; reverse D | Undercirculated; ± prominent bronchial vessels | Normal to small pulmonary trunk; ± cranial aortic bulge on lateral view |

*PDA*, Patent ductus arteriosus; *SAS*, subaortic stenosis; *PS*, pulmonic stenosis; *VSD*, ventricular septal defect; *ASD*, atrial septal defect; *T dys.*, tricuspid dysplasia; *M dys.*, mitral dysplasia; *T of F*, tetralogy of Fallot; *LAE*, left atrial enlargement; *LVE*, left ventricular enlargement; *L*, left; *RAE*, right atrial enlargement; *RVE*, right ventricular enlargement.

## Clinical Features

A left-to-right shunting PDA, discussed here, is by far the most common form; clinical features of reversed PDA are described on p. 165. The prevalence of PDA is higher in certain breeds of dogs, and a polygenic inheritance pattern is thought to be responsible (see Table 9-1). The incidence is approximately three times greater in female than male dogs. A PDA can be an isolated defect or it may occur in combination with other anomalies. Many animals with PDA are asymptomatic when first diagnosed, although reduced exercise ability, tachypnea, or cough is present in some cases. Characteristic physical examination findings include a continuous murmur heard best high at the left base (see p. 6), often with a precordial thrill, hyperkinetic (bounding, "waterhammer") arterial pulses, and pink mucous membranes.

## Diagnosis

Radiographic findings usually consist of cardiac elongation (left heart dilation), left atrial and auricular enlargement, and pulmonary overcirculation (Table 9-2). Often a bulge is evident in the descending aorta ("ductus bump") or main pulmonary trunk, or both (Fig. 9-3). The triad of all three bulges (i.e., pulmonary trunk, aorta, and left auricle), located in that order from the 1 to 3 o'clock position on a dorsoventral (DV) radiograph, is a classic finding but not always seen. There is also evidence of pulmonary edema in animals with left-sided heart failure. Characteristic ECG findings include wide P waves, tall R waves, and often, deep Q waves in leads II, aVF, and $CV_6LL$. Changes secondary to left ventricular enlargement may occur in the ST-T segment.

Echocardiography also shows left heart enlargement and dilation of the pulmonary trunk. Fractional shortening may be normal or decreased, and the E point–septal separation is often increased. The ductus itself may be difficult to visualize because of its location between the descending aorta and pulmonary artery. Views from the cranial left parasternal position are useful. Doppler studies document the presence of continuous, turbulent flow in the pulmonary artery (Fig. 9-4) and allow estimation of aortic to pulmonary artery pressure gradient. Cardiac catheterization is generally unnecessary, especially with the advent of Doppler echocardiography, unless an interventional procedure is planned. Catheterization findings include a higher oxygen content in the pulmonary artery than in the right ventricle (oxygen "step-up") and a wide aortic pressure pulse. Angiocardiography shows left-to-right shunting of opacified blood through the ductus (see Fig. 9-3, *C*).

## Treatment and Prognosis

Closure of the left-to-right ductus is recommended in affected animals, usually as soon as it is feasible. Surgical ligation, by one of several techniques, is successful in most cases, although a perioperative mortality of about 11% has been reported. Neither age nor weight appears to affect the outcome of surgery. Several methods of transcatheter PDA occlusion have also been described; these involve placement of wire coils with attached thrombogenic tufts or another vascular occluding device within the ductus. Vascular access is usually via the femoral artery, although some have used a venous approach to the ductus. Experience with and availability of transcatheter PDA occlusion are increasing; such techniques offer a much less invasive alternative to surgical ligation. However, not all cases are suitable for nonsurgical PDA closure. A normal life span can be expected after uncomplicated ductal closure. The concurrent mitral regurgitation usually resolves after ductus ligation or occlusion if the valve is structurally normal.

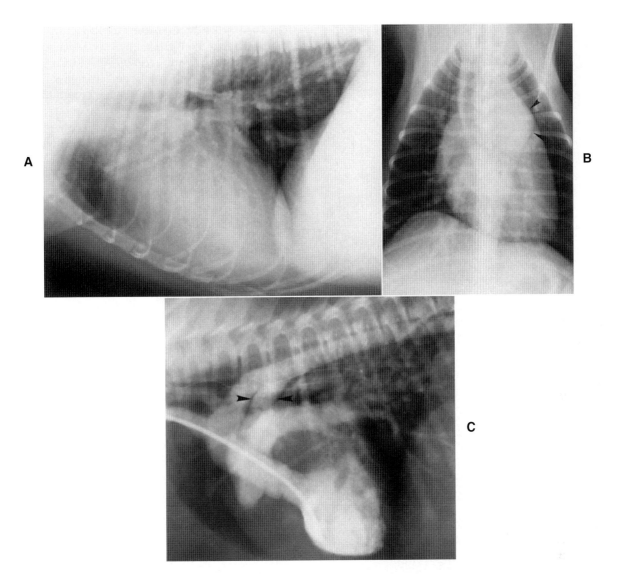

**FIG 9-3**
Lateral **(A)** and dorsoventral *(DV)* **(B)** radiographs from a dog with a patent ductus arteriosus. Note the large and elongated heart and prominent pulmonary vasculature. A large bulge is seen in the descending aorta on the DV view *(arrowheads* in **B**). **C,** Angiocardiogram obtained using a left ventricular injection outlines the left ventricle, aorta, patent ductus *(arrowheads),* and pulmonary artery.

Animals with congestive heart failure are treated with furosemide, an angiotensin-converting enzyme inhibitor, rest, and dietary sodium restriction (see Chapter 3). Digoxin is often used, because contractility tends to decline with time. Arrhythmias are treated as necessary.

If the ductus is not closed, the prognosis depends on the ductus size and the level of pulmonary vascular resistance. Congestive heart failure is the eventual outcome in most cases that do not undergo ductal closure. More than 50% of affected dogs die within the first year. In animals with pulmonary hypertension and shunt reversal, ductal closure is contraindicated because the ductus acts as a "pop-off" valve for the high right-sided pressures in these cases. Ductal ligation in animals with reversed PDA produces no improvement and promotes the onset of right ventricular failure.

## VENTRICULAR OUTFLOW OBSTRUCTIONS

Obstruction to ventricular outflow can occur at the semilunar valve, just below the valve (subvalvular), or above the valve in the proximal great vessel (supravalvular). Stenosis below the aortic valve (subaortic) is most common on the left side. On the right, malformations of the pulmonary valve itself are most common in dogs and cats; narrowing below the valve

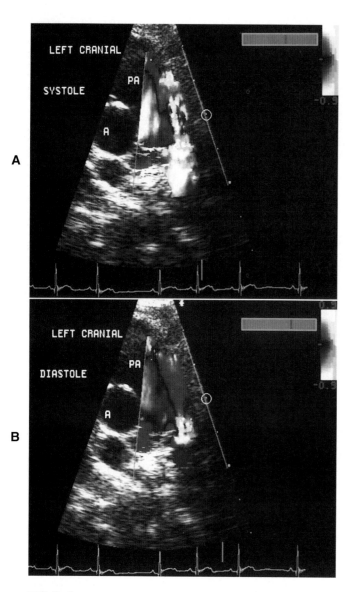

**FIG 9-4**
**A,** Continuous turbulent flow in the pulmonary artery is illustrated by this systolic and the following diastolic color flow Doppler frames from the left cranial parasternal position, optimized for the PA, in a 3-month-old female Keeshond. *A,* Ascending aorta; *PA,* main pulmonary artery. **B,** Turbulent flow in the pulmonary artery during diastole is illustrated by this color flow Doppler frame from the same dog and transducer position as in **A.** The diastolic flow disturbance in the PA is localized to the area where ductal flow enters from the descending aorta. *A,* Ascending aorta; *PA,* main pulmonary artery.

(infundibular area) resulting from muscular hypertrophy is a frequent accompaniment. Stenotic lesions impose a pressure overload on the affected ventricle, necessitating higher pressures and a slightly longer ejection time to move the stroke volume across the narrowed outlet. A systolic pressure gradient is then generated across the stenosis, and the magnitude of this gradient is related to the severity of the obstruction.

Concentric myocardial hypertrophy is the typical response to a systolic pressure overload, but some dilation of the af-

fected ventricle may also occur. Ventricular hypertrophy can impede diastolic filling (by increasing ventricular stiffness) or lead to secondary AV valve regurgitation. Heart failure results from high ventricular diastolic and atrial pressures. Cardiac arrhythmias also cause or contribute to the development of congestive failure. The combination of an outflow obstruction, paroxysmal arrhythmias, and/or inappropriate bradycardia secondary to ventricular baroreceptor stimulation can result in signs of low cardiac output. These are often associated with severe outflow tract obstruction and include exercise intolerance, syncope, and sudden death.

## SUBAORTIC STENOSIS

### Etiology and Pathophysiology

Subvalvular narrowing caused by a fibrous or fibromuscular ring is the most common type of aortic stenosis in dogs. SAS is thought to be inherited as an autosomal dominant trait with modifying genes that influence its phenotypic expression. The spectrum of SAS severity varies widely; three grades of SAS have been described in Newfoundland dogs. The mildest (grade I) is associated with no clinical signs or murmur, and only subtle subaortic fibrous tissue ridging is seen on postmortem examination. Dogs with moderate (grade II) SAS have only mild clinical and hemodynamic evidence of the disease and the postmortem finding of an incomplete fibrous ring below the aortic valve. Dogs with grade III SAS have severe disease and a complete fibrous ring around the outflow tract. Some cases have an elongated, tunnel-like obstruction. There may also be malformations of the mitral valve apparatus. Outflow tract narrowing and dynamic obstruction with or without a discrete subvalvular ridge have also been noted in Golden Retrievers. A dynamic left ventricular outflow tract obstruction may be important in other dogs as well. The obstructive lesion of SAS develops during the first several months of life, and there may be no audible murmur at an early age. In some dogs, no murmur is detected until 1 to 2 years of age, and the obstruction may continue to worsen beyond that age. Exercise or excitement generally increases the intensity of the murmur. Thus several factors make definitive diagnosis and genetic counseling to breeders problematic. SAS also occurs in cats; supravalvular lesions have been reported in this species as well.

The severity of the stenosis determines the degree of left ventricular pressure overload and resulting concentric hypertrophy. Coronary perfusion is easily compromised in animals with severe SAS. Capillary density may become inadequate as hypertrophy progresses, and high systolic wall tension with coronary narrowing can cause systolic flow to be reversed in small coronary arteries. These factors contribute to the development of myocardial ischemia and fibrosis. Clinical sequelae include arrhythmias, syncope, and sudden death. Many animals with SAS also have aortic or mitral valve regurgitation because of related malformations or secondary changes; this adds a volume overload to the left ventricle. Left-sided congestive heart failure results in some cases. Animals with SAS are predisposed to the development of aortic valve endocarditis because of jet lesion injury to the underside of the valve (see p. 146, and Fig. 8-4).

## Clinical Features

Certain larger breeds of dog are predisposed to this defect (see Table 9-1). A major challenge is the identification of subclinical and mildly affected carriers of the disease in the breeding population. Historical signs of fatigue, exercise intolerance or exertional weakness, syncope, or sudden death occur in about a third of dogs with SAS. With severe outflow obstruction, tachyarrhythmias or sudden reflex bradycardia and hypotension resulting from the activation of ventricular mechanoreceptors can cause low-output signs. Left-sided congestive heart failure can develop, usually in conjunction with concurrent mitral or aortic regurgitation, other cardiac malformations, or acquired endocarditis. Dyspnea is the most commonly reported sign in cats with SAS. Characteristic physical examination findings in dogs with moderate-to-severe stenosis include weak and late-rising femoral pulses *(pulsus parvus et tardus)*, a precordial thrill low on the left heart base, and the absence of a jugular pulse. There may be evidence of pulmonary edema or arrhythmias. A harsh systolic ejection murmur is heard at or below the aortic valve area on the left hemithorax. This murmur often radiates equally or more loudly to the right heart base because of the course of the aortic arch. Often the murmur is also heard over the carotid arteries, and it may even radiate to the calvarium. In mild cases a soft, poorly radiating ejection murmur at the left and sometimes right heart base may be the only abnormality noted during physical examination. Aortic regurgitation may produce a diastolic murmur at the left base or may be inaudible. Significant aortic regurgitation may cause the perceived arterial pulse strength to be increased.

## Diagnosis

Radiographic abnormalities (see Table 9-2) may be subtle, especially in dogs and cats with mild SAS. The left ventricle can appear normal or enlarged. A prominent cranial waist in the cardiac silhouette, especially on a lateral projection, and cranial mediastinal widening are manifestations of poststenotic dilation in the ascending aorta. The ECG is often normal, although there can be evidence of left ventricular hypertrophy (left axis deviation) or enlargement (tall complexes). Depression of the ST segment resulting from myocardial ischemia or changes secondary to hypertrophy may be present in leads II and aVF; exercise can induce further ischemic ST segment changes. Ventricular tachyarrhythmias are common.

Echocardiography reveals the extent of left ventricular hypertrophy and subaortic narrowing. A discrete ridge of tissue below the aortic valve is evident in many animals with moderate-to-severe disease (Fig. 9-5). Premature closure of the aortic valve, systolic anterior motion of the anterior mitral leaflet, and increased left ventricular subendocardial echogenicity (probably resulting from fibrosis) are common in animals with severe obstruction. Dilation of the ascending aorta and left atrial enlargement with hypertrophy may also be seen. Systolic turbulence originating below the aortic valve and extending into the aorta, as well as high peak systolic

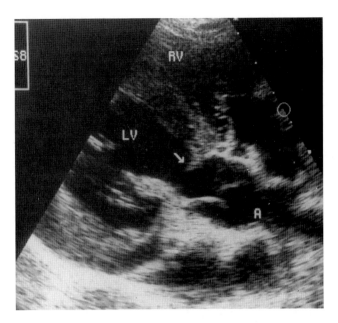

**FIG 9-5**
Echocardiogram from a 6-month-old German Shepherd Dog with severe subaortic stenosis. Note the discrete ridge of tissue *(arrow)* below the aortic valve creating a fixed outflow tract obstruction. *A,* Aorta; *LV,* left ventricle; *RV,* right ventricle.

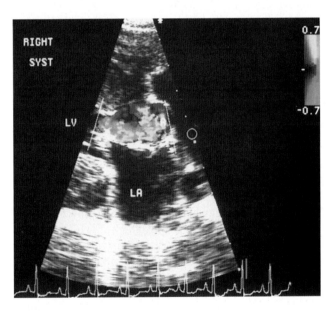

**FIG 9-6**
Color flow Doppler frame taken in systole from the right parasternal view of the left ventricular outflow tract in a 1-year-old Dalmatian with severe subaortic stenosis. Note the turbulent flow pattern (coded green and yellow) beginning in the outflow tract well below the aortic valve, as well as the thickened septum and left ventricular free wall. *A,* Aortic root; *LA,* left atrium; *LV,* area of the left ventricle.

outflow velocities, can be identified using Doppler echocardiography (Fig. 9-6). Many animals also show some degree of aortic or mitral regurgitation in color flow and spectral Doppler studies. Spectral Doppler studies are used to estimate the severity of the stenosis. Doppler-estimated systolic pressure gradients in unanesthetized animals are usually 40% to 50% higher than those recorded during cardiac catheterization, which is done under anesthesia. Peak estimated gradients of more than 100 to 125 mm Hg are associated with severe stenosis. The left ventricular outflow tract should be interrogated from more than one position to achieve the best possible alignment with blood flow. The subcostal (subxiphoid) position usually yields the highest velocity signals, although the left apical position may be better for this in some animals. Normal or equivocal M-mode and 2-D echocardiographic findings may be encountered in mildly affected animals. Likewise, the Doppler-estimated aortic outflow velocity may be equivocal in animals with mild SAS, especially if Doppler beam alignment with the left ventricular outflow is suboptimal. With optimal alignment, aortic root velocities of less than 1.7 m/sec are considered normal in unsedated dogs; velocities exceeding 2.0 to 2.2 m/sec are abnormal. Peak velocities between these values may indicate the presence of mild SAS, especially if there is other evidence of disease, such as disturbed flow in the outflow tract or ascending aorta and aortic regurgitation. A limitation of using the estimated pressure gradient to assess severity of outflow obstruction is the dependence of this gradient on blood flow. Factors causing sympathetic stimulation and increased cardiac output (e.g., excitement, exercise, fever) will increase outflow velocities, whereas myocardial failure, cardiodepressant drugs, and other causes of reduced stroke volume will decrease recorded velocities. Recently, calculation of an indexed effective orifice area of the left ventricular outflow tract obstruction has been proposed as a way to address this concern (Belanger and colleagues, 2001). Cardiac catheterization and angiocardiography are currently used less commonly to diagnose or quantify the defect, but they are used in conjunction with balloon dilation of the stenotic area.

## Treatment and Prognosis

Various surgical techniques have been used to reduce an outflow obstruction in dogs with severe SAS; however, surgical palliation of this defect is difficult. Cardiopulmonary bypass and open-heart surgery are necessary to directly reach the lesion. Although surgical resection of the stenotic membrane can significantly reduce the left ventricular systolic pressure gradient and possibly improve exercise ability, no improvement in long-term survival was found compared to dogs not undergoing the procedure (Orton, 2000). Transcatheter balloon dilation of the stenotic area has reduced the measured gradient in some dogs, but partial restenosis may develop with time. Likewise, no survival benefit has been documented with this procedure.

β-Adrenergic blockers have been advocated to reduce the myocardial oxygen demand and minimize the frequency and severity of arrhythmias. Animals with a high pressure gradient, marked ST segment depression, frequent ventricular premature beats, or a history of syncope may be more likely to benefit from this therapy. Whether β-blockers prolong survival is unclear. Exercise should be restricted in animals with moderate-to-severe SAS. Prophylactic antibiotic therapy is indicated for dogs and cats with SAS prior to procedures with the potential to cause bacteremia (e.g., dentistry).

The prognosis in dogs and cats with severe stenosis (catheterization pressure gradient of more than 80 mm Hg or a Doppler gradient of more than 100 to 125 mm Hg) is guarded. More than 50% of severely affected dogs die suddenly before the age of 3 years (Kienle and colleagues, 1994). The overall prevalence of sudden death in dogs with SAS appears to be just over 20%. Infective endocarditis and congestive heart failure may be more likely to develop later. Atrial and ventricular arrhythmias and worsened mitral regurgitation are complicating factors. Dogs with mild stenosis (e.g., a catheterization gradient of less than 35 mm Hg or a Doppler gradient of less than 60 to 70 mm Hg) are more likely to be asymptomatic and live longer.

## PULMONIC STENOSIS

### Etiology and Pathophysiology

Although some cases of pulmonic stenosis result from simple fusion of the valve cusps, dysplasia of the pulmonic valve is more common. Dysplastic valves have variably thickened, asymmetric, and partially fused valve leaflets with a hypoplastic valve annulus. Right ventricular hypertrophy and secondary dilation result. Severe ventricular hypertrophy can promote the development of myocardial ischemia and its sequelae. The high-velocity blood flow across the stenotic valve creates turbulence in the main pulmonary trunk and a post-stenotic dilation of this area. Right atrial dilation resulting from secondary tricuspid insufficiency and an increased right ventricular filling pressure predisposes to the development of atrial arrhythmias and congestive failure. The combination of PS and a patent foramen ovale or ASD can result in right-to-left shunting at the atrial level; however, this is rare in dogs and cats. A single anomalous coronary artery, thought to contribute to the development of outflow obstruction, has been described in association with PS in some English Bulldogs and a Boxer. In such cases, palliative surgical procedures and balloon valvuloplasty have caused death secondary to transection or avulsion of the major left coronary branch.

### Clinical Features

PS is more common in small breeds of dogs (see Table 9-1). Many dogs with PS are asymptomatic at the time of diagnosis, although signs of right-sided congestive failure or a history of exercise intolerance or syncope may exist. However, even in animals with considerable stenosis, these signs may not develop until the animal is several years old. Physical examination findings characteristic of moderate-to-severe stenosis include a prominent right precordial impulse, a thrill high at the left base, normal to slightly diminished femoral pulses, pink mucous membranes, and, occasionally, jugular pulses. On auscultation, a systolic ejection murmur is best heard high at the left base. The murmur may radiate cranioventrally and to the right in some cases but usually is not heard over the carotid arteries. An early systolic click is sometimes identified and probably results from abrupt checking of a fused valve at the onset of ejection. The murmur of secondary tricuspid insufficiency may also be heard, and arrhythmias may be present in some cases.

## Diagnosis

Radiographic findings typically seen in animals with PS are outlined in Table 9-2. Marked right ventricular hypertrophy often causes the cardiac apex to be shifted to the left and dorsad. The heart may appear as a "reverse D" shape on a DV or ventrodorsal (VD) view. A variably sized pulmonary trunk bulge (poststenotic dilation) is best seen at the 1 o'clock position on a DV or VD view (Fig. 9-7), but the size of the post-

stenotic dilation does not correlate with the severity of the pressure gradient. Dilation of the caudal vena cava is also seen in some animals.

ECG features include a right ventricular hypertrophy pattern, right axis deviation, and sometimes a right atrial enlargement pattern (P pulmonale) or tachyarrhythmias. Echocardiographic findings characteristic of moderate-to-severe stenosis include right ventricular hypertrophy and enlargement. The interventricular septum often appears flattened as the high right ventricular pressure pushes it toward the left (Fig. 9-8, *A*). Right atrial enlargement is frequently seen. A thickened, asymmetric, or otherwise malformed pulmonic

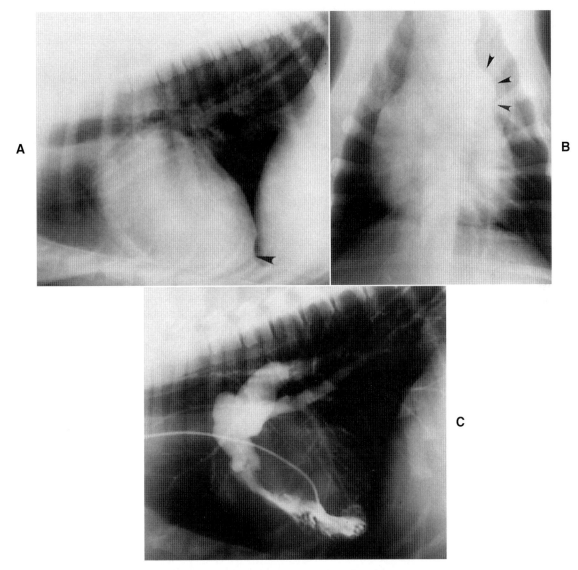

**FIG 9-7**
Lateral **(A)** and dorsoventral *(DV)* **(B)** radiographs from a dog with pulmonic stenosis, showing right ventricular enlargement (apex elevation on lateral view [*arrowheads* in **A**] and reverse D configuration on DV view) along with a pulmonary trunk bulge (*arrowheads* in **B**) seen on a DV view. **C,** An angiocardiogram using a selective right ventricular injection demonstrates poststenotic dilation of the main pulmonary trunk and pulmonary arteries. The thickened pulmonic valve is closed in this diastolic frame.

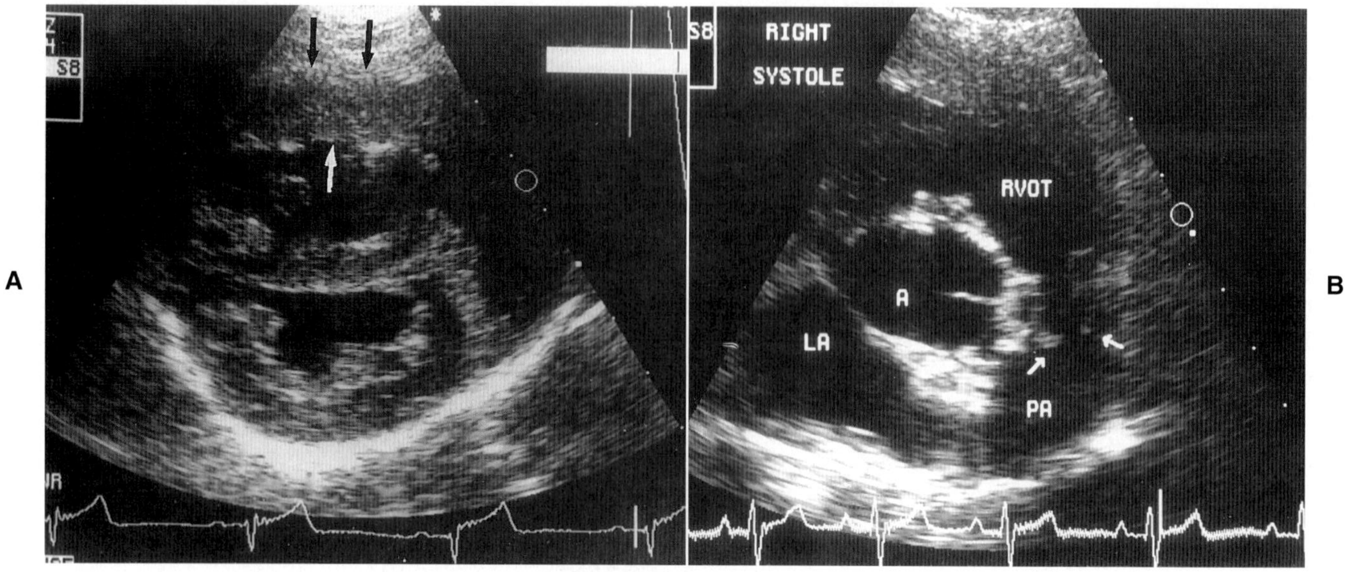

**FIG 9-8**
Echocardiograms from two dogs with severe pulmonic stenosis. **A,** A right parasternal short-axis view at the ventricular level in a 4-month-old male Samoyed shows right ventricular hypertrophy *(arrows)* and enlargement; high right ventricular pressure flattens the septum toward the left in this diastolic frame. **B,** Thickened, fused leaflets and systolic doming of the malformed pulmonary valve *(arrows)* are seen in this 10-month-old male English Bulldog. *A,* Aorta; *LA,* left atrium; *PA,* pulmonary artery; *RVOT,* right ventricular outflow tract.

valve usually can be identified (Fig. 9-8, *B*), although the outflow area may be narrow and difficult to visualize clearly. Poststenotic dilation of the main pulmonary trunk may also be appreciated. Pleural effusion and prominent right heart dilation often accompany secondary congestive failure. Paradoxical septal motion may be noted in such cases as well. Doppler echocardiographic evaluation along with anatomic findings can provide an estimate of lesion severity. The pressure gradient across the stenotic valve, the right heart filling pressure, and anatomic features can also be determined by cardiac catheterization and angiocardiography. Again, Doppler-estimated systolic pressure gradients in unanesthetized animals are usually 40% to 50% higher than those recorded during cardiac catheterization. PS is generally considered mild if the Doppler-derived gradient is less than 50 mm Hg and severe if it exceeds (80 to) 100 mm Hg.

## Treatment and Prognosis

The palliation of severe and sometimes moderate stenosis by balloon valvuloplasty is recommended, especially if infundibular hypertrophy is not excessive. Although it is unclear whether intervention truly improves long-term survival, it has reduced or eliminated clinical signs in severely affected animals. Balloon valvuloplasty is done in conjunction with cardiac catheterization and involves dilating the stenotic valve using a specially designed balloon catheter. The procedure is more likely to be successful in dogs with simple fusion of the pulmonic valve cusps. However, most dogs with PS have dysplastic valves, which are more difficult to dilate effectively. Various surgical procedures have been used to palliate moderate-

to-severe PS in dogs as well. Usually balloon valvuloplasty is attempted before surgical procedures because it is thought to be less risky. However, in animals with a single anomalous coronary artery, all these procedures are contraindicated. Normal coronary anatomy can be verified using echocardiography or angiography.

Exercise restriction is generally recommended, especially for animals with moderate-to-severe stenosis. A β-blocker may be helpful if right ventricular infundibular hypertrophy is prominent. Signs of congestive heart failure are managed medically. The prognosis in animals with PS is variable and depends on the severity of the stenosis. Those with mild PS may have a normal life span, but animals with severe stenosis often die within 3 years of diagnosis. Sudden death or the onset of congestive heart failure is common. The prognosis is considerably worse in animals that also have tricuspid regurgitation, atrial fibrillation or other tachyarrhythmias, or congestive heart failure.

## INTRACARDIAC SHUNTS

The volume of blood flow across an intracardiac shunt is related to the size of the defect and the pressure gradient across it. In most cases, blood flows from left to right and causes pulmonary overcirculation. Therefore blood volume and cardiac output increase in response to the partial diversion of blood away from the systemic circulation. The side of the heart doing the most work becomes volume overloaded. If right heart pressures increase as a result of pulmonary hypertension or a concurrent PS, shunt flow may equilibrate or reverse (i.e., become right to left).

## VENTRICULAR SEPTAL DEFECT

### Etiology and Pathophysiology

Most VSDs are located high in the membranous part of the septum, just below the aortic valve on the left and under the septal tricuspid leaflet on the right; however, they can also occur in other locations in the interventricular septum. In cats especially, a VSD may be part of an endocardial cushion defect (see p. 151). VSDs impose a volume overload on the lungs, left atrium, left ventricle, and right ventricular outflow tract. Small defects may be clinically insignificant. However, moderate-to-large defects tend to cause the left heart, which does most of the work, to dilate; left-sided congestive heart failure can result. Very large VSDs cause both ventricles to function as a common chamber and induce right ventricular dilation and hypertrophy. Secondary pulmonary hypertension is more likely to develop in animals with very large shunts. Aortic regurgitation resulting from diastolic valve leaflet prolapse occurs in some animals with VSD. Presumably this happens because the deformed septum provides inadequate anatomic support for the aortic root. Depending on the regurgitant volume, a significant additional hemodynamic burden may be placed on the left ventricle.

### Clinical Features

Exercise intolerance and evidence of left-sided congestive failure are the most common clinical manifestations of VSD, although many animals are asymptomatic at the time of diagnosis. Characteristic physical examination findings include a holosystolic murmur heard loudest at the cranial right sternal border (corresponding to the direction of shunt flow). A large shunt volume can cause relative or functional PS with a systolic ejection murmur at the left base. If the VSD is associated with aortic regurgitation, a corresponding diastolic decrescendo murmur may be heard at the left base.

### Diagnosis

The radiographic findings in animals with a VSD vary (see Table 9-2). Large shunts cause left heart enlargement and pulmonary overcirculation. However, right ventricular enlargement occurs in the presence of large shunts and increased pulmonary vascular resistance. A large shunt volume may also cause the main pulmonary trunk to be prominent. The ECG may be normal or suggestive of left atrial or ventricular enlargement; in some cases, the presence of disturbed intraventricular conduction is indicated by the finding of "fractionated" or splintered QRS complexes. The finding of a right ventricular enlargement pattern usually indicates the presence of a very large defect, pulmonary hypertension, a right ventricular outflow tract obstruction, or an endocardial cushion defect, although it may also result from a right bundle branch block.

Echocardiography reveals left heart dilation (with or without right ventricular dilation) in dogs and cats with large

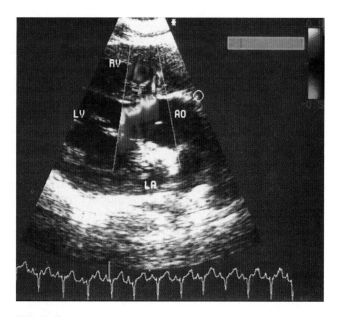

**FIG 9-9**
Color flow Doppler frame in early systole from the right parasternal view of the left ventricular outflow tract. A small, membranous ventricular septal defect is illustrated by the turbulent flow pattern from LV to RV just below the aorta *(green arrow)* in this 3-month-old Sharpei. *AO,* Aortic root; *LA,* left atrium; *LV,* left ventricle; *RV,* right ventricle.

shunts. Larger defects usually can be visualized just below the aortic valve in the right parasternal long-axis plane, optimized for the left ventricular outflow tract. The septal tricuspid leaflet is located to the right of the defect. Sometimes echo "dropout" occurs at the thin membranous septum, mimicking a VSD. Suspected defects should be scanned in more than one plane and the animal carefully examined to determine whether there is supporting clinical evidence and a murmur. Doppler (or echo-contrast) studies usually demonstrate the shunt flow (Fig. 9-9).

Cardiac catheterization, oximetry, and angiocardiography allow measurement of intracardiac pressures, can indicate the presence of an oxygen step-up at the level of the right ventricular outflow tract, and can show the pathway of abnormal blood flow.

### Treatment and Prognosis

Dogs and cats with a small-to-moderate defect can have a relatively normal life span. Occasionally, the defect closes spontaneously within the first 2 years of life. Closure can result from myocardial hypertrophy around the VSD or a seal formed by the septal tricuspid leaflet or a prolapsed aortic leaflet. Left-sided congestive heart failure is likely to develop in animals with a large septal defect, although pulmonary hypertension with shunt reversal develops in some instead, usually at an early age.

Definitive therapy for VSD requires cardiopulmonary bypass or hypothermia and intracardiac surgery. Large left-to-right shunts are sometimes palliated by placing a constrictive band around the pulmonary trunk to create a mild supravalvular PS. This causes right ventricular systolic pressure to rise in response to the increased outflow resistance. Consequently, less blood shunts from left to right ventricles. Obviously, however, an excessively tight band can cause right-to-left shunting (functionally analogous to a T of F). Animals in which left-sided heart failure develops are managed medically. Palliative surgery should not be attempted in the presence of pulmonary hypertension and shunt reversal.

## ATRIAL SEPTAL DEFECT

High ASDs (ostium secundum) are more common in dogs; defects low in the interatrial septum (ostium primum) are likely to be part of the endocardial cushion defect complex in cats. Sinus venosus–type defects are rare; these are located high in the atrial septum near the entry of the cranial vena cava. ASDs are often associated with other cardiac anomalies. In most cases, blood shunts from the left to the right atrium, resulting in a volume overload to the right heart. If PS or pulmonary hypertension is also present, right-to-left shunting and cyanosis may occur.

### Clinical Features

The clinical history for animals with an ASD is usually rather nonspecific. Physical examination findings may be unremarkable in a dog or cat with an isolated ASD, whereas large left-to-right shunts are associated with a murmur indicative of relative PS and fixed splitting of the second heart sound ($S_2$) (i.e., no respiratory variation). Rarely a soft diastolic murmur indicative of relative tricuspid stenosis may be audible.

### Diagnosis

Radiographically, right heart enlargement with or without pulmonary trunk dilation is found in animals with severe shunts (see Table 9-2). Pulmonary circulation may appear to be increased unless high pulmonary resistance has developed. The left heart is not enlarged unless another defect such as mitral insufficiency is present. The ECG may be normal, or it may show right ventricular and atrial enlargement patterns. Cats with an endocardial cushion defect may have right ventricular enlargement and a left axis deviation.

Echocardiography may show the presence of right atrial and ventricular dilation, with or without paradoxical interventricular septal motion. Large ASDs can be visualized, although the thinner fossa ovalis region of the interatrial septum can be confused with a septal defect because echo dropout also occurs here. Doppler echocardiography may identify smaller shunts that cannot be visualized on 2-D examination. Cardiac catheterization may show an oxygen step-up at the level of the right atrium, and the shunt may be delineated after the injection of contrast material into the pulmonary artery.

### Treatment and Prognosis

Large shunts can be treated surgically, similarly to VSDs. Otherwise, animals are managed medically if congestive heart failure develops. The prognosis is variable and depends on the shunt size, whether other defects are present, and the animal's pulmonary vascular resistance.

## ATRIOVENTRICULAR VALVE MALFORMATIONS

### MITRAL DYSPLASIA

Congenital malformations of the mitral valve apparatus include shortened or overly elongated chordae tendineae, direct attachment of the valve cusp to a papillary muscle, thickened or cleft or shortened valve cusps, prolapse of valve leaflets, upwardly displaced or malformed papillary muscles, and excessive dilation of the valve annulus. Mitral valve dysplasia is most common in large-breed dogs and also occurs in cats (see Table 9-1). Valvular regurgitation is the predominant functional abnormality, and it may be severe. The pathophysiology and sequelae are usually the same as those in animals with acquired mitral regurgitation (see p. 139).

Stenosis of the mitral valve orifice is uncommon and coexists with regurgitation. Obstruction to ventricular filling increases the left atrial pressure and can precipitate the development of pulmonary edema.

Except for the young age of the affected animal, the clinical signs seen in most animals with mitral dysplasia are similar to those seen in older dogs with severe degenerative mitral valve disease. Exercise intolerance, respiratory signs of left-sided congestive heart failure, anorexia, and atrial arrhythmias (especially atrial fibrillation) commonly develop in such animals. The systolic murmur of mitral regurgitation is heard at the left apex.

The radiographic, ECG, echocardiographic, and catheterization findings are similar to those seen in patients with severe acquired mitral insufficiency. Echocardiography can identify specific malformations of the mitral apparatus.

Therapy consists of medical management of the signs of congestive heart failure. The prognosis is poor. Surgical valve reconstruction or replacement may be possible.

### TRICUSPID DYSPLASIA

The malformations of the tricuspid valve and its support structures in animals with tricuspid dysplasia are similar to those seen in animals with mitral valve dysplasia. In some cases the tricuspid valve is displaced ventrally into the ventricle (an Ebstein-like anomaly). The prevalence of ventricular preexcitation (Wolff-Parkinson-White syndrome) may be increased in such animals. Tricuspid dysplasia is most frequently diagnosed in large-breed dogs; it may occur more often in males. The pathophysiologic features are the same as those of severe acquired tricuspid regurgitation. Progressive increases in right atrial and ventricular end-diastolic pressures eventually result in right-sided congestive failure. Tricuspid stenosis is rare.

The historical signs and clinical findings are similar to those seen in dogs with advanced degenerative tricuspid disease. Initially the animal may be asymptomatic or mildly exercise intolerant. However, exercise intolerance, abdominal

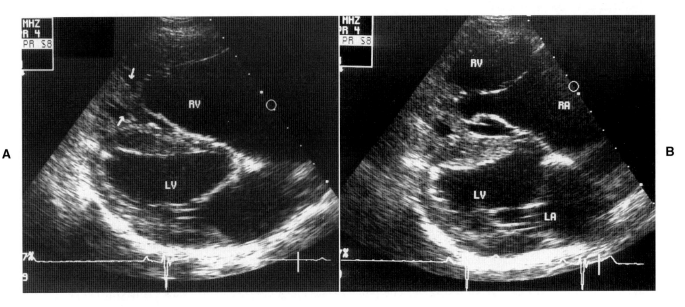

**FIG 9-10**

Right parasternal long-axis echocardiogram from a 1-year-old male Labrador Retriever with tricuspid valve dysplasia in diastole **(A)** and systole **(B).** The valve annulus appears to be ventrally displaced; the leaflet tips are tethered to a malformed, wide papillary muscle (*arrows* in **A**). Wide leaflet tip separation in systole **(B)** caused severe tricuspid regurgitation and clinical congestive heart failure. *LA,* Left atrium; *LV,* left ventricle; *RA,* right atrium; *RV,* right ventricle.

distention resulting from ascites, dyspnea resulting from pleural effusion, anorexia, and cardiac cachexia frequently develop. Physical examination features include the murmur of tricuspid regurgitation (not always audible) and jugular vein pulsations. Jugular vein distention, muffled heart and lung sounds, and ballotable abdominal fluid are present in animals with congestive heart failure.

Right atrial and ventricular enlargement is visible radiographically. The heart shadow may be quite round, similar to that seen with pericardial effusion or dilated cardiomyopathy. Distention of the caudal vena cava, pleural or peritoneal effusion, or hepatomegaly is often evident. The ECG usually shows right ventricular and occasionally right atrial enlargement patterns; a splintered QRS complex appearance is common. Atrial arrhythmias, including atrial fibrillation, may also be noted. Evidence for ventricular preexcitation is sometimes seen. Echocardiography depicts the often massive right heart dilation. Malformations of the valve apparatus can also be appreciated in multiple views (Fig. 9-10), although the left parasternal apical four-chamber view appears to be especially useful. Intracardiac electrocardiography is necessary to confirm the presence of Ebstein's anomaly, which is suggested by displacement of the tricuspid valve toward the right ventricle. Although this is rarely done, a ventricular electrogram recorded in the atrium above the tricuspid valve is diagnostic.

Congestive heart failure and arrhythmias are managed medically. Periodic thoracocentesis has been helpful in some animals with heart failure and pleural effusion that cannot be controlled with medication and diet. The prognosis is guarded to poor, especially if there is marked cardiomegaly. However, some dogs survive for several years.

## CARDIAC ANOMALIES CAUSING CYANOSIS

Cardiac malformations that allow unoxygenated blood to reach the systemic circulation result in hypoxemia. Visible cyanosis occurs when there are at least 5 g/dl of desaturated hemoglobin. Arterial hypoxemia stimulates the increased production of red blood cells and the development of polycythemia, which represents the body's attempt to carry more oxygen. However, blood viscosity and resistance to flow rise with the increases in the PCV. Severe polycythemia (a PCV of more than 65% or so) can cause microvascular sludging and poor tissue oxygenation, intravascular thrombosis, hemorrhage, stroke, and cardiac arrhythmias. A PCV of more than 80% develops in some animals. The possibility of a venous embolus crossing the shunt to the systemic circulation poses another danger in these cases. Some collateral blood flow to the lungs develops from the bronchial arteries of the systemic circulation. These small tortuous vessels may cause the overall radiographic opacity of the central pulmonary fields to be increased.

Anomalies that most commonly cause cyanosis in dogs and cats are T of F and pulmonary arterial hypertension secondary to a large PDA, VSD, or ASD. Other complex but uncommon anomalies, such as transposition of the great vessels or truncus arteriosus, also cause unoxygenated blood to reach the systemic circulation. Physical exertion tends to exacerbate right-to-left shunting and cyanosis because peripheral vascular resistance decreases with greater skeletal muscle blood flow. Despite the pressure overload on the right heart, congestive failure is rare, because the shunt provides a "pop-off" valve.

# TETRALOGY OF FALLOT

## Etiology and Pathophysiology

The anomalies that occur in T of F consist of VSD, PS, dextropositioning of the aorta, and right ventricular hypertrophy. The VSD is often quite large. The PS may involve the valve or infundibular area; sometimes the pulmonary artery is hypoplastic or atretic. The rightward shift of the aortic root causes it to override the interventricular septum and facilitates right ventricular-to-aortic shunting. Aortic anomalies also occur in some animals.

Right ventricular hypertrophy is secondary to the pressure overloads imposed by the PS and systemic arterial circulation. The volume of blood the right ventricle pumps into the aorta (by way of the VSD) depends on the degree of outflow resistance caused by the fixed PS compared with the degree of systemic arterial resistance, which can vary. A large volume may shunt from right to left, especially in response to exercise or other causes of decreased arterial resistance. The pulmonary vascular resistance is normal in animals with T of F.

## Clinical Features

A polygenic inheritance pattern for T of F has been identified in the Keeshond, although the defect also occurs in other dog breeds and in cats. A history of syncope, exertional weakness, dyspnea, cyanosis, and stunted growth is common. Physical examination findings vary with the relative severity of the disease components. Although cyanosis is seen at rest in some animals, others have pink mucous membranes; yet, cyanosis usually becomes evident with exercise in these animals. The precordial impulse on the right chest wall may be of equal intensity or stronger than that on the left. A precordial thrill may be palpable at the right sternal border or left basilar area, but this is an inconsistent finding. Jugular pulsation may be noted. Auscultation may reveal a holosystolic murmur at the right sternal border compatible with a VSD, or a systolic ejection murmur at the left base compatible with PS, or both. However, some animals have no audible murmur because the hyperviscosity associated with polycythemia diminishes blood turbulence and, therefore, murmur intensity.

## Diagnosis

Thoracic radiographs depict variable cardiomegaly, usually of the right heart (see Table 9-2). The pulmonary artery may appear small, although occasionally a bulge is evident. Pulmonary vascular markings are usually reduced, although a compensatory enhancement of the bronchial circulation will cause the overall pulmonary opacity to be increased. The malpositioned aorta appears to bulge cranially on lateral views. The thick right ventricle displaces the left heart dorsally, simulating left heart enlargement. The ECG typically indicates the presence of right ventricular hypertrophy, although a left axis deviation is occasionally seen in affected cats.

Echocardiography can show the VSD, a large aortic root shifted rightward and overriding the ventricular septum, some degree of PS, and right ventricular hypertrophy. Doppler studies reveal the right-to-left shunt and high-velocity stenotic pulmonary outflow jet. An echo-contrast study also can document the right-to-left shunt.

## Treatment and Prognosis

Definitive surgical repair of T of F requires open-heart surgery. Palliative procedures can increase pulmonary blood flow by surgically creating a left-to-right shunt. Anastomosis of a subclavian artery to the pulmonary artery and the creation of a window between the ascending aorta and pulmonary artery are two techniques that have been used successfully.

Periodic phlebotomy is recommended for dogs and cats with severe polycythemia and clinical signs associated with hyperviscosity (e.g., weakness, shortness of breath, seizures). A volume of blood is withdrawn (and sometimes replaced with isotonic fluid) to maintain the PCV at a level where clinical signs are minimal (see p. 166). Further reduction in the PCV can exacerbate signs of hypoxia. Alternatively, hydroxyurea might be tried to manage the polycythemia (see p. 1171). Some dogs with T of F are helped symptomatically by the use of β-adrenergic blockers. Although the exact mechanism of action in this setting is not clear, reductions in sympathetic tone, right ventricular contractility, right ventricular (muscular) outflow obstruction, and myocardial oxygen consumption, along with an increase in peripheral vascular resistance, are thought to be the benefits of β-blocker therapy in children with the disease. Exercise restriction is also important. Systemic vasodilating drugs should not be given.

The prognosis in animals with T of F depends on the degree of PS and polycythemia. Mildly affected animals or those that have undergone successful palliative surgical shunting procedures may live for about 4 to 7 years. However, progressive hypoxemia, polycythemia, and sudden death at an earlier age are common.

# PULMONARY HYPERTENSION WITH SHUNT REVERSAL

## Etiology and Pathophysiology

Pulmonary hypertension develops in a relatively small percentage of dogs and cats with shunts. The congenital lesions that are usually associated with the development of pulmonary hypertension are PDA, VSD, an endocardial cushion defect or a common AV canal, ASD, and an aorticopulmonary window. Normally the low-resistance pulmonary vascular system can accept a large increase in blood flow without pulmonary arterial pressure increasing significantly. It is not clear why pulmonary hypertension develops in some animals, but the associated defect in such animals is usually large. The normally high fetal pulmonary resistance may not regress in these animals, or their pulmonary vascular system may react abnormally to initially high left-to-right shunt flow. In any case, irreversible histologic changes develop that increase vascular resistance in the pulmonary arteries. These include intimal thickening, medial hypertrophy, and characteristic plexiform lesions. As pulmonary vascular resistance rises, pulmonary artery pressure increases and the volume of blood shunted from left to right diminishes. If right heart and pulmonary pressures exceed those of the systemic circulation, the shunt reverses direction and unoxygenated blood flows into the aorta. It appears these changes develop before the animal reaches 6 months of age, although exceptions may occur. The term *Eisenmenger's physiology* refers to the severe pulmonary hypertension and shunt reversal that develop.

Right-to-left shunts caused by pulmonary hypertension cause pathophysiologic and clinical sequelae similar to those produced by T of F. The major difference is that the impediment to pulmonary flow occurs at the level of the pulmonary arterioles rather than at the pulmonic valve. Hypoxemia, right ventricular hypertrophy and enlargement, polycythemia and its consequences, increased shunting with exercise, and cyanosis can occur. Likewise, right-sided congestive failure is uncommon but may develop in response to secondary myocardial failure or tricuspid insufficiency. The right-to-left shunt may allow venous emboli to cross into the arterial system, resulting in stroke or other arterial embolization.

## Clinical Features

The history and clinical presentation of animals with pulmonary hypertension and shunt reversal are similar to those associated with T of F. Exercise intolerance, shortness of breath, syncope (especially with exercise or excitement), seizures, and sudden death are common. Cough and hemoptysis may also occur. Cyanosis may be evident only during exercise or excitement. Classically, cyanosis of the caudal mucous membranes alone (differential cyanosis) is caused by reversed PDA. In this case, normally oxygenated blood flows to the cranial body by way of the brachycephalic trunk and left subclavian artery (from the aortic arch), whereas the rest of the body receives desaturated blood through the ductus, located in the descending aorta (Fig. 9-11, *B*). Rear limb weakness is an accompanying clinical sign in animals with reversed PDA. Intracardiac shunts cause equally intense cyanosis throughout the body.

A murmur typical of the underlying defect or defects may be present. However, often no murmur or only a very soft systolic murmur is heard because of the increased viscosity of the blood resulting from polycythemia. There is no continuous murmur with reversed PDA. In pulmonary hypertension, the $S_2$ may be loud and "snapping" or split. A gallop sound is occasionally heard. Other subtle physical examination findings include a pronounced right precordial impulse and jugular pulsations.

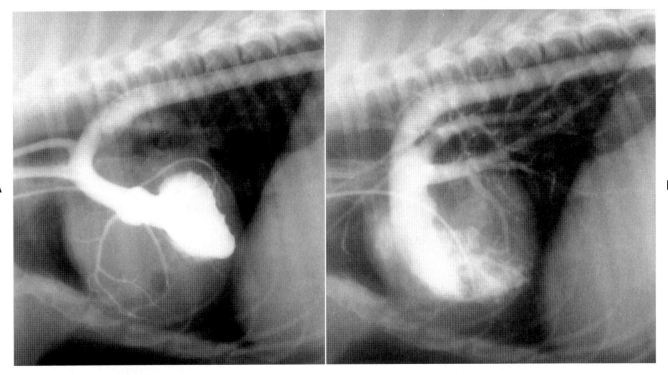

**FIG 9-11**
Angiocardiograms from an 8-month-old female Cocker Spaniel with patent ductus arteriosus, pulmonary hypertension, and shunt reversal. The left ventricular injection **(A)** shows the dorsal displacement of the left ventricle by the enlarged right ventricle. Note the diluted appearance of radiographic contrast solution in the descending aorta (mixed with nonopacified blood from the ductus) and the prominent right coronary artery. The right ventricular injection **(B)** illustrates the right ventricular hypertrophy and pulmonary trunk dilation secondary to severe pulmonary hypertension. Opacified blood courses through a large ductus into the descending aorta.

## Diagnosis

Thoracic radiographs often reveal right heart enlargement, a prominent pulmonary trunk, and tortuous, proximally widened pulmonary arteries. A bulge in the descending aorta may be seen in dogs with reversed PDA. The left heart in animals with a reversed PDA or VSD may be enlarged as well. The ECG usually indicates the existence of right ventricular and sometimes right atrial enlargement, with a right axis deviation. The echocardiogram substantiates the right ventricular hypertrophy and may reveal the anatomic defect and a widened pulmonary trunk. Doppler or an echo-contrast study can confirm the presence of an intracardiac right-to-left shunt. Reversed PDA flow can be shown by imaging the abdominal aorta during venous echo-contrast injection. Measurement of the peak velocity of a pulmonic or tricuspid regurgitation jet, if present, allows the estimation of pulmonary artery or right ventricular (and in the absence of PS, pulmonary artery) pressures, respectively. Cardiac catheterization findings can confirm the diagnosis and quantify the pulmonary hypertension and systemic hypoxemia (see Fig. 9-11).

## Treatment and Prognosis

Therapy has been limited mainly to exercise restriction and periodic phlebotomy to minimize signs of hyperviscosity. To manage this secondary polycythemia, RBC mass reduction to maintain the PCV at about 62% has previously been recommended. Removal of 5 to 10 ml blood/kg body weight and replacement with an equal volume of isotonic fluid can accomplish this. However, it is questionable whether the PCV alone should be used to guide treatment. Phlebotomy done only upon recurrence of physical manifestations of hyperviscosity (such as rear limb weakness, shortness of breath, or lethargy) is reasonable and was successful in several recently reported reversed PDA cases (Cote and colleague, 2001). In the technique described, 10% of the patient's circulating blood volume was removed initially without replacement fluids. This volume (in milliliters) was calculated as 8.5% × body weight (kg) × 1000 g/kg × 1 ml/g. After 3 to 6 hours of cage rest, an additional volume of blood was removed if the patient's initial PCV was over 60%. As described by Cote and Ettinger, an additional 5% to 10% of circulating blood volume was removed if the PCV was 60% to 70%, or an additional 10% to 18% was withdrawn if the initial PCV was over 70%. Preliminary experience using chronic hydroxyurea therapy (40 to 50 mg/kg PO q48h or 3×/week) suggests this may be a useful alternative to periodic phlebotomy (Moore and colleague, 2001) (see Chapter 86, Erythrocytosis). A CBC and platelet count should be monitored weekly or biweekly to start. A target PCV between 54% and 60% is suggested. Possible adverse effects include anorexia, vomiting, bone marrow hypoplasia, alopecia, and pruritus. The dose can be divided and given twice a day on treatment days, or administered twice a week, or given at a dosage of less than 40 mg/kg, depending on the patient's response. Surgical closure of the shunt is contraindicated. Vasodilating drugs tend to have systemic effects that are equal to or greater than their effects on the pulmonary arterial system, therefore they are of little benefit and possibly detrimental. The prognosis is generally poor in animals with pulmonary hypertension and shunt reversal, but some cases have done well for years with periodic phlebotomy.

# OTHER CARDIOVASCULAR ANOMALIES

## VASCULAR RING ANOMALIES

Various malformations of vessels arising from the embryonic aortic arches can occur. These may entrap the esophagus, and sometimes the trachea, within a vascular ring over the heart base. The most common vascular ring anomaly in the dog is the persistent right aortic arch, which encloses the esophagus dorsally and to the right with the aortic arch, to the left with the ligamentum arteriosum, and ventrally with the base of the heart. Other vascular ring anomalies have also been reported. Additional vascular anomalies, such as a left cranial vena cava or PDA, sometimes coexist with a vascular ring anomaly. Vascular ring anomalies are rare in cats.

Clinical signs of regurgitation and stunted growth commonly develop within 6 months of weaning in affected animals, because the vascular ring prevents the normal passage of solid food through the esophagus. The esophagus dilates cranial to the ring and may retain food. Occasionally the esophagus dilates caudal to the stricture as well, indicating that altered esophageal motility may also be a factor. Respiratory signs such as cough, wheezing, and cyanosis usually signal secondary aspiration pneumonia, although a double aortic arch may cause stridor and other respiratory signs secondary to tracheal stenosis. The animal may appear clinically normal, although thin, but generally becomes progressively debilitated. In some animals a dilated cervical esophagus (containing food or gas) can be palpated at the thoracic inlet. Fever and respiratory signs often accompany aspiration pneumonia. Thoracic radiographs usually show a widened cranial mediastinum and ventral displacement of the trachea, with or without evidence of aspiration pneumonia. A barium swallow allows visualization of the esophageal stricture over the heart base and cranial esophageal dilation (with or without caudal esophageal dilation).

Therapy involves surgical division of the ligamentum arteriosum or of another vessel if the anomaly is not a persistent right aortic arch. Recently, a thoracoscopic technique has been reported (Isakow and colleagues, 2000). Medical management consists of giving frequent, small, semisolid or liquid meals in an upright position for an indefinite time. Some dogs experience persistent regurgitation despite successful surgery, which indicates the presence of a permanent esophageal motility disorder (see Chapter 31, Disorders of the Oral Cavity, Pharynx, and Esophagus).

## COR TRIATRIATUM

Cor triatriatum is an uncommon malformation caused by the division of the right (dexter) or left (sinister) atrium into two chambers by an abnormal membrane. There are several reports of cor triatriatum dexter in dogs; cor triatriatum sinister has only been rarely described (cat). The intraatrial membrane of cor triatriatum dexter results from failure of the embryonic right sinus venosus valve to regress. The caudal vena cava and coronary sinus empty into the caudal right atrial (RA) chamber, and the tricuspid orifice is within the cranial RA chamber. Obstruction to venous flow through the opening in the abnormal membrane results in higher pressures within the caudal vena cava and the structures that it drains.

Large and middle-sized breeds of dog are most often affected. Development of persistent ascites at an early age is the most prominent clinical sign. Exercise intolerance, lethargy, distended cutaneous abdominal veins, and sometimes diarrhea have also been reported. Neither a cardiac murmur nor jugular venous distension are features of this anomaly.

Thoracic radiographs show a distended caudal vena cava without generalized cardiomegaly. The diaphragm may be displaced cranially with massive ascites. The ECG is generally normal. Echocardiography will reveal the abnormal membrane with a prominent caudal RA chamber and vena cava. Doppler studies allow estimation of the intra-RA pressure gradient and visualization of the flow disturbance.

Successful therapy requires enlarging the membrane orifice or excising the abnormal membrane to remove flow obstruction. A surgical technique using inflow occlusion, with or without hypothermia, allows excision of the membrane or manual breakdown of the membrane using a valve dilator. Percutaneous balloon dilation of the membrane orifice is a much less invasive option and works well as long as a large enough balloon is used. The simultaneous placement of several balloon dilation catheters can be successful in larger dogs.

## ENDOCARDIAL FIBROELASTOSIS

Endocardial fibroelastosis is a congenital abnormality characterized by diffuse fibrosis and elastic thickening of the endocardium. It is reported more commonly in cats, especially Burmese and Siamese, but has also been observed rarely in dogs. Left-sided or biventricular heart failure commonly develops early in life. The murmur of mitral regurgitation may be present. Criteria for LV and LA enlargement are seen on radiographs, ECG, and echocardiogram. Evidence of reduced LV myocardial function and increased stiffness may be present. Definitive antemortem diagnosis may be difficult.

## OTHER VASCULAR ANOMALIES

Various venous anomalies have been described but are usually not clinically relevant. The persistent left cranial vena cava is a fetal venous remnant; it courses lateral to the left AV groove and empties into the coronary sinus of the caudal right atrium. It causes no clinical signs but may complicate surgical exposure of other structures at the left heart base. Portosystemic venous shunts are common and can lead to the development of hepatic encephalopathy as well as other signs (see p. 531). These malformations are thought to be more prevalent in the Yorkshire Terrier, Pug, Miniature and Standard Schnauzer, Maltese, Pekingese, Shih Tzu, and Lhasa Apso breeds.

## Suggested Readings

GENERAL REFERENCES

Adin DB et al: Balloon dilation of cor triatriatum dexter in a dog, *J Vet Intern Med* 13:617, 1999.

Bonagura JD et al: Congenital heart disease. In Fox PR et al, editors: *Textbook of canine and feline cardiology,* ed 2, Philadelphia, 1999, WB Saunders, p 471.

Buchanan JW: Causes and prevalence of cardiovascular disease. In Kirk RW et al, editors: *Current veterinary therapy XI,* Philadelphia, 1992, WB Saunders.

Fossum TW et al: Cor triatriatum and caval anomalies, *Semin Vet Med Surg* 9:177, 1994.

Isakow K et al: Video-assisted thoracoscopic division of the ligamentum arteriosum in two dogs with persistent right aortic arch, *J Am Vet Med Assoc* 217:1333, 2000.

Kornreich BG et al: Right atrioventricular valve malformation in dogs and cats: an electrocardiographic survey with emphasis on splintered QRS complexes, *J Vet Intern Med* 11:226, 1997.

Lombard CW et al: Pulmonic stenosis and right-to-left atrial shunt in three dogs, *J Am Vet Med Assoc* 194:71, 1989.

Muldoon MM et al: Long-term results of surgical correction of persistent right aortic arch in dogs: 25 cases (1980-1995), *J Am Vet Med Assoc* 210:1761, 1997.

Nimmo-Wilkie JS et al: Pulmonary vascular lesions associated with congenital heart defects in three dogs, *J Am Anim Hosp Assoc* 17:485, 1981.

Tidholm A: Retrospective study of congenital heart defects in 151 dogs, *J Small Anim Pract* 38:94, 1997.

VanGundy T: Vascular ring anomalies, *Compend Contin Educ* 11:36, 1989.

Wright KN et al: Clinical spectrum of congenital tricuspid valve malformations in an extended family of Labrador retrievers, *J Vet Intern Med* 15:280, 2001 (abstract).

VENTRICULAR OUTFLOW TRACT OBSTRUCTIONS

Abbott JA et al: Aortic valve disease in Boxers with physical and echocardiographic findings of aortic stenosis, *J Vet Intern Med* 15:307, 2001 (abstract).

Belanger MC et al: Usefulness of the indexed effective orifice area in the assessment of subaortic stenosis in the dog, *J Vet Intern Med* 15:430, 2001.

Bonagura JD: Balloon valvuloplasty for congenital aortic stenosis, *Proceedings of the 19th ACVIM Forum,* Denver, 2001, p 154.

Bonagura JD: Problems in the canine left ventricular outflow tract, *J Vet Intern Med* 15:427, 2001 (editorial).

Buchanan JW: Pulmonic stenosis caused by single coronary artery in dogs: four cases (1965-1984), *J Am Vet Med Assoc* 196:115, 1990.

Buchanan JW: Pathogenesis of single right coronary artery and pulmonic stenosis in English bulldogs, *J Vet Intern Med* 15:101, 2001.

Buoscio DA et al: Clinical and pathological characterization of an unusual form of subvalvular aortic stenosis in four golden retriever puppies, *J Am Anim Hosp Assoc* 30:100, 1994.

Bussadori C et al: Balloon valvuloplasty in 30 dogs with pulmonic stenosis: effect of valve morphology and annular size on initial and 1-year outcome, *J Vet Intern Med* 15:553, 2001.

DeLellis LA et al: Balloon dilation of congenital subaortic stenosis in the dog, *J Vet Intern Med* 7:153, 1993.

Fingland RB et al: Pulmonic stenosis in the dog: 29 cases, *J Am Vet Med Assoc* 189:218, 1986.

Green BA et al: Relationship between severity of subvalvular aortic stenosis and ventricular ectopia in young Newfoundland dogs, *J Vet Intern Med* 15:280, 2001 (abstract).

Kienle RD et al: The natural history of canine congenital subaortic stenosis, *J Vet Intern Med* 8:423, 1994.

Kittleson M et al: Letter to the editor, *J Vet Intern Med* 6:250, 1992.

Lehmkuhl LB et al: Comparison of transducer placement sites for Doppler echocardiography in dogs with subaortic stenosis, *Am J Vet Res* 55:192, 1994.

Monnet E et al: Open resection for subvalvular aortic stenosis in dogs, *J Am Vet Med Assoc* 209:1255, 1996.

Nakayama T et al: Progression of subaortic stenosis detected by continuous wave Doppler echocardiography in a dog, *J Vet Intern Med* 10:97, 1996.

Orton EC et al: Influence of open surgical correction on intermediate-term outcome in dogs with subvalvular aortic stenosis: 44 cases (1991-1998), *J Am Vet Med Assoc* 216:364, 2000.

Pyle RL: Interpreting low-intensity cardiac murmurs in dogs predisposed to subaortic stenosis, *J Am Anim Assoc* 36:379, 2000 (editorial).

Ristic JME et al: A retrospective study of 26 dogs with pulmonic stenosis, *J Vet Intern Med* 15:280, 2001 (abstract).

CARDIAC SHUNTS

Birchard SJ et al: Results of ligation of patent ductus arteriosus in dogs: 201 cases (1969-1988), *J Am Vet Med Assoc* 196:2011, 1990.

Buchanan JW: Patent ductus arteriosus, *Semin Vet Med Surg* 9:168, 1994.

Cote E et al: Long-term clinical management of right-to-left ("reversed") patent ductus arteriosus in 3 dogs, *J Vet Intern Med* 15:39, 2001.

Fox PR et al: Nonsurgical transcatheter coil occlusion of patent ductus arteriosus in two dogs using a preformed Nitinol snare delivery technique, *J Vet Intern Med* 12:182, 1998.

Grifka RG et al: Transcatheter occlusion of a patent ductus arteriosus in a Newfoundland pup using the Gianturco-Grifka vascular occlusion device, *J Vet Intern Med* 10:42, 1996.

Miller MW et al: Percutaneous catheter occlusion of patent ductus arteriosus. *Proceedings of the 13th ACVIM Forum,* Lake Buena Vista, FL, 1995, p 308.

Moore KW et al: Hydroxyurea for treatment of polycythemia secondary to right-to-left shunting patent ductus arteriosus in 4 dogs, *J Vet Intern Med* 15:418, 2001.

Orton EC et al: Open surgical repair of tetralogy of Fallot in dogs, *J Am Vet Med Assoc* 219:1089, 2001.

Oswald GP et al: Patent ductus arteriosus and pulmonary hypertension in related Pembroke Welsh Corgis, *J Am Vet Med Assoc* 202:761, 1993.

Sisson D et al: Ventricular septal defect accompanied by aortic regurgitation in five dogs, *J Am Anim Hosp Assoc* 27:441, 1991.

Schneider M et al: Transvenous embolization of small patent ductus arteriosus with single detachable coils in dogs, *J Vet Intern Med* 15:222, 2001.

Stokhof AA et al: Transcatheter closure of patent ductus arteriosus using occluding spring coils, *J Vet Intern Med* 14:452, 2000.

# CHAPTER 10

# Heartworm Disease

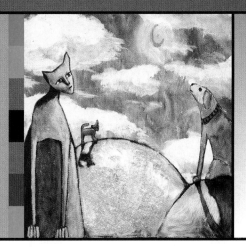

## CHAPTER OUTLINE

HEARTWORM LIFE CYCLE, 169
PATHOPHYSIOLOGY, 169
DIAGNOSTIC TESTING, 170
    Serologic tests, 170
    Detection of microfilariae, 171
HEARTWORM DISEASE IN DOGS, 171
HEARTWORM DISEASE IN CATS, 180

## HEARTWORM LIFE CYCLE

The life cycle of the heartworm *(Dirofilaria immitis)* is as follows: A mosquito ingests microfilariae (first-stage larvae [$L_1$]) from an infected host animal. The $L_1$ must molt twice within the mosquito in order to mature; therefore microfilariae passed to another dog by blood transfusion or across the placenta do not develop into adult worms. It takes approximately 2 to 2.5 weeks for infective $L_3$ larvae to develop within the mosquito. Infective larvae enter the new host when the mosquito takes a blood meal. The $L_3$ larvae travel within the subcutis of the new host, molting into the $L_4$ stage in about 9 to 12 days and then into the $L_5$ stage. The young worms enter the vascular system approximately 100 days after infection, migrating preferentially to the peripheral pulmonary arteries of the caudal lung lobes. It takes at least 5 and usually more than 6 months before an infection becomes patent and gravid female worms release microfilariae. Thus a puppy younger than 6 months with circulating microfilariae most likely received them transplacentally and does not have patent heartworm disease.

Various species of mosquitoes throughout the world can transmit the infection. The disease is widespread in the United States but is particularly prevalent along the eastern and gulf coasts and in the Mississippi River valley. Heartworm disease has been found in animals in all 50 states, although few cases are encountered in western desert states. Sporadic cases are encountered in other areas of the United States and in Canada. Heartworm transmission is limited by climatic conditions. For the $L_1$ larvae to mature to the infective stage within a mosquito, the average daily temperature must be more than 64° F for about 1 month. In most areas of the United States heartworm transmission peaks in July and August.

## PATHOPHYSIOLOGY

Heartworm disease is an important cause of pulmonary hypertension (cor pulmonale). The adult worms live mainly in the pulmonary arteries, where their presence incites the formation of reactive vascular lesions that precipitate pulmonary hypertension. Within days after young adult heartworms enter the caudal pulmonary arteries, pathologic changes begin to occur in these vessels. Although large worm burdens may be associated with severe disease, it appears that the host-parasite interaction is more important than the worm number alone in the development of clinical signs. Little or no correlation has been found between pulmonary vascular resistance and the number of worms present. Low worm burdens can cause serious lung injury and greater increases in pulmonary vascular resistance if the cardiac output is high. Exercise exacerbates the pulmonary vascular pathology because of the associated increase in pulmonary blood flow. If there are few worms, the caudal pulmonary arteries are the preferred site. As the worm burden increases, some migrate toward and into the heart. The migration of worms to the caudal vena cava has been associated with heavy worm burdens. Occasionally, mechanical occlusion of the right ventricular outflow tract, tricuspid valve, venae cavae, or pulmonary arteries occurs when there is a massive number of worms (caval syndrome).

Villous myointimal proliferation of the pulmonary arteries containing heartworms is the characteristic lesion. The heartworm-induced changes begin with endothelial cell swelling, widening of intercellular junctions, increases in endothelial permeability, and the development of periarterial edema. Endothelial sloughing results in the adhesion of activated white blood cells and platelets. Various trophic factors stimulate the migration and proliferation of smooth muscle cells within the media and into the intima. Villous proliferation

TABLE 10-1

Adult Heartworm Antigen Test Kits

| TEST TYPE | SAMPLE REQUIRED | PRODUCT NAME | SPECIES | MANUFACTURER |
|---|---|---|---|---|
| ELISA | P, S | DiroCHEK | B | Synbiotics |
| ELISA | P, S | PetChek HTWM PF | B | IDEXX |
| ELISA | P, S, WB | Snap Canine, Heartworm PF | B | IDEXX |
| ELISA | P, S, WB | Canine Snap 3DX* | D | IDEXX |
| Hemagglutination | WB | VetRED | D | Synbiotics |
| Immunochromatography | P, S, WB | Witness HW | D | Synbiotics |

*ELISA,* Enzyme-linked immunosorbent assay; *B,* approved for both dogs and cats; *D,* approved for dogs only; *P,* plasma; *S,* serum; *WB,* whole blood.
*Tests for HW Ag, *E. canis* Ab, and Lyme Ab.

of the intima occurs by 3 to 4 weeks after the arrival of adult worms. These proliferations, consisting of smooth muscle and collagen with an endothelium-like covering, cause the lumen of the smaller pulmonary arteries to narrow. These changes within the pulmonary arteries induce still further endothelial damage and the formation of proliferative lesions. Endothelial damage leads to the development of thrombosis as well as a perivascular tissue reaction. Periarterial edema may be severe enough to cause radiographically apparent interstitial and alveolar infiltrates. Partial lung consolidation develops in some animals. Dead worms appear to incite a more intense host response and worsen the pulmonary disease. Experimentally, heartworm extract causes mast cell degranulation and histamine release (Kitoh and colleagues, 2001). Worm fragments and thrombi cause embolization and further reaction, which eventually leads to fibrosis. Arterial embolization and infarction, fibrosis, and hypersensitivity pneumonitis can all contribute to the development of parenchymal lung lesions. The resistance to pulmonary blood flow is increased in the diseased, narrowed vessels, which in turn reduces affected lung lobe perfusion, raises pulmonary arterial pressure, and puts a strain on the right side of the heart. Alveolar hypoxia resulting from areas of lung consolidation exacerbates the already high pulmonary resistance.

The villous proliferation (and worm distribution) is most severe in the caudal and accessory lobar arteries. Affected pulmonary arteries lose their normal tapered peripheral branching appearance and appear blunted or pruned. Aneurysmal dilation and peripheral occlusion may occur. The vessels become tortuous and proximally dilated as the increased pulmonary vascular resistance demands higher perfusion pressures. The right ventricle dilates and then hypertrophies as higher systolic pressures are required. Chronic pulmonary hypertension can cause right ventricular myocardial failure and signs of right-sided congestive failure, especially in conjunction with secondary tricuspid insufficiency.

Chronic hepatic congestion secondary to heartworm disease can cause permanent liver damage and cirrhosis. Circulating immune complexes or possibly microfilarial antigens can produce glomerulonephritis. Renal amyloidosis has also been associated with heartworm disease in dogs but is rare.

Occasionally, aberrant worms can cause embolization of the brain, eye, or other systemic arteries.

## DIAGNOSTIC TESTING

### SEROLOGIC TESTS

**Heartworm antigen tests.** The American Heartworm Society recommends that adult heartworm antigen (Ag) tests be used as the primary method of screening for the disease in dogs. These Ag test kits are quite accurate and provide greater overall sensitivity than microfilaria tests. The monthly heartworm preventive drugs promote occult infections by virtually eliminating circulating microfilariae. Circulating Ag is generally detectable by about 6.5 to 7 months after infection. So there is no reason to test puppies younger than 7 months.

Commercially available test kits are immunoassays that detect circulating heartworm Ag from the adult female reproductive tract. Most are enzyme-linked immunosorbent assays (ELISAs), although a hemagglutination-based kit and an immunochromatographic assay are also available (Table 10-1). These tests are generally very specific and have a good sensitivity. Positive results are consistently obtained in the presence of at least three female worms 7 to 8 months or older. Most kits do not detect infections less than 5 months old, and male worms are not detected. Most serum/plasma kits often can detect infections with one live female worm. But because the adult worm burden is low in cats and there is greater probability of male unisex infections, false-negative test results are more likely in this species.

It is important to follow the manufacturer's directions carefully for best results. Weakly positive test results should be rechecked using a repeat test or a different Ag test kit, a microfilaria test, or thoracic radiographs, or a combination of these. False-positive test results usually stem from technical error; false-negative results usually are caused by a low worm burden, the presence of only immature female worms, a male unisex infection, or a cold test kit. It is possible to estimate the amount of circulating Ag using the ELISA and colloidal gold tests.

**Heartworm antibody tests for cats.** ELISA antibody (Ab) tests using either recombinant Ag (HESKA Solo Step FH Ab, HESKA Lab Ab [HESKA, Fort Collins, Colo]; Witness FHW Ab, ASSURE/FH Ab [Synbiotics, San Diego, Calif]) or heartworm Ag extracted and purified from an equal weight of male and female worms (Diagnostics Lab Ab; Animal Diagnostics, St. Louis, Mo) are commercially available for cats. These tests are used to screen for feline heartworm disease; they have minimal to no cross-reactivity with gastrointestinal (GI) parasitic infections. The Ab tests provide greater sensitivity than Ag tests since larvae of either gender can provoke a host immune response. The specificity of the Ab tests for heartworm disease is of some concern, however, because serum Ab to both immature and adult worms is detected as early as 60 days after infection. Some immature heartworm larvae never develop into adults. Therefore a positive Ab test indicates exposure to migrating larvae as well as adults, not the presence of adult heartworms specifically. A positive antibody test should be supported by other evidence of heartworm disease before a definitive diagnosis is made. The concentration of Ab does not appear to correlate with the number of worms present, nor with severity of clinical disease or radiographic signs. It is also unclear how long circulating Ab remains after elimination of heartworm infection.

False-negative Ab tests also occur fairly frequently (in an estimated 3% to 14% of cases), usually in association with a single worm. This is of concern because the worm burden in cats is frequently low. Therefore a negative heartworm Ab test suggests one of the following: (1) no heartworm infection, (2) infection less than 60 days old, or (3) a concentration of immunoglobulin G (IgG) Ab against the Ag used in making the test that is too low to be detected. If clinical findings suggest heartworm disease but the Ab test is negative, serologic testing should be repeated using a different Ab test and a heartworm Ag test. Chest radiographs and a 2-D echocardiogram are also recommended. The Ab test can also be repeated in a few months.

## DETECTION OF MICROFILARIAE

Tests for circulating microfilariae are no longer recommended for routine heartworm screening, as noted above. However, they may be used to confirm heartworm disease in some antigen-positive cases and to determine if microfilaricide therapy is needed. Microfilaria testing is still important if diethylcarbamazine (DEC) is used as a heartworm preventive (see p. 179); but the macrolide preventive drugs, which are given monthly, reduce and eliminate microfilaremia by impairing the reproductive function of female and possibly also male worms. Most dogs receiving these drugs become amicrofilaremic by the sixth monthly dose. However, an estimated 75% to 90% of heartworm-positive dogs that are not treated monthly with a macrolide have circulating microfilariae. The remaining so-called occult infections, in which there are no circulating microfilariae, can result from an immune response that destroys the microfilariae within the lung (true occult infection), unisex infection, the presence of sterile heartworms, or the presence of only immature worms

### TABLE 10-2

**Morphologic Differentiation of Microfilariae**

| SMEAR | DIROFILARIA IMMITIS | DIPETALONEMA RECONDITUM |
|---|---|---|
| Fresh smear | Few to large numbers<br>Undulate in one place | Usually small numbers<br>Move across field |
| Stained smear* | Straight body<br>Straight tail | Curved body<br>Posterior extremity hook ("button-hook" tail); inconsistent finding |
| | Tapered head<br>>290 μm long<br>>6 μm wide | Blunt head<br><275-280 μm long<br><6 μm wide |

*Size criteria given for lysate prepared using 2% formalin (modified Knott's test); microfilariae tend to be smaller with lysate of filter tests. Width and morphology are the best discriminating factors.

(prepatent infection). Occult infections are frequently associated with severe signs of disease. Low numbers of microfilariae and diurnal variations in the number of circulating microfilariae in peripheral blood can also cause microfilaria test results to be falsely negative. Circulating microfilariae are rarely found in cats with heartworm disease.

Concentration tests involving the use of at least 1 ml of blood are recommended to detect microfilariae in peripheral blood. The nonconcentration tests are not recommended because low numbers of microfilariae are more likely to be missed. Nonconcentration tests include a fresh wet blood smear or a spun-hematocrit-tube buffy coat examination. Concentration tests are done using either a Millipore filter or the modified Knott's technique. Both techniques lyse the red blood cells and fix any existing microfilariae. The modified Knott's test, which is cheaper but more time-consuming, concentrates the microfilariae by centrifugation, whereas the filter test (Evsco, Beuna, N.J.) concentrates the microfilariae by filtration. The microfilariae of *D. immitis* should be differentiated from those of *Dipetalonema reconditum* (Table 10-2). A concentration test should be used to evaluate dogs with positive serologic findings or signs suggestive of heartworm disease and to assess the efficacy of microfilaricide treatment. An occasional false-positive microfilaria test result occurs in animals with microfilariae but no live adult worms.

## HEARTWORM DISEASE IN DOGS

Heartworm disease in dogs has no specific age or breed predilection. Most affected dogs are between 4 and 8 years old, but the disease is also commonly diagnosed in dogs under 1 year of age (but older than 6 months) as well as in geriatric animals. Male dogs are affected two to four times as

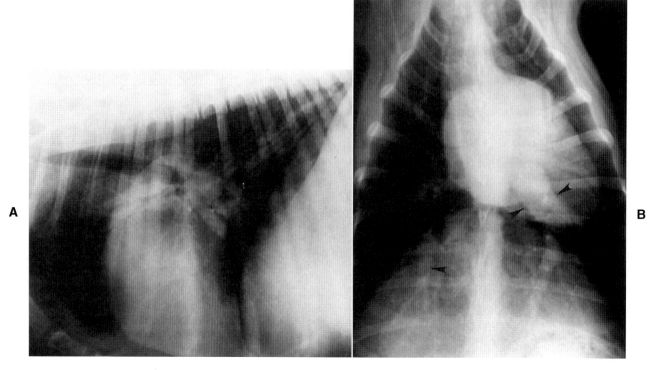

**FIG 10-1**
**A,** Lateral and, **B,** dorsoventral (DV) radiographs from a German Shepherd with advanced heartworm disease. Enlargement of pulmonary arteries is seen, especially on DV view (*arrowheads* in **B**).

often as female dogs. Large-breed dogs and those primarily living outdoors are at much greater risk of infection than small-breed or indoor dogs. The length of the hair coat does not appear to affect the risk of infection.

## Clinical Features

Many dogs are asymptomatic when the disease is diagnosed by a positive routine screening test result. Dogs with occult disease or those that have not been routinely tested are more likely to have advanced pulmonary arterial disease and clinical signs. Symptomatic dogs often have a history that includes exertional dyspnea, fatigue, syncope, cough, hemoptysis, shortness of breath, weight loss, or signs of right-sided congestive heart failure. A change in or the loss of a dog's bark has sometimes been reported. The physical examination findings may be normal in early or mild disease. Severe disease is frequently associated with poor body condition, tachypnea or dyspnea, jugular vein distention or pulsations, ascites, or other evidence of right-sided heart failure. Increased or abnormal lung sounds (wheezes, crackles), a loud and often split second heart sound ($S_2$), an ejection click or murmur at the left base, a murmur of tricuspid insufficiency, or cardiac arrhythmias are variably heard on auscultation. Severe pulmonary arterial disease and thromboembolism can be associated with epistaxis, disseminated intravascular coagulation (DIC), thrombocytopenia, and possibly hemoglobinuria; the latter is also a sign of the caval syndrome.

Occasionally, aberrant worm migration to the central nervous system (CNS), eye, femoral arteries, subcutis, peritoneal cavity, and other sites occurs and causes related signs. Several cases of systemic arterial migration causing hindlimb lameness, paresthesia, and ischemic necrosis have been described. Worm and thrombus extraction via femoral arteriotomies, along with adulticide therapy, has been successful in some cases, but limb amputation may be necessary.

## Diagnosis

Thoracic radiograph findings may be normal early in the disease, although marked changes develop rapidly in dogs with heavy worm burdens. Characteristic findings include right ventricular enlargement, a pulmonary trunk bulge, and centrally enlarged and tortuous lobar pulmonary arteries with peripheral blunting (Fig. 10-1). The caudal lobar arteries, which are usually the most severely affected, are best evaluated on a dorsoventral (DV) view; the width of these vessels is normally no larger than the ninth rib (at its intersection with the vessels). On a lateral view, the width of the cranial right lobar artery at its intersection with the fourth rib is no larger than the most narrow diameter of that rib in normal dogs. Enlargement of lobar pulmonary arteries (without concurrent venous distention) is strongly suggestive of heartworm disease. An enlarged caudal vena cava also may be present; a normal maximal caval width of $0.75 \pm 0.03 \times$ the length of the fifth thoracic vertebra has been reported (Lit-

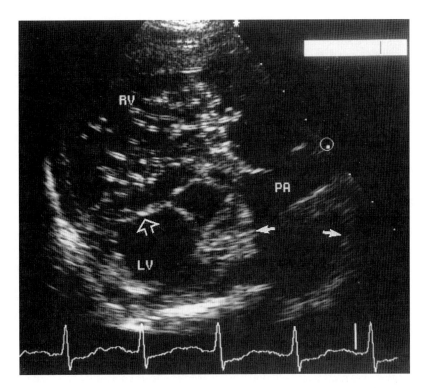

**FIG 10-2**
Echocardiogram from a 9-year-old, male, mixed-breed dog with caval syndrome. The transducer is in the right parasternal short-axis position at a level just below the aorta. The image shows the enlarged and hypertrophied right ventricle and its outflow tract. Many small, bright, parallel echoes are apparent in the body of the right ventricle *(RV)* in this diastolic frame and are caused by a clump of heartworms entangled in the tricuspid valve apparatus. Note also the widened main pulmonary artery segment typical of pulmonary hypertension *(small arrows)*. The interventricular septum is flattened and pushed toward the left ventricle *(LV)* by high right ventricular pressure *(open arrow)*. The LV itself is small, because the heartworms obstruct blood flow through the right side of the heart. *PA,* Main pulmonary artery.

ster and colleagues, 2001). The finding of patchy pulmonary interstitial or alveolar infiltrates suggestive of infarction, edema, pneumonia, or fibrosis also is common. These pulmonary opacities may be mainly perivascular. Right-sided heart failure resulting from heartworm disease is associated with radiographic evidence of severe pulmonary arterial disease and right-sided heart enlargement.

The electrocardiogram (ECG) is usually normal, but advanced disease may cause a right axis deviation or an arrhythmia. Dogs with heartworm-induced congestive heart failure almost always have the ECG features of right ventricular enlargement. Tall P waves occasionally occur, suggesting right atrial enlargement. Echocardiographic findings in dogs with advanced heartworm disease include right ventricular and atrial dilation, right ventricular hypertrophy, paradoxic septal motion, a small left side of the heart, and pulmonary artery dilation. Heartworms located in peripheral pulmonary arteries cannot be seen on echocardiograms. Heartworms within the heart, the main pulmonary artery and its bifurcation, and venae cavae appear as small, bright parallel echoes (Fig. 10-2). Suspected caval syndrome can be quickly con-

firmed by echocardiography. Secondary right-sided heart failure may be evidenced by pleural or pericardial effusion or ascites.

Eosinophilia, basophilia, and monocytosis are inconsistent findings in the complete blood count (CBC); fewer than 50% of dogs with heartworm disease have eosinophilia. Mild regenerative anemia is present in less than 30% of cases and is thought to result from hemolysis. Thrombocytopenia may be identified secondary to platelet consumption in the pulmonary arterial system, especially after adulticide treatment; DIC can also occur in dogs with advanced disease. The immune response to the heartworms produces a polyclonal gammopathy. A mild-to-moderate elevation in liver enzyme activity and sometimes azotemia may occur. Proteinuria is present in 20% to 30% of affected dogs, especially those with advanced disease. Hypoalbuminemia may develop in severely affected animals.

## Pretreatment Evaluation

All dogs should undergo a thorough history and physical examination before the start of treatment. Thoracic radiographs provide the best overall assessment of the status of pulmonary arterial and parenchymal disease and are useful for estimating prognosis. The risk of postadulticide pulmonary thromboembolism is increased in dogs with preexisting clinical and radiographic signs of severe pulmonary vascular disease, especially in those with right-sided heart failure or a high worm burden. In young, asymptomatic dogs the inclusion of a CBC, blood urea nitrogen or creatinine measurement, and urinalysis yields a sufficient database. A more complete serum chemistry profile, in addition to thoracic radiographs, CBC, and urinalysis, is recommended for middle-age and older dogs or those with clinical signs. A platelet count is advised in animals with radiographically severe pulmonary arterial disease. Urine protein loss is quantified or a urine protein/creatinine ratio is calculated if hypoalbuminemia or proteinuria is detected. Mild-to-moderate increases in liver enzyme activities may be caused by hepatic congestion but do not preclude therapy with melarsomine. Liver enzyme activities usually return to normal within 1 to 2 months of heartworm treatment. Aspirin is not recommended as a routine preadulticide treatment in most dogs because of the lack of convincing evidence of a beneficial antithrombotic effect. It is unclear whether dogs with severe pulmonary arterial disease benefit from aspirin therapy given for 1 to 2 weeks before the start of adulticide treatment.

## Adulticide Therapy in Dogs

The organic arsenical compounds melarsomine dihydrochloride and thiacetarsamide are the only effective heartworm adulticides. Melarsomine is the drug of choice. Thiacetarsamide, the adulticide used for many years, is no longer being manufactured but may still be available. Strict rest should be enforced for 4 to 6 weeks after adulticide therapy to reduce the sequelae of adult worm death and pulmonary thromboembolism (see p. 176). The rest period for working dogs should probably be longer, because increased pulmonary blood flow in response to exercise exacerbates pulmonary capillary bed damage and subsequent fibrosis.

Heartworm Ag testing should be repeated 3 to 4 months after adulticide therapy. If therapy was completely successful, the test should be negative. The decision to repeat treatment in a dog with persistent antigenemia is guided by the animal's overall health, performance expectations, and age. Complete worm kill is probably not necessary; even if some adult heartworms survive, pulmonary arterial disease improves considerably after adulticide therapy.

**Melarsomine.** Melarsomine (Immiticide; Merial, Iselin, N.J.) is a more effective adulticide than thiacetarsamide, although it does not appear to be associated with a greater risk of thromboembolism and pulmonary hypertension. It is effective against both immature and mature heartworms; male worms are easier to kill. The worm kill can be controlled by adjusting the dose. Melarsomine is rapidly absorbed from the intramuscular (IM) injection site. Unchanged drug and a major metabolite are rapidly eliminated in the feces; a minor metabolite is excreted in urine. The drug should be given by deep IM injection into the epaxial lumbar muscles (L3 to L5

region), exactly as recommended by the manufacturer. The lumbar muscle site provides good vascularity and lymphatic drainage with minimal fascial planes. Further, gravity may help prevent drug from leaking into subcutaneous tissues, where it can cause more irritation. The drug does cause a local reaction at the injection site; this is clinically noticeable in about one third of treated dogs. Coughing or gagging and (less often) dyspnea after treatment may be related to the heartworm disease itself, although pulmonary congestion is reported as a toxic effect of overdosing. Most clinical signs noted in dogs treated with melarsomine have been behavioral (e.g., tremors, lethargy, unsteadiness and ataxia, restlessness), respiratory (panting, shallow breathing, labored respirations, crackles), or injection-site related (edema, redness, tenderness, vocalization, increased aspartate aminotransferase and creatine kinase activities). Injection site reactions are generally mild to moderate and completely healed within 4 (to 12) weeks, but occasionally these reactions are severe. The manufacturer reports that firm nodules can persist indefinitely at the sites. General signs of lethargy, depression, and anorexia occur in about 15% or fewer dogs; other adverse effects, including fever, vomiting, and diarrhea, occur occasionally. Adverse effects in animals receiving recommended doses are generally mild. Hepatic and renal changes have not proved clinically relevant in animals receiving recommended doses of melarsomine. Overall melarsomine causes less systemic toxicity than thiacetarsamide.

An overdose of melarsomine can cause pulmonary inflammation, edema, and death. The pathophysiology of the pulmonary toxicity is unclear. During toxicity studies, three times the recommended dose caused collapse, severe salivation, vomiting, respiratory distress, stupor, and death in some dogs. Some clinical reversal of toxicity resulting from an overdose of melarsomine can be achieved with the administration of BAL (British Anti-Lewisite, dimercaprol) at a dose of 3 mg/kg IM. This will also decrease adulticide activity, however.

A classification of disease severity is useful in guiding therapy (Table 10-3). Dogs with mild (class 1) to moderate (class 2) disease are given the standard therapy. Dogs with severe disease (class 3), or those in class 2 in which a more conservative approach is desired, are treated with the alternative dosing regimen. Dogs with caval syndrome (class 4) should not be given adulticide treatment until worms are surgically removed (see p. 177). Serologic test results are negative in approximately 80% or more of dogs with mild-to-moderate heartworm disease 4 months after melarsomine treatment. If the dog remains antigen-positive at this time, the treatment can be repeated. Seroconversion approaches 100% if the treatment series is repeated.

Melarsomine is available as a sterile lyophilized powder in 50-mg vials. The rehydrated product is fully stable for 24 hours if kept refrigerated in the dark. In the standard therapy (Table 10-4), two doses of 2.5 mg/kg are given IM 24 hours apart. The manufacturer's administration instructions should be followed carefully. Dogs with severe disease are treated with an alternative protocol (see Table 10-4) designed to partially reduce the worm burden with an initial injection, fol-

TABLE 10-3

**Classification of Heartworm Disease Severity in Dogs**

| CLASS | CLINICAL SIGNS | RADIOGRAPHIC SIGNS | CLINICOPATHOLOGIC ABNORMALITIES |
|---|---|---|---|
| 1 (mild) | None; or occasional cough, fatigue on exercise, or mild loss of condition | None | None |
| 2 (moderate) | None; or occasional cough, fatigue on exercise, or mild to moderate loss of condition | Right ventricular enlargement and/or some pulmonary artery enlargement; ± perivascular and mixed alveolar/interstitial opacities | ± Mild anemia (PCV, 20%-30%); ± proteinuria (2+ on dipstick) |
| 3 (severe) | General loss of condition or cachexia; fatigue on exercise or mild activity; occasional or persistent cough; ± dyspnea; ± right-sided heart failure | Right ventricular ± atrial enlargement; moderate to severe pulmonary artery enlargement; perivascular or diffuse mixed alveolar/interstitial opacities; ± evidence of thromboembolism | ± Anemia (PCV, <30%); ± proteinuria (≥2+ on dipstick) |
| 4 (very severe) | Caval syndrome (see text, p. 177) | | |

*PCV,* Packed cell volume.

lowed by the standard adulticide regimen 1 month later. The risk of massive pulmonary thromboembolism and death resulting from an initially heavy worm kill is reduced with this protocol.

**Thiacetarsamide.** Thiacetarsamide is an older agent that may still be available, although melarsomine has many advantages over it. Thiacetarsamide (Caparsolate) is a 1% (10 mg/ml) solution that must be stored under refrigeration and protected from light; a yellow-orange discoloration and the formation of precipitates are signs that the drug has deteriorated. Because the drug is extremely caustic, meticulous intravenous (IV) injection is required; a butterfly catheter with saline flush is recommended. In the usual treatment protocol, a dose of 2.2 mg/kg (0.22 ml/kg) of thiacetarsamide sodium is given twice daily for 2 days. During and after adulticide treatment, the dog should be carefully reevaluated for signs of thiacetarsamide toxicity. Clinical signs of arsenic hepatotoxicity or nephrotoxicity include acute depression, anorexia, repeated emesis, icterus, fever, diarrhea, and death. Vomiting after administration is relatively common, but the treatment can continue if no other adverse signs occur and the animal's appetite is good. Complete anorexia, icterus, and persistent vomiting are indications to halt treatment.

**Other considerations.** Microfilaricide therapy is not recommended before adulticide treatment. The decision to withhold adulticide therapy in some asymptomatic dogs is controversial. The presence of concurrent disease or the animal's age may be factors in this decision, especially if thiacetarsamide therapy is being considered. An inactive dog with a low worm burden may not show clinical signs before the worms die naturally. However, the possibility of worsening pulmonary disease or other sequelae (e.g., glomerulonephritis) developing in the future, and thus increasing the

TABLE 10-4

**Checklist for Melarsomine (Immiticide) Adulticide Therapy**

**Before Initiating Treatment**

1. Confirm diagnosis.
2. Pretreatment evaluation and management.
3. Determine class (severity) of disease (see Table 10-3).
4. Determine Immiticide treatment regimen.

**Standard Treatment Regimen (for Class 1 and Most Class 2 Dogs)**

1. Draw Immiticide, 2.5 mg/kg, into a syringe; attach a fresh, sterile 23-gauge needle: 1 inch (2.5 cm) long for dogs <10 kg or 1.5 inch (3.75 cm) long for dogs >10 kg.
2. Give by deep intramuscular injection into lumbar (epaxial) musculature in the L3 to L5 region; avoid subcutaneous leakage.
3. Repeat steps 1 and 2 at 24 hours after first dose; use opposite side for injection.
4. Enforced rest for 4 to 6 weeks minimum; symptomatic treatment as needed.

**Alternate Treatment Regimen (for Class 3 and Some Class 2 Dogs)**

1. Symptomatic treatment as needed; enforced rest.
2. When condition is stable, administer *one* dose of 2.5 mg/kg as described above in the standard treatment regimen.
3. Continue enforced rest and symptomatic treatment as needed.
4. One month later, administer two more doses, 24 hours apart, according to the standard treatment regimen.

risks of adulticide therapy, must be considered. Active dogs are probably more likely to become symptomatic in the future, even if they have a low worm burden. If adulticide therapy is not provided, the dog should at least receive a macrolide to stop further worm development and disease transmission to other animals (by reducing the microfilaremia).

The use of other drugs, such as levamisole or stibophen, as adulticides is not recommended, especially with the availability of melarsomine. Levamisole does not consistently kill adult heartworms, although it is somewhat effective against male worms and may sterilize adult female worms.

## Pulmonary Thromboembolic Complications of Adulticide Therapy

Pulmonary arterial disease worsens from 5 to 30 days after adulticide therapy and is especially severe in previously symptomatic dogs. It occurs because dead and dying worms cause thrombosis and pulmonary artery obstruction, with exacerbation of platelet adhesion, myointimal proliferation, villous hypertrophy, granulomatous arteritis, perivascular edema, and hemorrhage. Obstructed pulmonary blood flow and high vascular resistance further increase right ventricular strain and oxygen consumption. Poor cardiac output, hypotension, and myocardial ischemia may result. Pulmonary hypoperfusion, hypoxic vasoconstriction and bronchoconstriction, pulmonary inflammation, and fluid accumulation can lead to the development of serious ventilation/perfusion abnormalities. Severe pulmonary thromboembolization is most likely to occur 7 to 17 days after adulticide therapy. As expected, the caudal and accessory lung lobes are most commonly and severely affected. Endothelial changes regress within 4 to 6 weeks, and pulmonary hypertension and arterial disease begin to resolve over the next several months. Eventually, pulmonary arterial pressure and the contour of the proximal pulmonary arteries normalize, although some fibrosis may remain around distal arteries.

Clinical signs include depression, fever, tachycardia, tachypnea or dyspnea, cough, hemoptysis, and sometimes right-sided heart failure, collapse, or death. Pulmonary crackles heard on auscultation result from interstitial and alveolar pulmonary inflammation and fluid accumulation. Focal lung consolidation can cause areas of muffled lung sounds. Patchy alveolar infiltrates with air bronchograms may be seen on thoracic radiographs, especially near the caudal lobar arteries. A CBC may show thrombocytopenia or a regenerative left shift.

Treatment of pulmonary thromboembolism includes strict rest (cage confinement) and glucocorticoid therapy to reduce pulmonary inflammation (prednisone, 1 to 2 mg/kg/day initially, then tapering). Supplemental oxygen therapy is recommended to reduce hypoxia-mediated pulmonary vasoconstriction. A bronchodilator (e.g., aminophylline, 10 mg/kg orally [PO], IM, or IV q8h; or theophylline, 9 mg/kg PO q6-8h), judicious fluid therapy (if there is evidence of cardiovascular shock), and cough suppressants may be useful. Antibiotics have been given empirically; however, they are of questionable benefit unless there is evidence of a concurrent bacterial infection. Hydralazine has been observed to reduce pulmonary vascular resistance experimentally, and some dogs seem to respond clinically to diltiazem. Systemic hypotension and tachycardia must be prevented in animals receiving a vasodilator. Aspirin is no longer recommended because there is no convincing evidence that it has a beneficial antithrombotic effect. It is unclear whether aspirin can help counteract the effects of prostaglandin-induced vasoconstriction. In cases of severe thromboembolism, the use of heparin (sodium heparin, 200 to 400 U/kg administered subcutaneously [SC] q8h, or calcium heparin, 50 to 100 U/kg SC q8-12h) can be considered. However, excessive bleeding could be a serious adverse effect of such therapy. Low–molecular weight heparin might provide a safer alternative to unfractionated heparin, but more veterinary experience with these products is needed before recommendations can be made (see p. 135).

## Treatment of Dogs with Complicated Heartworm Disease

**Pulmonary complications.** Immune-mediated pneumonitis occurs in some dogs, because inflammatory cells surround microfilariae trapped in the lungs. Allergic or eosinophilic pneumonitis has been noted in 10% to 15% of dogs with occult heartworm disease. The clinical manifestations of heartworm pneumonitis include a progressively worsening cough, crackles heard on auscultation, tachypnea or dyspnea, and sometimes cyanosis, weight loss, and anorexia. Eosinophilia, basophilia, and hyperglobulinemia are inconsistent findings; results of serologic tests for adult heartworm are usually positive. Diffuse interstitial and alveolar infiltrates that may resemble those seen in dogs with pulmonary edema or blastomycosis, especially in the caudal lobes, are commonly seen on radiographs. There is frequently no clinically relevant cardiomegaly or pulmonary lobar artery enlargement. A sterile eosinophilic exudate with variable numbers of well-preserved neutrophils and macrophages is typical on tracheal wash cytologic studies. Therapy with glucocorticoids (prednisone, 1 to 2 mg/kg/day initially) usually results in rapid and marked improvement. Prednisone given in gradually tapered doses (to 0.5 mg/kg every other day) can be continued as needed and does not appear to adversely affect the adulticide efficacy of melarsomine.

Pulmonary eosinophilic granulomatosis is an uncommon syndrome that has been associated with heartworm disease, although some affected dogs are heartworm-negative. A hypersensitivity reaction to heartworm antigens or immune complexes, or both, is thought to contribute to its pathogenesis. Pulmonary granulomas consist of a mixed population of mononuclear and neutrophilic cells, with many eosinophils and macrophages. A proliferation of bronchial smooth muscle within granulomas and an abundance of alveolar cells in the surrounding area are common findings; lymphocytic and eosinophilic perivascular infiltrates may also occur. Eosinophilic granulomas involving the lymph nodes, trachea, tonsils, spleen, gastrointestinal tract, and liver or kidneys may occur concurrently. The clinical signs of pulmonary eosinophilic granulomatosis are similar to those seen in the setting of eosinophilic pneumonitis. Variable clinicopathologic findings include leukocytosis, neutrophilia, eosinophilia, basophilia, monocytosis, and hyperglobulinemia. In some cases an exudative, primarily eosinophilic pleural effusion develops. Radiographic findings include multiple pulmonary nodules of varying size and location with mixed alveolar and interstitial pulmonary infiltrates; hilar and mediastinal lymphadenopathy may also be present. Eosinophilic granulomatosis associated with heartworm disease is treated initially with prednisone (1 to 2 mg/kg q12h); however, additional cytotoxic therapy may be needed as well (see Chapter 22). Not all dogs respond completely and relapse is common, especially when therapy is reduced or discontinued. The response to immunosuppressive drugs after relapse may be poor. Therapy for adult heartworms and microfilariae is given when pulmonary disease abates.

Severe pulmonary arterial disease is likely in dogs with long-standing heartworm infections, in those with many adult worms, and in active dogs. The clinical signs include severe cough, exercise intolerance, tachypnea or dyspnea, episodic weakness, syncope, weight loss, ascites, and death. Radiographic evidence of marked enlargement, tortuosity, and blunting of pulmonary arteries are common. Pulmonary parenchymal infiltrates can lead to the development of hypoxemia; these should be treated with prednisone, as just described, until resolved. Alternate-day, low-dose prednisone (e.g., 0.5 mg/kg) should have beneficial antiinflammatory effects, although long-term high doses of a corticosteroid may reduce pulmonary blood flow, enhance the risk of thromboembolism, and inhibit resolution of the vascular disease. Thrombocytopenia resulting from platelet consumption and hemolysis may occur in dogs with severe pulmonary arterial disease and thromboembolism; hence the platelet count and packed cell volume should be monitored. DIC develops in some dogs. Conservative therapy with oxygen, prednisone, and a bronchodilator (e.g., theophylline), as already outlined (see p. 176), helps to improve oxygenation and decrease pulmonary artery pressures in dogs with severe heartworm disease.

After initial stabilization of the animal's condition, the alternative melarsomine protocol can be started. The mortality in dogs with severe heartworm disease given melarsomine has been estimated to be 10%. This is similar to the mortality in dogs managed by strict cage confinement for 1 to more than 2 weeks before and 3 to 4 weeks after thiacetarsamide treatment. However, melarsomine-treated dogs can be confined at home with minimal pretreatment and posttreatment hospitalization. Under similar conditions, the survival rate in severely affected dogs treated with thiacetarsamide has historically been 53%. Aspirin should be avoided if hemoptysis is present. Prophylactic antibiotics are sometimes recommended because of the potential for devitalized pulmonary tissue and secondary bacterial infections to develop.

**Right-sided congestive heart failure.** Severe pulmonary arterial disease and pulmonary hypertension can cause right ventricular failure. Typical signs of right-sided congestive failure include jugular venous distention or pulsation, ascites, syncope, exercise intolerance, and arrhythmias.

Pleural or pericardial effusion can develop, and other signs secondary to pulmonary arterial and parenchymal disease may also be present. Treatment is the same as that for dogs with severe pulmonary arterial disease, with the addition of furosemide (1 to 2 mg/kg/day), an angiotensin converting enzyme inhibitor (e.g., enalapril), and a sodium-restricted diet. The use of digoxin in this setting is controversial.

**Caval syndrome.** The shocklike condition known as the (vena) caval syndrome occurs when venous inflow to the heart is obstructed by a mass of worms. Other terms for this condition have included postcaval syndrome, acute hepatic syndrome, liver failure syndrome, dirofilarial hemoglobinuria, and vena cava embolism. Although adult heartworms prefer to live in the pulmonary arteries and right ventricle, as the worm burden increases, the number of adult worms migrating to the right atrium and caudal vena cava rises. Factors other than worm burden alone are probably also involved in the development of the caval syndrome. The vena caval syndrome is more likely to occur in animals in geographic areas where heartworm disease is enzootic. It has been estimated that this complication develops in 15% to 20% of dogs with heartworm disease.

Most affected dogs have no history of heartworm-related signs. Acute collapse is common, often accompanied by anorexia, weakness, tachypnea or dyspnea, pallor, hemoglobinuria, and bilirubinuria. A tricuspid insufficiency murmur, jugular distention and pulsations, weak pulses, a loud and possibly split $S_2$, and a cardiac gallop rhythm are often found. Sometimes coughing or hemoptysis and ascites occur. Tricuspid insufficiency and partial occlusion of the right ventricular inflow tract caused by the physical presence of the worms, in conjunction with pulmonary hypertension, lead to the development of right-sided congestive signs and poor cardiac output.

Clinicopathologic findings can include microfilaremia, Coombs' test–negative fragmentation hemolytic anemia (resulting from red blood cell trauma), azotemia, abnormal liver function, increased liver enzyme activities, and, often, DIC. Intravascular hemolysis causes hemoglobinemia and hemoglobinuria. Right-sided heart and pulmonary artery enlargement is evident on thoracic radiographs. The ECG usually indicates the presence of right ventricular enlargement. Echocardiography reveals a mass of worms entangled at the tricuspid valve and in the right atrium and venae cavae (see Fig. 10-2). Right ventricular dilation and hypertrophy, paradoxic septal motion, and a small left ventricle are also features. Unless treated, most dogs die within 24 to 72 hours from cardiogenic shock complicated by metabolic acidosis, DIC, and anemia.

Surgical removal of the worms from the vena cava and right atrium as soon as possible after presentation is the only effective therapy. A right jugular venotomy is performed with the dog lightly sedated, if necessary, and using local anesthesia. The dog is restrained in left lateral recumbency. Long alligator forceps, an endoscopic basket retrieval instrument, or a horsehair brush device is used to grasp and withdraw the heartworms through the jugular vein incision. The instrument is gently passed down the vein into the right atrium. It may be necessary to manipulate the animal's head and neck to pass the instrument beyond the thoracic inlet. Retrieval of as many worms as possible is the goal, with five to six unsuccessful attempts in sequence the end point. Survival in excess of 50% to 80% has been reported for dogs undergoing this procedure. Right auricular cannulation performed via a thoracotomy to remove worms in very small dogs has recently been described. Additional information on these procedures is found in the Suggested Readings. Supportive care, including cautious IV fluid administration, is given during and after surgical worm removal. Central venous pressure monitoring helps in assessing the effectiveness of worm removal and fluid therapy. Treatment with digoxin or sodium bicarbonate is usually not necessary, but broad-spectrum antibiotic treatment is recommended. Platelet counts should be monitored and thrombocytopenia managed as discussed in Chapter 89. Other therapy for DIC may include heparin (see Chapter 89). Severe pulmonary thromboembolism and renal or hepatic failure are associated with poor outcome. Within a few weeks after stabilization of the dog's condition, an adulticide is given to eliminate the remaining worms.

Use of a flexible alligator forceps with fluoroscopic guidance has been advocated as a way to reduce the worm burden in the main pulmonary artery and lobar branches before the start of adulticide therapy. This procedure should reduce the risk for postadulticide thromboembolism in heavily infected dogs. However, the heavy sedation or anesthesia required for the procedure also entails some risk.

**Other complications.** Azotemia, severe proteinuria, or both develop in some dogs with heartworm disease. Prerenal azotemia should be corrected with fluid therapy before the start of adulticide treatment. The outcome of adulticide therapy may not be adversely affected in the presence of mild-to-moderate azotemia and proteinuria without hypoalbuminemia. However, glomerular disease secondary to immune complex deposition or amyloidosis may be associated with severe hypoproteinemia, nephrotic syndrome, or renal tubular damage. Loss of antithrombin III, as well as other proteins, may augment the risk for thromboembolism in these animals. There may also be an exaggerated immune response to the dead worms. Although melarsomine should not adversely affect compromised renal function, the other concerns remain. Dogs with nephrotic syndrome or severe azotemia with proteinuria are poor candidates for thiacetarsamide therapy.

## Microfilaricide Therapy

Ivermectin and milbemycin have been used effectively as microfilaricidal drugs, although neither is approved by the U.S. Food and Drug Administration for this purpose. Treatment for microfilariae is generally administered 3 to 4 weeks after adulticide therapy. The rapid death of many microfilariae within 3 to 8 (and occasionally 12) hours of the first dose can cause systemic effects, including lethargy, inappetence, salivation, retching, defecation, pallor, and tachycardia. Usually such adverse effects are mild. However, dogs with high numbers of circulating microfilariae occasionally experience circulatory collapse that responds to glucocorticoid therapy (e.g., prednisolone sodium succinate, 10 mg/kg, or dexamethasone, 1 mg/kg IV) and IV fluid administration (e.g., 80 ml/kg over 2 hours) if these are instituted immediately. It is recommended that animals be closely observed for 8 to 12 hours after initial microfilaria treatment with either macrolide. An additional benefit of both drugs is that they prevent new infection.

Ivermectin (Ivomec or Heartgard; Merial, Iselin, N.J.) is an avermectin with efficacy against a variety of nematode and arthropod parasites. It is administered in a single dose of 0.05 mg/kg PO (50 μg/kg), which is higher than the preventive dose. This dose is also safe for Collies. Multiple Heartgard 30 tablets can be used to equal the necessary dose. If the concentrated livestock product is used, dilution and dose calculation must be done carefully to prevent overdose. One milliliter of ivermectin (10 mg/ml) diluted in 9 ml of propylene glycol can be given PO at a dose of 1 ml/20 kg of body weight.

A standard heartworm preventive dose (0.5 to 1.0 mg/kg) of milbemycin oxime (Interceptor; Novartis Animal Health, Greensboro, N.C.) is an alternative to ivermectin. Adverse reactions resulting from rapid microfilaria death are more likely in response to milbemycin therapy in dogs with high numbers of microfilariae. Treatment with either drug can be repeated every 2 weeks until microfilariae are no longer found; usually one or two doses are sufficient.

Moxidectin and selamectin are also known to be microfilaricidal, but there is inadequate clinical experience with them for this purpose. Other drugs that have been used as microfilaricides include levamisole and fenthion; but since they are less effective than ivermectin and milbemycin, must be given for a longer period, and have frequent adverse effects they are not recommended.

## Heartworm Prevention

Heartworm prophylaxis is indicated for all dogs living in endemic areas. Because sustained warm, moist conditions are important for heartworm disease transmission, the time of year when infection is possible is limited in most parts of the United States. Transmission is limited to only a few months in the most northern part of the United States; year-round transmission is thought possible only in the far southern edge of the continental United States. It appears that monthly preventive therapy is necessary only from June through October or November for animals in most of the United States and from April through November or December for animals in the southern one third of the United States. Year-round monthly preventive therapy is probably prudent at the southernmost edge.

Several macrolide drugs are currently available for preventing heartworm disease: the avermectins (ivermectin, selamectin) and the milbemycins (milbemycin oxime, moxidectin). Diethylcarbamazine (DEC) is also still available as a preventive agent. Preventive therapy can begin at 6 to 8 weeks of age. Before chemoprophylaxis is started for the first time, dogs old enough to have been previously infected should be tested for circulating antigen and (if DEC is to be used) microfilariae. Retesting for circulating antigen should be done periodically; usually every 2 to 3 years is adequate. The avermectins and milbemycins induce neuromuscular paralysis and death in nematode (and arthropod) parasites by interacting with membrane chloride channels. These agents have a wide margin of safety in mammals.

Ivermectin (Heartgard 30) is effective in preventing heartworm infections if given monthly in doses of 6 to 12 μg/kg and is safe in Collies. Although these small doses block the maturation of $L_3$ and $L_4$ larvae, the drug is not effective against adult heartworms. Ivermectin can be given to dogs that are not free of microfilariae, although the manufacturer recommends that it be given to microfilaria-negative dogs. The drug is completely effective against infectious larvae acquired 2 to 3 months before the drug is administered; it is somewhat effective in preventing heartworm development in dogs infected 4 months before monthly treatment begins. Prolonged monthly administration (e.g., after 16 months) of ivermectin alone or in combination with pyrantel pamoate has a moderate level of efficacy against adult heartworms. Heartgard is also marketed in a feline formulation for heartworm and hookworm control. Heartgard Plus has the addition of pyrantel pamoate and also controls roundworm and hookworm infection in dogs.

Milbemycin oxime (Interceptor) is effective for preventing heartworm infection as well as for controlling hookworm infection. Doses of 0.5 to 1.0 mg/kg given every 30 days provide complete protection against infection if the therapy is started within 2 to 3 months of potential exposure to infected mosquitoes. There is no contraindication to its use in Collies. Interceptor is not effective against adult *D. immitis*. The drug is not marketed as a microfilaricide; a shocklike reaction has occurred after milbemycin oxime administration in a small number of dogs with high circulating microfilaria counts. The drug does not appear to have adverse effects on reproduction. A combination of milbemycin oxime with lufenuron (Sentinel; Novartis Animal Health, Greensboro, N.C.) is also marketed for dogs for protection against heartworms, fleas, roundworms, hookworms, and whipworms.

Selamectin (Revolution; Pfizer Animal Health, Exton, Pa) effectively prevents heartworm disease, kills adult fleas and prevents flea eggs from hatching, and controls ear mites in both dogs and cats. This drug also controls American dog tick infestation as well as feline hookworm and roundworm infections. Selamectin is applied topically at the base of the neck between the shoulder blades; the recommended dose is 6 mg/kg. Efficacy is not affected by bathing or swimming 2 hours or longer after application. Besides virtually complete disappearance of microfilariae in heartworm-positive dogs by 4 months after initiating treatment, at least a 39% reduction in adult worm burden by 18 months of treatment was recently reported (Dzimianski and colleagues, 2001). The drug is safe at the unit dose range of 6 to 12 mg/kg in ivermectin-sensitive Collies, in heartworm-positive dogs and cats, and in breeding animals.

Moxidectin (ProHeart; Fort Dodge Animal Health, Fort Dodge, Iowa) is also a safe and effective monthly heartworm preventive for dogs. The recommended minimum dose is 3 μg/kg given to dogs older than 8 weeks of age. It is safe at the recommended dose in ivermectin-sensitive Collies. The manufacturer recommends use only in heartworm-negative dogs. Experimentally, significant microfilaricidal activity occurs by the third month at 15 μg/kg/mo. Sustained-release moxidectin (ProHeart 6) is available as a subcutaneously injected suspension of drug-impregnated organic polymer microspheres. Its protective effects last at least 6 months after injection at the recommended dose; it is also effective against canine hookworm infections. ProHeart 6 is recommended for use in dogs 6 months of age or older at a dose of reconstituted suspension of 0.05 ml/kg (moxidectin, 0.17 mg/kg) SC. This product must be reconstituted at least 30 minutes before and mixed again immediately before injection. Transient, localized inflammatory reactions occur in some animals at the injection site. Other signs including vomiting, diarrhea, lethargy, weight loss, and seizures have occasionally been reported. ProHeart 6 is safe for ivermectin-sensitive Collies.

Diethylcarbamazine or DEC (Filaribits; Pfizer, Exton, Pa; Nemacide; Boehringer Ingelheim, St. Joseph, Mo) has been used for more than 30 years for the prevention of heartworm disease. This drug is given in a dose of 3 mg/kg (6.6 mg/kg of the 50% citrate) once per day. Several formulations are available. The drug is thought to affect the $L_3$ to $L_4$ molting stage of the heartworm that occurs 9 to 12 days after infection. In areas of the United States with cold winters, the drug can be discontinued 2 months after a killing frost and reinstituted 1 month before mosquito season in the spring. Before beginning (or restarting) DEC treatment, dogs must be negative for microfilariae (see p. 171). Puppies 6 months of age and older should also be tested for microfilariae. Annual microfilaria tests are strongly recommended, even in areas where the drug is given year-round. To be effective, DEC must be given daily; however, even with rigorous attention to this schedule, occasional treatment failures have occurred. If a lapse of less than 6 weeks in DEC administration has occurred, one dose of a monthly preventive drug should restore protection. If DEC has not been administered for more than 8 weeks, monthly chemoprophylaxis should be extended for 1 year.

Dogs with microfilariae should not be given DEC, because adverse reactions of variable severity can occur with each dose. Such reactions can progress to hypovolemic shock and death. Although dogs with low numbers of microfilariae may experience no reaction, adverse reactions to DEC have occurred in dogs with higher numbers of microfilariae. Reactions usually begin within the first hour after the drug is given. A depressed attitude, lethargy, and reduced responsiveness occur initially and are variably followed by vomiting, diarrhea, or defecation. Later, bradycardia, a weak femoral pulse, and diminished heart sounds occur. Finally shock develops, with pallor, cool extremities, a slowed capillary refill time, tachycardia, tachypnea, and poor arterial pulses. Recumbency, hepatomegaly, hypersalivation, and death usually follow. Abnormal clinicopathologic findings include leukocytosis, thrombocytopenia, and high liver enzyme activities.

Therapy consisting of high doses of IV dexamethasone (at least 2 mg/kg), fluids, and other supportive measures has been used to combat the hypovolemia and shock. Atropine is given for the control of severe bradycardia. Dogs experiencing this microfilaria-induced reaction either show clinical improvement within 3 to 5 hours or die.

Dogs with occult heartworm disease may be given DEC, because adverse reactions do not occur in the absence of circulating microfilariae. Dogs that are receiving DEC prophylaxis and that are subsequently discovered to have circulating microfilariae should continue to be given the drug during adulticide and microfilaricide therapy to prevent reinfection. DEC is safe in heartworm-negative dogs, although vomiting and depression occasionally occur after drug administration in such dogs. Reproductive abnormalities caused by DEC have not been substantiated, despite anecdotal reports to the contrary. The combination of DEC and oxibendazole (Filaribits-Plus; Pfizer, Exton, Pa), which has been marketed for heartworm and hookworm prevention, has been rarely associated with acute and chronic periportal hepatitis. This potentially fatal association is thought to be an idiosyncratic reaction. The concurrent administration of phenobarbital may increase the toxic potential of this drug combination.

Periodic retesting is an important part of heartworm prophylaxis. After the first year of monthly prophylaxis, a heartworm antigen test should be done to confirm the dog's negative status. If preventive therapy has been given as scheduled, retest intervals longer than 1 year may be sufficient. When DEC is used as a preventive, yearly microfilaria testing is important before DEC is reinstituted. Supplemental antigen testing is also recommended.

## HEARTWORM DISEASE IN CATS

The overall prevalence of heartworm disease in cats is thought to be 5% to 20% of that in dogs in the same geographic area. Reported prevalences range from 0% to more than 15%. Cases have been identified in most of the midwestern and eastern states and in California. Infected cats generally have fewer adult worms than infected dogs because heartworms mature more slowly, fewer numbers of infective larvae mature to adults, and the adult life span is shorter in cats. However, live worms can persist for 2 to 3 years. Heartworm-infected cats generally have less than eight adult worms in the right ventricle and pulmonary arteries, and most cats have only one or two worms. Yet even one adult worm can cause death. Unisex infections are common. Most cats have no or only a brief period of microfilaremia. Aberrant worm migration is also more common in cats than in dogs and complicates necropsy confirmation of infection. Aberrant sites have included the brain, subcutaneous nodules, body cavities, and occasionally, a systemic artery.

The pathophysiologic changes occur in two stages. Immature worms at 4 to 6 months after infection stimulate activation of pulmonary intravascular macrophages, which are specialized phagocytic cells located in the pulmonary capillary beds of cats, but not dogs. When stimulated, these macrophages cause acute inflammation in the pulmonary arteries and lung tissue. This phase is fatal in some cats. In those that survive, the acute inflammation subsides. Vascular injury causes myointimal proliferations and muscular hypertrophy in affected pulmonary arteries. These lesions tend to be focal, so clinically relevant pulmonary hypertension usually does not develop. Dead and degenerating worms cause recrudescence of pulmonary inflammation and thromboembolism. Disease is most severe in the caudal lung lobes. Villous proliferation, thrombi, or dead heartworms have been identified as causing caudal lobar arterial obstruction. However, the adult worms themselves are more likely to obstruct arteries in cats than in dogs because of their relative size. The bronchopulmonary circulation in cats is thought to prevent pulmonary infarction. Interstitial lung disease occurs as in dogs, but cats have more extensive alveolar type 2 (surfactant-producing) cell hyperplasia, which can interfere with alveolar $O_2$ exchange. Adventitial and perivascular inflammatory cell infiltrates consisting mainly of eosinophils and neutrophils are also seen. The parenchymal lesions probably play an important role in the development of acute respiratory distress in many cats 4 to 9 months after infection. Although some cats recover, sudden death can occur, and this is usually associated with the existence of degenerating worms in the pulmonary arteries. The presence of markedly dilated areas in the muscular pulmonary arteries suggests pulmonary hypertension; however, secondary right ventricular hypertrophy and right-sided congestive failure are uncommon.

### Clinical Features

Recent clinical reports suggest that male gender is not a risk factor for heartworm infection in cats, in contrast to previous experimental findings (Atkins and colleagues, 2000). Strictly indoor housing is not protective; about one third of infected cats in some reports lived only indoors. Most reported cases have occurred in cats 3 to 6 years of age, although cats of any age are susceptible. Domestic Short Hair cats seem to be overrepresented. The infection is self-limiting in some cats. Severe clinical signs are usually associated with the arrival of $L_5$ parasites in the pulmonary arteries (5 to 6 months after infection) and with thromboembolism after the death of one or more worms. Some have reported more cases diagnosed in fall and winter, presumably after infection in the spring, whereas others have noted fewer cases in the last quarter of the year (Atkins and colleagues, 2000).

Clinical signs are variable and may be transient or nonspecific. Respiratory signs occur in over half of symptomatic cats, especially dyspnea and/or paroxysmal cough. Other historical complaints include lethargy, anorexia, vomiting, syncope, other neurologic signs, and sudden death. However, heartworm disease is sometimes an incidental finding. Auscultation may reveal pulmonary crackles, muffled lung sounds (resulting from pulmonary consolidation or pleural fluid accumulation), tachycardia, or occasionally, a cardiac gallop sound or murmur. Sudden death is more likely in cats than in dogs and is thought to result from thromboembolism and acute respiratory distress. Chronic vomiting is the only sign in some cats; others have vomiting and respiratory or other signs. Pleural effusion from right-sided heart failure as well as syncope appears to be less common in cats than in dogs. Chylothorax and ascites have occasionally been associated with heartworm disease in this species. Pneumothorax occurs rarely. Caval syndrome develops in a few cats. Although heartworms usually cause significant pulmonary vascular disease, some cats have no clinical signs. The sudden onset of neurologic signs, often in association with anorexia and lethargy, is common during aberrant worm migration. These signs include seizures, dementia, apparent blindness, ataxia, circling, mydriasis, and hypersalivation. Only rarely do cardiopulmonary and neurologic signs coexist.

## Diagnosis

Heartworm disease is usually more difficult to diagnose in cats than in dogs. Serologic testing, thoracic radiographs, echocardiography, and occasionally, microfilaria testing are helpful but are not uniformly definitive. Feline heartworm antibody tests are often used for screening; but, although they are fairly sensitive tests, they are not specific for adult heartworms (see p. 171). The ELISA-based antigen tests (see p. 171) are highly specific in detecting adult heartworm infection, but their sensitivity depends on the gender, age, and number of worms. Serologic test results may be negative early in the infection although the cat may have clinical signs. Antigen test results are negative during the first 5 months after infection and can be variably positive at 6 to 7 months; infections with mature female worms should be detected after 7 months. False-negative results to heartworm antigen tests are more likely in cats because of the low worm burdens common in this species; also, a longer time is required for cats to become antigen-positive. Antigen test results are also negative in the presence of infections with only male worms. Acute death and severe clinical signs can still occur in antigen-negative cats. Further, a postmortem diagnosis can be difficult if the worms are located in distal pulmonary arteries or aberrant sites. Occasionally an antigen test result is positive in a cat in which no worms are found postmortem. Spontaneous worm death, worms missed during evaluation of the lungs, and ectopic infection are likely reasons for this.

Thoracic radiograph findings often suggest the presence of heartworm disease but may not correlate with clinical signs or results of serologic tests. Such findings may include pulmonary artery enlargement with or without visible tortuosity and pruning, right ventricular or generalized cardiac enlargement, and diffuse or focal pulmonary bronchointerstitial infiltrates. Pulmonary hyperinflation can sometimes be evident. Changes in the pulmonary artery and right side of the heart are typically more subtle in cats than in dogs. It has been found experimentally that arteries enlarge within a few weeks to 7 months of adult worm transplantation. Cranial pulmonary artery enlargement especially may regress thereafter. The DV view is best for evaluating the caudal lobar arteries, which appear more frequently abnormal on radiographs. The right caudal lobar artery may be more promi-

nent; however, a left caudal pulmonary artery of 1.6 or higher × the width of the ninth rib at the ninth intercostal space was reported as the most discriminating radiographic finding for separating heartworm-infected from noninfected cats (Schafer and colleague, 1995). The main pulmonary artery segment is not usually visible on DV or ventrodorsal views in cats, because it is located more medially than it is in dogs. Considerable right-sided heart enlargement is more likely in the presence of signs of right-sided heart failure (e.g., pleural effusion). Thoracocentesis may be necessary to evaluate the heart, pulmonary vasculature, and lung parenchyma if pleural effusion is present. Ascites occurs in some cats with heartworm disease (it is rare in cats with heart failure resulting from cardiomyopathy). Both allergic pneumonitis and pulmonary thromboembolism result in pulmonary infiltrates; focal perivascular and interstitial changes are more common than diffuse infiltrates. Radiographs are normal in a small minority of heartworm-infected cats. Pulmonary arteriography performed using a large-bore jugular vein catheter may confirm a suspected diagnosis of heartworm disease in a cat with a false-negative antigen test result and normal echocardiogram. Morphologic changes in the pulmonary arteries are outlined, and worms appear as linear filling defects.

Echocardiography is a useful diagnostic test and has allowed visualization of worms in 40% to 78% of positive cats (DeFrancesco and colleagues, 2001). Higher numbers of worms increase the chance of identification with echocardiography. Echocardiographic findings may be normal unless worms are located in the heart, main pulmonary artery segment, or proximal left and right pulmonary arteries. Worms are seen in the pulmonary arteries more often than in right-sided heart chambers, so an index of suspicion and careful interrogation of these structures are important.

Only about 33% to 43% of infected cats have peripheral eosinophilia, usually from 4 to 7 months after infection; in most cases, however, the eosinophil count is normal. Basophilia is uncommon. Mild nonregenerative anemia is present in about one third of cases. Advanced pulmonary arterial disease and thromboembolism may be accompanied by neutrophilia (sometimes with a left shift), monocytosis, thrombocytopenia, and DIC. Hyperglobulinemia, the most common biochemical abnormality, occurs inconsistently. The prevalence of glomerulopathies in cats with heartworm disease is unknown but does not appear to be high.

Tracheal wash or bronchoalveolar lavage cytologic specimens may show an eosinophilic exudate suggestive of allergic or parasitic disease, similar to that found with feline asthma or pulmonary parasites. Experimentally this has been found to occur between 4 and 8 months after infection. Later in the disease, tracheal wash cytologic specimens show a nonspecific chronic inflammation or the findings are unremarkable. Thus the absence of an eosinophilic exudate does not exclude a diagnosis of heartworm disease. Pleural fluid from heartworm-induced right-sided heart failure is generally a modified transudate, although chylothorax occasionally develops.

The ECG is often normal, although most cats with heartworm-induced right-sided heart failure have changes suggestive of right ventricular enlargement. Congenital heart disease or a right bundle branch block with or without cardiomyopathy should also be considered. Arrhythmias appear to be uncommon. Advanced pulmonary arterial disease and congestive heart failure are more likely to cause ventricular tachyarrhythmias.

A low and transient (1 to 2 months in duration) microfilaremia occurs in about 50% of infected cats approximately 6.5 to 7 months after infection. Thus microfilaria concentration test results are usually negative. Despite this, a concentration test may still be valuable in individual cats. Three to five milliliters, rather than 1 ml, of blood should be used to increase the probability of detecting microfilariae.

## Treatment of Cats with Heartworm Disease

**Medical therapy and complications.** Adulticide therapy is not recommended in light of the high prevalence of severe complications in this species, the fact that cats are not significant reservoirs for the transmission of heartworm disease to other animals, and the possibility of spontaneous cure because of the shorter life span of heartworms in cats. No difference in survival was found between cats not given adulticide and those receiving thiacetarsamide in a retrospective clinical study (Atkins and colleagues, 2000). A more conservative approach for infected cats is to use prednisone as needed, with a monthly heartworm preventive drug but no adulticide treatment. It is recommended that serologic tests be obtained every 6 to 12 months to monitor infection status. Antigen-positive cats usually become negative within 4 to 5 months of worm death. It is unclear how long Ab tests remain positive. Serial thoracic radiographs and echocardiograms are also useful for monitoring cats in which these tests have been abnormal. Radiographically evident interstitial infiltrates usually respond to diminishing doses of prednisone (e.g., 2 mg/kg/day, reduced gradually during 2 weeks to 0.5 mg/kg q48h, then discontinued after 2 more weeks). This treatment can be repeated periodically if respiratory signs recur.

Severe respiratory distress and death may occur at any time, especially after spontaneous or adulticide-induced worm death. Pulmonary thromboembolism is more likely to be fatal in cats than in dogs. Clinical signs of pulmonary thromboembolism include fever, cough, dyspnea, hemoptysis, pallor, pulmonary crackles, tachycardia, and hypotension. Supportive radiographic findings include poorly defined, rounded or wedge-shaped areas of interstitial (with or without alveolar) opacities that obscure associated pulmonary vessels. Supportive care for acutely ill cats can include IV glucocorticoids, fluid therapy, a bronchodilator, and supplemental $O_2$. Diuretics are not indicated. Aspirin or other nonsteroidal antiinflammatory drugs (NSAIDs) have not been shown to produce benefit and may exacerbate pulmonary disease. Aspirin therapy is therefore currently not recommended for cats with heartworm disease.

Right-sided congestive heart failure develops in some cats with severe pulmonary arterial disease. Cough, pulmonary parenchymal disease, or evidence of thromboembolic events may occur inconsistently. Dyspnea resulting from pleural fluid accumulation and jugular venous distention or pulsation are common. The presence of right ventricular enlargement is usually indicated by radiographs and ECG. Therapy directed at controlling the signs of heart failure includes thoracocentesis as needed, cage confinement, and cautious furosemide therapy (e.g., 1 mg/kg q12-24h). An angiotensin converting enzyme inhibitor may be helpful (see p. 64). Digoxin therapy is not generally recommended. The nature of other supportive care is guided by the cat's clinical progress and clinicopathologic abnormalities.

The caval syndrome, although rare, has been reported, with the successful removal of adult worms accomplished through a jugular venotomy.

An adulticide is the therapy of last resort for stable cats that continue to manifest clinical signs despite prednisone treatment. Potentially fatal thromboembolism is possible even with only one worm present. About one third of adulticide-treated cats are expected to have thromboembolic complications; a higher risk is expected for heavily infected cats. Adulticide should not be given only on the basis of a positive antigen, antibody, or microfilaria test result. Thiacetarsamide (Caparsolate) has been used in combination with prednisone and extremely close monitoring for 2 weeks. It has been given to dogs at 2.2 mg/kg IV twice daily for 2 days, and prevention of drug extravasation is essential. Cats eliminate the drug more slowly than dogs. Anorexia, profound depression, nausea, and vomiting frequently occur after each thiacetarsamide dose and may preclude completion of therapy. A sometimes fatal respiratory distress syndrome with fulminant noncardiogenic pulmonary edema has developed in some cats after thiacetarsamide, possibly related to arteriolar dilation and toxic effects of arsenic on microvascular integrity. Pretreatment with an antihistamine and soluble glucocorticoid before the start of thiacetarsamide therapy has been suggested, but the efficacy of this is unknown. There is very little clinical experience with melarsomine (Immiticide) in cats. Results of serologic tests done to detect adult worm antigen should be negative within 3 to 4 months if adulticide therapy has been successful, but the time required for the seroconversion of antibody titers is thought to be much longer.

**Surgical therapy.** Although technically challenging, several approaches have been described for removal of adult heartworms from cats. Worms in the right atrium and vena cava can be reached via right jugular venotomy using small alligator forceps, endoscopic grasping or basket retrieval forceps, or other device (Brown and colleague, 1998; Borgarelli and colleagues, 1997; Rawlings and colleagues, 1994). Right thoracotomy and atriotomy have also been used successfully. Worms in the pulmonary artery have been extracted using a left thoracotomy and pulmonary arteriotomy. There is concern about potentially fatal anaphylactic reactions associated with worm breakage during these procedures. For this reason, pretreatment with a glucocorticoid and antihistamine has been suggested. It is unclear whether pretreatment for several days with heparin reduces thromboembolic events associated with surgical worm removal.

## Microfilaricide and Preventive Therapy

Microfilaricide therapy is usually not necessary since microfilaremia is brief, but ivermectin and milbemycin should be effective in this setting.

Preventive medication is recommended for cats in endemic areas. Selamectin (Revolution), ivermectin (Heartgard for cats), and milbemycin oxime (Interceptor Flavor Tabs for cats) are marketed in the United States for heartworm prevention in cats (see p. 178). Selamectin is used at the same dose as for dogs (6 to 12 mg/kg, topically). Ivermectin is given PO at 24 μg/kg monthly, which is four times the dose used in dogs. Milbemycin oxime's minimum recommended dose is 2 mg/kg, which is about twice the dose used in dogs. Ivermectin and milbemycin oxime are labeled as safe for kittens 6 weeks of age or older; selamectin is recommended for cats 8 weeks of age or older. It is recommended that an antigen test be performed before initiating prophylaxis if infection could have occurred 8 months or more before. DEC has also been given to cats in doses similar to those used in dogs, with no apparent adverse effects, although daily administration makes it less convenient.

## Suggested Readings

### GENERAL

Knight DH et al: 1999 Guidelines for the diagnosis, prevention, and management of heartworm *(Dirofilaria immitis)* infection in dogs, http://www.heartwormsociety.org.

Knight DH et al: 1999 Guidelines for the diagnosis, treatment and prevention of heartworm *(Dirofilaria immitis)* infection in cats, *Vet Therapeutics* 2:78, 2001, http://www.heartwormsociety.org.

McCall JW et al: Evaluation of the performance of canine antigen test kits licensed for use by veterinarians and canine antigen tests conducted by diagnostic laboratories. In *Proceedings of the 10th Annual Heartworm Symposium*, San Antonio, 2001 (abstract).

McTeir TL et al: Features of adult heartworm antigen test kits. In *Proceedings of the 1995 Heartworm Symposium, American Heartworm Society*, Washington, DC, p 115.

Rawlings CA et al: Surgical removal of heartworms, *Semin Vet Med Surg* 9:200, 1994.

### HEARTWORM DISEASE IN THE DOG

Atkins CE et al: Pathophysiologic mechanism of cardiac dysfunction in experimentally induced heartworm caval syndrome in dogs: an echocardiographic study, *Am J Vet Res* 49:403, 1988.

Atkins CE et al: Acute effect of hydralazine administration on pulmonary artery hemodynamics in dogs with chronic heartworm disease, *Am J Vet Res* 55:262, 1994.

Atwell RB et al: Effective reversal of induced arsenic toxicity using BAL therapy. In *Proceedings of the 1989 Heartworm Symposium, American Heartworm Society*, Washington, DC, p 155.

Beal MW et al: Respiratory failure attributable to moxidectin intoxication in a dog, *J Am Vet Med Assoc* 215(12):1813, 1999.

Carastro SM et al: Intraocular dirofilariasis in dogs, *Compend Cont Educ* 14:209, 1992.

Case JL et al: A clinical field trial of melarsomine dihydrochloride (RM340) in dogs with severe (class 3) heartworm disease. In *Proceedings of the 1995 Heartworm Symposium, American Heartworm Society*, Washington, DC, p 243.

Dillon AR et al: Influence of number of parasites and exercise on the severity of heartworm disease in dogs. In *Proceedings of the 1995 Heartworm Symposium, American Heartworm Society*, Washington, DC, p 113.

Dzimianski MT et al: The safety of selamectin in heartworm infected dogs and its effect on adult worms and microfilariae. In *Proceedings of the 10th Annual Heartworm Symposium*, San Antonio, 2001 (abstract).

Frank J et al: Systemic arterial dirofilariasis in five dogs. *J Vet Intern Med* 11:189, 1997.

Jackson RF et al: Surgical treatment of the caval syndrome of canine heartworm disease, *J Am Vet Med Assoc* 171:1065, 1977.

Kitagawa H et al: Comparison of laboratory test results before and after surgical removal of heartworms in dogs with vena caval syndrome, *J Am Vet Med Assoc* 213:1134, 1998.

Kitoh K et al: Role of histamine in heartworm extract-induced shock in dogs, *Am J Vet Res* 62:770, 2001.

Kuntz CA et al: Use of a modified surgical approach to the right atrium for retrieval of heartworms in a dog, *J Am Vet Med Assoc* 208:692, 1996.

Litster A et al: Comparison of radiographic cardiac size in dogs with heartworm disease with reference values using the vertebral heart scale method. In *Proceedings of the 10th Annual Heartworm Symposium*, San Antonio, 2001 (abstract).

Lok JB et al: Activity of an injectable, sustained-release formulation of moxidectin administered prophylactically to mixed breed dogs to prevent infection with *Dirofilaria immitis*, *Am J Vet Res* 62:1721, 2001.

McCall JW et al: Evaluation of ivermectin and milbemycin oxime efficacy against *Dirofilaria immitis* infections of three and four months' duration in dogs, *Am J Vet Res* 57:1189, 1996.

Miller MW et al: Clinical efficacy of melarsomine dihydrochloride (RM340) and thiacetarsamide in dogs with moderate (class 2) heartworm disease. In *Proceedings of the 1995 Heartworm Symposium, American Heartworm Society*, Washington, DC, p 233.

Rawlings CA et al: Postadulticide pulmonary hypertension of canine heartworm disease: successful treatment with oxygen and failure of antihistamines, *Am J Vet Res* 51:1565, 1990.

Rawlings CA et al: Pulmonary thromboembolism and hypertension after thiacetarsamide vs melarsomine dihydrochloride treatment of *Dirofilaria immitis* infection in dogs, *Am J Vet Res* 54:920, 1993.

Vezzoni A et al: Reduction of post-adulticide thromboembolic complications with low dose heparin therapy. In *Proceedings of the 1989 Heartworm Symposium, American Heartworm Society*, Washington, DC, p 73.

### HEARTWORM DISEASE IN THE CAT

Atkins C et al: Prevalence of heartworm infection in cats with signs of cardiorespiratory abnormalities, *J Am Vet Med Assoc* 212:517, 1998.

Atkins C et al: Heartworm infection in cats: 50 cases (1985-1997), *J Am Vet Med Assoc* 217:355, 2000.

Borgarelli M et al: Surgical removal of heartworms from the right atrium of a cat, *J Am Vet Med Assoc* 211(1):68, 1997.

Brown WA et al: Surgical teatment of feline heartworm disease. In *Proceedings of the 16th Annual ACVIM Scientific Forum*, San Diego, 1998, p 88.

DeFrancesco TC et al: Use of echocardiography for the diagnosis of heartworm disease in cats: 43 cases (1985-1997), *J Am Vet Med Assoc* 218:66, 2001.

Dillon AR et al: Feline heartworm disease: correlations of clinical signs, serology, and other diagnostics—results of a multi-center study, *Vet Therapeutics* 1:176, 2000.

Glaus TM et al: Surgical removal of heartworms from a cat with caval syndrome, *J Am Vet Med Assoc* 206:663, 1995.

Mansour AE et al: Epidemiology of feline dirofilariasis. In *Proceedings of the 1995 Heartworm Symposium, American Heartworm Society,* Washington, DC, p 87.

McCall JW et al: Utility of an ELISA-based antibody test for detection of heartworm infection in cats. In *Proceedings of the 1995 Heartworm Symposium, American Heartworm Society,* Washington, DC, p 127.

Rawlings CA: Pulmonary arteriography and hemodynamics during feline heartworm disease: effects of aspirin, *J Vet Intern Med* 4:285, 1990.

Schafer M et al: Cardiac and pulmonary artery mensuration in feline heartworm disease, *Vet Radiol Ultrasound* 36:499, 1995.

Selcer BA et al: Radiographic and 2-D echocardiographic findings in eighteen cats experimentally exposed to *D. immitis* via mosquito bites, *Vet Radiol Ultrasound* 37:37, 1996.

Snyder PS et al: Performance of serologic tests used to detect heartworm infection in cats, *J Am Vet Med Assoc* 216:693, 2000.

Turner JL et al: Thiacetarsamide in healthy cats: clinical and pathological observations, *J Am Anim Hosp Assoc* 27:275, 1991.

# CHAPTER 11

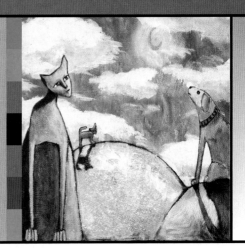

# Pericardial Diseases and Cardiac Tumors

## CHAPTER OUTLINE

GENERAL CONSIDERATIONS, 185
PERICARDIAL EFFUSION, 185
   Pericardiocentesis, 191
CONGENITAL PERICARDIAL DISORDERS, 192
   Peritoneopericardial diaphragmatic hernia, 192
   Other pericardial anomalies, 192
CONSTRICTIVE PERICARDIAL DISEASE, 194
CARDIAC TUMORS, 194

## GENERAL CONSIDERATIONS

Cardiac function can be disrupted by diseases involving the pericardium and intrapericardial space. Although there are few overt clinical consequences of removing a normal pericardium, this structure helps balance the output of the right and left ventricles and limits acute distension of the heart. The pericardium anchors the heart in place and provides a barrier to infection or inflammation from adjacent tissues; it is attached to the great vessels at the heart base. The pericardium is a closed serous sac, enveloping the heart so completely that the sac's lumen is reduced to a tiny space. The portion directly adhered to the heart is the *visceral pericardium,* or *epicardium,* which is composed of a thin layer of mesothelial cells. This layer reflects back over itself at the base of the heart, where the great vessels originate, to line the outer fibrous parietal layer. A small amount (~0.25 ml/kg body weight) of clear, serous fluid is normally contained between these layers and serves as a lubricant. Excess or abnormal fluid accumulation is the most common pericardial disorder, and it occurs most often in dogs. Other acquired and congenital pericardial diseases are infrequently seen. Acquired pericardial diseases are uncommon in cats; but of these, pericardial effusion from feline infectious peritonitis is most often identified. Pericardial effusions secondary to congestive heart failure (especially hypertrophic cardiomyopathy), lymphoma, systemic infections, and rarely renal failure are also found in cats.

## PERICARDIAL EFFUSION

### Etiology

In dogs, most pericardial effusions are serosanguineous or sanguineous and are of neoplastic or idiopathic origin. Transudates, modified transudates, and exudates are found occasionally in both dogs and cats.

**Hemorrhage.** Hemorrhagic effusions are common in dogs. The fluid usually appears dark red, with a packed cell volume (PCV) of over 7%, a specific gravity over 1.015, and a protein concentration of 3 to 6 g/dl. Mostly red blood cells are found in cytologic analysis, but reactive mesothelial, neoplastic, or other cells may be seen. The fluid does not clot unless hemorrhage was very recent. In general, middle-aged, large-breed dogs are most likely to have idiopathic, "benign" hemorrhagic effusion. Dogs older than 7 years are likely to have neoplastic hemorrhagic effusion.

Hemangiosarcoma is by far the most common neoplasm causing hemorrhagic pericardial effusion in dogs; it is uncommon in cats. Hemorrhagic pericardial effusion also results from various heart base tumors, pericardial mesotheliomas, and rarely, from metastatic carcinomas. Hemangiosarcomas (see Chapter 84) usually arise from the right atrial wall, especially in the auricular area. Chemodectoma is the most common heart base tumor; it arises from chemoreceptor cells at the base of the aorta. Other heart base tumors include thyroid, parathyroid, lymphoid, and connective tissue neoplasms. Pericardial mesotheliomas also occur uncommonly in dogs and cats. Lymphoma involving various parts of the heart is seen more often in cats than in dogs.

Idiopathic (benign) pericardial effusion has been described most frequently in medium- to large-breed dogs. The Golden Retriever, German Shepherd Dog, Great Dane, and Saint Bernard may be predisposed. Although dogs of any age can be affected, the median age is 6 to 7 years. More cases have been reported in males than females. Evidence of only mild pericardial inflammation with diffuse fibrosis and focal hemorrhage is common. Fibrosis in layers of varying maturity has been described, suggesting an episodic process. Constrictive pericardial disease is a potential sequela.

Less common causes of intrapericardial hemorrhage include left atrial rupture secondary to severe mitral insufficiency (see p. 141), coagulopathy (e.g., caused by ingestion of warfarin-type rodenticides), penetrating trauma (including iatrogenic laceration of a coronary artery during pericardiocentesis), and uremic pericarditis.

**Transudates.** Pure transudates are clear, with a low cell count (<1500 cells/μl), specific gravity (<1.012), and protein content (<2.5 g/dl). Modified transudates may appear slightly cloudy or pink tinged; cellularity (~1500 to 5000 cells/μl) and total protein concentration (~3 g/dl or slightly above) are higher than those of a pure transudate. Transudative effusions can be caused by congestive heart failure, pericardioperitoneal diaphragmatic hernias (see p. 192), hypoalbuminemia, pericardial cysts, and toxemias that increase vascular permeability (including uremia). Usually these conditions are associated with small volumes of pericardial effusion, and cardiac tamponade rarely develops.

**Exudates.** Exudates appear cloudy to opaque or serofibrinous to serosanguineous. They are characterized by a high nucleated cell count (usually >7000 cells/μl), protein concentration (usually much higher than 3 g/dl), and specific gravity (>1.015). Cytologic findings are related to the etiology. Exudative pericardial effusions are rarely found in small animals. Infectious pericarditis has been reported, usually related to plant awn migration, bite wounds, or extension of pleural or mediastinal infections. Various aerobic and anaerobic bacteria, actinomycosis, coccidioidomycosis, disseminated tuberculosis, and rarely, systemic protozoal infections have been identified. Sterile exudative effusions have occurred in association with leptospirosis, canine distemper, and idiopathic pericardial effusion in dogs and with feline infectious peritonitis and toxoplasmosis in cats. Chronic uremia occasionally causes a sterile, serofibrinous or hemorrhagic effusion.

## Pathophysiology

Unless intrapericardial pressure rises to equal or exceed cardiac filling pressure, fluid accumulation within the pericardial space does not cause clinical signs. When intrapericardial pressure is low, cardiac filling and output remain relatively normal. If fluid accumulates slowly, the pericardium can distend enough to accommodate the increased volume while low pressure is maintained. However, because the pericardium is relatively noncompliant, rapid fluid accumulation or very large effusions cause a steep rise in the intrapericardial pressure-volume relationship. Pericardial fibrosis and thickening further limit the compliance of this tissue.

Very large pericardial effusions occasionally cause clinical signs by virtue of their size, even in the absence of cardiac tamponade (see below). Lung and/or tracheal compression can cause dyspnea and cough; esophageal compression can cause dysphagia or regurgitation.

**Cardiac tamponade.** Cardiac tamponade develops when pericardial fluid accumulation raises intrapericardial pressure above the cardiac diastolic pressure. The external compression on the heart progressively limits filling, and cardiac output falls. Eventually, pressures in all cardiac chambers and great veins equilibrate during diastole. The neurohumoral compensatory mechanisms of heart failure are activated as tamponade develops. Although cardiac contractility is not directly affected by pericardial effusion, reduced coronary perfusion during tamponade can impair both systolic and diastolic functions. Low cardiac output, arterial hypotension, and poor perfusion of other organs as well as the heart can ultimately lead to cardiogenic shock and death. The rate of fluid accumulation and the distensibility of the pericardial sac determine whether and how quickly cardiac tamponade develops. Rapid fluid accumulation of even small volumes can markedly raise intrapericardial pressure because the pericardium can stretch only slowly. A large volume of pericardial fluid implies a gradual process. Cardiac tamponade is relatively common in dogs but rare in cats.

Pulsus paradoxus is an exaggerated respiratory variation in arterial blood pressure that occurs as a result of cardiac tamponade, although it may not be readily discernible using digital palpation of the femoral pulse. Inspiration reduces intrapericardial and right atrial pressures, thereby facilitating right heart filling and pulmonary blood flow. Simultaneously, left heart filling is reduced because more blood is held in the lungs and the interventricular septum bulges leftward from the inspiratory increase in right ventricular filling; consequently, left heart output and systemic arterial pressure decrease during inspiration. In patients with cardiac tamponade and pulsus paradoxus, the variation in systolic arterial pressure is usually greater than 10 mm Hg.

## Clinical Features

Clinical findings in patients with cardiac tamponade reflect poor cardiac output and usually right-sided congestive heart failure. Signs may be nonspecific (e.g., lethargy, weakness, poor exercise tolerance, inappetence) before obvious ascites develops. Rapid accumulation of even small volumes of fluid (50 to 100 ml) can cause acute tamponade, shock, and death. In such cases, jugular venous distention, hypotension, and pulmonary edema may be evident without notable radiographic signs of cardiomegaly or pleural and peritoneal effusions.

Gradual pericardial fluid accumulation results in signs of congestive heart failure because of compensatory volume retention and the direct effects of impaired cardiac filling. Signs of right-sided congestive heart failure predominate because of the right heart's thin wall and low pressures, although signs of biventricular failure may occur. Historical findings of weakness, exercise intolerance, abdominal enlargement, tachypnea, syncope, and cough are typical. Significant loss of lean body mass occurs in some chronic cases (Fig. 11-1). Jugular vein distention and/or positive hepatojugular reflux, hepatomegaly, ascites, labored respiration, and weakened femoral pulses are common physical examination findings. A palpable decrease in arterial pulse strength during inspiration (see pulsus paradoxus, above) might be discernable. High sympathetic tone causes sinus tachycardia, pale mucous membranes, and prolonged capillary refill time. The precordial impulse is attenuated by large pericardial fluid volumes. Auscultation reveals muffled heart sounds in animals with

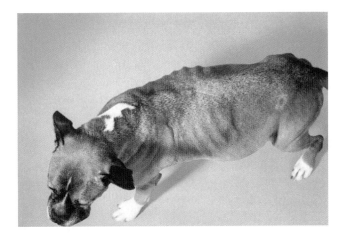

**FIG 11-1**
Older male Boxer with chronic cardiac tamponade and right-sided congestive heart failure secondary to chemodectoma. The abdomen is greatly distended with ascites; chronic loss of lean body mass is evident along the spine, pelvis, and rib cage.

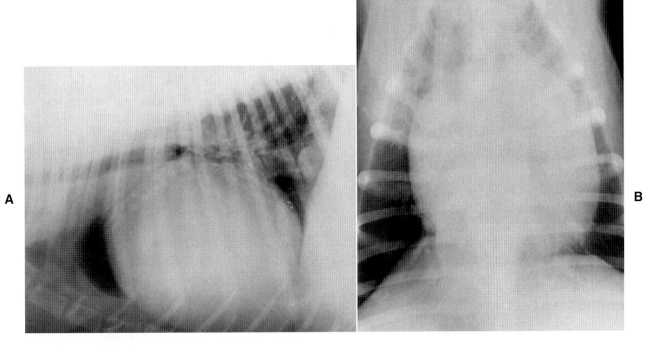

A

B

**FIG 11-2**
Lateral **(A)** and dorsoventral **(B)** radiographs from a mixed-breed dog with large pericardial effusion. Note globoid shape of cardiac silhouette and distended caudal vena cava **(A).**

moderate-to-large pericardial effusions and muffled ventral lung sounds in those with pleural effusion. Although pericardial effusion does not cause a murmur, concurrent cardiac disease may do so. Fever may be associated with infectious pericarditis, and rarely, a pericardial friction rub might be heard. Central venous pressure (CVP) elevation above 10 to 12 cm H$_2$O is common; normally CVP is less than 8 cm H$_2$O. Whenever the jugular veins are difficult to assess or it is unclear whether right heart filling pressures are elevated, CVP should be measured. Large pleural effusions should be drained prior to CVP measurement not only to stabilize the patient but also to minimize artifactual elevation of CVP. Pleural effusion and ascites are also common signs in cats with cardiac tamponade.

## Diagnosis

**Radiography.** Pericardial fluid accumulation enlarges the cardiac silhouette (Fig. 11-2). Massive pericardial effusion causes the classic globoid-shaped cardiac shadow seen on both radiographic views. However, this totally round heart shadow is not observed in many cases. Smaller fluid accumulations allow various cardiac contours to be identified, especially dorsally. Other findings associated with tamponade include pleural effusion, caudal vena cava distention, hepatomegaly, and ascites. Pulmonary opacities compatible with edema and distended pulmonary veins are less frequently noted. The presence of pleural effusion without jugular venous distention, an increased CVP, and ascites, however, suggests a disease other than cardiac tamponade and right

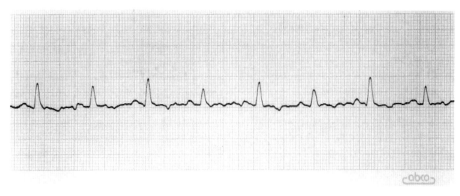

**FIG 11-3**
Electrical alternans is evident on this lead II ECG from a 10-year-old male English Bulldog with a large pericardial effusion. Note also the small voltage QRS complexes and sinus tachycardia (heart rate about 170 beats/min).

heart failure. Some heart base tumors cause deviation of the trachea or a soft tissue mass effect. Metastatic lung lesions are common in dogs with hemangiosarcoma. Fluoroscopy demonstrates diminished to absent motion of the cardiac shadow because the heart is surrounded by fluid.

Angiocardiography is currently used only rarely for the diagnosis of pericardial effusion and cardiac tumors because of the wide availability of echocardiography (see below); however, it typically reveals increased endocardial-to-pericardial distance. Cardiac neoplasms can cause displacement of normal structures, filling defects, and vascular "blushing" (opacification of excessive, abnormal tumor-associated vessels).

Echocardiography has also essentially replaced the use of pneumopericardiography in the evaluation of patients with pericardial effusion. Pneumopericardiography employs carbon dioxide or air injected into the drained pericardial sac to outline the heart. Radiographs are taken from different orientations, but the left lateral and dorsoventral views are most helpful. These views allow the injected gas to outline the right atrial and heart base areas, respectively, where tumors are most common.

**Electrocardiography.** Although there are no pathognomonic electrocardiographic (ECG) findings, the following abnormalities are suggestive of pericardial effusion: diminished amplitude of QRS complexes ($<1$ mV in dogs), electrical alternans, and ST segment elevation (epicardial injury current). Electrical alternans is a recurring alteration in the size of the QRS complex (or sometimes the T wave) with every other beat (Fig. 11-3). It results from physical swinging of the heart back and forth within the pericardium and is most often associated with a large volume of pericardial fluid. Electrical alternans may be most evident at heart rates between 90 and 140 beats/min and/or in the standing position. Sinus tachycardia is common in association with cardiac tamponade. Atrial or ventricular tachyarrhythmias may also occur.

**Echocardiography.** Echocardiography is highly sensitive for detecting even small volumes of pericardial fluid. Because pericardial fluid is sonolucent, pericardial effusion appears as an echo-free space between the bright parietal pericardium and the epicardium (Fig. 11-4). Abnormal cardiac wall motion and chamber shape, as well as intrapericardial or intracardiac mass lesions, can also be imaged. With large-volume pericardial effusions, the heart may appear to swing back and forth within the pericardial sac. Tamponade is manifested by diastolic compression/collapse of the right atrium and sometimes the right ventricle (Fig. 11-5), although other factors can contribute to this collapse. It is important to remember that the volume of the effusion is not the main determinant of hemodynamic compromise, but rather the intrapericardial pressure. The right ventricular and atrial walls are often well visualized and may appear hyperechoic because of the surrounding fluid. Better visualization of the heart base and mass lesions is generally obtained before pericardiocentesis is performed.

Sometimes pleural effusion, a markedly enlarged left atrium, a dilated coronary sinus, or persistent left cranial vena cava can be confused with pericardial effusion. Careful scanning from several positions helps to differentiate these conditions. Identification of the parietal pericardium in relation to the echo-free fluid helps to differentiate pleural from pericardial effusion. The pericardium is a relatively strong reflector of ultrasound; with progressive rejection of echoes, those echoes from the pericardium are usually the last to disappear. Most pericardial fluid accumulates near the cardiac apex because the pericardium adheres more tightly to the heart base; there is usually little fluid behind the left atrium. Furthermore, evidence of collapsed lung lobes or pleural folds can often be seen within the pleural effusion. Careful evaluation of all portions of the right atrium and auricle, right ventricle, ascending aorta, and pericardium itself is important to screen for neoplasia. The left cranial parasternal (and transesophageal) transducer positions are especially useful.

**Clinical pathology.** Hematologic and biochemical test results are generally nonspecific. The complete blood count (CBC) may suggest inflammation or infection. Cardiac hemangiosarcoma may be associated with a regenerative anemia,

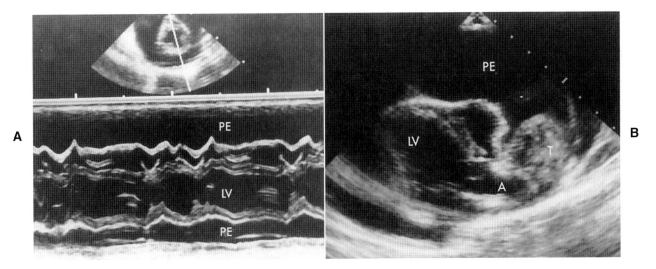

**FIG 11-4**
Echocardiographic examples of pericardial effusion. **A,** Short-axis M-mode view at mitral valve and chordal levels. Large echo-free (fluid) spaces are seen on either side of the heart; the right ventricular wall is clearly visualized. The small 2-D image above the M-mode shows the heart (transected by the M-mode cursor line) surrounded by pericardial fluid (which appears black on the image). **B,** Long-axis 2-D view from left parasternal position depicting a large heart base tumor and pericardial effusion in a Schnauzer. *PE,* Pericardial effusion; *T,* tumor mass; *LV,* left ventricle; *A,* aorta.

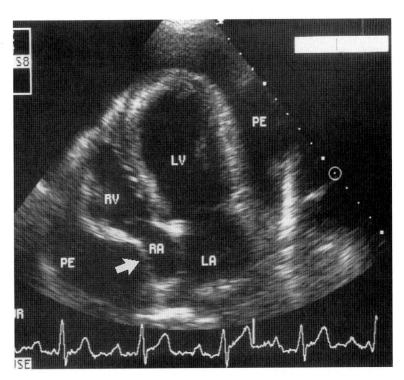

**FIG 11-5**
Diastolic compression of the right atrial wall *(arrow)* is evident in this left caudal four-chamber echocardiogram from a 3-year-old female Saint Bernard with cardiac tamponade. *LA,* Left atrium; *LV,* left ventricle; *PE,* pericardial effusion; *RA,* right atrium; *RV,* right ventricle.

increased numbers of nucleated red blood cells and schistocytes, and thrombocytopenia. Mild hypoproteinemia is seen in some cases of pericardial effusion. Cardiac enzyme activities may be elevated from ischemia or myocardial invasion; mild increases in liver enzyme activities and prerenal azotemia can occur secondary to heart failure. Pleural and peritoneal fluids in dogs and cats with cardiac tamponade are usually modified transudates.

Pericardiocentesis (see p. 191) usually yields a hemorrhagic effusion; less frequently the fluid is suppurative. Samples should be submitted for cytologic analysis and saved for possible bacterial (or fungal) culture. Nevertheless, differentiation of neoplastic effusions from benign hemorrhagic pericarditis is usually impossible on the basis of cytology alone. Reactive mesothelial cells within the effusion may closely resemble neoplastic cells; furthermore, chemodectomas and hemangiosarcomas may not shed cells into the effusion. However, neoplastic lymphoid cells are easily identified in dogs and cats with lymphoma. Thus echocardiography is useful for identifying mass lesions in many cases. Many neoplastic (and other noninflammatory) effusions have a pH of 7.0 or greater, whereas inflammatory effusions tend to have a lower pH. However, there appears to be too much overlap for pericardial pH to be used as a reliable discriminator. Pericardial fluid culture is done if cytology suggests an infectious-inflammatory cause. In some patients fungal titers (e.g., coccidioidomycosis) or other serologic tests are helpful. It is unclear at this time whether analysis of pericardial fluid for cardiac troponins or other substances will allow better differentiation of the underlying etiology.

## Treatment and Prognosis

It is important to differentiate cardiac tamponade from other causes of right-sided heart failure, because the treatment is very different. Positive inotropic drugs do not ameliorate the signs of tamponade; diuretics and vasodilators can further reduce cardiac output and exacerbate hypotension and shock. Pericardiocentesis is the therapeutic procedure of choice (see p. 191) and also provides diagnostic information. Most signs of congestive heart failure resolve after pericardial fluid has been removed, although a diuretic may be of limited value after pericardiocentesis in some animals. Pericardial effusions secondary to other diseases that cause congestive heart failure, congenital malformations, or hypoalbuminemia do not usually cause tamponade and often resolve with management of the underlying condition.

Dogs with idiopathic pericardial effusion are initially treated conservatively with pericardiocentesis and sometimes with a 1- to 2-week course of an antibiotic. After an infectious cause has been ruled out by pericardial fluid culture or cytologic analysis, a glucocorticoid is often used (e.g., oral prednisone, 1 mg/kg/day, tapered over 2 to 4 weeks); however, the efficacy of this therapy in preventing recurrent idiopathic pericardial effusion is not known. Periodic reevaluation of these dogs by radiography or echocardiography is advised to detect recurrence. Apparent recovery occurs after one or two pericardial taps in about half of affected dogs.

Cardiac tamponade recurs after a variable time span (days to years) in other cases.

Recurrent effusion that does not respond to repeated pericardiocenteses and antiinflammatory therapy is usually treated by surgical subtotal pericardiectomy. Removal of the pericardium ventral to the phrenic nerves allows pericardial fluid drainage to the larger absorptive surface of the pleural space. The less invasive technique of thoracoscopic partial pericardiectomy has also been used successfully to treat idiopathic and some cases of neoplastic pericardial effusion. Lateral and subxiphoid approaches have been described. Percutaneous balloon pericardiotomy also appears to be an effective and even less invasive option, although more experience is needed. This procedure, done under general anesthesia with fluoroscopic guidance, involves placing a needle or short catheter into the pericardial space, followed by a guide wire to assist replacement of the needle or catheter with a percutaneous sheath introducer for the balloon dilation catheter. The balloon is positioned so that, when inflated, it stretches the hole in the parietal pericardium. Although concerns exist that adhesions or fibrosis around smaller pericardiotomy openings may result in reaccumulation of fluid or increased risk of constrictive pericarditis, initial reports suggest that the pericardial window created by thoracoscopic or balloon dilation techniques may be as effective as subtotal pericardiectomy in preventing recurrent pericardial effusion.

Neoplastic pericardial effusions are also initially drained to relieve cardiac tamponade. Therapy may involve attempted surgical resection or surgical biopsy, a trial of chemotherapy (based on biopsy or clinicopathologic findings), or conservative therapy until episodes of cardiac tamponade become unmanageable. Specific information on chemotherapy is found in Chapters 79 and 84. Surgical resection of hemangiosarcoma is often not possible because of the size and extent of the tumor. However, small tumors involving only the tip of the right auricle have been successfully removed, and use of a pericardial patch graft may allow resection of larger masses involving the lateral right atrial wall. Partial pericardiectomy should avert recurrence of tamponade. Tumor dissemination throughout the thoracic cavity may be facilitated, but there appears to be no difference in survival time compared to pericardiocentesis alone for dogs with hemangiosarcoma or mesothelioma (Dunning and colleagues, 1998). The prognosis is poor for dogs with hemangiosarcoma (median survival of 2 to 3 weeks), although chemotherapy has been effective in some patients (see Chapter 84). Survival times for dogs with mesothelioma have been longer than for those with hemangiosarcoma.

Heart base tumors (e.g., chemodectoma) tend to be slow growing, locally invasive, and have a low metastatic potential. Partial pericardiectomy is recommended and may prolong survival for years. Percutaneous balloon pericardiotomy may also be an effective palliative procedure. Because of local invasion, complete surgical resection is rarely possible; attempts at aggressive resection are often met with severe bleeding and death. However, small, well-defined masses may be completely resectable. Surgical biopsy is indicated if chemotherapy is contemplated. Effusion secondary to myocardial lymphoma, usually easily diagnosed cytologically, often responds to pericardiocentesis and chemotherapy.

Infectious pericarditis should be treated aggressively with appropriate antimicrobial drugs as determined by microbial culture and sensitivity testing. Surgical therapy is likely to be more effective than continuous drainage with an indwelling pericardial catheter, and it also allows removal of penetrating foreign bodies. The prognosis is guarded. Even with successful elimination of infection, epicardial and pericardial fibrin deposition may lead to constrictive pericardial disease.

Pure hemorrhage into the pericardial space, whether from trauma, left atrial rupture, or a systemic coagulopathy, should be removed if signs of cardiac tamponade result. Only enough blood to control signs of tamponade should be removed, because continued drainage may predispose to further bleeding. The remaining blood is usually resorbed through the pericardium (autotransfusion). Surgery may be needed to stop continued bleeding or remove large clots. Dogs that survive an initial episode of intrapericardial bleeding from left atrial rupture still have a guarded to poor prognosis because of recurrent left atrial tears. Animals with intrapericardial hemorrhage of unclear cause should be evaluated for a coagulation disorder (see Chapter 89). When trauma-induced intrapericardial hemorrhage persists in an animal with normal hemostasis, surgical exploration is indicated.

**Complications.** Complications of diseases causing pericardial effusion relate to (1) sequelae of the fluid accumulation itself (e.g., cardiac tamponade and compression of surrounding structures [lung, esophagus, trachea]), (2) immediate effects of associated inflammatory processes (e.g., arrhythmias, local and systemic effects of infectious agents, further fluid formation), (3) pericardial fibrosis and subsequent constrictive pericarditis, (4) sequelae of neoplastic processes (e.g., further bleeding, metastases, local invasion and obstruction, seeding of the pleura, loss of function), and (5) complications of pericardiocentesis (see below). Overly aggressive surgical attempts to remove cardiac tumors or the entire pericardial sac can be fatal, and partial pericardiectomy may enhance intrathoracic dissemination of certain tumors such as mesothelioma and carcinoma.

## PERICARDIOCENTESIS

Pericardiocentesis is the treatment of choice for initial stabilization of animals with cardiac tamponade. Administration of diuretics or vasodilators without pericardiocentesis may cause further hypotension and cardiogenic shock. Pericardiocentesis is a relatively safe procedure when carefully performed. Removal of even small amounts of pericardial fluid can markedly decrease intrapericardial pressure in animals with tamponade.

Pericardiocentesis from the right side minimizes the risk of trauma to the lungs (because of the cardiac notch) and major coronary vessels (which are located mostly on the left). The need for sedation depends on the clinical status and temperament of the animal. The animal is usually placed in left lateral or sternal recumbency for more secure restraint, espe-

cially if the animal is weak or excitable. Sometimes needle pericardiocentesis can be successfully performed on the standing animal, but the risk of injury is increased if the animal suddenly moves. An elevated echocardiography table with a large cutout can also be used with good success. The animal is then placed in right lateral recumbency and the tap is performed from underneath. An advantage is that fluid moves to the right side with gravity; if adequate space is not available for wide sterile skin preparation or needle/catheter manipulation, this approach is not advised. Echo guidance can be used but is not necessary unless the effusion is of very small volume or appears compartmentalized. An ECG monitor should be in place during pericardiocentesis because needle/catheter contact with the heart commonly induces ventricular arrhythmias.

A variety of equipment can be used for pericardiocentesis. A butterfly needle/catheter (19 to 21 gauge) or appropriately long hypodermic or spinal needle attached to extension tubing is adequate in emergency situations. Alternatively, an over-the-needle catheter chosen according to patient size (e.g., 12- to 16-gauge catheter 4 to 6 inches long for large dogs, down to a 20-gauge catheter 1½ to 2 inches long for small dogs or cats) reduces the risk of cardiopulmonary laceration during fluid aspiration. A few extra small side holes can be smoothly cut near the tip of larger catheters to facilitate flow. During initial catheter placement the extension tubing is attached to the needle stylet. After the catheter has been advanced into the pericardial space, the extension tubing is reattached directly to the catheter. For all methods a three-way stopcock is placed between the tubing and a collection syringe.

The skin is shaved over a wide area of the right precordium (from about the third to the seventh intercostal space and from the sternum to the costochondral junction) and surgically prepared. Sterile gloves and aseptic technique are used for the procedure. The puncture site is located by palpating for where the cardiac impulse is strongest (usually between the fourth and sixth ribs just lateral to the sternum). Local anesthesia is necessary when using large catheters and recommended for needle pericardiocentesis. Lidocaine (2%) is infiltrated with sterile technique at the skin puncture site, into underlying intercostal muscles, and into the pleura. A small stab incision can be made in the skin to allow catheter entry. Intercostal vessels just caudal to each rib must be avoided when entering the chest. Once the needle has penetrated the skin, the operator's assistant should apply gentle negative pressure to the attached syringe as the operator slowly advances the needle toward the heart. It sometimes helps to aim the tip of the needle toward the animal's opposite shoulder. The tubing is observed so that fluid will be seen as soon as it is aspirated. Pleural fluid (usually straw colored) may enter the tubing first. The pericardium creates increased resistance to needle advancement and may produce a subtle scratching sensation. Gentle pressure is used to advance the needle through the pericardium; a loss of resistance may be noted with needle penetration. If the needle contacts the heart, a marked scratching or tapping sensation is usually felt, the needle may move with the heartbeat, and ventricular premature complexes are provoked; the needle should be retracted slightly if cardiac contact occurs. Be careful to avoid excessive needle movement within the chest. When a catheter system is used, after the needle/stylet is well within the pericardial space, the catheter is advanced, the stylet removed, and the extension tubing attached to the catheter. Initial fluid samples are saved for cytologic and microbiologic culture, and then as much fluid as possible is aspirated.

Pericardial effusion usually appears quite hemorrhagic. It can be disconcerting to see dark, bloody fluid being aspirated from so near the heart. However, pericardial fluid can be differentiated from intracardiac blood in several ways. Unless the fluid is caused by very recent hemorrhage into the pericardium, it will not clot. The PCV of the fluid is usually much lower than that of peripheral blood (except in some dogs with hemangiosarcoma), and when spun in a hematocrit tube, the supernatant is xanthochromic (yellow tinged). As the pericardial fluid is drained, the ECG complexes increase in amplitude, tachycardia diminishes, and the animal often takes a deep breath and appears more comfortable.

## Complications

Complications of pericardiocentesis include (1) cardiac injury or puncture causing arrhythmias (the most common complication, but usually self-limiting when the needle is withdrawn), (2) coronary artery laceration with myocardial infarction or further bleeding into the pericardial space, (3) lung laceration causing pneumothorax and/or hemorrhage, and (4) dissemination of infection or neoplastic cells into the pleural space.

## CONGENITAL PERICARDIAL DISORDERS

### PERITONEOPERICARDIAL DIAPHRAGMATIC HERNIA

Peritoneopericardial diaphragmatic hernia (PPDH) is the most common pericardial malformation encountered in dogs and cats. It occurs when abnormal embryonic development (probably of the septum transversum) allows persistent communication between the pericardial and peritoneal cavities at the ventral midline. The pleural space is not involved. Other congenital defects may accompany PPDH, such as umbilical hernia, sternal malformations, and cardiac anomalies. Abdominal contents herniate into the pericardial space to a variable degree and cause associated clinical signs. Although the peritoneal-pericardial communication is not trauma induced, trauma can facilitate movement of abdominal contents through a preexisting defect.

The initial onset of clinical signs with PPDH can occur at any age (e.g., ages between 4 weeks and 15 years have been reported), but the majority of cases are diagnosed during the first 4 years of life, usually within the first year. In some animals, clinical signs never develop, and PPDH is diagnosed fortuitously. Males appear to be affected more frequently than females, and Weimaraners may be predisposed. The malfor-

mation is common in cats as well. Clinical signs are usually gastrointestinal or respiratory. Vomiting, diarrhea, anorexia, weight loss, abdominal pain, cough, dyspnea, and wheezing are most often reported; shock and collapse can also occur. Physical examination findings may include muffled heart sounds on one or both sides of the chest, displacement or attenuation of the apical precordial impulse, an "empty" feel on abdominal palpation (with herniation of many organs), and rarely signs of cardiac tamponade.

Thoracic radiography is often diagnostic or highly suggestive of PPDH. Characteristic findings include enlargement of the cardiac silhouette, dorsal tracheal displacement, overlap of the diaphragmatic and caudal heart borders, and abnormal fat and/or gas densities within the cardiac silhouette (Fig. 11-6, *A* and *B*). A pleural fold is usually evident, extending between the caudal heart shadow and the diaphragm ventral to the caudal vena cava on lateral view. Gas-filled loops of bowel crossing the diaphragm into the pericardial sac, a small liver, and few organs within the abdominal cavity may also be seen. Echocardiography is useful in confirming the diagnosis in patients in which the diagnosis is equivocal (Fig. 11-7). A gastrointestinal barium series is diagnostic if stomach and/or intestines are in the pericardial cavity (Fig. 11-6, *C*). Fluoroscopy, nonselective angiography (especially if only falciform fat or liver has herniated), celiography, or pneumopericardiography also aid in diagnosis. ECG changes are inconsistent; decreased amplitude complexes and axis deviations caused by cardiac position changes sometimes occur.

Therapy involves surgical closure of the peritoneal-pericardial defect after viable organs have been returned to their normal location. The presence of other congenital abnormalities and the animal's clinical signs may influence the decision to operate. The prognosis in uncomplicated cases is excellent. Older animals without clinical signs may do well without surgery, especially because organs chronically adhered to the heart or pericardium may be traumatized during attempted repositioning.

## OTHER PERICARDIAL ANOMALIES

Pericardial cysts are rare anomalies thought to originate from abnormal fetal mesenchymal tissue development or from incarcerated omental or falciform fat from a small PPDH. The pathophysiologic signs and clinical presentation of these cases are similar to those of animals with pericardial effusion. The cardiac shadow may appear enlarged and deformed radiographically. Echocardiography or pneumopericardiography provides the diagnosis. Surgical removal of the cyst in conjunction with partial pericardiectomy has usually resulted in cure.

Congenital defects of the pericardium itself are extremely rare in dogs and cats; most are discovered incidentally on postmortem examination. Instances of partial (usually on the left side) and complete absence of the pericardium have been reported. A possible complication of partial absence of the pericardium is herniation of a portion of the heart; this could cause syncope, embolic disease, or sudden death. Echocardiography or angiocardiography should facilitate antemortem diagnosis.

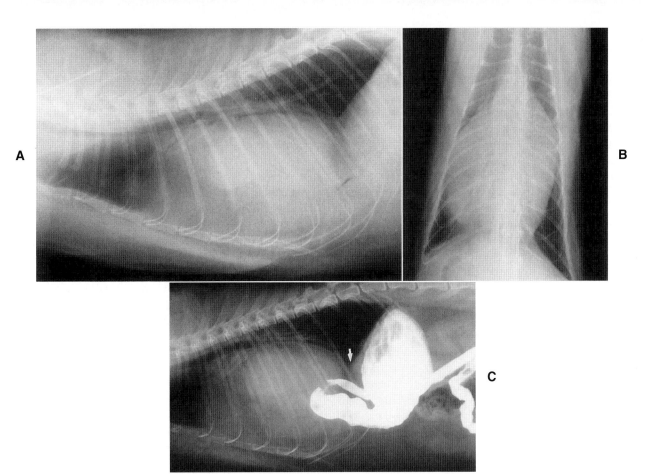

**FIG 11-6**
Lateral **(A)** and dorsoventral **(B)** radiographs from a 5-year-old male Persian cat with a congenital peritoneopericardial diaphragmatic hernia (PPDH). Note the greatly enlarged cardiac silhouette containing fat, soft tissue, and gas densities as well as tracheal elevation. There is overlap between the cardiac and diaphragmatic borders on both views. The presence of a portion of the stomach and duodenum within the pericardium is evident after barium administration **(C);** omental fat and liver are also present within the pericardial sac. In **C,** the dorsal pleural fold between the pericardium and diaphragm is best appreciated *(arrow)*.

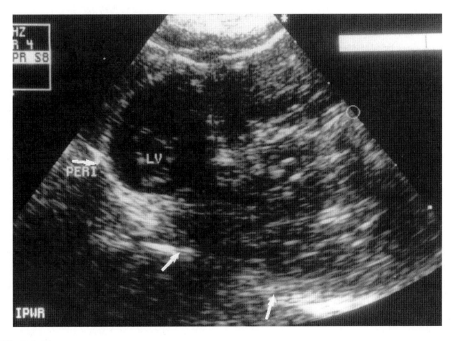

**FIG 11-7**
Right parasternal short-axis echocardiogram from a female Persian cat with peritoneo-pericardial diaphragmatic hernia (PPDH). The pericardium *(PERI)*, indicated by arrows, surrounds liver and omental tissue as well as the heart. *LV,* Left ventricle.

## CONSTRICTIVE PERICARDIAL DISEASE

Constrictive pericardial disease occurs occasionally in dogs, but rarely in cats, when a thickened visceral and/or parietal pericardium restricts ventricular diastolic distention. Chronic pericardial thickening and scarring create a rigid shell around the heart. This prevents normal cardiac filling and affects the function of both ventricles. Usually the entire pericardium is symmetrically involved. Fusion of the parietal and visceral pericardial layers will obliterate the pericardial space. In other cases, the visceral layer (epicardium) alone is involved; sometimes a small amount of pericardial effusion is present (constrictive-effusive pericarditis). Histopathologic examination of the pericardium usually reveals increased fibrous connective tissue and variable amounts of inflammatory and reactive infiltrates. The etiology of constrictive pericardial disease is often unknown. Acute inflammation with fibrin deposition and possibly varying degrees of pericardial effusion are thought to precede the development of constrictive pericardial disease. Specific causes identified in some dogs include recurrent idiopathic hemorrhagic effusion, infectious pericarditis (e.g., actinomycosis, mycobacteriosis, coccidioidomycosis), metallic foreign bodies in the pericardium, tumors, and idiopathic osseous metaplasia and/or fibrosis of the pericardium. Constrictive pericardial disease in people has been associated with prior viral or idiopathic pericardial effusions, tuberculosis, neoplastic infiltration, trauma, renal failure, immunologic disease, suppurative infections, and the use of certain drugs.

In advanced constrictive pericardial disease, ventricular filling is essentially limited to early diastole before ventricular expansion is abruptly curtailed. Any further ventricular filling is accomplished only at high venous pressures. Compromised filling reduces cardiac output. Compensatory mechanisms of heart failure cause fluid retention, tachycardia, and vasoconstriction.

### Clinical Features

Large to medium-sized middle-aged dogs are most often affected; males and German Shepherd Dogs may be at higher risk for this disorder. Clinical signs of right-sided congestive heart failure predominate. Historical complaints include abdominal distention (ascites), dyspnea or tachypnea, tiring, syncope, weakness, and weight loss. The signs can develop over weeks to months. Occasionally there is a history of pericardial effusion. Similar to cases of cardiac tamponade, ascites and jugular venous distention are the most consistent clinical findings. Weakened femoral pulses and muffled heart sounds are also found. An audible, diastolic pericardial knock, resulting from the abrupt deceleration of ventricular filling in early diastole, has been described but has not been commonly identified in dogs. A systolic murmur or click, probably caused by valvular disease not associated with the pericardial pathology, or a diastolic gallop sound may be heard.

### Diagnosis

Diagnosis of constrictive pericardial disease can be difficult. Typical radiographic findings include mild to moderate cardiomegaly, pleural effusion, and caudal vena cava distention. Reduced cardiac motion may be evident on fluoroscopy. Constrictive pericardial disease can produce subtle but suggestive echocardiographic changes, such as flattening of the left ventricular free wall in diastole and abnormal septal motion. The pericardium may appear thickened and intensely echogenic, but differentiation of this finding from normal pericardial echogenicity may be difficult. ECG abnormalities have included sinus tachycardia, P-wave prolongation, and small QRS complexes.

Invasive hemodynamic studies are the most diagnostic. CVPs over 15 mm Hg and high mean atrial and diastolic ventricular pressures are common. However, the classic early diastolic dip in ventricular pressure, followed by a mid-diastolic plateau, is not consistently seen in dogs with constrictive pericardial disease. Angiocardiography can be normal, or it may reveal atrial and vena caval enlargement and increased endocardial-pericardial distance.

### Treatment and Prognosis

Therapy for constrictive pericardial disease consists of surgical pericardiectomy. The procedure is often successful if only the parietal pericardium is involved. When visceral pericardial disease also contributes to the constriction, epicardial stripping is required. This additional procedure increases the difficulty and associated complications of surgery. Pulmonary thrombosis, sometimes massive, is reported to be a relatively common postoperative complication. Tachyarrhythmias are another complication of surgery. Moderate doses of diuretics may be helpful in the postoperative period, but positive inotropic and vasodilating drugs are not indicated. Without surgical intervention, the disease is progressive and ultimately fatal.

## CARDIAC TUMORS

Although the overall prevalence of cardiac tumors is low, the increased use of echocardiography has made their antemortem diagnosis more common. Cardiac tumors can cause severe clinical signs, although some are diagnosed fortuitously. It appears that cardiac tumors of all types occur at a rate of about 0.19% in dogs and less than 0.03% in cats. Dogs with cardiac tumors tend to be middle-aged or older. Over 85% of affected dogs are between 7 and 15 years of age; however, very old dogs (>15 years) have a surprisingly low prevalence. Reproductive status influences the relative risk for cardiac tumors in dogs, despite a similar frequency of occurrence in males and females overall. Neutered dogs have a greater relative risk, especially spayed females, which have a four to five times greater risk than intact females. Intact and neutered males also have a greater risk than intact females. Certain breeds of dog have a higher prevalence of cardiac tumor compared to the general population (Table 11-1). The age distribution of cats with cardiac tumors is different from dogs; about 28% are 7 years old or younger. Whether any effect of reproductive status on relative risk for cardiac tumors exists in cats is unknown.

TABLE 11-1

Dog Breeds with High Cardiac Tumor Incidence

| BREED | NUMBER WITH TUMOR | NUMBER IN DATABASE | RELATIVE RISK | 95% CI |
|-------|-------------------|--------------------|--------------|--------|
| Saluki | 6 | 401 | 7.75 | 3.92-15.38 |
| French Bulldog | 3 | 215 | 7.19 | 2.72-19.23 |
| Irish Water Spaniel | 2 | 168 | 6.13 | 1.81-20.83 |
| Flat-Coated Retriever | 4 | 534 | 3.85 | 1.54-9.62 |
| Golden Retriever | 215 | 32,940 | 3.73 | 3.26-4.27 |
| Boxer | 52 | 8496 | 3.22 | 2.47-4.18 |
| Afghan Hound | 12 | 2080 | 2.97 | 1.72-5.10 |
| English Setter | 21 | 3796 | 2.86 | 1.89-4.31 |
| Scottish Terrier | 16 | 3290 | 2.50 | 1.55-4.03 |
| Boston Terrier | 25 | 5225 | 2.47 | 1.68-3.62 |
| Bulldog | 24 | 5580 | 2.22 | 1.49-3.29 |
| German Shepherd Dog | 129 | 37,872 | 1.81 | 1.52-2.17 |

Modified from Ware WA et al: Cardiac tumors in dogs: 1982-1995, *J Vet Intern Med* 13:95, 1999.
*CI*, Confidence interval.

By far the most commonly reported cardiac tumor in dogs is hemangiosarcoma. Most are located in the right atrium and/or right auricle; some also infiltrate the ventricular wall. Hemangiosarcomas commonly are associated with hemorrhagic pericardial effusion and cardiac tamponade (see p. 186). Metastases have frequently occurred by the time of diagnosis. Golden Retrievers, German Shepherd Dogs, Afghan Hounds, Cocker Spaniels, English Setters, and Labrador Retrievers, among others, are at higher risk for this tumor.

Masses at the heart base are the second most frequently reported cardiac tumor in dogs. They are usually neoplasms of the chemoreceptor aortic bodies (alternately named chemodectoma, aortic body tumors, or nonchromaffin paragangliomas), ectopic thyroid tissue, or ectopic parathyroid tissue, or are of mixed-cell type. Heart base tumors tend to be locally invasive around the root of the aorta and surrounding structures; metastases to other organs have been reported but are rare. Chemodectomas are reported more frequently in brachycephalic dogs (e.g., Boxer, Boston Terrier, English Bulldog) but affect others as well. Clinical signs associated with heart base tumors are usually related to the development of pericardial effusion and cardiac tamponade.

Other primary tumors involving the heart are rare in dogs but have included myxoma, fibro(sarco)ma, rhabdomyo(sarco)ma, leiomyo(sarco)ma, chondro(sarco)ma, intracardiac ectopic thyroid tumors, and pericardial mesothelioma. Most cases involve right-heart structures. Metastatic tumors, including lymphoma, other sarcomas, and various carcinomas, may involve the heart as well.

The most common cardiac tumor type in cats is lymphoma, accounting for nearly one third of cases in a large database survey (Ware, 1995). Various (mostly metastatic) carcinomas are the next most common cardiac neoplasms in cats; hemangiosarcoma accounts for less than 9% of cases. Other tumors (such as aortic body tumor, fibrosarcoma, rhabdomyosarcoma) have been reported sporadically in cats.

## Clinical Features and Diagnosis

In general, clinical signs are referable to one or a combination of several pathophysiologic abnormalities. Many tumors cause pericardial effusion and cardiac tamponade (see above). Alternatively, the tumor itself can physically obstruct blood flow into or out of the heart, especially when the mass develops in an intracardiac location. An intrapericardial mass could both externally compress the heart and cause pericardial effusion. Finally, myocardial infiltration or ischemia can disrupt the cardiac rhythm or impair contractility. If the tumor is small or is located where cardiac function is not significantly impaired, clinical signs may be absent.

Cardiac tumors in dogs commonly affect the right side of the heart. Signs of right-sided congestive heart failure result from blood flow obstruction within the right atrium or ventricle or from cardiac tamponade. Syncope and weakness with exertion also result from cardiac tamponade, blood flow obstruction, arrhythmias, or impaired myocardial function secondary to cardiac tumors. Tachyarrhythmias of any type can occur; likewise, various conduction disturbances can result from tumor infiltration into the conduction system. Lethargy or collapse can occur in dogs with bleeding tumors (e.g., hemangiosarcoma) that may also be present in extracardiac locations.

Auscultation may reveal a murmur caused by intracardiac blood flow obstruction, a murmur of unrelated disease (e.g., degenerative mitral regurgitation), an arrhythmia, or muffled heart sounds (e.g., with large pericardial effusion). Auscultation is normal in some cases. Radiographic findings also can be quite variable; a normal cardiac silhouette, unusual cardiac bulge(s), a mass effect adjacent to the heart, or a "globoid" cardiac silhouette compatible with pericardial effusion can be found. Intrapericardial masses are obscured by pericardial effusion. Other radiographic findings, secondary to impaired cardiac filling, include pleural effusion, evidence of pulmonary edema, widening of the caudal vena cava (and/or pulmonary veins), hepatomegaly, or ascites. Dorsal deviation of the trachea and increased perihilar opacity are seen with some heart base tumors. Evidence of pulmonary metastases may be seen with some primary or secondary (metastatic) cardiac neoplasms. The ECG may be normal or show abnormalities reflective of the location and sequelae of the underlying disease.

Echocardiography can be used to identify cardiac masses and determine the presence or absence of pericardial effusion. Secondary changes in cardiac chamber size, shape, and ventricular function can also be detected. Doppler echocardiography allows qualitative and quantitative assessment of associated blood flow abnormalities. The presence of effusion facilitates identification of heart base tumors that extend into the pericardial space. Intracardiac masses are likewise accentuated by the echolucent intracardiac blood that surrounds them (Fig. 11-8). Assessment of the location, size, attachment (pedunculated or broad based), and extent (superficial or deeply invading adjacent myocardium) of the cardiac tumor(s) is valuable in determining whether surgical resection or biopsy may be possible. The identification of a suspected mass in more that one echocardiographic plane helps to avoid overinterpretation of artifacts. Images obtained from the left cranial parasternal transducer position can be especially useful in evaluating the ascending aorta, right auricle, and surrounding structures.

Cytologic analysis of any pericardial fluid is recommended; however, definitive diagnosis of neoplasia cannot usually be made based on cytologic findings alone. Cardiac lymphoma is more likely to be diagnosed based on pericardial fluid cytologic examination. Visualization of a cardiac mass using echocardiography, computed tomography, pneumopericardiography, angiography, or another modality is usually necessary for definitive diagnosis of neoplasia; a pericardial fluid pH measurement above 7.0 may be supportive. Hematologic and serum biochemical test results are generally nonspecific in dogs and cats with cardiac tumors. Cardiac enzyme activities may be high from ischemia or myocardial invasion; mild increases in serum alanine aminotransferase activity and azotemia can occur from congestive heart failure. Hemangiosarcoma is often associated with a regenerative anemia, increased number of nucleated red blood cells and schistocytes, leukocytosis, and thrombocytopenia. If present, pleural and peritoneal fluids are usually modified transudates.

## Treatment and Prognosis

Unfortunately, there are few good long-term options in most patients with a heart tumor. Management of cardiac tamponade was described earlier (see p. 190). Most signs of congestive heart failure resolve once the pericardial fluid has been removed. Conservative therapy (pericardiocentesis as needed, possibly with glucocorticoid administration to decrease inflammation) is used in some animals. Partial pericardiectomy or pericardiotomy can be helpful in animals with recurrent tamponade.

Surgical resection may be possible depending on tumor location, size, and invasiveness; tumors more likely to be resectable are those involving only the tip of the right auricular appendage or a pedunculated mass in a surgically accessible location. Intracardiac masses within the right side of the heart might be reached using venous inflow occlusion techniques and rapid cardiotomy; however, surgical access to lesions on the left side of the heart and large or medially attached masses on the right side of the heart would generally require cardiopulmonary bypass.

Surgical biopsy of a nonresectable mass may be helpful if chemotherapy is being contemplated. Although many cardiac tumors appear to be fairly unresponsive to chemotherapy, some are treated with short-term success. Some cardiac hemangiosarcomas respond to vincristine, doxorubicin, and cyclophosphamide combination chemotherapy for 3 to 9 months (see Chapter 84). Lymphoma should be treated using a standard protocol (see Chapter 82).

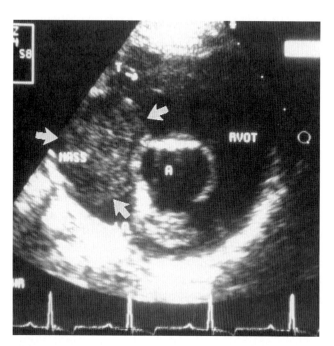

**FIG 11-8**

Right parasternal short-axis echocardiogram from an 8-year-old male Spitz with massive ascites. A large tumor *(MASS)*, indicated by arrows and attached to the interatrial septum, is contained within the right atrial lumen and partially obstructs the tricuspid orifice. Pericardial effusion was not present in this dog. *A,* Aorta; *LA,* left atrium; *T,* tricuspid valve; *RVOT,* right ventricular outflow tract.

## Suggested Readings

Aronsohn M: Cardiac hemangiosarcoma in the dog: a review of 38 cases, *J Am Vet Med Assoc* 187:922, 1985.

Aronsohn MG et al: Surgical treatment of idiopathic pericardial effusion in the dog: 25 cases (1978-1993), *J Am Anim Hosp Assoc* 35:521, 1999.

Aronson LR et al: Infectious pericardial effusion in five dogs, *Vet Surg* 24:402, 1995.

Berg J: Pericardial disease and cardiac neoplasia, *Semin Vet Med Surg* 9:185, 1994.

Berry CR et al: Echocardiographic evaluation of cardiac tamponade in dogs before and after pericardiocentesis: four cases (1984-1986), *J Am Vet Med Assoc* 192:1597, 1988.

Brisson BA et al: Use of pericardial patch graft reconstruction of the right atrium for treatment of hemangiosarcoma in a dog, *J Am Vet Med Assoc* 218:723, 2001.

Closa JM et al: Pericardial mesothelioma in a dog: long-term survival after pericardiectomy in combination with chemotherapy, *J Small Anim Pract* 40:383, 1999.

Dunning D et al: Analysis of prognostic indicators for dogs with pericardial effusion: 46 cases (1985-1996), *J Am Vet Med Assoc* 212:1276, 1998.

Edwards NJ: The diagnostic value of pericardial fluid pH determination, *J Am Anim Hosp Assoc* 32:63, 1996.

Fine DM et al: The pH of pericardial effusion does not reliably distinguish between idiopathic and neoplastic effusions, *J Vet Intern Med* 15:282, 2001 (abstract).

Jackson J et al: Thorascopic partial pericardiectomy in 13 dogs, *J Vet Intern Med* 13:529, 1999.

Miller MW et al: Pericardial disorders. In Ettinger SJ et al, editors: *Textbook of veterinary internal medicine,* ed 5, Philadelphia, 2000, WB Saunders, p 923.

Rush JE et al: Pericardial disease in the cat: a retrospective evaluation of 66 cases, *J Am Anim Hosp Assoc* 26:39, 1990.

Sidley JA et al: Percutaneous balloon pericardiotomy as a treatment for recurrent pericardial effusion in 6 dogs, *J Vet Intern Med* 16:541, 2002.

Sisson D et al: Diagnostic value of pericardial fluid analysis in the dog, *J Am Vet Med Assoc* 184:51, 1984.

Sisson D et al: Intrapericardial cysts in the dog, *J Vet Intern Med* 7:364, 1993.

Thomas WP et al: Detection of cardiac masses in dogs by two-dimensional echocardiography, *Vet Radiol* 25:65, 1984.

Vicari ED et al: Survival times of and prognostic indicators for dogs with heart base masses: 25 cases (1986-1999), *J Am Vet Med Assoc* 219:485, 2001.

Wallace J et al: A technique for surgical correction of peritoneal pericardial diaphragmatic hernia in dogs and cats, *J Am Anim Hosp Assoc* 28:503, 1992.

Ware WA: Cardiac neoplasia. In Bonagura JD, editor: *Kirk's current veterinary therapy XII,* Philadelphia, 1995, WB Saunders, p 873.

Ware WA et al: Cardiac tumors in dogs: 1982-1995, *J Vet Intern Med* 13:95, 1999.

Wright KN et al: Effusive-constrictive pericardial disease secondary to osseous metaplasia of the pericardium in a dog, *J Am Vet Med Assoc* 209:2091, 1996.

# CHAPTER 12

# Systemic Arterial Hypertension

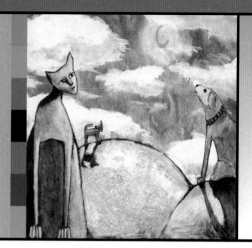

## CHAPTER OUTLINE

GENERAL CONSIDERATIONS, 198
BLOOD PRESSURE MEASUREMENT, 200
CLINICAL HYPERTENSION IN DOGS AND CATS, 201

## GENERAL CONSIDERATIONS

Hypertension is defined as abnormally high blood pressure, although the level at which arterial pressure becomes "abnormally high" is not clear-cut. Various factors, including time of day, can influence measurements of systolic, diastolic, and mean arterial blood pressure in healthy animals. Further, although some dogs and cats clearly have clinical disease caused by hypertension, many with "abnormally high" blood pressure measurements have no evidence of related pathology, although a predisposing disease condition may be present. Repeated blood pressure measurements over time along with careful clinical evaluation of the patient are indicated before making a diagnosis of hypertension. If antihypertensive therapy is indicated, close patient monitoring for efficacy, adverse effects, and deterioration of underlying conditions is warranted.

Various reports of direct and noninvasive blood pressure measurement in dogs and cats have been published. In general, blood pressures in normal, untrained, unanesthetized dogs and cats do not exceed 160/100 mm Hg (systolic/diastolic), although normal pressures in some breeds of dog (especially sight hounds) may fall above this range. Further, some normal animals have systolic pressures over 180 mm Hg when stressed or anxious; but generally, systolic pressures of 180 to 200/110 mm Hg are considered borderline or mildly increased. Arterial blood pressures greater than 200/110 are considered in the hypertensive range.

Differences in blood pressure related to age, breed, and gender as well as to disease have been identified in dogs, although some studies have not found similar age, gender, and body size effects (see Suggested Readings for further infor-

mation). There are conflicting reports as to whether blood pressures increase with age or whether systolic pressure in geriatric dogs is similar to that in younger dogs. Intact males may have higher pressures and intact females lower pressures than neutered animals. With regard to breed-related differences in the mean values for systolic, diastolic, and mean blood pressures, large- and giant-breed dogs generally have lower pressures than small-breed dogs, except for sight hounds. For example, Bodey and colleague (1996b) found mean values (mm Hg; systolic, diastolic, and mean pressure, respectively) for giant-breed dogs as a group of 121, 67, and 91; for Spaniels: 132, 74, and 98; and for sight hounds as a group: 146, 84, and 108. Mean values for all dogs were 133, 76, and 99. The higher blood pressures found in sight hounds appear to be functional and not associated with signs of disease.

Studies of arterial pressure measured noninvasively in normal cats have yielded variable pressure ranges. Differences in technique and study conditions no doubt contribute to this. One study using the oscillometric method in relatively calm cats found overall average pressures of 104/73 mm Hg (mean 84 mm Hg) and suggested an upper limit of normal blood pressure of 161/125 mm Hg (mean 138 mm Hg; Bartges and colleagues, 1995). Others have identified upper normal systolic pressures of 140 to 170 mm Hg and even 199 mm Hg in cats (Sparkes and colleagues, 1999). An age-related increase in blood pressure has been variably observed in cats.

### Etiology

Hypertension in dogs and cats is usually secondary rather than primary (idiopathic or essential hypertension). Primary (essential) hypertension is a diagnosis of exclusion and it is infrequently diagnosed in animals, although inherited essential hypertension has been documented in dogs.

Diseases associated with hypertension are listed in Table 12-1. There is a high prevalence of at least mild hypertension in cats with renal disease or hyperthyroidism. The hypertension associated with hyperthyroidism is reversible with effective treatment of this endocrine disease. Renal disease, especially that involving glomerular function, and hyperadrenocorticism are commonly associated with hypertension in dogs; diabetes mellitus, hypothyroidism, and liver disease also have been associated with higher arterial pressure. Transient hypertension can occur in association with drugs that cause vasoconstriction, including topical ocular phenylephrine. Hypertension also has been associated with obesity in dogs.

## Pathophysiology and Pathology

Blood pressure depends on cardiac output and peripheral vascular resistance. Blood pressure can be increased by conditions that raise cardiac output (by increasing heart rate and/or blood volume) or by those that increase vascular resistance. Normally, arterial blood pressure is maintained within narrow bounds by the actions of the autonomic nervous system (e.g., via arterial baroreceptors), various hormonal systems (e.g., renin-angiotensin system, vasopressin), blood volume regulation by the kidney, and other factors.

A chronic increase in blood pressure can result from enhanced sympathetic nervous activity or responsiveness (e.g., hyperthyroidism), increased catecholamine production (e.g., pheochromocytoma), or volume expansion secondary to increased sodium retention (e.g., renal failure, hyperaldosteronism, hyperadrenocorticism). Activation of the renin-angiotensin-aldosterone system with subsequent salt and water retention and vasoconstriction can result from intrarenal diseases (e.g., glomerulonephritis, chronic interstitial nephritis), enhanced production of angiotensinogen (e.g., hyperadrenocorticism), and extrarenal diseases that increase sympathetic nervous activity or interfere with renal perfusion (e.g., hyperthyroidism, renal artery obstruction). Other conditions can also cause or facilitate hypertension. Several mechanisms may contribute to the development of hypertension in dogs and cats with chronic renal failure: decreased glomerular filtration rate and reduced sodium excretion can increase blood volume, localized renal ischemia or reduced renal blood flow can activate the renin-angiotensin-aldosterone system, the production of vasodilating substances (e.g., prostaglandins, kallikreins) may decrease, and effects related to secondary hyperparathyroidism may be involved.

**Pathologic effects of hypertension.** High perfusion pressure can damage capillary beds. In most tissues, capillary pressure is regulated by vasoconstriction of arterioles that feed the capillaries, although this control may be inadequate because of underlying organ disease. The continued arteriolar constriction secondary to chronic hypertension leads to medial hypertrophy and other vascular remodeling changes that can further increase vascular resistance. These structural changes and vascular spasm can cause capillary hypoxia, tissue damage, hemorrhage, and infarction; variable signs of organ dysfunction then result (Table 12-2). Organs that are particularly vulnerable to damage by chronic hypertension and its associated vascular changes are the eye, kidney, heart, and brain. These

### TABLE 12-1

#### Diseases Associated with Hypertension

**Documented or Suspected Causes in Dogs and Cats**

Renal disease (tubular, glomerular, vascular)
Hyperadrenocorticism
Hyperthyroidism
Pheochromocytoma
Chronic anemia (cats)
High-salt diet
Diabetes mellitus
Liver disease
Obesity

**Other Diseases Associated with Hypertension in People***

Acromegaly
Inappropriate antidiuretic hormone secretion
Hyperviscosity/polycythemia
Renin-secreting tumors
Hyperaldosteronism
Hypercalcemia
Hypothyroidism with atherosclerosis
Hyperestrogenism
Coarctation of the aorta
Pregnancy
Central nervous system disease

*Essential hypertension in people is often associated with family history, high salt intake, smoking, or obesity.

### TABLE 12-2

#### Complications of Hypertension

**Ocular**

Blindness
Hemorrhage (retinal, vitreal, hyphema)
Retinal detachment
Glaucoma
Secondary corneal ulcers

**Neurologic**

Cerebrovascular accident
Seizures
Syncope

**Renal**

Polyuria/polydipsia
Further deterioration in renal function

**Cardiac**

Left ventricular hypertrophy (with or without failure)
Murmur

**Other**

Epistaxis

structures are often referred to as target-organs or end-organs. Increased systemic arterial pressure and vascular resistance increase the afterload stress on the heart and stimulate left ventricular hypertrophy. Vascular damage from chronic hypertension causes glomerulosclerosis and contributes to renal function deterioration in addition to causing increased vascular resistance. Thus chronic hypertension tends to perpetuate itself.

# BLOOD PRESSURE MEASUREMENT

Several methods can be used to measure systemic arterial blood pressure. Blood pressure measurement is easily performed in clinical practice given the availability of relatively accurate and inexpensive noninvasive techniques. Taking the average of multiple measurements (at least five) in succession is recommended to increase accuracy. High pressures should be confirmed by repeated measurement sessions before a diagnosis of hypertension is made. Anxiety related to the clinical setting may falsely increase blood pressure in some animals ("white-coat effect"). Using the least restraint possible in a quiet environment and allowing time (e.g., 10 to 15 minutes) for acclimatization are best for awake animals. A consistent technique is important.

## Direct Measurement

Direct arterial pressure measurement is performed by inserting a needle or fluid-filled catheter system, connected to a pressure transducer, directly into an artery. Direct arterial pressure measurement is considered the gold standard, although it requires more skill to obtain. In awake animals, the physical restraint and discomfort associated with arterial puncture can falsely increase blood pressure. For arterial pressure monitoring over a period of time, it is best to use an indwelling arterial line; the dorsal metatarsal artery is usually used for this approach. The pressure transducer must be placed at the level of the patient's right atrium to avoid falsely increasing or decreasing the measured pressure as a result of gravitational effects on the fluid within the connecting tubing. An electronic pressure monitor can provide continuous measurement of systolic and diastolic pressures and calculated mean pressure. The dorsal metatarsal artery or the femoral artery can be used for puncture with a small-gauge needle directly attached to a pressure transducer for occasional blood pressure measurement. To prevent hematoma formation, direct pressure should be applied to the arterial puncture site for several minutes after removal of the catheter or needle used for blood pressure measurement. Direct arterial pressure measurement is more accurate than indirect methods in hypotensive animals.

## Indirect Measurement

Several noninvasive methods are available to indirectly measure blood pressure. They use an inflatable cuff placed around a limb or the tail to occlude blood flow. Controlled release of cuff pressure is monitored to detect the return of flow. Doppler ultrasound and oscillometric methods are used most often in veterinary medicine. Both techniques can produce measurements that correlate fairly well with direct blood pressure measurement but are not exactly predictive of it. Although some studies have shown that indirect methods underestimate direct measurement by a variable degree, especially at higher pressures, others have found that measurements obtained by indirect methods were not consistently lower or higher than those obtained by direct methods. Indirect methods are most reliable in normotensive and hypertensive animals. In conscious cats, greater correlation with direct blood pressure measurement has been found using a Doppler ultrasonic flowmeter than with the oscillometric method (Brown and colleagues, 2001c).

Other methods, such as auscultation and arterial palpation, have been used to estimate blood pressure but are not recommended. The auscultatory method (similar to that used in people) is technically difficult because of the limb conformation of dogs and cats and is generally not used. Direct arterial palpation is not a reliable or accurate method to estimate blood pressure because pulse strength depends on the pulse pressure (systolic minus diastolic arterial pressure), not the absolute level of systolic or mean pressure. Pulse strength is also influenced by body conformation and other factors.

**Cuff size and placement.** The size of cuff used for indirect pressure measurement is important. The width of the inflatable balloon (bladder) within the cuff should be about 40% to 50% of the circumference of the extremity it encircles; the length of the balloon should cover at least 60% of this circumference. Some of the cuff inflation pressure goes toward tissue compression. Cuffs that are too narrow are more affected by this phenomenon and produce falsely increased pressure readings; cuffs that are too wide can underestimate blood pressure. Human pediatric and infant-sized cuffs (e.g., from Parks Medical Electronics, Inc., Aloha, Ore; Cardell Veterinary Products, Tampa, Fla), are used in dogs and cats. The cuff bladder should be centered over the target artery. Common cuff locations are midway between the elbow and carpus or in the tibial region; skeletal prominences are avoided. The cuff should encircle the limb snugly but not be excessively tight. Tape (not just the Velcro on the cuff) is used to secure the cuff in position.

**Oscillometric method.** An automated system for detecting and processing cuff pressure oscillation signals is commercially available for veterinary use (Cardell [formerly Dinamap] Veterinary Blood Pressure Monitor; Sharn, Inc., Tampa, Fla). With this system, the flow occlusion cuff is inflated to a pressure above systolic pressure and then slowly deflated by increments of 5 to 10 mm Hg while the microprocessor measures and averages the resulting pressure oscillation amplitudes. As cuff pressure approaches systolic blood pressure, oscillations in cuff pressure rapidly develop. Oscillations increase further at mean arterial pressure. As diastolic blood pressure is reached, the oscillations rapidly decrease. Mean pressure is measured as the lowest cuff pressure at which the averaged oscillations are greatest. Systolic and diastolic pressures are estimated at the pressures at which oscillation amplitude rapidly increases and decreases, respectively. Accurate results with this method depend on carefully following the directions for use and holding the animal very still. It is recommended that at least five readings be obtained, the lowest and highest be discarded, and the remaining measurements be averaged. Effective use of the oscillometric method may be difficult in very small animals.

**Doppler ultrasonic method.** This method uses the change in frequency between emitted ultrasound and returning echoes (from moving blood cells or vessel wall) to detect blood flow in a superficial artery. This frequency change, the Doppler shift, is converted into an audible signal. A small area of hair is clipped where the probe is to be placed. Ultrasonic coupling gel is applied to the flat Doppler flow probe to obtain an air-free interface with the skin. The probe must be held very still to minimize noise; it is often taped in place. When the flow-occluding cuff, attached to a sphygmomanometer, is inflated to a pressure above systolic blood pressure, flow stops and no audible signals are heard. Cuff inflation to a pressure 30 to 40 mm Hg above this is recommended. As the cuff is slowly deflated, the return of blood cell (or arterial wall) motion produces characteristic flow signals during systole.

One system used commonly in animals is designed to determine systolic pressure by detecting blood cell flow (Ultrasonic Doppler Flow Detector, Model 811; Parks Medical Electronics, Inc., Aloha, Ore). The probe is placed distal to the occluding cuff. Effective locations for pressure measurement include the dorsal metatarsal, common digital, and ventral coccygeal arteries. As the cuff is deflated, the pressure at which pulsatile blood flow first recurs (indicated by brief "swishing" sounds) is the systolic pressure. Sometimes a change in the flow sound from short and pulsatile to a longer, more continuous "swishing" can be detected as cuff pressure declines; the pressure at which this change occurs is an approximation of diastolic pressure. Diastolic blood pressure measurement is less accurate with this system because of the subjective nature of its determination. This change in flow sound may not be detectable, especially with small or stiff vessels. Although only systolic pressure is reliably estimated with this Doppler method, most animals are thought to have systolic rather than isolated diastolic hypertension. As with the oscillometric method, it may be difficult to obtain measurements in small or hypotensive animals with the Doppler method. Patient movement also interferes with measurement. Unlike the oscillometric technique, mean blood pressure is not measured.

## CLINICAL HYPERTENSION IN DOGS AND CATS

Clinical hypertension usually occurs in middle-aged to older dogs and cats, presumably because of their associated disease conditions. Some studies suggest that male dogs may be at higher risk than females. Cats with severe end-organ disease secondary to hypertension tend to be geriatric.

### Clinical Features and Diagnosis

Signs of hypertension relate to either the underlying or associated disease process (see related chapters in this text) or to end-organ damage caused by the hypertension itself. Blindness is the most common presenting complaint and usually results from acute retinal hemorrhage or detachment. Although the retina may reattach, sight does not return in most cases. Other ocular fundic changes secondary to hypertension include evidence of old retinal hemorrhages, hyperreflective scars, retinal edema, retinal atrophy, retinal arteriolar tortuosity, papilledema, and perivasculitis. Vitreal or anterior chamber hemorrhage, closed-angle glaucoma, and corneal ulceration can also occur.

Another common complaint in animals with hypertension is polyuria/polydipsia. This disorder is frequently associated with renal disease or hyperadrenocorticism in dogs and renal disease or hyperthyroidism in cats. Further, hypertension itself causes a so-called pressure diuresis. A soft systolic cardiac murmur is commonly auscultated in animals with hypertension. A gallop sound may also be heard, especially in cats; but clinical heart failure is uncommon. Epistaxis can result from vascular rupture in the nasal mucosa. Seizures, paresis, syncope, collapse, or other neurologic signs can be manifestations of cerebrovascular accidents (strokes) resulting from hypertensive arteriolar spasm or hemorrhage. It is unclear what percentage of hypertensive animals develop clinical signs related to their increased blood pressure.

Blood pressure measurement should be obtained not only whenever signs compatible with hypertension are found but also when a disease associated with hypertension is diagnosed. It is important to confirm a diagnosis of arterial hypertension by measuring blood pressure multiple times and on different days. A routine complete blood count (CBC), serum biochemical profile, and urinalysis are indicated in all hypertensive patients. Other tests are submitted as needed to rule out possible underlying diseases or complications. These tests might include various endocrine tests, thoracic and abdominal radiographs, ultrasonography (including echocardiography), electrocardiography, ocular examination, and serologic tests.

Thoracic radiographs in dogs and cats with chronic hypertension often reveal some degree of cardiomegaly. Other findings reported in cats include a prominent aortic arch and an undulating aorta, although these attributes are not thought to be pathognomonic for hypertension. Mild-to-moderate left ventricular hypertrophy may be identified on echocardiogram, although measurements within normal reference range are common (Snyder and colleagues, 2001; Nelson and colleagues, 1999). Aortic root dilation may also be identified with echocardiography (Nelson and colleagues, 1999).

### Therapy

Animals with severe hypertension and those with clinical signs presumed to be caused by hypertension should be treated. Measured blood pressure in these animals is generally over 200/110 mm Hg. Whether all dogs and cats with mild hypertension (e.g., repeatable systolic pressures of 170 to 200 mm Hg) benefit from specific antihypertensive treatment is not clear. The expense and time commitment required for long-term treatment and monitoring of such cases as well as the potential for adverse medication effects are considerations. The goal of therapy is to reduce blood pressure to below 170/100 mm Hg, since restoration of normal pressure is unlikely. Management of underlying or concurrent diseases is indicated in all patients (see related chapters in this text).

Several general treatment strategies may be beneficial. Reduced dietary sodium intake (e.g., ≤0.22% to 0.25% sodium on a dry matter basis) is advised for all cases. Even though this alone is not expected to normalize blood pressure, it may enhance the effectiveness of antihypertensive drugs. A high-salt diet has been implicated as a cause of feline hypertension, and salt sensitivity is associated with hypertension in some people; however, the prevalence of salt sensitivity in animals

with hypertension is unknown. Weight reduction is recommended for obese animals. Drugs that can potentiate vasoconstriction (e.g., phenylpropanolamine and other $\alpha_1$-adrenergic agonists) should be avoided. Glucocorticoids and progesterone derivatives should also be avoided when possible because steroid hormones can increase blood pressure. A diuretic (thiazide or furosemide; see Chapter 3) may help by reducing blood volume and sodium content, but a diuretic alone is rarely effective. Diuretics are avoided or used only with caution in azotemic animals. Serum potassium concentration should be monitored, especially in cats with chronic renal disease.

The ability to monitor blood pressure is important when antihypertensive drugs are prescribed. Serial measurements are needed to assess treatment efficacy and avoid hypotension. Adverse effects of antihypertensive therapy usually relate to hypotension, manifested by lethargy or ataxia, and reduced appetite. Several drugs have been used as antihypertensive agents in dogs and cats (Table 12-3). Usually one drug

 TABLE 12-3

**Drugs Used to Treat Hypertension**

| DRUG | DOG | CAT |
|------|-----|-----|
| **Diuretics (see also Chapter 3 and Table 3-6)** | | |
| Furosemide | 1-3 mg/kg q8-24h PO | 1-2 mg/kg q12-24h PO |
| Hydrochlorothiazide | 2-4 mg/kg q12h PO | 1-2 mg/kg q12h PO |
| **β-Adrenergic Blockers (see also Chapter 4 and Table 4-5)** | | |
| Atenolol | 0.2-1.0 mg/kg q12-24h PO (start low) | 6.25-12.5 mg/cat q(12-)24h PO |
| Propranolol | 0.1-1.0 mg/kg q8h PO (start low) | 2.5-10 mg/cat q8-12h PO |
| **Angiotensin Converting Enzyme Inhibitor (ACEI; see also Chapter 3 and Table 3-6)** | | |
| Enalapril | 0.5 mg/kg q24(-12)h PO | 0.25-0.5 mg/kg q24(-12)h PO |
| Captopril | 0.5-2.0 mg/kg q8-12h PO | 0.5-1.25 mg/kg q12-24h PO |
| **Calcium Entry Blocker** | | |
| Amlodipine besylate | 0.1-0.3(0.5) mg/kg q24(-12)h PO | 0.625 mg/cat q24(-12)h PO |
| **$\alpha_1$-Adrenergic Blockers** | | |
| Prazosin (see also Chapter 3) | Large dog: 1 mg q8-12h PO | Do not use |
| Phenoxybenzamine | 0.25-1.5 mg/kg q12h PO | 0.25-1.0 mg/kg q12h PO |
| **Agents used for Hypertensive Crisis** | | |
| Hydralazine (see also Chapter 3) | 0.5-2.0 mg/kg q12h PO | 2.5-10 mg/cat q12h PO |
| Nitroprusside (see also Chapter 3) | 0.5-1 μg/kg/min CRI (initial), to 5-15 μg/kg/min CRI | Same |
| Acepromazine | 0.05-0.1 mg/kg (up to 3 mg total) IV | Same |
| Intravenous propranolol | 0.02 mg/kg initially slow IV(to maximum 1 mg/kg) | Same |
| Esmolol | 200-500 μg/kg IV over 1 min, then 25-200 μg/kg/min CRI | Same |
| Phentolamine | 0.02-0.1 mg/kg IV bolus, followed by CRI to effect | Same |

*ACEI,* Angiotensin converting enzyme inhibitor; *CRI,* constant rate infusion.

at a time is administered, and the animal is monitored. It may take 2 or more weeks before a significant decrease in blood pressure is observed. The drugs most commonly used are angiotensin converting enzyme inhibitors (ACEIs), the calcium entry blocker amlodipine, and β-adrenergic blockers. In some cases, therapy with one agent is effective, but combination therapy may be needed for adequate blood pressure control in other animals. An ACEI is recommended as the initial agent to try in dogs. Amlodipine is recommended as first-line treatment for hypertension in cats, unless hyperthyroidism is the underlying cause. For hyperthyroid-induced hypertension, atenolol or another β-blocker is used first.

β-Adrenergic blockers may reduce blood pressure by decreasing heart rate, cardiac output, and renal renin release. Atenolol and propranolol have been used most often (see p. 91). A β-blocker is recommended for cats with hyperthyroid-induced hypertension, but β-blockers are often ineffective as monotherapy in cats with renal disease.

The ACEIs (e.g., enalapril, benazepril, captopril) diminish the production of angiotensin II, thereby reducing vascular resistance and volume retention (see p. 64). These agents have been more effective in dogs, although their effect depends on the degree of renin-angiotensin system activation underlying the hypertension. Hypertensive cats with chronic renal failure are often not responsive to ACEIs. Reduced renin activity may occur in some cats with end-stage renal disease (see Suggested Readings). However, ACEIs may help protect against hypertensive renal damage. ACEIs have been shown to reduce proteinuria and slow the progression of renal disease. Drugs that block angiotensin II receptors rather than ACE (e.g., candesartan, losartan) are also being used to treat hypertension in people, but veterinary experience with these agents is presently lacking.

Calcium entry blocking drugs (calcium channel blockers) as a group decrease free calcium ion concentration in arteriolar and cardiac muscle cells, resulting in vasodilation and reduced cardiac output (see p. 94). Some agents, such as amlodipine besylate, have mainly vasodilating effects. Amlodipine besylate is a long-acting dihydropyridine calcium entry blocker that has been used successfully and with minimal adverse effects as a single agent in cats. Besides its calcium-blocking effects, vasodilation may be mediated by nitric oxide release from blood vessels. Amlodipine's effects on blood pressure are thought to last at least 24 hours in cats. Amlodipine generally does not have significant effects on serum creatinine concentration or body weight in cats with chronic renal failure. Mild reduction in serum potassium concentration can be successfully treated with oral potassium supplementation. The usual amlodipine dose for a cat is 0.625 mg every 24 hours and can be given with or without food. The dose can be doubled in large cats or in those that do not respond to the lower dose. Alternatively, a β-blocker or ACEI can be added for cats that do not respond adequately to amlodipine alone. Amlodipine has also been effective in dogs (0.1 to 0.3 [to 0.5] mg/kg every 24 [to 12] hours); a lower dose is tried initially and titrated upward as

necessary over a period of days. Amlodipine besylate is available in 2.5-, 5-, and 10-mg tablets (Norvasc; Pfizer, New York, N.Y.). It is difficult to evenly split the tablets, as they can be compounded using lactose as a diluent.

$\alpha_1$-Adrenergic antagonists reduce peripheral vascular resistance by opposing the vasoconstrictive effects of these adrenergic receptors; they are especially useful for the treatment of hypertension caused by pheochromocytoma. The $\alpha_1$-blocker prazosin could be considered for use in large dogs (see p. 66). Phenoxybenzamine (Dibenzyline; Wellspring Pharm. Corp, Neptune, N.J.) is a noncompetitive α-blocker that has been used for pheochromocytoma-induced hypertension at 0.2 to 1.5 mg/kg q12h PO. A low dose is used initially and then titrated upward as necessary.

Adverse effects of antihypertensive therapy usually relate to hypotension. This is usually manifested by periods of lethargy or ataxia. Reduced appetite can be another adverse effect.

Emergency antihypertensive therapy is indicated in animals with acute retinal detachment and hemorrhage, encephalopathy or other evidence of intracranial hemorrhage, acute renal failure, or acute heart failure. Direct vasodilating drugs, such as hydralazine (see Table 12-3; also see p. 65) or nitroprusside, if constant rate infusion and adequate monitoring are available (see Table 12-3; also see p. 66), can be used for acute hypertensive crises. Intravenous propranolol (see Table 12-3; also see p. 91) or acepromazine (Table 12-3) has also been used. One of these agents can also be added to hydralazine therapy if it has not reduced blood pressure sufficiently within 12 hours. For hypertensive crisis caused by catecholamine excess (e.g., pheochromocytoma), the α-blocker phentolamine (Regitine; Bedford Labs, Bedford, Ohio) is used as an intravenous bolus (Table 12-3) followed by an infusion titrated to effect. A β-blocker may also be indicated for pheochromocytoma-induced tachyarrhythmias but should not be used alone or before an α-blocker to avoid exacerbation of hypertension by unopposed $\alpha_1$-receptors. Therapy with a calcium entry blocker, prazosin, or an ACEI by mouth may be effective for acute clinical hypertension of various causes, although parenteral therapy (or oral hydralazine) is advised in dogs and cats with severe hypertension.

In nonemergency cases, blood pressure monitoring to assess antihypertensive treatment efficacy is initially performed every 1 to 2 weeks. When satisfactory blood pressure control is attained, monitoring every 2 to 3 months is adequate. Initial control of blood pressure may take several weeks to months. Some animals respond initially but may become refractory to the same therapy later (Table 12-4).

Because most cases of hypertension are associated with severe underlying disease, the long-term prognosis is often guarded despite apparent response to antihypertensive drugs. It is important to be aware that some treatments for underlying disease can exacerbate hypertension, including fluid therapy, corticosteroids, and erythropoietin. Sodium loads should also be avoided, in both food and medications.

### TABLE 12-4

**Approach to the Hypertensive Patient**

| **Suspect Hypertension or Disease Associated with Hypertension (see Table 12-2, Text)** | **If Hypertension Confirmed—cont'd** |
|---|---|

**Suspect Hypertension or Disease Associated with Hypertension (see Table 12-2, Text)**

Measure BP (see text)
Use quiet environment
- Allow at least 5 to 10 minutes for patient to acclimate to environment (if animal easily stressed, have owner present when possible)
- Measure limb circumference and use appropriate-size cuff (use same cuff size for subsequent measurements as well)
- Use consistent measurement technique
- Take at least five BP readings; discard highest and lowest, average the remaining readings

Repeat BP measurements at other (one to three) times, preferably on different days, to confirm diagnosis of hypertension, except:
- If acute, hypertension-induced clinical signs (e.g., ocular hemorrhage, retinal detachment, neurologic signs) are present, begin therapy immediately (see p. 203; Table 12-3)

Screen for underlying disease(s) (see Table 12-1)
- Obtain in all patients: CBC, serum biochemistry tests, urinalysis
- Consider also, depending on individual patient presentation: endocrine testing, thoracic and abdominal radiographs, ocular examination, ECG, echocardiography, other tests as indicated

**If Hypertension Confirmed:**

Manage underlying disease(s)
Use reduced-sodium diet

**If Hypertension Confirmed—cont'd**

Begin initial antihypertensive drug therapy (see Table 12-3)
- Dogs: enalapril or other ACEI (but see p. 203 if pheochromocytoma-induced hypertension)
- Nonhyperthyroid cats: amlodipine
- Hyperthyroid cats: atenolol or other β-blocker
- If emergent therapy needed, see p. 203

Client education about the patient's disease(s) and potential complications, medication and reevaluation schedules, potential adverse effects of medication(s), and dietary concerns

**Patient Reevaluation**

Recheck BP in 1 to 2 weeks for clinically stable patients
- Sooner reevaluation advisable for unstable patients, although full effects of antihypertensive drugs may not yet be realized

Obtain other tests as indicated for the individual patient

Decide whether to continue therapy as before or adjust dose (up or down)

Continue weekly to biweekly BP monitoring and underlying disease management
- If BP control not achieved even with maximized dosage of initial agent, try alternative drug or piggyback two agents

When BP (and underlying disease) controlled, gradually increase time between recheck examinations
- Recheck no less frequently than every 2 to 3 months, because medication requirements may change

*ACEI,* Angiotensin converting enzyme inhibitor; *BP,* arterial blood pressure; *CBC,* complete blood count; *ECG,* electrocardiogram.

## Suggested Readings

Arnold RM: Pharm profile: amlodipine, *Comp Cont Educ* 23:558, 587, 2001.

Bartges JW et al: What is hypertension in cats? In *Proceedings of the 13th ACVIM Forum,* 1995, Lake Buena Vista, Fla, p 501.

Belew AM et al: Evaluation of the white coat effect in cats, *J Vet Intern Med* 13:134, 1999.

Binns SH et al: Doppler ultrasonographic, oscillometric sphygmomanometric, and photoplethysmographic techniques for noninvasive blood pressure measurement in anesthetized cats, *J Vet Intern Med* 9:405, 1995.

Bodey AR et al: Comparison of direct and indirect (oscillometric) measurements of arterial blood pressure in conscious dogs, *Res Vet Sci* 61:17, 1996a.

Bodey AR et al: Epidemiological study of blood pressure in domestic dogs, *J Small Anim Pract* 37:116, 1996b.

Bovee KC et al: Essential hereditary hypertension in dogs: a new animal model, *J Hypertens* 4:S172, 1986.

Brown SA: Systemic hypertension: management. In *Proceedings of the 19th ACVIM Forum,* Denver, 2001a, p 119.

Brown SA et al: Effects of the angiotensin converting enzyme inhibitor benazepril in cats with induced renal insufficiency, *Am J Vet Res* 62:375, 2001b.

Brown SA et al: Evaluation of Doppler ultrasonic and oscillometric estimation of blood pressure in cats, *J Vet Intern Med* 15:281, 2001c (abstract).

Crow DT et al: Doppler assessment of blood flow and pressure in surgical and critical care patients. In Bonagura JD, editor: *Kirk's current veterinary therapy XII,* Philadelphia, 1995, WB Saunders, p 113.

Hansen B: Blood pressure measurement. In Bonagura JD, editor: *Kirk's current veterinary therapy XII,* Philadelphia, 1995, WB Saunders, p 110.

Henik RA et al: Treatment of systemic hypertension in cats with amlodipine besylate, *J Am Anim Hosp Assoc* 33:226, 1997.

Jensen JL et al: Plasma renin activity and angiotensin I and aldosterone concentrations in cats with hypertension associated with chronic renal disease, *Am J Vet Res* 58:535, 1997.

Kallet AJ et al: Comparison of blood pressure measurements obtained in dogs by use of indirect oscillometry in a veterinary clinic versus at home, *J Am Vet Med Assoc* 210:651, 1997.

Kassab S et al: Blunted natriuretic response to a high-sodium meal in obese dogs, *Hypertension* 23:997, 1994.

Kobayashi DL et al: Hypertension in cats with chronic renal failure or hyperthyroidism, *J Vet Intern Med* 4:58, 1990.

Lane IF et al: Ocular manifestations of vascular disease: hypertension, hyperviscosity, and hyperlipidemia, *J Am Anim Hosp Assoc* 29:28, 1993.

Littman MP et al: Spontaneous systemic hypertension in dogs: five cases (1981-1983), *J Am Vet Med Assoc* 193:486, 1988.

Littman MP: Spontaneous systemic hypertension in 24 cats, *J Vet Intern Med* 8:79, 1994.

Maggio F et al: Ocular lesions associated with systemic hypertension in cats: 69 cases (1985-1998), *J Am Vet Med Assoc* 217:695, 2000.

Meurs KM et al: Comparison of the indirect oscillometric and direct arterial methods for blood pressure measurements in anesthetized dogs, *J Am Anim Hosp Assoc* 32:471, 1996.

Meurs KM et al: Arterial blood pressure measurement in a population of healthy geriatric dogs, *J Am Anim Hosp Assoc* 36:497, 2000.

Nelson OL et al: Echocardiographic and radiographic changes associated with systemic hypertension in cats, *J Vet Intern Med* 13:226, 1999 (abstract).

Ortega TM et al: Systemic arterial blood pressure and urine protein/creatinine ratio in dogs with hyperadrenocorticism, *J Am Vet Med Assoc* 209:1724, 1996.

Papanek PE et al: Chronic pressure-natriuresis relationship in dogs with inherited essential hypertension, *Am J Hypertens* 6:960, 1993.

Pascoe PJ et al: Arterial hypertension associated with topical ocular use of phenylephrine in dogs, *J Am Vet Med Assoc* 205:1562, 1994.

Remillard RL et al: Variance of indirect blood pressure measurements and prevalence of hypertension in clinically normal dogs, *Am J Vet Res* 52:561, 1991.

Snyder PS et al: Feline systemic hypertension. In *Proceedings of the 12th ACVIM Forum,* 1994, San Francisco, p 126.

Snyder PS et al: Effect of amlodipine on echocardiographic variables in cats with systemic hypertension, *J Vet Intern Med* 15:52, 2001.

Sparkes AH et al: Inter- and intraindividual variation in Doppler ultrasonic indirect blood pressure measurements in healthy cats, *J Vet Intern Med* 13:314, 1999.

Stepien RL et al: Clinical comparison of three methods to measure blood pressure in non-sedated dogs, *J Am Vet Med Assoc* 215:1623, 1999.

Stiles J et al: The prevalence of retinopathy in cats with systemic hypertension and chronic renal failure or hyperthyroidism, *J Am Anim Hosp Assoc* 30:564, 1994.

Taugner F et al: The renin-angiotensin system in cats with chronic renal failure, *J Comp Pathol* 115:239, 1996.

Turner JL et al: Idiopathic hypertension in a cat with secondary hypertensive retinopathy associated with a high-salt diet, *J Am Anim Hosp Assoc* 26:647, 1990.

## Drugs Used in Cardiovascular Disorders

| GENERIC NAME | TRADE NAME | DOG | CAT |
|---|---|---|---|
| **Diuretics** | | | |
| Furosemide | Lasix<br>Salix | 1 to 3 mg/kg q8-24h chronic PO; or 2 to 5 mg/kg q4 to 6h IV, IM, SC | 1 to 2 mg/kg q12h, up to 4 mg/kg q8-12h IV, IM, SC, PO |
| Spironolactone | Aldactone | 2 mg/kg q12h PO | 1 to 2 mg/kg q12h PO |
| Chlorothiazide | Diuril | 20 to 40 mg/kg q12h PO | Same |
| Hydrochlorothiazide | Hydrodiuril | 2 to 4 mg/kg q12h PO | 1 to 2 mg/kg q12h PO |
| Triamterene | Dyrenium | 2 (to 4) mg/kg/day PO | — |
| **ACEI & Other Vasodilators** | | | |
| Enalapril | Enacard<br>Vasotec | 0.5 mg/kg q(12-)24h PO | 0.25 to 0.5 mg/kg q(12-)24h PO |
| Captopril | Capoten | 0.5 to 2 mg/kg q8-12h PO (0.25 to 0.5 mg/kg initial dose) | 0.5 to 1.25 mg/kg q12-24 h PO |
| Benazepril | Lotensin | 0.25 to 0.5 mg/kg q24h PO | Same |
| Lisinopril | Prinivil<br>Zestril | 0.5 mg/kg q24h PO | 0.25-0.5 mg/kg q24h PO |
| Fosinopril | Monopril | 0.25-0.5 mg/kg q24h PO | — |
| Hydralazine | Apresoline | 0.5 to 2 mg/kg q12h PO (to 1 mg/kg initial)<br>For decompensated CHF: 0.5 to 1 mg/kg PO, repeat in 2-4h, then q12h | 2.5 (up to 10) mg per cat q12h PO |
| Amlodipine besylate | Norvasc | 0.05 to 0.3 (-0.5) mg/kg q(12-)24h PO | 0.625 mg/cat q(12-)24h PO |
| Prazosin | Minipress | Small dogs (<5 kg): do not use; medium dogs: 1 mg q8-12h PO; large dogs: 2 mg q8h PO | Do not use |
| Na⁺ nitroprusside | Nitropress | 0.5 to 1 μg/kg/min CRI (initial), to 5 to 15 μg/kg/min CRI | Same |
| Nitroglycerine ointment 2% | Nitrobid<br>Nitrol | ½ to 1½ inch q4-6h cutaneously | ¼ to ½ inch q4-6h cutaneously |
| Isosorbide dinitrate | Isordil<br>Titradose | 0.5 to 2 mg/kg q8h PO | — |
| Phenoxybenzamine | Dibenzyline | 0.25 (to 1.5) mg/kg q12h PO | 0.25 to 1.0 mg/kg q12h PO |
| Phentolamine | Regitine | 0.02 to 0.1 mg/kg IV bolus, followed by CRI to effect | Same |
| Acepromazine | | 0.05 to 0.1 mg/kg (up to 3 mg total) IV | Same |
| **Positive Inotropic Drugs** | | | |
| Digoxin | Cardoxin<br>Cardoxin LS<br>Lanoxin | Oral: dogs <22 kg: 0.011 mg/kg q12h; dogs >22 kg: 0.22 mg/m² q12h; or 0.005 mg/kg q12h; decrease by 10% for elixir. Max. 0.5 mg/day or 0.375 mg/day for Dobermans<br>IV loading: 0.01 to 0.02 mg/kg; give ¼ of total dose in slow boluses over 2 to 4h to effect | Oral: 0.007 mg/kg q48h<br>IV loading: 0.005 mg/kg—give ½ of total, then 1 to 2h later give ¼ dose bolus as needed |
| Digitoxin | Crystodigin | 0.02 to 0.03 mg/kg q8h (small dogs) to q12h (large dogs) | Do not use |
| Dopamine | Intropin | For CHF: 1 to 10 μg/kg/min CRI (start low)<br>For shock: 5-15 μg/kg/min CRI | 1 to 5 μg/kg/min CRI (start low) |
| Dobutamine | Dobutrex | 1 to 10 μg/kg/min CRI (start low) | Same |
| Amrinone | Inocor | 1 to 3 mg/kg initial bolus, IV; 10 to 100 μg/kg/min CRI | Same? |
| Milrinone | Primacor | 50 μg/kg IV over 10 min initially; 0.375 to 0.75 μg/kg/min CRI (humans) | Same? |

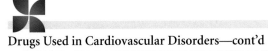

Drugs Used in Cardiovascular Disorders—cont'd

| GENERIC NAME | TRADE NAME | DOG | CAT |
|---|---|---|---|
| **Antiarrhythmic Drugs** | | | |
| *Class I* | | | |
| Lidocaine | Xylocaine | Initial boluses of 2 mg/kg slowly IV, up to 8 mg/kg; or rapid IV infusion at 0.8 mg/kg/min; if effective, then 25 to 80 µg/kg/min CRI (can also be used intratracheally for CPR) | Initial bolus of 0.25 to 0.5 mg/kg slowly IV, can repeat at 0.15 to 0.25 mg/kg in 5 to 20 min; if effective, 10 to 20 µg/kg/min CRI |
| Procainamide | Pronestyl Pronestyl SR Procan SR | 6 to 10 (up to 20) mg/kg IV over 5 to 10 min; 10 to 50 µg/kg/min CRI; 6 to 20 (up to 30) mg/kg q4-6h IM; 10 to 25 mg/kg q6h PO (sustained release: q6-8h) | 1 to 2 mg/kg slowly IV; 10 to 20 µg/kg/min CRI; 7.5 to 20 mg/kg q(6 to) 8h IM, PO |
| Quinidine | Quinidex Extentabs Quinaglute Dura-Tabs Cardioquin | 6 to 20 mg/kg q6h IM (loading dose 14 to 20 mg/kg); 6 to 16 mg/kg q6h PO; sustained action preps 8 to 20 mg/kg q8h PO | 6 to 16 mg/kg q8h IM, PO |
| Mexiletine | Mexitil | 4 to 10 mg/kg q8h PO | — |
| Tocainide | Tonocard | 10 to 20 (to 25) mg/kg q8h PO | — |
| Phenytoin | Dilantin | 10 mg/kg slow IV; 30 to 50 mg/kg q8h PO | Do not use |
| *Class II* | | | |
| Propranolol | Inderal | IV: initial bolus of 0.02 mg/kg slowly, up to max. of 0.1 mg/kg Oral: initial dose of 0.1 to 0.2 mg/kg q8h, up to max. of 1 mg/kg q8h | IV: Same Oral: 2.5 up to 10 mg per cat q8-12h |
| Atenolol | Tenormin | 0.2 to 1 mg/kg q12-24h PO (start low) | 6.25 to 12.5 mg per cat q(12-)24h PO |
| Esmolol | Brevibloc | 200 to 500 µg/kg IV over 1 min, followed by infusion of 25 to 200 µg/kg/min | Same |
| Metroprolol | Lopressor | 0.2 mg/kg initial dose q8h PO; up to 1 mg/kg q8h | — |
| Nadolol | Corgard | 0.2 mg/kg initial dose q8 to 12h PO; up to 1 mg/kg q8-12h | — |
| *Class III* | | | |
| Sotalol | Betapace | 1 to 3.5 mg/kg | — |
| Amiodarone | Cordarone | 10 mg/kg q12h PO for 7d; then 8 mg/kg q24h PO; 3 to 5 mg/kg slow IV | — |
| Bretylium | Bretylol | 2 to 6 mg/kg IV; may repeat in 1-2h (humans) | — |
| *Class IV* | | | |
| Diltiazem | Cardizem Cardizem-CD Dilacor XR | Initial dose 0.5 mg/kg q8h PO, up to 2 mg/kg; for atrial tachycardia, 0.5 mg/kg PO, followed by 0.25 mg/kg q1h to total of 1.5 (to 2 ) mg/kg or conversion; *or* 0.15 to 0.25 mg/kg over 2 to 3 min IV (can repeat q15 min until conversion or total of 0.75 mg/kg) | Same? For hypertrophic cardiomyopathy, 1 to 2.5 mg/kg q8h PO; sustained release Cardizem-CD: 10 mg/kg/day; Dilacor XR: 30 mg/cat/day |
| Verapamil | Calan Isoptin | Initial dose: 0.05 mg/kg slowly IV; can repeat q5 min, up to total of 0.15 (to 0.2) mg/kg; 0.5 to 2 mg/kg q8h PO | Initial dose 0.025 mg/kg slowly IV; can repeat q5 min, up to total of 0.15 (to 0.2) mg/kg; 0.5 to 1 mg/kg q8h PO |

*Continued*

Drugs Used in Cardiovascular Disorders—cont'd

| GENERIC NAME | TRADE NAME | DOG | CAT |
|---|---|---|---|
| **Anticholinergics** | | | |
| Atropine | | 0.02 to 0.04 mg/kg IV, IM, SC; can also be used intratracheally for CPR | Same |
| Glycopyrrolate | Robinul | 0.005 to 0.01 mg/kg IV, IM; 0.01 to 0.02 mg/kg SC | Same |
| Propantheline Br | Pro-Banthine | 3.73 to 7.5 mg q8-12h, PO | — |
| **Sympathomimetics** | | | |
| Isoproterenol | Isuprel | 0.045 to 0.09 μg/kg/min CRI | Same |
| Terbutaline | Brethine Bricanyl | 2.5 to 5 mg per dog q8-12h PO | 1.25 mg per cat q12h PO |
| **CPR Drugs** | | | |
| Epinephrine | Adrenaline Cl | (0.1 to) 0.2 mg/kg IV; 0.4 mg/kg IT (diluted with 2 to 5 ml sterile water or saline), q3-5min as needed; also can use IO (previously recommended: 0.1 to 0.5 mg/10 kg); 1:1000 = 1 mg/ml | Same |
| Methoxamine | Vasoxyl | 0.1 to 0.2 mg/kg IV; can use IT | Same |
| Metaraminol | | 0.1 to 0.2 mg/kg IV | Same |
| Mephentermine | | 0.1 to 0.5 mg/kg IV | Same |
| Phenylephrine | | 0.01 to 0.1 mg/kg IV | Same |
| Norepinephrine | Levophed | 0.01 to 0.1 mg/average dog | — |
| Dopamine | | 5 to 15 μg/kg/min CRI; can also use IO | 1 to 5 μg/kg/min CRI; can also use IO |
| Sodium bicarbonate | | 0.5 to 1.0 mEq/kg initial; up to 8 mEq/kg if prolonged arrest and/or CPR Do *not* give IT; can use IO | Same |
| CaCl (10%) | | 0.1 to 0.26 ml/kg IV (or 1.5 to 2 ml/dog) | Same |
| Ca gluconate (10%) | | 0.1 to 0.3 ml/kg IV; can use IO | Same |

Drugs Used in Cardiovascular Disorders—cont'd

| GENERIC NAME | TRADE NAME | DOG | CAT |
|---|---|---|---|
| **CPR Drugs—cont'd** | | | |
| Dexamethasone SP | | 4 mg/kg IV; can use IO | Same |
| Atropine | | 0.04 mg/kg IV, IM, IT, IO | Same |
| Lidocaine | | 2 mg/kg up to 8 mg/kg IV; see Table 4-5, can also use IT or IO | 0.25 to 0.5 mg/kg slowly IV; see Table 4-5, can also use IT or IO |
| **Drugs for Adult Heartworm Infections** | | | |
| Melarsomine | Immiticide | Follow manufacturer's instructions carefully; standard regimen: 2.5 mg/kg deep into lumbar muscles q24h for 2 doses. Alternate regimen: 2.5 mg/kg IM for 1 dose; 1 month later give standard regimen | — |
| Thiacetarsamide | Caparsolate | 2.2 mg/kg IV (0.22 ml/kg) q12h for 2 days | — |
| **Microfilaricide Therapy** | | | |
| Ivermectin | Ivomec Heartgard-30 | One dose (0.05 mg/kg) orally 3 to 4 weeks after adulticide therapy. Can repeat in 2 weeks | Same |
| Milbemycin oxime | Interceptor | One dose of 0.5 to 1.0 mg/kg PO; can repeat in 2 weeks | Same |
| **Heartworm Prevention** | | | |
| Ivermectin | Heartgard-30 | 0.006 to 0.012 mg/kg PO once a month | 0.024 mg/kg PO once a month |
| Milbemycin oxime | Interceptor | 0.5 (to 1.0) mg/kg PO once a month | 2 mg/kg PO once a month |
| Selamectin | Revolution | 6 to 12 mg/kg topically | Same |
| Moxidectin | ProHeart | 0.003 mg/kg once a month | |
| | ProHeart 6 | 0.17 mg/kg q6 months | |
| Diethylcarbamazine | Filaribits Nemacide | 3 mg/kg (6.6 mg/kg of 50% citrate) PO once a day | Same |

# C H A P T E R  13

# Clinical Manifestations of Nasal Disease

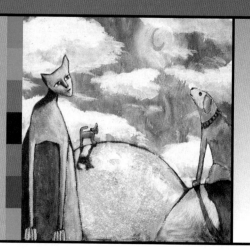

## CHAPTER OUTLINE

GENERAL CONSIDERATIONS, 210
NASAL DISCHARGE: CLASSIFICATION
AND DIAGNOSTIC APPROACH, 210
    Classification and etiology, 210
    Diagnostic approach, 211
SNEEZING: ETIOLOGY AND DIAGNOSTIC
APPROACH, 215
    Reverse sneezing, 215
STERTOR, 216
FACIAL DEFORMITY, 216

## GENERAL CONSIDERATIONS

The nasal cavity and paranasal sinuses have a complex anatomy and are lined by mucosa. Their rostral portion is inhabited by bacteria in health. Nasal disorders are frequently associated with mucosal edema, inflammation, and secondary bacterial infection. They are often focal or multifocal in distribution. These factors combine to make the accurate diagnosis of nasal disease a challenge that can be met only through a thorough, systematic approach.

Diseases of the nasal cavity and paranasal sinuses typically cause nasal discharge, sneezing, stertor (snoring or snorting sounds), facial deformity, systemic signs of illness (e.g., lethargy, inappetence, weight loss), or in rare instances, central nervous system signs. The most common clinical manifestation is nasal discharge. The general diagnostic approach to animals with nasal disease is included in the discussion of nasal discharge. Specific considerations related to sneezing, stertor, and facial deformity follow. Stenotic nares are discussed in the section on brachycephalic airway syndrome (Chapter 18, p. 248).

## NASAL DISCHARGE: CLASSIFICATION AND DIAGNOSTIC APPROACH

### Classification and Etiology

Nasal discharge is most commonly associated with disease localized within the nasal cavity and paranasal sinuses, although it may also develop with disorders of the lower respiratory tract, such as bacterial pneumonia and infectious tracheobronchitis, or systemic disorders, such as coagulopathies and systemic hypertension. Nasal discharge is characterized as serous, mucopurulent with or without hemorrhage, or purely hemorrhagic (epistaxis). Serous nasal discharge has a clear, watery consistency. Depending on the quantity and duration of the discharge, a serous discharge may be normal, may be indicative of viral upper respiratory infection, or may precede the development of a mucopurulent discharge. As such, many of the causes of mucopurulent discharge can initially cause serous discharge (Table 13-1).

Mucopurulent nasal discharge is typically characterized by a thick, ropey consistency and has a white, yellow, or green tint. A mucopurulent nasal discharge implies inflammation. Most intranasal diseases result in inflammation and secondary bacterial infection, making this sign a common presentation for most nasal diseases. Potential etiologies include infectious agents, foreign bodies, neoplasia, polyps, allergies, and extension of disease from the oral cavity (see Table 13-1). If mucopurulent discharge is present in conjunction with signs of lower respiratory tract disease, such as cough, respiratory distress, or auscultable crackles, the diagnostic emphasis is on evaluation of the lower airways and pulmonary parenchyma. Hemorrhage may be associated with mucopurulent exudate from any etiology, but significant and prolonged bleeding in association with mucopurulent discharge is usually associated with neoplasia or mycotic infections.

TABLE 13-1

**Differential Diagnoses for Nasal Discharge in Dogs and Cats**

### Serous Discharge

Normal
Viral infection
Early sign of etiology of mucopurulent discharge

### Mucopurulent Discharge with or without Hemorrhage

Viral infection
  Feline herpesvirus (rhinotracheitis virus)
  Feline calicivirus
Bacterial infection
Fungal infection
  *Aspergillus*
  *Cryptococcus*
  *Penicillium*
  *Rhinosporidium*
Nasal parasites
Foreign body
Neoplasia
  Carcinoma
  Sarcoma
  Malignant lymphoma
Nasopharyngeal polyp
Lymphocytic plasmacytic rhinitis
Allergic rhinitis
Extension of oral disease
  Tooth root abscess
  Oronasal fistula
  Deformed palate

### Pure Hemorrhagic Discharge (Epistaxis)

Nasal disease
  Acute trauma
  Acute foreign body
  Neoplasia
  Fungal infection
Systemic disease
  Coagulopathy
  Systemic hypertension
  Polycythemia
  Hyperviscosity syndrome
  Vasculitis

Persistent pure hemorrhage (epistaxis) can result from trauma, local aggressive disease processes (e.g., neoplasia, mycotic infections), systemic hypertension, or systemic bleeding disorders. Systemic hemostatic disorders that can cause epistaxis include thrombocytopenia, thrombocytopathies, von Willebrand's disease, rodenticide toxicity, and vasculitides. Ehrlichiosis and Rocky Mountain spotted fever can cause epistaxis through several of these mechanisms. Nasal foreign bodies may cause hemorrhage after entry into the nasal cavity, but the bleeding tends to subside quickly. Bleeding can also occur after aggressive sneezing from any cause.

## Diagnostic Approach

A complete history and physical examination can be used to prioritize the differential diagnoses for each type of nasal discharge (see Table 13-1). Acute and chronic diseases are defined by historical information regarding the onset of signs and by evaluating the overall condition of the animal. Acute processes, such as foreign bodies or acute feline viral infections, often result in a sudden onset of signs, including sneezing, and the animal's body condition is excellent. In chronic processes, such as mycotic infections or neoplasia, signs are present over a long period of time and the overall body condition can be deleteriously affected. A history of gagging or retching may indicate masses or foreign bodies in the caudal nasopharynx.

Unilateral and bilateral discharge are differentiated on the basis of both historical and physical examination findings. When nasal discharge is apparently unilateral, a cold microscope slide can be held close to the external nares to determine the patency of the side of the nasal cavity without discharge. Condensation will not be visible in front of the naris if airflow is obstructed, implying that the disease is actually bilateral. Although any bilateral process can initially cause signs from one side only and unilateral disease can progress to involve the opposite side, some generalizations can be made. Systemic disorders and infectious diseases tend to involve both sides of the nasal cavity, whereas foreign bodies, polyps, and tooth root abscessation tend to cause unilateral discharge. Neoplasia causes unilateral discharge initially but may progress to bilateral discharge following destruction of the nasal septum.

Ulceration of the nasal plane often occurs in dogs with nasal aspergillosis (Fig. 13-1). Polypoid masses protruding from the external nares in the dog are typical of rhinosporidiosis, and in the cat they are typical of cryptococcosis.

A thorough assessment of the head, including facial symmetry, teeth, gingiva, hard and soft palate, mandibular lymph nodes, and eyes, should be performed. Mass lesions invading beyond the nasal cavity can cause deformity of facial bones or the hard palate, exophthalmos, or inability to retropulse the eye. Pain on palpation of the nasal bones is typical of aspergillosis. Gingivitis, dental calculi, loose teeth, or pus in the gingival sulcus should raise an index of suspicion for oronasal fistulae or tooth root abscess, especially if unilateral nasal discharge is present. Foci of inflammation and folds of hyperplastic gingiva in the dorsum of the mouth should be probed for oronasal fistulae. A normal examination of the oral cavity does not rule out oronasal fistulae or tooth root abscess. The hard and soft palates are examined for deformation, erosions, or congenital defects such as clefts or hypoplasia. Mandibular lymph node enlargement suggests active inflammation or neoplasia, and fine-needle aspirates of enlarged or firm nodes are evaluated for organisms, such as *Cryptococcus,* and neoplastic cells (Fig. 13-2). A fundic examination should always be performed because active chorioretinitis can occur with cryptococcosis, ehrlichiosis, and malignant lymphoma (Fig. 13-3). Retinal detachment can occur with systemic hypertension or mass lesions extending into the bony orbit. With

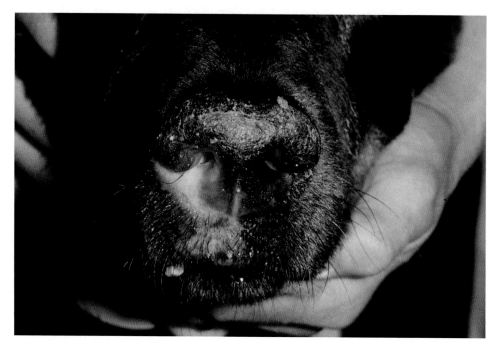

**FIG 13-1**
Depigmentation and ulceration of the planum nasale is suggestive of nasal aspergillosis. The visible lesions usually extend from one or both nares and are most severe ventrally. This dog has unilateral depigmentation and mild ulceration.

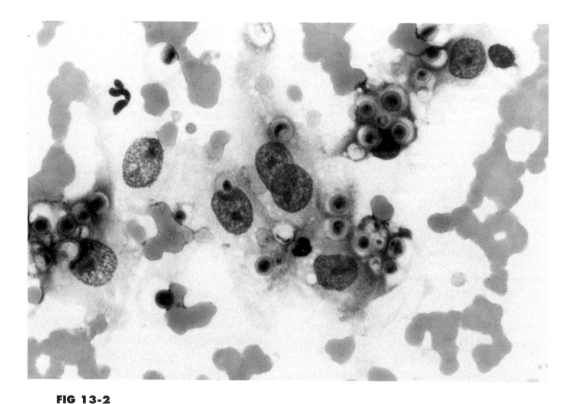

**FIG 13-2**
Photomicrograph of fine-needle aspirate of a cat with facial deformity. Identification of cryptococcal organisms provides a definitive diagnosis for cats with nasal discharge or facial deformity. Organisms can often be found in swabs of nasal discharge, fine-needle aspirates of facial masses, or fine-needle aspirates of enlarged mandibular lymph nodes. The organisms are variably sized, ranging from about 3 to 30 μm in diameter, with a wide capsule and narrow-based budding. They may be found intracellularly or extracellularly.

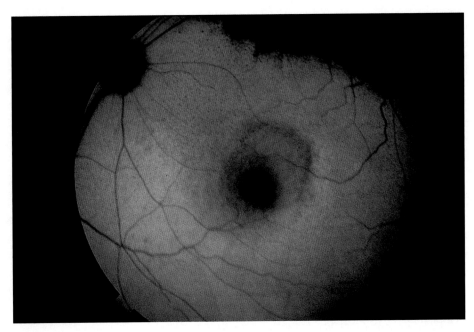

**FIG 13-3**
Fundic examination can provide useful information in animals with signs of respiratory tract disease. This fundus from a cat with chorioretinitis due to cryptococcosis has a large, focal, hyporeflective lesion in the area centralis. Smaller regions of hyporeflectivity were also seen. The optic disk is in the upper left-hand corner of the photograph. (Courtesy M. Davidson, North Carolina State University, Raleigh, N.C.)

epistaxis, identification of petechiae or hemorrhage in other mucous membranes, skin, ocular fundus, feces, or urine supports a systemic bleeding disorder. Note that melena may be present as a result of swallowing blood from the nasal cavity.

Diagnostic tests that should be considered for a dog or cat with nasal discharge are included in Table 13-2. The signalment, history, and physical examination findings dictate in part which diagnostic tests are ultimately required to establish the diagnosis. As a general rule, less invasive diagnostic tests are performed initially. A complete blood count (CBC) with platelet count, coagulation panel (i.e., activated clotting time or prothrombin and partial thromboplastin times), buccal mucosal bleeding time, and arterial blood pressure should be evaluated in dogs and cats with epistaxis. Von Willebrand's factor assays are performed in purebred dogs with epistaxis and in dogs with prolonged mucosal bleeding times. Determination of *Ehrlichia* spp. and Rocky Mountain spotted fever titers are indicated in regions of the country where potential exposure to these rickettsial agents exists. Testing for feline immunodeficiency virus (FIV) and feline leukemia virus (FeLV) should be performed in cats with chronic nasal discharge and potential exposure. Cats infected with FeLV may be predisposed to chronic infection with herpesvirus or calicivirus, whereas those with FIV may have chronic nasal discharge without concurrent infection with these upper respiratory viruses.

Most animals with intranasal disease have normal thoracic radiographs. However, thoracic radiographs can be useful in identifying primary bronchopulmonary disease, pulmonary involvement with cryptococcosis, and rare metastases from neoplastic disease. They may also be a useful preanesthetic screening test for animals that will require nasal imaging, rhinoscopy, and nasal biopsy.

Cytologic evaluation of superficial nasal swabs may identify cryptococcal organisms in cats (see Fig. 13-2). Nonspecific findings include proteinaceous background, moderate to severe inflammation, and bacteria. Tests to identify herpesvirus and calicivirus infections can be performed in cats with acute and chronic rhinitis. These tests are most useful in evaluating cattery problems rather than an individual cat (see Chapter 15).

Fungal titer determinations are available for aspergillosis in dogs and cryptococcosis in dogs and cats. The test for aspergillosis detects antibodies in the blood. A single positive test result suggests active infection by the organism; however, a negative titer does not rule out the disease. In either case, the result of the test must be interpreted in conjunction with results of nasal imaging, rhinoscopy, and nasal histology and culture.

The blood test of choice for cryptococcosis is the latex agglutination capsular antigen test (LCAT). Organism identification is usually possible in specimens from infected organs and is the method of choice for a definitive diagnosis. The LCAT is performed if cryptococcosis is suspected but an extensive search for the organism has failed. The LCAT is also performed in animals with a confirmed diagnosis as a means of monitoring therapeutic response (see Chapter 103).

TABLE 13-2

General Diagnostic Approach to Dogs and Cats with Chronic Nasal Discharge

| PHASE I (NONINVASIVE TESTING) | | | |
|---|---|---|---|
| **ALL PATIENTS** | **DOGS** | **CATS** | **DOGS AND CATS WITH HEMORRHAGE** |
| History | *Aspergillus* titer | Nasal swab cytologic evaluation (cryptococcosis) | Complete blood count |
| Physical examination | | Cryptococcal antigen titer | Platelet count |
| Thoracic radiographs | | Viral testing | Coagulation times |
| | |   Feline leukemia virus | Buccal mucoasl bleeding time |
| | |   Feline immunodeficiency virus | Rickettsial titers |
| | |   ± Herpesvirus | Arterial blood pressure |
| | |   ± Calicivirus | von Willebrand's factor assay |
| **PHASE II—ALL PATIENTS (GENERAL ANESTHESIA REQUIRED)** | | | |
| Nasal radiography or computerized tomography | | | |
| Oral examination | | | |
| Rhinoscopy: external nares and nasopharynx | | | |
| Nasal biopsy/histologic examination | | | |
| Deep nasal culture | | | |
|   Fungal | | | |
|   Bacterial | | | |
| **PHASE III—ALL PATIENTS (REFERRAL USUALLY REQUIRED)** | | | |
| Computerized tomography (if not previously performed) | | | |
| **PHASE IV—ALL PATIENTS (CONSIDER REFERRAL)** | | | |
| Repeat Phase II using computerized tomography | | | |
| Exploratory rhinotomy with turbinectomy | | | |

In general, nasal radiography or computerized tomography (CT), rhinoscopy, biopsy, and deep nasal cultures are required to establish a diagnosis of intranasal disease in most dogs and in cats in which acute viral infection is not suspected. These diagnostic tests are performed with the dog or cat under general anesthesia. Nasal radiographs or CT scans are obtained first, followed by oral examination and rhinoscopy, and then specimen collection. This order is recommended because the results of radiography or CT and rhinoscopy are often useful in the selection of biopsy sites. In addition, hemorrhage from biopsy sites could obscure or alter radiographic and rhinoscopic detail if the specimen were collected first. In dogs and cats suspected of having acute foreign body inhalation, rhinoscopy is performed first in the hopes of identifying and removing the foreign material. See Chapter 14 for more detail on nasal radiography, CT, and rhinoscopy.

The combination of radiography, rhinoscopy, and nasal biopsy has a diagnostic success rate of approximately 80% in dogs. Dogs with persistent signs in which a diagnosis cannot be obtained following the assessment described earlier require further evaluation. It is more difficult to evaluate the success rate for cats. High proportions of cats with chronic nasal discharge suffer from the effects of viral infection and are diagnosed only through exclusion. Cats are evaluated further only if signs suggestive of another disease are found during any part of their evaluation or if the clinical signs are progressive or intolerable to the owners.

Nasal CT is considered if not performed previously, and a diagnosis has not been made. CT provides excellent visualization of all of the nasal turbinates (Fig. 13-4) and may allow the identification of small masses that are not visible on nasal radiography or rhinoscopy. CT is also the technique of choice for determining the full extent of nasal tumors. In the absence of a diagnosis, nasal imaging (preferably CT), rhinoscopy, and biopsy can be repeated after a 1- to 2-month delay.

Exploratory rhinotomy with turbinectomy is the final diagnostic test. Surgical exploration of the nose allows direct visualization of the nasal cavity for the presence of foreign bodies, mass lesions, or fungal mats and for obtaining biopsies and culture specimens. The potential benefits of surgery, however, should be weighed against the potential complications associated with rhinotomy and turbinectomy. The Suggested Readings section offers information on the surgical procedure.

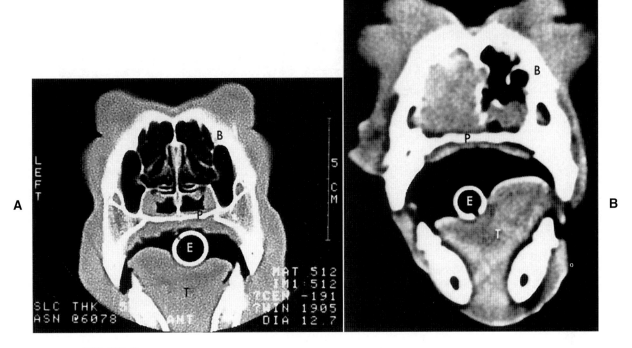

**FIG 13-4**
CT scans of nasal cavity of two different dogs. **A,** Normal nasal turbinates and intact nasal septum are present. **B,** Neoplastic mass is present within the left nasal cavity; it is eroding through the septum to involve the right side as well. *B,* Facial bones; *E,* endotracheal tube; *P,* hard palate; *T,* tongue.

## SNEEZING: ETIOLOGY AND DIAGNOSTIC APPROACH

A sneeze is an explosive release of air from the lungs through the nasal cavity and mouth. It is a protective reflex to expel irritants from the nasal cavity. Intermittent, occasional sneezing is considered normal. Persistent, paroxysmal sneezing should be considered abnormal. Disorders commonly associated with acute-onset, persistent sneezing include nasal foreign body and feline upper respiratory infection. The canine nasal mite, *Pneumonyssoides caninum,* and exposure to irritating aerosols are less common causes of sneezing. All the nasal diseases considered as differential diagnoses for nasal discharge are also potential causes for sneezing; however, animals with these diseases generally present with nasal discharge as the primary complaint.

The owners should be questioned carefully concerning the possible recent exposure of the pet to foreign bodies (e.g., rooting in the ground, running through grassy fields), powders, aerosols, or, in cats, exposure to new cats or kittens. Sneezing is an acute phenomenon that often subsides with time. A foreign body should not be excluded from the differential diagnoses just because the sneezing subsides. In the dog, a history of acute sneezing followed by the development of a nasal discharge is suggestive of a foreign body.

Other findings may help to narrow the list of differential diagnoses. Dogs with foreign bodies may paw at their nose. Foreign bodies are typically associated with unilateral, mucopurulent nasal discharge, although serous or serosanguineous discharge may be present initially. Foreign bodies in the caudal nasopharynx may cause gagging, retching, or reverse sneezing. The nasal discharge associated with reactions to aerosols, powders, or other inhaled irritants is usually bilateral and serous in nature. In cats, other clinical signs supportive of a diagnosis of upper respiratory infection, such as conjunctivitis and fever, may be present, as well as a history of exposure to other cats or kittens.

Dogs in which acute, paroxysmal sneezing develops should undergo prompt rhinoscopic examination (see p. 221). With time, foreign material may become covered with mucus or migrate deeper into the nasal passages, and any delay in performing rhinoscopy may interfere with the identification and removal of the foreign bodies. Nasal mites are also identified rhinoscopically. In contrast, cats sneeze more often as a result of acute viral infection rather than foreign body. Immediate rhinoscopic examination is not indicated unless there has been known exposure to a foreign body or the history and physical examination findings do not support a diagnosis of viral upper respiratory infection.

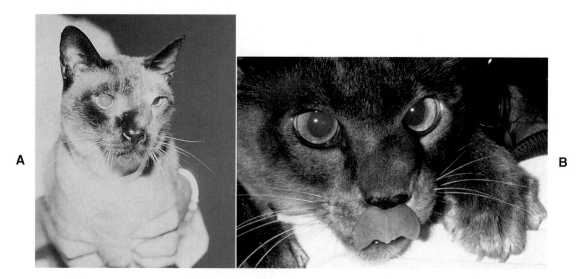

**FIG 13-5**
Facial deformity characterized by firm swelling over the maxilla in two cats. **A,** Deformity in this cat was the result of carcinoma. Notice the ipsilateral blepharospasm. **B,** Deformity in this cat was the result of cryptococcosis. A photomicrograph of the fine-needle aspirate of this swelling is provided in Fig. 13-2.

## REVERSE SNEEZING

Reverse sneezing is a paroxysm of noisy, labored inspiration initiated by nasopharyngeal irritation. Such irritation can be the result of a foreign body or viral infection. Epiglottic entrapment of the soft palate has been proposed as a cause. The majority of cases are idiopathic. Small-breed dogs are usually affected, and signs may be associated with excitement or drinking. The paroxysms last only a few seconds and do not significantly interfere with respiration. Although these animals usually display this sign throughout their life, the problem rarely progresses.

The diagnosis is generally made by a thorough history and physical examination. Generally, no treatment is needed because the episodes are self-limiting. Some owners report that massaging the neck shortens an ongoing episode or that administration of antihistamines decreases the frequency and severity of episodes, but controlled studies are lacking. Further evaluation for potential nasal or pharyngeal disorders is indicated if syncope, exercise intolerance, or other signs of respiratory disease are reported or if the reverse sneezing is severe or progressive.

## STERTOR

*Stertor* refers to coarse, audible snoring or snorting sounds associated with breathing. It indicates upper airway obstruc-tion. Stertor is most often the result of pharyngeal disease (see Chapter 16). Intranasal causes of stertor include obstruction caused by congenital deformities, masses, exudate, or blood clots. Evaluation for nasal disease proceeds as described for nasal discharge.

## FACIAL DEFORMITY

The most common causes of facial deformity adjacent to the nasal cavity are neoplasia and, in cats, cryptococcosis (Fig. 13-5). Visible swellings can often be evaluated directly through fine-needle aspiration or punch biopsy (see Fig. 13-2). If such an approach is not possible or is unsuccessful, then further evaluation proceeds as for nasal discharge.

### Suggested Readings

Bojrab MJ, editor: *Current techniques in small animal surgery,* ed 4, Baltimore, 1998, William & Wilkins.

Forbes SE et al: Evaluation of rhinoscopy and rhinoscopy-assisted mucosal biopsy in diagnosis of nasal disease in dogs: 119 cases (1985-1989), *J Am Vet Med Assoc* 201:1425, 1992.

Fossum TW: *Small animal surgery,* St Louis, 1997, Mosby.

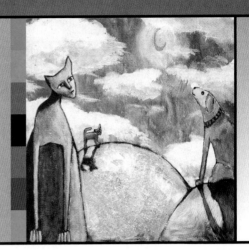

# CHAPTER 14

# Diagnostic Tests for the Nasal Cavity and Paranasal Sinuses

## CHAPTER OUTLINE

NASAL RADIOGRAPHY, 217
COMPUTERIZED TOMOGRAPHY, 221
RHINOSCOPY, 221
NASAL BIOPSY: INDICATIONS
AND TECHNIQUES, 224
    Nasal swab, 224
    Nasal flush, 224
    Pinch biopsy, 224
    Core biopsy, 225
    Turbinectomy, 225
    Complications, 225
NASAL CULTURES: SAMPLE COLLECTION
AND INTERPRETATION, 226

## NASAL RADIOGRAPHY

Nasal radiographs are frequently required in the diagnostic assessment of the animal with signs of intranasal disease. Nasal radiographs identify the extent and severity of disease, localize sites for biopsy within the nasal cavity, and help to prioritize the differential diagnoses. Radiographs rarely provide a definitive diagnosis and generally must be followed by rhinoscopy and nasal biopsy. Nasal radiographs should be obtained before, rather than after, these procedures for two reasons: (1) results of nasal radiographs help the clinician to direct biopsy instruments to the most abnormal regions, and (2) rhinoscopy and biopsy cause hemorrhage, which obscures radiographic detail.

The dog or cat must be anesthetized to prevent motion and facilitate positioning. Abnormalities are often subtle. At least four views should be taken: lateral, ventrodorsal, intraoral, and frontal sinus or skyline. Lateral-oblique views or dental films are also indicated in dogs and cats with possible tooth root abscess, and radiographs of the tympanic bullae are obtained in cats with suspected nasopharyngeal polyps. The intraoral view is particularly helpful for detecting subtle asymmetry between the left and right nasal cavities. The intraoral view is taken with the animal in sternal recumbency. The corner of a non-screen film is placed above the tongue as far into the oral cav-

ity as possible, and the radiographic beam is positioned directly above the nasal cavity (Figs. 14-1 and 14-2). The frontal sinus view is obtained with the animal in dorsal recumbency. Adhesive tape can be used to support the body and draw the forelimbs caudally, out of the field. The head is positioned perpendicular to the spine and the table by drawing the muzzle toward the sternum with adhesive tape. Endotracheal tube and anesthetic tubes are displaced lateral to the head to remove them from the field. A radiographic beam is positioned directly above the nasal cavity and frontal sinuses (Figs. 14-3 and 14-4). The frontal sinus view identifies disease involving the frontal sinuses, which in diseases such as aspergillosis or neoplasia may be the only area of disease involvement.

The tympanic bullae are best seen with an open-mouth projection in which the beam is aimed at the base of the skull (Figs. 14-5 and 14-6). The bullae are also evaluated individually by lateral-oblique films, offsetting each bulla from the surrounding skull.

Nasal radiographs are evaluated for increased fluid density, loss of turbinates, lysis of facial bones, radiolucency at the tips of the tooth roots, and the presence of radiodense foreign bodies (Table 14-1). Increased fluid density can be caused by mucus, exudate, blood, or soft tissue masses such as polyps, tumors, or granulomas. Soft tissue masses can appear localized, but the surrounding fluid often obscures their borders. A thin rim of lysis surrounding a focal density can represent a foreign body. Fluid density within the frontal sinuses may represent normal mucous accumulation caused by obstruction of drainage into the nasal cavity, extension of disease into the frontal sinuses from the nasal cavity, or primary disease involving the frontal sinuses.

Loss of the normal fine turbinate pattern in combination with increased fluid density within the nasal cavity can occur with chronic inflammatory conditions of any etiology. Early neoplastic changes can also be associated with an increase in soft tissue density and destruction of the turbinates (see Figs. 14-2 and 14-4). More aggressive neoplastic changes can include marked lysis or deformation of the vomer and/or facial bones. Multiple, well-defined lytic zones within the nasal cavity and increased radiolucency in the rostral portion of the nasal cavity suggest aspergillosis (Fig. 14-7). The vomer bone may be

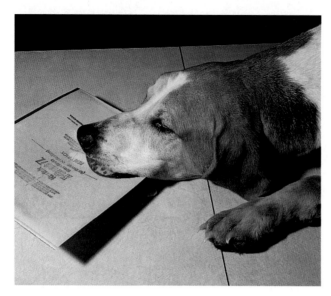

**FIG 14-1**
Positioning of a dog for intraoral radiographs.

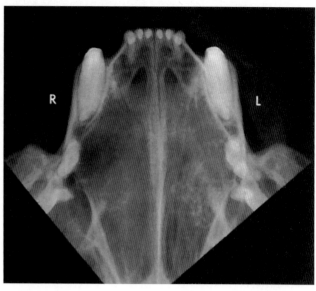

**FIG 14-2**
Intraoral radiograph of a cat with carcinoma. Normal fine turbinate pattern is visible on the left side *(L)* of nasal cavity and provides basis for comparison with the right side *(R)*. Turbinate pattern is less apparent on right side, and an area of turbinate lysis can be seen adjacent to the first premolar.

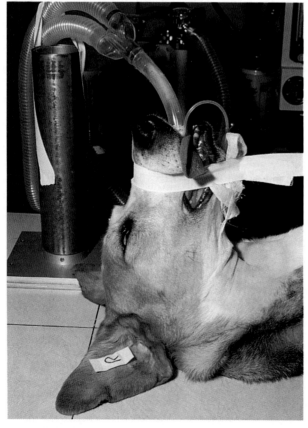

**FIG 14-3**
Positioning of a dog for frontal sinus radiographs. The endotracheal and anesthetic tubes are displaced laterally in this instance by taping them to an upright metal cylinder.

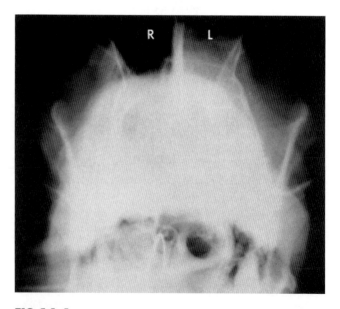

**FIG 14-4**
Frontal sinus view of a dog with a nasal tumor. The left frontal sinus *(L)* has increased soft tissue density compared with the air-filled sinus on the right side *(R)*.

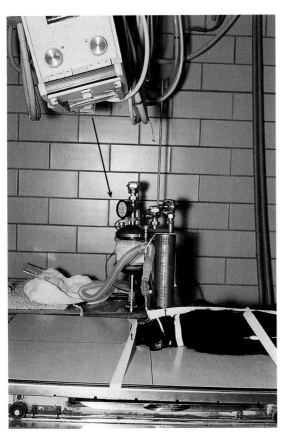

**FIG 14-5**
Positioning of a cat for open-mouth projection of the tympanic bullae. Beam *(arrow)* is aimed through the mouth toward the base of the skull. Adhesive tape *(t)* is holding head and mandible in position.

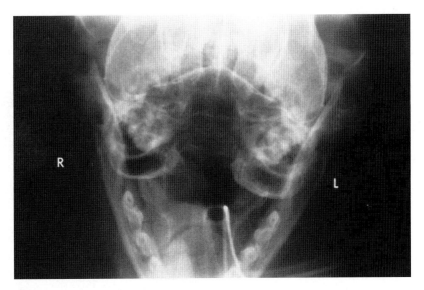

**FIG 14-6**
Radiograph obtained from a cat with nasopharyngeal polyp using the open-mouth projection demonstrated in Fig. 14-5. The left bulla has thickening of bone and increased fluid density, indicating bulla osteitis and probable extension of the polyp.

## Radiographic Signs of Common Nasal Diseases*

**Chronic Viral Rhinitis (Feline)**

Soft tissue opacity within nasal cavity, may be
 asymmetric
Mild turbinate lysis
Soft tissue opacity in frontal sinus(es)

**Nasopharyngeal Polyp**

Soft tissue opacity above soft palate
Soft tissue opacity within nasal cavity, usually unilateral
Mild turbinate lysis possible
Bulla osteitis: soft tissue opacity within bulla, thickening
 of bone

**Nasal Neoplasia**

Soft tissue opacity, may be asymmetric
Turbinate destruction
Vomer bone and/or facial bone destruction
Soft tissue mass external to facial bones

**Nasal Aspergillosis**

Well-defined lucent areas within the nasal cavity
Increased radiolucency rostrally
Increased soft tissue opacity may also be present
No destruction of vomer or facial bones, although signs
 often bilateral
Vomer bone may be roughened
Fluid density within the frontal sinus; frontal bones may
 be thickened or moth-eaten

**Cryptococcosis**

Soft tissue opacity, may be asymmetric
Turbinate lysis
Facial bone destruction
Soft tissue mass external to facial bones

**Lymphoplasmacytic Rhinitis**

Soft tissue opacity
Lysis of nasal turbinates, especially rostrally

**Allergic Rhinitis**

Increased soft tissue opacity
Mild turbinate lysis possible

**Tooth Root Abscesses**

Radiolucency adjacent to tooth roots, commonly apically

**Foreign Bodies**

Mineral and metallic dense foreign bodies readily
 identified
Plant foreign bodies: focal, ill-defined, increased soft
 tissue opacity
Lucent rim around abnormal tissue (rare)

*Note that these descriptions represent typical cases and are not specific findings.

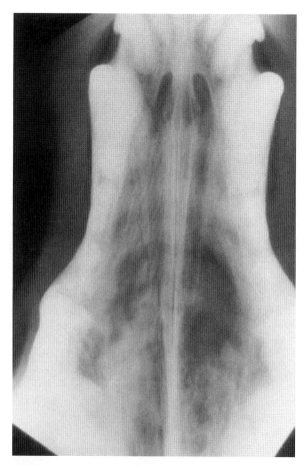

**FIG 14-7**
Intraoral radiograph of a dog with nasal aspergillosis. Focal
areas of marked turbinate lysis are present on both sides of
the nasal cavity. The vomer bone remains intact.

roughened but is rarely destroyed. Previous traumatic fracture of the nasal bones and secondary osteomyelitis can also be detected radiographically.

## COMPUTERIZED TOMOGRAPHY

Computerized tomography (CT) provides excellent visualization of the nasal turbinates, nasal septum, hard palate, and cribriform plate (see Fig. 13-4). It is more accurate than conventional radiography in assessing the extent of neoplastic disease, thus allows more accurate localization of mass lesions for subsequent biopsy than nasal radiography, and is instrumental for radiotherapy treatment planning. It may also identify the presence of lesions in animals with undiagnosed nasal disease when other techniques have failed.

## RHINOSCOPY

Rhinoscopy allows visual assessment of the nasal cavity through the use of a rigid or flexible fiberoptic endoscope or otoscopic cone. Rhinoscopy is used to visualize and remove foreign bodies; to grossly assess the nasal mucosa for the presence of inflammation, turbinate erosion, mass lesions, fungal plaques, and parasites; and to aid in the collection of nasal specimens for histopathologic examination and culture. Complete rhinoscopy always includes a thorough examination of the oral cavity and caudal nasopharynx, as well as visualization of the nasal cavity through the external nares.

The extent of visualization depends on the quality of the equipment and the outside diameter of the rhinoscope. A narrow (2- to 3-mm diameter), rigid fiberoptic endoscope provides the best visualization through the external nares (Fig. 14-8). Endoscopes without biopsy or suction channels are preferable because of their small outside diameter. Some of these systems are relatively inexpensive, including one model that can be attached to a standard otoscope handle for the light source (Fig. 14-9). Scopes designed for arthroscopy, cystoscopy, and sexing of birds also work well. In medium to large dogs, a flexible pediatric bronchoscope can be used. If an endoscope is not available, the rostral region of the nasal cavity can be examined with an otoscope. Human pediatric otoscopic cones (2- to 3-mm diameter) can be purchased for examining cats and small dogs.

General anesthesia is required for rhinoscopy. Rhinoscopy is usually performed immediately after nasal radiography or CT unless a foreign body is strongly suspected. The oral cavity and caudal nasopharynx should be assessed first. During the oral examination the hard and soft palates are visually examined and palpated for deformation, erosions, or defects, and the gingival sulci are probed for fistulae.

The caudal nasopharynx is evaluated for the presence of nasopharyngeal polyps, neoplasia, and foreign bodies. Foreign bodies, particularly grass or plant material, are commonly

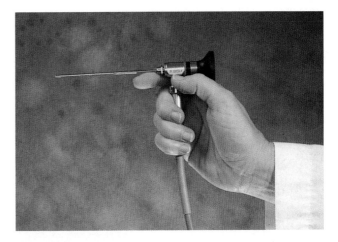

**FIG 14-8**
Rigid fiberoptic endoscope (diameter, 3 mm; length, 18 cm) for rhinoscopy. (Courtesy Richard Wolf Medical Instruments Corp., Vernon Hills, Ill.)

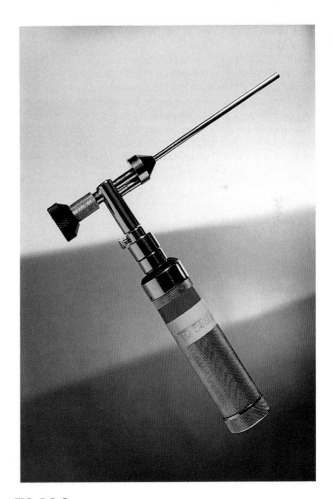

**FIG 14-9**
Rigid endoscope suitable for rhinoscopy that uses a standard otoscope handle as a light source. (Courtesy MDS, Inc., Brandon, Fla.)

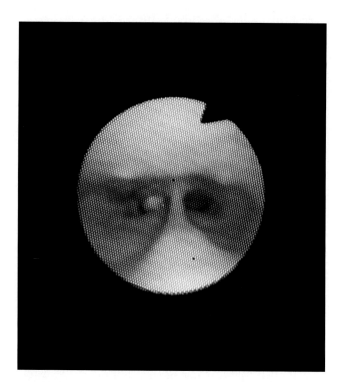

**FIG 14-10**
View of the internal nares obtained by passing a flexible bronchoscope around the edge of the soft palate in a dog with sneezing. A small white object is seen within the left nasal cavity adjacent to the septum. Note that the septum is narrow and the right internal naris is oval in shape and not obstructed. On removal, the object was found to be a popcorn kernel. The dog had an abnormally short soft palate, and the kernel presumably entered the caudal nasal cavity from the oropharynx.

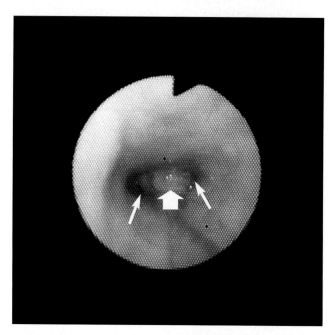

**FIG 14-11**
View of the internal nares *(thin arrows)* obtained by passing a flexible bronchoscope around the edge of the soft palate in a dog with nasal discharge. A soft tissue mass *(broad arrow)* is blocking the normally thin septum and is partially obstructing the airway lumens. Compare this view with the appearance of the normal septum and right internal naris in Fig. 14-10.

found in this location in cats and on occasion in dogs. The caudal nasopharynx is best visualized with a flexible fiberoptic endoscope that is passed into the oral cavity and retroflexed around the soft palate (Figs. 14-10 and 14-11). Alternatively, the caudal nasopharynx can be evaluated with the aid of a dental mirror, penlight, and spay hook, which is attached to the caudal edge of the soft palate and pulled forward to improve visualization of the area.

Rhinoscopy must be performed patiently, gently, and thoroughly to maximize the likelihood of identifying gross abnormalities while minimizing hemorrhage. The more normal side of the nasal cavity is examined first. The tip of the scope is lubricated and is passed through the naris with the tip pointed medially. Each nasal meatus is evaluated, beginning ventrally and working dorsally to ensure visualization should hemorrhage develop during the procedure. Each nasal meatus should be examined as far caudally as the scope can be passed without trauma.

Although the rhinoscope can be used to evaluate the large chambers of the nose, many of the small recesses cannot be examined, even with the smallest endoscopes. Thus disease or a foreign body can be missed if only these small recesses are involved. Swollen and inflamed nasal mucosa, hemorrhage

caused by the procedure, and the accumulation of exudate and mucus can also interfere with visualization of the nasal cavity. Foreign bodies and masses are frequently coated and effectively hidden by seemingly insignificant amounts of mucus, exudate, or blood. The tenacious material must be removed using a rubber catheter with the tip cut off attached to a suction unit. If necessary, saline flushes can also be used, although resulting fluid bubbles may further interfere with visualization. Some clinicians prefer to maintain continuous saline infusion of the nasal cavity using a standard intravenous administration attached to a catheter or, if available, the biopsy channel of the rhinoscope. The entire examination is done "under water." No catheter should ever be passed blindly into the nasal cavity beyond the level of the medial canthus of the eye to avoid entering the cranial vault through the cribriform plate. The clinician must be sure the endotracheal cuff is fully inflated and the back of the pharynx is packed with gauze to prevent aspiration of blood, mucus, or saline flush into the lungs.

The nasal mucosa is normally smooth and pink, with a small amount of serous to mucoid fluid present along the mucosal surface. Potential abnormalities visualized with the rhinoscope include inflammation of the nasal mucosa, mats of fungal hyphae (Fig. 14-12), mass lesions, erosion of the turbinates, foreign body, and rarely, nasal mites or *Capillaria* worms (Fig. 14-13 and Table 14-2).

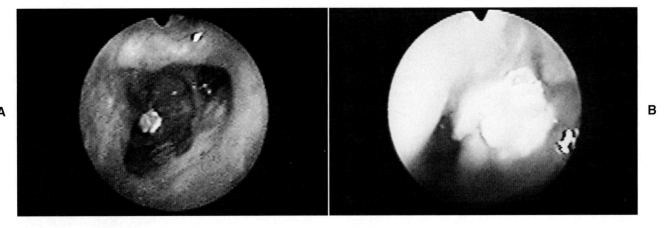

**FIG 14-12**
**A,** Rhinoscopic view through the external naris of a dog with aspergillosis showing loss of turbinates, a red-brown granulomatous mass, and a white fungal mat. **B,** A closer view of the fungal mat.

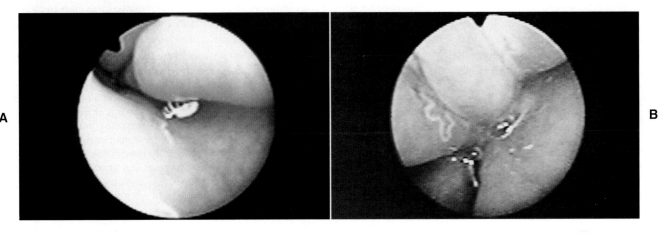

**FIG 14-13**
Rhinoscopic view through the external naris. **A,** A single nasal mite is seen in this dog with *Pneumonyssoides caninum*. **B,** A thin white worm is seen in this dog with *Capillaria boehmi (Eucoleus)*.

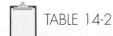 TABLE 14-2

**Differential Diagnoses for Gross Rhinoscopic Abnormalities in Dogs and Cats**

| | |
|---|---|
| **Inflammation (Mucosal Swelling, Hyperemia, Increased Mucus, Exudate)** | **Turbinate Erosion—cont'd** |
| Nonspecific finding; consider all differential diagnoses for mucopurulent nasal discharge (infectious, inflammatory, neoplastic) | Marked<br>  Neoplasia<br>  Aspergillosis<br>  Penicilliosis<br>  Cryptococcosis |
| **Mass** | **Fungal Plaques** |
| Neoplasia<br>Nasopharyngeal polyp<br>Cryptococcosis<br>Mat of fungal hyphae or fungal granuloma (aspergillosis, penicilliosis, rhinosporidiosis) | Aspergillosis<br>Penicilliosis |
| **Turbinate Erosion** | **Parasites** |
| Mild<br>  Feline herpesvirus<br>  Chronic inflammatory process | Mites: *Pneumonyssoides caninum*<br>Worms: *Capillaria boehmi (Eucoleus)*<br><br>**Foreign Bodies** |

The location of any abnormality should be noted, including the meatus involved (common, ventral, middle, dorsal), the medial-to-lateral orientation within the meatus, and the distance caudal from the naris. Exact localization is critical for directing instruments for the retrieval of foreign bodies or nasal biopsy should visual guidance become impeded by hemorrhage or size of the cavity.

## NASAL BIOPSY: INDICATIONS AND TECHNIQUES

Visualization of a foreign body or nasal parasites during rhinoscopy establishes a diagnosis. For many dogs and cats, however, the diagnosis must be based on cytologic, histologic, and microbiologic evaluation of nasal biopsy specimens. Nasal biopsy specimens should be obtained immediately after nasal radiography or CT and rhinoscopy while the animal is still anesthetized. These earlier procedures can help to localize the lesion, maximizing the likelihood of obtaining material representative of the primary disease process.

Nasal biopsy techniques include nasal swab, nasal flush, pinch biopsy, core biopsy, and turbinectomy. Fine-needle aspirates can be obtained from mass lesions as described in Chapter 77. The more aggressive, nonsurgical methods of specimen collection (i.e., pinch biopsy, core biopsy) are more likely to provide pieces of nasal tissue that extend beneath the superficial inflammation, which is common to many nasal disorders, than nasal swabs or flushes. In addition, the pieces of tissue obtained with the more aggressive methods can be evaluated histologically, whereas the material obtained with the less traumatic techniques may be suitable only for cytologic analysis. Histopathologic examination is preferred over cytologic examination in most cases because the marked inflammation that accompanies many nasal diseases makes it difficult to cytologically differentiate primary from secondary inflammation and reactive from neoplastic epithelial cells. Carcinomas can also appear cytologically as lymphoma and vice versa. For these reasons, the more traumatic biopsy techniques of pinch biopsy or core biopsy are preferred.

Regardless of the technique used (except for nasal swab), the cuff of the endotracheal tube should be inflated and the caudal pharynx packed with gauze sponges to prevent the aspiration of fluid. Intravenous crystalloid fluids (10 to 20 ml/ kg/hr plus replacement of estimated blood loss) are recommended during the procedure to counter the hypotensive effects of prolonged anesthesia and blood loss from hemorrhage following biopsy. Blood-clotting capabilities should be assessed before the more aggressive biopsy techniques are performed if there is any history of hemorrhagic exudate or epistaxis or any other indication of coagulopathy.

### NASAL SWAB

The least traumatic techniques are the nasal swab and nasal flush. Unlike the other collection techniques, nasal swabs can be collected from an awake animal. Nasal swabs are useful for

identifying cryptococcal organisms cytologically and should be collected early in the evaluation of cats with chronic rhinitis. Other findings are generally nonspecific. Exudate immediately within the external nares or draining from the nares is collected using a cotton-tipped swab. Relatively small swabs are available (e.g., Dacron swabs; Hardwood Products, Guilford, Me) that can facilitate specimen collection from cats with minimal discharge. The swab is then rolled on a microscope slide. Routine cytologic stains are generally used, although India ink can be applied to demonstrate cryptococcal organisms (see p. 1287).

### NASAL FLUSH

Nasal flush is a minimally invasive technique. A soft catheter is positioned in the caudal region of the nasal cavity via the oral cavity and internal nares, with the tip of the catheter pointing rostrally. With the animal in sternal recumbency and the nose pointed toward the floor, approximately 100 ml of sterile saline solution is forcibly injected in pulses by syringe. The fluid exiting the external nares is collected in a bowl and can be examined cytologically. A portion of it can also be filtered through a gauze sponge. Large particles trapped in the sponge can be retrieved and submitted for histopathologic analysis. These specimens are often insufficient for providing a definitive diagnosis.

### PINCH BIOPSY

Pinch biopsy is the author's preferred method of nasal biopsy. In the pinch biopsy technique, alligator cup biopsy forceps (minimum size, 2 × 3 mm) are used to obtain pieces of nasal mucosa for histologic evaluation (Figs. 14-14 and 14-15). Full-thickness tissue specimens are obtained, and guided specimen collection is more easily performed with this technique than with previously described methods. The biopsy forceps are passed adjacent to a rigid endoscope and directed to any gross lesions. After the first piece is taken, bleeding will prevent further visual guidance, so the forceps are passed blindly to the position identified during rhinoscopic examination (e.g., meatus involved and depth from external naris). If a mass is present, the forceps are passed in a closed position until just before the mass is reached. The forceps are then opened and passed a short distance further until resistance is felt. If lesions are not present grossly but are present radiographically, the biopsy instrument can be guided using the relationship of the lesion to the upper teeth. If a flexible scope is used, biopsy instruments can be passed through the biopsy channel of the endoscope. The resulting specimens are extremely small and may not be of diagnostic quality. Larger alligator forceps are preferred. Forceps should never be passed into the nasal cavity deeper than the level of the medial canthus of the eye without visual guidance to avoid penetrating the cribriform plate.

A minimum of six tissue specimens (using a 2 × 3 mm forcep) should be obtained from any lesion. If no localizable lesion is identified radiographically or rhinoscopically, multiple biopsies (usually 6 to 10) are obtained randomly from both sides of the nasal cavity.

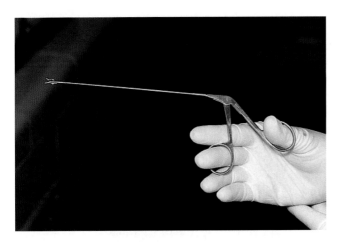

**FIG 14-14**
Alligator cup biopsy forceps.

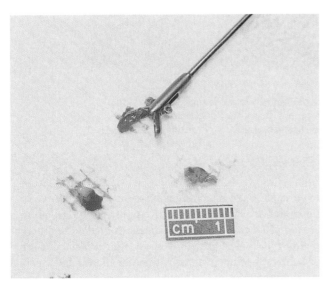

**FIG 14-15**
Relatively large pieces of nasal tissue are obtained using the alligator cup biopsy forceps.

## CORE BIOPSY

Core biopsy is an excellent method of tissue collection when a mass lesion is present. A large polypropylene male dog urinary catheter or the protective, relatively thin-walled, stiff plastic sleeve of certain spinal needles (e.g., B-D Spinal Needle; Becton Dickinson, Franklin Lakes, N.J.) is used (Fig. 14-16). To prepare the protective sleeve for use, the sleeve itself is removed and set aside. The syringe hub is disconnected from the spinal needle and is then reinserted into the protective sleeve to serve as a syringe adapter for the sleeve. The stylet is discarded. The tip of the sleeve or urinary catheter is cut at a sharp angle to aid in penetration of the mass. The sleeve or urinary catheter must be marked at the distance to the medial canthus of the eye to avoid inadvertently penetrating the cribriform plate. An empty 12-ml syringe is then attached to the

sleeve or urinary catheter, which is inserted into the nasal cavity until it rests against the mass. The catheter is then twisted on its longitudinal axis into the mass while simultaneous negative suction is applied with the syringe. When the sleeve or urinary catheter is removed, a core of tissue should be present within the lumen that can be submitted for histologic evaluation.

## TURBINECTOMY

Turbinectomy provides the best tissue specimens for histologic examination and allows the opportunity to remove abnormal or poorly vascularized tissues and to place drains for subsequent topical nasal therapy. Turbinectomy is performed through a rhinotomy incision and is a more invasive technique than the others previously described. Turbinectomy is a reasonably difficult surgical procedure that should be considered only when other less invasive techniques have failed to establish the diagnosis. Potential operative and postoperative complications include pain, excessive hemorrhage, inadvertent entry into the cranial vault, and recurrent nasal infections. Cats may be anorectic postoperatively. Placement of a gastrostomy tube (see p. 392) should be considered if necessary to provide a means for meeting nutritional requirements during the recovery period. See Suggested Readings in Chapter 13 for information on the surgical procedure.

## COMPLICATIONS

The major complication associated with nasal biopsy is hemorrhage. The severity of hemorrhage depends on the method used to obtain the biopsy, but even with aggressive techniques the hemorrhage is rarely life-threatening. When any technique is used, the floor of the nasal cavity is avoided to prevent damage to major blood vessels. For minor hemorrhage, the rate of administration of intravenous fluids should be increased and manipulations within the nasal cavity should be stopped until the bleeding subsides. Cold saline solution with or without diluted epinephrine (1:100,000) can be gently infused into the nasal cavity. Persistent severe hemorrhage can be controlled by packing the nasal cavity with umbilical tape. The tape must be packed through the nasopharynx, as well as through the external nares, or the blood will only be redirected. Similarly, placing swabs or gauze in the external nares only serves to redirect blood caudally. In the rare event of uncontrolled hemorrhage, the carotid artery on the involved side can be ligated without subsequent adverse effects. Rhinotomy should not be attempted. In the vast majority of animals only time or cold saline infusions are required to control hemorrhage. The fear of severe hemorrhage should not prevent the collection of good-quality tissue specimens.

Trauma to the brain is avoided by never passing any object into the nasal cavity beyond the level of the medial canthus of the eye without visual guidance. The distance from the external nares to the medial canthus is noted by holding the instrument or catheter against the face, with the tip at the medial canthus. The level of the nares is marked on the instrument or catheter with a piece of tape or marking pen. The object should never be inserted beyond that mark.

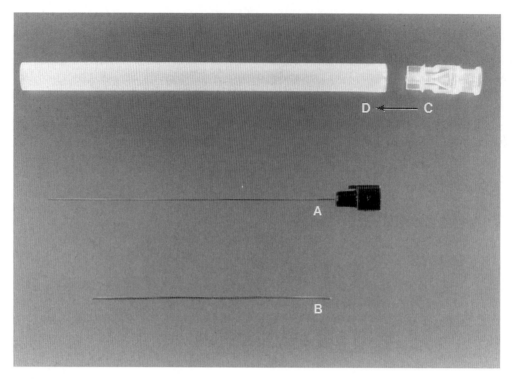

**FIG 14-16**
Preparing the sleeve of a spinal needle for core biopsy. The stylet *(A)* is removed. The spinal needle *(B)* is cut from the syringe hub *(C)*. The syringe hub is inserted back into the protective sleeve *(D)*. (B-D Spinal Needle courtesy Becton Dickinson and Co., Franklin Lakes, N.J.)

Aspiration of blood, saline solution, or exudate into the lungs must be avoided. A cuffed endotracheal tube should be in place during the procedure, and the caudal pharynx should be packed with gauze following visual assessment of the oral cavity and nasopharynx. The nose is pointed toward the floor over the end of the examination table, allowing blood and fluid to drip out from the external nares following rhinoscopy and biopsy. Finally, the caudal pharynx is examined during gauze removal and before extubation for visualization of continued accumulation of fluid. Gauze sponges are counted during placement and then recounted during removal so that none is inadvertently left behind.

## NASAL CULTURES: SAMPLE COLLECTION AND INTERPRETATION

Microbiologic cultures of nasal specimens are recommended but can be difficult to interpret. Aerobic and anaerobic bacterial cultures and fungal cultures can be performed on material obtained by swab, nasal flush, or tissue biopsy. According to Harvey (1984), the normal nasal flora can include *Escherichia coli; Staphylococcus, Streptococcus, Pseudomonas, Pasteurella,* and *Aspergillus* organisms; and a variety of other aerobic and anaerobic bacteria and fungi. Thus bacterial or fungal growth from nasal specimens does not necessarily reflect the cause of nasal signs.

A diagnosis of nasal aspergillosis or penicilliosis requires the presence of several supportive signs, and fungal cultures are indicated whenever fungal disease is one of the differential diagnoses. The growth of *Aspergillus* or *Penicillium* organisms is considered along with other clinical data, such as radiographic and rhinoscopic findings, and serologic titers. Fungal growth supports a diagnosis of mycotic rhinitis only when other data also support the diagnosis. The fact that fungal infection occasionally occurs secondary to nasal tumors should not be overlooked during initial evaluation and monitoring of therapeutic response.

Bacterial growth is generally either a normal finding or an abnormal overgrowth of normal flora secondary to another disease process. It is difficult or impossible to distinguish between these two situations on the basis of culture alone. Cultures should be performed on specimens collected deep within the nasal cavity because bacterial growth from superficial nasal swabs just inside the external nares is unlikely to represent abnormal growth. Deep specimens are difficult to collect without superficial contamination unless an expensive guarded catheter swab is used. Accepting some contamination, this author usually uses small sterile swabs carefully inserted deep into the nasal cavity. Tissue biopsy can be obtained for culture using sterilized biopsy forceps. The growth of many colonies of one or two types of bacteria more likely reflects abnormal growth, whereas the growth of many different organisms represents normal flora. The microbiology laboratory should be asked to report all growth. Otherwise the laboratory may report only one or two organisms that are more often pathogenic and provide misleading information about the relative purity of the culture. The presence of septic inflammation based on histologic examination of nasal specimens and a positive response to antibiotic therapy support a diagnosis of bacterial infection contributing to clinical signs. Although bacterial rhinitis is rarely a primary disease entity (see p. 238), improvement in nasal discharge may be seen if the bacterial component of the problem is treated; but the improvement is generally transient unless the underlying disease process can be corrected. Some animals in which a primary disease process is never identified or cannot be corrected (e.g., cats with feline viral rhinitis) respond well to long-term antibiotic therapy. Sensitivity data from bacterial cultures considered to represent significant infection may help in antibiotic selection. See p. 238 for further therapeutic recommendations.

## Suggested Readings

Codner EC et al: Comparison of computed tomography with radiography as a noninvasive diagnostic technique for chronic nasal disease in dogs, *J Am Vet Med Assoc* 202:1106, 1993.

Harvey CE: Therapeutic strategies involving antimicrobial treatment of the upper respiratory tract in small animals, *J Am Vet Med Assoc* 185:1159, 1984.

O'Brien RT et al: Radiographic findings in cats with intranasal neoplasia or chronic rhinitis: 29 cases (1982-1988), *J Am Vet Med Assoc* 208:385, 1996.

Padrid PA et al: Endoscopy of the upper respiratory tract of the dog and cat. In Tams TR, editor: *Small animal endoscopy,* ed 2, St Louis, 1999, Mosby, p 357.

Sullivan M et al: The radiological features of aspergillosis of the nasal cavity and frontal sinuses in the dog, *J Small Anim Pract* 27:167, 1986.

Sullivan M et al: The radiological features of sixty cases of intranasal neoplasia in the dog, *J Small Anim Pract* 28:575, 1987.

Tasker S et al: Aetiology and diagnosis of persistent nasal disease in the dog: a retrospective study of 42 cases, *J Small Anim Pract* 40:473, 1999.

Thrall DE et al: A comparison of radiographic and computed tomographic findings in 31 dogs with malignant nasal cavity tumors, *Vet Radiol* 30:59, 1989.

Willard MD et al: Endoscopic examination of the choane in dogs and cats: 118 cases (1988-1998), *J Am Vet Med Assoc* 215:1301, 1999.

Withrow SJ et al: Aspiration and punch biopsy techniques for nasal tumors, *J Am Anim Hosp Assoc* 21:551, 1985.

# CHAPTER 15

# Disorders of the Nasal Cavity

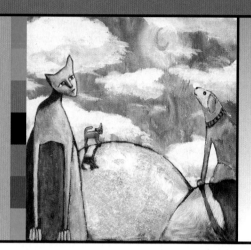

## CHAPTER OUTLINE

FELINE UPPER RESPIRATORY INFECTION, 228
NASOPHARYNGEAL POLYPS, 232
NASAL TUMORS, 233
NASAL MYCOSES, 235
    Cryptococcosis, 235
    Aspergillosis, 235
BACTERIAL RHINITIS, 238
NASAL PARASITES, 238
    Nasal mites, 238
    Nasal capillariasis, 238
LYMPHOPLASMACYTIC RHINITIS, 239
ALLERGIC RHINITIS, 239

## FELINE UPPER RESPIRATORY INFECTION

### Etiology

Upper respiratory infections (URIs) are common in cats. Feline herpesvirus (FHV), also known as feline rhinotracheitis virus, and feline calicivirus (FCV) cause nearly 90% of these infections. *Bordetella bronchiseptica* and *Chlamydophila felis* (previously, *Chlamydia psittaci*) are less commonly involved. Other viruses and *Mycoplasmas* may play a primary or secondary role, whereas other bacteria are considered secondary pathogens.

Cats become infected through contact with actively infected cats, carrier cats, and fomites. Cats that are young, stressed, or immunosuppressed are most likely to develop clinical signs. Infected cats often become carriers of FHV or FCV after resolution of the clinical signs. The duration of the carrier state is not known but may last from weeks to years. *Bordetella* can be isolated from asymptomatic cats, although the effectiveness of transmission of disease from such cats is not known.

### Clinical Features

Clinical manifestations of feline URI can be acute, chronic and intermittent, or chronic and persistent. Acute disease is the most common. The clinical signs of acute URI include fever, sneezing, serous or mucopurulent nasal discharge, conjunctivitis and ocular discharge, hypersalivation, anorexia, and dehydration. FHV can also cause corneal ulceration, abortion, and neonatal death, whereas FCV can cause oral ulcerations, mild interstitial pneumonia, or polyarthritis. *Bordetella* can cause cough and, in young kittens, pneumonia. Signs of *Chlamydophila* infection are usually limited to conjunctivitis.

Some cats that recover from the acute disease have periodic recurrence of acute signs, usually in association with stressful or immunosuppressive events. Other cats may have chronic, persistent signs, most notably a serous to mucopurulent nasal discharge. Chronic nasal discharge can result from persistence of an active viral infection or from irreversible damage to turbinates and mucosa by FHV; the latter predisposes the cat to frequent secondary bacterial infections.

### Diagnosis

Acute URI is usually diagnosed based on history and physical examination findings. The diagnosis of chronic URI is best made by eliminating other causes of chronic nasal discharge from the list of differential diagnoses (see Chapters 13 and 14).

Specific tests that are available to identify FHV, FCV, *Bordetella,* and *Chlamydophila* organisms include fluorescent antibody testing, virus isolation procedures or bacterial cultures, and serum antibody titers. Fluorescent antibody tests for FHV and FCV are performed on smears prepared from conjunctival scrapings, pharyngeal swabs, or tonsillar swabs or on impression smears from tonsillar biopsy specimens. Virus isolation tests can be performed on pharyngeal, conjunctival, or nasal swabs (using sterile swabs made of cotton) or on tissue specimens such as tonsillar biopsy specimens. Specimens are placed in viral transport media. Routine cytologic preparations of conjunctival smears can be examined for intracytoplasmic inclusion bodies suggestive of *Chlamydophila* infections, but these findings are nonspecific. Although routine bacterial cultures of the oropharynx can be used to identify *Bordetella,* the organism can be found in healthy and infected cats.

Demonstration of rising antibody titers against a specific agent over 2 to 3 weeks suggests active infection. Development of tests using polymerase chain reaction (PCR) to identify specific agents will likely improve the accuracy of testing in the near future. Regardless of the method used, close coordination with the pathology laboratory on specimen collection and handling is recommended for optimum results.

Tests to identify specific agents are particularly useful in cattery outbreaks in which the clinician is asked to recommend specific preventive measures (see p. 231). Multiple cats, both with and without clinical signs, should be tested when performing cattery surveys. Specific diagnostic tests are less useful for testing individual cats because their results do not alter therapy; false-negative results can occur if signs are the result of permanent nasal damage or if the specimen does not contain the agent. Positive results may merely reflect a carrier cat that has a concurrent disease process causing the clinical signs. The exception to this generalization is individual cats with suspected *Chlamydophila* infection, in which case specific effective therapy can be recommended.

## Treatment of Cats with Acute Signs

In most cats, URI is a self-limiting disease and treatment of cats with acute signs includes appropriate supportive care. Hydration and nutritional needs should be provided when necessary. Dried mucus and exudate should be cleaned from the face and nares. The cat can be placed in a steamy bathroom or a small room with a vaporizer for 15 to 20 minutes two or three times daily to help clear excess secretions. Severe nasal congestion is treated with pediatric topical decongestants such as 0.25% phenylephrine or 0.025% oxymetazoline. A drop is gently placed in each nostril daily for a maximum of 3 days. If longer therapy is necessary, the decongestant is withheld for 3 days before beginning another 3-day course to prevent possible rebound congestion after withdrawal of the drug. Another option for prolonged decongestant therapy is to alternate daily the naris treated.

Antibiotic therapy to treat secondary infection is indicated in cats with severe clinical signs. The initial antibiotic of choice is ampicillin (22 mg/kg q8h) or amoxicillin (22 mg/kg q8h to q12h), because they are often effective, are associated with few adverse reactions, and can be administered to kittens. If *Bordetella*, *Chlamydophila*, or *Mycoplasma* spp. is suspected, doxycycline (5 to 10 mg/kg q12h) or chloramphenicol (10 to 15 mg/kg q12h) should be used. Azithromycin (5 to 10 mg/kg q24h for 3 days, then q72h) can be prescribed for cats that are difficult to medicate.

*Chlamydophila* infection should be suspected in cats with conjunctivitis as the primary problem and in cats from catteries in which the disease is endemic. Oral antibiotics are administered for 3 weeks. In addition, chloramphenicol or tetracycline ophthalmic ointment should be applied at least three times daily and continued for a minimum of 14 days after the resolution of signs.

Corneal ulcers resulting from FHV are treated with topical antiviral drugs, such as trifluridine, idoxuridine, or adenine arabinoside. One drop should be applied to each affected eye five to six times daily for no longer than 2 to 3 weeks. Routine ulcer management is also indicated. Tetracycline or chloram-

phenicol ophthalmic ointment is administered two to four times daily. Topical atropine is used for mydriasis as needed to control pain. Treatment is continued for 1 to 2 weeks after epithelialization has occurred.

Topical and systemic corticosteroids are contraindicated in cats with acute URI or ocular manifestations of FHV infection. They can prolong clinical signs and increase viral shedding.

## Treatment of Cats with Chronic Signs

Cats with chronic persistent signs (e.g., nasal discharge, sneezing) often require management for years. Fortunately most of these cats are healthy in all other respects. Treatment strategies include facilitating drainage of discharge, controlling secondary bacterial infections, treating possible herpesvirus infection, reducing inflammation, and, as a last resort, turbinectomy and frontal sinus ablation (Table 15-1).

Keeping secretions moist, performing intermittent nasal flushes, and judicious use of topical decongestants facilitates drainage. Keeping the cat in a room with a vaporizer, for instance, during the night, can provide symptomatic relief by keeping secretions moist. Alternatively, drops of sterile saline can be placed into nares. Some cats have marked improvement in clinical signs for weeks after flushing of the nasal cavity with copious amounts of saline or dilute Betadine solution. General anesthesia is required, and the lower airways must be protected with an endotracheal tube, gauze sponges, and positioning of the head to facilitate drainage from the external nares. Topical decongestants, as described for acute

 TABLE 15-1

**Management Considerations for Cats with Chronic Upper Respiratory Tract Signs**

### Identify and Treat Underlying Diseases Whenever Possible
See Chapters 13 and 14 for diagnostic approach

### Facilitate Drainage of Discharge
Vaporizer treatments
Topical saline administration
Nasal cavity flushes under anesthesia
Topical decongestants

### Control Secondary Bacterial Infections
Long-term antibiotic treatment

### Treat Possible Herpesvirus Infection
Lysine treatment

### Reduce Inflammation, if Necessary
Oral prednisone treatment

### Surgical Intervention, as Last Resort
Turbinectomy
Frontal sinus ablation

management, also provide symptomatic relief during episodes of severe congestion.

Chronic antibiotic therapy may be required to manage secondary bacterial infections. Broad-spectrum antibiotics such as amoxicillin (22 mg/kg q12h) or trimethoprim-sulfadiazine (15 mg/kg q12h) are often successful. Chloramphenicol (10 to 15 mg/kg q12h) and doxycycline (5 to 10 mg/kg q12h) have activity against many bacteria and *Chlamydophila* and *Mycoplasma* organisms and can be effective in some cats when other drugs have failed. This author reserves fluoroquinolones for cats with documented resistant gram-negative infections. If a beneficial response to antibiotic therapy is seen within 1 week of its initiation, the antibiotic should be continued for at least 4 to 6 weeks. If a beneficial response is not seen, the antibiotic is discontinued. Note that the frequent stopping and starting of different antibiotics every 7 to 14 days is not recommended and may predispose the cat to resistant gram-negative infections. Cats that respond well during the prolonged course of antibiotics but that relapse shortly after discontinuation of the drug despite 4 to 6 weeks of relief are candidates for continuous long-term antibiotic therapy. Success can often be achieved with amoxicillin administered twice daily.

Treatment with lysine may be effective in cats with active herpesvirus infections. It has been postulated that excessive concentrations of lysine may antagonize arginine, a promoter of herpesvirus replication. Because the specific organism(s) involved is rarely known, trial therapy is initiated. Lysine (250 mg/cat q12h), obtained from health food stores, is added to food. A minimum of 4 weeks is necessary to assess success of treatment.

Cats with severe, persistent signs despite the previously described methods of supportive care may benefit from glucocorticoids to reduce inflammation. Risks are involved. Glucocorticoids may further predispose the cat to secondary infections, increase viral shedding, and mask signs of a more serious disease. Glucocorticoids should be prescribed only after a complete diagnostic evaluation has been performed to rule out other diseases (see Chapters 13 and 14). Prednisone is administered at a dose of 0.5 mg/kg every 12 hours. If a beneficial response is seen within 1 week, the dose is gradually decreased to the lowest dose that is still effective. A dose as low as 0.25 mg/kg every 2 to 3 days may be sufficient to control clinical signs. If a clinical response is not seen within 1 week, the drug should be discontinued.

Cats with severe or deteriorating signs despite conscientious care are candidates for turbinectomy and frontal sinus ablation, assuming a complete diagnostic evaluation to eliminate other causes of chronic nasal discharge has been performed (Chapters 13 and 14). Turbinectomy and frontal sinus ablation are difficult surgical procedures. Major blood vessels and the cranial vault must be avoided, and tissue remnants must not be left behind. Anorexia can be a postoperative problem; placement of a gastrostomy tube (see p. 392) provides an excellent means for meeting nutritional requirements if necessary after surgery. Complete elimination of respiratory signs is unlikely, but signs may be more easily managed. The reader is referred to surgical texts by Fossum or Bojrab for a description of the surgical techniques (see Suggested Readings).

## Prognosis

The prognosis for cats with acute URI is good. Chronic disease does not develop in most cats, and nearly all of those with chronic disease have a good quality of life with appropriate supportive care.

## Prevention in the Individual Pet Cat

Prevention of URI in all cats is based on avoiding exposure to the infectious agents (e.g., FHV, FCV, *Bordetella* and *Chlamydophila* organisms) and strengthening immunity against infection. Most household cats are relatively resistant to prolonged problems associated with URIs, and routine health care with regular vaccination using a subcutaneous product is adequate. Vaccination decreases severity of clinical signs resulting from URIs but does not prevent infection. Owners should be discouraged from allowing their cats to roam freely outdoors.

Subcutaneous modified-live virus vaccines for FHV and FCV are used for most cats and are available in combination with panleukopenia vaccine. These vaccines are convenient to administer, do not result in clinical signs when used correctly, and provide adequate protection for cats that are not heavily exposed to these viruses. These vaccines are not effective in kittens while maternal immunity persists. Kittens are usually vaccinated beginning at 8 to 10 weeks of age and again in 3 to 4 weeks. At least two vaccines must be given initially, with the final vaccine administered after the kitten is 12 weeks old. Thereafter, booster vaccinations are currently recommended every 1 to 3 years. A recent study indicates that detection of FHV and FCV antibodies in the serum of cats is predictive of susceptibility to disease and therefore may be useful in determining need for revaccination (Lappin and colleagues, 2002). Queens should be vaccinated before breeding.

Subcutaneous modified-live vaccines for FHV and FCV are safe but can cause disease if introduced into the cat by the normal oronasal route of infection. The vaccine should not be aerosolized in front of the cat. Vaccine inadvertently left on the skin after injection should be washed off immediately before the cat licks the area.

Modified-live vaccines should not be used in pregnant queens. Killed products are available for FHV and FCV that can be used in pregnant queens. Killed vaccines have also been recommended for cats with feline leukemia virus (FeLV) or feline immunodeficiency virus (FIV) infection.

Intranasal *Bordetella* and injectable *Chlamydophila* vaccines are also available, but these infections are not as common as FHV and FCV infections. Disease resulting from *Bordetella* infections occurs primarily in cats housed in crowded conditions. Further, these diseases can be effectively treated with antibiotics. Therefore such vaccines are recommended only for use in catteries or shelters where *Bordetella* or *Chlamydophila* is endemic.

## Prevention in Multiple-Cat Households

Multiple-cat household refers to situations in which cats are grouped together in high-density situations, including breeding catteries, humane rescue organizations, and private homes that have high numbers of cats and/or frequently acquire new additions. Chronic outbreaks of URI are common in these situations because of the large number of cats in a small area, frequent introduction of new cats, interactions between kittens and adults, and high levels of stress. Organisms are shed from not only clinically affected cats but also asymptomatic cats that are either chronic carriers, incubating infection, or have recently recovered. These factors result in exposure to high concentrations of organisms and to strains of organisms that are new to the household. The high stress level caused by grouping cats together and introducing new cats into the social order suppresses immunity to infection and predisposes to viral shedding.

Veterinarians must play an active role beyond providing vaccinations for multiple-cat households with chronic upper respiratory problems. A site visit by the veterinarian is essential. The protocols outlined are complex. Principles of disease prevention that are second nature to medical professionals are often not well understood by owners. The most careful history taking will not uncover every management practice that may be contributing to the persistence of viral exposure. The owner must perform accurate record keeping to identify potential carrier cats and to document the value of the professional services provided. Records are used to document decreased frequency, duration, and severity of infections as a result of the recommended strategies. In summary, one or more site visits, instruction in record keeping, and careful follow-up are essential for achieving success. Owners should have realistic expectations regarding control versus elimination of infections, should not expect a simple solution (i.e., "magic bullet"), and should expect to compensate the veterinarian for professional consultation.

Control of URIs in multiple-cat households is based on the same principles as defined for the individual pet cat: (1) avoiding exposure to the infectious agents and (2) strengthening immunity against infection (Table 15-2). These issues are addressed concurrently. Because these principles apply to any infectious disease situation, multiple-cat households that address these issues will also benefit from decreased incidence of other infectious diseases.

Minimizing exposure to infectious agents is achieved through housing arrangements and management practices. Ideally, all cats with a history of URI should be eliminated from the cattery because they may be carriers. However, such drastic measures are rarely practical or acceptable to the owner. Cats must be segregated to limit the extent of outbreaks and to facilitate in the identification of carrier cats. It may seem unrealistic to provide such segregated housing. Creative solutions can be found even for low-budget situations. For instance, a home can be divided into upstairs and downstairs, a neighbor involved in rescue can house all symptomatic cats, or cages can be grouped together and separated by solid partitions.

Kittens are kept separated, along with their queens before weaning, until 1 to 2 weeks after completion of the vaccination series. Quarantined animals that are new to the household should be isolated and observed for a minimum of 3 weeks. Ideally, new cats are already quarantined for several months as part of a FeLV prevention program (see p. 1284). Clinically ill cats are maintained in separate isolation facilities for at least 3 weeks after resolution of clinical signs.

It is essential that all handling of cats be performed in order of susceptibility: kittens first, healthy adults second, quarantined cats third, and clinically ill cats last. This order includes handling for cleaning, feeding, medicating, socializing, or any other interaction. Hands must be carefully washed between groups, and cleaning and feeding supplies must be kept separate or disinfected between groups. Interactions with cats in the reverse order for any reason are strictly avoided (e.g., going to the kitten area after a visit with clinically ill cats) (Fig. 15-1).

In breeding facilities, litters should be staggered to avoid having large numbers of highly susceptible kittens at the same time. Disease in young kittens may also be avoided through early weaning at 5 to 6 weeks of age. This strategy is limited to litters from queens with a history of recrudescent infection associated with pregnancy.

 TABLE 15-2

### Control of Upper Respiratory Infections in Multicat Households

| MINIMIZING EXPOSURE | STRENGTHENING IMMUNITY |
|---|---|
| Avoidance of overcrowding | Selective breeding for health |
| Segregation of cats into groups based on susceptibility to and likelihood of infection | Excellent nutrition |
| Handling of groups in order of susceptibility (most to least) | Control of internal and external parasites |
| Careful attention to cleanliness and disinfection | Control of retroviral infections |
| Adequate ventilation and humidity control | Vaccination |
| Staggered litters |     Routine protocols |
| Early weaning* |     Early vaccination programs* |

*Short-term measures to control severe outbreak only.

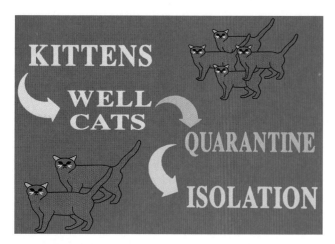

**FIG 15-1**

The order in which cats are fed, cleaned, and handled is strictly followed. Kittens are most susceptible to infection and are encountered first. Overtly ill cats are always visited last.

Principles of cleaning and disinfection should be reviewed. Thorough cleaning must precede disinfection. Housing and supplies should be examined for their ability to be thoroughly cleaned, and recommendations should be made for improvement.

Adequate ventilation must be provided. This aspect can be evaluated and corrected through consultation with an engineer. A minimum of 10 to 15 air exchanges per hour and less than 50% humidity in the room are standard recommendations. Minimally, the facilities should be subjectively assessed for odor, dust, and moisture. Even inexpensive modifications, such as window fans, can result in noticeable improvement in certain situations.

Strengthening immunity is an important adjunct in controlling signs of URI. Immunity is strengthened both generally and specifically. Selective breeding for healthy kittens, maintaining excellent nutrition, and eradicating controllable infections (e.g., FeLV, FIV, intestinal and external parasites) increase overall resistance to disease. Specific immunity is strengthened through vaccination. None of the available vaccines is known to completely prevent infection, nor are vaccines effective in eliminating the carrier state or in treating active disease. That is why other management strategies must be included for a program to be successful.

Households without major upper respiratory problems are advised to use routine vaccination protocols as described for the individual pet cat. The intensified vaccination schedules described in this chapter are useful in controlling outbreaks of disease, but chronic use should not be necessary. Continued reliance on an aggressive vaccination program should alert the veterinarian to problems addressed concerning minimizing exposure and strengthening overall immunity. The majority of the aggressive vaccination protocols are not according to product label, and owners should be so advised.

Households experiencing outbreaks among young kittens can begin vaccinations with a killed product at 4 or 5 weeks of age and repeat it at 6 or 7 weeks, respectively. Routine vaccination with a subcutaneous modified-live product is begun at 9 weeks of age. Intranasal vaccination against *Bordetella* or subcutaneous vaccination against *Chlamydophila* is indicated in households where one of these agents has been identified.

Intranasal modified-live vaccines for FHV and FCV are considered when subcutaneous products are inadequate. They are not as simple to administer as injectable vaccines, and upper respiratory signs can occur after vaccination. These signs tend to be self-limiting but are unacceptable to many owners. Intranasal vaccines are also more expensive than subcutaneous products. However, they induce a local immune response within 2 to 6 days of administration and can override interference by maternal immunity. These properties make them advantageous during outbreaks of disease and for rescue organizations with continuous new additions.

For humane organizations, new admissions should be vaccinated intranasally at the time of entry. In young kittens, vaccination is repeated after 12 weeks of age (but no sooner than 2 weeks after initial intranasal vaccination).

Households with uncontrollable outbreaks in young kittens can begin vaccination intranasally as young as 4 to 5 weeks of age. In severe situations with kittens affected at even younger ages, intranasal vaccines can be administered as early as 8 to 10 days of age at a reduced dose (one drop in each nostril). The series is completed with either intranasal vaccination at 9 and 12 weeks of age or subcutaneous vaccinations beginning at 6 to 7 weeks of age.

Whenever intranasal products are used, panleukopenia vaccines must still be administered by injection. The injectable FHV and FCV vaccines should not be used at the same time as the intranasal vaccine; thus the panleukopenia vaccine should be given without FHV and FCV included.

Readers with a specific interest in advising owners of multiple-cat households on the control of URIs are referred to articles by August, Pedersen, and Scott (see Suggested Readings).

## NASOPHARYNGEAL POLYPS

Nasopharyngeal polyps are benign growths that occur in kittens and young adult cats. Their origin is unknown, but they are often attached to the base of the eustachian tube. They can extend into the external ear canal, middle ear, pharynx, and nasal cavity. Grossly they are pink, polypoid growths, often arising from a stalk (Fig. 15-2). Their gross appearance can be mistaken for neoplasia.

### Clinical Features

Respiratory signs caused by nasopharyngeal polyps include stertorous breathing, upper airway obstruction, and serous-to-mucopurulent nasal discharge. Signs of otitis externa or otitis media/interna, such as head tilt, nystagmus, or Horner's syndrome, can also occur.

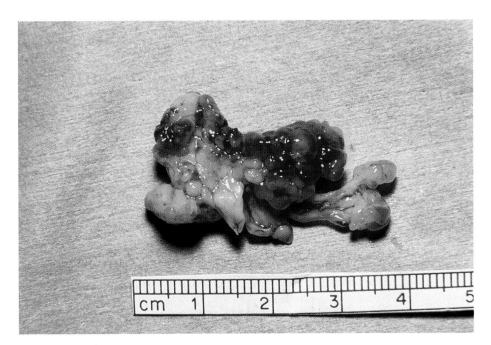

**FIG 15-2**
Nasopharyngeal polyp from a cat with chronic nasal discharge.

## Diagnosis

Identification of a soft tissue opacity above the soft palate radiographically and gross visualization of a mass in the nasopharynx, nasal cavity, or external ear canal support a tentative diagnosis of nasopharyngeal polyp. Complete evaluation of cats with polyps also includes a deep otoscopic examination and radiographs of the osseous bullae to determine the extent of involvement. The majority of cats with polyps have otitis media detectable radiographically as thickened bone or increased soft tissue opacity of the bulla (see Fig. 14-6). The definitive diagnosis is made by histopathologic analysis of tissue biopsy; the specimen is usually obtained during surgical excision. Nasopharyngeal polyps are composed of inflammatory tissue, fibrous connective tissue, and epithelium.

## Treatment

Treatment of nasopharyngeal polyps consists of surgical excision. Surgery is usually performed through the oral cavity. In addition, bullae osteotomy should be performed in cats with radiographic evidence of involvement of the osseous bullae. Rarely, rhinotomy is required for complete removal.

## Prognosis

The prognosis is excellent. Regrowth occurs at the same site if all abnormal tissue is not removed, with signs usually recurring within 1 year. Kapatkin and colleagues (1990) reported that 5 of 31 cats had regrowth of an excised polyp. Of the 5 cats with regrowth, 4 had not had bulla osteotomies. These findings show the importance of addressing involvement of the osseous bulla in cats with polyps.

## NASAL TUMORS

The majority of nasal tumors in the dog and cat are malignant. Adenocarcinoma, squamous cell carcinoma, and undifferentiated carcinoma are common nasal tumors in dogs. Lymphoma and adenocarcinoma are common in cats. Fibrosarcomas and other sarcomas also occur in both species. Benign tumors can include adenomas, fibromas, papillomas, and transmissible venereal tumors (the latter only in dogs).

### Clinical Features

Nasal tumors usually occur in older animals but cannot be excluded from the differential diagnosis of young dogs and cats. No breed predisposition has been consistently identified. Collies and Irish Setters were overrepresented in a report of malignant nasal tumors in dogs by Evans and colleagues (1989).

The clinical features of nasal tumors (usually chronic) reflect the locally invasive nature of these tumors. Nasal discharge is the most common complaint. The discharge can be serous, mucoid, mucopurulent, or hemorrhagic. One or both nostrils can be involved. With bilateral involvement, the discharge is often worse from one nostril compared with the other. For many animals the discharge is initially unilateral and progresses to bilateral. Sneezing may be reported. Obstruction of the nasal cavity by the tumor may cause decreased or absent air flow through one of the nares.

Deformation of the facial bones, hard palate, or maxillary dental arcade may be visible (see Fig. 13-5). Tumor growth extending into the cranial vault can result in neurologic signs. Growth into the orbit may cause exophthalmos or inability to retropulse the eye. Animals only rarely experience neurologic signs (e.g., seizures, behavior changes, abnormal mental status) or ocular abnormalities as the primary complaints (i.e., no signs of nasal discharge). Weight loss and anorexia may accompany the respiratory signs but are often absent.

## Diagnosis

A diagnosis of neoplasia is based on clinical features, and supported by typical abnormalities on radiographs or computerized tomograms (CTs) of the nasal cavity and frontal sinuses, or rhinoscopy. A definitive diagnosis requires histopathologic examination of a biopsy specimen, although fine needle aspirates of nasal masses may provide conclusive results. Radiographic and rhinoscopic abnormalities can reflect soft tissue mass lesions; turbinate, vomer bone, or facial bone destruction (see Figs. 14-2 and 14-4); or diffuse infiltration of the mucosa with neoplastic and inflammatory cells.

Biopsy specimens, including tissue from deep within the lesion, should be obtained in all patients for histologic confirmation. Nasal neoplasms frequently cause a marked inflammatory response of the nasal mucosa and in some patients secondary bacterial or fungal infection. A cytologic diagnosis of neoplasia must be accepted cautiously, taking into consideration concurrent inflammation and potentially marked hyperplastic and metaplastic change. Furthermore, in some cases the cytologic characteristics of lymphoma and carcinoma will mimic each other, which can lead to an erroneous classification.

Not all cases of neoplasia will be diagnosed on initial evaluation of the dog or cat. Radiographs, rhinoscopy, and biopsy may need to be repeated in 1 to 3 months in animals with persistent signs in which a definitive diagnosis has not been made. Repeated evaluation is particularly indicated for dogs with chronic nasal discharge, because, unlike cats, they do not develop chronic viral rhinitis. CT is a more sensitive technique for imaging nasal tumors than routine radiography and should be performed when available (see Fig. 13-4, *B*). Surgical exploration is occasionally necessary to obtain a definitive diagnosis.

Once a definitive diagnosis is made, determining the extent of disease can help to assess the feasibility of surgical or radiation therapy versus chemotherapy. Some information can be obtained from high-quality nasal radiographs, but CT is a more sensitive method for evaluating the extent of abnormal tissue. Aspirates of mandibular lymph nodes should be examined cytologically for evidence of local spread. Thoracic radiographs are evaluated, although pulmonary metastases are uncommon. Cytologic evaluation of bone marrow aspirates and abdominal radiographs or ultrasound are indicated for patients with lymphoma. Cats with lymphoma are also tested for FeLV and FIV.

## Treatment

Treatment of benign tumors should include surgical excision. Malignant nasal tumors can be treated with radiation therapy (with or without surgery) and/or chemotherapy. Palliative treatment can also be tried. The treatments of choice for cats with nasal lymphoma are chemotherapy using standard lymphoma protocols (see Chapter 82) or radiation therapy. Radiation therapy avoids the systemic adverse effects of chemotherapeutic drugs but may be insufficient if the tumor involves other organs.

Radiation therapy is the treatment of choice for most other malignant nasal tumors. Surgical debulking before radiation is recommended if orthovoltage radiation will be used. Surgery is not beneficial before megavoltage radiation (cobalt or linear accelerator), although there has been recent interest in surgical intervention after megavoltage radiation therapy.

Treatment of malignant nasal tumors with surgery alone does not result in prolonged survival times; it may indeed shorten survival times. It is doubtful that all abnormal tissue can be excised in the majority of cases. In one review, MacEwen and colleagues (1977) found a median survival time of 3 months for dogs undergoing surgery versus 5 months for the untreated dogs.

Chemotherapy can be attempted when radiation therapy has failed or is not a viable option. Carcinomas may be responsive to cisplatin, carboplatin, or multiagent chemotherapy. See Chapter 79 for a discussion of general principles for the selection of chemotherapy.

Treatment with piroxicam, a nonsteroidal antiinflammatory drug, can be considered for dogs with carcinoma for which radiation therapy is not elected. Partial remissions or improvement in clinical signs have been reported for some dogs with transitional cell carcinoma of the urinary bladder, oral squamous cell carcinoma, and several other carcinomas. Potential side effects include gastrointestinal ulceration (which can be severe) and kidney damage. For dogs with other types of tumors and cats, improvement of clinical signs may be seen with antiinflammatory doses of prednisone (0.5 to 1 mg/kg/d; tapered to lowest effective dose). Prednisone should not be given in conjunction with piroxicam.

## Prognosis

The prognosis for dogs and cats with untreated malignant nasal tumors is poor. Survival after diagnosis is usually only a few months. Euthanasia is often requested because of persistent epistaxis, anorexia and weight loss, neurologic signs, or labored respirations.

Radiation therapy can prolong survival and improve quality of life in some animals. The therapy is well tolerated by most animals, and in those that achieve remission the quality of life is usually excellent. Studies of dogs treated with megavoltage radiation, with or without surgical treatment, by Theon and colleagues (1993) and Henry and colleagues (1998) found median survival times of approximately 13 months. Survival rates for 1 and 2 years were 55% to 60% and 25% to 45%, respectively. A study by Evans and colleagues (1989) of dogs receiving orthovoltage radiation therapy after surgical debulking reported a median survival time of 16.5 months, a 1-year survival rate of 54% and a 2-year survival rate of 43%. More recently, Northrup and colleagues (2001) report a median survival time of approximately 7 months, a

1-year survival rate of 37% and a 2-year survival rate of only 17% in dogs treated with surgery and orthovoltage radiation.

Less information is available concerning prognosis in cats. According to Straw and colleagues (1986), six cats with malignant neoplasms (three with lymphoma) that received radiation therapy had a mean survival of 19 months. A study by Theon and colleagues (1994) of 16 cats with nonlymphoid neoplasia showed a 1-year survival rate of 44% and a 2-year survival rate of 17%.

## NASAL MYCOSES

### CRYPTOCOCCOSIS

*Cryptococcus neoformans* is a fungal agent that infects cats and less commonly dogs. It most likely enters the body through the respiratory tract and in some animals may disseminate to other organs. In cats, clinical signs usually reflect infection of the nasal cavity, central nervous system (CNS), eyes, or skin and subcutaneous tissues. In dogs, signs of CNS involvement are most common. The lungs are commonly infected in both species, but clinical signs of lung involvement (e.g., cough, dyspnea) are rare. Clinical features, diagnosis, and treatment of cryptococcosis are discussed in Chapter 103.

### ASPERGILLOSIS

*Aspergillus fumigatus* is a normal inhabitant of the nasal cavity in many animals. In some dogs and rarely cats it becomes a pathogen. The mold form of the organism can develop into visible fungal plaques that invade the nasal mucosa: "fungal mats." An animal that develops aspergillosis may have another nasal disease, such as neoplasia, foreign body, prior trauma, or immune deficiency that predisposes the animal to secondary fungal infection. Excessive exposure to *Aspergillus* organisms may explain the frequent occurrence of disease in otherwise healthy animals. Another type of fungus, *Penicillium,* can cause signs similar to those of aspergillosis.

#### Clinical Features

Aspergillosis can cause chronic nasal disease in dogs of any age or breed but is most common in young male dogs. Nasal infection is rare in cats. The discharge can be mucoid, mucopurulent with or without hemorrhage, or purely hemorrhagic. The discharge can be unilateral or bilateral. Sneezing may be reported. Features that are highly suggestive of aspergillosis are sensitivity to palpation of the face or depigmentation and ulceration of the external nares see (see Fig. 13-1). The lungs are rarely involved.

Systemic aspergillosis in dogs is generally caused by *Aspergillus terreus* and other *Aspergillus spp.* rather than *A. fumigatus.* It is an unusual, generally fatal, disease that occurs primarily in German Shepherd dogs. Nasal signs are not reported.

#### Diagnosis

No single test result is diagnostic for infection with aspergillosis. The diagnosis is based on the cumulative findings of a comprehensive evaluation of a dog with appropri-

ate clinical signs. In addition, aspergillosis can be an opportunistic infection, and underlying nasal disease must always be considered.

Radiographic signs of aspergillosis include well-defined lucent areas within the nasal cavity and increased radiolucency rostrally (see Fig. 14-7). Typically no destruction of the vomer or facial bones occurs, although the vomer bone may be roughened. Rarely, destruction of these bones and even the cribriform plate can occur in dogs with advanced disease. Increased fluid opacity may be present. Fluid opacity within the frontal sinus can represent a site of infection or mucus accumulation from obstructed drainage. In some patients the frontal sinus is the only site of infection.

Rhinoscopic abnormalities include erosion of nasal turbinates and fungal plaques, which appear as white-to-green plaques of mold on the nasal mucosa (see Fig. 14-12). Failure to visualize these lesions does not rule out aspergillosis. Confirmation that presumed plaques are indeed fungal hyphae can be achieved by cytology (Fig. 15-3) and culture of material collected by biopsy or swab under visual guidance.

*Aspergillus* organisms can generally be seen histologically in biopsy specimens of affected nasal mucosa after routine staining techniques, although special staining can be performed to identify subtle involvement. Neutrophilic, lymphoplasmacytic, or mixed inflammation is usually also present. Multiple biopsy specimens should be obtained because the mucosa is usually affected multifocally rather than diffusely. Invasion of fungal organisms into the nasal mucosa is indicative of infection.

Results of fungal cultures are difficult to interpret, unless the specimen is obtained from a visualized plaque. The organism can be found in the nasal cavity of normal animals, and false-negative culture results can also occur. A positive culture, in conjunction with other appropriate clinical and diagnostic findings, supports the diagnosis.

Positive serum antibody titers also support a diagnosis of infection. Although titers are indirect evidence of infection,

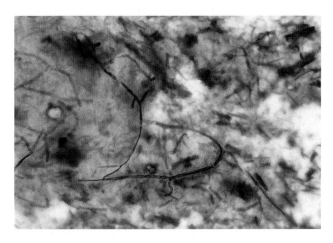

**FIG 15-3**
Branching hyphae of *Aspergillus fumigatus* from a swab of a visualized fungal plaque.

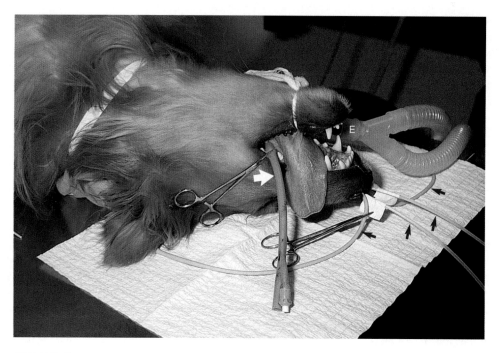

**FIG 15-4**

Dog with nasal mycotic infection prepared for 1-hour soak with clotrimazole. A cuffed endotracheal tube is in place *(E)*. A 24 Fr Foley catheter *(broad arrow)* is in the caudal nasopharynx. A 12 Fr Foley catheter *(narrow arrows)* is obstructing each nostril. A 10 Fr polypropylene catheter *(arrowheads)* is placed midway into each dorsal meatus for infusion of the drug. Laparotomy sponges are used to further pack the caudal nasopharynx, around the tracheal tube and the caudal oral cavity.

animals with *Aspergillus* organisms as a normal nasal inhabitant do not usually develop measurable antibodies against the organism. False-positive and false-negative results occur.

## Treatment

The current treatments of choice for nasal aspergillosis are topical clotrimazole, with a success rate of 85% to 90%, and oral itraconazole, with a success rate of 60% to 70%. Oral therapy is simpler to administer than topical therapy but is somewhat less successful, requires prolonged treatment, and is relatively expensive. Itraconazole is administered orally at a dose of 5 mg/kg every 12 hours and must be continued for 60 to 90 days or longer. See Chapter 103 for a complete discussion of this drug.

Successful topical treatment of aspergillosis was originally documented with enilconazole administered through tubes placed surgically into both frontal sinuses and both sides of the nasal cavity. The drug was administered through the tubes twice daily for 7 to 10 days. Subsequently, it was discovered that the over-the-counter drug clotrimazole was equally efficacious when infused through surgically placed tubes over a 1-hour period. During the 1-hour infusion, the dogs were kept under anesthesia and the caudal nasopharynx and external nares were packed to allow filling of the nasal cavity. It has since been demonstrated that good distribution of the drug can be achieved using a noninvasive technique (see the following text). Success with clotrimazole using this tech-

nique has been similar to that documented with infusion through surgically placed tubes.

The animal is anesthetized and oxygenated through a cuffed endotracheal tube. The dog is positioned in dorsal recumbency with the nose pulled down parallel with the table (Figs. 15-4 and 15-5). For a large-breed dog, a 24 Fr Foley catheter with a 5 ml balloon is passed through the oral cavity, around the soft palate, and into the caudal nasopharynx such that the bulb is at the junction of the hard and soft palates. The bulb is inflated with approximately 10 ml of air to ensure a snug fit. A laparotomy sponge is inserted within the oropharynx, caudal to the balloon and ventral to the soft palate to help hold the balloon in position and to further obstruct the nasal pharynx. Additional laparotomy sponges are packed carefully into the back of the mouth around the tracheal tube to prevent any drug that might leak past the nasopharyngeal packing from reaching the lower airways.

A 10 Fr polypropylene urinary catheter is passed into the dorsal meatus of each nasal cavity to a distance approximately midway between the external naris and the medial canthus of the eye. The correct distance is marked on the catheters with tape to prevent accidentally inserting the catheters too far during the procedure. A 12 Fr Foley catheter with a 5 ml balloon is passed adjacent to the polypropylene catheter into each nasal cavity. The cuff is inflated and pulled snugly against the inside of the naris. A small suture is placed across each naris lateral to the catheter to prevent balloon migra-

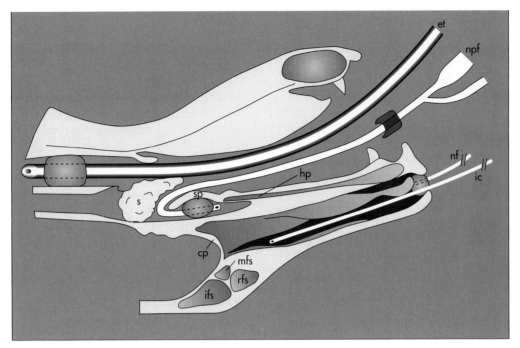

**FIG 15-5**
Schematic diagram of a cross section of the head of a dog prepared for 1-hour soak with clotrimazole: *et,* Endotracheal tube; *npf,* Foley catheter placed in caudal nasopharynx; *s,* pharyngeal sponges; *ic,* polypropylene infusion catheter; *nf,* rostral Foley catheter obstructing nostril; *hp,* hard palate; *sp,* soft palate; *cp,* cribriform plate; *rfs,* rostral frontal sinus; *mfs,* medial frontal sinus; *lfs,* lateral frontal sinus. (Reprinted with permission from Mathews KG et al: Computed tomographic assessment of noninvasive intranasal infusions in dogs with fungal rhinitis, *Vet Surg* 25:309, 1996.)

tion. A gauze sponge is placed between the endotracheal tube and the incisive ducts behind the upper incisors to minimize leakage.

A solution of 1% clotrimazole is administered through the polypropylene catheters. Approximately 30 ml is used for each side in a typical retriever-sized dog. Each Foley catheter is checked for filling during the initial infusion and is then clamped when clotrimazole begins to drip from the catheter. The solution is viscous, but excessive pressure is not required for infusion. Additional clotrimazole is administered during the next hour at a rate that results in approximately 1 drop every few seconds from each external naris. In the size dog described, approximately 100 to 120 ml will be used in total.

After the initial 15 minutes, the head is tilted slightly to one side and then the other for 15 minutes each and then back into dorsal recumbency for 15 minutes. After this hour of contact time, the dog is rolled into sternal recumbency with the head hanging over the end of the table and the nose pointing toward the floor. The catheters are removed from the external nares and the clotrimazole and resulting mucus are allowed to drain. Drainage will usually subside in 10 to 15 minutes. A flexible suction tip may be used to expedite this process. The laparotomy pads are then carefully removed from the nasopharynx and oral cavity and counted to ensure that all are retrieved. The catheter in the na-

sopharynx is removed. Any drug within the oral cavity is swabbed or suctioned.

Two potential complications of clotrimazole treatment are aspiration pneumonia and meningoencephalitis. Meningoencephalitis is generally fatal and results when clotrimazole and its carrier, polyethylene glycol (PEG), contact the brain through a compromised cribriform plate. It is difficult to determine the integrity of the cribriform plate before treatment without the aid of CT or magnetic resonance imaging, although marked radiographic changes in the caudal nasal cavity should increase concern. Fortunately, complications are not common.

Clinical signs generally resolve in 1 to 2 weeks. A second 1-hour soak is performed if signs persist after 2 weeks. Less common causes of persistent discharge are secondary bacterial rhinitis, extension of fungal infection beyond the nasal cavity (e.g., into the retrobulbar space), or inability of the clotrimazole to reach a completely obstructed frontal sinus. Trephination of the affected sinus, debulking of fungal granulomas, and intrasinus administration of clotrimazole is recommended if a frontal sinus granuloma is suspected based on radiography or CT.

## Prognosis

The prognosis for dogs with nasal aspergillosis has improved with the availability of new antifungal agents. For most animals a fair-to-good prognosis is warranted.

## BACTERIAL RHINITIS

Acute bacterial rhinitis caused by *Bordetella bronchiseptica* occurs occasionally in cats (see Feline Upper Respiratory Infection) and rarely in dogs (see Chapter 21, Canine Infectious Tracheobronchitis). It is possible that *Mycoplasma* can act as primary nasal pathogens. In the vast majority of cases, bacterial rhinitis is a *secondary* complication and not a primary disease process. Bacterial rhinitis occurs secondarily to almost all diseases of the nasal cavity. The bacteria that inhabit the nasal cavity in health are quick to overgrow when disease disrupts normal mucosal defenses. Antibiotic therapy often leads to clinical improvement, but the response is usually temporary. Therefore management of dogs and cats with suspected bacterial rhinitis should include a thorough diagnostic evaluation for an underlying disease process, particularly when signs are chronic.

### Diagnosis

Most dogs and cats with bacterial rhinitis have mucopurulent nasal discharge. No clinical signs are pathognomonic for bacterial rhinitis, and it is difficult to make a definitive diagnosis because of the diverse flora in the normal nasal cavity (see p. 226). Microscopic evidence of neutrophilic inflammation and bacteria is a nonspecific finding in the majority of animals with nasal signs. Bacterial cultures of swabs or nasal mucosa collected deep in the nasal cavity can be performed. The growth of many colonies of only one or two organisms may represent significant infection. Growth of many different organisms or small numbers of colonies probably represents normal flora. The microbiology laboratory should be requested to report all growth. Beneficial response to antibiotic therapy is often used to support a diagnosis of bacterial involvement.

### Treatment

The bacterial component of nasal disease is treated with antibiotic therapy. If growth obtained by bacterial culture is believed to be significant, sensitivity information can be used in selecting antibiotics. Anaerobic organisms can be involved. Broad-spectrum antibiotics that may be effective include amoxicillin (22 mg/kg q8h to q12h), trimethoprim-sulfadiazine (15 mg/kg q12h), chloramphenicol (50 mg/kg q8h for dogs; 10 to 15 mg/kg q12h for cats), or clindamycin (5.5 to 11 mg/kg q12h). Doxycycline (5 to 10 mg/kg q12h) or chloramphenicol is often effective against *Bordetella* and *Mycoplasma* organisms.

For acute infection or in cases in which the primary etiology (e.g., foreign body, diseased tooth root) has been eliminated, antibiotics are administered for 7 to 10 days. Chronic infections require prolonged treatment. Antibiotics are administered initially for 1 week. If a beneficial response is seen, the drug is continued for a minimum of 4 to 6 weeks. If signs recur after discontinuation of drug after 4 to 6 weeks, the same antibiotic is reinstituted for even longer periods.

If no response is seen after the initial 1 week of treatment, the drug should be discontinued. Another antibiotic can be tried, although further evaluation for another, as yet unidentified, primary disorder should be pursued. Further diagnostic evaluation is particularly warranted in dogs because, unlike cats, they do not have chronic sequelae from viral rhinitis. (Management recommendations for cats with feline URIs are provided early in this chapter.) Frequent stopping and starting of different antibiotics every 7 to 14 days is not recommended and may predispose the animal to the growth of resistant gram-negative infections.

### Prognosis

Bacterial rhinitis is usually responsive to antibiotic therapy. However, long-term resolution of signs depends on the identification and correction of any underlying disease process.

## NASAL PARASITES

### NASAL MITES

*Pneumonyssoides caninum* is a small, white mite approximately 1 mm in size (see Fig. 14-13, *A*). Most infestations are clinically silent, but some dogs may have moderate-to-severe clinical signs.

### Clinical Features and Diagnosis

A common clinical feature of nasal mites is sneezing, which is often violent. Head shaking, pawing at the nose, reverse sneezing, chronic nasal discharge, and epistaxis can also occur. These signs are similar to those caused by nasal foreign bodies. The diagnosis is made by visualizing the mites during rhinoscopy or by retrograde nasal flushing as described in Chapter 14. The mites can be easily overlooked in the retrieved saline solution; they should be specifically searched for with slight magnification or by placing dark material behind the specimen for contrast. Further, the mites are often located in the frontal sinuses and caudal nasal cavity. Marks and colleagues (1994) report the greatest success in identifying mites by flushing the nasal cavities with halothane in oxygen. The anesthetic mixture causes the mites to migrate to the caudal nasopharynx where the mites are visualized using an endoscope.

### Treatment

Milbemycin oxime (0.5 to 1 mg/kg, orally, every 7 to 10 days for three treatments) has been used successfully for treating nasal mites. Ivermectin has also been used for treatment (0.2 mg/kg administered subcutaneously and repeated in 3 weeks), but it is not safe for certain breeds. Any dogs in direct contact with the affected animal should also be treated.

### Prognosis

The prognosis for dogs with nasal mites is excellent.

### NASAL CAPILLARIASIS

Nasal capillariasis is caused by a nematode, *Capillaria boehmi* (*Eucoleus boehmi*), originally identified as a worm of the frontal sinuses in foxes. The adult worm is small, thin, and white and lives on the mucosa of the nasal cavity and frontal sinuses of dogs (see Fig. 14-13, *B*). The adults shed eggs that are swallowed and pass in the feces. Clinical signs include sneezing and mucopurulent nasal discharge, with or without hemorrhage. The diagnosis is made based on the identification of double operculated *Capillaria* eggs on routine fecal flotation (similar to the eggs of *Capillaria aerophila;* see Fig. 20-10) or visualizing adult worms during rhinoscopy. Treatments include ivermectin (0.2 mg/kg, orally, once) or fenbendazole (25 to 50 mg/kg q12h for 10 to 14 days). Success of treatment should be confirmed with repeated fecal examinations, in addition to resolution of clinical signs. Repeated treatments may be necessary, and reinfection is possible if exposure to contaminated soil continues.

## LYMPHOPLASMACYTIC RHINITIS

Lymphoplasmacytic rhinitis has been described in dogs but is an apparently uncommon cause of nasal disease. Infectious or neoplastic diseases of the nasal cavity, particularly aspergillosis or penicilliosis, can result in lymphoid reactivity and must be eliminated from the differential diagnosis before treatment for lymphoplasmacytic rhinitis is initiated.

### Clinical Features

Burgener and colleagues (1987) reported the disease in five dogs. There was no age or breed predisposition. Signs were typical of most nasal diseases and included sneezing and nasal discharge. The discharges were serous, mucopurulent, and hemorrhagic. Improvement was not seen with antibiotic therapy.

### Diagnosis

The definitive diagnosis of lymphoplasmacytic rhinitis is based on histologic examination of nasal biopsy specimens combined with negative findings for other diseases after an extensive diagnostic evaluation (see Chapters 13 and 14). Increased soft tissue opacity and lysis of nasal turbinates may be apparent radiographically. In Burgener, Slocombe, and Zerbe's report, abnormalities were confined to the rostral half of the nasal cavity. Bacterial or fungal cultures were positive in all patients, but organisms were believed to reflect normal flora based on lack of response to antimicrobial therapy. Masses, foreign bodies, and fungal plaques were not identified rhinoscopically.

Histologic examination of nasal biopsy specimens reveals infiltration of the nasal mucosa and submucosa with mature lymphocytes and plasma cells. Other inflammatory cells appear in lower numbers. Nonspecific abnormalities attributable to chronic inflammation, such as epithelial hyperplasia and fibrosis, can be seen.

### Treatment

Dogs with lymphoplasmacytic rhinitis are treated with immunosuppressive doses of prednisone (1 mg/kg q12h). A positive response is expected within 2 weeks, at which time the dose of prednisone is decreased gradually to the lowest effective amount. If no response to initial therapy occurs, the dose of prednisone can be doubled or other immunosuppressive drugs such as azathioprine can be added to the treatment regimen (see p. 1216, Immunosuppressive Therapy). If clinical signs worsen during treatment, the clinician should discontinue therapy and carefully reevaluate the dog for other diseases.

### Prognosis

The prognosis for lymphoplasmacytic rhinitis is not known because of the paucity of reported cases.

## ALLERGIC RHINITIS

### Etiology

The nasal cavity is an uncommon primary site for allergic disease in the dog and cat, and allergic rhinitis has not been well characterized in these species. However, dermatologists provide anecdotal reports of atopic dogs rubbing the face (possibly indicating nasal pruritus) and experiencing serous nasal discharge, in addition to dermatologic signs. Allergic rhinitis is generally considered to be a hypersensitivity response within the nasal cavity and sinuses to airborne antigens. Other antigens are capable of inducing a hypersensitivity response as well, and thus the differential diagnoses must include parasites, other infectious diseases, and neoplasia.

### Clinical Features

Dogs or cats with allergic rhinitis experience sneezing and/or serous or mucopurulent nasal discharge. Signs may be acute or chronic. Careful questioning of the owner may reveal a relationship between signs and potential allergens. For instance, signs may be worse during certain seasons; in the presence of cigarette smoke; or after the introduction of a new brand of kitty litter, new perfumes, cleaning agents, furniture, or fabric in the house. Debilitation of the animal is not expected.

### Diagnosis

Identifying a historical relationship between signs and a particular allergen and then achieving resolution of signs after removal of the suspected agent from the animal's environment confirms the diagnosis of allergic rhinitis. When this approach is not possible or successful, a thorough diagnostic evaluation of the nasal cavity is indicated (see Chapters 13 and 14). Nasal radiographs reveal increased soft tissue opacity with minimal or no turbinate destruction. Nasal biopsy reveals eosinophilic inflammation, characteristic of a hypersensitivity response. There should be no indication in any of the diagnostic tests of an aggressive disease process, parasites or other active infection, or neoplasia.

### Treatment

Removing the offending allergen from the animal's environment is the ideal treatment of allergic rhinitis. When this is not possible, a beneficial response may be achieved with antihistamines. Chlorpheniramine can be administered orally at a dose of 4 to 8 mg/dog every 8 to 12 hours or 2 mg/cat every 8 to 12 hours. Glucocorticoids can be used if antihistamines are unsuccessful. Prednisone is initiated at a dose of 0.25 mg/kg every 12 hours until signs resolve. The dose is then tapered to the lowest effective amount. If treatment is effective, signs will generally resolve within a few days. Drugs are continued only as long as needed to control signs.

## Prognosis

The prognosis for dogs and cats with allergic rhinitis is excellent if the allergen can be eliminated. Otherwise, the prognosis for control is good, but a cure is unlikely.

## Suggested Readings

August JR: The control and eradication of feline upper respiratory infections in cluster populations, *Vet Med* 85:1002, 1990.

Binns SH et al: Prevalence and risk factors for feline *Bordetella bronchiseptica* infection, *Vet Rec* 144:575, 1999.

Bojrab MJ, editor: *Current techniques in small animal surgery,* ed 4, Baltimore, 1998, Williams and Wilkins.

Bredal W et al: Use of milbemycin oxime in the treatment of dogs with nasal mite (*Pneumonyssoides caninum*) infection, *J Small Anim Pract* 39:126, 1998.

Burgener DC et al: Lymphoplasmacytic rhinitis in five dogs, *J Am Anim Hosp Assoc* 23:565, 1987.

Coutts AJ et al: Studies on natural transmission of *Bordetella bronchiseptica* in cats, *Vet Microbiol* 48:19, 1996.

Davidson AP et al: Treatment of nasal aspergillosis with topical clotrimazole. In Bonagura JD et al, editors: *Current veterinary therapy XII,* Philadelphia, 1995, WB Saunders, p 899.

Evans SM et al: Prognostic factors and survival after radiotherapy for intranasal neoplasms in dogs: 70 cases (1974-1985), *J Am Vet Med Assoc* 194:1460, 1989.

Evinger JV et al: Ivermectin for treatment of nasal capillariasis in a dog, *J Am Vet Med Assoc* 186:174, 1985.

Fossum TW: *Small animal surgery,* St Louis, 1997, Mosby.

Gunnarsson LK et al: Clinical efficacy of milbemycin oxime in the treatment of nasal mite infection in dogs, *J Am Anim Hosp Assoc* 35:81, 1999.

Harvey CE: Therapeutic strategies involving antimicrobial treatment of the upper respiratory tract in small animals, *J Am Vet Med Assoc* 185:1159, 1984.

Henry CJ et al: Survival in dogs with nasal adenocarcinoma: 64 cases (1981-1995), *J Vet Intern Med* 12:436, 1998.

Kapatkin AS et al: Results of surgery and long-term follow-up in 31 cats with nasopharyngeal polyps, *J Am Anim Hosp Assoc* 26:387, 1990.

Lappin MR et al: Use of serologic tests to predict resistance to feline herpesvirus 1, feline calicivirus, and feline parvovirus infection in cats, *J Am Vet Med Assoc* 220:38, 2002.

Maggs DJ et al: Effects of L-lysine and L-arginine on in vitro replication of feline herpesvirus type-1, *Am J Vet Res* 61:1474, 2000.

MacEwen EG et al: Nasal tumors in the dog: retrospective evaluation of diagnosis, prognosis, and treatment, *J Am Vet Med Assoc* 170:45, 1977.

Marks SL et al: *Pneumonyssoides caninum:* the canine nasal mite, *Compend Contin Educ Pract Vet* 16:577, 1994.

Mathews KG et al: Computed tomographic assessment of noninvasive intranasal infusions in dogs with fungal rhinitis, *Vet Surg* 25:309, 1996.

Northrup NC et al: Retrospective study of orthovoltage radiation therapy for nasal tumors in 42 dogs, *J Vet Intern Med* 15:183, 2001.

Parker NR et al: Nasopharyngeal polyps in cats: three case reports and a review of the literature, *J Am Anim Hosp Assoc* 21:473, 1985.

Pedersen NC: *Feline husbandry,* Goleta, Calif, 1991, American Veterinary Publications.

Richardson EF et al: Distribution of topical agents in the frontal sinuses and nasal cavity of dogs: comparison between current protocols for treatment of nasal aspergillosis and a new noninvasive technique, *Vet Surg* 24:476, 1995.

Schmidt BR et al: Evaluation of piroxicam for the treatment of oral squamous cell carcinoma in dogs, *J Am Vet Med Assoc* 218:1783, 2001.

Scott RW et al: Control of feline infectious diseases within multicat facilities, *Cornell Feline Health Center Inform Bull* 11:1, 1990.

Sharp N: Nasal aspergillosis. In Kirk RW, editor: *Current veterinary therapy X,* Philadelphia, 1989, WB Saunders, p 1106.

Speakman AJ et al: Antimicrobial susceptibility of *Bordetella bronchiseptica* isolates from cats and comparison of agar dilution and E-test methods, *Vet Microbiol* 54:53, 1997.

Straw RC et al: Use of radiotherapy for the treatment of intranasal tumors in cats: six cases (1980-1985), *J Am Vet Med Assoc* 189:927, 1986.

Tasker S et al: Aetiology and diagnosis of persistent nasal disease in the dog: a retrospective study of 42 cases, *J Small Anim Pract* 40:473, 1999.

Theon AP et al: Megavoltage irradiation of neoplasms of the nasal and paranasal cavities in 77 dogs, *J Am Vet Med Assoc* 202:1469, 1993.

Theon AP et al: Irradiation of nonlymphoproliferative neoplasms of the nasal cavity and paranasal sinuses in 16 cats, *J Am Vet Med Assoc* 204:78, 1994.

# CHAPTER 16

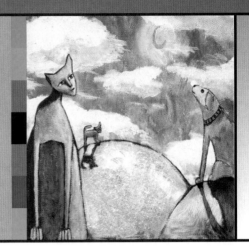

# Clinical Manifestations of Laryngeal and Pharyngeal Disease

## CHAPTER OUTLINE

CLINICAL SIGNS, 241
    Larynx, 241
    Pharynx, 241
DIFFERENTIAL DIAGNOSES FOR LARYNGEAL SIGNS
IN DOGS AND CATS, 242
DIFFERENTIAL DIAGNOSES FOR PHARYNGEAL
SIGNS IN DOGS AND CATS, 242

## CLINICAL SIGNS

### LARYNX

Diseases of the larynx result in similar clinical signs, most notably respiratory distress and stridor. Voice change is specific for laryngeal disease but is not always reported. Clients may volunteer that they have noticed a change in their dog's bark or cat's meow, but specific questioning may be necessary to obtain this important information. Localization of disease to the larynx can generally be achieved with a good history and physical examination. A definitive diagnosis is made through a combination of laryngoscopy, laryngeal radiography, and laryngeal biopsy.

Respiratory distress from laryngeal disease is due to airway obstruction. Although most laryngeal diseases are progressive over several weeks to months, animals typically present in acute distress. Dogs and cats are able to compensate for their disease initially through self-imposed exercise restriction. Often an exacerbating event occurs, such as exercise, excitement, or high ambient temperature, resulting in markedly increased respiratory efforts. These increased efforts lead to excess negative pressures on the diseased larynx, sucking the surrounding soft tissues into the lumen, and to laryngeal inflammation and edema. Obstruction to air flow becomes more severe, leading to even greater respiratory efforts (Fig. 16-1). The airway obstruction can ultimately be fatal.

A characteristic breathing pattern can often be identified on physical examination of patients in distress from extrathoracic (upper) airway obstruction, such as results from laryngeal disease (see Chapter 26). The respiratory rate is normal to only slightly elevated (often 30 to 40 breaths/min), which is particularly remarkable in the presence of overt distress. Inspiratory efforts are prolonged and labored, relative to expiratory efforts. The larynx tends to be sucked into the airway lumen as a result of negative pressure within the extrathoracic airways that occurs during inspiration, making inhalation of air more difficult. During expiration, pressures are positive in the extrathoracic airways, "pushing" the soft tissues open. Nevertheless, expiration may not be effortless. Some obstruction to air flow can occur during expiration with fixed obstructions, such as laryngeal masses. Even with the dynamic obstruction that results from laryngeal paralysis, in which expiration should be possible without any blockage to flow, resultant laryngeal edema and inflammation can interfere with normal expiration. On auscultation, referred upper airway sounds are heard and lung sounds are normal to increased.

Stridor, a high-pitched, audible wheezing sound, is sometimes heard during inspiration. It is audible without a stethoscope, although auscultation of the neck may aid in identifying mild disease. Stridor is produced by air turbulence through the narrowed laryngeal opening. Narrowing of the extrathoracic trachea less commonly produces stridor.

In patients that are not presented for respiratory distress (e.g., for patients with exercise intolerance or voice change), it may be necessary to exercise the patient to identify the characteristic breathing pattern and stridor associated with laryngeal disease.

Some patients with laryngeal disease have subclinical aspiration or overt aspiration pneumonia as a result of loss of normal protective mechanisms. Patients may have clinical signs reflecting aspiration, such as cough, lethargy, anorexia, fever, tachypnea, and abnormal lung sounds. See p. 304 for a discussion of aspiration pneumonia.

### PHARYNX

Space-occupying lesions of the pharynx can cause signs of upper airway obstruction as described for the larynx, but overt respiratory distress occurs only with advanced disease. More typical presenting signs of pharyngeal disease are stertor, reverse sneezing, gagging, retching, and dysphagia. Stertor is a loud, coarse sound such as that produced by snoring or snorting.

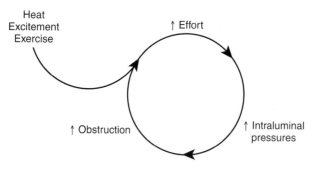

**FIG 16-1**
Patients with extrathoracic (upper) airway obstruction often present in respiratory distress as a result of a progressive worsening of airway obstruction following an exacerbating event.

TABLE 16-1

**Differential Diagnoses for Laryngeal Disease in Dogs and Cats**

Laryngeal paralysis
Laryngeal neoplasia
Obstructive laryngitis
Laryngeal collapse
Web formation
Trauma
Foreign body
Extraluminal mass
Acute laryngitis

Stertor results from excessive soft tissue in the pharynx, such as an elongated soft palate or mass, causing turbulent air flow. Reverse sneezing (see p. 215), gagging, or retching may occur from local stimulation from the tissue itself or from secondary secretions. Dysphagia occurs from physical obstruction, usually due to a mass. As with laryngeal disorders, a definitive diagnosis is made through a combination of visual examination, radiography, and biopsy of abnormal tissue. Visual examination includes a thorough evaluation of the oral cavity, larynx (see p. 243), and caudal nasopharynx (see p. 221).

## DIFFERENTIAL DIAGNOSES FOR LARYNGEAL SIGNS IN DOGS AND CATS

Differential considerations for dogs and cats with respiratory distress are discussed in Chapter 26.

Dogs are more commonly presented for laryngeal disease than cats and most often have laryngeal paralysis (Table 16-1).

TABLE 16-2

**Differential Diagnoses for Pharyngeal Disease in Dogs and Cats**

Brachycephalic airway syndrome
Elongated soft palate
Nasopharyngeal polyp
Foreign body
Neoplasia
Abscess
Granuloma
Extraluminal mass

Laryngeal neoplasia can occur in dogs or cats. Obstructive laryngitis is a poorly characterized inflammatory disorder. Other possible diseases of the larynx include laryngeal collapse (see Chapter 17, p. 245), web formation (adhesions or fibrotic tissue across the laryngeal opening, usually as a complication of surgery), trauma, foreign body, and extraluminal mass causing compression. Acute laryngitis is not a well-characterized disease in dogs or cats but presumably could result from viral or other infectious agents or excessive barking.

## DIFFERENTIAL DIAGNOSES FOR PHARYNGEAL SIGNS IN DOGS AND CATS

The most common pharyngeal disorders in dogs are brachycephalic airway syndrome and elongated soft palate (Table 16-2). Elongated soft palate is a component of brachycephalic airway syndrome and is discussed with this disorder on p. 248, but it often occurs in nonbrachycephalic dogs. The most common pharyngeal disorders in cats are lymphosarcoma and nasopharyngeal polyps (Allen and colleagues, 1999). Nasopharyngeal polyps, nasal tumors, and foreign bodies are discussed in the chapters on nasal diseases (see Chapters 13 to 15). Other differential diagnoses are abscess or granuloma, and extraluminal mass, causing compression.

### Suggested Readings

Allen HS et al: Nasopharyngeal diseases in cats: a retrospective study of 53 cases (1991-1998), *J Am Anim Hosp Assoc* 35:457, 1999.

Hendricks JC: Brachycephalic airway syndrome, *Vet Clin North Am Small Anim Pract* 22:1145, 1992.

Venker-Van Hangen AJ: Diseases of the larynx, *Vet Clin North Am Small Anim Pract* 22:1155, 1992.

# CHAPTER 17

# Diagnostic Tests for the Larynx and Pharynx

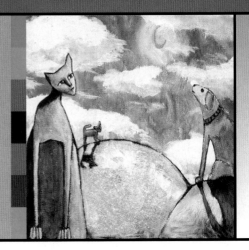

## CHAPTER OUTLINE

RADIOGRAPHY AND ULTRASONOGRAPHY, 243
LARYNGOSCOPY AND PHARYNGOSCOPY, 243

## RADIOGRAPHY AND ULTRASONOGRAPHY

Radiographs of the pharynx and larynx should be evaluated in animals with suspected upper airway disease. They are particularly useful in identifying radiodense foreign bodies such as needles, which can be embedded in tissues and may be difficult to find during laryngoscopy, and adjacent bony changes. Soft tissue masses and soft palate abnormalities may be seen, but apparent abnormal opacities are often misleading, particularly if there is any rotation of the head and neck, and overt abnormalities are often not identified. Abnormal soft tissue opacities or narrowing of the airway lumen identified radiographically must be confirmed with laryngoscopy or endoscopy and biopsy. Laryngeal paralysis cannot be detected radiographically.

A lateral view of the larynx, caudal nasopharynx, and cranial cervical trachea is usually obtained. The vertebral column interferes with airway evaluation on dorsoventral or ventrodorsal (VD) projections. In animals with abnormal opacities identified on the lateral view, a VD or oblique view may confirm the existence of the abnormality and allow further localization of it. When radiographs of the laryngeal area are obtained, the head is held with the neck slightly extended. Padding under the neck and around the head may be needed to avoid rotation. Radiodense foreign bodies are readily identified. Soft tissue masses that are within the airway or that distort the airway are apparent in some animals with neoplasia, granulomas, abscesses, or polyps, and elongated soft palate is sometimes detectable.

Ultrasonography provides another noninvasive imaging modality for evaluating the pharynx and larynx, and laryngeal motion can be assessed. Because air interferes with sound waves, accurate assessment of this area can be difficult. Nevertheless, ultrasonography was found to be useful in the diagnosis of laryngeal paralysis in dogs (Rudorf and colleagues, 2001). Localization of mass lesions and guidance of needle aspiration can also be performed.

## LARYNGOSCOPY AND PHARYNGOSCOPY

Laryngoscopy and pharyngoscopy allow visualization of the larynx and pharynx for assessment of structural abnormalities and function of the arytenoid cartilages and vocal cords. The procedures are indicated in any dog or cat with clinical signs that suggest upper airway obstruction or laryngeal or pharyngeal disease. It should be noted that patients with increased respiratory efforts resulting from upper airway obstruction might have difficulty during recovery from anesthesia. For a period of time between removal of the endotracheal tube and full recovery of neuromuscular function, the patient may be unable to maintain an open airway. Therefore laryngoscopy should not be undertaken in these patients unless the clinician is prepared to perform whatever surgical treatments may be indicated during the same anesthetic period.

The animal is placed in sternal recumbency. Anesthesia is induced and maintained with a short-acting injectable agent without prior sedation. Propofol, sodium thiopental, or sodium thiamylal is commonly used. Depth of anesthesia is carefully titrated, giving just enough drug to allow visualization of the laryngeal cartilages; some jaw tone is maintained, and spontaneous deep respirations occur. Gauze is passed under the maxilla behind the canine teeth, and the head is elevated by hand or by tying the gauze to a stand. This positioning avoids external compression of the neck (Fig. 17-1). Retraction of the tongue with a gauze sponge should allow visualization of the caudal pharynx and larynx. A laryngoscope is also helpful in illuminating this region and enhancing visualization.

The motion of the arytenoid cartilages is evaluated while the patient takes several deep breaths. An assistant is needed to identify inspiration and expiration by observing chest wall movements. Normally the arytenoid cartilages abduct symmetrically and widely with each inspiration and close on expiration (Fig.

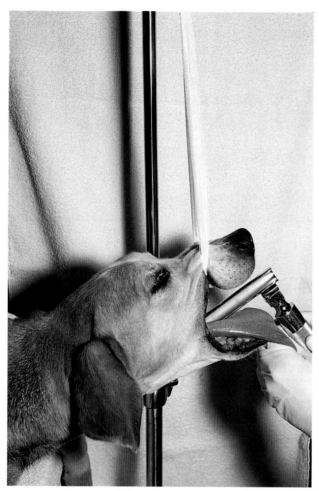

**FIG 17-1**
Dog positioned with the head held off the table by gauze passed around the maxilla and hung from an intravenous pole. The tongue is pulled out, and a laryngoscope is used to visualize the pharyngeal anatomy and laryngeal motion.

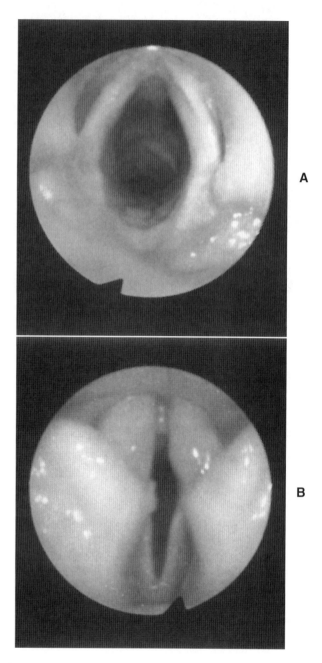

**FIG 17-2**
Canine larynx. **A,** During inspiration, arytenoid cartilages and vocal folds are abducted, resulting in wide symmetric opening to trachea. **B,** During expiration, cartilages and vocal folds nearly close the glottis.

17-2). Laryngeal paralysis resulting in clinical signs is usually bilateral. The cartilages are not abducted during inspiration but may be passively forced outward during expiration, resulting in paradoxical motion. If normal motion is not present, observation of the arytenoid cartilages should be continued as long as possible while the animal recovers from anesthesia. Effects of anesthesia and shallow breathing are the most common causes for an erroneous diagnosis of laryngeal paralysis.

After evaluation of laryngeal function, the plane of anesthesia is deepened, and the caudal pharynx and larynx are thoroughly evaluated for structural abnormalities, foreign bodies, or mass lesions; appropriate diagnostic samples should be obtained for histopathologic analysis and perhaps culture. The length of the soft palate should be assessed. The soft palate should normally extend to the tip of the epiglottis during inhalation. An elongated soft palate can contribute to signs of upper airway obstruction.

As described in Chapter 14, the caudal nasopharynx

should be evaluated for nasopharyngeal polyps, mass lesions, and foreign bodies. Needles or other sharp objects may be buried in tissue, and careful visual examination and palpation are required for detection.

Neoplasia, granulomas, abscesses, or other masses can occur within or external to the larynx or pharynx, causing compression or deviation of normal structures or both. Severe, diffuse proliferative thickening of the laryngeal mucosa can be caused by infiltrative neoplasia or obstructive laryngitis.

Biopsy specimens for histologic examination should be obtained from any lesions to establish an accurate diagnosis because the prognoses for these diseases are quite different. The normal diverse flora of the pharynx makes culture results difficult or impossible to interpret. Bacterial growth from abscesses or granulomatous lesions may represent infection.

Obliteration of most of the airway lumen by surrounding mucosa is known as *laryngeal collapse*. With prolonged upper airway obstruction, the soft tissues are sucked into the lumen by the increased negative pressure created as the dog or cat struggles to get air into its lungs. Eversion of the laryngeal saccules, thickening and elongation of the soft palate, and inflammation with thickening of the pharyngeal mucosa can occur. The laryngeal cartilages can become soft and deformed, unable to support the soft tissues of the pharynx. It is unclear whether this chondromalacia is a concurrent or secondary component of laryngeal collapse. Collapse most often occurs in dogs with brachycephalic airway syndrome but can also occur with any chronic obstructive disorder.

The trachea should be examined radiographically or visually with an endoscope if abnormalities are not identified on laryngoscopy in the dog or cat with signs of upper airway obstruction. For these animals, the laryngeal cartilages can be held open with an endotracheal tube for a cursory examination of the proximal trachea at the time of laryngoscopy if an endoscope is not available.

## Suggested Readings

Aron DN et al: Upper airway obstruction, *Vet Clin North Am Small Anim Pract* 15:891, 1985.

Rudorf H et al: The role of ultrasound in the assessment of laryngeal paralysis in the dog, *Vet Radiol Ultrasound* 42:338, 2001.

Wykes PM: Canine laryngeal diseases. I. Anatomy and disease syndromes, *Compend Cont Educ Pract Vet* 5:8, 1983.

# CHAPTER 18

## Disorders of the Larynx and Pharynx

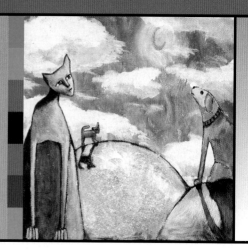

### CHAPTER OUTLINE

LARYNGEAL PARALYSIS, 246
BRACHYCEPHALIC AIRWAY SYNDROME, 248
OBSTRUCTIVE LARYNGITIS, 249
LARYNGEAL NEOPLASIA, 249

## LARYNGEAL PARALYSIS

*Laryngeal paralysis* refers to a failure of the arytenoid cartilages to abduct during inspiration, creating extrathoracic (upper) airway obstruction. The abductor muscles are innervated by the left and right recurrent laryngeal nerves. If clinical signs develop, both arytenoid cartilages are usually affected.

### Etiology

Potential causes of laryngeal paralysis are listed in Table 18-1. Laryngeal paralysis is most often idiopathic. Trauma or neoplasia involving the ventral neck can damage the recurrent laryngeal nerves directly or through inflammation and scarring. Masses or trauma involving the anterior thoracic cavity can also cause damage to the recurrent laryngeal nerves as they course around the subclavian artery (right side) or ligamentum arteriosum (left side). Dogs with polyneuropathymyopathy can be presented with laryngeal paralysis as the predominant clinical sign. Polyneuropathies in turn have been associated with immune-mediated diseases, endocrinopathies, or other systemic disorders (see Chapter 73). Congenital laryngeal paralysis has been documented in the Bouvier des Flandres and is suspected in Siberian Huskies and Bull Terriers. A laryngeal paralysis-polyneuropathy complex has been described in young Dalmations and Rottweilers. Anecdotally, there may be an increasing incidence of idiopathic laryngeal paralysis in older Golden and Labrador Retrievers, and in one study, 47 of 140 dogs (34%) with laryngeal paralysis were Labrador Retrievers (MacPhail and colleague, 2001). Laryngeal paralysis is uncommon in cats.

### Clinical Features

Laryngeal paralysis can occur at any age and in any breed, although the idiopathic form is most commonly seen in older, large-breed dogs. Clinical signs of respiratory distress and stridor are a direct result of narrowing of the airway at the arytenoid cartilages and vocal folds. The owner may also note a change in voice (bark or meow). Most patients are presented for acute respiratory distress, in spite of the chronic, progressive nature of this disease. Decompensation is frequently a result of exercise, excitement, or high environmental temperatures, resulting in a cycle of increased respiratory efforts, increased negative airway pressures sucking the soft tissue into the airway, and pharyngeal edema and inflammation leading to further increased respiratory efforts. Cyanosis, syncope, and death can occur. Dogs with respiratory distress require immediate emergency therapy.

Some dogs with laryngeal paralysis exhibit gagging or coughing with eating or have overt aspiration pneumonia, presumably resulting from concurrent pharyngeal dysfunction or a more generalized polyneuropathy-polymyopathy.

### Diagnosis

A definitive diagnosis of laryngeal paralysis is made through laryngoscopy (see p. 243). Movement of the arytenoid cartilages is observed during a light plane of anesthesia while the patient is taking deep breaths. In laryngeal paralysis, the arytenoid cartilages and vocal folds remain closed during inspiration and open slightly during expiration. The vocal folds may vibrate during inspiration and expiration, which should not be confused with the normal coordinated movement associated with breathing. Additional laryngoscopic findings may include pharyngeal edema and inflammation. The larynx and pharynx are also examined for neoplasia, foreign bodies, or other diseases that might interfere with normal function, and for laryngeal collapse (see p. 245).

Once a diagnosis of laryngeal paralysis is established, additional diagnostic tests should be considered to identify underlying or associated diseases, to rule out concurrent pulmonary problems (such as aspiration pneumonia) that may be contributing to the clinical signs, and to rule out concurrent

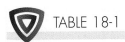 TABLE 18-1

## Potential Causes of Laryngeal Paralysis

**Idiopathic**

**Ventral Cervical Lesion**

Trauma to nerves
    Direct trauma
    Inflammation
    Fibrosis
Neoplasia
Other inflammatory or mass lesion

**Anterior Thoracic Lesion**

Neoplasia
Trauma
    Postoperative
    Other
Other inflammatory or mass lesion

**Polyneuropathy and Polymyopathy**

Idiopathic
Immune mediated
Endocrinopathy
    Hypothyroidism
    Hypoadrenocorticism
Other systemic disorder
    Toxicity
Congenital disease

 TABLE 18-2

## Diagnostic Evaluation of Dogs and Cats with Confirmed Laryngeal Paralysis

**Underlying Cause**

Thoracic radiographs
Cervical radiographs
Serum biochemical panel
Thyroid hormone evaluation
    Baseline $T_4$, free $T_4$, cTSH
    Thyroid-stimulating hormone stimulation test
Ancillary tests in select cases
    Evaluation for diffuse neuropathy-myopathy
        Electromyography
        Nerve conduction measurements
    Antinuclear antibody test
    Antiacetylcholine receptor antibody test
    Cortisol evaluation
        ACTH stimulation test

**Concurrent Pulmonary Disease**

Thoracic radiographs

**Concurrent Pharyngeal Dysfunction**

Evaluate gag reflex
Observe swallowing of food and water
Fluoroscopic observation of barium swallow

**Concurrent Esophageal Dysfunction**

Thoracic radiographs
Contrast-enhanced esophagram
Fluoroscopic observation of barium swallow

pharyngeal and esophageal motility problems (Table 18-2). The last mentioned is especially important if surgical correction for the treatment of laryngeal paralysis is being considered. If the diagnostic tests fail to identify a cause, idiopathic laryngeal paralysis is diagnosed.

## Treatment

In animals with respiratory distress, emergency medical therapy to relieve upper airway obstruction is indicated (see Chapter 26). Following stabilization and a thorough diagnostic evaluation, surgery is usually the treatment of choice. Even when specific therapy can be directed at an associated disease (e.g., hypothyroidism), complete resolution of clinical signs of laryngeal paralysis is rarely seen. Also, most cases are idiopathic, and signs are generally progressive.

Various laryngoplasty techniques have been described, including arytenoid lateralization (tie-back) procedures, partial laryngectomy, and castellated laryngoplasty. The goal of surgery is to provide an adequate opening for the flow of air, but not one so large that the animal is predisposed to aspiration and the development of pneumonia. Several operations to gradually enlarge the glottis may be necessary to minimize the chance of subsequent aspiration. The recommended initial procedure for most dogs and cats is unilateral arytenoid lateralization.

If surgery is not an option, medical management consisting of antiinflammatory doses of short-acting glucocorticoids (e.g., prednisone, 0.5 mg/kg q12h initially) and cage rest may reduce secondary inflammation and edema of the pharynx and larynx and enhance air flow.

## Prognosis

The overall prognosis for dogs with laryngeal paralysis treated surgically is fair to good. White (1989) reported on 62 dogs that underwent unilateral arytenoid lateralization, and more than 90% of owners considered the procedure successful 1 year after surgery. MacPhail and colleague (2001) reported a median survival time of 1800 days (nearly 5 years) for 140 dogs that underwent various surgical procedures, although the mortality rate from postoperative complications was high at 14%. The most common complication was aspiration pneumonia. A guarded prognosis is warranted for patients with signs of aspiration, dysphagia, megaesophagus, or systemic polyneuropathy or myopathy. Dogs with laryngeal paralysis as an early manifestation of generalized polymyopathy or polyneuropathy may have progression of signs.

## *BRACHYCEPHALIC AIRWAY SYNDROME*

The term *brachycephalic airway syndrome,* or *upper airway obstruction syndrome,* refers to the multiple anatomic abnormalities commonly found in brachycephalic dogs and, to a lesser extent, in short-faced cats such as Himalayans. These anatomic abnormalities include stenotic nares, elongated soft palate, everted laryngeal saccules, laryngeal collapse, and, in English Bulldogs, hypoplastic trachea. The severity of these abnormalities varies, and one or any combination of these abnormalities may be present in any given brachycephalic dog or short-faced cat (Fig. 18-1).

### Clinical Features

The abnormalities associated with the brachycephalic airway syndrome impair the flow of air through the extrathoracic (upper) airways and cause clinical signs of upper airway obstruction, including loud breathing sounds, stertor, increased inspiratory efforts, cyanosis, and syncope. Clinical signs are exacerbated by exercise, excitement, and high environmental

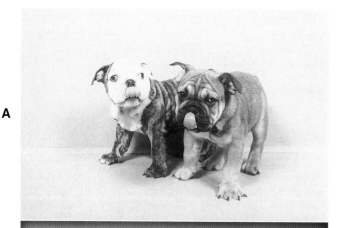

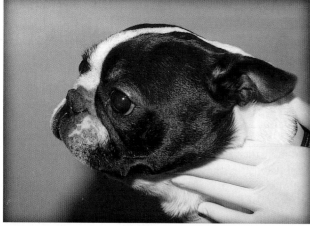

**FIG 18-1**
Two English Bulldog puppies **(A)** and a Boston Terrier **(B)** with brachycephalic airway syndrome. Abnormalities can include stenotic nares, elongated soft palate, everted laryngeal saccules, laryngeal collapse, and hypoplastic trachea.

temperatures. The increased inspiratory effort commonly associated with this syndrome may cause secondary edema and inflammation of the laryngeal and pharyngeal mucosae and enhance eversion of the laryngeal saccules, further narrowing the glottis, exacerbating the clinical signs, and creating a vicious cycle. As a result, some dogs may be presented with life-threatening upper airway obstruction requiring immediate emergency therapy.

### Diagnosis

A tentative diagnosis is made on the basis of the breed, clinical signs, and the appearance of the external nares. Stenotic nares are generally bilaterally symmetric, and the alar folds may be sucked inward during inspiration, thereby worsening the obstruction to air flow. Laryngoscopy (see Chapter 17) and radiographic evaluation of the trachea (see Chapter 20) are necessary to assess the number and severity of abnormalities and to thereby make a definitive diagnosis. Most other causes of upper airway obstruction (see Chapter 26, and Tables 16-1 and 16-2 on p. 242) can also be ruled in or out on the basis of the results of these diagnostic tests.

### Treatment

Therapy should be designed to minimize the factors that exacerbate the clinical signs (e.g., exercise, excitement, overheating) and to enhance the passage of air through the upper airways. Surgical correction of the anatomic defects is the treatment of choice. The specific surgical procedure selected depends on the nature of the existing problems and can include widening of the external nares and removal of excessive soft palate and everted laryngeal saccules. Correction of stenotic nares is a simple procedure and can lead to a surprising alleviation of the signs in affected animals. In affected puppies and kittens, stenotic nares can be safely corrected during routine ovariohysterectomy or castration, ideally before clinical signs develop. The soft palate should be evaluated at the same time and also corrected if elongated. Such early relief of obstruction should decrease the amount of negative pressure placed on the pharyngeal and laryngeal structures during inspiration and decrease progression of disease.

Medical management consisting of antiinflammatory doses of short-acting glucocorticoids (e.g., prednisone, 0.5 mg/ kg q12h initially) and cage rest may reduce the secondary inflammation and edema of the pharynx and larynx and enhance air flow, but it will not eliminate the problem. Emergency therapy may be required to alleviate the upper airway obstruction in animals presenting in respiratory distress (see Chapter 26).

### Prognosis

The prognosis depends on the severity of the abnormalities and the ability to surgically correct them. The prognosis after early surgical correction of the abnormalities is good for many animals. Laryngeal collapse (see p. 245) is a poor prognostic indicator. Permanent tracheostomy can be considered as a salvage procedure in animals with severe collapse. The clinical signs will progressively worsen if the underlying problems go uncorrected. A hypoplastic trachea is not surgically correctable, but there is no clear relationship between the degree of hypoplasia and morbidity or mortality.

## OBSTRUCTIVE LARYNGITIS

Nonneoplastic infiltration of the larynx with inflammatory cells can occur in dogs and cats, causing irregular proliferation, hyperemia, and swelling of the larynx. Clinical signs of an upper airway obstruction result. The larynx appears grossly neoplastic during laryngoscopy but is differentiated from neoplasia on the basis of the findings from the histopathologic evaluation of biopsy specimens. Inflammatory infiltrates can be granulomatous, pyogranulomatous, or lymphocytic-plasmacytic. Etiologic agents have not been identified.

This syndrome is poorly characterized and probably includes several different diseases. Some animals respond to glucocorticoid therapy. Prednisone (1.0 mg/kg given orally q12h) is used initially. Once the clinical signs have resolved, the dose of prednisone can be tapered to the lowest one that effectively maintains remission of clinical signs. Conservative excision of the tissue obstructing the airway may be necessary in animals with severe signs of upper airway obstruction or large granulomatous masses.

The prognosis varies, depending on the size of the lesion, the severity of laryngeal damage, and the responsiveness of the lesion to glucocorticoid therapy.

## LARYNGEAL NEOPLASIA

Neoplasms originating from the larynx are uncommon in dogs and cats. More commonly, tumors originating in tissues adjacent to the larynx, such as thyroid carcinoma and lymphoma, compress or invade the larynx and distort normal laryngeal structures. Clinical signs of extrathoracic (upper) airway obstruction result. Laryngeal tumors include carcinoma (squamous cell, undifferentiated, and adenocarcinoma), lymphoma, melanoma, mast cell tumors and other sarcomas, and benign neoplasia. Lymphoma is the most common tumor in cats.

### Clinical Features

The clinical signs of laryngeal neoplasia are similar to those of other laryngeal diseases and include noisy respiration, stridor, increased inspiratory efforts, cyanosis, syncope, and a change in bark or meow. Mass lesions can also cause concurrent dysphagia, aspiration pneumonia, or visible or palpable masses in the ventral neck.

### Diagnosis

Extralaryngeal mass lesions are often identified by palpation of the neck. Primary laryngeal tumors are rarely palpable and are best identified by laryngoscopy. Laryngeal radiographs, ultrasonography, or computed tomography can be useful in assessing the extent of disease. Differential diagnoses include obstructive laryngitis, nasopharyngeal polyp, foreign body, traumatic granuloma, and abscess. For a definitive diagnosis of neoplasia to be made, histologic or cytologic examination of a biopsy specimen of the mass must be done. A diagnosis of malignant neoplasia should not be made on the basis of the gross appearance alone.

### Treatment

The therapy used depends on the type of tumor identified histologically. Benign tumors should be excised surgically, if possible. Complete surgical excision of malignant tumors is rarely possible, although ventilation may be improved and time may be gained to allow other treatments such as irradiation or chemotherapy to become effective. Complete laryngectomy and permanent tracheostomy can be considered in select animals.

### Prognosis

The prognosis in animals with benign tumors is excellent if the tumors can be totally resected. Malignant neoplasms are associated with a poor prognosis.

### Suggested Readings

Aron DN et al: Upper airway obstruction, *Vet Clin North Am Small Anim Pract* 15:891, 1985.

Braund KG et al: Laryngeal paralysis-polyneuropathy complex in young Dalmatians, *Am J Vet Res* 55:534, 1994.

Burbridge HM: A review of laryngeal paralysis in dogs, *Br Vet J* 151:71, 1995.

Hendricks JC: Brachycephalic airway syndrome, *Vet Clin North Am Small Anim Pract* 22:1145, 1992.

MacPhail CM et al: Outcome of and postoperative complications in dogs undergoing surgical treatment of laryngeal paralysis: 140 cases (1985-1998), *J Am Vet Med Assoc* 218:1949, 2001.

Mahony OM et al: Laryngeal paralysis-polyneuropathy complex in young Rottweilers, *J Vet Intern Med* 12:330, 1998.

Schachter S et al: Laryngeal paralysis in cats: 16 cases (1990-1999), *J Am Vet Med Assoc* 216:1100, 2000.

White RAS: Unilateral arytenoid lateralisation: an assessment of technique and long term results in 62 dogs with laryngeal paralysis, *J Small Anim Pract* 30:543, 1989.

Withrow SJ: Tumors of the respiratory system. In Withrow SJ et al, editors: *Small animal clinical oncology*, Philadelphia, 1996, WB Saunders.

Wykes PM: Canine laryngeal diseases. I. Anatomy and disease syndromes, *Compend Contin Educ Pract Vet* 5:8, 1983.

# CHAPTER 19

# Clinical Manifestations of Lower Respiratory Tract Disorders

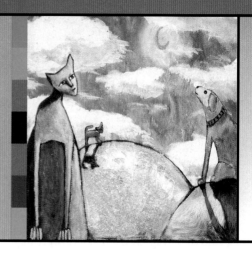

## CHAPTER OUTLINE

CLINICAL SIGNS, 250
    Cough, 250
    Exercise intolerance and respiratory distress, 251
DIAGNOSTIC APPROACH TO DOGS AND CATS
WITH LOWER RESPIRATORY TRACT DISEASE, 252
    Initial diagnostic evaluation, 252
    Further diagnostic evaluation, 253

## CLINICAL SIGNS

In this discussion, *lower respiratory tract disorders* refer to diseases of the trachea, bronchi, bronchioles, alveoli, and interstitium of the lung (Table 19-1). Terms do overlap, however, in that obstruction of the extrathoracic trachea often causes clinical signs of upper airway obstruction. Dogs and cats with diseases of the lower respiratory tract are commonly seen for evaluation of a cough. Lower respiratory tract diseases that interfere with the oxygenation of blood can result in respiratory distress, exercise intolerance, weakness, cyanosis, or syncope.

Nonspecific signs such as fever, anorexia, weight loss, and depression also occur and are the only presenting sign in some animals. In rare instances, potentially misleading signs, such as vomiting, can occur in animals with lower respiratory tract disease. Auscultation and thoracic radiography help to localize the disease to the lower respiratory tract in these animals. The two major presenting signs in animals with lower respiratory tract disease, cough and respiratory distress, can be further characterized by a careful history and physical examination.

### COUGH

A cough is an explosive release of air from the lungs through the mouth. It is generally a protective reflex to expel material from the airways, although inflammation or compression of the airways can also stimulate cough.

Classically, differential diagnoses for cough are divided into those that cause a productive cough and those that cause nonproductive cough. A productive cough results in the delivery of mucus, exudate, edema fluid, or blood from the airways into the oral cavity. A moist sound can often be heard during the cough. Animals rarely expectorate the fluid, but swallowing can be seen after a coughing episode. If expectoration occurs, clients may confuse the cough with vomiting. In human medicine, categorizing cough as productive or nonproductive is rarely difficult because the patient can report the coughing up of secretions. In veterinary medicine, recognition of a productive cough is more difficult. If the owner or veterinarian has heard or seen evidence that the cough is productive, it usually is. However, not hearing or seeing evidence of productivity does not rule out the possibility of its presence. Productive coughs are most commonly caused by inflammatory or infectious diseases of the airways or alveoli and by heart failure (Table 19-2).

Hemoptysis is the coughing up of foamy blood. Blood-tinged saliva may be observed within the oral cavity or dripping from the commissures of the mouth after a cough. Hemoptysis is an unusual clinical sign that most commonly occurs in animals with heartworm disease or pulmonary neoplasia. Less common causes of hemoptysis are mycotic infections, foreign bodies, severe congestive heart failure, thromboembolic disease, lung lobe torsion, and some systemic bleeding disorders, such as disseminated intravascular coagulation (see Table 19-2).

Intensity of cough is another quality that may be useful in prioritizing the differential diagnoses. Cough associated with airway inflammation (e.g., bronchitis) or airway collapse is often loud, harsh, and paroxysmal. The cough associated with tracheal collapse is often described as a "goose-honk." Cough resulting from tracheal disease can usually be induced by palpation of the trachea, although the concurrent involvement of deeper airways is possible. Cough associated with pneumonias and pulmonary edema is usually soft.

The association of coughing with temporal events can be helpful. Cough resulting from tracheal disease is exacerbated by pressure on the neck, such as pulling on the animal's collar. Cough caused by heart failure tends to occur more frequently at night, whereas cough caused by airway disease tends to occur more frequently upon rising from sleep or during and after exercise or exposure to cold air. The client's

## TABLE 19-1

**Differential Diagnoses for Lower Respiratory Tract Disease in Dogs and Cats**

### Disorders of the Trachea and Bronchi

Canine infectious tracheobronchitis
Collapsing trachea
Feline bronchitis
Allergic bronchitis
Canine chronic bronchitis
  Bronchiectasis
*Oslerus osleri* infection
Bronchial compression
  Left atrial enlargement
  Hilar lymphadenopathy
Tracheal tear
Neoplasia

### Disorders of the Pulmonary Parenchyma

Infectious diseases
  Viral pneumonia
    Canine distemper
  Bacterial pneumonia
  Protozoal pneumonia
    Toxoplasmosis
  Fungal pneumonia
    Blastomycosis
    Histoplasmosis
    Coccidioidomycosis
  Parasitic disease
    Heartworm disease
    Pulmonary parasites
      *Paragonimus* infection
      *Aelurostrongylus* infection
      *Capillaria* infection
      *Crenosoma* infection
Pulmonary infiltrates with eosinophils and other
  inflammatory diseases
Aspiration pneumonia
Pulmonary neoplasia
Pulmonary contusions
Pulmonary thromboembolism
Pulmonary edema

## TABLE 19-2

**Differential Diagnoses for Productive Cough in Dogs and Cats***

### Edema

Heart failure
Noncardiogenic pulmonary edema

### Mucus or Exudate

Canine infectious tracheobronchitis
Chronic bronchitis
Allergic bronchitis
Bacterial infection (bronchitis or pneumonia)
Parasitic disease
Aspiration pneumonia
Fungal pneumonia (severe)

### Blood (Hemoptysis)

Heartworm disease
Neoplasia
Fungal pneumonia
Thromboembolism
Severe heart failure
Foreign body
Lung lobe torsion
Systemic bleeding disorder

*These differential diagnoses should also be considered in patients with nonproductive cough.

of such compromise begin as mildly increased respirations and subtle decreased activity and progress through exercise intolerance (manifested as reluctance to exercise or respiratory distress with exertion) to overt respiratory distress at rest. Most owners will miss the early signs of increased respiratory rate and mild exercise intolerance. However, they can be taught to count the respiratory rate at home as an indicator of pulmonary function. The normal respiratory rate of a dog or cat without stress, at rest, is less than 20 respirations per minute. The stress of the veterinary hospital makes subtle increases difficult to detect, and a rate of up to 30 respirations per minute is generally considered normal during routine physical examination.

Cyanosis, in which normally pink mucous membranes are bluish, is a sign of severe hypoxemia and indicates that the increased respiratory effort is not sufficiently compensating for the degree of respiratory dysfunction. However, pallor of mucous membranes is a more common sign of acute hypoxemia resulting from respiratory disease. Cats normally have a minimally visible respiratory effort. Cats that show noticeable chest excursions or open-mouth breathing are severely compromised. Because of compensatory mechanisms, the ability of most pets to self-regulate their activity, and the inability of pets to communicate, many veterinary patients with compromised lung function arrive in overt respiratory distress. These patients require rapid physical assessment and immediate stabilization before further diagnostic testing, as discussed in Chapter 26.

perception of frequency may be biased by the times of day during which they have the most contact with their pets, often in the evenings and during exercise.

Surprisingly, cats with many of the disorders listed in Table 19-2 do not cough. In cats that cough, the index of suspicion for bronchitis, lung parasites, and heartworm disease is high.

## EXERCISE INTOLERANCE AND RESPIRATORY DISTRESS

Diseases of the lower respiratory tract can compromise the lung's function of oxygenating the blood through a variety of mechanisms (see Chapter 20, Blood Gas Analysis). Clinical signs

Physical examination findings that assist in localizing the cause of respiratory compromise to the lower respiratory tract, excluding the intrathoracic large airways, include: rapid and often shallow respirations; increased inspiratory or expiratory efforts, or both; and abnormal lung sounds on auscultation (see Chapter 26). Intrathoracic large airway obstruction generally results in normal to slightly increased respiratory rate; prolonged, labored expiration; and audible or auscultable expiratory sounds (see Chapter 26).

# DIAGNOSTIC APPROACH TO DOGS AND CATS WITH LOWER RESPIRATORY TRACT DISEASE

## INITIAL DIAGNOSTIC EVALUATION

The initial diagnostic evaluation of dogs or cats with signs of lower respiratory tract disease includes a complete history, physical examination, thoracic radiographs, and complete blood count (CBC). Further diagnostic tests are selected based on information obtained from these procedures; these include the evaluation of specimens collected from the lower respiratory tract, tests for specific diseases, and arterial blood gas analysis. Historical information was discussed in previous paragraphs.

### Physical Examination

A complete physical examination, including a fundic examination, is warranted to identify signs of disease that may be concurrently or secondarily affecting the lungs (e.g., systemic mycoses, metastatic neoplasia, megaesophagus). The cardiovascular system should be carefully evaluated. Mitral insufficiency murmurs are frequently auscultated in older, small-breed dogs brought to the clinician with the primary complaint of cough. Mitral insufficiency is often an incidental finding, but the clinician must consider both cardiac and respiratory tract diseases as differential diagnoses in these animals. Mitral insufficiency can lead to left atrial enlargement with compression of the mainstem bronchi, causing cough, or to congestive heart failure. Dogs in congestive heart failure are nearly always tachycardic. Other signs of heart disease include prolonged capillary refill time, weak or irregular pulses, abnormal jugular pulses, ascites or subcutaneous edema, gallop rhythms, and pulse deficits. Thoracic radiographs and occasionally echocardiography may be needed before cardiac problems can be comfortably ruled out as a cause of lower respiratory tract signs.

**Thoracic auscultation.** Careful auscultation of the upper airways and lungs is a critical component of the physical examination in dogs and cats with respiratory tract signs. Auscultation should be performed in a quiet location with the animal calm. Panting and purring do not result in deep inspiration, precluding evaluation of lung sounds. The heart and upper airways should be auscultated first. The clinician can then mentally subtract the contribution of these sounds from the sounds auscultated over the lung fields.

Initially, the stethoscope is placed over the trachea near the larynx. Discontinuous snoring or snorting sounds can be referred from the nasal cavity and pharynx as a result of obstructions stemming from structural abnormalities, such as an elongated soft palate or mass lesions, and excessive mucus or exudate. Wheezes, which are continuous high-pitched sounds, occur in animals with obstructive laryngeal diseases, such as laryngeal paralysis, neoplasia, inflammation, or foreign bodies. Discontinuous snoring sounds and wheezes are known as *stertor* and *stridor,* respectively, when they can be heard without a stethoscope. The entire cervical trachea is then auscultated for areas of high-pitched sounds caused by localized airway narrowing. Several breaths are auscultated with the stethoscope in each position, and the phase of respiration in which abnormal sounds occur is noted. Abnormal sounds resulting from extrathoracic disease are generally loudest during inspiration.

The lungs are auscultated next. Normally the lungs extend cranially to the thoracic inlet and caudally to about the seventh rib ventrally along the sternum and to approximately the ninth intercostal space dorsally along the spine. The cranioventral, central, and dorsal lung fields on both the left and right sides are auscultated systematically. Any asymmetry in the sounds between the left and right sides is abnormal.

Normal lung sounds have been described as a mixture of "bronchial" and "vesicular" sounds, although all sounds originate from the large airways. The bronchial sounds are most prominent in the central regions of the lungs. They are tubular sounds similar in character to those heard over the trachea, but they are quieter. Vesicular sounds are most prominent in the peripheral lung fields. They are soft and have been likened to a breeze blowing through leaves. These normal sounds are often described as "normal breath sounds."

Decreased lung sounds over one or both sides of the thorax occur in dogs and cats with pleural effusion, pneumothorax, diaphragmatic hernia, or mass lesions. Surprisingly, consolidated lung lobes and mass lesions can result in enhanced lung sounds because of the improved transmission of airway sounds from adjacent lobes. Abnormal lungs sounds are described as increased breath sounds (alternatively, harsh lung sounds), crackles, or wheezes. Increased breath sounds are a subtle finding, but are common in patients with pulmonary edema or pneumonia. *Crackles* are nonmusical, discontinuous noises that sound like paper being crumpled or bubbles popping. Diseases resulting in the formation of edema or an exudate within the airways (e.g., pulmonary edema, pneumonias, bronchitis) and some interstitial lung diseases, particularly interstitial fibrosis, can result in crackles. *Wheezes* are musical, continuous sounds that indicate the presence of airway narrowing. Narrowing can occur as a result of bronchoconstriction, bronchial wall thickening, exudate or fluid within the bronchial lumen, masses, or external airway compression. They are most commonly heard in cats with bronchitis. Wheezes caused by an intrathoracic airway obstruction are loudest during early expiration. Sudden snapping at the end of expiration can be heard in some dogs with intrathoracic tracheal collapse.

## Radiographs

Thoracic radiographs are indicated in dogs and cats with lower respiratory tract signs. Neck radiographs should also be obtained in animals with suspected tracheal disease. Radiography is perhaps the single most helpful diagnostic tool in the evaluation of dogs and cats with intrathoracic disease. It helps in localizing the problem to an organ system (i.e., cardiac, pulmonary, mediastinal, pleural), identifying the area of involvement within the lower respiratory tract (i.e., vascular, bronchial, alveolar, interstitial), and narrowing the list of potential differential diagnoses. It also helps in the formulation of a diagnostic plan (see Chapter 20). Additional diagnostic tests are necessary in most animals to establish a definitive diagnosis.

## Complete Blood Count

The CBC of patients with lower respiratory tract disease may show the anemia of inflammatory disease, polycythemia secondary to chronic hypoxia, or a white blood cell response characteristic of an inflammatory process of the lungs. The hematologic changes are insensitive, however, and an absence of abnormalities cannot be used as the basis for ruling out inflammatory lung diseases. For instance, only half of dogs with bacterial pneumonia have a neutrophilic leukocytosis and left shift.

Abnormalities are also not specific. For instance, eosinophilia is commonly encountered as a result of hypersensitivity or parasitic disease involving organs other than the lung.

## FURTHER DIAGNOSTIC EVALUATION

Based on results of the history, physical examination, thoracic radiographs, and CBC, a prioritized list of differential diagnoses is developed. Additional diagnostic tests (Fig. 19-1) are nearly always required to achieve a definitive diagnosis (necessary for optimal therapy and outcome). Selection of appropriate tests is based on the most likely differential diagnoses, the localization of disease within the lower respiratory tract (e.g., diffuse bronchial disease, single mass lesion), the degree of respiratory compromise of the patient, and the particular client's motivation for optimal care.

Invasive and noninvasive tests are available. Noninvasive tests have the obvious advantage of being nearly risk free but are usually aimed at confirming a specific diagnosis. Most patients with lower respiratory tract disease require collection of a pulmonary specimen for microscopic and microbiologic analysis to further narrow the list of differential diagnoses or to make a definitive diagnosis. Although the procedures for specimen collection from the lung are considered invasive, they carry varying degrees of risk, depending upon the procedure used and the degree of respiratory compromise of the patient. The risk is minimal in many instances.

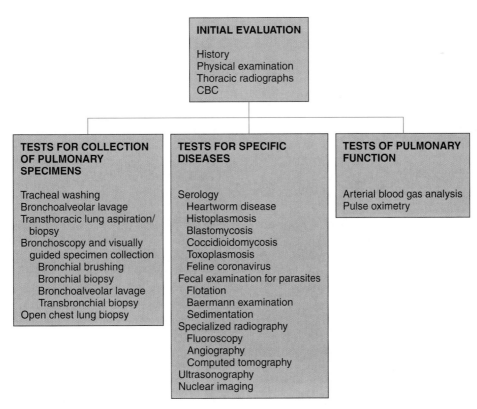

**FIG 19-1**

Diagnostic approach for dogs and cats with lower respiratory tract disease.

Noninvasive tests include serology for pulmonary pathogens, fecal examinations for parasites, and specialized radiographic techniques such as fluoroscopy, angiography, computerized tomograms (CTs), ultrasonography, and nuclear imaging. Techniques for collection of pulmonary specimens that can be performed without specialized equipment include tracheal wash, bronchoalveolar lavage, and transthoracic lung aspiration. Visually guided specimens can be collected during bronchoscopy. Bronchoscopy has the additional benefit of allowing visual assessment of the airways. If analysis of lung specimens and results of reasonable noninvasive tests do not provide a diagnosis in a patient with progressive disease, thoracotomy and lung biopsy are indicated.

Valuable information about patients with lower respiratory tract disease can also be obtained by assessing lung function through arterial blood gas analysis. Results are rarely helpful in making a final diagnosis, but they are useful in determining degree of compromise and in monitoring response to therapy. Pulse oximetry, a noninvasive technique to measure oxygen saturation of the blood, is particularly valuable in monitoring patients with respiratory compromise during anesthetic procedures or respiratory crises.

## Suggested Readings

Hamlin RL: Physical examination of the pulmonary system, *Vet Clin N Am Small Anim Pract* 30:1175, 2000.

Kotlikoff MI et al: Lung sounds in veterinary medicine. Part II. Deriving clinical information from lung sounds, *Compend Cont Ed Pract Vet* 6:462, 1984.

# CHAPTER 20

# Diagnostic Tests for the Lower Respiratory Tract

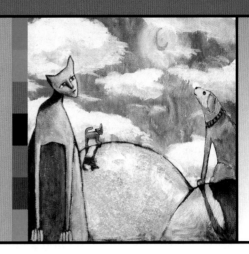

## CHAPTER OUTLINE

THORACIC RADIOGRAPHY, 255
    General principles, 255
    Trachea, 256
    Lungs, 256
ANGIOGRAPHY, 262
ULTRASONOGRAPHY, 262
COMPUTED TOMOGRAPHY AND MAGNETIC
RESONANCE IMAGING, 262
NUCLEAR IMAGING, 262
PARASITOLOGIC EVALUATION, 262
SEROLOGIC TESTS FOR PULMONARY
PATHOGENS, 264
TRACHEAL WASH, 264
NONBRONCHOSCOPIC BRONCHOALVEOLAR
LAVAGE, 270
TRANSTHORACIC LUNG ASPIRATION
AND BIOPSY, 274
BRONCHOSCOPY, 276
OPEN-CHEST LUNG BIOPSY
AND THORACOSCOPY, 281
BLOOD GAS ANALYSIS, 281
PULSE OXIMETRY, 285

## THORACIC RADIOGRAPHY

### GENERAL PRINCIPLES

Thoracic radiographs play an integral role in the diagnostic evaluation of dogs and cats with clinical signs related to the lower respiratory tract. They are also indicated for the evaluation of animals with vague, nonspecific signs of disease to detect occult pulmonary disease. Thoracic radiographs can be helpful in localizing disease processes, narrowing and prioritizing the differential diagnoses, determining the extent of disease involvement, and monitoring the progression of disease and response to treatment.

A minimum of two views of the thorax should be taken in all dogs and cats. Usually, right lateral and ventrodorsal (VD) views are preferred. The sensitivity of radiographs in the detection of lesions is improved if both right and left lateral views are obtained. These are indicated if disease of the right middle lung lobe, metastatic disease, or other subtle changes are suspected. The side of the lung away from the table is more aerated, thereby providing more contrast for soft-tissue opacities, and is slightly magnified compared with the side against the table. Dorsoventral (DV) views are taken to evaluate the dorsal pulmonary arteries in animals with suspected heartworm disease. The combination of DV and VD views has the same advantages as the combination of right and left lateral views in detecting subtle changes in the dorsally oriented vessels. DV, rather than VD, views are taken to minimize stress in animals in respiratory distress. Horizontal-beam lateral radiographs with the animal standing can be used to evaluate animals with suspected cavitary lesions or pleural effusion.

Careful technique is essential to ensure that thoracic radiographs are obtained that yield useful information. Poor technique can lead to either underinterpretation or overinterpretation of abnormalities. Appropriate film, settings, and development procedures should be used, and the films should be interpreted using proper lighting. The settings used are recorded so that the same technique can be used when obtaining future films, thereby allowing for more critical comparison of the progression of disease. The dog or cat should be restrained adequately to prevent movement, and a short exposure time is used.

Radiographs should be taken during maximum inspiration. Fully expanded lungs provide the most air contrast for soft-tissue opacities, and motion is also minimized during this phase of the respiratory cycle. Radiographic indications of maximum inspiration include widening of the angle between the diaphragm and vertebral column (representing maximal expansion of caudal lung lobes), a lucent region in front of the heart shadow (representing maximal expansion of the cranial lung lobes), flattening of the diaphragm, minimal contact between the heart and the diaphragm, and a well-delineated, nearly horizontal vena cava. Radiographs of the lungs obtained during phases of respiration other than peak inspiration are difficult to interpret. For example, incomplete expansion of the lungs can cause increased pulmonary opacities to be seen that appear pathologic, resulting in misdiagnosis.

Animals that are panting should be allowed to calm down before thoracic radiographs are obtained. A paper bag can be placed over the animal's muzzle to increase the concentration of carbon dioxide in the inspired air, causing the animal to take deeper breaths. It may be necessary to sedate some animals.

All structures within the thorax should be evaluated systematically in every animal. One reason for this is that extrapulmonary abnormalities may develop secondary to pulmonary disease and may be the only radiographic finding (e.g., subcutaneous emphysema after tracheal laceration). Conversely, the pulmonary system may be secondarily involved. For example, mass lesions such as tumors or abscesses may extend into the thoracic cavity, displacing the lung parenchyma medially. Excessive fat deposition can prevent full expansion of the lungs. Diaphragmatic hernias can appear as generalized or localized soft-tissue opacities that obscure the diaphragm-lung interface. A thorough evaluation of all structures on the radiographs enhances diagnostic accuracy and thus should always be done.

## TRACHEA

The trachea and, in young animals, the thymus are recognizable in the cranial mediastinum. Radiographs of the cervical trachea must also be taken in dogs and cats with suspected upper airway obstruction or primary tracheal disease, most notably tracheal collapse. When evaluating the trachea, it is important to obtain radiographs of the cervical portion during inspiration and of the thorax during both inspiration and expiration.

Only the inner wall of the trachea should be visible. If the outer wall of the trachea is identified, this is suggestive of pneumomediastinum. The trachea normally has a uniform diameter and is straight, deviating ventrally from the vertebral bodies on lateral views as it progresses toward the carina. It may appear elevated near the carina if the heart is enlarged or there is a pleural effusion. Flexion or extension of the neck may cause bowing of the trachea. On VD views, the trachea may deviate to the right of midline in some dogs. The tracheal cartilage becomes calcified in some older dogs and chondrodystrophic breeds.

The overall size and continuity of the tracheal lumen should also be evaluated. The normal tracheal lumen is nearly as wide as the laryngeal lumen. Hypoplastic tracheas have a lumen less than half the normal size (Fig. 20-1). Strictures and fractured cartilage rings can cause an abrupt, localized narrowing of the air stripe. Mass lesions in the tissues adjacent to the trachea can compress the trachea, causing a more gradual, localized narrowing of the air stripe. In animals with extrathoracic tracheal collapse, the tracheal air stripe is narrowed in the cervical region during inspiration. In animals with intrathoracic tracheal collapse, the air stripe is narrowed on thoracic films during expiration. Fluoroscopy, available primarily through referral centers, provides a more sensitive assessment of tracheal collapse. Finally, the air contrast of the trachea sometimes allows foreign bodies or masses to be vi-

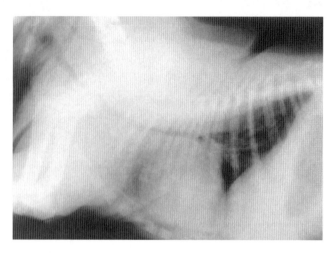

**FIG 20-1**
Lateral radiograph of a Bulldog with a hypoplastic trachea. The tracheal lumen is less than half the size of the larynx.

sualized within the trachea. Most foreign bodies lodge at the level of the carina or within the bronchi. The inability to radiographically identify a foreign body does not rule out the diagnosis, however.

## LUNGS

The clinician must be careful not to overinterpret lung abnormalities on thoracic radiographs. A definitive diagnosis is not possible in most animals, and microscopic examination of pulmonary specimens, further evaluation of the heart, or testing for specific diseases is necessary. The lungs are examined for the possible presence of four major abnormal patterns: vascular, bronchial, alveolar, and interstitial. Mass lesions are considered interstitial patterns. Lung lobe consolidation, atelectasis, pulmonary cysts, and lung lobe torsions are other potential abnormalities. Animals with severe respiratory distress but normal thoracic radiograph findings usually have thromboembolic disease or have suffered a very recent insult to the lungs, such as trauma or aspiration.

### Vascular Pattern

The pulmonary vasculature is assessed by evaluating the vessels to the cranial lung lobes on the lateral view and the vessels to the caudal lung lobes on the VD or DV view. Normally, the blood vessels should taper gradually from the left atrium (pulmonary vein) or right atrium (pulmonary arteries) toward the periphery of the lungs. Companion arteries and veins should be similar in size. Arteries and veins have a consistent relationship with each other and the associated bronchus. On lateral radiographs the pulmonary artery is dorsal and the pulmonary vein is ventral to the bronchus. On VD or DV radiographs the pulmonary artery is lateral and the pulmonary vein is medial to the bronchus. Vessels that are pointed directly toward or away from the x-ray beam are "end-on" and appear as circular nodules. They are distinguished from lesions by their association with a linear vessel and adjacent bronchus.

## TABLE 20-1

**Differential Diagnoses for Dogs and Cats with Abnormal Pulmonary Vascular Patterns on Thoracic Radiographs**

**Enlarged Arteries**

Heartworm disease
Thromboembolic disease
Pulmonary hypertension

**Enlarged Veins**

Left-sided heart failure

**Enlarged Arteries and Veins (Pulmonary Overcirculation)**

Left-to-right shunts
   Patent ductus arteriosus
   Ventricular septal defect
   Atrial septal defect

**Small Arteries and Veins**

Pulmonary undercirculation
   Cardiovascular shock
   Hypovolemia
      Severe dehydration
      Blood loss
      Hypoadrenocorticism
   Pulmonic valve stenosis
Hyperinflation of the lungs
   Feline bronchitis
   Allergic bronchitis

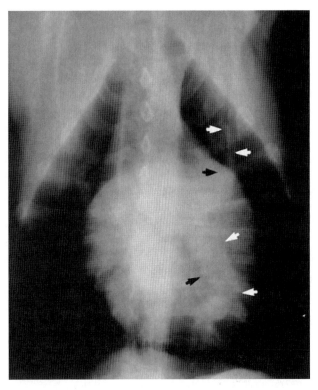

**FIG 20-2**
Dilation of pulmonary arteries is apparent on this ventro-dorsal view of the thorax in a dog with heartworm disease. The artery to the left caudal lung lobe is extremely enlarged. *Arrowheads* delineate the borders of the arteries to the left cranial and caudal lobes.

Abnormal vascular patterns generally involve an increase or decrease in the size of arteries or veins (Table 20-1). The finding of arteries larger than their companion veins indicates the presence of pulmonary hypertension or thromboembolism, most commonly caused by heartworm disease, a finding seen in both dogs and cats (Fig. 20-2). The pulmonary arteries often appear tortuous and truncated in such animals. Concurrent enlargement of the main pulmonary artery and right side of the heart may be seen in affected dogs. There may also be interstitial, bronchial, or alveolar infiltrates in cats and dogs with heartworm disease as a result of concurrent inflammation, edema, or hemorrhage.

Veins larger than their companion arteries indicate the presence of congestion resulting from left-sided heart failure. Pulmonary edema may also be present.

Dilation of both arteries and veins is an unusual finding, except in young animals. The finding of pulmonary overcirculation is suggestive of left-to-right cardiac or vascular shunts, such as patent ductus arteriosus and ventricular septal defects.

The finding of smaller than normal arteries and veins can indicate the presence of pulmonary undercirculation or hyperinflation. Undercirculation most often occurs in combination with microcardia resulting from hypoadrenocorticism or other causes of severe hypovolemia. Pulmonic stenosis may also cause radiographically visible undercirculation in

some dogs. Hyperinflation is associated with obstructive airway disease, such as feline bronchitis.

## Bronchial Pattern

Bronchial walls are normally most easily discernible radiographically at the hilus. They should taper and thin as they extend toward the periphery of each lung lobe. Bronchial structures are not normally visible radiographically in the peripheral regions of the lungs. The cartilage may be calcified in older dogs and chondrodystrophic breeds, making the walls more prominent but still sharply defined.

A bronchial pattern is caused by thickening of the bronchial walls or bronchial dilation. Thickened bronchial walls are visible as "tram lines" and "doughnuts" in the peripheral regions of the lung (Fig. 20-3). Tram lines are produced by airways that run transverse to the x-ray beam, causing the appearance of parallel thick lines with an air stripe in between. "Doughnuts" are produced by airways that are pointing directly toward or away from the beam, causing a thick circle to be seen radiographically, with the airway lumen creating the "hole." The walls of the bronchi tend to be indistinct. The finding of thickened walls indicates the presence of bronchitis and results from an accumulation of mucus or exudate along the walls within the lumens, an infiltration of inflammatory cells within the walls, muscular hypertrophy, epithelial hyperplasia,

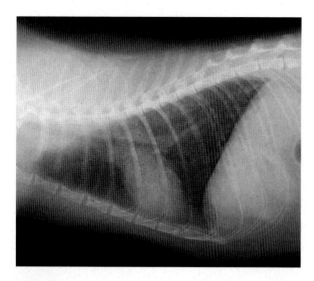

**FIG 20-3**
Lateral view of the thorax in a cat with allergic bronchitis, depicting a bronchial pattern. Thickened bronchial walls result in soft-tissue dense, parallel "tram lines" that extend into peripheral regions of the lungs.

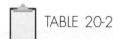

TABLE 20-2

**Differential Diagnoses for Dogs and Cats with Bronchial Patterns on Thoracic Radiographs\***

Feline bronchitis
Allergic bronchitis
Bacterial bronchitis
Canine chronic bronchitis
Bronchiectasis
Pulmonary parasites

*Bronchial disease can occur in conjunction with parenchymal lung disease. See Tables 20-3 to 20-5 for more differential diagnoses if mixed patterns are present.

or a combination of these changes. Potential causes of bronchial disease are listed in Table 20-2.

Chronic bronchial disease can result in irreversible dilation of the airways, which is termed *bronchiectasis*. It is identified radiographically by the presence of widened, nontapering airways (Fig. 20-4). Bronchiectasis can be cylindrical (tubular) or saccular (cystic). Cylindrical bronchiectasis is characterized by fairly uniform dilation of the airway. Saccular bronchiectasis additionally has localized dilations peripherally that can lead to a honey-comb appearance. All major bronchi are usually affected.

## Alveolar Pattern

Alveoli are not normally visible radiographically. Alveolar patterns occur when the alveoli are filled with fluid-dense material. The fluid opacity may be caused by edema, inflammation, hemorrhage, or neoplastic infiltrates, which generally originate from the interstitial tissues (Table 20-3). The fluid-filled alveoli are silhouetted against the walls of the airways they surround. The result is a visible stripe of air from the airway lumen in the absence of definable airway walls. This stripe is an air bronchogram (Fig. 20-5). If the fluid continues to accumulate, the airway lumen will eventually also become filled with fluid, resulting in the formation of solid areas of fluid opacity, or *consolidation.*

Edema most often results from left-sided heart failure (see Chapter 22). In dogs the fluid initially accumulates in the perihilar region and eventually the entire lung is affected. In cats patchy areas of edema can be present initially throughout the lung fields. The finding of enlarged pulmonary veins supports the cardiac origin of the infiltrates. Noncardiogenic edema is discussed in Chapter 22.

Inflammatory infiltrates can be caused by infectious agents, noninfectious inflammatory disease, or neoplasia. The location of the infiltrative process can often help establish a tentative diagnosis. For example, diseases of airway origin, such as most bacterial and aspiration pneumonias, primarily affect the dependent lung lobes (i.e., the right middle and cranial lobes and the left cranial lobe). In contrast, diseases of arterial origin, such as dirofilariasis and thromboemboli, primarily affect the caudal lung lobes. Localized processes involving only one lung lobe suggest the presence of a foreign body, neoplasia, abscess, granuloma, or lung lobe torsion.

Hemorrhage most often results from trauma. Thromboembolism, neoplasia, coagulopathies, and fungal infections can also cause hemorrhage into the alveoli.

## Interstitial Pattern

The pulmonary interstitial tissues confer a fine, lacy pattern to the pulmonary parenchyma of many dogs and cats as they age, in the absence of clinically apparent respiratory disease. They are not normally visible on inspiratory films in young adult animals.

Abnormal interstitial patterns are reticular (unstructured), nodular, or reticulonodular in appearance. A nodular interstitial pattern is characterized by the finding of roughly circular, fluid-dense lesions in one or more lung lobes. However, the nodules must be nearly 1 cm in diameter to be routinely detected. Interstitial nodules may represent active inflammatory, inactive inflammatory, or neoplastic lesions (Table 20-4).

Active inflammatory nodules often have poorly defined borders. Mycotic infections typically result in the formation of multiple, diffuse nodules. The nodules may be small (miliary) (Fig. 20-6) or large and coalescing. Parasitic granulomas are often multiple, although paragonimiasis can result in the formation of a single pulmonary nodule. Abscesses can form as a result of foreign bodies or as a sequela to bacterial pneumonia. Nodular patterns may also be seen on the radiographs obtained in animals with some eosinophilic lung diseases and other noninfectious inflammatory diseases.

Inflammatory nodules can persist as inactive lesions after the disease resolves. In contrast to active inflammatory nodules, however, the borders of inactive nodules are often well demarcated. Nodules may also become mineralized in some conditions, such as histoplasmosis. Well-defined, small, inac-

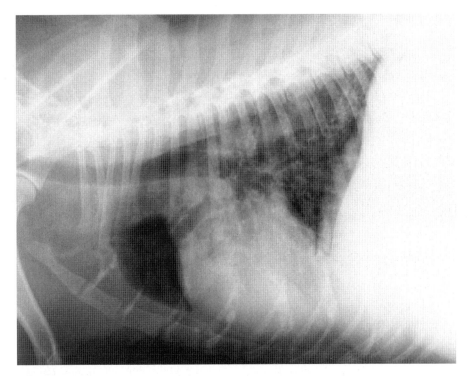

**FIG 20-4**
Lateral radiograph of a dog with chronic bronchitis and bronchiectasis. The airway lumens are greatly enlarged, and normal tapering of the airway walls is not seen.

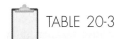 TABLE 20-3

**Differential Diagnoses for Dogs and Cats with Alveolar Patterns on Thoracic Radiographs***

**Pulmonary Edema**

**Severe Inflammatory Disease**

Bacterial pneumonia
Aspiration pneumonia

**Hemorrhage**

Pulmonary contusion
Thromboembolic disease
Neoplasia
Fungal pneumonia
Systemic coagulopathy

*Any of the differential diagnoses for interstitial patterns (Tables 20-4 and 20-5) can cause an alveolar pattern if associated with severe inflammation, edema, or hemorrhage.

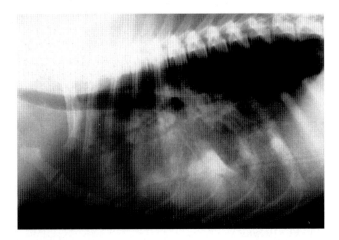

**FIG 20-5**
Lateral view of the thorax of a dog with aspiration pneumonia. An alveolar pattern is evidenced by the increased soft-tissue opacity with air bronchograms. Air bronchograms are bronchial air stripes without visible bronchial walls. This pattern is most severe in the ventral (dependent) regions of the lung.

tive nodules are sometimes seen in healthy older dogs without a history of disease. Radiographs taken several months later in these animals typically show no change in the size of these inactive lesions.

Neoplastic nodules may be singular or multiple (Fig. 20-7). They are often well defined, although secondary inflammation, edema, or hemorrhage can obscure the margins. There

is no radiographic pattern that is diagnostic for neoplasia. Lesions caused by parasites, fungal infections, and noninfectious inflammatory diseases can be indistinguishable from neoplastic lesions. In the absence of strong clinical evidence, malignant neoplasia must be confirmed cytologically or histologically. If this is not possible, radiographs can be obtained again 4 weeks later to evaluate for progression of disease.

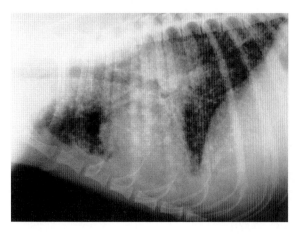

**FIG 20-6**
Lateral view of the thorax in a dog with blastomycosis. A miliary, nodular interstitial pattern is present. Increased soft-tissue opacity above the base of heart may be the result of hilar lymphadenopathy.

## TABLE 20-4

**Differential Diagnoses for Dogs and Cats with Nodular Interstitial Patterns**

**Mycotic Infection**

Blastomycosis
Histoplasmosis
Coccidioidomycosis

**Neoplasia**

**Pulmonary Parasites**

*Aelurostrongylus* infection
*Paragonimus* infection

**Abscess**

Bacterial pneumonia
Foreign body

**Pulmonary Infiltrates with Eosinophils**

**Miscellaneous Inflammatory Diseases**

**Inactive Lesions**

Neoplastic involvement of the pulmonary parenchyma cannot be totally excluded on the basis of thoracic radiograph findings, because malignant cells are present for a while before lesions reach a radiographically detectable size. The sensitivity of radiography in identifying neoplastic nodules can be improved by obtaining left and right lateral views of the thorax.

The reticular interstitial pattern is characterized by a diffuse, unstructured, "lacy" increase in the opacity of the pulmonary interstitium, which partially obscures normal vascular and airway markings. Reticular interstitial patterns frequently occur in conjunction with nodular interstitial patterns (also called *reticulonodular patterns*) and alveolar and bronchial patterns (Fig. 20-8).

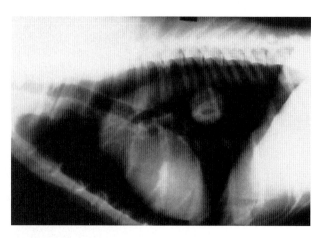

**FIG 20-7**
Lateral view of the thorax of a dog with malignant neoplasia. A well-circumscribed, solid, circular mass is present in the caudal lung field. Papillary adenocarcinoma was diagnosed after surgical excision.

The increased reticular interstitial opacity can result from edema, hemorrhage, inflammatory cells, neoplastic cells, or fibrosis within the interstitium (Table 20-5). The interstitial space surrounds the airways and vessels and is normally extremely small in dogs and cats. With the continued accumulation of fluid or cells, however, the alveoli can become flooded, and this produces an alveolar pattern. Visible focal interstitial accumulations of cells, or nodules, can also develop with time. Any of the diseases associated with alveolar and interstitial nodular patterns can cause a reticular interstitial pattern as long as the abnormal fluid or cells are present only in the interstitial space (see Tables 20-3 and 20-4). This pattern is also often seen in older dogs with no clinically apparent disease, presumably as a result of pulmonary fibrosis, further decreasing the specificity of the finding.

### Lung Lobe Consolidation

Lung lobe consolidation is characterized by a lung lobe that is entirely soft-tissue opacity. Consolidation occurs when an alveolar or interstitial disease process progresses to the point where the entire lobe is filled with fluid or cells. Common differential diagnoses for lung lobe consolidation are severe bacterial or aspiration pneumonia (essentially resulting in an abscess of the entire lobe), neoplasia, lung lobe torsion, and hemorrhage.

### Atelectasis

Atelectasis is also characterized by a lobe that is entirely soft-tissue opacity. In this instance the lobe is collapsed as a result of airway obstruction. All the air within the lobe has been absorbed and not replaced. It is distinguished from consolidation by the small size of the lobe and resultant shift in the heart toward the atelectatic lobe. Atelectasis is most commonly seen involving the right middle lobe of cats with bronchitis.

### Cavitary Lesions

Cavitary lung diseases include cysts and bullae. Cysts may be apparent as localized accumulations of air or fluid, often with a partially visible wall (Fig. 20-9). An air-fluid interface may be

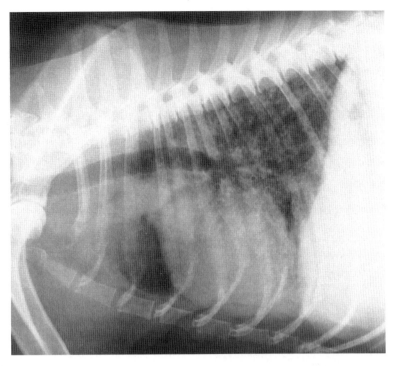

**FIG 20-8**
Lateral radiograph of a dog with pulmonary carcinoma. An unstructured interstitial pattern is present, as well as an increased bronchial pattern.

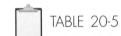 TABLE 20-5

**Differential Diagnoses for Dogs and Cats with Reticular (Unstructured) Interstitial Patterns**

**Pulmonary Edema (Mild)**

**Infection**

Viral pneumonia
Bacterial pneumonia
Toxoplasmosis
Mycotic pneumonia
Parasitic infection (more often bronchial or nodular interstitial pattern)

**Neoplasia**

**Pulmonary Fibrosis**

**Pulmonary Infiltrates with Eosinophils**

**Miscellaneous Inflammatory Diseases**

**Hemorrhage (Mild)**

visible using standing horizontal-beam projections. Cysts may be congenital, acquired, or idiopathic. They can be caused by *Paragonimus* infection, trauma, abscess, neoplasia, lung infarction (from thromboembolism), and granulomas. Bullae are most often a result of chronic airway disease (emphysema) and are rarely apparent radiographically.

Cavitary lesions may be discovered on thoracic radiographs of dogs and cats with spontaneous pneumothorax or incidentally. If pneumothorax is present, surgical excision is usually indicated (see Chapter 25). If inflammatory or neoplastic disease is suspected, further diagnostic testing is indicated. If the lesion is found incidentally, animals can be periodically reevaluated radiographically to determine whether the lesion is progressing or resolving. If the lesion does not resolve during the course of 1 to 3 months, surgical removal is considered for diagnostic purposes and to avoid potentially life-threatening spontaneous pneumothorax.

## Lung Lobe Torsion

Lung lobe torsion can develop spontaneously in deep-chested dogs or as a complication of a pleural effusion or pneumonectomy in dogs and cats. The right middle and left cranial lobes are most commonly involved. The lobe usually twists at the hilus, obstructing the flow of blood into and out of the lung lobe. Usually, venous drainage is obstructed before arterial flow, causing the lung lobe to become congested with blood. Over time, air is absorbed from the alveoli and atelectasis occurs.

Lung lobe torsion is difficult to identify radiographically. Severe bacterial or aspiration pneumonia resulting in consolidation of these same lobes is far more common and produces similar radiographic changes. The finding of pulmonary vessels or bronchi traveling in an abnormal direction is strongly suggestive of torsion. Unfortunately, pleural fluid, if not present initially, often develops and obscures the radiographic image of the affected lobe. Ultrasonography is often useful in detecting a torsed lung lobe. Bronchoscopy, bronchography, or thoracotomy is necessary to confirm the diagnosis in some animals.

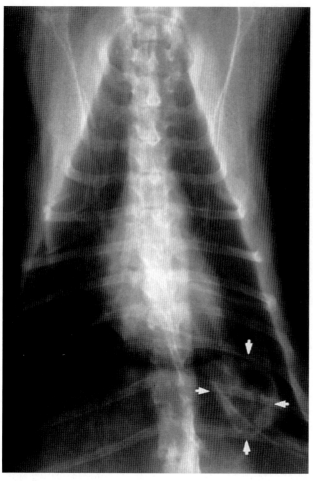

**FIG 20-9**
Ventrodorsal view of the thorax in a cat showing a cystic lesion *(arrowheads)* in the left caudal lung lobe.

## ANGIOGRAPHY

Angiography is used as a confirmatory test in cats with presumptive dirofilariasis but negative adult antigen blood test results and echocardiographic findings (see Chapter 10). Angiography is also used to confirm a diagnosis of thromboembolic disease. Obstructed arteries are blunted or do not show the normal gentle taper and arborization. Arteries may appear dilated and tortuous. There may also be localized areas of extravasated contrast agent. If several days have elapsed since the embolization occurred, however, lesions may no longer be identifiable; angiography should therefore be performed as soon as the disorder is suspected and the animal's condition is stabilized.

## ULTRASONOGRAPHY

Ultrasonography is used to evaluate pulmonary mass lesions adjacent to the body wall, diaphragm, or heart, and also consolidated lung lobes. Because air interferes with the sound waves, aerated lungs and structures surrounded by aerated lungs cannot be examined. The consistency of lesions often can be determined to be solid, cystic, or fluid filled. Some solid masses are hypolucent and appear to be cystic on ultrasonograms. Vascular structures may be visible, particularly with Doppler ultrasound, and this can be helpful in identifying lung lobe torsion. Ultrasonography can also be used to guide biopsy instruments into solid masses for specimen collection. It is also used for evaluating the heart in animals with clinical signs that cannot be readily localized to either the cardiac or respiratory systems. Using ultrasonography to evaluate animals with pleural disorders is discussed in Chapter 24.

## COMPUTED TOMOGRAPHY AND MAGNETIC RESONANCE IMAGING

Computed tomography (CT) and magnetic resonance imaging (MRI) are used routinely in human medicine for the diagnostic evaluation of lung disease. They are more sensitive and specific in the diagnosis of certain airway and parenchymal diseases. The application of these techniques to the diagnosis of specific canine and feline pulmonary diseases needs to be investigated.

These three-dimensional imaging techniques do provide helpful information in the preoperative evaluation of potential surgical candidates. The extent and location of disease and the potential involvement of other structures such as the major vessels can be assessed more accurately than with routine radiography.

## NUCLEAR IMAGING

Nuclear imaging can be used for the relatively noninvasive measurement of pulmonary perfusion and ventilation. Restrictions for handling radioisotopes and the need for specialized recording equipment limit the availability of these tools to specialty centers.

## PARASITOLOGIC EVALUATION

Parasites involving the lower respiratory tract are identified by direct observation, blood tests, cytologic analysis of respiratory tract specimens, or fecal examinations. *Oslerus osleri* reside in nodules near the carina, which can be identified bronchoscopically. Rarely, other parasites may be seen. Blood tests are often used to diagnose heartworm disease (see Chapter 10).

Larvae that may be present in fluid from tracheal or bronchial washings include *O. osleri*, *Aelurostrongylus abstrusus* (Fig. 20-10, *A*), and *Crenosoma vulpis*. Eggs that may be present include those of *Capillaria aerophila* and *Paragonimus kellicotti* (Fig. 20-10, *B* and *C*). Larvated eggs or larvae from *Filaroides hirthi* or *Aelurostrongylus milksi* can be present but are rarely associated with clinical signs. Larvated eggs can also be retrieved from *C. vulpis*. The more common organisms are described in Table 20-6.

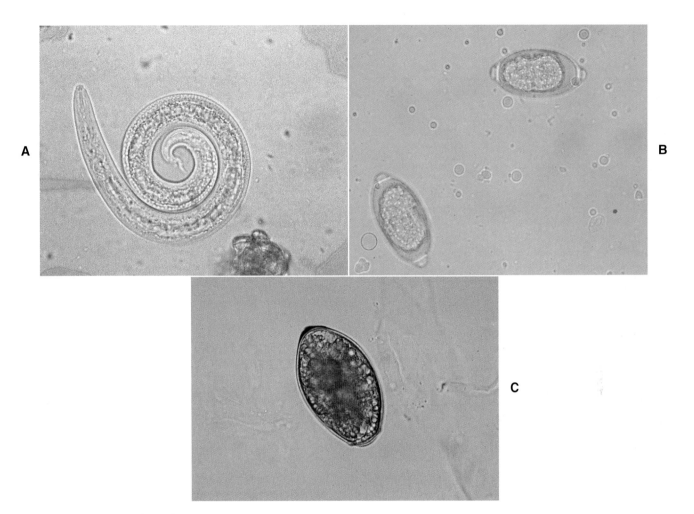

**FIG 20-10**
**A,** Larva of *Aelurostrongylus abstrusus.* **B,** Double operculated ova of *Capillaria* sp. **C,** Single operculated ova of *Paragonimus kellicotti.*

 TABLE 20-6

Characteristics of Eggs or Larvae from Respiratory Parasites

| PARASITE | HOST | STAGE | SOURCE | DESCRIPTION |
|---|---|---|---|---|
| *Capillaria aerophila* | Dog and cat | Egg | Routine flotation of feces, airway specimens | Barrel shaped, yellow, with prominent, transparent, asymmetric bipolar plugs; slightly smaller than *Trichuris* eggs; 60-80 μm × 30-40 μm |
| *Paragonimus kellicotti* | Dog and cat | Egg | High-density flotation or sedimentation of feces, airway specimens | Oval, golden-brown, single, operculated; operculum flat with prominent shoulders; 75-118 μm × 42-67 μm |
| *Aelurostrongylus abstrusus* | Cat | Larvae | Baermann technique for feces, airway specimens | Larvae with S-shaped tail; dorsal spine present; 350-400 μm × 17 μm; eggs or larvated eggs may be seen in airway specimens |
| *Oslerus osleri* | Dog | Larvae, egg | Tracheal wash, bronchial brushing of nodules, zinc sulfate flotation of feces | Larvae have S-shaped tail without dorsal spine; rarely found eggs are thin-walled, colorless, and larvated; 80 × 50 μm |
| *Crenosoma vulpis* | Dog | Larvae, larvated eggs | Baermann technique for feces (larvae), airway specimens (larvated eggs or larvae) | Larvae have tapered tail without severe kinks or spines; 250-300 μm |

## TABLE 20-7

**Sedimentation of Feces for Concentration of Eggs**

1. Homogenize 1 to 3 g of feces with water (at least 30 ml).
2. Pass through coarse sieve or gauze (250-μm mesh), washing debris remaining in sieve with fine spray of water.
3. Pour filtrate into conical urine flask and let stand for 2 minutes.
4. Discard most of supernate.
5. Pour remaining 12 to 15 ml into flat-bottomed tube and let stand for 2 minutes.
6. Draw off supernate.
7. Add 2 to 3 drops of 5% methylene blue.
8. Examine under low power.

Modified from Urquhart GM et al: *Veterinary parasitology,* New York, 1987, Churchill Livingstone.

## TABLE 20-8

**Baermann Technique for Concentration of Larvae**

1. Set up apparatus.
   a. Glass funnel supported in ring stand
   b. Rubber tube attached to bottom of funnel with a clamp
   c. Coarse sieve (250-μm mesh) placed in top of funnel
   d. Double-layer gauze on top of sieve
2. Place feces on gauze in funnel.
3. Fill funnel slowly with water to immerse feces.
4. Leave overnight at room temperature.
5. Collect water via rubber tube from neck of funnel in a small beaker.
6. Examine under low power.

Modified from Urquhart GM et al: *Veterinary parasitology,* New York, 1987, Churchill Livingstone.

The hosts of lung parasites generally cough up and swallow the eggs or larvae, which are then passed in the feces to infect the next host or an intermediate host. Fecal examination for eggs or larvae is a simple, noninvasive tool for the diagnosis of such infestations. However, because shedding is intermittent, parasitic disease cannot be included solely on the basis of negative fecal examination findings. Multiple (at least three) examinations should be performed in animals that are highly suspected of having parasitic disease. If possible, several days should be allowed to elapse between each collection of feces.

Routine fecal flotation can be used to concentrate eggs from *C. aerophila.* High-density fecal flotation (specific gravity [s.g.], 1.30 to 1.35) can be used to concentrate *P. kellicotti* eggs. Sedimentation techniques are preferred for concentrating and identifying *P. kellicotti* eggs, particularly if few eggs are present. Larvae are identified through the use of the Baermann technique. However, *O. osleri* larvae are insufficiently

motile for reliable identification with this technique, and zinc sulfate (s.g., 1.18) flotation is recommended. Even so, false-negative results are common. All of these techniques can be readily performed at minimal expense. Methods for sedimentation and the Baermann technique are described in Tables 20-7 and 20-8.

*Toxoplasma gondii* occasionally causes pneumonia in dogs and cats. Dogs do not shed *Toxoplasma* organisms in the feces, but cats may. However, the shedding of eggs is part of the direct life cycle of the organisms and does not correlate with the presence of systemic disease resulting from the indirect cycle. Infection is therefore diagnosed on the basis of the finding of tachyzoites in pulmonary specimens or indirectly on the basis of serologic findings.

Migrating intestinal parasites can cause transient pulmonary signs in young animals. Migration occurs primarily before the mature adults develop in the intestine, and eggs may therefore not be found in feces.

## SEROLOGIC TESTS FOR PULMONARY PATHOGENS

Serologic tests can detect a variety of pulmonary pathogens. Antibody tests provide only indirect evidence of infection, however. In general, they should be used only to confirm a suspected diagnosis, not to screen for disease. Whenever possible, identification of the infectious organisms is the preferred method of diagnosis. Tests available for common pulmonary pathogens include those for *Histoplasma, Blastomyces, Coccidiodomyces, Toxoplasma,* and feline coronavirus. These tests are discussed fully in Chapter 97. Antibody tests for dirofilariasis are also available and are used primarily to support the diagnosis of feline heartworm disease (see Chapter 10). Serum antigen tests for *Cryptococcus* (see Chapter 103) and adult heartworms are also available (see Chapter 10).

## TRACHEAL WASH

### Indications and Complications

Tracheal washing can yield valuable diagnostic information in animals with cough or respiratory distress resulting from disease of the airways or pulmonary parenchyma and in animals with vague presenting signs and pulmonary abnormalities detected on thoracic radiographs (i.e., most animals with lower respiratory tract disease). Tracheal washing is generally performed after results of the history, physical examination, thoracic radiography, and other routine components of the database are known.

Tracheal washing provides fluid and cells that can be used to identify diseases involving the major airways while bypassing the normal flora and debris of the oral cavity and pharynx. The fluid obtained is evaluated cytologically and microbiologically and therefore should be collected before the initiation of antibiotic treatment whenever possible. Tracheal washing is likely to provide a representative specimen in patients with bronchial or diffuse alveolar disease. It is less

TABLE 20-9

**Comparisons of Techniques for Collecting Specimens from the Lower Respiratory Tract**

| TECHNIQUE | SITE OF COLLECTION | SPECIMEN SIZE | ADVANTAGES | DISADVANTAGES | INDICATIONS |
|---|---|---|---|---|---|
| Tracheal wash | Large airways | Moderate | Simple technique<br>Minimal expense<br>No special equipment<br>Complications rare<br>Volume adequate for cytology and culture | Airway must be involved for specimen to represent disease | Bronchial and alveolar disease<br>Because of safety and ease, consider for any lung disease<br>Less likely to be representative of interstitial or small focal processes |
| Bronchoalveolar lavage | Small airways, alveoli, sometimes interstitium | Large | Simple technique<br>Nonbronchoscopic technique requires no special equipment and minimal expense<br>Bronchoscopic technique allows airway evaluation and directed sampling<br>Resultant hypoxemia is transient and responsive to oxygen supplementation<br>Safe for animals in stable condition<br>Large volume of lung sampled (millions of alveoli)<br>High cytologic quality<br>Large volume for analysis | General anesthesia required<br>Special equipment and expertise required for bronchoscopic collection<br>Not recommended for animals in respiratory distress<br>Capability to provide oxygen supplementation is required | Small airway, alveolar, or interstitial disease<br>Routine during bronchoscopy |
| Lung aspirate | Interstitium, alveoli when flooded | Small | Simple technique<br>Minimal expense<br>No special equipment<br>Solid masses adjacent to body wall: excellent representation with minimal risk | Potential for complications: pneumothorax, hemothorax, pulmonary hemorrhage<br>Relatively small area of lung sampled<br>Specimen adequate only for cytology<br>Specimen blood contaminated | Solid masses adjacent to chest wall (for solitary/localized disease, see also Thoracotomy/Lung Biopsy)<br>Diffuse interstitial disease |
| Thoracotomy/lung biopsy | Small airways, alveoli, interstitium | Large | Ideal specimen<br>Allows histologic examination in addition to culture | Relatively expensive<br>Requires expertise<br>Requires general anesthesia<br>Major surgical procedure | Localized process where excision may be therapeutic as well as diagnostic<br>Any progressive disease not diagnosed by less invasive methods |

likely to identify interstitial and focal disease processes. However, the procedure is inexpensive and minimally invasive, and this makes it reasonable to perform in most animals with lower respiratory tract disease if the risks of other methods of specimen collection are deemed too great. Potential complications are rare, and they include tracheal laceration, subcutaneous emphysema, and pneumomediastinum (Table 20-9). Cats with bronchitis can be treated with bronchodilators before the procedure (p. 292) to decrease the risk of bronchospasm.

## Techniques

Tracheal washing is performed using transtracheal or endotracheal techniques. Transtracheal washing is performed by passing a catheter into the trachea to the level of the carina through the cricothyroid ligament or between the tracheal rings in an awake or sedated animal. Endotracheal washing is performed by passing a catheter through an endotracheal tube in an anesthetized animal. The endotracheal technique is preferred in cats and very small dogs, although either technique can be used in any animal.

**Transtracheal technique.** Transtracheal wash fluid is collected using an 18- to 22-gauge through-the-needle intravenous catheter (e.g., Intracath; Becton-Dickinson, Sandy, Utah). The catheter should be long enough to reach the carina, which is located at approximately the level of the fourth intercostal space. The longest intravenous catheter available may be 12 inches (30 cm), which is long enough to reach from the cricothyroid ligament to the carina in most dogs. However, the catheter may need to be inserted between tracheal rings in giant-breed dogs to ensure that it reaches the carina. Alternatively, a 14-gauge, short, over-the-needle catheter is used to enter the trachea at the cricothyroid ligament and a 3.5F polypropylene male dog urinary catheter is passed

through the catheter into the airways. The ability of the urinary catheter to pass through the 14-gauge catheter should be tested each time before the procedure is performed.

The dog can sit or lie down, whichever is more comfortable for the animal and clinician. The dog is restrained with its nose pointing toward the ceiling at about 45 degrees from horizontal (Fig. 20-11, *A*). Overextension of the neck causes the animal to be more resistant. Dogs that cannot be restrained should be tranquilized.

The cricothyroid ligament is identified by palpating the trachea in the ventral cervical region and following it dorsally toward the larynx to the raised, smooth, narrow band of the cricoid cartilage. Immediately above the cricoid cartilage is a depression, and this is the cricothyroid ligament (Fig. 20-11, *B*). If the trachea is entered above the cricothyroid ligament, the catheter is passed dorsally into the pharynx and a nondiagnostic specimen is obtained. Such dorsal passage of the catheter often results in excessive gagging and retching.

Lidocaine is always injected subcutaneously at the site of entry. The skin over the cricothyroid ligament is prepared surgically, and sterile gloves are worn to pass the catheter. The needle of the catheter is held with the bevel facing ventrally. The skin over the ligament is then tented, and the needle is

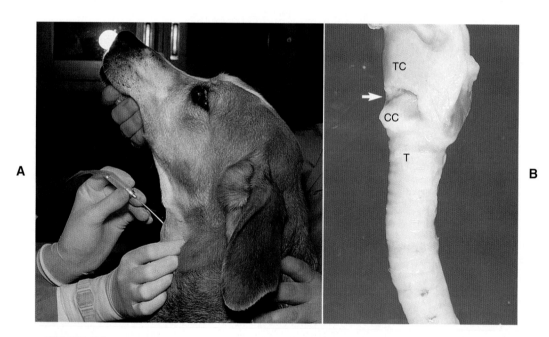

**FIG 20-11**
**A,** To perform a transtracheal wash, the animal is restrained in a comfortable position with the nose pointed toward the ceiling. The ventral neck is clipped and scrubbed, and the clinician wears sterile gloves. The cricothyroid ligament is identified as described in **B.** After an injection of lidocaine, the needle of the catheter is placed through the skin. The larynx is grasped firmly with the fingers and thumb at least 180 degrees around the airway. The needle can then be inserted through the cricothyroid ligament into the airway lumen. **B,** The lateral view of this anatomic specimen demonstrates the trachea and larynx in a position similar to that of the dog in **A.** The cricothyroid ligament *(arrow)* is identified by palpating the trachea *(T)* from ventral to dorsal until the raised cricoid cartilage *(CC)* is palpated. The cricothyroid ligament is the first depression above the cricoid cartilage. The cricothyroid ligament attaches cranially to the thyroid cartilage *(TC)*. The palpable depression above the thyroid cartilage (not shown) should not be entered.

passed through the skin. The larynx is stabilized with the nondominant hand. To properly stabilize it, the person should grasp at least 180 degrees of the circumference of the airway between the fingers and thumb. Failure to hold the airway firmly is the most common technical mistake made. Next, the tip of the needle is rested against the cricothyroid ligament and inserted through the ligament with a quick, short motion.

The hand stabilizing the trachea is then used to pinch the needle at the skin, with the hand kept firmly in contact with the neck, while the catheter is threaded into the trachea with the other hand. By keeping the hand holding the needle against the neck of the animal so that the hand, needle, and neck can move as one, the larynx or trachea is kept from being lacerated. Threading the catheter provokes coughing. There should be little or no resistance to the passage of the catheter. Elevating the hub of the needle slightly so that the tip points more ventrally or retracting the needle a few millimeters facilitates passage of the catheter if it is lodged against the opposite tracheal wall. The catheter itself should not be pulled back through the needle, because the tip can be sheared off within the airway by the cutting edge of the needle.

Once the catheter is completely threaded into the airway, the needle is withdrawn and the catheter guard is attached to prevent shearing of the catheter. The person restraining the

animal now holds the catheter guard against the neck of the animal so that movement of the neck will not dislodge the catheter. The head can be restrained in a natural position.

It is convenient to have four to six 12 ml syringes ready, each filled with 3 to 5 ml of 0.9% sterile preservative-free sodium chloride solution. The entire bolus of saline in one syringe is injected into the catheter. Immediately after this, many aspiration attempts are made. After each aspiration, the syringe must be disconnected from the catheter and the air evacuated without losing any of the retrieved fluid. Aspirations should be forceful and repeated at least five or six times so that small volumes of airway secretions that have been aspirated into the catheter are pulled the entire length of the catheter into the syringe.

The procedure is repeated using additional boluses of saline until a sufficient amount of fluid is retrieved for analysis. A total of 1.5 to 3 ml of turbid fluid is adequate in most instances. The clinician does not need to be concerned about "drowning" the animal with the infusion of the modest volumes of fluid described, because the fluid is rapidly absorbed into the circulation. Failure to retrieve adequate volumes of visibly turbid fluid can be the result of several technical difficulties, as outlined in Table 20-10.

The catheter is removed after sufficient fluid is collected. A sterile gauze sponge with antiseptic ointment is then

 TABLE 20-10

**Overcoming Problems with Tracheal Wash Fluid Collection**

| PROBLEMS | POTENTIAL CAUSES | REMEDIES |
|---|---|---|
| Poor or no return | Length of catheter within airway:<br>  Too far within airway can result in catheterization of a bronchus and loss of horizontal surface required to infuse, then recover, fluid.<br>  Not far enough within trachea leaves catheter tip in extrathoracic trachea, where surface is not horizontal. | Measure distance along path of trachea from cricothyroid ligament (transtracheal technique) or proximal end of endotracheal tube to fourth intercostal space for approximate distance to carina and ensure catheter reaches this position. |
| | Position of catheter tip when using stiff polypropylene urinary catheters: tip may be bent or curved such that it cannot rest on ventral surface of airway. | Physically straighten catheter before use. Once catheter is in position, rotate it along axis in several different positions until yield improves. |
| | Time delay between instillation and suction is too long. | Suction vigorously immediately after instillation of saline. |
| | Suction is not sufficiently vigorous. | Use a 12-ml syringe and suction with enthusiasm. |
| Recovery of only saline | Catheter is not placed far enough within trachea to exit endotracheal tube using endotracheal tube technique. | See first remedy (above). |
| | Too few suction attempts are performed to pull mucus through entire length of catheter. | Suction many, many times. Mucus that has only moved partway through catheter will be pushed back into airways with subsequent saline infusion. |
| Negative pressure | Catheter is kinked at neck (transtracheal technique). | Holder adjusts position to prevent kinking. |
| | Thick mucus is obstructing lumen of catheter. | Continue vigorous suction to retrieve this valuable material. If necessary, flush with more saline. If still unsuccessful, consider using a larger catheter. |
| | Catheter tip is flush against airway wall. | Move catheter slightly forward or backward, or rotate catheter. |

immediately placed over the catheter site, and a light bandage is wrapped around the neck. This bandage is left in place for several hours while the animal rests quietly in a cage. These precautions minimize the likelihood of subcutaneous emphysema or pneumomediastinum developing.

**Endotracheal technique.** The endotracheal technique is performed by passing a 3.5F male dog urinary catheter through a sterilized endotracheal tube. The animal is anesthetized with a short-acting intravenous agent to a sufficient depth to allow intubation. A short-acting barbiturate, propofol, or, in cats, a combination of ketamine and acepromazine or diazepam is effective. A sterilized endotracheal tube should be passed without dragging the tip through the oral cavity. The animal's mouth is opened wide with the tongue pulled out, a laryngoscope is used, and, in cats, sterile topical lidocaine is applied to the laryngeal cartilages to ease passage of the tube with minimum contamination.

The urinary catheter is passed through the endotracheal tube to the level of the carina (approximately the fourth intercostal space), maintaining sterile technique. The wash procedure is performed as described for the transtracheal technique. Slightly larger boluses of saline may be required, however, because of the larger volume of the catheter. Use of a catheter larger than 3.5F seems to reduce the yield of the wash except when secretions are extremely viscous.

## Specimen Handling

The cells collected in the wash fluid are fragile. The fluid is ideally processed within 30 minutes of collection, with minimal manipulation. Bacterial culture is performed on at least 0.5 to 1 ml of fluid. Fungal cultures are performed if mycotic disease is a differential diagnosis, and *Mycoplasma* cultures are considered for cats and dogs with bronchitis. Cytologic preparations are made from the fluid and any mucus within the fluid. Both fluid and mucus are examined because infectious agents and inflammatory cells can be concentrated in the mucus, but the proteinaceous material causes cells to clump and interferes with evaluation of the cell morphology. Mucus is retrieved with a needle, and squash preparations are made. Direct smears of the fluid itself can be made, but such specimens are often hypocellular. Sediment or cytocentrifuge preparations are generally necessary to make adequate interpretation possible. I do not recommend straining the fluid through gauze to remove the mucus, because infectious agents may be lost in the process. Routine cytologic stains are used.

Microscopic examination of slides includes the identification of cell types, qualitative evaluation of the cells, and an examination for infectious agents. Cells are evaluated qualitatively for evidence of macrophage activation, neutrophil degeneration, lymphocyte reactivity, and characteristics of malignancy. Epithelial hyperplasia secondary to inflammation should not be overinterpreted as neoplasia, however. Infectious agents such as bacteria, protozoa *(Toxoplasma gondii)*, fungi *(Histoplasma, Blastomyces,* and *Cryptococcus* organisms), and parasitic larvae or eggs may be present (Figs. 20-12 to 20-14; see also Fig. 20-10). Because only one or two organisms may be present on an entire slide, a thorough evaluation is indicated.

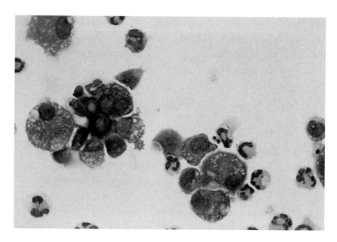

**FIG 20-12**
Photomicrograph of a *Blastomyces* organism from the lungs of a dog with blastomycosis. The organisms stain deeply basophilic, are 5 to 15 μm in diameter, and have a thick refractile cell wall. Often, as in this figure, broad-based budding forms are seen. The cells present are alveolar macrophages and neutrophils. (Bronchoalveolar lavage fluid, Wright stain.)

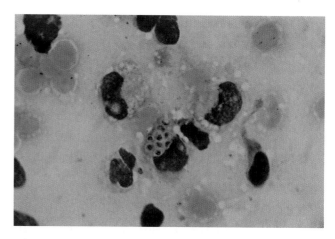

**FIG 20-13**
Photomicrograph of *Histoplasma* organisms from the lungs of a dog with histoplasmosis. The organisms are small (2 to 4 μm) and round, with a deeply staining center and a lighter-staining halo. They are often found within phagocytic cells: in this figure, an alveolar macrophage. (Bronchoalveolar lavage fluid, Wright stain.)

## Interpretation of Results

Normal tracheal wash fluid contains primarily respiratory epithelial cells. Few other inflammatory cells are present (Fig. 20-15). Occasionally macrophages are retrieved from the small airways and alveoli because the catheter was extended into the lungs beyond the carina or because relatively large volumes of saline were used. Most macrophages are not activated. In these instances the presence of macrophages does not indicate disease but rather reflects the acquisition of material from the deep lung (see Nonbronchoscopic Bronchoalveolar Lavage, p. 270).

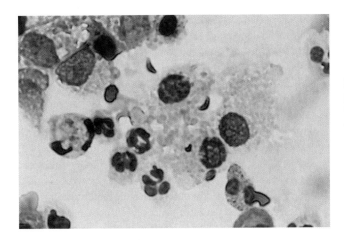

**FIG 20-14**
Photomicrograph of *Toxoplasma gondii* tachyzoites from the lungs of a cat with acute toxoplasmosis. The extracellular tachyzoites are crescent shaped with a centrally placed nucleus. They are approximately 6 μm in length. (Bronchoalveolar lavage fluid, Wright stain.)

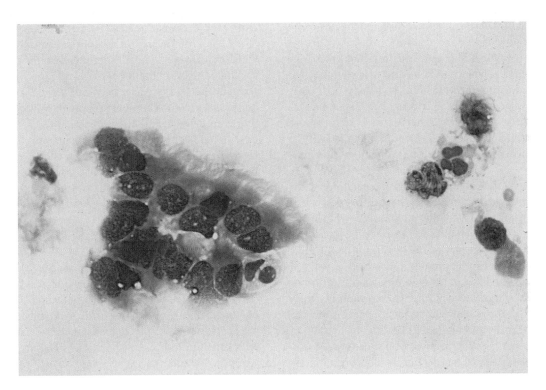

**FIG 20-15**
Tracheal wash fluid from a healthy dog showing ciliated epithelium and few inflammatory cells.

Slides are examined for evidence of overt oral contamination, which can occur during transtracheal washing if the catheter needle was inadvertently inserted proximal to the cricothyroid ligament. Rarely, dogs can cough the catheter up into the oropharynx. Oral contamination is indicated by the finding of numerous squamous epithelial cells, often coated with bacteria, and *Simonsiella* organisms. *Simonsiella* organisms are large basophilic rods that are frequently found stacked uniformly on each other along their broad side. Specimens with overt oral contamination generally do not provide accurate information about the airways, particularly with regard to bacterial infection.

Neutrophilic (suppurative) inflammation is common in bacterial infections. Before antibiotic therapy is initiated, the neutrophils may be (but are not always) degenerative, and organisms can often be seen. Neutrophilic inflammation can represent any acute inflammatory response. It can be caused by other infectious agents, chronic bronchitis, miscellaneous noninfectious inflammatory diseases, or even neoplasia. Some cats with bronchitis have neutrophilic inflammation rather than the expected eosinophilic response (see Chapter 21). The neutrophils in these instances are generally nondegenerative.

Eosinophilic inflammation reflects a hypersensitivity response, and common diseases resulting in eosinophilic inflammation include allergic bronchitis, parasitic disease, and eosinophilic lung disease. Parasites that affect the lung include primary lung worms or flukes, migrating intestinal parasites, and heartworms. Over time, mixed inflammation can occur in parasitized patients. It is occasionally possible for nonparasitic infections or neoplasia to cause eosinophilia, usually as part of a mixed inflammatory response.

Macrophagic (granulomatous) inflammation is characterized by the finding of increased numbers of activated macrophages, generally present as a component of mixed inflammation along with increased numbers of other inflammatory cells. Activated macrophages are vacuolated and have increased amounts of cytoplasm. This response is nonspecific unless an etiologic agent can be identified.

Lymphocytic inflammation alone is uncommon. Viral or rickettsial infection, noninfectious inflammatory diseases, and lymphoma are considerations in this setting.

True hemorrhage can be differentiated from a traumatic specimen collection by the presence of erythrophagocytosis and hemosiderin-laden macrophages. An inflammatory response is also usually present. Hemorrhage can be caused by neoplasia, mycotic infection, heartworm disease, thromboembolism, foreign body, lung lobe torsion, or coagulopathies. Minimal evidence of hemorrhage is seen in some animals with congestive heart failure.

Criteria of malignancy for making a diagnosis of neoplasia must be interpreted with extreme caution. Overt characteristics of malignancy must be present in many cells in the absence of concurrent inflammation for a definitive diagnosis to be made.

The finding of organisms in cytologic preparations without evidence of oral contamination indicates the presence of infection. The growth of any of the systemic mycotic agents in culture is also clinically significant, whereas the growth of bacteria in culture may or may not be significant, because low numbers of bacteria can be present in the large airways of healthy animals. In general, the cytologic identification of bacteria and their growth in culture without multiplication in enrichment broth are significant findings. Bacteria that are not seen cytologically and that grow only after incubation in enrichment media can result from several situations. For example, the bacteria may be causing infection but are not present in high numbers because of the prior administration of antibiotics or because of the collection of a poor-quality specimen. The bacteria may also be clinically insignificant and represent normal tracheal inhabitants or result from contamination during collection. Other clinical data must therefore be considered when interpreting such findings.

# NONBRONCHOSCOPIC BRONCHOALVEOLAR LAVAGE

## Indications and Complications

Bronchoalvelolar lavage (BAL) is considered for the diagnostic evaluation of patients with lung disease involving the small airways, alveoli, or interstitium that are not in respiratory distress (see Table 20-9). A large volume of lung is sampled by BAL (Figs. 20-16 and 20-17). The collected specimens are of large volume, providing more than adequate material for routine cytology, cytology involving special stains (e.g., Gram

stains, acid-fast stains), multiple types of cultures (e.g., bacterial, fungal, mycoplasmal), or other specific tests that might be helpful in particular patients (e.g., flow cytometry, polymerase chain reaction [PCR]). Cytologic preparations from BAL fluid are of excellent quality and consistently provide large numbers of well-stained cells for examination.

Although general anesthesia is required, the procedure is associated with few complications and can be performed repeatedly in the same animal to follow the progression of disease or observe the response to therapy. The primary complication of BAL is transient hypoxemia. The hypoxemia can generally be corrected with oxygen supplementation, but animals in respiratory distress in room air are not good candidates for this procedure. For patients with bacterial or aspiration pneumonia, tracheal washing routinely results in an adequate specimen for cytologic and microbiologic analysis and avoids the need for general anesthesia in these patients.

BAL is a routine part of diagnostic bronchoscopy, during which visually guided BAL specimens can be collected from specific, diseased lung lobes. However, nonbronchoscopic techniques (NB-BAL) have been developed that allow BAL to be performed with minimal expense in routine practice settings. Since visual guidance is not possible using these methods, they are used primarily for patients with diffuse disease. However, the technique described for cats probably samples the cranial and middle regions of the lung on the side of the cat placed against the table, whereas the technique described for dogs consistently samples one of the caudal lung lobes.

## Technique for NB-BAL in Cats

A sterile endotracheal tube and syringe adapter are used in cats to collect lavage fluid (Fig. 20-18; see also Fig. 20-17). Cats with bronchitis can be treated with bronchodilators before the procedure (p. 292) to decrease the risk of bronchospasm. The cat is premedicated with atropine (0.05 mg/kg subcutaneously) or glycopyrrolate (0.005 mg/kg subcutaneously) and anesthetized with ketamine and acepromazine or diazepam, given intravenously. The endotracheal tube is passed as cleanly as possible through the larynx to minimize oral contamination. To achieve sufficient cleanliness, the tip of the tongue is pulled out, a laryngoscope is used, and sterile lidocaine is applied topically to the laryngeal mucosa. The cuff is then inflated sufficiently to create a seal, but overinflation is avoided.

The cat is placed in lateral recumbency with the most diseased side, determined on the basis of physical and radiographic findings, against the table. Oxygen (100%) is administered for several minutes through the endotracheal tube. The anesthetic adapter is then removed from the endotracheal tube and replaced with a syringe adapter, avoiding contamination of the end of the tube or adapter. Immediately, a bolus of warmed, sterile 0.9% saline solution (5 ml/kg body weight) is infused through the tube over approximately 3 seconds. Immediately after infusion, suction is applied by syringe. Air is eliminated from the syringe, and several aspiration attempts are made until fluid is no longer recovered. The procedure is repeated using a total of two or three boluses of saline solution. The cat is allowed to expand its lungs between the infusions of

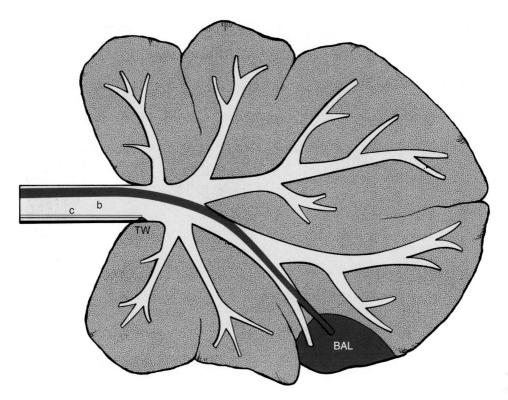

**FIG 20-16**
The region of the lower respiratory tract that is sampled by bronchoalveolar lavage *(BAL)* in comparison with the region sampled by tracheal wash *(TW)*. The solid black line *(b)* within the airways represents a bronchoscope or modified feeding tube. The open lines *(c)* represent the tracheal wash catheter. Bronchoalveolar lavage yields fluid representative of the deep lung, whereas tracheal wash yields fluid representative of processes involving major airways.

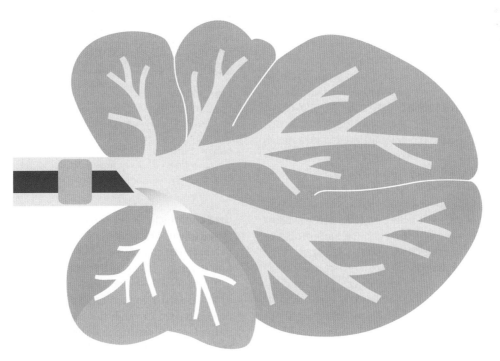

**FIG 20-17**
The region of the lower respiratory tract presumed to be sampled by nonbronchoscopic bronchoalveolar lavage in cats using an endotracheal tube.

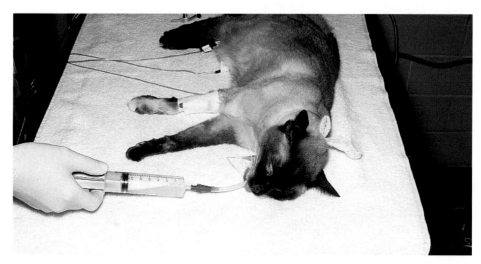

**FIG 20-18**
Bronchoalveolar lavage using an endotracheal tube in a cat. The fluid retrieved is grossly foamy because of the surfactant present. The procedure is performed quickly, because the airway is completely occluded during the infusion and aspiration of fluid.

saline solution. Following the last infusion, the syringe adapter is removed (because it greatly interferes with ventilation) and excess fluid is drained from the large airways and endotracheal tube by elevating the caudal half of the cat a few inches off of the table. At this point, the cat is cared for as described in Recovery of Patients Following BAL (p. 273).

### Technique for NB-BAL in Dogs

An inexpensive (<$2), 122-cm 16F Levin-type polyvinyl chloride stomach tube (Argyle stomach tube, Sherwood Medical, St. Louis) can be used in dogs to collect lavage fluid. The tube must be modified for successful NB-BAL. Sterile technique is maintained throughout. The distal end of the tube is cut off to remove the side openings. The proximal end is cut off to remove the flange and to shorten the tube to a length slightly greater than the distance from the open end of the dog's endotracheal tube to the last rib. A syringe adapter is placed within the proximal end of the tube (Fig. 20-19).

Recovery of BAL fluid can be improved by tapering the distal end of the tube. Tapering is readily achieved using a metal, single-blade, handheld pencil sharpener that has been autoclaved and is used only for this purpose (Fig. 20-19, A and B).

The dog is premedicated with atropine (0.05 mg/kg subcutaneously) or glycopyrrolate (0.005 mg/kg subcutaneously) and anesthetized using a short-acting protocol that will allow intubation, such as propofol, a short-acting barbiturate, or the combination of medetomidine and butorphanol. If the dog is of sufficient size to accept a size 6 or larger endotracheal tube, the dog is intubated with a sterile endotracheal tube placed as cleanly as possible to minimize oral contamination of the specimen. The modified stomach tube will not fit through a smaller endotracheal tube, so the technique must be performed without an endotracheal tube or a smaller stomach tube must be used. If no endotracheal tube is used, extreme care must be taken to minimize oral contamination in passing the modified stomach tube, and an appropriate-

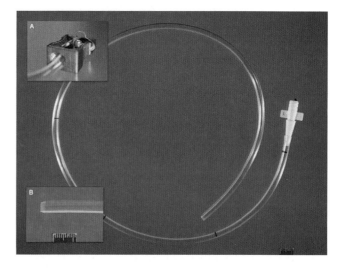

**FIG 20-19**
The catheter used for nonbronchoscopic bronchoalveolar lavage in dogs is a modified 16F Levin-type stomach tube. The tube is shortened by cutting off both ends. A simple pencil sharpener *(inset A)* is used to taper the distal end of the tube *(inset B)*. A syringe adapter is added to the proximal end. Sterility is maintained throughout.

sized endotracheal tube should be available to gain control of the airway in case of complications and for recovery. Results of a bacterial culture would need to be interpreted with caution because of unavoidable contamination.

Oxygen (100%) is provided through the endotracheal tube or by face mask for several minutes. The modified stomach tube is passed through the endotracheal tube using sterile technique until resistance is felt. The goal is to wedge the tube snugly into an airway and not butt against an airway division. Therefore the tube is withdrawn slightly, then passed again, until resistance is consistently felt at the same depth. Rotating the tube slightly during passage may help achieve a snug fit.

Remember that if the endotracheal tube is not much larger than the stomach tube, ventilation is restricted at this point and the procedure should be completed expediently.

For medium sized dogs and larger, two 35-ml syringes are prepared in advance, each with 25 ml of saline and 5 ml of air. While the modified stomach tube is held in place, a 25-ml bolus of saline is infused through the tube, followed by the 5 ml of air, by holding the syringe upright during infusion (Fig. 20-20). Gentle suction is applied immediately following infusion, using the same syringe. The tube may need to be withdrawn slightly if negative pressure is felt. The tube should not need to be withdrawn more than a few millimeters. If it is withdrawn too far, air rather than fluid will be recovered. The second bolus of saline is infused and recovered in the same manner, with the tube in the same position. The dog is recovered from the procedure as described in the following section.

In very small dogs, it is prudent to reduce the volume of saline used in each bolus, particularly if a smaller diameter stomach tube is used. Overinflation of the lungs with excessive fluid volumes should be avoided.

### Recovery of Patients Following BAL

Regardless of the method used, BAL causes a transient decrease in the arterial oxygen concentration, but this hypoxemia responds readily to oxygen supplementation. Where possible, patients are monitored with pulse oximetry (p. 285) before and throughout the procedure and during recovery. After the procedure, 100% oxygen is provided through an endotracheal tube for as long as the dog or cat will allow intubation. Several "sighs" are performed with the anesthesia bag to help expand any collapsed portions of lung. After extubation the mucous membrane color, pulses, and character of respirations are monitored closely. Crackles can be heard for several hours after BAL and are not cause for concern.

Treatment with oxygen supplementation is continued by mask, oxygen cage, or nasal catheter if there are any indications of hypoxemia. Bronchospasms are a reported complication of BAL in people, and bronchodilator therapy can be given if this occurs in animals. Premedication with bronchodilators is indicated in animals (particularly cats) where reactive airways are likely. It is rare that oxygen supplementation is necessary for more than 10 to 15 minutes after BAL, even in animals with diseased lungs; however, the ability to provide supplementation for longer periods is a prerequisite for the performance of this procedure.

### Specimen Handling

Successful BAL results in fluid that is grossly foamy, a result of the surfactant from the alveoli. Approximately 50% to 80% of the total volume of saline instilled is expected to be recovered. The fluid is placed on ice immediately after collection and is processed as soon as possible, with minimum manipulation to decrease cell lysis. For convenience, retrieved boluses can be combined for analysis; however, fluid from the first bolus usually contains more cells from the larger airways, and fluid from later boluses are more representative of the alveoli and interstitium.

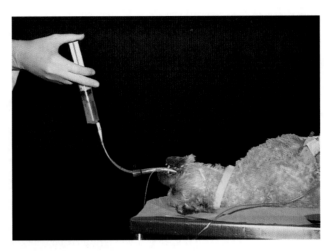

**FIG 20-20**
Bronchoalveolar lavage using a modified stomach tube in a dog. The tube is passed through a sterile endotracheal tube and lodged in a bronchus. A syringe preloaded with saline and air is held upright during infusion so that the saline is infused first, followed by the air.

The BAL fluid is analyzed cytologically and microbiologically. Nucleated cell counts are performed on undiluted fluid using a hemocytometer. Cells are concentrated onto slides for differential cell counts and qualitative analysis using sedimentation or cytocentrifugation techniques. Excellent-quality slides result that are stained using routine cytologic procedures. Differential cell counts are performed by counting at least 200 nucleated cells. Slides are scrutinized for evidence of macrophage activation, lymphocyte reactivity, neutrophil degeneration, and criteria of malignancy. All slides are examined thoroughly for possible etiologic agents, such as fungi, protozoa, parasites, and bacteria (see Figs. 20-10 and 20-12 to 20-14). As described for tracheal wash, visible strands of mucus can be examined for etiologic agents by squash preparation.

Approximately 5 ml of fluid is used for bacterial culture. Additional fluid is submitted for fungal culture if mycotic disease is among the differential diagnoses. *Mycoplasma* cultures are considered in cats and dogs with bronchitis.

### Interpretation of Results

Normal cytologic values for BAL fluid are inexact because of inconsistency in the techniques used and variability among individual animals of the same species. In general, total nucleated cell counts in normal animals are less than 400 to 500/$\mu$l. Differential cell counts for normal dogs and cats are listed in Table 20-11.

The same types of abnormal responses as described on p. 268 for tracheal wash fluid specimens may be seen in BAL fluid specimens and are suggestive of similar diseases, although, as previously noted, the specimens are from the deep lung rather than the airways. In addition, the normal cell population of macrophages must not be misinterpreted as being indicative of macrophagic or chronic inflammation (Fig. 20-21). As for all cytologic specimens, definitive diagnoses are made through the identification of organisms or

TABLE 20-11

### Differential Cell Counts from Bronchoalveolar Lavage Fluid from Normal Animals

| | BRONCHOSCOPIC BAL | | NONBRONCHOSCOPIC BAL | |
| **CELL TYPE** | **CANINE (%)*** | **FELINE (%)†** | **CANINE (%)‡** | **FELINE (%)§** |
|---|---|---|---|---|
| Macrophages | 70 ± 11 | 71 ± 10 | 81 ± 11 | 78 ± 15 |
| Lymphocytes | 7 ± 5 | 5 ± 3 | 2 ± 5 | 0.4 ± 0.6 |
| Neutrophils | 5 ± 5 | 7 ± 4 | 15 ± 12 | 5 ± 5 |
| Eosinophils | 6 ± 6 | 16 ± 7 | 2 ± 3 | 16 ± 14 |
| Epithelial cells | 1 ± 1 | — | — | — |
| Mast cells | 1 ± 1 | — | — | — |

*Mean ± SD, 6 clinically and histologically normal dogs. (From Kuehn NF: *Canine bronchoalveolar lavage profile*. Thesis for masters of science degree, West Lafayette, Ind, 1987, Purdue University.)

†Mean ± SE, 11 clinically normal cats. (From King RR et al: Bronchoalveolar lavage cell populations in dogs and cats with eosinophilic pneumonitis. In *Proceedings of the Seventh Veterinary Respiratory Symposium*, Chicago, 1988, Comparative Respiratory Society.)

‡Mean ± SD, 9 clinically normal dogs. (From Hawkins EC et al: Use of a modified stomach tube for bronchoalveolar lavage in dogs, *J Am Vet Med Assoc* 215:1635, 1999.)

§Mean + SD, 34 specific pathogen–free cats. (From Hawkins EC et al: Cytologic characterization of bronchoalveolar lavage fluid collected through an endotracheal tube in cats, *Am J Vet Res* 55:795, 1994.)

abnormal cell populations. Fungal, protozoal, or parasitic organisms may be present in extremely low numbers in BAL specimens, and the entire concentrated slide preparation therefore must be carefully scanned. Profound epithelial hyperplasia can occur in the presence of an inflammatory response and should not be confused with neoplasia.

If quantitative bacterial culture is available, growth of organisms at greater than $1.7 \times 10^3$ colony-forming units (CFU)/ml has been reported to indicate infection (Peeters and colleagues, 2000). In the absence of quantitative numbers, growth of organisms on a plate directly inoculated with BAL fluid is considered significant, whereas growth from fluid that occurs only following multiplication in enrichment broth may also be a result of normal inhabitants or contamination. Patients who are already receiving antibiotics at the time of specimen collection may have significant infection with few or no bacteria by culture.

### Diagnostic Yield

A retrospective study of BAL fluid cytologic analysis in dogs at referral institutions showed that BAL findings provided the basis for a definitive diagnosis in 25% of cases and were supportive of the diagnosis in an additional 50%. Only dogs in which a definitive diagnosis was obtained by any means were included. Definitive diagnoses were possible in those animals in which infectious organisms were identified or in those cases in which overtly malignant cells were present in specimens in the absence of marked inflammation. BAL has been shown to be more sensitive than radiographs in identifying pulmonary involvement with lymphosarcoma. Carcinoma was definitively identified in 57% of cases, and other sarcomas were not found in BAL fluid. Fungal pneumonia was confirmed in only 25% of cases, although organisms were found in 67% of cases in a previous study of dogs with overt fungal pneumonia.

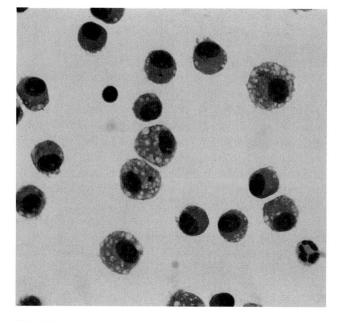

**FIG 20-21**
Bronchoalveolar lavage fluid from a normal dog. Note that alveolar macrophages predominate.

## TRANSTHORACIC LUNG ASPIRATION AND BIOPSY

### Indications and Complications

Pulmonary parenchymal specimens can be obtained by transthoracic needle aspiration or biopsy. Although only a small region of lung is sampled by these methods, collection can be guided by radiographic findings or ultrasonography to improve the likelihood of obtaining representative specimens. Potential complications include pneumothorax, hemothorax, and pulmonary hemorrhage. The procedures are not performed in animals with suspected cysts, abscesses, pulmonary hypertension, or coagulopathies. Severe complications are uncommon, but these procedures should not be performed unless the clinician is prepared to place a chest tube and otherwise support the animal if necessary.

Lung aspirates and biopsy specimens are indicated for the nonsurgical diagnosis of intrathoracic mass lesions that are in contact with the thoracic wall. The risk of complications in these animals is relatively low because the specimens can be collected without disrupting aerated lung. Obtaining aspirates or biopsy specimens from masses that are far from the body wall and near the mediastinum carries the additional risk of lacerating important mediastinal organs, vessels, or nerves. If a solitary, localized mass lesion is present, thoracotomy and biopsy should be considered, rather than transthoracic sampling, because this permits both the diagnosis of the problem and the potentially therapeutic benefits of complete excision (p. 281).

Transthoracic lung aspirates can be obtained in animals with diffuse interstitial pulmonary disease if findings from the previously described procedures have failed to provide the basis for a diagnosis. BAL should be considered before lung aspiration in animals that can tolerate the procedure, because it yields a larger specimen for analysis and, in my opinion, carries less risk than transthoracic aspiration in patients not having respiratory distress. Tracheal wash (if BAL is not possible) and appropriate ancillary tests are also generally indicated before lung aspiration in these patients, because they carry little risk.

## Techniques

The site of collection in animals with localized disease adjacent to the body wall is best identified with ultrasonography. If ultrasonography is not available, or if the lesion is surrounded by aerated lung, the site is determined on the basis of two radiographic views. The location of the lesion during inspiration in all three dimensions is identified by its relationship to external landmarks: the nearest intercostal space or rib, the distance from the costochondral junctions, and the depth into the lungs from the body wall. Fluoroscopy or computed tomography can also be used to guide the needle or biopsy instrument, if available.

The site of collection in animals with diffuse disease is a caudal lung lobe. The needle is inserted between the seventh to ninth intercostal spaces, approximately two thirds of the distance from the costochondral junctions to the spine.

The animal must be restrained for the procedure, and sedation or anesthesia is necessary in some. Anesthesia is avoided if possible, because the hemorrhage created by the procedure is not cleared as readily from the lungs in an anesthetized dog or cat. The skin at the site of collection is shaved and surgically prepared. Lidocaine is injected into the subcutaneous tissues and intercostal muscles to provide local anesthesia.

Lung aspiration can be performed with an injection needle, spinal needle, or a variety of thin-walled needles designed specifically for lung aspiration in people. Spinal needles are readily available in most practices, are sufficiently long to penetrate through the thoracic wall, and have a stylet. A 22-gauge, 1.5- to 3.5-inch (3.75- to 8.75-cm) spinal needle is adequate.

The clinician wears sterile gloves. The needle with stylet is advanced through the skin several rib spaces from the desired biopsy site. The needle and skin are then moved to the biopsy site. This is done because air is less likely to enter the thorax through the needle tract following the procedure if the openings in the skin and chest wall are not aligned. The needle is then advanced through the body wall to the pleura. The stylet is removed, and the needle hub is immediately covered by a finger to prevent pneumothorax until a 12-ml syringe can be placed on the hub. During inspiration the needle is thrust into the chest to a depth predetermined from the radiographs, usually about 1 inch (2.5 cm), while suction is applied to the syringe (Fig. 20-22). During insertion the needle can be twisted along its long axis in an attempt to obtain a core of tissue. The needle is then immediately withdrawn to the level of the pleura. The entire procedure takes only a second.

Several stabs into the lung can be made along different lines to increase the yield. After this has been done, the needle is withdrawn from the body wall, with a small amount of negative pressure maintained by the syringe.

It is unusual for the specimen to be large enough to enter the syringe. The needle is removed from the syringe, the syringe is filled with air and reattached to the needle, and the contents of the needle are then forced onto one or more slides. Grossly, the material is bloody in most cases. Squash preparations are made. Slides are stained using routine procedures and then evaluated cytologically. Increased numbers of inflammatory cells, infectious agents, or neoplastic cell populations are potential abnormalities. Alveolar macrophages are normal findings in parenchymal specimens and should not be interpreted as representing chronic inflammation. They should be carefully examined for evidence of phagocytosis of bacteria, fungi, or red blood cells and for signs of activation. Epithelial hyperplasia can occur in the presence of inflammation and should not be confused with neoplasia. Sometimes the liver is aspirated inadvertently, particularly in deep-chested dogs, yielding a population of cells that may resemble those from adenocarcinoma. However, hepatocytes typically contain bile pigment.

Bacterial culture is indicated in some animals, although the volume of material obtained is quite small. To increase sample volume, the procedure can be repeated or sterile saline can be injected into the lungs and aspirated back during the procedure.

Transthoracic lung core biopsies can be performed in animals with mass lesions. They are collected after an aspirate has proved to be nondiagnostic. Tru-cut instruments can be used to biopsy lesions adjacent to the chest wall. Smaller-bore, thin-walled lung biopsy instruments can be obtained from medical suppliers for human patients. These instruments

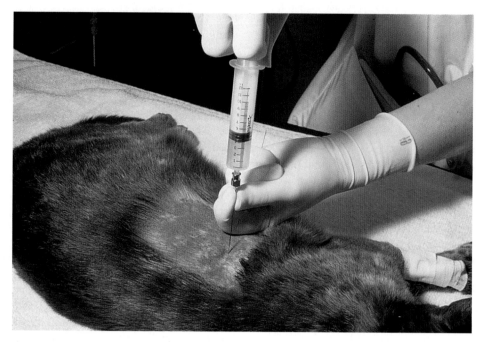

**FIG 20-22**
Transthoracic lung aspiration in a cat done with the use of a spinal needle. Note that sterile technique is used. Although this cat is under general anesthesia, this is not usually indicated.

collect smaller pieces of tissue but are less disruptive to normal lung. Ideally, sufficient material is collected for histologic evaluation. If not, squash preparations are made for cytologic studies.

## BRONCHOSCOPY

### Indications

Bronchoscopy is indicated for the evaluation of the major airways in animals with suspected structural abnormalities; for visual assessment of airway inflammation or pulmonary hemorrhage; and as a means of collecting specimens in animals with undiagnosed lower respiratory tract disease. Bronchoscopy can be used to identify structural abnormalities of the major airways, such as tracheal collapse, mass lesions, tears, strictures, lung lobe torsions, bronchiectasis, bronchial collapse, and external airway compression. Foreign bodies or parasites may be identified. Hemorrhage or inflammation involving the large airways may also be seen and localized.

Specimen collection techniques performed in conjunction with bronchoscopy are valuable diagnostic tools because they can obtain specimens from deeper regions of the lung than is possible with the tracheal wash technique, and visually directed sampling of specific lesions or lung lobes is also possible. Animals undergoing bronchoscopy must receive general anesthesia, and the presence of the scope within the airways compromises ventilation. Therefore bronchoscopy is contraindicated in animals with severe respiratory tract compromise unless the procedure is likely to be therapeutic (i.e., foreign body removal).

### Technique

Bronchoscopy of the airways is achieved using a small-diameter, flexible fiberoptic endoscope. A pediatric bronchoscope (4.8 mm outer diameter) with a biopsy channel that is 2 mm in diameter can be passed in most dogs and cats. Smaller scopes are useful for very small dogs and cats, but the collection of adequate biopsy specimens is not usually possible. Larger scopes can be used in large-breed dogs. The scope should be sterilized before use, according to the manufacturer's recommendations.

The dog or cat is premedicated with atropine or glycopyrrolate and anesthetized. Cats with bronchitis can be treated with bronchodilators before the procedure (p. 292) to decrease the risk of bronchospasm.

Injectable anesthetic agents can be used in any animal but are necessary for small dogs and cats, where passage of the scope through an endotracheal tube is not possible. The entire length of the trachea can be evaluated using this technique, the scope can be passed farther into the airways of very large dogs without an endotracheal tube in place, and leakage of anesthetic gases into the environment is avoided. Atropine or glycopyrrolate is used as a preanesthetic agent. In dogs a combination of hydromorphone as a preanesthetic agent, followed by diazepam (Valium) and propofol, can be used. In cats a combination of ketamine and diazepam or acepromazine is used to effect, and the larynx is anesthetized with a few drops of topical lidocaine.

The patient is preoxygenated for several minutes by delivering 100% oxygen through a face mask. Oxygen is delivered during the procedure either through the biopsy channel of the scope or through a soft feeding tube that is passed into the trachea. Manipulations must still be rapid in small dogs and cats, however, and the animal should be monitored closely. The bronchoscope is passed directly through the larynx while the animal's tongue is pulled out and the mouth opened wide to minimize contamination of the scope with oral debris. In medium- and large-sized dogs an endotracheal tube can be passed following assessment of the trachea, and oxygen can be delivered through the endotracheal tube during bronchoscopy as described here for inhalation anesthesia.

Inhalation anesthesia can be used except in small dogs and cats. The bronchoscope is passed through the endotracheal tube into the airways by means of an adapter that has a side port that allows it to be connected to the anesthesia machine. The adapter also has a diaphragm that allows the passage of the scope but lessens the escape of gases. The largest-diameter endotracheal tube possible should be used, because the scope obstructs part of the lumen. The endotracheal tube can be shortened to decrease its interference with visualization of the trachea, and it must be removed for the evaluation of the proximal trachea.

The animal is monitored closely throughout the procedure. The mucous membrane color, capillary refill time, pulse rate and quality, and respiratory rate are always checked. Pulse oximetry (p. 285) is valuable for detecting hypoxia. Blood pressure measurement, electrocardiography, and arterial blood gas analysis should be considered for high-risk animals.

The scope is lubricated with sterile, water-soluble lubricant before passage. Sterile gloves are worn to prevent contamination of the lower airways and collected specimens. The animal is positioned in sternal recumbency, and the head is elevated by placing a rolled-up towel under the mandibles until the oral cavity is parallel to the table at the level of the operator's eye. The scope must be protected from the teeth. Because manipulations within the airways can rouse a previously quiet animal, the mouth should be secured with a gag that is kept in place at all times.

In the normal animal a cross-section of the tracheal lumen is circular. The cartilaginous rings are just visible beneath the mucosa, and the dorsal tracheal membrane is taut (Fig. 20-23, *A*). The mucosa is uniformly pink, and blood vessels are seen through the thin epithelial surface. The carina, the division between the right and left mainstem bronchi, is a sharp division (see Fig. 20-24, *A*).

Each major bronchus is examined systematically, as is each branching bronchus, until the scope can no longer be advanced because of restrictions imposed by its length or diameter. The normal bronchial mucosa is pale pink and smooth. The cross-sections of the airway lumens are circular and remain open during respiration. The airway divisions are sharply defined. Gray-to-white glistening accumulations of mucus are scattered diffusely throughout the airways.

The entrances to the major bronchi are consistent in location with respect to the carina in the dog and cat, thus facilitating systematic examination (Fig. 20-24, *B* and *C*). The entrance to the right cranial bronchus is just beyond the carina, extending ventrolaterally from the right mainstem

bronchus. The right middle bronchus is beyond the entrance to the right cranial bronchus, and it is on the ventral floor of the main bronchus. The accessory lobe bronchus is just beyond the entrance to the right middle bronchus and extends medially from the main bronchus. Aiming directly caudal from this level is the right caudal bronchus.

The left cranial bronchus arises from the ventrolateral wall of the left mainstem bronchus just beyond the carina. It immediately divides into cranial and caudal branches. Aiming directly caudal is the left caudal bronchus.

A nomenclature for the major bronchi and their subdivisions is used to accurately describe bronchoscopic findings (Table 20-12). For example, a lesion found in the second dorsal branch of the right caudal lung lobe would be designated as being located in RB4D2. Such a system facilitates the discussion and reevaluation of lesions and their correlation with thoracic radiography.

Abnormalities that may be observed during bronchoscopy and their common clinical correlations are listed in Table 20-13. A definitive diagnosis may not be possible on the basis of the findings yielded by gross examination alone. Specimens are collected through the biopsy channel for cytologic, histopathologic, and microbiologic analysis. Bronchial specimens are obtained by bronchial washing, bronchial brushing, or pinch biopsy. Material for bacterial culture can be collected with guarded culture swabs. The deeper lung is sampled by BAL or transbronchial biopsy. Foreign bodies are removed with retrieval forceps.

### Bronchoscopic Bronchoalveolar Lavage

BAL is performed as a routine part of diagnostic bronchoscopy following thorough visual examination of the airways. Several lobes are lavaged in each animal to maximize the likelihood of identifying active disease. Specific lobes are selected on the basis of abnormal radiographic or bronchoscopic findings.

The bronchoscope is passed into the lobe to be lavaged until the tip is lodged in an airway. A snug fit must be achieved, or fluid recovery will be poor and the fluid will come from the airways rather than the deeper lung. Twenty-five milliliters of sterile 0.9% sodium chloride (saline) solution that has been warmed to body temperature is instilled by syringe into the lung through the biopsy channel of the scope. Immediately after this, gentle suction is applied to the syringe. If too much force is applied, however, the airway will collapse, and this will interfere with fluid return. Air is eliminated from the syringe, and additional suction attempts are made until no further fluid is obtained. A second 25-ml aliquot of saline is instilled into the lungs and retrieved with the scope in the same position. Other lobes are sampled in the same manner.

In cats it is often impossible to pass the scope beyond the left or right mainstem bronchi. In this instance three aliquots of saline solution, each with a volume of 5 ml/kg body weight, can be used. This volume is consistent with that described for NB-BAL in cats.

Other clinicians use 50 ml per lobe, divided into five 10-ml aliquots, in dogs and cats. This protocol is particularly useful for toy breed dogs or when using smaller-diameter

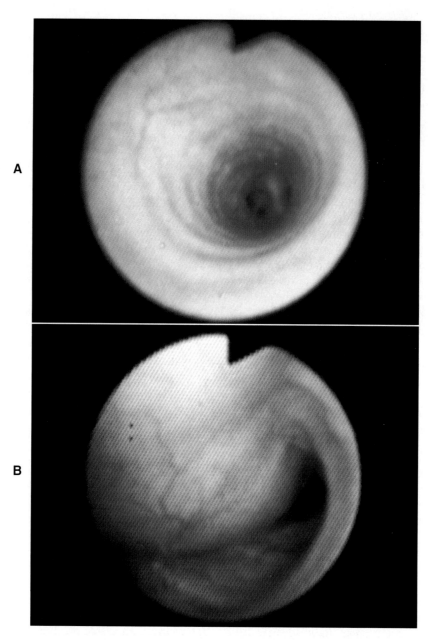

**FIG 20-23**
**A,** Bronchoscopic view of a normal trachea. Tracheal rings are visible beneath the mucosa, and the dorsal tracheal membrane is taut; the resulting lumen is circular. The carina is visible in the distance, with the right mainstem bronchus most apparent. **B,** Bronchoscopic view of a collapsing trachea. The dorsal tracheal membrane sags into the lumen of the airway, and the lumen is no longer circular.

bronchoscopes, where the volume of lung distal to the obstructed bronchus is relatively small.

Recovery of patients, specimen handling, interpretation, and diagnostic yield are the same as described previously for NB-BAL. Because nearly half of the dogs with radiographically diffuse lung disease are found to have cytologic differences in the BAL fluid collected from different lobes, ideally, BAL fluid collected from different lobes is analyzed separately. However, specimens from different lobes can be combined for the purpose of bacterial, fungal, or mycoplasmal culture.

## Transbronchial Lung Biopsy

Cup biopsy instruments are available for the collection of pinch biopsy specimens through the bronchial wall. A bronchoscope is used to guide the instrument, which is passed through the biopsy channel. Fluoroscopy can also be used for guidance after its initial introduction using a bronchoscope. The technique is most valuable for collecting tissue from intraluminal masses under direct bronchoscopic visualization. Bronchial wall tissue and a small volume of parenchymal tissue can be obtained by collecting pinches of tissue from sites

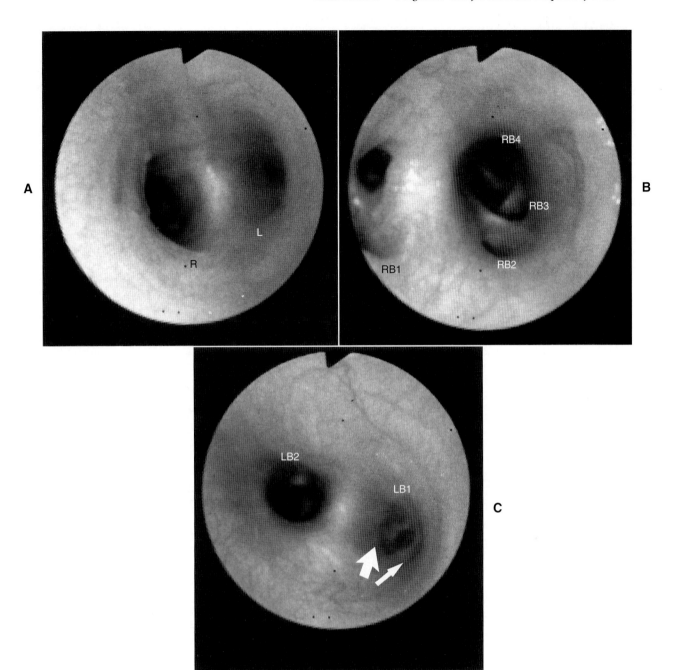

**FIG 20-24**
**A,** Bronchoscopic view of a normal carina, the division between the right *(R)* and left *(L)* mainstem bronchi. **B,** Bronchoscopic view at the entrance of the right mainstem bronchus. The right cranial bronchus *(RB1)* extends ventrolaterally just beyond the carina. The right middle bronchus *(RB2)* opens distal to the cranial bronchus and is located ventrally. The opening to the accessory lobe *(RB3)* is more distally located and is medially oriented. The right caudal bronchus *(RB4)* continues distally from the mainstem bronchus. **C,** Bronchoscopic view of the entrance to the left mainstem bronchus. The left cranial bronchus *(LB1)* is visible on the ventrolateral wall of the mainstem bronchus just beyond the level of the carina. It divides immediately into cranial *(narrow arrow)* and caudal *(broad arrow)* branches. The left caudal bronchus *(LB2)* continues distally from the mainstem bronchus.

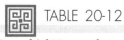

## TABLE 20-12

### Bronchial Nomenclature

| **Major Bronchi (Lobar Bronchi)** | |
| --- | --- |
| Right cranial bronchus | RB1 |
| Right middle bronchus | RB2 |
| Right accessory bronchus | RB3 |
| Right caudal bronchus | RB4 |
| Left cranial bronchus | LB1* |
| Left caudal bronchus | LB2 |

**Subdivisions (Segmental Bronchi) (Abbreviations Immediately Follow Major Bronchus and Subdivision Notations)**

Based on order of origination from major bronchus for all lobes except right middle

| | |
| --- | --- |
| First dorsal branch | D1 |
| Second dorsal branch | D2 |
| Etc. | |
| First ventral branch | V1 |
| Second ventral branch | V2 |
| Etc. | |

**Subdivisions (Segmental Bronchi) (Abbreviations Immediately Follow Major Bronchus and Subdivision Notations)—cont'd**

Based on order of origination from the major bronchus for the right middle lobe

| | |
| --- | --- |
| First rostral (cranial) branch | R1 |
| Second rostral (cranial) branch | R2 |
| Etc. | |
| First caudal branch | C1 |
| Second caudal branch | C2 |
| Etc. | |

**Further Divisions (Subsegmental Bronchi) (Abbreviations Immediately Follow Major Bronchus and Subdivision Notations)**

Based on order of origination from the segmental bronchus regardless of orientation: a, b, c, etc.

From Amis TC et al: Systematic identification of endobronchial anatomy during bronchoscopy in the dog, *Am J Vet Res* 47:2649, 1986.
*The bronchus to the caudal part of the left cranial lobe is identified as LB1V1.

## TABLE 20-13

### Bronchoscopic Abnormalities

| ABNORMALITY | CLINICAL CORRELATION |
| --- | --- |
| **Trachea** | |
| Hyperemia, loss of normal vascular pattern, excess mucus, exudate | Inflammation |
| Redundant tracheal membrane | Tracheal collapse |
| Flattened cartilage rings | Tracheal collapse |
| Uniform narrowing | Hypoplastic trachea |
| Strictures | Prior trauma |
| Mass lesions | Fractured rings, foreign body granuloma, neoplasia |
| Tears | Usually due to excessive endotracheal tube cuff pressure |
| **Carina** | |
| Widened | Hilar lymphadenopathy, extraluminal mass |
| Multiple raised nodules | *Oslerus osleri* |
| Foreign body | Foreign body |
| **Bronchi** | |
| Hyperemia, excess mucus, exudate | Inflammation |
| Collapse of airway during expiration | Chronic inflammation, weakened airway walls |
| Collapse of airway, inspiration and expiration, able to pass scope through narrowed airway | Chronic inflammation, weakened airway walls |
| Collapse of airway, inspiration and expiration, unable to pass scope through narrowed airway | Extraluminal mass lesions (neoplasia, granuloma, abscess) |
| Collapse of airway with "puckering" of mucosa | Lung lobe torsion |
| Hemorrhage | Neoplasia, fungal infection, heartworm, thromboembolic disease, coagulopathy, trauma (including foreign body related) |
| Single mass lesion | Neoplasia |
| Multiple polypoid masses | Usually chronic bronchitis; at carina, *Oslerus* |
| Foreign body | Foreign body |

of small airway division. The specimens are extremely small and fragile. Multiple biopsy specimens should be collected for histopathologic evaluation.

The primary complications associated with transbronchial biopsy are pulmonary hemorrhage and those associated with general anesthesia. Pneumothorax can occur but occurs less frequently than with transthoracic techniques.

## OPEN-CHEST LUNG BIOPSY AND THORACOSCOPY

Thoracotomy and surgical biopsy are performed in animals with progressive clinical signs of lower respiratory tract disease that has not been diagnosed using less invasive means. Although thoracotomy carries a greater risk than the previously mentioned diagnostic techniques, the modern anesthetic agents, surgical techniques, and monitoring capabilities now available have made this procedure routine in many veterinary practices. Analgesic drugs are used to manage the postoperative pain, and complication-free animals are discharged as soon as 2 to 3 days after surgery. Surgical biopsy provides excellent-quality specimens for histopathologic analysis and culture. Abnormal lung tissue, as well as accessible lymph nodes, are biopsied.

Excisional biopsy of abnormal tissue can be therapeutic in animals with localized disease. Removal of localized neoplasms, abscesses, cysts, and foreign bodies can be curative. The removal of large localized lesions can improve the matching of ventilation and perfusion, even in animals with evidence of diffuse lung involvement, thereby improving the oxygenation of blood and reducing clinical signs.

In practices where thoracoscopy is available, this less invasive technique can be used for initial assessment of intrathoracic disease. Similarly, a "mini" thoracotomy through a relatively small incision can be performed. If disease is obviously disseminated throughout the lungs such that surgical intervention will not be therapeutic, biopsies of abnormal tissue can be obtained with these methods via small incisions. For patients with questionable findings or apparently localized disease, thoracoscopy or "mini" thoracotomy can be transitioned to a full thoracotomy during the same anesthesia.

## BLOOD GAS ANALYSIS

### Indications

The measurement of partial pressures of oxygen ($PaO_2$) and carbon dioxide ($PaCO_2$) in arterial blood specimens provides information about pulmonary function. Venous blood analysis is less useful because venous blood is affected by cardiac function and peripheral circulation. Arterial blood gas measurements are indicated to document pulmonary failure, to differentiate hypoventilation from other causes of hypoxemia, to help determine the need for supportive therapy, and to monitor the response to therapy. Respiratory compromise must be severe for abnormalities to be measurable, because

of the tremendous mechanisms the body has that can compensate for disease states.

### Techniques

Arterial blood is collected using a 3 ml syringe and 25-gauge needle that have been flushed with heparin. The femoral artery is commonly used (Fig. 20-25). The animal is placed in lateral recumbency. The upper rear limb is abducted, and the rear limb resting on the table is restrained in a partially extended position. The femoral artery is palpated in the inguinal region, close to the abdominal wall, using two fingers. The needle is advanced into the artery between these fingers. The artery is thick walled and is loosely attached to adjacent tissues; thus the needle must be sharp and positioned exactly on top of the artery. A short, jabbing motion facilitates entry.

The dorsal pedal artery is useful for arterial collection in medium-sized and large dogs. The position of the artery is illustrated in Fig. 20-26.

Once the needle has penetrated the skin, suction is applied. On entry of the needle into the artery, blood should enter the syringe quickly, sometimes in pulses. Unless the animal is severely compromised, the blood will be bright red, as compared with the dark red of venous blood. Dark red blood or blood that is difficult to draw into the syringe may be from a vein. Mixed samples from both the artery and vein can also be collected accidentally, particularly from the femoral site.

After removal of the needle, pressure is applied to the puncture site for 5 minutes to prevent hematoma formation. Pressure is applied even after unsuccessful attempts if there is any possibility that the artery was entered.

All air bubbles are eliminated from the syringe. The needle is covered by a cork or rubber stopper, and the entire syringe is placed in crushed ice unless the blood specimen is to

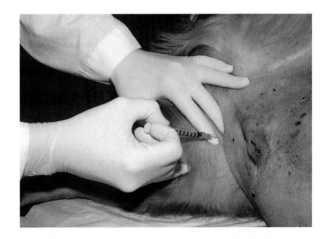

**FIG 20-25**
Position for obtaining an arterial blood specimen from the femoral artery. The dog is in left lateral recumbency. The right rear limb is being held perpendicular to the table to expose the left inguinal area. The pulse is palpated in the femoral triangle between two fingers to accurately locate the artery. The needle is laid directly on top of the artery, then stabbed into it with a short, jabbing motion.

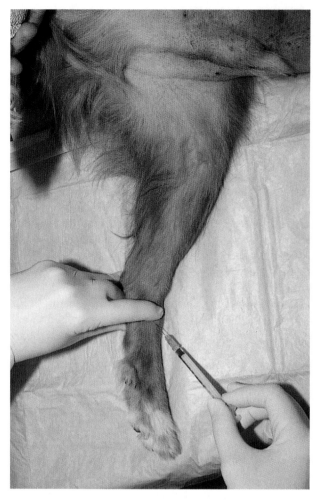

**FIG 20-26**
Position for obtaining an arterial blood specimen from the dorsal pedal artery. The dog is in left lateral recumbency, with the medial surface of the left leg exposed. A pulse is palpated just below the tarsus on the dorsal surface of the metatarsus between the midline and the medial aspect of the distal limb.

 TABLE 20-14

**Approximate Ranges of Arterial Blood Gas Values for Normal Dogs and Cats Breathing Room Air**

| MEASUREMENT | ARTERIAL BLOOD |
|---|---|
| $PaO_2$ (mm Hg) | 85-100 |
| $PaCO_2$ (mm Hg) | 35-45 |
| $HCO_3$ (mmol/L) | 21-27 |
| pH | 7.35-7.45 |

with normal mucous membrane characteristics being evaluated for exercise intolerance is unlikely to have a resting $PaO_2$ of 45 mm Hg. The collection of venous blood is a more likely explanation for this abnormal value.

Hypoxemia is present if the $PaO_2$ is below the normal range. The oxyhemoglobin dissociation curve describing the relationship between the saturated hemoglobin level and $PaO_2$ is sigmoid in shape, with a plateau at higher $PaO_2$ values (Fig. 20-27). Normal hemoglobin is almost totally saturated with oxygen when the $PaO_2$ is greater than 80 to 90 mm Hg, and clinical signs are unlikely in animals with such values. The curve begins to decrease more quickly at lower $PaO_2$ values. A value of less than 60 mm Hg corresponds to a hemoglobin saturation that is considered dangerous, and treatment for hypoxemia is indicated. (See Oxygen Content, Delivery, and Utilization [p. 284] for further discussion.)

In general, animals become cyanotic when the $PaO_2$ reaches 50 mm Hg or less, which results in a concentration of nonoxygenated (unsaturated) hemoglobin of 5 g/dl or more. Cyanosis occurs as a result of the increased concentration of nonoxygenated hemoglobin in the blood and is not a direct reflection of the $PaO_2$. The development of cyanosis depends on the total concentration of hemoglobin, as well as the oxygen pressure; cyanosis develops more quickly in animals with polycythemia than in animals with anemia. Acute hypoxemia resulting from lung disease more often produces pallor in an animal than cyanosis. Treatment for hypoxemia is indicated for all animals with cyanosis.

Determining the mechanism of hypoxemia is useful in selecting appropriate supportive therapy. These mechanisms include hypoventilation, diffusion abnormality, and inequality of ventilation and perfusion within the lung. Hypoventilation is the inadequate exchange of gases between the outside of the body and the alveoli. The $PaO_2$ and $PaCO_2$ are both affected by a lack of gas exchange, and hypercapnia occurs in conjunction with hypoxemia. Causes of hypoventilation are listed in Table 20-15.

Diffusion abnormalities alone do not result in clinically significant hypoxemia. Gas is normally exchanged between the alveoli and the blood by diffusing across the respiratory membrane. This membrane consists of the fluid lining the alveolus, alveolar epithelium, alveolar basement membrane, interstitium, capillary basement membrane, and capillary endothelium. Gases must also diffuse through plasma and red

be analyzed immediately. Specimens should be analyzed as soon as possible after collection. Minimal alterations occur in specimens stored on ice during the few hours required to transport the specimen to a human hospital if a blood gas analyzer is not available on site. Because of the availability of reasonably priced blood gas analyzers, in-office testing is now possible.

## Interpretation of Results

Approximate arterial blood gas values for normal dogs and cats are provided in Table 20-14. More exact values should be obtained for normal dogs and cats using the actual analyzer.

**$PaO_2$ and $PaCO_2$.** Abnormal $PaO_2$ and $PaCO_2$ values can result from technical error. The animal's condition and the collection technique are considered in the interpretation of blood gas values. For example, an animal in stable condition

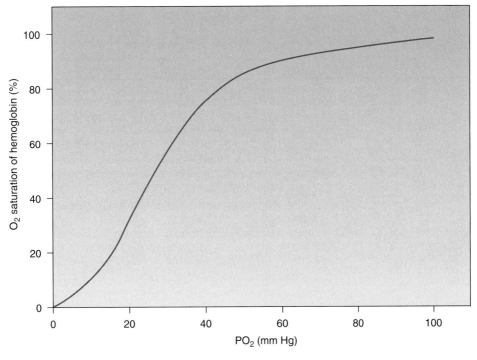

**FIG 20-27**
Oxygen-hemoglobin dissociation curve (approximation).

blood cell membranes. Functional and structural adaptations that facilitate diffusion between the alveoli and red blood cells provide an efficient system for this process, which is rarely affected by disease.

The ventilation and perfusion of different regions of the lung must be matched for the blood leaving the lung to be fully oxygenated. The relationship between ventilation ($\dot{V}$) and perfusion ($\dot{Q}$) can be described as a ratio ($\dot{V}/\dot{Q}$). Hypoxemia can develop if there are regions of lung with either a low or a high $\dot{V}/\dot{Q}$.

Poorly ventilated portions of lung with normal blood flow have a low $\dot{V}/\dot{Q}$. Regionally decreased ventilation occurs in most pulmonary diseases for reasons such as alveolar flooding, alveolar collapse, or small airway obstruction. The flow of blood past totally nonaerated tissue is known as a venous admixture or shunt ($\dot{V}/\dot{Q}$ of zero). The alveoli may be unventilated as a result of complete filling or collapse, resulting in physiologic shunts, or the alveoli may be bypassed by true anatomic shunts. Unoxygenated blood from these regions then mixes with oxygenated blood from ventilated portions of the lung. The immediate result is a decreased $Pa_{O_2}$ and an increased $Pa_{CO_2}$. The body responds to the hypercapnia by increasing ventilation, effectively returning the $Pa_{CO_2}$ to normal or even lower than normal. However, the increased ventilation cannot correct the hypoxemia, because blood flowing by ventilated alveoli is already maximally saturated.

Except where shunts are present, the $Pa_{O_2}$ can be improved in dogs and cats with lung regions with low $\dot{V}/\dot{Q}$s by providing supplemental oxygen therapy administered by face mask, oxygen cage, or nasal catheter. Positive-pressure ventilation may be necessary to combat atelectasis (see Chapter 27).

 TABLE 20-15

### Clinical Correlations of Blood Gas Abnormalities

**Decreased Pao$_2$ and Increased Paco$_2$**
**(Normal A-a Gradient)**

Venous specimen
Hypoventilation
  Airway obstruction
  Decreased ventilatory muscle function
    Anesthesia
    Central nervous system disease
    Polyneuropathy
    Polymyopathy
    Neuromuscular junction disorders (myasthenia gravis)
    Extreme fatigue (prolonged distress)
  Restriction of lung expansion
    Thoracic wall abnormality
    Excessive thoracic bandage
    Pneumothorax
    Pleural effusion
  Increased dead space (low alveolar ventilation)
    Severe chronic obstructive pulmonary
      disease/emphysema
End-stage severe pulmonary parenchymal disease
Severe pulmonary thromboembolism

**Decreased Pao$_2$ and Normal or Decreased Paco$_2$**
**(Wide A-a Gradient)**

Ventilation/perfusion ($\dot{V}/\dot{Q}$) abnormality
  Pulmonary parenchymal disease (see Table 19-1, p. 251)
  Lung lobe collapse
  Pulmonary thromboembolism

TABLE 20-16

**Relationships of Arterial Blood Gas Measurements**

| FORMULA | DISCUSSION |
|---|---|
| $PaO_2 \propto SaO_2$ | Relationship is defined by sigmoid oxygen-hemoglobin dissociation curve. Curve plateaus at greater than 90% $SaO_2$ with $PaO_2$ values greater than 80 mm Hg. Curve is steep at $PaO_2$ values of between 20 and 60 mm Hg. (Assuming normal hemoglobin, pH, temperature, and 2,3-diphosphoglycerate concentrations.) |
| $CaO_2 = (SaO_2 \times Hgb \times 1.34) + (0.003 \times PaO_2)$ | Total oxygen content of blood is greatly influenced by $SaO_2$ and hemoglobin concentration. In health, more than 60 times more oxygen is delivered by hemoglobin than is dissolved in plasma ($PaO_2$). |
| $PaCO_2 = PACO_2$ | These values are increased with hypoventilation at alveolar level and decreased with hypoventilation. |
| $PAO_2 = FIO_2 (P_B - P_{H_2O}) - PaCO_2/R$ on room air at sea level: $PAO_2 = 150$ mm Hg $- PaCO_2/0.8$ | Partial pressure of oxygen in alveolar air available for exchange with blood changes directly with inspired oxygen concentration and inversely with $PaCO_2$. R is assumed to be 0.8 for fasting animals. With normally functioning lungs (minimal $\dot{V}/\dot{Q}$ mismatch), alveolar hyperventilation results in increased $PAO_2$ and subsequently increased $PaO_2$, whereas hypoventilation results in decreased $PAO_2$ and decreased $PaO_2$. |
| $A\text{-}a = PAO_2 - PaO_2$ | A-a gradient quantitatively assesses $\dot{V}/\dot{Q}$ mismatch by eliminating contribution of alveolar ventilation and inspired oxygen concentration to measured $PaO_2$. Low $PaO_2$ with a normal A-a gradient (10 mm Hg in room air) indicates hypoventilation alone. Low $PaO_2$ with a wide A-a gradient ($>15$ mm Hg in room air) indicates a component of $\dot{V}/\dot{Q}$ mismatch. |
| $PaCO_2 \propto 1/pH$ | Increased $PaCO_2$ causes respiratory acidosis; decreased $PaCO_2$ causes respiratory alkalosis. Actual pH depends on metabolic ($HCO_3$) status as well. |

*A-a*, Alveolar-arterial oxygen gradient (mm Hg); *CaO_2*, oxygen content of arterial blood (ml of $O_2$/dl); *FIO_2*, fraction of oxygen in inspired air (%); *Hgb*, hemoglobin concentration (g/dl); *PaCO_2*, partial pressure of $CO_2$ in arterial blood (mm Hg); *PACO_2*, partial pressure of $CO_2$ in alveolar air (mm Hg); *PaO_2*, partial pressure of $O_2$ in arterial blood (mm Hg); *PAO_2*, partial pressure of $O_2$ in alveolar air (mm Hg); *P_B*, barometric (atmospheric) pressure (mm Hg); *P_{H_2O}*, partial pressure of water in alveolar air (100% humidified) (mm Hg); *pH*, negative logarithm of $H^+$ concentration (decreases with increased $H^+$); *R*, respiratory exchange quotient (ratio of $O_2$ uptake per $CO_2$ produced); *SaO_2*, amount of hemoglobin saturated with oxygen (%); *$\dot{V}/\dot{Q}$*, ratio of ventilation to perfusion of alveoli.

The ventilation of areas of lung with decreased circulation (a high $\dot{V}/\dot{Q}$) occurs in dogs and cats with thromboembolism. Initially there may be little effect on arterial blood gas values, because blood flow is shifted to unaffected regions of the lung. However, blood flow in the normal regions of the lungs increases with increasing severity of disease, and $\dot{V}/\dot{Q}$s are decreased enough that a decreased $PaO_2$ and a normal or decreased $PaCO_2$ occur, as described previously. Both hypoxemia and hypercapnia are seen in the setting of extremely severe embolization.

**A-a gradient.** Hypoventilation is differentiated from $\dot{V}/\dot{Q}$ abnormalities by evaluating the $PaCO_2$ in conjunction with the $PaO_2$. Qualitative differences are described in the preceding paragraphs: hypoventilation is associated with hypoxemia and hypercapnia, and $\dot{V}/\dot{Q}$ abnormalities are generally associated with hypoxemia and normocapnia or hypocapnia. It is possible to quantitate this relationship by calculating the alveolar-arterial oxygen gradient (*A-a* gradient), which factors out the effects of ventilation and the inspired oxygen concentration on $PaO_2$ (Table 20-16).

The premise of the *A-a* gradient is that $PaO_2$ (*a*) is nearly equal (within 10 mm Hg in room air) to the partial pressure of oxygen in the alveoli, $PAO_2$ (*A*), in the absence of a diffu-

sion abnormality or $\dot{V}/\dot{Q}$ mismatch. In the presence of a diffusion abnormality or $\dot{V}/\dot{Q}$ mismatch, the difference widens (greater than 15 mm Hg in room air). Examination of the equation reveals that hyperventilation, resulting in a lower $PaCO_2$, results in a higher $PAO_2$. Conversely, hypoventilation, resulting in a higher $PaCO_2$, results in a lower $PAO_2$. Physiologically the $PaO_2$ can never exceed the $PAO_2$, however, and the finding of a negative value indicates an error. The error may be in one of the measured values or in the assumed R value (see Table 20-16).

Clinical examples of the calculation and interpretation of the *A-a* gradient are provided in Table 20-17.

**Oxygen content, delivery, and utilization.** The commonly reported blood gas value $PaO_2$ reflects the pressure of oxygen dissolved in arterial blood. This value is critical for assessing lung function. However, the clinician must remember that other variables are involved in oxygen delivery to the tissues besides $PaO_2$ and that tissue hypoxia can occur in spite of a normal $PaO_2$. The formula for calculating the total oxygen content of arterial blood ($CaO_2$) is provided in Table 20-16. The greatest contribution to $CaO_2$ in health is oxygenated hemoglobin. In a normal dog ($PaO_2$, 100 mm Hg; hemoglobin, 15 g/dl), oxygenated hemoglobin accounts for

## TABLE 20-17

**Calculation and Interpretation of *A-a* Gradient: Clinical Examples**

*Example 1:* A healthy dog breathing room air has a $PaO_2$ of 95 mm Hg and a $PaCO_2$ of 40 mm Hg. His calculated $PAO_2$ is 100 mm Hg. ($PAO_2 = FIO_2 [P_B - P_{H2O}] - PaCO_2/R = 0.21 [765$ mm Hg $- 50$ mm Hg$] - [40$ mm Hg$/0.8]$.) The *A-a* gradient is 100 mm Hg $-$ 95 mm Hg $= 5$ mm Hg. This value is normal.

*Example 2:* A dog with respiratory depression due to an anesthetic overdose has a $PaO_2$ of 72 mm Hg and a $PaCO_2$ of 56 mm Hg in room air. His calculated $PAO_2$ is 80 mm Hg. The *A-a* gradient is 8 mm Hg. His hypoxemia can be explained by hypoventilation.

Later the same day, the dog develops crackles bilaterally. Repeat blood gas analysis shows a $PaO_2$ of 60 mm Hg and a $PaCO_2$ of 48 mm Hg. His calculated $PAO_2$ is 90 mm Hg. The *A-a* gradient is 30 mm Hg. Hypoventilation continues to contribute to the hypoxemia, but hypoventilation has improved. The widened *A-a* gradient indicates $\dot{V}/\dot{Q}$ mismatch. This dog has aspirated gastric contents into his lungs.

20 ml of $O_2$/dl, whereas dissolved oxygen accounts for only about 0.3 ml of $O_2$/dl.

The quantity of hemoglobin is routinely appraised by the complete blood count. It can also be estimated on the basis of the packed cell volume (by dividing the packed cell volume by 3). The oxygen saturation of hemoglobin ($SaO_2$) is dependent on the $PaO_2$, as depicted by the sigmoid shape of the oxygen-hemoglobin dissociation curve (see Fig. 20-17). However, the $SaO_2$ is also influenced by other variables that can shift the oxygen-hemoglobin dissociation curve to the left or right (e.g., pH, temperature, or 2,3-diphosphoglycerate concentrations) or interfere with oxygen binding with hemoglobin (e.g., carbon monoxide toxicity or methemoglobinemia). Some laboratories measure $SaO_2$.

Oxygen must also be successfully delivered to the tissues, and this depends on cardiac output and local circulation. Ultimately, the tissues must be able to effectively utilize the oxygen—a process interfered with in the presence of toxicities such as carbon monoxide or cyanide poisoning. Each of these processes must be considered when interpreting the blood gas values in an individual animal.

**Acid-base status.** The acid-base status of an animal can also be assessed using the same blood sample as that used to measure blood gases. Acid-base status is influenced by the respiratory system (see Table 20-16). Respiratory acidosis results if carbon dioxide is retained as a result of hypoventilation (see Table 20-15). If the problem persists for several days, compensatory retention of bicarbonate by the kidneys occurs. Excess removal of carbon dioxide by the lungs caused by hyperventilation results in respiratory alkalosis. Hyperventilation is usually an acute phenomenon, potentially caused by shock, sepsis, severe anemia, anxiety, or pain; therefore, compensatory changes in the bicarbonate concentration are rarely seen.

The respiratory system partially compensates for primary metabolic acid-base disorders, and this can occur quickly. Hyperventilation and a decreased $PaCO_2$ occur in response to metabolic acidosis. Hypoventilation and an increased $PaCO_2$ occur in response to metabolic alkalosis.

In most cases, acid-base disturbances can be identified as primarily respiratory or primarily metabolic in nature on the basis of the pH. The compensatory response will never be excessive and alter the pH beyond normal limits. An animal with acidosis (pH of less than 7.35) has a primary respiratory acidosis if the $PaCO_2$ is increased and a compensatory respiratory response if the $PaCO_2$ is decreased. An animal with alkalosis (pH of greater than 7.45) has a primary respiratory alkalosis if the $PaCO_2$ is decreased and a compensatory respiratory response if the $PaCO_2$ is increased.

If both the $PaCO_2$ and the bicarbonate concentration are abnormal, such that both contribute to the same alteration in pH, a mixed disturbance is present. For instance, an animal with acidosis, an increased $PaCO_2$, and a decreased $HCO_3$ has a mixed metabolic and respiratory acidosis.

## PULSE OXIMETRY

### Indications

Pulse oximetry is a method of monitoring the oxygen saturation of blood. The saturation of hemoglobin with oxygen is related to the $PaO_2$ by the sigmoid oxygen-hemoglobin dissociation curve (Fig. 20-27). Pulse oximetry is noninvasive, can be used to continuously monitor a dog or cat, provides immediate results, and is affordable for most practices. It is a particularly useful device for monitoring animals with respiratory disease that must undergo procedures requiring anesthesia. It can also be used in some cases to monitor the progression of disease or the response to therapy. More and more clinicians are using these devices for the routine monitoring of animals under general anesthesia, particularly if the number of personnel is limited, because alarms can be set to warn of marked changes in values.

### Methodology

Most pulse oximeters have a probe that is attached to a fold of tissue, such as the tongue, lip, ear flap, inguinal skin fold, toe, or tail (Fig. 20-28). This probe measures light absorption through the tissues. Other models measure reflected light and can be placed on mucous membranes or within the esophagus or rectum. Artifacts resulting from external light sources are minimized in the latter sites. Arterial blood is identified by the oximeter as that component which changes in pulses. Nonpulsatile absorption is considered background.

### Interpretation

Values provided by the pulse oximeter must be interpreted with care. The instrument must record a pulse that matches the palpable pulse of the animal. Any discrepancy between

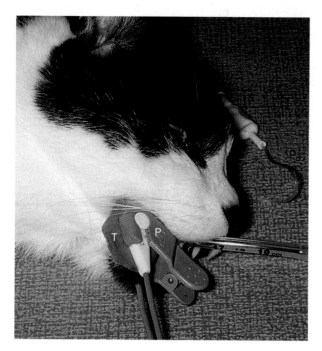

**FIG 20-28**
Monitoring oxygen saturation in a cat under general anesthesia using a pulse oximeter with a probe *(P)* clamped on the tongue *(T).*

the actual pulse and the pulse received by the oximeter indicates an inaccurate reading. Common problems that can interfere with the accurate detection of pulses include the position of the probe, animal motion (e.g., respirations, shivering), and weak or irregular pulse pressures (e.g., tachycardia, hypovolemia, hypothermia, arrhythmias).

The value measured indicates the saturation of hemoglobin in the local circulation. However, this value can be affected by factors other than pulmonary function, such as vasoconstriction, low cardiac output, and the local stasis of blood. Other intrinsic factors that can affect oximetry readings include anemia, hyperbilirubinemia, carboxyhemoglobinemia, and methemoglobinemia. External lights and the location of the probe can also influence results. Pulse oximetry readings of oxygen saturation are less accurate below values of 80%.

These sources for error should not discourage the clinician from using this technology, however, because changes in saturation in an individual animal provide valuable information. Rather, results must be interpreted critically.

The examination of the oxygen-hemoglobin dissociation curve (see Fig. 20-27) in normal dogs and cats shows that animals with $PaO_2$ values exceeding 85 mm Hg will have a hemoglobin saturation of greater than 95%. If $PaO_2$ values decrease to 60 mm Hg, the hemoglobin saturation will be approximately 90%. Any further decrease in $PaO_2$ results in a precipitous decrease in hemoglobin saturation, illustrated by the steep portion of the oxygen-hemoglobin dissociation curve. Ideally, then, hemoglobin saturation should be maintained at more than 90% by means of oxygen supplementation or ventilatory support (see Chapter 27) or the specific treatment of the underlying disease. However, because of the many variables associated with pulse oximetry, such strict guidelines are not always valid. In practice, a baseline hemoglobin saturation value is measured and subsequent changes in that value are then used to assess improvement or deterioration in oxygenation. Ideally, the baseline value is compared with the $PaO_2$ obtained from an arterial blood sample collected concurrently to ensure the accuracy of the readings.

## Suggested Readings

Amis TC et al: Systematic identification of endobronchial anatomy during bronchoscopy in the dog, *Am J Vet Res* 47:2649, 1986.

Bauer TG: Lung biopsy, *Vet Clin North Am Small Anim Pract* 30:1207, 2000.

Bowman DD et al: *Georgis' parasitology for veterinarians,* ed 6, Philadelphia, 1995, WB Saunders.

Hawkins EC et al: Bronchoalveolar lavage in the evaluation of pulmonary disease in the dog and cat, *J Vet Intern Med* 4:267, 1990.

Hawkins EC et al: Cytologic characterization of bronchoalveolar lavage fluid collected through an endotracheal tube in cats, *Am J Vet Res* 55:795, 1994.

Hawkins EC et al: Cytological analysis of bronchoalveolar lavage fluid in the diagnosis of respiratory tract disease in dogs: a retrospective study, *J Vet Intern Med* 9:386, 1995.

Hawkins EC et al: Use of a modified stomach tube for bronchoalveolar lavage in dogs, *J Am Vet Med Assoc* 215:1635, 1999.

Hendricks JC et al: Practicality, usefulness, and limits of pulse oximetry in critical small animal patients, *Vet Emerg Crit Care* 3:5, 1993.

Kneller SK: Thoracic radiography. In Kirk RW, editor: *Current veterinary therapy IX,* Philadelphia, 1986, WB Saunders.

Neath PJ et al: Lung lobe torsion in dogs: 22 cases (1981-1999), *J Am Vet Med Assoc* 217:1041, 2000.

Padrid PA et al: Tracheobronchoscopy of the dog and cat. In Tams TR, editor: *Small animal endoscopy,* ed 2, St Louis, 1999, Mosby.

Peeters DE et al: Quantitative bacterial cultures and cytological examination of bronchoalveolar lavage specimens from dogs, *J Vet Intern Med* 14:534, 2000.

Reinemeyer CR: Parasites of the respiratory tract. In Bonagura JD et al, editors: *Current veterinary therapy XII,* Philadelphia, 1983, WB Saunders.

Shaw DH et al: Eosinophilic bronchitis caused by *Crenosoma vulpis* infection in dogs, *Can Vet J* 37:361, 1996.

Suter PF: *Thoracic radiography,* Wettswil, Switzerland, 1984, Peter F Suter.

Teske E et al: Transthoracic needle aspiration biopsy of the lung in dogs with pulmonic disease, *J Am Anim Hosp Assoc* 27:289, 1991.

Urquhart GM et al: *Veterinary parasitology,* New York, 1987, Churchill Livingstone.

West JB: *Respiratory physiology: the essentials,* ed 3, Baltimore, 1985, Williams & Wilkins.

West JB: *Pulmonary pathophysiology: the essentials,* ed 4, Baltimore, 1992, Williams & Wilkins.

## CHAPTER 21

# Disorders of the Trachea and Bronchi

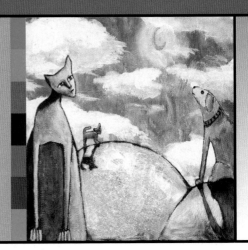

## CHAPTER OUTLINE

GENERAL CONSIDERATIONS, 287
CANINE INFECTIOUS TRACHEOBRONCHITIS, 287
COLLAPSING TRACHEA, 289
FELINE BRONCHITIS, 291
ALLERGIC BRONCHITIS, 295
CANINE CHRONIC BRONCHITIS, 295
*OSLERUS OSLERI,* 297

## GENERAL CONSIDERATIONS

Common diseases of the trachea and bronchi include canine infectious tracheobronchitis, collapsing trachea, feline bronchitis, allergic bronchitis, canine chronic bronchitis, and *Oslerus osleri* infection. Other diseases may involve the airways, either primarily or concurrently with pulmonary parenchymal disease. These diseases, such as bacterial infection, other parasitic infections, and neoplasia, are discussed in Chapter 22. Feline bordetellosis can cause signs of bronchitis (e.g., cough) but is more often associated with signs of upper respiratory disease (see Chapter 15, Feline Upper Respiratory Infections) or bacterial pneumonia (see Chapter 22, Bacterial Pneumonia).

## CANINE INFECTIOUS TRACHEOBRONCHITIS

### Etiology

Canine infectious tracheobronchitis, "kennel cough," is a highly contagious, acute disease that is localized in the airways. One or more infectious agents cause it, including canine adenovirus 2 (CAV2), parainfluenza virus (PIV), and *Bordetella bronchiseptica*. Other organisms may also be involved as secondary pathogens. In nearly all dogs the disease is self-limiting, with resolution of clinical signs in approximately 2 weeks.

### Clinical Features

Affected dogs are first seen because of the sudden onset of a severe productive or nonproductive cough, which is often exacerbated by exercise, excitement, or the pressure of the collar on the neck. Palpating the trachea can easily induce the cough. Gagging, retching, or nasal discharge can also occur. A recent history (i.e., within 2 weeks) of boarding, hospitalization, or exposure to a puppy or dog that has similar signs is common. Puppies recently obtained from pet stores, kennels, or humane societies have often been exposed to the pathogens.

Dogs with uncomplicated infectious tracheobronchitis do not show the signs of a systemic illness. Therefore dogs showing weight loss, persistent anorexia, or signs of involvement of other organ systems, such as diarrhea, chorioretinitis, or seizures, may have some other more serious disease, such as canine distemper or a mycotic infection. Although uncommon, respiratory complications can result from infectious tracheobronchitis. A secondary bacterial pneumonia can develop in very young puppies, immunocompromised dogs, and dogs that have preexisting lung abnormalities such as chronic bronchitis. Dogs with chronic airway disease or tracheal collapse can experience an acute, severe exacerbation of their chronic problems, and extended management may be necessary to resolve the signs associated with infection in these animals. *Bordetella* infection has been associated with chronic bronchitis, but which occurs first is not certain.

### Diagnosis

Uncomplicated cases of kennel cough are diagnosed based on the presenting signs. A clinicopathologic evaluation, including a complete blood count (CBC), thoracic radiographs, and tracheal wash fluid analysis, is indicated for dogs with signs suggestive of a more serious disease and for those with unresolving signs. The CBC and thoracic radiograph findings are unremarkable in dogs with uncomplicated tracheobronchitis. Evidence of acute inflammation is seen in tracheal wash fluid specimens. Bacterial culture of the fluid can be useful for identifying any bacteria involved in the disease, and concurrent antibiotic sensitivity information is helpful in selecting antibiotics.

## TABLE 21-1

### Common Cough Suppressants for Use in Dogs*

| AGENT | DOSAGE |
|-------|--------|
| Dextromethorphan | 1 to 2 mg/kg, q6-8h PO |
| Butorphanol | 0.5 mg/kg, q6-12h PO |
| Hydrocodone bitartrate | 0.25 mg/kg, q8-12h PO |

*Centrally acting cough suppressants are rarely, if ever, indicated for use in cats and can result in adverse reactions. The above dosages are for dogs only.

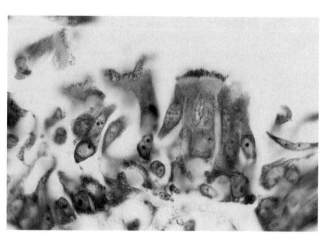

**FIG 21-1**
Photomicrograph of a tracheal biopsy from a dog infected with *Bordetella bronchiseptica*. The organisms are small, basophilic rods that are visible along the ciliated border of the epithelial cells. (Giemsa stain courtesy D. Malarkey.)

### Treatment

Uncomplicated infectious tracheobronchitis is a self-limiting disease. Rest for at least 7 days, specifically avoiding exercise and excitement, is indicated to minimize the continual irritation of the airways caused by excessive coughing. Cough suppressants are valuable for the same reason but should not be given if the cough is productive or if fluid is suspected to be accumulating in the lungs based on auscultation or thoracic radiograph findings.

A variety of cough suppressants can be used in dogs (Table 21-1). Dextromethorphan is a mild suppressant that is available in over-the-counter preparations. Cold remedies with additional ingredients such as antihistamines and decongestants should be avoided. Pediatric liquid preparations are palatable for most dogs, and the alcohol contained in them may also have a mild tranquilizing effect. Butorphanol and hydrocodone bitartrate are potent cough suppressants that can also be used in dogs. High doses can be sedating.

In theory, antibiotics are not indicated for most dogs with infectious tracheobronchitis for two reasons: (1) the disease is usually self-limiting and tends to resolve spontaneously, regardless of any specific treatment that is implemented, and (2) no antibiotic protocol has been proven to eliminate *Bordetella* organisms from the airways. In practice, however, antibiotics are often prescribed, and their use is justified based on the potential role of *Bordetella* in the disease. Consideration should be given to selecting an antibiotic based on its ability to reach the bronchial epithelium and airway secretions, because the bacteria are often present on the cilia of the respiratory epithelial cells (Fig. 21-1). Antibiotics that are effective against many *Bordetella* isolates include doxycycline (5 to 10 mg/kg q12h), chloramphenicol (50 mg/kg q8h), and amoxicillin with clavulanate (20 to 25 mg/kg q8h). Bacterial susceptibility data from tracheal wash fluid can be used to guide the selection of an appropriate antibiotic. Antibiotics are administered for 5 days beyond the time the clinical signs resolve or for at least 10 days.

Glucocorticoids should not be used. A field trial conducted by Thrusfield and colleagues (1991) failed to demonstrate any benefit of steroid therapy, either alone or in combination with antibiotics.

If clinical signs have not resolved within 2 weeks, further diagnostic evaluation is indicated. See Chapter 22 for the management of complicated cases of infectious tracheobronchitis with bacterial pneumonia.

### Prognosis

The prognosis for recovery from uncomplicated infectious tracheobronchitis is excellent.

### Prevention

Canine infectious tracheobronchitis can be prevented by minimizing an animal's exposure to organisms and through vaccination programs. Excellent nutrition, routine deworming, and avoidance of stress improve the ability of the dog to respond appropriately to infection without showing serious signs. To minimize exposure, dogs are kept isolated from puppies or dogs that have been recently boarded. Careful sanitation should be practiced in kenneling facilities. Caretakers should be instructed in the disinfection of cages, bowls, and runs, and anyone working with the dogs must wash their hands after handling each animal. Dogs should not be allowed to have face-to-face contact. Adequate air exchange and humidity control are necessary in rooms housing several dogs. Recommended goals are at least 10 to 15 air exchanges per hour and less than 50% humidity. An isolation area is essential for the housing of dogs with clinical signs of infectious tracheobronchitis.

Injectable and intranasal vaccines are available for the three major pathogens involved in canine infectious tracheobronchitis (i.e., CAV2, PIV, *B. bronchiseptica*). Injectable modified–live virus vaccines against CAV2 and PIV are adequate for most pet dogs. They are conveniently included in most combination distemper vaccines. Because maternal antibodies interfere with the response to the vaccines, puppies must be vaccinated every 2 to 4 weeks, beginning at 6 to 8 weeks of age and through 14 to 16 weeks of age. At least two vaccines must be given initially. Frequency of booster vaccination has traditionally been every year. Such frequent vaccination may not be necessary for most healthy, pet dogs (see Chapter 99).

Dogs at high risk for disease, such as those in kennels where the disease is endemic or those that are frequently boarded, may benefit from vaccines incorporating *B. bronchiseptica*. These vaccines do not prevent infection but aim to decrease clinical signs if infection occurs. Vaccines for *Bordetella* are available for parenteral and for intranasal administration. A study by Ellis and colleagues (2001) indicates that both forms of vaccine afford similar protection based on antibody titers, clinical signs, upper airway cultures, and histopathologic examination of tissues following exposure to organisms. The greatest benefit was achieved by administering both forms of vaccine sequentially at a 2-week interval. The dogs in this study were vaccinated between 14 to 18 weeks of age.

Intranasal *Bordetella* vaccines occasionally cause clinical signs, predominantly cough. The signs are generally self-limiting but are disturbing to most owners.

## COLLAPSING TRACHEA

The normal trachea is seen to be circular on cross section (see Fig. 20-23, *A*). An open lumen is maintained during all phases of respiration by the cartilaginous tracheal rings, which are connected by fibroelastic annular ligaments to maintain flexibility, thereby allowing movement of the neck without compromising the airway. The cartilaginous rings are incomplete dorsally. The dorsal tracheal membrane, consisting of the longitudinal tracheal muscle and connective tissue, completes the rings. Any narrowing of the trachea results in a greatly increased resistance to air flow and local turbulence, because the resistance to air flow is proportional to the reciprocal of the radius of the lumen to the fourth power. The term *tracheal collapse* refers to the narrowing of the tracheal lumen resulting from flattening of the cartilaginous rings, a redundancy of the dorsal tracheal membrane, or both. The condition can affect the extrathoracic trachea, the intrathoracic trachea, or both. Chronic bronchitis with collapse of the mainstem bronchi coexists in many dogs with intrathoracic tracheal collapse.

A credible theory of the pathogenesis of tracheal collapse is that certain dog are predisposed to collapse because of inherent abnormalities in their tracheal cartilage, but are initially asymptomatic. Dogs develop cough when an exacerbating problem develops. Once the cough begins, a cycle is started through chronic tracheal inflammation, changes in the tracheal mucosa, and perpetuation of cough.

### Clinical Features

Tracheal collapse is common in middle-aged toy and miniature dogs, although it can occur early in life and in large-breed dogs. Tracheal collapse is rare in cats; generally, it occurs secondarily to a tracheal obstruction such as a tumor or traumatic injury. Signs may occur acutely but then slowly

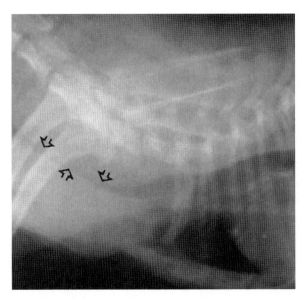

**FIG 21-2**
Lateral radiograph of the neck of a dog with collapsing trachea taken during inspiration. The extrathoracic airway stripe is severely narrowed *(arrows)*.

progress over months to years. The primary clinical feature is a nonproductive cough, described as a "goose honk." The cough is worse during excitement or exercise or when the collar exerts pressure on the neck. Eventually (usually after years of chronic cough) respiratory distress caused by obstruction to air flow may be brought on by exercise, overheating, or excitement. Systemic signs such as weight loss, anorexia, and depression are uncommon.

On physical examination the cough can often be elicited by palpation of the trachea. An end-expiratory snap or click may be heard during auscultation if intrathoracic collapse is present. In advanced cases or after exercise, increased inspiratory effort may be observed in dogs with extrathoracic collapse and increased expiratory effort observed in those with intrathoracic collapse.

History and physical examination should also emphasize a search for exacerbating or complicating disease. Possibilities include cardiac disease causing left atrial enlargement and bronchial compression or pulmonary edema; airway inflammation caused by bacterial infection, allergic bronchitis, exposure to smoke (e.g., from cigarettes, fireplaces), chronic bronchitis, or recent intubation; upper airway obstruction caused by elongated soft palate, stenotic nares, or laryngeal paralysis; and systemic disorders such as obesity or hyperadrenocorticism.

### Diagnosis

A collapsing trachea is most often diagnosed based on clinical signs and the findings from cervical and thoracic radiography. Radiographs of the neck to evaluate the size of the lumen of the extrathoracic trachea are taken during inspiration (Fig. 21-2), when narrowing caused by tracheal collapse is

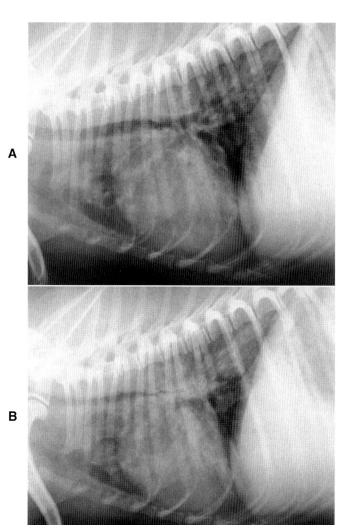

A

B

**FIG 21-3**

Lateral radiographs of a dog with intrathoracic tracheal collapse during inspiration **(A)** and expiration **(B)**. The distal trachea and mainstem bronchi are markedly narrowed during expiration. Evaluation of the pulmonary parenchyma should not be attempted using films exposed during expiration.

more evident because of negative airway pressure. Conversely, the size of the lumen of the intrathoracic trachea is evaluated on thoracic radiographs taken during expiration, when increased intrathoracic pressures make collapse more apparent (Fig. 21-3). Radiographs of the thorax should also be taken during inspiration to look for concurrent bronchial or parenchymal abnormalities. (See Chapter 20 for a further discussion of radiography.)

Alternatively, the trachea can be evaluated fluoroscopically or bronchoscopically (see Fig. 20-23, *B*). These methods are more sensitive for the diagnosis of collapsing trachea than routine radiography.

Tracheal washing or bronchoscopy with bronchoalveolar lavage (BAL) should be performed to identify the presence of airway inflammation and infection at the time of initial pre-

sentation or during exacerbation of signs. Cytologic analysis and bacterial culture are performed in all cases.

**Treatment**

Medical therapy is adequate treatment for most animals. In a study of 100 dogs by White and colleague (1994), medical therapy resulted in resolution of signs for at least 1 year in 71% of cases. Dogs that are overweight are placed on a weight-reducing diet. Harnesses should be used instead of collars, and owners should be counseled to keep their dogs from becoming overheated (e.g., they should not be left in a car). Excessive excitement should also be avoided. Sedatives such as phenobarbital are prescribed for some animals, and these can be administered before known stressful events.

In the absence of pneumonia, cough suppressants are used to control signs and disrupt the potential cycle of perpetuating cough (see Table 21-1). Cough suppressants can often be given with decreasing frequency over time and then discontinued, if the cough resolves. Bronchodilators may be beneficial in dogs with signs of chronic bronchitis (see p. 295). Antiinflammatory doses of glucocorticoids can be given for a short period during exacerbation of signs (prednisone, 0.5 to 1 mg/kg every 12 hours for 3 to 5 days, then tapered and discontinued over 3 to 4 weeks). Long-term use is avoided because of potential detrimental side effects, such as obesity. Dogs with signs referable to mitral insufficiency are managed for this disease (Chapter 8). Dogs with abnormalities causing upper airway obstruction are treated with corrective surgical procedures.

Antibiotics are not indicated for the routine management of a collapsing trachea. Dogs in which tracheal wash or BAL fluid analysis has revealed evidence of infection should be treated with appropriate antibiotics (selected based on the results of sensitivity testing). Because most antibiotics do not reach high concentrations in the airways, relatively high doses of antibiotics should be administered for several weeks, as described for canine chronic bronchitis (p. 295). Any other potentially related problems identified during the diagnostic evaluation are addressed.

Management of dogs in acute distress with signs of either extrathoracic airway obstruction or intrathoracic large airway obstruction is discussed in Chapter 26.

Surgical treatment of a collapsing trachea should be considered for animals that are no longer responsive to medical management, usually because of respiratory difficulty. The most common method of correction involves support of the trachea with an external splint. Procedures involving the use of modified syringe casings as a spiral splint, or polypropylene C-shaped splints, have been described. Dogs with extrathoracic collapse are better surgical candidates than those with intrathoracic collapse. Complications associated with intraluminal airway stents preclude their routine use.

**Prognosis**

In most dogs, clinical signs can be controlled with conscientiously performed medical management, with diagnostic evaluations performed during episodes of acute exacerbations of signs. Animals in which severe signs develop despite appropriate medical care have a guarded prognosis.

## FELINE BRONCHITIS

### Etiology

Bronchitis is a common cause of respiratory disease in cats and can result in cough, wheeze, and episodic respiratory distress. However, the term *feline bronchitis* or *feline asthma,* as applied to all cats with bronchial disease, belies the wide variety of pathologic processes that can affect individual cats. Clinically, the range in the severity of signs and the response to therapy shows this diversity.

Different combinations of factors that result in small airway obstruction, a consistent feature of feline bronchial disease, are present in each animal (Table 21-2). Some of these factors are reversible (e.g., bronchospasm, inflammation), and some are permanent (e.g., fibrosis, emphysema). The classification proposed by Moise and colleagues (1989b), which was formulated on the basis of similar pathologic processes that occur in people, is recommended as a way to better define bronchial disease in individual cats for the purpose of treatment recommendations and prognostication (Table 21-3). A cat can also have more than one type of bronchitis. Although it is not always possible to absolutely determine the type, or types, of bronchial disease present without sophisticated pulmonary function testing, routine clinical data (i.e., history and physical examination findings, thoracic radiographs, analysis of airway specimens, progression of signs) can be used to classify the disease in most cats.

Additional variations in signs from animal to animal occur as a result of the underlying cause. Feline bronchitis is not a specific disease but rather a descriptive diagnosis. In many cats, the bronchitis is idiopathic. However, some treatable diseases that can be associated with feline bronchitis should be considered in the diagnostic evaluation, and these include allergic bronchitis, bacterial or mycoplasmal infection, pulmonary parasites, and heartworm disease (Table 21-4).

### Clinical Features

Bronchitis can develop in cats of any age, although it most commonly develops in young adult and middle-aged animals. The major clinical feature is cough or episodic respiratory distress or both. The owners may report audible wheezing during an episode. The signs are often slowly progressive. Weight loss, anorexia, depression, or other systemic signs are not present. Owners should be carefully questioned regarding an association with exposure to potential allergens or irritants, such as new litter (usually perfumed), cigarette or fireplace smoke, carpet cleaners, or household items containing perfumes such as deodorant or hair spray. They should also be questioned about whether there has been any recent remodeling or any other change in the cat's environment, which could also be a source of allergens. Seasonal exacerbations are another sign of potential allergen exposure.

### TABLE 21-2

**Factors that Can Contribute to Small Airway Obstruction in Cats with Bronchial Disease**

Bronchoconstriction
Bronchial smooth muscle hypertrophy
Increased mucus production
Decreased mucus clearance
Inflammatory exudate in airway lumens
Inflammatory infiltrate in airway walls
Epithelial hyperplasia
Glandular hypertrophy
Fibrosis
Emphysema

### TABLE 21-3

**Classification of Feline Bronchial Disease**

**Bronchial Asthma**

Predominant feature: reversible airway obstruction primarily resulting from bronchoconstriction
Other common features: hypertrophy of smooth muscle; increased mucus production; eosinophilic inflammation

**Acute Bronchitis**

Predominant feature: reversible airway inflammation of short duration (<1-3 months)
Other common features: increased mucus production; neutrophilic or macrophagic inflammation

**Chronic Bronchitis**

Predominant feature: chronic airway inflammation (>2-3 months) resulting in irreversible damage (e.g., fibrosis)
Other common features: increased mucus production; neutrophilic, eosinophilic, or mixed inflammation; isolation of bacteria or *Mycoplasma* organisms causing infection or as nonpathogenic inhabitants; concurrent bronchial asthma

**Emphysema**

Predominant feature: destruction of bronchiolar and alveolar walls resulting in enlarged peripheral airspaces
Other common features: cavitary lesions (bullae); result of or concurrent with chronic bronchitis

Adapted from Moise NS et al: Bronchopulmonary disease. In Sherding RG, editor: *The cat: diseases and clinical management,* New York, 1989, Churchill Livingstone.

The physical examination findings result from small airway obstruction. Cats that are in distress show tachypnea, with increased respiratory efforts during expiration. Auscultation reveals expiratory wheezes, particularly during such episodes. Crackles are occasionally present. Physical examination findings may be unremarkable between episodes.

TABLE 21-4

**Differential Diagnoses (Etiologic) for Cats with Feline Bronchitis**

---

Allergic bronchitis
Pulmonary parasites
   *Aelurostrongylus abstrusus*
   *Capillaria aerophila*
   *Paragonimus kellicotti*
Heartworm disease
Bacterial bronchitis
Mycoplasmal bronchitis
Idiopathic feline bronchitis

---

## Diagnosis

A presumptive diagnosis of feline bronchitis is made based on the historical, physical examination, and thoracic radiographic findings. Findings from a tracheal wash or BAL fluid analysis can confirm the presence of airway inflammation, and one of these procedures is performed along with tests for heartworm disease and pulmonary parasitism to identify specific diseases that may be involved. Cats with bronchitis (particularly bronchial asthma) have been thought to have peripheral eosinophilia. However, this finding is neither specific nor sensitive and cannot be used to rule out or definitively diagnose feline bronchitis.

A bronchial pattern is generally seen on thoracic radiographs from cats with bronchitis (see Fig. 20-3). Increased reticular interstitial markings and patchy alveolar opacities can also be present. The lungs may be seen to be overinflated as a result of the trapping of air, and occasionally collapse (i.e., atelectasis) of the right middle lung lobe is seen. However, because clinical signs can precede radiographic changes and because radiographs cannot detect mild airway changes, thoracic radiographs can be normal in cats with bronchitis. Radiographs are also scrutinized for signs of specific diseases such as heartworm or pulmonary parasites.

The tracheal wash or BAL fluid cytologic findings are generally representative of the disease process and consist of increased numbers of inflammatory cells and an increased amount of mucus. Inflammation can be eosinophilic, neutrophilic, or mixed.

Although not a specific finding, eosinophilic inflammation is suggestive of a hypersensitivity response to allergens or parasites. Neutrophils should be examined for signs of the degeneration suggestive of bacterial infection. Slides should be carefully scrutinized for the presence of organisms, particularly bacteria and parasitic larvae or ova. Fluid should be cultured for bacteria, keeping in mind that the growth of organisms may or may not indicate the existence of true infection (Chapter 20). Cultures for *Mycoplasma* spp. can be helpful, but it is difficult to grow such organisms and the turnaround time for results is long.

 TABLE 21-5

**Common Bronchodilators for Use in Dogs and Cats**

---

**Methylxanthines**

Aminophylline
  Cat: 5 mg/kg PO q12h
  Dog: 11 mg/kg PO q8h
Oxtriphylline elixir (Choledyl, Parke-Davis)
  Dog: 14 mg/kg PO q8h
  Cat: None
Long-acting theophylline*
  Cat: 25 mg/kg q24h, in evening
  Dog: 10 mg/kg q12h†

**Sympathomimetics**

Terbutaline
  Cat: ⅛-¼ of 2.5 mg tablet/cat PO q12h, to start; or
    0.01 mg/kg SC, can repeat once
  Dog: 1.25-5 mg/dog PO q8-12h

---

From Bach JF et al: *Proceedings of the 20th Symposium of the Veterinary Comparative Respiratory Society,* Boston, 2002.
*Absorption of currently available products is unpredictable in dogs and cats. Monitoring of plasma concentrations is recommended.
†Theophylline SR, Inwood Laboratories, Inwood, N.Y.

Testing for heartworm disease should also be done (Chapter 10). Multiple fecal examinations using special concentrating techniques are performed to further evaluate young cats and cats with airway eosinophilia for the presence of pulmonary parasites (Chapter 20).

## Treatment

The condition of cats in acute respiratory distress should be stabilized before diagnostic tests are performed. Successful treatment includes administration of a bronchodilator, rapid-acting glucocorticoids, and oxygen supplementation. Terbutaline can be administered subcutaneously, avoiding stress (Table 21-5). Prednisolone sodium succinate (10 to 20 mg/kg intravenously) is the recommended glucocorticoid. If intravenous administration is too stressful, the drug can be given intramuscularly. After the drugs are administered, the cat is placed in a cool, stress-free, oxygen-enriched environment. See Chapter 26 for further discussion of cats with respiratory distress.

Once the cat's condition has been stabilized, diagnostic evaluation can proceed. Identifying any treatable underlying cause is a primary goal. Because of the difficulty in documenting *Mycoplasma* infection, a therapeutic trial of antibiotics should be considered. Either doxycycline (5 to 10 mg/kg every 12 hours) or chloramphenicol (10 to 15 mg/kg q12h) is administered for this purpose for 14 days. For cats that are difficult to medicate, azithromycin (5 to 10 mg/kg q24h for 3 days, then every 72 hours) can be tried.

The possibility of inhaled allergens being the cause of the problem should be pursued, particularly in cats with eosinophilic airway inflammation. Potential sources are determined through careful owner questioning (see Clinical features), after which the owner reevaluates the environment. Trial eliminations of possible allergens from the cat's environment should be performed. Potential reactions to smoke and litter perfumes should be tested, even in animals with no obvious association. Smoke can often aggravate signs because of its local irritating effects, even if it is not the primary allergen. The effect of litter perfumes can be evaluated by replacing the litter with sandbox sand or plain clay litter. Indoor cats may show improvement in response to measures taken to decrease the level of dusts, molds, and mildew in the home. Such measures include carpet, furniture, and drapery cleaning; cleaning of the furnace and the frequent replacement of air filters; and the use of an air cleaner. Any beneficial response to an environmental change is usually seen within 1 to 2 weeks.

**Glucocorticoids and bronchodilators.** Therapy with glucocorticoids, with or without bronchodilators, is necessary for most cats. Results can be quite dramatic. However, drug therapy can interfere with environmental testing; therefore the ability of the animal to tolerate a delay in the start of drug therapy must be assessed on an animal-by-animal basis. Glucocorticoids can relieve the clinical signs in most cats and may protect the airways from the detrimental effects of chronic inflammation. Short-acting products such as prednisone are recommended because the dose of drug can be tapered to the lowest effective amount. A dose of 0.5 mg/kg is administered every 8 to 12 hours initially, doubling it if signs are not controlled within 1 week. Once the signs are controlled, the dose is tapered. A reasonable goal is to administer 0.5 mg/kg or less every other day. Outdoor cats that cannot be treated frequently can be treated with depot steroid products, such as methylprednisolone acetate (10 mg/cat intramuscularly is effective for up to 4 weeks).

Cats that require relatively large amounts of glucocorticoids to control clinical signs, that react unfavorably to glucocorticoid therapy, or that suffer from periodic exacerbations of signs can benefit from bronchodilator therapy. The three major classes of bronchodilators are (1) methylxanthines, (2) sympathomimetics, and (3) parasympatholytics. Recommended doses of these drugs are listed in Table 21-5.

I prefer to use methylxanthines because they are effective and inexpensive, and because the plasma concentrations can be easily measured for the monitoring of difficult cases. Certain sustained-release formulations are effective in cats when given once daily. In addition to the relaxation of bronchial smooth muscles, their beneficial effects may include improved mucociliary clearance, decreased fatigue of respiratory muscles, and inhibition of release of mast cell mediators of inflammation. Potential adverse effects include gastrointestinal signs, cardiac arrhythmias, nervousness, and seizures. Serious adverse effects are extremely rare at therapeutic concentrations. The immediate-release forms (i.e., not sustained-release products) are rapidly absorbed after oral administration, so parenteral injection is rarely necessary. If they must be administered intravenously, the drug should be injected slowly.

A variety of methylxanthines are available; they are converted within the body into the active product theophylline.

Long-acting theophyllines provide the most convenient form of these drugs for owners, because they only need to be administered once daily to cats and twice daily to dogs. Dye and colleagues (1990) found two specific brands to have predictable absorption in dogs and cats: (1) Theo-Dur and (2) Slo-BID. Unfortunately, these brands are not currently available. Other brands that were investigated did not result in consistent blood concentrations in dogs and cats. It is reasonable to continue to prescribe long-acting theophyllines because of the convenience of infrequent dosing. However, routine monitoring of plasma theophylline concentrations is recommended when using these drugs.

The individual metabolism of all of the methylxanthines is variable, and plasma theophylline concentrations are also monitored in animals that respond poorly. Therapeutic peak concentrations, based on data from people, are 5 to 20 $\mu$g/ml.

Plasma for the determination of these concentrations should be collected 12 hours after the evening dosing of the long-acting products and 2 hours after short-acting products. Measurement of concentrations immediately before the next scheduled dose might provide useful information concerning duration of therapeutic concentrations.

Drugs being administered concurrently can also affect plasma concentrations. For example, fluoroquinolone and chloramphenicol administration can cause increased plasma theophylline concentrations and subsequent signs of toxicity. Doses of theophylline should be decreased by one third to one half, or sympathomimetic drugs should be used, if such drugs are given.

Sympathomimetic drugs are also effective bronchodilators. Terbutaline is selective for $B2$ adrenergic receptors, lessening its cardiac effects. Potential adverse effects include nervousness, tremors, hypotension, and tachycardia. It can be administered subcutaneously for the treatment of respiratory emergencies; it can also be administered orally. Note that the recommended oral dose for cats (one eighth to one fourth of a 2.5-mg tablet; see Table 21-5) is lower than the more commonly cited dose of 1.25 mg/cat. The subcutaneous dose is lower still: 0.01 mg/kg, repeated once in 5 to 10 minutes if necessary.

Administration of glucocorticoids (fluticasone propionate, Flovent) and bronchodilators (albuterol) to cats using metered dose inhalers (MDIs), as is routine in treating asthma in people, has been recommended by Padrid (2000). This route of administration offers the potential benefits of minimizing trips to the emergency clinic through the at-home administration of bronchodilators without injection and of minimizing systemic side effects, particularly of glucocorticoids. However, at this time, the administration of drugs to cats by MDI has many unknown variables. Particularly, it is not known how much drug reaches the lower airways and how much is retained on the oral and nasal mucosa. A drug administered by MDI is always deposited to some extent on the oral and nasal mucosa, even in people who can be taught techniques to maximize deposition into the lower airways. I believe it is potentially dangerous to administer potent glucocorticoids to cats by MDI. Unlike people, cats frequently have latent herpes infections and periodontal disease.

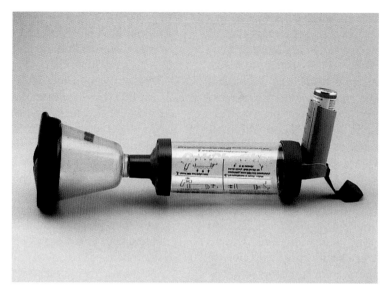

**FIG 21-4**
Apparatus for administering drugs by metered dose inhaler (MDI) to cats consisting of an anesthetic mask, spacer (OptiChamber, Respironics, Inc., Pittsburgh, Pa), and MDI (Ventolin, GlaxoSmithKline, Research Triangle Park, N.C.).

Administering glucocorticoids by MDI is not necessarily safer for these cats than systemic administration. Nevertheless, administration of glucocorticoids by MDI is a viable option for cats that are overtly intolerant of oral glucocorticoids. Administration of bronchodilators by MDI has not been shown to present a risk. Clinical response should indicate whether that route of administration of bronchodilators is being effective for an individual cat.

To administer drugs by MDI, a spacer must be used. Further, the breathing efforts of the cat must be sufficient to activate the one-way valve of the spacer. Padrid (2000) has found the Optichamber (Respironics Inc., Pittsburgh, Pa) to be effective. A small anesthetic mask, with rubber diaphragm, is attached to the spacer (Fig. 21-4).

Widening of the adapter of the anesthetic mask that is inserted into the spacer is necessary to create a snug fit. This is achieved simply by wrapping adhesive tape around the adapter. The cat is allowed to rest comfortably on a table. The client stands behind the cat and places the arms on either side to provide restraint. The MDI, attached to the spacer, is actuated (i.e., pressed) twice. The mask is placed immediately on the cat's face, covering the mouth and nose completely, and it is held in place while the cat takes 7 to 10 breaths, inhaling the drug into its airways.

Padrid (2000) recommends the following treatment schedule. Cats with mild daily symptoms should be given 220 μg of fluticasone propionate by MDI twice daily and albuterol by MDI as needed. The maximum effect of fluticasone is not expected until 7 to 10 days of treatment. For cats with moderate daily symptoms, treatment with MDI should be as described for mild symptoms; in addition, prednisone is administered orally for 10 days (1 mg/kg q12h for 5 days, then q24h for 5 days). For cats with severe symptoms, dexamethasone is administered once (2 mg/kg intravenously), albuterol

is administered by MDI every 30 minutes for up to 4 hours, and the cat is administered oxygen. Once stabilized, these cats are prescribed 220 μg of fluticasone propionate by MDI every 12 hours, and albuterol by MDI every 6 hours as needed. Oral prednisone is administered as needed.

**Other potential treatments.** Antihistamines are not recommended for treating feline bronchitis because histamine in some cats produces bronchodilation. However, work done by Padrid and colleagues (1995) has shown that the serotonin antagonist, cyproheptadine, has a bronchodilatory effect in vitro. A dose of 2 mg/cat orally every 12 hours can be tried in cats with signs that cannot be controlled with routine bronchodilator and glucocorticoid therapy. The client should be advised of the experimental nature of this, however.

Much interest has been shown among clients and veterinarians for the use of oral leukotriene inhibitors in cats (e.g., Accolate, Singulair, and Zyflo). However, the clinician should be aware that in people, leukotriene inhibitors are *less* effective in the management of asthma than glucocorticoids, and they are not used in the emergency management of the disease or for refractory cases. Their advantage for people lies in decreased side effects, compared with glucocorticoids, and ease of administration. To date, toxicity studies have not been performed on these drugs in cats. Further, there have been a few studies that suggest that leukotriene inhibition in cats would not be expected to be particularly effective because the part of the inflammatory cascade inhibited by the drugs is not a uniquely important part of the airway inflammation in feline bronchitis. Therefore their use in cats is not currently advocated. Further investigation into their potential role in treating feline bronchitis is certainly indicated.

The clinician should ask himself or herself the questions in Table 21-6, if cats fail to respond to glucocorticoid and bron-

## TABLE 21-6

**Considerations for Cats with Bronchitis that Fail to Respond to Glucocorticoid and Bronchodilator Therapy**

Is the cat receiving prescribed medication?
　Measure plasma theophylline concentrations.
　Trial therapy with repositol glucocorticoids.
Was an underlying disease missed on initial evaluation?
　Repeat diagnostic evaluation, including complete history
　　for potential allergens, thoracic radiographs, tracheal
　　wash fluid analysis, heartworm tests, and fecal
　　examinations for parasites. In addition, perform CBC,
　　serum biochemical analysis, and urinalysis.
　Trial therapy with anti-*Mycoplasma* drug.
　Trial environmental manipulations to minimize potential
　　allergen and irritant exposure.
Has a complicating disease developed?
　Repeat diagnostic evaluation as described above.

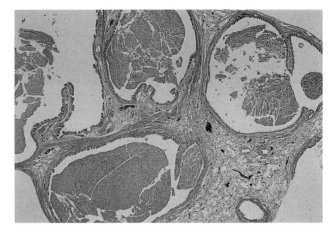

**FIG 21-5**
Photomicrograph of a lung biopsy from a dog with severe bronchiectasis. The airways are filled with exudate and are greatly dilated (H&E stain).

chodilator therapy or if exacerbation of signs occurs during chronic treatment.

### Prognosis

The prognosis for the control of clinical signs of feline bronchitis is good for most cats, particularly if extensive permanent damage has not yet occurred. Complete cure is unlikely unless an underlying cause can be eliminated; most cats require continued medication. Cats that have severe, acute asthmatic attacks are at risk for sudden death. Cats with persistent, untreated airway inflammation can develop the permanent changes of chronic bronchitis and emphysema.

## ALLERGIC BRONCHITIS

Allergic bronchitis involves an inflammatory response within the airways, usually to an inhaled antigen. The inflammatory response of the airways is typically eosinophilic, as shown by tracheal washings or BAL. Long-standing allergic bronchitis can result in the permanent changes recognized as chronic bronchitis. Feline allergic bronchitis was considered as part of the feline bronchitis complex just discussed.

The disease is less common in dogs and can result in acute or chronic cough. Rarely, respiratory distress and wheezing occur. Young to middle-aged dogs are most often affected, and the physical examination and radiographic findings reflect the presence of bronchial disease, as described in the following section on canine chronic bronchitis. Heartworm tests and fecal examinations for pulmonary parasites are performed to eliminate parasitism as the cause of the eosinophilic inflammation. In dogs less than 1 year of age, bronchoscopic evaluation for *O. osleri* should also be considered (p. 297).

Treatment consists of an attempt to identify and remove potential allergens from the environment and the administration of glucocorticoids and bronchodilators. Ways to

identify allergens are suggested in the section on feline bronchitis (p. 291). Glucocorticoid and bronchodilator treatment is discussed in the following section on canine chronic bronchitis.

Dogs and cats with allergic bronchitis should be treated aggressively in the hope of minimizing long-term airway inflammation and the resultant chronic bronchial changes. The response to therapy is often excellent, but continued treatment is usually necessary unless inciting allergens can be identified and eliminated.

## CANINE CHRONIC BRONCHITIS

### Etiology

Chronic bronchitis refers to long-term airway inflammation. There is generally a component of irreversible damage. Histologic changes of the airways include fibrosis, epithelial hyperplasia, glandular hypertrophy, and inflammatory infiltrates. Excessive mucus is present within the airways, and small airway obstruction and airway collapse occur. The cause is often not discovered, but long-standing inflammatory processes resulting from infections, allergies, or inhaled irritants can be at fault. Infections can also occur secondary to chronic bronchitis, making a cause-and-effect relationship difficult to determine.

Another potential complication of chronic bronchitis is bronchiectasis, or permanent dilation of the airways (see Fig. 20-4) (Fig. 21-5). Generally, all the major airways are dilated in this condition, but occasionally it is localized. Recurrent infections and overt pneumonia are common complications in dogs with bronchiectasis. Bronchiectasis is also a component of ciliary dyskinesia (i.e., immotile cilia syndrome).

### Clinical Features

Chronic bronchitis occurs most commonly in middle-aged or older, small-breed dogs. These breeds are also predisposed to the development of collapsing trachea and mitral insufficiency with left atrial enlargement causing compression of the mainstem bronchi. These diseases must be differentiated and their contribution to the development of the current clinical features determined for appropriate management to be implemented.

Dogs with chronic bronchitis are evaluated because of cough, which can be productive or nonproductive. The cough has usually slowly progressed over months to years, with no systemic signs of illness such as anorexia, weight loss, or lethargy. As the disease progresses, exercise intolerance becomes evident; then incessant coughing or overt respiratory distress is seen. Dogs with respiratory distress characteristically show marked expiratory efforts because of the narrowing and collapse of the intrathoracic airways.

Dogs are often seen because of a sudden exacerbation in the signs. The change in signs may result from transient worsening of the chronic bronchitis, perhaps after a period of unusual excitement, stress, or exposure to irritants or allergens; from a secondary complication, such as bacterial infection; or from the development of a concurrent disease. The client should be carefully questioned about the character of the cough and the progression of signs. Exacerbating and concurrent disorders that can contribute to worsening of cough are the same as those described for collapsing trachea (see p. 289), and relevant historic findings should be sought.

Increased breath sounds, wheezes, or crackles are auscultated in animals with chronic bronchitis. End-expiratory clicks caused by mainstem bronchial or intrathoracic tracheal collapse may be heard in animals with advanced disease. A prominent or split second heart sound occurs in animals with secondary pulmonary hypertension.

### Diagnosis

*Chronic bronchitis* has been defined as a cough occurring on most days of 2 or more consecutive months in the past year in the absence of other active disease. Therefore chronic bronchitis is diagnosed not only based on the clinical signs but also on the elimination of other diseases from the list of differential diagnoses. The existence of initiating or secondary inflammatory diseases complicates this simple definition.

A bronchial pattern with increased interstitial markings is typically seen on thoracic radiographs, although findings are frequently normal. Bronchiectasis is observed in some animals. An alveolar pattern, particularly with a dependent distribution, is suggestive of a complicating disease, such as infection (i.e., bacterial pneumonia).

Tracheal wash or BAL fluid should be collected at the time of the initial presentation and after an acute exacerbation of the signs. Neutrophilic or mixed inflammation and increased amounts of mucus are usually present. The finding of degenerative neutrophils indicates the possibility of a bacterial infection. Although not a specific finding, the finding of eosinophils is suggestive of a hypersensitivity reaction, as can occur with allergy, parasitism, or heartworm disease. Slides should be carefully examined for organisms (Chapter 20). Bacterial cultures are performed and the results interpreted as discussed in Chapter 20 (p. 268). Although the role of *My-*coplasma infections in these cases is not known, *Mycoplasma* cultures are also considered.

Bronchoscopy, with specimen collection, is performed in selected cases, primarily to help rule out other diseases. The maximum benefit of bronchoscopy is obtained early in the course of disease, before severe permanent damage has occurred and while the risk of the procedure is minimal. Gross abnormalities visualized by bronchoscopy include an increased amount of mucus, roughened mucosa, and hyperemia. Major airways may collapse during expiration as a result of weakened walls, and polypoid mucosal proliferation may be present. Bronchial dilatation is seen in animals with bronchiectasis.

Further diagnostic procedures are indicated to rule out other potential causes of chronic cough, and the selection of these depends on the presenting signs and the results of the previously discussed diagnostic tests. Diagnostic tests to be considered include heartworm tests, fecal examinations for pulmonary parasites, echocardiography, and systemic evaluation (i.e., CBC, serum biochemical panel, urinalysis). Echocardiography may reveal evidence of pulmonary hypertension secondary to chronic hypoxemia, including right heart enlargement (i.e., cor pulmonale).

*Ciliary dyskinesia,* having abnormal ciliary motion, is uncommon but should be considered in dogs with bronchiectasis or recurrent infection. Abnormalities exist in all ciliated tissues, and situs inversus (i.e., lateral transposition of the abdominal and thoracic organs, such that left-sided structures are found on the right and vice versa) is seen in 50% of such dogs. Dextrocardia occurring in association with chronic bronchitis is extremely suggestive of this disease. Sperm motility can be evaluated in intact male dogs. The finding of normal sperm motility rules out a diagnosis of ciliary dyskinesia. The disease is diagnosed based on the rate at which radioisotopes deposited at the carina are cleared and the findings from electron microscopic examination of bronchial biopsy, nasal biopsy, or sperm specimens.

### Treatment

Chronic bronchitis is managed symptomatically, with specific treatment possible only for underlying or complicating diseases that are identified. Each dog with chronic bronchitis is presented at a different stage of the disease, with or without concurrent cardiopulmonary disease and with or without secondary infection. Hence each dog must be managed individually. Ideally, medications are initiated one at a time to assess the most effective combination. It will likely be necessary to modify treatment over time.

Commonly used medications include bronchodilators, glucocorticoids, antibiotics, and cough suppressants. Airway hydration is maintained, and stimuli that may exacerbate signs are avoided.

Bronchodilators are discussed in the section on feline bronchitis (p. 293). The response to treatment may be less dramatic in dogs than that seen in some cats, however, because the airways of most dogs are less reactive than those of cats. Some long-acting theophylline preparations for people can be administered twice daily in dogs. Palatable elixirs suitable for toy breeds (e.g., oxtriphylline) are also available. The drug doses are different for dogs and cats (see Table 21-5). To measure the plasma theophylline concentrations in dogs, blood is obtained 4 to 5 hours after the administration of a long-acting product and 1.5 hours after the administration of other theophylline derivatives. Therapeutic peak concentrations, determined based on human data, are 5 to 20 µg/ml.

Glucocorticoids are often effective in controlling the signs of chronic bronchitis and may slow the development of permanent airway damage by decreasing inflammation and fibrosis. They may be particularly helpful in dogs with eosinophilic airway inflammation. Potential negative effects include an increased susceptibility to infection in dogs already impaired by decreased airway clearance; a tendency toward obesity, hepatomegaly, and muscle weakness that may adversely affect ventilation; and pulmonary thromboembolism. Therefore short-acting products are used, the dose is tapered to the lowest effective one (when possible, 0.5 mg/kg q48h or less), and the drug is discontinued if no beneficial effect is seen. Prednisone is initially given at a dose of 0.5 to 1.0 mg/kg every 12 hours, with a positive response expected within 1 week.

Antibiotics are prescribed for dogs with a bacterial infection, ideally selected based on results from the culture of tracheal or bronchial specimens and accompanying sensitivity data. *Bordetella* organisms are most commonly recovered, but a variety of gram-positive and gram-negative organisms can be found, making the antibiotic susceptibility difficult to predict. The ability of selected antibiotics to penetrate into the airway secretions to the site of infection must also be considered when selecting an antibiotic. Antibiotics that are likely to reach concentrations effective against susceptible organisms include doxycycline, chloramphenicol, fluoroquinolones, and probably amoxicillin with clavulanate. It is preferable to reserve fluoroquinolones for resistant infections. If an antibiotic is effective, a positive response is generally seen within 1 week. Treatment is then continued for at least 1 week beyond the time when the clinical signs stabilize, because complete resolution is unlikely in these animals.

Usually antibiotic treatment is necessary for 3 to 4 weeks and even longer if bronchiectasis or overt pneumonia is present. The use of antibiotics for the treatment of respiratory tract infections is discussed further in the section on canine infectious tracheobronchitis in this chapter (p. 287) and in the section on bacterial pneumonia in Chapter 22 (p. 299).

Cough suppressants are used cautiously because cough is an important mechanism to clear airway secretions. In some dogs, however, the cough is incessant and exhausting, or ineffective because of marked bronchial collapse. Cough suppressants can provide some relief in such animals and may even facilitate ventilation and decrease anxiety.

Although the doses given in Table 21-1 are the ones that provide prolonged effectiveness, less frequent administration (i.e., only during times of the day when coughing is most severe) may preserve some beneficial effect of cough. The most potent suppressants are hydrocodone and butorphanol.

Maintaining airway hydration is critical for facilitating mucociliary clearance. Systemic hydration must be maintained to ensure this, so diuretic therapy is avoided. Placing the animal in a steamy bathroom or in a room with a vaporizer daily can provide symptomatic relief, although the moisture does not reach far into the airways.

Nebulization will cause the moisture to reach deeper in the lungs. This technique is discussed further in the section on bacterial pneumonia in Chapter 22 (p. 299).

Exacerbating factors, either possible or proven, are avoided. Potential allergens are considered in dogs with eosinophilic inflammation and trial elimination pursued (see Feline Bronchitis, p. 292). Irritants such as smoke and perfumed products should be avoided in all dogs. Excitement or stress can cause an acute worsening of signs in some animals, and short-term tranquilization with acepromazine or sedation with phenobarbital can be helpful in relieving the signs. Weight loss should be attempted in obese animals. Routine dental prophylaxis may help maintain a healthy oral flora, some of which is normally aspirated into the airways.

Animals with localized bronchiectasis benefit from surgical removal of the affected lung lobe if signs are severe or if infections recur. The problem is generalized in most animals, and such animals are treated as for chronic bronchitis. These animals are particularly predisposed to the development of infection stemming from decreased airway clearance. Glucocorticoid therapy is avoided, or low doses are used.

## Prognosis

Chronic bronchitis is an irreversible process. The prognosis for the control of signs and a satisfactory quality of life in animals is good if the owners are conscientious about performing the medical management aspects of care, are willing to adjust treatment over time, and treat secondary problems as they occur.

# *OSLERUS OSLERI*

## Etiology

*Oslerus osleri* is an uncommon parasite of young dogs, usually those less than 2 years of age. The adult worms live at the carina and mainstem bronchi and cause a local, nodular inflammatory reaction with fibrosis. First-stage larvae are coughed up and swallowed. The main cause of infection in dogs appears to be through intimate contact with their dam as puppies.

## Clinical Features

Young affected dogs have an acute, nonproductive cough and occasionally wheezing. The dogs otherwise appear healthy, making the initial presentation indistinguishable from that of canine infectious tracheobronchitis. However, the cough persists and eventually airway obstruction occurs as a result of the formation of reactive nodules.

## Diagnosis

Nodules at the carina can occasionally be recognized radiographically. Cytologic examination of tracheal wash fluid in some dogs will show the characteristic ova or larvae, providing the basis for a definitive diagnosis (see Table 20-6). Rarely, larvae are found in fecal specimens using zinc sulfate (s.g. 1.18) flotation (preferred) or the Baermann technique (see Table 20-8).

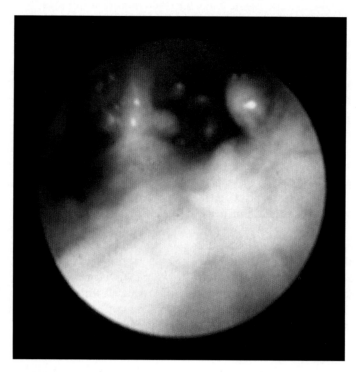

**FIG 21-6**
Bronchoscopic view of multiple nodules at the carina of a dog infected with *Oslerus osleri*.

The most sensitive diagnostic method is bronchoscopy, which enables the nodules to be readily seen (Fig. 21-6). Brushings of the nodules are obtained and immediately evaluated cytologically to detect the larvae. Material can be examined directly in saline solution or can be stained with new methylene blue. If a definitive diagnosis is not obtained from analysis of the brushings, biopsy specimens are obtained.

## Treatment

Treatment with ivermectin (400 μg/kg orally or subcutaneously) is recommended. The same dose is administered again every 3 weeks for 4 treatments. This treatment has not been extensively investigated, however, and is not an approved use of this drug. It cannot be administered to Collie breeds.

## Prognosis

The prognosis for dogs treated with ivermectin is good; the drug appears to be successful in eliminating infection in the limited number of dogs that have been treated.

## Suggested Readings

Bach JF et al: *Proceedings of the 20th Symposium of the Veterinary Comparative Respiratory Society,* Boston, 2002.

Buback JL et al: Surgical treatment of tracheal collapse in dogs: 90 cases (1983-1993), *J Am Vet Med Assoc* 208:380, 1996.

Dye JA et al: Chronopharmacokinetics of theophylline in the cat, *J Vet Pharmacol Ther* 13:278, 1990.

Dye JA et al: Feline bronchial disease. In Kirk RW et al, editors: *Current veterinary therapy XI,* Philadelphia, 1992, WB Saunders.

Ellis JA et al: Effect of vaccination on experimental infection with *Bordetella bronchiseptica* in dogs, *J Am Vet Med Assoc* 218:367, 2001.

Johnson LR: Tracheal collapse: diagnosis and medical and surgical treatment, *Vet Clin North Am Small Anim Pract* 30:1253, 2000.

Johnson LR et al: Clinical and microbiologic findings in dogs with bronchoscopically diagnosed tracheal collapse: 37 cases (1990-1995), *J Am Vet Med Assoc* 219:1247, 2001.

Koritz GD et al: Bioavailability of four slow-release theophylline formulations in the beagle dog, *J Vet Pharmacol Ther* 9:293, 1986.

McKiernan BC: Current uses and hazards of bronchodilator therapy. In Kirk RW et al, editors: *Current veterinary therapy XI,* Philadelphia, 1992, WB Saunders.

Moise NS et al: Bronchopulmonary disease. In Sherding RG, editor: *The cat: diseases and clinical management,* New York, 1989a, Churchill Livingstone.

Moise NS et al: Clinical, radiographic, and bronchial cytologic features of cats with bronchial disease: 65 cases (1980-1986), *J Am Vet Med Assoc* 194:1467, 1989b.

Outerbridge CA et al: Oslerus osleri tracheobronchitis: treatment with ivermectin in 4 dogs, *Can J Vet* 39:238, 1998.

Padrid PA et al: Cyproheptadine-induced attenuation of type-I immediate hypersensitivity reactions of airway smooth muscle from immune-sensitized cats, *Am J Vet Res* 56:109, 1995.

Padrid P: Feline Asthma: diagnosis and treatment, *Vet Clin North Am Small Anim Pract* 30:1279, 2000.

Randolf JF et al: Prevalence of mycoplasmal and ureaplasmal recovery from tracheobronchial lavages and of mycoplasmal recovery from pharyngeal swab specimens in cats with or without pulmonary disease, *Am J Vet Res* 54:897, 1993.

Thrusfield MV et al: A field investigation of kennel cough: efficacy of different treatments, *J Small Anim Pract* 32:455, 1991.

Wheeldon EB et al: Chronic respiratory disease in the dog, *J Small Anim Pract* 18:229, 1977.

White RAS et al: Tracheal collapse in the dog—is there really a role for surgery? A survey of 100 cases, *J Small Anim Pract* 35:191, 1994.

# CHAPTER 22

# Disorders of the Pulmonary Parenchyma

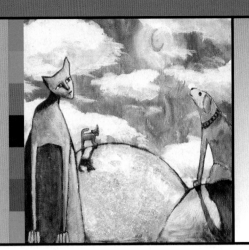

## CHAPTER OUTLINE

VIRAL PNEUMONIA, 299
BACTERIAL PNEUMONIA, 299
TOXOPLASMOSIS, 302
FUNGAL PNEUMONIA, 302
PULMONARY PARASITES, 302
    *Capillaria aerophila*, 303
    *Paragonimus kellicotti*, 303
    *Aelurostrongylus abstrusus*, 303
EOSINOPHILIC LUNG DISEASE (PULMONARY INFILTRATES WITH EOSINOPHILS AND EOSINOPHILIC PULMONARY GRANULOMATOSIS), 303
MISCELLANEOUS NONINFECTIOUS INFLAMMATORY LUNG DISEASES, 304
ASPIRATION PNEUMONIA, 304
PULMONARY NEOPLASIA, 307
    Lymphomatoid granulomatosis, 309
PULMONARY CONTUSION, 309
PULMONARY THROMBOEMBOLISM, 310
PULMONARY EDEMA, 312

## VIRAL PNEUMONIA

Several viruses can infect the lower respiratory tract, but rarely do signs of viral pneumonia predominate. The role of canine adenovirus 1 and parainfluenza virus in canine infectious tracheobronchitis has already been discussed (see p. 287). In dogs, canine distemper virus can also infect the respiratory epithelium. Clinical signs of pneumonia usually result from a secondary bacterial pneumonia. Infection of the gastrointestinal tract or central nervous system can also occur in dogs with distemper (see Chapter 102). In cats, calicivirus can cause pneumonia, but this manifestation of infection is rare. The dry form of feline infectious peritonitis can affect the lungs, but cats are generally seen because of signs of involvement of other organs. Feline infectious peritonitis is discussed in Chapter 102.

## BACTERIAL PNEUMONIA

### Etiology

The term *pneumonia* means inflammation of the lung, but the term is not specific for bacterial disease. A wide variety of bacteria can infect the lungs. Common bacterial isolates from dogs and cats with pulmonary infections include *Pasteurella* spp., *Klebsiella* spp., *Escherichia coli*, *Pseudomonas* spp., *Staphylococcus* spp., *Streptococcus* spp., and *Bordetella bronchiseptica* Anaerobic organisms can be part of mixed infections, particularly in animals with aspiration pneumonia or with lung lobe consolidation. *Mycoplasma* organisms have been isolated from dogs and cats with pneumonia, but their role is not known.

Bacteria can colonize the airways, alveoli, or interstitium. Infection limited to the airways and peribronchial tissues is called *bacterial bronchitis*. If all three regions are involved, the disease can be called either *bacterial bronchopneumonia* or *bacterial pneumonia*. Most cases of pneumonia result from bacteria entering the lungs via the airways, which causes a bronchopneumonia involving primarily the gravity-dependent cranial and ventral lung lobes (see Fig. 20-5). Bacteria that enter the lung through the hematogenous route usually cause pneumonia that assumes a caudal or diffuse pattern and marked interstitial involvement.

Bacterial pneumonia is a common lung disease, particularly in dogs, but a predisposing abnormality usually exists. Such abnormalities include decreased clearance of normally inhaled debris from the lungs, particularly in animals with chronic bronchitis, ciliary dyskinesia, or bronchiectasis; immunosuppression resulting from drugs, malnutrition, stress, endocrinopathies, or other infections, including feline leukemia virus infection, feline immunodeficiency virus infection, and canine distemper; the aspiration of ingested material or gastric contents resulting from a cleft palate, megaesophagus, or other causes of aspiration pneumonia (p. 304); the inhalation or migration of foreign bodies; and rarely, neoplasia or fungal or parasitic infections.

### Clinical Features

Dogs and cats with bacterial pneumonia are evaluated because of respiratory signs or systemic signs, or both. Respiratory signs can include cough (which is usually productive and soft), a bilateral mucopurulent nasal discharge, exercise intolerance, and respiratory distress. Cough is rare in cats with pneumonia. Systemic signs include lethargy, anorexia, fever, and weight loss. The animal may have a history of chronic airway disease or regurgitation. Cats, particularly kittens, from stressful housing situations (e.g., overcrowding) appear predisposed to develop pneumonia from *Bordetella* infections. Other potential predisposing factors, as listed in the preceding paragraph, are pursued through careful history taking.

Fever may be present on physical examination but is identified in only about half of patients. Crackles and, occasionally, expiratory wheezes may be auscultated, with the abnormal lung sounds often prominent over the cranioventral lung fields.

## Diagnosis

Bacterial pneumonia is diagnosed on the basis of the complete blood count (CBC), thoracic radiograph findings, and the results from tracheal wash fluid cytologic analysis and bacterial culture. A CBC showing neutrophilic leukocytosis with a left shift, neutropenia with a degenerative left shift, or moderate-to-marked neutrophil toxicity is supportive of bacterial pneumonia. A normal or stress leukogram is as likely to be found.

Abnormal patterns on thoracic radiographs vary with the underlying disease. The typical abnormality is an alveolar pattern, possibly with consolidation, that is most severe in the dependent lung lobes (see Fig. 20-5). Increased bronchial and interstitial markings are also often present. Infections secondary to foreign bodies can be localized to any region of the lung. An interstitial pattern alone may be present in animals with early or mild disease or in those with infections of hematogenous origin. A bronchial pattern alone may be present in animals with a primarily bronchial infection. Radiographs are also evaluated for the presence of megaesophagus.

Pulmonary specimens are evaluated cytologically and microbiologically to establish a definitive diagnosis and to provide guidance in antibiotic selection. To maximize the diagnostic yield, specimens should be collected before antibiotic therapy is initiated. In most cases a tracheal wash specimen is sufficient. Septic neutrophilic inflammation is typically found in animals with bacterial pneumonia, and growth of organisms on bacterial culture is expected.

A conscientious effort is also made to identify any underlying problems. In some animals, such as those with megaesophagus, the initiating cause is obvious. Further diagnostic tests are indicated in other animals, depending on the results of the clinicopathologic evaluation. These may include bronchoscopy to search for airway abnormalities or foreign bodies, conjunctival scrapings to look for distemper virus, serologic tests to determine whether the animal has a fungal infection, and hormonal assays to determine whether the animal has hyperadrenocorticism. Ciliary dyskinesia is discussed briefly in Chapter 21. The diagnostic evaluation for aspiration pneumonia is discussed on p. 304.

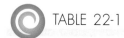 TABLE 22-1

**Therapeutic Considerations for Bacterial Pneumonia**

**Antibiotics**

Selected on basis of results from culture and sensitivity testing of pulmonary specimens

**Airway Hydration**

Maintain systemic hydration
Saline nebulization

**Physiotherapy**

Turning of recumbent animals every 1 to 2 hours
Mild exercise of animals in stable condition
Coupage

**Bronchodilators**

As needed, particularly in cats

**Oxygen Supplementation**

As needed

**AVOID**

Diuretics
Cough suppressants
Corticosteroids

## Treatment

**Antibiotics.** The treatment of bacterial pneumonia consists of antibiotics and appropriate supportive care, with follow-up evaluation (Table 22-1). Infections with gram-negative organisms and with multiple organisms occur in the majority of cases, which makes the susceptibility of organisms to specific antibiotics difficult to predict. Therefore antibiotics should be selected on the basis of susceptibility data from the cultures of pulmonary specimens. Cytologic characteristics of organisms (i.e., gram-staining characteristics and morphology) from pulmonary specimens can provide some initial guidance while culture results are pending.

The extent to which an antibiotic can penetrate into the airways is a potential concern, particularly in animals infected with marginally susceptible organisms, but antibiotics generally achieve concentrations within the pulmonary parenchyma equal to those in plasma. Nebulization of antibiotics is rarely indicated.

Antibiotics that can be initiated before susceptibility results are available include amoxicillin-clavulanate (20 to 25 mg/kg q8h), cephalexin (20 to 40 mg/kg q8h), or chloramphenicol (dogs, 50 mg/kg q8h; cats, 10 to 15 mg/kg q12h). Fluoroquinolones are reserved for animals with resistant gram-negative infections. Kittens from stressful environments suspected of having *Bordetella*-induced pneumonia should be treated with doxycycline (5 to 10 mg/kg q12h), fluoroquinolones, or amoxicillin-clavulanate while awaiting results of cultures. Doxycycline or a fluoroquinolone is more likely to be effective but has a greater potential for side effects in young kittens.

Animals with severe clinical signs or possible sepsis should be treated initially with intravenous antibiotics. Broad-spectrum coverage in animals with life-threatening infections can be achieved with imipenem (2 to 5 mg/kg q6-8h) or the combination of either ampicillin with sulbactam (50 mg/kg of combined drugs intravenously q8h) and a fluoroquinolone or ampicillin with sulbactam and an aminoglycoside (e.g., amikacin, 5 to 10 mg/kg q8h). Sulbactam is a beta-lactamase inhibitor, as is clavulanate, and the combination of ampicillin with sulbactam provides a drug with similar activity as amoxicillin-clavulanate in an intravenous formulation. If *Toxoplasma* or *Neospora* infection is among the differential diagnoses, the combination of a fluoroquinolone and clindamycin or a fluoroquinolone and azithromycin can be used.

Antibiotic treatment should be continued for at least 1 week beyond the time when the clinical signs resolve. Guidelines for patient monitoring are provided on p. 302.

**Airway hydration.** The drying of secretions results in increased viscosity and decreased ciliary function, which interfere with the normal clearance mechanisms of the lung. Thus the water content of airway secretions must be maintained and airways must be hydrated in animals with pneumonia. Animals with any evidence of dehydration should receive fluid therapy. Diuretics can cause dehydration, and their use is contraindicated in such animals.

Additional moisture for the airways can be provided through humidification or nebulization. Such therapy is particularly recommended for animals with areas of consolidation or with suspected decreased airway clearance, such as those with bronchiectasis. *Humidification* refers to the saturation of air with water vapor. Depending on the temperature, the volume of water that remains as vapor is limited. The moisture reaches only the nasal cavity and the proximal trachea. Vaporization is not effective in hydrating deeper regions of the lungs. However, the more proximal effect can still provide some relief, particularly in animals with nasal discharge. Humidification is convenient and can be achieved simply by placing the animal in a steamy bathroom or in a small room with an inexpensive vaporizer, which is readily available at pharmacies.

Nebulization is necessary to provide moisture deeper into the airways. Nebulizers generate small, variably sized droplets, with a diameter ranging from 0.5 to 5 μm being required to reach the deeper airways. Several types of nebulizers are available. Disposable jet nebulizers are readily available and inexpensive, and they can be attached to bottled oxygen or an air compressor (Fig. 22-1). The nebulized oxygen is delivered to the animal through a face mask. The particles can be seen as a mist.

Sterile saline solution is used as a nebulizing solution because it has mucolytic properties and is relatively nonirritating. Premedication with bronchodilators has been suggested as a way to reduce the bronchospasms, although I have not encountered problems using saline alone in dogs. It is recommended that nebulization be performed two to

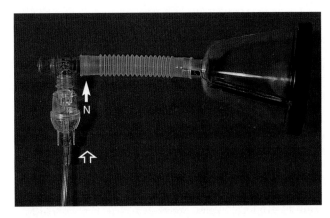

**FIG 22-1**
Disposable jet nebulizers are readily available and inexpensive. Sterile saline solution is placed in the nebulizer *(N)*. Oxygen enters the bottom of the nebulizer *(open arrow)*, and nebulized air exits the top *(closed arrow)*. Nebulized air is delivered to the animal with a face mask, as shown here, or it can be delivered into an enclosed cage.

six times daily for 10 to 30 minutes each time. Nebulization should be followed immediately by physiotherapy to promote the expectoration of exudate that may have increased in volume with rehydration. Nebulizers and tubing should be replaced after no more than 24 hours of use in actively infected patients.

**Physiotherapy.** Lying in one position impairs airway clearance, and lung consolidation can occur if one side remains dependent for prolonged periods. Therefore animals that are recumbent must be turned at least every 2 hours. Because activity causes animals to take deeper breaths and to cough, which promotes airway clearance, animals that are in a sufficiently stable condition and can tolerate the oxygen demands should be mildly exercised.

Physiotherapy is indicated after nebulization to promote coughing and to facilitate the clearance of exudate from the lungs. Mild exercise is used when possible. Otherwise, coupage is performed. To perform coupage, the person strikes the animal's chest over the lung fields with cupped hands. The action should be forceful but not painful and should be continued for 5 to 10 minutes if tolerated by the patient. Coupage may also be beneficial for animals with lung consolidation that are not receiving nebulization.

**Bronchodilators.** Bronchospasm can occur secondary to inflammation, particularly in cats. Bronchodilators are used in animals showing increased respiratory efforts, particularly if expiratory wheezes are auscultated. They are discontinued if clinical signs worsen or do not improve. Bronchodilators for cats are discussed on p. 293, and those for dogs are discussed on p. 296.

**Other treatment.** Expectorants are of questionable value in dogs and cats. Glucocorticoids are contraindicated in animals with bacterial pneumonia. Oxygen therapy (see Chapter 27) is provided if the clinical signs, arterial blood gas measurements, or pulse oximetry measurements indicate a need for it.

**Monitoring.** Dogs and cats with bacterial pneumonia should be closely monitored for signs of deteriorating pulmonary function. Respiratory rate and effort and the mucous membrane color are monitored at least twice daily. Thoracic radiographs and the CBC are evaluated every 24 to 72 hours. If the animal's condition does not improve within 72 hours, it may be necessary to alter treatment or collect additional pulmonary specimens. Animals showing improvement are sent home and evaluated again in approximately 2 weeks. If clinical and radiographic signs have resolved, antibiotic treatment is continued for an additional week.

The evidence of infection on initial radiographs can obscure that of focal disease processes such as neoplasia or foreign bodies, and focal opacities may not be apparent while an animal is receiving antibiotics. Therefore radiographs should be reevaluated approximately 1 week after antibiotic therapy has been discontinued in animals with recurrent infection or suspected localized disease. Persistence of localized disease after long-term antibiotic therapy is an indication for bronchoscopy or thoracotomy.

### Prognosis

Bacterial pneumonia responds readily to appropriate therapy. The prognosis is more guarded in animals with underlying problems that predispose them to infection. The likelihood of eliminating these problems must be taken into consideration when considering the prognosis.

Pulmonary abscess formation is a potential complication of bacterial pneumonia. Abscesses are seen as focal lesions on radiographs, and entire lobes may be involved. Horizontal-beam radiographs can be useful in determining whether the lesions are filled with fluid. Ultrasonography can also be helpful in characterizing areas of consolidation. Abscesses resolve in response to prolonged medical therapy in some animals, but if improvement is not observed or radiographic evidence of disease reappears after the discontinuation of therapy, surgical excision (i.e., lobectomy) is indicated.

## TOXOPLASMOSIS

The lungs are a common site of involvement in cats with toxoplasmosis. Thoracic radiographs typically show fluffy alveolar and interstitial opacities throughout the lungs in such animals. Less often, nodular interstitial or diffuse interstitial patterns, lung lobe consolidation, or a pleural effusion is seen. Organisms are rarely recovered from the lungs by tracheal wash. Bronchoalveolar lavage is more likely to retrieve organisms. Toxoplasmosis is a multisystemic disease and is discussed in detail in Chapter 104.

## FUNGAL PNEUMONIA

The common mycotic diseases that can involve the lungs are blastomycosis, histoplasmosis, and coccidioidomycosis. In most cases the organisms enter the body through the respiratory tract. The infection may be successfully eliminated without the animal showing clinical signs, or the animal may show only transient respiratory signs. The infection may also progress to cause disease involving the lungs alone or spread systemically to various target organs, or both processes may occur. Cryptococcal organisms also enter the body through the respiratory tract and can infect the lungs, particularly in cats. However, the presenting signs in cats are generally those of a nasal infection (see p. 235). Pulmonary signs are most often the primary presenting complaint in dogs with blastomycosis and cats with histoplasmosis.

Pulmonary mycoses are considered in the differential diagnoses of dogs or cats with progressive signs of lower respiratory tract disease, especially if they occur in conjunction with weight loss, fever, lymphadenopathy, chorioretinitis, or other evidence of multisystemic involvement. Thoracic radiographs typically show a diffuse, nodular, interstitial pattern of the lungs (see Fig. 20-6). The nodules are often miliary. The presence of this pattern in dogs with suspicious clinical signs supports a diagnosis of mycotic infection, but other diseases, including neoplasia, parasitic or atypical bacterial (e.g., mycobacterial) infections, and eosinophilic lung disease, can also produce similar patterns, so these must be borne in mind as well. Other potential radiographic abnormalities include alveolar and bronchointerstitial patterns and consolidated regions of the lung. Hilar lymphadenopathy can also occur, most commonly in animals with histoplasmosis. The lesions caused by histoplasmosis can also be calcified.

Organisms can occasionally be retrieved by tracheal wash. However, because of the interstitial nature of these diseases, bronchoalveolar lavage and lung aspiration are more likely to be successful. Fungal culture is probably more sensitive than cytologic analysis alone. An inability to find organisms in pulmonary specimens does not rule out the diagnosis of mycotic disease, however. A complete discussion of systemic mycoses is provided in Chapter 103.

## PULMONARY PARASITES

Several parasites can cause lung disease. Certain intestinal parasites, especially *Toxocara canis,* can cause transient pneumonia in young animals, usually those less than a few months of age, as the larvae migrate through the lungs. Infection with *Dirofilaria immitis* can result in severe pulmonary disease through inflammation and thrombosis (see Chapter 10). *Oslerus osleri* resides at the carina and mainstem bronchi of dogs and is discussed in Chapter 21, p. 297. The other primary lung larvae that are most commonly diagnosed are *Capillaria aerophila* and *Paragonimus kellicotti* in dogs and cats and *Aelurostrongylus abstrusus* in cats.

Infection occurs as a result of the ingestion of infective forms, often within intermediate or paratenic hosts, that subsequently migrate to the lungs. An eosinophilic inflammatory response often occurs within the lungs, causing clinical signs in some, but not all, infected animals. The definitive diagnosis is made on the basis of the identification of the characteristic eggs or larvae in respiratory or fecal specimens (see Chapter 20).

## CAPILLARIA AEROPHILA

*Capillaria aerophila* is a small nematode. Adult worms are located primarily beneath the epithelial surfaces of the large airways. Clinical signs develop in very few animals with *Capillaria* infections, and the disease is most often identified through the fortuitous identification of characteristic eggs during routine fecal examinations.

The rare animal that displays signs has signs of allergic bronchitis. Thoracic radiograph findings are generally normal, although a bronchial or bronchointerstitial pattern may be seen. Tracheal wash fluid can show eosinophilic inflammation. *Capillaria* is diagnosed by the finding of characteristic eggs in tracheal wash fluid or fecal flotation material (see Fig. 20-10, *B*).

Treatment is recommended for animals with clinical signs. Fenbendazole (25 to 50 mg/kg q12h for 14 days) is the treatment of choice for dogs and cats. Levamisole (8 mg/kg for 10 to 20 days) has also been used successfully in dogs. Ivermectin has been suggested for treatment, but an effective dosage has not been established. The prognosis in animals with the disease is excellent.

## PARAGONIMUS KELLICOTTI

*Paragonimus kellicotti* is a small fluke. Snails and crayfish are both necessary intermediate hosts, thus limiting the disease to animals that have been in the region of the Great Lakes, in the Midwest, or in the southern United States. Pairs of adults are walled off by fibrous tissue, usually in the caudal lung lobes, with a connection to an airway to allow for the passage of eggs. A local granulomatous reaction can occur around the adults, or a generalized inflammatory response to the eggs can occur.

Infection is more common in cats than in dogs. Some dogs and cats have no clinical signs. When clinical signs are present, they can be the same as those seen in animals with allergic bronchitis. Alternatively, signs of spontaneous pneumothorax can result from the rupture of cysts.

The classic radiographic abnormality is a solid or cavitary mass lesion, most commonly present in the right caudal lobe. Other abnormal patterns seen on thoracic radiographs can be bronchial, interstitial (reticular or nodular), or alveolar in nature, depending on the severity of the inflammatory response.

Infection is diagnosed definitively through the identification of the ova in fecal specimens, tracheal wash fluid, or other pulmonary specimens (see Fig. 20-10, *C*). Eggs are not always present, however, and a presumptive diagnosis is necessary in some cases.

Fenbendazole is used to treat paragonimiasis at the same dosage as that recommended for the treatment of capillariasis. Alternatively, praziquantel can be used at a dosage of 23 mg/kg every 8 hours for 3 days.

Thoracocentesis should be used to stabilize the condition of animals with pneumothorax. If air continues to accumulate within the pleural space, however, it may be necessary to place a chest tube and perform suction until the leak has been sealed (see p. 323). Surgical intervention is rarely required.

The response to treatment is monitored by thoracic radiographs and periodic fecal examinations. Treatment may have to be repeated in some cases. The prognosis is excellent.

## AELUROSTRONGYLUS ABSTRUSUS

*Aelurostrongylus abstrusus* is a small worm that infects the small airways and pulmonary parenchyma of cats. Snails or slugs serve as intermediate hosts. Most cats with infection have no clinical signs. Those cats that do are usually young. The clinical signs are those of feline bronchitis. The abnormalities seen on radiographs can also reflect bronchitis, although a diffuse miliary or nodular interstitial pattern is present in some cats. Eosinophilic inflammation may be apparent in peripheral blood and airway specimens.

A definitive diagnosis is made through the identification of larvae, which may be present in fecal specimens prepared using the Baermann technique (see Fig. 20-10, *A*) or in airway specimens obtained by tracheal washing or bronchoscopy. Multiple fecal specimens should be examined in suspected cases because the larvae are not always present.

Animals with clinical signs should be treated with fenbendazole at the same dosage as that used for the treatment of capillariasis. According to Kirkpatrick and colleague (1987), ivermectin at a dose of 0.4 mg/kg subcutaneously proved to be effective in one cat.

Antiinflammatory therapy with glucocorticoids alone often causes the clinical signs to resolve. However, eliminating the underlying parasitic disease is a preferable treatment goal, and glucocorticoid therapy may interfere with the effectiveness of the antiparasitic drugs. Bronchodilators may provide symptomatic relief and do so without interference with antiparasitic drug action. The prognosis in animals with the infection is excellent.

## EOSINOPHILIC LUNG DISEASE (PULMONARY INFILTRATES WITH EOSINOPHILS AND EOSINOPHILIC PULMONARY GRANULOMATOSIS)

*Eosinophilic lung disease* is a broad term describing inflammatory lung disease in which the predominant infiltrating cell is the eosinophil. Eosinophilic inflammation can involve primarily the airways or the interstitium. If airway signs predominate, the disease is considered to be allergic bronchitis (see Chapter 21, p. 295). Bronchitis is by far the most common eosinophilic lung disease seen in cats. Interstitial infiltration, with or without concurrent bronchitis, is sometimes referred to as *pulmonary infiltrates with eosinophils (PIEs)*. The term *eosinophilic bronchopneumopathy* is also used. These names by which the disorder goes are descriptive only and likely encompass a variety of hypersensitivity disorders of the lung. Eosinophilic pulmonary granulomatosis is a severe type of PIE seen in dogs and is characterized by the development of nodules and often hilar lymphadenopathy. It must be differentiated from a mycotic infection and neoplasia.

Because eosinophilic inflammation is a hypersensitivity response, an underlying antigen source is actively pursued in affected animals. Considerations include heartworms, pulmonary parasites, drugs, and inhaled allergens. Bacteria, fungi, and neoplasia can also induce a hypersensitivity response, but this response often is not the predominant finding. In many cases no underlying disease can be found. Eosinophilic pulmonary granulomatosis is strongly associated with heartworm disease.

### Clinical Features

Eosinophilic lung diseases are seen in young and older dogs. Affected dogs are evaluated because of slowly progressive respiratory signs, such as cough, increased respiratory efforts, and exercise intolerance. Systemic signs such as anorexia and weight loss are usually mild. Lung sounds are often normal, although crackles or expiratory wheezes can occur.

### Diagnosis

The finding of peripheral eosinophilia is included in some definitions of PIE, but it is not present in all animals with the disease, nor is it a specific finding. A diffuse interstitial pattern is seen on thoracic radiographs. Eosinophilic pulmonary granulomatosis results in the formation of nodules, usually with indistinct borders. These nodules can be quite large, and hilar lymphadenopathy may also be present. A patchy alveolar opacity and consolidation of the lung lobes can occur as well.

Pulmonary specimens must be examined to establish a diagnosis of PIE. In some cases of PIE, evidence of eosinophilic inflammation may be found in tracheal wash fluid. More aggressive techniques for collecting pulmonary specimens, such as bronchoalveolar lavage, lung aspiration, or lung biopsy, are required to identify the eosinophilic response in other cases. Other inflammatory cell populations are frequently present in lesser numbers in such specimens.

Potential antigen sources should be considered, and pulmonary specimens should be carefully examined for the presence of infectious agents and features of malignancy. Heartworm tests and fecal examinations for pulmonary parasites are indicated in all cases.

### Treatment

Any primary disease identified during the diagnostic evaluation of these animals is treated directly. Eliminating the source of the antigen that may be triggering the excessive immune response may result in a cure.

Antiinflammatory therapy with glucocorticoids is indicated for dogs in which an antigen source cannot be identified and for dogs with heartworm disease if the eosinophilic inflammation is causing respiratory compromise (see Chapter 10). Dogs with eosinophilic granulomatosis often require more aggressive immunosuppressive therapy.

Dogs are typically treated with glucocorticoids, such as prednisone, at an initial dosage of 1 to 2 mg/kg every 12 hours. Clinical signs and thoracic radiographs are used to monitor the animal's response to therapy, and initially these should be assessed every week. Once the clinical signs have resolved, the dosage of glucocorticoids is decreased to the lowest effective one. If signs have remained in remission for 3 months, discontinuation of therapy can be attempted. If signs are exacerbated by glucocorticoid therapy, immediate reevaluation to search for underlying infectious agents is indicated.

Dogs with large nodular (mass) lesions (eosinophilic granulomatosis) should be treated with a combination of glucocorticoids and a cytotoxic agent. Prednisone is administered to these animals at a dosage of 1 mg/kg every 12 hours, in combination with cyclophosphamide at a dosage of 50 mg/m$^2$ every 48 hours. Clinical signs and thoracic radiographs are evaluated every 1 to 2 weeks until remission is achieved. CBCs are also done every 1 to 2 weeks to detect excessive bone marrow suppression resulting from the cyclophosphamide. Attempts to discontinue therapy can be made after several months of remission. The cyclophosphamide may need to be discontinued earlier than this because long-term treatment is associated with sterile hemorrhagic cystitis. (See Chapter 80 for further discussion of the adverse effects of cyclophosphamide therapy.)

### Prognosis

A wide spectrum of disease is seen in terms of both the severity of the signs and the underlying causes. The prognosis is generally fair to good. However, the prognosis is guarded in dogs with severe eosinophilic pulmonary granulomatosis.

## MISCELLANEOUS NONINFECTIOUS INFLAMMATORY LUNG DISEASES

Idiopathic eosinophilic lung disease represents one form of noninfectious inflammatory lung disease. Other inflammatory lung diseases in which a cause cannot be identified are occasionally seen. The inflammatory infiltrates in such animals are generally interstitial. The lesions may represent a form of vasculitis, a component of systemic lupus erythematosus, immune complex disease, or some other hypersensitivity response. These diseases are rare, however, and not well documented. A lung biopsy must be performed for a definitive diagnosis to be made. A clinical diagnosis is made only after extensive testing has been done to rule out more common causes of lung disease, particularly infectious agents, and after there has been a prolonged positive response to immunosuppressive therapy. Lymphomatoid granulomatosis is a nodular interstitial disease that exhibits clinical signs similar to those seen in animals with eosinophilic pulmonary granulomatosis. It was initially considered to be a noninfectious inflammatory lung disease but is currently considered a form of neoplasia (p. 309).

## ASPIRATION PNEUMONIA

### Etiology

A small amount of fluid and bacteria is aspirated from the oropharynx into the airways of healthy animals, but normal airway clearance mechanisms prevent infection. Organisms from the oropharynx are thought to be the source of bacteria in many animals with bacterial pneumonia, specifically bronchopneumonia (p. 299). In humans such infection is termed *aspiration pneumonia*. In veterinary medicine the term *aspiration pneumonia* is generally used to refer to the inflammatory lung disease that occurs as a result of the inhalation of overt amounts of solid or liquid material into the lungs. The materials that are usually aspirated are stomach contents or food. Normal laryngeal and pharyngeal function prevents aspiration in healthy animals, although occasionally an excited puppy aspirates a foreign body. Otherwise, the presence of aspiration pneumonia in an animal of any age indicates an underlying predisposing abnormality (Table 22-2).

Aspiration pneumonia is a common complication of animals with regurgitation. Megaesophagus is the most common cause of regurgitation (Chapter 31, p. 410). Other causes of regurgitation (e.g., reflux esophagitis, esophageal obstruction) are less common. Another cause of aspiration pneumonia is localized or systemic neurologic or muscular disease affecting the normal swallowing reflexes of the larynx or pharynx.

## TABLE 22-2

**Underlying Causes of Aspiration Pneumonia in Dogs and Cats**

| ABNORMALITY | DISCUSSION IN TEXT (PAGE NO.) |
|---|---|
| **Esophageal Disorders** | |
| Megaesophagus | 410 |
| Reflux esophagitis | 412 |
| Esophageal obstruction | — |
| Myasthenia gravis (localized) | 1059 |
| Bronchoesophageal fistulae | — |
| **Localized Oropharyngeal Abnormalities** | |
| Cleft palate | — |
| Cricopharyngeal motor dysfunction | 409 |
| Laryngoplasty | 247 |
| Brachycephalic airway syndrome | 248 |
| **Systemic Neuromuscular Disorders** | |
| Myasthenia gravis | 1059 |
| Polyneuropathy | 1055 |
| Polymyopathy | 1062 |
| **Decreased Mentation** | |
| General anesthesia | — |
| Sedation | — |
| Post ictus | 1000 |
| Head trauma | — |
| Severe metabolic disease | — |
| **Iatrogenic*** | |
| Force-feeding | — |
| Stomach tubes | 391 |
| **Vomiting (In Combination with Other Predisposing Factors)** | 347 |

*Overzealous feeding, incorrect tube placement, or loss of lower esophageal sphincter competence because of presence of tube.

These reflexes can also be depressed in dogs or cats with abnormal levels of consciousness or in those that are anesthetized. Laryngeal paralysis does not always lead to the development of aspiration pneumonia, but aspiration can be a complication of therapeutic laryngoplasty. It can also occur in animals with abnormal pharyngeal anatomy resulting from mass lesions, the brachycephalic airway syndrome, or cleft palate. Bronchoesophageal fistulae are a rare cause of aspiration pneumonia.

Aggressive force-feeding, especially in mentally depressed animals, and improper placement of stomach tubes into the trachea are iatrogenic causes of aspiration pneumonia. Mineral oil administered to prevent hair balls can be a cause of aspiration pneumonia in cats, because the tasteless and odorless oil is poorly handled by the pharynx.

The damage to the lung resulting from aspiration can stem from chemical damage, obstruction of the airways, infection, and the resulting inflammatory response to each of these factors. Gastric acid causes severe chemical injury to the lower airways. Tissue necrosis, hemorrhage, edema, and bronchoconstriction ensue, and a marked acute inflammatory response is initiated. Hypoxemia resulting from decreased ventilation and compliance can be fatal.

Severe respiratory distress can occur from physical obstruction of the airways by the aspirated material. Most commonly only small airways are obstructed, but occasionally a large piece of food will obstruct a major airway. Obstruction is subsequently exacerbated by reflex bronchoconstriction and inflammation. Inhaled solid material initiates an inflammatory reaction that includes an abundance of macrophages. This response can become organized, resulting in the formation of granulomas.

Infection can occur in response to an initial aspiration of contaminated material, although acidic gastric contents are probably sterile. Regardless, the resultant damage to the lungs greatly predisposes the animal to the development of a secondary infection.

The inhalation of mineral oil elicits a chronic inflammatory response. The clinical signs in this setting are often mild, but in rare instances they can be severe. Radiographic abnormalities persist and can be erroneously interpreted as representing neoplastic lesions.

## Clinical Features

Dogs and cats with aspiration pneumonia are frequently first evaluated because of acute, severe respiratory signs. These animals may be in shock at presentation. Vomiting, regurgitation, or eating may have preceded the onset of distress by a few hours. Other patients are seen because of chronic intermittent or progressive signs of coughing or increased respiratory efforts, or show signs of the predisposing disease. Systemic signs such as fever, anorexia, and depression are common. The owners are carefully questioned about whether there are other signs of disease and whether force-feeding or medication administration has been attempted.

Crackles and wheezes are often auscultated, particularly over the dependent lung lobes. A thorough neuromuscular examination is performed in animals that are in a stable condition.

## Diagnosis

Aspiration pneumonia is usually diagnosed on the basis of the suggestive radiographic findings in conjunction with evidence of a predisposing condition. Thoracic radiographs typically show diffuse, increased interstitial opacities with alveolar flooding and consolidation of the dependent lung lobes (see Fig. 20-5, p. 259). Radiographic abnormalities may not be apparent until 12 to 24 hours after aspiration, however. Nodular interstitial patterns can be seen in chronic cases. Large nodules can form around solids; miliary nodules often form in animals that have aspirated mineral oil. Large airway obstruction is suspected if radiographs show a soft-tissue mass within large airways or show localized abnormalities, but these are unusual findings. A marked, diffuse alveolar pattern can be seen in dogs that have severe secondary edema (see Pulmonary Edema, p. 312).

The peripheral blood count can reflect the pulmonary inflammatory process, or it can be normal. Neutrophils are examined for the presence of toxic changes indicative of sepsis.

Tracheal washing is indicated for all animals that can tolerate the procedure to identify a complicating bacterial infection and obtain antibiotic susceptibility data. A marked inflammatory response characterized by a predominance of neutrophils is seen in cytologic specimens. Blood resulting from hemorrhage may be seen in specimens from animals in the acute period after aspiration. Bacteria may also be seen. Bacterial cultures should always be performed.

Bronchoscopy can be used to grossly examine the airways and detect and remove large solids. However, the likelihood of a large airway obstruction is very small, so bronchoscopy is performed only if there are clear signs of large airway obstruction (see Chapter 26) or if the animal is not conscious and therefore does not require general anesthesia for the procedure.

Blood gas analysis can be helpful in differentiating hypoventilation from ventilation-perfusion abnormalities (see Chapter 20, p. 281), although a combination of abnormalities exists in most animals with aspiration pneumonia. Animals with evidence of profound hypoventilation may have either a large airway obstruction or muscle weakness secondary to an underlying neuromuscular disorder such as myasthenia gravis. Blood gas analysis also assists in the therapeutic management of these animals and can be used effectively to monitor the response to therapy.

Diagnostic evaluation is indicated to identify potential underlying diseases (see Table 22-2). This may include a thorough oral and pharyngeal examination, contrast-enhanced radiographic studies to evaluate the esophagus, or specific neuromuscular tests (see Chapters 29 and 66).

## Treatment

Suctioning of the airways is helpful only for animals that aspirate in the hospital while already anesthetized or unconscious, when it can be performed immediately after aspiration. If a bronchoscope is available, suctioning can be performed through the biopsy channel, which affords visualized guidance. Alternatively, a sterile soft rubber tube attached to a suction pump can be passed blindly into the airways through an endotracheal tube. Excessive suction can result in lung lobe collapse. Therefore low-pressure, intermittent suction is used, followed by expansion of the lungs with several positive-pressure ventilations done using an anesthetic or Ambu bag. Airway lavage is contraindicated.

Animals in severe respiratory distress should be treated with fluid therapy, oxygen supplementation, bronchodilators, and glucocorticoids. Fluids are administered intravenously at high rates to treat shock (see Chapter 30) and should be continued after initial stabilization of the animal's condition to maintain systemic hydration, which is necessary to maximize the effectiveness of airway clearance mechanisms. However, overhydration must be avoided because of a tendency for pulmonary edema.

Oxygen supplementation (see Chapter 27) is initiated immediately in compromised animals. Positive-pressure ventilation is required for animals in severe respiratory distress that is unresponsive to oxygen therapy.

Bronchodilators (see pp. 293 and 296) can be administered to decrease bronchospasms and ventilatory muscle fatigue. They are most likely to be effective in cats. They are discontinued if no improvement is seen or clinical signs appear to worsen following their administration.

Rapid-acting glucocorticoids are administered for the treatment of shock. However, their use in the absence of shock is controversial. Although the antiinflammatory effects of glucocorticoids can be beneficial, they can interfere with normal defense mechanisms in tissues that have been severely compromised. Low doses of short-acting drugs such as prednisone (0.25 to 0.5 mg/kg q12h) can be given during the first 24 hours to control severe clinical signs but should then be discontinued.

Animals with a large airway obstruction can benefit from bronchoscopy and foreign body removal. However, routine bronchoscopy is not indicated because of the risk of the general anesthesia needed during the procedure and the infrequency of large airway obstructions.

Antibiotics are administered immediately in animals that are presented with overt systemic signs of sepsis. Selected antibiotics should have a broad spectrum of activity and be administered intravenously. Such drugs include imipenem or combinations of either ampicillin with sulbactam and a fluoroquinolone or ampicillin with sulbactam and an aminoglycoside (see Bacterial Pneumonia, p. 299).

A tracheal wash is performed in an animal without signs of sepsis as soon as the animal's condition is stable in order to document the presence of infection and to obtain antibiotic susceptibility data before initiation of antibiotics. This information is particularly valuable because prolonged treatment is often needed and also because it has been well proved in human medicine that resistant secondary infections can develop after aspiration in patients given antibiotics initially or on an empirical basis. As discussed for bacterial pneumonia, the high incidence of gram-negative and mixed infections make assumptions regarding antibiotic susceptibility prone to error. Pending results of culture, it is reasonable to initiate treatment with a penicillin with a beta-lactamase inhibitor (e.g., amoxicillin-clavulanate or ampicillin with sulbactam). Because infection can occur as a later complication in these patients, frequent monitoring with physical examination, CBC, and thoracic radiographs is necessary to detect any deterioration consistent with secondary infection. Tracheal wash is repeated if infection is suspected.

Further therapeutic and monitoring considerations are discussed in the section on bacterial pneumonia (p. 299). Underlying diseases are treated to prevent recurrence.

### Prognosis

Animals with mild signs of disease and a correctable underlying problem have an excellent prognosis. The prognosis is worse for animals with more severe disease or uncorrectable underlying problems.

## PULMONARY NEOPLASIA

Primary pulmonary tumors, metastatic neoplasia, and multicentric neoplasia can all involve the lungs. Lymphomatoid granulomatosis is a unique form of neoplasia and is discussed separately. Most primary pulmonary tumors are malignant. Carcinomas predominate and include adenocarcinoma, bronchoalveolar carcinoma, and squamous cell carcinoma. Small-cell carcinoma, or oat cell tumor, which occurs frequently in people, is rare in dogs and cats. Sarcomas and benign tumors are also rare.

The lungs are a common site for the metastasis of malignant neoplasia from other sites in the body, and even from primary pulmonary tumors. Neoplastic cells can be carried in the bloodstream and trapped in the lungs, where there is low blood flow and an extensive capillary network. Lymphatic spread or local invasion can also occur.

Multicentric tumors can involve the lungs. Such tumors include lymphoma, malignant histiocytosis, and mastocytoma.

Multiple tumors of different origins can occur in the same animal. That is, the presence of a neoplasm in one site of the body does not necessarily imply that the same tumor is also present in the lungs.

### Clinical Features

Neoplasms are most common in older animals but also occur in young adult animals. Tumors involving the lungs can produce a wide spectrum of clinical signs. These signs are usually chronic and slowly progressive, but peracute manifestations such as pneumothorax or hemorrhage can also occur.

Most signs reflect respiratory tract involvement. Infiltration of the lung by the tumor can cause oxygenation to be interfered with, leading to increased respiratory efforts and exercise intolerance. Mass lesions can compress airways, provoking cough and interfering with ventilation. Erosion through vessels can result in pulmonary hemorrhage. The blood loss can be sudden, resulting in acute hypovolemia and

anemia in addition to respiratory compromise. Edema, nonseptic inflammation, or bacterial infection can occur secondary to the tumor. Erosion through the airways can result in pneumothorax. A pleural effusion of nearly any character can form. In rare cases, the caudal or cranial venae cavae are obstructed, resulting in the development of ascites or head and neck edema, respectively.

Nonspecific signs in dogs and cats with pulmonary neoplasms can include weight loss, anorexia, depression, and fever. Gastrointestinal signs can be the primary complaint. Vomiting and regurgitation can be the presenting signs in cats in particular. Hypertrophic osteopathy secondary to thoracic mass lesions occurs in some animals. The presenting sign is often lameness.

Some animals with lung neoplasia have no clinical signs at all, and the tumor is discovered at the postmortem examination or as an incidental finding on thoracic radiographs. Animals with metastatic or multicentric lung neoplasia can be seen because of signs of tumor involvement in another organ.

Lung sounds may be normal, decreased, or increased. They are decreased over all lung fields in animals with pneumothorax or pleural effusion. Localized decreased or increased lung sounds can be heard over regions that are consolidated. Increased lung sounds consisting of crackles and wheezes occur in the setting of infiltration, inflammation, and airway obstruction. There can also be evidence of other organ involvement or hypertrophic osteopathy.

### Diagnosis

Neoplasia is definitively diagnosed through the histologic or cytologic identification of criteria of malignancy in populations of cells in pulmonary specimens (Fig. 22-2). Thoracic radiographs are commonly evaluated initially, and findings can support a tentative diagnosis of neoplasia. Radiographs can also identify the location of disease, and this information is used to select the most appropriate technique for specimen collection.

Good-quality radiographs, including both left and right lateral projections, should be evaluated. Primary pulmonary tumors can assume the appearance of localized mass lesions or a consolidation of entire lobes (see Fig. 20-7). Tumor margins are often distinct but can be indistinct as a result of inflammation and edema. Cavitation can be evident. In cats, primary lung tumors are often multifocal or diffuse, and the radiographic pattern may be suggestive of edema or pneumonia. Metastatic or multicentric disease results in a diffuse reticular interstitial pattern or a nodular interstitial pattern, or both (see Fig. 20-8). Hemorrhage, edema, inflammation, infection, and airway occlusion can produce alveolar patterns and consolidation. Lymphadenopathy, pleural effusion, or pneumothorax can also occur.

Nonneoplastic disease, including fungal infection, lung parasites, the aspiration of mineral oil, eosinophilic granulomatosis, atypical bacterial infections, and inactive lesions from previous disease, can produce similar radiographic abnormalities. Pulmonary specimens must be evaluated to establish

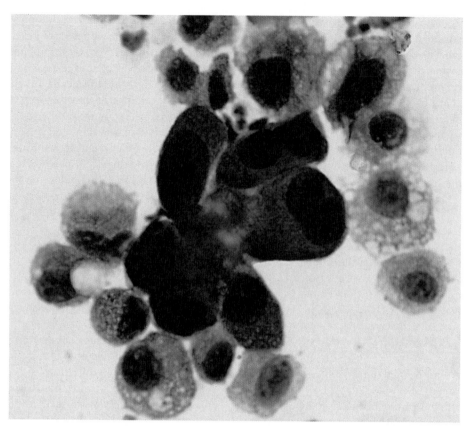

**FIG 22-2**
Bronchoalveolar lavage fluid from the dog whose lateral thoracic radiograph showing a severe, unstructured interstitial pattern is depicted in Fig. 20-8. Many clumps of deeply staining epithelial cells showing marked criteria of malignancy were seen. One such clump is shown here. A diagnosis of carcinoma was made. Note that a cytologic diagnosis of carcinoma should not be made if there is concurrent inflammation. The surrounding lighter-staining cells are alveolar macrophages, the normal predominant cell type in bronchoalveolar lavage fluid.

a diagnosis. Findings yielded by tracheal wash fluid analysis rarely result in a definitive diagnosis. It is generally necessary to evaluate lung aspirates, bronchoalveolar lavage fluid, or lung biopsy specimens to arrive at a definitive diagnosis.

It may be appropriate to delay pulmonary specimen collection in asymptomatic animals with multifocal disease or animals with significant unrelated problems. Rather, radiographs are obtained again in 4 to 6 weeks to document the progression of lesions. Such a delay is never recommended in dogs or cats with potentially resectable disease, however.

The confirmation of malignant neoplasia in other organs in conjunction with typical thoracic radiographic abnormalities is often adequate for making a presumptive diagnosis of pulmonary metastases. Overinterpretation of subtle radiographic lesions should be avoided. Conversely, the absence of radiographic changes does not eliminate the possibility of metastatic disease.

### Treatment

Solitary pulmonary tumors are treated by surgical resection. To obtain clear margins, usually the entire lung lobe that is involved must be excised. Lymph node biopsy specimens, as well as biopsy specimens from any grossly abnormal lung, are obtained for histologic analysis.

In animals with a large mass lesion, respiratory signs may abate after excision, even if metastatic lesions are present throughout the lungs. If the lesions cannot be removed surgically, chemotherapy can be attempted (see Chapter 79). No protocol is uniformly effective for the treatment of primary lung tumors.

Metastatic neoplasms of the lungs are treated with chemotherapy. In most animals, the initial protocol is determined by the expected sensitivity of the primary tumor. Unfortunately, metastatic neoplasms do not always have the same response to specific agents as the primary tumor.

Multicentric tumors are treated with standard chemotherapeutic protocols, regardless of whether the lungs are involved. Multicentric tumors are discussed in Chapter 81.

### Prognosis

The prognosis for animals with benign neoplasms is excellent, but these tumors are rare. The prognosis for animals with malignant neoplasia is potentially related to several variables, which include tumor histology, presence of regional lymph node involvement, and presence of clinical signs. Survival times of several years are possible following surgical excision. Ogilvie and colleagues (1989) reported that of 76 dogs with primary pulmonary adenocarcinoma, surgical excision resulted in remission (elimination of all macroscopic evidence of tumor) in 55 dogs. The median survival time of dogs that went into remission was 330 days, whereas the survival time in dogs that did not achieve remission was 28 days. Ten dogs remained alive at the completion of the study. McNiel and colleagues (1997) found that the histologic score of the tumor, presence of clinical signs, and regional lymph node metastases were significantly associated with the prognosis in 67 dogs with primary lung tumors. Median survival times for dogs with and without clinical signs were 240 and 545 days, respectively. Median survival times for dogs with and without lymph node involvement were 26 and 452 days, respectively. Median survival times for dogs with papillary carcinoma were 495 days, compared with 44 days for dogs with other histologic tumor types. Survival times ranged from 0 to 1437 days. A report of 21 cats with primary lung tumors found a median survival time of 115 days following surgery (Hahn and colleague, 1998). Cats with moderately differentiated tumors had a median survival time of 698 days (range of 13 to 1526 days), whereas cats with poorly differentiated tumors had a median survival time of 75 days (range of 13 to 634 days).

Animals with unresectable primary pulmonary malignant tumors or metastatic disease have a grave prognosis. The prognosis for animals with multicentric neoplasms is not known to depend on the presence or absence of pulmonary involvement.

## LYMPHOMATOID GRANULOMATOSIS

Lymphomatoid granulomatosis is characterized by infiltration with pleomorphic lymphoreticular and plasmacytoid cells around and into blood vessels, with accompanying eosinophils, neutrophils, lymphocytes, and plasma cells.

### Clinical Features

The presenting signs are similar to those of other diffuse pulmonary neoplasms (see previous discussion), although both young and old dogs are affected.

### Diagnosis

Thoracic radiographs in animals with lymphomatoid granulomatosis show increased interstitial opacities, often coalescing to form nodules of different sizes. Hilar lymphadenopathy is common. Cytologic preparations of tracheal wash fluid and other pulmonary specimens show a nonspecific mixed inflammatory response, often including lymphocytes, plasma cells, eosinophils, and mast cells. The radiographic and cytologic findings are similar to those found in animals with diseases such as eosinophilic pulmonary granulomatosis, metastatic or multicentric neoplasia, fungal infection, or atypical mycobacterial infection. Heartworm

tests, fungal titers, and cultures of pulmonary specimens are indicated to rule out other possible causes of these findings. A definitive diagnosis of lymphomatoid granulomatosis must be made on the basis of tissue biopsy findings, which necessitates a thoracotomy. Such specimens show an infiltration of atypical lymphoreticular cells surrounding and invading blood vessels, accompanied by eosinophils, lymphocytes, and plasma cells.

### Treatment

Dogs with lymphomatoid granulomatosis are treated with combination chemotherapy, as for lymphoma (see Chapter 82). Thoracic radiographs are taken every 1 to 2 weeks to monitor for the resolution of lesions.

### Prognosis

The treatment response in a large population of dogs has not been reported. Although not all dogs respond well to treatment, Postorino and colleagues (1989) reported that three of five dogs in their care were still in complete remission at 19, 27, and 32 months after treatment with prednisone and cyclophosphamide had been initiated.

## PULMONARY CONTUSION

### Etiology

Pulmonary contusion is caused by blunt trauma and is a common finding in animals that have been hit by cars. Hemorrhage into the interstitium and alveoli occurs, usually in localized regions of the lungs. Pneumothorax, hemothorax, and rib fractures can also occur. Thoracic involvement should be considered in any animal with evidence of severe trauma, even if there are no external signs of trauma in that region of the body.

### Clinical Features

Historical or physical examination evidence of trauma is generally present in animals with pulmonary contusions. Although increased respiratory efforts may be noted, pneumothorax, pain from rib fractures, cardiovascular shock, or neurologic damage may also affect breathing patterns. Crackles may be auscultated over the contused areas.

### Diagnosis

Pulmonary contusions are diagnosed on the basis of evidence of trauma and the finding of typical radiographic signs, although the latter may not be evident until almost a day after trauma. Large localized areas of alveolar and interstitial opacities are seen in such animals. The pleura, skeleton, and diaphragm should also be scrutinized for the presence of abnormalities.

### Treatment

Animals with pulmonary contusions receive treatment for trauma-related problems as indicated by clinical signs. The contusions themselves are not treated directly. Although antibiotics have been recommended to prevent infection in damaged tissue, they are more effectively used to treat animals that have developed actual signs of infection.

It is recommended that radiographs be obtained periodically to monitor the resolution of abnormalities. The frequency of this depends on the severity of the initial abnormalities and the clinical signs. Complications that may arise in animals with pulmonary contusions include a secondary bacterial infection, abscesses, lung lobe consolidation, and cavitary lesions. Bacterial infection is discussed on p. 299. Consolidated lung lobes are monitored radiographically for resolution for several months unless clinical signs of respiratory compromise persist, in which case lobectomy is performed. Cavitary lesions are also monitored for several months unless pneumothorax occurs. Most traumatic cysts will resolve during that time without requiring surgical excision.

### Prognosis

The prognosis for recovery from pulmonary contusions is excellent, provided that the animal's condition can be stabilized after the trauma. The possible complications of contusions noted earlier are rare.

## PULMONARY THROMBOEMBOLISM

The extensive, low-pressure vascular system of the lungs is a common site where emboli lodge. This is also because it is the first vascular bed through which thrombi formed in the systemic venous network or right ventricle pass. The respiratory signs can be profound and even fatal in dogs and cats. Hemorrhage, edema, and bronchoconstriction, in addition to the decreased blood flow, can contribute to the respiratory compromise. The attendant increased vascular resistance secondary to the physical obstruction by emboli and vasoconstriction results in pulmonary hypertension, which can ultimately lead to the development of right-sided heart failure.

Thromboemboli generally form as a result of disease in organs other than the lungs, and a search for the underlying cause of clot formation is therefore essential. Abnormalities predisposing to clot formation include venous stasis, turbulent blood flow, endothelial damage, and hypercoagulation. In addition to emboli originating from thrombi, emboli can consist of bacteria, parasites, neoplasia, or fat. Conditions that have been associated with the development of pulmonary emboli, and the pages where they are discussed, are listed in Table 22-3. The remainder of this discussion is limited to pulmonary thromboembolism (PTE).

### Clinical Features

Animals with PTE may have historical or physical examination findings related to the underlying disease. In many instances the predominant signs are peracute tachypnea and respiratory distress, which can lead to sudden death. Common presenting signs in dogs and cats include tachypnea, labored breathing, and lethargy or depression.

 TABLE 22-3

**Abnormalities Potentially Associated with Pulmonary Thromboembolism**

| ABNORMALITY | DISCUSSION IN TEXT (PAGE NO.) |
|---|---|
| Surgery | — |
| Severe trauma | — |
| Hyperadrenocorticism | 778 |
| Immune-mediated hemolytic anemia | 1160 |
| Hyperlipidemia | 822 |
| Glomerulopathies | 600 |
| Dirofilariasis and adulticide therapy | 169 |
| Cardiomyopathy | 106 |
| Endocarditis | 116 |
| Pancreatitis | 552 |
| Disseminated intravascular coagulation | 1195 |
| Hyperviscosity syndromes | — |
| Neoplasia | — |

Cardiovascular shock can occur. Milder or more chronic signs are possible. Crackles or wheezes are heard in some cases. A prominent or split-second heart sound may be heard if pulmonary hypertension develops.

### Diagnosis

Routine diagnostic methods do not provide information that can be used to make a definitive diagnosis of PTE. A high index of suspicion must be maintained, since this disease is frequently overlooked. The diagnosis is suspected on the basis of clinical signs, thoracic radiography, arterial blood gas analysis, echocardiography, and clinicopathologic data. Confirmation of the diagnosis is through angiography or nuclear perfusion scan findings.

PTE is suspected in dogs and cats with acute-onset, severe dyspnea, particularly if there are minimal or no radiographic signs of respiratory disease. In many cases of PTE, the lungs appear normal on thoracic radiographs in spite of the severe lower respiratory tract signs. When radiographic lesions occur, the caudal lobes are most often involved. Blunted pulmonary arteries, in some cases ending with focal or wedge-shaped areas of interstitial or alveolar opacities resulting from the extravasation of blood or edema, may be present. Areas of lung without a blood supply can appear hyperlucent. Diffuse interstitial and alveolar opacities and right-sided heart enlargement can occur. Pleural effusion is present in some cases and is usually mild. Echocardiography may show secondary changes (e.g., right ventricular enlargement, increased pulmonary artery pressures), underlying disease (e.g., heartworm disease, primary cardiac disease), or residual thrombi.

Arterial blood gas analysis can show hypoxemia to be mild or profound. Tachypnea leads to hypocapnia, except in severe cases, and the abnormal alveolar-arterial oxygen gradient (*A-a* gradient) supports the presence of a ventilation-perfusion disorder (see p. 281). A poor response to oxygen supplementation is supportive of a diagnosis of PTE.

Clinicopathologic evidence of a disease known to predispose animals to thromboemboli further heightens suspicion for this disorder. Unfortunately, measurements of clotting parameters are not helpful in making the diagnosis. In people, measurement of circulating D-dimers (a degradation product of cross-linked fibrin) is used as an indicator of the likelihood of PTE. It is not considered a specific test, so its primary value has been in the elimination of PTE from the differential diagnoses. However, even a negative result can be misleading in certain disease states and in the presence of small, subsegmental emboli. The usefulness of D-dimer measurement in veterinary medicine has not been well explored.

Angiography yields information on which to base a definitive diagnosis. Sudden pruning of pulmonary arteries or intravascular filling defects, as well as extravasation of dye, are characteristic findings. However, these changes may only be apparent for a few days after the event, so this test must be done early in the disease. Nuclear scans can provide evidence of PTE with minimal risk to the animal. Unfortunately, this technology is mostly available only at academic institutions.

Pulmonary specimens for histopathologic evaluation are rarely collected, except at necropsy. However, evidence of embolism is not always found at necropsy, because clots may dissolve rapidly after death. Therefore such tissue should be collected and preserved immediately after death. The extensive vascular network makes it impossible to evaluate all possible sites of embolism, and the characteristic lesions can also be missed.

## Treatment

Acutely, animals are treated for cardiovascular shock including high doses of rapid-acting glucocorticoids (e.g., prednisolone sodium succinate, 10 to 20 mg/kg intravenously). Animals should also receive immediate oxygen therapy (see Chapter 27).

Animals with suspected hypercoagulability are likely to benefit from anticoagulant therapy. Large clinical studies of the response of dogs or cats with PTE to anticoagulant therapy have not been described. Anticoagulant therapy is administered only to animals in which the diagnosis is highly probable. Dogs with heartworm disease suffering from post–adulticide therapy reactions usually are not treated with anticoagulants (see Chapter 10). Potential surgical candidates should be treated with great caution. Clotting times must be monitored frequently to minimize the risk of severe hemorrhage. General guidelines for anticoagulant therapy are provided here. However, more complete descriptions of anticoagulant therapy are available in the literature, and a current pharmacology text should be consulted before anticoagulants are used.

Initially heparin (200 to 300 U/kg subcutaneously q8h) is administered for anticoagulant therapy. The goal of heparin therapy is to maintain the partial thromboplastin time (PTT) at 1.5 to 2.5 times normal, which corresponds to approximately a 1.2 to 1.4 times increase above the normal activated clotting time (ACT). Clotting times are evaluated before and 2 hours after the administration of heparin, and the dosage is adjusted on the basis of the results. Low-molecular-weight heparin may provide a logistically easier and potentially safer means of heparinizing dogs and cats. Its use has not been studied extensively in dogs and cats with clinical disease.

Hemorrhage is a potential complication of heparin therapy. Protamine sulfate is a heparin antagonist that can be administered if bleeding is not adequately controlled after heparin treatment is discontinued. Some clinicians advocate gradually tapering the dosage of heparin over several days when discontinuing treatment to avert rebound hypercoagulation.

Heparin can be administered by the owner at home; however, long-term anticoagulation can be maintained with oral warfarin. Frequent monitoring of such animals is necessary, and dosage adjustments are common. The potential for drug interactions with all concurrent medications being administered must be investigated. An initial dosage of 0.1 to 0.2 mg/kg by mouth every 24 hours is prescribed for dogs, and a total of 0.5 mg every 24 hours is prescribed for most cats. The goal of therapy is to maintain a prothrombin time (PT) of 1.5 to 2 times normal or an international normalization ratio (INR) of 2.0 to 3.0. It appears that it is safer to use the INR than the PT for monitoring anticoagulation. The INR is calculated from the measured PT and corrects for the variable strength of the thromboplastin reagent used in the assay. The INR or the formula to calculate it can be obtained from the commercial laboratory or the supplier of in-office test kits. Heparin therapy can be discontinued once the desired prolongation has been reached. It may be possible to decrease the frequency of administration of oral warfarin to every 48 hours after several days of treatment.

Until the PT has stabilized, which takes a minimum of 5 days, clotting times are assessed daily. Subsequent examination of the animal and evaluation of clotting times are performed at least every 5 days, with the interval gradually increasing to every 4 to 6 weeks if consistent and favorable results are obtained.

Excessive hemorrhage is the primary complication of warfarin therapy. Plasma or vitamin $K_1$ (2 to 5 mg/kg/day, divided) can be used to treat uncontrollable hemorrhage. However, if vitamin K is used, further attempts at anticoagulation using warfarin cannot be made for several weeks.

Aspirin therapy for the treatment of PTE is controversial. This is because aspirin-induced alterations in local prostaglandin and leukotriene metabolism may be detrimental and an unpredictable increase in bleeding tendencies can occur if aspirin is given in combination with other anticoagulant drugs.

The use of fibrinolytic agents for the treatment of PTE in animals has not been well established. Recombinant tissue plasminogen activator has shown promise because it acts locally at sites of fibrin deposition.

Because of the serious problems associated with anticoagulant therapy, eliminating the predisposing problem must be a major priority.

## Prognosis

The prognosis depends on the severity of the respiratory signs and the ability to eliminate the underlying process. In general, a guarded prognosis is warranted.

## *PULMONARY EDEMA*

### Etiology

The same general mechanisms that cause edema elsewhere in the body cause edema in the pulmonary parenchyma. Major mechanisms are decreased plasma oncotic pressure, vascular overload, lymphatic obstruction, and increased vascular permeability. The disorders that can produce these problems are listed in Table 22-4.

The fluid initially accumulates in the interstitium. However, because the interstitium is a small compartment, the alveoli are soon involved. When profound fluid accumulation occurs, even the airways become filled. Respiratory function is further affected as a result of the atelectasis and decreased compliance caused by compression of the alveoli and decreased concentrations of surfactant. Airway resistance increases as a result of the luminal narrowing of small bronchioles. Hypoxemia results from ventilation-perfusion abnormalities.

### Clinical Features

Animals with pulmonary edema are seen because of cough, tachypnea, respiratory distress, or signs of the inciting disease. Crackles are heard on auscultation, except in animals with mild or early disease. Immediately preceding death from pulmonary edema, blood-tinged froth may appear in the trachea, pharynx, or nares. Respiratory signs can be peracute, as in *acute respiratory distress syndrome (ARDS),* or subacute, as in hypoalbuminemia. However, a prolonged history of respiratory signs (e.g., months) is not consistent with a diagnosis of edema. The list of differential diagnoses in Table 22-4 can often be greatly narrowed by obtaining a thorough history and performing a thorough physical examination.

### Diagnosis

Pulmonary edema in most dogs and cats is diagnosed on the basis of the finding of the typical radiographic changes in the lungs in conjunction with clinical evidence (from the history, physical examination, radiography, echocardiography, and serum biochemical analysis [particularly albumin concentration]) of a disease associated with pulmonary edema.

Early pulmonary edema assumes an interstitial pattern on radiographs that progresses to become an alveolar pattern. In dogs, edema caused by heart failure is generally more severe in the hilar region. In cats the increased opacities are more often patchy. Edema resulting from increased vascular permeability tends to be most severe in the dorsocaudal lung regions.

Radiographs should be carefully examined for signs of heart disease, venous congestion, PTE, pleural effusion, and mass lesions. Echocardiography is helpful in identifying pri-

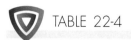

### TABLE 22-4

Possible Causes of Pulmonary Edema

**Decreased Plasma Oncotic Pressure**

Hypoalbuminemia
   Gastrointestinal loss
   Glomerulopathy
   Liver disease
   Iatrogenic overhydration
   Starvation

**Vascular Overload**

Cardiogenic
   Left-sided heart failure
   Left-to-right shunts
Overhydration

**Lymphatic Obstruction (Rare)**

Neoplasia

**Increased Vascular Permeability**

Inhaled toxins
   Smoke inhalation
   Gastric acid aspiration
   Oxygen toxicity
Drugs or toxins
   Snake venom
   Cisplatin in cats
Electrocution
Trauma
   Pulmonary
   Multisystemic
Sepsis
Pancreatitis
Uremia
Disseminated intravascular coagulation
Inflammation (infectious or noninfectious)*

**Miscellaneous Causes**

Thromboembolism
Upper airway obstruction
Near-drowning
Neurogenic edema
   Seizures
   Head trauma

*Inflammation is usually the prominent clinical abnormality, not edema.

mary cardiac disease if the clinical signs and radiographic findings are ambiguous.

Decreased oncotic pressure can be identified by the serum albumin concentration. Concentrations less than 1 g/dl are usually required before decreased oncotic pressure is considered to be the sole cause of the pulmonary edema. Pulmonary edema resulting purely from hypoalbuminemia is probably rare. In many animals, volume overload or vasculitis is a contributing factor. Plasma protein quantitation using a refractometer can indirectly assess albumin concentration in emergency situations.

Vascular permeability edema, or noncardiogenic pulmonary edema, can result in the full range of compromise, from minimal clinical signs that spontaneously resolve to the frequently fatal, fulminant process of ARDS. ARDS, or "shock lung," describes a syndrome of acute, rapidly progressive, pulmonary edema. In a review of 19 dogs with ARDS by Parent and colleagues (1996), the time of onset of dyspnea ranged from 0.5 to 48 hours (mean 4.5 hours) before admission, and the duration of dyspnea before death in dogs not mechanically ventilated ranged from 8 to 76 hours (mean 16 hours).

Pulmonary specimens from patients with vascular permeability edema are not cytologically unique, showing a predominantly neutrophilic response.

Arterial blood gas analysis and pulse oximetry in dogs and cats with pulmonary edema are useful for selecting and monitoring therapy. Hypoxemia is present, usually in conjunction with hypocapnia and a widened *A-a* gradient.

## Treatment

It is easier for the body to prevent edema fluid from forming than it is to mobilize existing fluid. The initial management of pulmonary edema should be aggressive. Once the edema has resolved, the body's own compensatory mechanisms become more effective and the intensity of therapeutic interventions can often be decreased.

All animals with pulmonary edema are treated with cage rest and minimal stress. Dogs and cats with significant hypoxemia should receive oxygen therapy (see Chapter 27). Positive-pressure ventilation is required in severe cases. Methylxanthine bronchodilators (see pp. 293 and 296) may also be beneficial in some patients. They are mild diuretics and also decrease bronchospasms and, possibly, respiratory muscle fatigue.

Diuretics are indicated for the treatment of most forms of edema but are not used in hypovolemic animals. Animals with hypovolemia actually require conservative fluid supplementation. If this is necessary to maintain the vascular volume in animals with cardiac impairment or decreased oncotic pressure, then positive inotropic agents or plasma infusions, respectively, are necessary.

Edema caused by hypoalbuminemia is treated with plasma or colloid infusions. However, the plasma protein concentrations do not need to reach normal levels for edema to decrease. Furosemide can be administered to more quickly mobilize the fluid from the lungs, but clinical dehydration and hypovolemia must be prevented. Diagnostic and therapeutic efforts are directed at the underlying disease.

The treatment of cardiogenic edema is discussed in Chapter 3.

Overhydration is treated by the discontinuation of fluid therapy. Furosemide is administered if respiratory compromise is present. If excessive volumes of fluid were not administered inadvertently, causes of fluid intolerance, such as oliguric renal failure, heart failure, and increased vascular permeability, must be sought.

Edema caused by increased vascular permeability is difficult to treat. In some cases, pulmonary compromise is mild and the edema transient. Routine supportive care with oxygen supplementation may be sufficient. Any active, underlying problem should be identified and corrected.

ARDS responds poorly to management. Ventilator therapy with positive end-expiratory pressure is indicated, and even with such aggressive support the mortality rate is high. Furosemide is generally ineffective in treating edema caused by increased vascular permeability, but because of limitations in our diagnostic capabilities it is reasonable to include this drug in the initial management of these patients. Glucocorticoids are of no clear benefit in these patients, but they are frequently given to animals with moderate to severe signs. Many novel therapies for ARDS have been studied in people, although to date, none have been shown to be consistently effective in improving outcome. Studies are ongoing. Examples of such therapies include endotoxin blockers, inhibitors of specific inflammatory mediators, inhaled nitrous oxide, antioxidant drugs, and surfactant replacement.

## Prognosis

The prognosis for an animal with pulmonary edema depends on the severity of the edema and the ability to eliminate or control the underlying problem. Aggressive management early in the course of edema formation improves the prognosis for an animal with any given disease. Animals with ARDS have a guarded to grave prognosis.

## *Suggested Readings*

Barsanti JA et al: Parasitic diseases of the respiratory tract. In Kirk RW, editor: *Current veterinary therapy VIII*, Philadelphia, 1983, WB Saunders.

Berry CR et al: Pulmonary lymphomatoid granulomatosis in seven dogs (1976-1987), *J Vet Intern Med* 4:15, 1990.

Bowman DD et al: Evaluation of praziquantel for treatment of experimentally induced paragonimiasis in dogs and cats, *Am J Vet Res* 52:68, 1991.

Bowman DD et al: *Georgis' parasitology for veterinarians,* ed 6, Philadelphia, 1995, WB Saunders.

Calvert CA et al: Pulmonary and disseminated eosinophilic granulomatosis in dogs, *J Am Anim Hosp Assoc* 24:311, 1988.

Clercx C et al: Eosinophilic bronchopneumopathy in dogs, *J Vet Intern Med* 14:282, 2000.

DeMonye W et al: Embolus location affects the sensitivity of a rapid quantitative D-dimer assay in the diagnosis of pulmonary embolism, *Am J Respir Crit Care Med* 165:345, 2002.

Drobatz KJ et al: Noncardiogenic pulmonary edema, *Compend Contin Educ Pract Vet* 16:333, 1994.

Drobatz KJ et al: Noncardiogenic pulmonary edema in dogs and cats: 26 cases (1989-1993), *J Am Vet Med Assoc* 206:1732, 1995.

Hahn KA et al: Primary lung tumors in cats: 86 cases (1979-1994), *J Am Vet Med Assoc* 211:1257, 1997.

Hahn KA et al: Prognosis factors for survival in cats after removal of a primary lung tumor: 21 cases (1979-1994), *Vet Surg* 27:307, 1998.

Johnson LR et al: Pulmonary thromboembolism in 29 dogs: 1985-1995, *J Vet Intern Med* 13:338, 1999.

Keyes ML et al: Pulmonary thromboembolism in dogs, *Vet Emerg Crit Care* 3:23, 1993.

Kirkpatrick CE et al: Use of ivermectin in treatment of *Aelurostrongylus abstrusus* and *Toxocara cati* infections in a cat, *J Am Vet Med Assoc* 190:1309, 1987.

LaRue MJ et al: Pulmonary thromboembolism in dogs: 47 cases (1986-1987), *J Am Vet Med Assoc* 197:1368, 1990.

McNiel EA et al: Evaluation of prognostic factors for dogs with primary lung tumors: 67 cases (1985-1992), *J Am Vet Med Assoc* 211:1422, 1997.

Norris CR et al: Pulmonary thromboembolism in cats: 29 cases (1987-1997), *J Am Vet Med Assoc* 215:1650, 1999.

Ogilvie GK et al: Prognostic factors for tumor remission and survival in dogs after surgery for primary lung tumor: 76 cases (1975-1985), *J Am Vet Med Assoc* 195:109, 1989.

Parent C et al: Clinical and clinicopathologic findings in dogs with acute respiratory distress syndrome: 19 cases (1985-1993), *J Am Vet Med Assoc* 208:1419, 1996.

Postorino NC et al: A syndrome resembling lymphomatoid granulomatosis in the dog, *J Vet Intern Med* 3:15, 1989.

Quinn DA et al: D-dimers in the diagnosis of pulmonary embolism, *Am J Respir Crit Care Med* 159:1445, 1999.

Reinemeyer CR: Parasites of the respiratory system. In Bonagura JD et al, editors: *Current veterinary therapy XII,* Philadelphia, 1995, WB Saunders.

Roudebush P: Bacterial infections of the respiratory system. In Greene CE, editor: *Infectious diseases of the dog and cat,* Philadelphia, 1990, WB Saunders.

Speakman AJ et al: Antimicrobial susceptibility of *Bordetella bronchiseptica* isolates from cats and a comparison of the agar dilution and E-test methods, *Vet Microbiol* 54:63, 1997.

Urquhart GM et al: *Veterinary parasitology,* New York, 1987, Churchill Livingstone.

# CHAPTER 23

# Clinical Manifestations of the Pleural Cavity and Mediastinal Disease

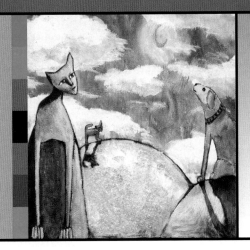

## CHAPTER OUTLINE

GENERAL CONSIDERATIONS, 315
PLEURAL EFFUSION: FLUID CLASSIFICATION
AND DIAGNOSTIC APPROACH, 315
    Transudates and modified transudates, 316
    Septic and nonseptic exudates, 317
    Chylous effusions, 317
    Hemorrhagic effusions, 317
    Effusions due to neoplasia, 318
PNEUMOTHORAX, 318
MEDIASTINAL MASSES, 318
PNEUMOMEDIASTINUM, 319

## GENERAL CONSIDERATIONS

Common abnormalities of the pleural cavity in the dog and cat include the accumulation of fluid (pleural effusion) or air (pneumothorax) in the pleural space. Mediastinal masses and pneumomediastinum are also discussed in this chapter. Respiratory signs caused by pleural disease result from interference with normal expansion of the lungs. Exercise intolerance is an early sign; ultimately overt respiratory distress occurs. Physical examination findings that assist in localizing the cause of respiratory compromise to the pleural space include increased respiratory rate, increased inspiratory effort relative to expiratory effort, increased abdominal excursions, and decreased lung sounds on auscultation (Chapter 26). In cats with mediastinal masses, decreased compressibility of the anterior thorax may be palpable. Thoracic radiography, thoracocentesis, or both, are performed to confirm the presence of pleural space disease.

Pulmonary thromboembolism (PTE) can cause a pleural effusion. The effusion is generally mild and may be an exudate or a modified transudate. PTE should be particularly considered as a diagnosis in patients whose respiratory efforts seem in excess of the volume of effusion (Chapter 22).

## PLEURAL EFFUSION: FLUID CLASSIFICATION AND DIAGNOSTIC APPROACH

The presence of pleural effusion in a dog or cat is usually confirmed by the findings from thoracic radiography or thoracocentesis (Chapter 24). In animals presented in respiratory distress with suspected pleural effusion, thoracocentesis is performed immediately to stabilize the animal's condition before radiographs are taken. Although thoracocentesis is more invasive than radiography, the potential therapeutic benefit of the procedure far outweighs the small risk of complications. Animals in stable condition at presentation can be evaluated initially with thoracic radiographs to confirm the presence and location of fluid before thoracocentesis is performed.

Ultrasonography is a valuable tool for the evaluation of patients with pleural effusion. If equipment is available on site, animals in critical condition can be examined ultrasonographically with minimal stress to both confirm the presence of fluid and direct needle placement for thoracocentesis. Ultrasonography is also useful in evaluating the thorax for the presence of mass lesions, hernias, and primary cardiac or pericardial disease. Because sound waves cannot pass through aerated lungs, any masses must be adjacent to the chest wall, heart, or diaphragm to be detected by ultrasound. The presence of pleural fluid facilitates the ultrasonographic evaluation of the chest. If the patient is stable, it is preferable to evaluate the thorax ultrasonographically before removing the pleural fluid.

Thoracic radiographs should be taken again after as much fluid or air as possible has been removed from the pleural space and the lungs have had time to reexpand. Full expansion of the lungs is required for accurate evaluation of the pulmonary parenchyma. The presence of fluid also obscures visibility of heart size and shape and mass lesions.

Cytologic analysis of pleural fluid obtained by thoracocentesis is indicated for the diagnostic evaluation of all animals with pleural effusion. Measurement of the protein concentration and total nucleated cell count, as well as the qualitative assessment of individual cells, are essential for classifying the fluid, formulating a diagnostic plan, and initiating appropriate therapy (Table 23-1). Types of pleural fluid include transudates and modified transudates, septic and nonseptic exudates, and chylous or hemorrhagic effusions. Effusions caused by neoplasia are also discussed. In addition to the inflammatory cell types in each cytologic category described later, mesothelial cells are generally present and are often reactive.

## TRANSUDATES AND MODIFIED TRANSUDATES

Pure transudates are fluids with low protein concentrations of less than 2.5 to 3 g/dl and low nucleated cell counts of less than 500 to 1000/µl. The primary cell types are mononuclear cells, comprised of macrophages, lymphocytes, and mesothelial cells. Modified transudates have a slightly higher protein concentration of up to 3.5 g/dl, nucleated cell counts of up to 5000/µl. The primary cell types include neutrophils as well as mononuclear cells.

Transudates and modified transudates form as a result of increased hydrostatic pressure, decreased plasma oncotic pressure, or a lymphatic obstruction. Increased hydrostatic pressure occurs in association with right-sided congestive heart failure or pericardial disease. Physical examination findings such as abnormal jugular pulses, gallop rhythms, arrhythmias, or murmurs support a diagnosis of heart disease. Heart sounds may be muffled in animals with pericardial ef-

fusions. Thoracic radiography (after fluid removal), electrocardiography, and echocardiography are indicated for cardiac evaluation (see Chapter 2).

Decreased plasma oncotic pressure is a result of hypoalbuminemia. Effusions secondary to hypoalbuminemia are pure transudates, having very low protein concentrations. Subcutaneous edema may be detected in dependent areas of the body. A decreased production of albumin causes hypoalbuminemia in patients with liver disease, and an increased loss of albumin causes it in patients with glomerulopathies or protein-losing enteropathies. The total protein concentration shown by refractometry at the time the packed cell volume is determined during the initial evaluation of the dog or cat can provide an early indication of hypoalbuminemia. Serum biochemical analysis provides an exact measurement of the albumin concentration. In general, albumin concentrations must be lower than 1.5 g/dl and are often less than 1 g/dl before transudation occurs due only to hypoalbuminemia.

Lymphatic obstruction can be caused by neoplasia and diaphragmatic hernias. Diaphragmatic hernias should be suspected in any animal with a history of trauma. The trauma may have been recent or may have occurred years ago. Although usually a modified transudate forms in the setting of a chronic diaphragmatic hernia, an exudative fluid can also be found. Diaphragmatic hernias are identified by radiography or ultrasonography. Occasionally it is necessary to orally administer barium and perform an upper gastrointestinal series or to intraperitoneally administer water-soluble

## TABLE 23-1

**Diagnostic Approach in Dogs and Cats with Pleural Effusion Based on Fluid Type**

| FLUID TYPE | COMMON DISEASE | DIAGNOSTIC TESTS |
|---|---|---|
| Pure and modified transudates | Right-sided heart failure | Evaluate pulses, auscultation, ECG, thor rad, echo |
| | Pericardial disease | See right-sided heart failure |
| | Hypoalbuminemia (pure transudate) | Serum albumin concentrations |
| | Neoplasia | Thor rad and US, CT, thoracoscopy, thoracotomy |
| | Diaphragmatic hernia | Thor rad and US |
| Nonseptic exudates | Feline infectious peritonitis (FIP) | Pleural fluid cytology is generally sufficient. In questionable cases available tests are many, but none has shown good specificity for diagnosing FIP. Consider systemic evaluation, ophthalmoscopic examination, serum or fluid electrophoresis, coronavirus antibody titer, PCR of tissues or effusion (see Chapter 102) |
| | Neoplasia | See Neoplasia above |
| | Diaphragmatic hernia | See Diaphragmatic hernia above |
| | Lung lobe torsion | Thor rad and US, bronchoscopy, thoracotomy |
| Septic exudates | Pyothorax | Gram staining, aerobic and anaerobic cultures, serial thor rad |
| Chylous effusion | Chylothorax | See Table 25-1 |
| Hemorrhagic effusion | Trauma | History |
| | Bleeding disorder | Systemic examination, coagulation tests (ACT, PT, PTT), platelet count |
| | Neoplasia | See Neoplasia above |
| | Lung lobe torsion | See Lung lobe torsion above |

*ACT,* Activated, clotting time; *CT,* computed tomography; *ECG,* electrocardiography; *echo,* echocardiography; *PCR,* polymerase chain reaction; *PT,* prothrombin time; *PTT,* partial thromboplastin time; *thor rad,* thoracic radiography; *US,* ultrasonography.

iodinated contrast media and perform peritoneography to confirm the presence of a diaphragmatic hernia. Normal imaging findings do not entirely rule out the existence of a tear in the diaphragm, however.

Neoplasia must be considered as a differential diagnosis for patients with any type of effusion, although it is rare for a pure transudate to develop. See Effusions Due to Neoplasia, below, for further discussion.

## SEPTIC AND NONSEPTIC EXUDATES

Exudates have a high protein concentration (greater than 3 g/dl) compared with that in transudates. Nucleated cell counts are also high (greater than 5000/μl). Cell types in nonseptic exudates include neutrophils, macrophages, eosinophils, and lymphocytes. The macrophages and lymphocytes may be activated, and typically the neutrophils are nondegenerative. There is no evidence of organisms. Differential diagnoses in animals with nonseptic exudates include feline infectious peritonitis (FIP), neoplasia, chronic diaphragmatic hernia, lung lobe torsion, and resolving septic exudates. Prior treatment with antibiotics in animals with a septic effusion can alter the characteristics of the neutrophil population in the fluid, making them appear nondegenerative, and decrease the number of organisms present in the fluid to an undetectable level. Therefore pleural fluid analysis should be performed before treatment is initiated so that a bacterial infection is not confused with a nonseptic process.

Cats with FIP can present with fever or chorioretinitis, in addition to respiratory signs (see Chapter 102). The pleural fluid protein concentration is often very high in such animals, approaching serum concentrations. It is common to see fibrin strands or clots in the fluid. Careful cytologic evaluation of the fluid is essential to differentiate FIP fluid from exudates caused by pyothorax or malignant lymphoma. The evaluation of animals for diaphragmatic hernia was described in the previous section (Transudates) and is described for neoplasia in a following section (Effusion due to Neoplasia).

Spontaneous lung lobe torsions are most common in dogs with deep, narrow thoracic cavities. In addition to causing an effusion, torsions can be seen in dogs and cats secondary to pleural effusion. Underlying pulmonary disease resulting in lobe atelectasis can also contribute to the development of torsion. Torsion should be considered in animals with a preexisting effusion or pulmonary disease if their condition suddenly deteriorates. Nonseptic exudates or hemorrhagic or chylous effusions develop as the blood and lymph vessels at the hilus are occluded by the rotating lung lobe. Signs of lung lobe torsion may be apparent on thoracic radiographs or ultrasonograms (see Chapter 20, p. 261). Bronchoscopy or thoracotomy is required to verify the condition in some animals.

Septic exudates often have extremely high nucleated cell counts (e.g., 50,000 to more than 100,000/μl), and degenerate neutrophils are the predominant cells. Bacteria can often be observed within neutrophils and macrophages, as well as extracellularly (see Fig. 25-1). The fluid may have a foul odor. Septic exudates are diagnostic for pyothorax. Pyothorax can occur spontaneously; secondary to wounds that penetrate

into the thoracic cavity through the chest wall or esophagus; secondary to migrating grass awns or other foreign bodies; or as an extension of bacterial pneumonia. A sterile technique should be used during thoracocentesis and chest tube placement in all animals with pleural effusion or pneumothorax to prevent iatrogenic infection.

Gram staining and both aerobic and anaerobic bacterial cultures with antibiotic susceptibility testing should be performed on the fluid. Culture and susceptibility testing provide valuable information that can be used for selecting appropriate antibiotics and monitoring therapy. Mixed bacterial infections are common. However, bacteria do not grow from cultures of all septic exudates. Gram staining provides immediate information that can be used to help select antibiotics and is helpful in cases in which bacteria cannot be grown from the fluid.

## CHYLOUS EFFUSIONS

Chylous effusions result from the leakage of material from the thoracic duct, which carries lipid-rich lymph from the body. Such leakage can be idiopathic, congenital, or secondary to trauma, neoplasia, cardiac disease, pericardial disease, dirofilariasis, lung lobe torsion, or diaphragmatic hernia. Chyle is usually grossly white and turbid, largely as a result of the chylomicrons in it that carry fats from the intestines. The fluid is occasionally blood tinged. It is also possible to obtain clear and colorless fluids, particularly in anorectic animals, but this is uncommon.

Chyle must be differentiated from other types of pleural effusions, especially nonseptic exudates. Chyle has moderate concentrations of protein, usually greater than 2.5 g/dl. The nucleated cell count is low to moderate, ranging from 400 to 10,000/μl. Early in the disease the predominant cell type is the small lymphocyte. A few neutrophils may also be present. With time, nondegenerative neutrophils become more predominant and there are fewer lymphocytes. Macrophages also increase in number with time, and plasma cells may be present.

A diagnosis of chylothorax is confirmed by measuring the concentrations of triglycerides in the pleural fluid and serum. Each specimen should be well mixed by the laboratory before a portion is analyzed because of the tendency for the lipid portion to rise to the surface. The triglyceride content in chyle is high compared with that in serum. Rarely, the test will need to be repeated after a meal in anorectic animals.

Most cases of chylothorax are idiopathic, but this diagnosis can be rendered only after the other disorders have been ruled out. Treatment is most likely to be successful if an underlying problem is identified and treated directly. See Chapter 25 for a complete discussion of chylothorax.

## HEMORRHAGIC EFFUSIONS

Hemorrhagic effusions are grossly red as a result of the large red blood cell content. Hemorrhagic effusions have greater than 3 g/dl of protein and more than 1000 nucleated cells/μl, with a distribution similar to that of peripheral blood. Over time the numbers of neutrophils and macrophages increase. Hemorrhagic effusions are readily distinguished from the recovery of peripheral blood through traumatic thoracocentesis by several features, except immediately following bleeding into the thorax. Hemorrhagic effusions have erythrophagocytosis and an inflammatory response on cytologic evaluation. The fluid does not clot, and the packed cell volume (PCV) is lower than that of peripheral blood.

Hypovolemia and anemia may contribute to the clinical signs of patients with hemothorax (Chapter 26). Hemothorax can result from trauma, systemic bleeding disorders, neoplasia, and lung lobe torsion. Respiratory distress caused by hemothorax can be the only clinical sign in animals with some bleeding disorders, including rodenticide intoxication. An activated clotting time and platelet count should be performed early in the evaluation of these animals, followed by more specific clotting tests (i.e., prothrombin time and partial thromboplastin time). Hemangiosarcoma of the heart or lungs is a common neoplastic cause of a hemorrhagic effusion, but malignant cells are rarely identified cytologically. Neoplastic effusions are discussed further in the next section.

## EFFUSIONS DUE TO NEOPLASIA

Neoplasia within the thoracic cavity can result in most types of effusion (modified transudates, exudates, chyle, or hemorrhagic effusion). Neoplasms may involve any of the intrathoracic structures, including the lungs, mediastinal tissues, pleura, heart, and lymph nodes. In some cases, neoplastic cells exfoliate from the tumor into the effusion, and an early diagnosis can be made through fluid cytology. This is often possible in patients with mediastinal lymphoma. Unfortunately, other than in cases of lymphoma, it can be difficult or impossible to establish a definitive diagnosis of neoplasia on the basis of cytologic findings in the pleural fluid alone. Inflammation can result in considerable hyperplastic changes of mesothelial cells that are easily confused with neoplastic cells. A cytologic diagnosis of neoplasia other than lymphoma should be made with extreme caution.

In the majority of cases, neoplastic cells are not present in the fluid or a cytologic diagnosis cannot be made. Thoracic radiography and ultrasonography should be performed to evaluate the thorax for evidence of neoplasia (Chapter 24). Ultrasonography can be used to differentiate localized accumulations of fluid from soft tissue masses. If soft tissue masses are detected, aspirates or biopsy specimens must be obtained for cytologic or histopathologic evaluation. A definitive diagnosis cannot be made on the basis of the radiograph findings or ultrasound images alone

Diffuse neoplastic infiltration of the pleura and some masses cannot be seen with these imaging techniques. Repeated thoracic radiography, computed tomography, thoracoscopy, or surgical exploration may be necessary in such cases.

## PNEUMOTHORAX

Pneumothorax is the accumulation of air in the pleural space. The diagnosis is confirmed by means of thoracic radiography

(see Fig. 24-2). The pleural cavity is normally under negative pressure, which helps to keep the lungs expanded in health. However, if an opening forms between the pleural cavity and the atmosphere or the airways of the lungs, air is transferred into the pleural space because of this negative pressure. A tension pneumothorax occurs if a one-way valve is created by tissue at the site of leakage, such that air can escape into the pleural space during inspiration but cannot reenter the airways or atmosphere during expiration. Increased intrapleural pressure and resultant respiratory distress occur quickly.

Leaks through the thoracic wall can occur after a traumatic injury or as a result of a faulty pleural drainage system. Air can also enter the thorax during abdominal surgery through a previously undetected diaphragmatic hernia. These causes are readily identified.

Pneumothorax from pulmonary air can occur after blunt trauma to the chest (traumatic pneumothorax) or as a result of existing pulmonary lesions (spontaneous pneumothorax). Traumatic pneumothorax occurs frequently, and the history and physical examination findings allow this to be diagnosed. Pulmonary contusions are often present in these animals.

Spontaneous pneumothorax occurs when preexisting pulmonary lesions rupture. Cavitary lung diseases include blebs, bullae, and cysts, which can be congenital or idiopathic or result from prior trauma, chronic airway disease, or *Paragonimus* infection. Necrotic centers can develop in neoplasms, thromboembolized regions, abscesses, and granulomas involving the airways, and these can rupture, allowing air to escape into the pleural space. Thoracic radiography should be performed to identify cavitary lesions in animals with spontaneous pneumothorax, although lesions are not always apparent.

Dogs and cats with pneumothorax and a recent history of trauma are managed conservatively. Cage rest, the removal of accumulating air by periodic thoracocentesis or by chest tube, and radiographic monitoring are indicated. If abnormal radiographic opacities persist without improvement for more than several days in trauma patients, further diagnostic tests should be performed as described in the section on spontaneous pneumothorax (Chapter 25).

## MEDIASTINAL MASSES

Mediastinal masses can cause inspiratory distress by displacing lung tissue and decreasing lung volume and as a result of the secondary pleural effusion that may develop. Additional clinical signs such as coughing, regurgitation, and facial edema may also be present. Neoplasia is the primary differential diagnosis. Lymphoma involving the mediastinum is common, particularly in cats. Other types of neoplasms include thymoma and rarely thyroid carcinoma, parathyroid carcinoma, and chemodectoma. Non-neoplastic mass lesions such as abscesses, granulomas, hematomas, and cysts are other possibilities.

Mediastinal masses in cats can often be palpated during gentle compression of the anterior thorax. Radiographically, mediastinal masses appear as soft tissue opacities in the anterior mediastinum (Fig. 23-1). However, it can be difficult to accurately identify a mediastinal mass if pleural fluid is present. Pleural fluid can both mimic the appearance of a mass and obscure its borders. Ultrasonography done before removal of the pleural fluid is helpful in identifying a mass and determining the extent to which surrounding structures are involved.

Thoracocentesis and fluid analysis should be performed in animals with pleural effusion. Lymphoma can frequently be diagnosed through the identification of malignant cells in the effusion. Transthoracic fine-needle aspiration or biopsy can be performed to obtain specimens for microscopic evaluation of the mass itself. Transthoracic biopsy specimens can be obtained relatively safely, particularly if the lesion is solid rather than cystic. Ultrasonography can be helpful in determining the consistency of the mass and can also be used to guide biopsy. Alternatively, sites for sampling can be determined from two radiographic views of the thorax. The dorsal mediastinal area and heart should be avoided when obtaining biopsy samples. Surgical exploration may be necessary to biopsy small lesions, cavitary lesions, and lesions adjacent to the heart or main blood vessels. Complete excision of the mass should be attempted at that time, unless lymphoma is diagnosed. Specific recommendations for the management of dogs and cats with mediastinal neoplasia are given in Chapter 81.

## PNEUMOMEDIASTINUM

Pneumomediastinum is identified radiographically. Subcutaneous emphysema or pneumothorax can occur concurrently or secondarily. Respiratory compromise most often results from pneumothorax. Mediastinal air commonly originates from rupture or tears in the trachea, bronchi, or alveoli. These leaks can occur as a result of bite wounds of the neck or sudden changes in intrathoracic pressure resulting from coughing, blunt trauma, or excessive respiratory efforts against obstructed airways. Potential iatrogenic causes include tracheal washing, tracheostomy, and endotracheal tube placement, usually due to excessive endotracheal tube cuff pressure. Air can also enter the mediastinum through esophageal tears, generally resulting from foreign bodies.

Strict cage rest is indicated for animals with pneumomediastinum to facilitate natural sealing of the tear. If air continues to accumulate, causing respiratory compromise, bronchoscopy should be performed to identify tracheal or bronchial lacerations that may require surgical repair.

### Suggested Readings

Anderson GI: Pulmonary cavitary lesions in the dog: a review of seven cases, *J Am Anim Hosp Assoc* 23:89, 1987.

Christopher MM: Pleural effusions, *Vet Clin North Am Small Anim Pract* 17:255, 1987.

Forrester SD et al: Pleural effusions: pathophysiology and diagnostic considerations, *Compend Contin Educ Pract Vet* 10:121, 1988.

Hardie EM et al: Tracheal rupture in cats: 16 cases (1983-1998), *J Am Vet Med Assoc* 214:508, 1999.

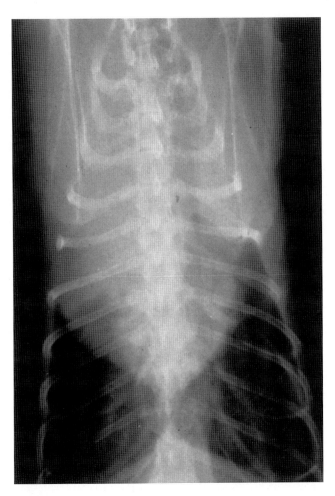

**FIG 23-1**
Ventrodorsal view of the thorax of a cat with an anterior mediastinal mass. Soft tissue opacity fills the anterior mediastinum and obscures the border of the heart.

# CHAPTER 24

# Diagnostic Tests for the Pleural Cavity and Mediastinum

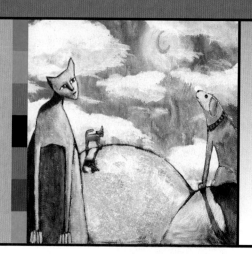

## CHAPTER OUTLINE

RADIOGRAPHY, 320
    Pleural cavity, 320
    Mediastinum, 320
ULTRASONOGRAPHY, 322
THORACOCENTESIS, 322
CHEST TUBES: INDICATIONS AND PLACEMENT, 323
THORACOSCOPY AND THORACOTOMY, 326

## RADIOGRAPHY

### PLEURAL CAVITY

The pleura surrounds each lung lobe and lines the thoracic cavity. It is not normally visible radiographically, and individual lung lobes cannot be distinguished. Abnormalities of the pleura and pleural cavity include pleural thickening, pleural effusion, and pneumothorax. The mediastinum in the dog and cat is not an effective barrier between the left and right side of the thorax, and effusion or pneumothorax is therefore usually bilateral.

### Pleural Thickening

Pleural thickening assumes the appearance of a thin, fluid-dense line between lung lobes where the pleura is perpendicular to the x-ray beam. These lines arc from the periphery toward the hilar region and are known as *pleural fissure lines.* The lines can occur as a result of prior pleural disease and subsequent fibrosis, mild active pleuritis, or low-volume pleural effusion. They can be an incidental finding in older dogs. Infiltration of the pleura with neoplastic cells generally results in effusion rather than thickening.

### Pleural Effusion

Pleural effusion is visible radiographically after about 50 to 100 ml has accumulated in the pleural cavity, depending on the size of the animal. An early effusion assumes the appearance of pleural fissure lines and can be confused with pleural thickening. As fluid accumulates, the lung lobes retract and

the lung lobe borders become rounded. Rounding of the caudodorsal angles of the caudal lung lobes is especially noticeable. The fluid silhouettes with the heart and diaphragm, obscuring their borders. The lungs float on top of the fluid, displacing the trachea dorsally and causing the illusion of a mediastinal mass or cardiomegaly (Fig. 24-1, *A).* As more fluid accumulates, the lung parenchyma appears abnormally dense as a result of incomplete expansion and eventually lung lobes collapse. Collapsed lobes should be examined carefully for evidence of torsion (see p. 261). Pockets of fluid accumulation or unilateral effusion indicates the possibility of concurrent pleural adhesions (Fig. 24-1, *B).*

Critical radiographic evaluation of intrathoracic structures, including the lungs, heart, diaphragm, and mediastinum, cannot be performed in animals with pleural effusion until the fluid has been removed. The interpretation of radiographs obtained in the presence of fluid is prone to error. An exception to this rule is the finding of gas-filled intestinal loops in the thorax, which is diagnostic for diaphragmatic hernia. Both left and right lateral views should be evaluated, in addition to a ventrodorsal view, to improve the sensitivity of detecting masses.

### Pneumothorax

Pneumothorax is the presence of air in the pleural space. If carefully sought, an air opacity without vessels or airways can be seen between the lung lobes and chest wall on radiographs. The lung parenchyma is often more dense than the air in the pleural space because of incomplete expansion. The heart is generally elevated above the sternum, with an air opacity between these two structures (Fig. 24-2). Radiographs should be examined carefully for evidence of possible causes of the pneumothorax, such as cavitary lesions or rib fractures (indicating trauma). To accurately evaluate the pulmonary parenchyma, the air must be removed and the lungs allowed to expand. Cavitary lesions are not always apparent radiographically.

### MEDIASTINUM

The cranial and caudal mediastinum contains the heart and great vessels, esophagus, lymph nodes, and associated sup-

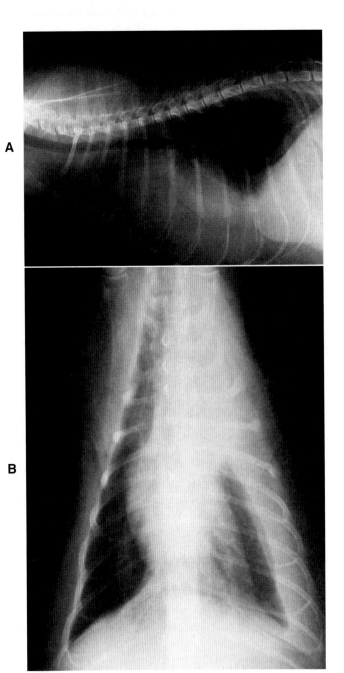

**FIG 24-1**
**A,** Lateral thoracic view of a cat with pleural effusion. See text.
**B,** Ventrodorsal view showing that the effusion is unilateral.

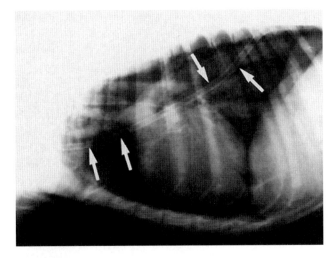

**FIG 24-2**
Lateral view of a dog with pneumothorax and pneumomediastinum. The pneumothorax is mild and is evidenced by elevation of the heart above the sternum. When high-intensity lighting was placed behind the original radiographs, retraction of lung borders could also be seen. It is possible to visualize the outer wall of the trachea and major blood vessels in the anterior mediastinum because of the pneumomediastinum. A chest tube placed to stabilize the dog's condition is also visible *(arrows)*.

port structures. Radiographic abnormalities involving the mediastinum include pneumomediastinum, alterations in size (e.g., mass lesions), displacement, and abnormalities involving the structures within the mediastinum (e.g., megaesophagus).

Pneumomediastinum is the accumulation of air in the mediastinum. If a pneumomediastinum is present, the outer wall of the trachea and the other cranial mediastinal structures, such as the esophagus, major branches of the aortic arch, and cranial vena cava, are contrasted against it (see Fig. 24-2). These structures are not normally visible.

Abnormal soft tissue opacities can occur in the cranial mediastinum, although concurrent pleural effusion often obscures such abnormalities. Localized lesions can represent neoplasia, abscesses, granulomas, or cysts (see Fig. 23-1). Less discrete disease can cause a general widening of the mediastinum that is seen to exceed the width of the vertebra on ventrodorsal views. Exudates, edema, hemorrhage, tumor infiltration, and fat can cause a widened mediastinum. Megaesophagus can often be observed in the cranial mediastinum, especially on lateral views.

The caudal vena cava and aorta are normally visible in the caudal mediastinum. The most common caudal mediastinal abnormalities are megaesophagus and diaphragmatic hernia. Megaesophagus is an important consideration in animals with respiratory signs because it is a common cause of aspiration pneumonia.

The mediastinum is normally located in the center of the thoracic cavity. In the setting of diseases, it can be shifted to one side, and this is identified by a shift in the position of the heart on ventrodorsal or dorsoventral views. Lung lobe collapse, lobectomy, and adhesions of the mediastinum to the chest wall can all cause the mediastinum to shift in the same direction. Space-occupying lesions can cause the mediastinum to shift in the opposite direction.

The lymph nodes and heart are mediastinal structures but are considered separately to ensure a careful evaluation. The sternal nodes are located immediately dorsal to the sternum near the thoracic inlet at the level of the first to third sternebrae (Fig. 24-3). Enlargement is seen on lateral views and has the appearance of a discrete mass lesion. The hilar

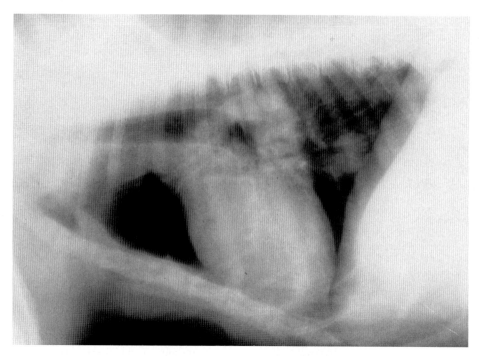

**FIG 24-3**
Lateral thoracic radiograph obtained in a dog with pulmonary neoplasia and sternal and hilar lymphadenopathy. The sternal node is the soft tissue opacity resting on the caudal half of the second sternebra. The hilar nodes are identified by the increased soft tissue opacity around the carina. Several discrete pulmonary nodules are also present.

nodes are located at the heart base around the carina. Enlargement is seen as a generalized increased soft tissue opacity in the perihilar region and is most easily seen on the lateral view. Common differential diagnoses for hilar lymphadenopathy are lymphoma and fungal infections (especially histoplasmosis). Other differential diagnoses include metastatic neoplasia, eosinophilic pulmonary granulomatosis, and mycobacterial infections. Any inflammatory disease can potentially cause lymphadenopathy. Other considerations in animals seen to have an increased perihilar opacity on radiographs include atrial enlargement and heart base tumors.

Evaluation of the heart is described in Chapters 1 and 2. Right-sided heart failure and pericardial effusion can cause pleural fluid accumulation.

## ULTRASONOGRAPHY

Ultrasonography is indicated in the diagnostic evaluation of dogs and cats with pleural effusion to search for masses, diaphragmatic hernia, lung lobe torsion, and cardiac disease. Mediastinal masses, masses involving the pulmonary parenchyma adjacent to the body wall, and masses extending into the thorax from the body wall may be identified and their echogenicity evaluated. Ultrasonography can also be used to guide biopsy instruments to the lesion, although biopsies can be safely done only on solid masses. Ultrasonography is also useful for directing needle placement during thoracocentesis in animals with localized accumulations of pleural fluid. Air interferes with the sound waves, so structures surrounded by aerated lung cannot be examined.

## THORACOCENTESIS

Thoracocentesis is indicated for the collection of diagnostic specimens in dogs and cats with pleural effusion, to remove pleural fluid or air to stabilize the condition of dogs and cats with impaired ventilation, and before radiographic evaluation of intrathoracic structures in dogs and cats with pleural fluid or air. Possible complications of thoracocentesis are pneumothorax caused by lung laceration, hemothorax, and iatrogenic pyothorax. Complications are extremely rare if careful technique is used.

Thoracocentesis is performed with the animal in a lateral or sternal recumbent position, whichever is less stressful. Fluid or air is usually present bilaterally throughout the pleural space and can be retrieved from the seventh intercostal space (ICS) by placing the needle approximately two thirds of the distance from the costochondral junction toward the spine. If initial attempts are unsuccessful, other sites are tried or the animal's position is changed. Fluid may be more successfully retrieved from gravity-dependent sites and air from nondependent sites. Thoracic radiographs are useful in choosing sides for thoracocentesis in the event of unilateral effusions. Ultrasonography is useful for guiding needle placement in patients where fluid collection proves difficult.

A local anesthetic can be administered at the site of thoracocentesis. Sedation is rarely required but may be useful for decreasing patient stress. The site is shaved and surgically prepared, and the procedure is performed using sterile technique. Most often, a butterfly catheter, three-way stopcock, and syringe are used. The removal of fluid or air by syringe is associated with movement of the syringe, and the tubing of the butterfly catheter prevents this movement from affecting the position of the needle within the thoracic cavity. Air and most fluids can be retrieved through a 21-gauge butterfly catheter. A larger catheter may be required to collect extremely viscous fluids, such as fluid from feline infectious peritonitis or pyothorax. The three-way stopcock is attached to the catheter to keep air from entering the thorax during emptying or changing of the syringe.

With the syringe snugly attached and the stopcock open between the catheter and syringe (closed to room air), the needle is advanced through the skin only. The needle and skin are then moved about two rib spaces to the actual collection site. This technique prevents air from entering the chest through the needle tract after the procedure. The needle is then advanced into the thorax immediately in front of the rib to avoid the intercostal vessels and nerves. The needle is held with a hand resting on the chest wall so that it will not move relative to the respirations or movement of the animal. Slight negative pressure can be applied to the catheter by the syringe so that entry into the pleural space is immediately identified by the recovery of fluid or air. It may be necessary to slightly reposition the needle to maintain the flow of fluid or air.

An alternative to a butterfly catheter is an intravenous over-the-needle catheter. In large dogs a 3¼- or 5¼-inch (8- or 13-cm) 14- to 16-gauge catheter can be used. These catheters are soft and less traumatic than butterfly catheters while in the pleural space and permit the animal to be repositioned or rolled to improve fluid or air removal. A few side holes can be added to the catheter using a surgical blade and sterile technique to increase the sites where fluid can enter. The holes should be spaced far apart, should not take up more than one third of the circumference of the catheter, and should have no rough edges because the catheter might then break off in the animal during removal. Extension tubing and a three-way stopcock are attached to the catheter immediately after placement.

After fluid specimens are saved for cytologic and microbiologic analysis, as much fluid or air as possible is removed, except in the event of a hemothorax (see Chapter 26).

## CHEST TUBES: INDICATIONS AND PLACEMENT

Chest tube placement is indicated for the management of dogs and cats with pyothorax (see Chapter 25) or with pneumothorax if air continues to accumulate despite several evacuations of the pleural cavity by needle thoracocentesis. Chest tubes keep fluid and air from accumulating in the pleural space until the underlying cause of the pleural disorder resolves. If possible, needle thoracocentesis and therapy for

shock are performed to stabilize dogs and cats in critical condition before chest tubes are placed.

The major complication of chest tubes is pneumothorax caused by a leak in the apparatus. Animals with chest tubes must be carefully monitored at all times to make sure they do not disrupt the tubing connections, pull the tube part of the way out of the chest so that there are fenestrations outside the body wall, or bite through the tubing. Any leaks in the system can result in a life-threatening pneumothorax within minutes. If an animal with a chest tube must be left unattended, the tube should be clamped off close to the body wall and should be well-protected by bandage material. Hemothorax, iatrogenic pyothorax, and pneumothorax caused by lung laceration can also occur, but these problems are generally prevented through the use of careful aseptic technique.

Pediatric chest tubes can be obtained from hospital supply companies. These tubes have multiple fenestrations, are calibrated along their length, and are radiopaque. For treating pyothorax, the tube should be as large as will fit between the ribs. The size of tube is less critical for control of pneumothorax. Before placement, the end of the tube is occluded with a syringe adapter, a three-way valve, and a hose clamp (Fig. 24-4, *A*).

Sterile technique is used during placement of the chest tube. In an animal with unilateral disease, the tube is placed in the involved side of the thorax. Either side can be used in an animal with bilateral disease. The lateral side of the animal over the caudal rib cage is shaved and surgically prepared. The animal is sedated, and a local anesthetic is placed subcutaneously at the tenth ICS and within the subcutaneous tissues, intercostal muscles, and pleura at the seventh ICS. The dorsoventral orientation is one half to two thirds the distance from the costochondral junction to the thoracolumbar musculature. This distance should correspond to the level where the ribs are maximally bowed.

The length of tube to be advanced into the chest must be determined from thoracic radiographs or by external landmarks on the animal. The tube should extend from the tenth ICS to the first rib. The fenestrations in the tube must not extend outside the point of exit from the pleural cavity.

A stab incision is made through the skin at the tenth ICS. A purse-string suture is then placed around the opening but is not tied. There is a stylet within some chest tubes made for humans. Smaller chest tubes are inserted with the aid of curved hemostats. The tip of the tube is grasped with the tip of the hemostats with the tube parallel to the body of the clamps (see Fig. 24-4, *B*).

The tube, with the stylet or hemostats, is then tunneled subcutaneously from the tenth to the seventh ICS. If hemostats are used, the tips are directed away from the animal's body (see Fig. 24-4, *C*). Once the tip reaches the seventh ICS, the stylet or hemostats are raised perpendicular to the chest wall. The palm of the hand is placed over the end of the stylet or the hemostat handles, and the tube is thrust through the body wall with one rapid motion (see Fig. 24-4, *D*). Once the tube has entered the pleural space, it is quickly advanced forward until the predetermined length has entered the chest while the stylet or hemostats are withdrawn (see Fig. 24-4, *E*).

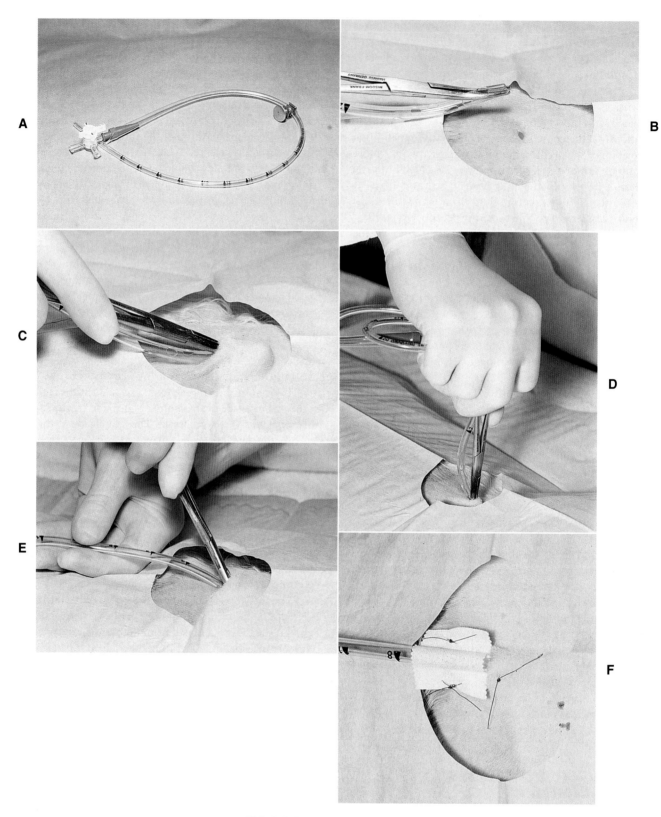

**FIG 24-4**
Placement of a chest tube. See text.

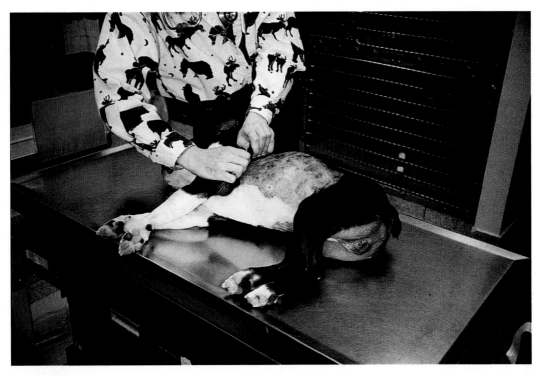

**FIG 24-5**
After an assistant pulls the skin forward, an incision can be made through the skin at the seventh intercostal space (ICS) and blunt dissection is used to reach the pleura. A chest tube can be popped into the pleural space with minimal trauma to the underlying lung. When the skin is released, the tube will course through a subcutaneous tunnel to prevent air leaks around the tube.

An alternative technique can be used to minimize trauma to the lungs caused when thrusting the tube through the body wall. In this technique, after the skin incision has been made and a purse-string suture placed, an assistant standing at the head of the animal draws the skin of the thorax cranially to pull the skin opening forward from the tenth to the seventh ICS (Fig. 24-5). With the skin held in this position, hemostats are used to bluntly dissect through the thoracic and intercostal musculature to the pleura. At this point the chest tube with the stylet or hemostats is easily popped through the pleura into the chest with minimal force. The tube is then advanced and the skin released.

Air will be sucked into the pleural cavity during tube placement regardless of the method used. This air must be immediately removed through the tube using a 35-ml syringe. The purse-string suture is then tied snugly around the tube. Immediately external to the skin entrance, the tube is attached to the body wall by suturing the tape that is formed as a butterfly around the tube to the skin on either side of it (Fig. 24-4, *F)* or by using a Chinese finger trap suture around the tube and attached to the skin. This prevents the chest tube from being withdrawn if tension is accidentally applied to the tubing. The opening in the skin is covered with a sterile sponge with antiseptic ointment. A light wrap is placed around the tube to hold it against the chest wall. The wrap must not be too tight so that it does not greatly decrease chest

wall compliance and increase the work of breathing in these compromised animals. The hose clamp is placed on the tube between the animal and the three-way valve to further protect against pneumothorax whenever suction is not being applied to the tube. An Elizabethan collar is always placed on the animal, because a single bite through the tube can be fatal.

Thoracic radiographs are taken to evaluate the tube position and the effectiveness of drainage. Two views must be evaluated. Ideally the tube should extend along the ventral aspect of the pleural space to the thoracic inlet. The most important sign of adequate tube placement is the absence of areas of persistent fluid or air accumulation. If areas of fluid or air persist, the tube may need to be replaced or a second tube placed in the opposite side.

Once a chest tube is in place and is determined to be in a satisfactory position, its position and the effectiveness of drainage must be monitored regularly by thoracic radiography, generally every 24 to 48 hours. The animal must also be monitored for the development of secondary complications. These include infection and the leakage of air. The bandage should be removed at least daily. The site where the tube enters the skin should be evaluated for signs of inflammation or subcutaneous emphysema. The tube and skin sutures should be examined for signs of motion. The skin around the tube is kept clean, and a sterile sponge is replaced over the entry site of the tube before rebandaging. Stopcock ports should be protected with sterile caps when not in use, and ports should be wiped with hydrogen peroxide before use.

# THORACOSCOPY AND THORACOTOMY

A definitive diagnosis for the cause of pleural effusion is sometimes elusive. In such cases, thoracoscopy or thoracotomy may be necessary to allow visual assessment of the thoracic cavity and the collection of specimens for histologic and bacteriologic analysis. Mesotheliomas and pleural carcinomatosis are often diagnosed through these methods.

## Suggested Readings

DeRycke LM et al: Thoracoscopic anatomy of dogs positioned in lateral recumbency, *J Am Anim Hosp Assoc* 37:543, 2001.

Suter PF: *Thoracic radiography,* Wettswil, Switzerland, 1994, Peter F Suter.

# CHAPTER 25

# Disorders of the Pleural Cavity

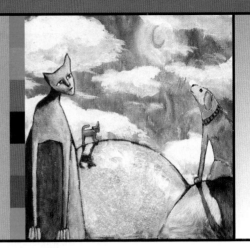

## CHAPTER OUTLINE

PYOTHORAX, 327
CHYLOTHORAX, 330
SPONTANEOUS PNEUMOTHORAX, 332
NEOPLASTIC EFFUSION, 332

## *PYOTHORAX*

### Etiology

Septic exudate in the pleural cavity is referred to as *pyothorax*. It is most often idiopathic in origin, particularly in cats. It can result from foreign bodies, puncture wounds through the chest wall, esophageal tears (usually from ingested foreign bodies), and extension of pulmonary infection. Thoracic foreign bodies are usually migrating grass awns. They are rare in cats and most common in sporting breeds of dogs in states, such as California, where there is a large concentration of fox-tail grasses.

### Clinical Features

Dogs and cats with pyothorax have clinical signs referable to pleural effusion and abscess formation. Signs may be acute or chronic. Tachypnea, decreased lung sounds, and increased abdominal excursions are typical of pleural effusion. In addition, fever, lethargy, anorexia, and weight loss are common. Animals may be presented in septic shock.

### Diagnosis

Pyothorax is diagnosed on the basis of the findings from thoracic radiography and the cytologic evaluation of pleural fluid. Thoracic radiographs are used to confirm the presence of pleural effusion and to determine whether the disease is localized, unilateral, or bilateral. In most animals, fluid is present throughout the pleural space. The finding of a localized accumulation of fluid indicates the possible presence of pleural fibrosis, mass lesions, or lung lobe torsion. Thoracic radiographs are taken again after removal of the fluid to evaluate the pulmonary parenchyma for evidence of underlying disease (e.g., bacterial pneumonia, foreign body) that may have caused the pyothorax. The identification of a septic exudate by pleural fluid analysis establishes the diagnosis of pyothorax.

Septic suppurative inflammation is a consistent finding in pleural fluid examined cytologically, except in animals that are receiving antibiotics (see Chapter 23; also Fig. 25-1). Pleural fluid is always evaluated by Gram staining and aerobic and anaerobic bacterial cultures. Anaerobes are usually present in the fluid and, in many dogs and cats, more than one type of bacteria are present. All of the types of bacteria involved may not grow in the laboratory in spite of cytologic evidence of their presence, possibly due to competition between organisms or an inhibitory effect of the exudative fluid. Organisms such as *Actinomyces* and *Nocardia* particularly do not grow well if specimens have been cultured using routine procedures. The absence of growth of bacteria does not rule out a diagnosis of pyothorax.

### Treatment

Medical therapy for pyothorax includes antibiotics, drainage of the pleural cavity, and appropriate supportive care (e.g., fluid therapy). At first, antibiotics are administered intravenously. The results of Gram staining and culture and sensitivity testing are helpful in selecting antibiotics. Generally, anaerobes and *Pasteurella* (a common isolate from cats with pyothorax) are susceptible to amoxicillin-clavulanate. Other gram negative organisms are often susceptible to amoxicillin-clavulanate, but their antibiotic susceptibilities are unpredictable. Unfortunately, this drug is not available for intravenous administration. Ampicillin with sulbactam, a different β-lactamase inhibitor, is an excellent substitute for intravenous use (50 mg/kg of combined drug q8h). Other drugs that have good activity against anaerobic organisms are chloramphenicol, metronidazole, and clindamycin. If metronidazole or clindamycin is used, additional gram-negative coverage is necessary and is achieved by adding a fluoroquinolone or aminoglycoside antibiotic to the treatment. Addition of one of these antibiotics may also be necessary in patients that fail to show improvement in clinical condition, complete

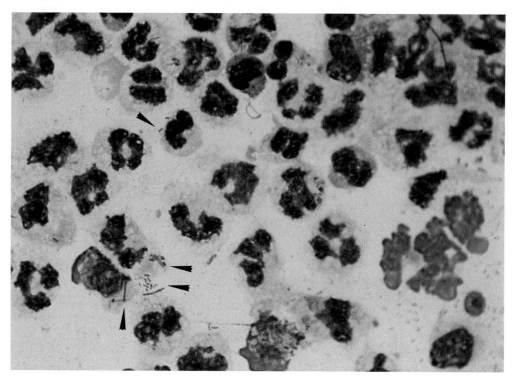

**FIG 25-1**
Cytologic preparation of a specimen of a pleural effusion from a cat with pyothorax. Degenerative neutrophils predominate, and intracellular and extracellular bacteria are prevalent *(arrowheads)*. Both rods and cocci are seen.

blood count (CBC), and fluid cytology within the first few days of treatment.

Oral antibiotics are used once significant improvement is noted, usually about the time of chest tube removal. Amoxicillin-clavulanate (20 to 25 mg/kg q8h PO) is used in patients that have responded to ampicillin with sulbactam. Oral antibiotic therapy is continued for an additional 4 to 6 weeks.

Drainage of the septic exudate is an essential part of the treatment of pyothorax. Although treatment with antibiotics alone often causes dramatic improvement in the animal's clinical condition initially, the signs generally recur, and complications of the prolonged infection, such as fibrosis or abscesses, are more likely (Fig. 25-2). Indwelling chest tubes provide the best drainage and can be used to keep the exudate from accumulating during the initial days of antibiotic therapy. Dogs and cats in critical condition at presentation are stabilized through the use of needle thoracocentesis and shock therapy before chest tube placement. Intermittent needle thoracocentesis is minimally effective for draining the pleural cavity and is not recommended for treatment unless the owner cannot afford the expense of chest tube management.

Chest tube placement and assessment of positioning are discussed in Chapter 24. Animals probably respond most rapidly to constant suctioning of the exudate from the chest, although intermittent suction is certainly adequate and often more feasible. Constant suction is applied with a suction pump and collection unit. Disposable, pediatric cage side collection units (e.g., Thora-Seal III, Sherwood Medical, St. Louis) are available through hospital supply companies. These units allow monitoring of collected fluid volume and adjustment of suction pressure. An initial suction pressure of 10 to 15 cm $H_2O$ is used, but more or less pressure may be necessary, depending on the viscosity of the pleural fluid and the collapsibility of the tubes. The collection systems must be carefully monitored for the occurrence of leaks or malfunctions that could cause a fatal pneumothorax.

Intermittent suction by syringe is ideally performed every 2 hours for the first days of treatment, with arrangements made for drainage to continue during the night. Within a few days the volume of fluid produced will decrease, and the interval can then be lengthened. If such intensive care is not possible, an effort should still be made to empty the chest of fluid at least once late in the evening to minimize the accumulation of exudate overnight.

Lavage of the chest cavity is performed twice daily. This consists of the removal of any fluid within the chest, followed by the slow infusion of warmed sterile saline solution into the chest. A volume of approximately 10 ml/kg of body weight is infused, but the infusion should be discontinued if any distress is noted. After this the animal is gently rolled from side to side, and the fluid then is removed. Sterile technique is used throughout the procedure. The volume recovered should be about 75% of the volume infused. If less fluid is re-

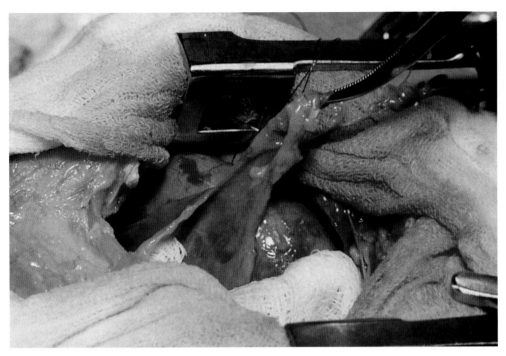

**FIG 25-2**
Pleural fibrosis evidenced by a markedly thickened pleura seen during thoracotomy in a cat with chronic pyothorax. Treatment with antibiotics alone was attempted, and several weeks later the cat's condition deteriorated. Fibrosis was too extensive to allow for routine drainage with chest tubes. Surgical debridement, several lobectomies, drainage through surgically placed tubes, and long-term antibiotic therapy resulted in a cure.

trieved, this may indicate that the chest tube is no longer providing adequate drainage.

Thoracic radiographs are taken every 24 to 48 hours to make sure the chest is being completely drained of fluid. Failure to monitor the effectiveness of drainage radiographically can lead to costly prolongation of the intensive care required for maintenance of the chest tube.

Serum electrolyte concentrations are also monitored. Many dogs and cats with pyothorax are dehydrated and anorectic at presentation and require intravenous fluid therapy. Supplementation of the fluid with potassium may be necessary.

The decision to discontinue drainage and remove the chest tube is based on the fluid volume and cytologic characteristics. The volume of fluid recovered should have decreased to less than 2 ml/kg/day. Slides of the fluid are prepared daily and evaluated cytologically. Bacteria should no longer be visible intracellularly or extracellularly. Neutrophils will persist but should no longer appear degenerate (Fig. 25-3). When these criteria have been met and no pockets of fluid are seen on thoracic radiographs, the chest tube is removed and the animal is monitored clinically for at least 24 hours for the development of pneumothorax or the recurrence of effusion. Thoracic radiographs can be taken to more sensitively evaluate the animal for these potential problems.

Thoracic radiographs are evaluated 1 week after removal of the chest tube and 1 week and 1 month after discontinua-tion of the antibiotic therapy. These radiographs are obtained so that a localized nidus of disease such as a foreign body or an abscess can be identified and also so that recurrence of a pyothorax can be detected before large volumes of pleural fluid accumulate. Such niduses are often invisible when large volumes of pleural fluid are present or while aggressive therapy is in progress.

Exploratory thoracotomy is indicated for the removal of a suspected nidus of infection and in those animals that do not respond to medical therapy. In the latter instance, surgery may be necessary to remove fibrotic and diseased tissue or a foreign body. A lack of response is evidenced by the continued need for a chest tube for longer than 1 week after the start of appropriate antibiotic treatment and drainage.

## Prognosis

Most cases of pyothorax are idiopathic. The prognosis for animals with pyothorax is good if it is recognized early and treated aggressively. Long-term complications such as pleural fibrosis and restrictive lung disease are uncommon.

Exploratory surgery is necessary to ensure complete resolution of the problem in dogs or cats with foreign bodies in the thoracic cavity. Radiolucent foreign bodies can be difficult to find, however, and the prognosis for pyothorax secondary to them is more guarded.

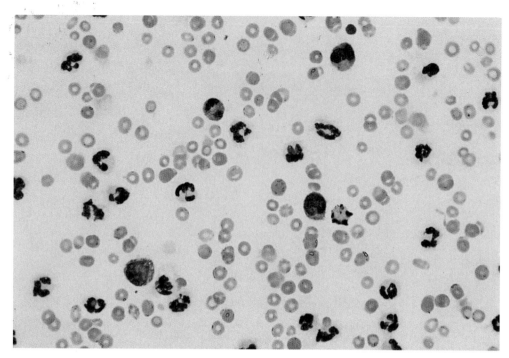

**FIG 25-3**
Cytologic preparation of a specimen of a pleural effusion from a cat being treated successfully for pyothorax with chest tube drainage and antibiotics. Compared with the fluid shown in Fig. 25-1, the nucleated cell count is low, the neutrophils are nondegenerative, organisms are not present, and mononuclear cells are appearing (Cytocentrifuge prep).

## CHYLOTHORAX

### Etiology

Chylothorax is the accumulation of chyle within the thoracic cavity. The chyle originates from the thoracic duct, which carries triglyceride-rich fluid from the intestinal lymphatics and empties into the venous system in the anterior thorax. The fluid also contains lymphocytes, protein, and fat-soluble vitamins. Thoracic duct rupture after thoracic trauma can result in transient chylothorax. However, most cases are not the result of a ruptured duct. Possible causes of nontraumatic chylothorax include generalized lymphangiectasia, inflammation, and obstruction of lymphatic flow. Flow can be obstructed for physical reasons, such as neoplasia, or as a result of increased venous pressures.

Chylothorax can be categorized as congenital, traumatic, or nontraumatic. Congenital chylothorax occurs in Afghan Hounds. A congenital predisposition may exist in animals in which chylothorax develops later in life. Traumatic events that induce chylothorax can be surgical (e.g., thoracotomy) or nonsurgical (e.g., being hit by a car). Neoplasia, particularly mediastinal lymphoma in cats, is a major nontraumatic cause of chylothorax. Tumors can invade or obstruct the thoracic duct. Other nontraumatic causes of chylothorax include cardiomyopathy, dirofilariasis, pericardial disease, and other causes of right-sided heart failure, lung lobe torsion, diaphragmatic hernia, and systemic lymphangiectasia. No underlying disease can be identified in most animals, and idiopathic chylothorax is diagnosed.

### Clinical Features

Chylothorax can occur in dogs or cats of any age. Afghan Hounds appear to be predisposed to the disorder. The primary clinical sign is respiratory distress typical of pleural effusion. Although the distress is often acute in onset, more subtle signs have generally been present for more than a month. Lethargy, anorexia, weight loss, and exercise intolerance are common. Cough can also occur.

### Diagnosis

Chylothorax is diagnosed on the basis of the documentation of pleural fluid on thoracic radiographs and the identification of chyle through cytologic and biochemical evaluation of pleural fluid obtained by thoracocentesis (see Chapter 23). Lymphopenia and panhypoproteinemia may be present in peripheral blood.

Once chylothorax has been diagnosed, further diagnostic tests are performed to identify potential underlying disease (Table 25-1). These tests include thoracic ultrasonography, echocardiography, microfilarial examination and adult antigen testing for heartworm disease, and, in cats, the measurement of thyroid hormone concentrations. Lymphangiography can be used to identify lymphangiectasia, sites of obstruction, and, rarely, sites of leakage from the thoracic

TABLE 25-1

Diagnostic Tests to Identify Underlying Diseases in Dogs and Cats With Chylothorax

---

**Complete Blood Count, Serum Biochemical Panel, Urinalysis**

Evaluate systemic status

**Cytologic Examination of Fluid**

Infectious agents
Neoplastic cells (especially lymphoma)

**Thoracic Radiographs (After Fluid Removal)**

Anterior mediastinal masses
Other neoplasia
Cardiac disease
Heartworm disease
Pericardial disease

**Ultrasonography (Ideally, in the Presence of Fluid)**

Anterior mediastinum
   Mass
Heart (echocardiography)
   Cardiomyopathy
   Heartworm disease
   Pericardial disease
   Congenital heart disease
Other fluid densities adjacent to body wall
   Neoplasia
   Lung lobe torsion

**Heartworm Antibody and Antigen Tests**

Heartworm disease

**Lymphangiography**

Preoperative and postoperative assessment of thoracic duct

---

duct. Lymphangiography is performed before the surgical ligation of lymphatics is attempted.

## Treatment

Thoracocentesis and appropriate fluid therapy are used to stabilize dogs and cats with chylothorax, as needed, at presentation. Electrolyte abnormalities may be present. A concerted effort is made to identify any underlying cause of the chylothorax so that it can be directly treated. Elimination of the underlying problem can result in resolution of the chylothorax, although medical management as described later for idiopathic chylothorax is generally required for several weeks or even months. The exception is chylothorax of traumatic origin, which generally resolves in 1 to 2 weeks.

A routinely successful treatment for idiopathic chylothorax has not been established. Because of the relatively poor success achieved with surgical treatment and the fact that spontaneous remission occurs in some cases, medical management of these cases is initially recommended. Thoracocentesis is performed as needed, based on the owner's observation of increased respiratory rate or effort or decreased activity or appetite. Initially, thoracocentesis may need to be performed every 5 to 15 days. The interval between thoracocenteses will gradually lengthen if the chylothorax is responsive to medical management. Ultrasound guidance of the needle during thoracocentesis is especially helpful in removing pockets of chyle from the pleural cavity, and by increasing the effectiveness of drainage, it can prolong the interval between thoracocenteses.

A low-fat, nutritionally complete diet is fed, such as Prescription Diet w/d (Hill's Pet Products, Topeka, Kan). In humans, medium-chain triglyceride oil is absorbed directly into the bloodstream, bypassing the lymphatics, and can be used as a fat supplement. Unfortunately, in dogs these triglycerides have been shown to enter the thoracic duct. Nevertheless, they can be added to the diet if additional calories are desired.

Medical management may be facilitated by the administration of rutin, a benzopyrone drug. Rutin has been used in humans for the treatment of lymphedema. It is thought to decrease the protein content of the effusion by affecting macrophage function. The resorption of effusion may thereby be enhanced and fibrosis of the pleura minimized. The drug is available over-the-counter at health food stores. A dose of 50 mg/kg given orally every 8 hours is currently being investigated by Fossum (1997). Clients should be warned that the effectiveness of rutin therapy has not been proved in clinical studies and that the dosage is merely extrapolated from that used in humans. Adverse reactions to the drug have not been noted.

Surgical management is considered if clinical signs have not improved within 2 to 3 months of medical therapy or if signs are intolerable. The surgical management of chylothorax includes thoracic duct ligation and the placement of drains. Unfortunately, thoracic duct ligation is successful in eliminating effusion in only about half of the cases, and drains commonly become nonfunctional within months of placement. If surgery is elected, multiple ligations of the thoracic duct and its collaterals are performed. The ducts are identified by lymphangiography before surgery, and this must be repeated after ligation to assess the success of ligation. In addition, pleuroperitoneal or pleurovenous shunts are placed or mesh is placed within the diaphragm to allow fluid to drain into the abdominal cavity. These drainage procedures provide a route for the leaking chyle to reenter the circulation without producing the respiratory compromise associated with pleural effusion.

## Prognosis

The prognosis is guarded unless the chylothorax was traumatically induced or the result of a reversible condition. Long-standing chylothorax can result in the development of pleural fibrosis, which in turn can lead to the pocketing of fluid, precluding adequate drainage and ultimately preventing expansion of the lungs. Surgical decortication of the lungs can be attempted, but the prognosis in animals who undergo this is poor.

## SPONTANEOUS PNEUMOTHORAX

In spontaneous pneumothorax, air leaks from the lungs into the pleural cavity in the absence of blunt trauma or a penetrating chest wound. It is much less common than traumatic pneumothorax. Underlying causes include pulmonary cavitary lesions (Chapter 23), pneumonia, thromboembolic disease resulting from dirofilariasis, abscesses, granulomas, and neoplasms. It occurs more commonly in dogs than in cats. Rapid, profound respiratory distress occurs in the subset of animals in which a tension pneumothorax develops.

Thoracocentesis is useful for initial stabilization of the animal's condition. If frequent thoracocentesis is needed to control the pneumothorax, a chest tube is placed (Chapter 24). Dogs and cats are evaluated for underlying disease with thoracic radiographs (repeated after full lung expansion), multiple fecal examinations for *Paragonimus* ova (see Chapter 20), heartworm tests, and possibly tracheal wash fluid analysis or bronchoscopy.

Patients with *Paragonimus* infections generally respond to medical treatment (Chapter 22). Otherwise, surgical therapy is indicated for most animals. In a review of 21 cases, Holtsinger and colleagues (1993) found that most dogs with spontaneous pneumothorax managed medically with chest tubes and suction ultimately required surgery during the initial hospitalization or upon subsequent recurrence of pneumothorax to resolve the problem. Because unobserved recurrence of spontaneous pneumothorax can be fatal, conservative treatment is felt to carry more risk than surgery. Further, a report of 64 cases by Puerto and colleagues (2002) showed that recurrence and mortality rates for dogs with spontaneous pneumothorax were lower in dogs that had surgery compared with dogs that were treated conservatively. A median sternotomy is generally recommended to allow exposure of all lung lobes, because it is often not possible to localize the disease preoperatively, and some diseases are multifocal. Abnormal tissue is evaluated histologically and microbiologically for a definitive diagnosis.

Conservative therapy consists of cage rest and chest tube placement with continuous suction (see Pyothorax, above). In large dogs a one-way Heimlich valve can be used rather than suction.

Regardless of the treatment used, recurrence is a possibility. Accurate diagnosis of the underlying lung disease and determination of the extent of involvement through a thoracotomy assist in determining the prognosis.

## NEOPLASTIC EFFUSION

Neoplastic effusions resulting from mediastinal lymphoma are treated with radiation or chemotherapy (see Chapter 81). Effusions due to mesothelioma or carcinoma of the pleural surfaces may respond to palliative therapy with intracavitary infusions of cisplatin or carboplatin (see Moore, 1992, in Suggested Readings). Placement of pleuroperitoneal shunts or intermittent thoracocentesis to alleviate the degree of respiratory compromise can also be considered to prolong life for patients that have no clinical signs beyond those resulting from the accumulation of pleural effusion.

### Suggested Readings

Fossum TW et al: Chylothorax in cats: 37 cases (1969-1989), *J Am Vet Med Assoc* 198:672, 1991.

Fossum TW et al: Chylothorax associated with right-sided heart failure in 5 cats, *J Am Vet Med Assoc* 204:84, 1994.

Fossum TW: *Small animal surgery,* St Louis, 1997, Mosby.

Holtsinger RH et al: Spontaneous pneumothorax in the dog: a retrospective analysis of 21 cases, *J Am Anim Hosp Assoc* 29:195, 1993.

Jonas LD: Feline pyothorax: a retrospective study of twenty cases, *J Am Anim Hosp Assoc* 19:865, 1983.

Kerpsack SJ et al: Evaluation of mesenteric lymphangiography and thoracic duct ligation in cats with chylothorax: 19 cases (1987-1992), *J Am Vet Med Assoc* 205:711, 1994.

Moore AS: Chemotherapy for intrathoracic cancer in dogs and cats, *Problems in Vet Med* 4:351, 1992.

Piek CJ et el: Pyothorax in 9 dogs, *Vet Q* 22:107, 2000.

Puerto DA et al: Surgical and nonsurgical management of and selected risk factors for spontaneous pneumothorax in dogs: 64 cases (1986-1999), *J Am Vet Med Assoc* 220:1670, 2002.

Turner WD et al: Continuous suction drainage for management of canine pyothorax: a retrospective study, *J Am Anim Hosp Assoc* 24:485, 1988.

Walker AL et al: Bacteria associated with pyothorax of dogs and cats: 98 cases (1989-1998), *J Am Vet Med Assoc* 216:359, 2000.

## CHAPTER 26

# Emergency Management of Respiratory Distress

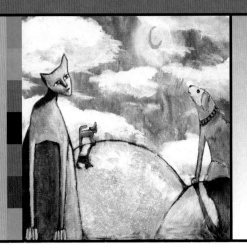

## CHAPTER OUTLINE

GENERAL CONSIDERATIONS, 333
LARGE AIRWAY DISEASE, 333
    Extrathoracic (upper) airway obstruction, 334
    Intrathoracic large airway obstruction, 335
PULMONARY PARENCHYMAL DISEASE, 335
PLEURAL SPACE DISEASE, 336

## GENERAL CONSIDERATIONS

Respiratory distress, or dyspnea, refers to an abnormally increased effort in breathing. Some authors prefer to use terms such as *hyperpnea* and *increased respiratory effort* in reference to this abnormality, because *dyspnea* and *distress* imply feelings that cannot be determined with certainty in animals. Difficulty breathing is extremely stressful for people and is likely so for dogs and cats as well. It is also physically exhausting to the animal as a whole and to the respiratory musculature specifically. Animals in respiratory distress at rest should be managed aggressively, and their clinical status should be frequently assessed.

A dog or cat in respiratory distress may show orthopnea, which is a difficulty in breathing in certain positions. Animals with orthopnea will assume a sitting or standing position with their elbows abducted and neck extended. Movement of the abdominal muscles that assist ventilation may be exaggerated. Cats normally have a minimal visible respiratory effort. Cats that show noticeable chest excursions or open-mouth breathing are severely compromised. Cyanosis, in which normally pink mucous membranes are bluish, is a sign of severe hypoxemia and indicates that the increased respiratory effort is not sufficiently compensating for the degree of respiratory dysfunction. Pallor of the mucus membranes is a more common sign of acute hypoxemia resulting from respiratory disease than is cyanosis.

Respiratory distress caused by respiratory tract disease most commonly develops as a result of large airway obstruction, severe pulmonary parenchymal disease (including pulmonary thromboembolism), pleural effusion, or pneumo-

thorax. Respiratory distress can also occur as a result of primary cardiac disease causing decreased perfusion, pulmonary edema, or pleural effusion (see Chapter 1). In addition, noncardiopulmonary causes of respiratory distress must be considered in animals with distress, including severe anemia, hypovolemia, acidosis, hyperthermia, and neurologic disease. Normal breath sounds may be increased in dogs and cats with these diseases, but crackles or wheezes are not expected.

A physical examination should be performed rapidly, paying particular attention to the breathing pattern, auscultatory abnormalities of the thorax and trachea, pulses, and mucous membrane color and perfusion. Attempts at stabilizing the animal's condition should then be made before initiating further diagnostic testing.

Dogs and cats in shock should be treated appropriately (see p. 387). Most animals in severe respiratory distress benefit from decreased stress and activity, placement in a cool environment, and oxygen supplementation. Cage rest is extremely important, and the least stressful method of oxygen supplementation should be used initially (see Chapter 27). An oxygen cage achieves both these goals, with the disadvantage that the animal is inaccessible. Sedation of the animal may be beneficial (Table 26-1). More specific therapy depends on the location and cause of the respiratory distress (Table 26-2).

## LARGE AIRWAY DISEASE

Diseases of the large airways result in respiratory distress by obstructing the flow of air into the lungs. For the purposes of these discussions, extrathoracic large airways (otherwise known as upper airways) include the pharynx, larynx, and trachea proximal to the thoracic inlet; intrathoracic large airways include the trachea distal to the thoracic inlet and bronchi. Animals presenting in respiratory distress caused by large airway obstruction typically have a markedly increased respiratory effort with a minimally increased respiratory rate (see Table 26-2). Excursions of the chest may be increased (i.e., deep breaths are taken). Breath sounds are often increased.

TABLE 26-1

Drugs Used to Decrease Stress in Animals with Respiratory Distress

**Upper Airway Obstruction: Decreases Anxiety and Lessens Respiratory Efforts, Decreasing Negative Pressure within Upper Airways**

| | | |
|---|---|---|
| Acepromazine | Dogs and cats | 0.05 mg/kg IV, SQ |
| Morphine | Dogs only, particular brachycephalic dogs | 0.1 mg/kg IV; repeat q3min to effect; duration, 1-4 hr |

**Pulmonary Edema: Decreases Anxiety; Morphine Reduces Pulmonary Venous Pressure**

| | | |
|---|---|---|
| Morphine | Dogs only | 0.1 mg/kg IV; repeat q3min to effect; duration, 1-4 hr |
| Acepromazine | Dogs and cats | 0.05 mg/kg IV, SQ; duration, 3-6 hr |

**Rib Fractures, After Thoracotomy, Other Trauma: Pain Relief**

| | | |
|---|---|---|
| Hydromorphone | Dogs | 0.05 mg/kg IV, IM; can repeat IV q3min to effect; duration, 2-4 hr |
| | Cats | 0.025-0.05 mg/kg IV, IM; can repeat IV q3min to effect but stop if mydriasis occurs; duration, 2-4 hr |
| Butorphanol | Cats | 0.1 mg/kg IV, IM, SQ; can repeat IV q3min to effect; duration, 1-6 hr |
| Buprenorphine | Dogs and cats | 0.005 mg/kg IV, IM; repeat to effect; duration, 4-8 hr |

*IV,* Intravenously; *SQ,* subcutaneously; *IM,* intramuscularly.

 TABLE 26-2

Localization of Respiratory Tract Disease by Physical Examination Findings in Dogs and Cats with Severe Respiratory Distress

| | LARGE AIRWAY DISEASE | | PULMONARY PARENCHYMAL DISEASE | | | PLEURAL SPACE DISEASE |
|---|---|---|---|---|---|---|
| | **EXTRATHORACIC (UPPER)** | **INTRATHORACIC** | **OBSTRUCTIVE** | **RESTRICTIVE** | **OBSTRUCTIVE AND RESTRICTIVE** | |
| Respiratory rate | N1-↑ | N ↑ | ↑↑↑ | ↑↑↑ | ↑↑↑ | ↑↑↑ |
| Relative effort | ↑↑↑ Inspiration | ↑↑ Expiration | ↑ Expiration | ↑↑ Inspiration | No difference | ↑ Inspiration |
| Audible sounds | Inspiratory stridor, stertor | Expiratory cough/wheeze | Rarely expiratory wheeze | None | None | None |
| Auscultable sounds | Referred upper airway sounds; ↑↑ breath sounds | Referred upper airway sounds; ↑↑ breath sounds | Expiratory wheezes or ↑↑ breath sounds; rarely, ↓ breath sounds with air trapping | ↑↑ Breath sounds; ± crackles | ↑↑ Breath sounds, crackles, and/or wheezes | ↓ Breath sounds |

↑, Slightly increased; ↑↑, increased; ↑↑↑, markedly increased; ↓, decreased; *N1,* normal. Normal respiratory rates for dogs and cats at rest are ≤20/min. In the hospital setting, rates of ≤30/min are generally accepted as normal.

# EXTRATHORACIC (UPPER) AIRWAY OBSTRUCTION

Patients with upper airway obstruction typically have the greatest breathing effort during inspiration, which is generally prolonged relative to expiration. Stridor or stertor is usually heard, generally during inspiration. A history of voice change may be present with laryngeal disease.

Laryngeal paralysis and brachycephalic airway syndrome are the most common causes of upper airway obstruction

(see Chapter 17). Other laryngeal and pharyngeal diseases are listed in Tables 16-1 and 16-2. Rarely, diseases of the extrathoracic trachea, such as foreign body, stricture, neoplasia, granuloma, hypoplasia, or tracheal collapse, result in respiratory distress.

Patients with upper airway obstruction usually present with acute distress in spite of the chronic nature of most of these diseases because of a vicious cycle of increased respirations leading to increased obstruction, as described in Chap-

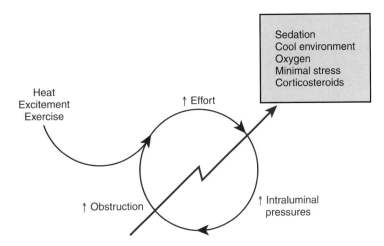

**FIG 26-1**
Patients with extrathoracic (upper) airway obstruction often present in acute respiratory distress because of a progressive worsening of airway obstruction following an exacerbating event. Medical intervention is nearly always successful in breaking this cycle and stabilizing the patient's respiratory status.

ter 16. This cycle can almost always be broken with medical management (Fig. 26-1). The patient is sedated (see Table 26-1) and provided a cool, oxygen-rich environment (oxygen cage). For dogs with pharyngeal disease, primarily brachycephalic airway syndrome, morphine is given. Otherwise, acepromazine is used. Subjectively, dogs with brachycephalic airway syndrome seem to have more difficulty maintaining a patent airway when sedated with acepromazine compared with morphine. Short-acting corticosteroids are thought by some to be effective in decreasing local inflammation (e.g., dexamethasone, 0.1 mg/kg intravenously [IV], or prednisolone sodium succinate, 10 to 20 mg/kg IV).

In rare cases, sedation and oxygen supplementation will not resolve the respiratory distress and the obstruction must be physically bypassed. Placement of an endotracheal tube is generally effective. A short-acting anesthetic agent is administered. Long and narrow endotracheal tubes with stylets should be available to pass by large or deep obstructions. If an endotracheal tube cannot be placed, a transtracheal catheter can be inserted distal to the obstruction (see Chapter 27). If a tracheostomy tube is needed, it can then be placed under controlled, sterile conditions. It is rarely necessary to perform a nonsterile emergency tracheostomy.

## INTRATHORACIC LARGE AIRWAY OBSTRUCTION

Respiratory distress caused by intrathoracic large airway obstruction is rare. Patients with intrathoracic large airway obstruction typically have the greatest breathing effort during expiration, which is generally prolonged relative to inspiration. The most common cause of intrathoracic large airway obstruction is collapse of the mainstem bronchi and/or intrathoracic trachea as a result of chronic bronchitis (see Chapter 21). A high-pitched, wheezing, coughlike sound is often heard during expiration in these patients, and crackles

or wheezes may be auscultated. Other differential diagnoses include foreign body, advanced *Oslerus* infection, tracheal neoplasia, tracheal stricture, and bronchial compression by extreme hilar lymphadenopathy.

Sedation, oxygen supplementation, and minimizing stress as described for the management of upper airway obstruction are often effective in stabilizing these patients as well. Dogs with end-stage bronchitis may benefit from bronchodilators and corticosteroids, and high doses of butorphenol or hydrocodone will provide cough suppression and sedation (see Chapter 21).

## PULMONARY PARENCHYMAL DISEASE

Diseases of the pulmonary parenchyma result in hypoxemia and respiratory distress through a variety of mechanisms, including the obstruction of small airways (obstructive lung disease; e.g., feline bronchial disease); decreased pulmonary compliance (restrictive lung disease, "stiff" lungs; e.g., pulmonary fibrosis); and interference with pulmonary circulation (e.g., pulmonary thromboembolism). The majority of patients with pulmonary parenchymal disease, such as those with pneumonias or pulmonary edema, develop hypoxemia through a combination of these mechanisms that contribute to $\dot{V}/\dot{Q}$ mismatch (see Chapter 20), including airway obstruction and alveolar flooding, and decreased compliance.

Animals presenting in respiratory distress caused by pulmonary parenchymal disease typically have a markedly increased respiratory rate (see Table 26-2). Patients with primarily obstructive disease, usually cats with bronchial disease, may have prolonged expiration relative to inspiration with increased expiratory efforts. Expiratory wheezes are commonly auscultated. Patients with primarily restrictive disease, usually dogs with pulmonary fibrosis, may have prolonged inspiration relative to expiration and effortless expiration. Crackles are commonly auscultated. Other patients, with a combination of these processes occurring, have increased efforts during both phases of respiration, shallow breathing, and crackles, wheezes, or increased breath sounds on auscultation. Differential diagnoses for dogs and cats with pulmonary disease are provided in Table 19-1.

Oxygen therapy is the treatment of choice for stabilizing dogs or cats with severe respiratory distress believed to be caused by pulmonary disease (see Chapter 27). Bronchodilators, diuretics, or glucocorticoids can be considered as additional treatments if oxygen therapy alone is not adequate.

Bronchodilators, such as short-acting theophyllines or β-agonists, are used if obstructive lung disease is suspected because they decrease bronchoconstriction. In combination with oxygen, they are the treatment of choice for cats with signs of bronchial disease (see Chapter 21). Subcutaneous terbutaline (0.01 mg/kg, SC; repeated in 5 to 10 minutes if necessary) is most often used in emergency situations. Bronchodilators are described in more detail in Chapter 21 (see pp. 293 and 296 and Table 21-5).

Diuretics, such as furosemide (2 mg/kg IV), are indicated for the management of pulmonary edema. However, potential complications of their use resulting from volume contraction and dehydration should be taken into consideration. Prolonged use of diuretics is contraindicated in animals with exudative lung disease or bronchitis, because systemic dehydration results in the drying of airways and airway secretions. The mucociliary clearance of airway secretions and contaminants is decreased, and airways are further obstructed with mucous plugs.

Glucocorticoids decrease inflammation. Rapid-acting formulations, such as prednisolone sodium succinate (10 to 20 mg/kg IV), are indicated for animals in severe respiratory distress caused by the following conditions: acute allergic bronchitis, feline bronchial disease, thromboembolism after adulticide treatment for heartworms, and respiratory failure soon after the initiation of treatment for pulmonary mycoses. Animals with other inflammatory diseases or acute respiratory distress syndrome may also respond favorably to glucocorticoid administration. Potential negative effects of corticosteroids must be considered before their use. For example, the immunosuppressive effects of these drugs can result in the exacerbation of an infectious disease. Although the use of short-acting corticosteroids for the acute stabilization of such cases probably will not greatly interfere with appropriate antimicrobial therapy, long-acting agents and prolonged administration should be avoided. Glucocorticoid therapy potentially interferes with the results of future diagnostic tests, particularly if lymphoma is a differential diagnosis. Appropriate diagnostic tests are performed as soon as the animal can tolerate the stress.

Broad-spectrum antibiotics are administered if there is evidence of sepsis (e.g., fever, neutrophilic leukocytosis with left shift and moderate to marked toxicity of neutrophils) or a high degree of suspicion of bacterial or aspiration pneumo-

nia. Note that airway specimens (usually tracheal wash) should be obtained for culture if at all possible before initiating broad-spectrum antibiotics in order to confirm the diagnosis of bacterial infection and to obtain susceptibility data. Specimens obtained after initiating antibiotics are often not diagnostic, even with continued progression of signs. However, airway sampling may not be possible in these unstable patients. If sepsis is suspected, blood and urine cultures may be useful. The diagnosis and treatment of bacterial and aspiration pneumonia are described in Chapter 22.

If the dog or cat does not respond to this management, it may be necessary to administer a short-acting anesthetic agent to allow the animal to be intubated and positive-pressure ventilation to be instituted and maintained (see Chapter 27) until a diagnosis can be established and specific therapy initiated.

## PLEURAL SPACE DISEASE

Pleural space diseases cause respiratory distress by preventing normal lung expansion. They are similar mechanistically to restrictive lung disease. Animals presenting in respiratory distress as a result of pleural space disease typically have a markedly increased respiratory rate (see Table 26-2). Relatively increased inspiratory efforts may be noted but are not always obvious. Decreased lung sounds on auscultation distinguish patients with tachypnea caused by pleural space disease from patients with tachypnea caused by pulmonary parenchymal disease. Increased abdominal excursions during breathing may be noted.

Most patients in respiratory distress from pleural space disease have pleural effusion or pneumothorax (see Chapter 23). Other differential diagnoses are diaphragmatic hernia and mediastinal masses. If pleural effusion or pneumothorax is suspected to be causing respiratory distress, needle thoracocentesis (see p. 322) should be performed immediately before further diagnostic testing is performed or any drugs are administered. Oxygen can be provided by mask while the procedure is performed, but successful drainage of the pleural space will quickly improve the animal's condition. Occasionally, emergency placement of a chest tube is necessary to evacuate rapidly accumulating air (see p. 323).

As much fluid or air should be removed as possible. The exception is in animals with hemothorax. Hemothorax is usually the result of trauma or rodenticide intoxication. The respiratory distress associated with hemothorax is often the result of acute blood loss, rather than an inability to expand the lungs. In this situation, as little volume as is needed to stabilize the animal's condition is removed. The remainder will be reabsorbed (autotransfusion), to the benefit of the animal. Aggressive fluid therapy is indicated.

### Suggested Reading

Hansen BD: Analgesic therapy, *Comp Cont Educ Pract Vet* 16:868, 1994.

# CHAPTER 27

# Ancillary Therapy: Oxygen Supplementation and Ventilation

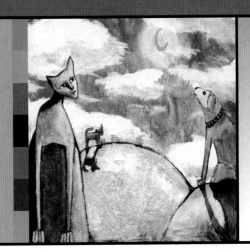

## CHAPTER OUTLINE

OXYGEN SUPPLEMENTATION, 337
    Oxygen masks, 337
    Oxygen hoods, 337
    Nasal catheters, 338
    Transtracheal catheters, 339
    Endotracheal tubes, 339
    Tracheal tubes, 339
    Oxygen cages, 340
VENTILATORY SUPPORT, 340

## OXYGEN SUPPLEMENTATION

Oxygen supplementation is generally indicated to maintain arterial blood oxygen pressures ($PaO_2$) at more than 60 mm Hg. Oxygen supplementation is indicated in every dog or cat with signs of respiratory distress or labored breathing. Cyanosis is another clear indication. Whenever possible, the cause of hypoxemia should be identified and specific treatment initiated as well. Assisted ventilation is indicated for animals with an inadequate arterial oxygen concentration despite supplementation and for animals with arterial carbon dioxide pressures exceeding 60 mm Hg (see p. 281).

The inhaled concentration of oxygen can be supplemented by the addition of 100% oxygen by mask, hood, nasal catheter, transtracheal catheter, endotracheal tube, tracheal tube, or oxygen cage. Administration of oxygen by nasal catheter is very well suited to most practices.

When administering 100% oxygen to an animal, consideration must be given to the anhydrous nature of pure oxygen and the toxic effects of oxygen in a high concentration. Because oxygen from tanks contains no water, drying of the airways can occur quickly, particularly if the nasal cavity has been completely bypassed by catheters or tubes. All animals with respiratory tract diseases should be systemically hydrated. Moisture must be added to the airways of animals receiving oxygen by catheter or tube for longer than a few hours. Ventilators designed for long-term use

have a heated humidifier incorporated into their design. Humidity exchange filters, which can also be attached to tracheal and endotracheal tubes, function by retaining moisture from exhaled air and adding it to inhaled air. These filters can support bacterial growth and must be replaced daily. Nebulization can also be used to add moisture to the airways. Less effective methods of hydration can be used if other options are not available, such as instillation of sterile 0.9% sodium chloride solution directly into tubes or catheters. Some water vapor can also be added to the oxygen by incorporating pass-over or bubble humidifiers in the system.

The inhalation of air with greater than 50% oxygen is toxic to the pulmonary epithelium. Pulmonary function deteriorates, and death can result. Air with greater than 50% oxygen is therefore not provided for longer than 12 hours. If higher concentrations are necessary to maintain adequate arterial oxygen concentrations, ventilatory support is initiated.

### OXYGEN MASKS

Oxygen masks are useful for short-term supplementation. The animal experiences minimal stress, and manipulations such as venous catheter placement and thoracocentesis can be performed. A snug fit is desirable to decrease the volume of dead space, and a relatively high flow rate is necessary (Table 27-1). A sterile eye ointment is applied to prevent desiccation of the corneas.

### OXYGEN HOODS

Oxygen hoods that can be placed over the animal's head are available. For some, the animals must be laterally recumbent and still, limiting the use of hoods to animals recovering from anesthesia, those that are severely depressed, and those that are heavily sedated (Fig. 27-1). Others have been fashioned that completely surround the animal's head and are attached around the neck. In some situations, oxygen hoods may be better tolerated than oxygen masks, and it may take less manpower to care for an animal in which one is being used than an animal with an oxygen mask. A means for escape of exhaled air must always be provided to prevent the buildup of $CO_2$ within the hood.

TABLE 27-1

Maximum Achievable Oxygen Concentrations and Associated Flow Rates for Various Methods of Supplementation

| METHOD OF ADMINISTRATION | MAXIMUM OXYGEN CONCENTRATION (%) | FLOW RATE (L/min)* |
|---|---|---|
| Mask | 50-60 | 8-12 |
| Nasal catheter | 50 | 6-8 |
| Transtracheal catheter | 30-40 | 1-2 |
| Endotracheal tube | 100 | 0.2 L/kg/min |
| Tracheal tube | 100 | 0.2 L/kg/min |
| Oxygen cage | 60 | 2-3* |

From Court MH et al: Inhalation therapy: oxygen administration, humidification, and aerosol therapy, *Vet Clin North Am Small Anim Pract* 15:1041, 1985.
*After cage is filled, flow is adjusted based on oxygen concentration as measured by oxygen sensor.

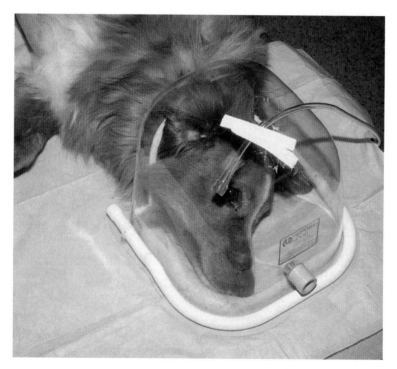

**FIG 27-1**
An oxygen hood can be used for recumbent animals as a substitute for an oxygen mask. In this patient, oxygen is being delivered through an opening in the top of the hood, and the light blue opening that will accommodate standard anesthesia tubing is left open for circulation of air. Regardless of the method used to increase the oxygen in inspired air, a means for escape of expired $CO_2$ is essential. (Courtesy Disposa-Hood, Utah Medical Products, Inc., Midvale, Utah.)

## NASAL CATHETERS

Nasal catheters can be used for long-term oxygen supplementation (Fig. 27-2). The animal is relatively free to move and is accessible for evaluation and treatment. Most animals tolerate the catheter well. Catheters can become obstructed with nasal secretions, however. Soft red rubber or infant feeding tubes or polyurethane catheters can be used. Tube size is based on patient size. In general, a 3.5 to 5 French tube is used for cats, and a 5 to 8 French tube is used for dogs.

The method of placement has been described by Fitzpatrick and colleague (1986). First, the length of tubing to be inserted into the nasal cavity is measured against the head of the animal. The tubing should reach the level of the carnassial tooth. Sedation is rarely necessary. A water-soluble lu-

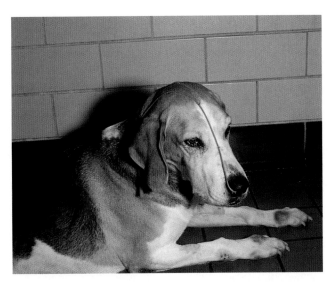

**FIG 27-2**
Dog with intranasal catheter in place for delivery of oxygen. The catheter is sutured to the muzzle less than 1 cm from its exit from the naris and is further anchored with sutures to the face so that it exits behind the animal's head. An Elizabethan collar is routinely used to prevent the animal from removing the catheter.

bricant or 0.2% lidocaine jelly is applied to the length of the catheter that will be within the nasal cavity. Next, 0.2% lidocaine is dripped gently into the nasal cavity through the naris with the animal's nose pointed upward. The catheter is then passed through the naris, initially aimed dorsomedially through the naris, then immediately ventromedially. Once the correct length of catheter has been inserted, it is gently bent beneath the lateral cartilage and sutured to the muzzle no farther than 1 cm caudal to the exit from the naris. The catheter can be further anchored to the face with sutures, traveling between the eyes to behind the animal's head. An Elizabethan collar is placed on the patient to prevent the animal from removing the catheter.

A sterile intravenous set can be connected to the catheter. The intravenous line can be attached to a half-filled bottle of sterile saline solution and positioned above the fluid level. Oxygen is then delivered through the bottle, below the fluid level, providing some moisture as the oxygen bubbles through the saline.

## TRANSTRACHEAL CATHETERS

Oxygen can be administered through a jugular catheter placed with a sterile technique through the trachea. This approach is particularly useful for the emergency stabilization of animals with an upper airway obstruction. Branditz and colleagues (1989) have described a method for cardiopulmonary resuscitation that can be performed by one person by administering oxygen at a high flow rate of 15 L/min through a tracheal catheter. In this method a large jugular catheter is placed as described for transtracheal washing (see p. 264).

## ENDOTRACHEAL TUBES

Endotracheal tubes are used to administer oxygen during surgical procedures and cardiopulmonary resuscitation. They can be used to bypass most upper airway obstructions for emergency stabilization. Pure oxygen can be administered for short periods. Longer supplementation requires the mixing of 100% oxygen with room air. Ventilation can be provided with a cuffed endotracheal tube. Trauma to the trachea is decreased through the use of high-volume, low-pressure cuffs and by inflating the cuff with the least pressure necessary to create a seal. If positive-pressure ventilation is not being used, the cuff can remain deflated.

Endotracheal tubes are not tolerated by alert animals, and for this reason tracheal tubes are preferred for long-term management. Conscious animals in which endotracheal tubes are used must be given sedatives, analgesics, paralyzing agents, or a combination of these drugs. The combination of hydromorphone and diazepam is adequate in some animals. Pentobarbital, administered intravenously to effect, can be added if necessary. The combination of ketamine and valium may be safer for the initial intubation of patients that are hypoxemic. Following intubation and improvement in hypoxemia, morphine and pancuronium can be given.

The cuff should be deflated when possible to minimize tracheal damage. The tube must be cleaned periodically to remove secretions (see recommendations for tracheal tube cleaning), and frequent flushing of the oral cavity is performed. Moisture must be added to the inspired gases, as previously discussed.

## TRACHEAL TUBES

Tracheal tubes are placed through the tracheal rings and are readily tolerated by conscious animals. It is rare that an animal requires an emergency tracheostomy. Nearly all such animals can be stabilized using other techniques. Thus tracheal tubes can be placed using a careful, sterile surgical technique. Tracheal tubes are generally used for the management of animals with an upper airway obstruction. Room air often contains adequate oxygen for use in animals with an upper airway obstruction once the obstruction has been bypassed.

The tube itself should have a diameter nearly as wide as the tracheal lumen and a length of five to 10 rings. It is necessary to use high-volume, low-pressure cuffs to prevent tracheal damage and subsequent stricture. Double-lumen tubes are ideal for this method. The inner tube can be removed for cleaning and replaced easily. Single-lumen tubes can also work and may be necessary in small animals.

Tracheal tubes are usually placed with the animal anesthetized with a short-acting agent. The trachea is exposed through a ventral midline incision made just beneath the larynx. The trachea is entered through an incision made a few rings below the cricoid cartilage, parallel to the trachea and perpendicular to the rings, and through just enough rings to allow passage of the tube. Either end of the incision can be widened with a small transverse incision. Stay sutures are placed on each side of the incision to facilitate placement of the tube initially, as well as replacement later if the tube is accidentally or intentionally removed. The tube is then inserted into the opening. With minimal pressure on the airway, it is tied with gauze around the neck of the animal. Few or no sutures are used to close the incision to prevent the collection of air subcutaneously. A gauze sponge with a slit cut in it and coated with antiseptic ointment can be placed over the incision and around the tube.

The tube must be monitored for obstruction and cleaned. The inner tube of double-lumen tubes can be easily removed for this purpose. The tube is cleaned every 30 to 60 minutes initially, with the interval increased as less secretions accumulate. A sterile technique is used when handling the tubes, and they must be replaced if they become contaminated.

Single-lumen tubes are difficult to remove and replace safely for the first few days unless stay sutures are left in place. Periodic cleaning can be performed with the tube in place. Sterile saline solution is instilled into the tube for this purpose. To perform suctioning, a sterile urinary catheter with several openings at the end is attached to a suction unit and passed through the tube. The trachea and tracheal tube are then suctioned to remove secretions. Suctioning is performed for short intervals to allow the lungs to reinflate. It is performed every few hours initially, then less frequently if secretions are not accumulating.

A smaller tube can be used once the animal is able to oxygenate adequately with room air. The tube can be removed when the animal can oxygenate by breathing around a small tube with the lumen obstructed. The incision is allowed to heal without suturing. The tip of the tube is cultured for bacteria.

Antibiotics are not administered prophylactically. An existing infection or infections that occur during therapy are treated on the basis of culture and sensitivity information.

## OXYGEN CAGES

Oxygen cages can provide an oxygen-enriched environment with minimal stress to animals. However, the animal is isolated from direct contact, which can be a disadvantage. Other environmental factors, such as humidity, temperature, and carbon dioxide concentration, must be monitored and controlled, or extreme stress and even death can occur. The animal is totally dependent on proper cage function. The ability of the cage to maintain the correct environment varies with the specific cage, as well as with each animal. Commercial cages are available for veterinary use. Incubators from human hospitals can be modified for small animals.

## *VENTILATORY SUPPORT*

The purposes of ventilatory support are to decrease the retention of carbon dioxide and to improve oxygenation. Ventilatory support is labor intensive and associated with complications, however. It is used when other means of respiratory support are not adequate.

The retention of carbon dioxide, or hypercapnia, occurs in animals that are unable to ventilate adequately. Spontaneous ventilation can be impaired by neurologic dysfunction, such as that which occurs in the settings of severe head trauma, polyneuropathies, and some toxicities. Ventilatory support is recommended in such animals if the $PaCO_2$ increases to more than 60 mm Hg. Hypoventilation caused by a pleural effusion or pneumothorax is treated by removing the fluid or air, not by positive-pressure ventilation. Hypoventilation caused by an upper airway obstruction is treated by establishing a patent airway.

Animals with cerebral edema, usually caused by trauma, may benefit from ventilatory support to maintain the $PaCO_2$ within 20 to 30 mm Hg. The resultant decrease in blood flow to the brain may decrease the total intracranial volume, thereby decreasing pressure on the brain.

Animals with severe lung disease may be unable to maintain adequate oxygenation without ventilatory support. Positive-pressure ventilation is routinely necessary for the management of patients with acute respiratory distress syndrome (ARDS) (p. 312). As previously noted, the long-term administration of air with an oxygen concentration greater than 50% results in serious lung damage. If the $PaO_2$ cannot be maintained at greater than 60 mm Hg without excessive oxygen supplementation, ventilatory support is indicated.

A form of positive-pressure ventilation is commonly used. The delivery of air by positive pressure is different from the normal inhalation of air by negative pressure. With positive pressure, the distribution of ventilation within the lungs is altered. The intrathoracic pressure increases each time the lungs are filled with air, which results in decreased venous return to the heart. Along with other effects, systemic hypotension results and can be severe enough to cause acute renal failure. Compliance of the lungs also decreases over time in animals receiving positive-pressure ventilation. As the lungs become stiffer, greater pressures are necessary to expand them. Careful monitoring of animals is essential during ventilation. Important variables to monitor include blood gas values, compliance, mucous membrane color, capillary refill time, pulse quality, arterial blood pressure, central venous pressure, lung sounds, and urine output. The extensive nursing care and monitoring required for these patients limits the use of long-term ventilatory support to large referral hospitals.

## *Suggested Readings*

Branditz FK et al: Continuous transtracheal oxygen delivery during cardiopulmonary resuscitation: an alternative method of ventilation in a canine model, *Chest* 95:441, 1989.

Court MH et al: Inhalation therapy: oxygen administration, humidification, and aerosol therapy, *Vet Clin North Am Small Anim Pract* 15:1041, 1985.

Fitzpatrick RK et al: Nasal oxygen administration in dogs and cats: experimental and clinical investigations, *J Am Anim Hosp Assoc* 22:293, 1986.

McKiernan BC: Principles of respiratory therapy. In Kirk RW, editor: *Current veterinary therapy VIII*, Philadelphia, 1983, WB Saunders, p 216.

Moon PF et al: Mechanical ventilation. In Kirk RW et al, editors: *Current veterinary therapy XI*, Philadelphia, 1992, WB Saunders, p 98.

## Drugs Used in Respiratory Disorders

| GENERIC NAME | TRADE NAME | DOGS (mg/kg*) | CATS (mg/kg*) |
|---|---|---|---|
| Acepromazine | — | 0.05 IV, IM, SQ (maximum, 4 mg) | 0.05 IV, IM, SQ (maximum, 1 mg) |
| Amikacin | Amiglyde | 5-10 IV, SQ q8h | Same |
| Aminophylline | — | 11 PO, IV, IM q8h | 5 PO, IV, IM q12h |
| Amoxicillin | Amoxi-tab, Amoxi-drop | 22 PO q8-12h | Same |
| Amoxicillin-clavulanate | Clavamox | 20-25 PO q8h | Same |
| Ampicillin | — | 22 PO, IV, SQ q8h | Same |
| Ampicillin-sulbactam | Unasyn | 50 mg/kg (combined) IV q8h | Same |
| Atropine | — | 0.05 SQ | Same |
| Azithromycin | Zithromax | 5-10 mg/kg PO q24h for 3 days, then q48-72h | 5-10 mg/kg PO q24h for 3 days, then q72h |
| Butorphanol | Torbutrol | 0.5 PO q6-12h (antitussive) | Not recommended |
| Cefazolin | — | 20-25 IM, IV q8h | Same |
| Cephalexin | Keflex | 20-40 PO q8h | Same |
| Chloramphenicol | — | 50 PO, IV, SQ q8h | 10-15 PO, IV, SQ q12h |
| Chlorpheniramine | Chlor-Trimeton | 4-8 mg/dog q8-12h | 2 mg/cat q8-12h |
| Clindamycin | Antirobe | 5.5-11 PO, IV, SQ q12h | Same |
| Cyclophosphamide | Cytoxan | 50 mg/m² PO q48h | Same |
| Cyproheptadine | Periactin | — | 2 mg/cat PO q12h |
| Dexamethasone | Azium | 0.1-0.2 IV q12h | Same |
| Dextromethorphan | — | 1-2 PO q6-8h | Not recommended |
| Diazepam | Valium | 0.2-0.5 IV | — |
| Diphenhydramine | Benadryl | 1 IM; 2-4 PO | Same |
| Doxycycline | — | 5-10 PO, IV q12h | Same |
| Enrofloxacin | Baytril | 10-20 PO, IV, SQ q24h | — |
| Fenbendazole (for lung worms) | Panacur | 25-50 mg/kg PO q12h for 14 days | Same |
| Furosemide | Lasix | 2 PO, IV, IM q8-12h | Same |
| Glycopyrrolate | — | 0.005 IV, SQ | Same |
| Heparin | — | 200-300 U/kg SQ q8h | Same |
| Hydrocodone bitartrate | Hycodan | 0.25 PO q8-12h | Not recommended |
| Hydromorphone | — | 0.05 IV, IM; can repeat IV q3min to effect; duration 2-4h | 0.025-0.05 IV, IM; can repeat IV q3min to effect; stop if mydriasis occurs |
| Imipenem-cilastin | Primaxin | 3-10 IV, q6-8h | Same |
| Itraconazole (for aspergillosis) | Sporanox | 5 PO q12h with food | — |
| Ivermectin | — | See text for specific parasites | See text for specific parasites |
| Ketamine | Ketaset, Vetalar | — | 2-5 IV |
| Lysine | — | — | 250 mg/cat PO q12h |
| Marbofloxacin | Zeniquin | 3-5.5 PO q24h | Same |
| Methylprednisolone acetate | Depo-Medrol | — | 10 mg/cat IM q2-4wk |
| Metronidazole | Flagyl | 10 PO q8h | 10 PO q12h |
| Milbemycin (for nasal mites) | Interceptor | 0.5-1 PO q7-10d for 3 treatments | — |
| Morphine | — | 0.1 IV; repeat q3min to effect; duration 1-4h | — |
| Oxtriphylline | Choledyl | 14 PO q8h | — |
| Oxymetazoline 0.025% | Afrin (0.025%) | — | 1 drop/nostril q24h for 3 days, then withhold for 3 days |
| Phenylephrine 0.25% | Neo-Synephrine (0.25%) | — | 1 drop/nostril q24h for 3 days, then withhold for 3 days |
| Praziquantel (for *Paragonimus*) | Droncit | 23 PO q8h for 3 days | Same |

*Unless otherwise noted.

*Continued*

Drugs Used in Respiratory Disorders—cont'd

| GENERIC NAME | TRADE NAME | DOGS (mg/kg*) | CATS (mg/kg*) |
|---|---|---|---|
| Prednisone | — | 0.25-2 PO q12h | Same |
| Prednisolone sodium succinate | Solu-Delta-Cortef | 10-20 IV | Same |
| Terbutaline | Brethine | 1.25-5 mg/dog PO q8-12h | ⅛-¼ of 2.5-mg tablet/cat q12h PO to start; 0.01 mg/kg SQ, repeat once in 5-10 min if necessary |
| Tetracycline | — | 22 PO q8h | Same |
| Tetracycline ophthalmic ointment | — | — | q4-8h |
| Theophylline (long-acting formulations)† | — | 10 PO q12h‡ | 25 PO q24h in evening |
| Trimethoprim-sulfadiazine | Tribrissen | 15-30 PO q12h | Same |
| Vitamin K₁ | Mephyton, Aquamephyton | 2-5 PO, SQ divided daily | Same |
| Warfarin | Coumadin | 0.1-0.2 PO q24h | 0.5 mg/cat |

From Bach JF et al: *Proceedings of the 20th Symposium of the Veterinary Comparative Respiratory Society,* Boston, 2002.

*Unless otherwise noted.

†Due to differences in available products, appropriate dosages are uncertain and therapeutic monitoring of animals should be performed (see p. 293).

‡Dog dosage is for theophylline SR (Inwood Laboratories, Inwood, N.Y.).

# CHAPTER 28

# Clinical Manifestations of Gastrointestinal Disorders

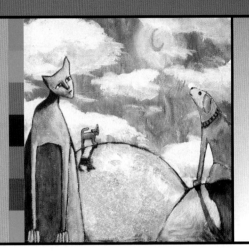

## CHAPTER OUTLINE

DYSPHAGIA, HALITOSIS, AND DROOLING, 343
DISTINGUISHING REGURGITATION FROM
VOMITING, 345
REGURGITATION, 346
VOMITING, 347
HEMATEMESIS, 351
DIARRHEA, 352
HEMATOCHEZIA, 355
MELENA, 356
TENESMUS, 356
CONSTIPATION, 357
FECAL INCONTINENCE, 358
WEIGHT LOSS, 358
ANOREXIA, 360
ABDOMINAL EFFUSION, 360
ACUTE ABDOMEN, 361
ABDOMINAL PAIN, 362
ABDOMINAL DISTENTION OR ENLARGEMENT, 363

## DYSPHAGIA, HALITOSIS, AND DROOLING

Dysphagia, halitosis, and drooling may coexist in many animals with oral disease. Dysphagia (i.e., difficulty in eating) usually results from oral pain, masses, foreign objects, trauma, neuromuscular dysfunction, or a combination of these (Table 28-1). Halitosis typically signifies an abnormal bacterial proliferation secondary to tissue necrosis, tartar, periodontitis, or the oral or esophageal retention of food (Table 28-2). Drooling occurs because animals are unable to or are in too much pain to swallow (i.e., pseudoptyalism); rarely animals produce excessive saliva (Table 28-3). Although any disease causing dysphagia may have an acute onset, one should usually first consider foreign objects or trauma as the cause in such an animal. The environment and vaccination history should also be assessed to determine whether rabies is a possibility.

The next step is a thorough oral, laryngeal, and cranial examination. This examination is often the most important diagnostic step, because most problems producing oral pain can be partially or completely defined on the basis of physical examination findings. Although this is ideally done without chemical restraint to allow pain to be detected, often the animal must be anesthetized for the oral examination to be performed adequately. A search for anatomic abnormalities, inflammatory lesions, pain, and discomfort should always be made. If pain is found, determine whether it occurs when the mouth is opened (e.g., retrobulbar inflammation), is associated with extraoral structures (e.g., muscles of mastication), or originates from the oral cavity. A search should also be made for fractures, lacerations, crepitus, masses, enlarged lymph nodes, inflamed or ulcerated areas, draining tracts, loose teeth, excessive temporal muscle atrophy, inability to open the mouth while the animal is under anesthesia, and ocular problems (e.g., proptosis of the eye, inflammation, or strabismus suggestive of retrobulbar disease). If oral pain is apparent but cannot be localized, retrobulbar lesions, temporomandibular joint disease, and posterior pharyngeal lesions should be considered. A concurrent clinicopathologic evaluation may be useful, especially if oral examination findings indicate the presence of systemic disease (e.g., lingual necrosis resulting from uremia, chronic infection secondary to hyperadrenocorticism).

Biopsies should be done of *mucosal lesions* (e.g., masses, inflamed or ulcerated areas) and *painful muscles* of mastication. Masses that do not disrupt the mucosa, especially those on the midline and dorsal to the larynx, can be difficult to discern and are sometimes only found by careful palpation. Fine-needle aspiration and cytologic evaluation are reasonable first steps for the diagnosis of masses. Fine-needle aspirates can only find disease; they cannot exclude disease. Subtle masses or those dorsal to the larynx may sometimes be aspirated more accurately with ultrasonographic guidance.

TABLE 28-1

## Causes of Dysphagia

### Oral Pain

Fractured bones or teeth
Trauma
Periodontitis or caries (especially cats)
Osteomyelitis
Other causes
  Retrobulbar abscess/inflammation
  Various other abscesses or granulomas of the oral cavity
  Temporal-masseter myositis
Stomatitis, glossitis, pharyngitis, gingivitis, tonsillitis, or sialoadenitis
  Immune-mediated disease
  Feline viral rhinotracheitis, calicivirus, leukemia virus, or immunodeficiency virus
  Lingual foreign objects, other foreign objects, or granulomas
  Tooth root abscess
  Uremia
  Miscellaneous causes
    Thallium
    Caustics
Pain associated with swallowing: esophageal stricture or esophagitis

### Oral Mass

Tumor (malignant or benign)
Eosinophilic granuloma
Foreign object (oral, pharyngeal, or laryngeal)
Sialocele

### Oral Trauma

Fractured bones
Soft tissue laceration
Hematoma

### Neuromuscular Disease

Oral, pharyngeal, or cricopharyngeal dysfunction
Various cranial nerve dysfunctions
Rabies
Tetanus
Localized myasthenia
Temporal-masseter myositis
Temporomandibular joint disease

TABLE 28-2

## Causes of Halitosis

### Bacterial Causes

Food retained in the mouth
  Anatomic defect allowing retention (exposed tooth roots, tumor, large ulcer)
  Neuromuscular defect allowing retention (pharyngeal dysphagia)
Food retained in the esophagus
Tartar or periodontitis
Damaged oral tissue
  Neoplasia/granuloma of mouth or esophagus
  Severe stomatitis/glossitis

### Eating Noxious Substances

Necrotic or odoriferous food
Feces

TABLE 28-3

## Major Causes of Drooling

### Ptyalism

Nausea
Hepatic encephalopathy (especially feline)
Seizure activity
Chemical or toxic stimulation of salivation (organophosphates, caustics, bitter drugs [e.g., atropine])
Behavior
Hyperthermia
Salivary gland hypersecretion

### Pseudoptyalism

Oral pain, especially stomatitis, glossitis, gingivitis, pharyngitis, tonsillitis, or sialoadenitis (see Table 28-1)
Oral or pharyngeal dysphagia (see Table 28-1)
Facial nerve paralysis

Multiple aspirations are usually done before a wedge or punch biopsy is done.

Incisional biopsy specimens must include generous amounts of submucosal tissues. Many oral tumors cannot be diagnosed on the basis of findings from superficial biopsy specimens because of superficial necrosis and inflammation caused by normal oral flora. Biopsies of these lesions are often not done aggressively because they bleed profusely and are hard to suture. Avoid major vessels (e.g., the palatine artery), and use silver nitrate to stop hemorrhage. It is better to have difficulty stopping hemorrhage after obtaining an adequate biopsy specimen than less difficulty stopping hemorrhage after obtaining a nondiagnostic specimen. If diffuse oral mucosal lesions are noted, search carefully for vesicles (e.g., pemphigus), and if these are found, remove them intact for histopathologic and immunofluorescent studies. If vesicles are not found, then at least two or three tissue samples representing a spectrum of new and old lesions should be submitted for analysis.

If oral examination findings are not helpful, plain oral and laryngeal radiographs are usually the best next steps. Oral cultures are rarely cost-effective, however, because the normal oral flora makes interpretation of the results difficult. Even animals with severe halitosis or stomatitis secondary to bacterial infection rarely benefit from bacterial culture, unless there is a draining tract or abscess.

*Halitosis* often accompanies dysphagia, in which case it is usually more productive to determine the cause of the dysphagia. If halitosis occurs without dysphagia, first be sure that the odor is abnormal and also check for the ingestion of odoriferous substances (e.g., feces). A thorough oral examination is still the most important test. Halitosis not attributable to an oropharyngeal lesion may be originating from the esophagus. Contrast-enhanced radiographs or esophagoscopy is a reasonable diagnostic alternative and may reveal the presence of tumors or retained food secondary to stricture or weakness. If the history and oral examination are unrevealing except for the finding of mild-to-moderate tartar accumulation, the teeth should be cleaned to try to alleviate the problem.

*Drooling* is usually caused by nausea, oral pain, or dysphagia. The approach to the diagnosis of oral pain and dysphagia is described under the appropriate headings. Nausea is considered under the heading of Vomiting.

Dysphagic animals without demonstrable lesions or pain may have neuromuscular disease. *Dysphagia of muscular origin* usually results from atrophic myositis (see p. 1062). Finding swollen, painful temporal muscles suggests acute myositis. The combination of severe temporal-masseter muscle atrophy and difficulty opening the mouth (even when the animal is anesthetized) is suggestive of chronic temporal-masseter myositis. Biopsy of affected muscles is indicated, but be sure that muscle tissue is retrieved; it is easy to obtain only fibrous scar tissue. It may help to have serum analyzed for antibodies to type 2M muscle fibers, a finding consistent with masticatory muscle myositis but not polymyopathy.

*Neurogenic dysphagia* is caused by disorders in the oral (i.e., also called *prehensile*), pharyngeal, or cricopharyngeal phases of swallowing (disorders of the latter two phases are discussed under Regurgitation). Rabies should always be considered, despite its relative rarity. After rabies is presumptively ruled out, cranial nerve deficits (especially deficits of cranial nerves V, VII, IX, XII) should be considered. Because the clinical signs vary depending on the nerve, or nerves, affected, a careful neurologic examination must be done.

Inability to pick up food or having food drop from the mouth while eating usually indicates a prehensile disorder. Dysphagia may be noticeable in dogs and cats with pharyngeal and cricopharyngeal dysfunction, but regurgitation is often more prominent. Dynamic contrast-enhanced radiographic studies (e.g., cinefluoroscopy or fluoroscopy) are best for detecting and defining neuromuscular dysphagia. If neuromuscular problems are seemingly ruled out by these radiographic studies, then anatomic lesions and occult causes of pain (e.g., soft tissue inflammation or infection) must be reconsidered.

## DISTINGUISHING REGURGITATION FROM VOMITING

Regurgitation is the expulsion of material (i.e., food, water, saliva) from the mouth, pharynx, or esophagus. It must be differentiated from vomiting (the expulsion of material from

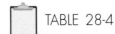 TABLE 28-4

**Aids to Differentiate Regurgitation from Vomiting***

| SIGN | REGURGITATION | VOMITING |
|---|---|---|
| Prodromal nausea† | No | Usually |
| Retching‡ | No | Usually |
| Material produced | | |
|   Food | ± | ± |
|   Bile | No | ± |
|   Blood | ± (undigested) | ± (digested or undigested) |
| Amount of material | Any amount | Any amount |
| Time relative to | | |
|   eating | Anytime | Anytime |
| Distention of cervi- | ± | No |
|   cal esophagus | | |
| Dipstick analysis | | |
|   of material | | |
|   pH | ≥7 | ≤5 or ≥8 |
|   Bile | No | ± |

*These are *guidelines* that often help distinguish vomiting from regurgitation. However, occasional animals will require plain and/or contrast-enhanced radiographs to distinguish between the two.
†May include salivation, licking lips, pacing, and an anxious expression. The owner may simply state that the animal is aware that it will soon "vomit."
‡These are usually forceful, vigorous abdominal contractions or dry heaves. This is not to be confused with gagging.

the stomach and/or intestines) and expectoration (the expulsion of material from the respiratory tract). Historical and physical examination findings sometimes allow these three to be differentiated (Table 28-4). Expectoration is generally associated with coughing at the time of the event. Animals that regurgitate and occasionally those that vomit may cough as a result of aspiration, but oral expulsion is not consistently correlated with coughing.

The criteria in Table 28-4 are only guidelines. Some animals that appear to be regurgitating are vomiting and vice versa. If one cannot distinguish between the two on the basis of the history and physical examination findings, one may use a urine dipstick to determine the pH and whether there is bilirubin in freshly "vomited" material. If the pH is less than 5, the material has originated from the stomach and probably resulted from vomiting. If the pH is more than 7 and there is no evidence of bilirubin, this is consistent with regurgitation. The presence of bilirubin indicates the material has originated from the duodenum (i.e., vomiting). A positive finding of blood in the urine dipstick test is not useful.

If vomiting and regurgitation still cannot be distinguished, plain and/or contrast-enhanced radiographs will usually detect any existing esophageal dysfunction. However, some esophageal disorders (e.g., hiatal hernia, partial stricture) are easily missed unless a careful radiographic technique is used.

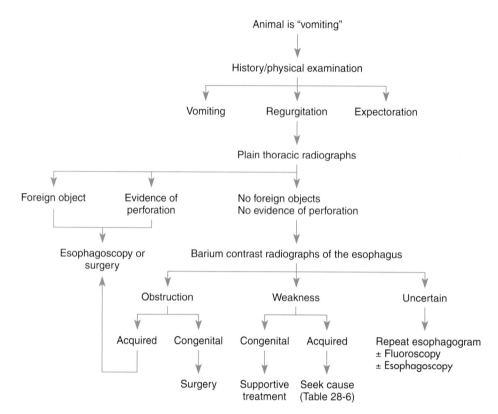

**FIG 28-1**
General diagnostic approach to regurgitation in the dog and cat.

## *REGURGITATION*

Once regurgitation is confirmed, the disease should be localized to the oral cavity, pharynx, or esophagus (Fig. 28-1). The history and observations of the pet eating should detect the signs of dysphagia (e.g., undue stretching or flexing of the neck during swallowing, repeated efforts at swallowing, food falling from the mouth during swallowing). Some animals with dysphagia associated with neuromuscular disorders have more difficulty swallowing liquids than solid foods, probably because it is easier to aspirate liquids. Attempts to swallow water may often produce coughing in these animals.

If a regurgitating animal is *dysphagic,* oral, pharyngeal, and cricopharyngeal dysfunctions should be considered; the latter two mimic each other. Cinefluoroscopic or fluoroscopic evaluation of swallowing during a barium meal is necessary to differentiate pharyngeal from cricopharyngeal dysfunction. If they are not accurately differentiated, inappropriate or detrimental therapy may be administered.

If the regurgitating animal is *not dysphagic,* esophageal dysfunction is tentatively diagnosed. The two main reasons for esophageal regurgitation are obstruction and muscular weakness. Plain and barium contrast–enhanced esophageal radiographs are the best tools for initially defining these problems. Although fluoroscopy is desirable, it is absolutely necessary in only a few animals with a partial loss of peristalsis,

segmental aperistalsis, gastroesophageal reflux, or sliding hiatal hernias. If the animal seems to be regurgitating but the contrast-enhanced radiographs fail to reveal esophageal dysfunction, either the assessment of regurgitation is wrong or there is occult disease (e.g., partial stricture of the esophagus, esophagitis, gastroesophageal reflux). Procedures involving the use of liquid barium sulfate may miss some lesions (e.g., partial strictures). Repeating contrast-enhanced esophagography using barium plus food or performing esophagoscopy is then recommended.

An *esophageal obstruction* is principally caused by foreign objects and vascular anomalies, although cicatrix, tumors, and achalasia of the lower esophageal sphincter may also be responsible (Table 28-5). Obstruction should be characterized as congenital or acquired and as intraluminal, intramural, or extraesophageal. Congenital obstructions are usually extraesophageal vascular ring anomalies. Acquired intraluminal obstructions are usually caused by foreign objects. However, always determine whether animals with esophageal foreign objects also have a partial esophageal stricture that has predisposed them to the obstruction. Endoscopy may be both diagnostic and therapeutic in these animals; thoracotomy is seldom needed for the management of cicatrix or intraluminal foreign objects.

*Esophageal weakness* may be congenital or acquired. *Congenital weakness* is of uncertain neurologic origin and should

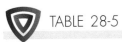

TABLE 28-5

### Causes of Esophageal Obstruction

**Congenital Causes**

Vascular ring anomaly
    Persistent fourth right aortic arch
    Other disorders

**Acquired Causes**

Foreign object
Cicatrix/stricture
Neoplasia
    Esophageal causes
        Carcinoma
        Sarcoma caused by *Spirocerca lupi*
        Leiomyoma of lower esophageal sphincter
    Extraesophageal cause
        Thyroid carcinoma
        Pulmonary carcinoma
Achalasia of the lower esophageal sphincter (rare)
Gastroesophageal intussusception (rare)

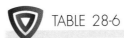

TABLE 28-6

### Causes of Esophageal Weakness

**Congenital Causes**

Idiopathic

**Acquired Causes**

Myasthenia (generalized or localized)
Hypoadrenocorticism
Esophagitis
    Persistent vomiting
    Hiatal hernia
    Gastroesophageal reflux
    Caustic ingestion
*Spirocerca lupi*
Myopathies/neuropathies
    Hypothyroidism (rare)
    Systemic lupus erythematosus
    Others
Miscellaneous causes
    Lead poisoning
    Chagas' disease
    Canine distemper
    Dermatomyositis (principally in Collies)
    Dysautonomia
Idiopathic

not be pursued diagnostically. *Acquired esophageal weakness* usually results from an underlying neuromuscular problem. Although an underlying cause is infrequently diagnosed, finding one potentially allows a permanent cure to be achieved, instead of supportive therapy being implemented that only treats symptoms. A complete blood count (CBC), serum biochemistry profile, urinalysis, determination of serum antibody titers to acetylcholine receptors, measurement of serum free thyroxine ($fT_4$) and endogenous canine thyroid-stimulating hormone (cTSH) concentrations, an adrenocorticotropic hormone (ACTH)–stimulation test, fecal examination for *Spirocerca lupi* ova, and determination of serum antinuclear antibody titers are performed to look for causes of acquired esophageal weakness (Table 28-6). One may also consider searching for lead intoxication (nucleated red blood cells and basophilic stippling in the CBC, serum and urine lead concentrations), canine distemper (retinal lesions), Chagas' disease (serum antibody titer), and neuropathy-myopathy (electromyography, nerve biopsy, muscle biopsy).

Esophagoscopy may detect esophagitis or small lesions (e.g., partial strictures) that contrast-enhanced esophagrams do not reveal. If esophagitis is found, look carefully for a hiatal hernia (sometimes only detected by chance on a plain or contrast-enhanced radiograph because some slide in and out of the thorax). After entering the stomach, retroflex the tip of the endoscope and examine the lower esophageal sphincter for leiomyomas. Gastroduodenoscopy is performed concurrently to look for gastric and duodenal reasons for gastroesophageal reflux or vomiting. If fluoroscopy is available, watch the lower esophageal sphincter for several minutes to note the frequency and severity of gastroesophageal reflux (normal animals will rarely show reflux).

## VOMITING

Vomiting is usually caused by (1) motion sickness, (2) the ingestion of emetogenic substances (e.g., drugs), (3) gastrointestinal tract obstruction, (4) abdominal (especially alimentary tract) inflammation or irritation, and (5) extragastrointestinal tract diseases that may stimulate the vagus nerve or the chemoreceptor trigger zone (Table 28-7). Occasionally, central nervous system (CNS) disease, behavior, and learned reactions to specific stimuli may cause vomiting. If the cause of the vomiting is not apparent from the history and physical examination findings, the next step depends on whether the vomiting is acute or chronic and whether there is hematemesis (Figs. 28-2 and 28-3). Remember that blood in vomitus may be fresh (i.e., red) or partially digested (i.e., "coffee grounds" or "dregs").

In animals with *acute vomiting without hematemesis*, first search for obvious causes (e.g., ingestion of a foreign body, intoxication, organ failure, parvovirus) as well as for fluid, electrolyte, or acid-base abnormalities or sepsis that require prompt, specific therapy. If the animal's condition seems

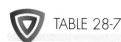

TABLE 28-7

Causes of Vomiting

| | |
|---|---|
| **Motion Sickness (Acute)** | **Gastrointestinal/Abdominal Inflammation (Acute or Chronic)** |
| **Emetogenic Substances (Acute)** | Inflammatory bowel disease (usually chronic) |
| Drugs: almost any drug can cause vomiting (especially drugs administered orally [PO]), but the following drugs most often seem to cause vomiting: | Gastritis with or without ulceration/erosion (acute or chronic) |
| Digoxin | Enteritis (acute) |
| Cyclophosphamide | Parvovirus |
| Cisplatin | Hemorrhagic gastroenteritis |
| Dacarbazine | Parasites (acute or chronic), especially *Physaloptera* |
| Adriamycin | Colitis (acute or chronic) |
| Erythromycin | |
| Tetracycline/doxycycline | **Extraalimentary Tract Diseases (Acute or Chronic)** |
| Amoxicillin + clavulanic acid | Uremia |
| Nonsteroidal antiinflammatory drugs | Adrenal insufficiency |
| Toxic chemicals | Hypercalcemia |
| | Hepatic insufficiency or disease |
| **Gastrointestinal Tract Obstruction (Acute or Chronic)** | Cholecystitis |
| Gastric outflow obstruction | Diabetic ketoacidosis |
| Benign pyloric stenosis | Pyometra |
| Foreign object | Peritonitis (acute or chronic) |
| Gastric antral mucosal hypertrophy | Pancreatitis (acute or chronic) |
| Neoplasia | |
| Nonneoplastic infiltrative disease (e.g., pythiosis) | **Miscellaneous Causes (Acute or Chronic)** |
| Gastric malpositioning | Dysautonomia |
| Gastric dilatation or volvulus (primarily see nonproductive retching) | Feline hyperthyroidism |
| Partial gastric dilatation/volvulus | Feline heartworm disease (?) |
| Intestinal | Postoperative nausea |
| Foreign object | Overeating |
| Nonlinear objects | Idiopathic hypomotility |
| Linear objects | Central nervous system disease |
| Neoplasia | Limbic epilepsy |
| Cicatrix | Tumor |
| Torsion/volvulus | Meningitis |
| Intussusception | Increased intracranial pressure |
| | Sialoadenitis/sialoadenosis |
| | Behavior |

stable and there is no obvious cause, then symptomatic treatment is often used for 1 to 3 days. If the animal is too sick for the clinician to take a chance on guessing wrong, or if the vomiting persists for 2 to 4 days after the start of symptomatic therapy, then more aggressive diagnostic testing is usually indicated.

Search for historical evidence of the ingestion of foreign objects, toxins, inappropriate food, or drugs. Physical examination is used to look for abdominal abnormalities (e.g., masses), linear foreign objects caught under the tongue, and evidence of extraabdominal disease (e.g., uremia, hyperthyroidism). Always consider the possibility of linear foreign bodies in vomiting cats, and carefully examine the base of the tongue. Chemical restraint of the animal (e.g., ketamine HCl, 2.2 mg/kg of body weight given intra-

venously) may be necessary to examine this area properly. The abdomen is palpated to search for masses or pain, but even careful palpation may miss intussusceptions in the craniodorsal area of the abdomen. It is reasonable to perform fecal examination for parasites, because they can be the cause of vomiting. If a cause cannot be found and the animal is not unduly ill, one may prescribe a therapeutic trial (e.g., pyrantel and a dietary trial; see pp. 389 and 402). Therapeutic trials must be designed so that the failure of a treatment allows the clinician to exclude at least one disease and then look for others.

If acute vomiting does not respond to symptomatic therapy or if the animal is so sick that one cannot take a chance on symptomatic therapy being ineffective, diagnostic tests are indicated. Animals with *acute or chronic vomiting without*

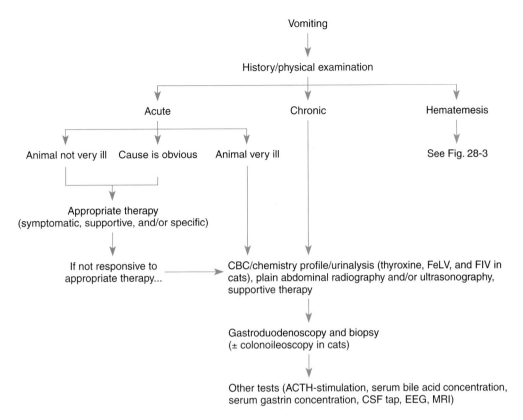

**FIG 28-2**
General diagnostic approach to vomiting in the dog and cat. *CBC,* Complete blood count;
*FeLV,* feline leukemia virus; *FIV,* feline immunodeficiency virus; *CSF,* cerebrospinal fluid;
*EEG,* electroencephalogram; *MRI,* magnetic resonance imaging.

*hematemesis* should undergo plain abdominal radiography or ultrasonography to look for problems such as an intestinal obstruction, foreign objects, masses, pancreatitis, peritonitis, poor serosal contrast in the region of the pancreas, free abdominal fluid, or free abdominal gas. Abdominal ultrasonography can be more revealing than plain radiographs. A CBC, serum biochemistry profile, and urinalysis are also indicated. In cats, one should test for feline leukemia virus, feline immunodeficiency virus, hyperthyroidism, and heartworm infection. It may be necessary to measure serum bile acid concentrations or perform an ACTH-stimulation test to identify hepatic or adrenal insufficiency, which may not be indicated by results of routine serum biochemistry profiles (i.e., normal hepatic enzyme activities and serum electrolyte concentrations).

If results of the CBC, chemistry profile, urinalysis, and plain abdominal imaging are not diagnostic, the next step is usually either contrast-enhanced abdominal radiography or endoscopy plus biopsy. Endoscopy is usually more cost-effective than contrast-enhanced radiography. During endoscopy, one should perform a biopsy of the stomach and duodenum, regardless of the gross mucosal appearance. In cats, endoscopic biopsy specimens of the ileum and ascending colon may be helpful in revealing

the cause of vomiting. If laparotomy is chosen over endoscopy, the entire abdomen should be examined and biopsy of the stomach, duodenum, jejunum, ileum, mesenteric lymph node, liver, and, in cats, the pancreas should be performed.

If the cause of vomiting is undiagnosed after biopsy, the basis for previously excluding the different diseases should be reviewed. Diseases can be inappropriately ruled out (or diagnosed) because one does not understand the limitations of certain tests. For example, dogs with hypoadrenocorticism may have normal electrolyte concentrations, inflammatory gastric and bowel disease may be localized to one area of the stomach or intestine and rarely causes significant changes in the white blood cell count, hyperthyroid cats may have normal serum thyroxine concentrations, dogs and cats with hepatic failure may have normal serum alanine aminotransferase and alkaline phosphatase activities, dogs and cats with pancreatitis may have normal serum amylase and lipase activities, and *Physaloptera* infections are almost never diagnosed on the basis of fecal examination results. Finally, the clinician may have to consider less common diseases that are more difficult to diagnose (e.g., idiopathic gastric hypomotility, occult CNS disease, limbic epilepsy).

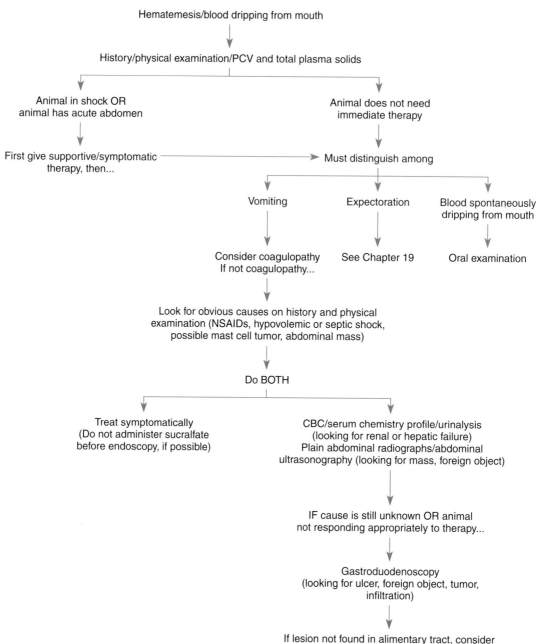

Hematemesis/blood dripping from mouth

History/physical examination/PCV and total plasma solids

Animal in shock OR
animal has acute abdomen

Animal does not need
immediate therapy

First give supportive/symptomatic
therapy, then...

Must distinguish among

Vomiting

Expectoration

Blood spontaneously
dripping from mouth

Consider coagulopathy
If not coagulopathy...

See Chapter 19

Oral examination

Look for obvious causes on history and physical
examination (NSAIDs, hypovolemic or septic shock,
possible mast cell tumor, abdominal mass)

Do BOTH

Treat symptomatically
(Do not administer sucralfate
before endoscopy, if possible)

CBC/serum chemistry profile/urinalysis
(looking for renal or hepatic failure)
Plain abdominal radiographs/abdominal
ultrasonography (looking for mass, foreign object)

IF cause is still unknown OR animal
not responding appropriately to therapy...

Gastroduodenoscopy
(looking for ulcer, foreign object, tumor,
infiltration)

If lesion not found in alimentary tract, consider
bronchoscopy and posterior nares examination

**FIG 28-3**
General diagnostic approach to hematemesis in the dog and cat. *PCV,* Packed cell volume; *CBC,* complete blood count.

# HEMATEMESIS

The clinician must distinguish hematemesis from other problems using the history and physical examination findings. Animals with oral lesions that have blood dripping from their lips do not have hematemesis. Likewise, hemoptysis (i.e., coughing up blood) is not hematemesis.

Hematemesis is usually caused by gastroduodenal ulceration and erosion (GUE). Although it is tempting to treat animals with hematemesis symptomatically with antacids, cytoprotective agents, or sucralfate, the preferable approach is to first check for shock (hypovolemic or septic) and an acute abdominal condition. This involves first checking the hematocrit and plasma total protein concentration to see whether a blood transfusion is necessary (see Fig. 28-3). The clinician should next try to determine the cause, whether it is a coagulopathy (uncommon), the ingestion of blood from another site (e.g., the respiratory tract), or GUE (Table 28-8). Historical and physical examination findings may help in ruling out a coagulopathy or respiratory tract disease as the cause. However, platelet counts and the clotting capability (e.g., activated clotting time or preferably a one-stage prothrombin time, partial thromboplastin time, buccal mucosal bleeding time) are preferred. Next look for obvious causes of GUE (e.g., acute gastritis, hemorrhagic gastroenteritis, ulcerogenic drugs [e.g., nonsteroidal antiinflammatory drugs], recent severe hypovolemic or septic shock, abdominal masses that may involve the gastric mucosa, cutaneous mast cell tumors). Remember that a mast cell tumor can grossly mimic almost any other benign or malignant neoplasm, especially lipomas.

If acute gastritis, nonsteroidal antiinflammatory drug–induced GUE, or shock is strongly suspected, one may treat the animal symptomatically for 3 to 5 days (see pp. 418 and 427) and see what effect this has in controlling clinical signs. However, if the cause is unknown, and especially if the vomiting or blood loss is severe or chronic, diagnostic tests (i.e., CBC, serum biochemistry profile, urinalysis, abdominal imaging) should be done (see Fig. 28-3). Evidence of renal and hepatic failure should also be sought. The stomach and duodenum should be imaged (e.g., plain and barium contrast–enhanced radiography or preferably abdominal ultrasonography) to look for alimentary tract infiltrations, foreign objects, and masses. Endoscopy is the most sensitive and specific means of finding and evaluating gastroduodenal ulcers and erosions. During endoscopy one can also do a biopsy of ulcers in an effort to rule out neoplasia or inflammatory bowel disease. Abdominal exploratory surgery may be performed instead of endoscopy, but it is easy to miss bleeding mucosal lesions when examining the serosal surface; intraoperative endoscopy (i.e., endoscopically examining the mucosal surface of the stomach and duodenum while the abdomen is opened) may be very useful in finding lesions that the surgeon cannot discern and thereby allowing for their resection.

If the source of bleeding cannot be found using gastroduodenoscopy, the clinician should consider possible bleeding sites beyond the reach of the endoscope; blood being

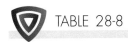

## TABLE 28-8

**Causes of Hematemesis**

**Coagulopathy (Uncommon Cause)**

Thrombocytopenia/platelet dysfunction
Clotting factor deficiency
Disseminated intravascular coagulation

**Alimentary Tract Lesion**

Gastrointestinal tract ulceration/erosion
  Infiltrative disease
    Neoplasia (especially older dogs)
    Pythiosis (younger dogs in the southeastern United States)
    Inflammatory bowel disease
  "Stress" ulceration
    Hypovolemic shock (common cause)
    Septic shock (i.e., systemic inflammatory response syndrome)
    After gastric dilatation or volvulus
    Neurogenic "shock"
  Hyperacidity
    Mast cell tumor
    Gastrinoma (rare)
  Iatrogenic causes
    Nonsteroidal antiinflammatory drug (very common cause)
    Corticosteroids (high-dose dexamethasone or any steroid that is combined with nonsteroidal antiinflammatory drugs)
  Other causes
    Hepatic disease
    Renal disease (not common)
    Hypoadrenocorticism
    Inflammatory diseases
  Foreign objects (rarely a primary cause but will worsen preexisting ulceration or erosion)
Gastritis
  Acute gastritis (very common cause)
  Hemorrhagic gastroenteritis
  Chronic gastritis
  *Helicobacter*-associated disease (questionable association with hematemesis in dogs and cats)
Esophageal disease (uncommon cause)
  Tumor
  Inflammatory disease (e.g., severe esophagitis)
  Trauma
Bleeding oral lesion
Gallbladder disease (rare)

**Extraalimentary Tract Lesion (Rare Cause)**

Respiratory tract disorders
  Lung lobe torsion
  Pulmonary tumor
  Posterior nares lesion

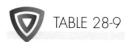

TABLE 28-9

### Causes of Acute Diarrhea

| | |
|---|---|
| **Diet** | **Infectious Causes—cont'd** |
| Intolerance/allergy | Bacterial causes |
| Poor-quality food |   *Salmonella* spp. |
| Rapid dietary change (especially in puppies and kittens) |   *Clostridium perfringens* |
| Bacterial food poisoning |   Verotoxin-producing *Escherichia coli* |
| |   *Campylobacter jejuni* |
| **Parasites** |   *Yersinia enterocolitica* |
| Helminths |   Various other bacteria |
| Protozoa | Rickettsial infection |
|   *Giardia* |   Salmon poisoning |
|   *Tritrichomonas* | |
|   *Coccidia* | **Other Causes** |
| | Hemorrhagic gastroenteritis |
| **Infectious Causes** | Intussusception |
| | "Irritable bowel syndrome" |
| Viral causes | Ingestion of "toxins" |
|   Parvovirus (canine, feline) |   "Garbage can" intoxication (spoiled foods) |
|   Coronavirus (canine, feline) |   Chemicals |
|   Feline leukemia virus (including infections secondary to it) |   Heavy metals |
|   Feline immunodeficiency virus (specifically infections secondary to it) |   Various drugs (antibiotics, antineoplastics, anthelmintics, anti-inflammatories, digitalis, lactulose) |
|   Various other viruses (e.g., rotavirus, canine distemper virus) | Acute pancreatitis (diarrhea usually modest component of clinical signs) |
| | Hypoadrenocorticism |

swallowed from a lesion in the mouth, posterior nares, trachea, or lungs; hemorrhage from the gallbladder; or an intermittently bleeding gastric or duodenal lesion.

## DIARRHEA

*Diarrhea* refers to feces containing excessive water. Fecal mucus is principally caused by large bowel disorders and is discussed under chronic large bowel diarrhea. The best approach to the assessment of animals with diarrhea is to first distinguish acute from chronic problems.

*Acute diarrhea* is usually caused by diet, parasites, or infectious diseases (Table 28-9). Dietary problems are often detected by history; parasites by history and fecal examinations; and infectious diseases by history (i.e., evidence of contagion or exposure), CBC, fecal enzyme-linked immunosorbent assay for canine parvoviral antigen, and the exclusion of other causes. If acute diarrhea becomes unduly severe or persistent, additional diagnostic tests are recommended. The approach used is similar to that adopted for the assessment of animals with chronic diarrhea.

Animals with *chronic diarrhea* should first be examined for evidence of parasites; multiple fecal examinations looking for nematodes, *Giardia*, and *Tritrichomonas* are indicated. Next it should be determined whether the diarrhea is small

or large intestinal in origin. History is the best tool (Table 28-10). Failure to lose weight almost always indicates the presence of large bowel disease; weight loss usually indicates the presence of small bowel disease, although some large bowel diseases (e.g., pythiosis, histoplasmosis, malignancy) may cause weight loss. Animals with weight loss resulting from large bowel disease usually have obvious signs of colonic involvement (i.e., fecal mucus, marked tenesmus, hematochezia). If there is tenesmus, ascertain whether it was present when the disease began; if tenesmus did not begin until late in the course, it may simply be due to perineal scalding or anal soreness resulting from chronic irritation.

Chronic small intestinal diarrhea can be segregated into maldigestion, non–protein-losing malabsorptive disease, and protein-losing malabsorptive disease. *Maldigestion* is principally caused by exocrine pancreatic insufficiency (EPI) and rarely causes significant hypoalbuminemia (i.e., serum albumin concentration of 2.2 g/dl or less if the normal range is 2.5 to 4.4 g/dl). Film digestion tests for fecal trypsin activity, Sudan staining of feces for undigested fats, and fat absorption tests yield many false-negative and false-positive results. The most sensitive and specific test for EPI is measuring the serum trypsin-like immunoreactivity (TLI) (see p. 562), which is indicated in dogs with chronic small intestinal diarrhea. EPI is rare in cats, but if suspected, an fTLI (feline TLI) is recommended.

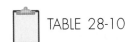

TABLE 28-10

**Differentiation of Chronic Small Intestinal from Large Intestinal Diarrheas**

| SIGN | SMALL INTESTINAL DISEASE | LARGE INTESTINAL DISEASE |
|---|---|---|
| Weight loss* | Expected | Rare* |
| Polyphagia | Sometimes | Rare to absent |
| Frequency of bowel movements | Often near normal | Sometimes very increased |
| Volume of feces | Often increased | Sometimes decreased (because of the increased frequency) |
| Blood in feces | Melena (rare) | Hematochezia (sometimes†) |
| Mucus in feces | Uncommon | Sometimes |
| Tenesmus | Uncommon (but may occur later in chronic cases) | Sometimes |
| Vomiting | May be seen | May be seen |

*Failure to lose weight or condition is the most reliable indication that an animal has large bowel disease. However, animals with colonic histoplasmosis, pythiosis, lymphoma, or similar infiltrative diseases may have weight loss despite large bowel involvement.
†Hematochezia becomes much more important as a differentiating feature in animals that are losing weight. Its presence in such animals confirms the presence of large bowel involvement (either by itself or in combination with small bowel disease) despite weight loss.

Diagnosing EPI by treating the animal and evaluating its response or nonresponse to therapy is not recommended, and if the animal has apparently responded to pancreatic enzyme supplementation, the enzymes should be repeatedly withheld and then readministered to be sure that it is the enzymes that are responsible for the improvement in the animal's stool characteristics. A false-positive diagnosis of EPI results in the unnecessary supplementation of expensive enzymes. Second, some dogs with EPI do not respond when enzymes are added to their diet. If EPI is incorrectly ruled out in such a case, then unnecessary endoscopies or operations often result. Antibiotic-responsive enteropathy (ARE) may be responsible for causing such a failure to respond to proper enzyme supplements and dietary changes. Therefore one should definitively diagnose or rule out EPI before proceeding with other diagnostic tests or treatments.

*Malabsorptive* intestinal disease may be protein-losing (PLE) or non–protein-losing. The serum albumin concentration will usually be markedly decreased (i.e., 2.1 g/dl or less; normal, 2.5 to 4.4 g/dl) in the former but not in the latter (Fig. 28-4); hypoglobulinemia may develop in patients with PLE. Diarrhea only occurs if the absorptive capacity of the colon is exceeded. Therefore a dog or cat can be losing weight because of small intestinal malabsorption and not have diarrhea (see the section on Weight Loss). If an animal has marked hypoproteinemia not resulting from protein-losing nephropathy, hepatic insufficiency, or skin lesions, then PLE must be the main consideration.

In patients with non–protein-losing malabsorptive disease, the clinician may perform additional diagnostic tests (e.g., intestinal biopsy) or design therapeutic trials (i.e., elimination diet for dietary intolerance, antibiotics for ARE) depending on how ill the patient is. If a therapeutic trial is performed, be sure that it is done properly (e.g., long enough, correct dose) so that it will almost certainly succeed if the animal has the suspected disease. However, if PLE is suspected, ultrasonography and intestinal biopsy are preferred because PLE usually requires prompt, appropriate therapy.

If diagnostic tests are chosen instead of a therapeutic trial, one may next search for ARE (in dogs) or proceed to gastroduodenoscopy or colonoscopy. ARE cannot reliably be diagnosed on the basis of quantitated duodenal culture or serum concentrations of vitamin $B_{12}$ (cobalamin) and folate (see p. 378). Decreased serum cobalamin plus increased serum folate concentrations are probably specific for ARE but are of dubious sensitivity. Duodenal mucosal cytologic and histologic findings can rarely be used to diagnose ARE. One usually treats ARE if it is found; however, it can be hard to diagnose.

The final diagnostic step is usually intestinal biopsy, because the findings typically determine the cause of PLE and non–protein-losing enteropathies (Tables 28-11 and 28-12). Absorptive tests and barium contrast–enhanced radiographs are rarely helpful and do not eliminate the requirement for biopsy. Abdominal ultrasonography may be diagnostic if it shows lymphadenopathy or intestinal infiltrates that can be aspirated percutaneously. Laparotomy or endoscopy is typically performed to obtain biopsy specimens. If ultrasonography reveals a localized lesion that cannot be reached with an endoscope, then laparotomy is recommended. Otherwise, endoscopy is quicker and safer than laparotomy. Endoscopic biopsy specimens can be nondiagnostic if the endoscopist has not been carefully trained in taking biopsy specimens. If laparotomy is performed in hypoalbuminemic animals, it may be prudent to use nonabsorbable suture material and/or perform intestinal patch grafting. The presence of distended intestinal lymphatics or lipogranulomas is suggestive of lymphangiectasia. If a cause is not shown by intestinal biopsy specimens, the main possible reasons for this are that the specimens were inadequate (i.e.,

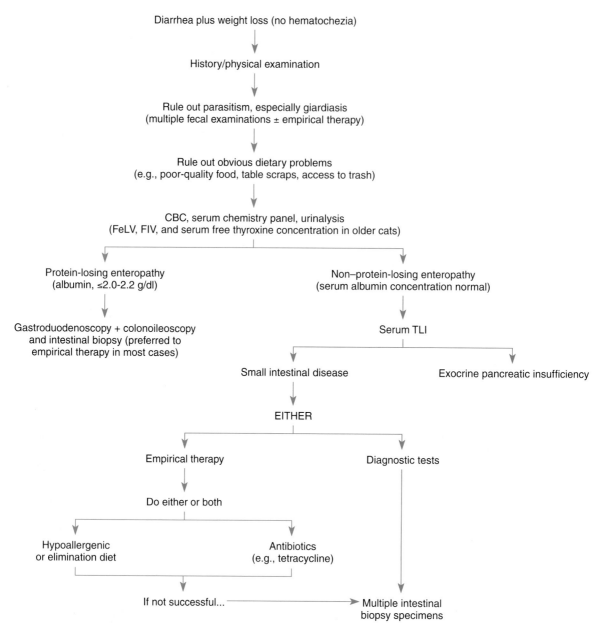

**FIG 28-4**
General diagnostic approach to small intestinal diarrhea in the dog and cat. *CBC,* Complete blood count; *FeLV,* feline leukemia virus; *FIV,* feline immunodeficiency virus, *TLI,* trypsin-like immunoreactivity.

not deep enough, from the wrong place, too much artifact), the animal has occult giardiasis, the animal has ARE, or the animal has a dietary intolerance.

Animals with *chronic large intestinal diarrhea* (Table 28-13) or fecal mucus should first undergo a digital rectal examination to search for mucosal thickening or proliferation. The rectum is the most common site of canine colonic neoplasia, and finding obvious mucosal lesions indicates the need for biopsy rather than a therapeutic trial. If the rectal mucosa seems normal and the animal has not lost weight or become hypoalbuminemic, one may first try therapeutic trials. However, multiple fecal examinations looking for whipworms, *Giardia,* and

*Tritrichomonas* are appropriate. Therapeutic trials usually consist of high-fiber diets, hypoallergenic diets, antibiotics to control clostridial colitis, or treatment for whipworms.

Additional diagnostic tests that may be done instead of therapeutic trials principally include obtaining biopsy specimens of the colonic mucosa by colonoscopy, fecal cultures, and assays for clostridial toxins. Fecal cultures for specific pathogens (e.g., *Salmonella* spp.) should be done if the history indicates the possibility of a contagious disorder or if the animal is not responding to seemingly appropriate therapy. Fecal examinations and cultures should be done before the animal receives enemas or intestinal lavage solutions.

## TABLE 28-11

**Major Causes of Malabsorptive Disease**

**Dog**

Food intolerance or allergy
Parasitism: giardiasis
Antibiotic-responsive enteropathy
Inflammatory bowel disease
    Lymphocytic-plasmacytic enteritis
    Eosinophilic enteritis
    Idiopathic villus atrophy
    Purulent enteritis
Neoplastic bowel disease: lymphoma
Pythiosis

**Cat**

Food intolerance or allergy
Parasitism: giardiasis
Inflammatory bowel disease: lymphocytic-plasmacytic
    enteritis
Neoplastic bowel disease: lymphoma

## TABLE 28-12

**Major Causes of Protein-Losing Enteropathy***

**Dog**

Severe inflammatory bowel disease (common)
    Lymphocytic-plasmacytic enteritis
    Eosinophilic enteritis
Alimentary tract lymphoma (especially common)
Alimentary tract histoplasmosis
Intestinal lymphangiectasia
Chronic intussusception (especially young dogs)
Alimentary tract hemorrhage (e.g., ulceration or erosion,
    neoplasia, parasites)
Unusual enteropathies (e.g., chronic purulent enteropathy,
    severe ectasia of mucosal crypts, severe mucosal
    edema)
Massive hookworm or whipworm infestation

**Cat**

Alimentary tract lymphoma
Severe inflammatory bowel disease: lymphocytic-
    plasmacytic enteritis
Alimentary hemorrhage (e.g., neoplasia)

*Except for lymphangiectasia, these diseases do not consistently
produce protein-losing enteropathy; however, when protein-losing
enteropathy exists, these are the most common causes.

If the results of these tests are not diagnostic, the clinician
must consider three main possibilities. First, the biopsy specimens may not be representative of the entire colonic mucosa
(i.e., biopsy of other areas of the colon must be done). If the
disease is localized to the region of the ileocolic valve, it will

## TABLE 28-13

**Major Causes of Chronic Large Intestinal Diarrhea**

**Dog**

Dietary intolerance or allergy
Parasitism
    Whipworms
    *Giardia*
    *Tritrichomonas*
Clostridial colitis
Functional disorder (so-called irritable bowel syndrome)
Histoplasmosis
Pythiosis
Inflammatory bowel disease
    Lymphocytic-plasmacytic colitis
    Eosinophilic colitis
    Chronic ulcerative colitis
    Histiocytic ulcerative colitis (principally Boxer dogs)
Neoplasia
    Lymphoma
    Adenocarcinoma

**Cat**

Dietary intolerance or allergy
Inflammatory bowel disease: lymphocytic-plasmacytic
    colitis
Functional disorder (so-called irritable bowel syndrome)
Feline leukemia virus infection (including infections
    secondary to it)
Feline immunodeficiency virus infection (specifically
    infections secondary to it)

be necessary to use a flexible endoscope to reach the area. Second, the pathologist may not have recognized the lesions.
This occasionally happens, especially if animals have colonic
histoplasmosis or neoplasia. Third, there may be no mucosal
infiltrates. This may occur in animals with a dietary intolerance or allergy, clostridial colitis, chronic giardiasis, or irritable bowel syndrome, all common problems in dogs.

## HEMATOCHEZIA

The diagnostic assessment of animals with *hematochezia*
(fresh blood in the feces) should be approached in the same
way as that for animals with large bowel diarrhea (see p. 352).
Coagulopathies (rarely a cause of rectal bleeding only) and
focal bleeding lesions in the distal part of the colon, rectum,
or perineal region should also be considered in such animals
(Table 28-14). Acute hematochezia may also result from
trauma. The presence of streaks of blood on the outside of
otherwise normal feces usually indicates the presence of a distal colonic or rectal lesion, whereas if the blood is mixed into
the feces, this implies that bleeding is higher in the colon.

A thorough digital rectal examination is the best initial
step (even if anesthesia is necessary). Express each anal sac

TABLE 28-14

**Major Causes of Hematochezia***

| **Dog** |
| --- |
| Parasitism |
|   Whipworms |
|   Hookworms (overwhelming infection) |
| Dietary intolerance or allergy |
| Clostridial colitis |
| Histoplasmosis |
| Pythiosis |
| Neoplasia |
|   Rectal adenocarcinoma |
|   Rectal polyp |
|   Colorectal leiomyoma or leiomyosarcoma |
| Intussusception |
|   Ileocolic |
|   Cecocolic |
| Hemorrhagic gastroenteritis |
| Parvoviral enteritis |
| Inflammatory bowel disease |
| Colonic trauma |
|   Foreign objects |
|   Automobile accident associated |
| Anal sacculitis |
| Coagulopathy |
| **Cat** |
| Dietary intolerance or allergy |
| Inflammatory bowel disease (especially lymphocytic-plasmacytic) |
| Parasitism: *Coccidia* |

*These diseases do not consistently produce hematochezia; however, when hematochezia is present, these are the most common causes.

 TABLE 28-15

**Major Causes of Melena***

| **Dog** |
| --- |
| Hookworms |
| Gastroduodenal tract ulceration/erosion (see Table 28-8) |
| Gastric or small intestinal tumor |
|   Lymphoma |
|   Adenocarcinoma |
|   Leiomyoma or leiomyosarcoma |
| Ingested blood |
|   Oral lesions |
|   Nasopharyngeal lesions |
|   Pulmonary lesions |
|   Diet |
| Coagulopathies |
| **Cat (Rare)** |
| Small intestinal tumor |
|   Lymphoma |
|   Duodenal polyps |
|   Other tumors (adenocarcinoma, mast cell tumor) |
| Coagulopathies: vitamin K deficiency (intoxication or resulting from malabsorption) |

*These diseases do not consistently produce melena; however, if melena is present, these are the most common causes.

repeatedly, and examine the contents. If the problem is chronic and results of these tests are uninformative, then colonoscopy and biopsy are usually indicated. An excellent barium enema is usually inferior to a good endoscopic examination. Biopsy specimens should include the submucosa, or some neoplastic lesions will be missed. Hematochezia is rarely severe enough to cause anemia; however, a CBC can be performed to look for and evaluate the cause of anemias.

## MELENA

*Melena* is defined by finding coal tar black (not dark) feces. It is often absent in animals with alimentary tract hemorrhage, but when present, it is strongly suggestive of upper alimentary tract bleeding or the ingestion of blood (Table 28-15). A CBC is indicated to look for iron deficiency anemia (i.e., microcytosis, hypochromasia, thrombocytosis). However, mea-

suring the total serum iron concentration and the total iron-binding capacity plus staining the bone marrow for iron are more definitive tests for iron deficiency anemia. Diagnostic imaging, especially ultrasonography, is useful when looking for bleeding lesions (e.g., an intestinal tumor). GUE often does not cause vomiting. Gastroduodenoscopy is the most sensitive test for GUE. If the results of endoscopy are nondiagnostic, contrast-enhanced radiography may detect small intestinal lesions beyond the reach of the endoscope. If imaging reveals a lesion beyond the reach of the endoscope, exploratory laparotomy is required. One may elect to immediately perform surgery, but it is easy to miss bleeding mucosal lesions when examining the serosa or palpating the bowel. Intraoperative endoscopy is recommended.

## TENESMUS

*Tenesmus* (ineffectual or painful straining at urination or defecation) and *dyschezia* (painful or difficult elimination of feces from the rectum) are principally caused by obstructive or inflammatory distal colonic or urinary bladder or urethral lesions (Table 28-16). Colitis, constipation, perineal hernias, prostatic disease, and cystic/urethral disease are the most common causes of tenesmus. Most rectal masses and strictures cause hematochezia; however, some do not disrupt the colonic mucosa and only cause tenesmus.

TABLE 28-16

**Major Causes of Tenesmus and/or Dyschezia**

| Dog | Dog—cont'd |
|---|---|
| Perineal inflammation or pain: anal sacculitis | Colonic/rectal obstruction—cont'd |
| Rectal inflammation/pain |   Pelvic fracture |
|   Perianal fistulae |   Other pelvic canal masses |
|   Tumor |   Rectal foreign object |
|   Proctitis (either primary disease or secondary to diarrhea or prolapse) | **Cat** |
|   Histoplasmosis/pythiosis | Urethral obstruction |
| Colonic/rectal obstruction | Rectal obstruction |
|   Rectal neoplasia |   Pelvic fracture |
|   Rectal granuloma |   Perineal hernia |
|   Perineal hernia | Constipation |
|   Constipation | Abscess near rectum |
|   Prostatomegaly | |

The first goal (especially in cats) is to distinguish lower urinary tract from alimentary tract disease. In cats, tenesmus secondary to a urethral obstruction is often misinterpreted as constipation. By observing the animal it may be possible to determine whether the animal is attempting to urinate or defecate. Palpate the bladder (i.e., a distended urinary bladder indicates an obstruction; a small, painful bladder indicates inflammation), perform a urinalysis, and, if necessary, catheterize the urethra to determine whether it is patent.

If one suspects tenesmus resulting from alimentary tract disease, the abdomen and rectum should be palpated and the anus and perineal areas visualized. One should not assume that constipation, if present, is causing the tenesmus. Severe pain (e.g., that resulting from proctitis) may make the animal refuse to defecate and cause secondary constipation. Most strictures, perineal hernias, masses, enlarged prostates, pelvic fractures, and rectal tumors can be detected during a digital rectal examination. One may need to use two fingers to detect partial strictures when examining large dogs. Perianal fistulae are usually visible but may be detected only as perirectal thickenings. Express the anal sacs, and examine their contents. Finally, evaluate the feces to determine whether they are excessively hard or have abnormal contents (e.g., hair, trash).

A biopsy should be done of any mass, stricture, or infiltrative lesion found by rectal examination. A rectal scraping is sometimes sufficient (e.g., histoplasmosis), but biopsy specimens that include the submucosa are usually preferred. Fine-needle aspiration should be performed if the biopsy is of an extracolonic mass, because abscesses occasionally occur in extracolonic locations.

If the clinician is confused by the findings from a physical examination, observing the animal defecate may help define the underlying process. Animals with inflammation often continue to strain after defecating, whereas a constipated animal strains before feces are produced. Tenesmus that occurs when an animal is in a squatting position often results from colitis, whereas tenesmus that occurs when an animal is in a semiwalking or partial squatting position usually results from constipation.

## CONSTIPATION

*Constipation* (the infrequent and difficult evacuation of feces) and *obstipation* (intractable constipation) have several causes (Table 28-17). The initial use of symptomatic therapy is often successful, but it is preferable to look for causes, because some problems that are initially treatable may become irreversible if symptomatic therapy masks the signs for too long.

A search of the history for iatrogenic, dietary, environmental, or behavioral causes should be done. Feces should be examined to determine whether they contain plastic, bones, hair, popcorn, or other such material. Physical and rectal examinations are done to search for rectal obstruction or infiltration. Plain pelvic radiographs can help show whether the animal has anatomic abnormalities or a previously undetected colonic obstruction (e.g., prostatomegaly, enlarged sublumbar lymph node). Ultrasonography is the preferred technique when looking for infiltrates. A CBC, serum biochemistry panel, and urinalysis may reveal causes of colonic inertia (e.g., hypercalcemia, hypokalemia, hypothyroidism).

Colonoscopy is indicated if one suspects an obstruction too orad to be detected by digital examination. Ultrasound-guided fine-needle aspiration of infiltrative colonic lesions sometimes yields diagnostic findings, but colonoscopy (especially rigid) allows a more reliable biopsy specimen to be obtained. If a thorough diagnostic work-up fails to identify a cause in a patient with a grossly dilated colon, then idiopathic megacolon may be present.

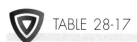

TABLE 28-17

Causes of Constipation

| **Iatrogenic Causes** | **Colonic Obstruction—cont'd** |
|---|---|
| Drugs | Intraluminal and intramural disorders—cont'd |
| Opiates | Cicatrix |
| Anticholinergics | Rectal foreign body |
| Carafate (sucralfate) | Congenital stricture |
| Barium | Extraluminal disorders |
| | Tumor |
| **Behavioral/Environmental Causes** | Granuloma |
| Change in household/routine | Abscess |
| Soiled litter box/no litter box | Healed pelvic fracture |
| House training | Prostatomegaly |
| Inactivity | Prostatic or paraprostatic cyst |
| | Sublumbar lymphadenopathy |
| **Refusal to Defecate** | |
| Behavioral | **Colonic Weakness** |
| Pain in rectal/perineal area (see Table 28-16) | Systemic disease |
| Inability to assume position to defecate | Hypercalcemia |
| Orthopedic problem | Hypokalemia |
| Neurologic problem | Hypothyroidism |
| | Chagas' disease |
| **Dietary Causes** | Localized neuromuscular disease |
| Excessive fiber in dehydrated animal | Spinal cord trauma |
| Abnormal diet | Pelvic nerve damage |
| Hair | Dysautonomia |
| Bones | Chronic, massive dilatation of the colon causing irreversible stretching |
| Indigestible material (e.g., plants, plastic) | of the colonic musculature |
| | |
| **Colonic Obstruction** | **Miscellaneous Causes** |
| Pseudocoprostasis | Severe dehydration |
| Deviation of rectal canal: perineal hernia | Idiopathic megacolon (especially cats) |
| Intraluminal and intramural disorders | |
| Tumor | |
| Granuloma | |

## *FECAL INCONTINENCE*

Fecal incontinence is caused by neuromuscular disease (e.g., cauda equina syndrome, lumbosacral stenosis) or a partial rectal obstruction. Severe, irritative proctitis may cause urge incontinence. Animals with rectal obstructions continually try to defecate because the anal canal is filled with feces. Proctitis is suspected on the basis of rectal examination findings and confirmed by proctoscopy and biopsy findings. Neuromuscular disease is suspected if an abnormal anal reflex is found, usually in conjunction with other neurologic defects in the anal, perineal, hindlimb, or coccygeal region. Defects in the coccygeal region are discussed in Chapter 72.

## *WEIGHT LOSS*

Weight loss is usually caused by one of several categories of problems (Table 28-18). If other problems with more defined lists of differentials (e.g., ascites, vomiting, diarrhea, polyuria-polydipsia) are also present, they should be investigated first. If there are no such concurrent problems that allow "quick" localization of the disease, the clinician should then determine what the animal's appetite was when the weight loss *began* (Fig. 28-5). Any disease can cause anorexia if the animal becomes too ill. Weight loss despite a good appetite usually indicates maldigestion, malabsorption, or excessive utilization (e.g., hyperthyroidism, lactation) or inappropriate loss (e.g., diabetes mellitus) of calories.

The animal's history should be reviewed for evidence of dietary problems, dysphagia, regurgitation, vomiting, or increased use of calories (e.g., lactation, work, extremely cold temperature). Signalments suggestive of particular diseases (e.g., hyperthyroidism in older cats, hepatic failure in younger dogs with signs of portosystemic shunts) should be recognized. Remember that diarrhea may be absent in animals with severe small intestinal disease.

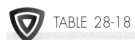

TABLE 28-18

Causes of Weight Loss

| | |
|---|---|
| **Food** | **Malassimilation—cont'd** |
| Not enough (especially if there are multiple animals) | Organ failure—cont'd |
| Poor quality or low caloric density |    Renal failure |
| Inedible |    Adrenal failure |
| **Anorexia (see Table 28-19)** | **Cancer Cachexia** |
| **Dysphagia (see Table 28-1)** | **Excessive Utilization of Calories** |
| **Regurgitation/Vomiting (i.e., losing enough calories to account for weight loss; see Tables 28-5 to 28-7)** | Lactation |
| | Increased work |
| | Extremely cold environment |
| **Maldigestive Disease** | Pregnancy |
| Exocrine pancreatic insufficiency (usually but not always associated with diarrhea) | Increased catabolism resulting from fever/inflammation |
| | Hyperthyroidism |
| **Malabsorptive Disease** | **Increased Loss of Nutrients** |
| Small intestinal disease (may be associated with normal stools) | Diabetes mellitus |
| | Protein-losing nephropathy |
| | Protein-losing enteropathy |
| **Malassimilation** | **Neuromuscular Disease** |
| Organ failure | Lower motor neuron disease |
|    Cardiac failure | |
|    Hepatic failure | |

Physical examination is performed to identify abnormalities that might help localize the problem to a particular body system (e.g., nasal disease preventing normal olfaction, dysphagia, arrhythmia suggestive of cardiac failure, weakness suggestive of neuromuscular disease, abnormally sized or shaped organs, abnormal fluid accumulations). Retinal examination may identify inflammatory or infiltrative diseases, especially in cats.

A CBC, serum biochemistry profile, and urinalysis should be done next to search for evidence of inflammation, organ failure, or a paraneoplastic syndrome. Cats should be tested for circulating feline leukemia virus antigen and antibodies to feline immunodeficiency virus. Serum $T_4$ and $fT_4$ concentrations should be determined in older cats. If clinical pathology data are not helpful, then thoracic radiographs are obtained because one cannot rule out significant thoracic disease on the basis of physical examination findings alone. Thoracic radiographs should include left and right lateral views (some masses can only be seen on one lateral view). Abdominal imaging can be helpful if the animal cannot be palpated well. Most cats and some dogs can be palpated well enough that abdominal radiographs are not cost-effective early in the work-up. However, abdominal ultrasonography may reveal lesions that cannot be palpated (plain radiographs reveal such lesions less frequently).

If the cause of weight loss remains unknown after these steps have been taken, additional tests are necessary. Perform daily physical examinations; they are often the best means of localizing the problem. Fever of unknown origin may be noted (see Chapter 95). Organ function testing (e.g., serum bile acid concentrations, ACTH-stimulation testing, serum TLI) is reasonable. Likewise, if serum $T_4$ and $fT_4$ concentrations are normal in a cat with suspected hyperthyroidism, the serum $T_4$ and $fT_4$ concentrations should be rechecked or a triiodothyronine-suppression test performed (see Chapter 51). If the means are available, nuclear scintigraphy of the thyroid glands with technetium-99 is very sensitive in detecting hyperthyroidism.

If the cause of weight loss still remains undiagnosed, consider performing gastric and intestinal biopsy (preferably endoscopically). If a laparotomy is performed instead, the entire abdomen should be examined, multiple biopsy samples of the alimentary tract obtained, and biopsy of the liver and mesenteric lymph nodes done. Biopsy of the pancreas should also be done in cats.

Other possible diagnostic tests include tests to evaluate the CNS (i.e., cerebrospinal fluid analysis, electroencephalography, computed tomography, magnetic resonance imaging; animals that are anorectic as a result of severe CNS disease do not always have obvious cranial nerve deficits or seizures) and peripheral nerves and muscles (i.e., electromyography, muscle or nerve biopsies; sometimes the weakness associated with neuropathies and myopathies is mistaken for lethargy) (see Chapter 66). If the cause of the weight loss still remains undiagnosed and the history and physical examination findings are still noncontributory, then occult cancer becomes a major differential diagnosis. In such cases, one may have to wait until the cancer (or other problem) progresses enough to be detected.

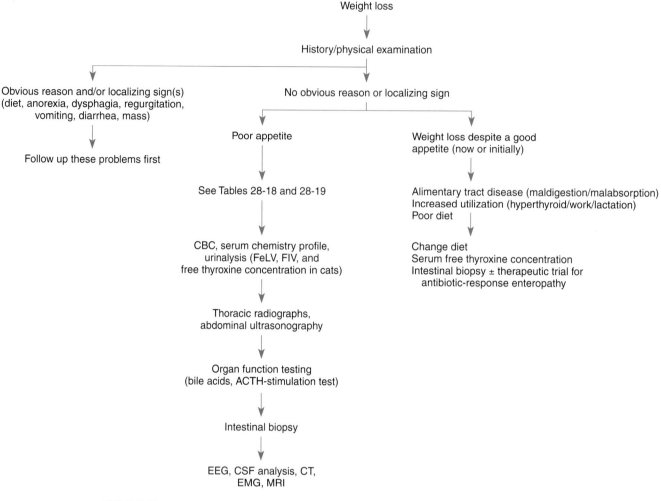

**FIG 28-5**
General diagnostic approach to weight loss in the dog and cat. *CBC,* Complete blood count; *FeLV,* feline leukemia virus; *FIV,* feline immunodeficiency virus; *ACTH,* adrenocorticotropic hormone; *EEG,* electroencephalography; *EMG,* electromyography; *CT,* computerized tomography; *CSF,* cerebrospinal fluid; *MRI,* magnetic resonance imaging.

Causes of weight loss that are particularly difficult to diagnose include feline hyperthyroidism with normal serum $T_4$ and $fT_4$ concentrations, gastric disease not causing vomiting, intestinal disease not causing vomiting or diarrhea, hepatic disease with normal serum alanine aminotransferase or alkaline phosphatase activities, occult inflammatory disease, hypoadrenocorticism with normal serum electrolyte concentrations, occult cancer, "dry" feline infectious peritonitis, and CNS disease without cranial nerve deficits or seizures.

## ANOREXIA

The approach to the diagnostic evaluation of animals with anorexia of uncertain cause is similar to that for animals with weight loss (see Fig. 28-5), and the differential diagnoses are also similar (Table 28-19). Inflammatory disease is often detected by the CBC or the finding of fever (see Chapter 95).

Gastric disease may produce anorexia without vomiting. Cancer cachexia (with anorexia as the predominant sign) may stem from relatively small tumors that are not grossly detectable, although this is rare. Finally, CNS disease must be considered whenever there is altered mentation. However, altered mentation may resemble the depression and lethargy commonly seen in animals with other diseases.

## ABDOMINAL EFFUSION

Abdominal effusion is usually caused by hypoalbuminemia, portal hypertension, or peritoneal inflammation. Effusions resulting from alimentary tract disorders are primarily caused by PLE or alimentary tract rupture (i.e., septic peritonitis). Some animals with PLE have normal stools, with ascites being the presenting complaint. Malignant tumors may obstruct lymphatic flow or increase vascular permeability, causing

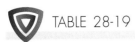

TABLE 28-19

**Major Causes of Anorexia**

**Inflammatory Disease**

Bacterial infections
Viral infections
Fungal infections
Rickettsial infections
Protozoal infections
Sterile inflammation
    Immune-mediated disease
    Neoplastic disease
    Pancreatitis

**Alimentary Tract Disease**

Gastric or intestinal disease
Dysphagia (especially resulting from pain)

**Nausea (stimulation of the medullary vomiting center for any reason, even if it is not sufficient to cause vomiting, especially gastric or intestinal disease)**

**Metabolic Disease**

Organ failure (e.g., kidney, adrenal, liver, heart)
Hypercalcemia
Diabetic ketoacidosis
Hyperthyroidism (usually causes polyphagia, but some cats have apathetic hyperthyroidism)

**Cancer Cachexia**

**Anosmia**

**Central Nervous System Disease**

**Psychologic Causes**

**Fever**

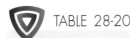

TABLE 28-20

**Major Causes of Acute Abdomen**

**Septic Inflammation**

Septic peritonitis resulting from any cause but especially a perforated or devitalized hollow viscus
Perforating linear foreign body
Ruptured gallbladder resulting from cholecystitis
Abscess
    Pancreatic
    Splenic
    Hepatic
    Prostatic
    Renal
    Pyometra

**Nonseptic Inflammation**

Pancreatitis
Iatrogenic inflammation: surgical sponge

**Organ Distention or Obstruction**

Gastric dilatation or volvulus
Mesenteric volvulus
Intussusception
Incarcerated obstruction
Intestinal obstruction resulting from many causes

**Ischemia**

Torsion of spleen, testicle, or other organ

**Other Causes of Abdominal Pain (see Table 28-21)**

**Abdominal Hemorrhage**

Abdominal neoplasia
Trauma
Coagulopathy

**Abdominal Neoplasia**

modified transudates to form or nonseptic peritonitis to develop. Modified transudates usually result from hepatic or cardiac disease or from malignant conditions. For further information on abdominal effusions, see Chapters 35 and 36.

## ACUTE ABDOMEN

*Acute abdomen* refers to various abdominal disorders producing shock (hypovolemic or septic), sepsis, or severe pain (Table 28-20). Causes may include alimentary tract obstruction or leakage, vascular compromise (e.g., congestion, torsion, volvulus, ischemia), inflammation, neoplasia, or sepsis. The approach to the diagnostic evaluation of this problem is determined by the severity of the clinical signs (Fig. 28-6).

Shock and gastric dilatation or volvulus (GDV) must be identified and treated immediately. Once these conditions are eliminated, the next major decision is whether to perform exploratory surgery or initiate medical therapy. Animals with abdominal masses, foreign objects, bunched-up

loops of painful small intestine (e.g., linear foreign body), or spontaneous septic peritonitis should undergo surgery as soon as supportive therapy has made the risk of anesthesia acceptable. If the cause of the acute abdomen is uncertain, it can be difficult to determine whether surgery is indicated. Surgery is not necessarily beneficial and may even be detrimental to animals with conditions such as pancreatitis, parvoviral enteritis, pyelonephritis, prostatitis, or cholecystitis. Typically, abdominal imaging (plain abdominal radiography or ultrasonography) and clinical pathologic studies (CBC, chemistry panel) should be performed before one decides to do a laparotomy. Ultrasound studies usually reveal changes detected radiographically as well as others (e.g., infiltration) that radiographs cannot detect. Radiographs may reveal spontaneous pneumoperitoneum, abdominal masses, foreign objects, alimentary tract obstruction, gastric or mesenteric torsion (these require surgical treatment), or free peritoneal fluid (this requires abdominocentesis and

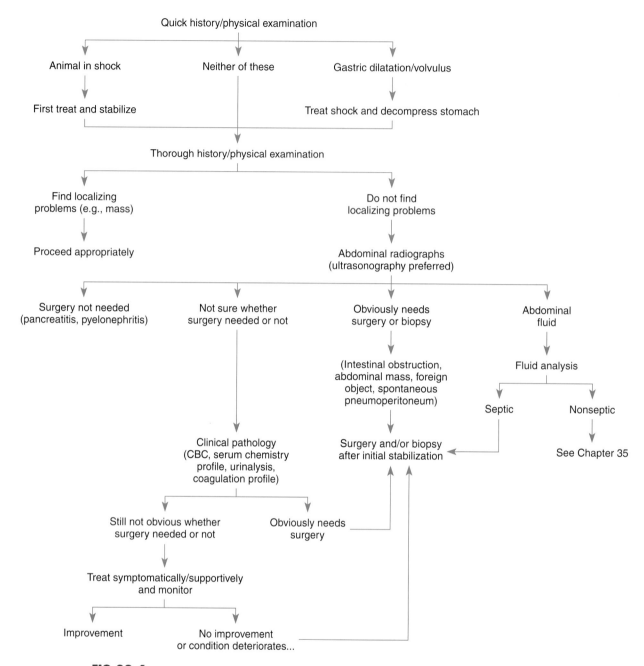

**FIG 28-6**
General diagnostic approach to acute abdomen in the dog and cat. *CBC,* Complete blood count.

fluid analysis for management). A barium series is seldom useful.

If optimal medical therapy is being given and the animal's condition is clearly deteriorating or does not improve after 2 to 5 days of therapy, or if the animal continues to have excruciating pain, it is often appropriate to recommend exploratory surgery. Inform the client that you may discover the animal has a disorder not surgically correctable (e.g., pancreatitis) or that nothing abnormal may be found. In the latter case, do a biopsy of various abdominal organs and then treat the animal symptomatically while awaiting biopsy results.

## ABDOMINAL PAIN

"Abdominal" pain must first be determined to be abdominal and not extraabdominal in origin (e.g., thoracolumbar pain is often erroneously assessed as being abdominal in origin). An animal with true abdominal pain may show obvious discomfort (e.g., paces or repeatedly assumes different positions, repeatedly looks at or licks its abdomen) and may whine, growl, or snap if the abdomen is touched. Some dogs stretch out and assume a "praying" position (i.e., the position of relief). Other animals have inconspicuous signs (e.g., the animal grunts or

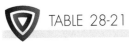

TABLE 28-21

### Causes of Abdominal Pain

| | |
|---|---|
| **Poor Palpation Technique** | **Peritoneum** |
| **Musculoskeletal System** | Peritonitis (common) |
| Fractures |   Septic |
| Intervertebral disk disease (common) |     Nonseptic (e.g., uroabdomen) |
| Diskospondylitis (common) | Adhesions |
| Abscesses | **Urogenital System** |
| **Gastrointestinal Tract** | Pyelonephritis |
| Gastrointestinal ulcer | Lower urinary tract infection |
| Foreign object | Nonseptic cystitis (common in cats) |
| Neoplasm | Cystic or ureteral obstruction or rupture (common, especially after trauma) |
| Adhesions | Urethritis or obstruction (common) |
| Intestinal ischemia | Metritis |
| Intestinal spasm | Uterine torsion (rare) |
| See also Table 28-20 under Organ distention | Neoplasm |
|   or obstruction | Testicular torsion (rare) |
| | Prostatitis (common) |
| **Hepatobiliary Tract** | Mastitis (does not cause true abdominal pain but mimics abdominal pain) |
| Hepatitis | **Miscellaneous Causes** |
| Cholelithiasis or cholecystitis | Adrenalitis (associated with hypoadrenocorticism) |
| **Pancreas** | Heavy metal intoxication |
| Pancreatitis (common) | Vasculopathy |
| |   Rocky Mountain spotted fever vasculitis |
| **Spleen** |   Infarct |
| Torsion (uncommon) | Autonomic (abdominal) epilepsy |
| Rupture | Iatrogenic causes |
| Neoplasm |   Misoprostol |
| Infection |   Bethanechol |
| |   Postoperative cause (especially if animal has a tight suture line) |

tries to walk away when palpated, the abdomen is tensed) that are easily missed. On the other hand, a poor or rough abdominal palpation technique in normal animals may elicit a guarding response that can mimic abdominal pain. The main causes of abdominal pain are listed in Table 28-21.

If abdominal pain occurs, the next step is to determine the source. If the pain is originating from within the abdominal cavity, the diagnostic approach depends on its severity, the progression of disease, and whether there are any obvious causes. The steps taken in diagnosing the cause of abdominal pain are similar to those taken in an animal with acute abdomen (see p. 361). Some causes of abdominal pain can be difficult to diagnose (e.g., acute pancreatitis, localized peritonitis).

## ABDOMINAL DISTENTION OR ENLARGEMENT

Abdominal distention or enlargement may be associated with an acute abdomen, but they are typically separate problems. It is best to believe clients who claim there is abdominal enlargement until good cause is found to disbelieve them. There are six main causes of abdominal distention (Table 28-22).

The first concern is whether an acute abdomen is present (e.g., GDV, septic peritonitis, hemoabdomen plus shock). After an acute abdomen is ruled out, it should be possible to classify the enlargement on the basis of the physical examination and abdominal imaging (i.e., radiography or ultrasonography) findings, per Table 28-22. Obesity and pregnancy should be obvious. Specimens of free abdominal fluid should be obtained and analyzed as described in Chapter 36. Biopsy should be done of abdominal masses and enlarged organs, unless there is a reason not to (e.g., hepatomegaly caused by severe right-sided heart failure). Fine-needle aspiration is usually safe, although the leakage of septic contents or implantation of neoplastic cells may occur. Ultrasonography helps determine the potential for hemorrhage or leakage (e.g., cyst, mass with ultrasonographic characteristics of hemangiosarcoma). The finding of a spontaneous pneumoperitoneum indicates the presence of alimentary tract rupture or septic peritonitis and is an indication for immediate surgical exploration. A hollow viscus dilated with gas may

TABLE 28-22

## Causes of Abdominal Enlargement

**Tissue**

Pregnancy

Hepatomegaly (infiltrative or inflammatory disease, lipidosis, neoplasia)

Splenomegaly (infiltrative or inflammatory disease, neoplasia, hematoma)

Renomegaly (neoplasia, infiltrative disease, compensatory hypertrophy)

Miscellaneous neoplasia

Granuloma (e.g., pythiosis)

**Fluid**

Contained in organ(s)

    Congestion resulting from torsion, volvulus, or right-sided heart failure

        Spleen

        Liver

    Cysts

        Paraprostatic cyst

        Perinephric cyst

        Hepatic cyst

    Hydronephrosis

    Intestines or stomach (resulting from obstruction or ileus)

    Pyometra

**Fluid—cont'd**

Free in abdomen

    Transudate, modified transudate, exudate, blood, chyle

**Gas**

Contained in organ(s)

    Stomach (gastric dilatation or volvulus)

    Intestines (resulting from obstruction)

    In parenchymatous organs (e.g., liver) resulting from infection with gas-producing bacteria

Free in abdomen

    Iatrogenic (after laparoscopy or laparotomy)

    Alimentary tract or female reproductive tract rupture

    Bacterial metabolism (peritonitis)

**Fat**

Obesity

Lipoma

**Weak Abdominal Muscles**

Hyperadrenocorticism

**Feces**

---

indicate obstruction (i.e., gastric dilatation, intestinal obstruction) or physiologic ileus (see pp. 372 and 424; Figs. 29-5 and 32-4). Surgery is indicated if an obstruction seems likely. If abdominal musculature weakness is suspected, one should test for hyperadrenocorticism. Results of a CBC, serum biochemistry panel, and urinalysis are used to determine if specific organ involvement (e.g., hyperadrenocorticism) is likely. Contrast-enhanced alimentary or urinary tract radiographs may be useful in selected cases, although by using ultrasonography, often these procedures are unnecessary.

## Suggested Readings

DeBowes LJ: Ptyalism. In Ettinger SJ et al, editors: *Textbook of veterinary internal medicine,* ed 5, Philadelphia, 2000, WB Saunders.

Guilford WG et al: *Small animal gastroenterology,* ed 3, Davis, Calif, 1996, WB Saunders.

Guilford WG: Melena and hematochezia. In Ettinger SJ et al, editors: *Textbook of veterinary internal medicine,* ed 5, Philadelphia, 2000, WB Saunders.

Jones B: Constipation, tenesmus, dyschezia, and fecal incontinence. In Ettinger SJ et al, editors: *Textbook of veterinary internal medicine,* ed 5, Philadelphia, 2000, WB Saunders.

Tams TR: *Handbook of small animal gastroenterology,* Philadelphia, 1996, WB Saunders.

Tams TR: Diarrhea. In Ettinger SJ et al, editors: *Textbook of veterinary internal medicine,* ed 5, Philadelphia, 2000, WB Saunders.

Twedt DC: Vomiting. In Ettinger SJ et al, editors: *Textbook of veterinary internal medicine,* ed 5, Philadelphia, 2000, WB Saunders.

Willard MD et al: Gastrointestinal, pancreatic, and hepatic disorders. In Willard MD et al, editors: *Small animal clinical diagnosis by laboratory methods,* ed 3, Philadelphia, 1999, WB Saunders.

# CHAPTER 29

# Diagnostic Tests
# for the Alimentary Tract

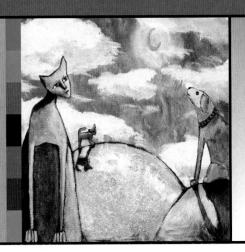

## CHAPTER OUTLINE

PHYSICAL EXAMINATION, 365
ROUTINE LABORATORY EVALUATION, 365
    Complete blood count, 365
    Serum biochemistry profile, 366
    Urinalysis, 366
FECAL PARASITIC EVALUATION, 366
FECAL DIGESTION TESTS, 366
MISCELLANEOUS FECAL ANALYSES, 367
BACTERIAL FECAL CULTURE, 367
CYTOLOGIC EVALUATION OF FECES, 368
RADIOGRAPHY OF THE ALIMENTARY TRACT, 368
ULTRASONOGRAPHY OF THE ALIMENTARY
TRACT, 368
IMAGING OF THE ORAL CAVITY, PHARYNX,
AND ESOPHAGUS, 368
    Indications, 368
    Indications for imaging of the esophagus, 369
IMAGING OF THE STOMACH AND SMALL
INTESTINE, 371
    Indications for radiographic imaging of the abdomen
        without contrast media, 371
    Indications for ultrasonography of the stomach and
        small intestines, 374
    Indications for contrast-enhanced gastrograms, 374
    Indications for contrast-enhanced studies of the small
        intestine, 376
    Indications for barium contrast enemas, 376
PERITONEAL FLUID ANALYSIS, 377
DIGESTION AND ABSORPTION TESTS, 378
SERUM CONCENTRATIONS OF VITAMINS, 378
OTHER SPECIAL TESTS FOR ALIMENTARY TRACT
DISEASE, 379
ENDOSCOPY, 379
BIOPSY TECHNIQUES AND SUBMISSION, 384
    Fine-needle aspiration biopsy, 384
    Endoscopic biopsy, 384
    Full-thickness biopsy, 385

## PHYSICAL EXAMINATION

Routine physical examination is the first step in evaluating animals with alimentary tract disease, although oral examination is sometimes skipped in uncooperative animals. However, if oral disease is a possibility, then one must thoroughly examine the mouth, even if it requires the use of chemical restraint. A good example of this is a vomiting cat with a possible linear foreign body. Methodically identify individual organs during abdominal palpation. In dogs the small intestine, large intestine, and urinary bladder can usually be found (unless there is an abdominal effusion, abdominal pain, or obesity). In cats both kidneys are palpable. In both species one can usually detect splenomegaly, hepatomegaly, intestinal or mesenteric masses, and intestinal foreign objects. Abdominal pain may be subtle; some animals will cry out during gentle palpation, whereas many just tense their abdomen (i.e., guarding) or try to move away. A rough palpation technique can cause a normal animal to tense up or vocalize during palpation, mimicking the reaction of an animal with abdominal pain. Light, careful palpation permits the definition of as much of the internal abdominal contents as possible. If sufficient abdominal fluid is present to prevent meaningful abdominal palpation, ballottement of the abdomen can be done, and this should reveal the existence of a fluid wave.

During a rectal examination, the examiner should be able to identify and evaluate the colonic mucosa, anal sphincter, anal sacs, pelvic canal bones, muscular support for the rectum, urogenital tract, and luminal contents. However, it is particularly easy to misinterpret mucosal polyps as mucosal folds and to miss partial strictures that are large enough to easily allow a single digit to pass through.

## ROUTINE LABORATORY EVALUATION

### COMPLETE BLOOD COUNT

Complete blood counts (CBCs) are especially important in animals at risk for neutropenia (e.g., suspected parvoviral enteritis, severe sepsis), infection (e.g., aspiration pneumonia), or anemia (e.g., pale mucous membranes, melena, hematemesis) and also in those that have fever, weight loss, or anorexia resulting from an occult cause. Only evaluate absolute numbers of the different types of white blood cells (WBCs), not the percentages, because an animal may have an abnormal percentage of a particular WBC and yet have a normal absolute number of cells (and vice versa). If the animal is anemic, evaluate the CBC for evidence of iron deficiency (e.g., hypochromasia, microcytosis, thrombocytosis, increased red blood cell distribution width). Iron deficiency anemia resulting from gastrointestinal tract disease is less common in cats than in dogs.

A *platelet count* is recommended if blood loss is suspected. Platelet numbers can be estimated from correctly made blood smears (i.e., a dog should have an average of 8 to 30 platelets per oil immersion field; finding 1 platelet per field suggests a platelet count of approximately 15,000 to 20,000/μl). Coagulation panels may reveal the presence of unsuspected coagulopathies (e.g., disseminated intravascular coagulation). Activated clotting times are crude estimates of the intrinsic clotting pathway; partial thromboplastin times are more sensitive.

## SERUM BIOCHEMISTRY PROFILE

Serum biochemistry profiles that include alanine transaminase and alkaline phosphatase activities, as well as the blood urea nitrogen, creatinine, total protein, albumin, sodium, potassium, calcium, phosphorus, magnesium, bilirubin, and glucose concentrations, are important in animals with severe vomiting, diarrhea, ascites, unexplained weight loss, or anorexia. Knowing what these values are is crucial to correctly diagnosing the animal's problem and appropriately treating it. However, one cannot predict the changes that will occur or the magnitude of the changes in a particular animal, even when the cause of the disease is known. The total carbon dioxide concentration is not as definitive as blood gas analysis but helps define the acid-base status, which also cannot be accurately predicted.

The albumin concentration is typically more useful than the total protein concentration. However, hyperglobulinemia, which has many causes (e.g., heartworms, chronic dermatitis, ehrlichiosis) in a hypoalbuminemic dog can cause the serum protein concentration to be normal. Severe hypoalbuminemia (i.e., less than 2.0 g/dl) is important diagnostically; it is more commonly found in animals with infiltrative alimentary tract disease, parvoviral diarrhea, intestinal lymphangiectasia, gastrointestinal blood loss, or ascites.

Ill animals (especially those receiving multiple drugs) are at risk for secondary renal or hepatic failure. Very young and very small animals easily become hypoglycemic if they cannot eat or absorb ingested nutrients. Finally, finding hypercalcemia or hypoalbuminemia may provide a clue to the underlying problem (i.e., make some disorders more likely) in animals with weight loss or anorexia.

## URINALYSIS

Urinalysis is required to accurately evaluate renal function and, in conjunction with the urine protein:creatinine ratio, to help identify the cause of hypoalbuminemia. Urine should always be obtained before fluid therapy is begun.

## FECAL PARASITIC EVALUATION

*Fecal flotation* is indicated in almost every animal with alimentary tract disease or weight loss, especially in puppies and kittens. Even if it is not the primary problem, parasitism may cause additional debilitation. Concentrated salt or sugar solutions are typically used for fecal flotation. The former are usually superior; however, incorrectly made solutions may not force heavier ova (i.e., whipworms) to float. On the other hand, concentrated salt solutions can distort *Giardia* cysts, making identification difficult. A zinc sulfate flotation solution is preferred for detecting nematode ova and *Giardia* cysts. It is best to centrifuge the mixture to promote the separation of cysts from the fecal matter. Some parasites intermittently shed small numbers of ova or cysts, necessitating repeated fecal analyses for diagnosis. Whipworm and *Giardia* infections can be especially difficult to diagnose.

The ova of the most common tapeworm species are contained in segments and are not found by flotation techniques. *Nanophyetus salmincola* (the fluke that transmits salmon poisoning) is detected by many flotation solutions, although sedimentation examinations are required to detect most other fluke ova. Cryptosporidiosis can be detected by flotation techniques, but higher magnification ($\times1000$) must be used. One should send the feces to a laboratory that is familiar with this coccidium and is able to perform special procedures to detect it. ELISA methodology is more sensitive than fecal examination for finding cryptosporidia.

*Direct fecal examination*, although convenient, is not sensitive and should not replace flotation techniques. However, occasionally amebiasis, strongyloidiasis, and whipworm infections missed by flotation procedures can be detected in this way. Motile *Giardia* and *Tritrichomonas* trophozoites may be found if the feces are very fresh and the smear is adequately diluted with saline solution. Direct examination seems about half as sensitive as zinc sulfate flotation techniques in detecting giardiasis.

*Fecal sedimentation* is time-consuming and offers no advantage in detecting common gastrointestinal tract parasites. However, it does detect fluke ova missed by other techniques, especially the ova of *Eurytrema* spp., *Platynosomum* spp., and *Amphimerus* spp.

Feces may be preserved by mixing equal volumes of feces and 10% neutral buffered formalin or by using commercially available kits. Polyvinyl alcohol is used in the latter, and feces preserved in this manner can be examined weeks to months later. These techniques are especially useful if one cannot immediately examine feces for protozoal cysts.

## FECAL DIGESTION TESTS

Examining feces for undigested food particles by staining thin fecal smears with the Sudan stain (for fat) or iodine (for starch and muscle fibers) is of dubious value. Although the finding of excessive amounts of undigested fecal fat is suggestive of exocrine pancreatic insufficiency (EPI), this test has many false-positive and false-negative results. If EPI is a differential diagnosis, serum trypsin-like immunoreactivity (TLI) is a better way to confirm the diagnosis (see later discussion, Digestion and Absorption Tests).

*Fecal analysis for proteolytic activity* (i.e., the fecal trypsin content) also tests for EPI. Qualitative estimates (e.g., fecal film digestion, fecal gelatin digestion) are unreliable. Quantitative analysis is seldom needed because the TLI test is easier and more pleasant to perform. It is rarely necessary to quantitate fecal proteolytic activity to diagnose EPI caused by pancreatic duct obstruction, something TLI does not detect. In this test, feces are collected for 3 consecutive days and stored frozen until sent to the laboratory.

*Quantitated fecal fat analysis* is seldom indicated. Although sensitive for detecting fat malabsorption and maldigestion, it is expensive and unpleasant to perform and does not differentiate malabsorption from EPI.

*Fecal occult blood* analyses are seldom useful because most pets eat meat by-products that cause a positive reaction. False-positive reactions may also be produced by cimetidine, oral iron preparations, and some vegetables. Furthermore, the sensitivity of different techniques varies, making it difficult to accurately compare results. Finally, blood is often not distributed homogeneously throughout the feces, and a negative result could stem from a sampling error (especially in animals with lower intestinal tract problems).

If analysis for fecal occult blood is desired, feed the animal a meat-free diet for 3 to 4 days before performing the test. Tests using the reagents benzidine or orthotoluidine to detect hemoglobin tend to be very sensitive (and hence less specific), whereas those using guaiac are less sensitive (and thus more specific). A sensitive and specific fluorometric method has been validated in dogs. Repeated testing may be necessary to demonstrate intermittent bleeding.

## MISCELLANEOUS FECAL ANALYSES

*Enzyme-linked immunosorbent assays* (ELISAs) can be used to detect various antibodies or antigens. The test for canine parvovirus seems to be very specific. However, virus may not be shed for the first 24 to 48 hours, and the test may need to be repeated in 2 to 3 days if initial results are negative in a dog strongly suspected of having parvoviral infection. In addition, although dogs with parvoviral diarrhea initially shed large amounts of virus, fecal shedding decreases substantially during the ensuing 7 to 14 days. A repeatedly negative test result therefore does not rule out parvoviral infection, but necessitates a consideration of other acute, febrile gastroenteritides (e.g., salmonellosis). This test is particularly valuable if there are epidemiologic considerations (e.g., breeding kennel).

An ELISA for detecting a *Giardia*-specific antigen in human feces (ProSpecT/Microplate ELISA assay for Giardia, Alexon, Inc., Sunnyvale, Calif) appears useful but has not been shown to clearly be more accurate than multiple zinc sulfate flotation examinations.

An ELISA for detecting cryptosporidial antigens in feces (ProSpecT Cryptosporidium Microplate Assay) appears to be more sensitive than fecal examinations. Rotavirus can also be detected in feces by ELISA. However, the finding is of uncertain significance in dogs, and the test has not been validated in these animals.

*Electron microscopy* can be used to identify various viral particles (e.g., coronavirus, astrovirus) in feces. Because the ELISA is usually adequate for detecting parvovirus, electron microscopy is rarely needed. However, it is indicated if other test results are not diagnostic and there are epidemiologic considerations. Fecal samples for electron microscopy analysis should be obtained early in the disease, because fecal viral concentrations may decrease dramatically within 7 to 14 days after the onset of signs. Furthermore, some delicate viruses (e.g., coronavirus) degenerate quickly, and the feces from animals suspected of having such an infection must be handled appropriately if meaningful results are to be obtained. Always contact your laboratory for instructions on sample handling.

An *assay for bacterial toxins* in feces may help implicate specific bacteria as causing diarrhea. Tests for *Clostridium perfringens* enterotoxin (Clostridium Perfringens Enterotoxin Test, TechLab Blacksburg, Va) and *Clostridium difficile* (ImmunoCard Toxin A, Meridan Diagnostics, Cincinnati, Ohio) toxins have been used for dogs. A single negative test result does not rule out either disease; one may need to perform the test two or three times before finding the toxin. Furthermore, not all animals that test positive for clostridial toxins have clinical signs of disease.

## BACTERIAL FECAL CULTURE

*Fecal culture* is seldom indicated in small animals unless a contagious disease is suspected or other test findings (e.g., endoscopy and biopsy) are nondiagnostic. Specific culture techniques for the detection of each pathogen are recommended. Therefore, contact the laboratory before submitting feces, tell them specifically what to culture for, and follow their instructions regarding the handling of specimens. Remember that fecal culture cannot be used to diagnose antibiotic-responsive enteropathy (ARE).

The pathogens most likely to be cultured from feces from small animals are *C. perfringens, C. difficile, Salmonella* spp., *Campylobacter jejuni, Yersinia enterocolitica,* and verotoxin-producing strains of *Escherichia coli.* These *E. coli* strains are often sorbitol negative. Confirmation of verotoxin production requires the use of either the polymerase chain reaction technique or a bioassay. *Aeromonas* spp. and *Plesiomonas* spp. may also cause diarrhea. However, the mere presence of any of these bacteria in an animal's feces does not confirm that they are causing disease. Culture results must be correlated with clinical signs and the results of other laboratory tests.

*Salmonella* spp. are best cultured by inoculating at least 1 g of fresh feces into an enrichment medium and subsequently a selective medium specific for *Salmonella* spp. One can sometimes culture *Salmonella* from the colonic mucosa in dogs with negative fecal findings. Recently a polymerase chain reaction technique has been used in the evaluation of equine feces and may be useful for the evaluation of canine and feline feces. To culture *C. jejuni,* very fresh feces must be inoculated onto selective media and incubated at approximately 40° C instead of 37° C. If inoculation is to be delayed, special transport media should be used, not routine commercial transport devices (e.g., culturette swabs).

*Candida* spp. are occasionally cultured from feces. The finding is often of uncertain significance, but the organisms may cause problems in some animals (e.g., those receiving chemotherapy).

## CYTOLOGIC EVALUATION OF FECES

Fecal cytologic evaluations may identify etiologic agents or inflammatory cells. In this method a thin, air-dried smear is stained with Gram's or a Romanowsky-type stain (e.g., Diff-Quick). The latter identifies cells better than Gram's stain does.

Finding excessive numbers of spore-forming bacteria (e.g., more than 3 to 4 per ×1000 field) was once thought to suggest clostridial colitis (see Fig. 33-1). However, recent work has found that the presence of spores is neither specific nor sensitive for clostridial colitis.

Short, curved, gram-negative rods (i.e., "commas" or "sea gull wings") are suggestive of campylobacteriosis. The larger spirochetes, which are often plentiful in diarrheic feces, are not *C. jejuni* and are of questionable pathogenicity. Although cytologic preparations are not critically analyzed in diarrheic small animals, fecal cytologic analysis for *Campylobacter* spp. is a specific, albeit insensitive, method in people. Fungal organisms (e.g., *Histoplasma capsulatum, Candida* spp.) are rarely found by fecal examination; cytologic examination of mucosal scrapings or histologic examination of biopsy specimens is usually necessary to diagnose histoplasmosis.

The finding of leukocytes in feces indicates the presence of a transmural colonic inflammation instead of just a superficial mucosal inflammation. However, a definitive diagnosis of a particular cause is not possible.

## RADIOGRAPHY OF THE ALIMENTARY TRACT

Imaging (i.e., radiography, ultrasonography) allows structures to be evaluated that cannot be adequately assessed during physical examination (e.g., esophagus, stomach) and may detect abnormalities missed by abdominal palpation (e.g., gastric mass, foreign object, splenic parenchymal mass). Plain radiographs should always be obtained before contrast-enhanced radiographs because (1) the former may yield diagnostic findings, (2) contrast-enhanced radiographs may be contraindicated, and (3) plain radiographs are needed to ensure a correct radiographic technique during the contrast

procedure. Contrast-enhanced radiographs may be able to delineate structures (e.g., a gastric outflow tract obstruction) that plain radiographs cannot.

Radiographs are generally useful in the diagnostic workup of animals with dysphagia, regurgitation, vomiting, abdominal mass or distention, abdominal pain, or acute abdomen. They are occasionally helpful in animals with constipation, weight loss, or anorexia of unknown cause, but other tests are usually indicated first in such animals and often render imaging unnecessary. Radiographic findings are rarely diagnostic in dogs or cats with diarrhea or copious abdominal effusion.

## ULTRASONOGRAPHY OF THE ALIMENTARY TRACT

Ultrasonography may be done in combination with or instead of radiography; however, it is extremely operator dependent. It is often useful in animals with an acute abdomen, abdominal effusion, vomiting, weight loss, or anorexia of unknown cause and also in those with an abdominal mass, distention, or pain. Ultrasonography can identify pancreatitis, infiltrations in various organs, and intussusceptions that radiography misses. Furthermore, effusions, which render radiographs useless, enhance ultrasonographic contrast. Ultrasonography can be more informative than radiography when determining whether an animal with an acute abdomen requires surgery. Finally, ultrasonography can be used to guide the percutaneous aspiration and biopsy of intraabdominal lesions that would otherwise necessitate surgery or laparoscopy.

### Techniques

A 5 MHz probe is probably the most utilitarian. Hair should be clipped so that there is no trapped air that could compromise the quality of the image. Fluid can be infused into the abdomen or stomach to improve the evaluation, but this is infrequently needed.

### Findings

The thickness, echodensity, and homogeneity of organs (e.g., liver, spleen, intestine, stomach, mesenteric lymph nodes, masses) may be assessed. Intraparenchymal infiltrates "invisible" to radiography may also be found. The particular ultrasonographic findings seen in specific disorders of the alimentary tract are discussed in subsequent chapters dealing with the disorders.

## IMAGING OF THE ORAL CAVITY, PHARYNX, AND ESOPHAGUS

### INDICATIONS

Any animal with dysphagia, oral pain, halitosis of unknown cause, or a swelling or mass should undergo imaging. If dysphagia of neuromuscular origin is suspected, dynamic studies (i.e., fluoroscopy) are recommended. Ultrasonography is particularly informative in the evaluation of any infiltrates or masses.

## Techniques

Anesthesia is necessary so that animals can be properly positioned for radiographs of the skull. Lateral, dorsoventral (DV), and oblique views are used if one is looking for foreign objects or fractures. Open-mouth ventrodorsal (VD) views and end-on views of the nose may also be helpful. However, dynamic studies (i.e., fluoroscopy, cinefluoroscopy) are necessary if one is looking for dysphagia of neuromuscular origin. These studies are performed by feeding conscious animals various forms of barium (i.e., liquid, paste, and mixed with food).

## Findings

Foreign objects, fractures, bone lysis, soft tissue masses or densities, and emphysema are commonly found. The bone surrounding the tooth roots should be examined for evidence of lysis and the temporomandibular joints for signs of arthritis. Remember the bilateral symmetry of the skull; compare one side with the other when evaluating the VD projection. When performing contrast-enhanced or dynamic studies, watch for the aspiration of barium, the strength with which the bolus is propelled into the esophagus, and the synchronization of the opening of the cricopharyngeal muscle with the pharyngeal phase of swallowing.

## INDICATIONS FOR IMAGING OF THE ESOPHAGUS

Indications for evaluating the esophagus include regurgitation (including pharyngeal dysphagia), pain when swallowing, unexplained recurrent pneumonia, and thoracic masses of undetermined origin. A barium contrast-enhanced esophagram is necessary unless plain films reveal the presence of an esophageal foreign object, evidence of esophageal perforation (e.g., a pleural effusion or pneumothorax), or an obvious hiatal hernia. Even if megaesophagus is present, a barium contrast procedure will show whether there is an obstruction at the lower esophageal sphincter (rare) or cricopharyngeal incompetence (worsens prognosis). Ultrasonography is seldom useful for dogs and cats with esophageal disease, unless there is a thoracic mass.

## Techniques

Liquid barium is the best contrast agent for esophageal studies; it provides excellent detail and, if aspirated, is not as noxious as paste or food. Be sure not to administer drugs that affect esophageal motility (e.g., xylazine, ketamine, anesthesia). The animal should take several swallows of barium from a syringe, after which right lateral and VD views are quickly obtained. If possible, perform fluoroscopy immediately after the animal has swallowed the barium to assess esophageal motility and look for gastroesophageal reflux and esophageal-pharyngeal reflux (i.e., cricopharyngeal incompetence). Radiographs may be taken if a lesion is found fluoroscopically. If fluoroscopy is not available, multiple radiographs (usually lateral projections) are taken in rapid succession, beginning very shortly (e.g., 5 to 10 seconds) after swallowing.

Barium paste is acceptable if liquid is not available. However, the aspiration of paste is generally more detrimental to the animal. Hypertonic, iodine-contrast agents do not achieve as good contrast as barium and cause severe problems if aspirated. Iohexol is a safe, albeit expensive, water-soluble iodine contrast agent that is not hypertonic. If radiographic studies performed with barium liquid or paste do not detect an abnormality in an animal in which esophageal disease is strongly suspected, the study should be repeated using a mixture of barium and food (both canned food and dry kibble). Such studies may detect partial strictures or muscular weakness not found in previous studies.

If barium is retained in the esophagus but little or none enters the stomach, the animal should be held in a vertical position so that gravity facilitates the migration of barium into the stomach. If barium readily enters the stomach, this indicates that there is no lower esophageal sphincter obstruction. If a hiatal hernia is suspected but not seen, a lateral radiograph of the caudal thorax may be taken while the abdomen is manually compressed. This is done to try to force the stomach to herniate into the thorax so that the hernia can be demonstrated.

If esophageal disease seems likely but is not found by static radiographs, fluoroscopic studies are required. The esophagus may need to be observed for several minutes (or longer) before some abnormalities (e.g., gastroesophageal or esophageal-pharyngeal reflux) occur. In animals with marginal esophageal disease, fluoroscopy may be necessary to document that primary or secondary esophageal waves are present but not readily stimulated.

If an esophageal perforation is suspected (e.g., septic pleuritis or mediastinitis, pneumomediastinum or pneumothorax), an iodine contrast medium (preferably iohexol) may be used. However, the only purpose of such a study is to localize the perforation. If one already knows where the leakage is likely to be (e.g., there is a bone foreign body in the esophagus), radiographs are of dubious value; exploratory surgery would be a better option in this instance.

## Findings

Esophageal dilation, foreign objects, soft tissue densities, spondylosis suggestive of spirocercosis, and hiatal hernia may often be identified on plain films. An air-filled esophagus is not always diagnostic of pathologic esophageal weakness. Although it is tempting to use plain radiograph findings as the basis for the diagnosis of esophageal disease when there is an "obvious" abnormality, it is easy to misinterpret plain films or miss abnormalities that a barium contrast-enhanced study reveals. Even the finding of a dilated, gas-filled esophagus on plain thoracic films does not definitively diagnose "megaesophagus." Rarely animals seen to have a dilated, air-filled esophagus on plain films are found to have normal esophageal function when evaluated with barium contrast-enhanced radiographs (Fig. 29-1). Likewise, the appearance of an accumulation of

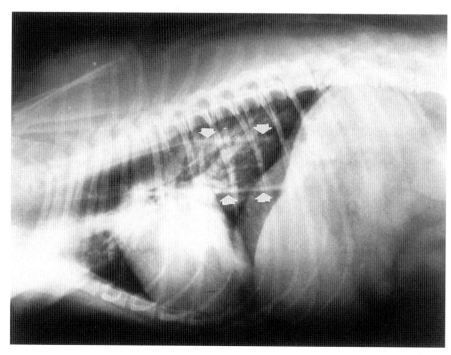

**FIG 29-1**
Lateral thoracic radiograph from a dog that was seen because of coughing. Note the dilated, air-filled esophagus in the caudal thorax *(arrows)*. Lateral radiograph and contrast-enhanced esophagram (with fluoroscopy) obtained 2 days later documented normal esophageal size and function.

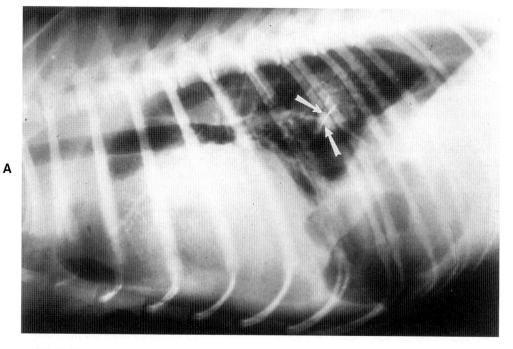

**FIG 29-2**
**A,** Lateral thoracic radiograph from a dog with a foreign object in the esophagus *(arrows)*. Note the concomitant pleural effusion. A chicken bone had perforated the esophagus, and septic pleuritis was present. (**A** from Allen D, editor: *Small animal medicine*, Philadelphia, 1991, JB Lippincott.)

*Continued*

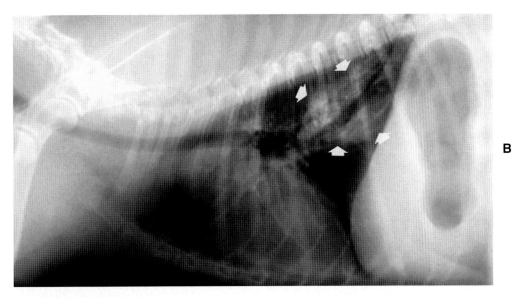

B

**FIG 29-2, cont'd**
**B,** Lateral thoracic radiograph from a dog with a pork bone in the esophagus. The density representing the bone *(arrows)* is more diffuse than was seen in **A** and looks more like a pulmonary parenchymal density than a bone.

foodlike material in the classic location for a vascular ring anomaly may be caused by a localized esophageal weakness or a thymic cyst.

Many foreign objects in the esophagus (e.g., bones) can be seen on plain radiographs. However, excellent radiographic technique is necessary, because some bones (especially poultry bones) as well as rawhide treats are relatively radiolucent (Fig. 29-2). An esophageal perforation sometimes causes pneumothorax, emphysematous mediastinitis, or a pleural or mediastinal effusion.

Contrast-enhanced esophagrams should be considered in animals with suspected esophageal disease and in those with unidentified thoracic masses, because many esophageal tumors radiographically resemble pulmonary parenchymal masses (see Fig. 31-5). Contrast-enhanced esophagrams may also show that structures that seemingly involve the esophagus actually do not. An obstruction is suggested on contrast-enhanced esophagrams if the barium column terminates abruptly as it travels caudally; weakness causes contrast to be retained throughout the esophagus (Fig. 29-3). A partial obstruction is suggested by the retention of barium-impregnated food but not of liquid or paste (see Fig. 31-4).

A barium contrast study may reveal malpositioning (e.g., hiatal hernia; see Fig. 31-2). However, the finding of a properly positioned structure on one study does not ensure that it will stay properly positioned (e.g., some hiatal hernias slide in and out of the diaphragm and may be normally positioned when the radiograph is taken). Gastroesophageal reflux and esophagitis may also be difficult to diagnose radiographically. Barium may adhere to a severely diseased mucosa, but less severe esophagitis may not be detected. In addition, normal dogs may have an episode of gastro-esophageal reflux during a contrast study, whereas dogs with pathologic gastroesophageal reflux may not have reflux during the examination.

If the animal is believed to be regurgitating but the barium contrast-enhanced radiographs are unrevealing, either the assessment of regurgitation is wrong or there is occult disease, in which case reexamination of the esophagus with fluoroscopy or endoscopy must be done.

## IMAGING OF THE STOMACH AND SMALL INTESTINE

### INDICATIONS FOR RADIOGRAPHIC IMAGING OF THE ABDOMEN WITHOUT CONTRAST MEDIA

Indications for plain abdominal radiography may include vomiting, acute abdomen, constipation, abdominal pain, enlargement, distention, or a mass. Plain radiographs are rarely beneficial in animals with a marked abdominal effusion (the fluid obliterates serosal detail) or with chronic diarrhea. Plain radiography is often not as cost-effective when the abdomen can be palpated thoroughly (i.e., many cats) as when the area is difficult to examine (e.g., large or obese animals or animals in pain). In vomiting animals, plain abdominal radiographs are most useful in detecting meager amounts of abdominal fluid or alimentary tract dilation resulting from obstruction, foreign objects, or masses.

### Techniques

Always obtain two radiographic views, usually right lateral and VD projections. Cleansing enemas may improve the

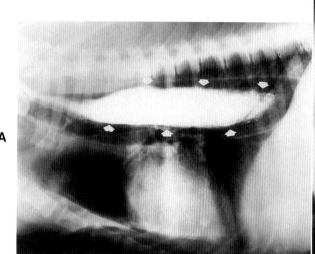
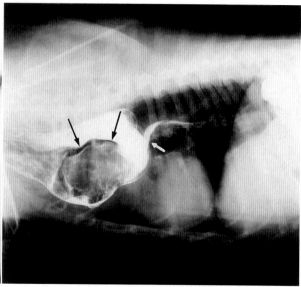

**FIG 29-3**
**A,** Lateral thoracic contrast-enhanced esophagram from a dog with generalized esophageal weakness. Note that barium is retained throughout the length of the esophagus *(arrows).*
**B,** Lateral thoracic contrast-enhanced radiograph of a dog with an esophageal obstruction caused by a vascular ring anomaly. The column of barium stops abruptly *(short arrow)* in front of the heart, a finding characteristic of a persistent fourth aortic arch. A filling defect is also displacing barium in the dilated portion of the esophagus *(long arrows).* (Courtesy Dr. Phillip F. Steyn, Colorado State University, Fort Collins, Colo.)

diagnostic usefulness of radiographs; however, a critically ill animal or one with an acute abdomen generally should not have an enema unless plain radiographs show it is necessary.

## Findings

Plain abdominal radiographs may detect masses, foreign objects, a gas- or fluid-distended hollow viscus, misshapen or emphysematous parenchymal organs, pneumoperitoneum, abdominal effusions, and displaced organs suggestive of a mass or adhesion.

A gastric outflow tract obstruction can be difficult to diagnose on the basis of plain radiograph findings unless there is marked gastric distention (Fig. 29-4) or foreign objects are seen. However, gastric dilation, especially with volvulus, is easily recognized (see Fig. 32-4). Radiolucent gastric foreign objects may be seen if swallowed air outlines them.

An intestinal obstruction is usually easier to diagnose on the basis of plain radiograph findings than is a gastric obstruction; obstructed intestines typically become distended with air, fluid, or ingesta. However, intestinal distention (i.e., ileus) may be caused by inflammation (i.e., adynamic or physiologic ileus) as well as obstruction (i.e., mechanical, occlusive, or anatomic ileus). Anatomic ileus (i.e., obstruction) typically produces a nonuniform intestinal distention with a greater degree of distention than is seen with physiologic ileus (Fig. 29-5). If "stacking" of the distended intestines or sharp bends and turns in the dilated intestines are seen, this also suggests the presence of an anatomic ileus. Lateral radio-

graphs obtained with the animal standing rarely aid in differentiating anatomic from physiologic ileus. Even experienced radiologists occasionally misdiagnose physiologic ileus as representing an obstruction. Thus diseases producing severe inflammation (e.g., parvoviral enteritis) may clinically and radiographically mimic an intestinal obstruction.

Special types of intestinal obstruction are associated with unique radiographic findings. If the entire intestinal tract is uniformly distended with gas (Fig. 29-6) and the clinical signs fit, mesenteric volvulus may be diagnosed. If marked intestinal distention is found but is very localized and seems out of place (e.g., has herniated), a strangulated or incarcerated intestinal obstruction (see Fig. 33-8) should be considered.

Linear foreign bodies may cause a much different radiographic pattern. They rarely produce gas-distended bowel loops. Instead, they tend to cause the intestines to bunch together, and sometimes small gas bubbles are present (see Fig. 33-9). This occurs because the intestines "gather" around the linear foreign object as they try to propel it abroad. Such bunching usually prevents the intestines from filling with gas. Sometimes pleated (i.e., "accordian-like") intestines can be seen on plain radiographs.

It is difficult to determine the thickness of intestines on plain radiographs. Animals with diarrhea and an increased amount of intestinal fluid are often misdiagnosed as having thickened intestinal walls.

There are other important radiographic findings. Decreased serosal contrast is due to either lack of fat or excessive

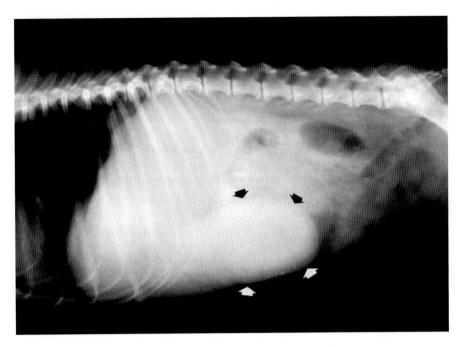

**FIG 29-4**
Plain lateral radiograph from a dog with gastric outflow obstruction. Note the dilated stomach protruding past the costal arch *(arrows)*.

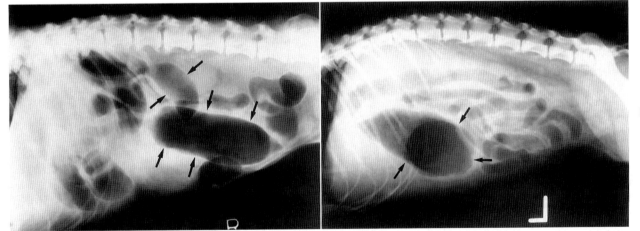

**FIG 29-5**
**A,** Plain lateral abdominal radiograph from a dog with an intestinal obstruction causing intestinal distention. Note the markedly increased diameter of the small intestinal lumen *(arrows)*. **B,** Plain lateral abdominal radiograph from a dog with peritonitis causing physiologic ileus. Note the lesser degree of small intestinal distention compared with that in **A.** The large gas-filled structure is the gastric pylorus *(arrows)*. (Courtesy Dr. Kenita Rogers, Texas A&M University, College Station, Tex.)

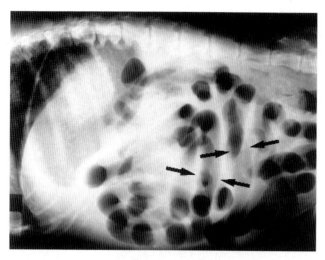

**FIG 29-6**
Lateral abdominal radiograph from a dog that had an acute onset of vomiting, abdominal pain, and shock. There is a uniform intestinal distention that is not as great as that in Fig. 29-5, *A*. However, distention is more than that seen in Fig. 29-5, *B*. Some intestinal loops have assumed a vertical orientation *(arrows)*, which suggests the existence of an obstruction. This dog had a mesenteric volvulus. (Courtesy Dr. Susan Yanoff, U.S. Military.)

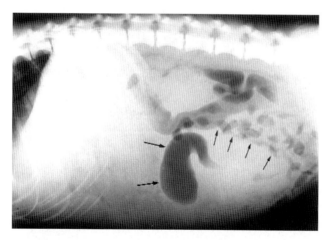

**FIG 29-7**
Lateral abdominal radiograph from a dog with a large granuloma caused by pythiosis. Small intestinal loops are displaced dorsally and caudally *(small arrows)*. The border of the mass is not discernible except where it displaces small intestinal loops. The finding of a dilated intestinal loop *(long arrows)* is consistent with obstruction.

abdominal fluid (see Chapter 36). Fig. 29-7 shows an example of a mass displacing intestines. Pneumoperitoneum is diagnosed if one can easily see both the thoracic and abdominal surfaces of the diaphragm or the serosal surfaces of the liver, stomach, or kidneys (see Fig. 34-1, *A*). Pneumoperitoneum may also be documented by the finding of only a few gas bubbles in the peritoneal cavity (see Fig. 34-1, *B*).

## INDICATIONS FOR ULTRASONOGRAPHY OF THE STOMACH AND SMALL INTESTINES

Ultrasonography usually reveals almost any soft tissue change that plain radiographs detect, plus infiltrations that radiographs cannot detect. Ultrasonography is useful for detecting intussusceptions, pancreatitis, abdominal infiltrative disease, and small amounts of effusion not seen radiographically; for evaluating the hepatic parenchyma; and for identifying abdominal neoplasia in animals with a substantial effusion. Ultrasonography is much more revealing than radiography in animals with minimal body fat that have little or no radiographic contrast in the abdomen. However, very dehydrated animals may be difficult to image. The skill of the ultrasonographer determines the usefulness of the technique.

### Technique

Before ultrasonography is performed, the abdominal hair usually should be clipped to improve the quality of the examination. In animals with minimal hair, this is not necessary. Because air in the stomach or intestines limits the usefulness of ultrasonography, exercise or drugs (e.g., some narcotics) that cause hyperventilation and enemas should be avoided prior to the examination.

### Findings

Ultrasonography should detect almost any soft tissue change that plain radiographs detect, plus gastric and intestinal infiltrates (Fig. 29-8, *A*), intussusceptions (Fig. 29-8, *B*), enlarged lymph nodes (Fig. 29-8, *C*), masses (Fig. 29-8, *D*), some radiolucent foreign objects, and small amounts of free peritoneal fluid that radiographs cannot detect. If tissue infiltrates are found, they can sometimes be aspirated by the fine-needle technique, using ultrasonography for guidance.

## INDICATIONS FOR CONTRAST-ENHANCED GASTROGRAMS

Contrast-enhanced gastrography is principally performed in vomiting animals when ultrasound studies and plain abdominal radiographs are unrevealing. It is primarily used to detect a gastric outflow tract obstruction and gastric masses.

### Technique

The animal should not be allowed to eat for at least 12 hours (preferably 24 hours), and feces should be removed with enemas. Plain radiographs should be obtained immediately before the contrast-enhanced films to verify that the abdomen has been properly prepared and the radiographic technique is correct and to determine if the diagnosis cannot be made on the basis of the plain radiograph findings. Liquid barium sulfate is then administered (8 to 10 ml/kg in small dogs and cats and 5 to 8 ml/kg in large dogs). Iohexol can be administered (i.e., 700 to 875 mg I/kg, which is about 1¼ to 1½ ml/lb). The agent should be administered via a stomach tube to ensure adequate gastric filling and optimal evaluation of the stomach. The animal should not receive motility-altering drugs (e.g., xylazine, parasympatholytics), which delay outflow.

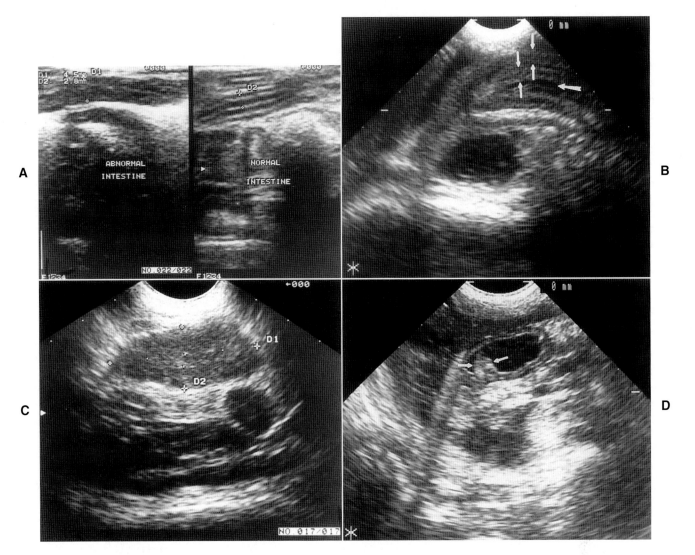

**FIG 29-8**
**A,** Ultrasonographic image of two sections of small intestine from a cat with an alimentary tract lymphoma. The normal intestine on the right is 2.8 mm thick (see the two "+'s" noted as D2), whereas the abnormal intestine on the left is 4.5 mm thick (D1) because of neoplastic infiltrates. **B,** Ultrasonographic image of an ileocolic intussusception that was not obvious on plain abdominal radiographs. There are two intestinal walls *(small arrows)* seen on each side of the lumen *(large arrow).* **C,** An enlarged mesenteric lymph node in a dog caused by lymphoma, seen by ultrasonography. The lymph node was not detected on radiographs or by abdominal palpation. **D,** Ultrasound image of the gastric antrum from a dog with benign gastric polyps. One polyp can be seen *(arrows)* protruding into the gastric lumen. (Courtesy Dr. Linda Homco, Cornell University, Ithaca, N.Y.)

Immediately after barium administration, radiographs are taken in the left and right lateral plus DV and VD projections. Radiographs in the lateral and DV projections should be obtained again at 15 and 30 minutes and perhaps also at 1 to 3 hours. The right lateral view causes barium to pool in the pylorus, the left lateral view causes it to pool in the gastric body, the DV view causes it to pool along the greater curvature, and the VD view allows better evaluation of the pylorus and antrum. Double-contrast gastrograms provide more detail and are often more informative than single-contrast gastro-grams. They are performed by giving barium via a stomach tube, then removing most of the barium through the same tube and insufflating the stomach with gas until it is mildly distended.

If available, fluoroscopy is best performed immediately after administration of the barium. It can be used to evaluate gastric motility, gastric outflow, and the maximal opening size of the pylorus. If the animal is fed barium mixed with food (only recommended if gastric outflow tract obstruction is suspected despite normal liquid barium study findings), gastric emptying will be markedly delayed compared with that seen when the animal is fed liquid barium.

## Findings

Gastric emptying is considered delayed if liquid barium does not enter the duodenum 15 to 30 minutes after administration or if the stomach fails to almost completely empty a liquid barium meal in 3 hours (see Fig. 32-2). Luminal filling defects (e.g., growths and radiolucent foreign objects), ulcers, pyloric lesions preventing gastric emptying, and infiltrative lesions may be seen using this method (see Fig. 32-2, *C*). However, normal peristalsis, ingesta, or gas bubbles may resemble an abnormality; therefore a change must be seen on *at least* two separate films before one can diagnose disease.

Contrast-enhanced gastrograms are not as sensitive as endoscopy for detecting gastric ulceration, and they cannot detect erosions. Ulcers are documented radiographically if barium is seen to enter the gastric or duodenal wall or if a persistent spot of barium is identified in the stomach long after the organ has emptied itself of the contrast agent (see Fig. 32-6). The duodenum should be scrutinized in a search for constrictions and infiltrative lesions, because many vomiting animals have disease there (e.g., inflammatory bowel disease, tumors) rather than in the stomach (see Chapter 33).

## INDICATIONS FOR CONTRAST-ENHANCED STUDIES OF THE SMALL INTESTINE

Vomiting is the principal reason for performing contrast studies of the upper small intestine. Contrast-enhanced radiographs are particularly useful for distinguishing anatomic from physiologic ileus. Orad obstructions are easier to demonstrate than aborad ones if the contrast medium is administered orally. If a very aborad obstruction is suspected (e.g., ileocolic intussusception), a barium enema (or preferably ultrasonography) is better than an upper gastrointestinal contrast series. Although linear foreign objects usually produce subtle findings on plain radiographs, they often cause a classic "pleating" of the intestines to be seen on contrast films (see Fig. 33-9, *C*).

Animals with diarrhea seldom benefit appreciably from contrast studies of the intestines. This is because normal radiographic findings do not exclude the presence of severe intestinal disease, and even if radiographic findings indicate the presence of infiltrative disease, it is still necessary to obtain a biopsy specimen to determine the cause. Contrast series are sometimes useful if the clinician is trying to decide whether to perform abdominal surgery. However, it is usually more cost-effective to perform endoscopy (or even surgery) and skip the contrast-enhanced radiographs.

Use of iodinated contrast agents (preferably iohexol) is reasonable if an alimentary tract perforation is suspected. However, if spontaneous septic peritonitis is strongly suspected, it is usually far better to perform a thorough exploratory laparotomy than contrast-enhanced radiography.

## Technique

Liquid barium sulfate is administered as described for contrast-enhanced gastrography. Lateral and VD radiographs should be obtained immediately and then 30, 60, and 120 minutes after barium administration. Additional films are obtained as necessary. The study is completed once contrast has reached the colon. If chemical restraint is absolutely necessary, acetylpromazine may be used. Fluoroscopy is rarely needed for these studies.

Hypertonic iodinated contrast agents are inferior to barium for small intestinal studies. This is because they decrease the intestinal transit time and can cause considerable fluid shifts by osmotically drawing fluid into the gastrointestinal tract. Although they are safer in the setting of perforation, the advantages of their use rarely outweigh the disadvantages. Although iohexol is safer and produces better detail than the hypertonic iodinated compounds, it is more expensive.

## Findings

In a complete intestinal obstruction, the barium column cannot advance beyond a certain point. A partial obstruction may be denoted by delayed passage past a certain point (there may or may not be dilation of the intestines orad to this point) or constriction of the lumen. Because it is easy to overinterpret contrast-enhanced radiographs of the intestines, changes must be seen on *at least* two different films taken at different times before a disease is diagnosed.

"Enteritis" is often diagnosed if a fine "brush border" in the lumen is found. However, this finding actually results from the barium normally distributing itself among villi, not from enteritis. Infiltration is denoted by scalloped margins (sometimes called *thumb-printing*); such a pattern (Fig. 29-9, *A*) may be seen in the setting of neoplasia (e.g., lymphoma), inflammatory bowel disease (e.g., lymphocytic-plasmacytic or eosinophilic enteritis), fungal infection (e.g., histoplasmosis), or parvoviral enteritis. However, its absence does not rule out the presence of infiltrative disease. Focal dilations not caused by obstruction (i.e., diverticula) are rare and usually represent a localized neoplastic infiltrate (Fig. 29-9, *B*). In rare instances, unsuspected intestinal blind loops or short-bowel syndromes may be detected. Motility problems may cause slowed passage of the contrast through the alimentary tract.

## INDICATIONS FOR BARIUM CONTRAST ENEMAS

If flexible colonoscopy is available, there is seldom any need for barium enemas. If only rigid colonoscopy is available, barium enemas are used to evaluate the ascending and transverse colon, areas inaccessible to rigid scopes. If colonoscopy is unavailable, a barium enema may be useful for looking for infiltrative lesions (e.g., rectal-colonic neoplasia causing hematochezia), a partial or complete obstruction, or ileocolic or cecocolic intussusception. It can also evaluate the colon orad to a near-complete rectal obstruction to determine whether there are more infiltrative lesions or obstructions besides the one palpated near the rectum.

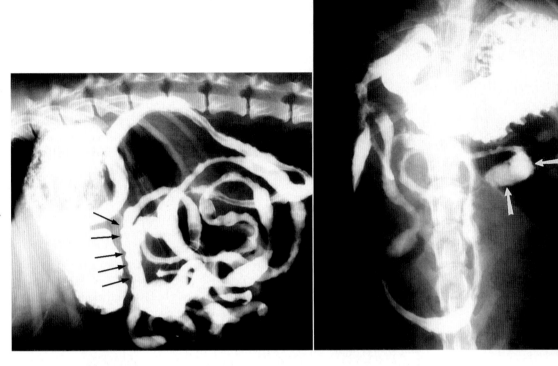

**FIG 29-9**
**A,** Lateral contrast-enhanced radiograph from a dog with duodenal lymphoma. Note the scalloped appearance to the margin of the small intestine *(arrows)*. **B,** Ventrodorsal projection shows a section of small intestine to be dilated *(arrows)*. This dilation was seen on repeated films. There was no obstruction; the dilation was caused by neoplastic infiltration of the intestine.

## Technique

The colon must be emptied and cleaned by enemas or alimentary tract lavage solutions, or both. The animal should be anesthetized and a balloon-tipped catheter placed in the colon. The balloon is then inflated so that barium cannot leak out the rectum. Seven to 10 ml of liquid barium/kg at body temperature is infused into the colon until it is uniformly distended, and lateral and VD radiographs are obtained. The colon may then be emptied of barium and insufflated with air to achieve a double-contrast barium enema, which provides greater detail. If too much barium is administered, the ileum may fill with the contrast agent, obscuring colonic detail and making the study less useful.

## Findings

Barium enemas unreliably detect mucosal disease (i.e., ulcers, inflammation). If the animal has been properly prepared, they can reveal intraluminal filling defects representing ileocolic or cecocolic intussusception (see Fig. 33-10), proliferative colonic neoplasia (e.g., polyps, adenocarcinoma), extraluminal compression denoted by smooth-surfaced displacement of the barium from the colonic lumen (Fig. 29-10, *A*), and infiltrative disease (i.e., a roughened, partial obstruction or an "ap-

ple core" lesion) (Fig. 29-10, *B*). However, it is imperative that a change be found on *at least* two films to be sure it is not an artifact.

## PERITONEAL FLUID ANALYSIS

Fluid analysis is discussed in detail on p. 491. The fluid is obtained by performing abdominocentesis with a syringe and needle. If this fails to retrieve fluid, fluid is obtained with a multifenestrated catheter (e.g., a dialysis catheter, a sterile teat cannula, or an 18-gauge cephalic catheter with additional holes cut with a scalpel). It is sometimes best to allow fluid to drain out of the catheter without applying negative pressure.

If peritoneal inflammation is suspected but abdominal fluid cannot be retrieved, a diagnostic peritoneal lavage may be performed. In this method a sterile catheter (preferably with multiple fenestrations) is inserted into the abdomen and warm, sterile physiologic saline solution (20 ml/kg) is administered rapidly. The abdomen is massaged vigorously for 1 to 2 minutes, and then some of the fluid is aspirated. The aspirate is evaluated cytologically.

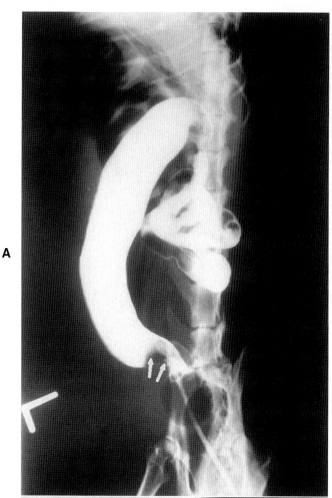

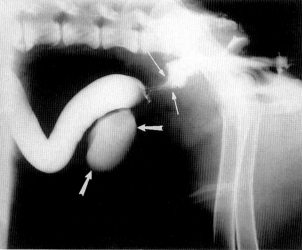

**FIG 29-10**
**A,** Oblique view of a constipated cat that has received a barium enema. Note the smooth filling defect caused by an extraluminal band of fibrous connective tissue *(arrows)*.
**B,** Lateral view of a dog that had a barium enema. There is circumferential narrowing with roughened borders *(thin arrows)* that is in distinction to the rest of the colon. This dog had infiltrative adenocarcinoma, which caused an obstruction. The urinary bladder is also seen as a result of the previous contrast procedure *(thick arrows)*.

## DIGESTION AND ABSORPTION TESTS

Exocrine pancreatic function may be tested by measuring fecal proteolytic activity (not recommended), fat absorption with and without pancreatic enzymes (not recommended), or serum TLI (recommended).

*Fat absorption testing* is simple but of questionable sensitivity and specificity. In this test, fat (e.g., 3 ml of corn oil/kg) is administered orally to a nonlipemic, fasting animal, and the blood is checked for lipemia every 1 to 2 hours for up to 5 hours by examining the plasma in a microhematocrit tube. If the plasma becomes obviously lipemic, EPI (and perhaps severe malabsorption) is tentatively ruled out. If lipemia does not occur, the test is repeated but with pancreatic enzyme powder added to the fat before it is administered. If lipemia then develops, the tentative diagnosis is EPI. If lipemia still does not occur, then malabsorptive disease is tentatively diagnosed. There should be an obvious lipemia before one can say that fat has been absorbed.

*Serum TLI* is the most sensitive and specific test for EPI, plus it is convenient (i.e., submit 1 ml of refrigerated serum obtained after an overnight fast) and readily available. The TLI assay detects circulating proteins produced by a normally functioning exocrine pancreas and is even valid in animals receiving pancreatic enzyme supplements orally. Pancreatitis, renal failure, and severe malnutrition may increase the serum TLI concentrations, but this rarely causes results to be misinterpreted. However, if EPI is caused by obstruction of the pancreatic ducts (apparently rare) as opposed to acinar cell atrophy (common), the serum TLI test may not detect maldigestion. In such cases, a quantitative fecal proteolytic assay is required.

Normal dogs have serum TLI activities of 5.2 to 35 μg/L. Values of less than 2.5 μg/L confirm a diagnosis of EPI. Normal cats have higher values (28 to 115 μg/L). The serum TLI assay is primarily indicated in dogs with chronic small intestinal diarrhea or chronic weight loss of unknown origin. Feline EPI is rare, therefore the test is seldom necessary in cats. Although principally used to detect EPI, serum TLI values substantially greater than normal are suggestive of pancreatitis.

## SERUM CONCENTRATIONS OF VITAMINS

*Serum concentrations of cobalamin and folate* are sometimes measured in animals with chronic small intestinal diarrhea or chronic weight loss. These tests may provide evidence of antibiotic-responsive enteropathy (ARE) or severe small intestinal mucosal disease. Dietary cobalamin is absorbed in the intestine, principally the ileum. When ARE is present, bacteria sometimes bind cobalamin and prevent its absorption, decreasing the serum concentrations. Cobalamin concentrations are usually decreased in dogs with EPI, possibly because of the high incidence of ARE in such animals. Severe mucosal disease, especially in the region of the ileum, may also cause serum cobalamin concentrations to be decreased, ostensibly because of malabsorption of the vitamin. Perhaps the major indication for this test is to look for evidence of intestinal disease in the patient with weight loss of uncertain cause. If the serum cobalamin is low, there is a high likelihood that small intestinal disease is responsible for the weight loss. B-complex vitamin supplementation is a reason for an increased serum cobalamin concentration.

Dietary folate is absorbed in the small intestine. If there are many bacteria in the upper small intestine, these sometimes synthesize and release folate, causing the serum concentrations to be increased. Likewise, severe intestinal mucosal disease may decrease absorption, causing lower serum concentrations. B-complex vitamin supplementation may increase serum folate concentrations.

Bright light degrades cobalamin, therefore samples should be frozen and kept in the dark during storage and transport. Although the specificity of a combination of decreased serum cobalamin and increased folate concentrations is high for ARE, the sensitivity is questionable because animals with ARE have been found, which have normal concentrations of these vitamins.

## OTHER SPECIAL TESTS FOR ALIMENTARY TRACT DISEASE

*Intestinal permeability testing* can be performed to determine the presence or absence of small intestinal disease. A solution with 2 to 5 sugars is administered after a fast, and either a blood sample or a urine sample is obtained (usually 6 hours later). The ratio and amounts of various sugars are determined, and from this one may ascertain whether there is normal or increased permeability of the small intestines. Finding increased permeability seems to be a reliable marker of small intestinal disease, but at this time one cannot diagnose a patient with increased small intestinal permeability as having a particular disease. Currently, the major value to such testing seems to be (1) determining that a patient with clinical signs of uncertain cause has small intestinal disease and (2) evaluating response to therapy in difficult to manage patients.

*Serum gastrin concentrations* are measured in animals with signs suggestive of gastrinoma (i.e., chronic vomiting, weight loss, and diarrhea in older animals, especially if there is concurrent esophagitis or duodenal ulceration). Gastrin is normally produced by pancreatic and alimentary tract G cells. It stimulates gastric acid secretion and is trophic for the gastric mucosa. Serum for assay of gastrin is harvested from an animal after an overnight fast and rapidly frozen.

The serum gastrin concentration may be increased in animals with gastrinoma, a gastric outflow tract obstruction, renal failure, short-bowel syndrome, or atrophic gastritis and in those receiving antacid therapy (e.g., $H_2$-receptor antagonist and proton pump inhibitors). Resting serum gastrin concentrations may vary, with occasional values in the normal range in animals with gastrinoma. Provocative testing is more sensitive in establishing the diagnosis than baseline serum gastrin concentrations and should be considered in dogs suspected of having gastrinoma but with normal baseline serum gastrin concentrations. The dog may be fed a meat-based meal and the serum gastrin concentrations measured 5, 15, 30, 45, and 60 minutes later. Alternatively, sequential serum gastrin concentrations can be determined after intravenous injection of secretin or calcium (gastrinoma is associated with paradoxic increases in the serum gastrin concentration; see Chapter 52).

*Testing for urease activity in gastric mucosa* is sometimes done if one is looking for a *Helicobacter* sp., a bacterium with strong urease activity. To perform this, one or preferably two fresh pieces of gastric mucosa are placed into urease agar and observed for up to 24 hours. If these urease-producing bacteria are present, their enzyme will split the urea in the agar into ammonia and the pH indicator in the agar will change from amber to pink (sometimes this occurs within 15 minutes). Tubes of urease agar may be obtained from microbiologic supply houses. There are also special kits designed to detect *Helicobacter* spp. In dogs and cats, there is no good evidence that this test is more advantageous than special staining (e.g., Warthin-Starry) of multiple gastric biopsy specimens.

*Antibodies to acetylcholine receptors* should be measured if one is looking for a cause of dysphagia or esophageal weakness that could be of neuromuscular origin (see p. 1059). Serum is obtained and sent to a laboratory that can perform a validated assay for the species being evaluated. Increased titers to such antibodies are strongly suggestive of a myasthenia-like disease, even if there are no systemic signs. False-positive results are rare. Testing can be done by Dr. Diane Shelton (Comparative Neuromuscular Laboratory, Basic Science Building, University of California at San Diego, La Jolla, CA 92093-0612).

Measurement of *antibodies to 2M muscle fibers* can be helpful in dogs with suspected masticatory muscle myositis (see p. 1062). These antibodies are typically not found in dogs with polymyositis, whereas most dogs with masticatory myositis have them. Serum is required for the test and can be sent to Dr. Diane Shelton for testing.

## ENDOSCOPY

Endoscopy is often cost-effective if radiographic and ultrasonographic findings have been nondiagnostic in animals with chronic vomiting, diarrhea, or weight loss. It permits rapid exploration of selected sections of the alimentary tract and mucosal biopsy without the need for a thoracotomy or laparotomy. Although excellent for detecting morphologic changes (e.g., masses, ulcers, obstruction), it is insensitive for revealing abnormal function (e.g., esophageal weakness).

Rigid endoscopy is easier to perform and less expensive than flexible endoscopy, and it provides excellent biopsy samples. Flexible endoscopes can be used to examine structures that cannot be inspected with a rigid endoscope. However, flexible instruments are expensive, and it takes time to become proficient at using them. In addition, even a trained clinician using an excellent scope is limited by how far the instrument can be advanced. Furthermore, tissue samples obtained through a flexible endoscope may have artifacts or may be too small to yield diagnostic findings unless one's technique is excellent.

*Esophagoscopy* is indicated in dogs and cats with suspected or confirmed esophageal masses, obstruction, esophagitis, or regurgitation that is difficult to diagnose. Animals must be anesthetized for the procedure.

Esophageal tumors (Fig. 29-11), foreign objects (Fig. 29-12), inflammation (Figs. 29-13 and 29-14), and obstructions caused by cicatrix (Fig. 29-15) are readily diagnosed using esophagoscopy. Foreign objects and cicatrix are preferentially treated endoscopically to avoid postoperative morbidity. Esophagoscopy may also show partial obstructions not detected by contrast esophagrams. It is important in such procedures to enter the stomach and retroflex the scope's tip to view the lower esophageal sphincter area to detect leiomyomas (Fig. 29-16) or other easily missed lesions. If esophageal mucosal biopsy specimens are desired, flexible endoscopes are typically inadequate for obtaining them unless there is a tumor, because the esophageal lumen is covered with squamous epithelium, which cannot be pulled off with typical flexible endoscopic forceps.

Although esophagoscopy may occasionally detect esophageal weakness (Fig. 29-17), it is not sensitive for detecting this and other selected disorders (e.g., diverticula, hiatal hernia). Not all foreign objects can be safely removed endoscopically, and one must guard against rupturing a diseased esophagus while trying to extract an object. Finally, care must be taken to avoid creating a potentially fatal tension pneumothorax in animals with an esophageal perforation.

Although flexible endoscopy is easier to perform, rigid endoscopy may be more useful in removing foreign objects because a rigid endoscope can protect the esophagus from laceration during extraction of the object. Care must be taken to maintain the animal's esophagus as straight as possible during extraction. If a flexible endoscope is used, it is often helpful to pass it through a rigid scope or tube that has been passed through the cricopharyngeal sphincter; this may facilitate passage of the foreign object through the sphincter.

*Gastroduodenoscopy and biopsy* are indicated in animals with vomiting, apparent gastroduodenal reflux, or small intestinal disease. It is more sensitive and specific than radiography for detecting mucosal ulcers (Fig. 29-18), erosions (Fig. 29-19), tumors (Fig. 29-20), and inflammatory lesions (Figs. 29-21 to 29-23). Endoscopy is also quicker and less stressful to the animal than exploratory laparotomy. Many foreign objects in the gastrointestinal tract (Fig. 29-24) can be removed using endoscopy, and multiple biopsy specimens can be ob-

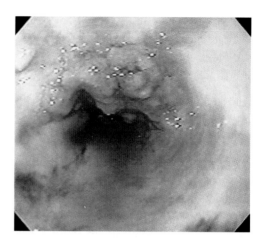

**FIG 29-11**
Endoscopic view of a polypoid mass in the esophagus of a Chow. This represents an adenocarcinoma.

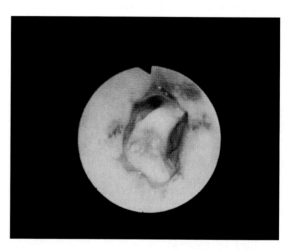

**FIG 29-12**
Endoscopic view of the esophagus of a dog with a chicken neck bone lodged in it. The bone was ultimately removed with a rigid scope and alligator forceps.

tained without danger to the animal. Occasionally, unexpected diagnoses (e.g., *Physaloptera* infection) (Fig. 29-25) may be found. It may be necessary to use endoscopes with outer diameters of 9 mm or less in dogs and cats weighing less than 4 to 5 kg. Whenever possible, a scope with a 2.8-mm biopsy channel should be used to obtain larger specimens and allow the use of better foreign object retrieval devices.

The stomach needs to be empty when gastroduodenoscopy is performed, which usually necessitates at least a 24-hour fast; many animals undergoing gastroscopy may not empty their stomachs as rapidly as normal. During the procedure the stomach must be adequately inflated with air to allow thorough evaluation of its mucosa. Suction must be available to remove secretions or air. The endoscopist must inspect the mucosa methodically to avoid missing lesions. It is particularly easy to miss lesions (e.g., ulcers or *Physa-*

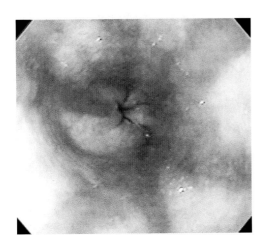

**FIG 29-13**
Endoscopic view of the lower esophageal sphincter of a dog with moderately severe reflux esophagitis secondary to vomiting. Note the hyperemic areas.

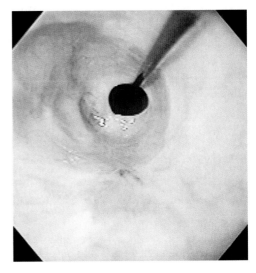

**FIG 29-15**
Endoscopic view of the same site as in Fig. 29-13, but 10 days later. A narrowing of the lumen is obvious; this is due to cicatrix formation. A guide wire has been passed through the cicatrix in preparation for balloon dilation.

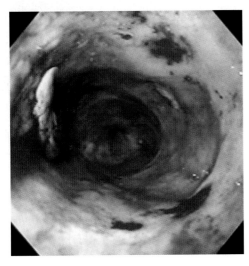

**FIG 29-14**
Endoscopic view of the distal esophagus of a dog with severe esophagitis secondary to a bone foreign body. Note the white plaque in the 9 o'clock position that is due to pressure necrosis from the foreign body.

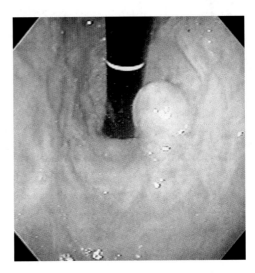

**FIG 29-16**
View of the lower esophageal sphincter (as seen from the stomach) of a dog with a leiomyoma. This lesion was causing vomiting and regurgitation and would easily have been missed if a careful, methodical examination had not been carried out.

*loptera*) just inside the pylorus. Biopsy specimens of the gastric and duodenal mucosa should always be obtained, because normal findings seen on visual examination do not rule out the presence of severe mucosal disease. Like esophagoscopy, gastroscopy is not sensitive in identifying functional problems (i.e., gastric hypomotility).

*Proctoscopy or colonoscopy* is indicated in dogs and cats with chronic large bowel disease unresponsive to appropriate dietary, antibacterial, or anthelmintic therapies. Colonos-

copy is more sensitive and definitive, yet comparable in cost to plain and contrast-enhanced radiography. Proctoscopy is used in animals with obvious rectal abnormalities (e.g., stricture felt on digital rectal examination). However, colonoscopy is usually preferred because it allows a more thorough evaluation of the colon. Rigid biopsy forceps obtain excellent tissue samples, which allows the identification of most lesions, including submucosal ones. Biopsy instruments used with flexible endoscopes do not obtain as deep a biopsy

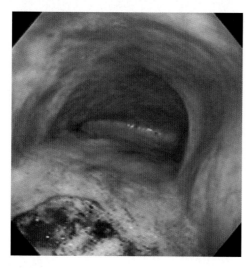

**FIG 29-17**
Endoscopic view of a dog with a megaesophagus. Note that the lumen is dilated and that there is substantial food material accumulation.

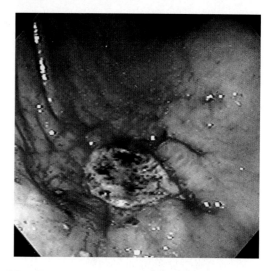

**FIG 29-18**
Endoscopic view of a gastric ulcer on the greater curvature in a Chow dog. Note that it is obvious that the mucosa is eroded to the level of the submucosa.

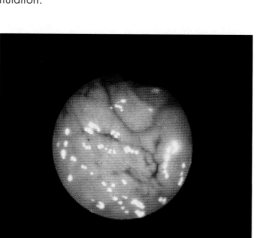

**FIG 29-19**
Endoscopic view of the gastric mucosa of a dog's stomach that has obvious bleeding. This dog had received nonsteroidal drugs, and the bleeding represented erosions that could not be detected with radiographs or ultrasonography. (From Fossum T, editor: *Small animal surgery,* St Louis, 1997, Mosby.)

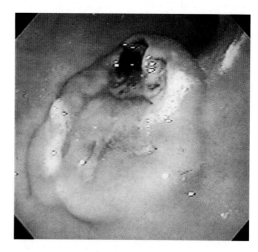

**FIG 29-20**
Endoscopic view of the stomach of a dog with an obvious mass in the greater curvature. This is an ulcerated leiomyosarcoma that was successfully removed.

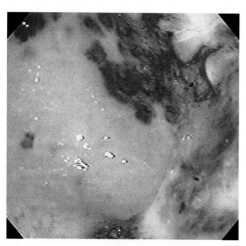

**FIG 29-21**
Endoscopic view of the stomach of a cat with diffuse inflammation, erosion, and ulceration of unknown cause.

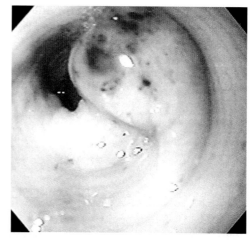

**FIG 29-22**
A focal gastritis near the pylorus of a dog. Note the reddened spots on the lesion, which were responsible for intermittent hematemesis.

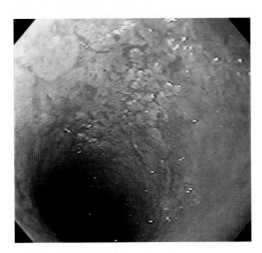

**FIG 29-23**
The duodenum of a dog with marked inflammatory bowel disease. Note the pseudomembrane-like appearance, which suggests severe disease.

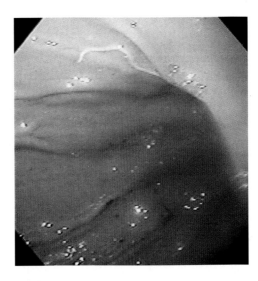

**FIG 29-25**
Endoscopic view of the greater curvature of the stomach of a dog with a *Physaloptera* attached.

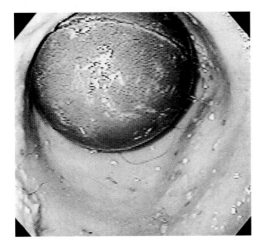

**FIG 29-24**
Endoscopic view of the antrum of a dog with a ball foreign object that has been present for months and was not detected on plain radiographs or by ultrasonography.

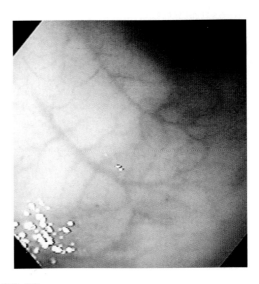

**FIG 29-26**
Endoscopic view of a normal colon in a dog, showing typical submucosal blood vessels. Inability to see such blood vessels may suggest inflammatory infiltrates.

specimen but are adequate for obtaining specimens from mucosal lesions.

Proctoscopy and colonoscopy are easier to perform, require less animal restraint, and do not always require the more expensive flexible equipment that other endoscopic procedures do. The colon must be clean to allow proper inspection of the mucosa. All food should be withheld for at least 24 hours before the procedure; a mild laxative (e.g., bisacodyl) should be administered the night before the procedure; and several copious warm water enemas should be given the night before and the morning of the procedure. Proctoscopy requires less cleaning than colonoscopy. Commercial intestinal lavage solutions (e.g., GoLytely, Colyte) clean the colon better than en-

emas and are particularly useful in larger dogs, those that will be undergoing ileoscopy (which necessitates a very clean ileocolic area), and animals in pain that resist enemas. The lavage solution must be given to the animal repeatedly and may rarely cause gastric dilation or volvulus.

Sedation plus manual restraint can often be used instead of anesthesia; however, many animals undergoing colonoscopy have colonic or rectal irritation, and anesthesia is usually preferred. Suction should be available in case the colon has not been adequately prepared.

Normal colonic mucosa is smooth and glistening, and the submucosal blood vessels can be seen (Fig. 29-26); enema tubes may cause linear artifacts. The colon should distend to

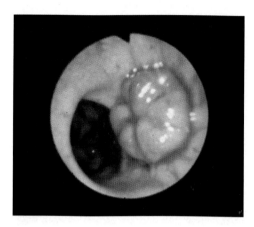

**FIG 29-27**
Normal ileocolic valve region in a dog. The ileocolic valve is the mushroomlike structure, and the opening below it is the cecocolic valve.

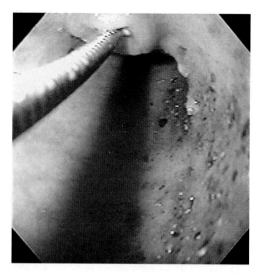

**FIG 29-29**
Same site as in Fig. 29-28. A biopsy instrument has been blindly passed into the ileum because the scope cannot be advanced through the narrow orifice.

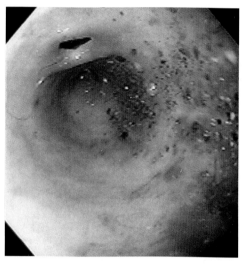

**FIG 29-28**
Endoscopic view of a normal ileocolic valve region from a cat. The blind pouch is the cecum, and the small opening above it is the ileocolic valve.

a uniform diameter, but it may have bends. If a flexible scope is used, the clinician should identify and inspect the ileocolic valve and the cecum (Figs. 29-27 and 29-28). Always biopsy the mucosa; normal gross findings do not rule out the presence of significant disease. Strictured areas with relatively normal appearing mucosa are usually caused by a submucosal lesion, in which case biopsying must be aggressive enough to ensure that submucosal tissue is included in the specimen. Cytologic studies are sensitive in detecting histoplasmosis or prototothecosis and may be useful in detecting some neoplasms and eosinophilic colitis.

An adult or a pediatric human sigmoidoscope is usually adequate for rigid colonoscopy. The tip of the rigid biopsy forceps should have a shearing action (i.e., one part of the tip should fit into the other when it is closed, thus acting like a pair of scissors) instead of a clamshell (also called "double spoon") action in which the edges of the top and bottom jaws simply meet.

*Ileoscopy* is principally indicated in dogs with diarrhea and in cats with vomiting or diarrhea. It is usually performed during flexible colonoscopy and requires thorough colonic cleansing so that the ileocolic valve can be visualized. It is difficult or impossible to enter the ileum of most cats (because of size), but one can often pass biopsy forceps through the ileocolic valve and blindly biopsy the ileal mucosa (Fig. 29-29). Ileoscopy is not as consistently beneficial as gastro-duodenoscopy or colonoscopy, although it is valuable in some cases.

## BIOPSY TECHNIQUES AND SUBMISSION

### FINE-NEEDLE ASPIRATION BIOPSY
Fine-needle aspiration or core biopsy of enlarged lymph nodes, abdominal masses, and infiltrated abdominal organs may be guided by abdominal palpation or ultrasonography if the structure can be held stationary. A 23- to 25-gauge needle is typically used so that any inadvertent intestinal or vascular perforation is insignificant (see Chapter 77).

### ENDOSCOPIC BIOPSY
Rigid endoscopy usually provides excellent biopsy samples of the descending colon (i.e., large specimens that include the full thickness of the mucosa, including some muscularis mucosa), but the stomach and small intestine cannot be biopsied with this equipment. Flexible endoscopes can reach most

areas of the alimentary tract, but the tissue samples obtained with these scopes may not always be deep enough to allow submucosal lesions to be diagnosed. Ideally the tissue to be biopsied is visualized; however, the clinician may pass the biopsy forceps through the pylorus or ileocolic valve and biopsy the duodenum or ileum blindly if the tip of the endoscope cannot be advanced into these areas.

Not all laboratories are adept at processing and interpreting these samples. Endoscopic biopsy specimens obtained with forceps through a 2-mm endoscope channel are often sufficient for the diagnosis of mucosal diseases of the alimentary tract. However, endoscopes with 2.8-mm biopsy channels allow the retrieval of substantially larger and deeper tissue samples.

When intestinal or gastric mucosa is biopsied, the tissue sample must be handled carefully to minimize artifacts and distortion. The tissue should be carefully removed from the biopsy forceps with a 25-gauge needle. A squash preparation of one tissue specimen can be evaluated cytologically, and the remaining samples are fixed in formalin and evaluated histologically. It is often helpful to have the cytology slides evaluated by a pathologist familiar with gastrointestinal cytology. Cytologic preparations of the gastric mucosa may show adenocarcinoma, lymphoma, inflammatory cells, or large numbers of spirochetes (see Fig. 32-1). Cytologic studies of the intestinal mucosa may show eosinophilic enteritis, lymphoma, histoplasmosis, or prototheccosis, and occasionally giardiasis, bacteria, or *Heterobilharzia* organisms. The absence of cytologic findings suggestive of these disorders does not rule them out, but finding them cytologically is diagnostic.

Tissue that is submitted for histopathologic analysis should be oriented on the surface of paper or similar material such that the submucosal side is on the material and the luminal side is away from the material. This orientation should be discussed with the pathology laboratory. After all of the tissue samples from an area have been gathered, the material is placed upside down in 10% neutral buffered formalin so that the tissue is fixed in a standard configuration that aids the pathologist in embedding the samples. It is imperative to place tissues from different locations in different vials of formalin; each vial should be properly labeled so that the pathologist can correctly identify the area evaluated. Do not allow small tissue samples to dry out or be damaged while waiting to place them in formalin.

Two common problems with endoscopically obtained tissue samples are that the sample is too small or there is excessive artifact. In particular, a lymphoma is sometimes relatively deep in the mucosa (or is submucosal), and a superficial biopsy specimen may then only show a tissue reaction above the tumor, resulting in a misdiagnosis of inflammatory bowel disease. Multiple biopsy specimens should be obtained until there are at least five to eight samples of excellent size and depth (i.e., the full thickness of mucosa). It is important to contact the pathologist and determine whether the quality of the tissue samples was adequate and if the severity of the histologic lesions found is consistent with the clinical signs.

## FULL-THICKNESS BIOPSY

If endoscopy is not available, abdominal surgery is needed to perform gastric and intestinal biopsies. Full-thickness biopsy specimens obtained surgically can have fewer artifacts than those obtained endoscopically; however, the clinician must consider the pros and cons of surgery in a potentially debilitated or ill animal. If surgery is performed, maximum benefit should be obtained from the procedure; the entire abdomen should be examined (i.e., literally from the beginning of the stomach to the end of the colon plus all parenchymal organs). Biopsy specimens should be obtained from all obviously abnormal structures. Biopsy specimens of the stomach, duodenum, jejunum, ileum, mesenteric lymph nodes, and liver (and the pancreas in cats) should be obtained, regardless of how normal these organs appear, unless an obvious lesion is found (e.g., a large tumor). However, it is a mark of wisdom to not assume that a grossly impressive lesion is responsible for the clinical signs; it is wise to biopsy even when the diagnosis is "obvious." Dehiscence is a concern if the serum albumin concentration is less than 1.5 g/dl, but the use of nonabsorbable suture material and serosal patch grafting over intestinal suture lines minimizes the risk. The clinician should consider whether gastrostomy or enterostomy feeding tubes should be placed in emaciated animals before exiting the abdomen.

### Suggested Readings

Baez JL et al: Radiographic, ultrasonographic, and endoscopic findings in cats with inflammatory bowel disease of the stomach and small intestine: 33 cases (1990-1997), *J Am Vet Med Assoc* 215:349, 1999.

Chandler ML et al: Radiopaque markers to evaluate gastric emptying and small intestinal transit time in healthy cats, *J Vet Intern Med* 11(6):361, 1997.

Cook AK et al: Effect of diet on results obtained by use of two commercial test kits for detection of occult blood in feces of dogs, *Am J Vet Res* 53:1749, 1992.

Goggin JM et al: Ultrasonographic measurement of gastrointestinal wall thickness and the ultrasonographic appearance of the ileocolic region in healthy cats, *J Am Anim Hosp Assoc* 36:224, 2000.

Guilford WG et al: *Small animal gastroenterology,* ed 3, Davis, Calif, 1996, WB Saunders.

Hall EJ et al: Diseases of the small intestine. In Ettinger SJ et al, editors: *Textbook of veterinary internal medicine,* ed 5, Philadelphia, 2000, WB Saunders.

Harvey HJ: Complications of small intestinal biopsy in hypoalbuminemic dogs, *Vet Surg* 19:289, 1990.

Jergens AE et al: Endoscopic biopsy specimen collection and histopathologic considerations. In Tams TR, editor: *Small animal endoscopy,* ed 2, Philadelphia, 1999, Mosby.

Jergens AE et al: Diseases of the large intestine. In Ettinger SJ et al, editors: *Textbook of veterinary internal medicine,* ed 5, Philadelphia, 2000, WB Saunders.

Jinbo T et al: Immunological determination of faecal haemoglobin concentrations in dogs, *Vet Res Commun* 22:193, 1998.

Konde LJ et al: Radiology and sonography of the digestive system. In Tams TR, editor: *Handbook of small animal gastroenterology,* Philadelphia, 1996, WB Saunders.

Marks SL et al: Evaluation of methods to diagnose *Clostridium perfringens*–associated diarrhea in dogs, *J Am Vet Med Assoc* 214: 357, 1999.

Newell SM et al: Sonography of the normal feline gastrointestinal tract, *Vet Radiol Ultra* 40:40, 1999.

Shelton GD et al: Acquired myasthenia gravis: selective involvement of esophageal, pharyngeal, and facial muscles, *J Vet Intern Med* 4:281, 1990.

Tams TR, editor: *Handbook of small animal gastroenterology,* Philadelphia, 1996, WB Saunders.

Vaden SL et al: Evaluation of intestinal permeability and gluten sensitivity in Soft-Coated Wheaten Terriers with familial protein-losing enteropathy, protein-losing nephropathy, or both, *Am J Vet Res* 61:518, 2000.

Weinstein WM: Mucosal biopsy techniques and interaction with the pathologist, *Gastrointest Endosc Clin N Am* 10(4):555, 2000.

Willard MD et al: Gastrointestinal, pancreatic, and hepatic disorders. In Willard MD et al, editors: *Small animal clinical diagnosis by laboratory methods,* ed 3, Philadelphia, 1999, WB Saunders.

Williams DA: Exocrine pancreatic disease and pancreatitis. In Ettinger SJ et al, editors: *Textbook of veterinary internal medicine,* ed 5, Philadelphia, 2000, WB Saunders.

# CHAPTER 30

# General Therapeutic Principles

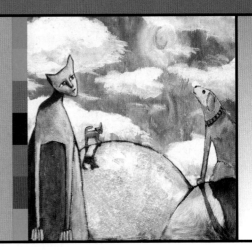

## CHAPTER OUTLINE

FLUID THERAPY, 387
DIETARY MANAGEMENT, 389
    Special nutritional supplementation, 390
    Diets for special enteral support, 395
    Parenteral nutrition, 396
ANTIEMETICS, 396
ANTACID DRUGS, 397
INTESTINAL PROTECTANTS, 398
DIGESTIVE ENZYME SUPPLEMENTATION, 398
MOTILITY MODIFIERS, 398
ANTIINFLAMMATORY AND ANTISECRETORY
DRUGS, 399
ANTIBACTERIAL DRUGS, 401
ANTHELMINTIC DRUGS, 401
ENEMAS, LAXATIVES, AND CATHARTICS, 402

## FLUID THERAPY

Fluid therapy is primarily used to treat shock, dehydration, and electrolyte and acid-base disturbances. The vomiting of gastric contents (even if does not stem from a gastric outlet obstruction) inconsistently produces a classic hypokalemic, hypochloremic metabolic alkalosis. The loss of intestinal contents classically produces hypokalemia, with or without acidosis. Vomiting animals are often assumed to be hypokalemic; however, animals with hypoadrenocorticism or anuric renal failure may be hyperkalemic. One cannot accurately predict the nature of electrolyte and acid-base changes on the basis of clinical parameters; hence, serum electrolyte concentrations must be measured. If these data are not available or if fluid therapy must be started before they are available, physiologic saline solution plus 20 mEq potassium chloride per liter is a reasonable therapeutic choice (see Chapter 55), assuming that the fluids are administered at one to two times the maintenance requirement. A lead II electrocardiographic (ECG) tracing may be evaluated to ensure that moderate to severe hyperkalemia is unlikely (see p. 833).

It is rarely necessary to administer bicarbonate, because reexpanding the vascular compartment and improving peripheral perfusion help alleviate lactic acidosis (a common cause of acidosis in small animals). Bicarbonate or lactated Ringer's solution should not be used if alkalosis seems likely (e.g., vomiting of gastric origin).

*Parenteral fluid administration* is indicated if the animal is significantly hypovolemic or if you cannot depend on the absorption of enteral fluids because of problems such as severe intestinal disease, obstruction, vomiting, or ileus. Shock necessitates the intravenous (IV) administration of fluids, even if a venous cutdown is necessary. Catheters are easy to insert in peripheral veins but often do not last as long as properly placed jugular catheters (i.e., 3 days versus more than 1 week, respectively). Intramedullary administration may be used if IV administration is desired but a catheter cannot be established. To do this, a large-bore hypodermic needle or a bone marrow aspiration needle (preferable) can be inserted through the femur (trochanteric fossa), the tibia, the wing of the ilium, or the humerus. Fluids can be administered by the intramedullary route at a maintenance rate or faster. Intraperitoneal administration is acceptable but repletes the intravascular compartment more slowly than IV or intramedullary techniques.

Dogs in shock, such as those with tachycardia, poor peripheral perfusion, cool extremities, a prolonged capillary refill time, a weak femoral pulse, or tachypnea, may receive up to 88 ml of isotonic crystalloids per kilogram IV during the first hour. Sometimes this "maximum" rate must be exceeded to reestablish adequate peripheral perfusion. Also, remember that septic shock initially causes brick red oral mucous membranes, warm extremities, and a strong, bounding femoral pulse before the signs of classic shock occur. Large dogs in severe shock, such as those with a gastric volvulus, may require two simultaneous 16- to 18-gauge cephalic catheters and IV bags placed in pneumatic compression devices to achieve this flow rate. It is easier to overhydrate cats; one should therefore monitor cats carefully when rapidly administering fluids. In general, one should not exceed 55 ml/kg for the initial dose of fluids for cats in shock. Lactated Ringer's solution or physiologic saline solution is commonly used for treating shock. However, be sure that fluids to be administered rapidly for shock do not contain too much potassium since cardiotoxicity can occur.

*Hypertonic saline solution* (i.e., 7%) may be used to treat severe hypovolemic or endotoxic shock. Relatively small volumes (i.e., 4 to 5 ml/kg delivered over 10 minutes) seem to be as effective as larger volumes of isotonic crystalloids. Hypertonic solutions shift fluid from the intracellular and interstitial compartments into the intravascular compartment and stimulate vascular reflexes. Hypertonic solutions generally should not be used in animals with hypernatremic dehydration, cardiogenic shock, or renal failure. Uncontrolled hemorrhage may also be a contraindication to their use. One may readminister hypertonic saline solution in 2 ml/kg aliquots until a total of 10 ml/kg has been given or until the serum sodium concentration is 160 mEq/L or more. After administering hypertonic saline solution, one may continue to administer other fluids, but at a reduced rate (e.g., 10 to 20 ml/kg/hr), until shock is controlled. A mixture of 7% saline solution plus dextran 70 has a longer duration of action than hypertonic saline solution alone. This combination may be administered at a rate of 3 to 5 ml/kg over 5 minutes. Dextran is rarely associated with allergic reactions or renal failure but should be used carefully or not at all in animals with coagulopathies.

Colloids (e.g., *hetastarch*) are also useful in treating shock. Like hypertonic saline solution, colloids draw water from the interstitial compartment into the vascular compartment; however, their effects last longer and do not increase the total body sodium load. Relatively small volumes are administered quickly (i.e., 5 to 10 ml/kg, maximum of 20 ml/kg in 1 day), and one must reduce the subsequent rate of IV fluid administration to prevent hypertension. Colloids should be used with caution in animals with bleeding tendencies.

Dehydrated animals are treated by replacing the estimated fluid deficit. To do this, first the degree of dehydration must be estimated. Prolonged skin tenting is usually first noted at 5% to 6% dehydration. However, any dog or cat that has lost weight may show skin tenting, whereas obese animals and those with peracute dehydration often do not show skin tenting, regardless of the severity of dehydration. Dry, tacky oral mucous membranes usually indicate 6% to 7% dehydration. However, dehydrated, nauseated animals may have moist oral mucous membranes, whereas well-hydrated, panting or dyspneic animals have dry mouths. Multiplying the estimated percentage of dehydration by the animal's weight (in kilograms) determines the liters required to replace the deficit. This amount is typically replaced over 2 to 8 hours, depending on the animal's condition. However, the fluid delivery rate should generally not exceed 88 ml/kg/hr. In general, it is better to overestimate rather than underestimate the fluid deficit, unless the animal has congestive heart failure, anuric or oliguric renal failure, severe hypoproteinemia, severe anemia, or pulmonary edema. It is usually easier to harm cats than dogs by excessive fluid administration.

Subcutaneous (SQ) fluid administration, although not ideal, is acceptable if the animal is not in shock, absorbs the fluids, and accepts repeated SQ administration. Multiple SQ depots of 10 to 50 ml each are given, depending on the animal's size. Dependent areas should be checked for the presence of unabsorbed fluids before administering more fluid. Severely dehydrated animals may not absorb SQ fluids as rapidly as desired, making initial IV administration more desirable.

Maintenance fluids should be administered once fluid deficits have been replaced. Approximately 60 ml of fluid per kilogram of body weight is required daily for maintenance, which is a little excessive for large-breed dogs. It is important to choose the correct fluid to prevent electrolyte imbalances, especially hypokalemia. In general, potassium should be supplemented if the animal is anorectic or vomiting, has diarrhea, or is receiving prolonged or intense fluid therapy (see guidelines for administration in Table 30-1). Monitor (e.g., ECG or plasma potassium determinations) the animal for the development of iatrogenic hyperkalemia, and do not administer more than 0.5 mEq/kg/hr. Oral (PO) potassium supplementation is often more effective than parenteral supplementation if the animal is not vomiting. Cats receiving fluids IV often initially show a decrease in their serum potassium concentrations, even if the fluids contain 40 mEq or more of potassium chloride per liter.

Ongoing losses are typically estimated from the observation of vomiting, diarrhea, and urination; however, it is common to underestimate losses. Weighing the animal regularly can be used as a way to estimate the adequacy of maintenance fluid therapy. A progressive weight loss implies inadequate fluid therapy in the face of an ongoing fluid loss (e.g., vomiting, diarrhea). Use a scale that is accurate enough to detect changes of tenths of a pound, and always use the same scale. A change of 1 lb (0.45 kg) represents approximately 500 ml of water.

The development of inspiratory pulmonary crackles, a systolic heart murmur, a gallop rhythm, or edema (especially cervical) indicates the animal is overhydrated. The central venous pressure is excellent for detecting excessive fluid administration; however, it is rarely necessary to measure it, except in an-

 TABLE 30-1

**General Guidelines for Potassium Supplementation of IV Fluids**

| PLASMA POTASSIUM CONCENTRATION (mEq/L) | AMOUNT OF KCl TO ADD TO FLUIDS GIVEN AT MAINTENANCE RATES* (mEq/L) |
| --- | --- |
| 3.7-5.0 | 10-20 |
| 3.0-3.7 | 20-30 |
| 2.5-3.0 | 30-40 |
| 2.0-2.5 | 40-60 |
| ≤2.0 | 60-70 |

*Do not exceed potassium, 0.5 mEq/kg/hr, except in animals in hypokalemic emergencies and then only with constant, close electrocardiogram (ECG) monitoring. Be sure to routinely monitor plasma potassium concentrations whenever administering fluids with more than 30 to 40 mEq of potassium per liter.

imals with severe cardiac or renal failure and those receiving aggressive fluid therapy. The central venous pressure is normally less than 4 cm $H_2O$ and generally should not exceed 10 to 12 cm $H_2O$, even during aggressive fluid therapy.

*Rehydration therapy* PO makes use of the facilitated intestinal absorption of sodium. The co-administration of a monosaccharide (e.g., dextrose) or amino acid with sodium speeds up sodium absorption and subsequent water uptake. This approach works if the animal can ingest oral fluids (i.e., it is not vomiting) and the intestinal mucosa is functional (i.e., there is reasonable villus function). Absorption primarily occurs in the mature epithelium near the villus tip.

A variety of products are commercially available, and there are also recipes for making these solutions. However, the veterinary products (e.g., Ritrol; Nutramax Labs, Edgewood Minn) are often superior for use in animals. Failure to follow instructions may lead to the development of severe hypernatremia. Many dogs and cats with acute enteritis not caused by severe parvoviral enteritis can usually receive rehydration fluids PO.

The type of *fluid therapy used in hypoproteinemic animals* depends on the degree of hypoalbuminemia. Excessive fluids can dilute and further decrease the serum albumin concentration and plasma oncotic pressure, causing ascites, edema, diminished peripheral perfusion, or a combination of these. Careful calculation of the fluid needs and ongoing losses is therefore necessary. In animals with severe hypoalbuminemia (e.g., serum albumin of 1.5 g/dl or less), a plasma transfusion (plasma, 6 to 10 ml/kg, initially) may be considered to improve the oncotic pressure. A common mistake is to give inadequate amounts of plasma; approximately one half of the administered albumin will ultimately reside in the interstitial space. Therefore the serum albumin concentration should be measured 8 to 12 hours after the transfusion to ensure that enough plasma was administered. Further, animals with severe protein-losing enteropathies and nephropathies rapidly excrete the supplemented protein, making repeated transfusions necessary if the plasma albumin concentration is to be maintained. It can therefore be very expensive to replenish albumin in large, hypoalbuminemic dogs. Human albumin has been used instead of canine plasma, but glomerulonephritis is a potential complication. Hetastarch (5 to 20 ml/kg/day) and dextran 70 may be used in place of plasma or albumin. Hetastarch (supplied as a 6% solution) may persist in the intravascular space longer than albumin and help maintain the plasma oncotic pressure in animals with severe protein-losing enteropathies. If hetastarch is used, one must be careful to decrease the rate of fluid administration to avoid the development of hypertension.

## DIETARY MANAGEMENT

Symptomatic or specific dietary therapy is often important in animals with gastrointestinal tract problems. Symptomatic therapy usually involves the use of bland, easily digested diets, whereas specific therapy typically involves the use of elimination or hypoallergenic diets, diets with a highly restricted fat content, fiber-supplemented diets, or a combination of these.

*Bland, easily digested diets* are indicated in animals with acute gastritis or enteritis. Food for such diets is available commercially (Table 30-2) or can be homemade. It usually consists of boiled poultry or lean hamburger, low-fat cottage cheese, boiled rice, boiled potatoes, or combinations of these. Boiled chicken or turkey or fish and green beans may be useful in cats. A typical mixture is one part boiled chicken or cottage cheese and two parts boiled potato. The low-fat content makes digestion easier. These diets also tend to be low in lactose, which helps prevent maldigestion. Frequent, small amounts of these foods are usually fed until the diarrhea resolves, and then the diet is gradually changed back to the previous one. This diet may be continued after the event is over; however, if a homemade diet is used long-term, it must be nutritionally balanced (especially for puppies and kittens).

These easily digested diets usually also help prevent vomiting because they are low in fat and fiber (both delay emptying) and high in complex carbohydrates. Extremely hyperosmolar diets should be avoided (e.g., do not use concentrated sugar solutions or honey), because they also may delay gastric emptying.

*Hypoallergenic and elimination diets* are indicated if a dietary allergy (i.e., an immune-mediated hypersensitivity to a dietary component) or intolerance (i.e., a non–immune-mediated problem) is suspected, respectively. Both types of diets will henceforth be referred to as *elimination diets*. These diets may be composed of the same ingredients found in bland diets; however, they must be formulated so that the animal is fed food that it either has not eaten before (and hence could not be responsible for causing allergy or intolerance) or that is very unlikely to provoke allergy or intolerance (e.g., potatoes). Commercial elimination diets are available; however, it may be best to first try a homemade one if the clients are willing to prepare it. Examples of homemade elimination diets are described in Table 30-3.

Elimination diets must be used for at least 6 (and preferably 8 or more) weeks before their efficacy can accurately be determined. It is critical that no other foods or treats be given to the animal during this time; this includes pills, toys, and medications with flavorings. If the signs resolve during this

 TABLE 30-2

**Examples of Commercial Bland\* Diets**

Hill's Prescription Diet i/d
Iams Eukanuba Low-Residue-Adult
Purina CNM EN-Formula
Select Care Canine Sensitive Formula
Waltham/Pedigree Canine Low Fat
Waltham/Whiskas Feline Selected Protein

\*"Bland" refers to easily digestible diets that often contain less fat than is found in many pet foods.
This list is a partial list for the purpose of showing examples of such diets. It is not an all-inclusive list of such diets.

TABLE 30-3

### Examples of Homemade, Hypoallergenic* Diets

1 part boiled white chicken or turkey meat without the skin + 2 parts boiled or baked potato (without the skin)
1 part boiled or broiled white fish without the skin + 2 parts boiled or baked potato (without the skin)
1 part boiled mutton, venison, or rabbit without the skin + 2 parts boiled or baked potato (without the skin)
1 part drained, low-fat cottage cheese + 2 parts boiled or baked potato (without the skin)

A *nonflavored* vitamin supplement may be given three times per week.
Rice can be substituted for potato, but most dogs and cats seem to digest potato easier than rice.
These diets are not balanced but are adequate for 3 to 4 months of use in mature animals. If growing animals are being fed such a diet, then a nutritionist must be consulted to determine how much dicalcium phosphate to add.
*Hypoallergenic refers to a diet specially formulated for a given animal, one that does not expose the animal to potential allergens that it has eaten in the past. Therefore one must obtain a careful dietary history to determine what will or will not constitute a hypoallergenic diet for a particular animal.

time, the diet should be continued for at least 4 to 6 more weeks to ensure that it is the diet that is responsible and not a spontaneous fluctuation of the disease. If the diet seems effective, a more convenient commercial diet may then be substituted for the homemade one. If the homemade diet is to be continued, appropriate vitamins, minerals, and fatty acids should be added to balance it, per Remillard and colleague (1989).

*Partially hydrolyzed diets* (Purina HA; Nestle Purina, St. Louis, Mo; Hill's z/d; Hill's Pet Products, Topeka, Kan) have been formulated in an attempt to eliminate proteins large enough to cause immunologic reactions (i.e., make a diet that is hypoallergenic for all animals). Although these diets are not hypoallergenic for all animals, many dogs and cats will not have allergic reactions to them, plus the partially hydrolyzed proteins may make them easier for diseased alimentary tracts to digest and absorb.

*Elemental diets* (e.g., Vivonex TEN; Novartis Nutrition, Minneapolis, Minn) are diets in which the nutrients are supplied as amino acids and simple sugars. These diets are hypoallergenic, but more importantly they are extremely easy to digest and absorb when there is major small intestinal disease. Further, diseased intestines have increased permeability, which allows luminal contents to leak into the mucosa. Such leakage may be an important mechanism perpetuating intestinal inflammation. The amino acids and simple sugars found in elemental diets do not elicit an inflammatory reaction when they enter the interstitium; thus they do not contribute to perpetuation of the inflammatory response in the intestines. The elemental diets prepared for people (e.g.,

Vivonex TEN) typically have less protein than desired for veterinary patients. Therefore we typically supplement protein when mixing up this diet by adding 350 ml of water plus 250 ml of 8.5% amino acids (for injection) instead of 600 ml of water. Adding 1 to 2 ml of a flavored vitamin syrup often makes it palatable. If the animal will not drink this formulation, it may be administered via nasoesophageal tube.

*Ultra–low-fat diets* are indicated in animals with intestinal lymphangiectasia. Because long-chain fatty acids enter lacteals and are reesterified, removing them from the diet therefore prevents the dilatation and rupture of lacteals and the subsequent intestinal lymphatic loss. Medium-chain triglycerides (MCTs) were once recommended as supplements to such diets at a dose of 1 to 2 ml/kg of body weight. MCTs are absorbed into the portal blood without going through the lacteals and thoracic duct. However, they have an unpleasant taste, so small amounts (e.g., 1 tsp/lb of food) should be added to the diet. Otherwise the animal may refuse to eat the food. Using a highly digestible, ultra–low-fat diet usually eliminates the need for supplementing MCTs.

*Fiber supplementation* may help many dogs and cats with large (and rarely small) intestinal diseases.

Fiber is classified as soluble or insoluble; however, these are artificial categories. Many fibers actually have both soluble and insoluble characteristics. Processing also alters characteristics of the fiber (e.g., coarse wheat bran has effects different from those of finely ground bran). Insoluble fiber is poorly digested or metabolized by bacteria and ultimately produces more stool bulk. Some insoluble fibers apparently "normalize" colonic myoelectrical activity and help prevent spasms. Soluble fiber is metabolized by bacteria into short-chain volatile fatty acids, which are trophic to colonic mucosa; it may also slow the small intestinal absorption of nutrients.

Fiber-enriched diets may ameliorate diarrhea in many animals with large bowel disease (especially those with minimal inflammation) and lessen constipation not caused by obstruction or pain. Such a diet should be fed for at least 2 weeks, although most animals that respond do so within the first week. A commercial high-fiber diet may be used, or fiber may be added to the current diet. Psyllium hydrocolloid (Metamucil) or coarse, unprocessed wheat bran may be added to the pet's diet in the amount of 1 to 2 tsp or 1 to 4 tbsp per can of food, respectively. Some cats will not eat these diets or fiber supplements; however, canned pumpkin pie filling is effective and usually acceptable to cats; 1 to 3 tbsp may be given daily. Be sure the animal maintains adequate water intake, lest the increased dietary fiber produce obstipation. If too much fiber is fed, there may be excessive stool, which the owner then mistakes for continued large bowel disease.

## SPECIAL NUTRITIONAL SUPPLEMENTATION

Refusal to ingest adequate calories necessitates special nutritional supplementation. Daily nutritional requirements should be calculated to avoid underfeeding. Approximately 60 kcal/kg/day is reasonable for the maintenance needs of

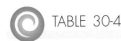

## TABLE 30-4

### Calculation of Nutritional Needs and Formulations of Parenteral Solutions

Actual body weight = _____ kg

**Basal Energy Requirement**

30 (weight in kg) + 70 = _____ kcal/day
However, if <2 kg or >25 kg, use 70 (weight in kg)$^{0.75}$

**Maintenance Energy Requirement**

| Adjustment factors: | Dogs | Cats |
|---|---|---|
| Cage rest | (1.25) | (1.1) |
| After surgery | (1.3) | (1.12) |
| Trauma | (1.5) | (1.2) |
| Sepsis | (1.7) | (1.28) |
| Severe burn | (2.0) | (1.4) |

**BASAL REQUIREMENT × ADJUSTMENT FACTOR =**

_____ kcal/day

**Protein Requirement**

4 g/kg in adult dogs
6 g/kg in cats and hypoproteinemic dogs
If there is renal failure, use 1.5 g/kg in dogs *or* 3 g/kg in cats

_____ g/day

Solution formulation:

_____ g of protein necessitates _____ ml of an 8.5% or 10% amino acid solution (85 or 100 mg of protein/ml, respectively). Determine the calories derived from the protein (4 kcal/g of protein), and subtract this from the daily caloric needs. Supply the remaining calories with glucose and lipid. _____ kcal needed.
Provide at least 10%, and preferably 40%, of caloric needs with lipid emulsion. A 20% lipid emulsion has 2 kcal/ml. Do not use in lipemic animals; use with caution in animals with pancreatitis.
_____ ml needed. Provide remainder of calories with 50% dextrose, which has 1.7 kcal/ml. _____ ml needed.
Use one half the calculated amount of solution on the first day, and increase it to the calculated amount on the second day, if hyperglycemia, lipemia, azotemia, or hyperammonemia does not occur. Either use amino acid solution with electrolytes or add electrolytes so that the solution has sodium, 35 mEq/L; chloride, 35 mEq/L; potassium, 42 mEq/L; magnesium, 5 mEq/L; and phosphate, 15 mmol/L. These concentrations may be adjusted as needed, depending on the animal's serum electrolyte concentrations. Add multiple vitamins and trace elements (especially zinc and copper) that are formulated for parenteral nutrition solutions.

mature dogs and cats that are not lactating or losing a significant amount of energy or protein. More exact calculations are recommended if the animal has severe disease or ongoing fluid and nutritional losses (Table 30-4).

In some animals, simply sending the animal home, warming the food, or feeding them palatable diets (e.g., chicken baby food in dogs) ensures adequate caloric intake. One can attempt force-feeding by manually placing food in the animal's mouth; however, this seldom works in severely anorexic animals.

Cyproheptadine (2 to 4 mg per cat) stimulates some cats to eat, especially those with mild anorexia. However, cyproheptadine seldom induces a severely anorectic cat (e.g., one with severe hepatic lipidosis) to ingest adequate calories. Diazepam rarely causes acute feline hepatic failure. Megestrol acetate is an excellent appetite stimulant but occasionally causes diabetes mellitus, reproductive problems, or tumors. Appetite stimulants are usually less effective in dogs than in cats.

Tube feeding is a more reliable way to ensure that adequate calories are ingested. *Intermittent orogastric tube* feeding is useful for animals that only need nutritional support for a relatively short time, although it may be used longer in orphaned puppies and kittens. It is typically done two or three times daily, with the animal restrained and using a mouth gag. A tube is measured and marked to correspond to the length from the tip of the nose to the midthoracic region. The tube is then carefully inserted through a mouth gag to the premarked point. If the animal coughs or is dyspneic, the tube may have entered the trachea and should be repositioned. It is safest if the tube is flushed with water before the warmed gruel is administered. The gruel should be given over several seconds or 1 minute. Because relatively large-diameter tubes can be used, homemade gruels may be administered in this way. The major disadvantage is the need to physically restrain the animal, which may detest the procedure. Placing an indwelling tube (see following discussion) circumvents this problem.

*Nasoesophageal tubes* are indicated in animals that need nutritional support and have a functional esophagus, stomach, and intestines. They are easy to place, but they are difficult to maintain in animals that are vomiting. To place them, after instilling a few drops of lidocaine solution in one nostril, a sterile polyvinyl chloride, polyurethane, or silicone tube (the diameter depends on the animal's size, but 5F to 12F is typical) is lubricated with sterile, water-soluble jelly and inserted into the ventromedial portion of the nostril. The animal's head is restrained in a position comparable to its normal carriage, and the tube is inserted until the tip is just beyond the thoracic inlet. If difficulty is encountered in passing the tube, the tip should be withdrawn, redirected, and advanced again. If the clinician is unsure whether the tube is in the esophagus, thoracic radiographs should be obtained or several milliliters of sterile saline solution should be instilled into the tube to see if this provokes coughing.

Tape is applied to the tube to secure it, and then the tape is glued or sutured as needed to the skin along the dorsal aspect of the nose. Do not allow the tube to touch sensory vibrissae because the animal will not tolerate it. An Elizabethan collar may have to be placed on some animals to prevent them from pulling the tube out. Only small-diameter tubes (e.g., 5F) can be used in small dogs and cats, which limits the rate of administration and necessitates the use of commercial liquid diets (Table 30-5) instead of homemade gruels. Flush the tube with water after each feeding to prevent occlusion. Long-term acceptance is typical, but rhinitis occurs in some animals.

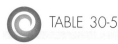

TABLE 30-5

**Selected Enteral Diets**

| DIET | COMMENTS |
|---|---|
| Ensure HN* | Polymeric diet |
| Osmolite HN* | Polymeric diet; contains MCT |
| Clinical Care Feline Diet† | Polymeric diet; contains taurine and reduced lactose |
| Clinical Care Canine Diet† | Polymeric diet; contains reduced lactose |
| Jevity* | Polymeric diet; contains taurine, fiber, carnitine, and MCT |
| Peptamen‡ | Oligomeric diet; contains taurine and MCT |
| Vital HN* | Oligomeric diet; contains MCT |
| Vivonex§ | Elemental diet; high in carbohydrates, low in protein and fat ‖ |

*MCT,* Medium-chain triglyceride.
*Ross Laboratories, Columbus, Ohio.
†Abbott Animal Health, North Chicago, Ill.
‡Nestle Nutrition, Deerfield, Ill.
§Novartis Nutrition, Minneapolis, Minn.
‖To increase protein content, reconstitute one packet of powder with 350 ml water plus 250 ml of 8.5% amino acids for injection.

Some dogs and cats do not tolerate nasoesophageal tubes and continually pull them out. However, they are usually effective for short-term therapy (e.g., 1 to 10 days), and some animals tolerate them for weeks.

*Pharyngostomy* and *esophagostomy tubes* are indicated in animals with a functional esophagus, stomach, and intestines that require nutritional support but do not tolerate nasoesophageal or intermittent tube feeding. Vomiting can make it difficult to maintain these tubes, but they can be used for weeks to months.

To place a pharyngostomy tube, the animal is anesthetized and a finger is inserted through the mouth so that the tip of the finger is caudal to the epihyoid bone and as dorsal and as close to the cricopharyngeal sphincter as possible. The tip of the finger is then pushed laterally, and a skin incision is made over this spot. Hemostats are used to bluntly dissect through to the pharynx. A soft latex or rubber catheter (18F to 22F, urinary) is then inserted into the opening and into the esophagus. In general, the tip of the catheter should end in the midthoracic esophagus. The tube is secured with traction sutures and the area bandaged. Some infection at the site is common, and routine cleansing and bandage changes are necessary. Systemic antibiotics are not typically needed. An Elizabethan collar may be used if the animal tries to remove the tube. To remove the tube, simply cut the sutures and pull it out. The opening will close spontaneously over the next 1 to 4 days. Pharyngostomy tubes effectively bypass oral lesions. Advantages of these tubes include easy placement, easy removal, and minimal complications if they have been prop-

erly inserted (i.e., they cannot cause peritonitis as gastrostomy or enterostomy tubes can). However, it is easy to place them such that they cause gagging and regurgitation (i.e., if they touch the larynx, especially in cats and small dogs). Take care not to disrupt vessels or nerves when using scissors or a scalpel during the dissection. Because pharyngostomy tubes are larger than nasoesophageal tubes, homemade gruels can be fed through them.

Esophagostomy tube placement is similar to that of pharyngostomy tubes. The animal is placed in right lateral recumbency, the mouth is held open, and a long right-angle hemostat is placed through the cricopharyngeal sphincter. The tip of the hemostat is then forced up to show where to make the incision in the left cervical region. The incision should be made midway between the cricopharyngeal sphincter and the thoracic inlet. The tip of the hemostat is forced up through the esophagus and the nick in the skin; the tip of a feeding tube is then grasped and pulled into the esophagus and out the mouth so that the flared end of the catheter (i.e., where the syringe will be attached) is left protruding from the neck. The distal end of the catheter is then redirected down the esophagus with a rigid colonoscope or other device. Esophagostomy tubes cannot cause gagging but are otherwise similar to pharyngostomy tubes.

*Gastrostomy tubes* bypass the mouth and esophagus in animals with a functional stomach and intestines. They can also be used when nasoesophageal, pharyngostomy, esophagostomy, or intermittent gastric tubing is unacceptable. Vomiting is not a contraindication. Surgery, endoscopy, or special devices designed for gastrostomy tube placement are necessary to place them.

The use of dedicated devices for the placement of gastrostomy tubes has made the procedure easier and readily available (Fig. 30-1). To place gastrostomy tubes using these devices, position the anesthetized animal in right lateral recumbency and surgically prepare the area behind the last rib on the left abdominal wall. The device is then blindly and carefully advanced down the esophagus until the tip is in the stomach and can be seen pushing against the skin behind the last rib. The plunger on the handle is advanced until the trocar in the tip penetrates the skin and can be seen. In the tip of the trocar is a hole in which a suture (e.g., No. 1 or 2 polyamide or other nonabsorbable material) is tied. The device is then withdrawn from the animal, bringing one end of the suture with it. In the meantime, another person grasps the other end of the suture firmly so that it cannot pass into and be lost in the stomach. The end of the suture that was brought out through the mouth is now passed retrograde through the sheath of an 18-gauge over-the-needle IV catheter or a disposable pipette tip of similar diameter. A mushroom-type catheter (usually 18F to 24F) is prepared by cutting off the syringe end. The clinician then attaches the suture that has been pulled out through the mouth to this end of the catheter using a needle to pass the suture through the catheter and make a mattress suture pattern. The end of the mushroom catheter tip that has just been attached to the suture is then inserted into the flared end of the IV catheter or disposable

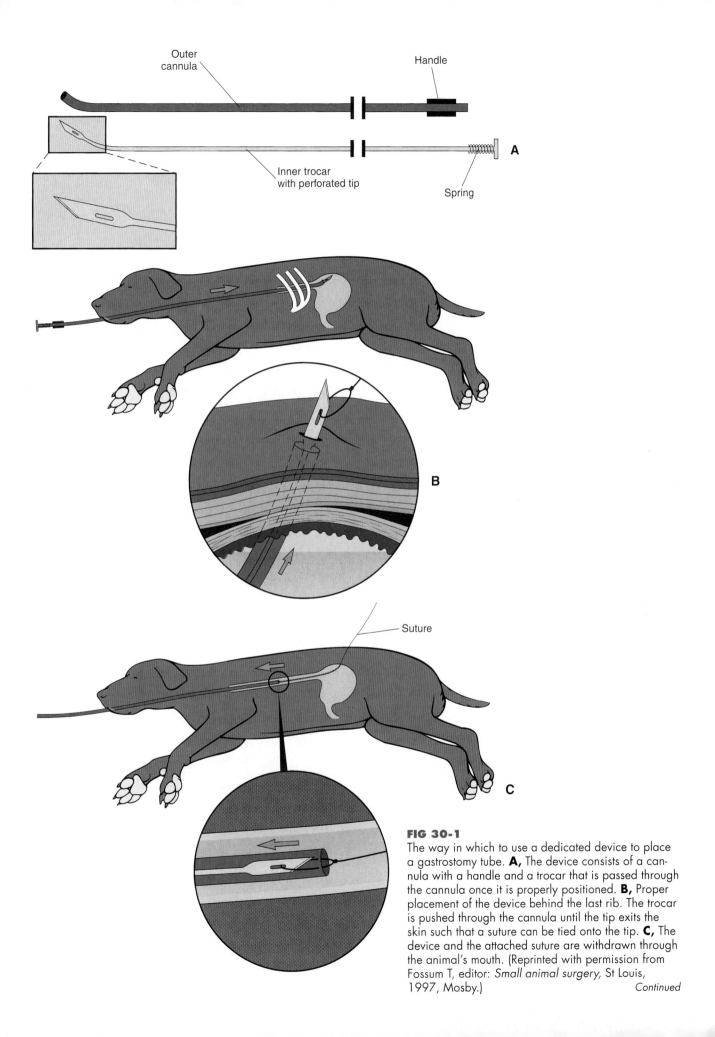

Outer
cannula

Handle

Inner trocar
with perforated tip

Spring

**A**

**B**

Suture

**C**

**FIG 30-1**
The way in which to use a dedicated device to place
a gastrostomy tube. **A,** The device consists of a cannula with a handle and a trocar that is passed through
the cannula once it is properly positioned. **B,** Proper
placement of the device behind the last rib. The trocar
is pushed through the cannula until the tip exits the
skin such that a suture can be tied onto the tip. **C,** The
device and the attached suture are withdrawn through
the animal's mouth. (Reprinted with permission from
Fossum T, editor: *Small animal surgery,* St Louis,
1997, Mosby.)

*Continued*

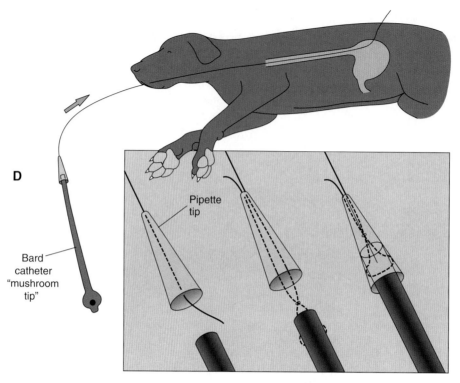

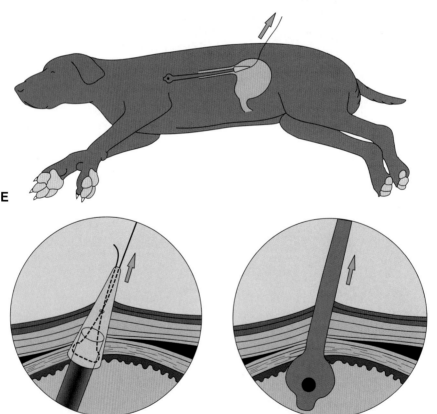

**FIG 30-1, cont'd**
**D,** The way in which to use a dedicated device to place a gastrostomy tube. The tip of the suture that exits the mouth is attached to the cut end of a mushroom-tip catheter. **E,** The other end of the suture is pulled so that the tip of the catheter exits the skin. It is pulled until the mushroom tip is snugly against the gastric mucosa and the stomach is held against the abdominal wall. (Reprinted with permission from Fossum T, editor: *Small animal surgery*, St Louis, 1997, Mosby.)

pipette tip. The other person then begins to pull on the end of the suture where it enters the abdominal wall, thus pulling the cut tip of the mushroom catheter into the stomach. The modified end of the mushroom catheter that was inserted into the disposable pipette tip is thus pulled out of the stomach through the same hole previously made by the trocar. Traction is placed on the mushroom catheter until the mushroom head is securely placed against the gastric mucosa, which is pulled next to the abdominal wall. (Take care not to pull the mushroom tip of the catheter out of the stomach.) The catheter is held in place by an outer flange and/or traction sutures (do not have so much pressure on the gastric mucosa that avascular necrosis results), and the area is bandaged lightly.

Gastrostomy tubes allow the administration of thick gruels and are often tolerated for weeks to years. Either home-made gruels or commercial liquid diets (see Table 30-5) may be used. These tubes must be left in place for at least 7 to 10 days to allow an adhesion to form between the stomach and the abdominal wall, which will prevent gastric leakage into the peritoneal cavity when the tube is removed. They are often used in cats that do not tolerate pharyngostomy or nasogastric tubes. The tube should be flushed with water and air after each feeding. Although the entire caloric requirement may be administered as soon as the tube is placed, it is often better to start with one half the daily requirement and work up to the complete nutritional needs over 1 to 3 days. If the tube becomes plugged, it can sometimes be unplugged by using flexible endoscopy forceps or by instilling a fresh carbonated beverage into the tube. When the tube is to be removed, sufficient traction is applied to the catheter so that the mushroom tip collapses and passes through the stomach and skin incision. The fistula usually closes spontaneously in 1 to 4 days. The major risk of using such tubes is leakage and peritonitis, which are rare but potentially catastrophic.

*Low-profile gastrostomy tubes* can be used if a stoma has been established by a routine gastrostomy tube. The major advantage of such tubes is that they may replace routine gastrostomy tubes that are disintegrating or have been inadvertently pulled out, and they may be placed without anesthesia or a surgical/endoscopic procedure. Typically, light sedation or analgesia is all that is needed. However, in order to use the preexisting stoma, the low-profile gastrostomy tube must be place within 12 hours of removing the old gastrostomy tube, or another tube (e.g., a red latex male urinary catheter) must be inserted into the stoma as quickly as possible to prevent the old stoma from closing.

*Enterostomy tubes* are indicated in animals with functional intestines when the stomach must be bypassed (e.g., recent gastric surgery). Laparotomy or laparoscopy is generally needed to place these tubes. A 12-gauge needle is used to puncture the antimesenteric border of the intestine, and a sterile 5F plastic catheter is advanced aborally through the needle until approximately 15 cm extends into the intestinal lumen. The 12-gauge needle is removed, and a purse-string suture is placed to prevent the catheter from moving freely. The needle is then used in the same manner to make a path-

way for the catheter to exit through the abdominal wall. The antimesenteric border of the intestine is sutured to the abdominal wall so that the sites where the tube enters the intestine and exits the abdomen are opposed. Traction sutures are used to secure the catheter.

One may try to place a jejunostomy tube by first placing a gastrostomy tube and then inserting a jejunostomy tube through the gastrostomy tube. Next, one directs the jejunostomy tube into the duodenum with a flexible endoscope. Alternatively, one can use a guidewire placed in the duodenum via an endoscope to feed the jejunostomy tube through the gastrostomy tube and into the duodenum.

The small diameter of enterostomy tubes often necessitates the administration of commercial liquid diets (see Table 30-5), which are best infused at a constant rate. The rate necessary to administer daily caloric needs is calculated. A one-half–strength feeding solution is administered at one half the calculated rate on the first day. On the second day the rate of administration is increased to the calculated rate, but a one-half–strength solution is still used. On the third day a full-strength solution is administered at the calculated rate. If diarrhea occurs, the rate of administration can be decreased or fiber (e.g., psyllium) can be added to the liquid diet. The tube should be left in place for 7 to 10 days, if possible, to allow adhesions to develop around the area and prevent leakage. When enteral feeding is no longer necessary, the clinician simply removes the sutures and pulls the catheter out.

## DIETS FOR SPECIAL ENTERAL SUPPORT

Commercial diets (see Table 30-5) may be used for enteral support. Diets containing glutamine (e.g., blended canned diets or diets with crystalline glutamine added), which is critical for small intestinal mucosal nutrition, may be beneficial. (Glutamine also appears to stimulate the intestinal absorption of salt and water.) If the feeding tube diameter is sufficient, blended commercial diets, which are less expensive and still effective, can be used. A gruel made by blending one can of feline p/d (Hill's Pet Products; Topeka, Kan) plus 1½ C (0.35 L) of water provides approximately 0.9 kcal/ml and is useful for dogs and cats. Elemental diets may be better than blended gruels in animals with intestinal disease. However, some elemental diets (e.g., Vivonex; Novartis Nutrition, Minneapolis, Minn) do not have as much protein as desired for dogs and cats (see Table 30-5); therefore one may replace some of the water used in mixing the elemental diet with 8.5% amino acids for injection (e.g., 350 ml water + 250 ml 8.5% amino acids). When feeding cats, be sure sufficient taurine is present in the diet.

Nasoesophageal, pharyngostomy, esophagostomy, and gastrostomy tubes are usually used for bolus feeding. Animals that have been anorectic for days to weeks should usually start by receiving small amounts (e.g., 3 to 5 ml/kg) every 2 to 4 hours. The amount is gradually increased and the frequency decreased until the animal is receiving its caloric needs in three or four daily feedings. One can expect to ultimately administer at least 22 to 30 ml/kg at each feeding to most dogs and cats. Larger volumes may be given if they do not cause vomiting or distress.

TABLE 30-6

Selected Antiemetic Drugs

| DRUG | DOSAGE* |
| --- | --- |
| **Peripherally Acting Drugs** | |
| Kaopectate | 1-2 ml/kg PO q8-12h |
| Bismuth subsalicylate (Pepto-Bismol) | 1 ml/kg PO q8-24h (dogs only) |
| Anticholinergic drugs | |
|     Propantheline (Pro-Banthine) | 0.25-0.5 mg/kg PO q8h |
|     Aminopentimide (Centrine) | 0.01-0.03 mg/kg SQ or IM q8-12h (dogs only) |
| | 0.02 mg/kg SQ or IM q8-12h (cats only) |
| **Centrally Acting Drugs** | |
| Phenothiazine derivatives | |
|     Chlorpromazine (Thorazine) | 0.3-0.5 mg/kg IM q8h |
|     Prochlorperazine (Compazine) | 0.1-0.5 mg/kg IM q6-8h |
| Metoclopramide (Reglan) | 0.25-0.5 mg/kg PO, IM, or IV q8h |
| | 1-2 mg/kg/day, constant IV infusion |
| Ondansetron (Zofran) | 0.1-0.2 mg/kg SQ q8h |
| Trimethobenzamide (Tigan) | 3 mg/kg PO or IM q8h (dogs only) |
| Antihistamine | |
|     Diphenhydramine (Benadryl) | 2-4 mg/kg PO q8h |
| | 1-2 mg/kg IM q8-12h |
| Narcotics | Not usually recommended as antiemetics, although some are quite effective after producing an initial episode of vomiting |

*Dosages are for both dogs and cats unless otherwise specified.

Enterostomy tubes are usually used for constant-rate feeding, which best involves the use of an enteral feeding pump. Begin by feeding the animal a one-half–strength diet at one half the rate that will ultimately be needed to meet the caloric needs. If diarrhea does not result after 24 to 36 hours, increase the flow rate to what will ultimately be needed. If diarrhea still does not occur, then change the diet from one-half strength to full strength. Constant infusion of these same diets may be done through gastrostomy and esophagostomy tubes in animals that readily vomit when fed food in boluses (e.g., some cats with severe hepatic lipidosis).

## PARENTERAL NUTRITION

*Parenteral nutrition* is indicated if the animal's intestines cannot reliably absorb nutrients. It is the most certain method of supplying nutrition to such animals; however, it is expensive and can be associated with metabolic and infectious complications. A central IV line is dedicated to the administration of total parenteral nutrition solution only (i.e., the piggybacking of other solutions and the obtaining of blood samples are forbidden). Double-lumen jugular catheters allow the administration of parenteral nutrition and fluids through the same catheter and are recommended. The aseptic placement and management of the catheter are the best protection against catheter-related sepsis. Antibiotic prophylaxis does not replace proper management and is ineffective in preventing infections. The daily caloric and protein requirements are determined (see Table 30-4), and the customized solution is administered by constant IV infusion. The clinician must routinely monitor the animal's weight; rectal temperature; and serum sodium, chloride, potassium, phosphorous, and glucose concentrations (and the urine for glucosuria). The feeding solution is adjusted to prevent or correct serum imbalances. Partial parenteral nutrition is similar but (1) aims to supply approximately 50% of caloric needs; (2) has a lower osmolality than total parenteral nutrition (TPN) solutions that allows administration via a peripheral vein and; (3) is intended to be used for approximately a week with the goal to get a severely ill or emaciated patient "over the hump" before starting enteral nutrition. If parenteral nutrition is used, the animal should also receive some feedings PO, if possible, to help prevent intestinal villous atrophy.

## ANTIEMETICS

Antiemetics are indicated for symptomatic therapy in many animals with acute vomiting or if vomiting is contributing to morbidity (e.g., discomfort or excessive fluid and electrolyte losses). Peripherally acting drugs (Table 30-6) are less effective than centrally acting ones but may suffice in animals with minimal disease. Some of these drugs are given orally, but this is an untrustworthy route in nauseated animals. Parasympatholytics (e.g., atropine, aminopentamide) have been used extensively. Although they are given parenterally and may have some central activity, they are seldom effective in animals with severe vomiting.

If it is important to halt the vomiting, a centrally acting drug should be administered parenterally. Suppositories are convenient, but their absorption is erratic.

*Phenothiazine derivatives* (e.g., prochlorperazine [Compazine]) are especially effective. They inhibit the chemoreceptor trigger zone and, in higher doses, the medullary vomiting center. Antiemesis is usually achieved at doses that do not produce marked sedation. However, chlorpromazine causes vasodilation and can decrease peripheral perfusion in a dehydrated animal. Phenothiazines also lower the seizure threshold in animals with epilepsy.

*Metoclopramide* (Reglan) inhibits the chemoreceptor trigger zone and increases gastric tone and peristalsis, both of which inhibit emesis. Rarely, animals experience apparent hallucinations or show other unusual behavior. The drug is excreted in the urine, and severe renal failure makes adverse effects (e.g., psychotic behavior) more likely. It rarely worsens vomiting, perhaps because it causes excessive gastric contractions. The liquid form of metoclopramide given PO is often not accepted by cats. Because of its prokinetic activity, the drug is contraindicated in animals with a gastric or duodenal obstruction. Metoclopramide may be more effective in animals with severe vomiting if given IV at a dosage of 1 to 2 mg/kg/day by constant-rate infusion.

*Ondansetron* (Zofran) is a serotonin receptor antagonist. Developed for use in people with vomiting resulting from chemotherapy, it is effective in some animals in which vomiting is not controlled with phenothiazines or metoclopramide (e.g., those with severe canine parvoviral enteritis). It is not effective in all vomiting animals, especially those with alimentary tract obstructions.

*Narcotics*, such as fentanyl, oxymorphone, and butorphanol, may cause vomiting initially, but vomiting is usually inhibited once the drug penetrates to the medullary vomiting center. *Trimethobenzamide* (Tigan) and *antihistamines* are effective in some animals but generally are untrustworthy antiemetics in dogs and cats.

## ANTACID DRUGS

Antacid drugs (Table 30-7) are indicated when it is appropriate to lessen gastric acidity (e.g., ulcer disease; acid hypersecretion resulting from renal failure, mast cell tumor, or gastrinoma). Although they are not antiemetics, they may diminish vomiting if gastric hyperacidity is responsible for it.

*Antacids*, which titrate the gastric acidity, are over-the-counter preparations that are typically of limited efficacy because of the way they are administered. Compounds containing aluminum or magnesium tend to be more effective and do not cause the gastric acid rebound that sometimes occurs in response to calcium-containing antacids. Antacids should be administered every 4 to 6 hours PO to ensure continued control of gastric acidity; however, this may cause diarrhea, especially in animals receiving magnesium-containing compounds. Hypophosphatemia, although unlikely, is possible after extensive aluminum hydroxide administration. Hypermagnesemia, also unlikely, is possible in dogs and cats with renal failure given magnesium-containing compounds. These types of antacids

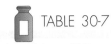 TABLE 30-7

**Selected Antacid Drugs**

| DRUG | DOSAGE* |
|---|---|
| **Acid Titrating Drugs** | |
| Aluminum hydroxide (many names) | 5-10 ml PO q4-6h |
| Magnesium hydroxide (many names) | 5-10 ml PO q4-6h (dogs), q8-12h (cats) |
| **Gastric Acid Secretion Inhibitors** | |
| H₂ receptor antagonists | |
|   Cimetidine (Tagamet) | 5-10 mg/kg PO, IM, or IV q6-8h |
|   Ranitidine (Zantac) | 2 mg/kg PO or IV q8-12h (dogs only) 2.5 mg/kg IV or 3.5 mg/kg PO q12h (cats only) |
|   Famotidine (Pepcid, Pepcid AC) | 0.5 mg/kg PO or IM q12-24h |
| Proton pump inhibitor | |
|   Omeprazole (Prilosec) | 0.7-1.5 mg/kg PO q12-24h (dogs only) |

*Dosages are for both dogs and cats unless otherwise specified.

may also interfere with the absorption of other drugs (e.g., tetracycline, cimetidine).

*Histamine₂ (H₂) receptor antagonists* are indicated when it is important to control gastric acidity. They act by preventing histamine from stimulating the gastric parietal cell. Cimetidine (Tagamet) is effective but should be given three or four times per day to achieve best results; it inhibits hepatic cytochrome P-450 enzymes, thereby slowing the metabolism of some drugs. Ranitidine (Zantac), famotidine (Pepcid), and nizatidine (Axid) are as or more effective if administered one or two times per day and do not affect hepatic enzyme activity as much as cimetidine does. The H₂ antagonists are now available as over-the-counter preparations. The main indication for these drugs is the treatment of gastric and duodenal ulcers. Some clinicians use them prophylactically to try to prevent ulceration associated with stress and the use of some nonsteroidal antiinflammatory drugs (NSAIDs), but they are most effective in treating existing ulcers. Nizatidine and ranitidine have prokinetic effects on the stomach. Very rarely these drugs may cause bone marrow suppression, central nervous system problems, or diarrhea. Parenteral administration, especially the rapid IV injection of ranitidine, may cause nausea, vomiting, or bradycardia.

*Omeprazole* (Prilosec) and *lansoprazole* (Prevacid) are proton pump inhibitors that block the final common pathway of gastric acid secretion. This is the most effective class of drugs for decreasing gastric acid secretion. Omeprazole is a noncompetitive inhibitor primarily used in animals with severe gastroesophageal reflux or gastrinomas (diseases in which H₂ antagonists are often inadequate). It is uncertain whether most animals with gastric ulcer benefit from the enhanced blockade of gastric acid secretion this drug provides, as compared with H₂ receptor antagonist therapy.

## INTESTINAL PROTECTANTS

Intestinal protectants (Table 30-8) include drugs and inert adsorbents such as kaopectate and barium sulfate contrast media. Many people believe that inert adsorbents hasten clinical relief in animals with minor inflammation, possibly because they "coat" the mucosa or adsorb toxins. They probably make fecal consistency more normal simply by increasing fecal particulate matter. Inert adsorbents do not have a proven efficacy in the treatment of gastritis or enteritis. It is inappropriate to rely on these drugs alone in very sick animals.

*Sucralfate* (Carafate) is principally indicated for animals with gastroduodenal ulceration or erosion but might also be useful for those with esophagitis (especially if administered as a slurry). It does not appear to effectively prevent NSAID-induced ulceration but may help prevent stress ulceration. Sucralfate is a nonabsorbable, sulfated sucrose complex that protects denuded mucosa by adhering tightly to it. It also inhibits peptic activity and may alter prostaglandin synthesis and the actions of endogenous sulfhydryl compounds. The dose is extrapolated from humans on the basis of the animal's weight. A large initial dose (e.g., 2 to 4 g) may be used in animals with severe bleeding. Although no supportive data are available for dogs and cats, sucralfate and $H_2$ antagonists are often used concurrently in animals with severe gastrointestinal tract ulceration or erosion. However, because sucralfate may adsorb other drugs, other orally administered drugs should be given 1 to 2 hours before or after sucralfate administration. Although an acidic pH promotes optimal activity, sucralfate seems reasonably effective at pHs occurring after $H_2$ receptor antagonist therapy. There are no absolute contraindications to the use of sucralfate. The biggest disadvantage is that it must be given orally, and many animals that need it are vomiting. Sucralfate's major adverse effect is constipation.

*Misoprostol* (Cytotec) is a prostaglandin $E_1$ analog used to help prevent NSAID-induced gastroduodenal ulceration. The drug is primarily used in dogs that require NSAIDs but in which NSAIDs cause anorexia or vomiting. Use of NSAIDs that have a higher risk of causing gastrointestinal tract problems (e.g., naproxen) may also be an indication. The major adverse effects of misoprostol seem to be abdominal cramping and diarrhea, which usually disappear after 2 to 3 days of therapy. Pregnancy may be a contraindication. There is evidence that misoprostol may have immunosuppressant properties, especially in combination with other drugs.

## DIGESTIVE ENZYME SUPPLEMENTATION

*Pancreatic enzyme supplementation* is indicated to treat exocrine pancreatic insufficiency; however, it is often used empirically without justification in animals with diarrhea. There are many products that vary greatly in their potency. Although pills may work, powdered preparations tend to be more effective; enteric-coated pills are particularly ineffective. Viokase-V (A.H. Robins Co., Richmond, Va) and Pancreazyme (Daniels Pharmaceuticals, St. Petersburg, Fla) are particularly efficacious products in dogs. The powder should be mixed with the food (approximately 1 to 2 tsp per meal), but allowing the mixture to "incubate" before feeding has not been found beneficial. Fat is the main nutrient that must be digested in animals with exocrine pancreatic insufficiency, and feeding them a low-fat diet may ameliorate diarrhea. Antacid or antibiotic therapy, or both, may occasionally be necessary to prevent gastric acidity or small intestinal bacteria from rendering the enzyme supplementation ineffective. Occasionally a stomatitis or diarrhea develops in dogs receiving large amounts of enzyme supplementation.

## MOTILITY MODIFIERS

*Drugs that prolong the intestinal transit time* are principally used to symptomatically treat diarrhea. Although infrequently needed, they are indicated if the diarrhea causes excessive fluid or electrolyte losses or owners demand control of

 TABLE 30-8

Selected Gastrointestinal Protectants and Cytoprotective Agents

| DRUG | DOSAGE* | COMMENT |
|---|---|---|
| Sucralfate (Carafate) | 0.5-1 g (dog) or 0.25 g (cat) PO 3-4 times daily, depending on animal's size; may administer 2-4 g as a "loading" dose in dogs with severe alimentary tract hemorrhage | Potentially constipating, absorbs some other orally administered drugs, primarily used to treat existing ulcers |
| Misoprostol (Cytotec) | 2-5 µg/kg PO 3 times daily (dogs only) | May cause diarrhea/abdominal cramps, primarily used to prevent ulcers, not for use in pregnant animals |
| Kaopectate | 1-2 mg/kg PO 4-8 times daily | Questionable efficacy |

*Dosages are for both dogs and cats unless otherwise specified.

the diarrhea at home. Opiates (Table 30-9) increase resistance to flow by augmenting segmental contraction. They tend to be more effective than parasympatholytics, which paralyze motility in the intestines (i.e., create ileus). Both classes of drugs have antisecretory effects. Cats do not tolerate narcotics as well as dogs, so opiates should be avoided in this species, although loperamide may be used carefully.

*Loperamide* (Imodium) is available as an over-the-counter drug. However, this opiate is so effective at decreasing intestinal flow that it theoretically increases the risk for bacterial proliferation in the intestinal lumen, thus potentially initiating or perpetuating disease, which is actually very rare in clinical practice. An overdose can cause narcotic intoxication (i.e., collapse, vomiting, ataxia, hypersalivation), which requires treatment with narcotic antagonists.

*Diphenoxylate* (Lomotil) is similar to loperamide but tends to be somewhat less effective. It has more potential for toxicity than loperamide. However, some dogs respond to it but not to loperamide. This drug should not be used in cats.

*Drugs that shorten the transit time* (prokinetic drugs) empty the stomach or increase intestinal peristalsis or both. *Metoclopramide* is a prokinetic drug that is only effective in the stomach and the proximal duodenum. However, it can be administered parenterally. Adverse effects are mentioned under the section on antiemetics. *Cisapride* stimulates normal motility from the lower esophageal sphincter to the anus. It is usually effective unless the tissue has been irreparably damaged (e.g., megacolon in cats). Primarily used for the treatment of con-

stipation, it may also be used for the management of gastroparesis (in which it is usually more effective than metoclopramide) and small intestinal ileus. It has rarely been reported to be beneficial in dogs with megaesophagus. Cisapride is no longer available from human pharmacies but is typically available from veterinary pharmacies. It is only available as an oral preparation. It has few significant adverse effects, although intoxication with large doses may cause diarrhea, muscular tremors, ataxia, fever, aggression, and other central nervous system signs. *Erythromycin* stimulates motilin receptors and enhances gastric motility at doses less than required for antibacterial activity (i.e., 2 mg/kg). It may also increase intestinal motility. *Nizatidine* and *ranitidine* are $H_2$ receptor antagonists that also have gastric prokinetic effects at routinely used doses. *Bethanechol* (Urecholine) is an acetylcholine analog that stimulates intestinal motility and secretion. It produces strong contractions that can cause pain or injure the animal; hence it is infrequently used, except for increasing urinary bladder contractions. Obstruction of an outflow area can be a contraindication to the use of prokinetic drugs, because vigorous contractions against such a lesion may cause pain or perforation. Obstruction of the urinary outflow tract is also a contraindication to the use of bethanechol.

*Pyridostigmine* (Mestinon) inhibits acetylcholinesterase and is used to treat myasthenia gravis (see p. 1059). It is used for the treatment of acquired megaesophagus associated with the formation of antibodies to acetylcholine receptors. It must be used cautiously, since overdose can cause toxicity accompanied by signs of parasympathetic overload (e.g., vomiting, miosis, diarrhea). Azathioprine (with or without steroids) seems to be a better long-term treatment for myasthenia gravis than pyridostigmine.

## TABLE 30-9

### Selected Drugs Used to Treat Diarrhea Symptomatically

| DRUG | DOSAGE* |
|---|---|
| **Intestinal Motility Modifiers** | |
| Anticholinergic drugs | |
| Methscopolamine (Pamine) | 0.3-1.0 mg/kg PO q8h (dogs only) |
| Propantheline (Pro-Banthine) | 0.25-0.5 mg/kg PO q8-12h |
| Opiates | |
| Diphenoxylate (Lomotil) | 0.05-0.2 mg/kg PO q8-12h (dogs only) |
| Loperamide (Imodium) | 0.1-0.2 mg/kg PO q8-12h (dogs only) 0.08-0.16 mg/kg PO q12h (cats only) |
| Paregoric | 0.05-0.06 mg/kg PO q12h (dogs only) |
| **Antiinflammatory/Antisecretory Drug** | |
| Bismuth subsalicylate (Pepto-Bismol) | 1 ml/kg PO q8-12h (dogs only) for 1-2 days |

*Dosages are for both dogs and cats unless otherwise specified.

## ANTIINFLAMMATORY AND ANTISECRETORY DRUGS

Intestinal antiinflammatory or antisecretory drugs or both are indicated for lessening the fluid losses resulting from diarrhea or for controlling intestinal inflammation that is unresponsive to dietary or antibacterial therapy.

*Bismuth subsalicylate* (Pepto-Bismol) is an over-the-counter antidiarrheal agent that is effective in many dogs with acute enteritis (see Table 30-9), probably because of the antiprostaglandin activity of the salicylate moiety. The main disadvantages are that the salicylate is absorbed (warranting its cautious use in cats or in dogs receiving other nephrotoxic drugs), it turns stools black (which mimics melena), and it must be administered orally (many animals dislike its taste). Bismuth is bactericidal for certain organisms (e.g., *Helicobacter* spp.).

*Octreotide* (Sandostatin) is a synthetic analog of somatostatin that inhibits alimentary tract motility and the secretion of gastrointestinal hormones and fluids. It has had limited use in dogs and cats but might be helpful in a few animals with intractable diarrhea or pancreatitis.

*Salicylazosulfapyridine* (*sulfasalazine* [Azulfidine]) is indicated for animals with considerable colonic inflammation, not for the empiric treatment of undefined diarrhea. This drug is generally not beneficial in animals with small intestinal problems. It is a combination of sulfapyridine and 5-aminosalicylic acid. The colonic bacteria split the molecule, and the 5-aminosalicylic acid (probably the active moiety) is subsequently deposited on diseased colonic mucosa. Dogs generally receive 50 to 60 mg/kg, divided into three times daily, but not to exceed 3 g/day. Sulfasalazine may be effective at lower-than-expected doses if used in combination with glucocorticoids. Empirically, 20 to 40 mg/kg/day, sometimes divided into twice-daily doses, is often tolerated by cats, but they must be closely observed for the development of salicylate intoxication (i.e., lethargy, anorexia, vomiting, hyperthermia, tachypnea). Some cats that vomit or become anorectic may tolerate the medication if it is given in enteric-coated tablets. Many dogs with colitis respond to therapy in 3 to 5 days. However, the drug should be given for 2 weeks before deciding that it is ineffective. If signs of colitis resolve, the dose of the drug should be gradually reduced. If the animal cannot be weaned off the drug entirely, the lowest effective dose should be used and the animal monitored regularly for the development of drug-induced adverse effects (especially those resulting from the sulfa drug). Sulfasalazine may cause transient or permanent keratoconjunctivitis sicca. Other possible complications include cutaneous vasculitis, arthritis, bone marrow suppression, diarrhea, and any other problem associated with sulfa drugs or NSAIDs.

*Olsalazine* and *mesalamine* contain or are metabolized to 5-aminosalicylic acid but do not have the sulfa, which is responsible for most of sulfasalazine's adverse effects. In people they are as effective as sulfasalazine but safer. Olsalazine and mesalamine have been used effectively in dogs. They are given in a dose generally about one half that of sulfasalazine. Keratoconjunctivitis sicca has also been found in dogs receiving mesalamine.

*Corticosteroids* are specifically indicated in animals with chronic alimentary tract inflammation (e.g., moderate-to-marked lymphocytic, plasmacytic, or eosinophilic inflammatory bowel diseases) that is not responsive to well-designed elimination diets. Relatively high doses (i.e., prednisolone, 2.2 mg/kg/day) are often used initially, which cats typically tolerate well. If PO administration is a problem in a cat, long-lasting steroid injections may be tried. Sometimes dexamethasone is effective when prednisolone is not, but dexamethasone seems to have more adverse effects than prednisolone. The response may be rapid or may take weeks.

*Corticosteroids* are often beneficial in cats with inflammatory bowel disease, but may worsen ulcerative colitides or lymphocytic-plasmacytic colitis in some dogs. Further, iatrogenic Cushing's syndrome is more of a problem in dogs. Finally, it is important to have a histologically based diagnosis before using high-dose prednisolone therapy, because some diseases that mimic steroid-responsive lymphocytic colitis (e.g., histoplasmosis) are absolute contraindications to corticosteroid therapy. Although more common in the southeastern United States and the Ohio River Valley, histoplasmosis has been found in almost every state.

*Retention enemas* of corticosteroids or 5-aminosalicylic acid are sometimes indicated in animals with severe distal colitis. The dose is estimated from the human dose. These enemas place large doses of an antiinflammatory agent directly on the affected area while minimizing systemic effects. Although effective in controlling the clinical signs, their administration is unpleasant for both clients and animals. Further, the active ingredient may be absorbed if there is substantial inflammation and increased mucosal permeability (i.e., animals receiving corticosteroid enemas can become polyuric and polydipsic). Therapeutic retention enemas are typically used in conjunction with other antiinflammatory therapy and then only until the clinical signs are controlled and other therapy (e.g., sulfasalazine, diet) becomes effective. The contraindications to their use are the same as those to the systemic administration of the active ingredient of the enema.

*Budesonide* is an orally administered steroid designed to have minimal systemic side effects because it is eliminated by first-pass metabolism in the liver. This drug has been used for inflammatory bowel disease (IBD) and hepatic disease in people, and it has recently been used in dogs and cats with similar problems. Iatrogenic hyperadrenocorticism has been anecdotally reported in some veterinary patients.

*Immunosuppressive* therapy (e.g., azathioprine, chlorambucil) is indicated in animals with severe inflammatory bowel disease that is unresponsive to corticosteroid and dietary therapy. It is also used in animals with severe disease in which it is in the animal's best interest to use aggressive therapy initially. These drugs should only be used if the diagnosis has been confirmed histopathologically. Immunosuppressive therapy can be more efficacious than corticosteroid therapy alone and allows corticosteroids to be given at lower doses and for shorter periods, thereby decreasing their adverse effects. However, the possibility of adverse effects from these drugs usually limits their use to animals with severe disease. The reader is referred to Chapter 93 for additional information on immunosuppressive therapy.

*Azathioprine* (Imuran) is commonly used in dogs (50 mg/m$^2$ daily or every other day) with severe alimentary tract lymphocytic-plasmacytic infiltrates. A lower dose (0.3 mg/kg every other day) has been used in cats with similar disease but is not recommended due to the risk for myelotoxicity. For smaller animals a 50-mg azathioprine tablet is typically crushed and suspended in a liquid (e.g., 15 ml of a vitamin supplement) to allow more accurate dosing. The suspension must be mixed well before each dosing. In both species it may take 2 to 5 weeks before the beneficial effects of this drug are seen.

In cats the major side effect of azathioprine is neutropenia caused by myelosuppression. If the neutrophil count decreases to less than 2000/μl, therapy should be stopped or the dose decreased. Side effects in dogs may include hepatic disease, pancreatitis, and bone marrow suppression.

Alkylating agents such as chlorambucil (Leukeran) are used for the same reasons as azathioprine. Chlorambucil, however, appears to have fewer adverse effects than azathioprine. A reasonable starting dose in cats is 1 mg twice weekly for cats weighing less than 7 lb (3 kg) and 2 mg twice weekly for cats weighing more than that. Beneficial effects may not be seen for 4 to 5 weeks. If a response is seen, the dose should then be decreased very slowly over the next 2 to 3 months. The animal should be monitored for myelosuppression. Stronger alkylating agents such as cyclophosphamide are seldom used for the management of nonneoplastic gastrointestinal tract disease.

## ANTIBACTERIAL DRUGS

In dogs and cats with gastrointestinal problems, antibiotics are primarily indicated if aspiration pneumonia, fever, a leukogram suggestive of sepsis, severe neutropenia, antibiotic-responsive enteropathy, clostridial colitis, symptomatic *Helicobacter* gastritis, or perhaps hematemesis or melena is found or suspected. Animals with an acute abdomen may reasonably be treated with antibiotics while the nature of the disease is being defined. However, most animals with enteritis or gastritis of unknown cause do not benefit from antibiotic therapy. In general, the routine use of antimicrobials in animals with alimentary tract disorders is not recommended, unless the animal is at high risk for infection or a specific disorder is being treated.

Nonabsorbable aminoglycosides (e.g., neomycin) are often used to "sterilize" the intestines. However, they do not kill anaerobic bacteria, which are the predominant type found there. Further, there are a plethora of viral and dietary causes of acute enteritis that are not responsive to antibiotics. Thus aminoglycosides given PO are not indicated unless a specific infection (e.g., campylobacteriosis) is being considered. Some data suggest that neomycin is effective against *Giardia*.

Broad-spectrum antibiotics effective against anaerobes (e.g., tetracycline) may be used for the treatment of antibiotic-responsive enteropathy. Metronidazole may also be used for this purpose (see later discussion) but has not been as successful in my hands. Inappropriate therapy with some of these drugs may hypothetically eliminate enough resident bacteria that overgrowth of pathogenic bacteria in the colon occurs. However, this is rarely a clinical problem in dogs and cats. One should treat for at least 2 weeks before deciding that therapy has been unsuccessful.

Occasionally pets have enteritis caused by a specific bacterium. However, even this is not necessarily an indication for antibiotics. Clinical signs resulting from some bacterial enteritides (e.g., salmonellosis, enterohemorrhagic *Escherichia. coli*) generally do not resolve more quickly when the animal is treated with antibiotics, even those to which the bacteria are sensitive.

Dogs and cats with viral enteritis but without obvious systemic sepsis may reasonably be treated with antibiotics if secondary sepsis is likely to occur (e.g., those with neutropenia or severe hemorrhagic diarrhea). First-generation cephalosporins (e.g., cefazolin) are often effective for such use.

If *systemic or abdominal sepsis* is suspected to have originated from the alimentary tract (e.g., septicemia caused by parvoviral enteritis, perforated intestine), broad-spectrum antimicrobial therapy is indicated. Antibiotics with a good aerobic gram-positive and anaerobic spectrum of action (e.g., ampicillin, 20 mg/kg given IV four times daily, or clindamycin, 10 mg/kg given IV three times daily) combined with antibiotics with excellent activity against most aerobic bacteria (e.g., amikacin, 25 mg/kg given IV once daily or enrofloxacin, 15 mg/kg given IV once daily) are often effective. To improve the anaerobic spectrum, especially if a cephalosporin is used instead of ampicillin, the clinician may include metronidazole (10 mg/kg given IV two or three times daily). Alternatively, a second-generation cephalosporin (e.g., cefoxitin, 22 mg/kg given IV three or four times daily) may be used. In general, it takes at least 48 to 72 hours before one can see whether the therapy will be effective.

*Helicobacter* gastritis may be treated with various combinations of drugs. Currently the combination of an antacid (i.e., famotidine or omeprazole; see Table 30-7) and a macrolide (i.e., erythromycin or azithromycin; see table of Drugs Used in Gastrointestinal Disorders, p. 469) or amoxicillin seems to be very effective. Adding metronidazole may enhance efficacy. However, some patients seem to respond to erythromycin or amoxicillin as a sole agent. If high doses of erythromycin (22 mg/kg given twice daily) cause vomiting, the dose may be lowered to 10 to 15 mg/kg given twice daily. A 10- to 14-day course of treatment appears to be adequate for most animals, although recurrence seems the rule.

*Metronidazole* is a "miscellaneous" drug that is commonly used in animals with inflammatory bowel disease. It has antimicrobial activity against anaerobic bacteria (which predominate in the gastrointestinal tract) and protozoa (e.g., *Giardia*). It also seems to have some effect on the immune system, as shown by its apparent beneficial effects in people with Crohn's disease. The usefulness of metronidazole in dogs and cats with inflammatory bowel disease (10 to 15 mg/kg given twice daily) is suspected but unproved. Adverse effects are uncommon but may include salivation (because of its taste), vomiting, central nervous system abnormalities (e.g., seizures), and perhaps neutropenia. These adverse effects usually resolve after withdrawing the drug. Cats sometimes accept oral suspensions better than the 250-mg tablets, which must be cut and taste badly. Some cats with inflammatory bowel disease respond to metronidazole better than they do to corticosteroids. Occasionally dogs with colitis do likewise.

## ANTHELMINTIC DRUGS

Anthelmintics are frequently prescribed for dogs and cats with alimentary tract disease, even if parasitism is not the primary problem. It is often reasonable to use these drugs

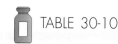

TABLE 30-10

Selected Anthelmintics

| DRUG | DOSAGE* (PO) | USE | COMMENTS |
|------|-------------|-----|----------|
| Albendazole (Valbazen) | 25 mg/kg q12h for 3 days (dogs only)<br>25 mg/kg q12h for 5 days (cats only) | G | May cause leukopenia in some animals. Do not use in early pregnancy. Not approved for use in dogs. |
| Fenbendazole (Panacur) | 50 mg/kg for 3 days | H/R/W/G | Not approved for cats but can be used for 3-5 days in cats to eliminate *Giardia*. Give with food. |
| Furazolidone | 4.4 mg/kg q12h for 5 days | G | — |
| Metronidazole (Flagyl) | 50 mg/kg for 5-10 days (dogs only)<br>25-50 mg/kg for 5 days (cats only) | G | Rarely see neurologic signs |
| Pyrantel (Nemex) | 5 mg/kg, repeat in 7-10 days (dogs only)<br>20 mg/kg, once only (cats only) | H/R/P | Give after meal |
| Ivermectin | 200 µg/kg (dogs only) | H/R/P | Do not use in Collies, Shelties, Border Collies, or Australian Shepherds. Use with caution in Old English Sheepdogs. Only approved for use as heartworm preventive. |
| Milbemycin (Interceptor) | 0.5 mg/kg, monthly | H/R/W | Not approved for use in cats |
| Praziquantel (Droncit) | 5 mg/kg for dogs >6.8 kg<br>7.5 mg/kg for dogs <6.8 kg<br>6.3 mg/kg for cats <1.8 kg<br>5 mg/kg for cats >1.8 kg | T | 10 mg/kg for juvenile *Echinococcus* spp. |
| Episprantel (Cestex) | 5.5 mg/kg for dogs<br>2.75 mg/kg for cats | T | — |
| Selamectin (Revolution) | 6 mg/kg topical for cats | H/R | Not approved for use in dogs |
| Sulfadimethoxine (Albon) | 50 mg/kg on day 1, then 27.5 mg/kg q12h for 9 days | C | — |
| Trimethoprim-sulfadiazine (Tribrissen) | 30 mg/kg for 10 days | C | May cause dry eyes, arthritis, cytopenia, hepatic disease |

*G, Giardia; H, hookworms; R, roundworms; W, whipworms; P, Physaloptera; T, tapeworms; C, coccidia.*
*Dosages are for both dogs and cats unless otherwise specified.*

empirically for the treatment of suspected parasitic infections in animals with acute or chronic diarrhea. Selected anthelmintics are listed in Table 30-10.

## ENEMAS, LAXATIVES, AND CATHARTICS

*Enemas* are classified as either cleansing or retention.

*Retention enemas* are given so that the material administered stays in the colon until it exerts its desired effects (e.g., antiinflammatory retention enemas are used in animals with inflammatory bowel disease, water in obstipated animals). Obstipated animals may require frequent administrations of modest volumes of water (e.g., 20 to 200 ml, depending on the animal's size) so that the water stays in the colon and gradually softens the feces. Avoid overdistending the colon or administering drugs that may be absorbed and produce undesirable effects. Suspected or pending colonic rupture is a

contraindication to the use of enemas; however, this is difficult to predict. Neurosurgical animals (e.g., those that have had a hemilaminectomy) receiving corticosteroids (e.g., dexamethasone) may be at increased risk for colonic perforation. Animals with colonic tumors or that have recently undergone colonic surgery or biopsy should not receive enemas either, unless there is an overriding reason.

*Cleansing enemas* are designed to remove fecal material. They involve the repeated administration of large volumes of warm water (with or without Castile soap). In dogs the water is administered by gravity flow from a bucket or bag held above the animal. The tube is gently advanced as far as it will easily go into the colon. Fifty to one-hundred milliliters is tolerated by most small dogs, 200 to 500 ml by medium-size dogs, and 1 to 2 L by large dogs. Care should be taken to avoid overdistending or perforating the colon. Enemas are usually administered to cats with a soft canine male urinary catheter and a 50-ml syringe. If fluid is administered too quickly, how-

TABLE 30-11

Selected Laxatives, Cathartics, Stool-Softening Agents, and Bulking Agents

| DRUG | DOSAGE (PO) | COMMENTS |
|---|---|---|
| Bisacodyl (Dulcolax) | 5 mg (small dogs and cats) 10-15 mg (larger dogs) | Do not break tablets |
| Coarse wheat bran | 1-3 tbsp/454 g of food | |
| Canned pumpkin pie filling | 1-3 tbsp/day (cats only) | Principally for cats |
| Dioctyl sodium sulfosuccinate (Colace) | 10-200 mg q8-12h (dogs only) 50 mg q12-24h (cats only) | Be sure animal is not dehydrated when treating |
| Lactulose (Cephulac) | 1 ml/5 kg q8-12h, then adjust dose as needed (dogs only) 5 ml q8h, then adjust dose as needed (cats only) | Can cause severe osmotic diarrhea |
| Psyllium (Metamucil) | 1-2 tsp/454 g of food | Be sure animal has enough water, or constipation may develop |

ever, the cat will usually vomit. A suspected or pending colonic perforation is also a contraindication to a cleansing enema.

*Hypertonic enemas* are potentially dangerous and should be used cautiously (if at all), because they can cause massive, fatal fluid and electrolyte shifts (i.e., hyperphosphatemia, hypocalcemia, hypokalemia, hyperkalemia). This is especially true for cats, small dogs, and any animal that cannot quickly evacuate the enema because of obstipation.

*Cathartics* and *laxatives* (Table 30-11) should only be used to augment defecation in animals that are not obstructed. They are not routinely indicated in small animals, except perhaps as part of lower bowel cleansing before contrast-enhanced abdominal radiography or endoscopy.

*Irritative laxatives* (e.g., bisacodyl) stimulate defecation rather than soften feces. They are often used before colonoscopic procedures and in animals that are reluctant to defecate because of an altered environment. They are probably not appropriate for long-term use because of the dependence and colonic problems noted in people that have used them inappropriately. A glycerin suppository or a lubricated match stick is often an effective substitute for an irritative laxative. These objects are carefully placed in the rectum to stimulate defecation.

*Bulk and osmotic laxatives* include a variety of preparations: various fibers (especially the soluble ones), magnesium sulfate, lactulose, and, in milk-intolerant animals, ice cream or milk. They promote the fecal retention of water and are indicated in animals that have overly hard stools not caused by the ingestion of foreign objects. These laxatives are more appropriate for long-term use than are the irritative cathartics. Larger doses may be needed in cats because they retain fluids better than dogs do.

*Fiber* is a bulking agent that is incorporated into the food and can be used indefinitely. Commercial diets relatively high in fiber may be used, or existing diets may be supplemented with fiber (see pp. 736 and 754). It is important to supply adequate amounts of water so that the additional fiber does not cause the formation of harder-than-normal stools. Too much fiber may cause excessive stool or inappetence resulting from decreased palatability (a danger for fat cats at risk for hepatic lipidosis). Fiber should not be given to animals with a partial or complete alimentary tract obstruction, because impaction may occur.

*Lactulose* (Cephulac) was designed to control signs of hepatic encephalopathy, but it is also a very effective osmotic laxative. It is a disaccharide that is split by colonic bacteria into unabsorbed particles. Lactulose is particularly useful for animals that refuse to eat high-fiber diets. The dose necessary to soften feces must be determined in each animal, but 0.5 or 5 ml may be given two or three times per day to small and large dogs, respectively. Cats often need higher dosages (e.g., 5 ml three times daily). If gross overdosing occurs, so much water can be lost that hypernatremic dehydration ensues. There are no obvious contraindications to the use of lactulose.

## Suggested Readings

Boothe DM: Gastrointestinal pharmacology. In Boothe DM, editor: *Small animal clinical pharmacology and therapeutics,* Philadelphia, 2001, WB Saunders.

Day TK: Shock syndromes in veterinary medicine. In DiBartola SP, editor: *Fluid therapy in small animal practice,* ed 2, Philadelphia, 2000, WB Saunders.

Dimski DS: Therapy of inflammatory bowel disease. In Bonagura JD, editor: *Current veterinary therapy XII,* ed 12, Philadelphia, 1995, WB Saunders.

Hall EJ et al: Diseases of the small intestine. In Ettinger SJ et al, editor: *Textbook of veterinary internal medicine,* ed 5, Philadelphia, 2000, WB Saunders.

Hall JA et al: Gastric prokinetic agents. In Bonagura JD, editor: *Current veterinary therapy XIII,* ed 13, Philadelphia, 2000, WB Saunders.

Jergens AE: Acute diarrhea. In Bonagura JD, editor: *Current veterinary therapy XII,* ed 12, Philadelphia, 1995, WB Saunders.

Jergens AE et al: Diseases of the large intestine. In Ettinger SJ et al, editors: *Textbook of veterinary internal medicine,* ed 5, Philadelphia, 2000, WB Saunders.

Marks SL et al: Nutritional management of diarrheal diseases. In Bonagura JD, editor: *Current veterinary therapy XIII,* ed 13, Philadelphia, 20005, WB Saunders.

Reinemeyer CR: Canine gastrointestinal parasites. In Bonagura JD, editor: *Current veterinary therapy XII,* ed 12, Philadelphia, 1995, WB Saunders.

Remillard RL et al: Dietary and nutritional management of gastrointestinal diseases, *Vet Clin North Am* 19:797, 1989.

Remillard RL et al: Assisted feeding in hospitalized patients: enteral and parenteral nutrition. In Hand MS et al, editors: *Small animal clinical nutrition,* ed 4, Topeka, Kan, 2000, Mark Morris Institute.

Remillard RL: Parenteral nutrition. In DiBartola SP, editor: *Fluid therapy in small animal practice,* ed 2, Philadelphia, 2000, WB Saunders.

Schertel ER et al: Hypertonic fluid therapy. In DiBartola SP, editor: *Fluid therapy in small animal practice,* ed 2, Philadelphia, 2000, WB Saunders.

Simpson KW et al: Fluid and electrolyte disorders in gastrointestinal, pancreatic, and hepatic disease. In DiBartola SP, editor: *Fluid therapy in small animal practice,* ed 2, Philadelphia, 2000, WB Saunders.

Volmer PA: Cisapride toxicosis in dogs, *Vet Hum Toxicol* 38:118, 1996.

## CHAPTER 31

# Disorders of the Oral Cavity, Pharynx, and Esophagus

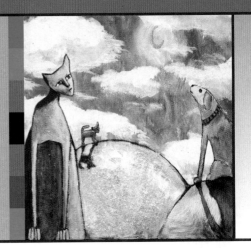

## CHAPTER OUTLINE

MASSES, PROLIFERATIONS, AND INFLAMMATION
OF THE OROPHARYNX, 405
    Sialocele, 405
    Sialoadenitis/sialoadenosis/salivary gland necrosis, 405
    Neoplasms of the oral cavity in dogs, 406
    Neoplasms of the oral cavity in cats, 407
    Feline eosinophilic granuloma, 407
    Gingivitis/periodontitis, 407
    Stomatitis, 408
    Feline lymphocytic-plasmacytic gingivitis/
      pharyngitis, 408
DYSPHAGIAS, 409
    Masticatory muscle myositis/atrophic myositis, 409
    Cricopharyngeal achalasia/dysfunction, 409
    Pharyngeal dysphagia, 409
ESOPHAGEAL WEAKNESS/
MEGAESOPHAGUS, 410
    Congenital esophageal weakness, 410
    Acquired esophageal weakness, 411
    Esophagitis, 412
    Hiatal hernia, 412
    Dysautonomia, 412
ESOPHAGEAL OBSTRUCTION, 413
    Vascular ring anomalies, 413
    Esophageal foreign objects, 414
    Esophageal cicatrix, 414
    Esophageal neoplasms, 415

## MASSES, PROLIFERATIONS, AND INFLAMMATION OF THE OROPHARYNX

### SIALOCELE
#### Etiology
Sialoceles are accumulations of saliva in subcutaneous tissues caused by salivary duct obstruction and/or rupture and subsequent leakage of secretions into subcutaneous tissues. Most cases are probably traumatic, but some are idiopathic.

#### Clinical Features
A large, usually painless swelling is found under the jaw or tongue or occasionally in the pharynx. Oral cavity sialoceles may cause dysphagia, whereas those located in the pharynx often produce gagging or dyspnea. If traumatized, sialoceles may bleed or cause anorexia due to discomfort.

#### Diagnosis
Aspiration with a large-bore needle reveals thick fluid with some neutrophils. The fluid usually resembles mucus, strongly suggesting its salivary gland origin. Contrast radiographic procedures (contrast sialograms) sometimes define which gland is involved.

#### Treatment
The mass is opened and drained, and the salivary gland responsible for the secretions must be excised.

#### Prognosis
The prognosis is excellent if the correct gland is removed.

### SIALOADENITIS/SIALOADENOSIS/ SALIVARY GLAND NECROSIS

#### Etiology
The etiology is unknown, but the condition apparently has occurred as an idiopathic event as well as secondary to vomiting/regurgitation.

#### Clinical Features
The condition may cause a painless enlargement of one or more salivary glands (usually the submandibular). If there is substantial inflammation, animals may be dysphagic. There appears to be a syndrome in which noninflammatory swelling is associated with vomiting that is responsive to phenobarbital therapy.

#### Diagnosis
Biopsy and cytology or histopathology confirm that the mass is salivary tissue and determine whether inflammation or necrosis is present.

## Treatment

If there is substantial inflammation and pain, surgical removal seems most efficacious. If the patient is vomiting, a search should be made for an underlying cause. If a cause is found, it should be treated and the size of the salivary glands monitored. If no other cause for vomiting can be found, phenobarbital may be administered at anticonvulsant doses (see Chapter 69, p. 1001).

## Prognosis

The prognosis is usually excellent.

## NEOPLASMS OF THE ORAL CAVITY IN DOGS

### Etiology

Most soft tissue masses of the oral cavity are neoplasms, and most of these are malignant (i.e., melanoma, squamous cell carcinoma, fibrosarcoma). However, acanthomatous epulides, fibromatous epulides (classically in Boxers), oral papillomatosis, and eosinophilic granulomas (e.g., in Siberian Huskies and Cavalier King Charles Spaniels) also occur.

### Clinical Features

The most common signs of tumors of the oral cavity are halitosis, dysphagia, bleeding, or a growth protruding from the mouth. Papillomatosis and fibromatous periodontal hyperplasia are benign growths that may cause discomfort when eating and occasionally cause bleeding, mild halitosis, or tissue protrusion from the mouth. The biologic behaviors of the different tumors are presented in Table 31-1.

### Diagnosis

A thorough examination of the oral cavity (which may require that the animal be under anesthesia) usually reveals a mass involving the gingiva, although the tonsillar area, hard palate, and tongue can also be affected. Diagnosis requires cytologic or histopathologic analysis, although papillomatosis and epulis may be strongly suspected from their gross appearance. The preferred diagnostic approach in a dog with a mass of the oral cavity is to perform an incisional biopsy and to obtain thoracic and skull radiographs of the affected area. If malignancy is a diagnostic consideration, thoracic radiographs should be obtained to evaluate for metastases (seldom seen but a very poor prognostic sign if present), and maxillary and mandibular radiographs should be obtained to check for bony involvement. Fine-needle aspiration of regional lymph nodes, even if they appear normal, is indicated to detect metastases. Melanomas may be amelanotic and can cytologically resemble fibrosarcomas or carcinomas. Biopsy and subsequent histopathologic analysis may be required for a definitive diagnosis.

 TABLE 31-1

Some Characteristics of Selected Oral Tumors

| TUMOR | TYPICAL APPEARANCE/LOCATION | BIOLOGIC BEHAVIOR | PREFERRED THERAPY |
|---|---|---|---|
| **Squamous Cell Carcinoma** | | | |
| Gingiva | Fleshy or ulcerated/on rostral gingiva | Malignant, locally invasive | Wide surgical resection on rostral gingiva ± radiation |
| Tonsil | Fleshy or ulcerated/on one or both tonsils | Malignant, commonly spreads to regional lymph nodes | None (chemotherapy may be of some benefit) |
| Tongue margin (dog) | Ulcerated/on margin of tongue | Malignant, locally invasive | Surgical resection of tongue/ radiotherapy |
| Base of tongue (cat) | Ulcerated/at base of tongue | Malignant, locally invasive | None (radiotherapy of tongue and/or chemotherapy may be used palliatively) |
| **Malignant Melanoma** | Grey or black; can be smooth, usually fleshy/on gum or palate | Very malignant, early metastases to lungs | None (resection and/or radiation are palliative but rarely curative); carboplatin and radiation might help |
| **Fibrosarcoma** | Pink and fleshy/on palate or gums | Malignant, very invasive locally | Wide surgical resection (chemotherapy and/or radiation may be of some value) |
| **Acanthomatous Epulis** | Pink and fleshy/on gum or rostral mandible | Malignant, locally invasive | Surgical resection ± radiation |
| **Fibromatous Epulis** | Pink, fleshy, solitary or multiple/on gums | Benign | Nothing or surgical resection |
| **Papillomatosis** | Pink or white, cauliflower-like, multiple/seen anywhere | Benign | Nothing or surgical resection |

## Treatment/Prognosis

The preferred therapeutic approach in dogs with confirmed malignant neoplasms of the oral cavity and lack of clinically detectable metastases is wide, aggressive surgical excision of the mass and surrounding tissues (e.g., mandibulectomy, maxillectomy). Enlarged regional lymph nodes should be excised and evaluated histopathologically, even if they are cytologically negative for neoplasia. Early complete excision of gingival or hard palate squamous cell carcinomas, fibrosarcomas, acanthomatous epulides, and (rarely) melanomas may be curative. Acanthomatous epulis and ameloblastomas may respond to radiation therapy alone (complete surgical excision is preferred), and squamous cell carcinomas or fibrosarcomas with residual postoperative disease may benefit from postoperative adjunctive radiation therapy. Lingual squamous cell carcinomas affecting the base of the tongue and tonsillar carcinomas have a very poor prognosis; complete excision or irradiation usually causes severe morbidity. Melanomas metastasize early and have a very guarded prognosis. Chemotherapy is usually not beneficial in dogs with squamous cell carcinoma, acanthomatous epulis, and melanoma, but an oncologist should be consulted about new protocols that may provide some benefit. There are anecdotal reports of piroxicam being beneficial for patients with squamous cell carcinoma. Combination chemotherapy may be beneficial in some dogs with fibrosarcoma (see Chapter 79). Radiotherapy plus hyperthermia has been successful in some dogs with oral fibrosarcoma.

Papillomatosis usually resolves spontaneously, although some of the masses may have to be resected if they interfere with eating. Fibromatous epulides may be resected if they cause problems.

## NEOPLASMS OF THE ORAL CAVITY IN CATS

### Etiology

Tumors of the oral cavity are less common in cats than in dogs, but they are usually squamous cell carcinomas, which are diagnosed and treated as described for dogs. However, eosinophilic granulomas (which have a much better prognosis) are relatively common in cats and can closely mimic carcinoma.

### Clinical Features

Dysphagia, halitosis, anorexia, and/or bleeding are common features of these tumors.

### Diagnosis

A large, deep biopsy specimen is needed because it is crucial to differentiate malignant tumors from eosinophilic granulomas. The superficial aspect of many masses of the oral cavity is ulcerated and necrotic as a result of the proliferation of normal oral bacterial flora, making it difficult to interpret this part of the mass.

## Treatment

Surgical excision is desirable. Radiation therapy and/or chemotherapy may benefit cats with incompletely excised squamous cell carcinomas not involving the tongue or tonsil.

## Prognosis

In general, the prognosis for cats with squamous cell carcinomas of the tongue or tonsil is guarded to poor (see Chapter 84).

## FELINE EOSINOPHILIC GRANULOMA

### Etiology

The cause is uncertain.

### Clinical Features

Feline eosinophilic granuloma complex includes indolent ulcer, eosinophilic plaque, and linear granuloma; however, it is not certain that these diseases are related. Indolent ulcers are classically found on the lip or oral mucosa of middle-aged cats. Eosinophilic plaque usually occurs on the skin of the medial thighs and abdomen. Linear granuloma is typically found on the posterior aspect of the rear legs of young cats but may also occur on the tongue, palate, and oral mucosa. Severe oral involvement of an eosinophilic ulcer or plaque typically produces dysphagia, halitosis, and/or anorexia. Cats with eosinophilic granulomas of the mouth may have concurrent cutaneous lesions.

### Diagnosis

An ulcerated mass may be found at the base of the tongue or on the hard palate, the glossopalatine arches, or anywhere else in the mouth. A deep biopsy specimen of the mass is necessary for accurate diagnosis. Peripheral eosinophilia is inconsistently present.

### Treatment

High-dose corticosteroid therapy (oral prednisolone, 2.2 to 4.4 mg/kg/day) often controls these lesions. Sometimes cats are best treated with methylprednisolone acetate injections (20 mg every 2 to 3 weeks as needed) instead of oral prednisolone. Although effective, megestrol acetate may cause diabetes mellitus, mammary tumors, and uterine problems and probably should not be used except under extreme constraints. Chlorambucil might prove useful in resistant cases.

### Prognosis

The prognosis is good, but the lesion can recur.

## GINGIVITIS/PERIODONTITIS

### Etiology

Bacterial proliferation and toxin production, usually associated with tartar buildup, destroy normal gingival structures and produce inflammation. Immunosuppression due to feline leukemia virus (FeLV) and feline immunodeficiency virus (FIV) can predispose some cats to this disease.

## Clinical Features

Dogs and cats may be affected. Many are asymptomatic, but halitosis, oral discomfort, refusal to eat, dysphagia, drooling, and tooth loss may occur.

## Diagnosis

Visual examination of the gums reveals hyperemia around the tooth margins. Gingival recession may reveal tooth roots.

## Treatment

Supragingival and subgingival tartar should be removed, and the crowns should be polished. Antimicrobial drugs effective against anaerobic bacteria (e.g., amoxicillin, clindamycin, metronidazole; see table, Drugs Used in Alimentary Tract Disorders, p. 469) may be used before and after cleaning teeth. Regular brushing of the teeth and/or oral rinsing with a veterinary chlorhexidine solution formulated for that purpose helps to prevent recurrence.

## Prognosis

The prognosis is good with proper therapy.

## STOMATITIS

### Etiology

There are many causes of canine and feline stomatitis (Table 31-2). The clinician should always consider the possibility of immunosuppression with secondary stomatitis (e.g., FeLV, FIV, diabetes mellitus, hyperadrenocorticism).

### Clinical Features

Most dogs and cats with stomatitis have thick, ropey saliva, severe halitosis, and/or anorexia caused by pain. Some animals are febrile and lose weight.

### Diagnosis

A thorough oral examination usually requires that the animal be under anesthesia. Stomatitis is diagnosed by gross observation of the lesions, but an underlying cause should be sought. Biopsy is routinely indicated, as are routine clinical pathology data and radiographs of the mandible and maxilla, including the tooth roots.

### Treatment

Therapy is both symptomatic (to control signs) and specific (i.e., directed at the underlying cause). Thorough teeth cleaning and aggressive antibacterial therapy (i.e., systemic antibiotics effective against aerobes and anaerobes, cleansing oral rinses with antibacterial solutions such as chlorhexidine) often help. In some animals, extracting teeth that are associated with the most severely affected areas may help. Bovine lactoferrin has been reported to ameliorate otherwise resistant lesions in cats.

### Prognosis

The prognosis depends on the underlying cause.

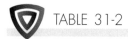 **TABLE 31-2**

**Common Causes of Stomatitis**

Renal failure
Trauma
   Foreign objects
   Chewing or ingesting caustic agents
   Chewing on electrical cords
Immune-mediated disease
   Pemphigus
   Lupus
Upper respiratory viruses (feline viral rhinotracheitis, feline calicivirus)
Infection secondary to immunosuppression (feline leukemia virus, feline immunodeficiency virus)
Tooth root abscesses
Severe periodontitis
Osteomyelitis
Thallium intoxication

## FELINE LYMPHOCYTIC-PLASMACYTIC GINGIVITIS/PHARYNGITIS

### Etiology

An idiopathic disorder, feline lymphocytic-plasmacytic gingivitis might be caused by feline calicivirus or any stimulus producing sustained gingival inflammation. Cats appear to have an excessive oral inflammatory response that can produce marked gingival proliferation.

### Clinical Features

Anorexia and/or halitosis are the most common signs. Affected cats grossly have reddened gingiva around the teeth and/or posterior pillars of the pharynx. The gingiva may be obviously proliferative in severe cases and bleed easily. Dental neck lesions often accompany the gingivitis. Teeth chattering is also occasionally seen.

### Diagnosis

Biopsy of affected (especially proliferative) gingiva is needed for diagnosis. Histologic evaluation reveals a lymphocytic-plasmacytic infiltration. Serum globulin concentrations may be increased.

### Treatment

Currently, there is no reliable therapy for this disorder. Proper cleaning and polishing of teeth and antibiotic therapy effective against anaerobic bacteria may help. High-dose corticosteroid therapy (prednisolone, 2.2 mg/kg/day) is often useful. In some severe cases, multiple tooth extractions may alleviate the source of the inflammation. However, extraction of the canine and carnassial teeth should be avoided. Immunosuppressive drugs such as chlorambucil also may be tried in obstinate cases.

## Prognosis

The prognosis is guarded; severely affected animals often do not respond well to therapy.

# DYSPHAGIAS

## MASTICATORY MUSCLE MYOSITIS/ATROPHIC MYOSITIS

### Etiology

Masticatory muscle myositis/atrophic myositis is an idiopathic, immune-mediated disorder that affects the muscles of mastication in dogs. The syndrome has not been reported in cats.

### Clinical Features

In the acute stages the temporalis and masseter muscles may be swollen and painful. However, most dogs are not presented until the muscles are severely atrophied and the mouth cannot be opened.

### Diagnosis

Atrophy of the temporalis and masseter muscles plus inability to open the dog's mouth while it is anesthetized allows one to establish a presumptive diagnosis. Muscle biopsy of the temporalis and masseter muscles provides confirmation. Antibodies to type 2M fibers strongly supports this diagnosis.

### Treatment

High-dose prednisolone therapy (2.2 mg/kg/day) with or without azathioprine (50 mg/m² every 24 hours) is usually curative. Once control has been achieved, the prednisolone and azathioprine are administered every 48 hours and then the dose of prednisolone is tapered to avoid adverse effects. However, this tapering must be done slowly to prevent recurrence (see Chapter 93 on Immunosuppressive Drugs). If needed, a gastrostomy tube may be used until the animal can eat.

### Prognosis

The prognosis is usually good, but continued medication may be needed.

## CRICOPHARYNGEAL ACHALASIA/ DYSFUNCTION

### Etiology

The cause of cricopharyngeal achalasia/dysfunction is uncertain but is usually congenital. There is an incoordination between the cricopharyngeus muscle and the rest of the swallowing reflex, which produces obstruction at the cricopharyngeal sphincter during swallowing (i.e., the sphincter does not open at the proper time).

### Clinical Features

Primarily seen in young dogs, cricopharyngeal achalasia rarely occurs as an acquired disorder. The major sign is regurgitation immediately after or concurrent with swallowing. Some animals become anorexic, and severe weight loss may occur. Clinically this condition may be indistinguishable from pharyngeal dysfunction.

### Diagnosis

Definitive diagnosis requires fluoroscopy or cinefluoroscopy while the animal is swallowing barium. A young animal that is regurgitating food immediately on swallowing is suggestive of the disorder, but pharyngeal dysphagia with normal cricopharyngeal sphincter function occasionally occurs as an apparently congenital defect and must be differentiated from cricopharyngeal disease.

### Treatment

Cricopharyngeal myotomy is curative. The clinician must be careful to avoid causing cicatrix at the surgery site. Esophageal function in the cranial esophagus must be evaluated before this surgery is considered (see Pharyngeal Dysphagia, below).

### Prognosis

The prognosis is good if cicatrix does not occur postoperatively.

## PHARYNGEAL DYSPHAGIA

### Etiology

Pharyngeal dysphagia is primarily an acquired disorder, and neuropathies, myopathies, and junctionopathies (e.g., localized myasthenia gravis) seem to be the main cause. Inability to form a normal bolus of food at the base of the tongue and/or propel the bolus into the esophagus is often associated with lesions of cranial nerves IX or X. Simultaneous dysfunction of the cranial esophagus may cause food retention just caudal to the cricopharyngeal sphincter.

### Clinical Features

Although pharyngeal dysphagia principally is found in older animals, young animals occasionally have transient signs. Pharyngeal dysphagia often clinically mimics cricopharyngeal achalasia; regurgitation is associated with swallowing. Pharyngeal dysphagia sometimes causes more difficulty swallowing fluids than solids. Aspiration (especially associated with liquids) is common because the proximal esophagus is often flaccid and retains food, predisposing to later reflux into the pharynx.

### Diagnosis

Fluoroscopy or cinefluoroscopy while the animal is swallowing barium is required for diagnosis. An experienced radiologist is needed to reliably distinguish pharyngeal dysphagia from cricopharyngeal dysphagia. In the former, the animal does not have adequate strength to properly push boluses of food into the esophagus, whereas in the latter the animal has adequate strength but the cricopharyngeal sphincter stays shut or opens at the wrong time during swallowing, thereby preventing normal movement of food from the pharynx to the proximal esophagus.

## Treatment

Although cricopharyngeal myotomy is curative for animals with cricopharyngeal achalasia, it may be disastrous for animals with pharyngeal dysphagias because it allows food retained in the proximal esophagus to more easily reenter the pharynx and be aspirated. One must either bypass the pharynx (e.g., gastrostomy tube) or resolve the underlying cause (e.g., treat or control myasthenia gravis).

## Prognosis

The prognosis is guarded because it is often difficult to find and treat the underlying cause, and the dog or cat is prone to progressive weight loss and recurring aspiration pneumonia.

# ESOPHAGEAL WEAKNESS/ MEGAESOPHAGUS

## CONGENITAL ESOPHAGEAL WEAKNESS
### Etiology

The cause of congenital esophageal weakness (i.e., congenital megaesophagus) is unknown. There is no evidence of demyelination or neuronal degeneration, and vagal efferent innervation appears to be normal.

## Clinical Features

Primarily found in dogs, affected animals are usually presented because of "vomiting" (actually regurgitation) with or without weight loss. However, coughing and other signs of aspiration tracheitis and/or pneumonia are common and may be seen without "vomiting."

## Diagnosis

The clinician usually first determines from the history that regurgitation is more likely than vomiting (see p. 345). Then, radiographically finding generalized esophageal dilation that is not associated with obstruction (see Fig. 29-3, *A*), the clinician can presumptively diagnose esophageal weakness. Diverticula in the cranial thorax caused by esophageal weakness occur occasionally and can be easy to confuse with vascular ring obstruction (Fig. 31-1). Congenital rather than acquired disease is suspected if the regurgitation and/or aspiration began when the pet was very young. If clinical features have been relatively mild or intermittent, the diagnosis might not be made until the animal is older, but consideration of the history should suggest that signs have been present since the animal was young. Endoscopy is not as useful as contrast radiographs for diagnosing this disorder. Collies may have dermatomyositis, which also causes esophageal weakness. Some breeds seemingly are at increased risk (e.g., Miniature Schnauzers, Great Danes, Dalmatians).

## Treatment

Congenital esophageal weakness currently cannot be cured or resolved by medical therapy, although cisapride (0.25 mg/ kg) seemingly ameliorates signs in rare cases. Conservative dietary management is used to try to prevent further dilation and aspiration. Classically the animal is fed a gruel from an

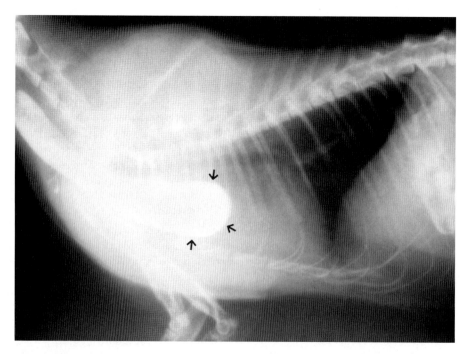

**FIG 31-1**
Lateral contrast thoracic radiograph of a cat. Note large diverticulum suggestive of obstruction *(arrows)*. This cat had generalized esophageal weakness without obstruction.

elevated platform that requires the pet to stand on its rear legs. In this manner the cervical and thoracic esophagus is nearly vertical when food is ingested, which allows gravity to aid food passing through the esophagus and into the stomach. This position should be maintained for 5 to 10 minutes after eating and drinking. If the dog cannot stand, it may be backed into a corner, forced to sit on its haunches, and have its front legs lifted while the corner prevents the dog from falling over. Feeding several small meals a day also helps to avoid esophageal retention.

Some animals do better if fed dry dog food free choice throughout the day from such a platform. One cannot predict whether a given dog will respond better to gruel or dry dog food. Therefore trial and error are necessary to determine the diet that works best for a particular animal. In some dogs the dilated esophagus may partially return to normal size and function. Even if the esophagus remains dilated, some dogs may be managed by dietary change and lead a good quality life.

Gastrostomy tubes bypass the esophagus and can provide some relief from regurgitation and/or aspiration. However, animals may still regurgitate saliva and, if there is gastroesophageal reflux, may also regurgitate food. Some animals with gastrostomy tubes respond well for periods of time.

### Prognosis

The prognosis is guarded; some animals respond well, and some continue to have severe regurgitation and/or aspiration despite all treatment efforts. Aspiration pneumonia is the major cause of death.

## ACQUIRED ESOPHAGEAL WEAKNESS

### Etiology

Acquired esophageal weakness in dogs is usually caused by a neuropathy, myopathy, or junctionopathy (e.g., myasthenia gravis) (see Table 28-6). German Shepherds, Golden Retrievers, and Irish Setters might have increased risk. In cats, gastroesophageal reflux and hiatal hernia seem to be more common causes.

### Clinical Features

Acquired esophageal weakness primarily occurs in dogs. The animals usually are presented because of "vomiting" (actually regurgitation), but some present with a cough and little or no obvious regurgitation (e.g., regurgitated material is sometimes reswallowed or reeaten by the animal). Severe weight loss may occur if the dog regurgitates most of its food.

### Diagnosis

The initial diagnostic step is to document that regurgitation is occurring instead of vomiting (see p. 345). Acquired esophageal weakness is usually diagnosed by finding generalized esophageal dilation without evidence of obstruction on plain and contrast radiographs (see Fig. 29-3, *A*). The severity of clinical signs does not always correlate with the magnitude of radiographic changes. Some symptomatic

animals have apparently mild retention in the orad cervical esophagus, just behind the cricopharyngeus muscle. It is important to rule out lower esophageal spasm and stricture, which, though very rare, radiographically mimic esophageal weakness but require surgical treatment. Radiographs should also be evaluated for evidence of gastroesophageal reflux, which may benefit from prokinetic therapy (e.g., cisapride).

It is important to search for underlying causes of acquired esophageal weakness (see Table 28-6). The presence of antibodies to acetylcholine receptors (indicative of myasthenia gravis) should be evaluated in dogs. "Localized" myasthenia may affect only the esophagus and/or oropharyngeal muscles. An adrenocorticotropic hormone (ACTH)–stimulation test is indicated to look for otherwise occult hypoadrenocorticism (even if serum electrolyte concentrations are normal). Serum thyroxine, free thyroxine, and thyroidstimulating hormone (TSH) concentrations may reveal hypothyroidism, which can rarely be associated with neuromuscular dysfunction. Tests of thyroid gland function must be interpreted carefully because of potential confusion due to the euthyroid sick syndrome (see p. 702). Electromyography may reveal generalized neuropathies or myopathies. Dysautonomia occurs occasionally and is suspected based on clinical signs (i.e., dilated colon, dry nose, dilated pupils, keratoconjunctivitis sicca, and/or bradycardia that responds poorly to atropine). Other causes are rarely found (see Table 28-6). If an underlying cause cannot be found, the disease is termed *idiopathic acquired esophageal weakness* (i.e., idiopathic acquired megaesophagus).

### Treatment

Dogs with acquired megaesophagus caused by localized myasthenia gravis, hypoadrenocorticism, or hypothyroid myopathy often respond to appropriate therapy (see Chapters 53, 73, and 74). Localized myasthenia seems to ultimately respond best to immunosuppressive therapy (e.g., azathioprine or perhaps mycophenolate mofetil), although pyridostigmine may help initially. Gastroesophageal reflux may respond to prokinetic and antacid therapy (cisapride at 0.25 mg/kg and omeprazole at 0.7 to 1.5 mg/kg are preferred). If the disease is idiopathic, conservative dietary therapy as described for congenital esophageal weakness is the only recourse. Although some dogs with congenital esophageal weakness regain variable degrees of esophageal function, this is exceedingly rare in those with idiopathic acquired esophageal weakness. Calcium channel blocking agents (e.g., nifedipine) have also been used but are of dubious value. Cisapride may help occasional animals with idiopathic megaesophagus, probably when there is concurrent gastroesophageal reflux. Severe esophagitis may cause secondary esophageal weakness, which resolves after appropriate therapy (see below). Gastrostomy tubes diminish the potential for aspiration, ensure positive nitrogen balance, and help to treat esophagitis if present. Some dogs benefit from long-term gastrostomy tube use; however, others continue to regurgitate and aspirate as a result of severe gastroesophageal reflux.

## Prognosis

All animals with acquired esophageal weakness are at risk for aspiration pneumonia and sudden death. If the underlying cause can be treated and the esophageal dilation and weakness can be resolved, the prognosis is good because the risk of aspiration is eliminated. The prognosis is guarded if the animal with idiopathic megaesophagus responds to dietary management (it is still at risk) and very poor if the animal does not respond to this protocol.

# ESOPHAGITIS

## Etiology

Esophagitis is principally caused by gastroesophageal reflux, persistent vomiting of gastric acid, esophageal foreign objects, and caustic agents. Pills (e.g., tetracycline) may stick in the esophagus if not washed down with water or food and are suspected of having caused severe esophagitis in cats.

## Clinical Features

Regurgitation is expected, although anorexia and drooling may predominate if swallowing is painful. If a caustic agent is ingested, the mouth and tongue are often hyperemic and/or ulcerated, and anorexia is the primary sign.

## Diagnosis

A history of vomiting followed by both vomiting and regurgitation suggests esophagitis secondary to excessive exposure to gastric acid. This sign may occur in parvoviral enteritis and in various other disorders. Plain and contrast radiographs may reveal hiatal hernias, gastroesophageal reflux, or esophageal foreign bodies. Contrast esophagrams do not reliably detect esophagitis; esophagoscopy with or without biopsy is needed to establish a diagnosis.

## Treatment

Decreasing gastric acidity, preventing reflux of gastric contents into the esophagus, and protecting the denuded esophagus are the hallmarks of treatment. $H_2$ receptor antagonists (see Table 30-7) may be used, but omeprazole is superior for decreasing gastric acidity, a critical factor in these animals. Metoclopramide stimulates gastric emptying, resulting in less gastric volume to reflux into the esophagus, but cisapride (0.25 to 0.5 mg/kg) tends to be more effective. Sucralfate (particularly suspensions) might protect denuded esophageal mucosa (see Table 30-8), but its usefulness is unknown. Antibiotics effective against anaerobes (e.g., amoxicillin, clindamycin; see table, Drugs Used in Alimentary Tract Disorders, p. 469) seem reasonable. A gastrostomy feeding tube helps to protect the esophagus while the mucosa is healing and ensures a positive nitrogen balance. Corticosteroids (e.g., prednisolone, 1.1 mg/kg/day) may be administered to try to prevent cicatrix, but their efficacy is dubious. Hiatal hernias may need to be surgically repaired.

## Prognosis

The prognosis depends on the severity of the esophagitis and whether an underlying cause can be identified and controlled.

Early, aggressive therapy helps to prevent cicatrix formation and allows a better prognosis.

# HIATAL HERNIA

## Etiology

Hiatal hernia is a diaphragmatic abnormality that allows part of the stomach to prolapse into the thoracic cavity. In severe cases, it allows gastroesophageal reflux. The condition may be congenital or acquired.

## Clinical Features

Sharpei dogs seem to be predisposed to this disorder. Regurgitation is the primary sign in symptomatic individuals, but some animals are asymptomatic.

## Diagnosis

Plain or positive-contrast esophagrams may reveal gastric herniation into the thorax (Fig. 31-2); however, herniation may be intermittent and difficult to detect. It is sometimes necessary to put pressure on the abdomen during the radiographic procedure to cause displacement of the stomach during the study. Hiatal hernias are occasionally found endoscopically.

## Treatment

If the hiatal hernia is symptomatic at an early age, surgery is more likely to be required to correct it. If signs of hiatal hernia first appear later in life, aggressive medical management of gastroesophageal reflux (e.g., cisapride, omeprazole) is often sufficient. If medical management is not successful, surgery can be considered.

## Prognosis

The prognosis is often good after surgical repair (congenital cases) or aggressive medical management (acquired cases).

# DYSAUTONOMIA

## Etiology

Dysautonomia in dogs and cats is an idiopathic condition that causes loss of autonomic nervous system function.

## Clinical Features

Clinical signs vary substantially. Megaesophagus and subsequent regurgitation are common (not invariable); however, dysuria and a distended urinary bladder, mydriasis and lack of pupillary light response, dry mucus membranes, weight loss, constipation, vomiting, poor anal tone, and/or anorexia are all reported. There appear to be geographic areas (e.g., Missouri and surrounding states) that currently have an increased incidence of the disease.

## Diagnosis

Dysautonomia is usually first suspected clinically by finding dysuria, dry mucus membranes, and abnormal pupillary light responses. Radiographs revealing distention of multiple ar-

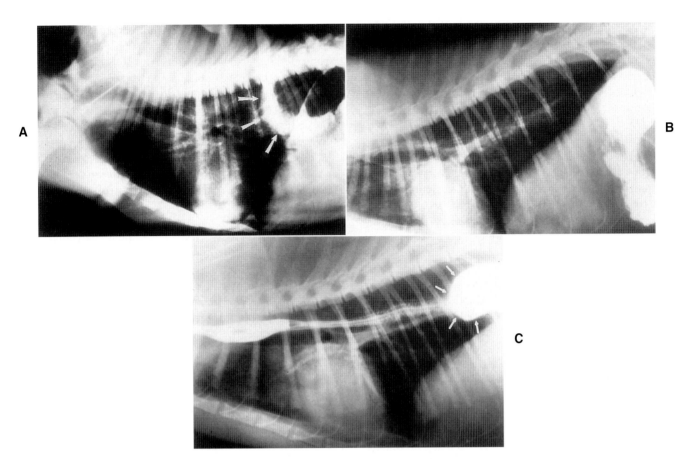

**FIG 31-2**
**A,** Lateral radiograph of a dog with a hiatal hernia showing the gastric shadow extending cranial to the diaphragm *(arrows).* **B,** Lateral view of contrast esophagram of a cat with hiatal hernia. There is no evidence of hernia on this radiograph because it has apparently slid back into the abdomen. **C,** Lateral view of contrast esophagram of the cat in **B.** The body of the stomach has now slid into the thoracic cavity *(arrows),* confirming that a hiatal hernia is present. (**A,** Courtesy Dr. Russ Stickle, Michigan State University, East Lansing, Mich. **B** and **C,** Courtesy Dr. Royce Roberts, University of Georgia, Athens, Ga.)

eas of the alimentary tract (e.g., esophagus, stomach, small intestine) also are suggestive. A presumptive, antemortem diagnosis is usually made by observing the effects of pilocarpine on pupil size after 1 to 2 drops of 0.05% pilocarpine are placed in one eye only. Finding that the treated eye rapidly constricts whereas the untreated eye does not is consistent with dysautonomia. Similarly, finding that a dysuric dog with a large urinary bladder can urinate after administration of 0.04 mg bethanechol/kg SQ is also suggestive (although not all affected animals respond). Definitive diagnosis requires histopathology of autonomic ganglia, which can only be obtained at necropsy.

### Treatment

Treatment is palliative. Bethanechol can be given (1.25 to 5 mg once daily) to aid in urinary evacuation. The urinary bladder should be expressed as needed. Gastric prokinetics (e.g., cisapride) may help lessen vomiting. Antibiotics may be administered for aspiration pneumonia secondary to megaesophagus.

## ESOPHAGEAL OBSTRUCTION

### VASCULAR RING ANOMALIES
#### Etiology

Vascular ring anomalies are congenital defects. An embryonic aortic arch persists, which traps the esophagus in a ring of tissue. Persistent right fourth aortic arch (PRAA) is the most commonly recognized vascular anomaly (see Chapter 9).

#### Clinical Features

Vascular ring anomalies occur in both dogs and cats. Regurgitation is the most common presenting complaint, although signs of aspiration may occur. Clinical features often begin shortly after the animal eats solid food for the first time. Some animals have relatively minor clinical signs and are not diagnosed until they are several years old.

#### Diagnosis

Definitive diagnosis is usually made by contrast esophagram (see Fig. 29-3, *B*). Typically the esophagus cranial to the heart is dilated, whereas the esophagus caudal to the heart is normal. Rarely the entire esophagus is dilated (the result of concurrent megaesophagus) except for a narrowing at the base of the heart. Endoscopically, the esophagus has an extramural narrowing (Fig. 31-3) (i.e., not a mucosal proliferation or scar) near the base of the heart.

### Treatment

Surgical resection of the anomalous vessel is necessary. Conservative dietary management (i.e., gruel diet) by itself is inappropriate because the dilation will persist and probably progress. In particular, the animal will be at risk for foreign body occlusion at the site of the PRAA. Dietary therapy may benefit some animals postoperatively.

### Prognosis

The prognosis may be influenced by how severely the esophagus is dilated. Although there are exceptions, the more severe the preoperative dilation, the more likely regurgitation will continue postoperatively. Therefore, although most pets benefit from surgery, a guarded prognosis is appropriate. If a postsurgical stricture occurs, esophageal ballooning or a second surgical procedure may be considered.

## ESOPHAGEAL FOREIGN OBJECTS

### Etiology

Almost anything may lodge in the esophagus, but objects with sharp points (e.g., bones, fishhooks) are probably most common. Most obstructions occur at the thoracic inlet, the base of the heart, or immediately in front of the diaphragm.

### Clinical Features

Dogs are more commonly affected because of their less discriminating eating habits. Regurgitation or anorexia secondary to esophageal pain is common. Acute onset of regurgitation (as opposed to vomiting) is suggestive of esophageal foreign body. Clinical signs depend on where the obstruction occurs, whether it is complete or partial, and whether esophageal perforation has occurred. Complete obstructions cause regurgitation of solids and liquids, whereas partial obstructions may allow passage of liquids to the stomach. If an esophageal foreign object is impinging on airways, acute dyspnea may occur. Esophageal perforation usually causes fever and anorexia; dyspnea may occur as the result of pleural effusion or pneumothorax. Subcutaneous emphysema rarely occurs.

### Diagnosis

Plain thoracic radiographs reveal most esophageal foreign bodies (see Fig. 29-2), although the clinician may have to search carefully to find poultry bones. It is also important to look for evidence of esophageal perforation (i.e., pneumothorax, pleural effusion, fluid in the mediastinum). Esophagrams are rarely necessary or helpful; esophagoscopy is diagnostic and typically therapeutic.

### Treatment

Foreign objects are best removed endoscopically unless (1) they are too firmly lodged to pull free or (2) radiographs suggest perforation. Thoracotomy is indicated in these two situations, although in rare cases perforations may be treated medically. Objects that refuse to move should not be pulled on vigorously because of the risk of creating or enlarging a perforation. An object should be pushed into the stomach only when the clinician is confident that further esophageal disease is unlikely (e.g., there are no sharp edges on the other side of the foreign object). During the procedure the esophagus should be insufflated carefully to avoid rupturing weakened areas or causing tension pneumothorax. After an object has been removed, the esophageal mucosa should be reexamined endoscopically to evaluate the damage caused by the object. Thoracic radiographs should be repeated to look for pneumothorax, an indication of perforation. Treatment after foreign body removal may include antibiotics, antacids, prokinetic agents, gastrostomy feeding tube, and/or corticosteroids (prednisolone, 1.1 mg/kg/day), depending on residual damage. Perforation usually requires thoracotomy to clean out septic debris and close the esophageal defect.

### Prognosis

The prognosis for animals with esophageal foreign bodies without perforation is usually good, but the presence of perforation warrants a guarded prognosis depending on the severity of thoracic contamination. Cicatrix formation with obstruction is possible if substantial mucosal damage occurs.

## ESOPHAGEAL CICATRIX

### Etiology

Prior esophagitis from any cause may produce a stricture. Severe, deep inflammation of the esophagus (e.g., subsequent to foreign bodies or severe gastroesophageal reflux) is usually required for cicatrix to occur.

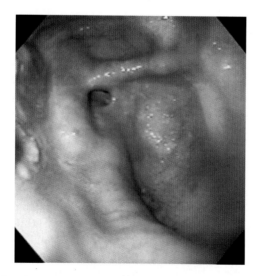

**FIG 31-3**
Endoscopic view of an esophageal lumen constricted by an extramural vascular ring anomaly.

## Clinical Features

Esophageal cicatrix occurs in both dogs and cats. The main sign is regurgitation (especially of solids). Some animals are clinically anorexic due to pain experienced when food becomes lodged at the stricture by forceful esophageal peristalsis.

## Diagnosis

Partial obstructions can be difficult to diagnose. Positive-contrast esophagrams (often using barium mixed with food) are needed (Fig. 31-4). Esophagoscopy is definitive, but a partial stricture may not be obvious in large dogs unless a large-diameter endoscope is used and the esophagus is carefully inspected after being dilated.

## Treatment

Treatment consists of correcting the suspected cause (e.g., esophagitis) and/or widening the stricture by ballooning or bougienage. Surgical resection should be avoided because iatrogenic strictures at the anastomotic site are common. Ballooning is less traumatic, has less chance of perforation, and may be accomplished during esophagoscopy. Angioplasty catheters or esophageal dilation balloons are more useful than Foley catheters because the former are less likely to slide to one side of the obstruction during inflation. After the esophagus has been dilated, antibiotics and/or corticosteroids (prednisolone, 1.1 mg/kg/day) are often administered to help to prevent infection and stricture reformation; however, their efficacy is unknown. If esophagitis is present, it should be treated aggressively. Some animals are cured after one ballooning, whereas others require multiple procedures.

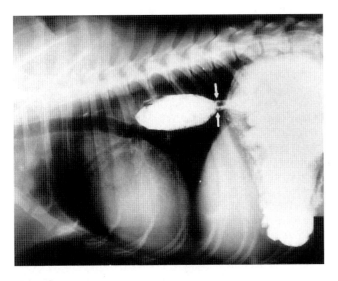

**FIG 31-4**
Lateral contrast esophagram using liquid barium mixed with moist food. Partial stricture *(arrows)* is preventing the bolus from readily entering the stomach. This stricture was not detected with barium paste, even when viewed fluoroscopically. However, when the barium-food mixture was used, the stricture was obvious and material was retained for minutes before passing. Endoscopically there was a band of fibrous connective tissue at this spot.

Early identification and appropriate treatment of high-risk animals (i.e., those with severe esophagitis or following foreign object removal) help to decrease the likelihood of stricture formation. Resolving esophagitis decreases inflammation and lessens fibrous connective tissue formation. The efficacy of corticosteroids is uncertain, but they are worth trying in selected cases.

## Prognosis

The shorter the length of esophagus involved and the sooner the corrective procedure is performed, the better the prognosis. Animals with extensive, mature stricture and/or continuing esophagitis often need repeated dilatory procedures and have a more guarded prognosis. Most animals with benign esophageal strictures can be helped. Long-term gastrostomy tubes may be needed in some animals.

# ESOPHAGEAL NEOPLASMS

## Etiology

Primary esophageal sarcomas in dogs are often due to *Spirocerca lupi*. Primary esophageal carcinomas are of unknown etiology. Leiomyomas and leiomyosarcomas are found at the lower esophageal sphincter in older dogs. Thyroid carcinomas and pulmonary alveolar carcinomas may invade the esophagus in dogs. Squamous cell carcinomas are the most common esophageal neoplasm in cats.

## Clinical Features

Dogs and cats with primary esophageal tumors may be asymptomatic until the tumor is far advanced, and these animals are diagnosed fortuitously when thoracic radiographs are obtained for other reasons. Regurgitation, anorexia, and/or fetid breath may occur if the tumor is large or causes esophageal dysfunction. If the esophagus is involved secondarily, clinical signs may result from esophageal dysfunction or tumor effects on other tissues.

## Diagnosis

Plain thoracic radiographs may reveal a soft tissue density in the caudal lung fields. These tumors may be difficult to radiographically discern from pulmonary lesions and usually require contrast esophagrams to make this distinction (Fig. 31-5). Esophagoscopy easily finds intraluminal and intramural masses (Fig. 31-6) or strictures and is sensitive in finding extraluminal masses causing esophageal stricture (i.e., the endoscopist will not be able to normally distend the esophageal lumen). Retroflexing the tip of an endoscope while it is within the stomach is the best method of identifying lower esophageal sphincter leiomyomas and leiomyosarcomas.

## Treatment

Surgical resection is rarely curative (except for leiomyomas at the lower esophageal sphincter) because of the advanced nature of most esophageal neoplasms when they are diagnosed. Resection may be palliative. Photodynamic therapy may be beneficial in dogs and cats with small superficial esophageal neoplasms.

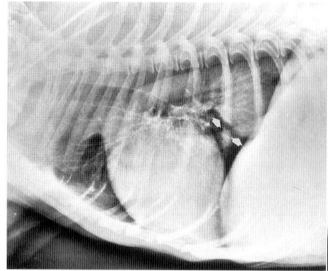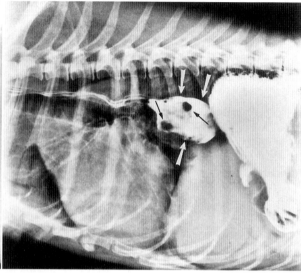

**FIG 31-5**
**A,** Lateral thoracic radiograph of a dog with a previously unsuspected mass *(arrows)* not obviously associated with the esophagus. **B,** Contrast esophagram in the same dog demonstrates that the esophagus is dilated *(large arrows)* and that there are intra-esophageal filling defects *(small arrows)* in this dilated area. This dog had a primary esophageal carcinoma. (**A** from Allen D, editor: *Small animal medicine,* Philadelphia, 1991, JB Lippincott.)

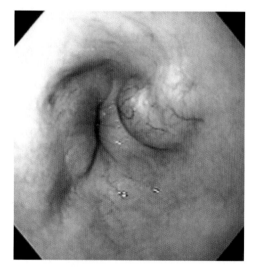

**FIG 31-6**
Endoscopic view of the lower esophageal sphincter of a dog. There is an intramural mass protruding into the lumen at 3 o'clock to the sphincter.

## Prognosis

The prognosis is usually poor.

### *Suggested Readings*

Boydell P et al: Sialadenosis in dogs, *J Am Vet Med Assoc* 216:872, 2000.

DeBowes LJ: Feline stomatitis and faucitis. In Bonagura JD, editor: *Current veterinary therapy XIII,* Philadelphia, 2000, WB Saunders.

Galatos AD et al: Gastro-oesophageal reflux during anaesthesia in the dog: the effect of preoperative fasting and premedication, *Vet Rec* 137:479, 1995.

Gaynor AR et al: Risk factors for acquired megaesophagus in dogs, *J Am Vet Med Assoc* 211(11):1406, 1997.

Graham JP et al: Esophageal transit of capsules in clinically normal cats, *Am J Vet Res* 61:655, 2000.

Harai BH et al: Endoscopically guided balloon dilation of benign esophageal strictures in 6 cats and 7 dogs, *J Vet Intern Med* 9(5): 332, 1995.

Holland CT et al: Vagal esophagomotor nerve function and esophageal motor performance in dogs with congenital idiopathic megaesophagus, *Am J Vet Res* 57(6):906, 1996.

Joffe DJ et al: Ulcerative eosinophilic stomatitis in three Cavalier King Charles Spaniels, *J Am Anim Hosp Assoc* 31:34, 1995.

Longshore RC et al: Dysautonomia in dogs: a retrospective study, *J Vet Intern Med* 10(3):103, 1996.

Lorinson D, Bright RM: Long-term outcome of medical and surgical treatment of hiatal hernias in dogs and cats: 27 cases (1978-1996), *J Am Vet Med Assoc* 213:381, 1998.

Mears EA et al: Canine megaesophagus. In Bonagura JD, editor: *Current veterinary therapy XIII,* Philadelphia, 2000, WB Saunders.

Melendez LD et al: Conservative therapy using balloon dilation for intramural, inflammatory esophageal strictures in dogs and cats: a retrospective study of 23 cases, *Eur J Compar Gastroenterol* 3:31, 1998.

Melendez LD et al: Suspected doxycyline-induced esophagitis with esophageal stricture formation in three cats, *Fel Pract* 28:10, 2000.

Michels GM et al: Endoscopic and surgical retrieval of fishhooks from the stomach and esophagus in dogs and cats: 75 cases (1977-1993), *J Am Vet Med Assoc* 207(9):1194, 1995.

Moses L et al: Esophageal motility dysfunction in cats: a study of 44 cases, *J Am Anim Hosp Assoc* 36:309, 2000.

Muldoon MM et al: Long-term results of surgical correction of persistent right aortic arch in dogs 25 cases: 1980-1995, *J Am Vet Med Assoc* 210(12):1761, 1997.

Niles JD et al: Resolution of dysphagia following cricopharyngeal myectomy in six young dogs, *J Small Anim Pract* 42:32, 2001.

O'Brien DP et al: Diagnosis and management of dysautonomia in dogs. In Bonagura JD, editor: *Current veterinary therapy XIII,* Philadelphia, 2000, WB Saunders.

Rendano VT et al: Impaction of the pharynx, larynx, and esophagus by avian bones in the dog and cat, *Vet Radiol* 29(3):213, 1988.

Rolfe DS et al: Chronic regurgitation or vomiting caused by esophageal leiomyoma in three dogs, *J Am Anim Hosp Assoc* 30:425, 1994.

Sato R et al: Oral administration of bovine lactoferrin for treatment of intractable stomatitis in feline immunodeficiency virus (FIV)-positive and FIV-negative cats, *Am J Vet Res* 57:1443, 1996.

Schroeder H et al: Salivary gland necrosis in dogs: a retrospective study of 19 cases, *J Small Anim Pract* 39:121, 1998.

Spielman BL et al: Esophageal foreign body in dogs: a retrospective study of 23 cases, *J Am Anim Hosp Assoc* 28:570, 1992.

Stickle R et al: Radiographic evaluation of esophageal function in Chinese Shar-pei pups, *J Am Vet Med Assoc* 201(1):81, 1992.

Tenorio AP et al: Chronic oral infections of cats and their relationship to persistent oral carriage of feline calici-, immunodeficiency, or leukemia viruses, *Vet Immun Immunopathol* 29:1, 1991.

Watrous BJ: Dysphagia and regurgitation. In Anderson NV, editor: *Veterinary gastroenterology,* ed 2, Philadelphia, 1992, Lea & Febiger.

White SD et al: Plasma cell stomatitis-pharyngitis in cats: 40 cases (1973-1991), *J Am Vet Med Assoc* 200(9):1377, 1992.

Willard MD et al: Esophagitis. In Bonagura JD, editor: *Current veterinary therapy XIII,* Philadelphia, 2000, WB Saunders.

# CHAPTER 32

# Disorders of the Stomach

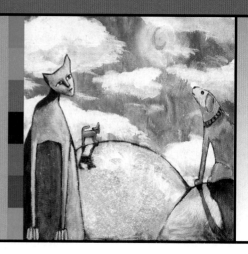

## CHAPTER OUTLINE

GASTRITIS, 418
    Acute gastritis, 418
    Hemorrhagic gastroenteritis, 419
    Chronic gastritis, 419
    *Helicobacter*-associated disease, 420
    *Physaloptera rara*, 420
    *Ollulanus tricuspis*, 421
GASTRIC OUTFLOW OBSTRUCTION/GASTRIC STASIS, 421
    Benign muscular pyloric hypertrophy (pyloric stenosis), 421
    Gastric antral mucosal hypertrophy, 421
    Gastric foreign objects, 423
    Gastric dilation/volvulus, 424
    Partial or intermittent gastric volvulus, 426
    Idiopathic gastric hypomotility, 427
    Bilious vomiting syndrome, 427
GASTROINTESTINAL ULCERATION/EROSION, 427
INFILTRATIVE GASTRIC DISEASES, 428
    Neoplasms, 428
    Pythiosis, 429

## GASTRITIS

### ACUTE GASTRITIS

**Etiology**

Ingestion of spoiled or contaminated foods, foreign objects, toxic plants, chemicals, and/or irritating drugs (e.g., non-steroidal antiinflammatory drugs [NSAIDs]) are common causes of acute gastritis. Infectious, viral, and bacterial causes are not well identified in dogs and cats but probably exist.

**Clinical Features**

Dogs are more commonly affected because of their less discriminating eating habits. Signs usually consist of acute onset of vomiting; food and bile are typically vomited, although small amounts of blood may be present. Affected animals are typically uninterested in food and may or may not feel sick. Fever and abdominal pain are uncommon.

**Diagnosis**

Unless the animal was seen eating some irritative substance, acute gastritis is usually a diagnosis of exclusion based on history and physical examination findings. Abdominal radiographs and/or clinical pathologic data are indicated if the animal is severely ill or if other disease is suspected. Once alimentary foreign body, obstruction, parvoviral enteritis, uremia, diabetic ketoacidosis, hypoadrenocorticism, hepatic disease, hypercalcemia, and pancreatitis are considered unlikely, acute gastritis is a reasonable tentative diagnosis. If the vomiting resolves after 1 to 2 days of symptomatic and supportive therapy, the tentative diagnosis is considered correct, although pancreatitis must still be considered (see p. 552). Gastroscopy in such animals might reveal bile or gastric erosions/hyperemia.

Because acute gastritis is a diagnosis of exclusion and its signs are suggestive of various other disorders (e.g., foreign bodies, intoxication), good history taking and physical examination are mandatory. The owner should monitor the pet, and if the animal's condition worsens or if it does not improve within 1 to 3 days, imaging, a complete blood count (CBC), a serum biochemistry profile, and urinalysis are indicated.

**Treatment**

Therapy principally consists of parenteral fluid therapy; withholding food and water for 24 hours often suffices to control vomiting. If the vomiting persists or is excessive, or if the animal becomes depressed because of the vomiting, central-acting antiemetics (e.g., prochlorperazine, metoclopramide, ondansetron) may be administered parenterally (see p. 396). When feeding begins, small amounts of cool water are offered frequently. If the animal drinks without vomiting, small amounts of a bland diet (e.g., one part cottage cheese and two parts potato; one part boiled chicken and two parts potato) are offered. Antibiotics and corticosteroids are rarely indicated.

## Prognosis

The prognosis is excellent as long as fluid and electrolyte balance is maintained.

## HEMORRHAGIC GASTROENTERITIS

### Etiology

The cause of hemorrhagic gastroenteritis is uncertain but may represent an immune-mediated reaction involving the gastrointestinal (GI) tract.

### Clinical Features

Hemorrhagic gastroenteritis occurs in dogs and is more severe than acute gastritis, typically causing profuse hematemesis and/or hematochezia. Classically occurring in smaller breeds that have not had access to garbage, this disorder has an acute course that rapidly produces an ill animal. In severe cases the animal may be moribund by the time of presentation to the hospital.

### Diagnosis

These animals are typically hemoconcentrated (i.e., packed cell volume [PCV] ≥55%) with normal plasma total protein concentrations. The acute onset of typical clinical signs plus marked hemoconcentration allows a presumptive diagnosis. Thrombocytopenia and renal or prerenal azotemia may be seen in severely affected animals.

### Treatment

Aggressive fluid therapy is begun to treat or prevent shock, disseminated intravascular coagulation (DIC) secondary to hypoperfusion, and renal failure secondary to hypovolemia. Parenteral antibiotics (e.g., ampicillin, chloramphenicol; see Drugs Used in Gastrointestinal Disorders, p. 469) are used because of fear that intestinal anaerobes are proliferating, but their value is uncertain.

### Prognosis

The prognosis is good for most animals that are presented in a timely fashion. Inadequately treated animals may die of circulatory collapse, DIC, and/or renal failure.

## CHRONIC GASTRITIS

### Etiology

There are several types of chronic gastritis (e.g., lymphocytic/plasmacytic, eosinophilic, granulomatous, atrophic). Lymphocytic-plasmacytic gastritis might be an immune and/or inflammatory reaction to a variety of antigens. *Helicobacter* organisms might be responsible for such a reaction in some animals (especially cats). *Physaloptera rara* has seemingly been associated with a similar reaction in some dogs. Eosinophilic gastritis may represent an allergic reaction, probably to food antigens. Atrophic gastritis may be the result of chronic gastric inflammatory disease and/or immune mechanisms. *Ollulanus tricuspis* may cause granulomatous gastritis in cats.

### Clinical Features

Anorexia and/or vomiting are the most common signs in affected dogs and cats. The frequency of vomiting varies from once weekly to many times per day. Some animals have only anorexia, ostensibly from low-grade nausea.

### Diagnosis

Clinical pathologic findings are not diagnostic, although eosinophilic gastritis inconsistently causes peripheral eosinophilia. Imaging sometimes documents mucosal thickening, but that sign is inconsistent and nondiagnostic. Diagnosis requires gastric mucosal biopsy, and endoscopy is the most cost-effective method of obtaining these samples. Biopsy of the stomach should always be performed, regardless of the visual mucosal appearance. It must be remembered that enteritis is far more common than gastritis (which is why duodenal biopsies are usually more important than gastric biopsies). Gastric lymphoma can be surrounded by lymphocytic inflammation, and obtaining inappropriately superficial biopsy specimens may result in an incorrect diagnosis of inflammatory disease. Appropriate use of a scope with a 2.8 mm biopsy channel will usually prevent this misdiagnosis (unless the tumor is in the muscular layers of the stomach). Meaningful histopathologic interpretation of alimentary tissue can be difficult; the clinician should not hesitate to request a second histologic opinion. If *Ollulanus tricuspis* is suspected, vomitus or gastric washings should be examined for the parasites, but they might also be found in gastric biopsy specimens. *Physaloptera* organisms are visible endoscopically.

### Treatment

Lymphocytic-plasmacytic gastritis sometimes responds to dietary therapy (low-fat, low-fiber, elimination diets) alone (see p. 389). If such therapy is inadequate, corticosteroids (e.g., prednisolone, 2.2 mg/kg/day) can be used concurrently. Even if corticosteroids are required, dietary therapy may ultimately allow one to decrease their dose (or even discontinue them), thus avoiding glucocorticoid adverse effects. If corticosteroid therapy is necessary, the dose should be gradually decreased to find the lowest effective dose. However, the dose should not be tapered too quickly after obtaining a clinical response or the clinical signs may return and be more difficult to control than they were initially. In rare cases, azathioprine or similar drugs will be necessary (see Chapter 93). Sometimes concurrent use of $H_2$-receptor antagonists is beneficial. Ulceration should be treated as discussed here.

Canine eosinophilic gastritis usually responds well to a *strict* elimination diet. If dietary therapy alone fails, corticosteroid therapy (e.g., prednisolone, 1.1 to 2.2 mg/kg/day) in conjunction with diet is usually effective.

Atrophic gastritis and granulomatous gastritis are more difficult to treat than lymphocytic-plasmacytic or canine eosinophilic gastritis. Diets low in fat and fiber (e.g., one part cottage cheese and two parts potato; one part boiled chicken and two parts potato) may help control signs. Atrophic gastritis may respond to antiinflammatory, antacid, and/or prokinetic therapy; the latter is designed to keep the stomach empty, especially at night. Granulomatous gastritis is uncommon in dogs and cats and does not respond well to diet or corticosteroid therapy.

### Prognosis

The prognosis for dogs and cats with lymphocytic-plasmacytic gastritis is often good with appropriate therapy. Lymphoma has been suggested to develop in cats with lymphocytic gastritis; however, it is possible that the original diagnosis of lymphocytic gastritis was incorrect or that lymphoma developed independently of the gastritis.

The prognosis for treated canine eosinophilic gastritis is also typically good. Feline eosinophilic gastritis can be a component of hypereosinophilic syndrome, which typically responds poorly to treatment. Hypereosinophilic syndrome has a guarded prognosis.

## HELICOBACTER-ASSOCIATED DISEASE

### Etiology

There are several bacteria in the genus *Helicobacter*. *Helicobacter pylori* is the principal spirochete found in human gastric mucosa, whereas *Helicobacter felis* and *Helicobacter heilmannii (Gastrospirillum hominis)* may be the principal gastric spirochetes in dogs and cats. However, *H. pylori* has also been found in cats.

### Clinical Features

People with symptomatic *H. pylori* infections usually develop ulceration and gastritis with neutrophilic infiltrates. This bacteria also causes a lymphocytic lesion in people that is indistinguishable from lymphoma but that can be cured with antibiotic therapy. Dogs and cats with gastric *Helicobacter* infections may have nausea, anorexia, and/or vomiting associated with lymphocytic and occasionally neutrophilic infiltrates; however, most dogs and cats with gastric *Helicobacter* infections are asymptomatic. Because so many infected animals are asymptomatic, cause-and-effect has not been clearly established between *Helicobacter* organisms and canine or feline gastric disease. Cats colonized with *H. pylori* seem to have more severe histologic lesions than those with *H. felis,* which in turn can have more severe lesions than those with *H. heilmannii.* There seems to be reasonable anecdotal evidence that some ill animals with gastric *Helicobacter* infections have their signs resolve when the organism is eliminated. Whether the "cure" is due to eliminating *Helicobacter* organisms or something else is uncertain, but it seems reasonable to assume that *Helicobacter* organisms cause disease in some animals.

### Diagnosis

Gastric biopsy is currently required for a diagnosis of *Helicobacter* infection. The organisms are easy to identify if the pathologist is looking for them and uses special stains (e.g., Giemsa, Warthin-Starry). The bacteria are not uniformly distributed throughout the stomach, and it is best to obtain biopsy specimens from the body, fundus, and antrum. One may also diagnose this infection by cytologic evaluation of the gastric mucosa (Fig. 32-1) or by looking for gastric mucosal urease activity (see Chapter 29). Because of the uncertain pathogenicity of *Helicobacter* spp, one is advised to first eliminate other, better explanations for the animal's clinical signs before deciding that a *Helicobacter* organism is causing disease.

### Treatment

A combination of metronidazole, omeprazole (or an H$_2$-receptor antagonist such as famotidine), and an antibiotic such as amoxicillin or a macrolide (see Drugs Used in Gastrointestinal Disorders, p. 469) seems to be the best approach in human medicine and, until there are data to the contrary, may be assumed to be optimal for veterinary patients. Anecdotally, some animals seem to respond to just erythromycin or amoxicillin. Azithromycin has fewer side effects than erythromycin and appears to be very effective for treating *Helicobacter.* Therapy should probably be for at least 10 days.

### Prognosis

Animals with apparent *Helicobacter*-associated disease seem to respond well to treatment and have a good prognosis. However, because cause-and-effect is uncertain, any animal that does not respond to therapy should be reexamined carefully to determine if other diseases are present. Recurrence of infection after treatment seems common.

## PHYSALOPTERA RARA

### Etiology

*Physaloptera rara* is a nematode that has an indirect life cycle; cockroaches and beetles are the intermediate hosts.

### Clinical Features

Primarily found in dogs, one parasite can cause intractable vomiting. The vomiting usually does not resolve with anti-

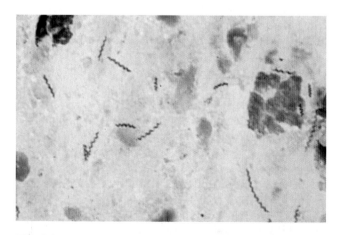

**FIG 32-1**
Air-dried smear of gastric mucosa obtained endoscopically and stained with Diff-Quick. Numerous spirochetes are seen. The affected dog was vomiting because of an ulcerated leiomyoma, and the spirochetes did not appear to be causing disease in this animal. (Magnification ×1000.)

emetics. Vomitus may or may not contain bile, and the animals otherwise appear healthy.

## Diagnosis

Ova are seldom found in feces, because few eggs are passed. Furthermore, sodium dichromate or magnesium sulfate solutions are usually needed when trying to identify the eggs in feces. Most diagnoses are made when the parasites are found during gastroduodenoscopy (see Fig. 29-25). There may be only one worm causing clinical signs, and it can be difficult to find, especially if it is attached within the pylorus. Alternatively, empirical treatment (as described here) is reasonable.

## Treatment

Pyrantel pamoate or ivermectin is usually effective. If the parasite is found during endoscopy, it can be removed with forceps.

## Prognosis

The vomiting usually stops as soon as the worms are removed or eliminated.

## OLLULANUS TRICUSPIS

### Etiology

*Ollulanus tricuspis* is a nematode with a direct life cycle that is transmitted via vomited material.

### Clinical Features

Cats are the most commonly affected species, although dogs and foxes are occasionally infected. Vomiting is the principal clinical sign, but clinically normal cats may harbor the parasite. Gross gastric mucosal lesions may or may not be seen in infested, ill cats.

### Diagnosis

Cattery situations promote infection because the parasite is passed directly from one cat to another. However, occasionally cats with no known contact with other cats are infected. Looking for parasites in gastric washings or vomited material with a dissecting microscope is the best means of diagnosis. One occasionally sees the parasite in gastric mucosal biopsy specimens.

### Treatment/Prognosis

Therapy is uncertain, but oxfendazole (10 mg/kg PO q12h for 5 days) or fenbendazole might be effective. Occasionally animals have severe gastritis and become debilitated.

## GASTRIC OUTFLOW OBSTRUCTION/GASTRIC STASIS

### BENIGN MUSCULAR PYLORIC HYPERTROPHY (PYLORIC STENOSIS)
#### Etiology

The cause of benign muscular pyloric hypertrophy is uncertain, although some experimental research suggests that gastrin promotes the development of pyloric stenosis.

## Clinical Features

Benign muscular pyloric stenosis typically causes persistent vomiting in young animals (especially brachycephalic dogs and Siamese cats) but can be found in any animal. These animals usually vomit food shortly after eating. The vomiting is sometimes described as projectile. The animals are otherwise clinically normal, although some pets may lose weight. Some cats with pyloric stenosis vomit so much that secondary esophagitis and regurgitation occur, confusing the clinical picture. Hypochloremic, hypokalemic, metabolic alkalosis sometimes occurs, but it is inconsistent and nonspecific for gastric outflow obstruction.

## Diagnosis

Diagnosing pyloric stenosis requires first finding gastric outflow obstruction during barium contrast–enhanced radiographs (Fig. 32-2), gastroduodenoscopy, and/or exploratory surgery. Then infiltrative disease of the pyloric mucosa must be ruled out via biopsy. Endoscopically, one may see increased folds of normal-appearing mucosa at the pylorus. At surgery the serosa appears normal, but the pylorus is usually thickened when palpated. The surgeon can open the stomach and try to pass a finger through the pylorus to assess its patency. Ultrasonography can also be used to detect thickened pyloric musculature. Extraalimentary tract diseases causing vomiting (see Table 28-7) should also be eliminated.

## Treatment

Surgical correction is indicated. Pyloroplasty (e.g., a Y-U–plasty) is more consistently effective than pyloromyotomy. However, improperly performed pyloroplasty can cause perforation or obstruction. Furthermore, one should not routinely do a pyloric outflow procedure whenever an exploratory fails to reveal another cause of vomiting.

## Prognosis

Surgery should be curative, and the prognosis is good.

## GASTRIC ANTRAL MUCOSAL HYPERTROPHY

### Etiology

Antral mucosal hypertrophy is idiopathic. Gastric outflow obstruction is caused by excessive, nonneoplastic mucosa that occludes the distal gastric antrum (Fig. 32-3). This disorder is different from benign muscular pyloric stenosis, in which the mucosa is thrown up into folds secondary to the submucosal thickening.

### Clinical Features

Principally found in older, small-breed dogs, antral hypertrophy clinically resembles pyloric stenosis (i.e., animals usually vomit food, especially after meals).

### Diagnosis

Gastric outlet obstruction is diagnosed radiographically, ultrasonographically, or endoscopically; however, definitive

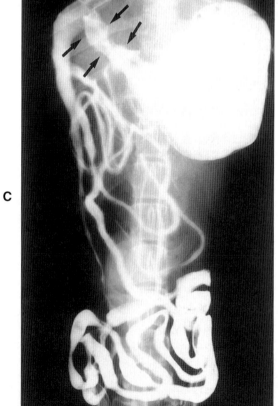

**FIG 32-2**
**A** and **B,** Ventrodorsal contrast radiographs of a dog with a gastric outflow obstruction. These radiographs were obtained approximately 3 hours after barium administration. There is inadequate gastric emptying despite obvious peristalsis. Note the smooth contour of barium in the antrum *(arrows),* which is in contrast to **C.** This is a case of pyloric stenosis. **C,** Dorso-ventral contrast radiographs of a dog with gastric adeno-carcinoma. The antrum has an irregular outline but is not distended *(arrows).* This failure to distend persisted on multiple radiographs and indicates an infiltrative lesion.

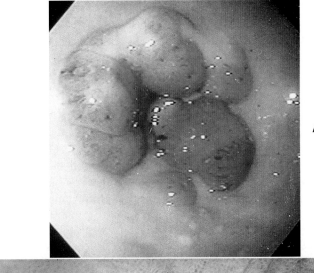

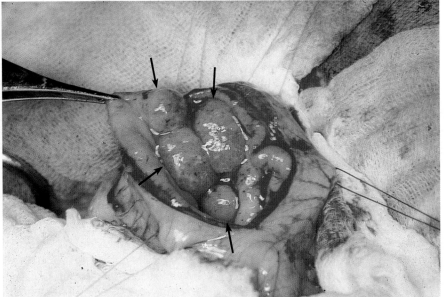

**FIG 32-3**
**A,** Endoscopic view of the pyloric region of a dog that has gastric antral mucosal hypertrophy. If biopsy is not performed, these folds may easily be mistaken for neoplasia. **B,** Intraoperative photograph of a dog's opened pylorus. Note the numerous folds of mucosa that are protruding *(arrows)* as a result of gastric antral mucosal hypertrophy.

diagnosis of antral mucosal hypertrophy requires biopsy. Endoscopically, the antral mucosa is redundant and may resemble a submucosal neoplasm causing convoluted mucosal folds. In some cases the mucosa will be obviously reddened and inflamed. However, the mucosa in dogs with antral hypertrophy is usually not as firm or hard as expected in those with infiltrative tumors. If antral mucosal hypertrophy is seen at surgery, there should be no evidence of submucosal infiltration or muscular thickening suggestive of neoplasia or benign pyloric stenosis, respectively. It is important to differentiate mucosal hypertrophy from these other diseases so that therapeutic recommendations are appropriate (e.g., gastric carcinomas typically have a worse prognosis, and surgery is not always indicated).

### Treatment

Antral mucosal hypertrophy is treated by mucosal resection, usually combined with pyloroplasty. Pyloromyotomy alone may be insufficient to resolve clinical signs from mucosal hypertrophy.

### Prognosis

The prognosis is excellent.

## GASTRIC FOREIGN OBJECTS

### Etiology

Objects that can pass through the esophagus may become a gastric or intestinal foreign object. Subsequently, vomiting may result from gastric outlet obstruction, gastric distention, or irritation. Linear gastric foreign objects may cause intestinal perforation with subsequent peritonitis and must be dealt with expeditiously (see Intestinal Obstruction, p. 452).

## Clinical Features

Dogs are affected more commonly than cats because of their less discriminating eating habits. Vomiting (not regurgitation) is a common sign, but some animals demonstrate only anorexia, whereas others are asymptomatic.

## Diagnosis

Acute onset of vomiting in an otherwise normal animal, especially a puppy, suggests foreign body ingestion. One might palpate an object during physical examination or see it during plain radiographic imaging. Contrast radiographs and endoscopy are the most reliable means of diagnosis. However, diagnosis can be difficult if the stomach is filled with food. Some diseases closely mimic obstruction caused by foreign objects; canine parvovirus may initially cause intense vomiting, during which time viral particles might not be detected in the feces. Hypokalemic, hypochloremic, metabolic alkalosis is consistent with gastric outflow obstruction; however, these changes can be absent in animals with gastric obstruction and present in animals without obstruction. Therefore although suggestive of gastric vomiting (or excessive furosemide therapy), these electrolyte changes are neither sensitive nor specific for gastric outflow obstruction.

## Treatment

Although small foreign objects that are unlikely to cause trauma may pass through the GI tract, most should be removed. Vomiting can be induced (e.g., apomorphine in the dog, 0.02 or 0.1 mg/kg IV or SC, respectively; hydrogen peroxide in the dog, 1 to 5 ml of 3% solution/kg PO; xylazine in the cat, 0.4 to 0.5 mg/kg IV) to eliminate gastric foreign objects if the clinician believes that the object will not cause problems during forcible ejection (i.e., it does not have sharp edges or points and is small enough to pass easily). If there is doubt as to the safety of this approach, the object should be removed endoscopically or surgically.

Before the animal is anesthetized for surgery or endoscopy, the electrolyte and acid-base status should be evaluated. Although electrolyte changes (e.g., hypokalemia) are common, one cannot accurately predict them. Hypokalemia predisposes to cardiac arrhythmias and should be corrected before anesthesia is induced.

Endoscopic removal of foreign objects requires a flexible endoscope and appropriate retrieval forceps (e.g., W-type coin forceps, loop, wire basket, rat-tooth forceps). The animal should always be radiographed just before being anesthetized to ensure that the object is still in the stomach. Laceration of the esophagus and entrapment of the retrieval forceps in the object should be avoided. If endoscopic removal is unsuccessful, gastrostomy should be performed.

## Prognosis

The prognosis is usually good unless the animal is debilitated or there is septic peritonitis secondary to gastric perforation.

# GASTRIC DILATION/VOLVULUS

## Etiology

The cause of gastric dilation/volvulus (GDV) is unknown but may involve abnormal gastric motility. Thoracic confirmation is correlated with risk; Irish Setters with a deeper thorax relative to width are more likely to experience GDV. Dogs with parents that had GDV may also be at increased risk. There are conflicting data on the effect of sex and speed of eating on risk, but eating once a day and eating from an elevated platform seem to increase risk. GDV occurs when the stomach dilates excessively with gas. The stomach may maintain its normal anatomic position (gastric dilation) or twist (GDV). In the latter situation the pylorus typically rotates from the right side of the abdomen below the body of the stomach to become positioned dorsal to the gastric cardia on the left side. If the stomach twists sufficiently, gastric outflow is obstructed and progressive distention with air results. Splenic torsion may occur concurrently if the stomach twists sufficiently. Massive gastric distention obstructs the hepatic portal vein and posterior vena cava, causing mesenteric congestion, decreased cardiac output, severe shock, and DIC. The gastric blood supply may be impaired, causing gastric wall necrosis.

## Clinical Features

GDV principally occurs in large- and giant-breed dogs with deep chests; it rarely occurs in small dogs or cats. Affected dogs typically retch nonproductively and may demonstrate abdominal pain. Marked anterior abdominal distention may be seen later. However, abdominal distention is not always obvious in large, heavily muscled dogs. Eventually, depression and a moribund state occur.

## Diagnosis

Physical examination findings (i.e., a large dog with a large tympanic anterior abdomen that is retching unproductively) allow presumptive diagnosis of GDV but do not permit differentiation between dilation and GDV; plain abdominal radiographs with the animal in right lateral recumbency are required. Volvulus is denoted by displacement of the pylorus and/or formation of a "shelf" of tissue in the gastric shadow (Fig. 32-4). It is impossible to distinguish between dilation and dilation/torsion on the basis of ability or inability to pass an orogastric tube.

## Treatment

Treatment consists of initiating aggressive therapy for shock (hetastarch or hypertonic saline infusion [see p. 388] may make treatment for shock quicker and easier) and then decompressing the stomach unless the patient is asphyxiating, in which case the stomach is decompressed first. Serum

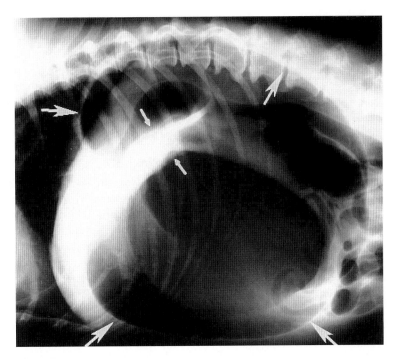

**FIG 32-4**
Lateral radiograph of a dog with GDV. The stomach is dilated *(large arrows)*, and there is a "shelf" of tissue *(small arrows)*, demonstrating that the stomach is malpositioned. Radiographs obtained from the right lateral position seem superior to those of other views in demonstrating this shelf. If the stomach were similarly distended but not malpositioned, the diagnosis would be gastric dilation.

electrolyte concentrations and acid-base status should be evaluated in all animals. Gastric decompression is usually performed with an orogastric tube, after which the stomach is lavaged with warm water to remove its contents. The stomach of dogs with dilation and many with GDV can be decompressed in this manner. Mesenteric congestion caused by the enlarged stomach predisposes to infection and endotoxemia, making systemic antibiotic administration reasonable (e.g., cefazolin, 20 mg/kg IV).

The orogastric tube should not be forced into the stomach against undue resistance, because it could rupture the lower esophagus. If the tube cannot be passed into the stomach, one may insert a large needle (e.g., a 3-inch, 12- to 14-gauge needle) into the stomach just behind the rib cage in the left flank to decompress the stomach (which usually causes some abdominal contamination) or perform a temporary gastrostomy in the left paralumbar area (i.e., the stomach wall is sutured to the skin, and then the stomach wall is incised to allow evacuation of accumulated gas and other contents). After the animal is stabilized, a second procedure is performed to close the temporary gastrostomy (if present), reposition the stomach, remove the spleen (if grossly infarcted), remove or invaginate devitalized gastric wall, and perform a gastropexy. Gastropexy (e.g., circumcostal, belt loop, tube gastrostomy) is recommended to help prevent recurrence of

torsion and may be correlated with prolongation of survival. Another option consists of immediately performing a laparotomy after decompressing the stomach but before stabilizing the animal. The decision as to whether to first stabilize the animal or immediately perform surgery is based on the condition of the dog at initial presentation and on whether the animal would be a considerably better anesthetic risk after stabilization.

If the dog has GDV (see Fig. 32-4), surgery is necessary to reposition the stomach; this is followed by gastropexy to prevent recurrence. This surgery should be performed as soon as the animal constitutes an acceptable anesthetic risk, because torsion (even when the stomach is deflated) impairs gastric wall perfusion and may cause necrosis. Areas of gastric wall necrosis should be resected, or preferably invaginated, to prevent perforation and abdominal contamination. In dogs with gastric dilation without torsion, gastropexy is optional and may be performed after the dog is completely recovered from the current episode. Gastropexy almost always prevents torsions but does not prevent dilation.

Postoperatively the animal should be monitored by electrocardiogram (ECG) for 48 to 72 hours. Lidocaine, procainamide, and/or soltolol therapy may be needed if cardiac arrhythmias diminish cardiac output (see Chapter 4). Hypokalemia is common and makes such arrhythmias refractory to medical control. Therefore hypokalemia should be resolved before antiarrhythmic therapy is initiated.

Prevention is difficult because the cause is unknown. Although preventing exercise after meals and feeding small meals of softened food intuitively seems useful, there are no data to confirm this speculation.

## Prognosis

The prognosis depends on how quickly the condition is recognized and treated. Mortality rates of 18% to 28% have been reported. Early therapy improves the prognosis, whereas preoperative cardiac arrhythmias, increased preoperative blood lactate concentrations, gastric wall necrosis, severe DIC, partial gastrectomy, and splenectomy seem to worsen the prognosis. Although rare, gastric dilation may recur after an appropriate gastropexy. Prophylactic gastropexy performed during other elective procedures (e.g., spay) may be elected for animals believed to be at increased risk for GDV.

## PARTIAL OR INTERMITTENT GASTRIC VOLVULUS

### Etiology

The causes for partial and intermittent gastric volvulus might be the same as for classic GDV.

### Clinical Features

Dogs with partial or intermittent volvulus do not have the life-threatening, progressive syndrome characterizing classic GDV. Although occurring in the same breeds as GDV, partial gastric volvulus usually produces a chronic, intermittent, potentially difficult-to-diagnose problem. It may occur repeatedly and spontaneously resolve; dogs may appear normal between bouts.

### Diagnosis

Occasionally the stomach maintains itself in a twisted position but does not fill with gas. Signs of gastric disease persist in such animals, and plain radiographs are usually diagnostic (Fig. 32-5). Intermittent torsion may necessitate repeated radiographs and/or contrast studies before it can be determined that the stomach is in an abnormal position. Endoscopic diagnosis may be especially difficult because it is possible to occasionally cause a temporary gastric volvulus by manipulating the gastroscope in an air-distended stomach. Therefore differentiation of spontaneous and iatrogenic volvulus can be difficult.

### Treatment

If diagnosed, surgical repositioning and gastropexy are usually curative.

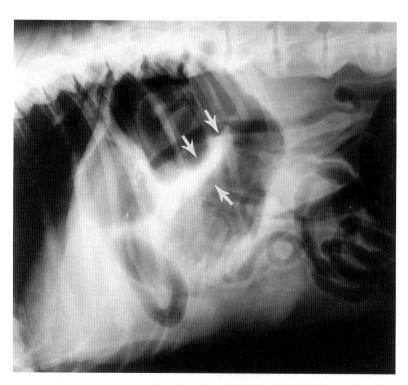

**FIG 32-5**
Lateral abdominal radiograph of an Irish Setter with chronic vomiting caused by gastric volvulus that did not cause dilation. A "shelf" of tissue *(arrows)* demonstrates that the stomach has twisted.

## Prognosis

The prognosis is usually good once the problem is identified and surgically corrected.

## IDIOPATHIC GASTRIC HYPOMOTILITY

### Etiology

Idiopathic gastric hypomotility refers to a syndrome characterized by poor gastric emptying and motility despite the lack of anatomic obstruction or inflammatory lesions.

### Clinical Features

Idiopathic gastric hypomotility has primarily been diagnosed in dogs. Affected dogs usually vomit food several hours after eating but otherwise feel well. Weight loss may or may not occur.

### Diagnosis

Fluoroscopic studies document decreased gastric motility, but diagnosis requires ruling out gastric outlet obstruction, infiltrative bowel disease, inflammatory bowel disease (IBD), and extraalimentary tract diseases (e.g., renal, adrenal, or hepatic failure; severe hypokalemia or hypercalcemia).

### Treatment

Metoclopramide (see Table 30-6) increases gastric peristalsis in some but not all affected dogs. Cisapride or erythromycin may be effective if metoclopramide fails. Diets low in fat and fiber promote gastric emptying and may be helpful.

### Prognosis

Dogs that respond to medical management have a good prognosis. Those that do not respond have a poor prognosis for cure, although they may still be acceptable pets.

## BILIOUS VOMITING SYNDROME

### Etiology

Bilious vomiting syndrome may be caused by gastroduodenal reflux that occurs when the dog's stomach is empty for long periods of time (e.g., during an overnight fast).

### Clinical Features

Bilious vomiting syndrome usually affects otherwise normal dogs that are fed once daily in the morning. Classically, the pet vomits bile-stained fluid once a day, usually late at night or in the morning just before eating.

### Diagnosis

One must rule out obstruction, GI inflammation, and extraalimentary tract diseases. Elimination of these disorders in addition to the history as described strongly suggests bilious vomiting syndrome.

### Treatment

Feeding the dog an extra meal late at night to prevent the stomach from being empty for long periods of time is often curative. If vomiting continues, then a gastric prokinetic may be administered late at night to prevent reflux.

### Prognosis

The prognosis is excellent. Most animals respond to therapy, and those that do not remain otherwise healthy.

## GASTROINTESTINAL ULCERATION/EROSION

### Etiology

There are several causes of gastrointestinal ulceration/erosion (GUE). Stress ulceration is caused by severe hypovolemic, septic, or neurogenic shock, such as occurs after trauma, surgery, and endotoxemia, but may occur with a variety of other illnesses. These ulcers are typically in the gastric antrum and/or duodenum.

NSAIDs (e.g., aspirin, phenylbutazone, ibuprofen, naproxen, piroxicam) are commonly administered to pets by their owners and are a major cause of canine GUE because these drugs have longer half-lives in dogs than in people. Any NSAID may be responsible, but naproxen, ibuprofen, and indomethacin are particularly dangerous to dogs. Flunixin meglumine also causes ulcers, especially if used in high doses or repeatedly. Concurrent use of more than one NSAID or use of an NSAID plus a corticosteroid (especially dexamethasone) increases the risk of GUE. Carprofen and etodolac (Etogesic) are NSAIDs with a lessened potential to cause GUE; however, GUE can still occur in a small number of animals taking these drugs. Use of NSAIDs in animals with poor visceral perfusion (e.g., cardiac failure, shock) also increases the risk of GUE. These ulcers are usually in the gastric antrum/pylorus and may be solitary or multiple. Steroids by themselves are seldom a problem unless dexamethasone is administered at a high dose or the animal is otherwise at increased risk for GUE (e.g., severely anoxic stomach due to anemia).

Mast cell tumors may release histamine (especially if radiation or chemotherapy is being used), which induces gastric acid secretion. Gastrinomas are APUDomas principally found in the pancreas. Usually occurring in older dogs and rarely in cats, these tumors secrete gastrin, which produces severe gastric hyperacidity, duodenal ulceration, esophagitis, and diarrhea.

Renal and hepatic failure may also cause GUE; the latter seems to be an important cause in dogs. Although foreign objects rarely cause GUE, they prevent healing and increase blood loss from ulcers. IBD may be associated with GUE in dogs, although most animals with IBD do not have these lesions. Gastric neoplasms and other infiltrative diseases (e.g., pythiosis) may also cause GUE (see p. 428).

### Clinical Features

GUE is more common in dogs than in cats. Anorexia can be the principal sign. If vomiting occurs, blood (i.e., fresh or digested) may or may not be present. Anemia and/or hypoproteinemia occasionally occur and cause signs (i.e., edema, pale mucous membranes, weakness, dyspnea) noted by the owner. Most dogs with even severe GUE do not demonstrate pain during abdominal palpation. Some ulcers perforate and seal over before generalized peritonitis occurs. In such cases a small abscess may develop at the site, causing abdominal pain, anorexia, and/or vomiting.

## Diagnosis

A presumptive diagnosis of GUE is usually based on finding evidence of GI blood loss (e.g., hematemesis, melena, iron-deficiency anemia) in an animal without a coagulopathy. The history and physical examination may identify an obvious cause (e.g., stress, NSAID administration, mast cell tumor). Perforation may cause peritonitis and signs of an acute abdomen and sepsis. Mast cell tumors can resemble almost any cutaneous lesion; therefore *all* cutaneous masses or nodules should be evaluated cytologically. Hepatic and renal failure are usually diagnosed from the CBC, serum biochemistry profile, and urinalysis. Contrast radiographs are diagnostic for foreign objects and sometimes for GUE (Fig. 32-6). Ultrasonography may be useful in detecting gastric thickening (such as would be seen in infiltrated lesions) and/or mucosal defects. Endoscopy is the most sensitive and specific tool for diagnosing GUE (see Figs. 29-18 to 29-21) and, in conjunc-

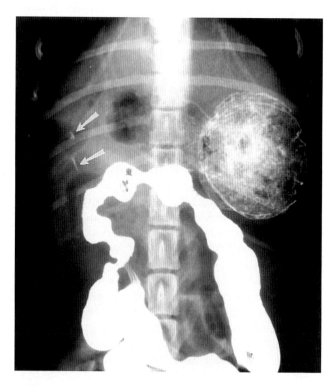

**FIG 32-6**
Contrast ventrodorsal radiograph of a dog with persistent vomiting. Note the small "sliver" representing retention of barium in the region of the pylorus *(arrows)*. This area of contrast persisted on several radiographs. Endoscopy and surgery confirmed a large ulcer that had perforated and spontaneously sealed. This radiograph demonstrates how difficult radiographic diagnosis of gastrointestinal ulceration can be.

tion with biopsy, can be used to diagnose tumors (see Fig. 29-20), foreign bodies (see Fig. 29-24), and inflammation that may cause ulcers. Endoscopic findings may also suggest a gastrinoma if multifocal duodenal erosion is found. Serum gastrin concentrations should be measured if a gastrinoma is suspected or if there are no other likely causes (see Chapter 52). Small abscesses on the gastric serosa caused by perforated ulcers that have sealed over (which is rare) require ultrasonography or exploratory surgery for diagnosis.

## Treatment

Therapy depends on the severity of GUE and whether an underlying cause is detected. Animals with suspected GUE that is not obviously life threatening (i.e., there is no evidence of severe anemia, shock, sepsis, severe abdominal pain, or severe depression) may first be treated symptomatically if the clinician believes that he or she knows the cause.

Symptomatic therapy (e.g., antacids, $H_2$-receptor antagonists, proton pump inhibitors, sucralfate, parenteral fluids, withholding food, parenteral nutrition [see Table 30-4]) is often successful. Additional therapy directed at the underlying etiology (i.e., NSAIDs, shock) is preferred, and any gastric foreign objects present must be removed. If appropriate medical therapy is unsuccessful after 5 to 6 days, or if the animal has life-threatening bleeding despite appropriate medical therapy, the ulcer(s) should usually be resected. The stomach should be examined endoscopically before surgery to determine the number and location of the ulcers; it is surprisingly easy to miss ulcers during laparotomy.

In animals with gastrinomas, $H_2$-receptor antagonist therapy is often palliative for months. Animals with high serum gastrin concentrations may require more potent and/or higher doses of $H_2$-receptor antagonists (e.g., famotidine) or the more potent proton pump inhibitors (i.e., omeprazole) (see Table 30-7).

Prevention of GUE is preferable to treatment. Sucralfate (Carafate) (see Table 30-8) or $H_2$-receptor antagonist (see Table 30-7) therapy helps to prevent GUE in some people and might help in dogs and cats. Misoprostol (see Table 30-8) is explicitly designed to prevent NSAID-induced ulceration and is more effective than $H_2$-receptor antagonists or sucralfate. However, it is not uniformly successful in preventing all NSAID-induced GUE.

## Prognosis

The prognosis is favorable if the underlying cause can be controlled and if therapy prevents perforation of the ulcer.

## *INFILTRATIVE GASTRIC DISEASES*

### NEOPLASMS
#### Etiology

Neoplastic infiltrations (e.g., adenocarcinoma, lymphoma, leiomyomas, and leiomyosarcomas in dogs; lymphoma in cats) may produce GUE through direct mucosal disruption. Gastric lymphoma is typically a diffuse lesion but can produce masses. Benign gastric polyps are of uncertain cause and significance. They seem to occur principally in the antrum.

## Clinical Features

Dogs and cats with gastric tumors are usually asymptomatic until the disease is advanced. Anorexia (not vomiting) is the most common sign. Vomiting caused by gastric neoplasia usually signifies advanced disease or gastric outflow obstruction. Adenocarcinomas are typically infiltrative and decrease emptying by impairing motility and/or obstructing the outflow tract. Weight loss is commonly caused by nutrient loss or cancer cachexia syndrome. Hematemesis occasionally occurs; leiomyomas often cause acute upper GI bleeding. Other gastric tumors often cause iron deficiency anemia even if GI blood loss is not obvious. Polyps rarely cause signs unless they obstruct the pylorus.

## Diagnosis

Iron deficiency anemia in a dog or cat without obvious blood loss suggests GI bleeding, often caused by a tumor. Plain and contrast imaging may reveal gastric wall thickening, decreased motility, and/or mucosal irregularities. The only sign of submucosal adenocarcinoma may be failure of one area to dilate (usually the antrum) (see Fig. 32-2, *C*). Ultrasound-guided aspiration of thickened areas in the gastric wall may produce cytologic preparations that are diagnostic for adenocarcinoma or lymphoma. Endoscopically, such areas may appear as multiple mucosal folds extending into the lumen without ulceration or erosion. Some tumors will be obvious endoscopically. When biopsy of such lesions is performed endoscopically, the sample must be obtained deep enough to ensure that submucosal tissue is included. Furthermore, scirrhous adenocarcinomas may be so dense that one cannot obtain diagnostic biopsy specimens with flexible endoscopic forceps. Mucosal lymphomas and adenocarcinomas often produce GUE, and tissue samples taken from the edge of the ulcer are usually diagnostic. Polyps are usually obvious endoscopically, but a biopsy specimen should always be obtained and evaluated to ensure that adenocarcinoma is not present.

## Treatment

Most adenocarcinomas are advanced before clinical signs are obvious, making complete surgical excision difficult or impossible. Leiomyomas and leiomyosarcomas are more likely to be resectable than adenocarcinomas. Gastroduodenostomy may palliate gastric outflow obstruction caused by an unresectable tumor. Chemotherapy is rarely helpful except for dogs and cats with lymphoma.

## Prognosis

The prognosis for adenocarcinomas and lymphomas is poor unless they are detected very early. Leiomyomas and leiomyosarcomas, if diagnosed relatively early, are often cured surgically. Seemingly, gastric polyps do not need to be resected unless they are causing outflow obstruction.

# PYTHIOSIS

## Etiology

Pythiosis is a fungal infection caused by *Pythium insidiosum*. This species is principally found in the Gulf coast area of the southeastern United States. Any area of the alimentary tract or skin may be affected; the stomach, duodenum, and colon are common sites. The fungus typically causes intense submucosal infiltration of fibrous connective tissue plus a purulent, eosinophilic, granulomatous inflammation causing GUE. Such infiltration prevents peristalsis, causing stasis.

## Clinical Features

Pythiosis principally affects dogs, typically causing vomiting, anorexia, diarrhea, and/or weight loss. Because gastric outflow obstruction occurs frequently, vomiting is common. Colonic involvement is suggested by the presence of tenesmus and hematochezia.

## Diagnosis

Diagnosis requires a biopsy sample that includes the submucosa. Such diagnostic biopsy specimens can be procured via rigid endoscopy; however, because of the dense nature of the infiltrate, a deep-enough sample can rarely be obtained by flexible endoscopy. Cytologic analysis of a tissue sample obtained by scraping an excised piece of submucosa with a scalpel blade may be diagnostic; fungal hyphae that do not stain and appear as "ghosts" with typical Romanowsky-type stains are strongly supportive of a diagnosis. The organisms can be sparse and difficult to find histologically, even in large tissue samples.

## Treatment

Complete surgical excision provides the best chance for cure. Itraconazole (5 mg/kg PO q12h) or liposomal amphotericin B (2.2 mg/kg/treatment) may benefit some animals.

## Prognosis

Pythiosis often spreads to or involves structures that cannot be surgically removed (e.g., root of the mesentery, pancreas surrounding the bile duct), resulting in a grim prognosis.

### *Suggested Readings*

Bellenger CR et al: Chronic hypertrophic pyloric gastropathy in 14 dogs, *Aust Vet J* 67(9):317, 1990.

Brockman DJ et al: Canine gastric dilation/volvulus syndrome in a veterinary critical care unit: 295 cases (1986-1992), *J Am Vet Med Assoc* 207(4):460, 1995.

Brourman JD et al: Factors associated with perioperative mortality in dogs with surgically managed gastric dilatation-volvulus: 137 cases (1988-1993), *J Am Vet Med Assoc* 108(11):1855, 1996.

de Papp E et al: Plasma lactate concentration as a predictor of gastric necrosis and survival among dogs with gastric dilatation-volvulus: 102 cases (1995-1998), *J Am Vet Med Assoc* 215:49, 1999.

Dow SW et al: Effects of flunixin and flunixin plus prednisone on the gastrointestinal tract of dogs, *Am J Vet Res* 51(7):1131, 1990.

Easton S: A retrospective study into the effects of operator experience on the accuracy of ultrasound in the diagnosis of gastric neoplasia in dogs, *Vet Radiol Ultrasound* 42:47, 2001.

Ellison GW: Gastric dilatation volvulus—surgical prevention, *Vet Clin North Am* 23(3):513, 1993.

Fonda D et al: Gastric carcinoma in the dog: a clinicopathological study of 11 cases, *J Small Anim Pract* 30:353, 1989.

Geyer C et al: Occurrence of spiral-shaped bacteria in gastric biopsies of dogs and cats, *Vet Rec* 133:18, 1993.

Glickman LT et al: A prospective study of survival and recurrence following the acute gastric dilation-volvulus syndrome in 136 dogs, *J Am Anim Hosp Assoc* 34:253, 1998.

Glickman LT et al: Incidence of and breed-related risk factors for gastric dilitation-volvulus in dogs, *J Am Vet Med Assoc* 216:40, 2000.

Glickman LT et al: Non-dietary risk factors for gastric dilatation-volvulus in large and giant breed dogs, *J Am Vet Med Assoc* 217:1492, 2000.

Guilford WG et al: *Small animal gastroenterology,* ed 3, Philadelphia, 1996, WB Saunders.

Hosgood G: Gastric dilatation-volvulus in dogs, *J Am Vet Med Assoc* 204(11):1742, 1994.

Lamb CR et al: Ultrasonographic appearance of primary gastric neoplasia in 21 dogs, *J Small Anim Pract* 40:211, 1999.

Leib MS et al: Endoscopic diagnosis of chronic hypertrophic pyloric gastropathy in dogs, *J Vet Intern Med* 7:335, 1993.

Matthiesen DT: Pathophysiology of gastric dilatation-volvulus. In Bojrab MJ, editor: *Disease mechanisms in small animal surgery,* ed 2, Philadelphia, 1993, Lea & Febiger, p 220.

Michels GM et al: Endoscopic and surgical retrieval of fishhooks from the stomach and esophagus in dogs and cats: 75 cases (1977-1993), *J Am Vet Med Assoc* 207(9):1194, 1995.

Miller RI: Gastrointestinal phycomycosis in 63 dogs, *J Am Vet Med Assoc* 186(5):473, 1985.

Neiger R et al: Gastric mucosal lesions in dogs with acute intervertebral disc disease: characterization and effects of omeprazole or misoprostol, *J Vet Intern Med* 14:33, 2000.

Neiger R et al: *Helicobacter* infection in dogs and cats: facts and fiction, *J Vet Intern Med* 14:125, 2000.

Otto G et al: Animal and public health implications of gastric colonization of cats by *Helicobacter*-like organisms, *J Clin Microbiol* 32:1043, 1994.

Penninck DG et al: Ultrasonography of gastric ulceration in the dog, *Vet Radiol Ultrasound* 38(4):308, 1997.

Penninck DG et al: Ultrasonography of canine gastric epithelial neoplasia, *Vet Radiol Ultrasound* 39:342, 1998.

Reimer ME et al: The gastroduodenal effects of buffered aspirin, carprofen and etodolac in healthy dogs, *J Vet Intern Med* 13:472, 1999.

Scanziani E et al: Gastric carcinoma in the Belgian Shepherd dog, *J Small Anim Pract* 32:465, 1991.

Scanziani E et al: Histologic and immunhistochemical detection of different *Helicobacter* species in the gastric mucosa of cats, *J Vet Diagn Invest* 13:3, 2001.

Schellenberg D et al: Influence of thoracic conformation and genetics on the risk of gastric dilatation volvulus in Irish setters, *J Am Anim Hosp Assoc* 34:64, 1998.

Schertel ER et al: Evaluation of a hypertonic saline dextran solution for treatment of dogs with shock induced by gastric dilatation volvulus, *J Am Vet Med Assoc* 210(2):226, 1997.

Spielman BL et al: Hemorrhagic gastroenteritis in 15 dogs, *J Am Anim Hosp Assoc* 29:341, 1993.

Stanton ME et al: Gastroduodenal ulceration in dogs, *J Vet Intern Med* 3:238, 1989.

Tams TR: Endoscopic removal of gastrointestinal foreign bodies. In Tams TR, editor: *Small animal endoscopy,* ed 2, St Louis, 1999, Mosby, p 247.

Thomas RC et al: Pythiosis in dogs and cats, *Compend Contin Educ* 20:63, 1998.

Walter MC et al: Chronic hypertrophic pyloric gastropathy as a cause of pyloric obstruction in the dog, *J Am Vet Med Assoc* 186(2):157, 1985.

Walter MC et al: Acquired antral pyloric hypertrophy in the dog, *Vet Clin North Am* 23(3):547, 1993.

Wilson RB et al: Chronic gastritis due to *Ollulanus tricuspis* infection in a cat, *J Am Anim Hosp Assoc* 26:137, 1990.

# CHAPTER 33

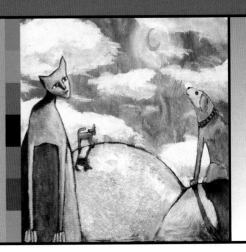

# Disorders
# of the Intestinal Tract

## CHAPTER OUTLINE

ABBREVIATIONS USED IN THE CHAPTER, 432
ACUTE DIARRHEA, 432
  Acute enteritis, 432
  Dietary-induced diarrhea, 433
INFECTIOUS DIARRHEA, 433
  Canine parvoviral enteritis, 433
  Feline parvoviral enteritis, 435
  Canine coronaviral enteritis, 436
  Feline coronaviral enteritis, 436
  Feline leukemia virus–associated panleukopenia, 436
  Feline immunodeficiency virus–associated diarrhea, 436
  Salmon poisoning, 437
  Campylobacteriosis, 437
  Salmonellosis, 437
  Clostridial diseases, 438
  Miscellaneous bacteria, 439
  Histoplasmosis, 439
  Prototothecosis, 430
ALIMENTARY TRACT PARASITES, 440
  Whipworms, 440
  Roundworms, 441
  Hookworms, 443
  Tapeworms, 443
  Strongyloidiasis, 444
  Coccidiosis, 444
  Cryptosporidia, 444
  Giardiasis, 445
  Trichomoniasis, 446
MALDIGESTIVE DISEASE, 446
  Exocrine pancreatic insufficiency, 446
MALABSORPTIVE DISEASES, 447
  Canine lymphocytic-plasmacytic enteritis, 447
  Canine lymphocytic-plasmacytic colitis, 448
  Feline lymphocytic-plasmacytic enteritis, 448
  Feline lymphocytic-plasmacytic colitis, 448
  Canine eosinophilic gastroenterocolitis, 448
  Feline eosinophilic enteritis/hypereosinophilic
    syndrome, 449
  Granulomatous enteritis/gastritis, 449
Immunoproliferative enteropathy in Basenjis, 449
Enteropathy in Sharpeis, 450
Antibiotic responsive enteropathy, 450
PROTEIN-LOSING ENTEROPATHY, 451
  Causes of protein-losing enteropathy, 451
  Intestinal lymphangiectasia, 451
  Protein-losing enteropathy in Soft-Coated Wheaten
    Terriers, 451
FUNCTIONAL INTESTINAL DISEASE, 452
  Irritable bowel syndrome, 452
INTESTINAL OBSTRUCTION, 452
  Simple intestinal obstruction, 452
  Incarcerated intestinal obstruction, 452
  Mesenteric torsion/volvulus, 453
  Linear foreign objects, 454
INTUSSUSCEPTION, 455
  Ileocolic intussusception, 455
  Jejunojejunal intussusception, 455
MISCELLANEOUS INTESTINAL DISEASES, 456
  Short bowel syndrome, 456
NEOPLASMS OF THE SMALL INTESTINE, 457
  Alimentary lymphoma, 457
  Intestinal adenocarcinoma, 457
  Intestinal leiomyoma/leiomyosarcoma, 458
INFLAMMATION OF THE LARGE INTESTINE, 458
  Acute colitis/proctitis, 458
  Chronic colitis, 458
INTUSSUSCEPTION/PROLAPSE OF THE LARGE
INTESTINE, 458
  Cecocolic intussusception, 458
  Rectal prolapse, 458
NEOPLASMS OF THE LARGE INTESTINE, 459
  Adenocarcinoma, 459
  Rectal polyps, 459
MISCELLANEOUS LARGE INTESTINAL
DISEASES, 460
  Pythiosis, 460
PERINEAL/PERIANAL DISEASES, 460
  Perineal hernia, 460
  Perianal fistulae, 461
  Anal sacculitis, 461

PERIANAL NEOPLASMS, 461

    Anal sac (apocrine gland) adenocarcinoma, 461

    Perianal gland tumors, 462

CONSTIPATION, 462

    Pelvic canal obstruction due to malaligned healing of old
        pelvic fractures, 462

    Benign rectal stricture, 462

    Dietary indiscretion leading to constipation, 463

    Idiopathic megacolon, 463

## *ABBREVIATIONS USED IN THE CHAPTER*

**ARE:** Antibiotic-responsive enteropathy (previously known as small intestinal bacterial overgrowth—IBO)

**CPV:** Canine parvovirus

**EGE:** Eosinophilic gastroenteritis

**EHEC:** Enterohemorrhagic *Escherichia coli*

**EPI:** Exocrine pancreatic insufficiency

**FeLV:** Feline leukemia virus

**FIV:** Feline immunodeficiency virus

**GDV:** Gastric dilation and volvulus

**GUE:** Gastric ulceration/erosion

**HES:** Hypereosinophilic syndrome

**IBD:** Inflammatory bowel disease

**IBS:** Irritable bowel syndrome

**IL:** Intestinal lymphangiectasia

**LPC:** Lymphocytic-plasmacytic colitis

**LPE:** Lymphoplasmacytic enteritis

**PCR:** Polymerase chain reaction

**PLE:** Protein-losing enteropathy

## *ACUTE DIARRHEA*

### ACUTE ENTERITIS
#### Etiology

Acute enteritis can be caused by infectious agents, poor diet, abrupt dietary changes, inappropriate foods, additives (e.g., chemicals), and/or parasites. Except for parvovirus, the cause is rarely diagnosed, because most affected animals spontaneously improve, although supportive therapy may be needed.

#### Clinical Features

Diarrhea of unknown cause occurs commonly, especially in puppies and kittens. Signs consist of diarrhea with or without vomiting, dehydration, fever, anorexia, depression, crying, and/or abdominal pain. Very young animals may become hypoglycemic and stuporous.

#### Diagnosis

History and physical and fecal examinations are used to identify possible causes. Fecal flotation (preferably with zinc sulfate flotation solution) and direct fecal examinations are always indicated because parasites may worsen the problem, even when they are not the main cause. The need for other diagnostic procedures depends on the severity of the illness and on whether there is risk of contagion. Clinically mild enteritis is usually treated symptomatically, with few diagnostic tests being performed. If the animal is febrile, has hemorrhagic stools, is part of an outbreak of enteritis, or is particularly ill, then additional tests (i.e., complete blood count [CBC] to identify neutropenia, fecal ELISA for canine parvovirus, serologic analysis for feline leukemia virus and feline immunodeficiency virus, blood glucose to identify hypoglycemia, and serum electrolytes to detect hypokalemia) are indicated. Abdominal radiographs and/or ultrasonograms should be evaluated if abdominal pain, masses, obstruction, or foreign body are suspected.

#### Treatment

Symptomatic therapy usually suffices. The cause is usually unknown or is a virus for which there is no specific therapy. The hallmark of symptomatic therapy is reestablishment of fluid, electrolyte, and acid-base homeostasis. Animals with severe dehydration (i.e., $\geq$8% to 10% as determined by sunken eyes; fast, weak pulse; and marked depression; or as detected by a history of significant fluid loss coupled with inadequate fluid intake) should receive intravenous fluids, whereas fluids administered orally or subcutaneously usually suffice for those less severely dehydrated. Potassium supplementation is usually indicated, but bicarbonate is rarely needed. Oral rehydration is useful in allowing home management of animals, especially when litters of young animals are affected. (See discussion on fluid, electrolyte, and acid-base therapy in Chapter 30 for details.)

Antidiarrheals are seldom necessary except when excessive fecal losses make maintenance of fluid and electrolyte balance difficult, but they are often requested by clients. Opiates are usually the most effective antidiarrheals. Bismuth subsalicylate (see Table 30-9) is useful in stopping diarrhea in dogs with mild to moderate enteritis. However, absorption of the salicylate may cause nephrotoxicity in some animals, and many dogs dislike the taste. Cats rarely need these medications. (See discussion on drugs that prolong intestinal transit time in Chapter 30.) If antidiarrheals are needed for more than 2 to 5 days, the animal should be carefully reassessed.

Severe intestinal inflammation often causes vomiting that is difficult to control. Central-acting antiemetics (e.g., prochlorperazine and metoclopramide; see Table 30-6) are more likely to be effective than peripheral-acting drugs. The animal must be well hydrated before receiving phenothiazine derivatives, which dilate blood vessels and can produce hypotension. If these antiemetics fail, ondansetron can be used.

Although food is typically withheld from animals with severe enteritis to "rest" their intestinal tract, such starvation may be detrimental to the bowel. Preventing any oral intake is occasionally necessary in animals in which eating causes severe vomiting or explosive diarrhea with substantial fluid loss. Recent data suggest that children who continue eating during episodes of acute enteritis recover sooner and have less weight loss than those who do not. Therefore if feeding does not make the pet's vomiting and diarrhea *much* worse, feeding small amounts of food is preferable to withholding food. Bowel starvation is to be avoided, if possible. Bowel "rest" consists of frequent, small feedings of easily digested, nonirritative foods (e.g., cottage cheese, boiled chicken, potato). If food is withheld, it should be reoffered as soon as possible. Some animals with severe enteritis may need parenteral nutrition to establish a positive nitrogen balance.

If the animal is febrile or neutropenic or has systemic inflammatory response syndrome (i.e., septic shock), broad-spectrum systemic antibiotics (e.g., β-lactam antibiotic plus an aminoglycoside) are indicated (see Drugs Used in Gastrointestinal Disorders, p. 469). The clinician should observe for hypoglycemia during septic shock, especially in young animals. Adding dextrose (2.5% to 5%) to the intravenous fluids or administering an intravenous bolus of 50% dextrose (2 to 5 ml/kg) may be necessary to counter hypoglycemia. Flunixin meglumine (1 mg/kg IV) seems helpful in treating septic shock; however, it may cause severe gastric ulceration and impair renal blood flow.

If the cause of the diarrhea is unknown, the clinician should assume it to be infectious and disinfect the premises accordingly. Bleach diluted in water (i.e., 1:32) destroys parvovirus and many other infectious agents causing diarrhea. Animals must not be injured by inappropriate contact with such disinfectants. Personnel coming in contact with the animals, cages, and litter should wear protective clothing (e.g., boots, gloves, gowns) that can be discarded or disinfected when leaving the area.

After the enteropathy appears to be clinically resolved, the animal is gradually returned to its normal diet over a 5- to 10-day period. If this change is associated with more diarrhea, then the switch is postponed for another 5 days.

## Prognosis

The prognosis depends on the animal's condition and can be influenced by its age and other gastrointestinal (GI) problems. Very young or emaciated animals and those with septic shock or substantial intestinal parasite burdens have a more guarded prognosis. Intussusception may occur secondary to acute enteritis, thus worsening the prognosis.

## DIETARY-INDUCED DIARRHEA

### Etiology

Dietary causes of diarrhea are common, especially in young animals. Poor-quality ingredients (e.g., rancid fat), bacterial enterotoxins or mycotoxins, allergy or intolerance to ingredients, or inability of the animal to digest normal foods are common causes. The latter mechanism revolves around intestinal brush border enzymes that are produced in response to the presence of substrates (e.g., disaccharidases). If the diet is suddenly changed, some animals (especially puppies and kittens) are unable to digest or absorb certain nutrients until the intestinal brush border adapts to the new diet. Other animals may never be able to produce the necessary enzymes (e.g., lactase) to digest certain nutrients (e.g., lactose).

### Clinical Features

Diet-induced diarrhea occurs in both dogs and cats. The diarrhea tends to reflect small intestinal dysfunction (i.e., there is usually no fecal blood or mucus) unless there is colonic involvement. The diarrhea usually starts shortly after the new diet is initiated (e.g., 1 to 3 days) and is mild to moderate in severity. Affected animals infrequently have other signs unless parasites or complicating factors are present.

### Diagnosis

History and physical and fecal examinations are used to eliminate other common causes. If diarrhea occurs shortly after a suspected or known dietary change (e.g., after the pet is brought home), a tentative diagnosis of diet-induced disease is reasonable. However, the pet may also be showing the first clinical signs of an infection it recently acquired. The animal should always be checked for intestinal parasites because they may contribute to the problem even when they are not the principal cause.

### Treatment

A bland diet (e.g., potato plus boiled skinless chicken) fed in multiple, small feedings (see p. 389) usually causes resolution of the diarrhea in 1 to 3 days. Once the diarrhea resolves, the diet can be gradually changed back to the pet's regular diet.

### Prognosis

The prognosis is usually excellent, unless a very young animal with minimal nutritional reserves becomes emaciated, dehydrated, or hypoglycemic.

## INFECTIOUS DIARRHEA

### CANINE PARVOVIRAL ENTERITIS
### Etiology

There are two types of parvoviruses that infect dogs. Canine parvovirus-1 (CPV-1), also known as "minute virus of canines," is a relatively nonpathogenic virus that sometimes is associated with gastroenteritis, pneumonitis, and/or myocarditis in very young puppies. Canine parvovirus-2 (CPV-2) is responsible for classic parvoviral enteritis. CPV-2 usually causes signs 5 to 12 days after the dog is infected via the fecal-oral route, and it preferentially invades and destroys rapidly dividing cells (i.e., bone marrow progenitors, intestinal crypt epithelium).

### Clinical Features

The virus has mutated since it was first recognized, and the most recently recognized CPV-2b may be more pathogenic in some dogs. CPV-2b can also infect cats. The clinical syndrome is similar to that seen with earlier strains and depends on the virulence of the virus, the size of the inoculum, and the host's defenses. Doberman Pinschers, Rottweilers, Pit Bulls, and Labrador Retrievers may be more susceptible than other breeds. Viral destruction of intestinal crypts may produce villus collapse, diarrhea, vomiting, intestinal bleeding, and subsequent bacterial invasion; however, some animals have mild or even subclinical disease. Many dogs are initially presented because of depression, anorexia, and/or vomiting (which can resemble foreign object ingestion), not for diarrhea. Diarrhea is often absent for the first 24 to 48 hours of illness and may not be bloody if and when it does occur. Intestinal protein loss may occur secondary to inflammation, causing hypoalbuminemia. Vomiting is usually a prominent finding and may be severe enough to cause esophagitis. Damage to bone marrow progenitors may produce transient or prolonged neutropenia, making the animal susceptible to serious bacterial infection, especially if a damaged intestinal tract allows bacteria access to the body. Fever and/or septic shock (i.e., systemic inflammatory response syndrome) are common in severely ill dogs but are often absent in less severely affected animals. Puppies that are infected *in utero* or before 8 weeks of age may develop myocarditis.

## Diagnosis

Diagnosis is often tentatively made on the basis of history and physical examination findings. Neutropenia is suggestive but is neither sensitive nor specific for canine parvovirus enteritis; salmonellosis or any overwhelming infection can cause similar changes in the CBC. Regardless of whether or not diarrhea occurs, infected dogs shed large numbers of viral particles in the feces (i.e., $>10^9$ particles/g). Therefore ELISA for CPV-2 in the feces is the best diagnostic test. Vaccination with a modified live parvoviral vaccine may cause a weak positive result for 5 to 15 days after vaccination. However, the ELISA results may be negative if the assay is performed early in the clinical course of the disease, and one should not hesitate to repeat this test in dogs that seem likely to have parvoviral enteritis but that initially have negative findings. Shedding decreases rapidly and may be undetectable 10 to 14 days after infection. The real advantage to testing is that either a presumptive diagnosis of parvoviral enteritis is confirmed or other diseases that can mimic parvovirus but require different therapy (e.g., salmonellosis, intussusception) must be considered. Electron microscopic evaluation of feces detects the presence of the virus; however, CPV-1 (which is usually nonpathogenic except perhaps in neonates) is morphologically indistinguishable from CPV-2. If the dog dies, there are typical histologic lesions (i.e., crypt necrosis) and fluorescent antibody techniques that can be used to establish a definitive diagnosis.

## Treatment

Treatment of canine parvoviral enteritis is fundamentally the same as for any severe, acute, infectious enteritis (see p. 432). Fluid and electrolyte therapy is used in combination with antibiotics (Table 33-1). Most dogs will live if they can be supported long enough. However, very young puppies, dogs in severe septic shock, and certain breeds seem to have more problems and may have a more guarded prognosis. Mistakes include inadequate fluid therapy (common), overzealous fluid administration (especially in dogs with severe hypoproteinemia), unrecognized sepsis, and unsuspected concurrent GI disease (e.g., parasites, intussusception).

If the serum albumin concentration is less than 2.0 g/dl, plasma should be administered. Colloids such as hetastarch may be substituted for plasma, but they do not contain antibodies that might be beneficial. Antibiotic therapy is needed if there is evidence of infection (i.e., fever, septic shock) or the risk of infection is great (i.e., severe neutropenia). If the animal is neutropenic but afebrile, the administration of a first-generation cephalosporin is reasonable. If the animal is in septic shock (i.e., systemic inflammatory response syndrome), then an antibiotic combination with a broad aerobic and anerobic spectrum is recommended (e.g., ampicillin plus amikacin). Caution should be used when administering enrofloxacin to young, large-breed dogs lest cartilage damage occur. Renal perfusion must be maintained with fluid therapy when using aminoglycosides. Human granulocyte colony–stimulating factor (G-CSF) (5 µg/kg q24h) has been used to increase neutrophil numbers, but there is no evidence that it makes any difference in outcome. Severe, intractable vomiting complicates therapy and may require administration of prochlorperazine, metoclopramide, or ondansetron (see Table 30-6). If esophagitis occurs, $H_2$-receptor antagonists and liquid sucralfate (carafate) may be useful (see Tables 30-7 and 30-8). A bland diet can be administered once vomiting has ceased for 18 to 24 hours. If necessary, total parenteral nutrition can be lifesaving for patients persistently unable to hold down oral food. If total parenteral nutrition is not acceptable because of financial reasons, then partial parenteral nutrition may be helpful. The dog should be kept away from other susceptible animals for 2 to 4 weeks after discharge, and the owner should be conscientious about the disposal of feces. Vaccination of other dogs in the household should be considered.

When trying to prevent the spread of parvoviral enteritis, it is important to remember that (1) parvovirus persists for long periods of time (i.e., months) in the environment, making it difficult to prevent exposure; (2) asymptomatic dogs may shed virulent CPV-2 in their feces; (3) maternal immunity can destroy the vaccine virus, and maternal immunity sufficient to inactivate vaccine virus may persist in some puppies up to 18 weeks of age; and (4) dilute bleach (1:32) is one of the few readily available disinfectants that kills the virus.

Vaccination of pups should generally commence at 5 to 8 weeks of age (preferably with a high-antigen-density vaccine). High-density vaccines may be effective in some animals given a single injection after 12 weeks of age; however, if an inactivated vaccine is administered, it may be best to give a second injection so that immunity is prolonged. In general, the last vaccination should be administered as per the manufacturer's recommendations (usually between 12 and 20 weeks of age). Animals considered at risk often receive vaccinations until 18 weeks of age. Annual revaccination is generally recommended for parvovirus, although it is possible that vaccination every 3 years may be sufficient after the initial series as a puppy. Adults that were previously unvaccinated usually receive two doses 2 to 4 weeks apart. There is no strong evidence that parvoviral vaccination should be given separately from modified-live canine distemper vaccinations. However, modified-live vaccinations should not be administered before 5 weeks of age or to dogs incubating or affected with distemper.

TABLE 33-1

General Guidelines for Treatment of Canine Parvoviral Enteritis*

**Fluids†**

A history of decreased intake plus increased loss such as vomiting and/or diarrhea confirms dehydration, regardless of whether or not dog appears to be dehydrated

Administer balanced electrolyte solution with 20-40 mEq potassium chloride/L

Dogs with very mild cases may receive subcutaneous fluids (intravenous fluids still preferred), but watch for sudden worsening of the disease

Dogs with moderate to severe cases should receive fluids via intravenous or intramedullary route

Add 2.5%-5% dextrose to the IV fluids if dog has been hypoglycemic or is at risk (e.g., septic shock)

Administer plasma or hetastarch if dog has serum albumin ≤2.0 g/dl

**Antibiotics†**

Administer to febrile or severely neutropenic dogs

Prophylactic antibiotics for nonfebrile neutropenic patients (e.g., cefazolin)

Antibiotics for febrile, neutropenic patients (e.g., ampicillin and amikacin)

**Antiemetics**

Prescribe as needed:
  Prochlorperazine (first choice)
  Metoclopramide
  Ondansetron (for intractable vomiting when dog does not respond to other medications)

**Flunixin Meglumine (Controversial)**

Sometimes used for patients with severe systemic inflammatory response syndrome (i.e., septic shock)

Use once but not with concurrent corticosteroids; repeated dosing or excessive doses can cause life-threatening gastro-duodenal ulceration and bleeding; sometimes severe ulceration with or without bleeding occurs even with modest doses

Do not use in severely dehydrated dogs

**Anthelmintics**

Use pyrantel if dog does not vomit it
Ivermectin is also acceptable

**Dogs with Secondary Esophagitis**

If regurgitation occurs in addition to vomiting, administer:
  $H_2$-receptor antagonists (injectable preferred)
  Sucralfate (Carafate) slurry

**Special Nutritional Therapy**

Administer total parenteral nutrition if prolonged anorexia occurs; if cannot use total parenteral nutrition, recommend partial parenteral nutrition

Try to feed dog small amounts as soon as feeding does not cause major exacerbation in vomiting

**Monitor Physical Status**

Physical examination (1-3 times per day depending on severity of signs)

Body weight (1-2 times per day to assess changes in hydration status)

Potassium (every 1-2 days depending on severity of vomiting/diarrhea)

Serum protein (every 1-2 days depending on severity of signs)

Glucose (every 4-12 hours in dogs that have septic shock or were initially hypoglycemic)

Packed cell volume (every 1-2 days)

White blood cell count: either actual count or estimated from a slide (every 1-2 days in febrile animals)

*The same guidelines generally apply to dogs with other causes of acute enteritis/gastritis.
†Usually the first considerations when an animal is presented.

If parvoviral enteritis develops in one dog in a multiple-dog household, it is reasonable to administer booster vaccinations to the other dogs, preferably using an inactivated vaccine in case they are incubating the infection at the time of immunization. If the client is bringing a puppy into a house with a dog that has recently had parvoviral enteritis, it may be best if the puppy is kept elsewhere until it has received its immunizations.

## Prognosis

Dogs treated in a timely fashion with proper therapy typically live, especially if they survive the first 4 days of clinical signs. Intussusception may be a sequela and cause persistent diar-rhea in pups recovering from the viral infection. Dogs that have recovered from CPV-2 enteritis develop long-lived immunity that may be lifelong. Whether immunization against CPV-1 will ever be needed is unknown.

## FELINE PARVOVIRAL ENTERITIS

### Etiology

Feline parvoviral enteritis (feline distemper, feline pan-leukopenia) is caused by a parvovirus distinct from CVP-2b. However, CPV-2b can infect cats and is thought to be able to cause disease.

## Clinical Features

Signs are similar to those described for dogs with parvoviral enteritis.

## Diagnosis

Diagnosis is similar to that stated for canine parvovirus. The ELISA used to detect fecal canine parvovirus has been anecdotally reported to cross-react with feline parvovirus.

## Treatment

Cats with parvoviral infection are treated as described for dogs with the disease. The major differences are in regard to immunization: parvoviral vaccine seems to engender a better protective response in cats than in dogs.

## Prognosis

As for dogs, many affected cats live if overwhelming sepsis is prevented and they can be supported long enough.

## CANINE CORONAVIRAL ENTERITIS

### Etiology

Canine coronaviral enteritis occurs when coronavirus invades and destroys mature cells on the intestinal villi. Because intestinal crypts remain intact, villi regenerate faster in dogs with coronaviral enteritis than in dogs with parvoviral enteritis; bone marrow cells are not affected.

### Clinical Features

Coronaviral enteritis is typically much less severe than classic parvoviral enteritis and rarely causes hemorrhagic diarrhea, septicemia, or death. Older dogs may be infected in addition to younger dogs. Signs may last approximately 3 to 20 days, and small or very young dogs may die from dehydration or electrolyte abnormalities if they are not properly treated. Dual infection with parvovirus may produce a high incidence of morbidity and mortality.

### Diagnosis

Because canine coronaviral enteritis is usually much less severe than many other enteritides, it is seldom definitively diagnosed. Most dogs are treated symptomatically for acute enteritis until they improve. Electron microscopic examination of feces obtained early in the course of the disease can be diagnostic. However, the virus is fragile and easily disrupted by inappropriate handling of the feces. A history of contagion and eliminating other causes are reasons to suspect canine coronaviral enteritis.

### Treatment

Fluid therapy, motility modifiers (see Chapter 30), and time should resolve most cases of coronaviral enteritis. Symptomatic therapy (see p. 432) is usually successful except perhaps for very young animals. A vaccination is available but of uncertain value except perhaps in animals at high risk of infection (e.g., those in infected kennels or dog shows).

## Prognosis

The prognosis for recovery is usually good.

## FELINE CORONAVIRAL ENTERITIS

The severity of feline coronaviral enteritis seems to be age related. Adults are often asymptomatic, whereas kittens may have mild, transient diarrhea and fever. Deaths are rare, and the prognosis for recovery is excellent. There is no vaccine available. This disease is important because (1) affected animals seroconvert and may become positive on feline infectious peritonitis serologic analysis and (2) mutation by the feline coronavirus may be the cause of feline infectious peritonitis.

## FELINE LEUKEMIA VIRUS–ASSOCIATED PANLEUKOPENIA

### Etiology

Feline leukemia virus (FeLV)–associated panleukopenia is a nonneoplastic disease caused by FeLV. The exact pathogenesis is unknown, but the intestinal lesion histologically resembles that produced by feline parvovirus. The bone marrow and lymph nodes are not consistently affected as in cats with parvoviral enteritis. These animals might have parvoviral infections that cannot be easily detected.

### Clinical Features

Chronic weight loss, vomiting, and diarrhea are common. The diarrhea often has characteristics of large bowel disease.

### Diagnosis

Finding FeLV infection in a cat with chronic diarrhea is suggestive of this disorder. The chronic course helps to differentiate it from parvoviral enteritis. Some cats are also neutropenic. Biopsy of the intestines eliminates other causes.

### Treatment

Symptomatic therapy (fluid/electrolyte therapy, antibiotics, antiemetics, and/or highly digestible bland diets as needed) plus elimination of other problems that compromise the intestines (e.g., parasites, poor diet) may be beneficial.

### Prognosis

This disease has a very poor prognosis because of other FeLV-related complications.

## FELINE IMMUNODEFICIENCY VIRUS–ASSOCIATED DIARRHEA

### Etiology

Feline immunodeficiency virus (FIV) can be associated with severe, purulent colitis. The pathogenesis is unclear and may involve multiple mechanisms.

### Clinical Features

Severe large bowel disease is common and can occasionally result in colonic rupture. These animals generally act ill, whereas many cats with chronic large bowel disease due to inflammatory bowel disease (IBD) or dietary intolerance seemingly feel fine.

### Diagnosis

Detection of antibodies to FIV plus severe, purulent colitis allows presumptive diagnosis.

### Treatment

Therapy is supportive (e.g., fluids/electrolytes, antiemetics, antibiotics, and/or highly digestible bland diets as needed).

### Prognosis

The long-term prognosis is very poor, although some cats can be maintained for months.

## SALMON POISONING

### Etiology

Salmon poisoning is caused by *Neorickettsia helminthoeca*. Dogs are infected when they eat fish (primarily salmon) infected with a fluke *(Nanophyetus salmincola)* that carries the rickettsia. The rickettsia spreads to the intestines and most lymph nodes, causing inflammation. This disease is principally found in the Pacific northwestern United States because the snail intermediate host for *N. salmincola* lives there.

### Clinical Features

Dogs, not cats, are affected. The severity of signs varies and may include fever, anorexia, vomiting, generalized lymphadenopathy, and/or diarrhea. The diarrhea is typically small bowel but may become bloody. Inappropriate therapy may result in death.

### Diagnosis

Presumptive diagnosis is usually based on the animal's habitat plus a history of recent consumption of raw fish or exposure to streams or lakes. Finding *Nanophyetus* spp. ova in the stool or rickettsia in fine-needle aspirates of enlarged lymph nodes is confirmatory.

### Treatment

Treatment consists of symptomatic control of dehydration, vomiting, and diarrhea and elimination of the rickettsia and fluke. Tetracycline, oxytetracycline, doxycycline, or chloramphenicol (see Chapter 98) eliminates the rickettsia. The fluke is killed with praziquantel (see Table 30-10).

### Prognosis

The prognosis depends on the clinical severity at the time of diagnosis. Most dogs respond favorably to tetracyclines and supportive therapy. The key to success is awareness of the disease. Untreated salmon poisoning has a poor prognosis.

## CAMPYLOBACTERIOSIS

### Etiology

Campylobacteriosis is caused by *Campylobacter jejuni*. The organism prefers high temperatures (i.e., 39° to 41° C); hence poultry is probably a reservoir. This organism is found in the intestinal tract of some healthy dogs and cats.

### Clinical Features

Campylobacteriosis is principally diagnosed in young animals in crowded conditions (e.g., kennels, humane shelters) or as a nosocomial infection. Mucoid diarrhea (with or without blood), anorexia, and/or fever are the primary signs. Campylobacteriosis tends to be self-limiting in dogs, cats, and people; however, it occasionally causes chronic diarrhea. This bacterium may cause enteritis during recovery from canine parvoviral enteritis.

### Diagnosis

*C. jejuni* has special culture requirements, and the laboratory must use specific techniques for isolation. The fecal sample must be submitted promptly, or appropriate transport media must be used (not culturettes). Occasionally, classic *Campylobacter* forms may be found during cytologic examination of a fecal smear (i.e., "commas," "seagull wings"), but the sensitivity of this examination is uncertain in the dog. Because this bacterium may be cultured from normal dogs and cats, diagnosis requires more than just growing the organism from feces. Appropriate clinical signs, history, and/or response to therapy are needed to confirm that *C. jejuni* is responsible for disease.

### Treatment

If campylobacteriosis is suspected, erythromycin (10 to 15 mg/kg PO q8h) or neomycin (20 mg/kg PO q12h) is usually effective. Tetracycline may also be a good therapeutic choice, but β-lactam antibiotics (i.e., penicillins, cephalosporins) are often ineffective. The length of treatment necessary for cure is uncertain. The animal should be treated for at least 1 to 3 days beyond resolution of clinical signs; however, antibiotic therapy may not eradicate the bacteria, and reinfection is likely in kennel conditions. Chronic infections may require prolonged therapy (e.g., weeks).

This bacterium is potentially transmissible to people. It has been estimated that more than 5% of cases of human campylobacteriosis originate from dogs and cats. Infected dogs and cats should be isolated, and individuals working with the animal or its environment or wastes should wear protective clothing and wash with disinfectants.

### Prognosis

With appropriate antibiotic therapy the prognosis for recovery is good.

## SALMONELLOSIS

### Etiology

There are numerous *Salmonella* serotypes that may cause disease. The bacteria may originate from animals shedding the organism (e.g., infected dogs and cats) or from contaminated foods (especially poultry and eggs).

## Clinical Features

*Salmonella* spp. are seldom confirmed to cause canine or feline GI disease, even though the bacteria are often present in the colon and/or mesenteric lymph nodes. *Salmonella* spp. may produce acute or chronic diarrhea, septicemia, and/or sudden death, especially in very young or geriatric animals. Salmonellosis in young animals can produce a syndrome that closely mimics parvoviral enteritis (one reason why ELISA testing for parvovirus is useful). The fact that salmonellosis occasionally develops during or after canine parvoviral enteritis makes the situation more confusing.

## Diagnosis

Culture of *Salmonella* spp. from the blood confirms septicemia. Diagnosis of GI salmonellosis requires culture of the organism from the feces or mucosa, appropriate clinical signs, elimination of other causes (e.g., parvovirus), and response to therapy. However, *Salmonella* may be cultured from normal animals; therefore, definitive diagnosis can be difficult. Successful fecal culture often necessitates use of enrichment and/or selective media. Identification by polymerase chain reaction (PCR) can be a sensitive method of diagnosis.

## Treatment

If salmonellosis is diagnosed, treatment depends on the animal's clinical signs. Septicemic animals should receive supportive therapy and parenteral antibiotics as determined by susceptibility testing, but quinolones, potentiated sulfa drugs, and chloramphenicol are often good initial choices (see Drugs Used in Gastrointestinal Disorders, p. 469). Animals with diarrhea may need only supportive therapy; antibiotics are of dubious value and might promote a carrier state. Infected animals might be public health risks and should be isolated from other animals, at least until they are asymptomatic. Even when signs disappear, reculturing of feces is reasonable to ensure that shedding has stopped. Individuals in contact with the animal, its environment, and its waste should wear protective clothing and wash with disinfectants such as phenolic compounds and bleach (1:32 dilution).

## Prognosis

The prognosis is usually good in animals with only diarrhea but guarded in septicemic dogs and cats.

## CLOSTRIDIAL DISEASES

### Etiology

*Clostridium perfringens* and *Clostridium difficile* can be found in clinically normal dogs but appear to cause diarrhea in some. For *C. perfringens* to produce disease, the bacteria must possess the ability to produce toxin, and environmental conditions must be such that spores are produced.

### Clinical Features

*C. perfringens* may produce an acute, bloody, self-limiting nosocomial diarrhea or a chronic large bowel diarrhea (with or without blood or mucus). This clostridial disease is primarily recognized in dogs. Disease associated with *C. difficile* is poorly characterized in small animals.

## Diagnosis

*C. perfringens* cannot be reliably diagnosed by finding spore-forming bacteria on fecal smears (Fig. 33-1) or by detecting enterotoxin by reversed passive latex agglutination (RPLA). These diagnostic tests are of uncertain sensitivity and specificity in dogs. Currently, ELISA methodology to detect fecal enterotoxin appears to hold promise. Successful treatment with tylosin, a drug to which *C. perfringens* is almost uniformly sensitive, or amoxicillin is typically used as a basis for tentative diagnosis.

*C. difficile* is hard to culture from feces. Diarrhea produced by this bacterium has been diagnosed by using commercial laboratory kits to find *C. difficile* toxin in feces in addition to seeing a response to therapy with metronidazole. However, the toxin assay appears to have the potential for false-positive and false-negative results.

## Treatment

If *C. perfringens* colitis is suspected, the animal may be treated with antimicrobials active against the bacteria (e.g., tylosin, amoxicillin). Some animals are cured after a 1- to 3-week course of therapy. However, antibiotic treatment does not necessarily eliminate the bacteria, and many dogs need indefinite therapy. Tylosin (20 to 80 mg/kg/day, divided, twice a day) or amoxicillin (22 mg/kg q12h) seems to be effective and yet has minimal adverse effects in these animals. Some animals can eventually be maintained with once daily or every other day antibiotic therapy. Some dogs with chronic large bowel diarrhea seemingly caused by *C. perfringens* respond well to fiber-supplemented diets that may alter the colonic microenvironment. The prognosis is good, and there is no obvious public health risk, although there is anecdotal evidence of transmission between people and dogs.

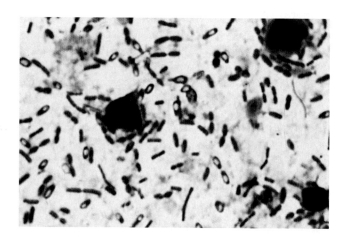

**FIG 33-1**
Photomicrograph of air-dried canine feces stained with Diff-Quick. Numerous spores are seen as clear vacuoles in darkly stained rods. (Magnification ×1000.)

If disease caused by *C. difficile* is suspected, supportive fluid and electrolyte therapy may be necessary depending on the severity of signs. Metronidazole should be effective in killing this bacterium, but one must be sure to use a high enough dose to achieve adequate metronidazole concentrations in the feces. Vancomycin is often used to treat people with this disease.

## Prognosis

The prognosis is excellent in dogs with diarrhea due to *C. perfringens* but uncertain for those cases caused by *C. difficile*.

## MISCELLANEOUS BACTERIA

### Etiology

*Yersinia enterocolitica, Aeromonas hydrophila,* and *Plesiomonas shigelloides* may cause acute or chronic enterocolitis in dogs and/or cats, as well as in people. However, these bacteria (especially the latter two) are uncommonly diagnosed in the United States. *Y. enterocolitica* is primarily found in cold environments and in pigs, which may serve as a reservoir. It is also a cause of food poisoning because of its ability to grow in cold temperatures. Enterohemorrhagic *Escherichia coli* (EHEC) may seemingly be associated with canine and feline diarrhea, although it does not appear to be especially common.

### Clinical Features

Small bowel diarrhea may be caused by any of these bacteria. Yersiniosis usually affects the colon and produces chronic large bowel diarrhea. Affected people report substantial abdominal pain.

### Diagnosis

Persistent diarrhea that cannot be diagnosed by routine means (e.g., fecal examination, mucosal biopsy), and apparently infectious diarrhea (i.e., multiple animals and/or people affected) are reasons to culture feces. Animals with persistent colitis, especially those that are in contact with pigs, may reasonably be cultured for *Y. enterocolitica*. If the clinician suspects yersiniosis, the laboratory must be told because specific enrichment and selection procedures are recommended. Although it is advantageous to tell the laboratory if *Aeromonas* or *Plesiomonas* spp. are suspected, it does not seem as critical as with *Campylobacter, Yersinia,* or *Salmonella* spp. If EHEC is suspected, it is helpful to screen *E. coli* isolates (which are expected in any fecal culture) for the ability to ferment sorbitol and then serotype the strains and/or use probes to see if the isolates can produce verotoxins (also called *Shiga-like toxins*). These toxins may also be detected in the feces.

### Treatment

Therapy is supportive. The affected animal should be isolated from other animals. People in contact with the animal and/or its environment and wastes should wear protective clothing and clean themselves with disinfectants. Although antibiotics intuitively seem indicated, their use has not shortened clinical disease caused by EHEC. Nonetheless, appropriate antibiotics as determined by culture and sensitivity are used (e.g., *Y. enterocolitica* is often sensitive to tetracyclines). The preferred length of antibiotic therapy is uncertain, but treatment should probably be continued for 1 to 3 days beyond clinical remission.

## Prognosis

The prognosis is uncertain but seems to be good if the bacteria can be identified by culture and the infection treated appropriately.

## HISTOPLASMOSIS

### Etiology

Caused by *Histoplasma capsulatum,* histoplasmosis is a mycotic infection that may affect the GI, respiratory, and/or reticuloendothelial systems, as well as the bones and eyes. Principally found in animals from the Mississippi and Ohio River valleys, it occurs in other areas as well.

### Clinical Features

Alimentary tract involvement is primarily found in dogs; diarrhea (with or without blood or mucus) and weight loss are the most common signs. The lungs, liver, spleen, lymph nodes, bone marrow, bones, and/or eyes may also be affected. Symptomatic alimentary involvement is much less common in cats; respiratory dysfunction (e.g., dyspnea, cough), fever, and/or weight loss are more common.

In GI histoplasmosis, the colon is usually the most severely affected segment. Diffuse, severe, granulomatous, ulcerative mucosal disease can produce bloody stool, intestinal protein loss, intermittent fever, and/or weight loss. Small intestinal involvement occasionally occurs. The disease may smolder for long periods of time, causing mild to moderate, nonprogressive signs. Occasionally histoplasmosis causes focal colonic granulomas or is present in grossly normal-appearing colonic mucosa.

### Diagnosis

Diagnosis requires finding the yeast cytologically (Fig. 33-2) or histologically; sometimes one technique detects it and the other does not. Dogs from endemic areas with chronic large bowel diarrhea are suspect. However, protein-losing enteropathy is common in dogs with severe histoplasmosis, and hypoalbuminemia in dogs with large bowel disease is suggestive of the disease, regardless of where the animal is from.

Rectal examination sometimes reveals thickened rectal folds, which can easily be scraped with a dull curette or syringe cap to obtain material for cytologic preparations. Evaluation of colonic biopsy specimens is usually diagnostic, but special stains may be necessary. Mesenteric lymph node samples or repeated colonic biopsy is rarely required. Fundic examination occasionally reveals active chorioretinitis. Abdominal radiographs might reveal hepatosplenomegaly, and thoracic radiographs sometimes demonstrate pulmonary

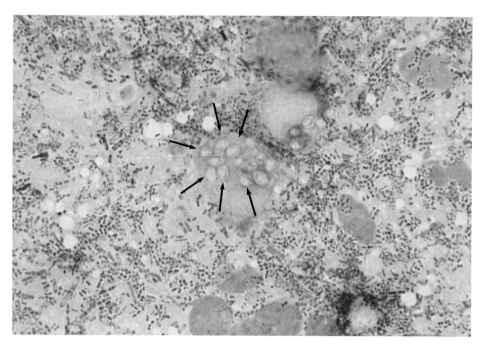

**FIG 33-2**
Cytologic preparation of a colonic mucosal scraping demonstrating *Histoplasma capsulatum*. Note the macrophage with numerous yeasts in the cytoplasm *(arrows)*. (Wright-Giemsa stain; magnification ×400.) (From Allen D, editor: *Small animal medicine*, Philadelphia, 1991, JB Lippincott.)

involvement (e.g., miliary interstitial involvement and/or hilar lymphadenopathy). Cytologic evaluation of hepatic or splenic aspirates may be diagnostic. The CBC rarely reveals yeasts in circulating white blood cells. Thrombocytopenia may occur. Cytologic examination of bone marrow or of buffy coat smears may reveal the organism. Serologic tests and fecal culture for the yeast are untrustworthy, especially in cats.

### Treatment

It is crucial to look for histoplasmosis before beginning empiric corticosteroid therapy for suspected canine colonic IBD. Corticosteroid therapy lessens host defenses and may allow a previously treatable case to rapidly progress and kill the animal. Itraconazole by itself or preceded by amphotericin B is often effective (see p. 1289). Treatment should be continued long enough (i.e., at least 4 to 6 months) to lessen chances for relapse.

### Prognosis

Many dogs can be cured if treated relatively early. Multiple organ system involvement worsens the prognosis. Involvement of the central nervous system (CNS) is also indicative of a poor prognosis.

## PROTOTHECOSIS

### Etiology

*Prototheca zopfii* is an alga that invades tissue. It appears to be acquired from the environment, and some type of deficiency in the host's immune system might be needed for the organism to produce disease.

### Clinical Features

Affecting dogs and occasionally cats, protothecosis principally involves the skin, colon, and eyes but may disseminate throughout the body. Collies may be overrepresented. Colonic involvement causes bloody stools and other signs of colitis much like histoplasmosis. Protothecosis is much less common than histoplasmosis, and the GI form primarily affects dogs.

### Diagnosis

Diagnosis requires demonstrating the organism via cytologic evaluation (Fig. 33-3) or histopathologic analysis of colonic biopsy specimens.

### Treatment

Most drugs work inconsistently. High doses of amphotericin B (administered via liposomes) might be useful.

### Prognosis

The prognosis for disseminated disease is poor because no treatment consistently works.

## ALIMENTARY TRACT PARASITES

### WHIPWORMS
#### Etiology

*Trichuris vulpis* is principally found in the eastern United States. Animals acquire the infection by ingesting ova; the adults burrow into the colonic and cecal mucosa and may cause inflammation, bleeding, and intestinal protein loss.

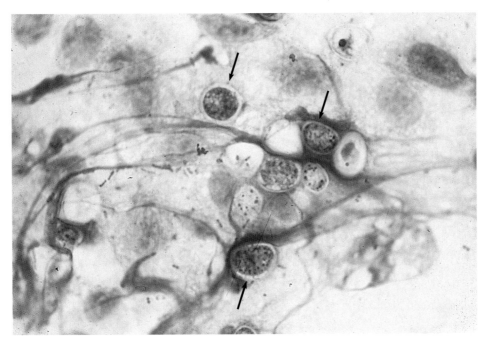

**FIG 33-3**
Cytologic preparation of a colonic mucosal scraping demonstrating *Prototheca* spp. Note the bean-shaped structures that have a granular internal structure and appear to have a halo *(arrows)*. (Wright-Giemsa stain; magnification ×1000.) (Courtesy Dr. Alice Wolf, Texas A & M University.)

## Clinical Features

Dogs and rarely cats acquire whipworms, which produce a wide spectrum of mild to severe colonic disease, including hematochezia and protein-losing enteropathy. Severe trichuriasis may cause severe hyponatremia and hyperkalemia, mimicking hypoadrenocorticism. The marked hyponatremia might be responsible for the CNS signs (e.g., seizures) sometimes attributed to whipworm infections. Whipworms generally do not affect cats as severely as dogs.

## Diagnosis

*T. vulpis* should always be sought in dogs with bloody stools or other colonic disease. Diagnosis is made through finding ova (Fig. 33-4) in the feces or seeing the adults at endoscopic evaluation. However, these ova are relatively dense and float only in properly prepared flotation solutions. Furthermore, ova are shed intermittently and sometimes can be found only if multiple fecal examinations are performed.

## Treatment

Because of the potential difficulty in diagnosing *T. vulpis,* it is reasonable to empirically treat dogs with chronic large bowel disease with fenbendazole or other appropriate drugs (see Table 30-10) before proceeding to endoscopy. If a dog is treated for whipworms, it should be treated again in 3 months to kill worms that were not in the intestinal lumen at the time of the first treatment. The ova persist in the environment for long periods.

## Prognosis

The prognosis for recovery is good.

# ROUNDWORMS

## Etiology

Roundworms are common in dogs (*Toxocara canis* and *Toxascaris leonina*) and cats (*Toxocara cati* and *Toxascaris leonina*). Dogs and cats can obtain roundworms from ingesting the ova (either directly or via paratenic hosts). *T. canis* is often obtained transplacentally from the mother; *T. cati* may use transmammary passage, and *T. leonina* can use intermediate hosts. Tissue migration of immature forms can cause hepatic fibrosis and significant pulmonary lesions. Adult roundworms live in the small intestinal lumen and migrate against the flow of ingesta. They can cause inflammatory infiltrates (e.g., eosinophils) in the wall of the intestine.

## Clinical Features

Roundworms may cause or contribute to diarrhea, stunted growth, a poor haircoat, and poor weight gain, especially in young animals. Runts with "potbellies" suggest severe roundworm infection. Sometimes roundworms gain access to the stomach, in which case they may be vomited. If parasites are numerous, they may obstruct the intestines or bile duct.

## Diagnosis

Diagnosis is easy because ova are produced in large numbers and are readily found by fecal flotation (Fig. 33-5; see also Fig.

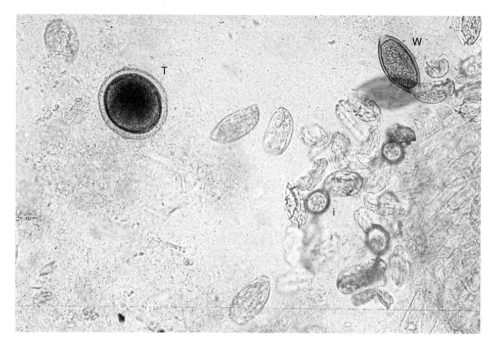

**FIG 33-4**
Photomicrograph of a fecal flotation analysis from a dog, demonstrating characteristic ova from whipworms *(W)*, *Toxocara canis (T)*, and *Isospora* spp. *(I)*. The remaining ova are those of an unusual tapeworm, *Spirometra* sp. (Magnification ×250.) (Courtesy Dr. Tom Craig, Texas A & M University.)

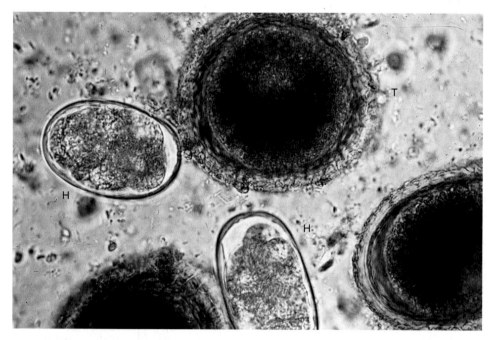

**FIG 33-5**
Photomicrograph of a fecal flotation analysis from a dog demonstrating characteristic ova from hookworms *(H)* and *Toxocara canis (T)*. (Magnification ×400.) (Courtesy Dr. Tom Craig, Texas A & M University.)

33-4). Occasionally neonates develop clinical signs of round-worm infestation but ova cannot be found in the feces. Transplacental migration results in large worm burdens, causing signs in these animals before the parasites mature and produce ova.

## Treatment

Various anthelmintics are effective (see Table 30-10), but pyrantel is especially safe for young dogs and cats, particularly those with diarrhea. Affected animals should be re-treated at 2- to 3-week intervals to kill roundworms that were initially in tissues and have migrated into the intestinal lumen since the last treatment.

High-dose fenbendazole therapy (i.e., 50 mg/kg/day from day 40 of gestation until 2 weeks postpartum) reduces the somatic roundworm burden in bitches and lessens transplacental transmission to puppies. No data exist concerning the efficacy or safety of similar treatment in the queen. Newborn puppies can be treated with fenbendazole (100 mg/kg for 3 days), which kills more than 90% of prenatal larvae. This treatment can be repeated 2 to 3 weeks later. Preweaning puppies should be treated at 2, 4, 6, and 8 weeks of age to lessen contamination of the environment because *T. canis* and *T. cati* pose a human health risk (i.e., visceral and ocular larval migrans). Preweaning kittens should be treated at 6, 8, and 10 weeks of age.

## Prognosis

The prognosis for recovery is good unless the animal is already severely stunted when treated, in which case it may never attain its anticipated body size.

## HOOKWORMS

### Etiology

*Ancylostoma* spp. and *Uncinaria* spp. are more common in dogs than in cats. Infestation is usually via ingestion of the ova or through transcolostral transmission; freshly hatched larvae may also penetrate the skin. The adults live in the small intestinal lumen, where they attach to the mucosa. Plugs of intestinal mucosa and/or blood is ingested, depending on the worm species. In severe infestations, hookworms may be found in the colon.

### Clinical Features

Dogs are more severely affected than cats. Young animals may have life-threatening blood loss or iron-deficiency anemia, melena, frank fecal blood, diarrhea, and/or failure to thrive. Older dogs rarely have disease solely from hookworms, but these worms may still contribute to disease caused by other intestinal problems.

### Diagnosis

Finding ova in the feces is diagnostic (see Fig. 33-5) and easy because hookworms are prolific egg producers. However, 5- to 10-day-old puppies may be exsanguinated by transcolostrally obtained hookworms before ova appear in the feces. Such prepatent infections rarely occur in older animals

that have received a sudden, massive exposure. Diagnosis is suggested by signalment and clinical signs in these animals. Iron deficiency anemia in a puppy or kitten free of fleas is highly suggestive of hookworm infestation.

### Treatment

Various anthelmintics are effective (see Table 30-10). Treatment should be repeated in approximately 3 weeks to kill parasites entering the intestinal lumen from the tissues. In anemic puppies and kittens, blood transfusions may be lifesaving.

High-dose fenbendazole therapy (see treatment for roundworms) in bitches reduces transcolostral transmission to puppies. Hookworms are a potential human health hazard (i.e., cutaneous larval migrans). Use of heartworm preventives containing pyrantel or milbemycin helps to minimize hookworm infestations.

### Prognosis

The prognosis is good in mature dogs and cats but guarded in severely anemic puppies and kittens. If the puppies or kittens are severely stunted in their growth, they may never attain their anticipated body size.

## TAPEWORMS

### Etiology

Several tapeworms infect dogs and cats, the most common being *Dipylidium caninum*. Tapeworms usually have an indirect life cycle; the dog or cat is infected when it eats an infected intermediate host. Fleas and lice are intermediate hosts for *D. caninum*, whereas wild animals (e.g., rabbits) are intermediate hosts for some *Taenia* spp.

### Clinical Features

Aesthetically offensive, tapeworms are rarely pathogenic in small animals, although *Mesocestoides* spp. can reproduce in the host and cause disease (e.g., abdominal effusion). The most common sign in infested dogs and cats is anal irritation associated with shed segments "crawling" on the area. Typically, the owner sees motile tapeworm segments on the feces and requests treatment. Occasionally a segment enters an anal sac and causes inflammation. Very rarely, large numbers of tapeworms cause intestinal obstruction.

### Diagnosis

*Taenia* spp. and especially *D. caninum* eggs are typically confined in segments not detected by routine fecal flotations. *Echinococcus* spp. and some *Taenia* spp. ova may be found in the feces. Tapeworms are usually diagnosed when the owner reports tapeworm segments (e.g., "rice grains") on feces or the perineal area.

### Treatment

Praziquantel and episprantel are effective against all species of tapeworms (see Table 30-10). Prevention of tapeworms involves controlling the intermediate hosts (i.e., fleas and lice for *D. caninum*). *Echinococcus* spp. are a human health hazard.

# STRONGYLOIDIASIS

## Etiology

*Strongyloides stercoralis* principally affects puppies, especially those in crowded conditions. These parasites produce motile larvae that penetrate unbroken skin or mucosa; thus the animal may be infested from its own feces even before the larvae are evacuated from the colon. In this manner, animals can quickly acquire large parasitic burdens. Most animals are infested after being exposed to fresh feces containing the motile larvae. Humane shelters and pet stores are likely sources for infestation.

## Clinical Features

Infested animals usually have mucoid or hemorrhagic diarrhea and are systemically ill (e.g., lethargy). Respiratory signs (i.e., verminous pneumonia) occur if parasites penetrate the lungs.

## Diagnosis

*S. stercoralis* is diagnosed by finding the larvae in fresh feces, either by direct fecal examination or by Baermann sedimentation. *Strongyloides* larvae must be differentiated from *Oslerus* spp. larvae. The feces must be fresh. If they are old, hookworm larvae (which resemble those of *Strongyloides* spp.) may hatch from the ova.

## Treatment

Fenbendazole (when used for 5 days instead of 3) (see Table 30-10), thiabendazole, and ivermectin are effective anthelmintics. This disease is a human health hazard because larvae penetrate unbroken skin. Immunosuppressed people are at great risk for severe disease after being infected.

## Prognosis

The prognosis is guarded in young animals with severe diarrhea and/or pneumonia.

# COCCIDIOSIS

## Etiology

*Isospora* spp. are principally found in young cats and dogs. The pet is usually infested by ingesting infective oocysts from the environment. The coccidia invade and destroy villous epithelial cells.

## Clinical Features

Coccidia may be clinically insignificant (especially in an asymptomatic, older animal), or they may be responsible for mild to severe diarrhea, sometimes with blood. A kitten or puppy may lose enough blood to require a blood transfusion, but that is rare.

## Diagnosis

Coccidiosis is diagnosed by finding oocysts on fecal flotation examination (see Fig. 33-4); however, repeated fecal examinations may be needed, and small numbers of oocysts do not ensure that the infestation is insignificant. These oocysts should not be confused with giardial cysts. If a necropsy is performed, multiple areas of the intestine should be sampled because the infection may be localized to one area. Occasionally *Eimeria* oocysts will be seen in the feces of dogs that eat deer or rabbit excrement.

## Treatment

If coccidia are believed to be causing a problem, sulfadimethoxine or trimethoprim-sulfa should be administered for 10 to 20 days (see Table 30-10). The sulfa drug does not eradicate the coccidia but inhibits it so that body defense mechanisms can reestablish control. Amprolium (50 mg PO q24h 3 to 5 days) can be used in puppies but is not approved for use in dogs; it is potentially toxic in cats. Toltrazuril (15 mg/kg q24h for 3 days) has been found to decrease oocyst shedding, at least temporarily.

## Prognosis

The prognosis for recovery is usually good unless there are underlying problems that allowed the coccidia to become pathogenic in the first place.

# CRYPTOSPORIDIA

## Etiology

Cryptosporidosis is caused by the coccidian *Cryptosporidium parvum*. Animals become infested when they ingest the sporulated oocysts. These oocysts originate from infested animals but may be carried in water. Thin-walled oocysts are produced, which can rupture in the intestine and produce autoinfection. The organism infests the brush border of small intestinal epithelial cells and causes diarrhea.

## Clinical Features

Diarrhea is the most common clinical sign in dogs and cats, although many infested cats are asymptomatic. Dogs with diarrhea are usually under 6 months of age, but a similar age predilection has not been recognized for cats.

## Diagnosis

Diagnosis requires finding the oocysts or a positive ELISA. *C. parvum* is the smallest of the coccidians and is easy to miss on fecal examination. Examination should be performed at ×1000 magnification. Use of acid-fast stains on fecal smears and fluorescent antibody techniques improves sensitivity. It is best to submit the feces to a laboratory experienced in diagnosing cryptosporidiosis. The laboratory must be warned that the feces may contain *C. parvum*, which is potentially infective for people. The ELISA is more sensitive than fecal examination.

## Treatment/Prognosis

There are no known reliable treatments. Immunocompetent people and cattle often spontaneously eliminate the infestation, but whether small animals do so is unknown. Most young dogs with diarrhea associated with cryptosporidiosis die or are euthanized. Many cats have asymptomatic infestations, and those with diarrhea have an unknown prognosis.

## GIARDIASIS

### Etiology

Giardiasis is caused by a protozoan, *Giardia* sp. Animals are infected when they ingest cysts shed from infected animals, often via water. Organisms are principally found in the small intestine, where they interfere with digestion through uncertain mechanisms. In people, *Giardia* organisms may occasionally ascend into the bile duct and cause hepatic problems.

### Clinical Features

Giardiasis is principally a problem of dogs, but cats are occasionally infected. Signs vary from mild to severe diarrhea, which may be persistent, intermittent, or self-limiting. Typically the diarrhea is "cow patty"-like, without blood or mucus; however, there is substantial variation. Some animals experience weight loss; others do not.

### Diagnosis

Giardiasis is diagnosed by finding motile trophozoites (Fig. 33-6) in fresh feces or duodenal washes, by finding cysts with fecal flotation techniques, or by finding giardial proteins in feces using an ELISA. Zinc sulfate solutions seem to be the best medium for demonstrating cysts (especially when cen-trifugal flotation is performed) because other solutions may distort them. At least three fecal examinations should be performed over the course of 7 to 10 days before discounting giardiasis. Washes of the duodenal lumen (performed endoscopically or surgically by instilling and then retrieving 5 to 10 ml of physiologic saline solution from the duodenal lumen) or cytologic evaluation of the duodenal mucosa occasionally reveal *Giardia* organisms when other techniques do not.

### Treatment

Because of the occasional difficulty in finding *Giardia* organisms (especially in animals that have had various symptomatic antidiarrheal medications), response to treatment is often the retrospective basis of diagnosis (see Table 30-10). This approach has limitations. Quinacrine is effective but no longer available. Metronidazole has few adverse effects and seems reasonably effective (approximately 85% cured after 7 days of therapy). However, clinical response to metronidazole therapy may result from the drug's antianaerobic activity and/or its effects on the immune system. Furazolidone (5 days of therapy) is probably as effective as metronidazole and comes as a suspension, making it easier to treat infected kittens. Albendazole (3 days of therapy in dogs, 5 days of therapy in cats) and fenbendazole (5 days of therapy in dogs or cats) are also effective, and recent data suggest that oral neomycin may be useful. However, none of these drugs is 100% effective, meaning that failure to respond to drug therapy does not rule out giardiasis.

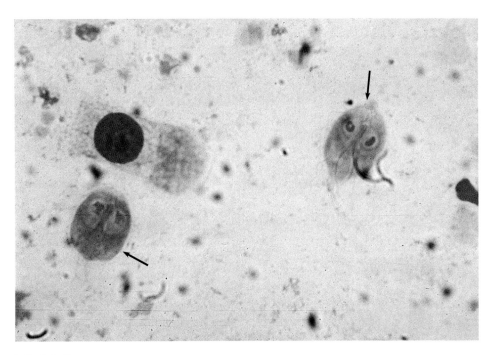

**FIG 33-6**
*Giardia* trophozoites *(arrows)* in a canine fecal smear that has been stained to enhance internal structures. (Magnification ×1000.) (Courtesy Dr. Tom Craig, Texas A & M University.)

There are several reasons why it is difficult to eliminate *Giardia* spp. First, *Giardia* organisms seemingly may become resistant to some drugs. Second, immunodeficiency (e.g., IgA deficiency) or concurrent host disease may make it difficult to eliminate the organism. Third, reinfection is easy because giardial cysts are rather resistant to environmental influences and relatively few are needed to reinfect a dog or person. Quaternary ammonium compounds and pine tars are effective disinfectants for the premises. Fourth, sometimes other protozoal agents (e.g, *Tritrichomonas*) are mistaken for *Giardia*.

## Prognosis

The prognosis for recovery is usually good, although in some cases the organisms are difficult to eradicate. It is uncertain whether people may occasionally be infected with *Giardia* organisms shed from dogs.

## TRICHOMONIASIS

### Etiology

Trichomoniasis in cats appears to be caused by *Tritrichomonas foetus/suis*. Animals are probably infected by the fecal-oral route.

### Clinical Features

Trichomoniasis typically is associated with large bowel diarrhea, which rarely contains blood or mucus. Cats are typically otherwise normal, although there may be anal irritation. The diarrhea may spontaneously resolve or may persist for long periods (e.g., months).

### Diagnosis

Diagnosis requires identifying the motile trophozoite, which necessitates timely examination of fresh feces diluted with warm saline solution. *Tritrichomonas* trophozoites are often mistakenly identified as *Giardia* trophozoites (Fig. 33-7).

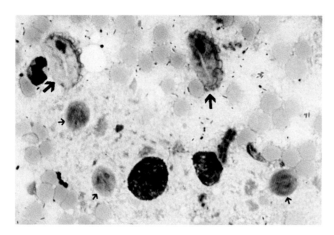

**FIG 33-7**
Comparison of *Giardia* trophozoites *(small arrows)* and *Tritrichomonas* trophozoites *(large arrows)* in a smear that has been stained to enhance internal structures. Note that the *Tritrichomonas* trophozoites are larger and have one large undulating membrane. (Magnification ×1000.) (Courtesy Dr. Tom Craig, Texas A & M University.)

### Treatment/Prognosis

There is not currently a treatment recognized to be effective in resolving feline trichomoniasis. Many cats improve somewhat while receiving various antibiotic therapies. If trichomoniasis is diagnosed, it is still important to look for other causes of diarrhea (e.g., *Clostridium perfringens*, diet, *Cryptosporidium* spp.) because treatment for one of these other causes often allows the patient to resolve the diarrhea. Most cats will eventually resolve the clinical signs of trichomoniasis, although diarrhea may recur if the patient undergoes "stressful" events (e.g., elective surgery).

## MALDIGESTIVE DISEASE

### EXOCRINE PANCREATIC INSUFFICIENCY
#### Etiology

Canine exocrine pancreatic insufficiency (EPI) is primarily caused by pancreatic acinar cell atrophy. German Shepherd Dogs seem overrepresented, suggesting a congenital or hereditary predisposition. Most animals are relatively young (e.g., 1 to 5 years of age) when clinical signs manifest. Repeated bouts of acute pancreatitis or smoldering subclinical chronic pancreatitis may destroy the pancreas and cause EPI, but this mechanism seems less common, except perhaps in Schnauzers.

#### Clinical Features

EPI is principally found in dogs and rarely in cats. Chronic small intestinal diarrhea, a ravenous appetite, and weight loss are classic findings. Steatorrhea (i.e., slate gray stools) is rarely seen, and animals occasionally have weight loss without diarrhea.

#### Diagnosis

The diarrhea is first classified as a small bowel problem (because of the weight loss and the nature of the diarrhea if present). Physical examination and routine clinical pathologic findings are not diagnostic. Once parasitic and dietary causes are eliminated, pancreatic exocrine function should be tested. The most sensitive and specific test for canine EPI is measurement of serum trypsin–like immunoreactivity (TLI) (i.e., low activity in affected dogs). If the TLI is just above the range diagnostic of EPI, it may be indicative of a patient that will develop EPI relatively soon. However, this is not consistent and the TLI should be rechecked in 4 to 12 months. Measurement of serum lipase and amylase activities is useless.

Response to pancreatic enzyme supplementation is commonly used as a diagnostic tool but has several shortcomings. First, disappearance of diarrhea associated with enzyme supplementation may be fortuitous. Many dogs have been treated with pancreatic enzyme supplements for long periods and at substantial cost because of the erroneous conclusion that resolution of the diarrhea was the result of enzyme supplementation. If pancreatic enzymes are believed to be responsible for clinical improvement, they should be withdrawn to see if the diarrhea recurs. Second, failure to respond to enzyme supplementation does not rule out EPI. Some enzyme preparations are inferior (e.g., many tablet and capsule formulations). Furthermore, dogs with EPI may have concurrent bacterial problems or be eating high-fat diets, which hinder efficacy of the enzyme supplements. Most dogs with EPI that I have diagnosed have been referred after failure to respond to empirical enzyme supplementation.

### Treatment

The animal should be fed a relatively low-fat diet (e.g., 15% of fat on a dry matter basis) with pancreatic enzymes added (see p. 563). Although some tablet formulations are effective, powder preparations are usually better. Preincubation of the enzyme with the food is not necessary. Most dogs show clinical response (i.e., resolution of diarrhea) within 1 week. If the animal does not respond well to appropriate therapy, one may need to also treat for bacterial problems (see p. 450) and/or use $H_2$-receptor antagonists (pancreatic enzymes may be inactivated in acidic environments).

### Prognosis

The prognosis is usually good, although dogs require lifelong therapy. More information on EPI can be found in Chapter 40.

## MALABSORPTIVE DISEASES

Inflammatory bowel disease (IBD) refers to *idiopathic* intestinal inflammation; therefore it is a diagnosis of exclusion. IBD can affect any portion of the canine or feline intestine. Although the cause of IBD is unknown, it is speculated to be a generic intestinal response to bacterial and/or dietary antigens. The clinical and histologic features of IBD can closely resemble those of alimentary lymphoma (see p. 457).

### CANINE LYMPHOCYTIC-PLASMACYTIC ENTERITIS

#### Clinical Features

Lymphocytic-plasmacytic enteritis (LPE) is the most commonly diagnosed canine IBD. Chronic small intestinal diarrhea is common, but some dogs have weight loss with normal stools. If the duodenum is severely affected, vomiting may be the major sign, and diarrhea can be either mild or absent. Protein-losing enteropathy occurs in dogs with the more severe forms.

#### Diagnosis

No physical examination or historic or clinical pathologic findings are diagnostic of canine LPE, although severe LPE may cause hypoalbuminemia with or without hypoglobulinemia. Endoscopic findings may be suggestive of infiltrative disease. Elimination of known causes plus histologic examination of intestinal mucosa is required for diagnosis. Mucosal cytologic evaluation is often unreliable because lymphocytes and plasma cells are normally present in intestinal mucosa. The pathologist must be experienced in this area because diagnosis of LPE is subjective and biopsy samples are frequently overinterpreted. Depending on the pathologist, "mild" LPE may refer to normal tissue. A description of "moderate" or "severe" LPE may be reason to have more confidence in the diagnosis, al-

though there is substantial inconsistency among pathologists. It can be difficult to distinguish a well-differentiated lymphocytic lymphoma from severe LPE, even with full-thickness samples. If the biopsy specimens are of marginal quality (either from the standpoint of size or artifacts present), it is easy to mistakenly diagnose LPE instead of lymphoma if the latter is causing a secondary tissue reaction. However, some animals with intense dietary reactions have biopsy findings that resemble lymphoma.

#### Treatment

Elimination diets and antibiotics should usually be included in the treatment regimen for LPE in case the "IBD" is actually dietary intolerance or antibiotic-responsive enteropathy (ARE), respectively (see p. 450). This is especially true for dogs with "mild" IBD. Homemade hypoallergenic diets are optimal, although the partially hydrolyzed diets and commercial hypoallergenic diets are often helpful. Elemental diets can be invaluable in severely emaciated or severely hypoproteinemic patients with severe inflammation, as a way to feed the patient and the intestinal mucosa without causing more mucosal irritation. Other therapy depends on the severity of the LPE. Moderate to severe canine LPE (i.e., more marked inflammatory infiltrates, especially if associated with hypoalbuminemia) usually requires dietary change, antibiotics (e.g., tetracycline), high-dose corticosteroid therapy (e.g., prednisolone, 2.2 mg/kg/day), metronidazole, and sometimes azathioprine. When severe LPE is being treated, azathioprine administration should be initiated at the same time as the other drugs and then a decision whether to continue it should be based on the animal's response over the first 2 to 3 weeks of treatment (i.e., before azathioprine causes a clinical effect). (See Chapter 79 for more information on these therapeutic modalities.) In severe cases, cyclophosphamide or cyclosporine might be considered. Failure of a dog to respond to "appropriate" therapy can be the result of inadequate therapy, owner noncompliance, or misdiagnosis (i.e., diagnosing LPE when the problem is lymphoma).

If the animal clinically responds to the above therapy, it should be continued without change for 2 to 4 more weeks to ensure that the clinical improvement is the result of the therapy and not a nonrelated, transient improvement. Once the clinician is convinced that the prescribed therapy is effective, the animal should be slowly weaned from the drugs, starting with those that have the greatest potential for adverse effects. Attempts should be made to maintain the pet on every-other-day corticosteroid and azathioprine therapy. If that regimen is successful, then the lowest effective dose of each should be slowly determined. Only one change should be made at a time, and the dose should not be decreased more frequently than once every 2 to 3 weeks, if possible. Dietary and antibiotic therapy are usually the last to be altered.

#### Prognosis

The prognosis for dogs with LPE seemingly depends on the severity of the infiltrate, the presence of hypoalbuminemia, the animal's body condition, and the need for immunosuppressive drug therapy. Most animals will at least need to be on a special diet for the rest of their lives. Many with moderate to severe disease will need prolonged medical therapy, which should be tapered cautiously. Iatrogenic Cushing's syndrome should be avoided. Severely affected animals may initially benefit from enteral or parenteral nutritional therapy. Although the relationship is unclear, LPE has been suggested to be a potentially prelymphomatous lesion in some dogs (see Immunoproliferative Enteropathy in Basenjis); however, this is very uncertain. If a dog with a prior diagnosis of LPE is later diagnosed as having lymphoma, it may be just as likely that either the initial diagnosis of IBD was wrong (i.e., the patient had lymphoma) or that the lymphoma developed independently of the IBD.

## CANINE LYMPHOCYTIC-PLASMACYTIC COLITIS

### Clinical Features

Lymphocytic-plasmacytic colitis (LPC) typically causes large bowel diarrhea (i.e., soft stools with or without blood or mucus; no appreciable weight loss). In general, these dogs are fundamentally healthy except for soft stools.

### Diagnosis

Biopsy is required for diagnosis. The pathologist must be experienced because it is easy to overinterpret tissues and diagnose LPC when other causes (e.g., *Clostridium* colitis, dietary intolerance, dietary fiber insufficiency) are responsible. In my practice, symptomatic canine LPC is rare, although many animals have been initially diagnosed as having it before referral.

### Treatment

A surprisingly large number of dogs initially diagnosed with LPC respond to hypoallergenic diets, fiber-supplemented diets, and/or tylosin. Sulfasalazine (Azulfidine), mesalamine, or olsalazine may be used in dogs with moderate to severe LPC. Corticosteroids and/or metronidazole may be effective by themselves and/or allow lower does of sulfasalazine to be successful.

### Prognosis

The prognosis for dogs with LPC tends to be better than for those with LPE because weight loss rarely occurs.

## FELINE LYMPHOCYTIC-PLASMACYTIC ENTERITIS

### Clinical Features

Feline LPE principally causes vomiting, but weight loss, diarrhea, and/or anorexia may also occur. Diarrhea and protein-losing enteropathy are less common than in dogs with LPE.

### Diagnosis

Biopsy and elimination of other known causes of the clinical signs are required for diagnosis.

### Treatment

Highly digestible elimination diets may be curative if the "IBD" is actually food intolerance, and therapeutic diets should always be used if the cat will eat them. High doses of corticosteroids are typically also administered because of their beneficial effects and the cat's resistance to iatrogenic hyperadrenocorticism. Low-dose metronidazole (10 to 15 mg/kg PO q12h), either alone or in combination with corticosteroids and diet, may also be effective. Chlorambucil is reserved for cats with biopsy-proven, severe LPE that does not respond to other therapy (see Chapter 79) or for cats with well-differentiated lymphoma. Enteral or parenteral nutritional supplementation may be useful in emaciated cats (see Chapter 30). There is anecdotal evidence that parenteral administration of cobalamin to cats with severely decreased serum concentrations may aid or be necessary for remission of diarrhea. Budesonide is a locally acting steroid that has been used in some patients with difficult-to-control IBD.

If the cat responds to this therapy (and most do), the elimination diet should be continued while the medications are gradually tapered one at a time.

### Prognosis

Because cats tolerate corticosteroids better than dogs, the prognosis is usually good. If the animal is emaciated, the prognosis is guarded. As for dogs, it is not at all clear that feline LPE is a premalignant lesion.

## FELINE LYMPHOCYTIC-PLASMACYTIC COLITIS

In my practice, LPC is much more common in cats than in dogs. Hematochezia is the most common clinical sign, and diarrhea is the second most common sign. LPC may occur by itself or concurrently with LPE. High-fiber and hypoallergenic diets are often beneficial; in fact, most "intractable" feline LPC cases seen in my practice are ultimately determined to be dietary related. Most cats with LPC respond well to prednisolone and/or metronidazole, and sulfasalazine is rarely needed. The prognosis is usually good.

## CANINE EOSINOPHILIC GASTROENTEROCOLITIS

### Etiology

Canine eosinophilic gastroenterocolitis (EGE) is usually an allergic reaction to dietary substances (e.g., beef, milk) and as such is not IBD. However, the clinical signs do not always respond to dietary change and may represent true IBD in some dogs. It is less common than LPE or LPC in this species.

### Clinical Features

Small and/or large intestinal diarrhea and weight loss are common. Vomiting may occur in dogs with gastric or duodenal involvement. German Shepherd Dogs seem to be overrepresented. Some dogs also have concurrent eosinophilic respiratory tract disease, and cutaneous dietary allergies may also be seen.

### Diagnosis

Biopsy is required for diagnosis because there are no reliable historical, physical examination, or clinical pathologic findings in this disorder. Although peripheral eosinophilia is consistent with EGE, it is not always present. Cytologic evaluation of mucosal impression smears from intestinal biopsy specimens may reveal numerous eosinophils (i.e., 1 to 3/high-power field).

## Treatment

A strict hypoallergenic diet (e.g., fish and potato, turkey and potato) often causes resolution of the signs. Partially hydrolyzed diets may also be helpful, but they are not a panacea. It is important to always determine what the dog was fed previously. If signs do not resolve with dietary therapy, the addition of corticosteroid therapy is usually curative. Animals usually respond better to elimination diets than to corticosteroids. If corticosteroids are needed, they should be slowly withdrawn after clinical signs resolve to determine if they are still needed. Sometimes an animal initially responds to dietary management but relapses while still eating this diet because it becomes allergic to one of the ingredients. This situation necessitates administration of another elimination diet. In some animals that are very prone to developing such intolerances, switching back and forth from one elimination diet to another at 2-week intervals helps to prevent this relapse from happening. (See Chapter 30 for more information on these therapies.)

## Prognosis

The prognosis is usually good, although some dogs are sensitive to many foods and are difficult to maintain in remission.

## FELINE EOSINOPHILIC ENTERITIS/ HYPEREOSINOPHILIC SYNDROME

### Etiology

Some cats have eosinophilic enteritis as part of a hypereosinophilic syndrome (HES). The cause of feline HES is unknown, but immune-mediated and neoplastic mechanisms may be responsible. Less severely affected cats without HES seem to have a condition similar to canine EGE.

### Clinical Features

Small intestinal diarrhea, vomiting, and/or weight loss are the principal signs in cats with HES.

### Diagnosis

Intestinal biopsy is necessary for diagnosis. Mucosal cytologic analysis sometimes establishes a presumptive diagnosis, and peripheral eosinophilia, although inconsistent, may be suggestive of this disorder. Severe feline eosinophilic enteritis, which is rare, is usually caused by HES. Intestinal eosinophilic infiltrates are the most common finding in HES, although splenic, hepatic, lymph node, and bone marrow infiltrates and peripheral eosinophilia are common.

### Treatment

High-dose corticosteroid therapy (i.e., prednisolone, 4.4 to 6.6 mg/kg/day) has been used with little success in cats with HES. Cats with eosinophilic enteritis not caused by HES often respond favorably to elimination diets plus corticosteroid therapy.

### Prognosis

The prognosis is guarded to poor for cats with HES. Cats with the less severe syndrome may have a fair prognosis.

## GRANULOMATOUS ENTERITIS/GASTRITIS

Canine granulomatous enteritis/gastritis is uncommon, and it can be diagnosed only histopathologically. Clinical signs are similar to those of other forms of IBD. Although compared to Crohn's disease in people, the two are dissimilar. If the disease is localized, surgical resection should be considered. If it is diffuse, corticosteroids, metronidazole, antibiotics, azathioprine, and dietary therapy should be considered. Too few cases have been described and treated to allow generalizations. The prognosis is poor.

Feline granulomatous enteritis is a rare IBD that causes weight loss, protein-losing enteropathy, and perhaps diarrhea; it also requires histopathologic confirmation. Affected cats seem to respond to high-dose corticosteroid therapy, but attempts to reduce the dose of glucocorticoids may cause recurrence of clinical signs. The prognosis is guarded.

## IMMUNOPROLIFERATIVE ENTEROPATHY IN BASENJIS

### Etiology

Immunoproliferative enteropathy in Basenjis principally involves the small intestine. It is an intense lymphocytic-plasmacytic small intestinal infiltrate often associated with villous clubbing, mild lacteal dilation, gastric rugal hypertrophy, lymphocytic gastritis, and/or gastric mucosal atrophy. It probably has a genetic basis or predisposition, and intestinal bacteria may play an important role.

### Clinical Features

The disease tends to be a severe form of LPE that waxes and wanes, particularly as the animal is stressed (e.g., traveling, disease). Weight loss, small intestinal diarrhea, vomiting, and/or anorexia are commonly seen. Most affected Basenjis start showing clinical signs by 3 to 4 years of age.

### Diagnosis

Marked hypoalbuminemia and hyperglobulinemia are common, especially in advanced cases. The early stages of the disease resemble many other intestinal disorders. In advanced cases the clinical signs are so suggestive that a presumptive diagnosis is often made without biopsy. However, because other diseases (e.g., lymphoma, histoplasmosis) may mimic immunoproliferative enteropathy, alimentary tract biopsy is recommended before aggressive immunosuppressive therapy is begun.

### Treatment

Therapy may include highly digestible, elimination, or elemental diets, antibiotics for ARE (see Antibiotic Responsive

Enteropathy), high-dose corticosteroids, metronidazole, and azathioprine. Response to therapy is variable, and affected dogs that respond are at risk for relapse, especially if stressed.

Although a genetic basis is suspected, not enough is known to be able to confidently recommend a breeding program. Performing biopsy of the intestines of asymptomatic dogs to identify animals in which the disease will develop is dubious because clinically normal Basenjis may have lesions similar to those of dogs with diarrhea and weight loss, although the changes tend to be milder.

### Prognosis

Many affected animals die 2 to 3 years after diagnosis. The prognosis is poor for recovery, but some dogs can be maintained for prolonged periods of time with careful monitoring and care. In a few dogs, lymphoma later develops.

## ENTEROPATHY IN SHARPEIS

### Etiology

Chinese Sharpeis have a poorly characterized enteropathy that may be unique to them or may be a severe form of IBD. Sharpeis and German Shepherd Dogs often have serum IgA deficiency (which may be associated with ARE), and both breeds are recognized for having many GI problems.

### Clinical Features

Diarrhea and/or weight loss (i.e., small intestinal dysfunction) are the main clinical signs.

### Diagnosis

Small intestinal biopsy is necessary for diagnosis. Eosinophilic and lymphocytic-plasmacytic intestinal infiltrates are typically found. Serum cobalamin and folate concentrations may help to identify ARE (see Antibiotic Responsive Enteropathy).

### Treatment

The animal is treated for IBD (i.e., elimination diets and immunosuppressive drugs) and ARE.

### Prognosis

Affected Sharpeis have a guarded prognosis.

## ANTIBIOTIC RESPONSIVE ENTEROPATHY

### Etiology

Antibiotic responsive enteropathy (ARE) is a syndrome in which the duodenum and/or jejunum are contaminated with excessive numbers of bacteria (i.e., usually $>10^5$ colony forming units/ml) and the host has an abnormal response to these bacteria. The host response is important, as seen by the fact that some dogs have comparable numbers of bacteria in their small intestine (i.e., $\geq 10^7$ to $10^8$/ml of fasting fluid) without clinical signs. Likewise, normal cats may have similarly high numbers of bacteria in their proximal small intestine. The bacteria may be present because of (1) an anatomic defect allowing retention of food (e.g., a partial stricture or an area of

hypomotility), (2) other diseases (e.g., intestinal mucosal disease), (3) impaired host defenses (i.e., hypochlorhydria, IgA deficiency, $H_2$-receptor antagonist therapy decreasing gastric acidity), or (4) no identifiable reason. Bacteria causing ARE are usually present in mixed culture, and they probably gain access to the alimentary tract by being swallowed (i.e., originating from the oral cavity or in the food). Therefore any species of bacteria may be present, but *Escherichia coli,* enterococci, and anaerobes such as *Clostridium* spp. seem to be especially common in symptomatic dogs. Enterocytes are damaged by deconjugation of bile acids, fatty acid hydroxylation, and generation of alcohols. Anaerobic bacteria might cause worse problems than aerobic bacteria because of the enzymes they produce.

### Clinical Features

ARE can be found in any dog. Clinical signs are principally diarrhea and/or weight loss, although vomiting may also occur.

### Diagnosis

Most of the diagnostic tests for ARE have uncertain sensitivity. Multiple, quantitative duodenal fluid cultures are the "gold standard," but these cultures are difficult to obtain in most private practices. Breath hydrogen analysis is easier, but it is limited to institutes with proper equipment and can be unreliable. Serum cobalamin and folate concentrations seem reasonable as screening tools, but although specific, are not as sensitive as desired. Duodenal mucosal cytologic evaluation occasionally detects bacteria; however, this test has poor sensitivity. Finally, bacteria are rarely found on histopathologic sections of affected intestines. Because of the difficulty in diagnosing ARE, many clinicians treat and observe for response.

### Treatment

Because of the difficulty in diagnosing ARE, therapy is reasonable whenever this disorder is suspected. Therapy consists of antibiotics plus removing potential causes (e.g., blind or stagnant loops of intestine). Because mixed bacterial populations are expected, broad-spectrum antibiotics effective against aerobic and anaerobic bacteria are recommended. Tetracycline (22 mg/kg q12h), tylosin, and amoxicillin (22 mg/kg q12h) are usually effective. The dose of tylosin for ARE has not been established by critical studies, but 10 to 80 mg/kg twice daily in the food has seemingly been effective.

Occasionally a pure culture of a specific bacteria will be found in the duodenum, such that a specific antibiotic is required. However, such cases appear to be rare. The minimum treatment time for animals with ARE is 2 to 4 weeks. Because there may be an underlying cause that cannot be corrected, some animals need long-term to indefinite antibiotic therapy.

### Prognosis

The prognosis is usually good for control of ARE, but the clinician must be concerned with possible underlying causes.

# PROTEIN-LOSING ENTEROPATHY

## CAUSES OF PROTEIN-LOSING ENTEROPATHY

Although protein-losing enteropathy (PLE) is usually discussed with intestinal lymphangiectasia, any disease that produces alimentary inflammation, infiltration, congestion, or bleeding can produce PLE or gastropathy (see Table 28-12). IBD and alimentary tract lymphoma are particularly common causes in adult dogs, whereas hookworms and chronic intussusception are common causes in very young dogs. When IBD is responsible, it is usually a severe form of LPE, although EGE or granulomatous disease may be responsible. Immunoproliferative enteritis of Basenjis, gastrointestinal ulceration/erosion, and bleeding tumors can also produce PLE. Cats infrequently have PLE, but when it occurs, it is usually caused by LPE or lymphoma. Therapy should be directed at managing the underlying cause.

## INTESTINAL LYMPHANGIECTASIA

### Etiology

Intestinal lymphangiectasia (IL) is a disorder of the intestinal lymphatic system of dogs. Lymphatic obstruction causes dilation and rupture of intestinal lacteals with subsequent leakage of lymphatic contents (i.e., protein, lymphocytes, and chylomicrons) into the intestinal submucosa, lamina propria, and lumen. Although these proteins may be digested and resorbed, excessive loss exceeds the intestine's ability to resorb them, thus resulting in hypoproteinemia. Leakage of lymphatic fat into the intestinal wall may cause granuloma formation, which exacerbates lymphatic obstruction. Not reported in cats, there are many potential causes in dogs (e.g., lymphatic obstruction, pericarditis, infiltrative mesenteric lymph node disease, infiltrative intestinal mucosal disease, congenital malformations). However, most cases of IL are idiopathic.

### Clinical Features

Breed predilections for IL are not documented, but Yorkshire Terriers, Soft-Coated Wheaten Terriers, and Lundehunds appear to be at higher risk than other breeds. Wheaten Terriers seemingly also have an unusually high incidence of protein-losing nephropathy. The first sign of disease caused by IL may be small intestinal diarrhea or transudative ascites. Diarrhea is inconsistent and may occur late in the course of the disease, if at all. Intestinal lipogranulomas (i.e., white nodules in the intestinal serosa) are sometimes found at surgery, but it is uncertain whether they are secondary to fat leaking out of dilated lymphatic vessels or represent the cause of the IL.

### Diagnosis

Clinical pathologic evaluation is not diagnostic, but hypoalbuminemia and hypocholesterolemia are expected. Although panhypoproteinemia is classically attributed to PLE, animals that were initially hyperglobulinemic may lose most of their serum proteins and still have normal serum globulin concentrations. Lymphopenia is common but inconsistent. Diagnosis requires histologic evaluation of intestinal mucosa; cytologic analysis is rarely helpful. Feeding the animal fat the night before the biopsy seems to make lesions more obvious, and classic endoscopic lesions may be seen in duodenal mucosa. Endoscopic biopsies are often diagnostic but surgical biopsies are sometimes required. If full-thickness surgical biopsies are performed, serosal patch grafting and nonabsorbable suture material decrease the risk of dehiscence and peritonitis. IL may be localized to one area of the intestines (e.g., the ileum) and may be missed during surgery or endoscopy.

### Treatment

The underlying cause of IL is rarely determined, necessitating reliance on symptomatic therapy. An ultra-low-fat diet restricted in long-chain fatty acids helps to prevent further intestinal lacteal engorgement and subsequent protein loss. Prednisolone (1.1 mg/kg/day) sometimes lessens inflammation around the lipogranulomas and improves lymphatic flow.

Monitoring serum albumin concentration may be the best way of assessing response to therapy. If the animal improves with dietary therapy, it should probably be fed that diet indefinitely. If prednisolone is also needed, it is reasonable to gradually decrease the dose after clinical control is attained and to eventually try to maintain the dog on dietary therapy alone.

### Prognosis

The prognosis is variable, but most dogs respond well to ultra-low-fat diets, although some require prednisolone in addition to the diet. Relatively few dogs die despite dietary and prednisolone therapy.

## PROTEIN-LOSING ENTEROPATHY IN SOFT-COATED WHEATEN TERRIERS

### Etiology

Soft-Coated Wheaten Terriers (SCWTs) have a predisposition to PLE and protein-losing nephropathy. The cause is uncertain, although food hypersensitivity has been reported to be present in some affected dogs.

### Clinical Features

Individual dogs may have PLE or protein-losing nephropathy or both. Typical clinical signs may include vomiting, diarrhea, weight loss, and ascites. Affected dogs are often middle aged when diagnosed.

### Diagnosis

Panhypoproteinemia and hypocholesterolemia are common, as with any PLE. Histopathology of intestinal mucosa may reveal lymphangiectasia, lymphangitis, or supposedly IBD.

### Treatment/Prognosis

Treatment is typically as for lymphangiectasia and/or IBD. The prognosis appears guarded to poor for clinically ill animals, with most dying within a year of diagnosis.

# FUNCTIONAL INTESTINAL DISEASE

## IRRITABLE BOWEL SYNDROME

### Etiology

Irritable bowel syndrome (IBS) is a disease of people that is characterized by diarrhea, constipation, and/or cramping (usually of the large intestines) in which an organic lesion cannot be identified. It is an idiopathic large bowel disease in which all known causes of diarrhea have been eliminated and a "functional" disorder is presumed. Although this syndrome has not been clearly defined in veterinary medicine, many dogs with chronic large bowel diarrhea seem to have a comparable syndrome (i.e., parasites, diet, bacteria, and mucosal inflammation have seemingly been eliminated). Although it is speculative, there are probably various causes of this syndrome in dogs.

### Clinical Features

Chronic large bowel diarrhea is the principal sign. Fecal mucus is common, blood in the feces is infrequent, and weight loss is very rare. Some dogs with IBS are small breeds that are heavily imprinted on a single family member. Clinical signs may develop following separation of the dog from the person. Other dogs with IBS are nervous and high-strung (e.g., police or guard dogs, especially German Shepherd Dogs). Some dogs have no apparent initiating cause.

### Diagnosis

Diagnosis consists of eliminating known causes by physical examination, clinical pathologic data, fecal analysis, colonoscopy/biopsy, and appropriately performed therapeutic trials.

### Treatment

Treatment with fiber-supplemented diets (i.e., ≥7% to 9% fiber on a dry matter basis) is often helpful (see p. 390). Many animals must receive fiber chronically to prevent relapse. Anticholinergics occasionally are useful (e.g., propantheline, 0.25 mg/kg; or dicyclomine, 0.15 mg/kg up to q8h, as needed).

### Prognosis

The prognosis is good; in most animals the signs are controlled by diet or medical management.

# INTESTINAL OBSTRUCTION

## SIMPLE INTESTINAL OBSTRUCTION

### Etiology

Simple intestinal obstruction (i.e., the intestinal lumen is obstructed but without peritoneal leakage, severe venous occlusion, or bowel devitalization) is usually caused by foreign objects. Infiltrative disease and intussusception may also be responsible.

### Clinical Features

Simple intestinal obstructions usually cause vomiting with or without anorexia, depression, or diarrhea. Abdominal pain is uncommon. The more orad the obstruction is, the more frequent and severe the vomiting tends to be. If the intestine becomes devitalized and septic peritonitis results, the obstruction becomes complicated and the animal may be presented in a moribund state or in septic shock.

### Diagnosis

Abdominal palpation, plain abdominal radiographs, or ultrasonographic imaging can be diagnostic if they reveal a foreign object, mass, or obviously obstructive ileus (see Fig. 29-5, *A*). Masses or dilated intestinal loops may be found with either technique. Abdominal ultrasonography tends to be the most sensitive technique (unless the intestines are filled with gas) and can reveal dilated or thickened intestinal loops that are not obvious on radiographs and palpation (e.g., poor serosal contrast caused by abdominal fluid or lack of abdominal fat). If it is difficult to distinguish the obstruction from physiologic ileus, abdominal contrast radiographs may be considered; barium sulfate is better than hypertonic iodine contrast agents.

Finding a foreign object is usually sufficient to establish a diagnosis. If an abdominal mass or an obvious obstructive ileus is found, a presumptive diagnosis of obstruction is made, and ultrasonography or exploratory surgery should be planned. Aspirate cytologic evaluation of masses may be used to diagnose some diseases (e.g., lymphoma) before surgery.

### Treatment

Once intestinal obstruction is diagnosed, the clinician should perform routine preanesthetic laboratory tests (serum electrolyte and acid-base abnormalities are common in vomiting animals), stabilize the animal, and promptly proceed to surgery. Vomiting of gastric origin classically produces a hypokalemic, hypochloremic metabolic alkalosis and paradoxical aciduria, whereas vomiting caused by intestinal obstruction may produce metabolic acidosis and varying degrees of hypokalemia. However, these changes cannot be accurately predicted even when the cause of the vomiting is known, making serum electrolyte and acid-base determinations important.

### Prognosis

If septic peritonitis is absent and massive intestinal resection is not necessary, the prognosis is usually good.

## INCARCERATED INTESTINAL OBSTRUCTION

### Etiology

Incarcerated intestinal obstruction refers to a loop of intestine trapped or "strangulated" as it passes through a hernia (e.g., abdominal wall, mesenteric) or similar rent. The entrapped intestinal loop quickly dilates, accumulating fluid in which bacteria flourish and release endotoxins. Septic shock occurs rapidly. This is a true surgical emergency, and animals deteriorate quickly if the entrapped loop is not removed.

## Clinical Features

Dogs and cats with incarcerated intestinal obstruction typically have acute vomiting, abdominal pain, and progressive depression. Palpation of the entrapped loop often causes severe pain and occasionally vomiting. On physical examination, "muddy" mucous membranes and tachycardia may be noted, suggesting endotoxic shock.

## Diagnosis

A presumptive diagnosis is made by finding a distended, painful intestinal loop, especially if the loop is contained within a hernia. Radiographically, a markedly dilated segment of intestine is detected (Fig. 33-8) that is sometimes obviously outside the peritoneal cavity. Otherwise, an obviously strangulated loop of intestine will be found at exploratory surgery.

## Treatment

Immediate surgery plus aggressive therapy for endotoxic shock (i.e., fluids, antibiotics, and possibly nonsteroidal antiinflammatory drugs [NSAIDs] as needed) is indicated. Devitalized bowel should be resected, with care taken to avoid spillage of septic contents into the abdomen.

## Prognosis

The prognosis is guarded. Rapid recognition and prompt surgery are needed to avoid mortality.

# MESENTERIC TORSION/VOLVULUS

## Etiology

In mesenteric torsion/volvulus, the intestines twist about the root of the mesentery, causing severe vascular compromise. Much of the intestine is typically devitalized by the time surgery is performed.

## Clinical Features

This uncommon cause of intestinal obstruction principally occurs in large dogs (especially German Shepherd Dogs). Mesenteric torsion is denoted by an acute onset of severe nausea, retching, vomiting, abdominal pain, and depression. Bloody diarrhea may or may not occur. Abdominal distention is not as evident as in animals with gastric dilation/volvulus (GDV).

## Diagnosis

Abdominal radiographs are often diagnostic and typically show widespread, uniform ileus (see Fig. 29-6).

## Treatment

Immediate surgery is necessary. The intestines must be properly repositioned, and devitalized bowel must be resected.

## Prognosis

The prognosis is extremely poor; most animals die despite heroic efforts. Animals that live may develop short bowel syndrome if massive intestinal resection was necessary.

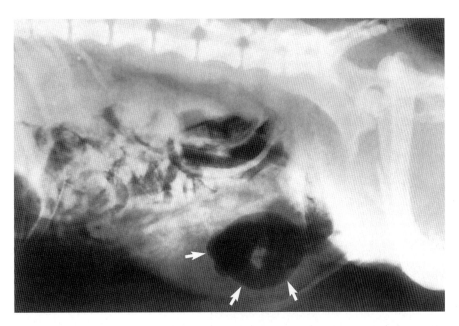

**FIG 33-8**
Lateral abdominal radiograph of a dog with a ruptured prepubic tendon and incarcerated intestinal obstruction. Note the dilated section of intestine in the area of the hernia *(arrows)*. (From Allen D, editor: *Small animal medicine,* Philadelphia, 1991, JB Lippincott.)

# LINEAR FOREIGN OBJECTS

## Etiology

Numerous objects can assume a linear configuration in the alimentary tract (e.g., string, thread, nylon stockings, cloth). The foreign object lodges or "fixes" at one point (e.g., the base of the tongue, pylorus) while the rest trails off into the intestines. The small intestine seeks to propel the object aborally via peristaltic waves and in this manner gathers around it and becomes pleated. As the intestines continue trying to propel it aborally, the linear object cuts or "saws" into the intestines, often perforating them at multiple sites on the antimesenteric border. Fatal peritonitis can result.

## Clinical Features

Linear foreign objects appear to be more frequent in cats than in dogs. Vomiting food, bile, and/or phlegm is common, but some animals are anorectic or depressed. A few (especially dogs with chronic linear foreign bodies) can be relatively asymptomatic for days to weeks while the foreign body continues to embed itself in the intestines.

## Diagnosis

The history may be suggestive of a linear foreign body (e.g., the cat was playing with cloth or string). Bunched, painful intestines are occasionally detected by abdominal palpation. The object is sometimes seen lodged at the base of the tongue; however, failure to find a foreign object at the base of the tongue does not eliminate linear foreign body as a diagnosis. Even when such objects lodge under the tongue, they can be very difficult to find despite a careful, thorough oral examination; some become embedded in the frenulum. If necessary, chemical restraint (e.g., ketamine, 2.2 mg/kg IV) should be used to allow adequate oral examination.

Foreign objects lodged at the pylorus and trailing off into the duodenum must be diagnosed by imaging or endoscopy. The objects themselves are infrequently seen radiographically and only rarely produce dilated intestinal loops suggesting anatomic ileus; pleating of the intestines around the object prevents the intestines from dilating. Plain radiographs may reveal small gas bubbles in the intestines, especially in the region of the duodenum, and obvious intestinal pleating may occasionally be seen (Fig. 33-9). If barium contrast radio-

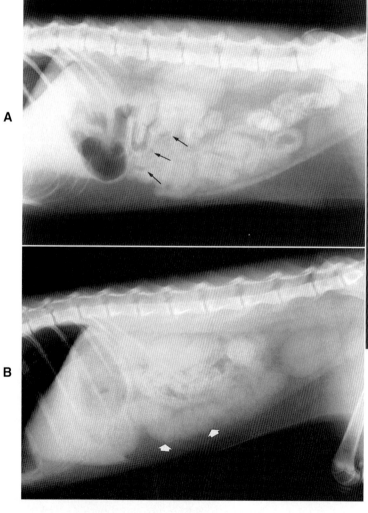

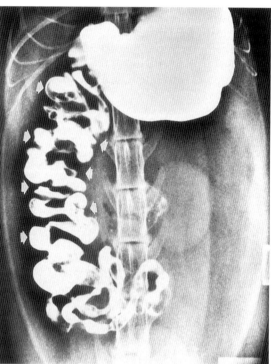

**FIG 33-9**

**A,** Plain abdominal radiograph of a cat with a linear foreign body lodged at the pylorus. Note the small gas bubbles in the mass of intestines *(arrows)*. **B,** Plain abdominal radiograph of a cat with a linear foreign body. Note the obviously pleated small bowel *(arrows)*. **C,** Contrast radiograph of a cat with a linear foreign body. Note the pleated, bunched pattern of intestines *(arrows)*. (**A** from Allen D, editor: *Small animal medicine,* Philadelphia, 1991, JB Lippincott.)

graphs are performed, they typically reveal a pleated or bunched intestinal pattern, which is diagnostic of linear foreign body. Finally, these objects are sometimes seen endoscopically lodged at the pylorus.

### Treatment

If the animal is otherwise healthy, if the linear foreign object has been present for only 1 or 2 days, and if it is fixed under the tongue, the object may be cut loose to see if it will now pass through the intestines without further problem. Surgery is indicated if the animal does not feel better 12 to 24 hours after the object is cut free from its point of fixation.

If there is doubt about how long the object has been present, or if it is fixed at the pylorus, surgery is a safer therapeutic approach. Endoscopic removal occasionally succeeds, but the clinician must be careful because it is easy to rupture devitalized intestine and cause peritonitis. If one can pass the tip of the endoscope to near the aboral end of the object and pull it out by grabbing the aboral end, surgery may sometimes be avoided. Abdominal surgery is often needed to remove linear foreign objects.

### Prognosis

The prognosis is usually good if severe septic peritonitis is absent and massive intestinal resection is unnecessary. If a linear foreign object has been present a long time, it may embed itself in the intestinal mucosa, making intestinal resection necessary. When massive intestinal resection is necessary, short bowel syndrome can result, which has a guarded to poor prognosis.

## INTUSSUSCEPTION

Intussusception is a telescoping of one intestinal segment (the intussusceptum) into an adjacent segment (the intussuscipiens). It may occur anywhere in the alimentary tract, but ileocolic intussusceptions (i.e., the ileum entering the colon) seem more common.

### ILEOCOLIC INTUSSUSCEPTION

#### Etiology

Ileocolic intussusceptions seem to be associated with active enteritis (especially in young animals), which ostensibly disrupts normal motility and promotes the smaller ileum to intussuscept into the larger colon. However, ileocolic intussusception may occur in animals with acute renal failure, leptospirosis, prior intestinal surgery, and other problems.

#### Clinical Features

Acute ileocolic intussusception causes obstruction of the intestinal lumen and congestion of the intussusceptum's mucosa. Scant bloody diarrhea, vomiting, abdominal pain, and a palpable abdominal mass are common. Chronic ileocolic intussusceptions typically produce less vomiting, abdominal pain, and hematochezia. These animals often have intractable diarrhea and are typically hypoalbuminemic as a result of protein loss from the congested mucosa. PLE in a young dog without hookworms or a puppy that seems to be having an unexpectedly hard time recovering from parvoviral enteritis should prompt suspicion of chronic intussusception.

### Diagnosis

Palpation of an elongated, obviously thickened intestinal loop establishes a presumptive diagnosis; however, some infiltrative diseases produce similar findings. Ileocolic intussusceptions that are short and do not extend far into the descending colon may be especially difficult to palpate because they are under the rib cage. Occasional intussusceptions "slide" in and out of the colon and can be missed during abdominal palpation. If the intussusception protrudes as far as the rectum, it may resemble a rectal prolapse. Therefore if tissue is protruding from the rectum, the clinician should carefully palpate around it to ascertain that a fornix exists (i.e., it is a rectal prolapse), to avoid missing the more important diagnosis of intussusception (in which a fornix cannot be found).

Plain abdominal radiographs infrequently allow the diagnosis of ileocolic intussusceptions because they usually cause minimal intestinal gas accumulation. A properly performed barium contrast enema may reveal a characteristic colonic filling defect caused by the intussuscepted ileum (Fig. 33-10). Abdominal ultrasonography is quick and reasonably accurate for detecting intussusceptions (see Fig. 29-8, *B*). Flexible colonoscopic examination is also definitive because it will allow visualization of the intussuscepted intestine extending into the colon (Fig. 33-11).

A reason for the intussusception (e.g., parasites, mass, enteritis) should always be sought. Fecal examination for parasites and evaluation of full-thickness intestinal biopsy specimens obtained at the time of surgical correction of the intussusception should be performed. In particular, the tip of the intussuscepted bowel (i.e., the intussusceptum) should be examined for a mass lesion, which could have served as a focus and allowed the intussusception to occur. Additional diagnostic tests may be warranted depending on the history, physical examination findings, and results of clinical pathologic evaluation.

### Treatment

Intussusceptions must be treated surgically. Acute ones may be reduced or resected, whereas chronic ones usually must be resected. Recurrence (in the same or a different site) is common unless the intestines are surgically plicated.

### Prognosis

The prognosis is often good if septic peritonitis has not occurred and the intestines do not reintussuscept.

### JEJUNOJEJUNAL INTUSSUSCEPTION

#### Etiology

The causes of jejunojejunal intussusception are probably the same as those for ileocolic intussusception.

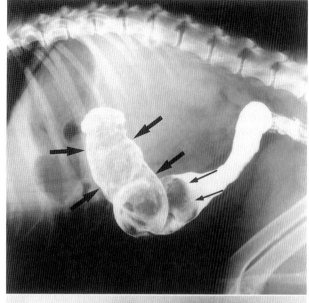

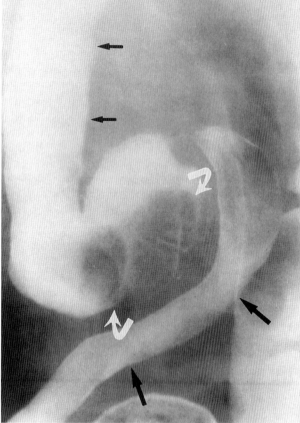

**FIG 33-10**
**A,** Lateral radiograph taken during a barium enema of a dog. Contrast medium outlines the end of a large ileocolic intussusception *(thin arrows)*. Note that barium does not fill up the normally positioned colonic lumen because of a long filling defect *(large arrows)*. **B,** Spot radiograph taken during a barium enema of a dog. The colon is descending on the left *(short arrows)*, and the ileum *(long arrows)* is entering the colon. There is an area in which barium is displaced, representing an intussuscepted cecum *(curved arrows)*. (**A** courtesy Dr. Alice Wolf, Texas A & M University.)

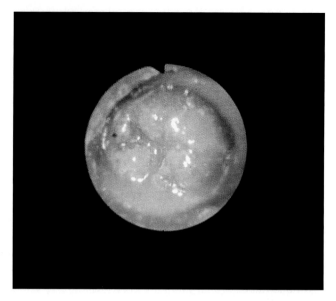

**FIG 33-11**
Endoscopic view of the ascending colon of a dog with an ileocolic intussusception. Note the large, "hot dog"–like mass in the colonic lumen, which is the intussusception.

## Clinical Features

Signs of intestinal obstruction (vomiting) and/or abdominal pain are the principal findings. Acute jejunojejunal intussusceptions usually do not cause hematochezia. Mucosal congestion can be more severe than that in ileocolic intussusception; intestinal devitalization eventually occurs, and bacteria and their toxins gain access to the peritoneal cavity. In severe cases the intestine may rupture as a result of ischemia.

## Diagnosis

Diagnosis is the same as for ileocolic intussusception. However, jejunojejunal intussusceptions may be easier to palpate because of their location. Furthermore, plain abdominal radiographs may be more likely to demonstrate obstructive ileus (i.e., gas-distended bowel loops) because the obstruction is not so far aborad. Abdominal ultrasonography is the preferred method of diagnosis.

## Treatment/Prognosis

Treatment and the prognosis are the same as for ileocolic intussusception.

# MISCELLANEOUS INTESTINAL DISEASES

## SHORT BOWEL SYNDROME
### Etiology

Short bowel syndrome is typically an iatrogenic disorder caused by resection of more than 75% to 90% of the small intestine. The remaining intestine is unable to adequately digest and absorb nutrients. Large numbers of bacteria may reach the upper small intestines, especially if the ileocolic valve is removed. Rarely, short bowel syndrome may be caused by congenital defects. However, not all animals with substantial small intestinal resections develop this syndrome. In general, dogs and cats seem better able than people to tolerate loss of a large percentage of small intestine.

## Clinical Features

Affected animals usually have severe weight loss and intractable diarrhea (typically without mucus or blood), which often occurs shortly after eating. Undigested food particles are often seen in the feces.

## Diagnosis

A history of substantial resection in conjunction with the clinical signs is sufficient for diagnosis. It is wise to determine how much small intestine is left by performing barium contrast radiographs; estimates made at surgery can be surprisingly inaccurate.

## Treatment

If the animal cannot maintain its body weight with oral feedings alone, total parenteral nutrition is needed until intestinal adaptation has occurred and treatments have become effective in controlling clinical signs. It is important to continue to feed the animal to stimulate intestinal mucosal hypertrophy. The diet should be highly digestible (e.g., low-fat cottage cheese, potato) and should be fed in small amounts, at least three to four times per day. Opiate antidiarrheals (e.g., loperamide), and $H_2$-receptor antagonists may be useful in lessening diarrhea and decreasing gastric hypersecretion. Antibiotics might be needed to control the large bacterial populations now present in the small intestine (p. 450).

## Prognosis

If intestinal adaptation occurs, the animal may eventually be fed a near normal diet. However, some animals will never be able to resume regular diets, and others die despite all efforts. Animals that are initially malnourished seem to have a worse prognosis than those that are well nourished. Some dogs and cats do better than one would intuitively expect them to do despite the loss of approximately 85% of the small intestines.

# NEOPLASMS OF THE SMALL INTESTINE

## ALIMENTARY LYMPHOMA
### Etiology

Lymphoma is a neoplastic proliferation of lymphocytes (see Chapter 82). It may be caused by FeLV in cats, but the etiology in dogs is unknown. LPE has been suggested to be pre-lymphomatous in some animals, but malignant transformation of LPE to lymphoma seems rare. Lymphoma often affects the intestines, although extraintestinal forms (e.g., lymph nodes, liver, spleen) are more common in dogs (see Chapter 82). Alimentary lymphoma appears to be more common in cats than in dogs. Malabsorption, diverticuli, and/or

intestinal obstruction may occur in association with the intestinal forms.

## Clinical Features

Chronic, progressive weight loss, anorexia, small intestinal diarrhea, and/or vomiting may occur. Alimentary lymphoma may cause nodules, masses, diffuse intestinal thickening due to infiltrative disease (see Fig. 29-9, *A*), dilated sections of intestine that are not obstructed (see Fig. 29-9, *B*), and/or focal constrictions. It may also be present in grossly normal-appearing intestine; PLE may also occur. Mesenteric lymphadenopathy (i.e., enlargement) is typical but not invariable. Extraintestinal abnormalities (e.g., peripheral lymphadenopathy) are inconsistently found in dogs and cats with alimentary lymphoma.

## Diagnosis

Diagnosis requires demonstration of neoplastic lymphocytes, which may be obtained by fine-needle aspiration, imprint, or squash cytologic preparations. However, histopathologic evaluation of intestinal biopsy specimens is the most reliable diagnostic method. If endoscopic biopsy samples are obtained, a poor sample or one that is not deep enough may cause the erroneous diagnosis of LPE instead of lymphoma. Occasionally, neoplastic lymphocytes are found only in the serosal layer and full-thickness surgical biopsy specimens are necessary, but this seems uncommon. Animals with extremely well-differentiated lymphocytic lymphoma may be impossible to distinguish from those with LPE, even with multiple full-thickness biopsy samples. In this case, diagnosis depends on finding lymphocytes in organs where they should not be found (e.g., liver) or in performing immunohistochemical stains to determine if the lymphoid population is monoclonal. Paraneoplastic hypercalcemia occasionally occurs but is neither sensitive nor specific for lymphoma.

## Treatment

Chemotherapy can prolong survival in cats with alimentary lymphoma. An appropriate treatment protocol is outlined in Chapter 82.

## Prognosis

The long-term prognosis is very poor, but some cats with well-differentiated intestinal lymphoma will live years with therapy.

# INTESTINAL ADENOCARCINOMA

Intestinal adenocarcinoma is more common in dogs than in cats. It typically causes diffuse intestinal thickening or focal circumferential mass lesions. Primary clinical signs are vomiting caused by intestinal obstruction and weight loss. Diagnosis requires demonstrating neoplastic epithelial cells either by cytologic or histopathologic evaluation. Endoscopy, surgery, and ultrasound-guided fine-needle aspiration may be diagnostic. Scirrhous carcinomas have very dense fibrous connective tissue that often cannot be obtained for a biopsy specimen with a flexible endoscope; therefore surgery is sometimes required in order to obtain diagnostic biopsies. The prognosis is good if complete surgical excision is possible, but metastases to regional lymph nodes are common by the time of diagnosis. Postoperative adjuvant chemotherapy does not appear to be beneficial.

## INTESTINAL LEIOMYOMA/ LEIOMYOSARCOMA

Intestinal leiomyomas and leiomyosarcomas are connective tissue tumors that usually form a distinct mass and are primarily found in the small intestine and stomach of older dogs. Primary clinical signs are intestinal hemorrhage, iron deficiency anemia, and obstruction. They can also cause hypoglycemia as a paraneoplastic effect. Diagnosis requires demonstration of neoplastic cells. Evaluation of ultrasound-guided fine-needle aspirate may be diagnostic, but these tumors do not exfoliate as readily as many carcinomas or lymphomas, and biopsy is often necessary. Surgical excision may be curative if there are no metastases. Metastases make the prognosis poor, although the conditions of some animals are palliated by chemotherapy.

## INFLAMMATION OF THE LARGE INTESTINE

### ACUTE COLITIS/PROCTITIS
#### Etiology

Acute colitis has many causes (e.g., bacteria, diet, parasites). The underlying cause is seldom diagnosed because this problem tends to be self-limiting. Acute proctitis probably has similar causes but may also be secondary to passage of a rough foreign object that traumatizes the rectal mucosa.

#### Clinical Features

More common in dogs than in cats, animals with acute colitis often feel good despite the presence of large bowel diarrhea (i.e., hematochezia, fecal mucus, tenesmus). Vomiting occurs infrequently. The major clinical signs of acute proctitis are constipation, tenesmus, hematochezia, dyschezia, and/or depression.

#### Diagnosis

Rectal examination is important; animals with acute colitis may have rectal discomfort and/or hematochezia. Eliminating obvious causes (e.g., diet, parasites) and resolving the problem with symptomatic therapy allows the establishment of a presumptive diagnosis. Colonoscopy and biopsy are definitive but seldom needed.

Rectal examination of animals with acute proctitis may reveal roughened, thick, and/or obviously ulcerated mucosa. Proctoscopy and rectal mucosal biopsy are definitive but seldom required.

#### Treatment

Symptomatic therapy is necessary because acute proctitis and colitis are usually idiopathic. Withholding food for 24 to 36 hours lessens the severity of clinical signs. The animal should then be fed small amounts of a bland diet (e.g., cottage cheese and rice) with or without fiber. After resolution of the clinical signs, the animal may be maintained on this diet or gradually returned to its original one. Areas of anal excoriation should be cleansed, and an antibiotic-corticosteroid ointment should be applied. Most animals recover within 1 to 3 days. For proctitis, broad-spectrum antimicrobial therapy effective against anaerobic bacteria, and stool softeners may also be used.

#### Prognosis

The prognosis for idiopathic disease is good.

### CHRONIC COLITIS

For a discussion of chronic colitis, see p. 448.

## INTUSSUSCEPTION/PROLAPSE OF THE LARGE INTESTINE

### CECOCOLIC INTUSSUSCEPTION
#### Etiology

Cecocolic intussusception, in which the cecum intussuscepts into the colon, is rare. The cause is unknown, although some suggest that whipworm-induced typhlitis may be responsible.

#### Clinical Features

Primarily occurring in dogs, intussuscepted cecums can bleed to the point where some dogs become anemic. Hematochezia is the major sign. It does not lead to intestinal obstruction and infrequently causes diarrhea.

#### Diagnosis

Cecocolic intussusception is rarely palpated during physical examination. Flexible endoscopy, ultrasonography, and barium enema (see Fig. 33-10, *B*) usually reveal the intussusception.

#### Treatment

Typhlectomy is curative, and the prognosis is good.

### RECTAL PROLAPSE
#### Etiology

Rectal prolapse usually occurs secondary to enteritis or colitis in young animals. They begin to strain because of rectal irritation, and eventually some or all of the rectal mucosa prolapses. Mucosal exposure increases irritation and perpetuates straining, which promotes prolapse. Hence a positive feedback cycle is initiated. Rectal prolapse may also be seen in Manx cats, which may be predisposed to it.

#### Clinical Features

Dogs and cats (especially juveniles) are affected. The presence of colonic or rectal mucosa extending from the anus is obvious during the physical examination.

#### Diagnosis

The diagnosis is based on physical examination. Rectal examination is needed to differentiate rectal prolapse from an intussusception protruding from the rectum (see p. 455).

## Treatment

Treatment consists of resolving the original cause of straining if possible, repositioning the rectal mucosa, and preventing additional straining. A well-lubricated finger is used to reposition the mucosa. If it readily prolapses after being replaced, a purse-string suture in the anus is used for 1 to 3 days to hold it in position. The subsequent rectal opening must be large enough so that the animal can defecate. Occasionally an epidural anesthetic is needed to prevent repeated prolapse. If the everted mucosa is so irritated that straining continues, kaolin (Kaopectate) retention enemas may provide relief. If a massive prolapse is present, or if the rectal mucosa is irreversibly damaged, resection may be necessary.

## Prognosis

The prognosis is usually good, but some cases tend to recur.

## NEOPLASMS OF THE LARGE INTESTINE

### ADENOCARCINOMA
#### Etiology

The cause of adenocarcinoma is unknown. Contrary to adenocarcinoma in people, relatively few colonic adenocarcinomas in dogs are documented to arise from polyps. These tumors can extend into the lumen or be infiltrative and produce a circumferential narrowing.

### Clinical Features

Principally found in dogs, colonic and rectal adenocarcinomas are more common in older animals. Hematochezia is common. Infiltrative tumors are likely to cause tenesmus and/or constipation secondary to obstruction.

### Diagnosis

Finding carcinoma cells is necessary for a diagnosis. Histopathologic evaluation is often preferable to cytologic analysis because dysplasia may be present, resulting in a false-positive diagnosis of carcinoma. Relatively deep biopsies obtained with rigid biopsy forceps are usually required to diagnose submucosal carcinomas. Because most colonic neoplasms arise in or near the rectum, digital examination is the best screening test. Colonoscopy is required for masses further orad. Imaging is used to detect sublumbar lymph node or pulmonary involvement (i.e., metastases).

### Treatment

Complete surgical excision is curative; however, most tumors cannot be completely excised because of their location in the pelvic canal, extent of local invasion, and/or tendency to metastasize to regional lymph nodes.

### Prognosis

The prognosis for unresectable adenocarcinoma is poor. Preoperative and intraoperative radiotherapy may be palliative for some dogs with nonresectable colorectal adenocarcinomas.

## RECTAL POLYPS
### Etiology

The cause of rectal polyps is unknown.

### Clinical Features

Principally found in dogs, hematochezia (which may be considerable) and tenesmus are the primary clinical signs. Obstruction is rare.

### Diagnosis

Usually detected during rectal examination, careful palpation often reveals a relatively larger mass with a narrow attachment to the underlying mucosa. Some adenomatous polyps resemble sessile adenocarcinomas because they are so large that the attachment cannot be readily discerned. Occasionally multiple, small polyps may be palpated throughout one segment of the colon, usually within a few centimeters of the rectum (Fig. 33-12). Histopathology is required for diagnosis and to distinguish polyps from malignancies.

### Treatment

Complete surgical excision is curative. If possible, a thorough endoscopic or imaging evaluation of the colon should be done before surgery to be certain additional polyps are not present. If they are incompletely excised, polyps return and must be excised again. Multiple polyps within a defined area may necessitate segmental colonic mucosal resection.

### Prognosis

Most canine rectal and colonic polyps do not result in carcinoma *in situ*, possibly because they are diagnosed relatively sooner than colonic polyps in people. The prognosis is good.

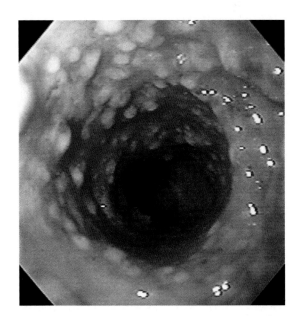

**FIG 33-12**
Endoscopic view of the distal colon of a dog that has multiple benign polyps. Biopsy is necessary to determine that these are not inflammatory or malignant.

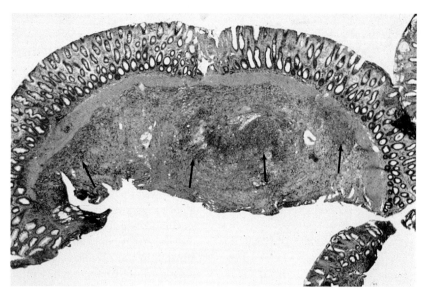

**FIG 33-13**
Photomicrograph of a colonic biopsy specimen. The mucosa is intact, but granulomas below the mucosa *(arrows)* contain fungal hyphae. These granulomas would not be found by superficial mucosal sampling. These granulomas are caused by pythiosis.

## MISCELLANEOUS LARGE INTESTINAL DISEASES

### PYTHIOSIS
**Etiology**

As discussed in Chapter 32, pythiosis is caused by *Pythium insidiosum.*

**Clinical Features**

Pythiosis of the large bowel usually occurs at or near the rectum. However, it can involve any area of the intestinal tract. Rectal lesions often cause partial obstruction. Fistulae may also develop, resembling perianal fistulae. The dog may be presented for constipation and/or hematochezia. Animals with advanced disease often lose weight. Rarely there will be infarction of mucosa or vessels with subsequent ischemia. Cats are rarely affected.

**Diagnosis**

Because the lesion is submucosal and very fibrotic, rigid biopsy forceps are necessary to obtain deep, diagnostic samples that include substantial amounts of submucosa (i.e., where the organism is found) (Fig. 33-13). Special stains (e.g., Warthin-Starry) are needed to find the organism. Sometimes the organism cannot be found, but a suggestive pyogranulomatous, eosinophilic inflammation is present. A serologic test shows promise (Dr. Grooters, Louisiana State University, Baton Rouge, La).

**Treatment**

Complete surgical excision is preferred. No medication has consistently been effective, although itraconazole or liposomal amphotericin B might be beneficial in some dogs.

**Prognosis**

The prognosis is poor unless the lesion can be completely excised.

## PERINEAL/PERIANAL DISEASES

### PERINEAL HERNIA
**Etiology**

Perineal hernia occurs when the pelvic diaphragm (i.e., coccygeus and levator ani muscles) weakens and allows the rectal canal to deviate laterally.

**Clinical Features**

This condition is principally found in older intact male dogs (especially Boston Terriers, Boxers, Corgis, and Pekingeses); cats are rarely affected. Most animals present because of dyschezia, constipation, or perineal swelling; however, urinary bladder herniation into this defect may cause severe postrenal uremia with depression and vomiting.

**Diagnosis**

Digital rectal examination should detect rectal deviation, lack of muscular support, and/or a rectal diverticulum. The clinician should check for retroflexion of the urinary bladder into the hernia. If such herniation is suspected, it can be confirmed by ultrasonography, radiographs, catheterizing the bladder, or aspirating the swelling (after imaging) to see if urine is present.

**Treatment**

Animals with postrenal uremia constitute an emergency; the bladder should be emptied and repositioned, and intravenous fluids should be administered (see p. 647). The preferred treatment is surgical reconstruction of the muscular support; however, surgery may fail, and clients should be prepared for the fact that their pet may require additional reconstructive procedures.

## Prognosis

The prognosis is fair to guarded.

## PERIANAL FISTULAE

### Etiology

The cause of perianal fistulae is unknown. Impacted anal crypts and/or anal sacs have been hypothesized to become infected and rupture into deep tissues. An immune-mediated mechanism is likely to be involved, as seen by the clinical response to immunosuppressive drugs.

### Clinical Features

Perianal fistulae occur in dogs and are more common in breeds with a sloping conformation and/or a broad base to the tail head (e.g., German Shepherd Dogs). There are typically one or more painful draining tracts around the anus. Animals are usually presented because of constipation (due to the pain), odor, rectal pain, and/or rectal discharge.

### Diagnosis

Diagnosis is made by physical and rectal examination. Draining tracts are sometimes absent, but granulomas and abscesses can be palpated per the rectum. Rectal pythiosis rarely mimics perianal fistulae.

### Treatment

Surgical excision and/or electrofulguration of the draining tracts were once recommended. However, many affected dogs are cured with immunosuppressive (e.g., cyclosporine, 5 mg/kg q12h; azathioprine, 50 mg/m² q48h; topical 0.1% tacrolimus) therapy with or without antibacterial (e.g., metronidazole, erythromycin) drugs. Generally, only one of the immunosuppressive drugs is used, and administering ketoconazole (5 mg/kg PO q12h) may allow a lower dose of cyclosporine to be effective, thus decreasing the client's cost. If cyclosporine is used, one should monitor therapeutic blood levels of the drug to ensure that the dose is correct for that patient. Hypoallergenic diets may also be beneficial. Rarely, animals will not respond to medical therapy and will require surgery. Surgery may cause fecal incontinence. Postoperative care is important and consists of keeping the area clean. Fecal softeners are sometimes useful.

### Prognosis

Many patients are treated successfully. However, the prognosis is guarded, and repeated medical care or surgeries may be needed.

## ANAL SACCULITIS

### Etiology

The anal sac becomes infected, resulting in an abscess or cellulitis.

### Clinical Features

Anal sacculitis is relatively common in dogs and occasionally occurs in cats. Small dogs (e.g., Poodles, Chihuahuas) probably have a higher incidence of this disorder than other breeds. Mild cases cause irritation (i.e., "scooting," licking, or biting the area). Anal sacs occasionally bleed onto the feces. Severe cases can have obvious pain, swelling, and/or draining tracts. Dyschezia or constipation may develop because the animal refuses to defecate. Fever may occur in dogs and cats with severe anal sacculitis.

### Diagnosis

Physical and rectal examination is usually diagnostic. The anal sacs are often painful; the sac contents may appear purulent, bloody, or normal but increased in volume. In severe cases it may be impossible to express the affected sac. If the sac ruptures, the fistulous tract is usually in a 4-o'clock or 7-o'clock position in relation to the anus. Occasionally there is an obvious abscess.

### Treatment

Mild cases require only that the anal sac be expressed and an aqueous antibiotic-corticosteroid preparation be infused; this regimen is usually necessary only once. Infusion with saline solution may aid in expressing impacted sacs. If clients express the anal sacs at home, they can often prevent impaction and reduce the likelihood of severe complications.

Abscesses should be lanced, drained, flushed, and hot packed; systemic antibiotics should also be administered. Hot packs also help soft spots form in early abscesses. If the problem recurs, is severe, or is nonresponsive to medical therapy, affected sacs can be resected.

### Prognosis

The prognosis is usually good.

## PERIANAL NEOPLASMS

### ANAL SAC (APOCRINE GLAND) ADENOCARCINOMA

#### Etiology

Anal sac adenocarcinomas are derived from the apocrine glands and are usually found in older female dogs.

#### Clinical Features

An anal sac or pararectal mass can often be palpated, but some are not obvious. Paraneoplastic hypercalcemia causing anorexia, weight loss, vomiting, and polyuria-polydipsia is common. Occasionally constipation occurs as a result of the hypercalcemia or perineal mass. Metastatic sublumbar lymphadenopathy occurs early in the course of the disease, but metastases to other organs are rare.

#### Diagnosis

Cytologic and/or histopathologic evaluation is necessary to establish a diagnosis. Hypercalcemia in an older female dog should lead to careful examination of both anal sacs and pararectal structures. Abdominal ultrasonography may reveal sublumbar lymphadenopathy.

### Treatment

Hypercalcemia, if present, must be treated (see Chapter 55). The tumor should be removed, but these tumors have often metastasized to regional lymph nodes by the time of diagnosis. Palliative chemotherapy (see Chapter 79) may be beneficial in some dogs.

### Prognosis

The prognosis is guarded.

## PERIANAL GLAND TUMORS

### Etiology

Perianal gland tumors arise from modified sebaceous glands. Perianal gland adenomas have testosterone receptors.

### Clinical Features

Perianal gland adenomas are often sharply demarcated, raised, and red and may be pruritic. Commonly found around the anus and base of the tail, they may be solitary or multiple and can occur over the entire back half of the dog. Male hormones appear to stimulate their growth, and they are often found in older male dogs (especially Cocker Spaniels, Beagles, and German Shepherd Dogs). Pruritus may lead to licking and ulceration of the tumor. Perianal gland adenocarcinomas are rare; they are usually large, infiltrative, ulcerated masses with a high metastatic potential.

### Diagnosis

Cytologic and/or histopathologic evaluation is needed for diagnosis, but neither reliably distinguishes malignant from benign masses. Finding metastases (e.g., regional lymph nodes, lungs) is the most certain method of diagnosing malignancy.

### Treatment

Surgical excision is preferred for benign or solitary tumors that have not metastasized. Neutering is recommended for dogs with adenomas. Radiation is recommended for multicentric and some malignant tumors. Chemotherapy (vincristine adriamycin cyclophosphamide [VAC] protocol) is helpful in dogs with adenocarcinomas (see Chapter 79).

### Prognosis

The prognosis is good for benign lesions but guarded for malignant lesions.

## CONSTIPATION

Constipation may be caused by any perineal or perianal disease that causes pain (e.g., perianal fistulae, perineal hernia, anal sacculitis), obstruction, or colonic weakness. It may also be caused by other disorders (see Table 28-17).

## PELVIC CANAL OBSTRUCTION DUE TO MALALIGNED HEALING OF OLD PELVIC FRACTURES

### Etiology

Prior trauma (e.g., automobile-associated injuries) is a common cause of pelvic canal obstruction in cats because they frequently sustain pelvic trauma that heals if they are allowed to rest. Cats appear clinically normal once the fractures heal, but the diminution of the pelvic canal can produce megacolon and/or dystocia.

### Diagnosis

Digital rectal examination should be diagnostic. Radiographs will further define the extent of the problem.

### Treatment

Constipation caused by minimal pelvic narrowing may be controlled with stool softeners, but orthopedic surgery is needed to widen very narrow pelvic canals. The prognosis depends somewhat on how severely the colon has been distended. Unless the colon is massively stretched out of shape, it can often resume function if it is kept empty and allowed to regain its normal diameter. Prokinetic drugs such as cisapride (0.25 mg/kg PO q8-12h) may stimulate peristalsis; however, prokinetic drugs must not be used if there is residual obstruction.

### Prognosis

The prognosis depends on the severity and chronicity of colonic distention and the success of surgery in widening the pelvic canal.

## BENIGN RECTAL STRICTURE

### Etiology

The cause is uncertain but may be congenital.

### Clinical Features

Constipation and tenesmus are the principal clinical signs.

### Diagnosis

Digital rectal examination detects a stricture, although this sign can be missed if a large dog is palpated carelessly or if the stricture is beyond reach. Proctoscopy and evaluation of a deep biopsy specimen (i.e., including submucosa) of the stricture are needed to confirm that the lesion is benign and fibrous as opposed to neoplastic or fungal.

### Treatment

In some animals, simple dilation via balloon or retractor will tear the stricture and allow normal defecation; other animals require surgery. Owners should be warned that strictures may re-form during healing and that surgery can rarely cause incontinence. Corticosteroids (prednisolone, 1.1 mg/kg/day) might impede stricture re-formation.

### Prognosis

The prognosis is guarded to good.

# DIETARY INDISCRETION LEADING TO CONSTIPATION

## Etiology

Eating inappropriate foods or other materials (e.g., paper, popcorn, hair, bones) is common in dogs. Excessive dietary fiber supplements can cause constipation if the animal becomes dehydrated.

## Diagnosis

Dietary causes are common in dogs that eat trash. Dietary indiscretion is best diagnosed by examining fecal matter retrieved from the colon.

## Treatment

Controlling the pet's eating habits, adding appropriate amounts of fiber to the diet, and feeding a moist diet (especially in cats) help to prevent constipation. Repeated retention and cleansing (*not* hypertonic) enemas may be needed. Manual disruption of hard feces should be avoided; however, if it is necessary, the animal should be anesthetized to help prevent colonic trauma during the procedure, and sponge forceps or curved hemostats should be used to mechanically break apart the feces. It often helps to insert a rigid colonoscope up to the fecal mass and then insert a tube with a vigorous stream of running water at body temperature issuing from the tip. This will soften the fecal mass and wash away debris that breaks off.

## Prognosis

The prognosis is usually good. The colon should function normally after cleansing unless the distention has been prolonged and severe.

# IDIOPATHIC MEGACOLON

## Etiology

The cause is unknown but may include behavior (i.e., refusal to defecate) or altered colonic neurotransmitters.

## Clinical Features

Idiopathic megacolon is principally a feline disease, although dogs are occasionally affected. Affected animals may be depressed and anorectic and are often presented because of infrequent defecation.

## Diagnosis

Diagnosis requires palpating a massively dilated colon (not one just filled to normal capacity) plus elimination of dietary, behavioral, metabolic, and anatomic causes. Abdominal radiographs should be evaluated if proper abdominal palpation cannot be performed.

## Treatment

Impacted feces must be removed. Multiple warm water retention and cleansing enemas over 2 to 4 days usually work. Future fecal impaction is prevented by adding fiber to a moist diet (e.g., Metamucil, pumpkin pie filling), making sure clean litter is always available, and using osmotic laxatives (e.g., lactulose) and/or prokinetic drugs (e.g., cisapride). Lubricants are not helpful, because they do not change fecal consistency. Bisacodyl is seldom as useful as lactulose. If this conservative therapy fails or is refused by the client, subtotal colectomy is indicated. Cats typically have soft stools for a few weeks postoperatively, some for the rest of their lives.

## Prognosis

The prognosis is fair to guarded. Many cats respond well to conservative therapy if treated early.

## *Suggested Readings*

Baez JL et al: Radiographic, ultrasonographic, and endoscopic findings in cats with inflammatory bowel disease of the stomach and small intestine: 33 cases (1990-1997), *J Am Vet Med Assoc* 215:349, 1999.

Barr SC et al: Evaluation of two test procedures for diagnosis of giardiasis in dogs, *Am J Vet Res* 53(11):2028, 1992.

Barr SC et al: Efficacy of fenbendazole against giardiasis in dogs, *Am J Vet Res* 55(7):988, 1994.

Barrs VR et al: Intestinal obstruction by trichobezoars in five cats, *J Fel Med Surg* 1:199, 1999.

Basher AWP et al: Conservative versus surgical management of gastrointestinal linear foreign bodies in the cat, *Vet Surg* 16(2):135, 1987.

Bellenger CR et al: Intussusception in 12 cats, *J Small Anim Pract* 35:295, 1994.

Breitschwerdt EB: Immunoproliferative enteropathy of basenjis, *Semin Vet Med Surg* 7:153, 1992.

Brinson RR et al: Diarrhea associated with severe hypoalbuminemia: a comparsion of a peptide-based chemically defined diet and standard enteral alimentation, *Crit Care Med* 16(2):130, 1988.

Brown C et al: An outbreak of enterocolitis due to *Campylobacter* spp. in a Beagle colony, *J Vet Diagn Invest* 11:374, 1999.

Cairo J et al: Intestinal volvulus in dogs: a study of four clinical cases, *J Small Anim Pract* 40:136, 1999.

Coyne MJ: Seroconversion of puppies to canine parvovirus and canine distemper virus: a comparison of two combination vaccines, *J Am Anim Hosp Assoc* 36:137, 2000.

Couto CG: Gastrointestinal neoplasia in dogs and cats. In Kirk RW et al, editors: *Current veterinary therapy IX,* Philadelphia, 1992, WB Saunders, p 595.

Dennis JS et al: Lymphocytic/plasmacytic gastroenteritis in cats: 14 cases (1985-1990), *J Am Vet Med Assoc* 200(11):1712, 1992.

Dennis JS et al: Lymphocytic/plasmacytic colitis in cats: 14 cases (1985-1990), *J Am Vet Med Assoc* 202:313, 1993.

Doherty D et al: Intestinal intussusception in five postparturient queens, *Vet Rec* 146:614, 2000.

Dow SW et al: Clinical features of salmonellosis in cats: six cases (1981-1986), *J Am Vet Med Assoc* 194(10):1464, 1989.

Epe C et al: Investigations into the prevention of neonatal *Ancyclostoma caninum* infections in puppies by application of moxidectin to the bitch, *J Vet Med* 46:361, 1999.

Evans KL et al: Gastrointestinal linear foreign bodies in 32 dogs: a retrospective evaluation and feline comparison, *J Am Anim Hosp Assoc* 30:445, 1994.

Feinstein RE et al: Chronic gastroenterocolitis in nine cats, *J Vet Diagn Invest* 4:293, 1992.

Ferguson JF: Triple pelvic osteotomy for the treatment of pelvic canal stenosis in a cat, *J Small Anim Pract* 37:495, 1996.

Fisher MA et al: Efficacy of fenbendazole and piperazine against developing stages of toxocara and toxascaris in dogs, *Vet Rec* 132:473, 1993.

Foley JE et al: Outbreak of fatal salmonellosis in cats following use of a high-titer modified-live panleukopenia virus vaccine, *J Am Vet Med Assoc* 214:67, 1999.

Gabor LJ et al: Clinical and anatomical features of lymphosarcoma in 118 cats, *Aust Vet J* 76:725, 1998.

Gookin JL et al: Experimental infection of cats with *Tritrichomonas foetus, Am J Vet Res* 62:1690, 2001.

Graham JP et al: Ultrasonographic features of canine gastrointestinal pythiosis, *Vet Radiol Ultrasound* 41:273, 2000.

Griffiths LG et al: Cyclosporin as the sole treatment for anal furunculosis: preliminary results, *J Small Anim Pract* 40:569, 1999.

Hall EJ et al: Survey of the diagnosis and treatment of canine exocrine pancreatic insufficiency, *J Small Anim Pract* 32:613, 1991.

Harkin KR et al: Association of perianal fistula and colitis in the German shepherd dog: response to high-dose prednisone and dietary therapy, *J Am Anim Hosp Assoc* 32:515, 1996.

Hart JR et al: Lymphocytic-plasmacytic enterocolitis in cats: 60 cases (1988-1990), *J Am Anim Hosp Assoc* 30:505, 1994.

Hill SL et al: Prevalence of enteric zoonotic organisms in cats, *J Am Vet Med Assoc* 216:687, 2000.

Hosgood G et al: Perineal herniorrhaphy: perioperative data from 100 dogs, *J Am Anim Hosp Assoc* 31:331, 1995.

Hoskins JD: Canine parvovirus: the evolving syndrome, *Infect Dis Bull* 1:1, 1995.

Hoskins JD: Neonatal diarrhea in puppies and kittens. In Bonagura JD, editor: *Current veterinary therapy XIII,* ed 13, Philadelphia, 2000, WB Saunders.

Houston DM et al: Risk factors associated with parvovirus enteritis in dogs: 283 cases (1982-1991), *J Am Vet Med Assoc* 208(4):542, 1996.

Jergens AE et al: Idiopathic inflammatory bowel disease in dogs and cats: 84 cases (1987-1990), *J Am Vet Med Assoc* 201(10):1603, 1992.

Jergens AE et al: Diseases of the large intestine. In Ettinger SJ et al, editors: *Textbook of veterinary internal medicine,* ed 5, Philadelphia, 2000, WB Saunders, p 1238.

Jordan HE et al: Endoparasitism in dogs: 21,583 cases (1981-1990), *J Am Vet Med Assoc* 203(4):547, 1993.

Kawashima K et al: *Salmonella* carriers among cats derived from Kanagawa prefecture, *J Jpn Vet Med Assoc* 43:679, 1990.

Kimmel SE et al: Hypomagnesemia and hypocalcemia associated with protein-losing enteropathy in Yorkshire terriers: five cases (1992-1998), *J Am Vet Med Assoc* 217:703, 2000.

Larson LJ et al: Comparison of selected canine vaccines for their ability to induce protective immunity against canine parvovirus infection, *Am J Vet Res* 58(4):360, 1997.

Leib MS et al: Endoscopic aspiration of intestinal contents in dogs and cats: 394 cases, *J Vet Intern Med* 13:191, 1999.

Leib MS: Treatment of chronic idiopathic large-bowel diarrhea in dogs with a highly digestible diet and soluble fiber: a retrospective review of 37 cases, *J Vet Intern Med* 14:27, 2000.

Littman MP et al: Familial protein-losing enteropathy and protein-losing nephropathy in Soft Coated Wheaten Terriers: 222 cases (1983-1997), *J Vet Intern Med* 14:68, 2000.

Lutz H et al: Panleukopenia-like syndrome of FeLV caused by co-infection with FeLV and feline panleukopenia virus, *Vet Immun Immunopathol* 46:21, 1995.

Mahoney OM et al: Alimentary lymphoma in cats: 28 cases (1988-1993), *J Am Vet Med Assoc* 207(12):1593, 1995.

Marks SL et al: Evaluation of methods to diagnose *Clostridium perfingens*–associated diarrhea in dogs, *J Am Vet Med Assoc* 214: 357, 1999.

Mathews KA et al: Randomized controlled trial of cyclosporine for treatment of perianal fistulas in dogs, *J Am Vet Med Assoc* 211(10):1249, 1997.

Matthiesen DT et al: Subtotal colectomy for the treatment of obstipation secondary to pelvic fracture malunion in cats, *Vet Surg* 20(2):113, 1991.

McDonough PL et al: Diagnosing emerging bacterial infections: salmonellosis, campylobacteriosis, clostridial toxicosis, and helicobacteriosis, *Semin Vet Med Surg* 11:187, 1996.

McPherron MA et al: Colorectal leiomyomas in seven dogs, *J Am Anim Hosp Assoc* 28(1):43, 1992.

McReynolds CA et al: Regional seroprevalence of *Cryptosporidium parvum*–specific IgG of cats in the United States, *Vet Parasitol* 80:187, 1999.

Meyer EK: Adverse events associated with albendazole and other treatments used for treatment of giardiasis in dogs, *J Am Vet Med Assoc* 213:44, 1998.

Miller WW et al: Cecal inversion in eight dogs, *J Am Anim Hosp Assoc* 20:1009, 1984.

Misseghers BS et al: Clinical observations of the treatment of canine perianal fistulas with topical tacrolimus in 10 dogs, *Can Vet J* 41:623, 2000.

Mochizuki M et al: Feline coronavirus participation in diarrhea of cats, *J Vet Med Sci* 61:1071, 1999.

Nash JM et al: Enteroplication in cats, using suture of n-butyl cyanoacrylate adhesive, *Res Vet Sci* 65:253, 1998.

Nemzek JA et al: Mesenteric volvulus in the dog: a retrospective study, *J Am Anim Hosp Assoc* 29:357, 1993.

Oakes MG et al: Enteroplication for the prevention of intussusception recurrence in dogs: 31 cases (1978-1992), *J Am Vet Med Assoc* 205(1):72, 1994.

Olson ME et al: Preliminary data on the efficacy of *Giardia* vaccine in puppies, *Can Vet J* 38:777, 1997.

Pratelli A et al: Fatal canine parvovirus type-1 infection in pups from Italy, *J Vet Diagn Invest* 11:365, 1999.

Reinemeyer CR et al: Comparison of the efficacies of three heartworm preventives against experimentally induced infections with *Ancylostoma caninum* and *Toxocara canis* in pups, *J Am Vet Med Assoc* 206:1710, 1995.

Rewerts JM et al: CVT update: diagnosis and treatment of parvovirus. In Bonagura JD, editor: *Current veterinary therapy XIII,* ed 13, Philadelphia, 2000, WB Saunders.

Rosin E et al: Subtotal colectomy for treatment of chronic constipation associated with idiopathic megacolon in cats: 38 cases (1979-1985), *J Am Vet Med Assoc* 193(7):850, 1988.

Roth L et al: Comparisons between endoscopic and histologic evaluation of the gastrointestinal tract in dogs and cats: 75 cases (1984-1987), *J Am Vet Med Assoc* 196(4):635, 1990.

Rutgers HC et al: Small intestinal bacterial overgrowth in dogs with chronic intestinal disease, *J Am Vet Med Assoc* 206:187, 1995.

Schrader SC: Pelvic osteotomy as a treatment for obstipation in cats with acquired stenosis of the pelvic canal: six cases (1978-1989), *J Am Vet Med Assoc* 200(2):208, 1992.

Shealy PM et al: Canine intestinal volvulus: a report of nine new cases, *Vet Surg* 21(1):15, 1992.

Sherding RG et al: Intestinal histoplasmosis. In Kirk RW et al, editors: *Current veterinary therapy XI,* ed 11, Philadelphia, 1992, WB Saunders, p 609.

Simpson JW et al: Long-term management of canine exocrine pancreatic insufficiency, *J Small Anim Pract* 35:133, 1994.

Steinberg H et al: Primary gastrointestinal lymphosarcoma with epitheliotropism in three shar-pei and one boxer dog, *Vet Pathol* 32:423, 1995.

Tauni MA et al: Outbreak of *Salmonella typhimurium* in cats and humans associated with infections in wild birds, *J Small Anim Pract* 41:339, 2000.

Turk J et al: Enteric *Clostridium perfringens* infection associated with parvoviral enteritis in dogs: 74 cases (1987-1990), *J Am Vet Med Assoc* 200(7):991, 1992.

Twedt DC: *Clostridium perfringens*–associated diarrhea in dogs, *Proc Am Coll Vet Intern Med* 11:121, 1993.

Villeneuve V et al: Efficacy of oxfendazole for the treatment of giardiasis in dogs: experiments in dog breeding kennels, *Parasitology* 7:221, 2000.

Weichselbaum RC et al: Comparison of upper gastrointestinal radiographic findings to histopathologic observations: a retrospective study of 41 dogs and cats with suspected small bowel infiltrative disease (1985 to 1990), *Vet Radiol Ultrasound* 35(6):418, 1994.

Welches CD et al: Perineal hernia in the cat: a retrospective study of 40 cases, *J Am Anim Hosp Assoc* 28:431, 1992.

Wiberg ME et al: Exocrine pancreatic atrophy in German shepherd dogs and rough-coated Collies: an end result of lymphocytic pancreatitis, *Vet Pathol* 36:530, 1999.

Wiberg ME et al: Serum trypsin-like immunoreactivity measurement for the diagnosis of subclinical exocrine pancreatic insufficiency, *J Vet Intern Med* 13:426, 1999.

Willard MD et al: Intestinal crypt lesions associated with protein-losing enteropathy in the dog, *J Vet Intern Med* 14:298, 2000.

Williams DA: Exocrine pancreatic disease and pancreatitis. In Ettinger SJ et al, editors: *Textbook of veterinary internal medicine*, ed 5, Philadelphia, 2000, WB Saunders, p 1345.

Zajac AM et al: Giardia infection in a group of experimental dogs, *J Small Anim Pract* 33:257, 1992.

Zajac AM et al: Efficacy of fenbendazole in the treatment of experimental giardia infection in dogs, *Am J Vet Res* 59(1):61, 1998.

Zwahlen CH et al: Results of chemotherapy for cats with alimentary malignant lymphoma: 21 cases (1993-1997), *J Am Vet Med Assoc* 213:1144, 1998.

# CHAPTER 34

# Disorders of the Peritoneum

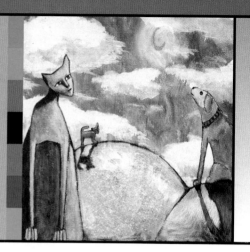

## CHAPTER OUTLINE

INFLAMMATORY DISEASES, 466
  Septic peritonitis, 466
  Sclerosing, encapsulating peritonitis, 468
HEMOABDOMEN, 468
  Abdominal hemangiosarcoma, 468
MISCELLANEOUS PERITONEAL DISORDERS, 469
  Abdominal carcinomatosis, 469
  Feline infectious peritonitis, 469

## INFLAMMATORY DISEASES

### SEPTIC PERITONITIS
#### Etiology

Spontaneous septic peritonitis is usually caused by alimentary tract perforation or devitalization caused by neoplasia, ulceration, intussusception, foreign objects, or dehiscence of suture lines. Septic peritonitis can also develop after abdominal gunshot wounds, surgery, or hematogenous spread from elsewhere.

#### Clinical Features

Septic peritonitis occurs more frequently in dogs than in cats. If it occurs secondary to suture line dehiscence, it classically manifests 3 to 6 days postoperatively. Affected animals are usually depressed, febrile, and vomiting and may have abdominal pain (if they are not too depressed to respond). Abdominal effusion is usually mild to modest in amount. Signs usually progress rapidly until septic shock (i.e., systemic inflammatory response syndrome) occurs. However, some animals with septic peritonitis may have mild vomiting, slight fever, and copious volumes of abdominal fluid and feel relatively well.

#### Diagnosis

Most animals with septic peritonitis have small amounts of abdominal fluid that cannot be detected by physical examination but that decrease serosal detail on plain abdominal radiographs (much like what is seen in animals with a lack of body fat). Ultrasonography is a sensitive means for detecting such small fluid volumes. Free peritoneal gas strongly suggests alimentary tract leakage (Fig. 34-1) or infection with gas-forming bacteria (unless there has been recent abdominal surgery). Ultrasonography may detect masses responsible for such leakage. Neutrophilia is common in dogs and cats with septic peritonitis but is nonspecific for this disorder.

Abdominocentesis (with or without diagnostic peritoneal lavage) is indicated if free abdominal fluid is detected or if septic peritonitis is suspected. Retrieved fluid is examined cytologically and cultured. If fluid is difficult to retrieve, it may be obtained at surgery instead, but this approach is not preferred.

Severely degenerative neutrophils, bacteria (especially if phagocytized by white blood cells), or fecal contents in abdominal fluid are diagnostic for septic peritonitis (Fig. 34-2). However, fecal contents and bacteria are often not seen despite severe infection. Prior antibiotic use may greatly suppress bacterial numbers and the percentage of neutrophils demonstrating degenerative changes. Finally, mild degeneration of neutrophils in abdominal fluid is expected after recent abdominal surgery.

#### Treatment

Animals with spontaneous septic peritonitis usually have an alimentary tract leak and should be surgically explored as soon as they are stable. A preanesthetic complete blood count (CBC), serum biochemistry profile, and urinalysis are desirable; however, surgery should not be delayed even if the laboratory results are. At surgery a careful search should be made for intestinal or gastric defects. Biopsy of tissue surrounding a perforation should be performed to search for underlying neoplasia or inflammatory bowel disease (IBD). After the defect is corrected, the abdomen should be repeatedly lavaged with large volumes of warm crystalloid solutions to dilute and remove debris and bacteria. The abdomen cannot be adequately lavaged via a drain tube or even a peritoneal dialysis catheter except in the mildest cases. Adhesions re-form quickly; they should not be broken down unless it is necessary to examine the intestines. Intestines should be resected only if they are truly devitalized. Intestines are sometimes unnecessarily removed because of adhesions, resulting in short bowel syndrome (see p. 456), which has substantial morbidity.

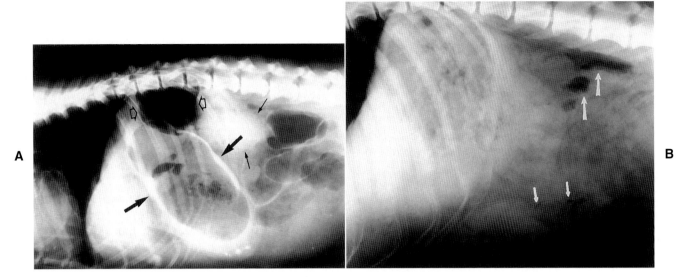

**FIG 34-1**
**A,** Plain lateral abdominal radiograph of a dog. Visceral margins of kidney *(small solid arrows)* and stomach *(large solid arrows)* are outlined by negative contrast (i.e., air). In addition, there are pockets of free air in the abdomen *(open arrows)*. This dog had a gastric ulcer that spontaneously perforated. **B,** Plain lateral radiograph of a dog with a splenic abscess. There are air bubbles in the region of the spleen *(short arrows)* and free gas in the dorsal peritoneal cavity *(long arrows)*.

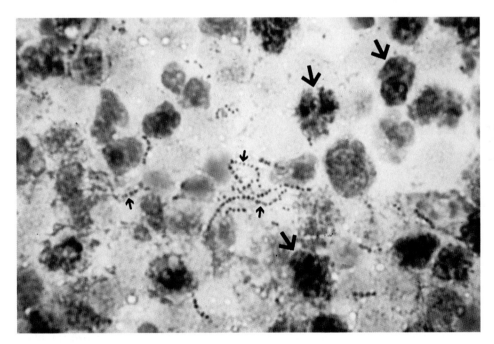

**FIG 34-2**
Photomicrograph of peritoneal exudate from a dog with septic peritonitis. Note bacteria *(small arrows)* and neutrophils that have degenerated so much that it is difficult to identify them as neutrophils *(large arrows)*. (Wright's stain; magnification ×1000.) (Courtesy Dr. Claudia Barton, Texas A & M University.)

Substantial abdominal contamination may require protracted drainage. Penrose drains are inadequate for this purpose. If drainage is imperative, open abdominal drainage is preferred and is accomplished by using a nonabsorbable suture to close the abdomen except for a 6 to 8 cm opening at its most dependent aspect. This open incision is covered with sterile absorbent dressings (e.g., a sterile sanitary napkin held in place by sterile cast padding and sterile gauze) that are changed as needed, usually two to four times per day initially. Eventually only one change per day will be needed. When the dressing is changed, a sterile, gloved hand should explore the opening to ensure that omentum and intestines have not blocked the site. This dressing change regimen is continued until abdominal drainage decreases and most or all of the peritoneal contamination is gone. Then a second surgery is performed to close the abdomen. Sometimes the opening will close spontaneously. The abdomen should be recultured at the time of the second surgery. Although time-consuming, this technique is extremely effective in animals with severe peritoneal contamination (e.g., that caused by feces, food, barium).

Systemic antimicrobial therapy should consist of broad-spectrum and parenteral antibiotics. Combinations of a β-lactam drug (e.g., ampicillin) plus an aminoglycoside (e.g., amikacin) plus metronidazole are reasonable (see Drugs Used in Gastrointestinal Disorders, p. 469). Administration of the entire daily aminoglycoside dose in one injection is safer and probably as or more effective than administering smaller doses two to three times daily. Enrofloxacin may be substituted for the aminoglycoside. Cefoxitin, a second-generation cephalosporin (22 mg/kg q6-8h), is almost as effective as a β-lactam drug plus an aminoglycoside. Fluid and electrolyte support helps to prevent aminoglycoside-induced nephrotoxicity. Hypoalbuminemia can occur, especially if open abdominal drainage is used.

## Prognosis

The prognosis depends on the cause of the leak (e.g., perforations may be caused by malignancies) and the animal's condition when it is diagnosed. Septic shock and disseminated intravascular coagulation (DIC) worsen the prognosis.

## SCLEROSING, ENCAPSULATING PERITONITIS

### Etiology

Reported causes include bacterial infection, steatitis, and fiberglass ingestion. This form of peritonitis is rare.

### Clinical Features

Sclerosing, encapsulating peritonitis is a chronic condition in which abdominal organs are covered and encased in heavy layers of connective tissue. Typical clinical signs usually include vomiting, abdominal pain, and ascites. During exploratory surgery the lesions may mimic those of a mesothelioma. Analysis of abdominal fluid usually reveals red blood cells, mixed inflammatory cells, and macrophages. Diagnosis is confirmed by surgical biopsy of the thick covering of the abdominal organs.

### Treatment

Antibiotics with or without corticosteroids may be tried. Removal of underlying causes (e.g., steatitis in cats) is desirable, but such causes are rarely found.

### Prognosis

Most affected animals die despite therapeutic attempts.

## HEMOABDOMEN

Most red effusions are blood-tinged transudates, not hemoabdomen. Hemoabdomen is usually indicated by a fluid with a hematocrit greater than or equal to 10% to 15%. Blood in the abdominal cavity is either iatrogenic (i.e., occurs during abdominocentesis) or represents spontaneous disease. Clots or platelets in the sample mean that the bleeding is iatrogenic or is currently occurring near the site of the abdominocentesis. Hemoabdomen is usually the result of a bleeding neoplasm (e.g., hemangiosarcoma, hepatoma), coagulopathy (e.g., rodenticide intoxication), or trauma (e.g., automobile-associated injury). History, physical examination, coagulation studies, and/or abdominal ultrasonography usually establish the diagnosis. It should be noted that thrombocytopenia may cause or be caused by abdominal bleeding.

## ABDOMINAL HEMANGIOSARCOMA

### Etiology

Abdominal hemangiosarcoma often originates in the spleen (see p. 1142). It can spread throughout the abdomen by implantation, causing widespread peritoneal seepage of blood, or it can metastasize to distant sites (e.g., liver, lungs).

### Clinical Features

Abdominal hemangiosarcoma is principally found in older dogs, especially German Shepherd Dogs and Golden Retrievers. Anemia, abdominal effusion, and periodic weakness or collapse from poor peripheral perfusion are common presenting complaints.

### Diagnosis

Ultrasonography is the most sensitive test for splenic and hepatic masses, especially when there is copious abdominal effusion. Radiographs may reveal a mass if there is minimal free peritoneal fluid. Abdominocentesis typically reveals hemoabdomen but not neoplastic cells. Definitive diagnosis requires biopsy (via laparotomy) because splenic hematoma, hemangioma, and widespread accessory splenic tissue masquerade as hemangiosarcoma but have a much better prognosis. Two or more large tissue samples should always be submitted, and the clinician should be prepared to request recuts; hemangiosarcoma may be difficult to find histologically. Fine-needle biopsy (especially fine-needle core biopsy) is sometimes diagnostic. However, there is the risk of inducing life-threatening hemorrhage, and the patient must be watched closely after the procedure for evidence of hypovolemia.

### Treatment

Solitary masses should be excised. Chemotherapy may be palliative for some animals with multiple masses; chemotherapy is also indicated as an adjuvant postoperative treatment modality (see p. 1143).

### Prognosis

The prognosis is poor because the tumor metastasizes early.

# MISCELLANEOUS PERITONEAL DISORDERS

## ABDOMINAL CARCINOMATOSIS
### Etiology

Abdominal carcinomatosis refers to widespread, miliary peritoneal carcinomas that may have originated from various sites; intestinal and pancreatic adenocarcinomas are common neoplasms that may result in carcinomatosis.

### Clinical Features

Weight loss may be the predominant complaint, although some animals are presented because of obvious abdominal effusion.

### Diagnosis

Physical examination and radiography rarely help to establish the diagnosis. Ultrasonography may reveal masses or infiltrates if they are large enough; however, small, miliary lesions can be missed by ultrasound. Fluid analysis reveals a nonseptic exudate or a modified transudate; epithelial neoplastic cells are occasionally found (see Chapter 36). Laparoscopy or abdominal exploratory surgery with histologic examination of biopsy specimens is usually needed for diagnosis.

### Treatment

Intracavitary chemotherapy has been palliative for some animals, although generally there is no effective treatment for this disorder. Cisplatin (50 to 70 mg/m$^2$ every 3 weeks) and 5-fluorouracil (150 mg/m$^2$ every 2 to 3 weeks) are frequently effective in decreasing fluid accumulation in dogs with carcinomatosis but should not be used in cats; carboplatin (150 to 200 mg/m$^2$ every 3 weeks) may be effective in cats.

### Prognosis

The prognosis is guarded to poor.

## FELINE INFECTIOUS PERITONITIS

Feline infectious peritonitis (FIP) is a viral disease of cats, which is discussed in detail in Chapter 102. Only the abdominal effusion of FIP is discussed here. Although a major cause of feline abdominal effusion, FIP is not the only cause. Furthermore, not all cats with FIP have effusions. FIP effusions are classically pyogranulomatous (i.e., macrophages and nondegenerate neutrophils) with a relatively low nucleated cell count (i.e., ≤10,000/μl). However, some cats with FIP have effusions that primarily contain neutrophils. A nonseptic exudate in a nonazotemic cat suggests FIP until proven otherwise.

### Suggested Readings

Allen DA et al: Prevalence of small intestinal dehiscence and associated clinical factors: a retrospective study of 121 dogs, *J Am Anim Hosp Assoc* 28(1):70, 1992.

Culvenor JA: Peritonitis following intestinal anastomosis and enteroplication in a kitten with intussusception, *Aust Vet J* 75(3):175, 1997.

Day MJ et al: A review of pathological diagnoses made from 87 canine splenic biopsies, *J Small Anim Pract* 36:426, 1995.

Drobatz KJ et al: Feline hemoperitoneum: 16 cases (1986-1993), *J Vet Emerg Crit Care* 5:93, 1997.

Greenfield CL et al: Open peritoneal drainage for treatment of contaminated peritoneal cavity and septic peritonitis in dogs and cats: 24 cases (1980-1986), *J Am Vet Med Assoc* 191(1):100, 1987.

Hardie EM et al: Sclerosing encapsulating peritonitis in four dogs and a cat, *Vet Surg* 23:107, 1994.

Hosgood G et al: Generalized peritonitis in dogs: 50 cases (1975-1986), *J Am Vet Med Assoc* 193(11):1448, 1988.

King LG: Postoperative complications and prognostic indicators in dogs and cats with septic peritonitis: 23 cases (1989-1992), *J Am Vet Med Assoc* 204(3):407, 1994.

Kyles AE et al: Foreign body intestinal perforation and intra-abdominal abscess formation as a complication of enteroplication in a dog, *Vet Rec* 143:112, 1998.

Lanz OI et al: Surgical treatment of septic peritonitis without abdominal drainage in 28 dogs, *J Am Anim Hosp Assoc* 37:87, 2001.

Merlo M et al: Radiographic and ultrasonographic features of retained surgical sponge in eight dogs, *Vet Radiol Ultrasound* 41:279, 2000.

Sharpe A et al: Intestinal haemangiosarcoma in the cat: clinical and pathological features of four cases, *J Small Anim Pract* 41:411, 2000.

Sparkes AH et al: An appraisal of the value of laboratory tests in the diagnosis of feline infectious peritonitis, *J Am Anim Hosp Assoc* 30:345, 1994.

## Drugs Used in Gastrointestinal Disorders

| GENERIC NAME | TRADE NAME | DOSE FOR DOGS | DOSE FOR CATS |
|---|---|---|---|
| Albendazole | Valbazen | 25 mg/kg PO q12h for 3-4 days | Same for 5 days |
| Aluminum hydroxide | Amphojel | 10-30 mg/kg; PO q6-8h | Unknown |
| Amikacin | Amiglyde | 20-25 mg/kg IV q24h | Same |
| Aminopentamide | Centrine | 0.01-0.03 mg/kg PO, IV, SQ q8-12h | 0.02 mg/kg PO, SQ q8-12h |
| Amoxicillin | | 22 mg/kg PO, IM, SQ, q12h | Same |
| Amphotericin B | Fungizone | 0.1-0.5 mg/kg IV q2-3d; watch for toxicity | 0.1-0.3 mg/kg IV q2-3d; watch for toxicity |

| GENERIC NAME | TRADE NAME | DOSE FOR DOGS | DOSE FOR CATS |
|---|---|---|---|
| Amphotericin B (lipid complex or liposomal) | Abelcet AmBisome | 1.1-3.3 mg/kg/treatment IV; watch for toxicity | 0.5-2.2 mg/kg/treatment IV; not approved, watch for toxicity |
| Ampicillin | | 22 mg/kg IV, q6-8h | Same |
| Amprolium | | 50 mg/kg (puppies) for 3-5 days (not approved) | Do not use |
| Apomorphine | | 0.02-0.04 mg/kg IV; 0.04-0.1 mg/kg SQ | Do not use |
| Atropine | | 0.02-0.04 mg/kg IV, SQ q6-8h; 0.2-0.5 mg/kg IV, IM for organophosphate toxicity | Same |
| Azathioprine | Imuran | 50 mg/m² PO q24h (not approved) | 0.3 mg/kg PO q2d (not approved and not recommended) |
| Azithromycin | Zithromax | 10 mg/kg PO q12-24h (not approved) | 5 mg/kg PO q24h (not approved) |
| Bethanechol | Urecholine | 5-15 mg total dose PO q8h | 1.2-5 mg total dose PO |
| Bisacodyl | Dulcolax | 5-15 mg total dose PO as needed | 5 mg total dose PO q24h |
| Bismuth subsalicylate | Pepto-Bismol | 1 ml/kg PO q8-12h for 1-2 days | Do not use |
| Cefazolin | Ancef | 20-25 mg/kg IV, IM, SQ q6-8h | Same |
| Cefoxitin | Mefoxin | 22-30 mg/kg IV, IM, SQ q6-8h (not approved) | Unknown, probably the same |
| Chlorambucil | Leukeran | Not used for IBD | 1 mg twice weekly for cats <3.5 kg; 2 mg twice weekly for cats >3.5 kg (not approved) |
| Chloramphenicol | | 50 mg/kg PO, IV, SQ q8h | Same, but q12h |
| Chlorpromazine | Thorazine | 0.3-0.5 mg/kg IV, IM, SQ q8-12h for vomiting | Same |
| Cimetidine | Tagamet | 5-10 mg/kg PO, IV, SQ q6-8h | Same |
| Cisapride | Propulsid | 0.25-0.5 mg/kg PO q8-12h | 2.5-5 mg total dose PO q8-12h (1 mg/kg maximum dose) |
| Clindamycin | Antirobe | 11 mg/kg PO q8h | Same |
| Cyproheptadine | Periactin | Not used for anorexia | 2-4 mg total dose |
| Dexamethasone | Azium | 0.05-0.1 mg/kg IV, SQ, PO q24h for inflammation | Same |
| Diazepam | Valium | Not used for anorexia | 0.2 mg IV |
| Dicyclomine | Bentyl | 0.15 mg/kg PO q8h | Unknown |
| Dioctyl sodium sulfosuccinate | Colace | 10-100 mg total dose PO, depending on weight, q8-12h | 10-25 mg total dose PO q12-24h |
| Diphenhydramine | Benadryl | 2-4 mg/kg PO; 1-2 mg/kg IV, IM q8h | Same |
| Diphenoxylate | Lomotil | 0.05-0.2 mg/kg PO q8-12h | Do not use |
| Doxycycline | Vibramycin | 10 mg/kg PO q24h | 2.5-5 mg/kg PO q12h |
| Enrofloxacin | Baytril | 2.5-20 mg/kg PO q12h | Same |
| Episprantel | Cestex | 5.5 mg/kg PO once | 2.75 mg/kg PO once |
| Erythromycin | | 11-22 mg/kg PO q8h (for antimicrobial action); 1 mg/kg PO q8h (for prokinetic activity) | Same |
| Famotidine | Pepcid | 0.5-1.0 mg/kg PO, IV q12-24h | Same (not approved) |
| Fenbendazole | Panacur | 50 mg/kg PO q24h for 3-5 days | Not approved, but probably the same as for dogs |
| Flunixin meglumine | Banamine | 1 mg/kg IV for septic shock | Not recommended |
| Furazolidone | Furoxone | 4.4 mg/kg PO q12h for 5 days for giardiasis | Same |
| Itraconazole | Sporanox | 5 mg/kg PO q12h | Same |
| Ivermectin | | 200 µg/kg SQ (not in Collies or other sensitive breeds) for intestinal parasites | 250 µg/kg SQ |
| Kaopectate | | 1-2 ml/kg PO q8-12h | Same |
| Ketamine | | Not used | 1-2 mg/kg IV for 5-10 minutes of restraint |
| Ketoconazole | Nizoral | 10-20 mg/kg PO q24h | Same (usually divided dose) |
| Lactulose | Cephulac | 0.2 ml/kg PO q8-12h, then adjust (not approved) | 5 ml total dose PO q8h (not approved) |

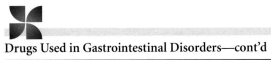

Drugs Used in Gastrointestinal Disorders—cont'd

| GENERIC NAME | TRADE NAME | DOSE FOR DOGS | DOSE FOR CATS |
|---|---|---|---|
| Loperamide | Imodium | 0.1-0.2 mg/kg PO q8-12h (not approved) | 0.08-0.16 mg/kg PO q12h (not approved) |
| Magnesium hydroxide | Milk of Magnesia | 5-10 ml total dose PO q6-8h (antacid) | 5-10 ml total dose PO q8-12h (antacid) |
| Megestrol acetate | Ovaban | Not recommended | Not recommended |
| Mesalamine | Pentasa | 10-20 mg/kg PO q12h (not approved) | Not recommended |
| Methscopolamine | Pamine | 0.3-1 mg/kg PO q8h | Unknown |
| Methylprednisolone acetate | Depo-Medrol | 1 mg/kg IM q1-3wk | 10-40 mg total dose IM q1-3wk |
| Metoclopramide | Reglan | 0.25-0.5 mg/kg IV, PO, IM q8-24h 1-2 mg/kg/day, CRI | Same (not approved) |
| Metronidazole | Flagyl | 25-50 mg/kg PO q24h for 5-7 days for giardiasis; 10-15 mg/kg PO q12h for IBD | 25-50 mg/kg PO q24h for 5 days for giardiasis |
| Milbemycin | Interceptor | 0.5 mg/kg PO monthly | Not approved |
| Misoprostol | Cytotec | 2-5 µg/kg PO q8h (not approved) | Unknown |
| Neomycin | Biosol | 10-20 mg/kg PO q6-12h | Same |
| Nizatidine | Axid | 5 mg/kg PO q24h (not approved) | Unknown |
| Olsalazine | Dipentum | 10 mg/kg PO q12h (not approved) | Unknown |
| Omeprazole | Prilosec | 0.7-1.5 mg/kg PO q12-24h (not approved) | Same (not approved) |
| Ondansetron | Zofran | 0.5-1 mg/kg PO; 0.1-0.2 mg/kg IV q8-24h (not approved) | Unknown |
| Oxazepam | Serax | Not used for anorexia | 2.5 mg total dose PO |
| Oxytetracycline | | 22 mg/kg PO q12h | Same |
| Pancreatic enzymes | Viokase-V Pancreazyme | 1-3 tsp/454 g of food | Same |
| Paregoric | Corrective mixture | 0.05 mg/kg PO q12h (not approved) | Not recommended |
| Piperazine | | 44-66 mg/kg PO once | Same |
| Praziquantel | Droncit | See manufacturer's recommendations | See manufacturer's recommendations |
| Prednisolone | | 1-2 mg/kg PO, IV, SQ, q24h or divided, for antiinflammatory effects | Same |
| Prochlorperazine | Compazine | 0.1-0.5 mg/kg IM q8-12h | 0.13 mg/kg IM q12h (not approved) |
| Propantheline | Pro-Banthine | 0.25-0.5 mg/kg PO q8-12h (not approved) | Same (not approved) |
| Psyllium hydrocolloid | Metamucil | 1-2 tsp/454 g of food | Same |
| Pyrantel pamoate | Nemex | 5 mg/kg PO | 20 mg/kg PO |
| Pyridostigmine | Mestinon | 0.5-2 mg/kg PO q8-12h | Not used |
| Rantidine | Zantac | 2 mg/kg PO, IV, IM, q8-12h (not approved) | 2.5 mg/kg IV; 3.5 mg/kg PO bid |
| Selemectin | Revolution | 6 mg/kg topically (not approved) | 6 mg/kg topical |
| Sucralfate | Carafate | 0.5-1 g q6-8h, depending on size | 0.25 g q6-12h |
| Sulfadimethoxine | Albon | 50 mg/kg PO first day, then 27.5 mg/kg PO q12h for 9 days | Same |
| Sulfasalazine | Azulfidine | 10-15 mg/kg PO q6-8h | Not recommended, but 7.5 mg/kg PO q12h is used |
| Tetracycline | | 20 mg/kg PO q8-12h | Same |
| Thiabendazole | Omnizole | 50 mg/kg PO q24h for 3 days (not approved) | Unknown |
| Toltrazuril | Baycox | 5-20 mg/kg PO q24h (dogs) | Unknown (cats) |
| Trimethobenzamide | Tigan | 3 mg/kg IM q8h (not approved) | Unknown |
| Trimethoprim-sulfadiazine | Tribrissen | 30 mg/kg PO q24h for 10 days | Same as for dogs |
| Tylosin | Tylan | 20-40 mg/kg PO q12-24h in food | Same |
| Vitamin B$_{12}$ | None | 100-200 mg PO q24h or 0.25-1.0 mg IM, SQ q7d (dogs) | 50-100 mg PO q24h (cats) |
| Xylazine | Rompun | 1.1 mg/kg IV; 2.2 mg/kg SQ, IM | 0.44 mg/kg IM or IV for emesis |

# CHAPTER 35

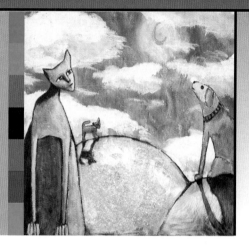

# Clinical Manifestations of Hepatobiliary Disease

## CHAPTER OUTLINE

GENERAL CONSIDERATIONS, 472
ABDOMINAL ENLARGEMENT, 472
    Organomegaly, 472
    Abdominal effusion, 474
    Abdominal muscular hypotonia, 476
JAUNDICE, BILIRUBINURIA, AND CHANGE IN FECAL COLOR, 476
HEPATIC ENCEPHALOPATHY, 479
COAGULOPATHIES, 481
POLYURIA AND POLYDIPSIA, 482

## GENERAL CONSIDERATIONS

Clinical signs of hepatobiliary disease in cats and dogs can be extremely variable, ranging from anorexia and weight loss to abdominal effusion, jaundice, and hepatic coma (Table 35-1). However, none of these signs are pathognomonic for hepatobiliary disease, and they must be distinguished from identical signs caused by disease of other organ systems. The severity of the clinical sign does not necessarily correlate with the prognosis or with the degree of liver injury, although several of these signs are often seen together in dogs and cats with end-stage hepatic disease (e.g., ascites, metabolic encephalopathy from hepatocellular dysfunction and acquired portosystemic venous shunting, bleeding). At the opposite end of the spectrum of hepatobiliary disease, there may be no clues for the presence of a hepatic disorder except for abnormal screening test results obtained before an elective anesthetic procedure.

## ABDOMINAL ENLARGEMENT

### ORGANOMEGALY

Abdominal enlargement may be the presenting complaint of owners of cats and dogs with hepatobiliary disease, or it may be noted during physical examination. Organomegaly, fluid expansion of the peritoneal space, or poor abdominal muscle tone is usually the cause of this abnormality.

Enlarged organs that most often account for increased abdominal size are the liver, the spleen (see Chapter 90), and occasionally the kidneys (see Chapter 41). Normally, the liver is palpable just caudal to the costal arch along the ventral body wall in the cat and dog, but it may not be palpable at all (Fig. 35-1). Inability to palpate the liver, especially in dogs, does not automatically mean it is abnormally small. In lean cats it is possible to palpate the diaphragmatic surface of the liver. In cats or dogs with pleural effusion or other diseases that expand thoracic volume, the liver may be displaced caudally and appear to be enlarged.

The pattern of liver enlargement may be generalized or focal, depending on the cause. Infiltrative and congestive disease processes or those that stimulate hepatocellular hypertrophy or mononuclear-phagocytic cell hyperplasia tend to result in smooth or slightly irregular, firm, diffuse hepatomegaly. Focal or asymmetrical hepatic enlargement is often seen with proliferative or expansive diseases that form solid or cystic mass lesions. Examples of such diseases are listed in Table 35-2.

Smooth, generalized hepatosplenomegaly may be associated with nonhepatic causes, such as increased intravascular hydrostatic pressure (passive congestion) secondary to right-sided congestive heart failure or pericardial disease. In rare instances, hepatic vein occlusion (Budd-Chiari syndrome) results in similar findings. Hepatosplenomegaly in icteric dogs or cats may be attributable to benign mononuclear-phagocytic cell hyperplasia and extramedullary hematopoiesis secondary to immune-mediated hemolytic anemia or to infiltrative processes such as lymphoma, systemic mast cell disease, or myeloid leukemia.

Another cause of hepatosplenomegaly is primary hepatic parenchymal disease with sustained intrahepatic portal hypertension. In dogs and cats with this disease, the liver is usually firm and irregular on palpation (the spleen can be enlarged and congested from portal hypertension). For conditions that involve primarily the spleen, see Chapter 90.

TABLE 35-1

## Clinical Signs and Physical Examination Findings in Cats and Dogs with Hepatobiliary Disease

**General, Nonspecific**

Anorexia
Depression
Lethargy
Weight loss
Small body stature
Poor or unkempt haircoat
Nausea, vomiting
Diarrhea
Dehydration

**More Specific but not Pathognomonic**

Abdominal enlargement (organomegaly, effusion, or muscular hypotonia)

**More Specific but not Pathognomonic—cont'd**

Jaundice, bilirubinuria, acholic feces
Metabolic encephalopathy
   Behavioral changes (aggression, dementia, hysteria)
   Circling, ataxia, staggering, aimless pacing, head pressing,
     cortical blindness
   Intermittent hypersalivation
   Tremors
   Generalized seizures
   Coma
Coagulopathies
Polydipsia, polyuria

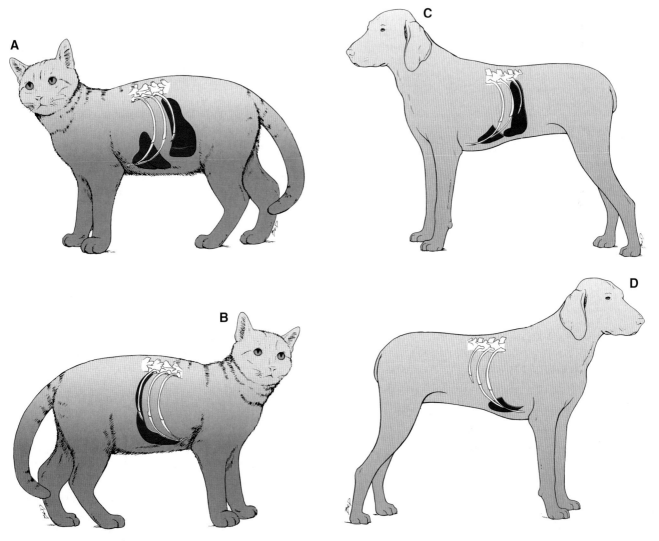

**FIG 35-1**
Position of the liver and spleen (variable) in the normal cat (**A** and **B**) and dog (**C** and **D**) during abdominal palpation with the animal standing.

TABLE 35-2

## Differential Diagnoses for Changes in Hepatic Size

| DIAGNOSIS | SPECIES |
|---|---|
| **Hepatomegaly** | |
| ***Generalized*** | |
| Infiltration | |
| Primary or metastatic neoplasia | C, D |
| Chronic hepatitis complex | D |
| Cholangitis | C |
| Extramedullary hematopoiesis* | C, D |
| Mononuclear-phagocytic cell hyperplasia* | C, D |
| Amyloidosis (rare) | C, D |
| Passive congestion* | |
| Right-sided heart failure | C, D |
| Pericardial disease | D |
| Caudal vena cava obstruction | D |
| Caval syndrome | D |
| Budd-Chiari syndrome (rare) | C, D |
| Hepatocellular hypertrophy | |
| Lipidosis | C (moderate to marked), D (mild) |
| Hypercortisolism (steroid hepatopathy) | D |
| Anticonvulsant drug therapy | D |
| Acute extrahepatic bile duct obstruction | C, D |
| Acute hepatotoxicity | C, D |
| ***Focal or asymmetric*** | |
| Primary or metastatic neoplasia | C, D |
| Nodular hyperplasia | D |
| Chronic hepatic disease with fibrosis and nodular regeneration | D |
| Abscess(es) (rare) | C, D |
| Cysts (rare) | C, D |
| **Microhepatia (Generalized Only)** | |
| Reduced hepatic mass† | |
| Chronic hepatic disease with progressive loss of hepatocytes | D |
| Decreased portal blood flow with hepatocellular atrophy | |
| Congenital portosystemic shunt | C, D |
| Intrahepatic portal vein hypoplasia | D |
| Chronic portal vein thrombosis | D |
| Hypovolemia | |
| Shock? | ? |
| Addison's disease | D |

*Concurrent splenomegaly likely.
†Loss of portal blood flow to one lobe can cause the lobe to atrophy.
*C*, Primarily cats; *D*, primarily dogs; *C, D*, cats and dogs.

## ABDOMINAL EFFUSION

The origin of abdominal effusion in cats and dogs with hepatobiliary disease is determined by chemical and cytologic analysis of a fluid specimen, the results of which reflect the mechanism of formation (Fig. 35-2). The term *ascites* is reserved for fluid of low protein content and low cell count and is usually related to disorders of hepatic or cardiovascular origin. A small amount of effusion is suspected when abdominal palpation yields a "slippery" sensation during physical examination. Moderate-to-large–volume effusion is frequently conspicuous but may distend the abdomen so much that details of abdominal organs are obscured during palpation. Whether there is small- or large-volume effusion, the general pathogeneses of third-space fluid accumulation (excessive formation by increased venous hydrostatic pressure, decreased intravascular oncotic pressure, or altered vascular permeability and insufficient resorption), singly or in combination, apply to cats and dogs with hepatobiliary diseases. On the basis of cell and protein content, abdominal fluids are classified by standard criteria as transudates (moderate-to-low cellularity with moderate-to-low protein concentration) or exudates (high cellularity and protein concentration; see Chapter 36).

Intrahepatic portal venous hypertension is the most common mechanism leading to ascites in companion animals with hepatobiliary diseases. Whether abdominal effusion forms or not depends on the site, rate, and degree of defective venous outflow. Sustained resistance to intrahepatic portal blood flow at the level of the portal triad favors exudation of fluid from more proximal (in the direction of portal blood flow; i.e., intestinal) lymphatics into the abdominal cavity. The fluid is generally of low protein content and is hypocellular. Inflammatory or neoplastic cellular infiltrates or fibrosis in this region of the liver are the pathologic processes most often responsible for this type of effusion. Sinusoidal obstruction caused by regenerative nodules, collagen deposition, or cellular infiltrates causes effusion of a fluid composed of a mixture of hepatic and intestinal lymph that has a variable protein content and generally low cell count.

Prehepatic portal venous occlusion or the presence of a large arteriovenous fistula, leading to portal venous volume overload, and associated high intrahepatic vascular resistance triggered by increased portal flow also produce a low-protein, hypocellular effusion, as would diffuse mesenteric lymphatic obstruction associated with lymphoma. Examples of causes of portal venous occlusion include intraluminal obstructive masses (e.g., thrombus), extraluminal compressive masses (e.g., mesenteric lymph node, neoplasm), and portal vein hypoplasia or atresia.

Venous congestion from disease of the major hepatic veins and/or distally (i.e., thoracic caudal vena cava, heart; posthepatic venous congestion) increases formation of hepatic lymph, which exudes from superficial hepatic lymphatics. Because the endothelial cell–lined sinusoids are highly permeable, hepatic lymph is of high protein content. Abdominal effusion formed under these conditions is more likely to develop in dogs than in cats. Reactive hepatic veins that behave as postsinusoidal sphincters have been identified in dogs and are speculated to add to venous outflow impingement. Certain concurrent factors in dogs (and rarely cats) with hepatic parenchymal failure such as hypoalbuminemia ($\leq$1.5 g/dl), an altered rate of peritoneal resorption, or sodium and water retention may further enhance movement of fluid into the peritoneal space. Perivenular pyogranulomatous infiltrates in the

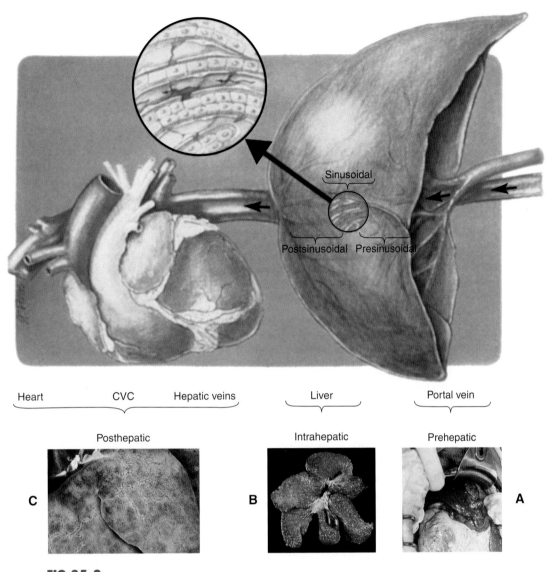

**Heart**  **CVC**  **Hepatic veins**  **Liver**  **Portal vein**

Posthepatic  Intrahepatic  Prehepatic

C  B  A

**FIG 35-2**
Mechanisms of abdominal fluid accumulation associated with altered portal and hepatic blood flow and clinical correlates. PREHEPATIC: arteriovenous fistula **(A)** or portal vein obstruction or hypoplasia; INTRAHEPATIC, presinusoidal: periportal fibrosis or portal venule hypoplasia; INTRAHEPATIC sinusoidal: cellular infiltrates or collagen **(B)**; INTRAHEPATIC postsinusoidal: central (terminal hepatic) venular fibrosis; POSTHEPATIC (passive congestion): obstruction of hepatic veins or intrathoracic caudal vena cava, right-sided heart failure **(C)** or pericardial disease. Arrows indicate direction of venous blood flow. (From Johnson SE: Portal hypertension. I. Pathophysiology and clinical consequences, *Compend Contin Educ* 9:741, 1987.)

visceral and parietal peritoneum of cats with the effusive form of feline infectious peritonitis increase vascular permeability and promote exudation of straw-colored, protein-rich fluid into the peritoneal space. Typically the fluid is of low-to-moderate cellularity, with a pleomorphic cell population of neutrophils and macrophages, and with a moderate-to-high protein concentration.

Hepatobiliary malignancies or other intraabdominal carcinomas that have disseminated to the peritoneum can elicit an inflammatory reaction, with subsequent exudation of lymph and fibrin. The fluid may be serosanguineous, hemorrhagic, or chylous in appearance. Regardless of the gross appearance of the fluid, the protein content is variable, and the

fluid is likely to contain exfoliated malignant cells if the primary neoplasm is a carcinoma, mesothelioma, or lymphoma.

Extravasation of bile from a ruptured biliary tract elicits a strong inflammatory response and stimulates transudation of lymph by serosal surfaces. The damaging component of bile has been identified as bile acids in experimental animal models. Unlike with most other causes of abdominal effusion associated with hepatobiliary disease, there may be evidence of cranial abdominal or diffuse abdominal pain identified during physical examination in cats and dogs with bile peritonitis. The fluid appears characteristically dark orange, yellow, or green, and the predominant cell type is the healthy neutrophil, except when the biliary tract is infected. Because normal bile is sterile,

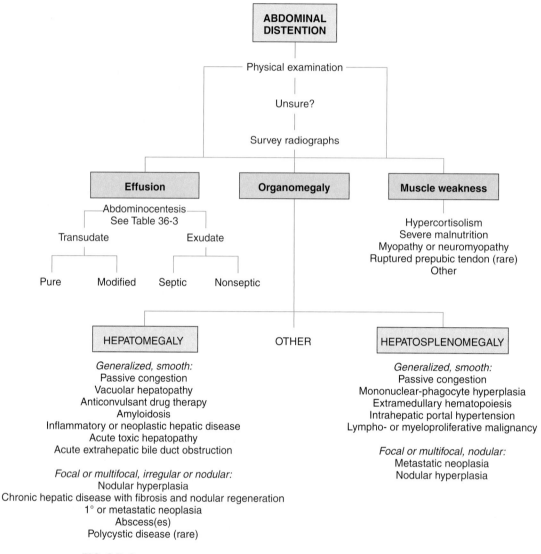

**FIG 35-3**
Algorithm for initial evaluation of the cat or dog with abdominal distention.

the initial phase of bile peritonitis is nonseptic, but unless treatment is initiated rapidly, secondary infection, usually with anaerobes, may become life-threatening.

## ABDOMINAL MUSCULAR HYPOTONIA

The presence of a distended abdomen in the absence of organomegaly or abdominal effusion suggests abdominal muscular hypotonia. Either the catabolic effects of severe malnutrition or excess endogenous or exogenous corticosteroids reduce muscular strength, giving the appearance of an enlarged abdomen. In both cats and dogs with hyperadrenocorticism, the combination of generalized hepatomegaly (mild and associated with diabetes mellitus in cats), redistribution of fat stores to the abdomen, and muscular weakness causes abdominal distention.

On the basis of physical examination, the problem of abdominal enlargement should be refined to the level of organomegaly, abdominal effusion, or poor muscular tone, as shown in Fig. 35-3. Additional tests are required to obtain a definitive diagnosis.

## JAUNDICE, BILIRUBINURIA, AND CHANGE IN FECAL COLOR

By definition, jaundice in cats and dogs is the yellow staining of serum or tissues by an excessive amount of bile pigment or bilirubin; the terms *jaundice* and *icterus* may be used interchangeably. Because the normal liver has the ability to take up and excrete a large amount of bilirubin, there must be either a large, persistent increase in the production of bile pigment (hyperbilirubinemia) or a major impairment in bile excretion (cholestasis with hyperbilirubinemia) before jaundice is detectable as yellow-stained tissues (serum bilirubin concentration $\geq 2$ mg/dl) or serum (serum bilirubin concentration $\geq 1.5$ mg/dl).

In normal animals, bilirubin is a waste product of heme protein degradation. The primary source of heme proteins is senescent erythrocytes, with a small contribution by myoglobin and heme-containing enzyme systems in the liver. After phagocytosis by cells of the mononuclear-phagocytic system, primarily in the bone marrow and spleen, heme oxygenase opens

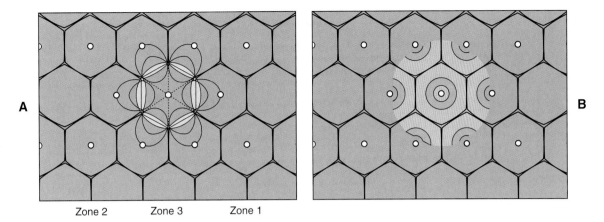

**FIG 35-4**
**A,** Rappaport scheme of the hepatic functional lobule (acinus), organized according to biochemical considerations (1958). For example, zone 1 cells are responsible for protein synthesis, urea and cholesterol production, gluconeogenesis, bile formation, and cytogenesis; zone 2 cells also produce albumin and are actively involved in glycolysis and pigment formation; and zone 3 cells are the major site of liponeogenesis, ketogenesis, and drug metabolism. **B,** Outdated theory of hepatic functional lobule as first proposed in 1833. The apparent hexagonal boundaries have little to do with functional arrangement.

the protoporphyrin ring of hemoglobin, forming biliverdin. Biliverdin reductase converts biliverdin to fat-soluble bilirubin IXa, which is released into the circulation, where it is bound to albumin for transport to hepatic sinusoidal membranes. After uptake, transhepatocellular movement, and conjugation to various carbohydrates, conjugated bilirubin, now water-soluble, is excreted into the bile canaliculi. Conjugated bilirubin is then incorporated into micelles and stored with other bile constituents in the gallbladder until it is discharged into the duodenum. After arrival in the intestine, conjugated bilirubin undergoes bacterial deconjugation and then reduction to urobilinogen, with most urobilinogen being resorbed into the enterohepatic circulation. A small fraction of urobilinogen is then excreted in the urine, and a small portion remains in the intestinal tract to be converted to stercobilin, which imparts normal fecal color.

Inherited abnormalities of bilirubin metabolism have not been identified in cats and dogs; thus, in the absence of massive increases in bile pigment production by hemolysis, jaundice is attributable to impaired excretion of bilirubin (and usually other constituents of bile) by diffuse intrahepatic hepatocellular or biliary disease or by interrupted delivery of bile to the duodenum. The inability to take up, intracellularly process, or excrete bilirubin into the bile canaliculi (the rate-limiting step) is the mechanism of cholestasis believed to be operational in many primary hepatocellular diseases. Jaundice is more likely to be a clinical feature if the liver disorder involves primarily the periportal (zone 1) hepatocytes (Fig. 35-4) than if the lesion involves centrilobular (zone 3) hepatocytes. Inflammation and swelling of larger intrahepatic biliary structures could similarly delay bile excretion.

Obstruction of the bile duct near the duodenum results in increased intraluminal biliary tract pressure, interhepatocellular regurgitation of bile constituents into circulation, and jaundice. If only one of the hepatic bile ducts exiting the liver is blocked or if only the cystic duct exiting the gallbladder is obstructed for some reason, there may be biochemical clues for localized cholestasis, such as high serum alkaline phosphatase activity; however, the liver's overall ability to excrete is preserved and jaundice does not ensue. Traumatic or pathologic biliary tract rupture allows leakage of bile into the peritoneal space and some absorption of bile components. Depending on the underlying cause and the time elapsed between biliary rupture and diagnosis, the degree of jaundice may be mild to moderate. If biliary rupture has occurred, the total bilirubin content of the abdominal effusion is greater than that of serum.

Reference ranges for serum total bilirubin concentrations in dogs and cats may vary from laboratory to laboratory, but most published resources agree that concentrations over 0.3 mg/dl in cats and 0.6 mg/dl in dogs are abnormal. When results of laboratory tests are assessed, species differences in the formation and renal processing of bilirubin between cats and dogs must be taken into account. Canine renal tubules have a low resorptive threshold for bilirubin. Dogs (males to a greater extent than females) have the necessary renal enzyme systems to process bilirubin to a limited extent, therefore bilirubinuria (up to 2+ to 3+ reaction by dipstick analysis) may be a normal finding in canine urine specimens of specific gravity greater than 1.025. Cats do not have this ability, and they have a ninefold higher tubular absorptive capacity for bilirubin than dogs. Bilirubinuria in cats is associated with hyperbilirubinemia and is always pathologic. Because unconjugated and most conjugated bilirubin is albumin-bound in circulation, only the small amount of non–protein-bound conjugated bilirubin is expected to appear in the urine in physiologic and pathologic states. In dogs with hepatobiliary disease, increasing bilirubinuria often precedes the development of hyperbilirubinemia and clinical jaundice, and may be the first sign of illness detected by owners.

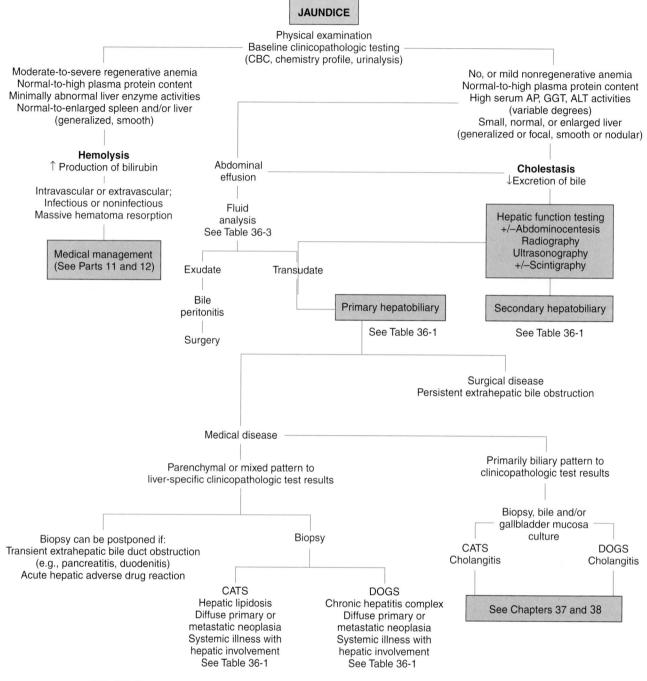

**FIG 35-5**
Algorithm for preliminary evaluation of the icteric cat or dog. *AP,* Alkaline phosphatase; *GGT,* γ-glutamyltransferase; *ALT,* alanine transaminase.

Several nonhepatobiliary disorders impede bilirubin excretion by poorly understood means. Jaundice with evidence of hepatocellular dysfunction but minimal histopathologic changes in the liver has been described in septic human and canine patients. Certain products released by bacteria, such as endotoxin, are known to reversibly interfere with bile flow. As yet unexplained mild hyperbilirubinemia (≤2.5 mg/dl) may also be detected in about 20% of hyperthyroid cats. Experimental investigations of thyrotox-

icosis in laboratory animals have demonstrated increased production of bilirubin, which has been proposed to be associated with increased degradation of hepatic heme proteins. There is no histologic evidence of cholestasis at the light microscopic level in affected cats, and the hyperbilirubinemia resolves with return to euthyroidism. Guidelines for initial evaluation of the icteric cat or dog are given in Fig. 35-5. Finally, lipemia is a common cause of pseudohyperbilirubinemia in dogs.

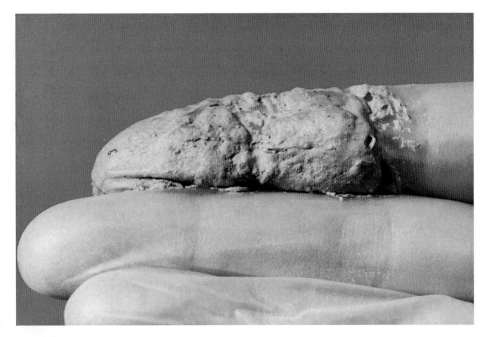

**FIG 35-6**
Acholic feces from a 7-year-old spayed female Collie dog with a strictured bile duct and complete bile duct obstruction 3 weeks after recovery from severe acute pancreatitis.

Acholic feces result from total absence of bile pigment in the intestine (Fig. 35-6). Only a small amount of bile pigment is needed to be changed to stercobilin and yield normal fecal color, therefore bile flow into the intestine must be completely discontinued in order to form acholic feces. Interruption of the normal enterohepatic recycling of dietary pigment derived from plant chlorophyll may also explain the pale appearance of acholic feces. In addition to appearing pale from lack of stercobilin and other pigments, acholic feces are pale because of steatorrhea from lack of bile acids to facilitate fat absorption. Mechanical diseases of the extrahepatic biliary tract (e.g., unremitting complete extrahepatic bile duct obstruction [EBDO], traumatic bile duct avulsion from the duodenum) are the most common causes of acholic feces in cats and dogs. Total inability to take up, conjugate, and excrete bilirubin because of generalized hepatocellular failure is theoretically possible. However, because the functional organization of the liver is heterogeneous (see Fig. 35-4) and because primary hepatic diseases do not affect all hepatocytes uniformly, the overall ability of the liver to process bilirubin may be altered, although it is usually preserved. A condition has been reported rarely in cats with severe cholangitis in which bile flow ceases. Under these circumstances, "bile" consists of only clear, viscous biliary epithelial secretions, and this may result in the production of acholic feces. A similar finding, known as "white bile syndrome," has been associated with prolonged total biliary obstruction and is thought to be the result of resorption of bile pigments. The true frequency of "white bile" in cats or dogs with severe cholestasis is not known.

## HEPATIC ENCEPHALOPATHY

Signs of abnormal mentation and neurologic dysfunction develop in dogs and cats with serious hepatobiliary disease as a result of exposure of the cerebral cortex to absorbed intestinal toxins that have not been removed by the liver. Substances that have been implicated as important in the genesis of hepatic encephalopathy (HE), singly or in combination, are ammonia, mercaptans, short-chain fatty acids, skatoles, indoles, and aromatic amino acids. Either there is marked reduction in functional hepatic mass or portal blood flow has been diverted by the development of portosystemic venous anastomoses, thus preventing detoxification of gastrointestinal (GI) toxins. Portosystemic shunting can occur via the presence of a macroscopic vascular pattern that results from a congenital vascular miscommunication or by a complex of acquired "relief valves" that open in response to sustained portal hypertension secondary to severe primary hepatobiliary disease (Fig. 35-7). Intrahepatic, microscopic portosystemic shunting or widespread hepatocellular inability to detoxify noxious enteric substances accounts for HE when an abnormal portal vascular pattern cannot be demonstrated. Rarely, if congenital portovascular anomalies and severe primary hepatobiliary disease with acquired shunting have been ruled out, congenital urea enzyme cycle deficiencies and organic acidemias, in which ammonia cannot be degraded to urea, are considered. Urinary tract infection with urea-splitting organisms (e.g., *Staphylococcus, Proteus*) could cause transient hyperammonemia and signs of HE if marked urine stasis is also present. Animals with systemic diseases having hepatic manifestations do not undergo sufficient loss of hepatic mass or change in hepatic blood flow to develop signs of HE.

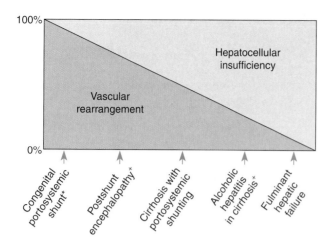

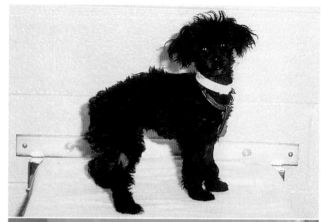

A

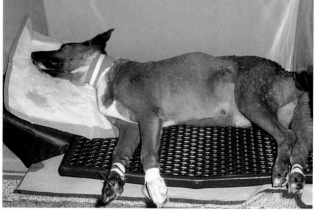

B

**FIG 35-7**
Spectrum of hepatic encephalopathy in cats and dogs ranging from pure vascular to pure hepatocellular causes. *, Clinically relevant only in dogs and cats; †, clinically relevant only in human patients. (Modified from Schafer DF et al: Hepatic encephalopathy. In Zakim D et al, editors: *Hepatology: a textbook of liver disease*, Philadelphia, 1990, WB Saunders.)

 TABLE 35-3

**Encephalotoxins Believed to Be Involved in the Pathogenesis of Hepatic Encephalopathy**

Ammonia*
Amino acid neurotransmitters (γ-aminobutyric acid, L-glutamate)
Benzodiazepine receptors and endogenous benzodiazepines
Aromatic amino acids*
Methionine, converted to mercaptans*
Skatoles*
Octopamine
Indoles*
Tryptophan
Serotonin

*Intestinal origin.

**FIG 35-8**
Two dogs with similar fasting plasma ammonia concentrations, emphasizing the lack of correlation between plasma ammonia content and severity of encephalopathic signs.
**A,** Female Miniature Poodle with congenital portosystemic shunt. The plasma ammonia concentration was 454 μg/dl.
**B,** Male mixed-breed dog with chronic hepatic failure and acquired portosystemic shunting. The plasma ammonia concentration was 390 μg/dl.

The pathogenesis of this reversible abnormality in cerebral metabolism currently is incompletely understood. Multiple factors are likely involved, including accumulation of encephalotoxins (Table 35-3), shifts in plasma amino acid composition, and increased cerebral sensitivity to biochemical changes associated with hepatic failure. Ammonia generated from endogenous and exogenous protein catabolism and endogenous urea diffused into the colon is an important, although not singular, cerebral toxin in HE. The severity of clinical signs does not correlate with the magnitude of hyperammonemia (Fig. 35-8), therefore other toxins, such as mercaptans and short-chain fatty acids, are thought to act synergistically with ammonia to alter cerebral neurotransmitter and membrane physiology. The molar ratio of branched chain amino acids (BCAA) (leucine, isoleucine, valine) to aromatic amino acids (AAA) (phenylalanine, tyrosine) is disturbed in dogs and cats with hepatic failure, approaching 2:1 or less (normal is approximately 2.2:1 to 4.8:1). Because of increased BCAA use, possibly stimulated by hyperammonemia-induced glucagon release, and diminished AAA degradation, there is a relative excess of AAAs, favoring the formation of various false and inhibitory neurotransmitters in the brain. It is not clear, however, whether these false and inhibitory neurotransmitters are important in the genesis of HE. Regardless of the mechanisms involving changes in BCAAs and AAAs, human patients with HE improve clinically when the normal serum ratio of BCAA to AAA is restored. Similar improvement is observed after administration of a mixture of BCAA to dogs made encephalopathic by intravenous infusion of tryptophan and phenylalanine.

Recent investigations of the pathogenesis of HE have focused on several areas, one of which is the role of a specific inhibitory neurotransmitter, γ-aminobutyric acid (GABA). One theory suggests that the normally small amounts of GABA present in the brain, combined with substances with GABA-like activity absorbed from the intestine into portal blood, act to disrupt the normal balance of excitatory and inhibitory neurotransmitters, resulting in neural depression and signs of HE. Studies to date have not documented alterations in brain concentrations of GABA or in GABA receptor binding in animal models of HE. The most recent hypothesis for the cause of HE concerns an as yet unidentified endogenous benzodiazepine, the concentration of which has been shown by some investigators to be increased in human patients with HE. Among other supportive evidence, some studies of both animal models and human patients with HE have shown transient improvement in signs after administration of benzodiazepine antagonists. Although endogenous benzodiazepine substances were found in the portal blood of dogs with congenital portosystemic shunt in one study (Aronson and colleagues, 1997), they were not found in the cerebrospinal fluid of dogs with created portocaval shunt in another study (Meyer and colleagues, 1998). It is unlikely that a single gut-derived, protein-based substance will be determined to be the putative encephalotoxin in animals with HE; an interaction among several seems more plausible.

Subtle, nonspecific signs of HE in cats and dogs that could be noted at any time and that represent chronic or subclinical HE include anorexia, depression, weight loss, lethargy, nausea, fever, hypersalivation, intermittent vomiting, and diarrhea. Certain events might precipitate an acute episode of HE with severe neurologic signs. During feeding, a large load of nutrients, especially protein, and enteric toxins (AAA, short-chain fatty acids, mercaptans generated from methionine) is delivered rapidly into the portal circulation for hepatic detoxification. Major GI hemorrhage is another source of protein that could account for an episode of acute HE. Drugs that require hepatic biotransformation to an inactive metabolite could bring about HE if given to an animal so predisposed. Other conditions such as azotemia, metabolic alkalosis, hypokalemia, dehydration, infection, and constipation could also precipitate HE and cause a previously stable animal to decompensate. Nearly any central nervous system (CNS) sign may be observed in cats and dogs with HE: trembling, ataxia, hysteria, dementia, marked personality change (usually toward aggressiveness), circling, head pressing, cortical blindness, or seizures (see Table 35-1). Most dogs and cats with HE have symmetrical CNS signs. There have been isolated instances in which animals with hyperammonemia have had asymmetrical, localizing neurologic signs that have regressed with appropriate treatment for HE.

## COAGULOPATHIES

Because of the integral role of the liver in hemostasis, hemorrhagic tendencies can be a presenting sign in cats and dogs with severe hepatobiliary disease. Despite the fact that most coagulation proteins and inhibitors, except for von Wille-

 TABLE 35-4

**Coagulation Proteins and Inhibitors Synthesized by the Liver**

Proteins C and S
Antithrombin
Fibrinogen
Plasminogen
Vitamin K–dependent factors
    II (prothrombin)
    VII
    IX
    X
Factor V
Factor XI
Factor XII
Factor XIII

brand's factor (vWF) and possibly factor VIII, are synthesized in the liver (Table 35-4), the overall frequency of clinical sequelae of disturbances in hemostasis is low. Inability to synthesize vitamin K–dependent factors (II, VII, IX, and X) because of the absence of bile acid–dependent fat absorption secondary to complete EBDO or a transected bile duct from abdominal trauma can cause clinically apparent bleeding. Subclinical and clinical coagulopathies are also noted in animals with severe diseases of the hepatic parenchyma. Some animals with severe hepatic disease and relatively unremarkable results of routine coagulation tests have high serum activity of proteins induced by vitamin K antagonism (PIVKA) that could impart bleeding tendencies. In early studies of the mechanism of impaired coagulation after partial hepatectomy in dogs, following surgical removal of 70% of the hepatic mass, dogs achieved significant alterations in plasma clotting factor concentrations without spontaneous hemorrhage. Having severe hepatic parenchymal disease predisposes a dog or cat not only to changes in coagulation factor activity from hepatocellular dysfunction, but also to disseminated intravascular coagulation (DIC) (see Chapter 89). In dogs with acute hepatic necrosis, some clinicians have observed thrombocytopenia thought to be associated with increased platelet use or sequestration.

Other than noticeable imbalances in coagulation factor activity, the only other mechanism by which bleeding might occur in a cat or dog with severe hepatic disease is portal hypertension–induced vascular congestion and fragility. In such cases, which are expected considerably more often in dogs than in cats because of the types of hepatobiliary diseases they acquire, the common site affected is the upper GI tract (stomach, duodenum); therefore hematemesis and melena are common bleeding presentations. In contrast to human patients, in whom fragile esophageal varices develop and can burst, causing severe and often fatal hemorrhage, the mechanism of GI hemorrhage in companion animals is unknown but is suspected to be related to poor mucosal perfusion and reduced

TABLE 35-5

**Mechanisms of Polyuria and Polydipsia in Cats and Dogs with Serious Hepatocellular Dysfunction**

Altered sense of thirst (possible manifestation of hepatic encephalopathy)—primary polydipsia with compensatory polyuria

Increased secretion of ACTH, leading to hypercortisolemia and altered threshold for ADH release

Delayed aldosterone degradation, leading to secondary hyperaldosteronism and sodium retention

Altered function of portal vein osmoreceptors

Loss of renal medullary concentrating gradient associated with low blood urea concentration

Delayed cortisol degradation

Persistent hypokalemia

*ACTH,* Adrenocorticotropic hormone; *ADH,* antidiuretic hormone.

epithelial cell turnover. Hypergastrinemia was observed in dogs made cirrhotic under experimental conditions and was theorized to have been provoked by excess serum bile acid concentrations. More recent studies have not borne out this theory. Although GI lesions identified at necropsy in other experimental investigations and in canine patients with hepatic failure may be true ulcers, they are not consistently associated with hypergastrinemia.

## POLYURIA AND POLYDIPSIA

Increased thirst and volume of urination can be clinical signs of serious hepatocellular dysfunction (Table 35-5). Several factors are suspected to contribute to polydipsia and polyuria, which are seen primarily in dogs, and rarely in cats, with marked hepatic dysfunction. Altered sense of thirst may be a manifestation of HE. Excess secretion of adrenocorticotropic hormone stimulated by abnormal neurotransmitters leads to excess cortisol secretion and altered threshold for antidiuretic hormone release in dogs with HE. Secondary hyperaldosteronism from delayed excretion of aldosterone, which is accomplished normally by the liver, leads to sodium retention and increased water intake with compensatory polyuria. Changes in the function of portal vein osmoreceptors that stimulate thirst without

hyperosmolality are also thought to be partly responsible for polydipsia. Loss of the renal medullary concentrating gradient for urea because of inability to produce urea from ammonia would first cause polyuria and then compensatory polydipsia. Delayed cortisol excretion and persistent hypokalemia may also contribute to the renal concentrating defect. Investigation of polydipsia in dogs with congenital portosystemic shunt has identified partial renal concentrating ability in response to water deprivation, with resolution of polydipsia when normal portal blood flow was reestablished.

### Suggested Readings

Aronson LR et al: Endogenous benzodiazepine activity in the peripheral and portal blood of dogs with congenital portosystemic shunts, *Vet Surg* 26:189, 1997.

Badylak SF: Coagulation disorders and liver disease, *Vet Clin North Am Small Anim Pract* 18:87, 1988.

Bunch SE: Abdominal effusion. In Ford RB, editor: *Clinical signs and diagnosis in small animal practice,* New York, 1988, Churchill Livingstone, p 521.

Center SA et al: PIVKA clotting times in dogs with suspected coagulopathies. *Proceedings of the 16th ACVIM Forum,* San Diego, Calif, 1998, p 704.

Center SA et al: PIVKA clotting time in clinically ill cats with suspected coagulopathies, *Proceedings of the 16th ACVIM Forum,* San Diego, Calif, 1998, p 704.

Hess PR et al: Management of portal hypertension and its consequences, *Vet Clin North Am Small Anim Pract* 25:461, 1995.

Johnson SE: Portal hypertension. I. Pathophysiology and clinical consequences, *Compend Contin Educ* 9:741, 1987.

Johnson SE: Portal hypertension. II. Clinical assessment and treatment, *Compend Contin Educ* 9:917, 1987.

Maddison JE: Newest insights into hepatic encephalopathy, *Eur J Compar Gastroenterol* 5:17, 2000.

Meyer HP et al: No benzodiazepine activity in cerebrospinal fluid of dogs with chronic hepatic encephalopathy, *Proceedings of the 16th ACVIM Forum,* San Diego, Calif, 1998, p 705.

Sutherland RJ: Biochemical evaluation of the hepatobiliary system in dogs and cats, *Vet Clin North Am Small Anim Pract* 19:899, 1989.

Rothuizen J et al: Chronic glucocorticoid excess and impaired osmoregulation of vasopressin release in dogs with hepatic encephalopathy, *Domest Anim Endocrinol* 12:13, 1995.

Rothuizen J: History, physical examination, and signs of liver disease. In Ettinger SJ et al, editors: *Textbook of veterinary internal medicine,* ed 5, Philadelphia, 2000, WB Saunders, p 1272.

Wright KN et al: Peritoneal effusion in cats: 65 cases (1981-1997), *J Am Vet Med Assoc* 214:375, 1999.

# CHAPTER 36

# Diagnostic Tests for the Hepatobiliary System

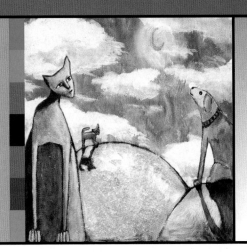

## CHAPTER OUTLINE

DIAGNOSTIC APPROACH, 483
DIAGNOSTIC TESTS, 485
    Complete blood count, 485
    Tests to assess status of the hepatobiliary system, 486
    Tests to assess function of the hepatobiliary system, 487
    Urinalysis, 490
    Fecal evaluation, 491
    Abdominocentesis/fluid analysis, 491
    Coagulation tests, 492
DIAGNOSTIC IMAGING, 492
    Survey radiography, 492
    Ultrasonography, 494
    Scintigraphy, 499
LIVER BIOPSY, 499

## DIAGNOSTIC APPROACH

Because the liver is physiologically and anatomically diverse, no single test adequately identifies liver disease or its underlying cause. For this reason, a battery of tests must be used to assess the hepatobiliary system. A reasonable package of screening tests recommended for an animal suspected of having hepatobiliary disease includes a complete blood count (CBC), serum biochemical profile, urinalysis, fecal analysis, and survey abdominal radiographs or ultrasonography. Results of these tests may suggest evidence of hepatobiliary disease that can be confirmed by other, more specific tests. The need for other laboratory tests (e.g., abdominocentesis, coagulation profile) is determined by each animal's history and physical examination findings.

Of the recommended screening tests for hepatobiliary disease, the serum biochemistry profile offers specific information regarding the distribution and activity or status (e.g., hyperbilirubinemia, enzyme activities) of a hepatobiliary disorder and an estimate of the degree of functional impairment (e.g., inadequate protein synthesis, altered toxin excretion). Determining hepatic functional capacity adds a mean-

ingful dimension to the diagnostic evaluation and permits construction of a reasonable list of differential diagnoses and tentative assignment of prognosis. It is important to remember that some hepatobiliary diseases are characterized by subtle changes in enzyme activity in association with severe functional disturbance, and some have high enzyme activities and normal functional indices. Because of the large reserve capacity of the liver, detection of global hepatic functional impairment by conventional means is not possible until there is at least 55% loss of hepatic mass. The recommended serum biochemistry profile includes albumin, urea nitrogen, bilirubin, cholesterol, and glucose concentrations, which are used to assess the ability of the liver to synthesize proteins, detoxify protein degradation products, excrete organic anions and other substances, and help to maintain euglycemia, respectively. Development of automated methods for laboratory analysis has made measurement of many substances in the blood easy; these laboratory analytic methods are available at competitive prices through commercial laboratories or as in-house test kits. For this reason, there is no excuse for excluding a multiple component serum biochemistry profile from the initial diagnostic plan for a cat or dog suspected of having hepatobiliary disease.

A sensitive, although relatively nonspecific, test of hepatobiliary function is determination of fasting and postprandial serum bile acid concentrations. Serum bile acid concentrations are measured if there are persistent liver-specific serum biochemical abnormalities.

Results of laboratory evaluation reflect one point in time in a spectrum of dynamic changes. If the test results are equivocal and the clinical signs are vague, sequential evaluation may be necessary to allow time for the disease to be fully expressed.

By using a combination of history, physical examination findings, and results of screening and hepatobiliary-specific laboratory tests, the clinician should be able to describe the disorder as active or quiescent; characterize the pattern of hepatobiliary disease as primarily hepatocellular, primarily biliary, or mixed hepatobiliary; and estimate the degree of hepatobiliary dysfunction. From this same information, an animal may be described clinically as having *hepatic disease,* with evidence of hepatic abnormalities such as high liver enzyme activities and hepatomegaly, or *hepatic failure,* in which there is a state of multiple function loss. Some primary hepatic diseases may progress to failure; most secondary hepatic diseases do not (Table 36-1). Use of the term *failure* often inappropriately connotes a poor prognosis. If the underlying cause can be removed (e.g., complete ligation of a single congenital extrahepatic portosystemic shunt [PSS]), full recovery is possible. Most important, before an accurate prognosis can be given, a complete evaluation must be conducted, including, for most primary hepatobiliary diseases, a liver biopsy.

TABLE 36-1

### Clinically Relevant Hepatobiliary Diseases

| | PRIMARY | SECONDARY |
| --- | --- | --- |
| **Common** | | |
| Cat | Idiopathic lipidosis | Secondary lipidosis |
| | | Lymphoproliferative or metastatic neoplasia (including FeLV-related) |
| | | Hyperthyroidism |
| | | Feline infectious peritonitis |
| Dog | Chronic hepatitis complex | Acute pancreatitis |
| | Congenital portosystemic venous anomaly | Extrahepatobiliary sepsis |
| | Drug-/toxin-induced hepatopathy | Vacuolar hepatopathy (hypercortisolism, diabetes mellitus, hypothyroidism, hyperlipidemia-associated in Miniature Schnauzers, other adrenal steroid?) |
| | | Right-sided congestive heart failure |
| | | Metastatic neoplasia |
| **Less Common** | | |
| Cat | Cholangitis complex | Toxoplasmosis |
| | Extrahepatic bile duct obstruction | Histoplasmosis |
| | Congenital portosystemic venous anomaly | |
| Dog | Biliary tract disease, all kinds | Leptospirosis |
| | Primary neoplasia | Canine distemper |
| | Intrahepatic portal vein hypoplasia | Histoplasmosis |
| | | Rocky Mountain spotted fever |
| | | Ehrlichiosis |
| | | Babesiosis |
| **Rare** | | |
| Cat | Drug-/toxin-induced hepatopathy | Leptospirosis |
| | Hepatic or biliary cysts | Extrahepatobiliary sepsis (?) |
| | Liver flukes (except in predatory Florida cats) | Abscess(es) |
| | Primary neoplasia | |
| | Venoocclusive disease | |
| | Peliosis hepatis | |
| | Biliary cirrhosis | |
| | Intrahepatic arteriovenous fistula | |
| | Intrahepatic portal vein hypoplasia | |
| | Massive necrosis, all causes | |
| Dog | Infectious canine hepatitis | Amyloidosis |
| | Hepatic or biliary cysts | Hepatocutaneous syndrome (superficial necrolytic dermatitis) |
| | Inherited glycogen storage disease | Abscess(es) |
| | Amyloidosis | |
| | Peliosis hepatitis | |
| | Destructive cholangiolitis | |
| | Venoocclusive disease | |
| | Intrahepatic arteriovenous fistula | |
| | Massive necrosis, all causes | |

*FeLV,* Feline leukemia virus.

## DIAGNOSTIC TESTS

### COMPLETE BLOOD COUNT

There are few changes in blood cells that suggest hepatobiliary disease. Most are changes in erythrocytes (red blood cells [RBCs]) associated with fragmentation or changes in cell size or membrane composition (Fig. 36-1). Microcytosis (mean cell volume [MCV] <60 fl in canine breeds other than the Japanese Akita or Shiba Inu) with normochromia or slight hypochromia (mean cell hemoglobin concentration: 32 to 34 g/dl) is a rather common finding in dogs with congenital PSS (≥60%); it is less common in cats with congenital PSS (≤30%). Most affected animals are not anemic. The cause of microcytosis, which has also been observed with less frequency in dogs with chronic hepatic failure and acquired PSS, is poorly understood. Although absolute iron deficiency is the most common cause of microcytosis in dogs, several recent studies of iron and copper status have eliminated this cause in dogs with congenital PSS. Because iron stores seem adequate (obviating the need for iron administration), investigators

have theorized that hyperammonemia interferes with iron incorporation into hemoglobin or that there is a defect in iron transport. Regardless of the mechanism, delay in attaining the full complement of hemoglobin causes RBC precursors to undergo an extra cell division, resulting in smaller than normal RBCs. Studies pursuing other explanations of disturbed hemoglobin synthesis, such as pyridoxine (B$_6$) deficiency, have not been undertaken. The change in RBC size is reversible upon restoration of portal blood flow. If anemia is also present, microcytosis must be distinguished from anemia of inflammatory disease, which can occasionally cause small RBCs and relative iron deficiency, or from iron deficiency anemia associated with chronic gastrointestinal blood loss (see Chapter 85).

Strongly regenerative anemia, with macrocytosis, high reticulocyte count, and normal to slightly increased serum protein concentration in a jaundiced dog, especially if spherocytes are also identified, indicates hemolytic anemia and increased bilirubin formation as the cause of jaundice. Cats and dogs with hemolytic anemia typically also have high serum

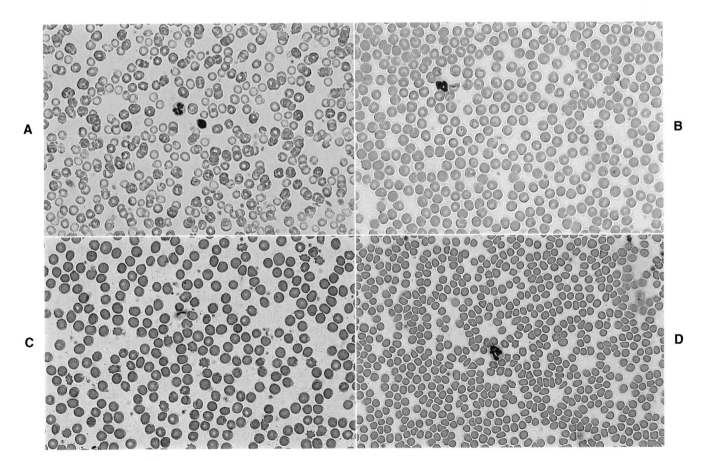

**FIG 36-1**
Erythrocyte morphologic changes often associated with hepatobiliary disease in cats and dogs (Wright-Giemsa stain). **A,** Microcytic red blood cells (mean corpuscular volume [MCV] = 45 fl) from dog with congenital portosystemic shunt; compare the microcytic RBCs with the size of a nearby normal small lymphocyte 6 to 9 μm in diameter. **B,** Normal canine red blood cells (MCV = 70 fl) for comparison. **C,** Acanthocytes from dog with severe chronic hepatic passive congestion. **D,** Poikilocytes from cat with cholangitis.

liver enzyme activities and bile acid concentrations, pointing to hepatic consequences developing secondary to the effects of marked hemolysis, such as hypoxia and thromboembolism.

Certain RBC morphologic changes are considered to be consistent with serious hepatobiliary disease and are related to alterations in lipoprotein metabolism and irregularities in RBC membrane structure. Acanthocytes, leptocytes, and codocytes (target cells) are good examples (see Fig. 36-1). Poikilocytosis of unknown pathogenesis is a consistent finding in cats with congenital PSS and occasionally with other feline hepatobiliary diseases. Fragmented RBCs or schistocytes constitute an expected finding in animals with disseminated intravascular coagulopathy (DIC); hemangiosarcoma is considered when an inappropriate number of nucleated RBCs is also detected. Mild to moderate nonregenerative anemia is common in cats with many different illnesses, including those of the hepatobiliary tract.

Few changes in the leukon are expected in cats or dogs with hepatobiliary disease except when an infectious agent is present as the initiating event (histoplasmosis, bacterial cholangitis, or leptospirosis in dogs) or when infection has complicated a primary hepatobiliary disorder (e.g., gram-negative sepsis in a dog with cirrhosis, septic bile peritonitis). Neutrophilic leukocytosis is likely in such cases, whereas pancytopenia is typical of disseminated histoplasmosis and severe toxoplasmosis in cats, and of early infectious canine hepatitis.

## TESTS TO ASSESS STATUS OF THE HEPATOBILIARY SYSTEM

### Serum Enzyme Activities

Liver-specific serum enzyme activities are included routinely in screening serum biochemistry panels and are regarded as markers of hepatocellular and biliary injury and reactivity. Marked hepatic disease can be present in patients with nominal serum enzyme activity, so finding normal values should not preclude further investigation, especially if there are clinical signs or other laboratory test results that suggest hepatobiliary disease. Increased serum activity of enzymes normally located in hepatocyte cytosol in high concentration reflects structural or functional cell membrane injury that would allow these enzymes to escape or leak into the blood. The two enzymes found to be of most diagnostic use in cats and dogs are alanine transaminase (ALT; glutamic-pyruvic transaminase [GPT]) and aspartate transaminase (AST; glutamic-oxaloacetic transaminase [GOT]). Because ALT is found principally in hepatocytes and AST (also located within hepatocyte mitochondria) has a wider tissue distribution, ALT is the enzyme selected to most accurately reflect hepatocellular injury. Less is known about the behavior of AST in various hepatobiliary diseases in companion animals, although some studies have indicated that AST is a more reliable indicator of liver injury in cats. Several recent studies have demonstrated mild to moderately high serum ALT activity (without histologic or biochemical evidence of liver injury), in addition to expected high serum activities of muscle-specific creatine kinase and AST, in dogs with skeletal muscle necrosis.

In general, the magnitude of serum ALT and AST activity

elevation approximates the extent, but not the reversibility, of hepatocellular injury. Rather than clinical relevance being assigned to absolute values for ALT or AST activity (e.g., serum ALT activity of 200 IU/L is *worse* than 100 IU/L), the values should be assessed in terms of number of fold elevations from normal. Twofold to threefold elevations in serum ALT activity are associated with mild hepatocellular lesions, fivefold to tenfold elevations are seen with moderately severe lesions, and greater than tenfold increases suggest marked hepatocellular injury.

Other enzyme activities can also be used as markers of hepatocellular injury, including arginase, sorbitol dehydrogenase, glutamate dehydrogenase, and lactate dehydrogenase, but they offer little diagnostic advantage over ALT, and methods to measure these enzyme activities are not always commercially available. Because of the location of arginase within mitochondria, its activity may be a more precise index of the severity of a hepatic lesion, as results of studies of experimentally induced hepatic disease in dogs have shown.

Serum enzyme activities that reflect new synthesis and release of enzyme in response to certain stimuli are alkaline phosphatase (AP) and γ-glutamyltransferase (GGT). Bile retention (i.e., cholestasis) is the strongest stimulus for accelerated production of these enzymes. Unlike ALT and AST, AP and GGT are in low concentration in hepatocytes and biliary epithelium and are membrane-associated, so their simply leaking out of damaged cells does not account for increased serum activity. Measurable AP activity is also detectable in nonhepatobiliary tissues of cats and dogs (including osteoblasts, intestinal mucosa, renal cortex, and placenta), but serum activity in healthy adult cats and dogs arises only from the liver, with some contribution by the bone isoenzyme in young, rapidly growing dogs and in kittens less than 15 weeks old. The half-life of feline AP is shorter than that of canine AP; thus serum activity is relatively lower in cats than in dogs with a similar degree of cholestasis. Markedly high serum AP activity of bone origin (mean total serum AP values more than fivefold higher than those in nonaffected individuals, with only the bone isoenzyme detected) was identified in certain healthy juvenile (7 months old) members of a family of Siberian Huskies (Lawler and colleagues, 1996). This change is believed to be benign and familial and should be considered when results of serum AP activity are interpreted in this breed.

Certain drugs, the most common of which are anticonvulsants (specifically, phenytoin, phenobarbital, and primidone) and corticosteroids, can elicit striking increases (up to 100-fold) in serum AP activity (and to a lesser extent GGT activity) in dogs but not in cats. There usually is no other clinicopathologic or microscopic evidence of cholestasis (i.e., hyperbilirubinemia). Anticonvulsant drugs stimulate production of AP identical to the normal liver isoenzyme; GGT activity does not change. Pharmacologic levels of corticosteroids administered orally, by injection, or topically reliably provoke a unique AP isoenzyme that is separable from the others by electrophoretic and immunoassay techniques. This characteristic is useful when interpreting high total serum AP activity in a dog with subtle clinical signs suggestive of iatrogenic or naturally occurring hypercortisolism. The corticosteroid AP isoenzyme has recently become a component of routine canine serum biochemistry profiles at several veterinary colleges and commercial laboratories. Serum GGT activity rises similarly in response to corticosteroid influence but less spectacularly. Preliminary studies and clinical experience suggest that some dogs given anticonvulsants long term, as well as dogs with chronic nonadrenal illnesses and presumably greater than physiologic circulating cortisol concentrations, may also have abnormally high serum AP activity of the corticosteroid variant.

Serum AP and GGT activities tend to be parallel in cholestatic hepatopathies of cats and dogs, although they are much less dramatic in cats. Because simultaneous measurement of serum AP and GGT may aid in differentiating seemingly benign drug-induced effects from nonicteric cholestatic hepatic disease in dogs, assessing serum AP and GGT activities together may also offer clues to the type of hepatic disorder in cats. Both enzymes are in low concentration in feline liver tissue compared with that in the canine liver and have short half-lives, so relatively smaller increases in serum activity, especially of GGT, are important signs of the presence of hepatic disease in cats. In cats, a pattern of high serum AP activity with less strikingly abnormal GGT activity is most consistent with hepatic lipidosis, although extrahepatic bile duct obstruction (EBDO) must also be considered.

## TESTS TO ASSESS FUNCTION OF THE HEPATOBILIARY SYSTEM

### Serum Albumin Concentration

The liver is virtually the only source of albumin production in the body; thus hypoalbuminemia could be a manifestation of hepatic inability to synthesize this protein. Causes other than lack of hepatic synthesis (i.e., massive glomerular or gastrointestinal loss, bleeding) must be considered before ascribing hypoalbuminemia to hepatic insufficiency. Renal protein loss can be detected presumptively by routine urinalysis. Consistent identification of positive protein dipstick reactions, especially in dilute urine with inactive sediment, justifies further evaluation by at least measurement of random urine protein/creatinine ratio (normal ratio is <1 in cats and dogs; see p. 586). If proteinuria is ruled out, diseases that cause gastrointestinal protein loss should be considered; however, these diseases usually result in equivalent loss of globulins and thus panhypoproteinemia, which is not typical of hypoproteinemia of hepatic origin. In fact, globulin concentrations frequently are normal to increased in dogs and cats with chronic inflammatory hepatic disease. Because the plasma half-life of albumin is long in cats and dogs (8 to 10 days) and there must be loss of approximately 80% of functioning hepatocytes before hypoalbuminemia is expressed, the finding of hypoalbuminemia indicates severe chronic hepatic insufficiency. Hypoalbuminemia of any cause is unusual in cats except in those with nephrotic syndrome. When serum protein concentrations are interpreted, it should be remembered that total protein values for young cats and dogs are lower than those for adults, and that puppy serum albumin concentration is similar to that in adults, whereas kitten serum albumin concentration is lower than that in adult cats.

### Serum Urea Nitrogen Concentration

Formation of urea as a means of detoxifying ammonia derived from intestinal sources takes place only in the liver. Despite this apparent advantage as a specific measure of hepatic function, serum urea concentration is commonly affected by several nonhepatic factors. Prolonged restricted protein intake because of complete anorexia or intentional reduction in protein intake for therapeutic purposes (e.g., chronic renal failure; urate, cystine, or struvite urolithiasis) is the most common cause of low blood urea nitrogen (BUN) content. As always, reference ranges should be considered for each species when interpreting BUN values. For example, a BUN concentration of 12 mg/dl is well within normal limits for dogs but is subnormal for cats. Marginally normal BUN values can be further decreased by medullary washout associated with sustained polydipsia and polyuria. If low BUN values are noted in a cat or dog with normal water intake and a good appetite for a diet with the appropriate protein content for the species (on a dry matter basis: 22% for dogs, 35% to 40% for cats), then the possibility of hepatic inability to convert ammonia to urea should be investigated.

### Serum Bilirubin Concentration

Because of the large reserve capacity of the mononuclear-phagocytic system and liver to process bilirubin (e.g., 70% hepatectomy will not cause jaundice), hyperbilirubinemia can occur only from greatly increased production or decreased excretion of bile pigment. Specific inborn errors of bilirubin uptake, conjugation, and excretion have not been documented in cats or dogs. Increased production of bilirubin from RBC destruction arises from intravascular or extravascular hemolysis and rarely from resorption of a large hematoma. Under these circumstances in dogs, serum bilirubin concentrations are usually lower than 10 mg/dl. Values usually do not increase above 10 mg/dl unless there is a concurrent flaw in bilirubin excretion. This has been borne out clinically in studies of dogs with immune-mediated hemolytic anemia in which high liver enzyme activities are observed, even before treatment with corticosteroids, and moderately delayed bilirubin excretion has been documented. It has been proposed that cholestasis results from liver injury associated with hypoxia. Therefore, because increased production *and* decreased excretion of bilirubin occur in dogs with severe hemolysis, serum bilirubin concentrations can be as high as 35 mg/dl. Icterus in cats with pure hemolytic disease is an inconsistent finding and mild if present; specific bilirubin concentrations associated with experimentally induced or naturally occurring hemolytic diseases in cats are not available.

Nearly all diseases associated with hyperbilirubinemia in cats and dogs are characterized by a mixture of conjugated and unconjugated bilirubinemia, so quantifying the two fractions by use of van den Bergh's test achieves little in discriminating primary hepatic or biliary disease versus nonhepatobiliary disease in a clinical setting. This lack of benefit in using van den Bergh's test may relate to the time between onset of illness and examination, which is usually at least several days. Under conditions of acute massive hemolysis, the total serum bilirubin concentration may consist primarily of the unconjugated form initially. As hemolysis continues, the liver is able to take up and conjugate bilirubin, accounting for a combination of unconjugated and conjugated bilirubin.

Because RBC membrane changes are often a component of many primary hepatobiliary disorders, accelerated RBC destruction often contributes to high serum bilirubin content. In such cases, there is strong clinicopathologic evidence of cholestasis (high serum AP and GGT activities with moderate to high ALT activity), and, if there is anemia, it is mild and poorly regenerative. Hyperbilirubinemia is attributed primarily to hemolysis when there is moderate to marked anemia with strong evidence of regeneration and minimal changes in serum markers of cholestasis.

### Serum Cholesterol Concentration

Total cholesterol concentration is included in serum chemistry profiles by many commercial laboratories but affords useful information for only a limited number of hepatobiliary diseases. High total cholesterol values are observed in cats and dogs with severe intrahepatic cholestasis involving bile ducts or EBDO because of impaired excretion of free cholesterol into the bile and subsequent regurgitation into the blood. An abnormal lipoprotein, lipoprotein X, appears in the blood of dogs with EBDO.

Low total serum cholesterol concentrations have been noted in dogs with chronic severe hepatocellular disease and frequently in cats and dogs with congenital PSS. It has been speculated that hypocholesterolemia is a sign of markedly altered intestinal absorption of (and increased use of) cholesterol for bile acid synthesis when the enterohepatic recirculation of bile acids is disturbed, as occurs with PSS. In other hepatobiliary diseases of cats and dogs, the total cholesterol values vary considerably within the reference range. Normal values in 4-week-old kittens are higher than those for adults; 8-week-old puppy reference ranges are the same as those for adults.

### Serum Glucose Concentration

Hypoglycemia is an unusual event associated with hepatobiliary disease in dogs and especially in cats. Lost capacity to maintain normal serum glucose concentrations occurs in animals with acquired chronic progressive hepatobiliary disease when 20% functional hepatic mass or less is remaining. This inability to maintain normal serum glucose concentrations is presumably caused by the loss of hepatocytes with functioning gluconeogenic and glycolytic enzyme systems and impaired hepatic degradation of insulin. Hypoglycemia is often a near-terminal event in dogs with chronic progressive hepatobiliary disease. In striking contrast is the frequent observation of hypoglycemia in dogs with congenital PSS. In either case, if hypoglycemia is identified and confirmed by repeating the test using sodium fluoride tubes if necessary, and if nonhepatic causes (functional hypoglycemia, sepsis, insulinoma or other neoplasm producing an insulin-like substance, Addison's disease; see Chapter 53) are excluded, either a primary hepatic tumor (e.g., hepatocellular carcinoma) or severe generalized hepatopathy is suspected.

### Serum Electrolyte Concentrations

Serum electrolyte measurements facilitate supportive care of cats and dogs with hepatobiliary disease but give no particular hints as to the character of the disorder. The most common abnormality is hypokalemia, which is attributed to a combination of excessive renal and gastrointestinal losses, reduced intake, and secondary hyperaldosteronism in dogs and cats with severe chronic hepatobiliary disease. Metabolic alkalosis, presumptive evidence of which might be abnormally high serum total carbon dioxide content confirmed by blood gas analysis, is usually caused by overzealous diuretic therapy in dogs with chronic hepatic failure and ascites. Hypokalemia and metabolic alkalosis potentiate each other and may also worsen signs of HE by promoting persistence of readily membrane-diffusible ammonia ($NH_3$).

### Serum Bile Acid Concentrations

Recent validation of rapid, technically simple methods for serum bile acid (SBA) analysis in cats and dogs has provided a sensitive, variably specific test of hepatocellular function and the integrity of the enterohepatic portal circulation. "Primary" bile acids (i.e., cholic, chenodeoxycholic) are synthesized only in the liver, where they are conjugated with various amino acids (primarily taurine) before secretion into the bile. Bile is stored in the gallbladder, where it is concentrated until, under the influence of cholecystokinin, it is released into the duodenum. After facilitating fat absorption in the small intestine, the primary bile acids are efficiently absorbed into the portal vein and returned to the liver for reuptake and resecretion into the bile. A small percentage of primary bile acids that escapes resorption is converted by intestinal bacteria to "secondary" bile acids (i.e., deoxycholic, lithocholic), some of which are also resorbed into the portal circulation. Absorption of bile acids by the intestine is extremely efficient, but hepatic extraction from portal venous blood is not. This accounts for small concentrations of cholic, chenodeoxycholic, and deoxycholic acids that are released into the peripheral blood of healthy cats and dogs in the fasting state (total $<5$ μmol/L by enzymatic method and 5 to 10 μmol/L by radioimmunoassay [RIA]). During a meal, a large load of bile acids is delivered to the intestine and portal circulation for recycling; postprandial values in normal dogs and cats may increase up to threefold to fourfold over fasting values (15 μmol/L with the enzymatic method for cats and dogs; 25 μmol/L with the RIA method for dogs). Normal values for juvenile animals are similar to adult reference ranges. Abnormally high fasting and/or postprandial SBA concentrations reflect disturbance in hepatic secretion into the bile or at any point along the path of portal venous return to the liver and hepatocellular uptake. Low SBA concentrations may be attributable to small intestinal (ileal) malabsorption of bile acids but might be difficult to interpret because both fasting and postprandial SBA concentrations may not be measurable in healthy animals.

The standard way to assess SBA concentrations is to collect a 3-ml blood sample in a serum tube after the animal was fasted for 12 hours. Feeding a small amount of food that is normal in fat content (approximately 27% fat [dry matter basis] in dogs) is a form of endogenous challenge or tolerance test that stimulates gallbladder contraction and discharge of bile acids into the intestine; 2 hours after the meal, another 3-ml blood sample is collected. Collective experience indicates that the likelihood of precipitating an episode of HE during this part of the test is extremely low, even in predisposed animals. After the serum is harvested, the samples may be refrigerated for several days or frozen almost indefinitely before assay.

Recent studies of SBAs have confirmed their value in detecting clinically relevant hepatobiliary disease requiring definitive diagnostic testing in cats and dogs, especially in anicteric animals with equivocal clinical signs and unexplained high liver enzyme activity. There continues to be controversy as to whether a fasting or postprandial value alone is sufficient or whether fasting and postprandial measurements are required. If only one sample can be obtained (and the animal will eat or can tolerate being force-fed a small meal), the postprandial value is most useful to determine the presence or absence, but not the type of clinically relevant hepatobiliary disease in most cats and dogs. Current recommendations state that for animals suspected of having acquired hepatobiliary disease, biopsy is needed when postprandial SBA concentration using the enzymatic method exceeds 20 $\mu$mol/L in cats and 25 $\mu$mol/L in dogs. No pattern of preprandial and postprandial values is pathognomonic for any particular hepatic disorder, although it is safe to make certain generalizations. Magnitude of elevation above 20 $\mu$mol/L in cats and 25 $\mu$mol/L in dogs roughly correlates with the severity, but not the reversibility, of the hepatobiliary disorder. The change between the fasting value and the postprandial value likely corresponds to portosystemic shunting, either microscopic (intrahepatic) or macroscopic. There is so much overlap in fasting and postprandial SBA patterns among primary hepatobiliary diseases that no particular statement can be made regarding the specific causative hepatobiliary disease. In general, secondary hepatic diseases cause more modest hepatobiliary dysfunction (SBA values <100 $\mu$mol/L).

For the diagnosis of congenital PSS, fasting and postprandial SBA determinations are recommended in order to enhance detection ability, because it is relatively common for fasting values to be well within normal limits and for postprandial values to be as high as tenfold to twentyfold higher than normal postprandial values.

Now that simplified methods for SBA measurement have been developed (i.e., enzymatic, RIA) and are accessible, determination of total SBA has become a convenient, practical test of hepatobiliary function in cats and dogs. Some reference laboratories use an adapted enzymatic method, a commercial enzymatic kit (Enzabile; Nyegaard and Co., Olso, Norway), or a commercial RIA (Conjugated Bile Acids Solid Phase Radioimmunoassay Kit $^{125}$I; Becton Dickinson, Orangeburg, N.Y.). Each yields comparable diagnostic results, although the sample size needed for the RIA assay is quite small (50 $\mu$l) compared with the enzymatic method (400 to 500 $\mu$l). Because the measurement of fasting and postprandial SBA concentrations assesses the same functions as the ammonium chloride ($NH_4Cl$) tolerance test without potentially dangerous consequences, it is the preferred test. As with any specially requested test, the laboratory chosen should use methods verified for clinical use in the target species and be able to provide reference ranges.

Several factors may affect SBA values and therefore their interpretation. One aspect of the SBA challenge test that has not been standardized is the feeding step. The ideal quantity and composition of the test meal have not been determined. Size of the test meal and therefore consumption of the entire meal or only part of the meal may affect gastric emptying. Delayed gastric emptying could cause the peak SBA concentration to occur later than 2 hours. Hastened or delayed intestinal transit time or the presence of intestinal disease (especially of the ileum) may also impede and blunt peak absorption of the test meal. It is likely that fat content of the test meal is important because fat is the primary stimulus for the small intestinal mucosa to secrete cholecystokinin, which causes gallbladder contraction. Expulsion of bile during periodic physiologic gallbladder contraction between meals may complicate interpretation of the fasted sample result.

Several questions remain to be answered regarding the clinical use of SBA measurement in cats and dogs. For example, can the "challenge" phase be improved by use of exogenous cholecystokinin instead of a meal? Preliminary results indicate that an intravenous injection of cholecystokinin will stimulate gallbladder contraction in healthy cats, but research in cats with hepatobiliary disease is still needed and the compound is rather cost-prohibitive. Also, investigation of individual SBA profiles in cats and dogs with various hepatobiliary diseases has provided interesting information but no clear and specific profile for any one disease. Can sequential SBA values be used to more precisely monitor a cat's or dog's progress? Until these and other questions are answered, use of SBA analysis is limited to measuring total serum values as a sensitive and relatively specific screening test for the presence or absence of clinically significant hepatobiliary disease. Additional diagnostic testing must always follow to identify the specific cause.

## Plasma Ammonia Concentration

One test that is not included in a standard screening battery of tests but is available through special reference or human hospital laboratories is plasma ammonia concentration. Fasting plasma ammonia is measured in any cat or dog with historic or physical examination findings suggestive of HE. Signs of HE (see Table 35-1), whether they have a congenital or acquired basis, appear the same. Quantifying plasma ammonia concentration is important not only for confirmation of HE, although normal fasting values in animals with hepatobiliary disease are relatively common, but also for providing baseline data and evaluating response to treatment. Some investigators have suggested that arterial ammonia concentrations may more accurately represent blood ammonia status in dogs with hepatobiliary disease than venous measurements because skeletal muscle can metabolize ammonia. High plasma ammonia concentration usually indicates reduced hepatic mass available to process ammonia and/or the presence of portosystemic shunting, which disrupts presentation of ammonia to the liver for detoxification.

Fasting plasma ammonia values for normal dogs are 100 mg/dl or less, and 90 mg/dl or less for normal cats. At least 6 hours of fasting should precede sample collection. Samples must be collected into iced ammonia-free heparinized tubes and spun immediately in a refrigerated centrifuge. Plasma must be removed within 30 minutes so that values will not be spuriously elevated by hemolysis because RBCs contain two to three times the ammonia concentration of plasma. To obtain accurate values, feline plasma can be frozen at $-20°$ C and assayed within 48 hours; canine plasma must be assayed within 30 minutes.

If signs are compatible with HE at the time of sample collection, a single fasting sample will suffice. Challenging such an animal with ammonium chloride ($NH_4Cl$) would provide no further information and could have devastating consequences. If there are no signs of HE and results of other tests are equivocal, an ammonium chloride challenge test can be performed. Three approaches are available (Table 36-2); two use a solution of $NH_4Cl$ dissolved in water, and one uses the same dose packed in gelatin capsules. With each of the techniques, plasma ammonia is measured before and 30 minutes after administration. To administer the substance by stomach tube, a 10% solution is used at a dose of 0.1 g/kg (1 ml/kg, maximum 3 g total dose). Some animals vomit after $NH_4Cl$ administration, making interpretation of the postsample results difficult because the entire administered dose of $NH_4Cl$

may not have been absorbed. For the rectal approach, the same dose of a 5% solution is used (i.e., 2 ml/kg) given by enema catheter and deposited as proximally into the colon as possible. The final method, in which $NH_4Cl$, 0.1 g/kg contained within gelatin capsules, is given directly by mouth, seems technically easiest to perform. All approaches have comparable success in detecting hyperammonemia; plasma values after $NH_4Cl$ administration in normal animals do not exceed a twofold increase over baseline values. An exaggerated response most commonly indicates congenital or acquired direct communication of the portal vasculature with the systemic circulation (portosystemic shunting) so that hepatic detoxification of ammonia to urea cannot occur. Alternatively, an exaggerated response may result from massive acute or chronic loss of functional hepatocytes, leaving insufficient overall enzymatic capability to degrade ammonia.

## URINALYSIS

Common findings in urinalysis consistent with hepatobiliary disease include excessive bilirubinuria in a nonanemic dog ($\geq 2+$ in urine of specific gravity $\leq 1.025$), presence of bilirubin in the urine of cats, and ammonium biurate crystalluria in properly processed urine specimens (Fig. 36-2). In dogs, excessive bilirubinuria may precede the onset of hyperbilirubinemia and jaundice. Small numbers of bilirubin crystals may be found in concentrated urine specimens from normal dogs, but ammonium biurate crystals are not found in freshly voided urine. Hyperammonemia combined with excess uric acidemia from diminished hepatic conversion to allantoin exceeds the renal threshold and favors precipitation of crystals, especially in alkaline urine. Their presence in the urine may fluctuate, but alkalinizing the urine specimen with a few drops of sodium or potassium hydroxide may augment the likelihood of identifying ammonium biurate crystals during sediment examination.

Measurement of urinary urobilinogen by dipstick analysis has traditionally been used to assess the patency of the extrahepatic biliary system. So many factors influence detection of

 TABLE 36-2

**Summary of Techniques for Ammonium Chloride Challenge Testing\* in the Diagnosis of Hyperammonemia**

| ROUTE | DOSE OF NH₄Cl |
|---|---|
| **Oral** | |
| Via stomach tube | 0.1 g/kg as a 10% solution (1 ml/kg, maximum 3-g total dosage) |
| Via gelatin capsule | 0.1 g/kg |
| **Rectal** | Give cleansing enema first; 0.1 g/kg as a 5% solution (2 ml/kg) |

\*Test should be preceded by at least a 6-hour fast; blood samples should be collected for plasma ammonia concentration before and at 30 minutes after NH₄Cl administration.

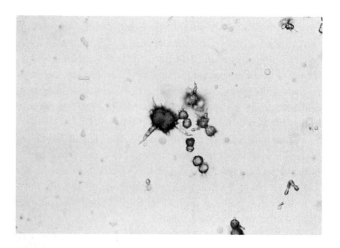

**FIG 36-2**
Ammonium biurate crystals in the urine of a dog with a congenital portosystemic shunt.

urobilinogen in the urine (e.g., intestinal flora and transit time, renal function, urine pH and specific gravity, exposure of the urine specimen to light) that the test is now considered to be of minimal value in diagnosing EBDO. If urine samples are obtained serially and processed properly, repeated absence of urobilinogen suggests, but is not diagnostic of, complete EBDO.

Consistently dilute urine (specific gravity as low as 1.005) may be a feature of congenital PSS and severe hepatocellular diseases. Urine specific gravity must also be interpreted in light of concurrent drug therapy, such as administration of diuretics, corticosteroids, or anticonvulsants.

## FECAL EVALUATION

Fecal specimen analysis rarely provides useful information in the evaluation of a dog or cat with suspected hepatobiliary disease, except for a change in appearance associated with two specific conditions. Absence of fecal pigment (acholic feces) and steatorrhea are consequences of chronic complete EBDO, and dark, orange-colored feces reflect increased bilirubin production and excretion after marked hemolysis.

## ABDOMINOCENTESIS/FLUID ANALYSIS

If abdominal fluid is detected during physical examination, abdominal radiography, or ultrasonography, a sample must always be obtained for analysis. For moderate to large volume effusion, simple needle paracentesis is sufficient to obtain 5 to 10 ml of fluid for gross inspection, determination of protein content, cytologic evaluation, and, in selected cases, special biochemical analysis. Larger volumes are removed using an over-the-needle–style catheter with extension tubing or a needle with attached tubing (E-Z infusion set) if clinical signs secondary to fluid accumulation are present (e.g., dyspnea)

or if removal of abdominal fluid is part of the treatment (e.g., bile peritonitis). Fluid analysis is one of the first steps in ruling out extrahepatic causes of abdominal effusion, such as right-sided heart failure or caval syndrome.

In dogs with chronic hepatic failure and sustained intrahepatic portal hypertension, abdominal fluid is usually a pure transudate with low cell count (<2500 cells/$\mu$l) and protein concentration (<2.5 g/dl), and a clear, minimally colored appearance; the specific gravity is usually less than 1.016. Early in the course of acquired chronic hepatic failure, abdominal fluid may have a higher protein content and be described as a modified transudate. Abdominal fluid in dogs with intrahepatic postsinusoidal venous obstruction (e.g., venoocclusive disease) or posthepatic venous obstruction (e.g., any cause of right-sided heart failure) can be any color but is typically red- or yellow-tinged, contains a low number of nucleated cells (<7000 cells/$\mu$l) and moderate amounts of protein ($\geq$2.5 g/dl), has specific gravity in the range of 1.010 to 1.033, and is classified as a modified transudate. Feline infectious peritonitis fluid and neoplastic effusions are also commonly classified as modified transudates or nonseptic exudates. Reactive mesothelial cells can be mistaken for carcinoma cells, emphasizing the need for experience in evaluating cytologic specimens. Exudates have high cell counts (>20,000 cells/$\mu$l) and protein content (>2.5 g/dl) and, on the basis of whether the inflammatory cells look toxic or contain ingested bacteria, are further classified as septic or nonseptic; specific gravity varies from 1.020 to 1.031. Septic exudates tend to have higher nucleated cell counts than nonseptic exudates. Fluid analysis provides additional clues to the origin of hepatobiliary disease and must not be overlooked. A guide to assessment of fluid analysis results is given in Table 36-3.

## TABLE 36-3

Characteristics of Abdominal Effusion in Hepatobiliary Disease

| | APPEARANCE | NUCLEATED CELL COUNT | PROTEIN CONTENT | SPECIFIC GRAVITY | EXAMPLE(S) |
|---|---|---|---|---|---|
| **Transudates** | | | | | |
| Pure | Clear, colorless | <2500/$\mu$l | <2.5 g/dl | <1.016 | Chronic hepatic failure with marked hypoalbuminemia, intrahepatic portal vein hypoplasia, chronic portal vein thrombosis |
| Modified | Serosanguineous, amber | <7000/$\mu$l | $\geq$2.5 g/dl | 1.010-1.031 | Chronic hepatic failure, right-sided heart failure, pericardial disease, caval syndrome, Budd-Chiari–like syndrome, feline infectious peritonitis |
| **Exudates** | | | | | |
| Septic | Cloudy; red, dark yellow, green | >20,000/$\mu$l | $\geq$2.5 g/dl | 1.020-1.031 | Perforated duodenal ulcer, bile peritonitis (fluid bilirubin concentration exceeds serum bilirubin concentration) |
| Nonseptic | Clear; red, dark yellow, green | <20,000/$\mu$l | $\geq$2.5 g/dl | 1.017-1.031 | Feline infectious peritonitis, neoplasia with serosal involvement, ruptured hemangiosarcoma, early bile peritonitis |

TABLE 36-4

Summary of First- and Second-Line Clinicopathologic Tests Useful in the Diagnosis of Hepatobiliary Disease

| SCREENING TEST | PRINCIPLE EXAMINED | COMMENTS |
|---|---|---|
| Serum ALT, AST activities | Integrity of liver cell membranes; escape from cells | Degree of increase roughly correlates with number of hepatocytes involved |
| Serum AP, GGT activities | Reactivity of liver cells and biliary epithelium to various stimuli; increased synthesis and release | Increase associated with intrahepatic or extrahepatic cholestasis or drug effect (dogs only): corticosteroids, anticonvulsants (AP only, not GGT) |
| Serum albumin concentration | Protein synthesis | Rule out other causes of low concentration (glomerular or intestinal loss); low value indicates ≥80% overall hepatic function loss |
| Serum urea concentration | Protein degradation and detoxification | With low values, rule out prolonged anorexia; dietary protein restriction; severe PU/PD; urea cycle enzyme deficiency (rare); congenital PSS; severe, acquired chronic hepatobiliary disease |
| Serum bilirubin concentration | Uptake and excretion of bilirubin | Rule out marked hemolysis first; if PCV is normal, intrahepatic or extrahepatic cholestasis is present |
| Serum cholesterol concentration | Biliary excretion, intestinal absorption, integrity of the enterohepatic circulation | High values compatible with severe cholestasis of any kind; low values suggest congenital PSS; anticonvulsant drug–induced change; severe, acquired chronic hepatobiliary disease; or severe intestinal malassimilation |
| Serum glucose concentration | Hepatocellular gluconeogenic or glycolytic ability | Low values indicate severe hepatocellular dysfunction or presence of a primary liver tumor |
| Plasma ammonia concentration | Integrity of the enterohepatic circulation, hepatic function and mass | High fasting or postchallenge values suggest congenital or acquired PSS or acute hepatocellular inability to detoxify ammonia to urea (massive necrosis) |
| Serum bile acid concentrations | Integrity of the enterohepatic circulation, hepatic function and mass | High fasting or postprandial values compatible with hepatocellular dysfunction, congenital PSS, or loss of hepatic mass |
| Coagulation profile | Hepatocellular function, adequacy of vitamin K stores | Abnormal values may indicate marked hepatocellular dysfunction, acute or chronic DIC, complete EBDO |

*ALT*, Alanine aminotransferase; *AST*, aspartate aminotransferase; *AP*, alkaline phosphatase; *GGT*, γ-glutamyltransferase; *PU/PD*, polyuria/polydipsia; *PSS*, portosystemic shunting; *PCV*, packed cell volume; *DIC*, disseminated intravascular coagulation; *EBDO*, extrahepatic bile duct obstruction.

## COAGULATION TESTS

Clinically relevant coagulopathies are unusual in cats and dogs with hepatobiliary disease except for those with acute hepatic failure, complete EBDO, or active DIC. It is more common to have subtle prolongation of activated partial thromboplastin time (APTT; 1.5 times normal), abnormal fibrin degradation products (10 to 40 or higher), and variable fibrinogen concentration (<100 to 200 mg/dl) in cats and dogs with severe parenchymal hepatic disease. Platelet numbers may be normal or low; mild thrombocytopenia (130,000 to 150,000 cells/μl) is usually associated with splenic sequestration or chronic DIC. More severe thrombocytopenia (≤100,000 cells/μl) would be expected in acute DIC or decompensated chronic DIC. Some animals with severe hepatic disease and relatively unremarkable routine coagulation test results have high serum activity of proteins induced by vitamin K antagonism (PIVKA) that could impart bleeding tendencies. Primary or metastatic cancer of the liver could also cause coagulopathy unrelated to loss of hepatocellular ability to make or degrade coagulation proteins.

A summary of laboratory tests for cats and dogs with hepatobiliary disease and interpretation of their results is given in Table 36-4.

## DIAGNOSTIC IMAGING

### SURVEY RADIOGRAPHY

Radiographic evaluation of the abdomen is used to complement physical examination findings and to confirm suspicions regarding the character and location of the hepatobiliary disease suggested by results of clinicopathologic examination. Survey radiographs provide subjective information regarding the size and shape of the liver (see Table 35-2). Optimally, the animal should have an empty gastrointestinal tract at the time the radiographs are obtained. In the normal dog in right lateral recumbency, the gastric axis is parallel to the ribs at the tenth intercostal space, and the caudoventral border of the liver (the left lateral liver lobe) appears sharp; the image is made possible by the contrasting fat-filled falciform ligament. In dog breeds with narrow, deep chests, the entire liver shadow may be contained within the caudal rib cage. In dogs with wide, shallow thoracic conformation, the liver may extend slightly beyond the costal arch. In the ventrodorsal view the borders of the liver are defined by the cranial duodenum and the gastric fundus; in this view, the gastric shadow is perpendicular to the spine. Immature animals have a relatively larger liver than do adults. The gallbladder and extrahepatic biliary tree are not visible radiographically in healthy animals.

Survey radiography is of minimal to no benefit if there is moderate to marked abdominal effusion, because the similar radiographic opacities of the liver and fluid preclude distinction of liver size and shape except by indirect assessment (e.g., malposition of a gas-filled stomach and duodenum). Poor abdominal detail in emaciated or very young animals lacking abdominal fat stores also makes detection of subtle hepatic changes difficult.

In cats and dogs with *generalized hepatomegaly,* the liver extends beyond the costal arch; it causes displacement of the gastric axis and pylorus caudally and dorsally in the lateral projection, and shifting of the gastric shadow caudally and to the left in the ventrodorsal view. In addition, the edges of the liver in the lateral view may appear rounded (Fig. 36-3). Occasionally the spleen and liver cannot be differentiated when they are in direct contact, as seen in the right lateral view. A ventrodorsal view would help to determine the size, shape, and position of each organ. Increased intrathoracic volume associated with deep inspiration, severe pleural effusion, or overinflation of the lungs may result in caudal displacement of the liver, giving the erroneous impression of hepatomegaly using other radiographic criteria.

Because the liver may be contained entirely within the rib cage in normal cats and dogs, *microhepatia* is more difficult to recognize than hepatomegaly. Changes in the angle of the gastric fundus in the right lateral projection (Fig. 36-4) could indicate a small hepatic shadow if the angle is more upright or perpendicular to the spine and especially if the stomach seems rather close to the diaphragm. The liver may also seem small in animals with traumatic diaphragmatic hernia and herniation of liver lobes into the thorax or in those with congenital peritoneopericardial hernia.

*Focal hepatic enlargement* is indicated by displacement of organs adjacent to the affected lobe. The most common radiographically detectable focal hepatic enlargement is that of the right lateral lobe, an example of which is shown in Fig. 36-5. In this case, the body and pyloric regions of the stomach are shifted dorsally (lateral view) and to the patient's left (ventrodorsal view); the gastric fundus remains in normal position. Shifting of the stomach to the left is normal in cats and should not be mistaken for right hepatomegaly. If the left lateral lobe or lobes are enlarged, the gastric fundus moves to the left and caudally; the lesser curvature of the stomach may appear indented. Primary or metastatic neoplasia, hyperplastic or regenerative nodules, and cysts most commonly account for focal hepatic en-

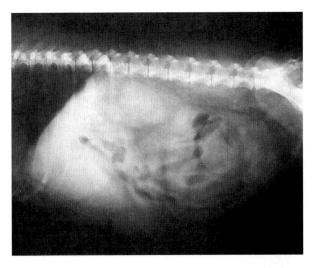

**FIG 36-3**
Lateral abdominal radiograph of an 8-year-old female Cairn Terrier with iatrogenic hypercortisolism demonstrating generalized hepatomegaly. Note that the liver extends beyond the costal arch and its edges are rounded.

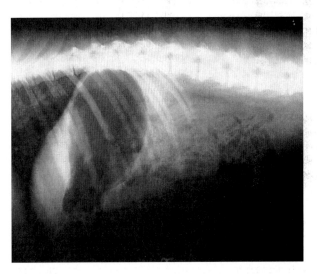

**FIG 36-4**
Lateral abdominal radiograph of a 3-year-old castrated male Dalmatian with microhepatia associated with congenital intrahepatic portosystemic shunt. The stomach is distended with gas, which provides contrast with the liver shadow. Note that the stomach appears very close to the diaphragm, implying reduced hepatic mass.

largement or for irregular liver margins without enlargement. If the gallbladder is massively enlarged because of EBDO, it may mimic a right cranial abdominal mass or an enlarged, rounded liver lobe.

Changes in hepatic radiographic opacity are rare and are usually associated with hepatic or biliary tract infection caused by gas-forming bacteria (patchy and/or linear areas of

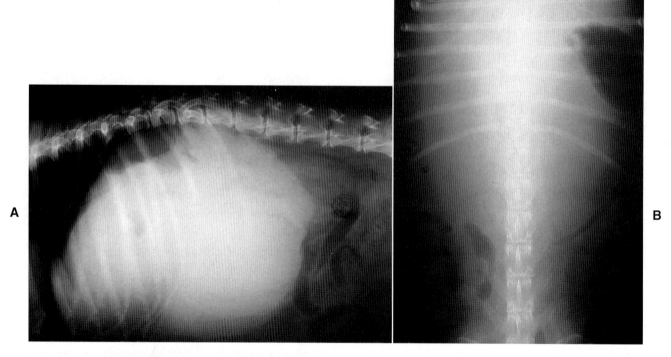

**FIG 36-5**
**A,** Lateral and, **B,** ventrodorsal abdominal radiographs of a 9-year-old spayed female mixed-breed dog with a hepatocellular carcinoma enlarging the right lateral liver lobe. The dog was also severely hypoglycemic.

decreased opacity) or mineralization (focal or diffuse spots of mineralization or mineralized biliary calculi).

With the advent of ultrasonography, contrast radiographic procedures are seldom needed to confirm the presence of hepatic masses, cholelithiasis, EBDO, congenital PSS, and other structural diseases. The contrast study that is still necessary to localize some types of congenital PSS and is achievable in private practice is portal venography. Acceptable approaches for this technique are splenoportography, operative mesenteric portography, and operative splenoportography. The two operative procedures require general anesthesia and a small abdominal incision; however, little sophisticated equipment is needed, and the procedures are associated with few complications. A 22-gauge catheter is placed in the splenic vein or a mesenteric vein (Fig. 36-6), and the resting portal venous pressure is measured with a water manometer (N = 6 to 13 cm $H_2O$). Portal pressure is measured as soon as possible in the procedure because prolonged anesthesia may complicate its interpretation. An injection of iodine-based contrast medium at a dose of 0.5 to 1 ml/kg is then quickly made. Lateral and possibly ventrodorsal and oblique radiographs are made at the end of the injection. Contrast medium given to a normal cat or dog should flow into the portal vein, enter the liver, and branch multiple times, opacifying the extrahepatic and intrahepatic portal vasculature. Diversion of the contrast medium into the systemic circulation indicates PSS (Fig. 36-7). Measurement of portal pressure and a liver biopsy can

be performed during the operative techniques; they are required to distinguish causes of acquired PSS from causes of congenital PSS, which is essential to rendering an accurate prognosis and developing the correct treatment plan. It may be necessary to repeat the contrast study after congenital PSS ligation if there is concern about the adequacy of the intrahepatic portal vasculature.

## ULTRASONOGRAPHY

A similarly noninvasive diagnostic modality that often complements abdominal radiography and offers a new dimension to hepatobiliary imaging is ultrasonography (US). Once restricted to veterinary colleges and research institutes, sonographic imaging has evolved to be within reach of the private practitioner. Refined technology and widespread availability of continuing education lectures and workshops have made US a feasible diagnostic tool for many contemporary veterinarians. Operating on the principle that a pulse of sound (echo) can be reflected when it passes through the interface between two different materials, US can detect differences between homogeneous liquids of low echogenicity such as blood and bile, and more heterogeneous echogenic structures made up of several soft tissues. Whereas abdominal effusion obscures abdominal detail on survey radiography, it enhances US detection of abnormalities. Bone and gas-filled organs reflect the sound beam completely (acoustic shadowing) so that structures beneath cannot be imaged by US. The proce-

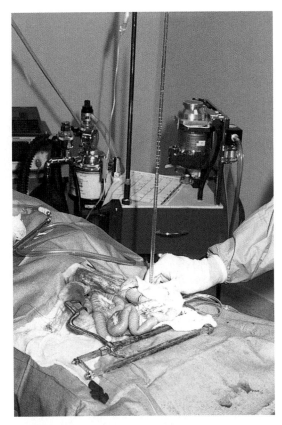

**FIG 36-6**
A 22-gauge intravenous catheter attached to an extension set, three-way stopcock, and water manometer has been placed in a mesenteric vein in preparation for intraoperative measurement of resting portal pressure. The catheter may also be secured in place and used for operative portal venography.

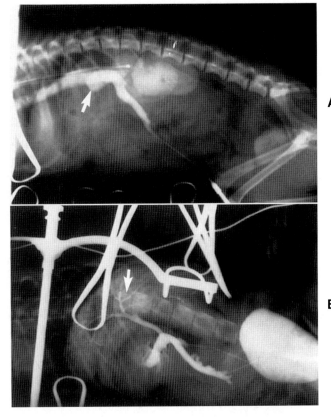

**FIG 36-7**
Operative mesenteric portal venography in an 11-month-old female Miniature Poodle with single extrahepatic portacaval shunt *(arrow)* before, **A,** and after, **B,** surgical correction (note improvement in hepatic portal blood flow *[arrow]* in **B).**

dure does not require that the animal be anesthetized, but the patient must be still, and good contact between the transducer and abdominal skin must be ensured by clipping the hair coat and applying acoustic coupling gel. Animals are usually positioned in dorsal or lateral recumbency. The hepatic parenchyma, gallbladder, large hepatic and portal veins, and adjacent caudal vena cava are all visible in the liver of the normal cat and dog. Unlike plain radiography, which requires two views to complete the study, US makes many slices through several planes to create a three-dimensional reconstruction of the target structures.

Performing US and interpreting the recorded images are a blend of technical skill and experience. Some diagnoses can be made quickly and confidently; others require comparison of images from sequential examinations. Dilated anechoic (black) vascular channels and echoic bile ducts can be identified, as well as localized accumulations of anechoic material that represents neoplastic masses (Fig. 36-8), cysts, or abscesses. Echoes that originate from within "cystic" areas correspond to cellular debris. Hyperechoic (bright) areas indicate increased fibrous tissue, mineralization, or gas pockets. Mixed patterns can be seen in association with parenchymal

neoplastic disease and with chronic hepatic disease with nodular regeneration. A dilated gallbladder may indicate prolonged anorexia, unless dilated bile ducts, particularly the common bile duct, are also seen, which supports EBDO (Fig. 36-9) or chronic cholangitis/cholangiohepatitis in cats. Intrahepatic or extrahepatic anomalous vessels have also been identified in animals with clinicopathologic evidence of severe chronic hepatobiliary disease or congenital PSS (Fig. 36-10). Use of Doppler color-flow imaging confirms the location of the suspicious vessel(s) and the direction of blood flow within. Doppler imaging can also provide supportive evidence of intrahepatic portal hypertension by allowing the assessment of the speed and direction of portal flow. Portal blood flow toward the liver (hepatopetal) is normal; away from the liver (hepatofugal) is abnormal. Whether the lesion is determined to be focal or diffuse, US can also be used as a guide to obtain diagnostic specimens for cytologic or histopathologic analysis. US has developed into a valuable and critically important adjunct to diagnosis of hepatobiliary disease of cats and dogs by allowing characterization of structural changes not possible by any other modality (Table 36-5) and by providing a way to obtain needle liver biopsy

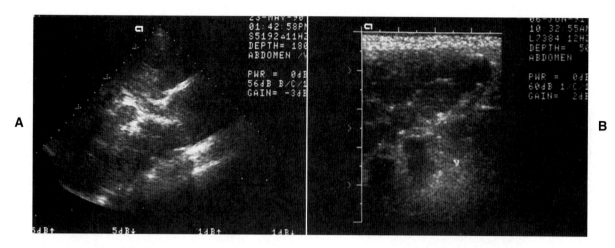

**FIG 36-8**

Ultrasonographic appearance of nodular lesions in liver. **A,** Hemangiosarcoma in an 8-year-old female Golden Retriever. **B,** Chronic hepatopathy with regenerative nodule formation and intralobular and interlobular fibrosis in a 10-year-old castrated male Cocker Spaniel that had received primidone followed by phenobarbital for 9.5 years. (Courtesy Dr. Kathy A. Spaulding, North Carolina State University, College of Veterinary Medicine.)

**FIG 36-9**

Ultrasonographic appearance of dilated gallbladder *(GB)* and cystic duct in a 5-year-old female Beagle with severe ulcerative duodenitis and extrahepatic bile duct obstruction. The extrahepatic bile duct was dilated and tortuous; its entire length could not be demonstrated in the same view. (Courtesy Dr. Kathy A. Spaulding, North Carolina State University, College of Veterinary Medicine.)

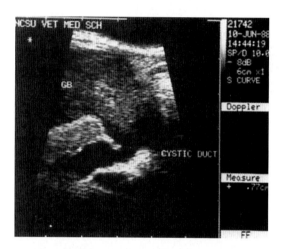

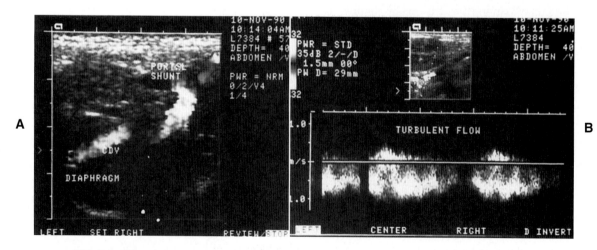

**FIG 36-10**

**A,** Ultrasonographic findings of abnormal vascular shadows in a 9-month-old male Himalayan cat with congenital extrahepatic portacaval shunt. **B,** Turbulent blood flow from the portal vein to the caudal vena cava is demonstrated by use of Doppler color-flow imaging. (Courtesy Dr. Kathy A. Spaulding, North Carolina State University, College of Veterinary Medicine.)

TABLE 36-5

Ultrasonographic Findings in Dogs and Cats with Hepatobiliary Diseases

| FINDING | POSSIBLE INTERPRETATIONS |
|---|---|
| **Parenchyma** | |
| ***Anechogenicity*** | |
| Focal | Cyst(s)—may be singular or multiple with septae; thin-walled |
| | Abscess(es)—may be poorly demarcated and have a heterogeneous echo pattern |
| | Hematoma(s)—appearance depends on maturity |
| | Lymphoma—may look like cyst if solitary |
| ***Hypoechogenicity*** | |
| Focal | Focal or multifocal neoplasia |
| | Regenerative nodule formation |
| | Extramedullary hematopoiesis |
| | Normal liver surrounded by hyperechoic liver |
| | Hematoma(s) |
| Diffuse | Abscess(es) or granuloma(s) |
| | Neoplastic or inflammatory cell infiltrates |
| | Passive congestion |
| | Hepatocellular necrosis |
| ***Hyperechogenicity*** | |
| Focal | Focal or multifocal neoplasia |
| | Mineralization (creates shadowing artifact) |
| | Fibrosis |
| | Gas (creates reverberation artifact) |
| | Hematoma or abscess |
| Diffuse | Fatty infiltration (attenuates the sound beam) |
| | Fibrosis |
| | Neoplastic or inflammatory cell infiltrates |
| | Steroid hepatopathy (dogs only) |
| **Tubular Structures—Biliary Tract** | |
| Dilated intrahepatic and extrahepatic bile ducts | Extrahepatic bile duct obstruction (see Table 37-2); persistent or recently relieved |
| | Severe cholangitis complex (cats) |
| | Choledochal cyst (rare) |
| Distended gallbladder | Normal (prolonged fasting) |
| Distended gallbladder and cystic duct | Cystic duct obstruction |
| Distended gallbladder and common bile duct | Extrahepatic bile duct obstruction (see Table 37-2); persistent or recently relieved |
| Focal areas of gravity-dependent hyperechogenicity within biliary tract or gallbladder that cause acoustic shadowing | Cholelithiasis |
| Focal areas of hyperechogenicity within gallbladder that settle to dependent portion of gallbladder when animal's position changes | "Sludged" or inspissated bile from severe cholestasis, prolonged anorexia, and dehydration |
| Stellate or "kiwi fruit" appearance to gallbladder | Gallbladder mucocele |
| Intraluminal echoic masses in gallbladder | Neoplasia (polyp, malignant neoplasm) |
| | Adherent inspissated bile |
| | Cystic hyperplasia (focal) |
| Apparent thickened gallbladder wall | Cholecystitis, cholangitis |
| | Infectious canine hepatitis |
| | Hypoalbuminemia with edema formation |
| | Abdominal effusion |
| | Neoplasia |

*Continued*

TABLE 36-5

Ultrasonographic Findings in Dogs and Cats with Hepatobiliary Diseases—cont'd

| FINDING | POSSIBLE INTERPRETATIONS |
|---|---|
| **Tubular Structures—Blood Vessels** | |
| Dilated hepatic veins and portal veins | Right-sided congestive heart failure<br>Pericardial disease<br>Intrathoracic caudal vena cava occlusion<br>Hepatic vein occlusion (Budd-Chiari syndrome) |
| Prominent hepatic arteries | Reduced portal blood flow |
| Distended portal vein with reduced velocity and flow | Portal hypertension of any cause (by Doppler) |
| Inapparent hepatic vessels | Cirrhosis<br>Severe fatty infiltration |
| Inapparent portal veins | Congenital portosystemic shunt<br>Portal vein thrombus<br>Intrahepatic portal vein hypoplasia |
| Aberrant vessel that communicates with systemic circulation | Intrahepatic or extrahepatic congenital portosystemic shunt |
| Connection between a portal vein and an artery within one or more liver lobes | Arterioportal venous fistula |
| Many tortuous veins clustered around left kidney and along colon | Acquired portosystemic shunts associated with portal hypertension |

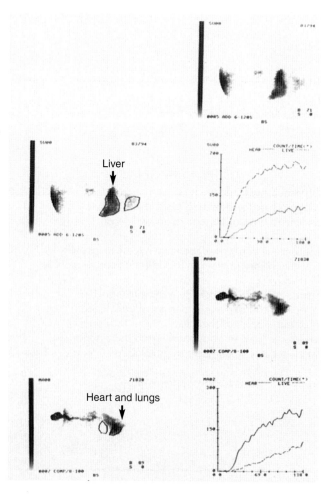

**FIG 36-11**
Transcolonic scintigraphy demonstrating the portal vascular path to the liver. **A,** Normal dog with isotope following a direct path to the liver and a small (5%) shunt fraction. **B,** Abnormal arrival of isotope in the heart and lungs of 1-year-old male Miniature Schnauzer with congenital portosystemic shunt and large (84%) shunt fraction. In each scan image, the dog's head is to the right. (Courtesy Dr. Lisa J. Forrest, North Carolina State University, College of Veterinary Medicine.)

specimens in a visualized manner without the need for general anesthesia.

## SCINTIGRAPHY

Other imaging modalities, such as scintigraphy (nuclear imaging), magnetic resonance imaging, and computed tomography, are available primarily through teaching or larger referral institutions. Of these three imaging modalities, scintigraphy has been evaluated most thoroughly for diagnosis of hepatobiliary disease in cats and dogs. The isotope selected most often for clinical use is technetium-99m ($^{99m}$Tc), which is incorporated into the radiopharmaceutical specific for the planned study. For example, $^{99m}$Tc bound to sulfur colloid, which is phagocytized by monocyte-macrophage cells of the liver and spleen, is given to assess liver mass. Images are made by collection of emissions from decaying isotope using a gamma camera focused over the animal's liver region and recorded on radiographic film. The isotope has a short (6-hour) half-life; thus, although the animal must be relatively isolated for 24 to 48 hours and urinary and fecal waste stored until radioactivity has fallen to background levels, there is minimal radiation hazard to the animal or involved personnel. To distinguish medical from surgical jaundice, $^{99m}$Tc is combined with disofenin (Hepatolite). After an intravenous injection of radiopharmaceutical, scintigraphic images are made sequentially over 3 hours to determine whether isotope has been taken up by the liver, excreted into the biliary tract, and expelled into the intestine. In cats and dogs with EBDO, no evidence of radiopharmaceutical is detected in the gallbladder or intestine.

Another application of scintigraphy is used in the diagnosis of PSS in cats and dogs. Following placement of pertechnetate labeled with $^{99m}$Tc into the descending colon, the vascular path taken by the isotope after absorption is plotted. Time/activity curves determine whether the isotope arrived in the liver first, which is normal, or in the heart and lungs, which is compatible with any kind of portal venous bypass of the liver (Fig. 36-11). This approach has the advantage of specifically evaluating the portal blood supply rather than the hepatic mass, which may or may not be reduced in animals with congenital PSS or primary hepatobiliary disease and acquired PSS. The test results do not provide anatomic detail but only evidence of the presence or absence of congenital *or* acquired portosystemic shunting. Transcolonic portal scintigraphy is most helpful in confirming the presence of congenital PSS in a cat or dog with atypical clinicopathologic test results, equivocal abdominal ultrasound findings (e.g., normal-sized liver, no identifiable vessel arising from the portal vein), and no evidence of portal hypertension, such as ascites.

## LIVER BIOPSY

### General Considerations

For many primary hepatobiliary diseases of cats and dogs, hepatic biopsy is needed to establish a final diagnosis and prognosis. In some cases, bile culture is also imperative. Biopsy is indicated to (1) explain abnormal results of hepatic status and/or function tests, especially if they persist for longer than 1 month; (2) explain hepatomegaly of unknown cause; (3) determine hepatic involvement in systemic illness; (4) stage neoplastic disease; (5) objectively assess response to therapy; or (6) evaluate progress of previously diagnosed, not specifically treatable disease. Percutaneous hepatic biopsy is *not* performed if there is a good chance that the disease can be corrected surgically, such as in EBDO or congenital PSS; instead, a specimen is obtained at the time of surgery to complete the diagnostic evaluation. Several approaches are available; choice is dictated by patient and operator considerations (Table 36-6). All cats and dogs undergoing hepatic biopsy are fasted at least 12 hours, regardless of the approach selected. In general, percutaneous needle core biopsy or aspiration (for cytologic analysis) of a single cavitary or solid lesion highly likely to be nonlymphoid cancer is avoided unless the owner is unwilling to permit surgery for complete resection (see Chapter 81). Fine-needle aspiration for cytologic analysis is advisable if multiple nodules are noted; metastatic cancer may have a similar ultrasonographic appearance as benign hyperplastic or regenerative nodules. However, an overall correlation of only 44% was found in one study comparing the cytologic diagnosis with the histopathologic diagnosis of neoplasia (Fondacaro and colleagues, 1999). In an especially small and/or firm fibrotic liver, it is difficult to obtain a biopsy specimen by percutaneous needle methods; small, fragmented specimens that are challenging to interpret are often the result (Fig. 36-12). There is less than a 40% correlation between 18-gauge needle biopsy and wedge biopsy for certain hepatobiliary diseases (i.e., chronic hepatitis/

## TABLE 36-6

**Patient and Operator Considerations for Hepatic Biopsy**

| PATIENT | OPERATOR |
|---|---|
| 1. Characteristics of the suspected hepatobiliary disorder: liver size (small, normal, enlarged); texture (fibrotic or friable); focal, multifocal, or diffuse distribution; presence of abdominal effusion | 1. Available equipment |
| 2. Clinical stability and suitability for anesthesia | 2. Experience with chosen technique |
| 3. Coagulation status | 3. Complication rate for chosen technique |
| | 4. Size of specimen needed |
| | 5. Access to reliable veterinary pathology laboratory |

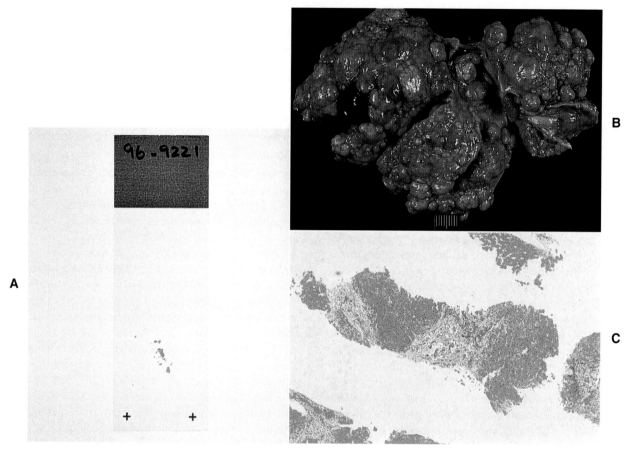

**FIG 36-12**
**A,** Liver specimen obtained percutaneously (with ultrasound guidance) from a dog with hepatic fibrosis and nodular regeneration, **B.** The specimen was difficult to obtain because the liver was firm and rubbery in texture. **C,** The resultant sample was difficult to interpret histologically.

cirrhosis, cholangitis, portovascular anomaly, fibrosis). If a needle technique is selected, the largest available instrument is used (preferably 14 gauge; minimum 16 gauge) to ensure samples adequate for examination.

The animal's coagulation status is determined before a liver biopsy is performed, regardless of the approach. Ideally a complete coagulation profile (one-stage prothrombin time [OSPT], APTT, fibrin degradation products, fibrinogen content, platelet count) is obtained; a platelet count and an activated clotting time, as a screening test of the intrinsic coagulation cascade, are also acceptable. Bleeding following ultrasound-guided biopsy is more likely if the platelet count is less than 80,000 cells/μl or if the OSPT (dogs) or APTT (cats) is prolonged (Bigge and colleagues, 2001). If possible, von Willebrand's factor is measured in susceptible breeds in advance of biopsy because results of standard coagulation tests are usually normal in affected dogs. A buccal mucosa bleeding time test provides indirect assessment of platelet function (see p. 1187). In dogs with von Willebrand's disease, desmopressin acetate (DDAVP) is given (1 μg/kg intranasal preparation subcutaneously) before surgery to enhance shift of von Willebrand's factor activity from endothelial cells to the plasma.

Mild abnormalities in coagulation test results do not preclude liver biopsy. In fact, results of routine coagulation tests may not correlate with liver bleeding times, as was found in one study of human patients. Liver biopsy is delayed if there is clinical evidence of bleeding or marked abnormalities in results of coagulation tests. Because animals with complete EBDO may be vitamin K–deficient (manifested by prolongation of both OSPT and APTT), treatment with vitamin $K_1$ (5 mg subcutaneously once or twice daily) is indicated for 1 or 2 days before surgery. Repeating the OSPT and APTT within 24 hours after administration of vitamin $K_1$ should demonstrate normal or near-normal values. If not, the dose can be adjusted and the procedure delayed. Although it may not seem rational to give vitamin $K_1$ to animals with severe parenchymal hepatic disease before surgery, it has been of benefit to some animals and, if given properly, can do no harm. These animals may have high serum activity of proteins induced by vitamin K antagonism (PIVKA) that could impart bleeding tendencies. If there has been minimal improvement in coagulation test results after vitamin $K_1$ has been administered, fresh frozen plasma is administered before biopsy. If bleeding is excessive during or after biopsy and

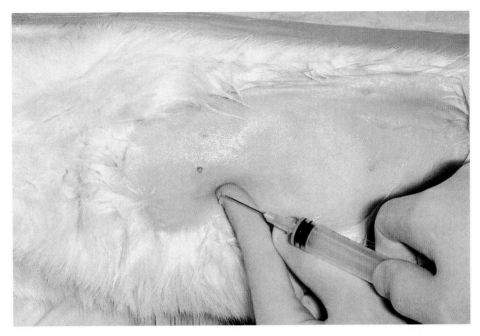

**FIG 36-13**
Four-year-old spayed female domestic short-haired cat with suspected hepatic lipidosis positioned in right lateral recumbency for blind fine-needle aspirate for cytology. With care taken to avoid the spleen, the needle is directed craniomedially into the liver.

cannot be controlled locally with direct pressure or application of clot-promoting substances, fresh whole blood or plasma is given (see Chapter 85 for transfusion guidelines).

## Techniques

*Percutaneous biopsy techniques* are used in dogs and cats with hepatomegaly and ultrasonographic evidence of diffuse, uniform hepatic parenchymal disease. A fine-needle aspirate of the liver for cytologic evaluation is often obtained first because evidence for certain disorders such as vacuolar hepatopathy (lipidosis, steroid hepatopathy) and lymphoid neoplasia can be presumptively identified by this method (Fig. 36-13).

Information gathered before biopsy must support the fact that the likelihood of acquiring a diagnostic sample without complications is high. A specimen procured from any area of the liver is considered representative of the disease. Because only a small stab incision large enough to accommodate the biopsy needle is needed (a No. 11 blade is the perfect choice for this purpose), healing in hypoalbuminemic animals is not compromised. If the operator is confident with the biopsy procedure, there is little time involved and only heavy sedation is required. If the results are nondiagnostic, a larger specimen is obtained, usually by laparoscopy or laparotomy, for histopathologic examination.

Biopsy can be performed *blindly* if the cat or dog has generalized hepatomegaly and the operator is confident of the path of the needle. The most common needle biopsy instruments used are the Tru-Cut (Baxter Healthcare Corporation, Deerfield, Ill) and Menghini (Baxter Healthcare Corporation, Deerfield, Ill) needles. With the latter two, which can be op-

erated with one hand, aspiration is used to sever and contain the specimen within the barrel of a 6- or 12-ml syringe. The Tru-Cut needle requires two hands to operate and relies on the tissue falling into the specimen trough and then being severed by the sharp outer cannula (Fig. 36-14). One-handed operatable versions of this instrument are also available (e.g., Temno [Bauer Medical, Inc., Clearwater, Fla] in 14-, 15-, and 16-gauge, 5-inch length; PGI EZ Core [Products Group International, Lyons, Colo] in 14- and 16-gauge, 3.6- and 6-inch lengths; Anchor Tru-Cut [Anchor Products Co., Addison, Ill], 14-gauge, 6-inch length; Fig. 36-15). These instruments are intended for single use and cost in the range of $20 to $30 each.

Biopsy can be done of any palpably enlarged lobe as long as care is taken to angle the needle to avoid puncturing the gallbladder. Most often, the animal is placed in right lateral recumbency for this purpose and biopsy of the left lateral lobe is done. Elevating the head and thorax slightly may assist in "presenting" the liver to the operator. Two or three complete core specimens are obtained; if indicated, one core specimen is placed in a sterile container for culture and sensitivity testing. Gently rolling a specimen on a slide for cytologic assessment is a good way to attempt to identify the disease process quickly and inexpensively. Each of the remaining core specimens is laid on a piece of stiff paper (e.g., filter paper) in correct orientation (Fig. 36-16) before immersion in fixative for histologic examination and/or special testing.

After biopsy, a small bandage is applied to keep the site clean during recovery, and the animal is placed in a position to allow body weight to compress the region of the biopsy

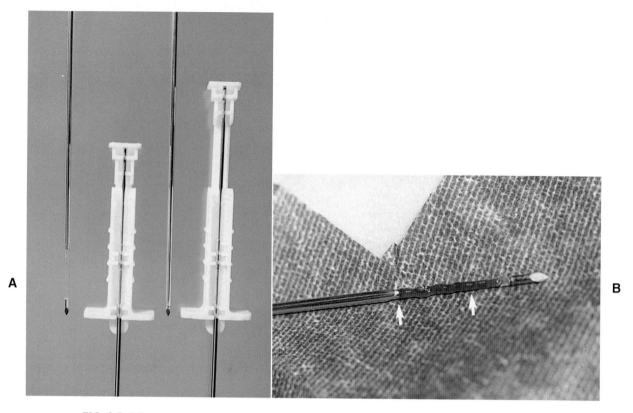

**FIG 36-14**
**A,** Tru-Cut biopsy needle with the specimen trough exposed *(left)* and then covered by the sharp outer cannula *(right)*. **B,** Liver tissue filling the specimen trough *(between arrows)*.

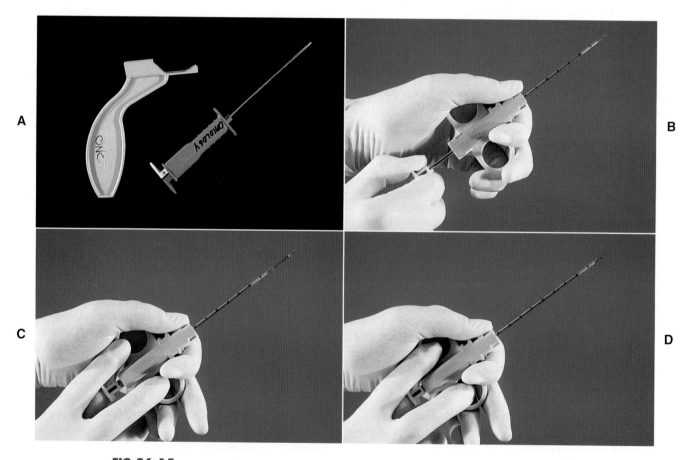

**FIG 36-15**
Single-use biopsy needles that enable the user to accurately position and operate the needle to obtain a specimen with one hand. **A,** Anchor Tru-Cut biopsy needle with pistol-grip device, PGI EZ Core biopsy needle; "cocked" **(B),** biopsy trough exposed **(C),** and fired **(D)** with tissue inside.

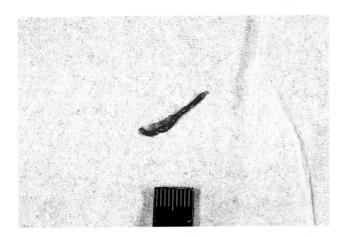

**FIG 36-16**
Needle biopsy specimen affixed to a stiff piece of paper to preserve orientation of the sample during formalin fixation for histopathologic examination.

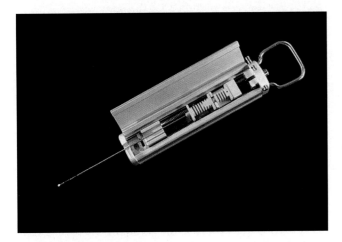

**FIG 36-17**
Biopsy gun instrument with accompanying biopsy needle used for obtaining liver specimens with ultrasound guidance.

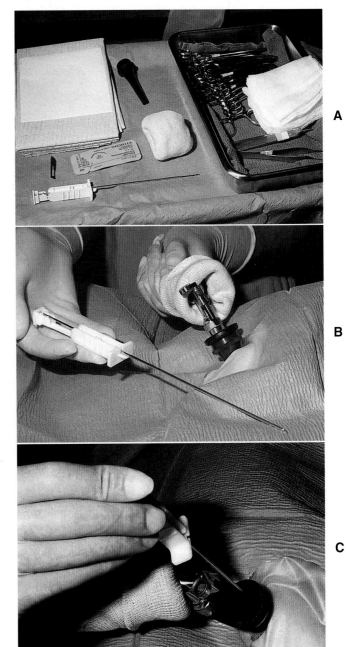

**FIG 36-18**
Modified laparoscopic approach for liver biopsy. **A,** Readily available materials needed for the procedure. **B,** A Tru-Cut biopsy needle is used for obtaining liver specimens. **C,** The liver is first inspected, and then the needle is passed through a sterile otoscope cone into the liver for tissue sampling. See Bunch and colleagues (1985) in Suggested Readings for further details on this procedure.

sites in the liver (e.g., left lateral recumbency). As long as the biopsy procedure proceeded smoothly and without unpleasant surprises (animal awake and struggling), only basic monitoring of mucous membrane color and the skin puncture site is needed. Naturally, if there is excessive hemorrhage or damage to other organs with this blind technique, detection and treatment may be delayed.

*Visualized percutaneous needle biopsy,* with the aid of either US (Fig. 36-17) or modified laparoscopic equipment (Fig. 36-18), allows selection of the site(s) and direct or indirect inspection after the biopsy. When properly performed, serious complications are few. In an animal in which diffuse or multifocal hepatobiliary disease is suspected, multiple biopsy specimens are obtained safely. General anesthesia is usually required for use of a modified laparoscope. Aspiration of the gallbladder for cytologic analysis and culture can be accomplished with US guidance or by laparoscopy. Bile leakage may occur, even if a small-gauge needle is used, so

attempts are made to completely evacuate the gallbladder. Some surgeons prefer to obtain bile during laparotomy when a purse-string suture can be applied to the aspiration site to prevent seepage. Large-volume abdominal effusion hinders direct inspection of the liver and associated structures and must be removed before laparoscopic biopsy is attempted.

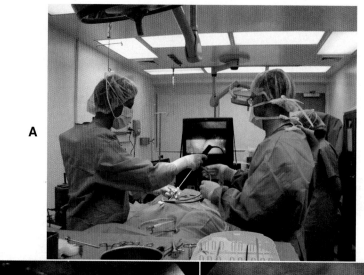

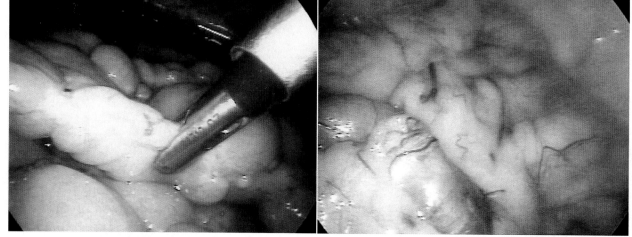

**FIG 36-19**
**A,** Laparoscopic liver biopsy. **B,** Tip of the biopsy instrument that is passed through one of the preplaced cannulas. **C,** Intraabdominal view of a dog with chronic hepatic disease and portal hypertension. Note the prominent, tortuous omental veins.

An *operative approach* (laparoscopy [Fig. 36-19], laparotomy) is preferred for liver biopsy if the liver is small, US equipment is not available, or the operator is not experienced with the above percutaneous needle methods. Laparotomy is perfectly acceptable for dogs and cats that are good anesthetic risks and allows thorough examination of the liver, biliary tract, and portal vein, as well as other abdominal structures such as lymph nodes. Bile can be acquired easily and safely. The procedure is more prolonged and healing complications may arise in severely hypoalbuminemic animals, notably those with intractable ascites, but larger samples for histopathologic examination and special staining techniques are obtainable (Fig. 36-20), and hemorrhage can be arrested directly. Use of nonabsorbable suture material and small cranial or flank incisions may lessen incision complications. Obviously this is the approach of choice for surgically correctable diseases; a liver biopsy specimen is obtained concurrently.

As for the percutaneous biopsy techniques, liver and/or bile specimens for microbiologic culture are aseptically processed first. Impression smears for cytologic analysis are then made by gently touching the specimen to a slide before placing it in fixative. Excess blood is removed by blotting the sample on gauze before slides are made. Abnormal populations of cells (e.g., mast cells, lymphoblasts) are readily detectable using rapid stain systems such as Diff Quik (Harleco, Gibbstown, N.J.). For routine processing and histopathologic examination, liver tissue specimens are submerged in buffered 10% formalin at a ratio of at least 10 parts formalin to 1 part tissue. Samples for copper histochemical staining or tissue quantification are harvested and fixed or preserved according to the specifications of the pathology laboratory selected to do the assays. Other special stains for infectious agents or fibrous tissue, amyloid, glycogen, and other metabolic products are available, and their use is discussed with the attending pathologist before the tissue specimen is obtained.

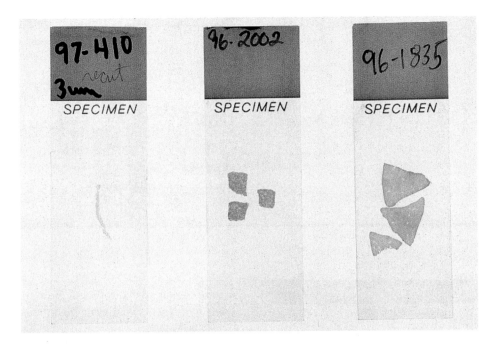

**FIG 36-20**
Comparison of liver specimens obtained by different methods and mounted on glass slides. These samples are adequate for histopathologic examination: percutaneous needle sample *(left)*; samples obtained intraoperatively by use of an 8 mm skin biopsy punch *(middle)* or removal of a wedge specimen *(right)*.

## Suggested Readings

Bigge LA et al: Correlation between coagulation profile findings and bleeding complications after ultrasound-guided biopsies: 434 cases (1993-1996), *J Am Anim Hosp Assoc* 37:228, 2001.

Boothe HW et al: Use of hepatobiliary scintigraphy in the diagnosis of extrahepatic biliary obstruction in dogs and cats: 25 cases (1982-1989), *J Am Vet Med Assoc* 201:134, 1992.

Bunch SE et al: A modified laparoscopic approach for liver biopsy in dogs, *J Am Vet Med Assoc* 187:1032, 1985.

Center SA: Serum bile acids in companion animal medicine, *Vet Clin North Am Small Anim Pract* 23:625, 1993.

Center SA: Pathophysiology and laboratory diagnosis of liver disease. In Ettinger SJ, editor: *Textbook of veterinary internal medicine*, ed 4, Philadelphia, 1995, WB Saunders, p 1261.

Center SA et al: PIVKA clotting times in dogs with suspected coagulopathies. In *Proceedings of the 16th Annual Forum, American College of Veterinary Internal Medicine,* San Diego, Calif, 1998, p 704.

Center SA et al: PIVKA clotting time in clinically ill cats with suspected coagulopathies. In *Proceedings of the 16th Annual Forum, American College of Veterinary Internal Medicine,* San Diego, Calif, 1998, p 719.

Cole T et al: Diagnostic comparison of needle biopsy and wedge biopsy specimens of the liver in dogs and cats, *J Am Vet Med Assoc* 220:1483, 2002.

Dial SM: Clinicopathologic evaluation of the liver, *Vet Clin North Am Small Anim Pract* 25:257, 1995.

Fondacaro JV et al: Diagnostic correlation of liver aspiration cytology with histopathology in dogs and cats with liver disease. In *Proceedings of the 17th Annual Forum, American College of Veterinary Internal Medicine,* Chicago, 1999, p 704.

Hardy RM: Hepatic biopsy. In Kirk RW, editor: *Current veterinary therapy VIII,* Philadelphia, 1983, WB Saunders, p 813.

Hess PR et al: Diagnostic approach to hepatobiliary disease. In Bonagura JD, editor: *Kirk's current veterinary therapy XIII,* Philadelphia, 2000, WB Saunders, p 659.

Kerwin SC: Hepatic aspiration and biopsy techniques, *Vet Clin North Am Small Anim Pract* 25:275, 1995.

Klaus E: Bleeding after liver biopsy does not correlate with indices of peripheral coagulation, *Dig Dis Sci* 26:388, 1981.

Koblik PD et al: Transcolonic sodium pertechnetate Tc 99m scintigraphy for diagnosis of macrovascular portosystemic shunts in dogs, cats, and pot-bellied pigs: 176 cases (1988-1992), *J Am Vet Med Assoc* 207:729, 1995.

Lawler DF et al: Benign familial hyperphosphatasemia in Siberian Huskies, *Am J Vet Res* 57:612, 1996.

Léveillé R et al: Complications after ultrasound-guided biopsy of abdominal structures in dogs and cats: 246 cases (1984-1991), *J Am Vet Med Assoc* 203:413, 1993.

Müller PB et al: Effects of long-term phenobarbital treatment on the liver in dogs, *J Vet Intern Med* 14:165, 2000.

Partington BP et al: Hepatic imaging with radiology and ultrasound, *Vet Clin North Am Small Anim Pract* 25:305, 1995.

Pechman RD Jr: The liver and spleen. In Thrall DR, editor: *Textbook of veterinary diagnostic radiology,* ed 2, Philadelphia, 1986, WB Saunders, p 391.

Roth L et al: Interpretation of liver biopsies, *Vet Clin North Am Small Anim Pract* 25:293, 1995.

Rothuizen J et al: Arterial and venous ammonia concentrations in the diagnosis of canine hepato-encephalopathy, *Res Vet Sci* 33:17, 1982.

Rothuizen J et al: Bilirubin metabolism in canine hepatobiliary and haemolytic disease, *Vet Q* 9:235, 1987.

Withrow SJ: Risks associated with biopsies for cancer. In Bonagura JD, editor: *Kirk's current veterinary therapy XII,* Philadelphia, 1995, WB Saunders, p 24.

# CHAPTER 37

# Hepatobiliary Diseases in the Cat

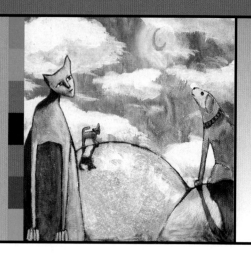

## CHAPTER OUTLINE

GENERAL CONSIDERATIONS, 506
HEPATIC LIPIDOSIS, 506
INFLAMMATORY HEPATOBILIARY DISEASE, 513
NEOPLASIA, 517
EXTRAHEPATIC BILE DUCT OBSTRUCTION, 518
CONGENITAL PORTOSYSTEMIC SHUNT, 520
ACUTE TOXIC HEPATOPATHY, 521
SECONDARY HEPATOBILIARY DISEASE, 523

## GENERAL CONSIDERATIONS

The clinical signs of most major hepatobiliary diseases in adult cats are similar. Other than nonspecific constitutional signs such as lethargy, anorexia, and weight loss, the most consistent clinical findings are jaundice and various degrees of hepatomegaly, regardless of the histologic lesion. Other signs observed less frequently include chronic intermittent vomiting, diarrhea, fever, abdominal effusion, and central nervous system (CNS) signs. The results of basic and specialized laboratory testing are often very similar also. Because of this overlap, subtle details of the history and hepatic biopsy assume an even greater role in the diagnostic evaluation of cats than of dogs with hepatobiliary disease. The feline hepatopathies (see Table 36-1) in this chapter are described in order of their frequency in clinical practice in the United States.

## HEPATIC LIPIDOSIS

### Etiology and Pathogenesis

Primary or idiopathic hepatic lipidosis has emerged within the past 10 years as the most common hepatic disease of cats in North America. Numerous factors have been proposed to be involved in its pathogenesis; high dietary protein catabolism is a species characteristic that could accelerate protein-calorie malnutrition in anorectic cats. Inadequate protein ingestion could lead to insufficiency of transport proteins necessary for hepatocellular secretion of triglycerides. The results of plasma amino acid analysis of cats with experimentally induced hepatic lipidosis suggest that deficiency of certain essential amino acids, such as arginine and methionine, may be the most crucial in the development of hepatic lipid accumulation. Other studies have suggested that disturbances in appetite, which is complexly regulated via CNS neurotransmitters, hormones, and cytokines, induce anorexia in a previously overeating obese cat. Carbohydrates in the diet in less than maintenance amounts encourage mobilization of fatty acids that are incompletely oxidized in the liver, enhancing lipid deposition. It is theorized that peripheral insulin resistance, commonly documented in obese human patients, may also contribute to hepatic lipid accumulation by allowing continued release of fatty acids from adipose tissue. Although this theory has never been documented, low-dose insulin therapy was once recommended for treatment of feline hepatic lipidosis, with inconclusive results. There is no evidence to support the theory that lipid collection is deleterious to hepatocytes; rather, it represents an expression of an as yet unidentified metabolic disturbance.

Cats may also become ill from hepatic lipidosis when they are anorectic and suffering from another illness (secondary hepatic lipidosis), such as diabetes mellitus, cardiomyopathy, neoplasia, neurologic disease, inflammatory hepatobiliary or intestinal disease, pancreatitis, feline infectious peritonitis (FIP), or chronic renal disease. The response of the liver to certain toxic agents is to accumulate lipid. In all of these instances, hepatic lipid accumulation should resolve, assuming the primary inciting illness is controlled and the cat's appetite returns to normal. Whether lipid deposition in hepatocytes occurs with or without a detectable cause, prolonged anorexia seems to be important in the genesis of this syndrome, and clinical illness develops after more than 50% of hepatocytes are affected.

### Clinical Features

Most affected cats are older than 2 years of age, but there does not appear to be a breed or gender predilection. Affected cats are commonly obese, are housed indoors, and have experienced a stressful event (e.g., introduction of a new pet into the household, abrupt dietary change) or an illness that causes them to become anorectic, and they lose weight rapidly. The initiating event is not always known; complete or near-complete anorexia for about 2 weeks precedes the development of jaundice, intermittent vomiting, and dehydration. Hepatic encephalopathy, most often manifested as depression and ptyalism, may be related to severe hepatocellular dysfunction or to arginine deficiency, to which the anorectic cat is predisposed. Cats are unable to synthesize arginine, which is needed to transform ammonia to urea (Krebs ornithine cycle), therefore they must depend on dietary sources. Previously obese cats have extensive loss of muscle mass but maintain certain fat stores, such as those in the falciform ligament and inguinal region. Cats with hepatic lipidosis and concurrent pancreatitis are often underweight.

## Diagnosis

A definitive diagnosis of hepatic lipidosis requires cytologic or histopathologic evaluation of a liver specimen. Typical clinicopathologic findings are those of cholestasis; total bilirubin concentrations range from normal (<0.3 mg/dl) to 20 mg/dl, with mild-to-moderate nonregenerative anemia. The serum hepatic enzyme pattern includes normal to moderately high (threefold to fivefold) alanine transaminase (ALT) activity and high (tenfold to fifteenfold) alkaline phosphatase (AP) activity, which approximates the level seen in cats with extrahepatic bile duct obstruction (EBDO). Serum γ-glutamyltransferase (GGT) activity is disproportionately low compared with that seen in other feline cholestatic hepatopathies. Serum GGT activity in cats with hepatic lipidosis is usually normal or only slightly elevated instead of greatly elevated as would be expected with other cholestatic hepatobiliary diseases. Fasting serum bile acid (SBA) concentrations are above normal limits in most cats. Blood cholesterol and glucose content may also be high but should not be confused with concentrations commonly observed in diabetic cats. Coagulation test abnormalities are noted more often in cats with concurrent hepatic lipidosis and acute pancreatitis.

Hepatomegaly may be confirmed by means of abdominal radiography. Ultrasonographic examination enables exclusion of other diseases with similar clinical features. The principal ultrasonographic feature of hepatic lipidosis is generalized hyperechogenicity; evidence of localized structural disease, such as mass lesions, or of dilated gallbladder and bile ducts suggestive of EBDO or cholangitis is absent. The presence of abdominal effusion and an irregular pancreas with low or mixed echogenicity suggest coexisting acute pancreatitis.

Additional diagnostic tests are performed to determine the presence of concurrent illnesses that could be causing protracted anorexia and secondary hepatic lipidosis. Tests are selected according to clues in the history, physical examination, and clinicopathologic and ultrasound evaluations. In addition to these tests (e.g., serum pancreatic lipase immunoreactivity in cats suspected of having pancreatitis [see Chapter 40]), microscopic examination of liver tissue is essential for diagnosis. Because percutaneous fine-needle aspiration for cytology is usually safe, quick, and easy to perform, it should be performed at the time of ultrasound examination and before needle or surgical biopsy is considered. Smears are stained with Wright's or quick hematology stains; Sudan III can be applied to unstained smears to confirm lipid vacuolation in hepatocytes. The vacuoles may be small or large, and there is a conspicuous absence of inflammatory or other cells in the primary or idiopathic form of hepatic lipidosis (Fig. 37-1). Cytologic findings correlate inconsistently with histopathologic findings, therefore if the results of diagnostic evaluation do not fit perfectly with a diagnosis of primary or idiopathic hepatic lipidosis, liver biopsy (see Chapter 36) is essential. The liver appears pale, friable, and yellow, with a prominent reticular pattern, when a visualized (laparoscopic or surgical) biopsy technique is used. Specimens are placed in buffered 10% formalin, in which they usually float, although lipid within hepatocytes will be removed by routine processing techniques. Special staining procedures using Oil red O applied to snap-frozen biopsy samples confirm that hepatocellular vacuolation is indeed lipid, but these procedures are not practical in a private practice setting. Routine staining with hematoxylin and eosin identifies clear vacuolation (most commonly caused by lipid accumulation in cats) in a majority of hepatocytes, with no particular zonal distribution. If there is no evidence either of illness in other body systems or of a single stressful event suspected of having initiated anorexia (e.g., new member brought into the household, sudden change in diet or environment), then hepatic lipidosis is considered to be primary or idiopathic.

## Treatment and Prognosis

Once a diagnosis of hepatic lipidosis has been made, the most important aspect of treatment is complete nutritional support, along with treatment of known concurrent and possibly precipitating illnesses. Published survival rates in earlier years suggested a dismal prognosis. Now that there are reliable

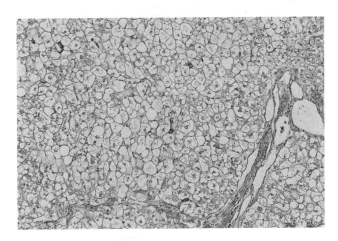

**FIG 37-1**
Photomicrograph of a liver specimen from a cat with severe idiopathic hepatic lipidosis (hematoxylin-eosin stain).

methods to ensure that nutritional requirements are met, recovery rates are improving to well over 60%.

Appetite stimulants such as diazepam (0.2 mg/kg IV q24h or q12h; avoid oral administration, see Acute Toxic Hepatopathy, p. 521), oxazepam (¼ of a 15 mg tablet PO q24h or q12h), and cyproheptadine (1 to 2 mg PO q12h or q8h) can be given to cats that are minimally affected and are still interested in eating one third to one half of their daily maintenance requirements. If the total daily nutritional needs are not being met with the assistance of appetite stimulants within 2 to 3 days, prompt use of aggressive nutritional support (i.e., tube feeding) will likely make a difference in whether the cat survives.

The results of recent studies of experimentally induced hepatic lipidosis indicate that a high-protein diet may hasten recovery. Severely affected cats are stabilized by attending to their fluid and electrolyte needs before anesthesia is considered for hepatic biopsy and/or feeding tube placement. During this time, nutritional support can be provided via nasoesophageal tube (Fig. 37-2) with one of several available liquid enteral diets, such as CliniCare Feline Liquid Diet, Abbott Laboratories, North Chicago, Ill (contains 1 kcal/ml). Cats with signs of hepatic encephalopathy are given a protein-restricted liquid enteral diet (CliniCare Feline Liquid Diet NF, Abbott Laboratories, North Chicago, Ill [contains about 1 kcal/ml]), with other medications added, if needed, to control signs (see Chapter 39).

First, the total number of calories to be fed daily is calculated on the basis of the current weight of the cat:

Maintenance energy requirement (MER) in calories =
$$1.4 \, (30 \, [\text{Body weight in kg}] + 70)$$

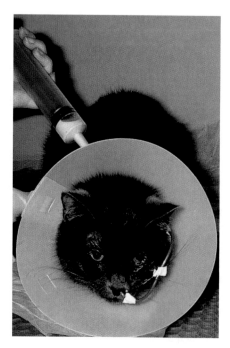

**FIG 37-2**
Nasoesophageal tube in place in a cat being fed a liquid enteral diet.

Then, one third of the daily requirement is administered in three to four meals on day 1; on day 2, the size of each meal is increased so that two thirds of the daily requirement is fed. The full complement of feedings is administered by day 3 (total daily needs split into three to four feedings) and can be continued for 5 to 7 days. When the cat is stable, a more permanent feeding system can be installed with the cat under general anesthesia. If necessary, hepatic biopsy can also be achieved during the same anesthetic episode, taking care to keep the total operative time short. Techniques for placing a midcervical esophagostomy (Fig. 37-3) or a gastrostomy tube with the assistance of an endoscope (Fig. 37-4) have been developed recently and are preferred over pharyngostomy tube placement. Several devices have also been developed to aid nonendoscopic placement of feeding tubes (Fig. 37-5). Feeding may begin the day after tube placement with a small amount of water (10 ml). Assuming there is no vomiting, bolus feeding may begin, using the calorie calculation and schedule described previously. The feeding tube should be aspirated before each feeding to ensure gastric emptying and flushed with a small bit of water after feeding to keep the tube patent. If the tube becomes plugged, a small amount of carbonated beverage is instilled, and 15 minutes later, another attempt is made to flush it.

The large bore of the French-pezzar mushroom-tip tube (Bard urological catheter, Bard Urological Division, Covington, Ga; 16 or 18 Fr; a Foley catheter should not be used) allows use of blenderized diets (Feline p/d or k/d, Hill's Pet Products, Topeka, Kan; a mixture of one can with 1½ cups water yields a slurry with 0.9 kcal/ml) for administration at home. Recently, several diets have been formulated to be fed as is, making home feeding even easier (a/d, Hill's Pet Products, Topeka, Kan [1.3 kcal/ml], or Maximum-Calorie, Eukanuba Veterinary Diets, The Iams Co., Dayton, Ohio [2.1 kcal/ml]) for the first 1 to 2 weeks. Feline k/d or Veterinary Diet NF (Ralston Purina Co., St. Louis) is preferred for initial treatment of cats with hepatic encephalopathy; the diet is gradually switched to a higher protein diet when signs of encephalopathy subside. Several other diets are made to be use warmed and undiluted (Feline a/d, Hill's Pet Products, Topeka, Kan, or Maximum Calorie, Eukanuba Veterinary Diet, The Iams Co., Dayton, Ohio). As yet, no information is available that suggests that taurine, carnitine, or arginine supplementation speeds recovery.

Additional treatments may be needed for some cats. Those that cannot tolerate full feeding because of gastroparesis, as indicated by vomiting, or repeated aspiration of more than 10 ml of food or fluid before feeding benefit from potassium supplementation if hypokalemic, or from administration of a promotility agent such as metoclopramide (0.2 to 0.5 mg/kg SQ or via tube q6-8h 15 to 20 minutes before feeding). Cisapride (0.5 mg/kg PO q8-12h) is a potent prokinetic agent but is no longer commercially available. Hypophosphatemia may develop during refeeding and, if severe, can cause hemolytic anemia. If the serum phosphate concentration is equal to or less than 2.0 mg/dl, supplementation is provided with potassium phosphate (0.015 mmol of phosphate/kg/hour added to 0.9%

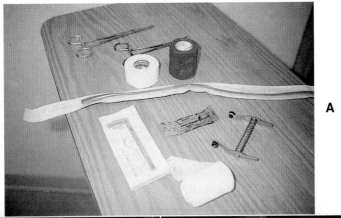

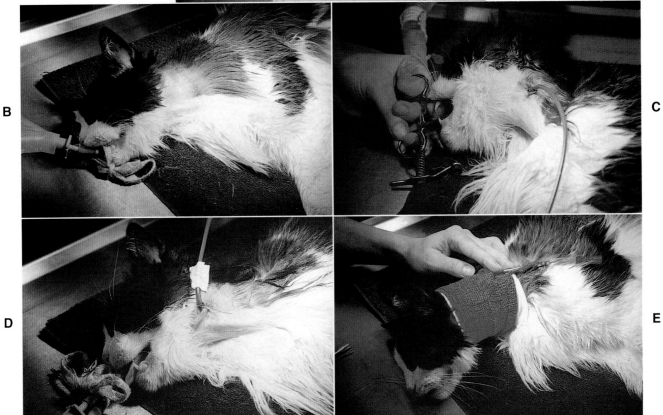

**FIG 37-3**
Feeding tube placed percutaneously in the midcervical esophagus. **A,** Materials needed for
the procedure: mouth speculum, No. 15 scalpel blade, curved forceps, needle holders, red
rubber feeding tube at least 10 Fr in size, suture, and bandage material. **B,** With the cat
under general anesthesia, the left lateral cervical area is clipped and prepared aseptically.
**C,** The curved forceps is introduced into the proximal esophagus. The overlying skin,
subcutaneous tissue, and esophagus are incised only enough to accommodate the feeding
tube, taking care to avoid the jugular vein, and the forceps tip is pushed through the
incision to grasp the tip of the feeding tube. **D,** The feeding tube is pulled out of the mouth,
reinserted into the esophagus with the tip in the distal one third of the esophagus, and
sutured to the skin to prevent dislodgment (note the position of the jugular vein). **E,** A
support wrap is placed around the neck. (Courtesy Dr. Sandra Albright, Raleigh, N.C.; see
Crowe and colleague (1997) in Suggested Readings for further details on the procedure.)

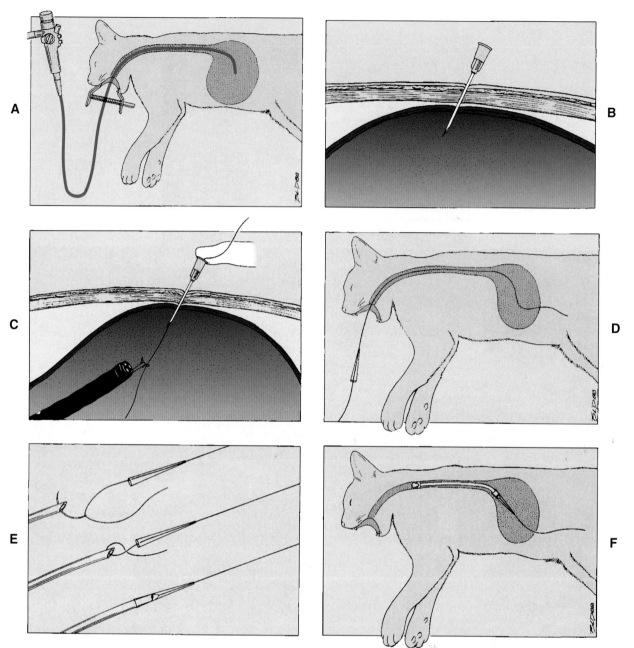

**FIG 37-4**

Endoscopically aided placement of a gastrostomy tube in a cat. The feeding tube is prepared by cutting off the end without the mushroom tip. Two flanges are constructed for the feeding tube; one is to be positioned on the feeding tube just above the mushroom tip (delete in small cats), the other outside the body wall. **A,** The cat is placed in right lateral recumbency, the endoscope is introduced, and the stomach is insufflated sufficiently to ensure contact of the stomach with the abdominal wall. **B,** Taking care that the spleen is displaced caudally, a sterilely gloved assistant pushes on the site for tube placement (caudal to the rib cage and in the dorsal two thirds of the flank) and pushes on the site with a finger, enabling the endoscopist to visualize it from the gastric lumen. While insufflation is maintained, the assistant introduces an 18-gauge, 1.5-inch needle or over-the-needle catheter through the body wall until the endoscopist can see the tip. **C,** Plain single, No. 0 nylon suture is threaded through the needle into the stomach and into the view of the endoscopist. Capping the end of the needle helps to maintain insufflation until the endoscopist grasps the suture with the aid of an endoscopic retrieval device. **D,** The nylon suture is pulled through the body wall by the endoscopist, and the needle is removed by the assistant. A disposable pipette or sharpened 3.5 Fr polypropylene urethral catheter is threaded onto the suture tip first. **E,** The nylon suture is attached firmly to the feeding tube, and the slanted tip of the feeding tube is pulled up snugly into the pipette tip. **F,** The assistant applies steady traction on the suture, pulling the feeding tube into the esophagus and stomach. (From Armstrong PJ et al: Enteral nutrition by tube, *Vet Clin North Am Small Anim Pract* 20:237, 1990.)

*Continued*

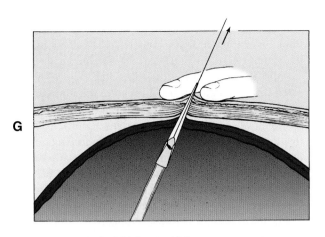

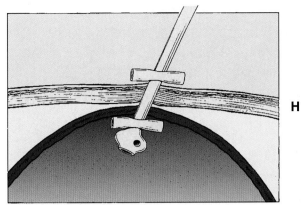

**FIG 37-4, cont'd**
**G,** When the pipette tip touches the stomach and body wall, counterpressure is applied to the body wall and the suture is pulled until the feeding tube is visible outside the body. A small relief incision in the skin allows the feeding tube to exit the skin more easily. **H,** The remaining flange is placed onto the feeding tube; a small piece of tape may be positioned on the tube just above the flange to prevent the flange from slipping. The tube is capped, and a support wrap is placed on the abdomen.

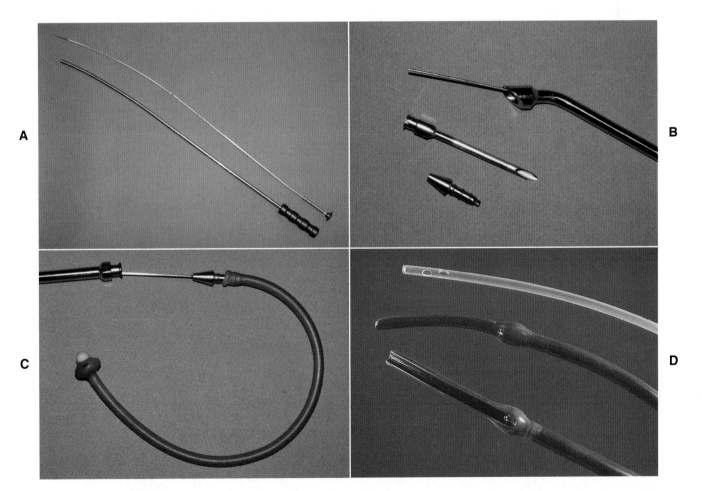

**FIG 37-5**
Devices manufactured to facilitate nonendoscopic placement of feeding tubes. **A,** ELD gastrostomy tube applicator, Jorgensen Laboratories, Inc., Loveland, Colorado. **B** and **C,** Gastrostomy tube introduction set, Cook Veterinary Products, Queensland, Australia. **D,** Esophageal feeding tube applicator, Firma Fixomed, Munich, Germany.

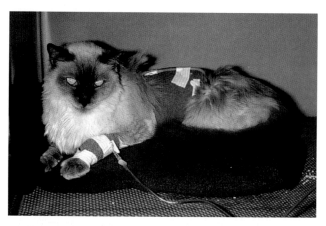

**FIG 37-6**
Gastrostomy tube in place in cat with chronic renal failure. Near-complete nutritional support was provided via tube gastrostomy for 4 months while the cat awaited a renal transplant.

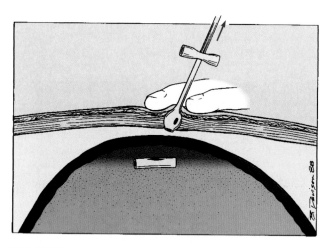

**FIG 37-7**
The gastrostomy tube is removed by steady traction on the tube with counterpressure on the body wall. (From Armstrong PJ et al: Enteral nutrition by tube, *Vet Clin North Am Small Anim Pract* 20:237, 1990.)

saline given IV over 6 to 12 hours or until the serum concentration is near the reference range). For cats with a coagulopathy, vitamin $K_1$ (0.5 mg/kg SQ q12h) is recommended.

Most cats tolerate feeding tubes well (Fig. 37-6) for the extended time needed to deliver total nutritional support (2 or more weeks); after minimal instruction, owners can feed their cats three to four times daily at home. In the event that the cat begins eating voluntarily after feeding tube placement, the tube should remain in place for at least 5 days before removal to ensure that an adequate seal has formed between the stomach and the body wall and that peritoneal contamination is prevented. Latex feeding tubes are adequate for most cats needing assisted feeding for less than 3 months; silicone feeding tubes have been left in place for up to 6 months with no complications. The support wrap for either feeding tube should be changed as needed. The gastric feeding tube should be removed by firm, consistent traction (Fig. 37-7), with the cat sedated if necessary, as soon as a normal appetite has resumed for at least 1 week. Esophagostomy tubes are removed after the retention sutures have been snipped. Neither ostomy site requires surgical closure or other special attention.

The cat with concurrent hepatic lipidosis and pancreatitis presents a special nutritional challenge because the preferred feeding methods for each of these conditions are diametrically opposed. Because pancreatitis can be difficult to diagnose in cats (see p. 560), its prevalence is currently unknown. There is no compelling information available to recommend a specific approach for the nutritional aspect of treatment. Enteral tube feeding distal to the pancreas, such as duodenostomy (Fig. 37-8; DeNovo and colleagues, 2001) or jejunostomy, has been successful in a small number of cats in our hospital and would seem to be the approach of choice.

There are no known permanent sequelae of hepatic lipidosis in cats that recover, and there is no reason to believe that the condition will recur. Because obesity and concurrent illnesses that can cause a cat to stop eating are important predisposing factors, these conditions should be avoided. The

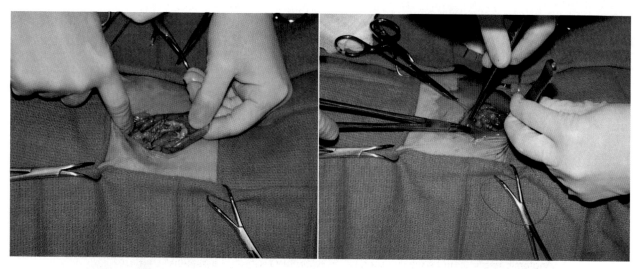

**FIG 37-8**
Placement of a feeding tube into the duodenum and jejunum via a right flank grid incision.

prognosis for cats with concurrent hepatic lipidosis and pancreatitis is guarded to grave.

## INFLAMMATORY HEPATOBILIARY DISEASE

### Pathogenesis and Etiology

Excluding hepatic lipidosis, clinically important acquired hepatic disease in cats tends to be more biliary in distribution than in dogs, in which most of the important hepatic diseases are primarily hepatocellular. *Cholangitis* (CH) is the term used to define a group of diseases characterized by inflammation of bile ducts, with bile duct proliferation and hyperplasia also observed as a nonspecific response to cholestasis. Because of the unusual anatomic relationship between the common bile duct and the major pancreatic duct in the cat (Fig. 37-9), ascension of substances such as bacteria from the duodenum or digestive enzymes from a subclinically inflamed pancreas has been postulated to be the reason that CH is more common in cats than in dogs. Inflammatory lesions of the duodenum, pancreas, and biliary tract are seen frequently in cats with CH, and until recently it was not known which came first or if they were even related. In a recent retrospective study of 78 cats, liver, intestinal, pancreatic, and renal tissues were examined for evidence of concurrent disease of these organs (Weiss and colleagues, 1996). More than 80% of cats with CH also had histologic findings of inflammatory bowel disease, and about half had changes consistent with mild pancreatitis, implying that the source or result of CH in some cats might be extension of inflammation to or from these organs.

There are several types of CH, based on histopathologic findings; a name is ascribed according to the predominant inflammatory cell type. Because the classification is somewhat controversial and heavily dependent on interpretation of hepatic biopsies, attempts are being made to standardize the terminology, thereby facilitating understanding of these conditions (Rothuizen, 2001). It is tempting to speculate that these conditions represent phases of a progressive biliary tract disorder that begins with acute inflammation in the extrahepatic bile ducts, changes in cytologic character from neutrophilic to lymphoplasmacytic or pleomorphic as the disease progresses, extends into the hepatic parenchyma, and possibly culminates in biliary cirrhosis, which is rare in cats. To date, there is insufficient evidence to state confidently that these are simply different manifestations of the same disease, therefore they should be considered separate entities. The following represents a summary of available published information about CH in cats.

### Clinical Features

Cats with CH have no particularly unique historic or physical examination features; many are male cats of any breed 4 years old or older. Histories of affected cats are chronic, with waxing and waning illness. Common presenting signs include anorexia, depression, weight loss, vomiting, diarrhea, dehydration, hepatomegaly, and jaundice. About half of affected cats have hyperglobulinemia; a few have been reported to have an IgG monoclonal gammopathy (Lucke and colleague, 1984).

#### Cholangiohepatitis

*Acute CH* was first described in five older cats, although a more recent study of 16 cats suggested a tendency toward the

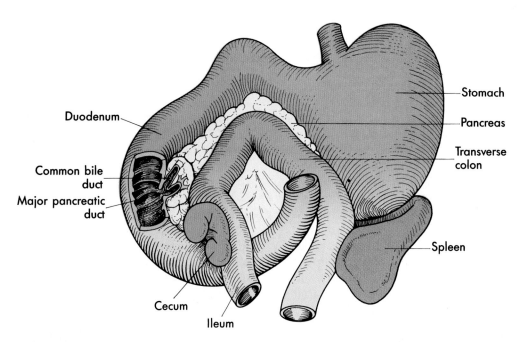

**FIG 37-9**
Anatomic relationship between pancreas, common bile duct, and duodenum in the cat. (From Strombeck DR: *Small animal gastroenterology*, Davis, Calif, 1979, Stonegate Publishing.)

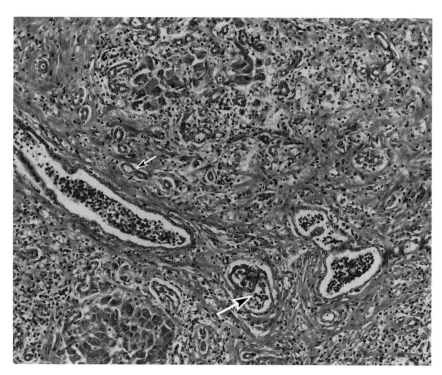

**FIG 37-10**
Photomicrograph of liver specimen from a cat with acute cholangitis. Notice the neutrophilic inflammation in and around bile ducts *(large arrow)*. Biliary ductular hyperplasia is also present *(small arrow)* (hematoxylin-eosin stain).

disease in younger and middle-aged animals (Gagne and colleagues, 1999; mean and median ages, 5.7 and 3.3 years, respectively). Clinical signs are typical of any feline chronic hepatobiliary disease except for the findings of a *relatively short period of illness (≤1 month), fever, and an inflammatory leukogram.* Serum liver enzyme activities are typical of a mixed pattern of parenchymal and biliary injury, with normal to twofold elevations of AP activity and as high as tenfold elevations of ALT activity. Most cats have an underlying disorder that could favor ascending bacterial invasion of the biliary tract by enteric bacteria. Examples include biliary anomaly (e.g., bilobed gallbladder), liver flukes, cholelithiasis, cholecystitis, pancreatitis, pancreatic periductal fibrosis, or duodenitis. Bile collected for bacterial culture most often yields enteric organisms, such as *Escherichia coli*, *Pseudomonas* sp., and *Enterococcus* sp.; results may be negative if antimicrobial therapy has already been initiated at the time of sampling. Consistent histologic features in the liver biopsy specimens from affected cats include dilated intrahepatic bile ducts containing an exudate of degenerate neutrophils and neutrophilic invasion of bile duct walls and adjacent periportal hepatocytes (Fig. 37-10). Imprints of the biopsy specimen and bile cytologic analysis can provide evidence of bacterial infection before results of histopathologic examination and culture are known.

*Chronic CH* may be a later stage of acute CH. Cats affected with chronic CH are generally older (Gagne and colleagues, 1999; mean and median ages, 9.7 and 9.0 years, respectively).

Histopathologically, there is a mixed cellular infiltrate of neutrophils, lymphocytes, and plasma cells in portal tracts around bile ducts. Bile duct hyperplasia and portal fibrosis are prominent features. Perhaps this form results from inappropriate treatment of acute CH or represents an immune-mediated response to initiating antigens from the intestine.

### Lymphocytic cholangitis

Lymphocytic cholangitis differs from acute and chronic CH clinically and histopathologically. Cats with lymphocytic cholangitis generally are young (6 months to 4 years old) to middle-aged (6 to 9 years) adults, and Persians appear to be overrepresented. In four studies comprising 47 cats with lymphocytic cholangitis, abdominal effusion of high protein content (>5 g/dl) was a presenting sign in 16 cats (35%). Serum biochemical findings are similar to those of cats with acute CH. Because affected cats often have hyperglobulinemia and abdominal effusion, they can be mistaken for having the more dismal effusive form of FIP. A liver biopsy, therefore, is essential in differentiating these two conditions. The hepatic lesion of lymphocytic cholangitis is characterized histologically by aggregates of inflammatory cells, predominantly lymphocytes but also smaller numbers of neutrophils, plasma cells, and eosinophils, in portal tracts and around bile ducts (Fig. 37-11). There is a variable degree of periductal fibrosis, and the lesion may progress to biliary cirrhosis. Occasionally the lumina of bile ducts are obliterated. Some affected cats have lymphocytic aggregates in the pancreas on postmortem examination, but this has not been reported in most cases.

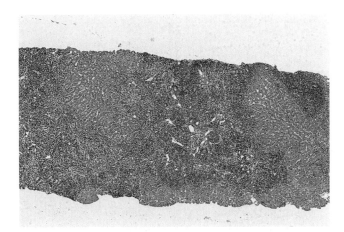

**FIG 37-11**
Photomicrograph of liver specimen from a cat with severe lymphocytic cholangiohepatitis. There is intense mononuclear cell infiltration in the portal tract *(center)*.

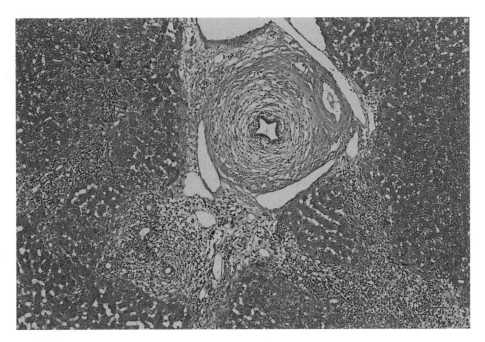

**FIG 37-12**
Photomicrograph of liver specimen from a cat with sclerosing cholangitis. The wall of the bile duct *(center)* is extensively thickened by fibrosis, but there is minimal inflammation (hematoxylin-eosin stain). (Courtesy Dr. Tom VanWinkle, University of Pennsylvania, School of Veterinary Medicine, Philadelphia, Pa.)

The typical hepatic lesion in cats with FIP is a multifocal pyogranulomatous reaction with evidence of vasculitis or perivasculitis.

### Sclerosing cholangitis

Thickened extrahepatic and/or intrahepatic bile ducts, characterized histologically by diffuse proliferative fibrosis of their walls, is typical of sclerosing cholangitis (Fig. 37-12), which is a rare condition of older cats (≥10 years); the gallbladder may also be involved. The result is the appearance of distended ducts with luminal narrowing to the point of near obliteration. The signs and clinicopathologic features are typical of severe chronic cholestasis, therefore diseases that cause mechanical bile duct obstruction must be excluded before this diagnosis can be considered (see Table 37-1 and p. 518, Extrahepatic Bile Duct Obstruction). Although there may be some pleomorphic cell infiltrates in affected portal regions similar to those seen in chronic CH, this is not a predominant finding. This condition has been likened to primary sclerosing cholangitis of humans, which is immunologically mediated. However, because it has been described only rarely in cats, it is difficult to make accurate comparisons, and it may indeed represent an advanced stage of lymphocytic cholangitis.

### Lymphocytic portal hepatitis

Three recent studies have described an inflammatory hepatopathy, commonly discovered in asymptomatic cats over 10 years of age of either gender, that is characterized by infiltration of portal areas by lymphocytes and to a lesser extent plasma cells, bile duct proliferation, and portal and bridging

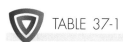

TABLE 37-1

Causes of Extrahepatic Bile Duct Obstruction

| EXTRALUMINAL COMPRESSIVE | INTRALUMINAL OBSTRUCTIVE |
| --- | --- |
| **Neoplasia**<br>Biliary<br>Pancreatic<br>Duodenal<br>**Stricture**<br>Following trauma, pancreatitis, or duodenitis<br>**Diaphragmatic hernia**<br>**Congenital anomalies** of the extrahepatic biliary tract (e.g., choledochal cyst)* | **Cholelithiasis**<br>Mixed composition<br>Pigment<br>Cholesterol (rare)<br>**Inspissated bile**<br>**Liver flukes** (*Platynosomum concinnum*, others)* |

*Cats only.

fibrosis. Although small numbers of lymphocytes and plasma cells (<10/portal area) are found in healthy young cats, large numbers (>10/portal area) are associated with many extra-hepatobiliary diseases, some of which might be merely coincidental. The hepatic histopathologic findings in this condition resemble a form of autoimmune or viral-associated chronic hepatitis in humans that rarely progresses called *chronic persistent hepatitis,* or it may represent a secondary or reactive hepatopathy. This condition appears to progress and cause illness in some cats, but it is not related to intercurrent intestinal or pancreatic inflammation. Further information is needed to determine the clinical relevance of this condition and whether specific treatment is indicated.

## Diagnosis

Although the major forms of inflammatory hepatic disease in cats may share similar clinical and clinicopathologic features typical of intrahepatic cholestasis (e.g., mild nonregenerative anemia, variable leukocytosis, high serum liver-specific enzyme activities, hyperbilirubinemia, high SBA concentration), a definitive diagnosis can be established only by hepatic biopsy (see Table 37-1). Radiographic findings are nonspecific; ultrasonographic examination may detect dilated intrahepatic and extrahepatic bile ducts and gallbladder, with shadowing that often represents "sludged" or inspissated bile (see Table 36-5). Also on ultrasound examination, the walls of portal veins appear less clearly identifiable in cats with lymphocytic portal hepatitis (LPH) compared with CH (Gagne and colleagues, 1999). Preliminary impressions of the cytologic nature of the infiltrate can be achieved by fine-needle aspiration, but percutaneous needle biopsy or surgical biopsy is essential for a definitive diagnosis. Bile for bacterial culture and sensitivity is best obtained from the gallbladder with ultrasound guidance or during exploratory laparotomy. The finding of "white bile" (bile completely devoid of bilirubin pigment; Fig. 37-13) denotes severe cholestasis and lack of hepatocellular ability to excrete bilirubin. Most often this observation has been made in association with the chronic forms of CH, but it has also been reported in acute CH; acholic feces are also expected in these cases.

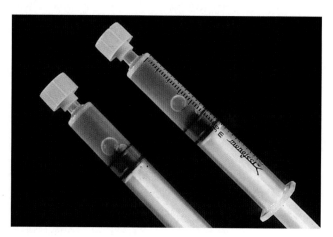

**FIG 37-13**
Syringe containing bile obtained at surgery from the gall-bladder of a cat with severe lymphocytic cholangitis *(left),* compared with a syringe filled with sterile water *(right).*

## Treatment and Prognosis

Because the major forms of CH in cats seem to be distinct at this time, specific treatment is dictated by the results of hepatic biopsy and bile culture. Until these are known, other clinical features, such as signalment and clinicopathologic findings, must guide treatment decisions. A good empiric antibiotic choice for acute CH, which is a septic process, is amoxicillin or cefazolin (22 mg/kg PO or IV q8h) until bile culture results are available. Addition of an aminoglycoside (amikacin) or a fluoroquinolone (marbofloxacin) is advised for cats suspected of having systemic involvement. In confirmed cases, specific antibiotic treatment should continue for at least 6 to 8 weeks. For cats with chronic CH, long-term antibiotic treatment is given first, followed by corticosteroids (see below) if no improvement is seen.

Some investigators have attempted to compare feline lymphocytic cholangitis to primary biliary cirrhosis or chronic destructive cholangitis in humans, a disease suspected to have a primary immunologic basis. Investigators have found no evidence of antibodies to mitochondria, smooth muscle, thyroid, or parietal cells in affected cats, and immunohistochemical staining of liver tissue specimens for nonspecific T and B lymphocyte markers, major histocompatibility complex Class II, and immunoglobulins revealed that the lymphocytes invading bile ducts were mostly T cells with aggregates of B cells. Although the resemblance is weak and until the underlying causes are better understood, treatment for lymphocytic cholangitis consists of modulating the histologic lesion with corticosteroids. The initial dose of corticosteroids is 2.2 mg/kg every 24 hours; prednisone is usually given orally. The decision as to when to decrease the dose depends on the individual patient; clinical, clinicopathologic, or histopathologic evidence of improvement usually indicates control of the disease. Some cats may benefit from a higher dose of prednisone (4 mg/kg PO q24h) or addition of metronidazole (7.5 mg/kg PO q12h) for its immunomodulatory effect, and some cats may fail to respond completely. Some investigators have attempted to use methotrexate in cats that have not responded to other immunosuppressive agents, prompted by reports of improvement in human patients with sclerosing cholangitis or primary biliary cirrhosis given this drug. Specific guidelines for the use of methotrexate and other immunosuppressive drugs (see Chapter 93), such as chlorambucil, have not been established.

Use of ursodeoxycholic acid (ursodiol) is a valuable adjunctive medical treatment for cats with chronic cholestatic hepatopathies. However, this and other choleretic agents should not be used in cats with EBDO. The actions of this drug are to stimulate bile flow, replace injurious bile acids in the circulating bile acid pool, and serve an antiinflammatory function. Investigations in normal cats indicate that a dose of 10 mg/kg given orally every 24 hours is safe for at least 3 months; controlled studies of safety and efficacy in cats with cholestatic hepatopathy have not been performed. Preparations are available only in 300-mg capsules; individual doses must be compounded, usually into small gelatin capsules.

Nutritional support is an important component of medical therapy for cats with CH. A balanced, high-protein (30% to 40% protein on a dry matter basis) maintenance diet is fed to cats that do not have signs of hepatic encephalopathy (HE) (see recommendations for treatment of hepatic lipidosis). For cats with HE, a combination of boiled rice and cottage cheese can be given over the short term, or a protein-restricted prescription diet (Feline k/d, Hill's Pet Products, Topeka, Kan, or Veterinary Diet NF, Ralston Purina Co., St. Louis) can be used (see p. 546). The preferred route of enteral feeding (e.g., appetite stimulation, nasoesophageal tube, esophagostomy or gastrostomy tube) depends on the degree and duration of anorexia. The reader is referred to the section on hepatic lipidosis for more information on this topic (see p. 506).

Long-term follow-up information on a large number of cats with CH is not available. On the basis of reported retrospective studies, the prognosis for cats with acute CH seems to be variable. Most cats that survive the initial period of treatment of 1 to 2 months have a good chance for cure and long-term survival. Because some cats with chronic CH, lymphocytic cholangitis, or LPH appear to live comfortably for months to years with or without corticosteroid therapy, the role of treatment in improving the quality of life in affected cats is less clear. A better understanding of the underlying cause or causes of chronic CH is needed.

## NEOPLASIA

### Etiology

*Primary* hepatobiliary neoplasms are rare in cats. Of those that cause clinical illness, cholangiocellular (bile duct) carcinoma (CC) and hepatocellular carcinoma (HC) are reported most often. The overall frequency of hepatobiliary neoplasia varies among surveys performed between 1951 and 1980, but a review at the Angell Memorial Animal Hospital (Carpenter and colleagues, 1987) concluded that neoplasms of the liver and biliary tract comprised 1.9% of all feline neoplasia (63 of 3248). Although some naturally occurring and experimental causes of primary hepatobiliary cancer in other species have been identified, causes in cats are not well understood. It is more common to document hepatic metastases from neoplasia arising from other tissues because of the liver's dual blood supply, lymphatic network, and close proximity to other abdominal organs. The most common lesions are hemolymphatic neoplasms such as lymphoma, myeloproliferative disease, systemic mast cell disease, and hemangiosarcoma; occasionally, the liver may appear to be the only site of involvement with these neoplasms. Hepatic metastases from malignancy of the mammary gland, pancreas, kidney, and gastrointestinal tract have also been observed in cats.

### Clinical Features

There is no particular breed predilection for hepatobiliary neoplasia, and most affected cats are over 10 years old, except for cats with feline leukemia virus (FeLV)–related disease. Male cats are predisposed to HC; females are predisposed to CC. Clinical signs are nonspecific and include lethargy, anorexia, weight loss, and abdominal distention from either hepatomegaly or effusion (ascites or hemoperitoneum). The finding of simultaneous pleural and peritoneal (or double) effusion suggests the presence of cancer in either cavity. Whether jaundice is present or not depends on the distribution of the neoplasm in the liver. Those involving intrahepatic or extrahepatic biliary structures or portal tracts would be expected to cause cholestasis. Neoplasm affecting the liver commonly causes organ enlargement, either in a firm diffuse or nodular (small, massive) pattern that is detectable by physical, radiographic, or ultrasonographic examination (see Figs. 36-5 and 36-8).

### Diagnosis

A suspicion for hepatic neoplasia may be gained from the physical examination findings, survey radiographs, and ultrasonographic characteristics of the liver. A definitive diagnosis requires cytologic or histopathologic evaluation of a liver specimen. Abnormal liver enzyme activities are common, but unless there is greater than 75% to 80% involvement with neoplasm, functional disturbances do not occur. Because the liver is most often involved secondarily in neoplastic processes, a careful search for a primary site is essential to the diagnostic evaluation. Certain relatively benign conditions such as hepatic cysts and bile duct adenomas must not be mistaken for malignant processes such as CC, which can be cystic.

### Treatment

Treatment of cats with hemolymphatic or metastatic hepatobiliary neoplasia is usually selected according to the cell type of the primary neoplasm. Surgical resection of a primary hepatobiliary neoplasm that is confined to one liver lobe and has not metastasized may result in prolonged (>1 year) disease-free survival. The size of the neoplasm is less important in determining the prognosis than the degree of invasiveness and the presence of regional or distant metastases. Investigational treatments such as hepatic dearterialization or chemotherapy combined with hyperthermia may be available through referral institutions.

### Prognosis

The prognosis for cats with benign hepatocellular or biliary tumors after resection is good; most cats are free of disease at least 1 year later. The prognosis for malignant neoplasia is generally grave because of the extent of involvement at the time of diagnosis. However, as discussed, complete resection of HC can result in prolonged survival.

## EXTRAHEPATIC BILE DUCT OBSTRUCTION

### Pathogenesis and Etiology

Extrahepatic bile duct obstruction is a syndrome with several different underlying causes. Causes of EBDO are categorized as extraluminal compressive or intraluminal obstructive lesions (see Table 37-1). Neoplasms arising from the extrahepatic biliary tract, pancreas, or proximal duodenum can compress the common bile duct (CBD) along its course or occlude its termination at the sphincter of Oddi. Severe inflammatory conditions of these same tissues could also result in obstruction or, once the active inflammatory phase has subsided, fibrosis of the CBD. Abdominal trauma from automobile accidents or penetrating wounds can lead to CBD avulsion or stricture or to entrapment of the liver and biliary tract in a diaphragmatic hernia. Congenital anomalies of the gallbladder or CBD are usually incidental findings but occasionally have been associated with EBDO.

Choleliths can be a cause of EBDO or an incidental finding. In cats (and dogs) with clinical features consistent with hepatobiliary disease, choleliths form most commonly as a result of altered local factors such as dehydration, bacterial infection, and infrequent gallbladder evacuation during periods of anorexia. In such instances, stones are greenish brown or black and are composed of a mixture of bilirubin,

cholesterol, calcium carbonate, and other metabolites. These stones may or may not be radiographically opaque, depending on how much mineral they contain (Fig. 37-14). They can be located in the gallbladder, CBD, or rarely in the cystic, hepatic, or interlobar ducts, and are visible with ultrasonography (US). Inspissated bile, which could be loosely termed a type of "pigment" stone, may be a complication of severe intrahepatic cholestasis from CH or hepatic lipidosis. Cholesterol stones form when the bile becomes supersaturated with cholesterol, the cholesterol monohydrate crystals are nucleated, and the gallbladder is incapable of complete emptying. These stones are the most common choleliths in metabolically predisposed human patients but form rarely in animals.

Liver fluke (*Platynosomum* spp., *Amphimerus pseudofelineus, Metametorchis intermedius*) infestations, reported most commonly in cats from Louisiana, Florida, and Hawaii, are most often subclinical but may be responsible for EBDO in severely affected cats. Two intermediate hosts, snails and lizards or freshwater fish (depending on the fluke species), are required for the infective stage of the liver fluke to develop. Cats acquire the infection by ingesting infected intermediate hosts. Histologic changes in the hepatobiliary system induced by liver fluke infestation are not unique, except occasionally in the cat with pleomorphic portal infiltrates consisting of eosinophils, lymphocytes, plasma cells, neutrophils, and macrophages. The diagnosis is made by finding fluke ova in feces prepared by the formalin-ether sedimentation technique (Table 37-2) in cats with compatible clinicopathologic findings or at surgery.

### Clinical Features

The clinical signs, clinicopathologic findings, and survey radiographic findings of cats with EBDO may be indistinguishable from those of other severe cholestatic hepatopathies (e.g., anorexia, depression, vomiting, jaundice, hepatomegaly), especially if obstruction is incomplete. A greatly distended gallbladder may be found by abdominal palpation.

### Diagnosis

EBDO is diagnosed by physical examination findings, results of standard laboratory testing, survey abdominal radiographs, US, and exploratory laparotomy. Studies of cats with experimental complete EBDO have shown high serum AP activity (up to fivefold) and striking increases in the serum ALT activity (tenfold to thirty-fourfold), fasting SBA concentration (up to 100-fold), and serum bilirubin concentration (up to 25 mg/dl). High serum GGT activity is also characteristic, with a similar or greater magnitude of elevation than that seen in the serum AP. Acholic feces, vitamin K–responsive coagulopathy, and persistent absence of urobilinogen in correctly processed urine specimens are persuasive evidence of complete bile duct obstruction. The most common location of obstruction is the CBD at or near the duodenum. Because bile flow into the intestine is impeded, the gallbladder and bile ducts proximal to the obstruction become distended and tortuous; these, along with generalized hepatomegaly, are dis-

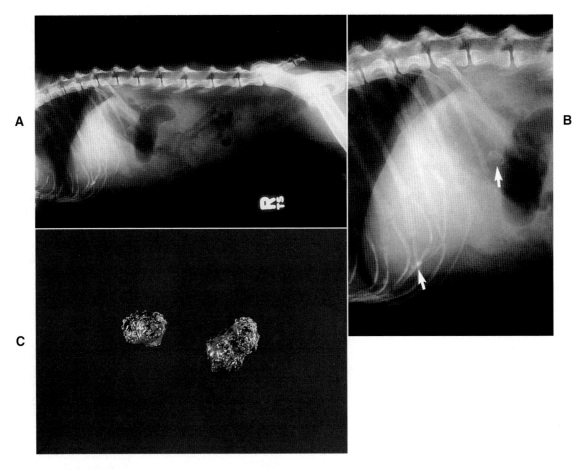

**FIG 37-14**
**A,** Lateral abdominal survey radiograph of a 13-year-old castrated male domestic short-haired cat with cholelithiasis and bacterial cholangitis. **B,** Collimated image demonstrating mineral opacities in a major bile duct and gallbladder *(arrows).* **C,** Choleliths removed from the bile duct.

 TABLE 37-2

Formalin-Ether Sedimentation Technique for Detecting *Platynosomum concinnum* Ova in Feces

| | |
|---|---|
| 1. Mix 1 g of feces in 25 ml saline; filter through a fine mesh screen. | 4. Add 3 ml of cold ether on top of solution and shake vigorously for 1 min. Centrifuge for 3 min at 1500 rpm. |
| 2. Centrifuge solution for 5 min at 1500 rpm; discard the supernate. | 5. Discard the supernate, resuspend the pellet in several drops of saline, and prepare slide of solution to examine microscopically. |
| 3. Resuspend the pellet with 7 ml of 10% neutral buffered formalin; let stand for 10 min. | |

From Bielsa LM et al: Liver flukes *(Platynosomum concinnum)* in cats, *J Am Anim Hosp Assoc* 21:269, 1985.

cernible ultrasonographically (see Fig. 36-9). Mild gallbladder distention associated with anorexia and infrequent evacuation should not be overinterpreted as indicative of EBDO. Secondary hepatic consequences of unrelieved EBDO observed on histologic examination of liver tissue are bile canalicular plugs, biliary epithelial hyperplasia, bile ductule multiplication, periportal fibrosis, and variable degrees of neutrophilic inflammation and necrosis.

## Treatment

A combined surgical and medical approach is usually needed for treatment of cats with EBDO. After the animal has been stabilized (fluid and electrolyte therapy, vitamin K supplementation), the immediate goals are to relieve obstruction surgically and to determine the underlying cause and remove it if possible. If the precipitating cause cannot be removed and bile flow reestablished easily (e.g., because of a nonresectable neoplasm or stricture), reconstructive procedures (i.e., chole-cystojejunostomy or cholecystoduodenostomy) may need to be performed. Because choleliths and inspissated bile can form secondary to primary hepatobiliary disease, liver and/or gallbladder biopsy, bile culture and cytologic examination, and stone analysis are important diagnostic aids.

Limited information from reports of liver fluke infestation in cats suggests that praziquantel may be effective. Several dosage regimens have been used in reported clinical cases, although a regimen of 20 mg/kg given orally or subcutaneously every 24 hours for 3 days is currently recommended. Because use of praziquantel in this situation is an extralabel application, owner consent is recommended.

The importance of supportive care postoperatively cannot be overemphasized. Attending to fluid, electrolyte, and nutritional needs is critical to a successful outcome. Biochemical abnormalities associated with EBDO should begin to subside immediately after surgery. Whether the trend continues toward normality will depend on whether the initiating cause has been addressed.

## CONGENITAL PORTOSYSTEMIC SHUNT

### Etiology and Pathogenesis

Diversion of portal blood flow around the liver by an anomalous vessel allows portal blood constituents direct access to the systemic circulation. The pathophysiologic effects are a result of the missed opportunity for the liver to extract deleterious substances (e.g., ammonia and other encephalotoxins, absorbed bacteria, endotoxins) and reduced total hepatic blood flow to some percentage less than the 80% normally provided by the portal vein. Because portal blood carries 50% of the oxygen delivered to the liver and contains important trophic factors, especially insulin, diminished portal blood flow results in poor hepatocyte growth and function. Several patterns of abnormal portosystemic vascular connections have been described in dogs, but the most common anomaly in cats is a single extrahepatic shunt arising from the gastric, splenic, or portal vein and joining with the caudal vena cava. Complete portacaval shunt with intrahepatic portal vein hypoplasia, as well as patent ductus venosus, has also been detected occasionally in cats. These defects probably result from failure of fetal venous communications to regress, perhaps caused by lack of the appropriate metabolic signals to trigger fetal vein closure. Because intrahepatic portal pressure is normally higher than caudal vena cava pressure, blood flow is diverted around the liver preferentially through these patent anomalous channels.

### Clinical Features

Male cats less than 3 years old seem to be predisposed, and mixed breed, Persian, and Himalayan cats are at increased risk. Typical clinical signs in both cats and dogs with congenital portosystemic shunts (PSS) are referable primarily to HE. Behavioral and obvious neurologic abnormalities (e.g., dementia, seizures, visual disturbances, ataxia) are common in

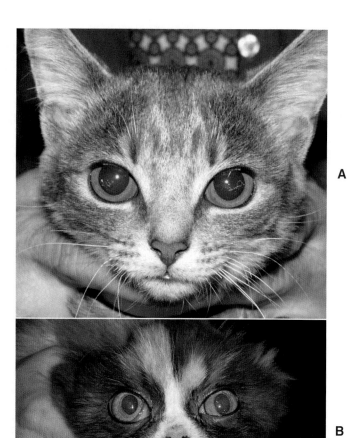

**FIG 37-15**
**A,** One-year-old spayed female domestic short-haired cat with a congenital portosystemic shunt. Notice the unusual color of the irises. **B,** Healthy Persian cat with similar colored irises for comparison.

both species. Interestingly, intermittent ptyalism is a more consistent finding in cats and may be a subtle manifestation of HE. The onset of signs correlates with meal ingestion about half the time. The severity of additional clinical signs, such as stunted growth, may be related to the size and location of the aberrant vessel. Less common historic features are recurrent urate urolithiasis, prolonged recovery from anesthesia or tranquilization because of delayed degradation of drugs, and improvement of behavioral and neurologic signs with antibiotic therapy. Most affected cats are underweight and some have renomegaly, but physical examination findings are otherwise nonspecific. Evidence of additional congenital defects, such as heart murmur or cryptorchidism, is also observed. Some clinicians have described a unique copper coloration to the irises in cats of non-Asian breed with congenital PSS (Fig. 37-15).

## Diagnosis

A suspicion for congenital PSS can be gained from evaluation of results of routine and liver-specific laboratory tests. The most common clinicopathologic abnormalities are postchallenge (food or ammonium chloride) hyperammonemia and high fasting and/or postprandial SBA concentrations. Low serum urea and creatinine concentrations, mild changes in liver enzyme activities, microcytosis, poikilocytosis, and low urine specific gravity are seen less often. Finding other clinicopathologic abnormalities typical of hepatic insufficiency, such as hypoalbuminemia and ammonium biurate crystalluria, is unreliable. Because congenital PSS is a pure vascular anomaly, evidence of striking hepatocellular injury is not characteristic unless there is a superimposing hepatic insult. Mild increases in serum AP activity might be attributable to accelerated bone turnover in cats presented at less than 6 months old. Subclinical hepatic organelle injury might also be the cause.

Diagnosis of congenital PSS is confirmed by US, transcolonic portal scintigraphy, or contrast portal venography (see p. 494), in addition to measurement of portal pressures and hepatic biopsy. Liver size in affected cats is normal to small. A hepatic biopsy specimen should be obtained to ensure that the hepatic histologic changes characteristic of congenital PSS are present: lobular hepatocellular atrophy, inconspicuous portal vein tributaries, arteriolar duplication, and, occasionally, mild lipidosis and vacuolar change. There should be minimal if any evidence of necrosis or inflammation.

## Treatment

Definitive treatment for congenital PSS is complete surgical ligation of the anomalous vessel, assuming there is adequate intrahepatic portal venous vasculature to accept redirected blood flow. This surgical procedure is best performed at referral centers or veterinary colleges. After the vessel has been ligated, portal venous pressures should not exceed 18 cm $H_2O$ (N = 6 to 15), and the abdominal organs should not appear dusky or congested after 5 to 10 minutes of observation. If this occurs, the ligature should be loosened or replaced to partially occlude the vessel to 50% to 75% of its original diameter. To evaluate the adequacy of intrahepatic portal perfusion, portography is repeated after shunt ligation. Partial improvement is expected after incomplete shunt ligation; cats that have had complete shunt ligation become clinically normal.

For cats with congenital PSS that cannot be completely occluded, applying a device that causes progressive narrowing of the shunt vessel over about 30 days (Ameroid constrictor, Research Instruments, Corvallis, Ore) (Fig. 37-16) may be an option. Preliminary experience in two cats was encouraging, although more recent published information in 12 cats describes complete success in only 3 cats and persistent, untreatable neurologic complications in 6 cats (Havig and colleague, 2002). Older cats (>5 years of age) or cats with preexisting neurologic signs may be at greater risk for a poor outcome following surgical treatment of congenital PSS.

Symptomatic management to control signs of chronic HE (see p. 546) preoperatively is wise and should continue for

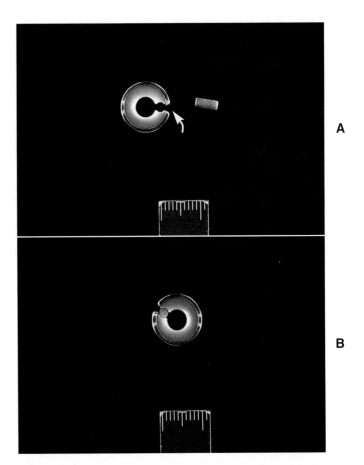

**FIG 37-16**
**A,** Ameroid constrictor (with an inner diameter of 3.5 mm) ready for placement around a congenital portosystemic shunt vessel. Notice the open slot *(arrow)*. **B,** After placement around the vessel, the "key" (plug) is placed into the slot to prevent dislodgment of the device.

approximately 1 month after corrective surgery. The same regimen is used for cats with inoperable PSS or for cats whose owners decline surgery. It is emphasized that symptomatic management is not a suitable long-term alternative to surgical correction. Signs of HE are less severe, but without restoration of portal blood flow, hepatic health continues to deteriorate, and CNS changes associated with poorly controlled HE may become permanent. Results of experimental studies have shown that dogs with created portacaval shunts can live comfortably for nearly 1 year free of signs of HE and maintain body weight while receiving a purified diet. Similar studies have not been performed in cats.

## ACUTE TOXIC HEPATOPATHY

### Pathogenesis and Etiology

By definition, toxic hepatopathy is hepatic injury directly attributable to exposure to environmental toxins or certain therapeutic agents. There are long lists that mention many

TABLE 37-3

**Therapeutic Agents or Environmental Toxins Observed to Cause Clinically Relevant Hepatic Injury**

| | DOSAGE | |
|---|---|---|
| | **CATS** | **DOGS** |
| **Therapeutic Agents** | | |
| Acetaminophen | 120 mg/kg | 200 mg/kg |
| Griseofulvin | X | — |
| Megesterol acetate | X | — |
| Ketoconazole | X | X |
| Phenazopyridine | X | — |
| Aspirin | >33 mg/kg/day | X |
| Primidone, phenytoin, phenobarbital | — | X |
| Glucocorticoids | — | X |
| Thiacetarsemide | — | X |
| Phenylbutazone | — | X |
| Mebendazole | — | X |
| Diethylcarbamazine-oxibendazole | — | X |
| Halothane, methoxyflurane | — | X |
| Trimethoprim-sulfa | — | X |
| Mibolerone | — | X |
| Naproxen | — | X |
| Carprofen | — | X |
| Tetracycline | X | — |
| Diazepam | X | — |
| Stanozolol | X | — |
| Nitrofurantoin | X | — |
| Amiodarone | X | — |
| Lomustine (CCNU) | — | X |
| **Environmental Toxins** | | |
| Pine oil + isopropanol | X | ? |
| Inorganic arsenicals (lead arsenate, sodium arsenate, sodium arsenite) | X | X |
| Thallium | X | X |
| Zinc phosphide | X | X |
| White phosphorus | X | X |
| *Amanita phalloides* (mushroom) | X | X |
| *Zamia floridana* (Cycad) | ? | X |
| Aflatoxin | X | X |
| Dry-cleaning fluid (trichlorethane) | X | X |
| Toluene | X | X |
| Phenols | X | X |
| Zinc | — | X |

*X*, Hepatotoxic; —, not known to be hepatotoxic; *?*, possibly hepatotoxic.

substances reported or suspected to be hepatotoxic in companion animals, but few of these are clinically relevant, especially in cats. Cats are particularly sensitive to phenolic toxicity because of their limited hepatic glucuronide transferase activity. A partial list of hepatotoxins is given in Table 37-3.

Complete information that could support meaningful conclusions about the frequency, character, and substances that consistently cause hepatotoxicity in cats is not available. Currently we must rely on anecdotal reports, clinical observations, and data accumulated by central agencies such as the National Animal Poison Control Center, Urbana, Ill (900-680-0000; $20 for the first 5 minutes, $2.95/minute thereafter, or 800-548-2423; $30 per case via credit card), and the U.S. Food and Drug Administration's Center for Veterinary Medicine, Washington, DC (the toll-free telephone number for reporting suspected adverse drug experiences is 1-888-FDA-VETS). In general, drug- or toxin-induced hepatic injury in cats is very unusual, and most reactions are acute (within 5 days of exposure). The character and severity of the toxic reaction depend on the characteristics of the substance and the species, as well as the dose and the duration of exposure.

Three therapeutic agents have recently been discovered to be hepatotoxic in certain cats: tetracycline (1 cat), diazepam (17 cats), and stanozolol (16 cats). Veterinarians have used these agents for years without known deleterious effects. For each drug, clinical and clinicopathologic signs of hepatotoxicosis developed within 13 days of daily oral administration at recommended dosages. The adverse hepatic reaction to tetracycline was serious but nonlethal, and the cat recovered completely after drug discontinuation and 6 weeks of supportive care (Kaufman and colleague, 1993). Histologic findings in the liver included centrilobular fibrosis, mild cholangiohepatitis, and mild lipid deposition in hepatocytes. For the cats that experienced diazepam-associated hepatic failure, the outcome was death in 16 of 17 despite intensive treatment. The oral dosages of diazepam that cats received primarily for inappropriate urination ranged from 1 mg every 24 hours to 2.5 mg every 12 hours. The histologic lesions in the liver were similar to those observed in the cat with tetracycline-associated hepatic injury but more severe: massive, predominantly centrilobular necrosis, suppurative cholangitis, and mild lipid vacuolation in some cats. Because of the severity of the lesions reported in cats apparently susceptible to diazepam-associated hepatic necrosis, serum liver enzyme activities are assessed during the window of days 3 to 5 of administration in cats given diazepam by mouth. Until there is more information that would improve understanding of this lethal and unpredictable hepatic reaction, use of other agents for control of behavior and elimination problems in cats is recommended. Cats that experienced an adverse reaction to stanozolol were healthy or had chronic renal failure (14 of 18 cats) or gingivitis/stomatitis (2 of 3 cats; Harkin and colleagues, 2000). Serum ALT activity was markedly increased in most cats given 1 mg orally every 24 hours for several months or 4 mg orally every 24 hours (and 25 mg IM once) for 3 weeks; all but one survived after the drug was discon-

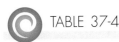 TABLE 37-4

Suggested Specific Treatments for Dogs and Cats Exposed to Hepatotoxins

| SUBSTANCE | TREATMENT |
|---|---|
| **Therapeutic Agents** | |
| Acetaminophen | 140 mg/kg *N*-acetylcysteine PO or IV as a 20% solution for a loading dose; continue at 70 mg/kg 6 hours later and q6h thereafter for a total of 7 treatments; ascorbic acid, 30 mg/kg PO q6h, should also be given |
| **Environmental Toxins** | |
| Inorganic arsenicals | 2.5-5 mg/kg BAL IM q4h for 2 days, then q12h until recovery; should be initiated within 36 hours of exposure |
| Thallium | 70 mg/kg diphenylthiocarbazone PO q8h; must be started within 24 hours of exposure; controversial |

*BAL,* British antilewisite.

tinued and intensive supportive care given. The histologic lesions were moderate to marked, diffuse centrilobular lipidosis and evidence of intrahepatic cholestasis (accumulation of bile and lipofuscin in hepatocytes and Kupffer cells).

The discriminatory eating habits of cats may account for the relatively uncommon occurrence of hepatotoxicity from ingested environmental toxins such as pesticides, household products, and other chemicals. It is certainly possible that many adverse hepatic reactions to drugs or toxic chemicals go unnoticed in cats because the first clinical signs of illness are vomiting and diarrhea, after which the medication is stopped. If the signs resolve, there usually is no further evaluation, and the medication is not readministered to prove that the substance caused the reaction.

### Diagnosis

Clinical evidence that suggests drug- or toxin-induced hepatic damage includes supportive history (e.g., known exposure), normal liver size to mild generalized tender hepatomegaly, laboratory test results consistent with acute liver injury (e.g., high serum ALT and/or AST activity, hyperbilirubinemia), and, if the exposure was nonlethal, recovery with discontinuation of the agent and specific or supportive care. There are no pathognomonic histologic changes in the liver, although necrosis with minimal inflammation and lipid accumulation are considered "classic" findings. Many times all clinical and clinicopathologic markers of a toxic liver insult are present, but the inciting chemical cannot be identified. In the case of hepatotoxicity from therapeutic agents, idiosyncratic reactions can occur (e.g., with tetracycline or diazepam), although drug overdose is usually the reason for liver injury.

### Treatment

In cats with suspected acute hepatotoxicity, the basic principles for treatment of toxicoses are applied: preventing further exposure and absorption, managing life-threatening cardiopulmonary and renal complications, hastening elimination of the substance, implementing specific therapy if possible, and providing supportive care. Because few hepatotoxins have specific antidotes (Table 37-4), the success of recovery often relies on time and aggressive supportive care.

## SECONDARY HEPATOBILIARY DISEASE

Several feline systemic illnesses have hepatic manifestations that may be identified by physical, clinicopathologic, or radiographic examination, but few signs can be attributed to clinically significant hepatic disease (see Table 36-1). In such cases, the hepatic lesion should recede with satisfactory treatment of the primary illness.

Metastatic neoplasia could be the underlying reason for abdominal enlargement from hepatomegaly or, rarely, malignant abdominal effusion. Some of the signs of hyperthyroidism, especially occasional vomiting, diarrhea, and weight loss, can resemble primary hepatobiliary disease. Thyrotoxic cats commonly have high liver enzyme activities; more than 75% of affected cats have high serum AP activity (twofold to twelvefold), although in cats it is not known whether this is of liver or bone origin or, as is true for hyperthyroid human patients, both. More than 50% of hyperthyroid cats have high serum ALT or aspartate transaminase (AST) activity (twofold to tenfold). Over 90% of affected cats have high serum activity of at least one of the enzymes AP, ALT, and AST. Approximately 3% are hyperbilirubinemic. Histopathologic changes are minimal, and there appears to be little functional disturbance. It is thought that malnutrition, hepatocellular hypoxia, and the direct effects of thyroid hormone on liver cells are responsible for these liver-related abnormalities. Hepatomegaly associated with mild-to-moderate lipid deposition is a common physical examination finding in cats with diabetes mellitus; a small number of cats may also be icteric. Mild-to-moderate increases in liver-specific enzyme activities are typical. More severe clinicopathologic abnormalities might be expected in cats with more severe hepatic lipidosis. Signs of hyperadrenocorticism that could be misinterpreted as those of primary hepatobiliary disease are a pendulous abdomen and hepatomegaly. In contrast to canine hyperadrenocorticism, it is unusual to identify high serum AP and ALT activities in hyperadrenocorticoid cats. Abnormal liver enzyme activities (especially serum ALT) are probably related to intercurrent diabetes mellitus, because these activities may resolve with management of the diabetic state alone.

Liver involvement is an important characteristic of several feline infectious diseases (see Chapters 101-104). Following ingestion or inhalation and replication of virulent strains of FIP virus, primary viremia leads to transport of virus throughout the body, including the liver, spleen, and lymph nodes. Virus is also localized in circulating mononuclear cells and within the walls of small vessels. Interaction among several variables, including host immunologic status and strain of virus, probably explains why there are several different clinical syndromes. Intense pyogranuloma formation, vasculitis, and serositis result from deposition of virus-infected mononuclear cells and virus-antibody complexes, allowing protein-rich fluid to escape into intercellular spaces and producing effusive FIP. Pyogranulomatous lesions in multiple tissues, including the liver and regional lymph nodes, are more typical of the noneffusive form of FIP.

Intracellular growth of *Toxoplasma gondii* during active clinical disease causes cell death in many tissues. Effects of delayed hypersensitivity reactions and immune-complex vasculitis also contribute to clinical illness. Infection of the lungs, liver, and CNS (including the eyes) is most commonly responsible for clinical signs. As would be expected, high serum ALT activity and hyperbilirubinemia commensurate with the degree of hepatocellular necrosis are the typical serum biochemical findings in cats with liver involvement. Cholangiohepatitis from infection of biliary epithelium has been noted occasionally in experimental and spontaneously occurring cases of toxoplasmosis in cats. The distribution of affected tissues in disseminated histoplasmosis often includes the lung, eye, bone marrow, spleen, lymph node, skin, bone, and liver.

## Suggested Readings

Armstrong PJ et al: Enteral nutrition by tube, *Vet Clin North Am Small Anim Pract* 20:237, 1990.

Armstrong PJ et al: Percutaneous endoscopic gastrostomy: a retrospective study of 54 clinical cases in dogs and cats, *J Vet Intern Med* 4:202, 1990.

Aronson LR et al: Acetaminophen toxicosis in 17 cats, *J Vet Emerg Crit Care* 6:65, 1996.

Beasley VR: Toxicology of selected pesticides, drugs, and chemicals, *Vet Clin North Am Small Anim Pract* 20:283, 1990.

Bielsa LM et al: Liver flukes (*Platynosomum concinnum*) in cats, *J Am Anim Hosp Assoc* 21:269, 1985.

Biourge VC et al: Effects of protein, lipid, or carbohydrate supplementation on hepatic lipid accumulation during rapid weight loss in obese cats, *Am J Vet Res* 55:1406, 1994.

Broussard JD et al: Changes in clinical and laboratory findings in cats with hyperthyroidism from 1983 to 1993, *J Am Vet Med Assoc* 206:302, 1995.

Carpenter JL et al: Tumors and tumorlike lesions. In Holzworth J, editor: *Diseases of the cat, medicine and surgery,* Philadelphia, 1987, WB Saunders, p 500.

Center SA et al: A retrospective study of 77 cats with severe hepatic lipidosis: 1975-1990, *J Vet Intern Med* 7:349, 1993.

Center SA et al: Fulminant hepatic failure associated with oral administration of diazepam in 11 cats, *J Am Vet Med Assoc* 209:618, 1996.

Cornelius LM et al: *CVT Update: Therapy for hepatic lipidosis. In Bonagura JD et al, editors: *Kirk's current veterinary therapy XIII,* Philadelphia, 2000, WB Saunders, p 686.

Crowe DT et al: Esophagostomy tubes for feeding and decompression: clinical experience in 29 small animal patients, *J Am Anim Hosp Assoc* 33:393, 1997.

Day MJ: Immunohistochemical characterization of the lesions of feline progressive lymphocytic cholangitis/cholangiohepatitis, *J Comp Pathol* 119:135, 1998.

DeNovo RE et al: Limited approach to the right flank for placement of a duodenostomy tube, *J Am Anim Hosp Assoc* 37:193, 2001.

Gagne JM et al: Histopathologic evaluation of feline inflammatory liver disease, *Vet Pathol* 33:521, 1996.

Gagne JM et al: Clinical features of inflammatory liver disease in cats: 41 cases (1983-1993), *J Am Vet Med Assoc* 214:513, 1999.

Harkin KR et al: Hepatotoxicity of stanozolol in cats, *J Am Vet Med Assoc* 217:681, 2000.

Havig M et al: Outcome of ameroid constrictor occlusion of single congenital extrahepatic portosystemic shunts in cats: 12 cases (1993-2000), *J Am Vet Med Assoc* 220:337, 2002.

Hughes D et al: The diagnosis and management of acute liver failure in dogs and cats, *Vet Clin North Am Small Anim Pract* 25:437, 1995.

Hughes D et al: Acute hepatic necrosis and liver failure associated with benzodiazepine therapy in six cats, 1986-1995, *J Vet Emerg Crit Care* 6:13, 1996.

Kaufman AC et al: Increased alanine transaminase activity associated with tetracycline administration in a cat, *J Am Vet Med Assoc* 202:628, 1993.

Levy JK et al: Feline portosystemic vascular shunts. In Bonagura JD et al, editors: *Kirk's current veterinary therapy XII,* Philadelphia, 1995, WB Saunders, p 743.

Lucke VM et al: Progressive lymphocytic cholangitis in the cat, *J Small Anim Pract* 25:249, 1984.

Rothuizen J: Seeking global standardization on liver disease, *J Small Anim Pract* 42:424, 2001.

Sparkes AH et al: Feline infectious peritonitis: a review of clinicopathological changes in 65 cases and a critical assessment of their diagnostic value, *Vet Rec* 129:209, 1991.

Steyn PF et al: Radiographic, epidemiologic, and clinical aspects of simultaneous pleural and peritoneal effusions in dogs and cats: 48 cases (1982-1991), *J Am Vet Med Assoc* 202:307, 1993.

Thamm DH: Hepatobiliary tumors. In Withrow RG et al, editors: *Small animal clinical oncology,* ed 3, Philadelphia, 2001, WB Saunders, p 327.

Weiss DJ et al: Characterization of portal lymphocytic infiltrates in feline liver, *Vet Clin Pathol* 24:91, 1995.

Weiss DJ et al: Relationship between feline inflammatory liver disease and inflammatory bowel disease, pancreatitis, and nephritis in cats, *J Am Vet Med Assoc* 209:1114, 1996.

# CHAPTER 38

# Hepatobiliary Diseases in the Dog

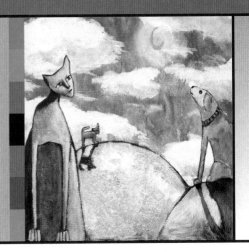

## CHAPTER OUTLINE

GENERAL CONSIDERATIONS, 525
CHRONIC HEPATITIS, 525
    Familial chronic hepatitis, 526
    Drug administration, 528
    Infectious agents, 529
    Idiopathic chronic hepatitis, 530
IDIOPATHIC HEPATIC FIBROSIS, 530
CONGENITAL PORTOVASCULAR DISORDERS
WITH NORMAL PORTAL PRESSURE, 531
    Congenital portosystemic shunt, 531
    Microvascular dysplasia, 531
CONGENITAL PORTOVASCULAR DISORDERS
WITH HIGH PORTAL PRESSURE, 533
    Hepatoportal fibrosis, 534
    Primary portal vein hypoplasia, 534
    Idiopathic noncirrhotic portal hypertension, 534
    Arterioportal fistula, 535
TREATMENT FOR CHRONIC LIVER DISORDERS, 535
    Prevention and treatment of copper excess, 535
    Glucocorticoids, 536
    Azathioprine, 537
    Antifibrotic agents, 537
    Dietary modification, 537
    Adjunctive treatments, 537
ACUTE TOXIC HEPATOPATHY, 537
BILIARY TRACT DISORDERS, 538
FOCAL HEPATIC LESIONS, 541
    Abscesses, 541
    Nodular hyperplasia, 542
NEOPLASIA, 542
SECONDARY HEPATIC DISEASE, 542
    Pancreatitis, 543
    Sepsis, 543
    Miscellaneous disorders, 543

## GENERAL CONSIDERATIONS

Although the clinical presentation of congenital canine hepatobiliary disease roughly parallels that in cats, acquired liver disorders in dogs are more diverse and thus are not predictably characterized by jaundice and hepatomegaly as in cats. Because of the heterogeneity of acquired canine hepatic diseases, more extensive and sometimes serial testing is required to reach a precise diagnosis. Hepatocytes are the target of injury in dogs, rather than the biliary epithelium, as is the case in cats; in addition, the clinical syndrome of hepatic failure with abdominal effusion, acquired portosystemic shunts (PSSs), and other complications of portal hypertension is observed frequently in dogs but rarely in cats. The following canine hepatopathies are addressed in order of likelihood in clinical practice (see Table 36-1). In dogs, chronic hepatopathies are much more common than acute hepatic diseases.

## CHRONIC HEPATITIS

The complexity of chronic hepatitis in dogs is just beginning to be appreciated and understood. Lack of adequate characterization of these diseases and the temptation to extrapolate directly from medical literature in human patients to say that some chronic hepatic diseases in dogs are identical to those long studied in human patients (e.g., chronic active hepatitis, chronic persistent hepatitis, chronic lobular hepatitis) have added to the confusion and may be preventing more progress being made in veterinary medicine. In fact, these terms have become obsolete in human medicine, and a reporting system using etiology, grade, and stage has been recommended for use by pathologists (Batts and colleague, 1995).

Chronic hepatitis in dogs comprises a spectrum of hepatic diseases that share similar historic, clinical, and possibly histopathologic features. Affected animals are ill for weeks to months with combinations of anorexia, weight loss, lethargy, polyuria and polydipsia, jaundice, abdominal effusion, signs of hepatic encephalopathy (HE), and hemorrhagic tendencies. Persistently high serum alanine transaminase (ALT) activity, with less strikingly abnormal serum alkaline phosphatase (AP) and γ-glutamyltransferase (GGT) activities early in the course of the disease, followed by evidence of multiple hepatocyte function loss late in the course (e.g., hypoalbuminemia, low blood urea nitrogen [BUN] concentration, high serum bile acid concentrations), is a typical clinicopathologic finding.

Occasionally, high serum liver enzyme activities are detected during routine evaluation before elective surgery in asymptomatic animals. In addition, there may be clinically relevant hepatic disorders in which liver enzyme activities are "silent" but there is other evidence of serious hepatic disease. A liver biopsy is crucial for accurate diagnosis and prognosis, although there is great overlap in histopathologic findings among these diseases (Table 38-1). With the use of routine staining methods (i.e., hematoxylin-eosin), histopathologic changes found in varying degrees include hepatocellular necrosis, mixed inflammatory cell infiltrates, fibrosis, biliary hyperplasia, and nodular regeneration. These changes involve primarily the portal and periportal regions, with involvement of lobular hepatocytes in some dogs. Depending on the time of diagnosis and the cause (Table 38-1; discussion of individual diseases to follow), it may be possible to reverse or control the process with specific therapy or at least to modulate its course with symptomatic treatment.

To better understand the role of the immune system in the development of idiopathic chronic hepatitis in dogs, two studies (Anderson and colleague, 1992; Weiss and colleagues, 1995) sought to determine the frequency of serum antibodies directed at cell nuclear material, smooth muscle mitochondria, and liver membrane in 21 and 24 dogs with histologically confirmed chronic hepatitis, respectively. Results of the studies were conflicting; one found low positive antinuclear antibody (ANA) titers (1:10 to 1:40) in 62% to 75% of all dogs with some kind of liver disorder. Dogs with chronic hepatitis could not be distinguished from dogs with neoplastic or degenerative disease by ANA titer. No other autoantibody was detected. The other study found antiliver membrane antibody titers in 50% of dogs with chronic hepatitis; dogs with positive titers had more severe clinicopathologic and histopathologic changes in the liver than antibody-negative dogs. These studies have demonstrated the presence of certain autoantibodies in dogs with chronic

hepatitis, but the clinical significance of these findings remains to be clarified.

Another study evaluated the proliferative response of mononuclear cells from dogs with chronic hepatitis and from dogs with other hepatic diseases to standard mitogens and to canine liver membrane protein (Poitout and colleagues, 1997). Members of both groups of dogs with chronic hepatopathies demonstrated proliferative responses compared with healthy dogs; the investigators concluded that cell-mediated processes are involved in dogs with chronic hepatitis, but it was not possible to determine whether the immune response was the cause or the consequence of liver injury.

## FAMILIAL CHRONIC HEPATITIS

### Bedlington Terriers

Familial chronic hepatitis has been recognized only since 1975, when observations by owners of Bedlington Terriers indicated that dogs of this breed were dying of liver disease at an unusually high rate. In 1977, Hardy and colleagues determined that the clinical, biochemical, and histopathologic features of this disease in Bedlington Terriers were strikingly similar to the hepatic component of Wilson's disease in humans, an inherited multisystemic disorder. The hepatic manifestations of this disease in dogs range from abnormal serum liver enzyme activities in asymptomatic individuals to cirrhosis with outward manifestations of hepatic failure. The fundamental metabolic error in Wilson's disease is accumulation of tissue copper (Cu) as the result of impaired biliary excretion. Because of these early investigations, knowledge of Cu hepatotoxicosis in Bedlington Terriers has been further refined.

The disease is inherited as an autosomal recessive trait, and signs of illness generally become evident in middle age. Severity of clinical signs, clinicopathologic test results, and hepatic histopathologic findings are directly related to the degree of hepatic Cu accumulation. Clinical signs usually do not de-

 TABLE 38-1

## Acquired Canine Hepatic Diseases Known Collectively as Chronic Hepatitis

| FAMILIAL | DRUG-ASSOCIATED | INFECTIOUS | IDIOPATHIC |
|---|---|---|---|
| **Copper Hepatotoxicosis**<br><br>Bedlington Terrier<br>Doberman Pinscher?<br>West Highland White Terrier<br>Dalmatian<br><br>**Other, Copper Accumulation Associated With Cholestasis?**<br><br>Skye Terrier<br>Doberman Pinscher?<br>Labrador Retriever?<br>Cocker Spaniel? | Diethylcarbamazine-oxibendazole<br>Anticonvulsants (phenytoin, primidone, phenobarbital)<br>Trimethoprim-sulfa? | Infectious canine hepatitis<br>Acidophil cell hepatitis (Great Britain)<br>Leptospirosis?<br>Subsequent to *Corynebacterium parvum* immunotherapy? | Chronic hepatitis<br>Lobular dissecting hepatitis |

velop until there is marked Cu accumulation in hepatocytes (approximately 2000 μg/g* of dry liver weight [DW]) after which lysosomes rupture and release Cu, damaging hepatocytes. Hemolytic anemia can occur if a large number of hepatocytes die suddenly and release Cu into the blood, but this is rare. Liver Cu concentration secondary to cholestatic hepatic disease from any cause infrequently exceeds 2000 μg/g.

In liver specimens stained with hematoxylin-eosin, histopathologic changes are not unique and range from multifocal necrosis with associated inflammatory reaction to more severe changes, including nodular regeneration, bile duct hyperplasia and fibrosis, and macronodular or micronodular cirrhosis. Special stains, such as Timm's silver sulfide, rubeanic acid, orcein, or rhodamine (Fig. 38-1), must be used to confirm that dark brownish eosinophilic granules within lysosomes contain Cu. Histochemical staining of liver biopsy or cytologic specimens can be used as a qualitative measure of liver Cu concentration, but quantitative assessment can be made only by spectrophotometric analysis using dried or wet liver specimens. Liver Cu concentration in normal juvenile and adult Bedlington Terriers is 91 to 358 μg/g DW or 10 to 40 μg/g wet weight (WW). Most affected (homozygous) dogs have liver Cu concentrations greater than 800 μg/g DW (grades 4, 5, and possibly 3 by cytologic methods), regardless of age at the time of biopsy.

Currently the only practical, widely available means of identifying affected homozygous dogs and asymptomatic carriers (purebred heterozygotes and Bedlington crosses) before the onset of signs is by hepatic Cu quantitation at 6 months of age and, if necessary, 10 to 12 months later. Carrier dogs have hepatic Cu concentrations in both specimens that are normal or slightly higher than normal (range: 400 to 700 μg/g DW; grades 1, 2, and possibly 3 by cytologic methods) but similar to one another. In affected dogs the hepatic Cu concentration

---

*μg/g = mg/kg = parts per million (ppm).

of the second specimen is much greater than that of the first, confirming progressive Cu retention. If there still is uncertainty, especially about dogs intended for breeding, test matings between known affected dogs and dogs in question, with liver specimens for hepatic Cu measurement obtained from all offspring, are necessary. If the dog in question were heterozygous for this trait, 50% of the offspring of such a test mating would be affected. Serial hepatic Cu determinations or test matings are recommended only for dogs intended for breeding; carrier and affected dogs should be neutered.

More recently, genetic analysis has been the focus of considerable interest. Several investigators have evaluated the use of a microsatellite marker in identifying affected dogs in the United States, United Kingdom, and Europe. As long as several related dogs are available for testing, this method will identify affected, heterozygous, and normal dogs. Researchers in the Netherlands have made considerable progress in identifying the putative gene causing Cu hepatotoxicosis, which will be very useful as a single diagnostic test.

Chronic hepatopathy characterized by Cu accumulation is also known to occur in other breeds, particularly the Doberman Pinscher (predominantly middle-aged females), West Highland White Terrier, Skye Terrier, and Dalmatian. Some dogs of these breeds have hepatic Cu accumulation but no clinical signs or histopathologic abnormalities. Although the genetics are yet to be clarified, a familial basis is strongly suspected.

## Doberman Pinschers

The Doberman Pinscher was first identified as having a breed-associated hepatopathy in 1982. Some investigators have attempted to equate this disease with the autoimmune type of chronic active hepatitis (CAH) in human patients to which it bears a weak resemblance. In both species signs of illness and biochemical markers of persistent hepatocellular injury are usually present for months. To reach a diagnosis of autoimmune CAH in a human patient, there must be strong evidence of autoantibody production directed at nuclear protein, smooth muscle, mitochondria, and several liver cell membrane antigens. Lupus cell phenomena are detected less frequently. Viral infection and drug-induced hepatic disease must also be excluded. The hepatic histopathologic features are not distinguishable from those associated with other causes of CAH, including chronic hepatitis B, C, and D viruses and many drugs. In some patients a cause cannot be identified. Regardless of the initiating event, immune-mediated reactions are directed toward altered hepatocytes; this may cause self-perpetuated injury.

Classic histopathologic lesions of CAH of any cause in humans are mononuclear cell portal inflammation with extension into adjacent parenchyma ("piecemeal necrosis") indicated by disruption of the limiting plate, which may extend to other lobules ("bridging necrosis"), and degrees of periportal fibrosis. Advanced CAH is characterized by cirrhosis with evidence of ongoing hepatocyte injury. On the basis of the hepatic histopathologic lesions typical of human CAH, veterinary investigators have been tempted to assume that the same

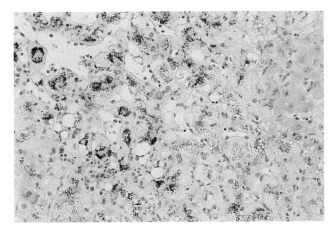

**FIG 38-1**
Photomicrograph of a liver specimen stained with rhodanine to identify copper granules (counterstained with Mayer's hematoxylin for cellular orientation).

disease exists in dogs. The history, results of routine clinicopathologic tests, and hepatic histopathologic lesions (Fig. 38-2) of Doberman Pinschers with this hepatopathy are similar to those of human patients with autoimmune CAH, but preliminary immunologic analysis of affected Doberman Pinschers has failed to reveal evidence of these markers. In addition to parenchymal, portal, and periportal inflammation, there is also pericentral inflammation in some dogs. Two studies of affected asymptomatic dogs (dogs with high serum ALT activity and histopathologic evidence of chronic hepatitis) agree that Doberman hepatopathy is progressive (van den Ingh and colleagues, 1988; Speeti and colleagues, 1998).

Hepatic Cu accumulation to the extent typical of Doberman Pinscher hepatopathy (450 to 3600 μg/g DW; reference range in healthy mixed-breed dogs, 200 to 400 μg/g DW) is not characteristic of human CAH. Cu accumulation in Doberman Pinscher hepatopathy is less well understood than in Bedlington Terrier Cu hepatotoxicosis. Results of serum biochemistry tests and histopathologic studies reveal more evidence of cholestasis in Doberman Pinschers than in affected Bedlington Terriers. Because the major route of Cu excretion is biliary, one possible explanation for high hepatic Cu content is that it is a consequence of cholestasis, although high hepatic Cu content has also been reported in Doberman Pinschers without evidence of cholestasis. Whether the specific error in Cu metabolism is a primary or secondary event in Doberman Pinschers with chronic hepatitis is currently not known. Unexplained excessive hepatic iron has also been observed in both Bedlington Terrier and Doberman Pinscher Cu-associated hepatopathies.

### West Highland White Terriers

On the basis of one study of 70 adult dogs and one puppy, hepatic disease associated with Cu retention in West High-

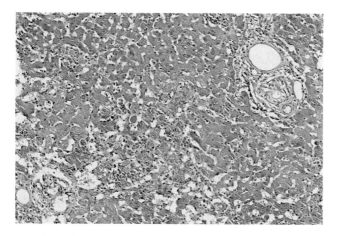

**FIG 38-2**
Photomicrograph of a liver specimen from a 3-year-old castrated male Doberman Pinscher with chronic hepatitis (hematoxylin-eosin). A portal area is to the right; note the diffuse mononuclear inflammatory cell infiltrates in the parenchyma. There also is extensive lobular disorganization. The liver Cu content was 2840 μg/g on a dry matter basis.

land White Terriers appears to differ from other familial hepatopathies. Liver Cu content does not increase progressively with age, but the reason for variable liver Cu content in affected dogs is not understood. The range of hepatic Cu content in affected dogs is 450 to 3500 μg/g DW, which is similar to that of affected Doberman Pinschers but lower than that of many affected Bedlington Terriers. Further information regarding the inheritance pattern, clinical course, and mechanism of Cu retention is not currently available.

### Skye Terriers

Familial hepatopathy in nine Skye Terriers of varying ages has been described as mild to moderate periportal and pericentral inflammation with intracanalicular cholestasis and Cu accumulation. Regenerative parenchymal nodules surrounded by fibrous connective tissue bands are seen in more chronic cases. The degree of Cu retention seems to correlate with the degree and duration of cholestasis. The cause is unknown but might relate to disturbed membrane bile transfer and transport systems.

### Dalmatians

Cu-associated liver injury has been reported in three case reports comprising 12 Dalmatian dogs. Clinical signs were nonspecific; anorexia, lethargy, vomiting, and diarrhea were the presenting complaints. The dogs ranged in age from 1.5 years to 10 years (median 5 years), with no gender predilection; two dogs were related. The predominant serum biochemical change was high ALT activity (up to elevenfold elevation), with mild increases in AP activity (normal to fivefold elevation). Histologic lesions in the liver included extensive necrosis of hepatocytes associated with moderate to marked numbers of neutrophils and macrophages involving primarily the periportal area (zone 1) in six dogs and the centrilobular area (zone 3) in four dogs. Liver Cu concentration was greater than 2000 μg/g DW in 7 of 11 dogs. Seven dogs were treated with a Cu chelator or zinc, but treatment made little difference, and most dogs died within 90 days of diagnosis.

## DRUG ADMINISTRATION

Long-term drug administration is a frequent cause of chronic hepatitis in humans. Heartworm prevention and treatment for osteoarthritis, central nervous system disorders, allergic or immune-mediated diseases, and cancer are the most common circumstances under which dogs given drugs long-term might develop chronic adverse hepatic reactions. The overall frequency of such reactions is low, and most are likely associated with unique susceptibility because of genetic differences in drug-metabolizing enzyme systems. Except for glucocorticoid hepatopathy, hepatic histopathologic lesions in dogs with drug-induced hepatotoxicity are not unique; presumptive diagnosis is usually based on careful examination of the history and improvement following discontinuation of drug therapy. Recreating the clinical syndrome by readministering the suspected drug is the only means to document that the reaction was drug-induced. This approach would be reasonable only for drugs for which there are no substitutes and for which the adverse hepatic reaction is not life-threatening.

## Heartworm Preventives

Soon after release of a product developed for heartworm and hookworm prevention for dogs (diethylcarbamazine-oxibendazole) (Filaribits Plus; Pfizer Animal Health, New York) in 1986, there were reports of illness characterized by depression, anorexia, weight loss, vomiting, polyuria and polydipsia, and icterus. Clinical signs were observed within weeks of starting drug administration and resolved, along with clinicopathologic abnormalities typical of acute hepatobiliary disease, shortly after discontinuation of the drug. In some dogs, evidence of persistent hepatobiliary disease was noted, perhaps related to continued drug administration past the onset of signs of illness. The current frequency of the subacute, and especially the chronic, forms of adverse hepatic reactions is not known. Serious hepatic injury is probably rather uncommon because of heightened awareness.

## Anticonvulsants

Of the anticonvulsants used for management of seizures in dogs today, primidone, alone or in combination with other anticonvulsants, has been reported to cause clinically relevant hepatic disease most often. High serum liver enzyme activities (AP, fivefold to eightfold increase; ALT, twofold to threefold increase) are common in dogs given anticonvulsant drugs. This finding probably represents a combination of drug-induced new enzyme synthesis (AP of liver origin) and low-grade hepatocellular injury (high ALT) that most animals tolerate without serious consequences. Serum GGT activity is usually normal except in dogs with clinically relevant hepatic injury. In a small fraction of treated dogs, especially those with seizures that become increasingly difficult to control and thus require higher than recommended dosages of drugs, serious hepatic injury may develop and progress to cirrhosis. Hepatic function testing (e.g., preprandial and postprandial serum bile acid [SBA] concentrations) must be used to determine if abnormal liver enzyme activity is associated with serious hepatic consequences. Chronic phenobarbital administration can cause similar changes, although no evidence of liver injury was documented in 12 healthy dogs given phenobarbital (5 to 6 mg/kg by mouth [PO] q12h) for 29 weeks (Müller and colleagues, 2000). Despite the observation of adverse hepatic reactions to other anticonvulsant drugs in human medicine, there is little information about hepatotoxicity associated with these medications, such as carbamazepine or valproic acid, in dogs. In dogs in which hepatotoxicity associated with phenobarbital or primidone develops, potassium bromide may be safely substituted for seizure control (see Chapter 69).

## Glucocorticoids

Continued administration of glucocorticoids to dogs causes a unique, now well-recognized chronic hepatopathy. Hepatomegaly and high serum liver enzyme activities (total AP, up to 100-fold increase; GGT, sixfold to tenfold increase; ALT, twofold to fourfold increase) are common, especially if prednisone has been given. Mild hepatic dysfunction demonstrated by high fasting SBA concentrations (up to 50 μmol/L in most cases; can be as high as 100 μmol/L) is gradually reversible on termination of glucocorticoid therapy, as are the histopathologic lesions. The classic histopathologic finding is not a necroinflammatory change but is vacuolation, which is believed to be caused by glycogen accumulation (Fig. 38-3). The distribution of the vacuoles depends on the duration of drug administration, with more diffuse involvement seen after weeks of treatment. Although the enzyme pattern appears to be compatible with cholestasis, the AP is a specific glucocorticoid-induced isoenzyme, and hyperbilirubinemia and histopathologic criteria of intrahepatic cholestasis are absent. Glucocorticoid hepatopathy is rarely severe enough to cause hepatic failure, although this finding has been reported anecdotally.

## Chemotherapeutic Drugs

Most chemotherapeutic agents commonly in use today cause little if any clinically relevant chronic hepatic injury. Glucocorticoid hepatopathy would be expected in dogs receiving prednisone. Other anticancer or immunosuppressive drugs, such as methotrexate, azathioprine, dacarbazine, and cytosine arabinoside, that are used in animals and known to be hepatotoxic in human patients are rarely responsible for serious hepatic consequences in dogs. Recently, lomustine (CCNU) has been identified as a relatively common hepatotoxin in dogs. Of these, azathioprine has been implicated most often. Severe hepatic injury in this case usually represents an idiosyncratic reaction or misadministration (e.g., daily, long-term use instead of every other day, short-term administration).

## INFECTIOUS AGENTS

Primary chronic hepatitis caused by infectious organisms seems to be unusual in dogs. Although the liver is often involved secondarily in many acute systemic illnesses (see Table 36-1), clinically relevant chronic sequelae are rare. Hepatic lesions similar to CAH in humans have been produced experimentally in partially immune dogs exposed to virulent canine adenovirus type I, which is responsible for infectious canine hepatitis (ICH). It is suspected that persistent inflammation occurs because of latent hepatic viral infection. The same pathogenesis could account for chronic hepatic lesions in dogs that have survived the acute phase of spontaneous ICH infection.

Chronic hepatitis suspected to be induced by a virus that can cause both acute and chronic hepatic disease in dogs has been recognized in Great Britain. The agent is believed to be a virus because clinical disease can be transmitted with bacteriologically sterile serum or liver homogenates from dogs free of ICH and canine adenovirus type II. The liver lesions contain unique cells not detected in other hepatic diseases of dogs termed *acidophil cells*. These cells are angular hepatocytes with acidophilic cytoplasm and a hyperchromatic condensed nucleus. To date, there have been no reports of this form of chronic hepatitis outside Great Britain.

Circumstantial evidence in one report supported the assumption that hepatic lesions typical of CAH seen in human

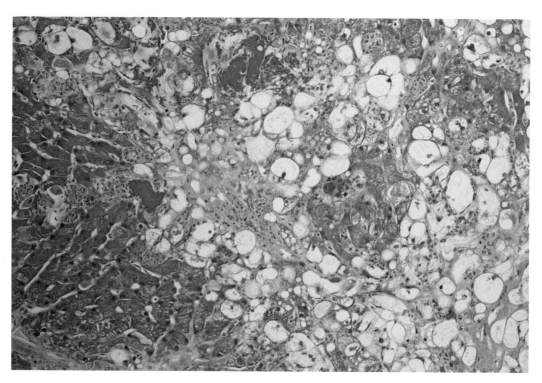

**FIG 38-3**
Photomicrograph of a liver specimen from a 5-year-old castrated male Schnauzer with iatrogenic hypercortisolism; note the presence of clear vacuoles within hepatocytes.

patients were caused by infection with *Leptospira interrogans* serovar *grippotyphosa* in five young American Foxhounds. Spirochetes were identified in the liver of four of the five dogs and were presumed to have initiated hepatocellular injury and subsequent immune-mediated responses. This is most unusual because chronic infection with leptospiras is usually limited to renal involvement. There have been no other reports of chronic hepatic disease following acute leptospirosis in dogs. Other reports of canine leptospirosis indicate that although some dogs may have clinical or biochemical evidence of hepatic involvement, the most common presenting syndrome currently is acute renal failure. The serovars implicated most often are *pomona, grippotyphosa,* and *autumnalis.*

## IDIOPATHIC CHRONIC HEPATITIS

Lobular dissecting hepatitis was first characterized in the veterinary literature in six relatively young dogs (7 months to 5 years of age) and possibly a seventh, by ascites and clinicopathologic test results consistent with hepatic failure. Multifocal inflammatory infiltrates, disturbance of lobular architecture by fine collagen and reticulin fibers that interrupt the limiting plate, and scanty inflammation and connective tissue deposition in portal tracts were the typical histopathologic features. Acquired PSSs developed secondary to intrahepatic portal hypertension. All six dogs died within 5 months of diagnosis despite supportive care, which implies that the prognosis for this disease based on a limited number of reported cases is extremely poor. Another dog with similar clinical and histopathologic findings was treated with corticosteroids as if for autoimmune hepatitis. The hepatic lesions improved but persisted for at least 8 months; during this time the dog had minimal clinical signs. In a more recent report, 21 juvenile and young adult dogs with this condition were described. Clinical, clinicopathologic, and histopathologic findings resembled those in the earlier report. Although details were not provided regarding treatment and outcome in this larger group of 21 dogs, the authors gave the impression that lobular dissecting hepatitis was a devastating disease that often had progressed irreversibly to cirrhosis by the time of diagnosis. The author is aware of isolated cases of lobular dissecting hepatitis in dogs that have survived comfortably for up to 6 years with supportive care, during which time clinicopathologic test results were normal and there was evidence of partial resolution of the lesions in sequential liver biopsies.

The most common form of chronic hepatitis in mixed-breed and purebred dogs other than those addressed previously is idiopathic chronic hepatitis.

## IDIOPATHIC HEPATIC FIBROSIS

Idiopathic hepatic fibrosis was recently described in 19 dogs, nine of which were German Shepherd Dogs and two of which were German Shepherd Dog crosses (Rutgers, 2000). Most dogs were anorexic and lethargic; and had microhepatia, ascites, and signs of HE. Clinicopathologic findings in most dogs included microcytosis and high serum AP activity; six dogs had mild hyperbilirubinemia. Three subtypes of fibrosis

## TABLE 38-2

**Clinical Features of Congenital Portosystemic Shunt in Cats and Dogs**

| | |
|---|---|
| Signalment | Less than 1 yr of age, either gender, purebred |
| History | Neurologic signs, often following a meal (dementia, circling, wall-hugging, personality change, seizures [rare]) |
| | Intermittent vomiting; sometimes diarrhea |
| | Preference for fruits and vegetables (especially dogs) |
| | Hypersalivation (especially cats) |
| | Apparent improvement in neurologic signs with antibiotic treatment |
| | Anesthetic or sedative intolerance |
| | Polydipsia/polyuria (less common) |
| | Recurrent urate urolithiasis in breeds other than the Dalmatian or English Bulldog |
| Physical examination | Small stature |
| | Bilateral renomegaly |
| | Poor or unkempt hair coat |
| | Other congenital anomalies |
| | Cystic calculi (especially in cats and older dogs) |
| | Cryptorchidism |
| | Copper-colored irises in non-Asian cat breeds |

were noted: central perivenous, diffuse pericellular, and periportal; there was no evidence of inflammation. All dogs received medical treatment for HE and ascites; some dogs received prednisolone, and some dogs received colchicine, each for antifibrotic effect. Response to treatment was variable; three dogs were euthanized shortly after diagnosis, but three were still alive 4 years later. Although the number of treated dogs was small, the authors' impression was that colchicine was of benefit and that further evaluation of a larger number of dogs is needed.

## CONGENITAL PORTOVASCULAR DISORDERS WITH NORMAL PORTAL PRESSURE

### CONGENITAL PORTOSYSTEMIC SHUNT
#### Etiology and Pathogenesis

Pathophysiologic sequelae of PSS (the most common portovascular anomaly) in the dog are similar to those in the cat (see p. 520) and result from reduced total hepatic blood flow and inability of the liver to extract noxious substances from the portal circulation. Many different patterns of portovascular anomalies have been described in dogs; the most common are single extrahepatic communications between the portal vein or one of the mesenteric veins and the caudal vena cava or azygous vein in small-breed dogs (see Fig. 36-7) and patent ductus venosus in large-breed dogs. Hypoplasia or aplasia of intrahepatic portal vasculature could complicate any of these anomalies, but it is unusual. A familial predisposition for single extrahepatic PSS is suspected in the Yorkshire Terrier, Miniature Schnauzer, Lhasa Apso, and Shih Tzu. Retrievers, Irish Setters, Irish Wolfhounds, and other large-breed dogs are predisposed to intrahepatic PSS.

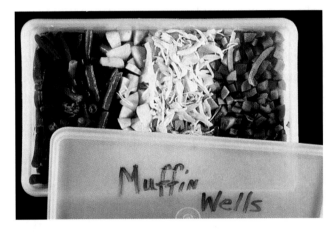

**FIG 38-4**
Plate of vegetables prepared by the owner of a 15-month-old castrated male Shih Tzu with a congenital portosystemic shunt for her dog to eat during hospitalization.

### Clinical Features

Similar to cats, common clinical signs in dogs with single intrahepatic or extrahepatic PSS are those of HE, not always related to meal ingestion, and/or gastrointestinal disturbance, such as vomiting, diarrhea, or pica (Table 38-2). Many dogs with PSS have a history of preferring fruits and vegetables to meat-containing diets (Fig. 38-4). Additional signs or presenting complaints are polyuria and polydipsia, urate urolithiasis, and anesthetic or sedative intolerance. Age range of affected dogs is 2 months to 10 years; most are presented when less than 1 year old, and there is no gender predilection. Physical examination findings include small stature, poor hair coat, and occasionally renal enlargement; neurologic signs (e.g., dementia, dullness) may or may not be apparent.

## Diagnosis

Definitive diagnosis of PSS is based on demonstration of an abnormal portal vein-to-systemic vein connection and characteristic hepatic histopathologic findings in dogs with clinical and clinicopathologic evidence of hepatic insufficiency. Clinicopathologic findings in more than 50% of affected dogs, regardless of the type of vascular anomaly, are microcytosis, hypoalbuminemia, mild increases in serum AP and ALT activities, hypocholesterolemia, low BUN concentration, postchallenge hyperammonemia, and normal or high fasting SBA with high postprandial SBA. The origin of serum AP activity is unknown; it could be of bone or liver origin, but subcellular hepatic organelle injury is also possible. The liver is frequently small. Because more types of vascular anomalies are observed in dogs than in cats and clinical signs and clinicopathologic test results often do not distinguish among them, additional noninvasive tests are often required to localize the anomaly. A study (Bostwick and colleague, 1995) comparing dogs with intrahepatic PSS versus dogs with extrahepatic PSS made no particularly surprising discoveries; dogs with intrahepatic PSS weighed more and had higher blood glucose and serum AP values than dogs with extrahepatic PSS. Combinations of ultrasonography, transcolonic scintigraphy, or contrast portal venography (Fig. 38-5) may therefore be needed to confirm the location of the anomalous vessel before surgical correction is attempted (see p. 492).

## Treatment and Prognosis

Occlusion of the anomalous vessel to restore normal portal blood flow is the treatment of choice. Surgical correction of both extrahepatic and intrahepatic PSSs is challenging and is best performed at referral centers or veterinary colleges. Por-

tal pressure, which is normal in dogs with congenital PSS, should be measured, and a liver biopsy specimen should be obtained in all dogs undergoing surgery. Dogs with single extrahepatic PSS that can be ligated completely without portal pressure exceeding 18 cm $H_2O$ have the best prognosis for a normal life span with excellent quality of life. Partial recovery is expected in dogs that have extrahepatic PSSs that cannot be totally occluded without causing fatal portal hypertension. Ligation of intrahepatic PSSs is technically more difficult than closure of extrahepatic PSSs. A nonsurgical technique has been introduced recently for gradual closure of intrahepatic PSS. With the dog under general anesthesia, a stainless steel coil, to which thrombogenic material is attached, is introduced with radiographic guidance into the shunt vessel via an introducer catheter in the left jugular vein. The procedure may need to be repeated several times, several weeks apart, until the shunt vessel is occluded. This technique is worth considering for dogs that are poor surgical risks.

Recently, generalized motor seizures as a postoperative complication were described in five dogs after ligation of single extrahepatic congenital PSS (Matushek and colleagues, 1990). Four of five dogs died or were euthanized because of intractable seizures; the surviving dog has residual neurologic abnormalities. Other than age (four of five were older than 18 months), there were no clinical findings, clinicopathologic abnormalities, or surgical observations that differed from those of other dogs that have undergone successful surgical attenuation of congenital PSSs. The authors suggested that dogs with congenital PSS diagnosed and treated surgically at an older age might be predisposed to seizures postoperatively. They propose that an altered brain metabolic state might exist as a result of chronic, perhaps subclinical HE, which decompensates when portosys-

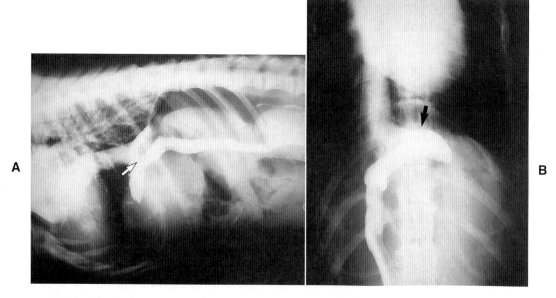

**FIG 38-5**

**A,** Lateral and, **B,** ventrodorsal views made during an operative mesenteric portal venogram in a 1-year-old female Great Dane delineating an intrahepatic portosystemic shunt *(arrows).*

temic shunting is stopped abruptly. Conversely, lack of signs of HE is a positive prognostic factor for complete ligation of single extrahepatic PSS in dogs.

Signs of HE are controlled medically (see p. 546) before surgery is scheduled, and these measures are continued for approximately 1 month after surgical correction. For dogs with partially occluded or inoperable PSS, symptomatic management is recommended for life. The current ability to manage clinical signs in dogs with congenital PSS primarily with diet is limited unless a purified diet is used, but it is no substitute for surgical correction. In a study of the long-term effects of surgically created end-to-side portacaval shunts in adult dogs, the diet used was a purified, carbohydrate-based diet formulated with a specific ratio of branched-chain amino acid to aromatic amino acid composition. Both dogs with created portacaval shunts and sham-operated dogs lived comfortably for nearly 1 year, free of signs of HE and weight loss. These diets are not made commercially, so they are inaccessible to owners. Another study evaluated 23 dogs with congenital PSS that did not have corrective surgery but had symptomatic treatment for at least 3 years. About one half of the dogs had been euthanized within 1 year of diagnosis, mostly because of uncontrollable HE (Watson and colleague, 1998), but nine dogs lived a reasonable quality of life for 3 to 8 years. Despite these encouraging findings, hepatic deterioration associated with poor portal blood flow progresses as long as the abnormal vascular pattern persists.

## MICROVASCULAR DYSPLASIA

### Etiology and Pathogenesis

Microvascular dysplasia (MVD) is the term currently given to a disorder in which there are clinical features of congenital PSS (including signalment, clinical signs, and clinicopathologic features), a macroscopic vascular anomaly cannot be identified, and there is microscopic evidence of disordered hepatic vasculature. This condition can occur as a singular anomaly or jointly with congenital PSS. In one breed (the Cairn Terrier), the site of anatomic abnormality has been identified as the terminal portal veins. In this breed, it is believed to be an autosomal, inherited trait; the specific mode of inheritance has not been established.

### Clinical Features

The same breeds that are predisposed to extrahepatic congenital PSS are those that have been described with MVD. Typical signs include vomiting, diarrhea, and HE, especially in dogs with both defects. Dogs with only MVD are somewhat older, and many have mild to no signs of illness. In the case of young purebred dogs that have been screened for congenital PSS before sale or that are ill for nonhepatic reasons, high SBA may be the only clinicopathologic finding.

### Diagnosis

Dogs with MVD alone may have some of the same clinicopathologic features of those with congenital PSS; some appear normal except for modest increases in SBA concentra-

tions. Unlike in dogs with congenital PSS, the liver is usually normal size. Contrast portography using repeated injections and multiple exposures might indicate altered perfusion of the smaller branches of the portal vasculature in one or more liver lobes but no evidence of a macroscopic shunt vessel. Results of transcolonic scintigraphy are normal. The histopathologic changes in the liver are considered identical to those of dogs with congenital PSS: decreased size of intrahepatic portal radicles, mild arteriolar duplication, mural hypertrophy of the central veins, some fibrosis, and Ito cell hypertrophy. Random juvenile intralobular blood vessels can also be seen in dogs with MVD or congenital PSS and may represent a compensatory response to decreased portal blood flow.

The most important aspects of identifying a dog with MVD are ruling out a surgically correctable PSS and obtaining a liver biopsy specimen for confirmation or exclusion of other hepatopathies. It is also important to remember that affected Cairn Terriers, and perhaps other breeds such as the Maltese, are usually asymptomatic for this condition, although they have clinicopathologic evidence of hepatic dysfunction.

### Treatment and Prognosis

There is no surgical remedy for MVD, so symptomatic management for HE (if present) is the only treatment. Affected dogs seem to live comfortably in good to excellent condition for at least 5 years without serious consequences (Christiansen and colleagues, 2000).

## CONGENITAL PORTOVASCULAR DISORDERS WITH HIGH PORTAL PRESSURE

Noncirrhotic portal hypertension describes a category of hepatopathies in human patients characterized by intraabdominal portal hypertension, a patent portal vein, and relatively unremarkable liver biopsy findings. Two unusual previously reported diseases of primarily young dogs (≤2.5 years) might be able to be grouped under this title: hepatoportal fibrosis and primary hypoplasia of the portal vein. Two more recent reports describe a syndrome resembling idiopathic noncirrhotic portal hypertension in four Doberman Pinschers, three of which were related, and a similar condition in 33 dogs of various breeds. Affected dogs do not consistently have signs of HE, commonly have microhepatia, and usually have ascites and clinicopathologic features compatible with hepatic failure. Multiple extrahepatic PSSs (Fig. 38-6) are characteristic. These disorders are also characterized by abnormal liver enzyme activities and microcytosis. Hepatic histopathologic changes are nearly indistinguishable from those in dogs with PSS or MVD. Considering the similarity of the cases and the histopathologic descriptions, it is possible that all three are variations of the same disorder, intrahepatic portal vein hypoplasia, and that the severity of signs and clinicopathologic changes relates to the degree of portal vasculature affected. Symptomatic treatment for ascites and HE (see pp. 549 and 546) is usually indicated.

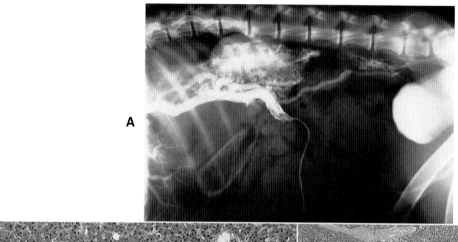

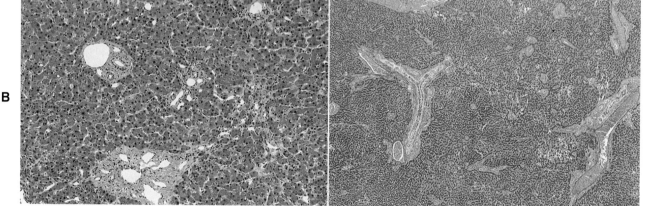

**FIG 38-6**
**A,** Operative mesenteric portal venogram in a 1-year-old male Pointer with noncirrhotic portal hypertension outlining the typical pattern of acquired portosystemic shunts. **B,** Photomicrograph of liver biopsy specimen from the same dog demonstrating hepatocellular atrophy, arteriolar duplication, and lack of necrosis or inflammation (hematoxylin-eosin). **C,** A trichrome stain demonstrates little fibrous tissue.

## HEPATOPORTAL FIBROSIS

Hepatoportal fibrosis was first described in Great Britain in three dogs with ascites that were 4 to 6 months old. The hepatic lesion is one of periportal fibrosis with portoportal bridging, leading to intrahepatic portal hypertension and acquired PSSs. All three dogs were euthanized soon after diagnosis; thus there is no further information about response to specific or supportive treatment in these three dogs. Another dog was reported to have responded well to treatment with colchicine (see p. 537) for 2.5 years and was euthanized for unrelated reasons.

## PRIMARY PORTAL VEIN HYPOPLASIA

Primary hypoplasia of the portal vein was described in 42 young dogs (van den Ingh and colleagues, 1995). The cause of the clinical and clinicopathologic findings of hepatic failure was believed to be associated with portal blood deprivation from an underdeveloped extrahepatic portal vein in 13 dogs and hypoplastic intrahepatic portal veins in the remaining 29 dogs. The conclusions on portal vein size were made subjectively by visually comparing portal veins from affected dogs with those of normal dogs. Specific treatment was not sug-

gested, but the authors remarked that affected dogs could remain in good health for a number of years with medical treatment for HE and ascites. The authors also remarked that they believed that three dogs they had previously reported as having hepatoportal fibrosis actually had portal vein hypoplasia.

## IDIOPATHIC NONCIRRHOTIC PORTAL HYPERTENSION

On the basis of two recent publications (De Marco and colleagues, 1998; Bunch and colleagues, 2001) describing a total of 37 dogs, idiopathic noncirrhotic portal hypertension is seen most often in purebred dogs 4 years of age or younger, of either gender, weighing over 10 kg. Individual cases had been described earlier but were included in reports of congenital PSS. Presenting signs include abdominal enlargement associated with effusion, gastrointestinal abnormalities, polydipsia and weight loss, and less consistently, signs of HE. Characteristic clinicopathologic abnormalities include microcytosis, evidence of hepatic dysfunction (e.g., hypoalbuminemia), and low urine specific gravity. Microhepatia, anomalous portacaval venous anastomoses, and hypoechogenic abdominal fluid are the notable abdominal ultrasound findings. The cause has not been identified, but the unifying thread among the theories is vascular malformation. One study concluded that affected dogs might live as long as 9 years after diagnosis with minimal symptomatic treatment for ascites and, for some, HE. A few dogs were euthanized because of problems related to persistent portal hypertension (e.g., duodenal ulceration, urate urolithiasis).

## ARTERIOPORTAL FISTULA

Intrahepatic arterioportal fistula, causing marked volume overload of the portal circulation resulting in portal hypertension, acquired PSSs, and ascites, is seen occasionally. Abdominal ultrasound with Doppler can usually detect the tortuous tubular structures representing the connection between an artery and overperfused portal vein or veins; sometimes the turbulent blood flow through the fistula can be auscultated through the body wall as a bruit. If only one lobe of the liver is affected, the lobe containing the arterioportal fistula can be removed surgically; assuming there is adequate intrahepatic portal vasculature, acquired PSSs regress once portal overcirculation subsides. More often, multiple liver lobes are involved making surgical cure impossible. Multiple microscopic hepatic arteriovenous fistulae were suspected to be the cause of similar signs and clinicopathologic findings in another young dog (Schermerhorn and colleagues, 1997); this condition would also be surgically incurable.

## TREATMENT FOR CHRONIC LIVER DISORDERS

Treatment for drug-induced chronic hepatitis is straightforward. Clinical signs and results of clinicopathologic tests should improve soon after drug administration is suspended. If complete resolution does not occur, liver biopsy is indicated to determine if other hepatic disease is present or if there are findings that would support the use of medication to modify persistent pathologic processes.

Treatment of dogs with other chronic hepatic diseases consists of supportive care, including use of modified diets (Table 38-3), and specific medications given to subdue the pathologic processes (e.g., Cu accumulation, mononuclear cell inflammation, fibrosis). Of the following therapeutic agents, only prednisone and *S*-adenosylmethionine (SAME) are approved for use in dogs. Specific therapy should address the underlying cause, if known. Overall prognosis is guarded to poor because for most chronic hepatic diseases the underlying cause cannot be eliminated.

## PREVENTION AND TREATMENT OF COPPER EXCESS

### Reduced Copper in the Diet

In Bedlington Terriers and other breeds with familial Cu hepatotoxicosis, progressive liver injury occurs unless dietary Cu intake is decreased and—most importantly—hepatic Cu is mobilized for urinary excretion. Decreasing Cu in the diet does not remove excess hepatic Cu but helps to slow further

TABLE 38-3

**Dietary Management of Chronic Hepatic Encephalopathy in Cats and Dogs**

| | COMMERCIAL* | HOME PREPARED† |
|---|---|---|
| Cats | l/d | 21 g cooked chicken liver<br>21 g cooked white chicken<br>98 g cooked white rice (no added salt)<br>8 g vegetable oil<br>0.7 g calcium carbonate<br>0.5 g iodized salt<br>0.5 g salt substitute (KCl) |
| Dogs | l/d | 78 g cooked regular beef<br>20 g large hard-boiled egg<br>237 g cooked rice (no added salt)<br>50 g white bread<br>3 g vegetable oil<br>1.5 g calcium carbonate<br>0.5 g iodized salt |
| | None | **24% protein (cat)‡**<br>1.5 cups low-fat (1%) cottage cheese<br>3 cups cooked rice (do not use instant rice)<br>1 oz cooked beef liver<br>1 tsp dicalcium phosphate<br>1 tsp corn oil<br>250 mg vitamin C<br>1 capsule B complex vitamins plus iron<br>**18% protein (dog)‡**<br>Same as above except use 1 cup low fat cottage cheese |

*g*, Gram; *oz*, ounce; *tsp*, teaspoon.
*Hill's Prescription Diets, Topeka, Kan. Composition (%) on a dry matter basis (canned/dry):

| | Protein | Carbohydrate | Fat | kcal/can or cup |
|---|---|---|---|---|
| Feline l/d | 31.7/31.8 | 37.9/37.4 | 23.3/23.4 | 164/505 |
| Canine l/d | 25.9/26.4 | 52.6/52.3 | 14.0/13.6 | 548/379 |

†From Hand MS et al: *Small animal clinical nutrition*, ed 4, Marceline, Mo, 2000, Walsworth Publishing Co. A balanced vitamin-mineral supplement should accompany each of these diets. Recipe is for daily feeding of a 4.5 kg cat (24.4% protein) or 18 kg dog (21.1% protein). Cats also need 250 to 500 mg taurine daily.
‡From Biourge V: *Nutrition support service*, School of Veterinary Medicine, University of California at Davis, 1991. Contains 1000 kcal of metabolizable energy. Calculate calorie requirements with the formula: $132 \times (\text{body weight [kg]})^{0.75}$.

accumulation. Completely eliminating Cu from the diet is impossible. Most commercial diets contain much greater quantities of Cu than the National Research Council recommends for dogs (i.e., 2 mg/g of dog food). The following diets can be used:

1. Certain commercial diets (Cornucopia Senior or Life; Cornucopia Natural Pet Foods, Huntington,

N.Y.; described as low in Cu but actual Cu content unknown)

2. Prescription diets (Canine l/d; Hill's Prescription Diets, Topeka, Kan; 4.5 to 4.9 mg/g diet on a dry matter basis) that contain lower concentrations of Cu
3. A homemade diet that does not contain organ meats, shellfish, or cereals (specifically described as low in Cu but has not been analyzed specifically for Cu content (Strombeck and colleagues, 1983) (see Table 38-3)

Snacks containing high Cu content foods, such as organ meats, shellfish, cereal, chocolate, nuts, dried fruit, legumes, and mushrooms, should be avoided.

## Reduced Intestinal Absorption of Copper

Administration of zinc (Zn) salts (preferably acetate or sulfate; 100 mg of elemental Zn PO q12h) has been found to be beneficial in the management of affected West Highland and Bedlington Terriers early in life before massive accumulation of hepatic Cu occurs. Zn is best absorbed without the presence of food. For dogs that tend to vomit with Zn administration, a small amount of tuna fish can be given with the Zn dose. Zn discourages absorption of Cu by stimulating the formation of metallothionein by the intestinal mucosa. Swallowed Cu (from dietary and gastrointestinal secretions) binds more avidly than Zn to this protein, sequestering it in mucosal cells that are eventually shed. This approach does not extract Cu from the liver, so its use is primarily preventive. The goal of treatment is to maintain serum Zn concentrations (measured every 2 to 3 months) in the range of 200 to 300 μg/dl and no greater than 600 μg/dl (well below toxic range); a single blood sample is drawn before the morning Zn dose. The dose may be reduced to 50 mg twice daily after about 3 months of treatment, assuming the plasma Zn concentration remains in the target range. If the serum concentration is below 150 μg/dl, the dose must remain in the range of 50 to 100 mg PO every 12 hours.

## Copper Chelation

In older dogs that have marked Cu accumulation, maximal benefit is derived from use of drugs that chelate Cu and promote its extraction from the liver, although studies of arge numbers of affected dogs have not been conducted. *D-Penicillamine*, 10 to 15 mg/kg PO every 12 hours 30 minutes before meals, is the drug most often recommended; it also has weak antifibrotic and antiinflammatory properties. Starting at the lower end of the dose range and increasing the dose after 1 week or dividing the dose and giving it more frequently can reduce the common adverse effects of vomiting and anorexia. Decreases in hepatic Cu concentration occur only after at least several months of therapy; thus rapid improvement cannot be expected in severely ill dogs. Use of D-penicillamine is recommended in West Highland White Terriers only when the liver Cu content is greater than or equal to 2000 μg/g DW. A decrease in liver Cu content of about 900 μg/g DW per year can be anticipated in dogs treated with D-penicillamine.

Another equally efficacious Cu chelator agent, trientine, may be used (10 to 15 mg/kg PO q12h 30 minutes before meals) in dogs that cannot tolerate D-penicillamine. It may not be immediately available and may require special ordering directly from the manufacturer (Merck & Co., 800-637-2579). A more potent related compound, 2,3,2-tetramine (7.5 mg/kg PO q12h), has been found to be as safe but is not currently available as a pharmaceutical. Additional therapy to modify hepatic inflammatory changes is not indicated.

Copper chelation treatment is continued until normal liver Cu concentration is reached, best determined by liver biopsy and Cu quantitation or cytologic estimate; this is to avoid Cu deficiency. The regimen can then be changed to a preventive protocol consisting of a Cu-restricted diet (see above) and Zn administration.

## GLUCOCORTICOIDS

Use of glucocorticoids for treatment of dogs with chronic hepatitis is rather controversial. Glucocorticoids are advocated for treatment of idiopathic autoimmune CAH in human patients for their antiinflammatory and antifibrotic effects. Certainly not all causes of chronic hepatitis in dogs are known to have an immune-mediated component that could justifiably be manipulated with glucocorticoids. On the basis of observations of a few individual dogs, there is reason to believe that glucocorticoids may be of greater benefit than Cu chelator therapy in some Doberman Pinschers and perhaps other breeds with Cu-associated hepatopathy of unknown mechanism.

Only one study (Strombeck and colleagues, 1988), performed retrospectively in 151 dogs with chronic hepatitis that aimed to identify predictors of survival and whether glucocorticoid therapy could improve survival time has been published. Case records were accepted for evaluation if the liver biopsy findings included increased numbers of mononuclear cells and fibroblasts and in some cases bile ductule proliferation. Attempts to specifically classify the liver disease in each case were not made. Because this study was retrospective, there were no criteria for selection as to which dogs received glucocorticoids or no treatment other than supportive care. The decision regarding whether to treat and with what regimen was made by the attending clinician. Initial hepatic histopathologic changes were more severe in the glucocorticoid-treated group, which presumably was the reason clinicians initiated therapy. Inflammatory cell infiltrates and necrosis, especially in the periportal region, were the major changes. The most valuable predictors of death within 1 week of diagnosis were low normal blood glucose concentration and prolonged one-stage prothrombin time. In dogs that lived longer than 1 week, those with hypoalbuminemia had shorter survival times than dogs with normal serum albumin content. Overall, dogs given glucocorticoids using a regimen resembling treatment of immune-mediated disease (prednisone: 1.1 mg/kg PO q12h for 7 to 10 days initially, then 1.1 mg/kg/day for 10 days, then 0.6 mg/kg/day until the disease was judged to be in remission) lived three times longer than those that were not given glucocorticoids. Among 58 dogs given glucocorticoids, liver biopsy was repeated to determine remission in 26 dogs. Improvement in clinical signs and clinicopathologic test results was used to assess treatment success in the remaining 32 dogs. The investigators did not specifically report the results of repeat clinicopathologic evaluations or liver biopsies in dogs treated with glucocorticoids. Histopathologic lesions progressed in dogs not given glucocorticoids.

The authors concluded that few clinicopathologic variables could be used to accurately predict the outcome in dogs with chronic hepatitis and that glucocorticoid treatment was indicated to prolong survival. Possible explanations for the success of glucocorticoid therapy were not put forth. The authors also recommended ascorbic acid (25 mg/kg/day PO), because of reduced capacity to produce ascorbic acid in dogs with hepatic insufficiency, and Zn supplementation to delay Cu absorption and hepatic deposition. Whether to give antiinflammatory or immunosuppressive doses also needs to be clarified. Although these preliminary results seem encouraging, there can be no specific guidelines for use of glucocorticoids in dogs with chronic hepatitis until controlled prospective studies have been conducted.

## AZATHIOPRINE

If a decision has been made to institute immunosuppressive therapy with prednisone and if remission of clinical signs, clinicopathologic abnormalities, and hepatic histopathologic lesions has been achieved, but there are unacceptable adverse effects of prednisone, combination immunosuppressive therapy can be used. Azathioprine, 50 mg/m$^2$ PO every 24 hours, initially given together, then later on alternate days with prednisone, 1 mg/kg/day PO, can be used to maintain remission and reduce adverse effects of glucocorticoids. Because of the potential for bone marrow toxicity associated with azathioprine administration, complete blood counts (CBCs) should be performed weekly or at least every other week during therapy. Treatment should be suspended for 5 to 7 days if the total neutrophil count is less than 2000 cells/$\mu$l or if the platelet count is less than 100,000 cells/$\mu$l. Once the hematologic abnormalities have resolved, azathioprine can be reinstituted at 75% of the original dose. Although this regimen is often recommended and used, studies have not been conducted to objectively determine its efficacy.

## ANTIFIBROTIC AGENTS

Antifibrotic agents can be chosen as the sole agent for dogs with a primarily fibrotic hepatopathy (e.g., idiopathic hepatic fibrosis). An antifibrotic agent can also be added to the treatment regimen of dogs with chronic hepatitis and a fibrotic component that are intolerant or nonresponsive to glucocorticoids, especially if they have clinical manifestations of portal hypertension (ascites and HE). Investigations of use of these drugs have been carried out in human patients and laboratory animal species but not in dogs. The drug used most often is *colchicine,* which inhibits collagen synthesis and enhances collagenase activity in vitro. Improvement in clinical signs and greater long-term survival rates have been clearly demonstrated by recent clinical trials of colchicine in human patients with cirrhosis of various causes. Hepatic histopathologic changes were improved in 60% of colchicine-treated pa-

tients who permitted repeat biopsy. The only undesirable adverse effect noted was diarrhea in a few patients, which, along with vomiting and abdominal discomfort, is one of the early signs of toxicity. Other adverse effects, such as renal injury, bone marrow suppression with prolonged use, myopathy, and peripheral neuropathy, have been reported infrequently. Some dogs benefit from colchicine with no adverse effects at an oral dose of 0.03 mg/kg/day. Similar to Cu chelator therapy, colchicine must be given for months to years to be of benefit.

## DIETARY MODIFICATION

Use of special diets for dogs with chronic hepatitis is aimed at providing sufficient nutrients and calories to support repair of hepatic tissue while minimizing aberrations in protein metabolism that induce or perpetuate HE. These diets, whether homemade or commercial prescription diets, are formulated to be highly digestible, contain high-quality protein in moderately restricted quantities, and rely on nonprotein sources for most of their calories. Reducing the metabolic loads on the liver (e.g., amino acid deamination, gluconeogenesis, lipid metabolism, bile secretion) can be aided by dietary therapy during the recovery phase (see Table 38-3 and p. 546).

## ADJUNCTIVE TREATMENTS

### Antioxidants

Several medications have been recommended for their free radical–scavenging capabilities. *Vitamin E* (400 to 500 IU/day PO as a water-soluble preparation) has been found to protect liver cells from Cu toxic injury and cholestatic concentrations of bile acids in laboratory studies and appears safe clinically. *S-adenosylmethionine* (Denosyl SD4; Nutramax Laboratories, Edgewood, Md; 20 mg/kg PO q24h after an overnight fast), a substance found naturally in most cells of the body, replenishes depleted glutathione stores, scavenges free radicals, and appears to protect liver cells from bile acid–induced injury in laboratory investigations. Because of its ability to restore glutathione, it may be of some benefit to animals with acute toxic hepatopathy, such as acetaminophen toxicity.

*Ursodiol* was first developed to dissolve gallstones in humans, but, along the way, other effects were discovered that could be beneficial to patients with chronic hepatitis of various kinds. It displaces injurious bile acids from the bile acid pool, protects liver cells from oxidant injury, increases bile flow, and modulates cytokine responses. It is safe at a dosage of 10 to 15 mg/kg PO every 24 hours, but its place in the treatment of dogs with chronic hepatitis is unknown.

## ACUTE TOXIC HEPATOPATHY

### Etiology and Pathogenesis

Drugs or environmental toxins with inherent ability to cause hepatic injury do so either by direct hepatocellular damage or by disturbance of hepatocellular homeostasis, which results in cell death. Such substances are in limited use today and exist mainly as pesticides, herbicides, cleaning agents, and plant toxins. Most clinically relevant adverse hepatic reactions observed in dogs involve chronic administration of therapeutic agents and are thought to result from individual susceptibility (idiosyncrasy) associated with differences in hepatic drug–metabolizing enzyme populations. Although accurate figures on the frequency of adverse hepatic drug reactions are not available, they are estimated to be quite low. A partial list of drugs and environmental toxins reported to be hepatotoxic in dogs is given in Table 37-3. Of these, certain antimicrobials (ketoconazole, trimethoprim-sulfa), anthelmintics (mebendazole, diethylcarbamazine-oxibendazole, thiacetarsamide), inhalation anesthetics (halothane, methoxyflurane), and analgesics (acetaminophen, naproxen, carprofen, phenylbutazone) have been incriminated more than once in unpublished reports to the Center of Veterinary Medicine in Washington, D.C., and in the scientific literature.

## Clinical Features

The clinical signs and clinicopathologic features of acute toxic hepatopathy are not distinct from other hepatopathies except in onset and perhaps in severity. Vomiting is a common sign. Host response is determined by interaction between the inherent characteristics of the host and the biologic behavior of the agent. Nutritional status and gender are important host factors; females seem to be more susceptible to toxic liver injury than males. Dose, duration of exposure, and chemical composition of the agent contribute to how toxicity is expressed by the host. Some agents cause hepatic injury rapidly, whereas others must accumulate after repeated exposure to cause illness. Although several patterns of drug-induced liver injury have been described in human patients (i.e., cytotoxic, cholestatic, or mixed), only the cytotoxic and mixed patterns have been recognized in dogs. Clinicopathologic test results are typical of mild, moderate, or severe hepatocellular damage, suggested by high serum ALT activity, and variable increases in serum AP activity. Jaundice is usually of hepatocellular rather than biliary tract origin. A liver biopsy is performed only if recovery is incomplete and other hepatobiliary diseases are suspected. Histopathologic lesions described thus far in acute to subacute drug-induced hepatopathy in dogs are centrilobular necrosis or periportal inflammation, either of which can be features of other hepatopathies. Because the clinicopathologic and hepatic histopathologic features of acute toxic hepatopathy can resemble other hepatic diseases, a careful, detailed history is the most valuable diagnostic test.

## Treatment and Prognosis

Most adverse hepatic reactions in dogs are believed to be idiosyncratic and therefore unpredictable; thus a high level of suspicion with prompt recognition is the best defense. It is possible that some chronic adverse hepatic drug reactions result from failure to recognize early signs of toxicity or from self-perpetuated injury that occurs despite discontinuation of drug administration. If there is reason to believe that a drug might be associated with hepatic disease, its administration should be suspended. Except for a few hepatotoxic agents for which there are specific antidotes (see Table 37-4), additional treatment for acute toxic hepatopathy is supportive (see p. 546). As soon as exposure to the offending agent is terminated, improvement in clinical signs and in results of repeat clinicopathologic testing should be evident. In cases of brief toxic exposure, complete recovery is likely to occur. If a large amount of hepatic mass has been seriously injured, residual hepatic insufficiency may persist after the acute phase of recovery.

## BILIARY TRACT DISORDERS

### Etiology and Pathogenesis

Disorders of the biliary tract are generally classified as primary diseases originating in the biliary tract itself or diseases of other organ systems that secondarily impact the biliary tract (see Fig. 35-5 and Table 36-1). The most common causes of secondary biliary tract disease are pancreatitis and sepsis arising from nonhepatobiliary sources. Rarely, certain drugs are believed to cause bile ductule injury (destructive cholangiolitis), such as sulfonamides.

Primary conditions that diffusely involve the bile ducts (cholangitis) and sometimes the gallbladder (cholecystitis) are common in cats but unusual in dogs. The clinical signs and diagnostic evaluation is identical to those for a cat suspected of having acute (bacterial) cholangitis (see p. 513). Mechanical obstruction is ruled out first, usually by ultrasonography, and then liver and bile and/or gallbladder mucosa specimens are obtained for histopathology and microbial culture and sensitivity testing, preferably before antibiotic treatment is initiated. If surgery is not an option because of owner constraints, liver and bile samples are obtained via ultrasonographic guidance. To minimize bile leakage, a 22-gauge needle with attached 12-ml syringe is used for cholecystocentesis (bile retrieval), and an attempt is made to evacuate the gallbladder. Risk of iatrogenic bile or septic peritonitis is greatest with a severely diseased gallbladder wall (determined ultrasonographically); surgical treatment is necessary in such cases. Enteric organisms similar to those found in cats, such as *Escherichia coli*, *Enterobacter* sp., *Klebsiella* sp., *Clostridium* sp. (which may be a gas-forming species causing emphysematous changes in the gallbladder wall visible radiographically), *Pseudomonas* sp., and rarely *Campylobacter jejuni*, are usually isolated. Choleliths can be found in association with cholecystitis or cholangitis; the cause and effect relationship is not always clear.

More common primary conditions of the biliary tract in dogs are those that require surgical intervention: extrahepatic bile duct obstruction (EBDO), bile peritonitis, and gallbladder mucocele. Similar to EBDO in cats (see p. 518), EBDO in dogs is a syndrome with several underlying causes, which are listed in Table 37-1. The most common causes in dogs are extraluminal inflammatory conditions, which may cause transient EBDO from mild periductal edema or permanent EBDO from severe inflammation and scarring. Bile duct injuries that heal and result in stricture formation several weeks later are also seen in dogs; the common bile duct (CBD) may be compressed when carried with the liver into the thorax in dogs with diaphragmatic hernia. Extraluminal compressive lesions, such as pancreatic, biliary, or duodenal neoplasms, are less common causes, and cholelithiasis as a cause of EBDO is rare. To be considered EBDO, a pathologic process must exist at the level of the CBD that impedes bile flow into the duodenum. Only if bile flow has been completely interrupted for several weeks do acholic feces, vitamin K–responsive coagulopathy, and repeated absence of urobilinogen in properly processed urine specimens occur. If obstruction is incomplete, these features are not present and the constellation of signs and clinicopathologic test results resembles those of other, nonobstructive biliary tract disorders.

Bile peritonitis results most often from abdominal trauma damaging the CBD (e.g., penetrating injury, horse kick, automobile accident) or pathologic rupture of a severely diseased gallbladder. Early signs of bile peritonitis are nonspecific, but with progression, jaundice, fever, and abdominal effusion are seen. When bile, which is normally sterile, comes in contact with the peritoneal surface, resultant cell necrosis and changes in permeability predispose to infection with bacteria that move across the intestinal wall. Hypovolemia and sepsis may occur in animals with undetected bile peritonitis.

Gallbladder mucocele was recently described in two reports totaling 16 dogs. Older dogs of various small breeds were most often presented for anorexia, lethargy, and vomiting. On abdominal ultrasound, the gallbladder had a very characteristic stellate appearance to the contents, resembling a cross section of kiwi fruit (Fig. 38-7). Gallbladder rupture occurred in about half of affected dogs, spilling some of the rubbery mucoid material into the abdomen. Enteric bacteria

were isolated from six of nine dogs that had microbial bile culture; infection was believed to be secondary to bile stasis in some dogs and could have been the initiating event in others. Mucosal hyperplasia and degrees of mural necrosis were common histopathologic findings in the gallbladder. It is believed to occur subsequent to cystic duct obstruction, allowing bile to be resorbed and stimulating excess mucous production. Cholecystectomy was curative.

## Clinical Features

Presenting clinical signs and clinicopathologic and physical examination findings of all these disorders may not differ greatly unless the underlying condition has caused EBDO or bile peritonitis. Regardless of the underlying disorder, typical clinical signs are jaundice, acute or chronic vomiting, anorexia, depression, weight loss, and occasionally vague cranial abdominal pain. Because of the protected location of the gallbladder in the abdomen, it is rarely possible to be able to palpate it in a dog with EBDO unless the gallbladder is greatly enlarged.

## Diagnosis

The pattern of clinicopathologic findings typical of biliary tract disorders is that of hyperbilirubinemia, high serum AP and GGT activities, high fasting and postprandial SBA concentrations, and less severe changes in serum ALT activity. Generally more severe cholestatic lesions are associated with more severe clinicopathologic changes. Fractionating the total bilirubin concentration into direct- and indirect-reacting components (i.e., the van den Bergh reaction) does not distinguish intrahepatic from extrahepatic cholestasis or obstructive from nonobstructive cholestasis. Radiographically there may be evidence of hepatomegaly and a mass effect in the area of the gallbladder on survey abdominal films. Gas shadows associated

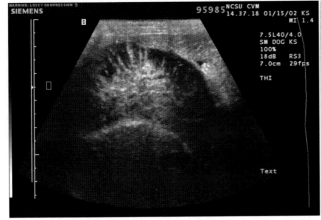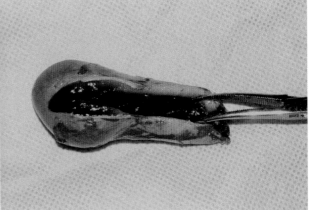

**FIG 38-7**
**A,** Ultrasonographic transverse image of the gallbladder of a dog with a mucocele; note the stellate pattern to the bile. The mucinous material does not move with change in patient position. **B,** Appearance of the gallbladder and contents after surgical removal. (Courtesy Dr. Kathy A. Spaulding, North Carolina State University, College of Veterinary Medicine.)

with the gallbladder and other biliary tract structures could be ascribed to ascending infection with gas-forming organisms. Findings consistent with acute pancreatitis as an underlying cause of EBDO are loss of serosal detail in the area of the pancreas as an indication of localized peritonitis, trapped pockets of gas in the duodenum, and duodenal displacement. Choleliths form in dogs in a manner similar to the way they form in cats (see p. 518), usually as a sequela to cholestasis and infection, but they may be found in asymptomatic dogs. These concretions are radiolucent unless they contain calcium, which occurs about 50% of the time. Inflammatory abdominal effusion is expected in dogs with bile peritonitis but not in those with most causes of EBDO (except for malignant effusion associated with pancreatic cancer).

The ability to differentiate medical from surgical causes of jaundice has been refined with the development of ultrasonography, although this imaging modality is certainly not foolproof. Dilated and tortuous hepatic bile ducts and CBD, as well as gallbladder distention, are convincing ultrasonographic evidence of EBDO at the CBD or sphincter of Oddi. When dilated biliary structures are seen, it might be difficult to distinguish EBDO that requires surgical intervention from resolving, transient EBDO associated with severe acute pancreatitis or from nonobstructive biliary disease (e.g., bacterial cholecystitis/cholangitis; Fig. 38-8) unless a source of obstruction is specifically identified (e.g., pancreatic mass, cholelith in the CBD). Prolonged fasting causes mild gallbladder enlargement because of delayed evacuation and should not be misinterpreted. In addition, cystic hyperplasia and epithelial polyp formation are common lesions in older dogs, not to be confused with choleliths in the gallbladder. A stellate appearance to the contents of the gallbladder is characteristic of gallbladder mucocele. Monitoring serum bilirubin concentrations to determine when to intervene surgically is not worthwhile because serum bilirubin concentration begins to decline over days to weeks, without relief of obstruction, in both cats and dogs with experimentally induced EBDO.

## Treatment and Prognosis

If the distinction between medical and surgical causes of jaundice is not clear, it is safer to proceed surgically to avoid excessive delays in diagnosis. Should a site of obstruction or biliary injury not be identified, at least tissue (i.e., liver, gallbladder mucosa) and bile specimens can be obtained for histopathologic and cytologic evaluation and bacterial culture and sensitivity testing.

Surgery is required in dogs with persistent EBDO, bile peritonitis, and gallbladder mucocele. It is possible to obtain liver and bile specimens in dogs with suspected nonobstructive biliary disease with ultrasonographic guidance or by laparoscopy, but risk of delayed bile leakage is higher with these techniques. Coagulation status and fluid and electrolyte needs should be addressed preoperatively. Use of bile acids to stimulate bile flow is contraindicated in dogs with EBDO. If there is clinical or subclinical coagulopathy, vitamin $K_1$ is administered (1 mg/kg SQ q24h) for 24 to 48 hours before and after surgery. Abdominal fluid is analyzed cytologically and cultured for aerobic and anaerobic bacteria. If surgery for bile peritonitis is to be delayed, peritoneal drainage should be established to remove noxious, bile-containing abdominal fluid and for lavage. Surgical goals are to relieve biliary obstruction or leakage and restore bile flow. Reconstructive procedures to divert bile flow can be performed if the cause of EBDO cannot be corrected. A liver biopsy specimen should be obtained in all cases. Typical hepatic histopathologic findings in early EBDO are canalicular bile plugs and bile ductular proliferation, with degrees of periportal inflammation and fibrosis in chronic cases. Confounding biliary infection incites a stronger inflammatory reaction in the periportal region.

A bile specimen is collected for cytologic analysis and aerobic and anaerobic bacterial cultures if choleliths are found or if the biliary structures appear thickened and inflamed. Because some bacterial agents have a predilection for the mucous membrane of the gallbladder, a specimen of gallbladder mucosa should also be obtained and submitted, along with the bile specimen, for microbial culture. Antibiotic therapy is started immediately after bile samples are obtained; ampicillin or amoxicillin (22 mg/kg intravenously [IV], subcutaneously [SQ], or PO q8h), first-generation cephalosporins (22 mg/kg IV or PO q8h), and metronidazole (7.5 to 15 mg/kg PO q8-12h; use lower dose when severe hepatobiliary dysfunction is present) are good empiric choices as single agents initially in animals without a long history of antibiotic administration.

The prognosis for dogs with EBDO or bile peritonitis depends on the underlying cause. If the cause can be addressed without surgical reconstruction, the prognosis is fair to good. If extensive biliary reconstruction is needed, the prognosis is guarded because of the potential for recurrent ascending bacterial infections and other complications.

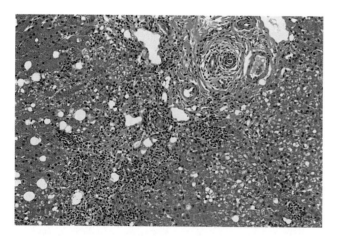

**FIG 38-8**
Photomicrograph of a liver biopsy specimen from a 6-year-old spayed female Doberman Pinscher with ascending bacterial cholangitis (hematoxylin-eosin). There is periductular fibrosis with mild to moderate mononuclear inflammation around bile ducts. *Escherichia coli* was isolated from the bile.

# FOCAL HEPATIC LESIONS

## ABSCESSES

### Etiology

Hepatic abscesses are usually the result of septic embolization from an abdominal site of bacterial infection. In puppies they are a consequence of omphalophlebitis, whereas in adult dogs they arise most often subsequent to inflammatory conditions of the pancreas or hepatobiliary system. Adult dogs with certain endocrine diseases, such as diabetes mellitus or hypercortisolism, are also at risk. Occasionally, infection arising from a location other than the abdominal cavity, such as the endocardium, lung, or blood, may disseminate to the liver, causing abscessation.

In a recent review (Farrar and colleagues, 1996) of 14 dogs with hepatic abscesses, aerobic bacteria were isolated in 9 of 10 cases in which material from the hepatic lesions was submitted for culture. Although the most common isolates were gram-negative organisms, *Staphylococcus* spp. were identified in two dogs. *Clostridium* sp. was the only isolate cultured anaerobically from abscess fluid in four of seven dogs.

### Clinical Features

The typical signalment and physical examination findings of a dog with hepatic abscesses depend on the underlying cause. Dogs over 8 years old are most often affected because the predisposing causes of liver abscesses are conditions seen more commonly in older dogs. Regardless of the initiating event,

anorexia, lethargy, and vomiting are consistent presenting complaints. Expected physical examination findings include fever, dehydration, and abdominal pain. Hepatomegaly may be detected in dogs with diabetes mellitus or hypercortisolism and in some dogs with primary hepatobiliary disease.

### Diagnosis

Neutrophilic leukocytosis with a left shift and high serum AP and ALT activities are dependable but nonspecific clinicopathologic abnormalities. Survey abdominal radiographs may reveal evidence of irregular hepatomegaly, mass, or gas opacity within the area of the hepatic parenchyma (Fig. 38-9), but ultrasonography is the imaging modality of choice. One or more hypoechoic or anechoic hepatic masses and perhaps a hyperechoic rim surrounding the mass or masses are characteristic findings. If there are multiple masses that would preclude surgical removal or if the owner declines surgery, fine-needle aspiration cytologic analysis of the contents of a representative lesion would distinguish an abscess from nodular hyperplasia, neoplasm (e.g., hemangiosarcoma), or granuloma. Ideally, material is obtained for cytologic analysis and aerobic and anaerobic bacterial culture from a representative lesion deep in the liver parenchyma to avoid abscess rupture and abdominal contamination. Abscess material is also obtained by this approach in animals having surgery so that antibiotic treatment can be initiated preoperatively. Results of the preliminary clinicopathologic and radiographic evaluation are scrutinized for

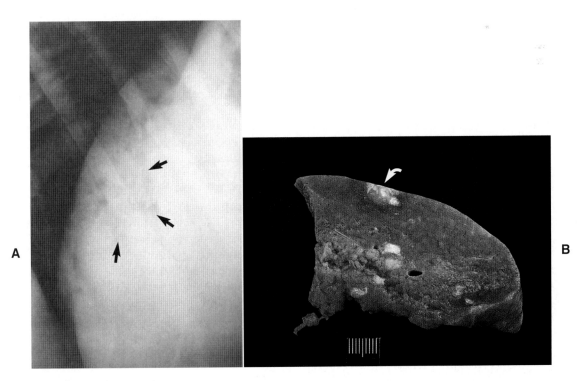

**FIG 38-9**
**A,** Lateral abdominal radiograph of a 1-year-old female Great Dane with a liver abscess *(arrows)* caused by *Clostridium* spp.; the cause was undetermined. **B,** Gross appearance of the resected liver lobe containing an abscess *(arrow)*.

evidence of previously mentioned associated or predisposing illnesses.

## Treatment and Prognosis

Treatment for liver abscesses consists of surgical removal of infected tissue, administration of appropriate antibiotics, supportive care, and resolution of underlying predisposing conditions. Infected liver tissue is removed, if possible, and submitted for histopathologic examination and bacterial culture, if not done preoperatively. Fluid, electrolyte, and acid-base abnormalities are addressed. Administration of a combination of antibiotics with a gram-negative and anaerobic spectrum is initiated until culture and sensitivity test results are available. Amikacin (10 mg/kg IV or intramuscularly [IM] q8h) or enrofloxacin (2.5 mg/kg IV or PO q12h) combined with metronidazole (10 mg/kg PO q8-12h or 7.5 mg/kg PO q8-12h for dogs with hepatic dysfunction) or clindamycin (10 mg/kg IV or PO q12h) is a good empiric choice. Surgery is not indicated in animals with multiple abscesses; ultrasound-guided centesis and abscess evacuation may be a reasonable adjunct to treatment. Antibiotic treatment is continued long term, usually for 6 to 8 weeks or until clinicopathologic and ultrasonographic indicators of septic abscessation are resolved. From the limited information available about this rare condition, it seems that with aggressive medical and surgical management, the prognosis for dogs with liver abscesses may not be as dismal as once thought.

## NODULAR HYPERPLASIA

Hepatic nodular hyperplasia is a benign condition of older dogs that does not cause clinical illness but may be misinterpreted as a more serious condition, such as primary or metastatic malignancy or regenerative nodules associated with cirrhosis. Affected dogs have high serum AP activity (usually 2.5-fold elevation but may be as high as fourteen-fold), which prompts investigation for hypercortisolism. There is no evidence of hepatic dysfunction on serum biochemical analysis. Most dogs have multiple macroscopic nodules found ultrasonographically or at surgery, ranging in size from 2 to 5 cm in diameter; some dogs have a single nodule. Micronodular change occurs much less frequently and would be identified in liver biopsy specimens. The lesion consists of increased numbers of normal to vacuolated hepatocytes with more mitotic figures and fewer binucleate cells than expected in normal liver; components of normal lobular architecture (e.g., portal tracts, central vein) remain. Adjacent parenchyma is compressed by growth of the nodules; fibrosis, necrosis, inflammation, and bile ductule hyperplasia are absent. Because the prognosis for each of these nodular conditions is different, and the margin of the lesion with adjacent hepatic tissue is important to include, wedge biopsy is recommended. Needle specimens are likely to be too small to confidently differentiate nodular hyperplasia from primary hepatocellular carcinoma or adenoma. The cause of this lesion is unknown; on the basis of experimental development of nodular hyperplasia in rodent species, some have speculated a dietary role (extremely low protein).

## NEOPLASIA

### Etiology

Primary hepatic neoplasms are rare in dogs; most types occur in older animals of any breed. Although certain chemicals can induce hepatic neoplasms experimentally, the cause of naturally occurring hepatic neoplasms is unknown. Gender predisposition for the most common types of primary hepatic cancer (hepatocellular carcinoma [HC], intrahepatic cholangiocellular [bile duct] carcinoma [CC]) varies with the reported study. Hepatocellular adenoma (HA) is observed less frequently in either gender. Primary sarcomas such as hemangiosarcoma account for a small fraction of primary hepatic neoplasms. Metastases to the liver by hematogenous routes from distant sites are much more common, arising from gastrointestinal, pancreatic, and mammary adenocarcinoma, and from splenic hemangiosarcoma. Liver involvement is also common in dogs with hemolymphatic disorders, such as lymphoma, myeloproliferative disorders, and mast cell neoplasia.

### Clinical Features

Clinical signs and physical examination findings are nonspecific except for diffuse or nodular hepatomegaly. The left liver lobes are often affected by HC, which can occur in three different patterns: massive (single, large nodule; most common), nodular (multiple smaller nodules), and diffuse (indistinct nodules throughout). Clinicopathologic test results are likewise not specific for neoplasia and may be normal, even in dogs with extensive involvement. Hypoglycemia has been described in association with HC in dogs; one report described a dog with acquired myasthenia gravis and CC. Invasion into adjacent hepatic parenchyma certainly identifies HC. Metastases from HC or CC usually occur early; the most common sites are regional lymph nodes, lung, and peritoneal surfaces. HA is a benign tumor that most often occurs as a single mass that is typically smaller than the massive form of HC but can be multifocal. Histologic features of HA are very similar to those of nodular hyperplasia except for the presence of a fine rim of reticulin surrounding the adenoma and lack of apparent normal architecture (i.e., few portal tracts, no central veins).

### Treatment and Prognosis

When a single large hepatic mass is identified, it can be very difficult to distinguish well-differentiated HC from nodular hyperplasia and HA. Surgical resection is the treatment of choice for primary hepatic neoplasms; other treatments are investigational at this time. The prognosis for HA is reportedly good, but the prognosis for dogs with HC is more variable. In a study of 18 dogs with HC that underwent partial hepatectomy, survival times greater than 1 year were observed in 11 of 18 dogs (Kosovsky, 1989).

## SECONDARY HEPATIC DISEASE

Hepatic involvement is a component of many canine systemic illnesses (see Table 36-1). The fact that hepatic involvement is present often lends support for a particular diagnosis when test results are equivocal. For most of these systemic illnesses, the hepatic manifestations regress after the primary illness resolves, and clinical and clinicopathologic evidence of serious hepatic insufficiency is not present. Should the hepatic component of systemic illness not resolve, primary hepatobiliary diseases should be considered.

## PANCREATITIS

Acute pancreatitis in dogs typically involves the liver by several mechanisms. Close proximity of the pancreas to the liver allows direct extension of inflammation to the liver. Injurious activated pancreatic enzymes enter common lymphatic drainage to cause more distant hepatic inflammation. The CBD is surrounded by pancreatic tissue so active pancreatic inflammation may cause transient or persistent EBDO. Patterns of liver enzyme activities in dogs with pancreatitis are typical of those found with a mixed hepatocellular and biliary tract insult: high serum AP and GGT with less striking ALT activity and variable serum bilirubin concentrations.

## SEPSIS

Cholestasis associated with sepsis of nonhepatobiliary origin is well-recognized in humans and has also been described in dogs. Gram-negative organisms are cultured most often, but gram-positive and mixed infections have also been reported. It is believed that bacterial endotoxin interacts with the bile secretory apparatus to impede bile secretion without relevant hepatocellular or biliary injury. Serum bilirubin concentration may exceed 30 mg/dl, fasting SBA concentration is high, and serum activities of liver-specific enzymes are only mildly to moderately altered; serum AP is usually more greatly increased than serum ALT.

## MISCELLANEOUS DISORDERS

Hepatomegaly associated with lipid or glycogen accumulation is a common physical examination finding in dogs with hypercortisolism, hypothyroidism, and diabetes mellitus. Chronic passive congestion from congestive heart failure or heartworm disease causes generalized hepatomegaly and ascites with normal to minimally abnormal serum liver enzyme activities. Acute hepatic necrosis may be a consequence of heat stroke or other type of thermal injury.

### Treatment and Prognosis

Secondary hepatobiliary diseases usually resolve with treatment of the systemic disorder; liver biopsy is not necessary. Because there rarely are serious hepatic sequelae with these diseases, no liver-specific treatment is indicated.

### Suggested Readings

Allen L et al: Clinicopathologic features of dogs with hepatic microvascular dysplasia with and without portosystemic shunts: 42 cases (1991-1996), *J Am Vet Med Assoc* 214:218, 1999.

Andersson M et al: Circulating autoantibodies in dogs with chronic liver disease, *J Small Anim Pract* 33:389, 1992.

Batts KP et al: Chronic hepatitis: an update on terminology and reporting, *Am J Surg Pathol* 19:1409, 1995.

Besso JG et al: Ultrasonographic appearance and clinical findings in 14 dogs with gallbladder mucocele, *Vet Radiol Ultrasound* 41:261, 2000.

Boothe HW et al: Multiple extrahepatic portosystemic shunts in dogs: 30 cases (1981-1993), *J Am Vet Med Assoc* 208:1849, 1996.

Bostwick DR et al: Intrahepatic and extrahepatic portal venous anomalies in dogs: 52 cases (1982-1992), *J Am Vet Med Assoc* 206:1181, 1995.

Brewer GJ et al: Use of zinc acetate to treat copper toxicosis in dogs, *J Am Vet Med Assoc* 201:564, 1992.

Bunch SE: Hepatotoxicity associated with pharmacologic agents in dogs and cats, *Vet Clin North Am Small Anim Pract* 23:659, 1993.

Bunch SE et al: Idiopathic noncirrhotic portal hypertension in dogs: 33 cases (1982-1998), *J Am Vet Med Assoc* 218:392, 2001.

Christiansen JS et al: Hepatic microvascular dysplasia in dogs: a retrospective study of 24 cases (1987-1995), *J Am Anim Hosp Assoc* 36:385, 2000.

Church EM et al: Surgical treatment of 23 dogs with necrotizing cholecystitis, *J Am Anim Hosp Assoc* 24:305, 1988.

Crawford MA et al: Chronic active hepatitis in 26 Doberman Pinschers, *J Am Vet Med Assoc* 187:1343, 1987.

Dayrell-Hart B et al: Hepatotoxicity of phenobarbital in dogs: 18 cases, *J Am Vet Med Assoc* 199:1060, 1991.

DeMarco J et al: A syndrome resembling idiopathic noncirrhotic portal hypertension in 4 young Doberman Pinschers, *J Vet Intern Med* 12:147, 1998.

Fahie MA et al: Extrahepatic biliary obstruction: a retrospective study of 45 cases (1983-1993), *J Am Anim Hosp* 31:478, 1995.

Farrar ET et al: Hepatic abscesses in dogs: 14 cases (1982-1994), *J Am Vet Med Assoc* 208:243, 1996.

Greene CE: Infectious canine chronic hepatitis and canine acidophil cell chronic hepatitis. In Greene CE, editor: *Infectious diseases of the dog and cat*, Philadelphia, 1998, WB Saunders, p 22.

Grooters AM et al: Hepatic abscesses in dogs, *Compend Cont Educ Pract Vet* 17:833, 1995.

Hardy RM: Chronic hepatitis in dogs: a syndrome, *Compend Cont Educ Pract Vet* 8:904, 1986.

Hardy RM et al: Chronic progressive hepatitis in Bedlington terriers (Bedlington liver disease). In Kirk RW, editor: *Current veterinary therapy IV*, Philadelphia, 1977, WB Saunders, p 995.

Hardy RM et al: Periportal chronic hepatitis associated with the use of a heartworm-hookworm preventive (diethylcarbamazine-oxibendazole) in 13 dogs, *J Am Anim Hosp Assoc* 25:419, 1989.

Harkin KR et al: Canine leptospirosis in New Jersey and Michigan: 17 cases (1990-1995), *J Am Anim Hosp Assoc* 32:495, 1996.

Harvey J et al: Complete ligation of extrahepatic congenital portosystemic shunts in nonencephalopathic dogs, *Vet Surg* 27:413, 1998.

Haywood S et al: Chronic hepatitis and copper accumulation in Skye Terriers, *Vet Pathol* 25:408, 1988.

Holmes NG et al: DNA marker C04107 for copper toxicosis in a population of Bedlington terriers in the United Kingdom, *Vet Rec* 142:351, 1998.

Hottinger HA et al: Long-term results of complete and partial ligation of congenital portosystemic shunts in dogs, *Vet Surg* 24:331, 1995.

Hultgren BD et al: Inherited, chronic, progressive hepatic degeneration in Bedlington Terriers with increased liver copper concentrations: clinical and pathologic observations and comparison with other copper-associated liver diseases, *Am J Vet Res* 47:365, 1986.

Hunt GB et al: Outcomes after extrahepatic portosystemic shunt ligation in 49 dogs, *Aust Vet J* 77:303, 1999.

Inoue S et al: Five cases of canine peliosis hepatis, *Jpn J Vet Sci* 50:565, 1988.

Jarrett WFH et al: A new transmissible agent causing acute hepatitis, chronic hepatitis and cirrhosis in dogs, *Vet Rec* 116:629, 1985.

Johnson CA et al: Congenital portosystemic shunts in dogs: 46 cases (1979-1986), *J Am Vet Med Assoc* 191:1478, 1987.

Johnson GF et al: Chronic active chronic hepatitis in Doberman pinschers, *J Am Vet Med Assoc* 180:1438, 1982.

Johnson GF et al: Cytochemical detection of inherited copper toxicosis in Bedlington terriers, *Vet Pathol* 21:57, 1984.

Johnson SE: Cholelithiasis and cholangitis. In Kirk RW, editor: *Current veterinary therapy X*, Philadelphia, 1989, WB Saunders, p 884.

Kirpensteijn J et al: Cholelithiasis in dogs: 29 cases (1980-1990), *J Am Vet Med Assoc* 202:1137, 1993.

Kosovsky JE et al: Results of partial hepatectomy in 18 dogs with hepatocellular carcinoma, *J Am Anim Hosp Assoc* 25:203, 1989.

Leveille CR et al: Pathophysiology and pharmacologic modulation of hepatic fibrosis, *J Vet Intern Med* 7:73, 1993.

MacPhail CM et al: Hepatocellular toxicosis associated with administration of carprofen in 21 dogs, *J Am Vet Med Assoc* 212:1895, 1998.

Matushek KJ et al: Generalized motor seizures after portosystemic shunt ligation in dogs: five cases (1981-1988), *J Am Vet Med Assoc* 196:2014, 1990.

Meyer HP et al: Progressive remission of portosystemic shunting in 23 dogs after partial closure of congenital portosystemic shunts, *Vet Rec* 144:333, 1999.

Müller PB et al: Effects of long-term phenobarbital treatment on the liver in dogs, *J Vet Intern Med* 14:165, 2000.

Napier P: Hepatic necrosis with toxic copper levels in a two-year-old Dalmatian, *Can Vet J* 37:45, 1996.

Newell SM et al: Gallbladder mucocele causing biliary obstruction in two dogs: ultrasonographic, scintigraphic, and pathological findings, *J Am Anim Hosp Assoc* 31:467, 1995.

Noaker LJ et al: Copper associated acute hepatic failure in a dog, *J Am Vet Med Assoc* 214:1502, 1999.

Partington BP et al: Transvenous coil embolization for treatment of patent ductus venosus in a dog, *J Am Vet Med Assoc* 202:281, 1993.

Phillips L et al: Hepatic microvascular dysplasia in dogs, *Prog Vet Neurol* 7:88, 1996.

Poitout F et al: Cell-mediated immune responses to liver membrane protein in canine chronic hepatitis, *Vet Immunol Immunopathol* 57:169, 1997.

Prause LC et al: Hepatic nodular hyperplasia. In Bonagura JD et al, editors: *Kirk's current veterinary therapy XIII*, Philadelphia, 2000, WB Saunders, p 675.

Proschowsky JF et al: Microsatellite marker C04107 as a diagnostic marker for copper toxicosis in the Danish population of Bedlington terriers, *Acta Vet Scand* 41:345, 2000.

Rolfe DS et al: Copper-associated hepatopathies in dogs, *Vet Clin North Am Small Anim Pract* 25:399, 1995.

Rutgers HC et al: Hepatic organelle pathology in dogs with congenital portosystemic shunts, *J Vet Intern Med* 5:351, 1991.

Rutgers HC: Hepatic fibrosis in the dog. In Bonagura JD et al, editors: *Kirk's current veterinary therapy XIII*, Philadelphia, 2000, WB Saunders, p 677.

Schaeffer MC et al: Long-term biochemical and physiologic effects of surgically placed portacaval shunts in dogs, *Am J Vet Res* 47:346, 1986.

Schall WD: Use of zinc acetate for the treatment and prevention of canine copper hepatotoxicosis. In Bonagura JD et al, editors: *Kirk's current veterinary therapy XII*, Philadelphia, 1995, WB Saunders, p 757.

Schermerhorn T et al: Characterization of a hepatoportal microvascular dysplasia in a kindred of Cairn Terriers, *J Vet Intern Med* 10:219, 1996.

Schermerhorn T et al: Suspected microscopic hepatic arteriovenous fistulae in a young dog, *J Am Vet Med Assoc* 211:70, 1997.

Seguin MA et al: Iatrogenic copper deficiency in a Bedlington terrier associated with long-term copper chelation treatment for copper storage disease, *J Am Vet Med Assoc* 218:1593, 2001.

Speeti M et al: Lesions of subclinical Doberman hepatitis, *Vet Pathol* 35:361, 1998.

Sterczer A et al: Fast resolution of hypercortisolemia in dogs with portosystemic encephalopathy after surgical shunt closure, *Res Vet Sci* 66:63, 1998.

Strombeck DR et al: Dietary therapy for dogs with chronic hepatic insufficiency. In Kirk RW, editor: *Current veterinary therapy VIII*, Philadelphia, 1983, WB Saunders, p 821.

Strombeck DR et al: Effects of corticosteroid treatment on survival time in dogs with chronic hepatitis: 151 cases (1977-1985), *J Am Vet Med Assoc* 193:1109, 1988.

Taboada J et al: Cholestasis associated with extrahepatic bacterial infection in five dogs, *J Vet Intern Med* 3:216, 1989.

Teske E et al: Cytological detection of copper for the diagnosis of inherited copper toxicosis in Bedlington terriers, *Vet Rec* 131:30, 1992.

Thornburg LP et al: Hereditary copper toxicosis in West Highland White Terriers, *Vet Pathol* 23:148, 1986.

Tobias KMS et al: Surgical techniques for extravascular occlusion of intrahepatic shunts, *Compend Cont Educ Pract Vet* 18:745, 1996.

Tobias KMS et al: Surgical approaches to single extrahepatic portosystemic shunts, *Compend Contin Educ Pract Vet* 20:593, 1998.

Twedt DC et al: Association of hepatic necrosis with trimethoprim sulfonamide administration in 4 dogs, *J Vet Intern Med* 11:20, 1997.

Twedt DC: A review of traditional and not so traditional therapies for liver disease. In *Proceedings of the 19th Annual ACVIM Forum*, Denver, 2001, p 610.

van de Sluis B et al: Identification of a new copper metabolism gene by positional cloning in a purebred dog population, *Hum Mol Genet* 11:165, 2002.

van den Ingh TSGAM et al: Congenital cystic disease of the liver in seven dogs, *J Comp Pathol* 95:405, 1985.

van den Ingh TSGAM et al: Chronic active hepatitis with cirrhosis in the Doberman Pinscher, *Vet Q* 10:84, 1988.

van den Ingh TSGAM et al: Destructive cholangiolitis in seven dogs, *Vet Q* 10:240, 1988.

van den Ingh TSGAM et al: Lobular dissecting hepatitis in juvenile and young adult dogs, *J Vet Intern Med* 8:217, 1994.

van den Ingh TSGAM et al: Circulatory disorders of the liver in dogs and cats, *Vet Q* 17:70, 1995.

van den Ingh TSGAM et al: Portal hypertension associated with primary hypoplasia of the hepatic portal vein in dogs, *Vet Rec* 137:424, 1995.

Vogt JC et al: Gradual occlusion of extrahepatic portosystemic shunts in dogs and cats using the ameroid constrictor, *Vet Surg* 25:495, 1996.

Watson PJ et al: Medical management of congenital portosystemic shunts in 27 dogs—a retrospective study, *J Small Anim Pract* 39:62, 1998.

Webb CB et al: Copper associated liver disease in Dalmatians: a review of 10 cases (1998-2001), *J Vet Intern Med* 2002 (in press).

Weiss DJ et al: Anti-liver membrane protein antibodies in dogs with chronic hepatitis, *J Vet Intern Med* 9:267, 1995.

Wohl JS: Canine leptospirosis, *Compend Cont Educ Pract Vet* 18: 1215, 1996.

Youmans KR et al: Cellophane banding for the gradual attenuation of single extrahepatic portosystemic shunts in eleven dogs, *Aust Vet J* 76:531, 1998.

# CHAPTER 39

# Treatment of Complications of Hepatic Failure

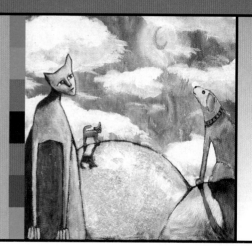

## CHAPTER OUTLINE

GENERAL CONSIDERATIONS, 546
HEPATIC ENCEPHALOPATHY, 546
    Chronic hepatic encephalopathy, 546
    Acute hepatic encephalopathy, 547
    Massive hepatic necrosis, 548
ASCITES, 549
COAGULOPATHY/GASTROINTESTINAL
HEMORRHAGE, 550
SEPSIS, 551

## GENERAL CONSIDERATIONS

The following problems are common in dogs with hepatic failure and are usually related to sudden or chronic progressive loss of functional hepatocyte mass, intrahepatic portal hypertension from primary hepatobiliary disease, portosystemic shunting (PSS), or a combination of these factors. The clinical syndrome of hepatic failure with abdominal effusion, acquired PSS, and other complications of portal hypertension is observed frequently in dogs but rarely in cats. Aggressive management of these problems is vital to achieve a reasonable quality of life for the patient and to enable hepatic recovery while specific therapy is taking effect or when the underlying cause cannot be eradicated.

## HEPATIC ENCEPHALOPATHY

### CHRONIC HEPATIC ENCEPHALOPATHY
**Treatment**

The goal of treatment in cats and dogs with hepatic encephalopathy (HE) is to restore normal neurologic function by decreasing formation of gut-derived encephalotoxins, eliminating precipitating factors, and correcting acid-base and electrolyte abnormalities. A combination of dietary protein restriction, locally acting agents that discourage formation of readily absorbable ammonia and hasten evacuation

of the intestinal tract, and antibiotics to suppress bacterial populations that generate ammonia and other gut-derived encephalotoxins is the standard approach for long-term management of chronic HE (Table 39-1). Whether treatment is given to control signs until corrective surgery can be scheduled, as for congenital PSS, or to control signs indefinitely, as for chronic hepatic failure and acquired PSS, the approach is basically the same. Controlled trials have not been conducted in animals to determine the optimal combination for each stage (mild, moderate, severe) of HE, therefore treatment must be individualized. In general, animals with chronic signs of HE undergo diet modification initially; medications are added if control of signs is inadequate.

**Diet.** The ideal diet for long-term management of HE should (1) be based primarily on carbohydrates as the energy source; (2) use highly digestible protein of high biologic value; (3) contain low levels of aromatic amino acids and methionine and high levels of branched chain amino acids (BCAA) and arginine; (4) have normal fat content (neither restricted nor supplemented); (5) have adequate concentrations of vitamins A, B, C, D, E, and K; and (6) be supplemented with potassium, calcium, and zinc. Prolonged stability and high palatability are also desirable features. Modified diets based on non-meat-based protein are available commercially in feline and canine formulations (Hill's Prescription Diets l/d, Topeka, Kan; Veterinary Diet NF, Ralston Purina Co., St. Louis) or can be prepared by owners (see Table 38-3). Homemade diets using milk-based protein such as low-fat cottage cheese are optimal, but they are inconvenient for many owners. Egg protein is a good source of arginine (especially for cats, which cannot synthesize their own), but it also contains more methionine, which may induce HE, than milk protein. Vegetable protein, such as soy, appears to be well tolerated and can also be incorporated. Quantities of vegetable protein required to provide all protein calories are often too bulky, but tofu, vegetables, and fruits can be used to supplement existing diets and as treats. The formulation of homemade diets should be tailored to the individual animal according to clinical signs and acceptance. Although protein restriction ameliorates the signs of HE, sufficient protein (on

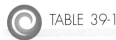

## TABLE 39-1

**Medical Management of Hepatic Encephalopathy**

**Acute**

Nothing by mouth
Fluids given intravenously
1. 0.45% saline solution in 2.5% dextrose with added potassium at a maintenance or 1.5 × maintenance rate
2. Add potassium according to serum electrolyte concentration, or use a safe concentration (20 mEq of potassium chloride per liter of administered fluids) until serum electrolyte results are available

Enemas every 6 hours
1. Warm water cleansing enemas
2. Retention enemas containing povidone-iodine (10%), neomycin sulfate (22 mg/kg), or lactulose (3 parts lactulose to 7 parts water at 20 ml/kg); instill into colon with aid of Foley catheter; leave in place for 15-20 min

Other
1. Flumazenil (0.02 mg/kg IV; efficacy unproven)
2. Branched-chain amino acid solutions
3. L-dopa
4. Ion exchange resins

**Chronic**

Protein-restricted diet (commercial or homemade)
Lactulose (cats: 2.5-5 ml PO q8h; dogs: 2.5-15 ml PO q8h)
Antibiotics
1. Metronidazole (7.5 mg/kg PO q12h)
2. Amoxicillin (22 mg/kg PO q12h)
3. Neomycin sulfate (20 mg/kg PO q8h)

a dry matter basis: about 20% for dogs, 30% to 35% for cats; or 2 [dogs] to 4 [cats] g/kg body weight/day) must be provided to curb endogenous protein catabolism and maintain muscle mass and body weight.

Some cats and dogs with chronic HE refuse a commercial or home-cooked protein-restricted diet. Feeding smaller meals frequently, adding seasoning such as garlic powder, warming the food, and providing positive reinforcement (e.g., a soothing voice, petting, interactive hand-feeding) may encourage voluntary intake of modified diets. Gradually mixing the new diet in with the animal's former regular diet over the course of 1 week may also result in acceptance of the new diet. If these measures fail and there is no evidence of another complication of hepatic failure (e.g., subclinical gastrointestinal ulceration) or other unrelated health problem, then two choices remain: continue to give the previous diet and rely more heavily on medical measures to control HE (i.e., antibiotics, increasing dosages of lactulose) or provide forced nutrition. Placing a feeding tube or initiating total parenteral nutrition is an aggressive step that should be reserved for animals that are likely to survive short-term and improve and that just need additional time. Tube esophagostomy is the

preferred approach; tube gastrostomy placed percutaneously is contraindicated in cats or dogs with ascites but would be acceptable if placed surgically (see Chapters 30 [dogs] and 37 [cats] for details).

**Lactulose.** The beneficial effects of the semisynthetic disaccharide lactulose (2.5 to 5 ml [cats] or 2.5 to 15 ml [dogs] PO q8h) in controlling HE are acidification of intestinal contents to trap ammonium and discourage formation of ammonia, and promotion of osmotic diarrhea. In addition, because lactulose is a carbohydrate, it provides a nonprotein substrate for bacteria, which diminishes generation of ammonia. The dose is adjusted until there are two to three soft stools per day; overdosing results in watery diarrhea. There are no known complications of chronic lactulose use in animals. Lactulose can also be given by enema in animals with acute HE (see below). Many cats and dogs object strongly to the sweet taste of lactulose; an attractive alternative is lactitol, which is a relative of lactulose. Used as a powder (500 mg/kg/day in three to four doses, adjusted to produce two to three soft stools daily) in controlled studies of human patients with chronic HE in Europe, lactitol was better tolerated than lactulose and at least as effective. Currently lactitol is available in the United States as a food sweetener, but it has not been studied in dogs and cats with HE.

**Antibiotic treatment.** If dietary therapy alone or in combination with lactulose is insufficient to control signs of HE, other medications may be added. Antibacterial drugs that are effective for anaerobic organisms (metronidazole, 7.5 mg/kg PO q8-12h; amoxicillin, 22 mg/kg PO q12h) and for gram-negative, urea-splitting organisms (neomycin sulfate, 20 mg/kg PO q12h) are preferable. There are few adverse effects of long-term use of neomycin, although nephrotoxicity and malabsorption have been observed rarely. The lowered dosage of metronidazole is given to avert neurotoxicity as a potential adverse effect of delayed hepatic excretion.

**Controlling precipitating factors.** Certain conditions, listed in order of frequency, are well known to accentuate or precipitate HE and should be avoided or treated aggressively when detected (Table 39-2).

## ACUTE HEPATIC ENCEPHALOPATHY

### Treatment

Acute HE is a true medical emergency. The same principles as those for management of chronic HE apply, but the steps are more aggressive (see Table 39-1). Nothing by mouth (NPO), administration of enemas, and intravenous fluid therapy constitute the basic therapeutic approach. Warm water cleansing enemas may be useful simply to remove colonic contents and prevent absorption of intestinal encephalotoxins. Povidone-iodine (10%) or neomycin sulfate liquid (20 mg/kg) may be added to decrease bacterial numbers. The most effective enema contains three parts lactulose to seven parts water at a total dose of 20 ml/kg. The solution is left in place, with the aid of a Foley catheter, as a retention enema for 15 to 20 minutes. For lactulose to be beneficial, the pH of the evacuated colon contents must be 6 or lower. These enemas can be given

TABLE 39-2

**Conditions that May Accentuate or Precipitate Hepatic Encephalopathy**

**Increased Generation of Ammonia in the Intestine**

High-protein diet (especially red meat)
Gastrointestinal hemorrhage
Azotemia (increased enterohepatic recirculation of urea)
Constipation
Infection (increased tissue catabolism and endogenous nitrogen load, decreased BCAA:AAA ratio)

**Movement of Ammonia Intracellularly in the Brain**

Metabolic alkalosis (favors formation of readily diffusible form of the ammonia molecule: $NH_3 + H^+ \leftrightarrow NH^{4+}$)
Hypokalemia (increased renal ammonia production)

**Excess Tranquilization**

Direct depressant action by heightened brain receptor sensitivity

**Use of Methionine-Containing Compounds**

Urinary acidifiers, "lipotrophic agents" (are converted to mercaptans)

**Use of Stored Blood for Transfusion**

High ammonia content

*BCAA,* Branched-chain amino acid; *AAA,* aromatic amino acid.

every 4 to 6 hours. Because lactulose is osmotically active, dehydration can occur if enemas are used too aggressively without careful attention to fluid intake. Fluids chosen for replacement of losses, volume expansion, and maintenance should not contain lactate, which is converted to bicarbonate, because alkalinizing solutions may precipitate or worsen HE by promoting formation of the more readily diffusible form of ammonia. Half-strength (0.45%) saline solution in 2.5% dextrose is a good empirical choice, with potassium added according to its serum concentration (see Table 55-2). Serum electrolyte values of dogs with HE are extremely variable; until serum electrolyte concentrations have been determined, 20 mEq KCl/L of administered fluids is a safe amount to add.

Because excess numbers of endogenous benzodiazepine (EBZ) receptors have been found in the brains of experimental animals and human patients with acute hepatic failure, use of EBZ receptor antagonists (e.g., flumazenil) has been explored clinically in human patients with refractory acute HE. Flumazenil has been studied only clinically in animals for its ability to reverse the action of benzodiazepine tranquilizers; 0.01 mg/kg administered intravenously successfully reversed the sedative effects of diazepam in dogs. Anecdotal experience in a small number of animals with severe HE at several institutions indicates that the product is safe and can rapidly and dramatically improve neurologic sta-

tus in some animals when given once intravenously at a dosage of 0.02 mg/kg; use of repeated injections has not been described. Two studies measured EBZ concentrations in the blood (peripheral and portal) or cerebrospinal fluid (CSF) of dogs with naturally occurring or created portacaval shunt. Although EBZs were found in the blood, they were not found in the CSF, putting into question the role of these substances in the development of chronic HE in dogs with PSS.

Other therapeutic approaches, such as use of BCAAs, either as dietary supplements or as an intravenous infusion; L-dopa; and ion exchange resins have been investigated in a laboratory setting and used in human patients with HE. Although preliminary results in human patients are encouraging, a shortage of pharmacologic data and controlled clinical trials, as well as lack of availability, preclude confident recommendations for use of these medications in animals at this time.

## MASSIVE HEPATIC NECROSIS

A condition that could be a cause of acute HE is massive hepatic necrosis. Called *fulminant hepatic failure* in human patients, this rare but well-known syndrome was recently redefined as rapidly progressive (2 weeks) massive liver cell injury causing necrosis and loss of confluent hepatic parenchyma. The most common causes are viruses or drugs. Clinical experience suggests that an analogous syndrome probably occurs in animals (Fig. 39-1). Examples in companion animals include severe toxic hepatopathy that follows oral administration of carprofen or trimethoprim-sulfa to a susceptible dog or diazepam to a susceptible cat, massive accidental dose of acetaminophen to a cat, ingestion of cycad palm seeds or several *Amanita phalloides* mushrooms by a dog, or severe feline hepatic lipidosis. More commonly, similar clinical signs are observed in animals with acute decompensation of long-term, stable, chronic hepatobiliary disease and severe HE precipitated by one of several factors (see Table 39-2). The prognosis is guarded in either case (true acute hepatic failure or decompensated chronic hepatic failure), but if there is sufficient hepatic mass to regenerate, animals can recover and survive at least the first few days and possibly longer.

Clinical signs are attributable to HE, vasogenic cerebral edema, coagulopathy, and sepsis. Failure to respond to treatment for HE or rapid central nervous system (CNS) deterioration is suggestive of brain edema, for which mannitol (1 g/kg of 20% solution administered IV over 30 minutes; repeated every 4 hours if needed) and furosemide (1 to 2 mg/kg IV q8h for three doses) are given; glucocorticoids are not indicated. Several controlled trials of glucocorticoid therapy in human patients with fulminant hepatic failure failed to demonstrate advantages over placebo, and serious adverse effects were associated with its use. Other complications of hepatic failure that can compound the animal's condition (i.e., hypoglycemia [see Chapter 52], hypokalemia [see Chapter 55], and gastrointestinal hemorrhage [see p. 550]) should also be treated aggressively. Mechanical hyperventilation to create hypocapnia may also assist in decreasing intracranial pressure.

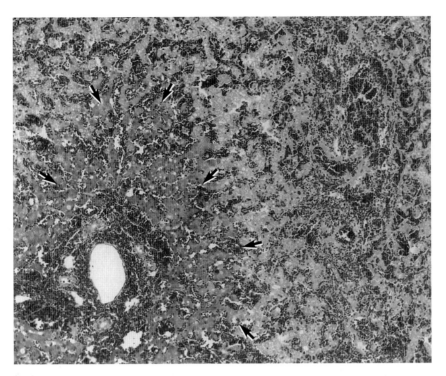

**FIG 39-1**
Photomicrograph of a liver specimen from a 2-year-old spayed female mixed-breed dog that died of acute hepatic necrosis believed to be associated with recent drug administration. Few viable hepatocytes surround a portal tract *(small arrows);* the pale, blood-filled spaces are dying hepatocytes (hematoxylin-eosin stain).

## ASCITES

### Pathogenesis

Accumulation of fluid in the peritoneal space as a result of sustained intrahepatic portal hypertension is common in dogs with chronic hepatic failure but is rarely seen in cats, except for some cats with lymphocytic cholangitis. Occasionally fluid collects in other third spaces such as the subcutaneous tissues or the pleural space; abdominal fluid travels to the pleural space, presumably through diaphragmatic lymphatic channels. The most important factors in the genesis of ascites in dogs with chronic hepatic failure are increased portal hydrostatic pressure and sodium-retaining mechanisms (e.g., secondary hyperaldosteronism, alterations in natriuretic factors, renal handling of sodium). Decreased plasma oncotic pressure from hypoalbuminemia associated with diminished hepatic synthesis, and to a lesser extent, from sequestration in abdominal fluid also contributes to the overall tendency to accumulate fluid.

### Treatment

Whether ascites is potentially dangerous for the dog with chronic liver failure, as is suspected in human patients with cirrhosis, is not known. Spontaneous bacterial peritonitis, a serious complication of cirrhosis in human patients, is rare in cirrhotic dogs. Treatment to control moderate to marked ascites is indicated if it is associated with respiratory embarrassment or anorexia because of a perceived sense of fullness.

**Diet.** A combination of dietary sodium restriction and diuretic therapy is usually needed to discourage sodium and fluid retention. The average sodium content in commercial diets for healthy dogs is approximately 0.3% to 0.4% (on a dry matter basis). Some protein-restricted commercial diets (Canine l/d, Hill's Pet Products, Topeka, Kan, 0.21% [canned or dry] sodium on a dry matter basis; Veterinary Diet NF-Formula, Ralston Purina Co., St. Louis, 0.24% [canned] and 0.22% [dry] sodium on a dry matter basis) and their home-cooked equivalents are also moderately reduced in sodium content but not as much as diets used in the management of congestive heart failure (e.g., Canine h/d, Hill's Pet Products, Topeka, Kan, 0.10% [canned] and 0.07% [dry] sodium on a dry matter basis; approximately 17% protein on a dry matter basis). The protein composition of the severely sodium-restricted diets is not optimal for control of HE, however.

**Diuretics.** If dietary sodium restriction alone is insufficient to control ascites after 5 to 7 days, diuretic therapy is added. The therapeutic aim is to achieve gradual diuresis that does not exceed the capacity to mobilize excess fluid; otherwise volume depletion will develop. Aldosterone antagonists such as spironolactone (beginning dose, 0.5 to 1 mg/kg PO q12h) are the agents of choice initially. The dose may be doubled for dogs that do not respond; these dogs probably have very high serum aldosterone activity. Potassium supplementation should not be given when higher doses of spironolactone are administered because the drug has potassium-sparing properties. If improvement is still not noted after 1 to 2 weeks at the higher spironolactone dose, a loop diuretic such as furosemide (1 mg/kg PO q12h initially) is added or substituted. Complications associated with well-intentioned but overzealous loop diuretic therapy, such as dehydration, azotemia, hypokalemia, and hyponatremia, are common and should be avoided. Measuring body weight (aim for about 0.5 kg for a 25 kg dog, or about 2% loss in body weight per day) combined with gradually decreasing abdominal girth is an objective means to assess the efficacy of diuretic therapy. Once ascites is under control, the dose of diuretic is reduced to the minimum necessary (daily or on alternate days) to keep the abdomen moderately diminished in size and pliable.

**Abdominocentesis.** For dogs that are refractory to dietary manipulation and pharmacologic diuresis, physical removal of fluid by abdominocentesis or with the aid of a shunt device containing a one-way valve (LeVeen or Denver shunt) can be accomplished. Serious consequences such as hypovolemia and renal failure have been reported in some human patients after rapid removal of large volumes of abdominal fluid. Similar complications have not been recorded in dogs with experimentally induced or spontaneously occurring chronic hepatic failure, but most clinicians prefer to avoid large-volume abdominocentesis in patients with a serum albumin concentration equal to or less than 2.0 g/dl. To slow reformation if removal of abdominal fluid is necessary (to provide symptomatic relief or in association with abdominal surgery), improvement in the plasma oncotic pressure is achieved temporarily by use of colloids such as hetastarch (20 ml/kg/day IV) or human albumin (12.5 g IV/20 kg lean body weight over 24 hours) around the time of fluid removal. Shunt devices that effectively transport ascitic fluid from a high intraabdominal pressure area to the low-pressure central venous system by use of tubing with a one-way valve are used in human patients with intractable ascites. Because of the high expense and complication rate of these devices and poor long-term prognosis for dogs with chronic hepatic failure, their application is limited.

## COAGULOPATHY/GASTROINTESTINAL HEMORRHAGE

### Pathogenesis

Aside from having a subclinical coagulopathy associated with altered synthesis and degradation of coagulation proteins from hepatocellular failure, as well as disseminated intravascular coagulopathy (DIC), dogs with chronic hepatic failure often have gastrointestinal bleeding. The frequency of gastrointestinal ulceration in dogs with various serious hepatobiliary diseases is high, although the pathogenesis is incompletely understood. Hypergastrinemia was reported in earlier studies of dogs with experimentally induced cirrhosis; it was thought that high peripheral blood bile acid concentrations stimulated excess gastrin secretion, but more recent investigations have not con-

firmed this finding. Unlike in human patients with cirrhosis who experience potentially life-threatening gastrointestinal hemorrhage from ruptured esophageal varices, gastrointestinal bleeding may occur in dogs with chronic hepatic failure as a result of a complex interaction involving mucosal hypoperfusion and enhanced release of gastric secretagogues. Whatever the underlying events, gastric acid–induced mucosal injury accounts for ulcer formation; the most common location is the duodenum.

### Clinical Features

Gastrointestinal hemorrhage can easily account for acute decompensation of a previously stable patient with chronic hepatic failure, because blood is an excellent protein source for bacterial generation of ammonia. Depending on the volume of blood lost, hypovolemia and azotemia, which also promote HE, can occur. Because the intestinal tract can hold a large volume of blood, and melena may not be seen for at least 24 hours, gastrointestinal hemorrhage should be suspected in any dog with chronic hepatic failure presented for signs of acute HE. Rectal examination may disclose evidence of melena in a dog that is anorectic and not defecating. Subclinical intestinal blood loss can be detected with a commercially available test that uses a fluorometric method for quantitative assay of fecal hemoglobin (Hemoquant, SmithKline Bioscience Laboratories, Van Nuys, Calif; normal fecal blood loss in dogs is 0.043 ml/kg/day). Vague cranial abdominal discomfort detected by abdominal palpation may indicate the presence of a gastrointestinal ulcer. Upper gastrointestinal contrast studies, endoscopy and/or ultrasonography may be needed for confirmation.

### Treatment

Treatment for gastrointestinal hemorrhage not caused by DIC consists of antiulcer medications. Until the ideal regimen is known, one of the $H_2$-receptor antagonists, ranitidine (2 mg/kg PO or IV q8h), or famotidine (0.5 mg/kg PO q12-24h) is usually combined with sucralfate (1 g/25 kg PO q6-8h). A more potent gastric acid inhibitor, omeprazole (0.7 mg/kg PO q24h), may be of benefit to dogs nonresponsive to $H_2$ receptor antagonists. If blood transfusion is needed, fresh whole blood or fresh packed red blood cells (RBCs) are used; stored RBCs elaborate ammonia, which could precipitate or worsen HE. Use of drugs that could cause gastrointestinal hemorrhage, such as corticosteroids or nonsteroidal antiinflammatory agents, should be avoided.

Coagulopathy from DIC in dogs with chronic hepatic failure is managed with heparin therapy if sufficient plasma antithrombin (AT) activity is present (>40%; see Chapter 89). It might be difficult to distinguish severe hepatic failure from DIC on the basis of plasma AT activity because values in each disease state can overlap considerably (hepatic failure: 30.8% ± 10.8%; DIC: 34.8% ± 20%; normal = 80% to 120%; Green, 1988). Because plasma AT activity may be low in both conditions, fresh whole blood or plasma transfusion with one dose of heparin (50 to 200 IU/kg) added to the unit of blood component is recommended. The dose of heparin given subcutaneously for maintenance may need to be lowered in some dogs with chronic hepatic failure if heparin degradation is compromised; this situation has been observed in isolated cases. Impaired heparin degradation is suspected if the activated partial thromboplastin time is excessively prolonged ($>1.5 \times$ normal) 2 hours after injection of a recommended dose; each subsequent dose is reduced by 20% until the target 2-hour postinjection activated partial thromboplastin time is reached ($1.5 \times$ normal).

## SEPSIS

The liver is an important site of removal of bacteria from the blood. Human patients with serious chronic hepatocellular disease have a high frequency of bacteremia arising from infection in various tissues (e.g., skin, lung, urinary tract, intestine). It was once thought that gram-negative organisms originating in the intestinal tract, especially accompanied by evidence of gastrointestinal hemorrhage, were the most common isolates. More recent studies of human patients have also implicated gram-positive bacteria from a number of non-digestive-tract sources. In such patients, hepatic mononuclear-phagocytic system phagocytosis is decreased, neutrophil function is abnormal, and serum bactericidal and opsonic activities are defective. Evidence of bacteria or endotoxin in the peripheral or portal blood or monocyte-macrophage dysfunction has not been convincingly demonstrated in dogs with congenital PSS or severe, induced hepatic disease and acquired PSS.

Similar investigations of the immunocompetency of dogs with chronic hepatocellular disease have not been carried out. It is reasonable to suggest that these animals are more susceptible to infection and that their owners should watch for this complication. If there are clinical signs or clinicopathologic findings compatible with sepsis (e.g., fever, leukocytosis with a left shift, and toxic neutrophils), specimens for anaerobic and aerobic bacterial culture should be collected. Blood is obtained for culture and sensitivity testing unless there is an obvious source of infection evident from diagnostic test results, such as a urinary tract infection, pyoderma, or pneumonia. In such cases samples of urine, skin lesions, or tracheal wash fluid are collected. Treatment with an antibiotic or a combination of antibiotics with broad-spectrum bactericidal activity and minimal nephrotoxicity is instituted until results are available. Amikacin (10 mg/kg IV, IM, or SQ q8h) combined with ampicillin or cefazolin (22 mg/kg IV q8h) is a good initial choice.

## Suggested Readings

Aronson LR et al: Endogenous benzodiazepine activity in the peripheral and portal blood of dogs with congenital portosystemic shunts, *Vet Surg* 26:189, 1997.

Grauer GF et al: Ascites, renal abnormalities, and electrolyte and acid-base disorders associated with liver disease, *Vet Clin North Am Small Anim Pract* 15:197, 1985.

Green RA: Pathophysiology of antithrombin III deficiency, *Vet Clin North Am Small Anim Pract* 18:95, 1988.

Hess PR et al: Management of portal hypertension and its consequences, *Vet Clin North Am Small Anim Pract* 25:461, 1995.

Howe LM et al: Endotoxemia associated with experimentally induced multiple portosystemic shunts, *Am J Vet Res* 58:83, 1997.

Howe LM et al: Detection of portal blood and systemic bacteremia in dogs with severe induced hepatic disease and multiple portosystemic shunts, *Am J Vet Res* 60:181, 1999.

Koblik PD et al: Technetium 99m sulfur colloid scintigraphy to evaluate reticuloendothelial system function in dogs with portosystemic shunts, *J Vet Intern Med* 9:374, 1995.

LaFlamme DP: Nutritional management of liver disease. In Bonagura JD et al, editors: *Kirk's current veterinary therapy XIII*, Philadelphia, 2000, WB Saunders, p 693.

Lemke KA et al: Ability of flumazenil, butorphanol, and naloxone to reverse the anesthetic effects of oxymorphone-diazepam in dogs, *J Am Vet Med Assoc* 209:776, 1996.

Meyer HP et al: No benzodiazepine activity in cerebrospinal fluid of dogs with chronic hepatic encephalopathy, *Proceedings of the 16th ACVIM Forum*, San Diego, 1998, p 705.

Papich MG: Antiulcer therapy, *Vet Clin North Am Small Anim Pract* 23:497, 1993.

Peterson SL et al: Endotoxin concentrations measured by a chromogenic assay in portal and peripheral venous blood in ten dogs with portosystemic shunts, *J Vet Intern Med* 5:71, 1991.

Stanton ME et al: Gastroduodenal ulceration in dogs: retrospective study of 43 cases and literature review, *J Vet Intern Med* 3:238, 1989.

Swalec Tobias KM et al: Evaluation of leukocytosis, bacteremia, and portal vein partial oxygen tension in clinically normal dogs and dogs with portosystemic shunts, *J Am Vet Med Assoc* 211:715, 1997.

Taboada J et al: Hepatic encephalopathy: clinical signs, pathogenesis, and treatment, *Vet Clin North Am Small Anim Pract* 25:337, 1995.

# C H A P T E R 40

# The Exocrine Pancreas

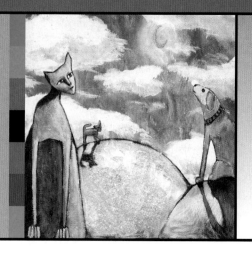

## CHAPTER OUTLINE

GENERAL CONSIDERATIONS, 552
ACUTE PANCREATITIS, 552
FELINE ACUTE PANCREATITIS—COMPARATIVE
ASPECTS, 560
RELAPSING AND CHRONIC PANCREATITIS, 560
EXOCRINE PANCREATIC INSUFFICIENCY, 560
EXOCRINE PANCREATIC NEOPLASIA, 564

## GENERAL CONSIDERATIONS

The major function of the exocrine pancreas is to secrete digestive enzymes and other substances that facilitate absorption of dietary nutrients and certain vitamins and minerals (Table 40-1). Clinical signs of pancreatic diseases, as they are known in cats and dogs, relate either to misplaced elaboration of activated digestive enzymes that results in tissue injury or to failure to secrete satisfactory amounts of digestive enzymes to maintain nutrient homeostasis. Because the clinical signs associated with these diseases are nonspecific (e.g., vomiting, diarrhea, polyphagia, weight loss), their pathophysiologies are discussed as they pertain to each specific pancreatic disease (Table 40-2).

## ACUTE PANCREATITIS

### Pathogenesis

The major digestive enzymes exist in pancreatic acinar cells in inactive forms (zymogens). After release into the intestinal lumen, they undergo peptide cleavage by enterokinase (also known as enteropeptidase; secreted by duodenal mucosal cells) on trypsinogen and by trypsin on other zymogens, which renders them able to initiate nutrient assimilation. Normally, a network of defense mechanisms prevents activity of these digestive enzymes on pancreatic tissue. That digestive enzymes exist as inactive precursors is of primary importance in averting autodigestion. Physical separation by packaging of zymogens in membrane-bound granules within acinar cells,

together with the distance between the site of enterokinase release and zymogens, prevents premature enzyme activation. The presence of enzyme inhibitors within the pancreas (pancreatic secretory trypsin inhibitor, $\alpha_1$-antitrypsin) and in the circulation ($\alpha_1$-antitrypsin, $\alpha_2$-macroglobulins) also inhibits inadvertent enzyme activation. Muscular sphincters in the pancreatic ducts block reflux of duodenal contents, which has been shown experimentally to incite pancreatic injury.

The event that initiates intrapancreatic enzyme activation is conversion of trypsinogen to trypsin. Several factors leading to trypsin activation have been elucidated in experimental canine and feline models of pancreatitis and are suspected to occur in the clinical setting. Pancreatitis induced experimentally by hyperstimulation with certain chemicals or by use of specific diets (high in methionine, low in choline) seems to more closely resemble the natural disease than other models. In these models it has been shown that, for an undetermined reason, zymogen granules fuse with protease-containing lysosomes, activating trypsinogen. From there, other digestive enzymes become activated and cause increases in capillary permeability and other direct pancreatic injury, as well as initiation of the vasoactive amine cascade. Trypsin, phospholipase A, elastase, lipase, and colipase are responsible for vascular injury and necrosis. Pancreatic inflammation can extend locally to the stomach, duodenum, and colon. Vasoactive polypeptides released into the systemic circulation from the inflamed pancreas cause the many systemic effects commonly associated with severe pancreatitis (i.e., hepatocellular necrosis, pulmonary edema, renal tubular degeneration, cardiomyopathy, hypotension, disseminated intravascular coagulopathy [DIC]). Severity of pancreatitis is the greatest when endogenous protease inhibitors have been consumed and pancreatic perfusion is poor.

Several factors have been implicated in the spontaneous development of acute pancreatitis (Table 40-3), which is more common in dogs than in cats. It is likely that more than one factor is involved.

### Clinical Features

Typically, middle-aged or older dogs of Terrier or nonsporting breeds, and domestic short-haired cats are affected with

TABLE 40-1

**Major Proteins and Other Substances Secreted by or Found in the Exocrine Pancreas**

| Digestive Enzymes (as Zymogens) | Digestive Enzymes (Intact) | Other |
|---|---|---|
| Trypsinogen | α-Amylase | Bicarbonate |
| Chymotrypsinogen | Lipase | Antibacterial factors |
| Proelastase | | Pancreatic secretory trypsin inhibitor |
| Procarboxypeptidases A and B | | $\alpha_1$-Antitrypsin |
| Procolipase | | |
| Prophospholipase A | | |

 TABLE 40-2

**Diseases of the Exocrine Pancreas**

| | | PRIMARY | SECONDARY |
|---|---|---|---|
| Common | Cat | Nodular hyperplasia (incidental finding in old cats) | Chronic pancreatitis (cholangitis, inflammatory bowel disease) |
| | Dog | Acute pancreatitis<br>Nodular hyperplasia (incidental finding in old dogs) | Acute pancreatitis (trauma: automobile accident, surgical; ischemia; hypercortisolism?; hyperlipoproteinemia; drugs) |
| Less common | Cat | Acute pancreatitis<br>Subclinical chronic pancreatitis | Acute pancreatitis (trauma; acute toxoplasmosis) |
| | Dog | Exocrine pancreatic insufficiency<br>Relapsing or chronic pancreatitis | Exocrine pancreatic insufficiency (protein/calorie malnutrition; duodenal hyperacidity; acute, severe or chronic, relapsing pancreatitis)<br>Chronic pancreatitis (diabetes mellitus; idiopathic hyperlipoproteinemia; hypercortisolism? |
| Rare | Cat | Exocrine pancreatic insufficiency<br>Pancreatic flukes (*Eurytrema procyonis*)<br>Pancreatic adenocarcinoma | Chronic pancreatitis (feline infectious peritonitis; toxoplasmosis) |
| | Dog | Pancreatic adenocarcinoma | Exocrine pancreatic insufficiency (pancreatic adenocarcinoma) |

 TABLE 40-3

**Factors Believed to be Involved in the Development of Acute Pancreatitis***

**Nutrition**

Obesity
High-fat diet

**Ischemia**

Hypovolemia
Vasoactive amine-induced vasoconstriction
Associated with DIC

**Hyperlipoproteinemia**

After ingestion of a large fatty meal
Idiopathic form in Miniature Schnauzers

**Drugs**

L-Asparaginase?
Azathioprine?

**Drugs—cont'd**

Other chemotherapeutic agents
Organophosphates
Corticosteroids (controversial)

**Duodenal Reflux**

Increased intraluminal pressure during severe vomiting

**Other**

Abdominal trauma
Hypercalcemia
Cholangitis (cats)
Infection (toxoplasmosis, feline infectious peritonitis)
Hyperadrenocorticism?

*DIC,* Disseminated intravascular coagulation.
*Uncommon in cats.

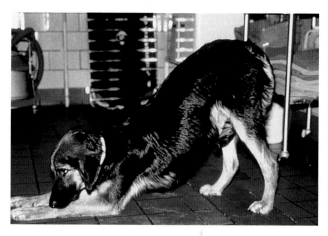

**FIG 40-1**
Dog exhibiting evidence of cranial abdominal pain by assuming the "position of relief." (Courtesy Dr. William E. Hornbuckle, Cornell University, College of Veterinary Medicine.)

acute pancreatitis. There is no gender predilection; neutered cats and dogs are predisposed. Regardless of breed or gender, most dogs affected by idiopathic acute pancreatitis are overweight. The history in dogs often includes recent ingestion of a large fatty meal. Drug history and evidence for intercurrent disease should be recorded during history taking.

Typical signs and physical examination findings are variable according to the stage of illness at presentation and can range from anorexia and depression with vague abdominal pain (Fig. 40-1) in mildly affected dogs to severe acute vomiting, hemorrhagic diarrhea, shock, and even death in more severely affected animals (Table 40-4). On the basis of histopathologic changes, mild pancreatic inflammation is often classified as edematous or interstitial, whereas more severe inflammation is categorized as hemorrhagic, necrotizing, or suppurative. The clinical features of acute pancreatitis roughly coincide with this classification, although the natural disease is best represented by a spectrum with the two basic forms as the extremes. Complications (Table 40-5) are more likely to occur in patients with severe acute pancreatitis, and specific diagnostic testing is required to confirm their existence.

## Diagnosis

The basic diagnostic approach for a cat or dog suspected of having pancreatitis consists of laboratory analysis (i.e., complete blood count [CBC], serum biochemistry profile, serum amylase and lipase activities [dogs only], urinalysis) and survey abdominal radiographs. Abdominal ultrasonography offers more convincing support for the presence of pancreatitis in dogs, especially if survey radiographs are inconclusive (see Diagnostic imaging, below); the sensitivity of ultrasonography for pancreatitis in cats is very low. A broad-based evaluation is necessary because the clinical features of acute pancreatitis are indistinguishable from those of other intestinal and extraintestinal disorders (e.g., acute enteritis or gastroenteritis, intestinal foreign body, acute toxic enteropathy

or hepatopathy, sepsis, peritonitis, pyometra) that cause an acute condition in the abdomen, and there is no single test that is pathognomonic for pancreatitis. Given the anatomic relationship between the pancreas and the liver in the cat (see Fig. 37-9) and the recently described frequency of concurrent cholangitis, inflammatory bowel disease, and pancreatitis in cats, it is not surprising that pancreatitis has not been recognized as a clinical entity more often. This fact may be related to a lower index of suspicion because of nonspecific signs and insensitive methods of detection in cats with pancreatitis.

**Complete blood count.** Evidence of dehydration (high packed cell volume [PCV] and plasma protein content) and leukocytosis are common abnormalities on the CBC in dogs with pancreatitis; leukocytosis is an inconsistent finding in cats. A stress leukogram is seen in mild cases, with greater leukocytosis and a mild to severe left shift observed in more severe cases. Platelet numbers are usually adequate unless DIC is present. The plasma may be lipemic and icteric. Cats with pancreatitis often have moderate nonregenerative anemia.

**Serum biochemistry profile.** The most helpful components of a serum biochemistry profile are concentrations of blood urea nitrogen (BUN), creatinine, glucose, albumin, calcium, and total bilirubin, as well as hepatic enzyme activities (alkaline phosphatase [AP], alanine transaminase [ALT]). Prerenal azotemia is found in more than 50% of cats and dogs with acute pancreatitis and is attributable to volume contraction from vomiting, lack of fluid intake, and extravasation of fluid into third spaces (abdominal cavity, interstitial space) from vascular injury. Renal azotemia and acute renal failure are uncommon but serious complications of severe pancreatitis that may be related to vasoactive amine-induced vasoconstriction or protracted hypovolemia. Release of glucagon in excess of insulin from an inflamed pancreas results in modest hyperglycemia (200 to 250 mg/dl) in up to 65% of cats and dogs with pancreatitis; stress may also be a contributing factor in cats. Hypoalbuminemia can result from vascular and peritoneal leakage. Hypocalcemia (after correction for albumin concentration) is thought to occur secondary to an acute shift of calcium into soft tissues, such as muscle, through altered membrane integrity in dogs. Hormonal mechanisms involving thyrocalcitonin and abnormal parathyroid responsiveness may also be involved. Deposition of calcium in plaques of saponified fat plays less of a role in hypocalcemia than was once thought. Extension of the pancreatic inflammatory process to the liver occurs directly because of close proximity of the two organs and indirectly as the activated digestive enzymes travel to the liver via common lymphatic pathways. High serum AP (twofold to fifteenfold increase) and ALT (normal to tenfold increase) activities are frequent findings in cats and dogs with pancreatitis; moderate hyperbilirubinemia (twofold to fivefold increase) is seen in 30% to 40% of affected dogs. Cats are more often icteric at presentation (about 65%). Higher serum AP and ALT activities and serum bilirubin concentration are observed with interruption of bile flow through the common bile duct by adjacent pancreatic inflammation (i.e., EBDO).

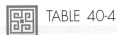

### TABLE 40-4

Presenting Clinical Signs and Physical Examination Findings in Dogs with Acute Pancreatitis

| MILD | MODERATE TO SEVERE |
|---|---|
| **Common Clinical Signs** | |
| Depression, anorexia, nausea (ptyalism, licking lips) | Depression, anorexia |
| Vomiting | Vomiting (possibly hematemesis) |
| Behavior indicating abdominal pain (position of relief) | Behavior indicating abdominal pain (position of relief) |
| **Other Clinical Signs** | |
| Diarrhea (can be large or small bowel) | Hematochezia/melena |
| | Jaundice |
| | Respiratory distress |
| | Shock |
| **Common Physical Examination Findings** | |
| Abdominal pain localized to the right cranial quadrant | Abdominal pain localized to the right cranial quadrant or generalized |
| Fever | Fever or hypothermia |
| Dehydration | Dehydration |
| | Hyperemic mucous membranes |
| | Tachycardia, tachypnea |
| **Other Physical Examination Findings** | |
| Weakness | Jaundice |
| | Abdominal effusion |
| | Mass effect in the region of the pancreas (inflamed pancreas with adhesions?) |
| | Petechiae or ecchymoses |
| | Cardiac arrhythmia |
| | Glossitis, glossal slough |

### TABLE 40-5

Complications of Severe Acute Pancreatitis in Dogs

| COMPLICATION | DIAGNOSTIC TEST(S) |
|---|---|
| **Medical** | |
| Cardiac arrhythmia (usually ventricular) | Lead II ECG, thoracic radiographs |
| DIC | Coagulation profile (OSPT, APTT, FDPs, fibrinogen concentration, platelet count), antithrombin III activity |
| Dyspnea (pleural effusion; pulmonary edema; pulmonary thromboembolism; pulmonary distress sydrome?) | Arterial blood gases, thoracic radiographs, radionuclide lung perfusion scan |
| Acute renal failure | Measurement of urine production, biochemical profile |
| Permanent diabetes mellitus | Hyperglycemia that persists beyond resolution of acute pancreatitis; measure serum insulin? |
| Nodular panniculitis | Biopsy |
| Sepsis | Blood cultures |
| **Surgical** | |
| Extrahepatic bile duct obstruction | Biochemical profile, coagulation profile, ultrasonography |
| Pancreatic abscess or pseudocyst | CBC, ultrasonography, aspiration for cytologic analysis and culture (ultrasound-guided or at surgery) |
| Intestinal obstruction (usually duodenal) | Abdominal radiographs and ultrasonography; upper gastrointestinal contrast study (if animal can tolerate barium orally) |

*ECG,* Electrocardiogram; *DIC,* disseminated intravascular coagulation; *OSPT,* one-stage prothrombin time; *APTT,* activated partial thromboplastin time; *FDPs,* fibrin degradation products; *CBC,* complete blood count.

Other serum biochemistry values may be abnormal but are even less specific. For example, hypercholesterolemia, with or without hypertriglyceridemia, is seen in cats and dogs with acute pancreatitis. However, fasting hyperlipidemia and persistent hyperglycemia in dogs other than Miniature Schnauzers with idiopathic hyperlipoproteinemia is highly suggestive of diabetes mellitus; the predominant change is hypertriglyceridemia. Electrolyte concentrations are useful in selecting the type of fluid to be administered and in determining the amount of potassium supplementation needed (see Tables 55-2 and 55-4); hypokalemia is common in cats.

**Serum amylase activity.** Serum total amylase activity is high in most dogs with pancreatitis (>80%); thus it could be considered a specific test for this disease. Similar to other serum enzyme activities, however, the value must be interpreted in light of its tissues of origin (primarily pancreas, also duodenal mucosa, with relatively smaller contributions by other regions of the digestive system and other nondigestive organs), mechanisms of serum activity increase, and means of enzyme elimination. Serum total amylase activity during health arises primarily from the pancreas and duodenal mucosa. The kidney is involved in clearance of serum enzyme in normal and pathologic states, so renal failure alone may cause high (2.5-fold to threefold increase) serum amylase activity. These factors make interpretation of serum amylase activity in a vomiting azotemic dog that much more difficult because severe duodenitis or a duodenal foreign body could cause an identical clinical picture. Separating the total serum amylase activity into organ-specific isoamylases improves the diagnostic accuracy of this test, especially in the 15% to 20% of dogs with pancreatitis that have normal total values. However, this test is not commercially available. Serum amylase activity is now considered an adequate screening test for pancreatitis in dogs (sensitivity about 62%, specificity about 57%; Mansfield and colleague, 2000) but is not a reliable indicator of pancreatic injury in cats.

**Serum lipase activity.** Lipase is said to have a more limited tissue distribution (primarily pancreas and gastric and duodenal mucosa) than amylase, and its serum activity has been promoted as a better test of accelerated release from the inflamed pancreas. Like amylase, lipase is eliminated by the kidney, and its activity can be high in dogs with azotemia (2.5-fold to threefold increase) and other extrapancreatic disorders. Glucocorticoid treatment (dexamethasone, prednisone) and manipulation of the pancreas during surgery can increase serum lipase activity (≥ threefold increase) in dogs without histopathologic changes in the pancreas, and high serum lipase activity has been associated with a variety of cancers and hepatobiliary diseases. Serum lipase activity in experimental canine models of acute pancreatitis roughly parallels that of serum amylase activity, although this is often not true for the natural disease. Many times one or the other is high, or both can be high or normal, and the magnitude of elevation does not correlate with the degree of pancreatic inflammation. Currently, serum lipase activity is considered an adequate screening test for pancreatitis in dogs (sensitivity about 73%, specificity about 55%; Mansfield and colleague,

2000). Serum lipase activity was high in one study of cats with experimental pancreatitis (Kitchell and colleagues, 1986) but is unreliable clinically.

**Urinalysis.** Urine for analysis should be obtained before fluids are administered to best assess the pathogenesis of azotemia. Other aspects of urinalysis that are valuable for establishing trends and comparing with serum values are glucose and bilirubin concentrations (i.e., no change, increasing, decreasing).

**Diagnostic imaging.** There are no pathognomonic radiographic signs of pancreatitis—only signs that are consistent with regional peritonitis. These signs include a ground-glass appearance in the right cranial quadrant of the abdomen; trapped gas pockets in the duodenum; and a mass effect of increased opacity in the area of the pancreas that displaces the duodenum laterally, widens the pyloroduodenal angle, and may delay gastric emptying (Fig. 40-2). Survey radiographs may be helpful in ruling out intestinal foreign body, which can cause vomiting, abdominal pain, high serum

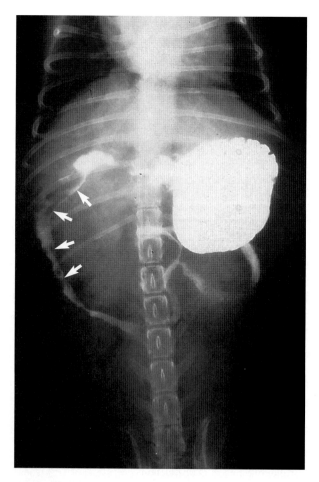

**FIG 40-2**
Ventrodorsal abdominal radiograph of a dog with acute pancreatitis. Contrast medium in the stomach and small intestine traces the path of the duodenum, which is displaced laterally. The duodenal lumen appears irregular, which is consistent with hypermotility.

amylase and lipase activities, and leukocytosis. Other disorders, such as severe duodenitis and duodenal ulcer, may cause radiographic changes similar to those of pancreatitis. These findings have not been described consistently in cats with pancreatitis.

As many as 50% of cats with pancreatitis have radiographically detectable fluid in body compartments. Of the cats that have evidence of fluid accumulation, most have serosanguineous fluid in both the pleural and abdominal cavities.

Ultrasonography is the preferred imaging technique for canine pancreatitis, yielding more specific information about the size, shape, and homogeneity of the pancreas than survey abdominal radiographs. The most consistent changes are a nonhomogeneous mass effect and hypoechogenicity in the area of the pancreas attributable to edema, hemorrhage, and inflammatory exudate (Fig. 40-3). There also may be evidence of hyperechoic peripancreatic fat and dilated bile ducts. Finding a more discrete homogeneous fluid-dense structure is compatible with abscess or pseudocyst formation, which are complications of severe pancreatitis. Similar changes are observed in some cats with pancreatitis.

**Other tests.** Acute pancreatitis is highly likely in a cat or dog with compatible signs and physical examination findings, leukocytosis, abnormal hepatic enzyme activities, and ultrasonographic evidence consistent with pancreatic inflammation, even if serum amylase and lipase activities are normal. Other tests are necessary if results are inconclusive. When abdominal effusion is present, abdominocentesis may furnish fluid for cytologic examination and specific biochemical analysis. Because acute pancreatitis is a type of chemical peritonitis, results of cytologic analysis are characteristically compatible with a nonseptic exudate. Amylase and lipase activities in the abdominal fluid are often higher than in the serum of dogs with pancreatitis, although severe duodenal inflammation or perforation may also yield the same result.

**Definitive tests.** Other diagnostic tests have been investigated in the search for a more specific, more sensitive, minimally invasive test for pancreatitis in cats and dogs. In addition to serum isoamylase separation, measurement of serum trypsinlike immunoreactivity (TLI), which is most often used for detection of exocrine pancreatic insufficiency (EPI; see p. 560), has been studied in experimentally created canine pancreatitis and has been of diagnostic benefit in about 50% of clinical cases in both cats and dogs. In such cases the value has been more than 100 $\mu$g/L in affected cats (reference range 12 to 82 $\mu$g/L) or more than 50 $\mu$g/L in affected dogs (reference range 5 to 35 $\mu$g/L), indicating inappropriate discharge of enzyme from the pancreas. The serum TLI value must be assessed in light of renal function because increases can occur with nonazotemic renal disease in dogs, but it appears to be a sensitive and clinically useful test in cats. Another accurate indicator of acute pancreatitis, low serum antiprotease ($\alpha_1$-antitrypsin, $\alpha_2$-macroglobulin) activities, has been documented in experimental canine pancreatitis models and carries therapeutic importance but is not available commercially. A highly sensitive and specific test for pancreatic injury, pancreatic lipase immunoreactivity (PLI), is available for dogs (cPLI, reference range 2.2 to 102.1 $\mu$g/L; http://www.cvm.

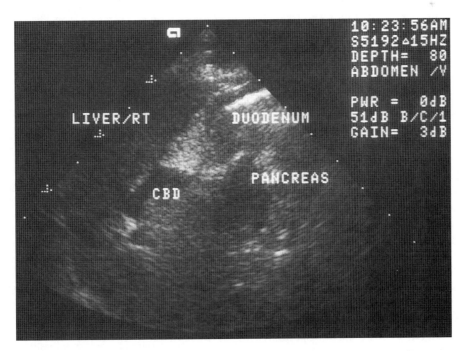

**FIG 40-3**
Abdominal ultrasonographic image of an enlarged, somewhat indistinct pancreas in a dog with acute pancreatitis. The common bile duct (CBD) is distended, and the duodenal wall is thickened.

tamu.edu/gilab/; Gastrointestinal Laboratory, Department of Small Animal Medicine & Surgery, College of Veterinary Medicine, Texas A&M University, College Station, TX 77843-4474, phone [979]862-2861, fax [979]862-2864, E-mail: gilab@cvm.tamu.edu) and will soon be available for cats. Currently, the drawback to routine use of all these tests is that they are offered only at certain laboratories; thus the results are not available rapidly enough to aid in immediate decision-making.

If the diagnosis is still elusive, exploratory laparotomy and pancreatic biopsy can be performed. Edema, hemorrhage, and plaques of peripancreatic fat necrosis are easily identifiable grossly as markers of pancreatic injury. Whether pancreatic biopsy causes pancreatitis is controversial. Manipulating a normal pancreas at surgery does not cause pancreatitis, but the trauma of obtaining a biopsy specimen from an already inflamed pancreas could exacerbate existing inflammation and further complicate the postoperative recovery of a cat or dog with pancreatitis.

## Treatment and Prognosis

Acute pancreatitis in cats and dogs should be considered a potentially devastating disease and should be treated aggressively. Goals of treatment include (1) removing the inciting cause if possible, (2) restoring and maintaining intravascular volume and pancreatic perfusion, (3) reducing pancreatic secretion, (4) relieving pain, (5) managing complications that delay complete recovery, and (6) providing nutritional support.

The backbones of treatment for mild or severe acute pancreatitis remain fluid therapy and nothing by mouth (NPO). Balanced electrolyte solutions are given in sufficient quantity to address dehydration and continuing losses and to meet maintenance needs during the period of NPO, which may be 48 to 72 hours or longer. Withholding food and water and administering all medications parenterally prevent gastric stimulation, which leads to pancreatic secretion. If possible, the sight and smell of food should be avoided because these also are factors in the initiation of pancreatic secretion.

**Treatment of mild pancreatitis.** For the mildly affected cat or dog that is minimally dehydrated and not azotemic, fluids may be given subcutaneously. At least 24 hours after the last episode of vomiting, small amounts of water and then bland food (low-salt meat baby food or low-fat cat or dog food [Feline w/d or Canine i/d; Hill's Pet Products, Topeka, Kan]) can be given four times daily. If water and food are tolerated without vomiting, the quantity of each may be gradually increased until the total daily requirements are being provided, usually over 5 or 6 days. No other medications (e.g., anticholinergics, antibiotics) are necessary. Recovery should be complete in about 7 days.

Overall prognosis for dogs with a single bout of mild pancreatitis is good. Dietary management using a diet low in fat, high in carbohydrates, and with a moderate level of protein (e.g., Canine i/d or w/d; Hill's Pet Products, Topeka, Kan) should be instituted indefinitely to prevent recurrence. Access to table scraps, food belonging to other pets in the household, and garbage should be strictly avoided. Cooked rice and cottage cheese may be added to prescription diets to encour-

age acceptance. Obese dogs should lose weight. Marked dietary fat restriction (Canine r/d; Hill's Pet Products, Topeka, Kan) may be required in dogs that have idiopathic hyperlipoproteinemia or that experience repeated confirmed bouts of pancreatitis.

**Treatment of severe pancreatitis.** The same principles of treatment apply to the more severely affected cat or dog (see Tables 40-4 and 40-5) but are more intensive (Table 40-6). Fluids should be given intravenously (IV), preferably with an indwelling catheter in a large-bore vein so that central venous pressure can be monitored. This monitoring of central venous pressure, along with measuring urine production, packed cell volume (PCV), plasma protein concentration, and body weight, ensures that fluid requirements are being met. Two of the most common mistakes in managing the care of a dog with acute severe pancreatitis are giving too few fluids (i.e., underhydration) and reinstituting oral feeding too soon.

A period of NPO of 5 days or longer may be necessary. If vomiting is protracted and not related to intestinal obstruction, central-acting antiemetics (chlorpromazine or prochlor-

## TABLE 40-6

**Summary of Treatment Recommendations for Dogs and Cats with Acute Pancreatitis***

### Mild Pancreatitis

NPO for 48 to 72 hours; provide fluids at rate to meet maintenance needs and replace ongoing losses using a balanced electrolyte solution by SQ or IV route

Give small amounts of water, then bland food (low-salt meat baby food or fat-restricted balanced pet food) four times daily beginning at least 24 hours after last episode of vomiting

If vomiting does not recur with feeding, gradually increase amount of food at each feeding until total daily requirements are being met in one or two feedings per day

Dogs susceptible to recurrent bouts of pancreatitis should receive a fat-restricted diet indefinitely, with no access to table scraps or garbage

### Severe Pancreatitis

NPO for at least 48 to 72 hours (if period of NPO exceeds 5 days, provide nutritional support by tube duodenostomy or jejunostomy or total parenteral nutrition)

Provide fluids to reverse dehydration, meet maintenance requirements, and replace ongoing losses using balanced electrolyte solution IV

Give fresh or fresh-frozen plasma to supply antiprotease activity

Administer broad-spectrum antibiotics parenterally

Use central-acting antiemetics if vomiting is profuse

Give analgesics for abdominal pain

Treat complications as they are detected (see Table 40-5)

*NPO,* Nothing by mouth; *SQ,* subcutaneous; *IV,* intravenous.
*More common in dogs than cats.

perazine), 0.25 to 0.5 mg/kg intramuscularly (IM) or subcutaneously (SQ) every 6 to 8 hours, may be given as long as intravascular volume is normal. Analgesics that cause few changes in pancreatic ducts or secretions are hydromorphone (0.03 to 0.05 mg/kg IM as needed) and butorphanol (0.055 to 0.11 mg/kg SQ q6-12h; dogs only). The total daily dose of each of these analgesics can also be given over 24 hours as a continuous IV infusion. Transfusion with fresh or fresh-frozen plasma has been shown to be beneficial in dogs with experimental acute pancreatitis by providing serum antiprotease activity, and it can be repeated if steady improvement is not seen.

Although bacteria do not play a primary role in canine acute pancreatitis, the necrotic pancreas is a good medium for bacterial growth. The frequency of pancreatic sepsis in dogs is not known, but the most common organisms retrieved from human patients are gram-negative bacteria (e.g., *Escherichia coli, Klebsiella pneumoniae*). In some dogs it may be difficult to differentiate severe pancreatitis from pancreatic or systemic gram-negative infection since clinical signs and hematologic changes (leukocytosis with a left shift and toxic neutrophil changes) are similar. In such cases cefotaxime (6 to 40 mg/kg IM or IV q6h) or trimethoprim-sulfamethoxazole (15 mg/kg IV q12h; must be diluted and given slowly in a central vein over 60 to 90 minutes) are good empiric choices because each penetrates the canine pancreas well. Enrofloxacin (2.5 to 5 mg IM or IV q12h) achieves good pancreatic concentrations and is effective against most pancreatic pathogens, so it also may be used in dogs. Other antibiotics traditionally recommended for gram-negative sepsis in dogs (e.g., amikacin and ampicillin or cephalothin) likely also reach therapeutic concentrations in the inflamed feline or canine pancreas. Insulin administration is not required for modest hyperglycemia unless ketosis develops or the hyperglycemia persists and steadily increases. If insulin is required, the regular formulation should be used every 6 hours at doses that maintain blood glucose concentration in the range of 150 to 200 mg/dl.

Other therapeutic approaches have been put forth for treatment of severe pancreatitis but are not of proven value. Some investigators advocate administration of heparin (50 to 75 IU/kg SQ q8-12h) to discourage thromboembolic tendencies, prevent DIC, and ensure pancreatic perfusion, but this approach has not been critically evaluated. Routine administration of corticosteroids is not recommended other than as emergency use for shock. Peritoneal lavage has been found to improve survival in dogs with experimentally created pancreatitis by removing toxic products and activated digestive enzymes. It has also been reported recently to be successful in preventing pancreatic sepsis that occurs after apparent recovery in human patients with severe acute pancreatitis, but because peritoneal lavage must be continued for 7 days, it may not be practical for most feline or canine patients.

In addition to PCV and plasma protein concentration, clinicopathologic tests that should be monitored daily include serum electrolytes and BUN or creatinine concentration. A CBC and complete biochemical profile should be performed every other day until favorable trends are established. If serum amylase and/or lipase activity is abnormal initially, this test can be repeated every other day.

IV fluid administration should be tapered and suspended and oral intake of food and water resumed only after vomiting has resolved. This may take 5 to 7 days or more. Hyperamylasemia/hyperlipasemia and high hepatic enzyme activities may persist for longer and, as long as they are approaching normal values, should not be the reason to continue to withhold food or keep an animal hospitalized. If vomiting recurs, a 24-hour period of NPO should be instituted. If the total time of NPO exceeds 5 days, total parenteral nutrition is instituted or a duodenal or jejunal feeding tube is placed surgically (see Chapter 37, p. 512). If a duodenal or jejunal feeding tube is placed, an elemental diet (Peptamen; Nestle Clinical Nutrition; or Feline or Canine CliniCare Liquid Diet; Abbott Laboratories, Deerfield, Ill [each contains 1 kcal/ml]) is fed via continuous infusion. The same plan for dietary management as that for mildly affected dogs should be followed after hospital discharge. Too little information exists to make recommendations for long-term management of cats with pancreatitis. Empirically, cats are managed in a similar fashion to dogs until results of studies dictate otherwise.

Complications (see Table 40-5) should be treated as they develop. Although there is no scheme devised for assignment of prognosis in dogs with severe acute pancreatitis, the greater the number of complications, the poorer the prognosis. Some complications (e.g., DIC, acute renal failure, cardiac arrhythmia) are managed medically. Common bile duct obstruction, from adjacent pancreatic edema and inflammation, is most commonly transient in cats and dogs with pancreatitis. Permanent bile duct obstruction that occurs after the acute phase of pancreatitis has resolved should be addressed surgically. Evidence for this includes progressive increases in serum AP and ALT activities, increasing hyperbilirubinemia, and ultrasonographic evidence of a dilated extrahepatic biliary tree. A recent review of 46 cats with acute pancreatitis concluded that cats with a plasma ionized calcium of 4 mg/dl or less must be assigned a grave prognosis (Kimmel and colleagues, 2001).

Three reports (Salisbury and colleagues, 1988; Edwards and colleagues, 1990; Hines and colleagues, 1996) described pancreatic masses (abscess, phlegmon, pseudocyst) in six dogs, seven dogs, and one cat, respectively, as a complication of severe acute pancreatitis. Surgical intervention 5 days to several weeks after the onset of illness from pancreatitis was required in all but one dog that recovered spontaneously; the cat and only three operated dogs survived. Reasons for surgical intervention and pancreatic debridement included (1) apparent recovery with relapse of signs or (2) persistent fever and leukocytosis with a left shift and toxic neutrophil changes beyond the time of expected recovery, along with physical examination, radiographic, or ultrasonographic evidence of a mass lesion in the area of the pancreas. Although each of these pancreatic mass lesions is usually sterile, specimens from the lesion should be obtained before surgery via ultrasound guidance if possible for bacterial culture and sensitivity testing. Surgery can be delayed or avoided in animals that have ultrasonographic findings of a mass lesion but are improving steadily with medical management. In such cases, ultrasound-guided drainage, which can be repeated if needed, is an acceptable alternative treatment.

## FELINE ACUTE PANCREATITIS— COMPARATIVE ASPECTS

The syndrome of pancreatitis as it is known in dogs occurs rarely in cats. In cats, pancreatitis is predominantly subclinical, occurring as a component of multisystemic disease, such as toxoplasmosis, or in association with inflammatory bowel disease. The same clinical signs and clinicopathologic features seen in dogs with acute pancreatitis have been noted in experimental models and in some of the reported natural cases of acute pancreatitis in cats, but they are more subtle. On the basis of pancreatic histopathologic changes, there appear to be at least two types of severe pancreatitis in cats (Hill and colleague, 1993): acute necrotizing (more common, similar to canine pancreatitis) and acute suppurative (less common). The acute suppurative form was seen more often in younger cats (mean age 3.5 years). Lethargy, anorexia, vomiting, dehydration, weight loss, jaundice, and hypothermia are typical presenting signs for cats with either form. Because the history and physical examination findings of cats with pancreatitis are nonspecific, antemortem diagnosis can be difficult. Similar diagnostic and treatment approaches to those for dogs with suspected pancreatitis are recommended for cats at this time, except for the duration of NPO. Because of the potential for hepatic lipidosis associated with a protracted period of NPO, institution of enteral tube feeding (i.e., via duodenostomy or jejunostomy) as soon as pancreatitis is diagnosed is recommended. Both forms of acute pancreatitis in cats are severe and may be difficult to recognize, so the prognosis for either type appears guarded at this time.

## RELAPSING AND CHRONIC PANCREATITIS

### Clinical Features and Diagnosis

Some cats and dogs appear to undergo repeated bouts of acute pancreatitis, with periods of recovery in between. Such cases could be considered to be relapsing pancreatitis.

Published information about chronic pancreatitis in dogs exists primarily in the contexts of experimental models and diabetes mellitus and in isolated case reports in which pancreatic involvement was incidental. Reports specifically describing chronic pancreatitis in dogs are lacking. About one third of the cats described as having acute necrotizing pancreatitis (Hill and colleague, 1993) also had histopathologic evidence of chronic pancreatitis, demonstrated by interstitial lymphoplasmacytic inflammation and fibrosis and acinar cell atrophy. Most cats with chronic pancreatitis are older domestic short-haired cats. Clinical signs in over 50% of affected cats include anorexia, weight loss, and intermittent vomiting. Results of physical examination are variable.

Diagnosis is made primarily by the combined findings of high serum TLI and characteristic microscopic features in pancreatic biopsy specimens, that is, interstitial mononuclear cell inflammation and fibrosis. Chronic pancreatitis can coexist with inflammatory hepatic and/or intestinal disease, all of which may have similar clinical signs. It is likely that chronic pancreatitis is identified infrequently in cats because the signs resemble those of inflammatory bowel disease and biopsy specimens are only obtained from the intestine.

Persistent, usually subclinical inflammation is believed to result in progressive loss of functional pancreatic tissue. After loss of about 85% of functional pancreatic tissue, EPI and diabetes mellitus may develop.

### Treatment and Prognosis

Relapsing pancreatitis and chronic pancreatitis are controlled primarily by strict nutritional management using a highly digestible diet with high fiber and limited fat content (see p. 558). With strict adherence to administration of a controlled diet, prognosis is good. Administration of pancreatic enzyme supplement is thought to relieve abdominal discomfort in human patients with chronic pancreatitis; this regimen seems worth a trial for the cat or dog with confirmed chronic pancreatitis. Administration of insulin and pancreatic enzyme supplements is clearly indicated for cats and dogs with undetected pancreatitis that has resulted in endocrine and exocrine insufficiency, respectively.

## EXOCRINE PANCREATIC INSUFFICIENCY

### Pathogenesis

Greater than 85% loss of pancreatic acinar ability to secrete digestive enzymes results in clinical signs of nutrient malassimilation. It was once thought that a single bout of severe acute pancreatitis or repeated bouts of less severe pancreatitis resulted in progressive loss of pancreatic acinar cell tissue. More recent studies indicate that this cause of EPI is uncommon and that heritable (in German Shepherd Dogs) or adult-onset (idiopathic, of any breed) pancreatic acinar atrophy is responsible for the majority of cases of canine EPI. The converse may be true of feline EPI; progressive destruction of acinar tissue associated with chronic, subclinical pancreatitis is suspected to be the most common cause, with occasional reported cases of pancreatic acinar cell atrophy.

Ingested nutrients are not biotransformed to absorbable forms in cats and dogs with EPI because of lack of intraluminal enzyme activity. Secondary changes in the intestinal mucosa are as important in the genesis of malassimilation; villous atrophy, inflammatory cell infiltrates, and alterations

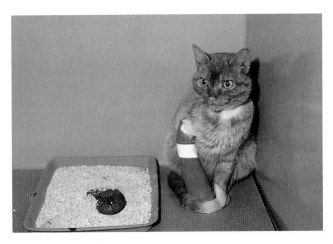

**FIG 40-4**
Four-year-old spayed female mixed-breed cat with exocrine pancreatic insufficiency (EPI). The cat was a strictly outdoor cat, so the owner did not complain of polyphagia or voluminous feces.

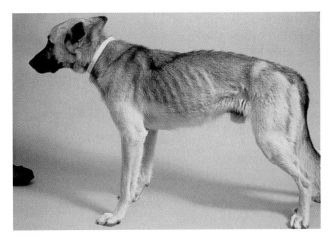

**FIG 40-5**
Physical appearance of a 2-year-old male German Shepherd Dog with exocrine pancreatic insufficiency (EPI). (Courtesy Dr. William E. Hornbuckle, Cornell University, College of Veterinary Medicine.)

in mucosal enzyme activity have all been identified in dogs with EPI. Multiple factors, including those of luminal, nutritional, and hormonal origin, are likely involved. Bacterial overgrowth is a common problem in dogs with EPI, perhaps because of absence of pancreatic secretions containing antibacterial properties, and it may account for many of the mucosal changes. In both experimentally induced and some naturally occurring cases of EPI, duodenal bacterial populations return to normal after pancreatic enzyme supplementation. Depending on the species of overgrown bacteria, changes of brush border enzyme activities, degrees of villous atrophy, and competition for ingested nutrients may occur. Malabsorption of cobalamin (vitamin $B_{12}$), perhaps related to bacterial overgrowth and other factors, and the fat-soluble vitamins A and E has been demonstrated in affected dogs, but there seem to be few clinical consequences. Almost all cats with EPI have vitamin $B_{12}$ deficiency from malabsorption. There is little information about the impact of EPI on vitamin K metabolism in cats and dogs. Vitamin K deficiency was reported in a cat with EPI; coagulopathy resolved with pancreatic enzyme supplementation.

## Clinical Features

Cats and dogs with EPI are typically presented by their owners for a chronic history of weight loss despite a vigorous, even ravenous, appetite. Owners may also describe pica and coprophagia. The character of the feces can be normal, soft and voluminous (Fig. 40-4), or watery. Affected German Shepherd Dogs are usually presented by 2 years of age (Fig. 40-5), whereas other breeds are usually middle-aged adults; there is no gender predilection. Rarely, affected animals may have prolonged bleeding after venipuncture because of severe malabsorption of fat-soluble vitamin K. There are few abnormal physical examination findings except for degrees of weight loss, poor-quality hair coat, and possibly oily staining

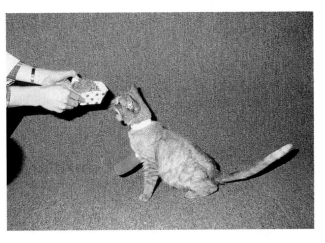

**FIG 40-6**
Four-year-old spayed female mixed-breed cat with exocrine pancreatic insufficiency (EPI) depicted in Fig. 40-4: alert, active, and hungry. (Courtesy Dr. P. Jane Armstrong, University of Minnesota, College of Veterinary Medicine.)

of the perineal region because of steatorrhea. Affected animals are bright, alert, and hungry (Fig. 40-6).

## Diagnosis

Results of standard clinicopathologic testing (CBC, chemistry profile, urinalysis) are usually normal. Some dogs have high serum ALT activity (twofold to threefold increase) because of disrupted small intestinal barriers and resultant hepatic inflammation, and many have hypocholesterolemia. At this point, results of history, physical examination, and diagnostic testing cannot differentiate primary small intestinal disease with malabsorption from EPI. Two screening tests, triglyceride challenge test and qualitative fecal analysis for the presence of trypsin activity and undigested food particles, can be

TABLE 40-7

## Screening Tests for Diagnosis of Exocrine Pancreatic Insufficiency

### Triglyceride Challenge Test

1. After a 12-hour fast, obtain serum sample, then give corn oil, 3 to 4 ml/kg PO
2. Measure serum triglyceride concentration at 0, 2, and 3 hours after corn oil (Fig. 40-7)
   a. Normal: twofold to threefold increase over baseline value in post–corn oil samples
   b. Abnormal: no change from baseline value in post–corn oil samples
3. If abnormal, repeat test the following day but add 2 tsp of pancreatic enzyme powder (Viokase-V) to dose of corn oil
   a. Pancreatic enzyme–responsive: twofold to threefold increase in serum triglyceride concentration over baseline value
   b. Not pancreatic enzyme–responsive: no change in serum triglyceride concentrations in post–corn oil serum samples; consider primary small intestinal disease (see Part 3: Digestive System Disorders)

### Qualitative Fecal Analysis

1. Fecal proteolytic (trypsin) activity
   a. Mix 1 ml of feces with 9 ml of 5% sodium bicarbonate; incubate with tubes of gelatin for 30 to 60 minutes at 37° C; perform test at least three times on each patient
   b. Normal: gelatin dissolves if trypsin is present and there are few intact striated muscle fibers seen on Wright's stained fresh fecal smears
2. Fecal amylase activity
   a. Stain fresh fecal smears with 2% Lugol's iodine solution
   b. Normal: few starch granules (blue-black in color) are present
3. Fecal lipase activity
   a. Stain fresh fecal smears with Sudan III
   b. Normal: few fat globules (red-orange in color) are present

*PO*, By mouth.

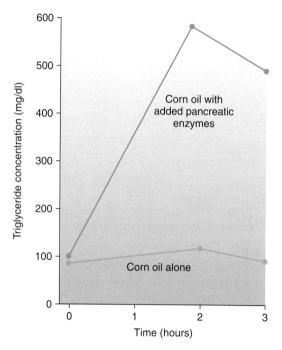

**FIG 40-7**
Results of triglyceride challenge in a 10-year-old spayed female English Springer Spaniel with EPI; serum trypsinlike immunoreactivity (TLI), 0.3 μg/L.

used to arrive at a presumptive diagnosis (Table 40-7). The triglyceride challenge test operates on the principle that dogs with EPI or primary small intestinal disease may have fat malabsorption and that the post–corn oil serum triglyceride concentrations will be similar to the fasting value in such cases. When the test is repeated with pancreatic enzyme powder (Viokase-V) added to the corn oil and the post–corn oil serum triglyceride concentrations rise at least twofold over baseline, a tentative diagnosis of EPI can be made (Fig. 40-7). These results alone, however, are not conclusive evidence for EPI because there can be both false-negative and false-positive results.

Qualitative assessment of fecal trypsin activity (see Table 40-7) is also subject to differences in technique, interpreta-

tion, and daily variation. Microscopic examination for evidence of intact striated muscle fibers, starch granules, and fat globules in feces is an imprecise, subjective diagnostic test for EPI but lends supportive information. If triglyceride malabsorption, persistent absence of trypsin activity measured serially in fresh fecal specimens, and repeated evidence of unprocessed nutrients in the feces by special staining techniques are present, a stronger case for EPI can be made, and specific treatment can be instituted while awaiting the results of definitive tests.

Now that assays have been validated for both species, the definitive test for EPI in cats and dogs is to measure serum TLI. Serum TLI measurement is not affected by feeding in healthy cats, but ideally the serum sample is collected after a 12-hour fast. TLI in serum reflects release of trypsinogen from pancreatic acinar cells, so subnormal values indicate inadequate pancreatic exocrine secretion. Normal values for dogs are 5 to 35 μg/L; values less than 2 μg/L are diagnostic of EPI, with the equivocal or nondiagnostic zone 2 to 5 μg/L. The normal range for serum TLI in cats is 12 to 82 μg/L; values less than 8 μg/L are consistent with a diagnosis of EPI, and values between 8 and 12 μg/L are equivocal. Protein content in the diet fed at the time the sample is collected may positively influence the serum TLI value (i.e., the higher or lower the protein content of the diet, the higher or lower the serum TLI value, respectively, presumably as a result of pancreatic adaptation). Despite the relationship between protein content of the diet and serum TLI, however, dogs with normal pancreatic function fed diets severely restricted in protein still have serum TLI values within the reference range.

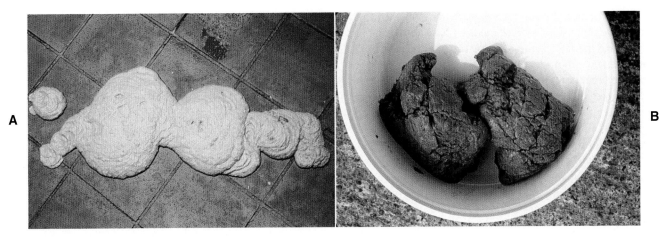

**FIG 40-8**
Appearance of feces from a dog with exocrine pancreatic insufficiency (EPI). **A,** Before and, **B,** after pancreatic enzyme supplementation. (Courtesy Dr. William E. Hornbuckle, Cornell University, College of Veterinary Medicine.)

Because there is no appreciable absorption of pancreatic proteases from the intestine, serum TLI can be determined accurately, even if pancreatic enzyme supplementation has been started.

Both assays for serum TLI are performed by the Gastrointestinal Laboratory, Department of Small Animal Medicine & Surgery, College of Veterinary Medicine, Texas A&M University, College Station, TX 77843-4474, phone (979)862-2861, fax (979)862-2864, E-mail: gilab@cvm.tamu.edu, http://www.cvm.tamu.edu/gilab/. Canine serum TLI assays can also be requested through certain reference laboratories that use a commercial kit (Canine TLI Radioimmunoassay; Diagnostic Products Corp., Los Angeles, Calif). Measuring serum TLI in cats and dogs has replaced other tests such as the N-benzoyl-L-tyrosyl-p-aminobenzoic acid (BT:PABA) absorption test, quantitative fecal proteolytic enzyme activity, and fecal fat quantitation because it is simple, specific, and sensitive. Pancreatic ductular obstruction is suspected in animals that have clinical findings consistent with EPI, normal triglyceride absorption when pancreatic enzyme powder is added to corn oil during the triglyceride challenge test, and a normal serum TLI value, and in which primary small intestinal disease has been ruled out. A specific clinically relevant example of this in cats is pancreatic fluke infestation (*Eurytrema procyonis*). If initial testing yields serum TLI values in the equivocal range, treating presumptively for EPI and repeating the test 1 to 2 months later are recommended.

Serum cobalamin (vitamin $B_{12}$) concentration is low in almost all cats and many dogs with EPI. This low value may be related to several factors including consumption by overgrown bacterial populations and lack of release of intrinsic factor from the pancreas, which binds with $B_{12}$ for ileal absorption.

## Treatment and Prognosis

The goals of therapy are to replace intraluminal pancreatic enzyme activity and to reverse nutritional imbalances. Several products are available in both powder and tablet formulation. Powder is preferred because of its higher enzyme concentration; 1 teaspoon contains six times the enzyme activity of one tablet. Most cats and dogs can be managed by adding 1 teaspoon (for a cat) to 2 teaspoons (for a 20-kg dog) of pancreatic enzyme powder (Viokase-V) or finely crushed nonenteric-coated tablets to each of two meals of balanced feline or canine ration. Some dogs, especially large-breed dogs, may need up to 2 teaspoons per meal, but more than that is not advantageous. It is not necessary to incubate the enzyme preparation with the ration before feeding. The feces should improve in appearance and volume immediately (Fig. 40-8), and the animal should steadily gain weight. The feeding regimen should be tailored to the individual animal to maintain optimal body weight. For cats and dogs that prefer a dry ration, the pancreatic enzyme powder or crushed tablets can be mixed with a small amount of water and stirred into the dry ration. For cats that refuse to eat food treated with pancreatic enzymes, the pancreatic enzyme powder or crushed tablets can be put into gelatin capsules for direct administration. Treatment is usually lifelong, although rare instances of dogs losing their requirement for pancreatic enzyme supplementation have been reported. No studies have been performed to determine the efficacy of the various human and veterinary pancreatic enzyme preparations. Until this information is available, it is recommended that only the powdered veterinary product be used. Some practitioners have observed that cats find a certain pancreatic enzyme preparation (Pancrezyme) more palatable than others; the enzyme content is the same as Viokase-V.

Some owners discontinue administering pancreatic enzyme powder because of expense; an economic alternative is use of raw bovine or swine pancreas (3 to 4 oz/20 kg per meal). This source of pancreatic enzymes is stable for 3 months when frozen at standard temperatures (−20° C), but it must be obtained from animals certified to be free of transmissible diseases.

Because pancreatic enzyme supplementation is very inefficient, several unsubstantiated methods have been proposed to enhance the effectiveness of this treatment if continued improvement is not seen. Use of $H_2$-receptor antagonists to diminish premature enzyme destruction by gastric acidity has been suggested. This approach should be reserved for particularly intractable cases because of expense and lack of clear benefit; fat absorption improved in experimental studies of dogs with induced EPI, although fecal weight remained unchanged. Changing the diet to one that is somewhat fat reduced and highly digestible, although based on a reasonable theory, has not been found to be particularly helpful in alleviating clinical signs; neither has addition of bile salts to the diet. High-fiber diets are not beneficial. Adding medium-chain triglycerides (MCT oil; 1 to 2 ml/kg/day PO) as a source of easily absorbable calories may improve weight gain. Vitamin deficiencies documented by measurement of blood concentrations should be corrected. Persistence of bacterial overgrowth in dogs may induce malabsorption, accounting for continued diarrhea despite adequate enzyme supplementation. Antibiotics (metronidazole [7.5 to 15 mg/kg PO q8-12h], tetracycline [22 mg/kg PO q8h], or tylosin [20 to 30 mg/kg/day with meals]) should be given for 6 weeks in such cases. Cats and dogs with low serum $B_{12}$ concentrations require supplementation weekly at first (100 to 250 μg for cats, 250 to 500 μg for dogs, SQ or IM) to normalize serum values; injections can then be given every 3 months. Serum $B_{12}$ concentration should be measured annually afterward.

Most cats and dogs respond to this regimen and have a favorable prognosis for a good-quality life. Recently an unusual complication of EPI, mesenteric torsion, was reported in 21 of 199 (10.5%) affected German Shepherd Dogs in Finland (Westermarck and colleague, 1989). All dogs died despite surgical intervention. The authors suspected that a motility disorder was the underlying cause. This devastating complication of EPI in dogs has not been noted in any other country.

# EXOCRINE PANCREATIC NEOPLASIA

Primary cancer of the exocrine pancreas (adenocarcinoma) is rare in dogs and cats. It is important to remember that it is seen in older animals (some investigators say that Airedale Terriers are overrepresented) and that affected animals may be presented most commonly with signs of pancreatitis or extrahepatic bile duct obstruction and rarely with signs of EPI. Common signs include lethargy, anorexia, and especially weight loss. A mass in the region of the pancreas may be detectable by abdominal palpation or survey radiography. Results of routine laboratory testing (i.e., CBC, serum biochemical profile, urinalysis) are usually compatible with the consequences of the neoplasm (e.g., EBDO) and are noncontributory to establishing the diagnosis. Wide fluctuations in serum glucose concentration have also been observed occasionally in cats and dogs with pancreatic exocrine neoplasms. Abdominal ultrasonography usually identifies a pancreatic mass and possibly metastases in the peripancreatic region and liver. Histopathologic examination of a biopsy specimen from the mass or cytopathologic examination of an aspirate specimen obtained with ultrasonographic guidance (Bennett and colleagues, 2001) is required for definitive diagnosis. The other primary differential diagnosis is chronic pancreatitis. These neoplasms are rapidly metastatic, and there is currently no successful treatment for disseminated disease. Surgical excision of the primary tumor may prolong disease-free survival, but most affected cats and dogs die within 6 months of diagnosis.

## Suggested Readings

Akol KG et al: Acute pancreatitis in cats with hepatic lipidosis, *J Vet Intern Med* 7:205,1993.

Bennett PF et al: Ultrasonographic and cytopathological diagnosis of exocrine pancreatic carcinoma in the dog and cat, *J Am Anim Hosp Assoc* 37:466, 2001.

Cook AK et al: Risk factors associated with acute pancreatitis in dogs: 101 cases (1985-1990), *J Am Vet Med Assoc* 203:673, 1993.

Edwards DF et al: Pancreatic masses in seven dogs following acute pancreatitis, *J Am Anim Hosp Assoc* 26:189, 1990.

Freeman L M et al: Nutritional support in pancreatitis: a retrospective study, *J Vet Emerg Crit Care* 5:32, 1995.

Gerhardt A et al: Comparison of the sensitivity of different diagnostic tests for pancreatitis in cats, *J Vet Intern Med* 15:329, 2001.

Hill RC et al: Acute necrotizing pancreatitis and acute suppurative pancreatitis in the cat: a retrospective study of 40 cases (1976-1989), *J Vet Intern Med* 7:25, 1993.

Hines BL et al: Pancreatic pseudocyst associated with chronic-active necrotizing pancreatitis in a cat, *J Am Anim Hosp Assoc* 32:147, 1996.

Kimmel SE et al: Incidence and prognostic value of low plasma ionized calcium concentration in cats with acute pancreatitis: 46 cases (1996-1998), *J Am Vet Med Assoc* 219:1105, 2001.

Kitchell BE et al: Clinical and pathologic changes in experimentally induced acute pancreatitis in cats, *Am J Vet Res* 47:1170, 1986.

Mansfield CS et al: Trypsinogen activation peptide in the diagnosis of canine pancreatitis, *J Vet Intern Med* 14:346, 2000.

Murtaugh RJ et al: Serum antiprotease concentrations in dogs with spontaneous and experimentally induced acute pancreatitis, *Am J Vet Res* 46:80, 1985.

Owens JM et al: Pancreatic disease in the cat, *J Am Anim Hosp Assoc* 11:83, 1975.

Rallis TS et al: Serum lipase activity in young dogs with acute enteritis or gastroenteritis, *Vet Clin Pathol* 25:65, 1996.

Rimaila-Parnanen E et al: Pancreatic degenerative atrophy and chronic pancreatitis in dogs: a comparative study of 60 cases, *Acta Vet Scand* 23:400, 1982.

Salisbury SK et al: Pancreatic abscess in dogs: six cases (1978-1986), *J Am Vet Med Assoc* 193:1104, 1988.

Simpson KW: Current concepts of the pathogenesis and pathophysiology of acute pancreatitis in the dog and cat, *Compend Cont Ed Pract Vet* 15:247, 1993.

Steiner JM et al: Diagnosis of canine and feline pancreatitis. In *Proceedings of the 20th Annual Forum, ACVIM,* Dallas, 2002, p 562.

Washabau RJ: Feline acute pancreatitis—important species differences. Proceedings of the European Society of Feline Medicine Symposium, *J Feline Med Surg* 3:95, 2001.

Westermarck E et al: Mesenteric torsion in dogs with exocrine pancreatic insufficiency: 21 cases (1978-1987), *J Am Vet Med Assoc* 195:1404, 1989.

Westermarck E et al: Role of low dietary fat in the treatment of dogs with exocrine pancreatic insufficiency, *Am J Vet Res* 56:600, 1995.

Willard MD et al: Duodenal foreign body mimicking acute pancreatitis, *J Am Anim Hosp Assoc* 29:351, 1993.

Williams DA: Exocrine pancreatic disease. In Ettinger SJ, editor: *Textbook of veterinary internal medicine*, ed 5, Philadelphia, 2000, WB Saunders, p 1345.

## Drugs Used in Hepatobiliary and Exocrine Pancreatic Disorders

| INDICATION | DRUG | TRADE NAME | DOSAGE |
|---|---|---|---|
| **Diagnostic** | | | |
| Detect hyperammonemia | $NH_4Cl$ | — | 0.1 g/kg<br>In gelatin capsules PO<br>As 10% solution PO<br>As 5% solution (per rectum) |
| Detect fat malabsorption | Corn oil (long-chain triglyceride) | — | 3-4 ml/kg PO |
| Determine portal venous anatomy | Iothalamate sodium | Conray 400; Mallinckrodt, St. Louis, Mo. | 0.5-1.0 ml/kg as a rapid injection |
| Confirm mechanical bile duct obstruction | Disofenin/[99mTc] | Heptolite; DuPont NEN Medical Products, North Billerica, Mass. | 1 µC IV once |
| Detect presence or absence of porto-systemic shunting | Pertechnetate/[99mTc] | — | 1 µC instilled into the descending colon once |
| **Therapeutic** | | | |
| Analgesic | Butorphanol | Torbugesic; Fort Dodge Animal Health, Fort Dodge, Iowa | 0.2-0.8 mg/kg SQ, IM, or IV q1-2h (D); 0.1-0.4 mg/kg SQ, IM, or IV q2-6h (C) |
| | Hydromorphone | — | 0.03-0.05 mg/kg IM prn |
| Antidote for acetaminophen toxicity | N-acetylcysteine | Mucomyst; Geneva Pharmaceuticals, Broomfield, Colo. | 140 mg/kg PO or IV as a 20% solution (loading dose), followed 6 hr later by 70 mg/kg PO or IV q6h for 7 treatments; also give ascorbic acid, 30 mg/kg PO q6h |
| Antidote for inorganic arsenical toxicity | Dimercaprol | BAL in oil | 2.5-5.0 mg/kg IM q4h for 2 days; then q12h until recovery |
| Antidote for thallium toxicity | Diphenylthio-carbozone | — | 70 mg/kg PO q8h (controversial) |
| Antiemetic | Chlorpromazine | Thorazine; GlaxoSmithKline, Research Triangle Park, N.C. | 0.25-0.5 mg/kg SQ or IM q6-8h |
| | Prochlorperazine | Compazine; GlaxoSmithKline, Research Triangle Park, N.C. | 0.25-0.5 mg/kg SQ or IM q6-8h |
| Antiinflammatory or antifibrotic | Azathioprine | Imuran; Prometheus Laboratories, San Diego, Calif. | 50 mg/m² PO q24h initially, then q48h |
| | Colchicine | Colchicine Tablets; Qualitest Pharmaceuticals, Huntsville, Ala. | 0.03 mg/kg/day PO |
| | Prednisone | — | 1.0 mg/kg PO q12h (D); 1.0-2.0 mg/kg PO q12h (C), then q24h, then q48h |
| | Ursodeoxycholic acid | Ursodiol; Teva Pharmaceuticals USA, Sellersville, Pa. | 10-15 mg/kg PO q24h |

*PO*, By mouth; *[99mTc]*, technetium-99m; *SQ*, subcutaneously; *IM*, intramuscularly; *prn*, as needed; *IV*, intravenously; *D*, dog; *C*, cat; *VWD*, von Willebrand's disease.

*Continued*

Drugs Used in Hepatobiliary and Exocrine Pancreatic Disorders—cont'd

| INDICATION | DRUG | TRADE NAME | DOSAGE |
|---|---|---|---|
| **Therapeutic—cont'd** | | | |
| Antimicrobial | Amikacin | — | 10 mg/kg IV or SQ q8h |
| | Ampicillin, amoxicillin | — | 22 mg/kg IV or PO q8h |
| | Cephalozin | — | 22 mg/kg IV q8h |
| | Cephalexin | — | 22 mg/kg PO q8h |
| | Cefotaxime | Claforan; Aventis Pharmaceuticals, Bridgewater, N.J. | 6-40 mg/kg IV or IM q6h |
| | Clindamycin | Antirobe; Pharmacia & Upjohn, Kalamazoo, Mich. | 10 mg/kg IV or PO q12h |
| | Enrofloxacin | Baytril; Bayer Corp., Shawnee Mission, Kan. | 2.5 mg/kg IV or PO q12h |
| | Marboflaxacin | Zeniquin; Pfizer Animal Health, Exton, Pa. | 2.75-5.5 mg/kg PO q24h |
| | Metronidazole | Metronidazole; Teva Pharmaceuticals USA, Sellersville, Pa. | 7.5-15 mg/kg PO q12h or q8h (use lower dose if severe hepatic dysfunction present) |
| | Praziquantel | Droncit; Bayer Corp., Shawnee Mission, Kan. | 20 mg/kg SQ q24h for 3 days |
| | Trimethoprim-sulfamethoxasole | Septra; Monarch Pharmaceuticals, Bristol, Tenn. | 15 mg/kg IV q12h |
| | Tylosin | Tylan 40; Elanco, Indianapolis, Ind. | 20-30 mg/kg/day PO |
| Antioxidants | Vitamin E | — | 400-500 IU/day PO (water-soluble form) |
| | S-adenosylmethionine | Denosyl SD4; Nutramax Laboratories, Edgewood, Md. | 20 mg/kg PO q24h (after an overnight fast) |
| Appetite stimulant | Cyproheptadine | Periacatin; Merck and Co., West Point, Pa. | 1-2 mg PO q12h or q8h |
| | Diazepam | Valium; Roche Laboratories, Nutley, N.J. | 0.2 mg/kg IV q12-24h |
| | Oxazepam | Oxazepam tablets; Geneva Pharmaceuticals, Broomfield, Colo. | 4 mg PO q24h or q12h |
| Caloric supplement | MCT oil | — | 1-2 ml/kg/day PO |
| Cupretic | D-Penicillamine | Cuprimine; Merck and Co., West Point, Pa. | 10-15 mg/kg PO q12h, 30 min before meal |
| | Trientine | Syprine; Merck and Co., West Point, Pa. | 10-15 mg/kg PO q12h, 30 min before meal |
| | Zinc acetate or sulfate | — | 5-10 mg/kg PO q12h |
| Diuresis | Furosemide | Lasix; Aventis Pharmaceuticals, Bridgewater, N.J. | 1-2 mg/kg IV q8h for 3 doses |
| Acute (massive hepatic necrosis) | Mannitol | — | 1 g/kg of 20% solution IV over 30 min; can repeat q4-6h for 3 additional doses |
| Chronic | Furosemide | Lasix; Aventis Pharmaceuticals, Bridgewater, N.J. | 1-2 mg/kg PO q12h or q8h initially, then q24h or q12h |
| | Spironolactone | Aldactone; Pharmacia & Upjohn, Kalamazoo, Mich. | 0.5-1 mg/kg PO q12h; can be doubled if no effect initially |

rugs

Drugs Used in Hepatobiliary and Exocrine Pancreatic Disorders—cont'd

| INDICATION | DRUG | TRADE NAME | DOSAGE |
|---|---|---|---|
| **Therapeutic—cont'd** | | | |
| Hemorrhagic tendency Intestinal | Cimetidine | Tagamet; GlaxoSmithKline, Research Triangle Park, N.C. | 5-10 mg/kg IV, SQ, or PO q8h |
| | Famotidine | Pepcid; Merck and Co., West Point, Pa. | 0.05 mg/kg PO q12h or q24h |
| | Ranitidine | Zantac; GlaxoSmithKline, Research Triangle Park, N.C. | 2 mg/kg IV or PO q12h |
| | Omeprazole | Prilosec; Merck and Co., West Point, Pa. | 0.7 mg/kg PO q24h |
| Generalized | Sucralfate | — | 1 g/25 kg PO q8h or q6h |
| | Desmopressin acetate for VWD | — | 1 µg/kg intranasal preparation SQ 1 hr preoperatively |
| | Heparin for DIC | — | (See Parts 11 and 12: Oncology; Hematology and Immunology) |
| | Vitamin K$_1$ | Vitamin K$_1$; Phoenix Pharmaceutical, Inc, St. Joseph, Mo. | 1 mg/kg SQ q24h |
| Hyperammonemia | Lactulose | — | 2.5-5 ml (C) or 2.5-15 ml (D) PO q8h, or as retention enema left in place 15-20 min (3 parts lactulose and 7 parts water, 20 ml/kg) |
| | Lactitol | Lacty; PURAC America, Lincolnshire, Ill. | 50 mg/kg PO q8h (estimate) |
| | Neomycin sulfate | Biosol; Pharmacia & Upjohn, Kalamazoo, Mich. | 20 mg/kg PO q8h |
| | Flumazenil | Romazicon; Roche Laboratories, Nutley, N.J. | 0.01-0.02 mg/kg IV once; can be repeated once 30 min later (used primarily for diazepam overdose) |
| Nutritional supplement | Elemental diet | CliniCare Liquid Diet; Abbott Laboratories, Chicago, Ill. | 1 kcal/ml |
| Stimulate gastric motility | Metoclopramide | Reglan; AH Robins, Richmond, Va. | 0.2-0.5 mg/kg PO, SQ, or IV 30 min before meal |
| | Cisapride | — | 0.5 mg/kg PO q8-12h |
| Other | Ascorbic acid | — | 25 mg/kg/day PO |
| | Heparin for pancreatitis | — | 50-75 IU/kg SQ q8-12h |
| | Pancreatic enzyme powder or crushed tablets | Viokase V; Fort Dodge Animal Health, Fort Dodge, Iowa  Pancrezyme; JPI Jones Animal Health, St. Louis, Mo.  Pancreatic Plus Powder; The Butler Co., Dublin, Ohio | 1-2 tsp mixed with each meal |
| | Vitamin B$_{12}$ | — | 100-250 µg SQ or IM q7days initially (C)  250-500 µg SQ or IM q30days (D) |

*PO,* By mouth; *$^{99m}$Tc,* technetium-99m; *SQ,* subcutaneously; *IM,* intramuscularly; *prn,* as needed; *IV,* intravenously; *D,* dog; *C,* cat; *VWD,* von Willebrand's disease.

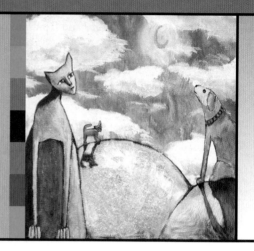

# CHAPTER 41

# Clinical Manifestations of Urinary Disorders

## CHAPTER OUTLINE

GENERAL CONSIDERATIONS, 568
 Pollakiuria and dysuria-stranguria, 568
 Urethral obstruction, 568
 Urinary tract infection, 568
 Transitional cell carcinoma, 570
 Urolithiasis, 570
 Feline lower urinary tract inflammation, 571
 Hematuria, 572
DISORDERS OF MICTURITION, 575
 Distended bladder, 576
 Small or normal-sized bladder, 576
 Geriatric incontinence, 577
POLYDIPSIA AND POLYURIA, 577
PROTEINURIA, 579
AZOTEMIA, 581
RENOMEGALY, 583

## GENERAL CONSIDERATIONS

This chapter begins with a discussion of urinary tract problems that are likely to be identified by pet owners (e.g., pollakiuria and dysuria-stranguria, hematuria, urinary incontinence, and polydipsia and polyuria). Problems that are usually identified on the basis of a physical exam, a minimum database or with imaging techniques, including proteinuria, azotemia, and renomegaly, are discussed subsequently.

## POLLAKIURIA AND DYSURIA-STRANGURIA

Inflammation of the lower urinary tract (LUTI) usually results in increased frequency of urination (pollakiuria) and difficult urination (dysuria) associated with straining (stranguria) (Fig. 41-1). LUTI in dogs is often caused by bacterial infection; in contrast, primary bacterial infection of the urinary tract is relatively rare in cats. Sterile inflammation of the urinary tract

(e.g., some cases of calcium oxalate urolithiasis, neoplasia, and idiopathic cystitis) can result in pollakiuria and dysuria-stranguria in both dogs and cats. When an animal has clinical signs suggestive of a lower urinary tract inflammation or obstruction, transabdominal palpation of the bladder may confirm the presence of a distended bladder, a thickened bladder wall, a bladder mass, or urolithiasis. If possible, urinary bladder palpation should be performed before and after voiding, because a full bladder may obscure intraluminal masses or uroliths. Digital rectal examination in smaller male and female dogs as well as cats often allows one to evaluate the trigone of the bladder and the pelvic urethra, in a search for masses or uroliths. Urinalysis, urine bacterial culture, ultrasonography of the bladder, and/or plain or contrast-enhanced radiography of the bladder and urethra will often demonstrate the cause of the pollakiuria and dysuria-stranguria. If systemic signs (e.g., depression, lethargy, anorexia, and vomiting) are present in animals with LUTI, a complete blood count (CBC) and serum biochemistry profile should also be obtained, and the kidneys, prostate, and uterus/uterine stump should be evaluated as a possible source of the inflammation.

## URETHRAL OBSTRUCTION

Urethral obstruction, either functional (e.g., reflex dyssynergia, urethral spasm) or anatomic (e.g., urolithiasis, granulomatous urethritis, neoplasia), usually causes pollakiuria, dysuria-stranguria, or both, with an attenuated or absent urine stream. A urethral catheter will pass relatively easily in patients with a functional obstruction, whereas an anatomic obstruction will result in "grating," difficult passage, or the inability to pass the catheter. If a complete urethral obstruction exists, the degree of postrenal azotemia and hyperkalemia should be assessed immediately. Hyperkalemia can cause life-threatening cardiac arrhythmias and should be treated promptly (see Fig. 41-1).

## URINARY TRACT INFECTION

Urine for bacterial culture may be obtained by antepubic cystocentesis, urinary bladder catheterization, or a mid-

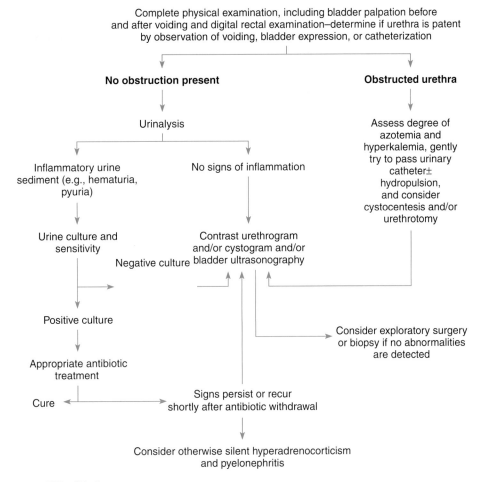

**FIG 41-1**
Diagnostic approach to pollakiuria and dysuria-stranguria (see also Fig. 41-7).

TABLE 41-1

**Numbers of Bacteria per Milliliter Considered Significant According to Method of Urine Collection in Dogs and Cats**

| COLLECTION METHOD | SIGNIFICANT | QUESTIONABLE | CONTAMINATION |
|---|---|---|---|
| Cystocentesis | >1000 | 100 to 1000 | <100 |
| Catheterization | >10,000 | 1000 to 10,000 | <1000 |
| Voided or expressed | >100,000 | 10,000 to 100,000 | <10,000 |

stream catch during voiding. However, the number of organisms isolated in a normal dog or cat varies according to the technique used (Table 41-1). Ideally, urine should be obtained by cystocentesis, and urine specimens should be plated within 30 minutes of collection. If this is not possible, the urine sample should be refrigerated, because bacteria may double their numbers in urine every 45 minutes at room temperature, resulting in false-positive culture findings. On the other hand, false-negative urine culture results may be obtained if the urine has been frozen or refrigerated for 12 to 24 hours or more.

Animals with recurrent urinary tract infections (UTIs) or a UTI that does not respond to appropriate antibiotic treatment should undergo ultrasonography or contrast-enhanced radiography in a search for underlying anatomic disorders. Bladder tumors or polyps, uroliths, pyelonephritis, prostatitis, and urachal remnants are common causes of recurrent or unresponsive UTIs. In some cases, systemic disorders such as hyperadrenocorticism, chronic renal insufficiency-failure, and diabetes mellitus may be associated with recurrent UTIs, as can long-term corticosteroid treatment. UTIs are discussed in greater depth in Chapter 45.

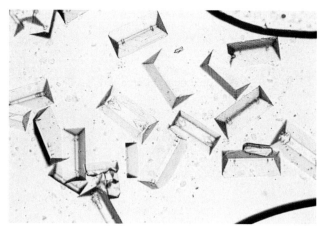

**FIG 41-2**
Struvite crystals in urine sediment. These crystals are normally colorless. (From Grauer GF: Canine urolithiasis. In Allen DG, editor: *Small animal medicine,* Philadelphia, 1991, JB Lippincott.)

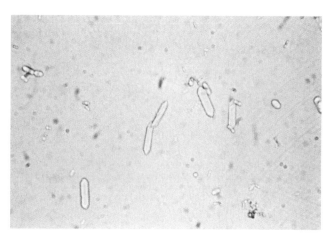

**FIG 41-3**
Monohydrate calcium oxalate crystals in urine sediment. These crystals are normally colorless. (From Grauer GF: Canine urolithiasis. In Allen DG, editor: *Small animal medicine,* Philadelphia, 1991, JB Lippincott.)

## TRANSITIONAL CELL CARCINOMA

Transitional cell carcinoma (TCC) is the most common malignant bladder tumor in dogs and should be suspected in older dogs with hematuria, pollakiuria, and dysuria-stranguria. TCCs are rare in cats, where they are usually detected as a diffuse thickening of the bladder wall during palpation or imaging. TCCs most frequently arise in the bladder trigone region; therefore rectal palpation can often detect their presence. Urinary bladder ultrasonography or double contrast–enhanced cystography will confirm that a bladder mass exists. In some cases, unilateral or bilateral hydroureter-hydronephrosis is observed as a result of obstruction of one or both ureters at the vesicoureteral junction. Tumor biopsy and histopathologic evaluation should be done to confirm the tumor type and stage and to direct the nature of specific treatment.

## UROLITHIASIS

Urinary bladder and urethral uroliths can often be palpated during abdominal or rectal examinations; however, a thickened, inflamed bladder wall may obscure small uroliths. In male dogs with dysuria, the urethra should be palpated subcutaneously from the ischial arch to the os penis in a search for urethral uroliths. Ultrasonography or plain or contrast-enhanced radiography of the urinary tract is necessary to confirm the presence of uroliths. Calcium oxalate and struvite uroliths are the most radiodense uroliths, whereas urate uroliths are relatively radiolucent, and contrast-enhanced radiographs may be required for their diagnosis. Silicate and cystine uroliths have an intermediate radiodensity.

Urinalysis findings in dogs and cats with urolithiasis often indicate the presence of urinary tract inflammation (e.g., hematuria, pyuria, increased numbers of epithelial cells, and proteinuria). The urine pH varies, depending on the stone type, whether there is a concurrent bacterial infection, and the animal's diet. In general, struvite uroliths are associated with an alkaline urine (especially if urease-producing bacteria are pres-

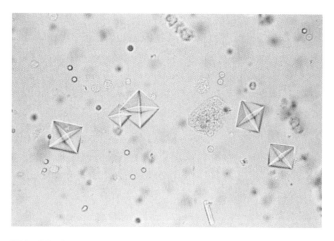

**FIG 41-4**
Dihydrate calcium oxalate crystals in urine sediment. These crystals are normally colorless. (From Grauer GF: Canine urolithiasis. In Allen DG, editor: *Small animal medicine,* Philadelphia, 1991, JB Lippincott.)

ent); cystine uroliths with an acidic urine; and oxalate, urate, and silicate uroliths with a neutral-to-acidic urine. Crystalluria may be observed, depending on the urine concentration, pH, and temperature. Although crystalluria may exist in the absence of uroliths, and uroliths may be present in the absence of crystalluria, if the two coexist, the identity of the crystals is usually the same as that of the urolith (Figs. 41-2 to 41-6). Exceptions do occur, however; for example, a urease-producing bacterial infection could generate struvite crystals in the presence of silicate or calcium oxalate uroliths. Bacterial urine culture and sensitivity testing should be performed in all animals with urolithiasis to identify and properly treat any concurrent UTI. If a cystotomy is performed to remove stones, a small piece of bladder mucosa or urolith should be submitted for bacterial culture. This is because urine may be sterile in dogs and cats that have

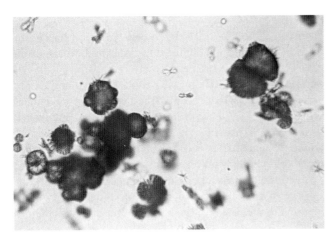

**FIG 41-5**
Ammonium biurate crystals in urine sediment. These crystals are normally dark yellow. (From Grauer GF: Canine urolithiasis. In Allen DG, editor: *Small animal medicine,* Philadelphia, 1991, JB Lippincott.)

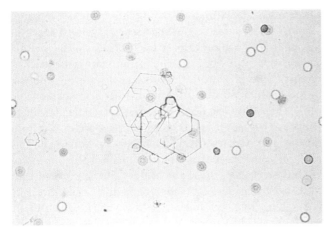

**FIG 41-6**
Cystine crystals in urine sediment. These crystals are normally clear to light yellow. (From Grauer GF: Canine urolithiasis. In Allen DG, editor: *Small animal medicine,* Philadelphia, 1991, JB Lippincott.)

previously been treated with antibiotics, whereas the stone or bladder mucosa may still harbor bacteria.

The animal's signalment, as well as the clinicopathologic and radiographic findings, are often helpful in determining the type of urolith (Table 41-2); however, a quantitative urolith analysis should be performed if uroliths are passed or removed surgically. Identification of the urolith type facilitates the use of specific measures to dissolve them or prevent their recurrence. Qualitative commercial kit analysis of uroliths is not recommended, because these kits do not detect silicic acid salts, frequently fail to detect calcium-containing uroliths, and yield false-positive results for uric acid more than half the time in animals with cystine uroliths. Quantitative urolith analysis, available at most teaching hospitals and reference laboratories, is recommended instead.

 TABLE 41-2

### Factors that May Aid in the Identification of Uroliths in Dogs

**Struvite**

- 80% to 97% of uroliths in female dogs are struvite.
- Uroliths in dogs less than 1 year of age are usually struvite.
- High incidence of concurrent urinary tract infection (especially *Staphylococcus* or *Proteus*).
- Urine is usually alkaline.
- Uroliths are radiodense.
- Increased prevalence occurs in Miniature Schnauzers, Miniature Poodles, Bichon Frises, Cocker Spaniels.

**Calcium Oxalate**

- Increased prevalence occurs in older male dogs (especially Miniature Schnauzers, Miniature Poodles, Yorkshire Terriers, Lhasa Apsos, Bichon Frises, and Shih Tzus).
- Urine is usually acidic to neutral.
- Uroliths are radiodense.
- Hypercalcemia may be a contributing factor.

**Ammonium Acid Urate**

- Increased prevalence occurs in male dogs (especially Dalmatians and English Bulldogs).
- Urine is usually acidic to neutral.
- Uroliths are relatively radiolucent.
- Increased incidence in dogs with severe hepatic insufficiency (e.g., portosystemic shunts in Miniature Schnauzers and Yorkshire Terriers).

**Silicate**

- Increased prevalence occurs in male dogs (especially German Shepherd Dogs, Golden Retrievers, and Labrador Retrievers).
- Urine is usually acidic to neutral.
- Urolith radiodensity is variable.
- High dietary intake of silicates probably predisposes (corn gluten and soybean hulls).

**Cystine**

- Increased prevalence occurs in male dogs (especially Dachshunds, Basset Hounds, English Bulldogs, Yorkshire Terriers, Irish Terriers, Chihuahuas, Mastiffs, and Rottweilers).
- Urine is usually acidic.
- Urolith radiodensity is variable.

Urolithiasis is discussed in greater detail in Chapters 46 and 47.

## FELINE LOWER URINARY TRACT INFLAMMATION

Cats with LUTI (often referred to as the *feline urologic syndrome, feline lower urinary tract inflammation* (FLUTI), or *feline interstitial cystitis;* see Chapter 47) usually are presented because of pollakiuria, dysuria-stranguria, microscopic or gross hematuria, and inappropriate voiding. In male cats with a urinary tract obstruction, the presenting signs depend on how long the obstruction has been present. Within the first 6 to 24 hours, most obstructed cats will make frequent attempts to urinate, pace, vocalize, hide under beds or behind couches, lick their genitalia, and display anxiety. If the obstruction is not relieved within 36 to 48 hours, characteristic clinical signs of postrenal azotemia, including anorexia, vomiting, dehydration, depression, weakness, collapse, stupor, hypothermia, acidosis with hyperventilation, or bradycardia, may be observed. Sudden death may also occur.

On physical examination, an unobstructed cat is apparently healthy, except for a small, easily expressible bladder. The bladder wall may be thickened, and palpation may cause the animal to void. Abdominal palpation may be painful to the unobstructed cat; however, the obstructed cat will always resent manipulation of the caudal abdomen unless he or she is severely depressed or comatose. The most significant physical examination finding in an obstructed cat is a turgid, distended bladder that is difficult or impossible to express. Care should be exercised in manipulating the distended bladder, however, because the wall has been injured by the increased intravesical pressure and is susceptible to rupture. In a male cat with a urethral obstruction, the penis may be congested and it may protrude from the prepuce. Occasionally a urethral plug is seen extending from the urethral orifice, and in some cases the cat may lick his penis until it becomes excoriated and bleeds.

A history of acute onset of pollakiuria, dysuria-stranguria, and hematuria in an otherwise healthy cat indicates the presence of the FLUTI syndrome. Physical examination should include digital rectal palpation of the caudal bladder and urethra in an attempt to determine whether there are masses or calculi, as well as abdominal palpation of the bladder before and after voiding to determine the residual urine volume and whether there are intraluminal masses or uroliths. The minimal diagnostic workup in cats with pollakiuria and dysuria-stranguria should always include a complete urinalysis. The urine should preferably be obtained by cystocentesis; however, if manipulation of the bladder during abdominal palpation results in voiding, a sample obtained from a clean tabletop may be used to assess urine pH and sediment.

An extensive diagnostic evaluation of the unobstructed cat is unwarranted if the urine is alkaline and there are struvite crystals in the sediment, because in most of these cases the urine is bacteriologically sterile, and clinical signs respond to dietary therapy. However, if clinical signs persist beyond 5 to 7 days of dietary therapy, a second urinalysis with urine culture and sensitivity, radiography of the abdomen, ultrasound and/or contrast-enhanced cystography-urethrography should be performed (Fig. 41-7). These should also be performed in a cat with signs of FLUTI if the urine is acidic and there are no struvite crystals, because dietary therapy in these cases will likely be ineffective.

## HEMATURIA

Hematuria, the abnormal presence of red blood cells in the urine, is frequently encountered in clinical veterinary medicine. Hematuria occurring in conjunction with pollakiuria and dysuria-stranguria is usually associated with LUTI. Conversely, hematuria that occurs in the absence of other clinical signs often originates from the upper urinary tract. Hematuria may be gross (macroscopic hematuria) or occult (microscopic hematuria). Occult hematuria (more than five red blood cells per high-power field) is often present in dogs and cats with pollakiuria and dysuria-stranguria. The diagnostic workup in dogs and cats with hematuria is directed toward identifying the origin of the hemorrhage, as well as the underlying disease.

In most cases hematuria is caused by inflammation, trauma, or neoplasia of the urogenital tract; however, hematuria may also be caused by bleeding disorders, strenuous exercise, heat stroke, or renal infarcts. The renal telangiectasia that occurs in Welsh Corgi dogs may also cause hematuria, as can the renal hematuria in Weimaraners. The timing of gross hematuria during voiding often provides clues to the source of the hemorrhage. Hematuria that occurs at the beginning of voiding (initial hematuria) is suggestive of hemorrhage originating from the lower urinary tract (bladder neck, urethra, vagina, vulva, penis, or prepuce). Extraurinary causes such as proestrus, metritis, pyometra, prostatic disease, or neoplasia of the genital tract may also cause initial hematuria (Table 41-3). Hematuria that occurs at the end of voiding (terminal hematuria) usually results from hemorrhage originating from the upper urinary tract (bladder, ureters, or kidneys). In this case the hemorrhage may be intermittent, which allows the red blood cells to settle in the bladder and be expelled with the last of the bladder contents. If hematuria occurs throughout voiding (total hematuria), the hemorrhage usually originates in the bladder, ureters, or kidneys. Pseudohematuria may be caused by myoglobin or hemoglobin, drugs, and natural or artificial food dyes in urine. In cases of pseudohematuria, the urine supernate remains discolored after centrifugation.

In dogs and cats with hematuria caused by inflammation, trauma, or neoplasia of the lower urinary tract, concurrent clinical signs usually include pollakiuria and dysuria-stranguria. Hematuria associated with upper urinary tract disease may be associated with systemic signs, including depression, lethargy, anorexia, vomiting, diarrhea, weight loss, and abdominal pain, or it may be asymptomatic. In some cases upper tract hemorrhage can result in the formation of blood clots in the bladder, with subsequent dysuria-stranguria. If hemorrhage from the genital tract is causing hematuria, spontaneous bleeding unassociated with voiding may also be observed. Additional signs indicating that the genital tract is the source of hemorrhage include a purulent vaginal or urethral discharge independent of voiding, behavioral changes (e.g., proestrus), or straining to defecate in association with a stilted gait (e.g., prostatic disease).

A complete physical examination often helps localize the source of the hematuria. If possible, the kidneys should be

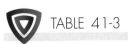

TABLE 41-3

Potential Causes of Hematuria

| URINARY CAUSES | EXTRAURINARY CAUSES |
|---|---|
| **Initial Hematuria** | |
| Urethral causes | Spontaneous bleeding unassociated with voiding may also occur with the following: |
| Trauma | |
| Infection | Prostatic: infection, cyst, abscess, tumor |
| Urolithiasis | Uterine: infection, tumor, proestrus, subinvolution |
| Neoplasia | Vaginal: tumor, trauma |
| Granulomatous urethritis | Preputial/penile: tumor, trauma |
| Bladder trigone region | |
| Neoplasia | |
| **Total or Terminal Hematuria** | |
| Pseudohematuria | |
| Kidney, ureter, bladder | Prostatic (see above) |
| Trauma | Bleeding disorders |
| Infection | Heat stroke |
| Urolithiasis | Exercise-induced |
| Tumor | |
| Parasitism | |
| Drug induced (cyclophosphamide) | |
| Feline lower urinary tract inflammation syndrome | |
| Renal infarct | |
| Renal telangiectasia | |
| Idiopathic renal hematuria | |

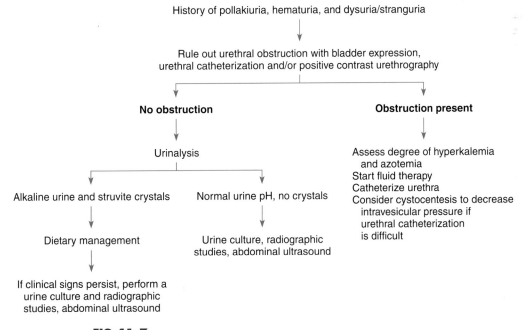

History of pollakiuria, hematuria, and dysuria/stranguria

↓

Rule out urethral obstruction with bladder expression, urethral catheterization and/or positive contrast urethrography

**No obstruction**                                      **Obstruction present**

↓                                                                        ↓

Urinalysis                                              Assess degree of hyperkalemia
                                                                and azotemia
                                                              Start fluid therapy
                                                              Catheterize urethra
Alkaline urine and struvite crystals    Normal urine pH, no crystals    Consider cystocentesis to decrease
                                                                intravesicular pressure if
↓                                             ↓                 urethral catheterization
Dietary management            Urine culture, radiographic    is difficult
                                      studies, abdominal ultrasound
↓

If clinical signs persist, perform a
urine culture and radiographic
studies, abdominal ultrasound

**FIG 41-7**
Diagnostic plan for feline lower urinary tract inflammation syndrome.

palpated and assessed in terms of their size, shape, consistency, and symmetry and for the presence of pain. The urinary bladder should be palpated before and after voiding, because, as already noted, a full bladder may obscure intraluminal masses, uroliths, or wall thickening. Observation of voiding should also be part of the physical examination and provides the opportunity to obtain a voided urine sample (Fig. 41-8). In addition, the timing of the hematuria can be confirmed and the character of the urine stream, as well as the presence or absence of dysuria, can be noted. Rectal palpation allows evaluation of the prostate in male dogs and of the pelvic urethra in dogs and cats of both sexes. The trigone region of the bladder can also be palpated rectally in small dogs and cats; this is facilitated by concurrent abdominal palpation, with the examiner pushing the bladder toward the pelvic inlet. In larger female dogs, digital vaginal palpation and the use of a vaginal speculum allow the urethral orifice to be evaluated; vaginal masses, strictures, and lacerations can be ruled in or out in this way. In male dogs, the perineal urethra should be palpated subcutaneously from the ischial arch to the os penis, and the penis should be extruded from the prepuce and examined to determine whether there are masses, signs of trauma, or urethral prolapse. Finally, catheterization of the urethra in dysuric animals allows assessment of urethral patency.

Comparison of urine obtained by cystocentesis with voided urine may help differentiate lower urinary tract or genital tract disease from upper urinary tract disease. Cystocentesis prevents the urine from being contaminated with bacteria, cells, and debris from the urethra, vagina, vulva, prepuce, or uterus; however, prostatic disease may alter the characteristics of urine obtained by cystocentesis (as a result of the reflux of fluid into the bladder). Abnormal urinalysis findings in urine collected by cystocentesis indicate involvement of the bladder, ureters, kidneys, or prostate. It should be remembered, however, that catheterization or bladder expression, and to a greater extent cystocentesis, may result in traumatic hematuria.

Urinalysis should be performed as soon as possible after urine collection. In addition to evaluating the urine sediment for red blood cells, the clinician should look for white blood cells, epithelial cells, tumor cells, casts, crystals, parasite ova, and bacteria. If urine remains at room temperature for more than 30 minutes, urease-producing bacteria can proliferate, resulting in an increase in the urine pH, which may cause red and white blood cells and casts to fragment and lyse and may alter the crystal composition. In addition, hyposthenuria can result in the lysis of red and white blood cells, and lysed red blood cells in urine may create confusion between hemoglobinuria and hematuria. Refrigeration is the easiest way to preserve the stability of a urine sample. Although overnight refrigeration is acceptable for urine to be used for bacterial culture samples, it is not recommended for urine intended for chemical and cellular analysis.

Reagent strips used to detect blood in urine do so by detecting the peroxidase-like activity of hemoglobin from lysed cells. The test can detect approximately 0.05 to 0.3 mg of hemoglobin per deciliter of urine (equivalent to 10,000 lysed red blood cells per milliliter of urine, or approximately three lysed red blood cells per high-power field). These reagent test strips can also show a positive reaction for blood in the presence of myoglobinuria.

A complete blood count and serum biochemistry profile should be evaluated in dogs and cats with hematuria and concurrent systemic signs. An inflammatory leukogram is compatible with metritis-pyometra, acute bacterial pyelone-

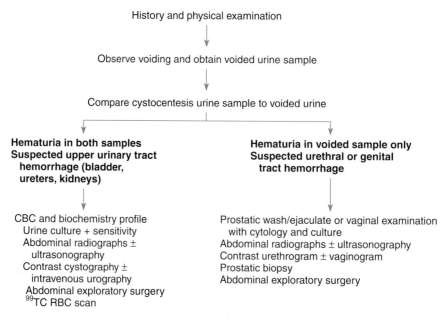

History and physical examination

↓

Observe voiding and obtain voided urine sample

↓

Compare cystocentesis urine sample to voided urine

**Hematuria in both samples**
**Suspected upper urinary tract**
**hemorrhage (bladder,**
**ureters, kidneys)**

↓

CBC and biochemistry profile
Urine culture + sensitivity
Abdominal radiographs ±
  ultrasonography
Contrast cystography ±
  intravenous urography
Abdominal exploratory surgery
$^{99}$TC RBC scan

**Hematuria in voided sample only**
**Suspected urethral or genital**
**tract hemorrhage**

↓

Prostatic wash/ejaculate or vaginal examination
  with cytology and culture
Abdominal radiographs ± ultrasonography
Contrast urethrogram ± vaginogram
Prostatic biopsy
Abdominal exploratory surgery

**FIG 41-8**
Diagnostic approach to dogs and cats with hematuria.

phritis, or prostatitis. Azotemia occurring in association with hematuria usually indicates the presence of renal parenchymal disease or a rent in the urinary excretory pathway; however, prerenal causes of azotemia should also be ruled out. If the blood loss caused by hematuria is severe or if signs of generalized bleeding exist, a hemostasis profile, platelet count, and bleeding time should be evaluated (see Chapter 89).

Plain and contrast-enhanced radiography, ultrasonography, and/or cystoscopy will often help show the location and cause of hematuria. In some cases, abdominal exploratory surgery and biopsy may be necessary to arrive at a diagnosis. Biopsy specimens may be obtained from the kidneys, bladder, and prostate gland; if indicated, individual ureteral catheterization through a cystotomy or visualization through a cystoscope may be performed to determine if renal hematuria is unilateral or bilateral.

## DISORDERS OF MICTURITION

Disorders of micturition include both urine retention and urine leakage (incontinence) problems. Incontinence, the inappropriate passage of urine, may be caused by congenital abnormalities or acquired disorders. In evaluating an animal with incontinence, it is helpful to determine whether the urinary bladder is distended, small, or normal-sized (Table 41-4). Incontinence associated with a distended bladder is usually caused by increased urethral resistance (paradoxic incontinence) or overflow associated with decreased bladder contractility. Conversely, incontinence associated with a small or normal-sized bladder is usually caused by bladder hypercontractility or decreased urethral resistance.

### Initial Evaluation

The age of onset, sexual status of the animal, age at neutering, current medications, and history of trauma or previous urinary tract disorders are important anamnestic points to cover when obtaining the history in an animal with any disorder of micturition. The physical examination should include an evaluation of the perineum for evidence of urine scalding or staining. Thorough palpation of the bladder to assess its size and wall thickness and a rectal examination to assess anal tone, the prostate gland, the pelvic urethra, and the trigone region of the bladder should be performed in all cases. A digital vaginal examination is indicated, and vaginoscopy may be used to help identify congenital defects (e.g., vaginal strictures, ectopic ureters) in larger female dogs.

A neurologic examination should include evaluation of the perineal and bulbospongiosus reflexes. The perineal reflex causes the anal sphincter to contract and the tail to ventroflex in response to pinching of the perineal skin. The bulbospongiosus reflex causes the anal sphincter to contract in response to gentle compression of the bulb of the penis or the vulva. Both of these reflexes are dependent on an intact pudendal nerve (sensory and motor) and intact sacral spinal cord segments S1-S3. If both reflexes are normal, the pudendal reflex arc is intact.

Dogs should be walked outside so that the voiding posture and urine stream size and character can be observed. Immediately after the animal has attempted to void, the bladder should be palpated to estimate the residual volume (normal residual volume is approximately 0.2 to 0.4 ml/kg). Catheterization to quantify the residual volume is indicated if a large bladder is palpable after voiding (in male dogs, behavioral urine marking can make it difficult to assess the true residual urine volume).

A urinalysis should be performed in all animals with urinary incontinence. If a bacterial urine culture is indicated, as noted earlier, cystocentesis is the preferred method of collection; however, dogs and cats with a distended bladder should ideally be catheterized to empty the bladder and to prevent urine from leaking from the cystocentesis site.

 TABLE 41-4

Causes of Urinary Incontinence and Associated Clinical Signs

| DISORDERS | CLINICAL SIGNS |
| --- | --- |
| **Large Bladder** | |
| Lower motor neuron lesions | Dribbling of urine; distended bladder that is easily expressed; history of trauma or surgery in pelvic region |
| Upper motor neuron lesions | Distended bladder that is difficult to express; paresis or paralysis may be present |
| Reflex dyssynergia | Often, large-breed male dog; distended bladder that is difficult to express but easy to catheterize; urine stream initiated and then interrupted |
| Outflow tract obstruction | Usually male animals; dysuria-stranguria, dribbling of urine; distended bladder that is difficult to express and catheterize |
| **Small Bladder** | |
| Urethral sphincter mechanism incompetence | Middle-aged or older neutered or spayed dogs; dribbling of urine usually occurs when animal is relaxed or asleep, normal voiding otherwise |
| Detrusor hyperreflexia/instability | Pollakiuria, dysuria-stranguria, hematuria, bacteriuria |
| Congenital abnormalities | Young animal; constant dribbling of urine may occur, voiding may be normal otherwise |

## Pharmacologic Testing and Treatment

Frequently the diagnosis of disorders of micturition (see Chapter 48) is based to some degree on the animal's response to pharmacologic testing and therapy. For example, detrusor hypocontractility should improve in response to a parasympathomimetic drug such as bethanechol, and urethral hypotonicity should respond to α-adrenergic agents such as phenylpropanolamine or hormone replacement therapy. Urethral hypertonicity is treated with α-sympatholytics (e.g., phenoxybenzamine) and striated muscle relaxants (e.g., diazepam). Detrusor hypercontractility often responds to treatment of the underlying inflammatory process (e.g., bacterial cystitis or urolithiasis); however, smooth muscle antispasmodics (e.g., oxybutynin) and parasympatholytics (e.g., propantheline) may be useful in cases of severe inflammation.

## DISTENDED BLADDER

Causes of incontinence that are usually associated with a distended bladder include neurogenic disorders (lower and upper motor neuron lesions and reflex dyssynergia) and urine outflow tract obstructive disorders (paradoxic incontinence) (see Table 41-4). If neurologic lesions or deficits are detected during a neurologic examination, the status of the bladder helps localize the lesion and helps classify the injury as an upper motor neuron (UMN) lesion (located above the fifth lumbar vertebral body) or a lower motor neuron (LMN) lesion (located at or below the fifth lumbar vertebral body). The most characteristic sign of an LMN lesion to the bladder is a distended bladder that is easily expressed. A LMN injury affecting innervation to the bladder creates both sphincter and detrusor hyporeflexia; if the lesion involves the S1-S3 spinal cord segments, both perineal and bulbospongiosus reflexes are absent.

Animals with UMN lesions to the bladder characteristically have a large, distended bladder that is difficult to express; the UMN lesion may also cause paresis or paralysis. In an animal with a UMN lesion, there is no voluntary control of micturition, and the urethral sphincter shows reflex hyperexcitability because there is a lack of inhibition to the somatic efferents in the pudendal nerve, making expression of the bladder difficult. With time, UMN bladders may develop reflex contraction and partial emptying in response to detrusor stretching. This "automatic" emptying occurs without control or sensation.

Reflex dyssynergia or detrusor-urethral dyssynergia is a condition observed primarily in larger breed male dogs. The cause is usually difficult to determine but may include any of several neurologic lesions of the spinal cord or autonomic ganglia. Reflex dyssynergia results from active contraction of the detrusor without relaxation of the internal or external urethral sphincters. Characteristic signs of reflex dyssynergia include a normal or near-normal initiation of voiding, followed by a narrowed urine stream. Urine may be delivered in spurts, or flow may be completely disrupted and the animal will often strain to produce urine. After a while, the dog lowers his leg and then often begins dribbling urine as he walks away. It is difficult to express urine from the bladder of a dog with reflex dyssynergia; however, urethral catheterization is usually easy.

Incontinence in an animal with urinary outflow tract obstruction is called *paradoxic incontinence*. It occurs because, when intravesical pressure exceeds the pressure within the urethra, urine usually leaks past the obstruction before a urethral or bladder rupture occurs. Clinical signs associated with an anatomic urethral obstruction include dribbling of urine, straining to urinate without producing urine, restlessness, and abdominal pain. The most common causes of urethral obstruction are calculi and neoplasia in dogs and urethral plugs in cats; however, urethral strictures and granulomatous urethritis can also create obstructions to urine flow. Any type of prostatic disease in dogs may cause an outflow tract obstruction. Older male dogs with benign prostatic hyperplasia may be evaluated because of stranguria and tenesmus; however, prostatic neoplasia and prostatic abscess formation are more likely causes of urinary outflow tract obstruction in such animals.

## SMALL OR NORMAL-SIZED BLADDER

Causes of urinary incontinence in animals with a small or normal-sized bladder include urethral sphincter mechanism incompetence (USMI), detrusor hyperreflexia or instability, and congenital abnormalities. Estrogen and testosterone are believed to contribute to the integrity of urethral muscle tone by increasing its responsiveness to α-adrenergic innervation. Thus middle-aged to older, spayed female dogs are prone to the development of incontinence associated with decreased estrogen concentrations. This incontinence is most pronounced when the animal is asleep or relaxed and often responds to estrogen replacement therapy. Less frequently, incontinence develops in male dogs after castration; the condition seems to occur most commonly in dogs castrated at an older age and often responds to intramuscular testosterone administration. Diagnosis of both processes is based on the history, physical examination, and urinalysis findings (no evidence of LUTI) and on the response to therapy. Frequently, α-adrenergic treatment (e.g., phenylpropanolamine) is also effective in male and female dogs with USMI incontinence and in severe cases may be combined with hormone replacement treatment. Testosterone treatment is contraindicated in dogs that were neutered because of behavioral, prostatic, or perineal problems. In these cases, α-adrenergic treatment should be used.

Detrusor hyperreflexia or instability is the inability to control voiding because of a strong urge to urinate. Inflammation of the bladder or urethra may create a sensation of bladder fullness, which triggers the voiding reflex. Clinical signs of this type of incontinence include pollakiuria, dysuria-stranguria, and frequently hematuria. Bacterial UTI is the most common cause in the dog, and sterile LUTI is the most common cause in cats. A urinalysis that reveals evidence of urinary tract infection or inflammation (e.g., bacteriuria, pyuria, or hematuria) initially supports a tentative diagnosis of urge or inflammatory incontinence. If clinical signs persist after appropriate treatment for the urinary tract inflammation has been initiated, further diagnostic testing, including ultrasonography, contrast-enhanced radiography, and/or cystoscopy are indicated, because infiltrative disease of the bladder (e.g., neoplasia, chronic cystitis), polyps, uroliths, or urachal remnants can also result in pollakiuria and stranguria. It should also be noted that detrusor hyperreflexia/instability may also be a primary or idiopathic disorder that is not associated with bladder or urethral inflammation.

Urinary incontinence in a young animal may be associated with a variety of congenital defects of the urinary and genital systems. The most common defects are ectopic ureters and vaginal strictures, but a patent urachus, urethrorectal and urethrovaginal fistulas, and female pseudohermaphroditism have also been associated with urinary incontinence. Ectopic ureters are most commonly observed in female dogs. Breeds at high risk for ectopic ureters include Siberian Huskies, Miniature and Toy Poodles, Labrador Retrievers, Fox Terriers, West Highland White Terriers, Collies, and Welsh Corgis. Ectopic ureters are rarely seen in cats, but the gender predisposition is reversed, with the prevalence higher in male than in female animals.

The most common clinical sign in an animal with ectopic ureters is a constant dribbling of urine, although dogs and cats with a unilateral ectopic ureter may void normally. Because 70% of ectopic ureters in dogs terminate in the vagina, vaginoscopy of the vagina may allow visualization of the opening of the ectopic ureter; however, the opening can be difficult to see, even if the vagina is fully distended with air. Intravenous urography and retrograde vaginourethrography are the diagnostic tests of choice for characterizing the defect. In contrast to the incontinence associated with ectopic ureters, that associated with a vaginal stricture is often intermittent, occurring with changes in body position. Vaginal strictures can be diagnosed using digital vaginal examination, vaginoscopy, or contrast-enhanced vaginography.

## GERIATRIC INCONTINENCE

Incontinence may also be caused by senility, decreased bladder capacity, or decreased mobility in senior animals. Polyuric-polydipsic disorders such as chronic renal insufficiency-failure and diabetes mellitus in senior animals also often exacerbate incontinence. Likewise, diuretic and corticosteroid therapy should be avoided in incontinent animals because of their negative effects on urine concentration.

## *POLYDIPSIA AND POLYURIA*

Increased thirst and urine production are frequent presenting complaints in small animals. Polydipsia and polyuria in the dog and cat have been defined as a water consumption greater than 100 ml/kg/day and a urine production greater than 50 ml/kg/day, respectively. However, it is possible for thirst and urine production to be within the normal range and yet be abnormal in individual animals. Polydipsia and polyuria usually coexist, and determining the primary component of the syndrome is one of the initial diagnostic considerations in an animal showing increased water consumption and urine production.

Thirst is stimulated primarily by osmotic factors. Hyperosmolality of the extracellular fluid usually occurs secondary to water loss, or it may result from the ingestion or intravenous infusion of hypertonic solutions. This hyperosmolality results in the dehydration of osmoreceptors, which stimulates thirst. Nonosmotic factors, including decreased arterial blood pressure, increased body temperature, pain, and certain drugs, can also stimulate thirst. Thirst is inhibited by expansion of the extracellular fluid volume, increased arterial blood pressure, drinking, and fullness of the stomach. Thirst is abnormally stimulated in animals with primary polydipsia, resulting in water consumption that exceeds physiologic need. Renal function in these animals is usually normal, and secondary polyuria occurs to rid the body of the excess water.

The kidneys maintain body fluid composition and volume by resorbing water and solutes from the glomerular filtrate. The resorption of solute in excess of water results in the formation of dilute urine. Conversely, the resorption of water in excess of solute results in the formation of concentrated urine. For concentrated urine to form, antidiuretic hormone (ADH) must be produced and released, and the renal tubules must be responsive to the ADH. For the latter to occur, the renal medullary interstitium must be hypertonic and at least one third of the total nephron population must be functional. ADH is synthesized in the supraoptic and paraventricular nuclei of the hypothalamus and is stored in the posterior pituitary gland. Its release is stimulated by the same factors that stimulate thirst. In the presence of ADH, the distal portion of the distal convoluted tubule and the collecting duct become permeable to water, and water is resorbed from the tubular lumen. The hypertonicity of the renal medullary interstitium produces the osmotic pressure that drives the water resorption. A primary polyuria associated with a relative or absolute lack of ADH is termed *central* or *pituitary diabetes insipidus,* whereas a polyuria caused by nonresponsiveness to ADH is termed *nephrogenic diabetes insipidus* (Table 41-5).

 TABLE 41-5

Potential Causes of Polydipsia and Polyuria

**Primary Polydipsia**

Psychogenic
Hepatic insufficiency or portosystemic shunt

**Primary Polyuria**

Pituitary diabetes insipidus
Nephrogenic diabetes insipidus
   Renal insufficiency or failure
   Hyperadrenocorticism
   Hypoadrenocorticism
   Hepatic insufficiency
   Pyometra
   Hypercalcemia
   Hypokalemia
   Postobstructive diuresis
   Diabetes mellitus
   Normoglycemic glucosuria
   Hyperthyroidism
   Iatrogenic or drug induced
   Renal medullary solute washout

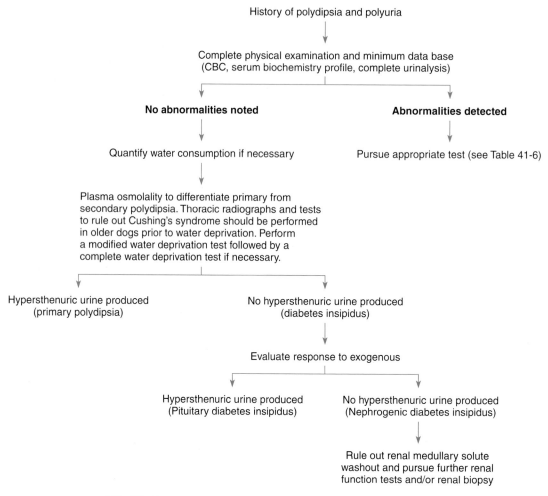

History of polydipsia and polyuria

↓

Complete physical examination and minimum data base
(CBC, serum biochemistry profile, complete urinalysis)

**No abnormalities noted**        **Abnormalities detected**

Quantify water consumption if necessary      Pursue appropriate test (see Table 41-6)

Plasma osmolality to differentiate primary from
secondary polydipsia. Thoracic radiographs and tests
to rule out Cushing's syndrome should be performed
in older dogs prior to water deprivation. Perform
a modified water deprivation test followed by a
complete water deprivation test if necessary.

Hypersthenuric urine produced      No hypersthenuric urine produced
(primary polydipsia)      (diabetes insipidus)

Evaluate response to exogenous

Hypersthenuric urine produced      No hypersthenuric urine produced
(Pituitary diabetes insipidus)      (Nephrogenic diabetes insipidus)

Rule out renal medullary solute
washout and pursue further renal
function tests and/or renal biopsy

**FIG 41-9**
Diagnostic approach to dogs and cats with polydipsia and polyuria.

Even though polydipsia and polyuria usually occur together, the owner may not be aware of one or both components, depending on their severity and how closely the animal is observed. Conversely, owners frequently confuse pollakiuria with polyuria. Polyuria is often manifested by nocturia, pollakiuria, and incontinence, whereas polydipsia is often manifested by a constantly empty water bowl and drinking from unusual sources, including toilets and puddles, and eating snow. It is relatively easy for most pet owners to measure water consumption, and this is a good way to confirm the presence of polydipsia.

A complete history and physical examination may indicate the underlying cause in animals with polydipsia and polyuria (Fig. 41-9); these include lymphadenopathy in dogs (lymphoma with hypercalcemia), perineal mass (anal sac adenocarcinoma with hypercalcemia), cataracts (diabetes mellitus), symmetric truncal alopecia (hyperadrenocorticism), vaginal discharge (pyometra), and small, irregular kidneys (chronic renal failure). A minimum workup consisting of a complete blood count, serum biochemistry profile, urinalysis, thoracic radiography, and abdominal radiography or ultrasonography may confirm or suggest a diagnosis in many animals with primary polyuria (e.g., hypercalcemia and mediastinal lymphadenopathy in dogs with lymphoma or increased serum alkaline phosphatase activity in dogs with hyperadrenocorticism). Frequently, further specific tests are necessary to confirm a diagnosis (e.g., lymph node aspiration or biopsy for lymphoma and an adrenocorticotropic hormone–stimulation test for hyperadrenocorticism [Table 41-6]).

The urine specific gravity may also be helpful in determining the underlying cause of the syndrome and in confirming whether the pet is actually polyuric. Urine specific gravity is usually divided into four ranges: hyposthenuric urine has a specific gravity of between 1.001 and 1.007; isosthenuric urine has the same specific gravity as plasma, 1.008 to 1.012; minimally concentrated urine has a specific gravity of between 1.013 and 1.030 in dogs and 1.013 and 1.035 in cats; and hypersthenuric urine has a specific gravity of more than 1.030 in dogs and more than 1.035 in cats. The animal's hydration status, serum urea nitrogen and creatinine concentrations, and current medications must be known in order to interpret random urine specific gravity values. For example, a normally hydrated dog may have a urine specific gravity in the isosthenuric range and a cat receiving furosemide may be somewhat dehydrated and

TABLE 41-6

Ancillary Diagnostic Tests That May Be Used to Evaluate Dogs and Cats with Polydipsia and Polyuria

| SUSPECTED DISORDER | FURTHER DIAGNOSTIC TESTS |
|---|---|
| Primary polydipsia | Plasma osmolality, modified water deprivation, rule out hepatic insufficiency or PSS |
| Pituitary diabetes insipidus | Plasma osmolality, modified water deprivation test, response to exogenous antidiuretic hormone |
| Nephrogenic diabetes insipidus | |
|   Renal insufficiency or failure | Serum urea nitrogen and creatinine concentrations, creatinine clearance, electrolyte fractional clearance, biopsy |
|   Hyperadrenocorticism | ACTH-stimulation test, dexamethasone-suppression test, urine cortisol/creatinine ratio |
|   Hypoadrenocorticism | Serum sodium/potassium ratio, ACTH-stimulation test |
|   Hepatic insufficiency or PSS | Serum bile acids preprandially and postprandially, abdominal ultrasonography ± Doppler, 99Tc scan (enema), portal angiography, biopsy |
|   Pyometra | Abdominal radiography or ultrasonography, vaginal cytology |
|   Hypercalcemia | Serum calcium concentrations (total and ionized), radiography, lymph node cytology or biopsy, bone marrow cytology, PTH/PTHrp assays |
|   Hypokalemia | Serum potassium concentration, potassium fractional clearance |
|   Glucosuria | Obtain concurrent serum glucose concentration |
|   Hyperthyroidism | Serum total and free thyroxine concentrations, triiodothyronine-suppression test, cardiac evaluation, 99Tc scanning |
|   Renal medullary solute washout | Repeat water deprivation and exogenous ADH testing after gradual water restriction and dietary salt and protein supplementation for 10 to 14 days |

*ACTH,* Adrenocorticotropic hormone; *ADH,* antidiuretic hormone; *PSS,* portosystemic shunt; *PTH,* parathyroid hormone; *PTHrp,* parathyroid hormone–related peptide.

still have minimally concentrated urine; however, normal dogs and cats should produce hypersthenuric urine in response to clinically detectable dehydration.

It is unusual for dogs and cats with polydipsia and polyuria to have a urine specific gravity consistently in the hypersthenuric range; this finding warrants the measurement of water consumption to confirm the polydipsia and polyuria. Animals with primary polydipsia or with central diabetes insipidus usually have urine specific gravities in the hyposthenuric range, whereas animals with nephrogenic diabetes insipidus are most likely to be isosthenuric or to have minimally concentrated urine. If the history, physical examination, and minimal diagnostic workup findings are unrewarding, specialized diagnostic tests, including determination of the plasma osmolality, water deprivation testing, and determination of the animal's response to exogenous ADH, may be necessary to arrive at a diagnosis (see Chapter 42 and Fig. 41-6).

## PROTEINURIA

Normally the urine of dogs and cats contains only a small amount of protein, because the selective permeability of the glomerular capillary wall restricts the filtration of most plasma proteins on the basis of protein weight and charge. Proteins with a molecular weight greater than 60,000 to 65,000 daltons are normally not present in large quantities in the glomerular filtrate (Table 41-7). The negatively charged glomerular capillary wall further impedes the passage of negatively charged proteins such as albumin. In addition,

 TABLE 41-7

Approximate Molecular Weights of Various Plasma Proteins

| PLASMA PROTEIN | MOLECULAR WEIGHT (DALTONS) |
|---|---|
| Insulin | 6000 |
| Parathyroid hormone | 9000 |
| Lysozyme | 14,000 |
| Myoglobin | 17,000 |
| Growth hormone | 22,000 |
| Bence Jones proteins (monomer) | 22,000 |
| Amylase | 50,000 |
| Hemoglobin | 64,500 |
| Antithrombin | 65,000 |
| Albumin | 69,000 |
| Immunoglobulin G | 160,000 |
| Immunoglobulin A (dimer) | 300,000 |
| Fibrinogen | 400,000 |
| Immunoglobulin M | 900,000 |

smaller-molecular-weight proteins, as well as those positively charged proteins that do pass through the glomerular capillary wall, are largely resorbed by the proximal tubular epithelial cells. Such resorbed proteins may be broken down and used by the epithelial cells or returned to the bloodstream. Protein resorption by tubular epithelial cells, however, has a transport maximum, and proteinuria ensues if that maximum is exceeded. Urine protein also results from the secretion of enzymes, mucoproteins, and immunoglobulins by tubular and lower urinary and genital tract epithelial cells. These secreted proteins may account for as much as 50% of the proteins that are normally present in urine.

When one first evaluates a cat or dog with proteinuria, it is important to identify its source. Proteinuria may be caused by physiologic or pathologic conditions (Table 41-8). Physiologic or benign proteinuria is often transient and abates when the underlying cause is corrected. Strenuous exercise, seizures, fever, exposure to extreme heat or cold, and stress are examples of conditions that may cause physiologic proteinuria. The pathophysiology of physiologic proteinuria is not completely understood; however, relative renal vasoconstriction, ischemia, and congestion are thought to be involved. Decreased physical activity may also affect urine protein excretion in dogs; one study showed that urinary protein loss is higher in dogs confined to cages than in dogs with normal activity. This is different from the postural or orthostatic proteinuria that occurs in people. In this latter condition, mild proteinuria occurs when the person is standing or active but diminishes when the person is recumbent.

Pathologic proteinuria may be caused by urinary or nonurinary abnormalities. Nonurinary disorders associated with proteinuria often involve the production of small-molecular-weight proteins that are filtered by the glomeruli and that subsequently overwhelm the resorptive capacity of the proximal tubule. Examples of this include the production of immunoglobulin light chains (Bence Jones proteins) by neoplastic plasma cells and the release of hemoglobin from damaged red blood cells, which then exceeds the binding capacity of haptoglobin. Renal congestion secondary to congestive heart failure can also result in pathologic nonurinary proteinuria, as can genital tract inflammation (e.g., prostatitis or metritis).

Pathologic urinary proteinuria may be renal or nonrenal in origin. Nonrenal proteinuria most frequently occurs in association with lower urinary tract inflammation or hemorrhage. Changes seen in the urine sediment usually reflect the underlying cause (e.g., urolithiasis, neoplasia, trauma, bacterial cystitis). On the other hand, renal proteinuria is most often caused by glomerular lesions. Glomerulonephritis and amyloidosis alter the selective permeability of the glomerular capillaries and frequently result in a proteinuria greater than 50 mg/kg/24 hours or urine protein/creatinine ratios greater than 3.0 (see Chapter 42). The occurrence of persistent proteinuria with a normal urine sediment or accompanied by hyaline cast formation is strongly suggestive of glomerular disease. Besides glomerular disease, renal proteinuria may be caused by inflammatory or infiltrative disorders of the kidney (e.g., neoplasia, pyelonephritis) or by tubular abnormalities that result in the decreased resorption of filtered protein (e.g., Fanconi's syndrome).

Proteinuria is routinely detected by semiquantitative methods, including the dipstick colorimetric test and the sulfosalicylic turbidimetric test. The dipstick test is inexpensive and easy to use; amino groups of proteins bind to the indicator incorporated in the filter paper on the dipstick and cause a color change. The color change is graded by comparing it to a standard, but the comparison is subjective. The dipstick test is most sensitive to albumin, because albumin has more free amino groups than globulins or Bence Jones proteins. False-positive results may be obtained if the urine is alkaline, if it has been contaminated with quaternary ammonium compounds, or if the dipstick is left in contact with the urine long enough to leach out the citrate buffer that is incorporated in the filter paper pad. False-negative results may occur in the setting of Bence Jones proteinuria or dilute or acidic urine. The dipstick test can detect approximately 30 to 1000 mg of protein per deciliter. The dipstick method is not affected by urine turbidity; however, the supernatant from centrifuged urine samples should ideally be used for all physiochemical analyses.

The sulfosalicylic acid test is performed by mixing equal quantities of urine supernate and 5% sulfosalicylic acid, and subjectively grading the turbidity that results from precipitation of protein on a 0 to 4+ scale. This test is also more sensitive to albumin than globulins, but Bence Jones proteinuria can be detected. False-positive results may occur if the urine contains radiographic contrast agents, penicillin, cephalosporins, sulfisoxazole, or the urine preservative thymol. The protein content may be overestimated with the sulfosalicylic acid test if uncentrifuged urine or turbid urine is analyzed. False-negative results may occur if the urine is markedly alkaline or diluted. Because the varying degrees of turbidity are not standardized, results may also vary among laboratories. This test can detect

## TABLE 41-8

**Classification of Proteinuria**

| TYPE | CAUSES |
|---|---|
| Physiologic | Strenuous exercise |
| | Seizures |
| | Fever |
| | Exposure to heat or cold |
| | Stress |
| | Decreased activity level (strict cage rest) |
| Pathologic | |
|   Nonurinary | Bence Jones proteinuria |
| | Hemoglobinuria or myoglobinuria |
| | Congestive heart failure |
| | Genital tract inflammation |
|   Urinary | |
|     Nonrenal | Cystourolithiasis |
| | Bacterial cystitis |
| | Trauma or hemorrhage |
| | Neoplasia |
| | Drug-induced cystitis (e.g., cyclophosphamide) |
|     Renal | Glomerular lesions |
| | Abnormal tubular resorption |
| | Renal parenchymal inflammation or hemorrhage |

approximately 5 to 5000 mg of protein per deciliter. Further information on such tests is contained in Chapter 42.

Proteinuria detected by these semiquantitative methods should always be interpreted in light of the urine specific gravity and urine sediment, because a significant amount of urine protein may be overlooked if urine is dilute. Conversely, a protein reaction of trace or 1+ may be normal in an animal with concentrated urine. For example, a 2+ proteinuria with a 1.010 urine specific gravity is suggestive of a much greater urine protein loss on a 24-hour basis than is a 2+ proteinuria with a 1.040 urine specific gravity. Because the urine protein concentration is frequently increased in animals with lower urinary tract inflammation or hemorrhage, proteinuria should also be assessed in the context of urine sediment changes indicative of inflammation or hemorrhage (e.g., bacteria and increased numbers of white and red blood cells and epithelial cells in the urine sediment). The evaluation of the animal with proteinuria is further discussed in Chapter 42.

Prerenal (physiologic and pathologic—nonurinary) and postrenal (pathologic urinary—nonrenal) proteinuria, as well as inflammatory renal proteinuria, can usually be identified on the basis of history and physical examination findings and the urine sediment changes. Renal proteinuria caused by abnormal tubular resorption is frequently accompanied by normoglycemic glucosuria and an abnormal urinary loss of electrolytes, which helps differentiate tubular from glomerular proteinuria. It is important to identify the source of the proteinuria, because the quantification of glomerular proteinuria can be a helpful prognostic tool, although it is not useful in animals with prerenal or postrenal proteinuria.

## AZOTEMIA

Azotemia is defined as increased concentrations of urea and creatinine (and other nonproteinaceous nitrogenous substances) in the blood. The interpretation of serum urea nitrogen and creatinine concentrations as a measure of renal function requires a knowledge of the production and excretion of these substances. Urea is synthesized in the liver from ammonia, which is in turn generated from the catabolism of ingested and endogenous proteins. Urea production is increased in the settings of a high dietary protein intake, upper gastrointestinal tract hemorrhage, and catabolic states that result in the breakdown of body proteins (e.g., corticosteroid administration). Conversely, urea production is decreased in the settings of a low dietary protein intake, decreased hepatic function, or decreased delivery of ammonia to the liver (e.g., portosystemic shunt). Urea has a small molecular weight (60 daltons) and is a permeate solute that readily diffuses throughout all body fluid compartments; its concentration is similar in intracellular and extracellular fluid and in plasma, serum, and blood. Urea that diffuses into the intestinal lumen is degraded by enteric organisms to ammonia, which is then reabsorbed into the portal circulation and again converted to urea by the liver. Urea is principally excreted by the kidneys; it is freely filtered through the glomeruli and passively re-

sorbed by the renal tubules. The tubular resorption of urea is increased when tubular flow rates and volumes are decreased. Conversely, the tubular resorption of urea is decreased and excretion increased in the presence of diuresis. Decreased renal blood flow (prerenal causes, such as dehydration or decreased cardiac output) and decreased excretion of urine (postrenal causes, such as urethral obstruction or ruptured bladder), as well as primary renal dysfunction, will result in decreased excretion of urea.

Creatinine is irreversibly formed by the nonenzymatic metabolism of creatine and phosphocreatine in muscle. Creatinine production is relatively constant and proportional to muscle mass; animals with a large muscle mass produce more creatinine each day than do animals with a small muscle mass. Muscle trauma and inflammation do not increase the production of creatinine. In comparison with the urea nitrogen concentration, the creatinine concentration is relatively unaffected by the dietary protein level; however, serum creatinine concentrations can increase after the ingestion of meat and the subsequent increased absorption of creatinine from the gastrointestinal tract. The molecular weight of creatinine is 113 daltons, therefore it diffuses throughout body fluid compartments more slowly than urea does. Some creatinine diffuses into the intestinal lumen, is degraded by enteric bacteria, and is excreted from the body in the feces; however, most creatinine is excreted by the kidneys. Creatinine is freely filtered by the glomeruli and is not significantly resorbed or secreted by the renal tubules. Because the production of creatinine is relatively constant, an increase in the serum creatinine concentration is indicative of decreased renal excretion. It is important to remember, however, that prerenal and postrenal factors influence renal function and, therefore, the excretion of creatinine. Disproportionate increases in blood urea nitrogen (BUN) relative to creatinine can be caused by high-protein diets, upper gastrointestinal hemorrhage, and increased tubular reabsorption of urea nitrogen associated with prerenal azotemia. Conversely, a disproportionately low BUN can be observed with decreased liver function, portosystemic shunts, low-protein diets, and prolonged diuresis.

Although increased production of urea may result in an increased BUN concentration, the production of creatinine is relatively stable. Therefore, when an animal presents with azotemia, decreased renal excretion should be the main diagnostic consideration. The decreased renal excretion of urea nitrogen and creatinine may result from extrarenal (prerenal and postrenal) or primary renal causes. Any condition that causes a decrease in renal blood flow may result in prerenal azotemia, and this includes hypovolemia (e.g., dehydration, hypoadrenocorticism), hypotension (e.g., anesthesia, cardiomyopathy), and aortic or renal arterial thrombus formation. Initially the kidneys are structurally and functionally normal in dogs and cats with prerenal azotemia, and they respond to the decreased renal blood flow by conserving water and sodium. Hypersthenuric urine (i.e., specific gravity greater than 1.030 in dogs and greater than 1.035 in cats) with a relatively low concentration of sodium and a high concentration

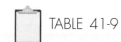

TABLE 41-9

**Differentiation of Prerenal Azotemia from Acute Renal Failure**

| INDICES | PRERENAL AZOTEMIA | ACUTE RENAL FAILURE |
|---|---|---|
| Urine specific gravity | Hypersthenuric | Isosthenuric or minimally concentrated |
| Fractional clearance of sodium (Urine$_{Na}$ × Serum $_{Cr}$/(Urine$_{Cr}$ × Serum$_{Na}$) | <1% | >2% |
| Urine creatinine-to-serum creatinine ratio | >20:1 | <10:1 |

of creatinine is produced (Table 41-9). Elimination of the underlying disorder (e.g., fluid therapy to correct hypovolemia) results in rapid resolution of the azotemia unless the underlying disorder has persisted long enough or is severe enough to have caused renal parenchymal damage.

Postrenal azotemia is usually caused by an obstruction to urine outflow or a rupture of the urine outflow tract. Similar to prerenal azotemia, in postrenal azotemia the kidneys are initially normal; however, the urine specific gravity varies, depending on the animal's hydration status. In patients with urethral obstruction, catheterization is difficult and dysuria and stranguria are common clinical signs. Rupture of the urinary tract usually involves the bladder or urethra, is more common in male than female animals, and frequently results in abdominal effusion or subcutaneous fluid accumulation. Fluid obtained by abdominocentesis is usually sterile and contains a higher concentration of creatinine than the serum does. Even though creatinine is a small molecule and equilibrates rapidly, the concentration of creatinine in the abdominal fluid will be higher than that of serum if the kidneys are producing urine that is draining into the abdomen. Positive contrast–enhanced urethrography or cystography is the best way to confirm a rupture of the urethra or bladder.

Renal azotemia occurs as a result of nephron loss or damage and is usually associated with renal failure. A diagnosis of renal azotemia is confirmed if the azotemia is persistently associated with isosthenuria or minimally concentrated urine (see Table 41-9). Inasmuch as urine is usually stored in the bladder for several hours, it is important not to evaluate the specific gravity of urine produced before the onset of the azotemia. For example, prerenal azotemia may occur in response to acute, severe dehydration; however, the animal may appear to have renal azotemia if the hypersthenuric urine being produced in response to the dehydration is diluted by a larger volume of previously formed, less concentrated urine. The differentiation of prerenal from renal azotemia can be a diagnostic challenge in some animals. Prerenal dehydration causing azotemia and accompanied by a decreased urine-concentrating ability can be confused with renal azotemia. Examples of conditions that can cause this syndrome include furosemide treatment, which causes dehydration, and hypercalcemia, which compromises the urine-concentrating ability and results in dehydration secondary to vomiting. Although fluid therapy is often implemented initially in animals with

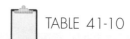

TABLE 41-10

**Differentiation of Acute from Chronic Renal Failure on the Basis of History, Clinical Signs, and Clinical Pathology Data**

| ACUTE RENAL FAILURE | CHRONIC RENAL FAILURE |
|---|---|
| History of ischemia or toxicant exposure | History of renal disease or polydipsia-polyuria |
| Normal or increased hematocrit value | Nonregenerative anemia |
| Swollen kidneys | Small, irregular kidneys |
| Hyperkalemia (with oliguria) | Normal or hypokalemia |
| More severe metabolic acidosis | Normal or mild metabolic acidosis |
| Active urine sediment | Inactive urine sediment |
| Good body condition | Weight loss |
| Relatively severe clinical signs for level of dysfunction | Relatively mild clinical signs for level of dysfunction |

either prerenal or renal azotemia to manage the dehydration, the prognosis is quite different. Frequently the response to fluid therapy is the best way to differentiate prerenal from renal azotemia; renal azotemia does not completely resolve in response to fluid therapy alone.

Renal failure is a state of decreased renal function in which azotemia and the inability to produce hypersthenuric urine persist concurrently. The treatment and prognosis vary for animals with acute and chronic renal failure; therefore it is important to distinguish between these two entities. Acute renal failure (ARF) develops within hours or days. Unique clinical signs and clinicopathologic findings often associated with ARF include enlarged or swollen kidneys, hemoconcentration, good body condition, an active urine sediment, relatively severe hyperkalemia and metabolic acidosis, and relatively severe clinical signs for the degree of azotemia (Table 41-10). Chronic renal failure (CRF) develops over a period of weeks, months, or years, and the clinical signs are often relatively mild for the magnitude of azotemia. Unique signs of CRF often include a history of weight loss and polydipsia-polyuria, poor body condition, nonregenerative anemia, small and irregular kidneys, and osseous fibrodystrophy caused by secondary renal hyperparathyroidism (see Table 41-10).

## RENOMEGALY

Renal enlargement is usually detected by physical examination or by abdominal radiography or ultrasonography. A quick rule of thumb is that the kidney length on abdominal radiographs should be approximately equivalent to 2.5 to 3.0 times the length of the second lumbar vertebra in cats and 2.5 to 3.5 times length of the second lumbar vertebra in dogs. Enlarged kidneys with a normal shape can be caused by edema, acute inflammation, diffusely infiltrating neoplastic disease, unilateral compensatory hypertrophy, trauma (intracapsular hemorrhage), or hydronephrosis. Enlarged, abnormally shaped kidneys may be caused by renal neoplasia, cysts, abscesses, hydronephrosis, or hematomas. Ultrasonography and intravenous urography can be used to further define kidney shape and reveal internal details. Ultrasonography is particularly useful for evaluating enlarged kidneys associated with fluid accumulation (e.g., hydronephrosis, abscesses, and perirenal and parenchymal cysts) and can also be used to guide fine-needle aspiration or needle biopsy of the affected kidney. Kidney biopsy is often necessary to confirm the cause of the renomegaly; however, biopsy is contraindicated if only one kidney is present or if a bleeding disorder, hydronephrosis, a cyst, or an abscess is suspected.

### Suggested Readings

Bartges JW: Discolored urine. In Ettinger SJ et al, editors: *Textbook of veterinary internal medicine*, ed 5, Philadelphia, 2000, WB Saunders, p 96.

Bartges JW et al: Clinical algorithms and data bases for urinary tract disorders. In Osborne CA et al, editors: *Canine and feline nephrology and urology*, Philadelphia, 1995, Williams & Wilkins, p 68.

Krawiec DR: Proteinuria. In Ettinger SJ et al, editors: *Textbook of veterinary internal medicine*, ed 5, Philadelphia, 2000, WB Saunders, p 100.

Lane IF: Urinary obstruction and functional urine retention. In Ettinger SJ et al, editors: *Textbook of veterinary internal medicine*, ed 5, Philadelphia, 2000, WB Saunders, p 93.

Lees GE: Incontinence, enuresis, dysuria, and nocturia. In Ettinger SJ et al, editors: *Textbook of veterinary internal medicine*, ed 5, Philadelphia, 2000, WB Saunders, p 89.

Meric SM: Polyuria and polydipsia. In Ettinger SJ et al, editors: *Textbook of veterinary internal medicine*, ed 5, Philadelphia, 1995, WB Saunders, p 85.

Osborne CA: Techniques of urine collection and preservation. In Osborne CA et al, editors: *Canine and feline nephrology and urology*, Philadelphia, 1995, Williams & Wilkins, p 100.

# CHAPTER 42

# Diagnostic Tests for the Urinary System

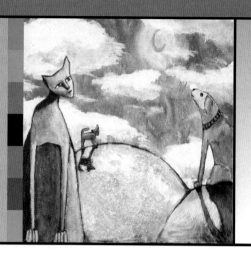

## CHAPTER OUTLINE

RENAL EXCRETORY FUNCTION, 584
    Glomerular filtration rate, 584
    Fractional clearance, 585
QUANTIFICATION OF PROTEINURIA, 586
PLASMA AND URINE OSMOLALITY, WATER
DEPRIVATION TEST, AND RESPONSE TO
EXOGENOUS ANTIDIURETIC HORMONE, 587
BLADDER AND URETHRAL FUNCTION, 588
BACTERIAL ANTIBIOTIC SENSITIVITY TESTING, 588
DIAGNOSTIC IMAGING, 589
CYSTOSCOPY, 596
RENAL BIOPSY, 598

## RENAL EXCRETORY FUNCTION

### GLOMERULAR FILTRATION RATE

Serum urea nitrogen and creatinine concentrations provide a crude index of the glomerular filtration rate (GFR). However, inasmuch as the creatinine concentration is influenced by fewer extrarenal variables and creatinine is not resorbed by the renal tubules, the serum creatinine concentration is a better index of GFR than the BUN. Nevertheless, azotemia resulting from impaired renal function is not detectable until approximately three fourths of the nephrons in both kidneys are nonfunctional. This percentage may be even higher in dogs and cats with chronic progressive renal disease, because the remaining viable nephrons often undergo compensatory hypertrophy. Therefore renal clearance and measurement of GFR can provide more accurate information about renal excretory function than the serum creatinine and urea nitrogen concentrations, especially early in renal disease, before three fourths of the nephrons have been destroyed.

Renal clearance is the rate at which a substance is completely cleared from a certain volume of plasma. Substances used to measure renal clearance must be freely filtered by the glomerulus (not protein-bound) and not affected by tubular resorption or secretion or by metabolism elsewhere in the body. In addition, the substance used must not alter renal function. The renal clearance of inulin is the gold standard method of determining GFR; however, it is difficult to measure the inulin concentration in plasma and urine. On the other hand, it is relatively easy to determine the renal clearance of creatinine, and therefore more practical. The renal clearance of creatinine can be calculated by multiplying the concentration of creatinine in urine by the rate of urine production and then dividing the product by the serum concentration of creatinine, as follows:

$$\text{Volume of plasma cleared (ml/min)} = \text{GFR (ml/min)} = \frac{(\text{Urine}_{Cr}[\text{mg/dl}] \times \text{Urine volume [ml/min]})}{\text{Serum}_{Cr}(\text{mg/dl})}$$

For example, if the urine creatinine concentration is 60 mg/dl, urine flow is 3 ml/min, and the serum creatinine concentration is 1.8 mg/dl, 100 ml of plasma is cleared of creatinine per minute. This value is divided by the animal's body weight in kilograms and expressed in milliliters per minute per kilogram. Note that prerenal and postrenal factors, as well as renal parenchymal lesions, influence plasma clearance.

The GFR can be calculated using the clearance of either endogenous or exogenous creatinine. Endogenous creatinine clearance, however, requires urine collection for a lengthy period (i.e., 24 hours) to minimize errors in the collection, thus necessitating the use of indwelling catheters, repeated urinary catheterization, or the use of metabolism cages for urine collection. Endogenous creatinine clearance is frequently used in the clinical setting to evaluate renal excretory function if renal dysfunction is suspected, but the serum urea nitrogen and creatinine concentrations are within normal ranges. Less commonly, endogenous creatinine clearance can be used to better quantify renal excretory function in animals with azotemia. A serum sample obtained approximately midway through the urine collection period and a well-mixed aliquot from the 24-hour urine sample are used to measure creatinine concentrations. The volume of urine collected is divided by 1440, the number of minutes in 24 hours (Table 42-1). One drawback to this method, however, is the fact that noncreatinine chromogens present in the serum falsely increase serum creatinine concentrations if the standard alkaline picrate method of analysis is used. In fact, noncreatinine chromogens can ac-

TABLE 42-1

**Calculation of Endogenous Creatinine Clearance, 24-Hour Urine Protein Excretion, and Urine Protein/Creatinine Ratio**

---

**Data**

Body weight = 20 kg
24-hour urine volume = 400 ml (4.0 dl)
Urine protein concentration = 650 mg/dl
Urine creatinine concentration = 110 mg/dl
Serum creatinine concentration = 1.9 mg/dl
Time—24 hours = 1440 minutes

**Calculations**

Endogenous creatinine clearance =

$$\frac{(\text{Urine}_{Cr}) \times (\text{Urine volume})}{(\text{Serum}_{Cr}) \times (\text{Time}) \times (\text{Body weight})}, \text{ or}$$

$$\frac{(110 \text{ mg/dl}) \times (400 \text{ ml})}{(1.9 \text{ mg/dl}) \times (1440 \text{ min}) \times (20 \text{ kg})} =$$

$$0.8 \text{ ml/min/kg}$$

24-hour urine protein excretion =

$$\frac{(650 \text{ mg/dl}) \times (4.0 \text{ dl})}{(20 \text{ kg})} = 130 \text{ mg/kg}$$

**Data**

Urine protein from random urine sample = 750 mg/dl
Urine creatinine from random urine sample = 120 mg/dl

**Calculation**

Urine protein/creatinine ratio =
$$(750 \text{ mg/dl})/(120 \text{ mg/dl}) = 6.25$$
$$6.25 \times 20 \text{ (linear regression conversion factor)} =$$
$$125 \text{ mg of urine protein/kg/24 hours}$$

---

count for a significant percentage of the total amount of chromagens in animals with serum creatinine concentrations within normal ranges. Because noncreatinine chromogens are not excreted in the urine, the calculated endogenous creatinine clearance can be falsely decreased. Despite this problem, endogenous creatinine clearance has been shown to closely approximate inulin clearance in dogs and cats. Normal values for endogenous creatinine clearance in the dog and cat are 2.8 to 3.7 and 2 to 3 ml/min/kg, respectively.

The clearance of exogenous creatinine can be determined over a relatively short period, and because the serum creatinine concentration is considerably increased, the effect of noncreatinine chromogens is largely negated. Measurement of exogenous creatinine clearance is most appropriate in nonazotemic animals. Initially a constant intravenous infusion of creatinine was used in the test; however, research has shown that a single subcutaneous injection of 100 mg of creatinine per kilogram of body weight (Sigma Chemicals, St. Louis) can be used instead. Urine is collected for 20 minutes, starting 40 minutes after the injection, and serum samples are obtained at the start and end of the collection period (the average of the two serum creatinine concentrations is used to calculate creatinine clearance). Because of the short collection period, it is important to rinse the bladder with a sterile saline solution at the start and end of the collection. To increase the accuracy of this technique, two 20-minute clearances can be calculated and averaged. Normal exogenous creatinine clearance values are 3.5 to 4.5 ml/min/kg in dogs and 2.4 to 3.3 ml/min/kg in cats.

Plasma clearance of iohexol, an iodinated radiographic contrast agent, has been shown to reliably estimate GFR in dogs and cats. Because calculation of iohexol clearance does not require urine collection, the procedure is less labor intensive and invasive compared with creatinine clearance. Plasma concentrations of iohexol can be determined at university teaching hospitals or specialized reference laboratories.

Renal scintigraphy using technetium 99m–labeled diethylenetriaminepentaacetic acid also allows the GFR to be evaluated and is available at several universities and major referral centers. This is a quick, noninvasive method that does not require urinary catheterization and has the advantage of being able to quantitatively evaluate individual kidney function. Disadvantages of this procedure include its limited availability, exposure of the animal to radioisotopes, and the need for radioisotope disposal.

## FRACTIONAL CLEARANCE

The clearance of various solutes in the urine may be compared with the clearance of creatinine in the urine to assess the degree of tubular resorption or secretion. Because the renal clearance of creatinine is relatively constant over time, expressing the renal clearance of a solute as a percentage of the clearance of creatinine gauges the body's attempt to conserve or excrete the solute. The fractional clearance (FC) of a solute (S) is the quotient of the urine/serum solute ratio divided by the urine/serum creatinine ratio ($[\text{Urine}_S/\text{Serum}_S]/[\text{Urine}_{Cr}/\text{Serum}_{Cr}]$). A timed urine collection is not necessary to determine the FC of a solute. Some solutes, including glucose and amino acids, are normally highly conserved, whereas electrolytes such as sodium, chloride, potassium, calcium, and phosphorus are variably conserved. In normal dogs and cats, the FCs of sodium, chloride, and calcium are less than 1%; however, the FCs of potassium and phosphorus are more variable and may be as high as 20% and 39%, respectively. The FC of electrolytes should be determined only after a 12- to 15-hour fast, because dietary intake and intestinal absorption can influence the renal excretion of electrolytes. When determining the FCs of predominantly intracellular electrolytes such as potassium, magnesium, and phosphorus, however, the previous diet may still affect the FC results, even after a 15-hour fast. The alternative is to feed the animal a standard diet for several days before the FC determination.

Examples of situations in which a knowledge of the FC of electrolytes may be helpful include (1) the diagnosis of primary hyperparathyroidism, in which the FC of phosphorus is increased; (2) the diagnosis of tubular dysfunction, such as Fanconi's syndrome, in which the FCs of all electrolytes are increased; and (3) the differentiation of prerenal azotemia, in which the FC of sodium is decreased, from acute renal failure, in which the FC of sodium is increased (>2%) (see Table 41-9). In addition, the FCs of electrolytes can be monitored on a daily basis in dogs and cats receiving potentially nephrotoxic drugs such as gentamicin. Twofold to threefold increases over baseline values can indicate the presence of tubular damage before overt azotemia occurs.

## QUANTIFICATION OF PROTEINURIA

If the results of the dipstick or sulfosalicylic acid test for proteinuria (see Chapter 41) indicate the presence of a significant proteinuria in light of the urine specific gravity, and the urine sediment examination findings are normal (i.e., renal proteinuria is suspected), urine protein excretion should be quantified. This helps to evaluate the severity of renal lesions and to assess the response to treatment or the progression of disease. The trichloroacetic acid-*N*-Ponceau S, Coomassie brilliant blue, or benzethonium chloride tests are the most common methods used to quantify urine protein and are available at referral centers and reference laboratories. The 24-hour collection of urine with the measurement of urine protein excretion in milligrams per kilogram per 24 hours has been the time-honored method for quantifying proteinuria, because errors caused by a variation in urine volume are minimized by a 24-hour collection (see Table 42-1). However, such collections require the use of a metabolism cage or of indwelling or repeated urinary catheterization, making the procedure cumbersome and expensive. In addition, incomplete collection of all urine produced during the 24-hour period results in errors.

Renal proteinuria occurs mainly as a result of lesions involving the glomerular capillary wall. However, by resorbing water from the glomerular filtrate, the renal tubules can markedly alter urine volume and therefore the protein concentration in a random urine sample. Inasmuch as creatinine is freely filtered through the glomeruli without significant secretion or reabsorption by the renal tubules, the concentration of creatinine in urine is a reflection of urine volume. By dividing the urine protein concentration (in milligrams per deciliter) by the urine creatinine concentration (in milligrams per deciliter), the effect of urine volume on the urine protein concentration is negated.

The urine protein/creatinine ratio in canine and feline urine samples has been shown to accurately reflect the quantity of protein excreted in the urine over a 24-hour period. This test has greatly facilitated the diagnosis of glomerulonephritis in small animals. Most studies have shown that normal urine protein excretion in dogs and cats is less than 10 to 20 mg/kg/24 hours. A regression-line equation allows for the urine protein/creatinine ratio, when multiplied by 20 (Lulich and colleague, 1990), to be converted to milligrams of protein per kilogram per 24 hours (see Table 42-1). Therefore a urine protein/creatinine ratio of less than 0.5 to 1 is considered normal in dogs and cats. A complete urinalysis should always be performed before or along with determination of the urine protein/creatinine ratio, because hematuria or pyuria may indicate the presence of nonglomerular proteinuria. If there is evidence of inflammation (e.g., pyuria, bacteriuria), the protein concentration should be measured again after successful treatment of the inflammatory disorder. The urine protein/creatinine ratio cannot be used to differentiate between glomerular proteinuria and proteinuria associated with lower urinary tract inflammation or hemorrhage.

No relationship appears to exist between urinary protein excretion and GFR in dogs with renal disease; however, the magnitude of the proteinuria does appear to correlate roughly with the nature of the glomerular lesion. In several studies, although there was overlap, urine protein excretion in dogs with glomerulonephritis was greater than that in dogs with glomerular atrophy or interstitial nephritis but lower than that in dogs with amyloidosis.

Recently an antigen capture enzyme-linked immunosorbent assay (ELISA) test for the detection of low levels of albumin in canine urine (microalbuminuria) has become commercially available (E.R.D.-Screen, Heska Corp., Fort Collins, Colo). Microalbuminuria is usually defined as a urine albumin concentration between 1.0 and 30 mg/dl. These are concentrations too low to be routinely detected by standard dipstick screening tests. It is interesting to note that the presence of microalbuminuria has been shown to be an accurate predictor of subsequent renal disease in human beings with both systemic hypertension and diabetes mellitus, and it has also been observed in human beings with systemic diseases that are associated with glomerulopathy. Studies in dogs have shown the prevalence of microalbuminuria in apparently healthy dogs and Soft-Coated Wheaten Terriers genetically predisposed to developing glomerular disease to be 19% and 76%, respectively (Jensen and colleagues, 2001; Vaden and colleagues, 2001). In additional studies, development of microalbuminuria preceded the development of overt albuminuria in dogs with experimentally induced heartworm disease (Grauer and colleagues, 2002) and in dogs with X-linked hereditary nephropathy (Lees and colleagues, 2002). Further study is necessary to determine whether microalbuminuria is an accurate predictor of overt proteinuria and renal disease in dogs and cats. If microalbuminuria does predict overt proteinuria and/or renal disease, this early detection tool should increase our ability to alter the disease's progression.

Urine and serum protein electrophoresis may help in identifying the source of the proteinuria and in establishing a prognosis. For example, proteinuria associated with hemorrhage into the urinary tract has an electrophoretic pattern very similar to that of serum. Early glomerular damage usually results principally in albuminuria; however, as the glomerular disease progresses, an increasing amount of globulin may be lost as well. Marked hypoalbuminemia and increased concentrations of larger-molecular-weight proteins in the serum indicate the presence of severe glomerular proteinuria and the nephrotic syndrome.

## PLASMA AND URINE OSMOLALITY, WATER DEPRIVATION TEST, AND RESPONSE TO EXOGENOUS ANTIDIURETIC HORMONE

Measurement of plasma osmolality may aid in the determination of the primary component of the polydipsia and polyuria syndrome. Normal plasma osmolality in dogs and cats is 280 to 310 mOsm/kg. Plasma osmolality in animals with a primary polydipsia is usually low (275 to 285 mOsm/kg), reflecting the dilutional effect of excessive water consumption. In contrast, animals with a primary polyuria often have high plasma osmolalities (305 to 315 mOsm/kg) because of their inability to concentrate urine and the resultant dehydration (see Fig. 41-9). However, there can also be considerable overlap in randomly obtained plasma osmolalities between animals with primary polydipsic and those with primary polyuric disorders.

Determination of a urine/plasma osmolality ratio allows a more precise determination of urine concentration than does urine specific gravity alone, because specific gravity measures the density of urine rather than the number of particles in solution. For example, moderate-to-marked glucosuria or proteinuria increases urine specific gravity more than the urine osmolality. In response to dehydration, normal dogs and cats should be able to form urine that is five to six times more concentrated than plasma. Plasma and urine osmolality may be determined using either a vapor pressure or freezing point depression osmometer, and measurement is available at a reasonable cost at human hospitals, veterinary teaching hospitals, and reference laboratories.

Water deprivation causes dehydration and plasma hyperosmolality and allows the neurohypophyseal-renal axis to be evaluated. Water deprivation tests are used to differentiate diabetes insipidus from primary polydipsia and should be performed only after other causes of polyuria and polydipsia have been ruled out on the basis of the findings from physical examination and a minimum database. It should be noted that water deprivation tests are potentially dangerous. They should therefore be performed only under close observation and after water intake has been gradually reduced (see later discussion), because failure to produce concentrated urine (i.e., diabetes insipidus) may result in severe dehydration and potential ischemic renal injury. Increases in plasma osmolality of 1% to 2% above normal stimulate the release of antidiuretic hormone (ADH), and normal kidneys should respond to this ADH by producing hypersthenuric urine. The water deprivation test is ended when the animal loses 5% of its body weight as a result of dehydration, becomes azotemic, becomes hyperosmolemic (plasma osmolality of greater than 320 mOsm/kg), or produces hypersthenuric urine (specific gravity of greater than 1.030 in dogs or greater than 1.035 in cats). It is important to obtain accurate baseline values and to make sure the bladder is emptied each time the urine specific gravity or osmolality is measured so that urine produced between evaluations is not diluted by previously formed urine. Plasma osmolality constitutes a good measure of hydration status during water deprivation, and in fact a water deprivation test may not be necessary if it is measured at baseline. The finding of a baseline plasma osmolality of 320 mOsm/kg or greater in a clinically nondehydrated dog or cat with hyposthenuria or isosthenuria indicates a failure of the neurohypophyseal-renal axis. Similarly, a water deprivation test should not be performed in an animal that is clinically dehydrated or azotemic and that has hyposthenuria, isosthenuria, or minimally concentrated urine, because these conditions already demonstrate a failure of the neurohypophyseal-renal axis. The time it takes to reach the end-point of a water deprivation test is variable; small dogs and cats may dehydrate within several hours, whereas significant dehydration may not occur in large dogs for 36 to 48 hours. Animals that fail to produce hypersthenuric urine in response to water deprivation have either pituitary or nephrogenic diabetes insipidus.

A pharmacologic dose of ADH may be administered to differentiate pituitary diabetes insipidus (lack of ADH) from nephrogenic diabetes insipidus (no response to ADH). Aqueous ADH (3 to 5 U given intramuscularly) is commonly used for diagnostic testing, although synthetic desmopressin acetate nasal spray, given as drops in the conjunctival sac, or an injectable preparation of desmopressin acetate, given subcutaneously (3 to 5 U), may also be used. The ADH should be administered immediately at the end-point of the water deprivation test, before water is made available, in animals that do not respond to water deprivation. It is important that the bladder be empty immediately before the administration of ADH so that the urine produced in response to ADH is not diluted by previously formed urine. Animals with pituitary diabetes insipidus usually respond by producing urine with greatly increased urine specific gravity within 1 to 2 hours. The absence of an increase in urine specific gravity in response to both water deprivation and exogenous ADH administration indicates the presence of nephrogenic diabetes insipidus.

Renal medullary hypertonicity may be lost after prolonged polyuria (primary or secondary). Therefore medullary washout may develop in animals with primary polydipsia or pituitary diabetes insipidus, making them appear to have nephrogenic diabetes insipidus. Water intake may be gradually reduced over 10 to 14 days to correct renal medullary washout before the water deprivation test is performed. In addition to gradually limiting the dog's or cat's water intake (10% reduction every other day until the animal is drinking 80 to 90 ml/kg/day), a lightly salted, high-protein diet should be fed to the animal to facilitate reestablishment of normal medullary tonicity. Water restriction should be discontinued if the animal becomes overly aggressive in its desire for water or becomes lethargic or weak. The response to water deprivation and, if necessary, the response to exogenous ADH should be evaluated after 10 to 14 days of this gradual water deprivation. The lack of a response to water deprivation and exogenous ADH administration after gradual water reduction indicates that nephrogenic diabetes insipidus unrelated to medullary washout is the cause of the polydipsia and polyuria.

## BLADDER AND URETHRAL FUNCTION

Several specialized diagnostic tests, including urethral pressure profilometry, cystometry, and uroflowmetry, may help categorize bladder and urethral function in dogs and cats with disorders of micturition. These tests are available at many referral centers. The urethral pressure profile (UPP) assesses the perfusion pressure or minimal distention pressure within the neck of the bladder and urethra during the storage phase of micturition. The functional urethral length (the length of the urethra that has a pressure greater than the intravesical pressure) and the maximal urethral closure pressure (the greatest urethral pressure minus the intravesical pressure) can be determined from a UPP. Electromyography may be combined with a UPP to define the portion of urethral resistance contributed to by periurethral striated muscle (external sphincter). The UPP can be used to assess urethral sphincter tone in animals with suspected urethral sphincter incompetence or functional urethral obstruction and urethral spasm. In addition, the UPP can be used to evaluate sphincter response to treatment with α-adrenergic drugs or estrogens. Finally, the UPP should be determined preoperatively to evaluate urethral sphincter function in dogs and cats with ectopic ureters and vaginal strictures due to the increased incidence of sphincter incompetence in animals with these congenital anomalies. A cystometrogram records changes in intravesical pressure during bladder filling and detrusor contraction. It evaluates the detrusor reflex, maximal detrusor contraction pressure, and bladder capacity and compliance in animals with suspected detrusor atony, instability, and decreased capacity or compliance. Uroflowmetry measures urine flow during the voiding phase of micturition and defines the relationship between urine flow and detrusor contraction. The presence of normal, increased, or decreased urethral resistance can be established with uroflowmetry.

## BACTERIAL ANTIBIOTIC SENSITIVITY TESTING

A previous study showed that results of in vitro susceptibility testing (disk-diffusion and Kirby-Bauer methods) correctly predicted the outcome of ampicillin therapy in 173 of 187 (92.5%) urinary tract infections (UTIs) caused by *Staphylococcus, Streptococcus, Proteus, Escherichia coli,* or *Klebsiella* organisms in dogs (Ling and colleagues, 1984). Likewise, disk-diffusion sensitivity results correctly predicted the outcome of trimethoprim-sulfa therapy in 239 of 283 (84%) UTIs caused by *E. coli, Klebsiella, Proteus, Streptococcus,* or *Staphylococcus* organisms in dogs (Ling and colleagues, 1984). However, because of differences in the serum and urine concentrations of antibiotics, in vivo sensitivity may exist even though disk-diffusion sensitivity testing has shown in vitro resistance. For example, the minimum inhibitory concentrations (MICs) of penicillin for staphylococcal organisms, including penicillinase-producing strains, are approximately 10 μg/ml. The average urine concentration of ampicillin when given in standard doses orally exceeds 300 μg/ml, whereas the expected serum concentration is only 1 to 2 μg/ml. High antibiotic concentrations in the urine frequently result in organism sensitivity, even if the disk-diffusion method indicates resistance. The general rule of thumb in interpreting MICs is that, if the MIC is 25% or less of the expected mean urine concentration (Table 42-2), the organism should be susceptible. If disk-diffusion sensitivity testing shows an organism infecting the urinary tract to be highly resistant to antibiotics (e.g., susceptible only to aminoglycosides), MIC sensitivity testing can be helpful in determining

## TABLE 42-2

Urine Concentration of Selected Antimicrobial Agents Determined in Healthy Dogs with Normal Renal Function

| ANTIBIOTIC | DOSAGE* | ROUTE | URINE CONCENTRATION (μg/ml; MEAN ± STANDARD DEVIATION) |
|---|---|---|---|
| Penicillin G | 40,000 U/kg q8h | PO | 294 ± 211 |
| Ampicillin | 25 mg/kg q8h | PO | 309 ± 55 |
| Amoxicillin | 11 mg/kg q8h | PO | 202 ± 93 |
| Tetracycline | 20 mg/kg q8h | PO | 138 ± 65 |
| Chloramphenicol | 33 mg/kg q8h | PO | 124 ± 40 |
| Sulfisoxazole | 22 mg/kg q8h | PO | 1466 ± 832 |
| Cephalexin | 30 mg/kg q12h | PO | 805 ± 421 |
| Trimethoprim/sulfa | 15 mg/kg q12h | PO | 55 ± 19 |
| Enrofloxacin | 2.5 mg/kg q12h | PO | 43 ± 12 |

*Dosages are the same for cats, except that the dosage or chloramphenicol in cats is 20 mg/kg q8h for 1 week.
*PO,* Orally.

whether alternative antibiotics will be efficacious. However, MIC sensitivity should not be used in animals with pyelonephritis or bladder infections with a thickened bladder wall, because drug concentrations in these tissues will be closer to serum concentrations than to urine concentrations.

## DIAGNOSTIC IMAGING

It is relatively difficult to visualize the kidneys on plain abdominal radiographs, with the right kidney usually being more difficult to visualize than the left because of its close association with the caudate lobe of the liver. It is even more difficult to visualize the kidneys in thin or emaciated animals, because the contrast provided by abdominal fat is lacking.

Plain abdominal radiographs, however, should be obtained to evaluate kidney number, location, size, shape, and radiographic density (Table 42-3). Kidney size is best estimated by comparing kidney length with the length of adjacent lumbar vertebrae; the kidneys should be approximately equivalent to 2.5 to 3 times the length of the second lumbar vertebra in cats and 2.5 to 3.5 times the length of the second lumbar vertebra in dogs. Canine kidneys are generally bean shaped, whereas feline kidneys are more spherical. The right kidney is approximately one-half length cranial to the left kidney in both cats and dogs, and the kidneys of cats are more moveable than those of dogs. Kidneys have a soft tissue or water density throughout and are more dense than the perirenal fat. Any radiopacity within the kidney is abnormal (Fig. 42-1). Ideally, patient preparation for radiographic evaluation of the

 **TABLE 42-3**

**Imaging Procedure and Potential Findings in Cats and Dogs with Urinary Disorders**

| PROCEDURE | POTENTIAL FINDINGS |
|---|---|
| Plain abdominal radiography | Radiopaque uroliths |
| | Increased or decreased kidney size |
| | Abdominal mass(es) |
| | Bladder distention |
| | Emphysematous cystitis |
| | Enlarged uterus |
| | Enlarged prostate |
| | Lymphadenopathy |
| Renal ultrasonography | Tissue architecture (diffuse versus focal disease, echodense versus echolucent lesions) |
| | Pyelonephritis |
| | Perirenal fluid, renal cysts, or abscesses |
| | Hydronephrosis, hydroureter |
| Excretory urography | Renal parenchymal filling defects |
| | Renal pelvic dilatation or filling defects |
| | Hydronephrosis or hydroureter |
| | Ureteral obstruction |
| | Ectopic ureter(s) |
| | Extravasation of contrast material |
| Contrast-enhanced cystography | Radiolucent uroliths |
| | Intraluminal mass(es) |
| | Wall thickening |
| | Urachal remnant |
| | Extravasation of contrast material |
| | Enlarged prostate |
| | Reflux of contrast material into ureters* |
| Bladder ultrasonography | Intraluminal masses (uroliths, blood clots, tumors, polyps) |
| | Wall thickening |
| | Prostatic lesions |
| | Sublumbar lymphadenopathy |
| Contrast-enhanced urethrography | Intraluminal filling defects |
| | Extraluminal compression |
| | Extravasation of contrast material |
| | Enlarged prostate |
| | Reflux of contrast material into prostate* |

*May be observed in normal dogs.

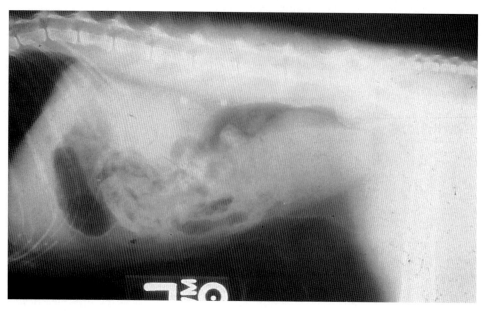

**FIG 42-1**
Plain film radiographic appearance of bilateral renal calculi in a cat. (Courtesy Dr. Phillip Steyn, Colorado State University, Fort Collins, Colo.)

urinary system should include withholding food for 24 hours and the administration of cleansing enemas the evening before and morning of (1 to 3 hours before) the evaluation.

Ultrasonography is used to evaluate renal tissue architecture if kidney abnormalities have been detected by physical examination (e.g., abnormal kidney size or shape), clinicopathologic findings (e.g., azotemia or proteinuria), or survey radiographs (e.g., abnormal kidney size, shape, or opacity or nonvisualization of a kidney). Ultrasonography can provide information about the internal detail of the kidneys. Normally the renal cortex is hypoechoic compared with the spleen, and the renal medulla is hypoechoic compared with the cortex (Fig. 42-2). The renal pelvis and diverticula are relatively hyperechoic. Relatively hypoechoic renal cortices can be observed in patients with acute tubular necrosis, polycystic kidney disease, abscesses, and the renal edema associated with acute renal failure. Conversely, relatively hyperechoic renal cortices are associated with end-stage renal failure, nephrocalcinosis, amyloidosis, feline infectious peritonitis, and calcium oxalate nephrosis secondary to ethylene glycol ingestion. Glomerular and tubulointerstitial disease can show a normal or hyperechoic echotexture, depending on chronicity. Renal lymphoma can make the renal cortices appear hypoechoic or hyperechoic (Fig. 42-3). Hydronephrosis and hydroureter are easily and noninvasively diagnosed on the basis of ultrasonographic findings (Fig. 42-4). Resistance to renal blood flow (resistive index), which can be calculated with the use of color flow Doppler imaging, is increased in several renal diseases.

An intravenous urogram (Table 42-4) can also aid in the evaluation of renal structures, specifically the renal vessels,

parenchyma, and pelvis, as well as the ureters (Fig. 42-5). Potential indications for intravenous urography include kidney abnormalities noted on plain radiographs or ultrasonograms, inability to visualize one or both kidneys on plain radiographs or ultrasonograms, and hematuria of suspected renal origin. In addition, intravenous urography qualitatively assesses individual kidney excretory function; therefore it should be performed before nephrectomy or nephrotomy. The utility of intravenous urography diminishes if azotemia exists, and good renal opacification becomes more difficult as azotemia increases. Intravenous urography should be avoided in dehydrated animals and in those receiving potentially nephrotoxic drugs.

If the ureters are normal, they cannot be visualized on plain radiographs. Normal ureters appear as radiopaque lines that extend from the kidneys to the trigone region of the bladder on intravenous urograms (see Fig. 42-5, *B*). The normal ureteral diameter is 1 to 2 mm, and apparent filling defects are frequently caused by peristaltic contractions that propel urine and contrast material to the bladder. Indications for intravenous urography to evaluate the ureters include suspected obstructive uropathy (Fig. 42-6), trauma (rupture or laceration), calculi, ectopic ureters (Fig. 42-7), neoplasia, and ureterocele.

The size, shape, and position of the urinary bladder can usually be evaluated and any radiopacities detected on plain abdominal radiographs and ultrasonograms (Fig. 42-8). However, retrograde contrast-enhanced radiographic studies are easy to perform and are used to visualize the entire bladder and its relationship to other structures in the posterior abdomen. Negative (air or carbon dioxide) or positive (iodinated

*Text continued on p. 595*

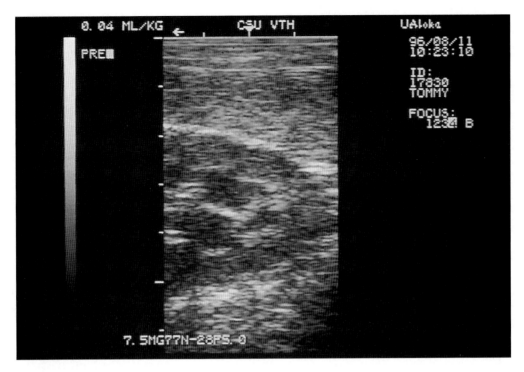

**FIG 42-2**
Ultrasonographic images of the kidney and spleen in a dog showing the increased echogenicity of the spleen *(upper right)* compared with the renal cortex. (Courtesy Dr. Robert Wrigley, Colorado State University, Fort Collins, Colo.)

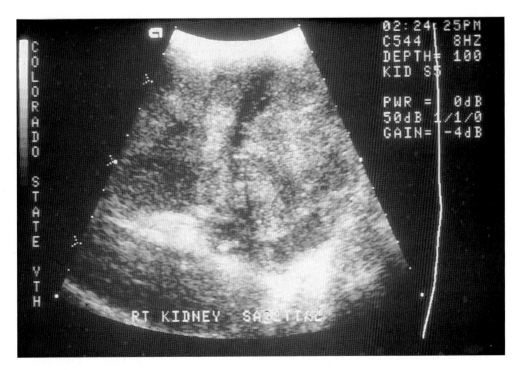

**FIG 42-3**
Ultrasonographic image of a feline kidney with lymphoma. (Courtesy Dr. Phillip Steyn, Colorado State University, Fort Collins, Colo.)

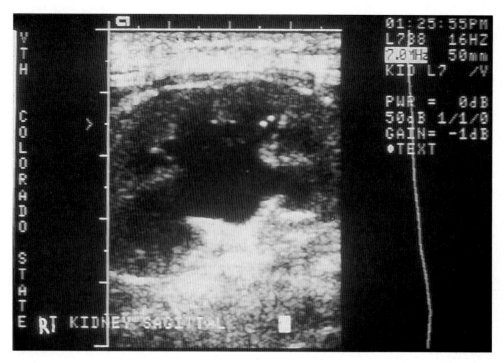

**FIG 42-4**
Ultrasonographic image of a hydronephrotic kidney. (Courtesy Dr. Phillip Steyn, Colorado State University, Fort Collins, Colo.)

TABLE 42-4

**Technique for Intravenous Urography**

1. Patient preparation
   No food for 24 hours; water available, free choice
   One or more enemas at least 2 hours before radiography
   Assess hydration status; do not proceed if animal is dehydrated
2. Evaluate survey radiographs for effectiveness of enemas
3. Use sedation only if necessary
4. Infuse contrast solution IV via jugular or cephalic vein as bolus injection
   400 mg of iodine per lb (0.45 kg) of body weight; dose can be doubled if renal function is poor
   Nonionic iodinated contrast solutions are safest but more expensive
5. Obtain abdominal radiographs as follows:
   Ventrodorsal views at 5 to 20 seconds, 5 minutes, 20 minutes, and 40 minutes after injection
   Lateral view at 5 minutes
   Oblique views at 3 to 5 minutes to assess ureteral termination in bladder

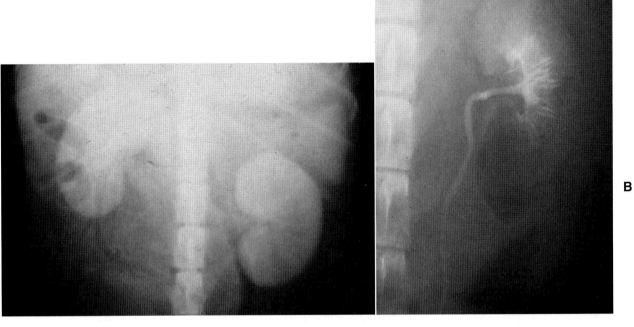

A                                                                                    B

**FIG 42-5**
Radiographic appearance of normal canine kidneys during **(A)** the nephrogram stage of an
intravenous pyelogram and **(B)** the pyelogram stage of an intravenous pyelogram.

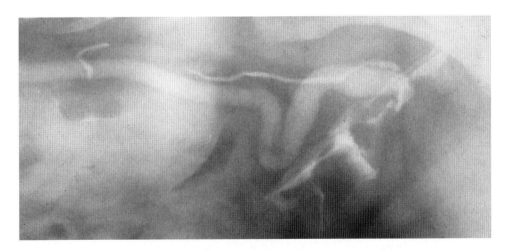

**FIG 42-6**
Intravenous pyelogram of a dog with a transitional cell carcinoma of the bladder and
unilateral hydroureter. (Courtesy Dr. Phillip Steyn, Colorado State University, Fort Collins,
Colo.)

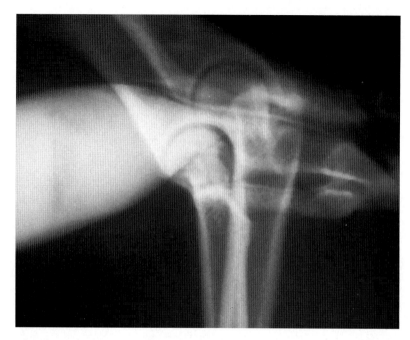

**FIG 42-7**
Intravenous pyelogram of a dog with a unilateral ectopic ureter. (Courtesy Dr. Phillip Steyn, Colorado State University, Fort Collins, Colo.)

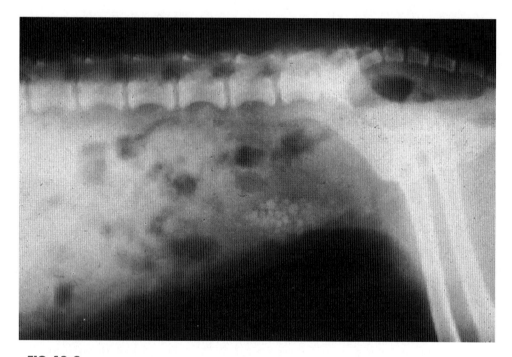

**FIG 42-8**
Appearance of radiopaque cystouroliths on plain film radiographs of a dog. (Courtesy Dr. Phillip Steyn, Colorado State University, Fort Collins, Colo.)

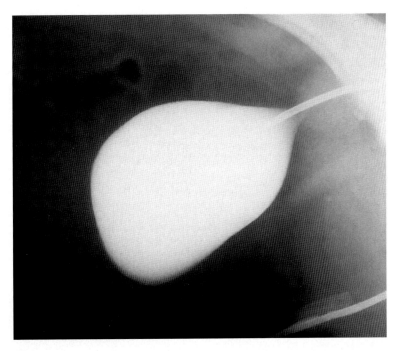

**FIG 42-9**
Positive contrast–enhanced cystogram in a male dog showing a small urachal remnant.
(Courtesy Dr. Phillip Steyn, Colorado State University, Fort Collins, Colo.)

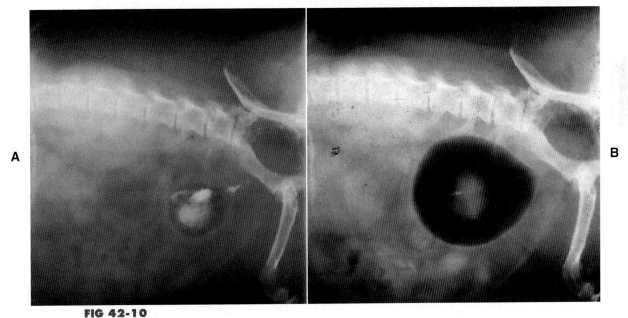

**FIG 42-10**
Double contrast–enhanced cystograms of a dog showing **(A)** insufficient distention of
the bladder with air, giving an artificial appearance of a thickened bladder wall, and
**(B)** proper distention of the bladder with negative contrast.

contrast medium) contrast material may be used for contrast-enhanced cystography (Fig. 42-9); however, double-contrast studies (bladder is filled with a positive-contrast medium that is removed and replaced with air or carbon dioxide) provide the best information about the bladder mucosal sur-face (Fig. 42-10). Abnormalities that may be identified by contrast-enhanced cystography include mucosal and mural lesions, luminal filling defects, urachal remnants, diver-ticuli, vesicoureteral reflux, extraluminal masses, and bladder tears.

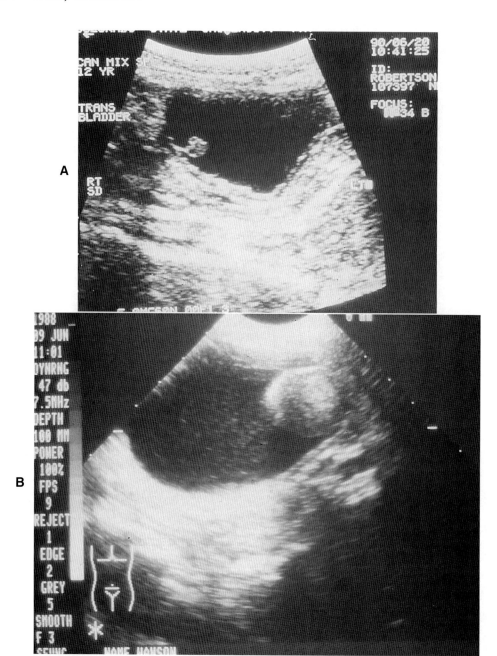

**FIG 42-11**
**A** and **B,** Ultrasonographic images of the bladders of dogs with benign polyps. (**A** courtesy Dr. Phillip Steyn, Colorado State University, Fort Collins, Colo.)

Ultrasonography can also be used to evaluate the urinary bladder, in most cases without the sedation and urinary catheterization required for contrast-enhanced cystography. It is particularly useful for differentiating intraluminal masses (e.g., calculi, blood clots, tumors, polyps) (Figs. 42-11 and 42-12). The prostate gland and sublumbar lymph nodes are also easily evaluated with ultrasonography. However, it may be less effective than contrast-enhanced cystography in detecting mucosal irregularities, small uroliths, and bladder rupture.

Similar to the ureters, the urethra is not routinely visualized on plain radiographs. Contrast-enhanced urethrography is most frequently performed in male dogs and cats to detect or rule out urethral obstruction or rupture (Figs. 42-13 and

42-14). It may be used to identify the presence and location of mucosal and mural lesions, luminal filling defects, strictures, an extramural compression, and urethral rupture or laceration.

Computerized tomography (plain and with contrast) is increasingly used for evaluation of renal pathology in university hospitals and other referral centers.

## CYSTOSCOPY

Cystoscopy is being used with increasing frequency in dogs and cats because it allows relatively noninvasive visualization and biopsy of the urethral and bladder mucosal surface. In

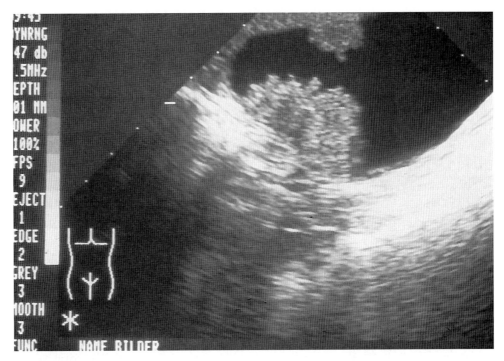

**FIG 42-12**
Ultrasonographic image of the bladder of a dog with a transitional cell carcinoma.

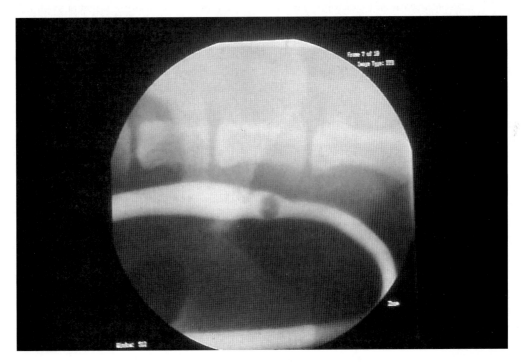

**FIG 42-13**
Positive contrast–enhanced urethrogram in a dog with an intraluminal urolith. (Courtesy Dr. Phillip Steyn, Colorado State University, Fort Collins, Colo.)

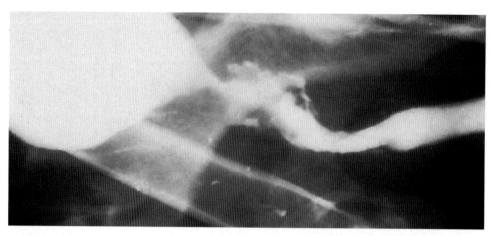

**FIG 42-14**
Positive contrast–enhanced urethrogram in a dog with an obstructive uropathy associated with prostatic neoplasia.

some cases, bladder mucosal lesions can be resected and uroliths removed or crushed by means of cystoscopy. Finally, it can be used to catheterize the ureters to obtain urine samples and perform retrograde pyelography. Cystoscopy is used to evaluate patients with lower urinary tract inflammation; to evaluate potential anatomic abnormalities in animals with recurrent urinary tract infections (e.g., urolithiasis, polyps, urachal remnants) and animals with urine retention or leakage; to evaluate and obtain a biopsy specimen of bladder or urethral masses; and to differentiate unilateral from bilateral renal hematuria.

## RENAL BIOPSY

The biopsy and histopathologic evaluation of renal tissue is a valuable diagnostic and prognostic tool. Renal biopsy should be considered if the diagnosis is in question (e.g., immune complex glomerulonephritis versus amyloidosis in dogs with proteinuria), if treatment may be altered on the basis of results (e.g., confirmation and culture of bacterial pyelonephritis), or if the prognosis may be altered on the basis of results (e.g., evidence of reversible tubular lesions in a dog or cat with acute tubular necrosis). A specific diagnosis is required in order to implement specific treatment in most animals with renal disease, and for a specific diagnosis to be obtained, frequently a biopsy must be done. In addition, the prognosis for animals with renal disease is most accurate if based on three variables: the severity of dysfunction, the response to treatment, and the renal histopathologic findings.

Renal biopsy should be considered only after less invasive tests have been done and the blood clotting ability has been assessed. Contraindications to renal biopsy include a solitary kidney, a coagulopathy, severe systemic hypertension, and renal lesions associated with fluid accumulation (e.g., hydronephrosis, renal cysts and abscesses). In addition, renal biopsy should not be attempted by inexperienced clinicians or in animals that are not adequately restrained.

Renal biopsy specimens can be obtained percutaneously using the keyhole technique or under laparoscopic or ultrasonographic guidance. Frequently the best way to obtain a specimen is at laparotomy when both kidneys can be visualized, because postbiopsy hemorrhage can then be accurately assessed and treated, and an adequate biopsy specimen assured. The cortical region of the kidney should be biopsied to obtain an adequate number of glomeruli in the specimen and to avoid renal nerves and major vessels in the medullary region. Most animals will have microscopic hematuria for 1 to 3 days after the biopsy procedure, and overt hematuria is not uncommon. Severe hemorrhage occurs less than 3% of the time and is almost always the result of faulty technique.

Care must be exercised when handling and fixing renal tissue to prevent artifactual changes. It is important to consult the histopathology laboratory before performing the biopsy to ensure that appropriate fixatives are used. When possible, immunofluorescent or immunohistochemical techniques and electron microscopy should be used to maximize the information gained from the biopsy specimen. Communication with the laboratory pathologist prior to biopsy will help determine which fixatives should be used and will maximize the utility of the biopsy sample.

### Suggested Readings

Bagley RS et al: The effect of experimental cystitis and iatrogenic blood contamination on the urine protein/creatinine ratio in the dog, *J Vet Intern Med* 5:66, 1991.

Brown SA et al: Evaluation of a single injection method, using iohexol, for estimating glomerular filtration rate in cats and dogs, *Am J Vet Res* 57:105, 1996.

Center SA et al: 24-Hour urine protein/creatinine ratio in dogs with protein-losing nephropathies, *J Am Vet Med Assoc* 187:820, 1985.

DiBartola SP et al: Urinary protein excretion and immunopathologic findings in dogs with glomerular disease, *J Am Vet Med Assoc* 177:73, 1980.

DiBartola SP: Clinical evaluation of renal function. The 16th Annual Waltham/OSU Symposium for the Treatment of Small Animal Diseases. Nephrology and Urology. Kal Kan Foods, Inc., 3250 East 4th Street, Vernon, CA, 90058. *Proc Waltham Symp Treat Small Anim Dis* 16:7, 1992.

Finco DR et al: Procedure for a simple method of measuring glomerular filtration rate in the dog, *J Am Anim Hosp Assoc* 18:804, 1982.

Finco DR et al: Exogenous creatinine clearance as a measure of glomerular filtration rate in dogs with reduced renal mass, *Am J Vet Res* 52:1029, 1991.

Finco DR et al: Endogenous creatinine clearance measurement of glomerular filtration rate in dogs, *Am J Vet Res* 54:1575, 1993.

Grauer GF et al: Estimation of quantitative proteinuria in the dog using the urine protein-to-creatinine ratio from a random, voided sample, *Am J Vet Res* 46:2116, 1985.

Grauer GF et al: Development of microalbuminuria in dogs with heartworm disease, *J Vet Intern Med* 16:352, 2002 (abstract).

Hardy RM et al: Water deprivation test in the dog: maximal normal values, *J Am Vet Med Assoc* 174:479, 1979.

Hardy RM et al: Aqueous vasopressin response test in clinically normal dogs undergoing water diuresis: technique and results, *Am J Vet Res* 43:1987, 1982.

Hardy RM et al: Repositol vasopressin response test in clinically normal dogs undergoing water diuresis: technique and results, *Am J Vet Res* 43:1991, 1982.

Jensen WA et al: Prevalence of microalbuminuria in dogs, *J Vet Intern Med* 15:300, 2001.

Konde LJ et al: Comparison of radiography and ultrasonography in the evaluation of renal lesions in the dog, *J Am Vet Med Assoc* 188:1420, 1986.

Labato MA et al: Plasma disappearance of creatinine as a renal function test in the dog, *Res Vet Sci* 50:253, 1991.

Lees GE et al: Persistent albuminuria precedes onset of overt proteinuria in male dogs with X-linked hereditary nephropathy, *J Vet Intern Med* 16:353, 2002 (abstract).

Ling GV et al: Canine urinary tract infections: a comparison of in vitro antimicrobial susceptibility test results and response to oral therapy with ampicillin or with trimethoprim sulfa, *J Am Vet Med Assoc* 185:277, 1984.

Lulich JP et al: Interpretation of protein-creatinine ratios in dogs with glomerular and nonglomerular disorders, *Compend Contin Educ* 12:59, 1990.

Miyamoto K: Use of plasma clearance of iohexol for estimating glomerular filtration rate in cats, *Am J Vet Res* 62:572, 2001.

Rogers KS et al: Comparison of four methods of estimating glomerular filtration rate in cats, *Am J Vet Res* 52:961, 1991.

Russo EA et al: Evaluation of renal function in cats using quantitative urinalysis, *Am J Vet Res* 47:1308, 1986.

Senior DF: Endoscopy. In Osborne CA et al, editors: *Canine and feline nephrology and urology,* Baltimore, 1995, Williams & Wilkins.

Vaden SL et al: Longitudinal study of microalbuminuria in Soft-Coated Wheaten Terriers, *J Vet Intern Med* 15:300, 2001.

# CHAPTER 43

# Glomerulonephropathies

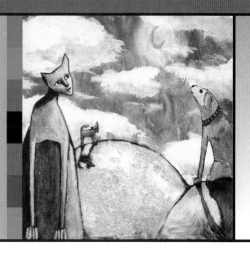

## CHAPTER OUTLINE

Etiology and pathophysiology, 600
Clinical features, 603
Diagnosis, 605
Treatment, 605
Prognosis, 607

Glomerulonephritis ([GN] inflammation of the glomerulus) is the most common type of glomerulonephropathy and is usually caused by immune complexes within the glomerular capillary walls. It is thought to be one of the major causes of chronic renal insufficiency or renal failure, and several studies have shown that the prevalence of glomerulonephritis in randomly selected dogs is as high as 50%. The deposition of amyloid within the glomeruli is another important, although less common, cause of glomerulonephropathy. A loss of plasma proteins, principally albumin, in the urine is the hallmark of glomerulonephropathy, and use of the urine protein/creatinine ratio to identify and quantify proteinuria has greatly facilitated the diagnosis of glomerular disease in cats and dogs (see p. 586).

## Etiology and Pathophysiology

Most glomerulonephropathies in dogs and cats are mediated by immunologic mechanisms. Immune complexes present in the glomerular capillary wall are usually responsible for initiating glomerular damage and proteinuria. For example, soluble circulating antigen-antibody complexes may be deposited or trapped in glomeruli if a mild antigen excess exists or if antigen and antibody molecules are present in approximately equal numbers (Fig. 43-1). On the other hand, if a large antibody excess exists, the resulting immune complexes tend to be large and insoluble and are rapidly removed from the circulation by phagocytic cells. Conversely, those complexes formed with a large antigen excess do not readily bind complement and have a reduced capacity to produce immunologic injury.

In contrast to the glomerular deposition of preformed complexes, immune complexes may also form *in situ* in the glomerular capillary wall (see Fig. 43-1). This occurs when circulating antibodies react with endogenous glomerular antigens or "planted," nonglomerular antigens in the glomerular capillary wall. Nonglomerular antigens may localize in the glomerular capillary wall as a result of an electrical charge interaction or a biochemical affinity with the glomerular capillary wall. Recent evidence indicates that immune complexes form *in situ* in dogs with glomerulonephritis associated with dirofilariasis (Grauer and colleagues, 1989).

Although antibodies directed against intrinsic glomerular basement membrane material have not been found in dogs and cats with naturally occurring glomerulonephritis, several infectious and inflammatory diseases have been associated with immune-mediated glomerular disease (Table 43-1). In many cases, however, the antigen source or underlying disease is not identified and, in such cases, the glomerular disease is referred to as *idiopathic*. It is not difficult to identify endogenous immunoglobulin or complement within glomeruli using various immunologic techniques, but the antigens associated with the immune complex are rarely identified within glomerular tissue.

After immune complexes have been formed or deposited in the glomerular capillary wall, several processes, including activation of the complement system, platelet adhesion and aggregation, infiltration with polymorphonuclear leukocytes, and activation of the coagulation system with fibrin deposition, contribute to glomerular damage (Fig. 43-2). Platelet adhesion and aggregation occur secondary to vascular endothelial damage or an antigen-antibody interaction. The platelets in turn exacerbate glomerular damage by releasing vasoactive and inflammatory substances (principally thromboxanes) and by activating the coagulation cascade. There is much evidence indicating that thromboxanes are important mediators of the inflammation and proteinuria associated with immune complex glomerulonephritis.

Similarly, angiotensin is thought to be involved in the pathogenesis of glomerulonephritis. Angiotensin II can be generated in the systemic circulation and delivered to the kidney, or it can be generated within the kidney by local conversion of angiotensin I. Angiotensin II contributes to intraglomerular hypertension and proteinuria via efferent arteri-

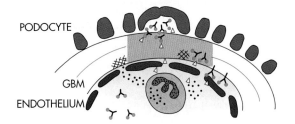

PODOCYTE

GBM

ENDOTHELIUM

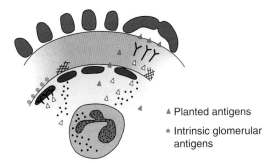

➤ Antibody
• Antigen
△ Complement
# Damaged GBM
⠐⠐ Lysosomal enzyme

▲ Planted antigens
• Intrinsic glomerular antigens

**FIG 43-1**
The two major types of immunologically mediated glomerular injury. Circulating soluble immune complexes have become trapped in the glomerular filter and have fixed complement. Chemotactic complement components have attracted neutrophils to the area. The release of oxygen free radicals and lysosomal enzymes from neutrophils has resulted in damage to the glomerulus *(top)*. Damage may also result from the attachment of autoantibodies directed against fixed intrinsic glomerular antigens *(bottom, left)*. Finally, damage may result from the attachment of antibodies directed against planted nonglomerular antigens *(bottom, right)*. *GBM,* Glomerular basement membrane; *PMN,* polymorphonuclear leukocyte. (From Chew DJ et al: *Manual of small animal nephrology and urology,* London, 1986, Churchill Livingstone.)

 TABLE 43-1

**Diseases Associated with Glomerulonephritis in Dogs and Cats**

| DOGS | CATS |
|---|---|
| **Infectious** | |
| Canine adenovirus I | Feline leukemia virus |
| Bacterial endocarditis | Feline immunodeficiency |
| Brucellosis | virus |
| Dirofilariasis | Feline infectious peritonitis |
| Ehrlichiosis | Mycoplasma polyarthritis |
| Leishmaniasis | Chronic bacterial infections |
| Pyometra | |
| Borelliosis | |
| Chronic bacterial infections (gingivitis, pyoderma) | |
| Rocky Mountain spotted fever | |
| Trypanosomiasis | |
| Septicemia | |
| Helicobacter? | |
| **Neoplasia** | **Neoplasia** |
| **Inflammatory** | |
| Pancreatitis | Pancreatitis |
| Systemic lupus erythematosus | Systemic lupus erythematosus |
| Other immune-mediated diseases | Other immune-mediated diseases |
| Prostatitis | Chronic skin disease |
| Hepatitis | |
| Inflammatory bowel disease | |
| **Other** | |
| Hyperadrenocorticism and long-term, high-dose corticosteroids? | Idiopathic |
| | Familial |
| | Nonimmunologic— hyperfiltration? |
| Idiopathic | Diabetes mellitus |
| Familial | |
| Nonimmunologic— hyperfiltration? | |
| Diabetes mellitus | |

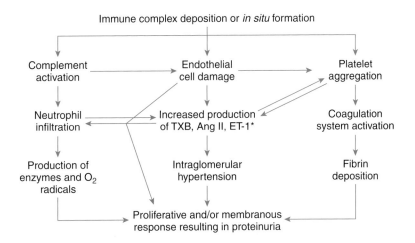

*\*TXB,* Thromboxane; *Ang II,* angiotensin II; *ET-1,* endothelin-1.

**FIG 43-2**
Glomerular response to the presence of immune complexes.

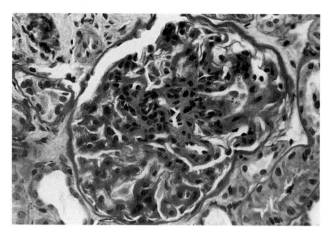

**FIG 43-3**
Membranoproliferative glomerulonephritis characterized by cellular proliferation, thickened capillary walls, and increased mesangial matrix. (PAS stain; original magnification ×400.) (From Grauer GF: The urinary system. In Allen DG, editor: *Small animal medicine*, Philadelphia, 1991, JB Lippincott.)

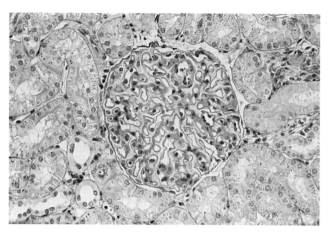

**FIG 43-4**
Membranous glomerulonephritis characterized by capillary basement membrane thickening. (Periodic acid–Schiff stain; original magnification ×400.) (From Grauer GF: The urinary system. In Allen DG, editor: *Small animal medicine*, Philadelphia, 1991, JB Lippincott.)

ole vasoconstriction and glomerular cell proliferation via its growth factor effects.

Cellular proliferation (proliferative GN) (Fig. 43-3), thickening of the glomerular basement membrane (membranous GN) (Fig. 43-4), and, eventually, hyalinization and sclerosis (Fig. 43-5) occur in the glomerulus as a result of this injury. The initial pathophysiologic consequence of a proliferative and/or membranous GN is proteinuria. Azotemia is not an early clinicopathologic finding. Azotemia occurs when more than three fourths of the nephrons are damaged and become nonfunctional.

Although glomerular amyloidosis is less common than GN, it is a progressive disease that also frequently leads to chronic renal failure. It is characterized by the extracellular deposition of nonbranching fibrillar proteins that stack into a specific β-pleated sheet conformation and exhibit green birefringence under polarized light when stained with Congo red (Fig. 43-6). Amyloidosis in dogs and cats is the reactive systemic form, in which amyloid may be deposited in several organs besides the kidneys. Reactive systemic amyloid deposits contain amyloid protein AA, which is an amino-terminal fragment of the acute-phase reactant protein, serum amyloid A protein (SAA), and is produced by hepatocytes in response to tissue injury. Cytokines (e.g., interleukins, tumor necrosis factor) released from macrophages after tissue injury stimulate hepatocytes to produce SAA. Amyloidosis is usually associated with an underlying inflammatory or neoplastic process; however, no predisposing factors can be identified in many dogs and cats with amyloidosis. Amyloidosis has been associated with cyclic neutropenia and with ciliary dyskinesia and recurrent respiratory tract infections in dogs. Renal amyloidosis is a familial disease in the Abyssinian cat; it results in medullary amyloid deposition as a part of systemic

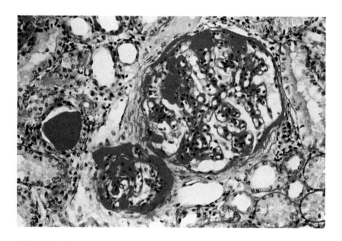

**FIG 43-5**
Advanced membranoproliferative glomerulonephritis. The large glomerulus shows hypercellularity with prominent focal accumulations of mesangial matrix material and thickened glomerular capillary walls. Adhesions to Bowman's capsule and periglomerular fibrosis are also present. The smaller glomerulus is sclerotic and obsolescent. Notice the hyaline cast in a tubule *(left)*. (Periodic acid–Schiff stain; original magnification ×400.) (From Grauer GF: The urinary system. In Allen DG, editor: *Small animal medicine*, Philadelphia, 1991, JB Lippincott.)

amyloidosis. A similar form of suspected familial medullary amyloidosis resulting in renal failure has been observed in Chinese Sharpei dogs. Intermittent fever that occurs in association with tibiotarsal joint swelling and that resolves regardless of treatment is often observed in these dogs. The staining characteristics of the amyloid in Chinese Sharpeis

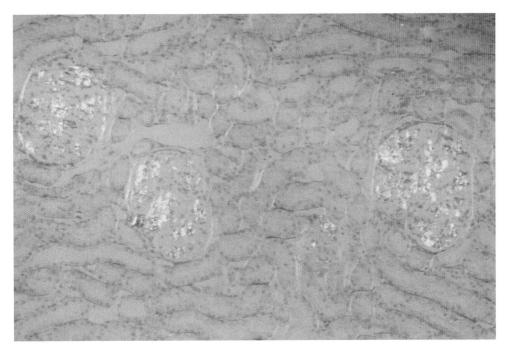

**FIG 43-6**
Typical appearance of glomerular amyloid (green birefringence) when renal tissue is stained with Congo red and viewed under polarized light.

indicate that the amyloid is an inflammatory type. This amyloidosis syndrome in Chinese Sharpeis is similar to that observed in people with familial Mediterranean fever. The medullary deposition of amyloid in Abyssinian cats and Chinese Sharpei dogs makes proteinuria uncommon; renal failure, however, is a common sequela.

Once a glomerulus has been irreversibly damaged by GN or amyloidosis, the entire nephron becomes nonfunctional and is replaced by fibrous scar tissue (see Fig. 43-4). As more and more nephrons become involved, glomerular filtration decreases and sodium retention and hypertension often occur. Remaining viable nephrons compensate for the decrease in toto numbers of glomeruli by increasing individual glomerular filtration rates (Fig. 43-7). This hyperfiltration, coupled with systemic hypertension and possibly a high dietary consumption of protein, if present, may contribute to the development of glomerular hyalinization and sclerosis. Hyperfiltration in remnant nephrons is thought to result in progressive nephron loss independent of the previously discussed immunologic glomerular disorders.

## Clinical Features

The clinical signs associated with mild-to-moderate urinary protein loss are usually nonspecific; examples include weight loss and lethargy, but many patients with low-grade proteinuria appear normal. However, if the protein loss is severe (serum albumin concentration of less than 1.5 or 1 g/dl),

edema or ascites, or both, often occur (Table 43-2). If the glomerular disease is extensive, such that three fourths of the nephrons are nonfunctional, renal failure and resultant azotemia, polydipsia-polyuria, anorexia, nausea, and vomiting may occur. Occasionally signs of an underlying infectious, inflammatory, or neoplastic disease may be the reason that prompts owners to seek veterinary care. Rarely, dogs may be evaluated because of acute dyspnea or severe panting caused by pulmonary thromboembolism (see below). In other rare cases, dogs may be presented because of acute blindness caused by retinal hemorrhage or detachment secondary to systemic hypertension.

A persistent proteinuria can lead to clinical signs of the nephrotic syndrome, the combination of marked proteinuria, hypoalbuminemia, ascites or edema, and hypercholesterolemia. The nephrotic syndrome is more common in dogs than in cats. Edema or ascites usually occurs as a result of the combination of decreased plasma oncotic pressure and increased aldosterone activity, causing sodium retention. However, the aldosterone concentrations may be normal or even low in nephrotic human patients, therefore treatment with angiotensin-converting enzyme inhibitors (ACEIs) may not prevent sodium retention. As a result, it has been hypothesized that intrarenal mechanisms independent of the circulating aldosterone concentration also contribute to the development of sodium retention in some cases. The hypercholesterolemia associated with the nephrotic syndrome

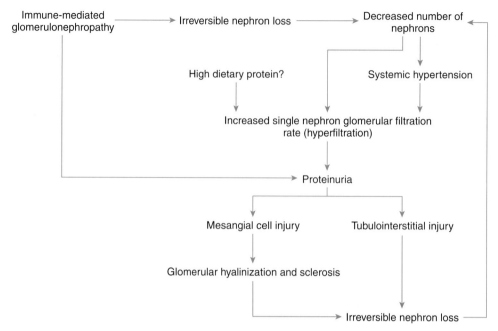

**FIG 43-7**
Proposed pathogenesis of progressive loss of nephrons secondary to a primary glomerulonephropathy.

TABLE 43-2

Signs Associated with Different Manifestations of Glomerular Disease

| MANIFESTATION | CLINICAL SIGNS | CLINICOPATHOLOGIC FINDINGS |
|---|---|---|
| Mild-to-moderate proteinuria* | Lethargy, mild weight loss, decreased muscle mass | Serum albumin 1.5-3.0 g/dl |
| Marked proteinuria (>3.5 g/day) | Severe muscle wasting, weight gain may occur, however, as result of edema or ascites | Serum albumin <1.5 g/dl, hypercholesterolemia |
| Renal failure | Depression, anorexia, nausea, vomiting, weight loss, polyuria-polydipsia | Azotemia, isosthenuria or minimally concentrated urine, hyperphosphatemia, nonregenerative anemia |
| Pulmonary thromboembolism | Acute dyspnea or severe panting | Hypoxemia; normal or low $P_{CO_2}$; fibrinogen >300 mg/dl; antithrombin <70% of normal |
| Retinal hemorrhage and/or detachment | Acute blindness | Systolic blood pressure >180 mm Hg |

*Microalbuminuria, as discussed in Chapter 42, may precede proteinuria and therefore be an early diagnostic tool.
$P_{CO_2}$, Partial pressure of carbon dioxide.

probably results from a combination of the decreased catabolism of proteins and lipoproteins and the increased hepatic synthesis of proteins and lipoproteins. This results in the accumulation of large-molecular-weight, cholesterol-rich lipoproteins, which are not as easily lost through the damaged glomerular capillary wall as are the smaller-molecular-weight proteins.

In addition to the clinical signs just described, systemic hypertension and hypercoagulability are frequent complications in dogs with nephrotic syndrome. Hypertension probably re-

sults from a combination of sodium retention, glomerular capillary and arteriolar scarring, decreased renal production of vasodilators, increased responsiveness to normal pressor mechanisms, and activation of the renin-angiotensin system. Hypertension has been associated with immune-mediated GN, glomerulosclerosis, and amyloidosis; in one study, 84% of dogs with glomerular disease were found to be hypertensive (Cowgill, 1991). Retinal changes, including hemorrhage, detachment, and papilledema, can be an indication of hypertension; the acute onset of blindness may be the presenting complaint in hypertensive dogs. Blood pressure measurement can help in the evaluation and management of animals with glomerular disease in that, by identifying and controlling hypertension, the progression of the glomerular disease as well as other target organ damage may be attenuated.

The hypercoagulability and thromboembolism associated with the nephrotic syndrome occur secondary to several abnormalities in the clotting system. In addition to a mild thrombocytosis, a hypoalbuminemia-related platelet hypersensitivity causes platelet adhesion and aggregation to increase proportional to the magnitude of the hypoalbuminemia. A loss of antithrombin (molecular weight of 65,000 daltons) in urine also contributes to the development of hypercoagulability. Antithrombin works in concert with heparin in playing a vital role in modulating thrombin activation and fibrin formation. Finally, altered fibrinolysis and increases in the concentration of large-molecular-weight clotting factors (fibrinogen and factors V, VII, VIII, and X) can lead to a relative increase in the concentration of clotting factors as opposed to those of regulatory proteins. The pulmonary arterial system is the most common destination for thromboemboli. Dogs with pulmonary thromboembolism are usually dyspneic, hypoxic, and hypocapnic but have minimal pulmonary parenchymal radiographic abnormalities (see p. 310). The treatment of pulmonary thromboembolism is difficult, often expensive, and frequently unrewarding; therefore early prophylactic treatment to prevent coagulation disorders is important (see later discussion).

### Diagnosis

Persistent, severe proteinuria with a normal urine sediment (hyaline casts may be observed) is the hallmark clinicopathologic sign of glomerulonephropathies. The urine protein/creatinine ratio is used to quantify the magnitude of the urine protein loss. Microalbuminuria may precede overt proteinuria in many cases (see section on proteinuria in Chapter 42). Protein-losing nephropathies are definitively diagnosed on the basis of renal cortical histopathologic findings. (See sections on proteinuria and renal biopsy in Chapters 41 and 42.)

### Treatment

The generation of immune complexes depends on the presence of antigen. Hence, the most important therapeutic approach for glomerular disease is the identification and treatment of underlying diseases (see Tables 43-1 and 43-3). Dirofilariasis, ehrlichiosis, borreliosis, and systemic lupus erythematosus are examples of treatable diseases that may cause glomerulonephritis. However, because an antigen source or underlying disease is frequently not identified or is impossible to eliminate, immunosuppressive drugs have been recommended for the treatment of animals with GN. Corticosteroids, azathioprine, cyclophosphamide, and cyclosporin have been used clinically or experimentally to prevent immunoglobulin production by B cells or to alter the function of T-helper or T-suppressor cells. Unfortunately no controlled clinical trials have shown the efficacy of immunosuppressive drugs in the treatment of GN in small animals. The

### TABLE 43-3

**Treatment Guidelines for Dogs and Cats with Glomerulonephritis**

1. Identify and eliminate any underlying diseases
2. Immunosuppressive treatment (usually not recommended for dogs)
   a. Cyclophosphamide, 50 mg/m² PO q48h (dogs) or 200 to 300 mg/m² PO q3wk (cats) or
   b. Azathioprine, 50 mg/m² PO q24h × 7 days, then q48h (dogs only) or
   c. Cyclosporin, 15 mg/kg PO q24h (dogs only)
   d. Prednisone, 1.0 to 2.0 mg/kg PO q12-24h (cats only)
3. Antiinflammatory-hypercoagulability treatment: aspirin, 0.5 to 5.0 mg/kg PO q12h (dogs); 0.5 to 5.0 mg/kg PO q48h (cats)
4. Supportive care
   a. Dietary: sodium restriction, high-quality–low-quantity protein
   b. Hypertension: dietary sodium reduction; ACEIs (e.g., enalapril, 0.5 mg/kg PO q12-24h, and benazepril, 0.25 to 0.5 mg/kg PO q24h; ACEIs often have antiproteinuric effects as well) and/or calcium channel blockers
   c. Edema and ascites: dietary sodium restriction; furosemide, 2.2 mg/kg PO q8-24h, if necessary

*ACEIs,* Angiotensin-converting enzyme inhibitors.

recently noted association of hyperadrenocorticism (and long-term exogenous corticosteroid therapy) with glomerulonephritis and thromboembolism in the dog, as well as the absence of a consistent response to the treatment of glomerular disease with corticosteroids, suggests that corticosteroids should probably not be used in dogs with glomerulonephritis (Center and colleagues, 1987). The exception would be a corticosteroid-responsive underlying disease such as systemic lupus erythematosus. Anecdotal clinical results indicate that corticosteroid treatment of GN may be more efficacious in cats than in dogs. If immunosuppressive drugs are used, the proteinuria should be quantified (urine protein/creatinine ratio) frequently to assess the effects of treatment. In many instances, immunosuppressive treatment will be of no benefit, and in some instances, immunosuppressive treatment may exacerbate the glomerular lesions and proteinuria. For specific information on immunosuppressive drugs, see Chapter 93.

There is increasing evidence that platelets and their arachidonic acid metabolites (thromboxanes) are integrally involved in the pathogenesis of GN. Beneficial responses to antiplatelet therapy, including thromboxane synthetase inhibitors, aspirin, indomethacin, dipyridamole, and platelet-activating factor antagonists, have been demonstrated in several studies performed in laboratory animals, dogs, and humans. The dosage appears to be important if nonspecific cyclooxygenase inhibitors such as aspirin are used. Low-dose aspirin therapy (0.5 to 5 mg/kg PO q12-24h for dogs and q48h for cats) can selectively inhibit the platelet cyclooxygenase–mediated production of thromboxane but has less effect on the formation of prostacyclin by endothelial cells. Similarly, in several studies conducted in mice, rats, rabbits, and dogs, thromboxane synthetase inhibitors and thromboxane receptor antagonists have been observed to attenuate experimental GN, as evidenced by decreased proteinuria, decreased glomerular cell proliferation and infiltration, decreased fibrin deposition, and preservation of the glomerular filtration rate. It is anticipated that thromboxane synthetase inhibitors and receptor antagonists will soon be marketed in this country for the treatment of bronchial asthma and coronary artery disease in people, and these drugs may also be useful in animals with proteinuric disease. In addition to antiplatelet therapy, the treatment of glomerular disease with prostaglandin analogs or dietary supplementation with marine (n-3) polyunsaturated fatty acids to enhance prostacyclin activity and decrease the production of thromboxanes and leukotrienes has also generally been observed to attenuate glomerular disease in several species; however, additional studies are necessary before specific treatment recommendations can be made for dogs.

Similar to the treatment of GN, the primary treatment for amyloidosis, if possible, should be the identification and treatment of any underlying inflammatory process. Dimethylsulfoxide (DMSO) has been shown to dissolve amyloid fibrils in vitro and in vivo in mice. It has been hypothesized that DMSO has a similar amyloid-dissolving effect in domestic animals. The antiinflammatory effects of DMSO may also serve to decrease production of the acute-phase reactant SAA and the inflammation associated with an underlying disease. Decreased urinary protein excretion was observed in one dog with amyloidosis treated with DMSO (Spyridakis and colleagues, 1986); however, the effects of the DMSO were difficult to determine, because two potential underlying causes (interdigital pyoderma and a Sertoli cell tumor) were eliminated prior to the DMSO treatment. The dosage of DMSO used in this dog was 80 mg/kg administered subcutaneously three times per week; the treatment was continued for more than a year without apparent adverse effects. Other studies assessing the effects of DMSO in dogs with amyloidosis, however, have shown the treatment to be ineffective.

Colchicine is another drug that is frequently mentioned for the treatment of amyloidosis. It prevents the production of SAA by hepatocytes and has been shown to prevent amyloidosis in humans and mice if used early in the disease. Although colchicine has been recommended to prevent medullary amyloidosis in Sharpei dogs with fever and tibiotarsal joint swelling, no controlled studies of its use in this setting have been performed. The dosage of colchicine that has been recommended for the prophylactic treatment of amyloidosis is 0.025 mg/kg given orally once daily. Increasing the dose to 0.025 mg/kg given orally twice a day may be considered if the animal tolerates the initial dose well for 2 weeks. However, adverse effects of colchicine may include bone marrow toxicity.

Inasmuch as glomerular amyloid deposition results in severe proteinuria, with its attendant effects, the disease is relentlessly progressive, resulting in chronic renal failure and uremia; as no specific treatment has proved to be effective, the prognosis for animals with renal amyloidosis is guarded to poor.

Supportive therapy is important in the management of cats and dogs with GN or amyloidosis and should be aimed at decreasing hypertension and edema and lowering the risk for thromboembolism. High-quality, reduced-quantity protein diets should be recommended in an attempt to decrease glomerular hyperfiltration and the nonimmunologic progression of the glomerular disease (see Chapter 44). Replacing the urine protein loss with supplemental dietary protein is not recommended, however, because it tends to exacerbate the proteinuria via increased intraglomerular pressures. Sodium-restricted diets (approximately 0.3% dry matter) are often recommended (although they are without proven benefit), and vasodilators and diuretics may be used as necessary. Although ACEIs may not prevent sodium retention in all nephrotic animals, they have been shown to decrease the proteinuria and intrarenal hypertension in many cases.

It was recently demonstrated that treatment with enalapril improves renal function and prolongs survival in male Samoyed dogs with hereditary nephritis (Grodecki and colleagues, 1997). This primary glomerular disease results in proteinuria and chronic renal failure before 1 year of age in affected dogs. In addition, in dogs that had undergone unilateral nephrectomies and had had experimentally induced diabetes mellitus, treatment with lisinopril was found to reduce the glomerular transcapillary hydraulic pressure and glomerular cell hypertrophy as well as the proteinuria (Brown and colleagues, 1993). Finally, in a prospective, placebo-controlled, double-blind study of dogs with naturally occurring, idiopathic GN, enalapril treatment decreased proteinuria and systolic blood pressure and prevented an increase in serum creatinine (Grauer and colleagues, 2000). The recommended dosage of enalapril is 0.5 mg/kg given orally every 12 to 24 hours.

Treatment with ACEIs probably decreases the proteinuria and preserves renal function in animals with glomerular disease by means of several mechanisms, in addition to decreasing intraglomerular hypertension and cellular proliferation. In rats, enalapril prevents the loss of glomerular heparan sulfate that can occur in glomerular disease. Heparan sulfate is a glycosaminoglycan-proteoglycan that contributes to the negative charge of the glomerular capillary wall, which in turn hinders the filtration of negatively charged proteins such as albumin. ACEIs are also thought to attenuate the proteinuria by decreasing the size of glomerular capillary endothelial cell pores in human beings. This attenuation of proteinuria alone may be renoprotective, inasmuch as a correlation between proteinuria and renal functional decline has been observed in human beings. In addition, the antiproteinuric and renal protective effects of ACEIs may be associated with improved lipoprotein metabolism. Lipid deposition in the glomerular mesangium can contribute to the development of proteinuria and glomerulosclerosis. In human beings with nephrotic-range proteinuria, ACEIs not only decrease the proteinuria but also reduce the plasma concentrations of low-density lipoprotein cholesterol and triglycerides.

With regard to anticoagulant treatment, it may be helpful to measure plasma antithrombin and fibrinogen concentrations. Dogs with antithrombin concentrations less than 70% of normal and fibrinogen concentrations greater than 300 mg/dl are candidates for such therapy. Antiplatelet drugs, heparin, and coumarins have been used for anticoagulant therapy. Inasmuch as antithrombin III deficiency is marked in some animals with protein-losing nephropathies, coumarins should be more effective than heparin in reducing hypercoagulability. Low-dose aspirin therapy is easily administered on an outpatient basis and does not require extensive monitoring, as does coumarin treatment. Because fibrin accumulation within the glomerulus is a frequent consequence of GN, anticoagulant treatment may serve a dual purpose.

It is important to monitor the protein/creatinine ratio after initiating immunosuppressive treatment. Immunosuppressive treatment could alter the ratio of antigen to antibody and exacerbate the glomerular lesions and the proteinuria (i.e., a decrease in antibody formation leading to a mild excess of antigen or equal amounts of antigen and antibody in the immune complexes), in which case treatment should be altered or discontinued.

In addition, the serum creatinine and urea nitrogen concentrations should be monitored in animals with GN, especially if antihypertensive treatment is used. In cases in which the glomerular filtration rate depends on sodium retention and volume expansion, treatment with ACEIs can be associated with a decrease in renal excretory function. Although, classically, proteinuria occurs before the onset of azotemia, glomerulonephritis can lead to chronic renal insufficiency and failure. With its development, the glomerular filtration rate decreases and the proteinuria therefore usually also decreases. Management guidelines for chronic renal failure are presented in Chapter 44.

## Prognosis

The prognosis for dogs and cats with immune-complex GN is fair to guarded unless the causative underlying disease can be identified and eliminated. Monitoring the urine protein/creatinine ratio and the serum urea nitrogen and creatinine concentrations during treatment helps in establishing the prognosis. The prognosis for animals with renal amyloidosis is poor because the disease tends to be progressive and there is no treatment of proven benefit.

## *Suggested Readings*

Brown SA et al: Long-term effects of antihypertensive regimens on renal hemodynamics and proteinuria, *Kidney Int* 43:1210, 1993.

Center SA et al: Clinicopathologic, renal immunofluorescent, and light microscopic features of glomerulonephritis in the dog: 41 cases (1975-1985), *J Am Vet Med Assoc* 190:81, 1987.

Cook AK et al: Clinical and pathological features of protein-losing glomerular disease in the dog: a review of 137 cases (1985-1992), *J Am Anim Hosp Assoc* 32:313, 1996.

Cowgill LD: Diagnosing systemic hypertension in dogs and cats, *Partners in Practice* (Hill's Pet Products) 4:2, 1991.

Dambach DM et al: Morphologic, immunohistochemical, and ultrastructural characterization of a distinctive renal lesion in dog putatively associated with *Borrelia burgdorferi* infection: 49 cases (1987-1992), *Vet Pathol* 34:85, 1997.

DiBartola SP et al: Clinicopathologic findings in dogs with renal amyloidosis: 59 cases (1976-1986), *J Am Vet Med Assoc* 195:358, 1989.

DiBartola SP et al: The pathogenesis of reactive systemic amyloidosis, *J Vet Intern Med* 3:31, 1989.

DiBartola SP et al: Familial renal amyloidosis in Chinese Shar Pei dogs, *J Am Vet Med Assoc* 197:483, 1990.

Grauer GF et al: Clinicopathologic and histologic evaluation of *Dirofilaria immitis*–induced nephropathy in dogs, *Am J Trop Med Hyg* 37:588, 1987.

Grauer GF et al: Effects of a specific thromboxane synthetase inhibitor on development of experimental *D. immitis* immune-complex glomerulonephritis in the dog, *J Vet Intern Med* 2:192, 1988.

Grauer GF et al: Experimental *Dirofilaria immitis*–associated glomerulonephritis induced in part by in situ formation of immune complexes in the glomerular capillary wall, *J Parasitol* 75:585, 1989.

Grauer GF: Glomerulonephritis, *Semin Vet Med Surg (Small Anim)* 7:187, 1992.

Grauer GF et al: Glomerular disease. In Ettinger SJ et al, editors: *Textbook of veterinary internal medicine,* ed 4, Philadelphia, 2000, WB Saunders, p 1662.

Grauer GF et al: Effects of enalapril vs placebo as a treatment for canine idiopathic glomerulonephritis, *J Vet Intern Med* 14:526, 2000.

Green RA et al: Hypercoagulable state in three dogs with nephrotic syndrome: role of acquired antithrombin III deficiency, *J Am Vet Med Assoc* 181:914, 1982.

Green RA et al: Hypoalbuminemia-related platelet hypersensitivity in two dogs with nephrotic syndrome, *J Am Vet Med Assoc* 186:485, 1985.

Grodecki K et al: Treatment of X-linked hereditary nephritis in Samoyed dogs with angiotensin-converting enzyme (ACE) inhibitor, *J Comp Pathol* 117:209, 1997.

Jaenke RS et al: Membranous nephropathy in the dog, *Vet Pathol* 23:718, 1986.

Lees GE et al: Glomerular ultrastructural findings similar to hereditary nephritis in 4 English Cocker Spaniels, *J Vet Intern Med* 11:80, 1997.

Longhofer SL et al: Effects of thromboxane synthetase inhibition on immune complex glomerulonephritis, *Am J Vet Res* 52:480, 1991.

MacDougall DF et al: Canine chronic renal disease: prevalence and types of glomerulonephritis in the dog, *Kidney Int* 29:144, 1986.

Minkus G et al: Familial nephropathy in Bernese Mountain Dogs, *Vet Pathol* 31:421, 1994.

Relford RL et al: Nephrotic syndrome in dogs: diagnosis and treatment, *Compend Contin Educ Pract Vet* 18:279, 1996.

Spyridakis L et al: Amyloidosis in a dog: treatment with dimethyl-sulfoxide, *J Am Vet Med Assoc* 189:690, 1986.

Vaden SL et al: The effects of cyclosporin versus standard care in dogs with naturally occurring glomerulonephritis, *J Vet Intern Med* 9:259, 1995.

# CHAPTER 44

# Renal Failure

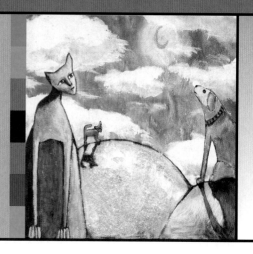

## CHAPTER OUTLINE

ACUTE RENAL FAILURE, 608
    Etiology and pathogenesis, 608
    Clinical features and diagnosis, 611
    Risk factors for renal failure, 611
    Monitoring patients at risk for renal failure, 613
    Treatment, 613
CHRONIC RENAL FAILURE, 615
    Etiology and pathogenesis, 615
    Clinical features and diagnosis, 616
    Treatment, 617

Renal failure occurs when approximately three fourths of the nephrons of both kidneys cease to function. Acute renal failure (ARF) results from an abrupt decline in renal function and is usually caused by an ischemic or toxic insult to the kidneys, although leptospirosis is reenergizing as an important infectious cause of ARF. Ischemic or toxicant-induced injury most frequently results in damage to the metabolically active epithelial cells of the proximal tubules and thick ascending loop of Henle, causing impaired regulation of water and solute balance. Nephrotoxicants interfere with essential tubular cell functions and cause cellular injury, swelling, and death. Renal ischemia causes cellular hypoxia and substrate insufficiency, which leads to the depletion of adenosine triphosphate (ATP) and cellular swelling and death. Vasoconstriction secondary to toxic or ischemic tubular epithelial injury further decreases glomerular filtration. It is important to note, however, that tubular lesions and dysfunction caused by toxic and ischemic insults may be reversible. In contrast, the nephron damage associated with chronic renal failure (CRF) is usually irreversible. Regardless of whether the underlying disease primarily affects the glomeruli, tubules, interstitial tissue, or renal vasculature, irreversible damage to any portion of the nephron renders the entire nephron nonfunctional. Irreversibly damaged nephrons are replaced by fibrous tissue, therefore a specific cause is rarely determined once end-stage kidney damage is present. CRF occurs over a period of weeks, months, or years and is a leading cause of death in dogs and cats. Once end-stage failure has occurred, improving renal function is usually not possible. The goal of treatment is to reduce the renal workload and the clinical signs associated with the decreased renal function, as well as preventing progression of the renal lesions and dysfunction.

Many different and sometimes confusing terms are used to describe renal function and its deterioration (Fig. 44-1):

- Renal disease implies the existence of renal lesions; it does not qualify the cause, severity, or distribution of the lesions or the degree of renal function.
- *Renal reserve* may be thought of as the percentage of "extra" nephrons; those not necessary to maintain normal renal function. Although it probably varies from animal to animal, it is greater than 50% in normal cats and dogs.
- *Renal insufficiency* begins when the renal reserve is lost. Animals with renal insufficiency outwardly appear normal but have a reduced capacity to compensate for stresses such as infection or dehydration and have lost urine concentrating ability.
- *Azotemia* is the increased concentration of urea nitrogen, creatinine, and other nonproteinaceous nitrogenous waste products in the blood.
- *Renal azotemia* denotes azotemia caused by renal parenchymal lesions.
- *Renal failure* is a state of decreased renal function that allows persistent abnormalities (azotemia and inability to concentrate urine) to exist; it refers to a level of organ function rather than a specific disease entity.
- *Uremia* is the presence of all urine constituents in the blood. It may occur secondary to renal failure or postrenal disorders, including urethral obstruction and urinary bladder rupture.
- The *uremic syndrome* is a constellation of clinical signs (e.g., gastroenteritis, acidosis, pneumonitis, osteodystrophy, and encephalopathy) that occur secondary to uremia.

## ACUTE RENAL FAILURE

### Etiology and Pathogenesis

The kidneys are susceptible to the effects of ischemia and toxicants because of their unique anatomic and physiologic features (Table 44-1). For example, the large renal blood flow

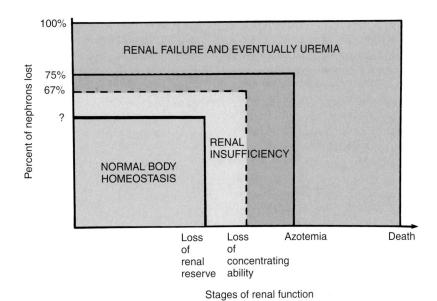

**FIG 44-1**
The stages of renal function. (From Grauer G et al: Chronic renal failure in the dog, *Compend Contin Educ Pract Vet* 3:1009, 1981.)

TABLE 44-1

**Factors that May Predispose the Kidney to Ischemia and Toxicant-Induced Injury**

The kidneys receive 20% of cardiac output; the cortex receives 90% of the renal blood flow.

The glomerular capillaries have a large surface area.

Proximal tubule and thick ascending loop of Henle cells have a high metabolic rate and are susceptible to hypoxia and nutrient deficiency.

Tubular secretion and resorption may concentrate toxicants within cells.

A countercurrent multiplier system may concentrate toxicants within the medulla.

Xenobiotic metabolism within the kidney may generate toxic metabolites (e.g., metabolism of ethylene glycol).

(approximately 20% of the cardiac output) results in the increased delivery of blood-borne toxicants to the kidney, as compared with that to other organs. The renal cortex is especially susceptible to toxicants because it receives 90% of the renal blood flow and contains the large endothelial surface area of the glomerular capillaries. Within the renal cortex, the epithelial cells of the proximal tubule and thick ascending loop of Henle are most frequently affected by ischemia and toxicant-induced injury because of their transport functions and high metabolic rates. Toxicants disrupt the metabolic pathways that generate ATP, and ischemia can rapidly deplete cellular ATP stores. With the resulting loss of energy, the sodium-potassium pump fails, leading to cell swelling and death. By resorbing water and electrolytes from the glomerular filtrate, tubular epithelial cells may be exposed to increasingly higher concentrations of toxicants. Toxicants that are either secreted or resorbed by tubular epithelial cells (e.g., gentamicin) may accumulate in high concentrations within these cells. Similarly, the countercurrent multiplier system may concentrate toxicants in the medulla. Finally, the kidneys also play a role in the biotransformation of many drugs and toxicants. This usually results in the formation of metabolites that are less toxic than the parent compound; however, in some cases (e.g., the oxidation of ethylene glycol to glycolate and oxalate), the metabolites are more toxic than the parent compound.

Table 44-2 presents a partial list of potential nephrotoxicants. It should be noted that toxic insults to the kidney are often caused by therapeutic agents, in addition to the better-known nephrotoxicants. Gentamicin and ethylene glycol are two of the most common causes of toxicant-induced ARF. Table 44-3 presents a partial list of ischemic causes of ARF.

In many cases, ARF inadvertently develops in the hospital setting in conjunction with the performance of diagnostic or therapeutic procedures. For example, ARF may be caused by hypotension and decreased renal perfusion associated with anesthesia and surgery or with the use of vasodilators or nonsteroidal antiinflammatory drugs (NSAIDs). Prolonged anesthesia with inadequate fluid therapy in older dogs and cats with preexisting, subclinical renal insufficiency is a frequent cause of renal ischemia and ARF in the hospital setting. Similarly, ARF frequently occurs in animals treated with potential nephrotoxicants such as gentamicin or amphotericin.

The kidneys can maintain adequate renal perfusion pressure by autoregulation as long as the mean arterial blood pressure exceeds approximately 60 to 70 mm Hg. Renal blood flow and perfusion pressure must be maintained for glomerular filtration and the cellular delivery of oxygen and nutrients to occur. Cellular swelling secondary to decreased sodium-potassium ($Na^+/K^+$) pump activity results from the osmotic extraction

### TABLE 44-2

**Partial List of Potential Nephrotoxicants in Dogs and Cats**

| Therapeutic Agents | Organic Compounds—cont'd |
|---|---|
| Antimicrobials | Chloroform |
|   Aminoglycosides | Pesticides |
|   Cephalosporins | Herbicides |
|   Nafcillin | Solvents |
|   Polymyxins | **Pigments** |
|   Sulfonamides | Hemoglobin |
|   Tetracyclines | Myoglobin |
| Antifungals | **Intravenous Agents** |
|   Amphotericin B | Radiographic contrast |
| Anthelmintics |   agents |
|   Thiacetarsamide | **Chemotherapeutic Agents** |
| Analgesics | Cisplatin |
|   Piroxicam | Methotrexate |
|   Ibuprofen | Doxorubicin |
|   Phenylbutazone | **Anesthetics** |
|   Naproxen | Methoxyflurane |
| **Heavy Metals** | **Miscellaneous Agents** |
| Lead | Hypercalcemia |
| Mercury | Snake venom |
| Cadmium | |
| Chromium | |
| **Organic Compounds** | |
| Ethylene glycol | |
| Carbon tetrachloride | |

### TABLE 44-3

**Partial List of Potential Causes of Decreased Renal Perfusion/Ischemia in Dogs and Cats**

Dehydration
Hemorrhage
Hypovolemia
Decreased oncotic pressure
Deep anesthesia
Increased blood viscosity
Sepsis
Shock/Vasodilation
Administration of nonsteroidal antiinflammatory agents, decreased renal prostaglandin formation
Hyperthermia
Hypothermia
Burns
Trauma
Renal vessel thrombosis or microthrombus formation
Transfusion reactions

of water from the extracellular space, causing the amount of water in the plasma to decrease. The consequences of a decreased amount of plasma water in the renal vasculature are erythrocyte aggregation and vascular congestion and stasis, which tend to potentiate and perpetuate decreased glomerular

blood flow and decreased oxygen and nutrient delivery. The common result of ischemic or toxicant-induced tubular cell swelling, injury, and death is nephron dysfunction leading to a decreased glomerular filtration rate (GFR).

In ARF, dysfunction and reduced glomerular filtration occur at the individual nephron level as a result of a combination of tubular obstruction, tubular backleak, renal arteriolar vasoconstriction, and decreased glomerular capillary permeability. Specifically, cellular debris within the tubule may inspissate and obstruct the flow of filtrate through the nephron. Alternatively, interstitial edema may compress and obstruct renal tubules. A "backleak" or abnormal reabsorption of filtrate occurs because of a loss of tubular cell integrity, allowing the filtrate to cross from the tubular lumen into the renal interstitium and subsequently the renal vasculature. Tubular backleak is facilitated by tubular obstruction due to the increased intratubular pressures proximal to the obstruction. The decreased resorption of solute and water by damaged proximal tubule segments results in the increased delivery of solutes and fluid to the distal nephron and macula densa in many nephrons, which causes afferent glomerular arteriole constriction. The exact mediator of this vasoconstriction is not known, but natriuretic factor, the renin-angiotensin system, and thromboxane may be involved. A decrease in the permeability of the glomerular capillary wall also leads to a reduction in glomerular filtration. For example, aminoglycosides have been shown to decrease both the number and size of fenestrae in glomerular capillary endothelial cells, thereby decreasing the surface area available for ultrafiltration. The impaired glomerular capillary permeability that occurs in ARF often persists after vasoconstriction and renal blood flow have been corrected.

ARF has three distinct phases: (1) initiation, (2) maintenance, and (3) recovery. During the initiation phase, therapeutic measures that reduce the renal insult can prevent the development of established ARF. The maintenance phase is characterized by the formation of tubular lesions and established nephron dysfunction. Although therapeutic interventions during the maintenance phase are often lifesaving, they usually do little to diminish the severity of existing renal lesions, improve function, or hasten recovery. In the recovery phase, renal lesions are repaired, and function improves. Tubular damage may be reversible if the tubular basement membrane is intact and viable epithelial cells are present. Although new nephrons cannot be produced and irreversibly damaged nephrons cannot be repaired, the functional hypertrophy of surviving nephrons may adequately compensate for the decrease in nephron numbers. Even if renal functional recovery is incomplete, adequate function may be reestablished.

Renal biopsy specimens from animals with ARF show proximal tubular cell degeneration, ranging from cloudy swelling to necrosis, with edema and mononuclear and polymorphonuclear leukocyte infiltration in the interstitium. Although these changes do not allow toxicant-induced ARF to be differentiated from ARF caused by ischemia, renal histologic findings are often helpful in establishing a prognosis. Evidence of tubular regeneration (e.g., flattened, basophilic epithelial cells with an irregular nuclear size; mitotic figures;

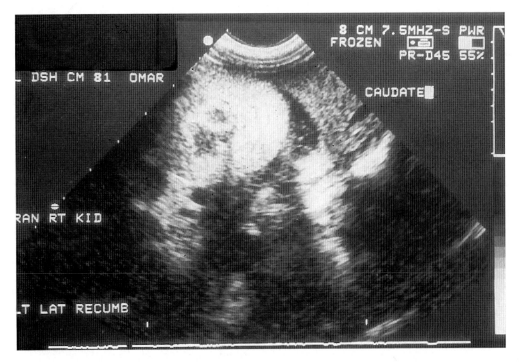

**FIG 44-2**
Ultrasonographic appearance of a kidney from a dog that ingested ethylene glycol. Notice the markedly increased renal cortical echogenicity. (Courtesy Dr. Phillip Steyn, Colorado State University, Fort Collins, Colo.)

high nuclear/cytoplasmic ratios) and the finding of generally intact tubular basement membranes are good prognostic findings. Conversely, large numbers of granular casts, extensive tubular necrosis, and interstitial mineralization and fibrosis with disrupted tubular basement membranes are poor prognostic signs. In addition to the renal histopathologic changes, the degree of functional impairment and, even more important, the response to therapy should be considered when formulating a prognosis.

## Clinical Features and Diagnosis

Clinical signs of ARF are often nonspecific and include lethargy, depression, anorexia, vomiting, diarrhea, and dehydration; occasionally uremic breath or oral ulcers may be present. A diagnosis of renal failure is confirmed if azotemia with concurrent isosthenuria or minimally concentrated urine persists. Prerenal dehydration and azotemia superimposed on an inability to concentrate urine (e.g., Addison's disease, hypercalcemia, or overzealous use of furosemide) initially mimics renal failure; however, in these cases, volume replacement results in resolution of the azotemia.

ARF occurs within hours or days of exposure to the insult. Unique clinical signs and clinicopathologic findings associated with ARF include enlarged or swollen kidneys, hemoconcentration, good body condition, an active urine sediment (e.g., granular casts, renal epithelial cells), and relatively severe hyperkalemia and metabolic acidosis (especially in the face of oliguria) (see Table 41-10). Clinical signs in an animal with ARF tend to be severe relative to those seen in an animal with CRF and the same magnitude of azotemia. Renal ultrasonographic findings in dogs and cats with ARF are usu-

ally nonspecific, with diffusely normal to slightly hyperechoic renal cortices. In animals with calcium oxalate nephrosis associated with ethylene glycol ingestion, the renal cortices can be very hyperechoic (Fig. 44-2). Doppler estimation of the resistive index in renal arcuate arteries is increased in many dogs with ARF; however, this method of evaluation must be more extensively correlated with the renal histopathologic changes before firm conclusions regarding the merits of the index can be drawn. Histopathologic examination of renal cortical biopsy specimens from animals with ARF will reveal varying degrees of tubular necrosis. Evidence of tubular epithelial regeneration can be observed as early as 3 days after the acute insult and is a positive prognostic indicator.

## Risk Factors for Renal Failure

Although the prevention of trauma (e.g., hit by car) that may lead to shock and the development of renal ischemia or exposure to nephrotoxicants outside the hospital relies on client education and environmental control, an important aspect of the prevention of hospital-acquired ARF is the identification of animals at increased risk. Several risk factors that predispose dogs to the development of gentamicin-induced ARF have been identified (Table 44-4); however, it is likely that many also predispose dogs and cats to the development of other types of toxicant-induced ARF, as well as ARF induced by ischemia. In many cases a combination of decreased renal perfusion or treatment with nephrotoxic agents in the context of more chronic, preexisting risk factors is responsible for the development of ARF in the hospital setting. Once the clinician detects predisposing risk factors, he or she can assess the risk-benefit ratio in individual cases in which an elective

TABLE 4-4

**Risk Factors for Acute Renal Failure**

Preexisting renal disease or renal insufficiency
Dehydration
Decreased cardiac output
Sepsis, pyometra
Disseminated intravascular coagulation (DIC)
Fever
Liver disease
Electrolyte abnormalities such as hypokalemia and
    hypercalcemia
Concurrent use of diuretics with potentially nephrotoxic
    drugs such as aminoglycosides
Concurrent use of potentially nephrotoxic drugs such as
    aminoglycosides, NSAIDs, and intravenous
    radiographic contrast agents
Decreased dietary protein
Diabetes mellitus

anesthetic procedure is considered or treatment with potentially nephrotoxic drugs is indicated. In some situations, predisposing risk factors can be eliminated or corrected before any potential renal insults occur.

Major categories of risk factors include disorders affecting renal perfusion, preexisting renal disease, electrolyte disturbances, treatment with nephrotoxic drugs, and dietary influences. Poor renal perfusion increases the risk of nephrotoxic and ischemic damage to the kidney. Dehydration and volume depletion are perhaps the most common causes of decreased renal perfusion. In human beings, volume depletion increases the hospitalized patient's risk of ARF by a factor of 10. Renal hypoperfusion has also been associated with decreased cardiac output, decreased plasma oncotic pressure, increased blood viscosity, and systemic vasodilation. In addition to decreased renal perfusion, volume depletion also leads to a decreased volume of distribution of nephrotoxic drugs and a decreased flow of tubular fluid. Decreased tubular flow in turn potentiates tubular resorption, which can increase the intratubular concentration of nephrotoxicants. From the standpoint of potentially nephrotoxic drugs, the use of NSAIDs can also be associated with decreased renal perfusion. For example, in animals with decreased cardiac output, decreased oncotic pressure, or dehydration, the maintenance of renal perfusion depends on prostaglandin-mediated renal vasodilation. If prostaglandin production is decreased by NSAID treatment, vasopressors that are not affected by the treatment (e.g., epinephrine, renin-angiotensin, norepinephrine) can cause severe and "unopposed" renal vasoconstriction that may result in ischemic tubular damage.

Preexisting renal disease and advanced age, which is often associated with some degree of decreased renal function, may increase the potential for nephrotoxicity produced by several mechanisms. For example, the pharmacokinetics of potentially nephrotoxic drugs may be altered in the face of decreased renal function. Specifically, the excretion of gentamicin has been shown to be decreased in partially nephrectomized dogs with subclinical renal dysfunction. Animals with renal insufficiency or advanced age may also have reduced urine concentrating ability and therefore a decreased ability to compensate for dehydration. Preexisting renal disease may also compromise the production of vasodilatory prostaglandins. The resulting unbalanced vasoconstriction could result in decreased renal perfusion.

Studies in dogs have shown that reduced dietary potassium intake exacerbates gentamicin-induced nephrotoxicity, possibly because potassium-depleted cells are more susceptible to necrosis. It is important to note that an adverse effect of high-dose gentamicin treatment in dogs is an increase in the urinary excretion of potassium. It is possible that this could result in potassium depletion (especially if it occurs in combination with anorexia or vomiting) and thus increase the risk of gentamicin-induced nephrotoxicity. Because potassium is primarily an intracellular cation, any patient with prolonged anorexia, vomiting, or diarrhea may have whole-body potassium depletion even if serum potassium concentrations are within the normal range.

The administration of potentially nephrotoxic drugs or drugs that may enhance nephrotoxicity obviously increases the risk of ARF. For example, the concurrent use of furosemide and gentamicin in dogs is associated with an increased risk of ARF and an increased severity of ARF, should it occur. Furosemide probably potentiates gentamicin-induced nephrotoxicity by causing dehydration, reducing the volume of distribution of gentamicin and increasing its renal cortical uptake. Fluid repletion minimizes but does not negate the additive effect of furosemide on gentamicin-induced nephrotoxicity in the dog, because furosemide facilitates the tubular uptake of gentamicin independent of hemodynamic changes. By means of similar mechanisms, furosemide has been shown to enhance radiocontrast agent and cisplatin-induced nephrotoxicity in human beings.

The use of NSAIDs can also increase the risk of ARF. Anesthesia, sodium or volume depletion, sepsis, congestive heart failure, the nephrotic syndrome, and hepatic disease are all conditions in which renal blood flow can become compromised, with decreased prostaglandin synthesis secondary to the administration of NSAIDs. If NSAIDs are used preoperatively to reduce postoperative pain, hydration status and blood pressure should be carefully monitored during surgery. Dogs appear to be particularly sensitive to newer NSAIDs such as ibuprofen and naproxen, which, in addition to ARF, may cause gastrointestinal tract ulceration. In theory, COX 2 inhibitors should have less effect on renal blood flow; however, comparative studies have not been performed in dogs. Recently concern has been raised about the use of nafcillin in combination with anesthesia and surgery; ARF developed postoperatively in seven dogs receiving nafcillin for antimicrobial prophylaxis associated with surgery (Pascoe and colleagues, 1996).

Studies in healthy dogs have shown that the quantity of protein fed before a nephrotoxic insult can significantly affect the degree of subsequent renal damage and dysfunction that occur. High-dietary-protein (27.3%) conditioning beginning 21 days before and continuing during gentamicin administration was found to reduce nephrotoxicity, enhance gentamicin clearance, and result in a larger volume of distribution compared with the findings in dogs fed medium (13.7%) or low levels of protein (9.4%) (Grauer and colleagues, 1994). In addition, creatinine clearance and the renal elimination of gentamicin were preserved throughout 7 days of treatment in dogs fed a high-protein diet, whereas these parameters decreased during the treatment period in dogs fed a medium- or low-protein diet. Although dietary protein conditioning may not be practical in the clinical setting, it is important to realize that anorectic animals may be at increased risk for ARF as a result of decreased protein intake.

Risk factors are additive, and any complication occurring in high-risk animals increases the potential for ARF. By virtue of their diseases, animals in shock or with acidosis, sepsis, or major organ system failure are at increased risk for ARF, and these are also the animals that are likely to require anesthesia or chemotherapy that is potentially damaging to the kidneys. For example, ARF is common in dogs with pyometra and *Escherichia coli* endotoxin–induced urine-concentrating defects. If fluid therapy is inadequate during anesthesia for ovariohysterectomy or during the recovery period, dehydration and decreased renal perfusion may result in ARF. Trauma, extensive burns, pancreatitis, diabetes mellitus, and multiple myeloma are examples of disorders associated with a high incidence of ARF in people. Additional clinical conditions that are thought to enhance the risk of ARF in dogs include vasculitis, fever, and prolonged anesthesia.

## Monitoring Patients at Risk for ARF

The recognition and appropriate management of renal injury in the initial phase of ARF are associated with improved prognosis; therefore animals receiving potentially nephrotoxic drugs and high-risk animals undergoing anesthesia should be monitored closely.

Urine production is an excellent parameter to monitor during anesthesia. Ideally, urine production should be greater than 2 ml/kg/hr. Increased urinary excretion of protein, glucose (normoglycemic glucosuria), or casts may be an early indication of renal tubular damage in animals receiving potentially nephrotoxic drugs. As an alternative to standard clinicopathologic tests, the detection and quantification of urine enzymes (enzymuria) have been used to recognize early nephrotoxicity in the dog. Inasmuch as most serum enzymes are not filtered by the glomerulus because of their large molecular weight, enzymuria can be an indication of renal tubular leakage or necrosis. Several enzymes originate from specific cellular organelles and thus can serve as markers for damage to a specific site. For example, γ-Glutamyl transpeptidase (GGT) originates from the proximal tubular brush border and *N*-acetyl glucosaminidase (NAG) is a lysosomal enzyme. Other substances (e.g., lysozyme and β₂-microglobulin) are released from numerous tissues and have molecular weights that allow glomerular filtration. Once in the glomerular filtrate,

## TABLE 44-5

**Hypothetical Comparison of the Glomerular Filtration Rate and Urine Production in Normal and Nonoliguric Acute Renal Failure States***

| | NORMAL (L/day) | ACUTE RENAL FAILURE (L/day) |
|---|---|---|
| Glomerular filtration rate | 100 | 10 |
| Tubular resorption | 99 | 7 |
| Urine production | 1 | 3 |

*These show the effect of tubular resorption on urine production in the face of decreased glomerular filtration.

these small-molecular-weight enzymes are normally extensively resorbed by the proximal tubule, so that virtually none appear in urine. However, decreased proximal tubular function results in increased urinary excretion of these small-molecular-weight enzymes. Enzymuria usually precedes other manifestations of nephrotoxic proximal tubular injury by several days. Recently the urine GGT/creatinine and NAG/creatinine ratios have been shown to accurately reflect 24-hour urine GGT and NAG excretion in dogs, if determined before the onset of azotemia (Grauer and colleague, 1995). Baseline urine GGT/creatinine and NAG/ creatinine ratios therefore should be determined in all dogs that are to receive potentially nephrotoxic drugs. Twofold to threefold increases in the GGT/creatinine or NAG/creatinine ratio over the baseline are suggestive of clinically relevant tubular damage. Drug therapy should be discontinued if this occurs.

## Treatment

The goals of treatment of established ARF are to eliminate renal hemodynamic disorders and alleviate water and solute imbalances to "buy time" for the nephrons to repair and hypertrophy. A positive response to therapy is indicated by a decrease in the serum creatinine concentration and an increase in urine production. Induction of diuresis facilitates the management of ARF by decreasing serum urea nitrogen and potassium concentrations and by lessening the likelihood of overhydration. Even though the GFR and renal blood flow may improve in response to diuresis, they are frequently unchanged, and the increased urine production is actually a result of decreased tubular resorption of filtrate (Table 44-5). Increased urine production alone does not indicate an improvement in GFR.

Treatment guidelines for ARF are listed in Table 44-6. Identification and elimination of any prerenal or postrenal abnormalities are essential. If renal damage is suspected, all potentially nephrotoxic drugs should be discontinued. Induction of emesis or gastric lavage should be considered in order to decrease the absorption of recently ingested toxicants. In addition, the use of gastrointestinal tract adsorbents and cathartics (activated charcoal and sodium sulfate) may be beneficial. Peritoneal dialysis can be used to decrease blood

TABLE 44-6

**Treatment Guidelines for Dogs and Cats with Acute Renal Failure**

Discontinue all potentially nephrotoxic drugs; consider measures to decrease absorption (e.g., induction of emesis and administration of activated charcoal and sodium sulfate).

Start specific antidotal therapy if applicable (e.g., alcohol dehydrogenase inhibitors for ethylene glycol).

Identify and treat any prerenal or postrenal abnormalities.

Start intravenous fluid therapy with normal saline solution or 0.45% saline solution in 2.5% dextrose:
  a. Rehydrate animal within 6 hours.
  b. Provide maintenance fluid and replace continuing fluid losses.

Assess volume of urine production.

Correct acid-base and electrolyte abnormalities; rule out hypercalcemic nephropathy.

If necessary, to increase urine production, provide mild volume expansion while monitoring urine volume, body weight, plasma total solids, hematocrit, and central venous pressure.

Administer vasodilators or diuretics, or both, if necessary, to increase urine production:
  a. Mannitol or
  b. Furosemide and dopamine

Base subsequent fluid volumes on urine production plus 20 ml/kg/24 hr.

Consider peritoneal dialysis if there is no response to above treatment; biopsy kidney at time of dialysis catheter placement.

Control hyperphosphatemia:
  a. Phosphate-restricted diet and, if necessary,
  b. Enteric phosphate binders

Treat vomiting and gastroenteritis with:
  a. Metoclopramide,
  b. Trimethobenzamide, or
  c. Chlorpromazine

Treat gastric hyperacidity with $H_2$ blockers.

Provide caloric requirements (70 to 100 kcal/kg/day).

 TABLE 44-7

**Hypothetical Examples of Daily Maintenance Fluid Requirements in Dogs and Cats**

| | NORMAL URINE PRODUCTION | OLIGURIC ARF | NONOLIGURIC ARF |
|---|---|---|---|
| Insensible loss (ml/kg) | 20 | 20 | 20 |
| Urine volume (ml/kg) | 40 | 10 | 160 |
| Total (ml/kg) | 60 | 30 | 180 |

*ARF,* Acute renal faliure.

assessed. Because approximately two thirds of normal maintenance fluid requirement results from the fluid loss in urine, oliguric and nonoliguric animals can have large variations in their fluid needs (Table 44-7). Measurement of the urine volume also facilitates the assessment of endogenous creatinine clearance, providing a more accurate estimate of GFR than does serum creatinine concentration alone. If indwelling urinary catheters are used to measure urine volume, strict aseptic technique and closed collection systems should be used. This is because uremic animals have depressed cellular immunity and phagocytic function, and infection can be life-threatening in these animals. Intermittent urinary bladder catheterization is usually preferable to indwelling catheterization for timed urine collections.

During rehydration, the animal's acid-base and electrolyte status should be evaluated and any abnormalities treated accordingly. Metabolic acidosis and hyperkalemia are common in animals with oliguric ARF; the acidosis is usually partially compensated for by a respiratory alkalosis. Bicarbonate therapy should be reserved for animals with a blood pH of 7.15 or less. However, such therapy must be carefully administered, because overzealous sodium bicarbonate therapy can produce ionized calcium deficits and sodium excesses, which may contribute to the development of hypervolemia in the oliguric animal. Hyperkalemia can cause cardiac conduction abnormalities and is the main life-threatening electrolyte disturbance that can occur in dogs and cats with ARF. Hyperkalemia is best diagnosed on the basis of serum potassium concentrations; however, bradycardia and the electrocardiographic finding of a decreased P-wave amplitude, an increased PR interval, widened QRS complexes, and tall, spiked T waves frequently occur in association with this electrolyte abnormality. If severe, hyperkalemia can cause atrial standstill, sinoventricular rhythms, ventricular tachycardia, fibrillation, and asystole. Hyperkalemia should be promptly treated with a slow intravenous bolus administration of sodium bicarbonate (1 to 2 mEq/kg) or with regular insulin (0.25 to 0.5 U/kg IV) followed by dextrose (4 ml of 50% dextrose per unit of insulin administered). Alternatively, calcium gluconate (0.5 to 1 ml of 10% solution per kilogram of body

concentrations of dialyzable toxicants (e.g., ethylene glycol and gentamicin), and diuresis with intravenous isotonic saline solution may help maintain renal perfusion and the excretion of toxicants. Fluid deficits should be replaced intravenously within 6 hours with 0.45% saline solution in 2.5% dextrose or with normal saline solutions. Maintenance fluid therapy and replacement of continuing fluid losses should be provided over a 24-hour period using 0.45% saline solution in 2.5% dextrose to prevent worsening of the hypernatremia and hyperkalemia. Oliguria is common in animals with ARF and was once thought to be a hallmark of the syndrome. However, because nonoliguric ARF is now being recognized with increasing frequency, urine production should be quantified so that maintenance fluid needs can be properly weight given slowly IV while monitoring the animal's electrocardiogram) may also be used to counteract the effects of hyperkalemia on cardiac conduction.

If there are no signs of overhydration and oliguria persists after apparent rehydration, mild volume expansion with 3% to 5% of the animal's body weight in fluid may be initiated, because dehydration of this magnitude is difficult to detect clinically (see Table 44-6). Monitoring body weight, the plasma total solid content, hematocrit value, and central venous pressure will help prevent overhydration. If fluid therapy alone fails to induce diuresis, either mannitol or a combination of dopamine and furosemide is the therapy of choice. If one regimen proves ineffective, the other may be tried. Dopamine and furosemide therapy is a better choice for overhydrated animals; however, it appears that this combination is more efficacious in the management of ischemic ARF than of toxicant-induced ARF. Furosemide may also potentiate gentamicin-induced nephrotoxicosis. Regardless of whether diuresis occurs, maintenance fluid requirements should be derived from the volume of urine produced (ins-and-outs fluid therapy) (see Table 44-7). If diuresis occurs, polyionic solutions (e.g., Normosol or lactated Ringer's solution) should be used to meet maintenance fluid requirements; potassium supplementation is often necessary and should be determined on the basis of the serum potassium concentrations (Table 44-8).

Provision of the daily caloric requirements is an important aspect of the conservative management of patients with renal failure. Because the body's energy requirements have a higher priority than does protein anabolism, endogenous proteins will be catabolized if caloric needs are not met. Endogenous protein catabolism not only causes weight loss and muscle wasting but also increases blood urea concentrations. Protein breakdown in humans with renal failure can be reduced by providing as little as 100 g of carbohydrate per day. Supplementation of essential amino acids in anephric dogs has also been shown to stabilize serum urea nitrogen concentrations and lengthen survival. Inappetence resulting from gastric hyperacidity and vomiting can usually be controlled by the administration of an $H_2$-receptor blocker (e.g., ranitidine) and antiemetics that act at the chemoreceptor trigger zone (trimethobenzamide or metoclopramide) (see discussion on treatment of CRF) (see also the table Drugs Used in Dogs and Cats with Urinary Tract Disorders at the end of this section). Food blended with water administered through a stomach tube may be tolerated by animals that are anorectic but not vomiting. Reduced-protein diets and enteric phosphate binders (aluminum hydroxide or aluminum carbonate) should be used to reduce serum urea nitrogen concentrations and combat hyperphosphatemia in uremic dogs and cats. In some instances, adequate (but not normal) renal function can be regained, and reduced-protein diets should probably be used on a continuous basis if the serum urea nitrogen concentration is more than 60 to 75 mg/dl.

Peritoneal dialysis should be considered in animals with severe, persistent uremia; acidosis; or hyperkalemia. Dialysis may also be used to treat overhydration and in some cases may hasten the elimination of toxicants. Renal biopsy should

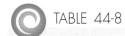

**TABLE 44-8**

**Potassium Supplementation Guidelines**

| MEASURED SERUM POTASSIUM CONCENTRATION (mEq/L) | AMOUNT OF KCl (mEq) TO BE ADDED TO EACH LITER OF FLUID ADMINISTERED* |
|---|---|
| 3.0-3.5 | 28 |
| 2.5-3.0 | 40 |
| 2.0-2.5 | 60 |
| <2.0 | 80 |

*Do not administer at a rate of more than 0.5 mEq/kg/hr.

be performed if the diagnosis is in doubt, if the animal does not respond to therapy within 3 to 5 days, or if peritoneal dialysis is being considered. The long-term prognosis for dogs and cats with ARF is usually fair to good if the animal survives the period of renal regeneration and compensation. It may take several weeks to months for renal function to improve, however. The severity of the azotemia and the histopathologic lesions, as well as the response to therapy, are the most important prognostic indicators early in ARF.

## CHRONIC RENAL FAILURE

### Etiology and Pathogenesis

Unlike ARF, the cause of CRF is usually difficult to determine. Because of the interdependence of the vascular and tubular components of the nephron, the end-point of irreversible glomerular or tubular damage is the same. A morphologic heterogeneity among nephrons exists in the chronically diseased kidney, with the changes ranging from severe atrophy and fibrous scar tissue replacement to marked hypertrophy. The histopathologic changes are not process-specific, therefore the cause is usually unknown. Nevertheless, recent studies have shown that primary glomerular disorders are a major cause of CRF in the dog. Because glomerular filtration *in toto* is uniformly reduced, CRF may be considered a single pathologic entity, although many diverse pathways can lead to this endpoint. Potential causes of CRF are listed in Table 44-9.

In progressive diseases that slowly destroy nephrons, intact nephrons undergo a compensatory hypertrophy. When renal failure finally occurs, the hypertrophied nephrons can no longer maintain adequate renal function. Renal lesions associated with CRF are usually irreversible and often progressive, therefore treatment of the CRF rarely improves renal function.

The pathophysiology of CRF can be considered at both the organ and systemic level. At the level of the kidney, the fundamental pathologic change that occurs is a loss of nephrons and decreased GFR. Reduced GFR in turn results in increased plasma concentrations of substances that are normally eliminated from the body by renal excretion. Many

TABLE 44-9

**Potential Causes of Chronic Renal Failure in Dogs and Cats**

**Immunologic Disorders**

Systemic lupus erythematosus
Glomerulonephritis
Vasculitis (e.g., feline infectious peritonitis)

**Amyloidosis**

**Neoplasia**

Primary
Secondary

**Nephrotoxicants**

**Renal Ischemia**

**Inflammatory or Infectious Causes**

Pyelonephritis
Leptospirosis
Renal calculi

**Hereditary and Congenital Disorders**

Renal hypoplasia or dysplasia
Polycystic kidneys
Familial nephropathies (Lhasa Apsos, Shih Tzus,
   Norwegian Elkhounds, Rottweilers, Bernese Mountain
   Dogs, Chow Chows, Newfoundlands, Bull Terriers,
   Pembroke Welsh Corgis, Chinese Sharpeis,
   Doberman Pinschers, Samoyeds, Golden Retrievers,
   Standard Poodles, Soft-Coated Wheaten Terriers,
   Cocker Spaniels, Beagles, Keeshonds, Bedlington
   Terriers, Cairn Terriers, Basenjis, Abyssinian cats)

**Urinary Outflow Obstruction**

**Idiopathic**

TABLE 44-10

**Substances that Can Increase in Concentration in the Plasma of Dogs and Cats with Renal Failure**

Amino acids
Ammonia
Aromatic and aliphatic amines
Creatinine
Cyclic adenosine monophosphate
Gastrin
Glucagon
Growth hormone
Guanidinium compounds
Indoles
Parathyroid hormone
Peptides
Phenols
Phosphate
Polyols
Purine and pyrimidine derivatives
Renin
Ribonuclease
Urea
Uric acid

substances have been shown to accumulate in plasma in the setting of renal failure (Table 44-10). The constellation of clinical signs known as the uremic syndrome is thought to occur, at least in part, as a result of increasing plasma concentrations of these substances. Components of the uremic syndrome include sodium and water imbalance, anemia, carbohydrate intolerance, neurologic disturbances, gastrointestinal tract disturbances, osteodystrophy, immunologic incompetence, and metabolic acidosis.

In addition to excreting metabolic wastes and maintaining fluid and electrolyte balance, the kidneys also function as endocrine organs and catabolize several peptide hormones. Therefore hormonal disturbances also play a role in the pathogenesis of CRF. For example, the decreased production of erythropoietin and calcitriol in animals with CRF contributes to the development of nonregenerative anemia and hyperparathyroidism, respectively. Conversely, decreased metabolism and increased concentrations of parathyroid hormone and gastrin contribute to the development of hyperparathyroidism and gastritis, respectively.

Part of the pathophysiologic changes that occur in CRF are brought about by compensatory mechanisms. The osteodystrophy of CRF occurs secondary to hyperparathyroidism, which develops in an attempt to maintain normal plasma calcium and phosphorus concentrations. Similarly, the GFR of intact hypertrophied nephrons increases in animals with CRF in an attempt to maintain adequate renal function; however, proteinuria and glomerulosclerosis in these individual nephrons, leading to additional nephron damage and loss, may be consequences of this hyperfiltration (Fig. 44-3).

## Clinical Features and Diagnosis

Unlike ARF, CRF develops over a period of weeks, months, or years, and its clinical signs are often relatively mild for the magnitude of the azotemia. Unique signs of CRF include a history of weight loss, polydipsia-polyuria, poor body condition, nonregenerative anemia, and small and irregularly shaped kidneys. A diagnosis of CRF is usually based on a combination of compatible historical, physical examination, and clinicopathologic findings. Plain radiographs can confirm the presence of small kidneys. Renal ultrasonography will usually show diffusely hyperechoic renal cortices with loss of the normal corticomedullary boundary. The increased cortical echogenicity results from replacement of the irreversibly damaged nephrons with fibrous scar tissue. Radiographic studies and ultrasonography can also help identify or rule out potentially treatable causes of CRF, such as pyelonephritis and renal urolithiasis. Renal biopsy is not routinely performed in animals with CRF unless the diagnosis is in question. Renal histopathologic preparations will show some combination of a loss of tubules with replacement

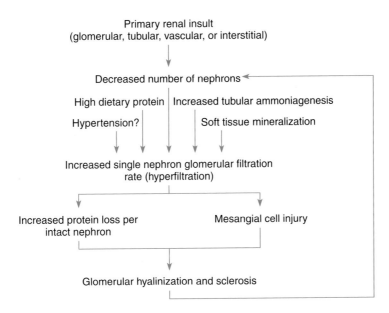

Primary renal insult
(glomerular, tubular, vascular, or interstitial)

Decreased number of nephrons

High dietary protein | Increased tubular ammoniagenesis

Hypertension? | Soft tissue mineralization

Increased single nephron glomerular filtration
rate (hyperfiltration)

Increased protein loss per
intact nephron | Mesangial cell injury

Glomerular hyalinization and sclerosis

**FIG 44-3**
Proposed pathogenesis of progressive loss of nephrons in chronic renal failure.

fibrosis and mineralization, glomerulosclerosis and glomerular atrophy, and foci of mononuclear cells (small lymphocytes, plasma cells, and macrophages) within the interstitium in association with fibrous scar tissue replacement.

## Treatment

The regenerative and hypertrophic nephron changes have had time to occur in an animal with CRF, yet the fact that renal failure has occurred indicates the inadequacy of these compensatory processes. Even though CRF is usually irreversible, the severity of clinical signs can generally be reduced with proper treatment (Table 44-11). In addition, treatment is directed at the amelioration of several disorders that may contribute to progression of renal failure (e.g., systemic hypertension, soft tissue mineralization).

In animals with CRF, polyuria and compensatory polydipsia occur as a result of a decrease in the urine concentrating ability. As the number of functional nephrons decreases, there is a compensatory increase in the GFR in each intact nephron, which in turn increases individual tubular flow rates and volumes. In addition, there is a decrease in the renal medullary sodium concentration gradient because of the decrease in the number of functional nephrons and thus in the number of sodium pumps. Decreased medullary hypertonicity decreases the medullary osmotic pressure gradient that drives the passive resorption of water from the distal tubules and collecting ducts when ADH is present. Because of the compensatory polydipsia, it is important that the animal with CRF always have water available for ad libitum consumption. Dehydration, as can occur in gastroenteritis, may cause a rapid and severe decline in renal function. If anorexia, vomiting, or diarrhea results in dehydration, fluid deficits should be aggressively replaced parenterally. The volume of fluids required is determined by the extent of dehydration and the maintenance and continuing fluid loss requirements of the patient. Daily maintenance fluid requirements in ani-

 TABLE 44-11

**Treatment Guidelines for Dogs and Cats with Chronic Renal Failure**

Discontinue all potentially nephrotoxic drugs.
Identify and treat any prerenal or postrenal abnormalities.
Rule out or identify any treatable conditions such as pyelonephritis and renal urolithiasis by means of radiography or ultrasonography.
Measure blood pressure; consider treatment with ACEIs or calcium channel blockers if animal has systemic hypertension.
Initiate dietary protein reduction if there is moderate to severe azotemia (blood urea nitrogen, ≥60 to 75 mg/dl).
If animal has hyperphosphatemia, start a phosphorus-restricted diet and add enteric phosphate binders; consider use of calcitriol.
Treat vomiting and gastroenteritis, if present, with:
  a. Metoclopramide,
  b. Trimethobenzamide, or
  c. Chlorpromazine
  d. H$_2$ blockers
Treat anemia, if present, with:
  a. Anabolic steroids
  b. Human recombinant erythropoietin
Provide caloric requirements (70 to 100 kcal/kg/day); consider the placement of a gastrostomy or esophagostomy tube if the animal is not vomiting.

mals with CRF are higher than those of normal animals because of polyuria. This polyuria also results in an increased loss of water-soluble vitamins B and C, which should be compensated for in the diet. If the patient with CRF is not able to drink enough to keep up with its urine output, daily subcutaneous fluids may be indicated. In many cases, owners are able to perform this treatment at home.

Salt should not be supplemented in animals with CRF in an attempt to maintain extracellular fluid volume and increase urine production. In fact, there is evidence that sodium intake should be reduced proportionate to the decrease in the GFR. In dogs with a reduced renal mass, a decrease in the dietary sodium intake causes urinary sodium excretion to be decreased without evidence of volume depletion or other adverse effects. It is thought that the maintenance of sodium excretion in animals with CRF represents an adaptation of individual intact nephrons and that the additional natriuresis associated with normal or high dietary sodium intake may have negative consequences.

Hypertension is common in dogs and cats with CRF, occurring in approximately 60% of these patients. Although the exact mechanism responsible for causing the hypertension is not known, a combination of glomerular capillary and arteriolar scarring, a decreased production of renal vasodilatory prostaglandins, an increased responsiveness to normal pressor mechanisms, and activation of the renin-angiotensin system may be involved. A reduction in dietary salt intake is often recommended as the first line of treatment; however, in many cases angiotensin-converting enzyme inhibitors (ACEIs) or calcium channel blockers may also be necessary to control the hypertension (Table 44-12). Hypertension may contribute to progressive nephron loss by causing further glomerular damage associated with intraglomerular hypertension. Recently, benazepril treatment in cats with surgically induced CRF sustained single nephron glomerular filtration (Brown and colleagues, 2001). Benazepril also reduced systemic hypertension and increased whole kidney glomerular filtration in these cats. Based on these results, ACEIs may be an effective treatment to slow the rate of progression of naturally occurring CRF in cats. Preliminary studies in dogs with the remnant kidney model of CRF also suggest that ACEIs may have beneficial effects.

The decreased renal sulfate and phosphate excretion secondary to decreased GFR in animals with CRF results in decreased hydrogen ion excretion and increased urinary bicarbonate loss. In addition, reduced protein intake (discussed in the following paragraph) may further compromise urinary acid excretion by decreasing renal ammoniagenesis. The am-

 TABLE 44-12

**Drugs used in Dogs and Cats with Acute and Chronic Renal Failure**

| DRUG | ACTION | DOSAGE |
|------|--------|--------|
| Amlodipine besylate (Norvasc) | Calcium antagonist | 2.5 mg/dog or 0.1mg/kg PO q24h (dog); 0.625 mg/cat/day PO (cat) |
| Aluminum hydroxide (Dialume Amphojel) | Enteric phosphate binder | 10-30 mg/kg q8h PO, with or immediately after meals |
| Benazepril (Lotensin) | Angiotensin-converting enzyme inhibitor | 0.25-0.5 mg/kg q24h |
| Chlorpromazine (Thorazine) | Antiemetic | 0.25-0.5 mg/kg q6-8h IM, SQ, PO, after rehydration only |
| Cimetidine (Tagamet) | H$_2$ blocker | 2.5-5.0 mg/kg q6-8h PO, IV, IM |
| Dopamine (Intropin) | Renal vasodilator | 2-10 µg/kg/min IV |
| Enalapril (Enacard) | Angiotensin-converting enzyme inhibitor | 0.25-0.5 mg/kg q12-24h PO (dog); 6.25 mg/cat q12h PO (cat) |
| Erythropoietin (,-HuEPO) (Epogen) | | Doses range from 35-50 u/kg three times/week to 400 u/kg/week IV, SQ (adjust dose to PCV of 30% to 35%) |
| Famotidine (Pepcid) | H$_2$ blocker | 0.5 mg/kg q12-24h IM, SQ, PO |
| Furosemide (Lasix) | Loop diuretic | 2-4 mg/kg q8-12h IV, PO |
| Hydralazine (Apresoline) | Arterial vasodilator | 0.5-2.0 mg/kg q8-12h PO (dog); 2.5-5.0 mg/cat q12-24h PO (cat) |
| Lisinopril (Prinivil, Zestril) | Angiotensin-converting enzyme inhibitor | 0.5 mg/kg PO q24h (dog) |
| Mannitol | Osmotic diuretic | 0.5-1.0 g/kg as 20% to 25% solution, slow IV bolus over 5-10 min |
| Metoclopramide (Reglan) | Antiemetic | 0.2-0.5 mg/kg q8-24h PO, SQ |
| Nandrolone decanoate (Deca-Durabolin) | Anabolic steroid | 1.0-1.5 mg/kg every week IM (dog); 1.0 mg/cat every week IM (cat) |
| Ranitidine (Zantac) | H$_2$ blocker | 2.0 mg/kg q24h PO, IV (dog); 2.5 mg/kg q12h IV, 3.5 mg/kg q12h PO (cat) |
| Sodium bicarbonate or potassium citrate | Alkalinization | 8-12 mEq/kg q12h PO |
| Trimethobenzamide (Tigan) | Antiemetic | 3.0 mg/kg q8h IM (dog) |

*PCV,* Packed cell volume.

monia produced from glutamine by the distal tubules combines with hydrogen ions within the tubular lumen to form ammonium ions, which are poorly lipid soluble (ion trapped). This results in the urinary excretion of acid. If dietary protein intake is reduced in dogs with CRF, less glutamine is available for ammonia production and therefore the urinary excretion of hydrogen ions may be decreased. At the same time, individual hypertrophied nephrons in dogs and cats with CRF may be capable of increased ammoniagenesis, which can have local toxic and inflammatory effects and contribute to progressive nephron destruction. Sodium bicarbonate or potassium citrate should therefore be cautiously supplemented at a dosage of 8 to 12 mEq/kg given orally twice a day to minimize the metabolic acidosis and lessen the stimulus for renal ammoniagenesis. It should be noted, however, that overzealous bicarbonate treatment may aggravate hypertension and create ionized calcium deficits. If the urine pH increases above 7.0 or the plasma bicarbonate concentration increases to more than 18 to 20 mEq/L, the amount of bicarbonate supplemented should be reduced or supplementation should be discontinued. Many protein-reduced prescription diets are already supplemented with potassium citrate to help decrease acidosis, and further supplementation may not be necessary.

A reduction in dietary protein intake has long been the cornerstone of management in dogs and cats with CRF. The benefits of this include decreased serum urea nitrogen and phosphorus concentrations. There are, however, potential undesirable effects associated with dietary protein reduction. Specifically, if dietary protein is restricted in relation to the animal's protein needs, reduced renal hemodynamics, protein depletion (decreased body weight, muscle mass, and serum albumin concentration), anemia, and acidosis can occur or be aggravated. Just as increased dietary protein intake results in increased glomerular filtration, restricted intake is often associated with a reduction in the GFR. The anemia of CRF is exacerbated because protein depletion further compromises erythrogenesis. Dietary protein restriction also decreases renal ammoniagenesis and therefore renal acid excretion.

Ideally, when dietary protein intake is reduced, all essential amino acid requirements are met without excesses by feeding the animal a reduced amount of high-biologic-value protein. Reduced intake also results in a decreased requirement for the renal clearance of phosphorus, urea, and other nitrogenous metabolites. In animals being fed protein-reduced diets, it must be kept in mind that the energy requirements of the body have a higher priority than protein anabolism does; therefore, if the available carbohydrates and fats are insufficient to meet caloric requirements, endogenous proteins are often broken down as a source of energy. The catabolism of endogenous proteins for this purpose increases the nitrogenous waste the kidney must then excrete and exacerbates the clinical signs of renal failure.

Researchers have established that the minimum protein requirements for dogs and cats with CRF are higher than those of normal animals. Ideally, dogs with CRF should receive a minimum of 2 to 2.2 g and cats a minimum of 3.3 to 3.5 g of protein per kilogram of body weight per day. A good recommendation to effectively achieve dietary protein reduction is to feed the maximum amount of high-biologic-value protein that the animal can tolerate at its level of renal function. *Reduced dietary protein intake* refers to decreased protein intake compared with a normal protein intake. Most commercial pet foods have a relatively high protein content. Restricting the dietary protein intake or feeding the animal less protein than is required should be avoided. A favorable response to this measure is a stable body weight and stable serum creatinine and albumin concentrations, with decreasing serum urea nitrogen and phosphorus concentrations. Most veterinary nephrologists recommend that dietary protein reduction be initiated when the animal's blood urea nitrogen concentration is between 60 and 80 mg/dl. Examples of commercially available diets that contain reduced-quantity, high-quality-protein include Hill's Prescription Diet k/d, Purina NF-formula diets, Iams early and advanced stage renal failure, and Waltham Veterinarium medium- and low-protein diets. Homemade reduced-protein diet recipes are also available (Table 44-13).

Management of the hyperphosphatemia that occurs in CRF is closely related to dietary protein reduction, inasmuch as protein-reduced diets are also phosphorus-reduced. Hyperphosphatemia in animals with CRF occurs as a result of decreased renal excretion of phosphate (Figs. 44-4 and 44-5). Concurrently, a decrease in the concentration of the active form of vitamin D decreases the intestinal absorption of calcium, which, in conjunction with the impaired tubular resorption of calcium, decreases the plasma concentrations of ionized calcium. Parathyroid hormone (PTH) production and release are stimulated by decreased plasma calcium and vitamin $D_3$ concentrations. Increasing PTH concentrations facilitate the renal excretion of phosphorus and increase serum calcium concentrations by increasing renal calcium resorption and calcium absorption from bones and the gastrointestinal tract. The consequences of this hyperparathyroidism, however, can be severe and include osteodystrophy, neuropathy, bone marrow suppression, and soft tissue mineralization. Soft tissue mineralization occurs predominantly in damaged tissue. If it occurs in renal tissue, irreversibly damaging nephrons, renal function will progressively decline. If the product of the serum calcium and phosphorus concentrations exceeds 50 to 70 mg/dl, the animal is at risk for soft tissue mineralization. Studies in cats with CRF have shown that normal dietary phosphorus intake is associated with the occurrence of microscopic renal mineralization and fibrosis and that these changes are prevented by decreasing the dietary phosphorus intake. Similar studies in dogs with CRF have shown that normal dietary phosphorus intake, as opposed to a reduced intake, is associated with a higher mortality rate. In addition to feeding the animal a phosphorus-reduced diet, enteric phosphate binders such as aluminum carbonate or aluminum hydroxide can be administered to help combat hyperphosphatemia (see Tables 44-6, 44-12, and Drugs Used in Dogs and Cats with Urinary Tract Disorders, p. 657). Enteric phosphate binders do not directly

TABLE 44-13

**Homemade Reduced-Protein Diet Recipes for Dog and Cats with Chronic Renal Failure***

| REDUCED PROTEIN DIET FOR DOGS | REDUCED PROTEIN DIET FOR CATS |
|---|---|
| ¼ lb ground beef (do not use lean ground chuck)<br>2 cups cooked white rice without salt<br>1 hard-cooked egg, finely chopped<br>3 slices white bread, crumbled<br>1 tsp (5 g) calcium carbonate<br>Also add a balanced supplement that fulfills the minimal daily requirement for all vitamins and trace minerals.<br>Cook beef in skillet, stirring until lightly browned. Stir in remaining ingredients and mix well. This mixture is somewhat dry, and its palatability can be improved by adding a little water (not milk). Keep covered in the refrigerator. Yield: 1¼ lb. | ¼ lb liver (beef, chicken, or pork only)<br>2 large hard-cooked eggs<br>2 cups cooked white rice without salt<br>1 tsp vegetable oil<br>1 tsp (5 g) calcium carbonate<br>¼ tsp potassium chloride (salt substitute)<br>Also add a balanced supplement that fulfills the minimal daily requirement for all vitamins and trace minerals and 250 mg of taurine/day.<br>Dice and braise the meat, retaining fat. Combine all ingredients and mix well. This mixture is somewhat dry, and its palatability may be improved by adding some water (not milk). Keep covered in the refrigerator. Yield: 1¼ lb. |

| Analysis | As Fed | Analysis | As Fed |
|---|---|---|---|
| Protein | 6.9% | Protein | 7.3% |
| Fat | 5.5% | Fat | 5.3% |
| Carbohydrate | 21.1% | Carbohydrate | 15.8% |
| Moisture | 65.5% | Moisture | 70.0% |
| Metabolizable energy | 750 kcal/lb | Metabolizable energy | 635 kcal/lb |

This diet supplies 17% protein calories, 30% fat calories, and 53% carbohydrate calories.

This diet supplies 21% protein calories, 35% fat calories, and 44% carbohydrate calories.

| Body Weight | Approximate Daily Feeding (lb) | Body Weight | Approximate Daily Feeding (lb) |
|---|---|---|---|
| 5 lb | ¼ | 5 lb | ¼ |
| 10 lb | ½ | 7-8 lb | ⅓ |
| 20 lb | 1 | 10 lb | ⅖ |
| 40 lb | 1½ | | |
| 60 lb | 2 | | |
| 80 lb | 2½ | | |
| 100 lb | 3 | | |

*Developed by Mark Morris Associates, Topeka, Kansas.

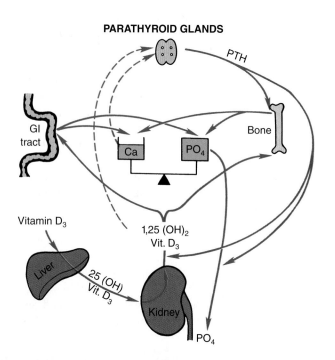

**FIG 44-4**

Some of the major interactions of plasma calcium *(Ca)*, phosphorus *(PO₄)*, parathyroid hormone *(PTH),* and vitamin D and its metabolites. The dashed arrow represents the inhibition of PTH release produced by the high plasma calcium and vitamin D concentrations. (From Harrington AR et al: *Renal pathophysiology,* New York, 1982, Wiley.)

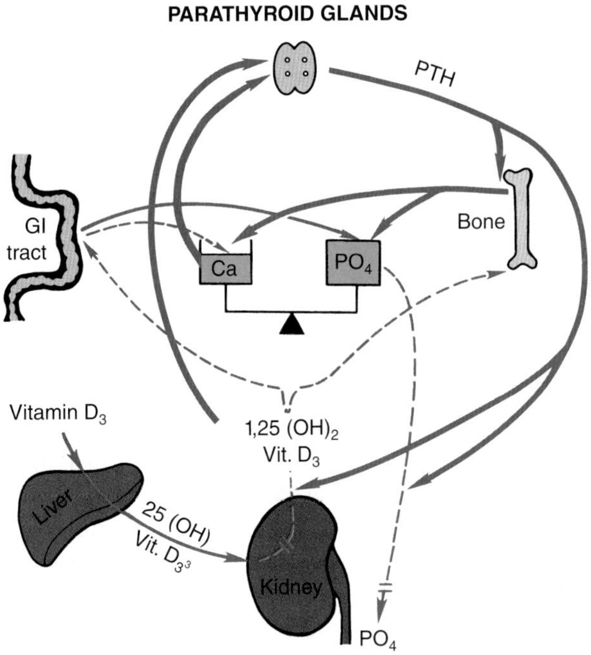

**PARATHYROID GLANDS**

**FIG 44-5**
The disturbed relationships among the plasma concentrations of calcium *(Ca)*, phosphorus *(PO$_4$)*, parathyroid hormone *(PTH)*, and vitamin D and its metabolites in chronic renal failure. Heavy lines represent the overstimulation of PTH release triggered by the decreased plasma vitamin D and calcium concentrations and the high concentrations of PTH acting on target organs. Dashed or interrupted lines indicate pathways that are at least partially inoperative or blocked in chronic renal failure. (From Harrington AR et al: *Renal pathophysiology,* New York, 1982, Wiley.)

lower the plasma phosphorus concentration, but rather bind phosphates in the intestinal tract and prevent their absorption. These agents are generally ineffective, however, if used with nonphosphorus-reduced diets.

A reduction in dietary phosphorus intake and the use of enteric phosphate binders usually lower but do not normalize serum PTH concentrations. The addition of ultra-low-dose (physiologic dose replacement) calcitriol treatment will generally further decrease serum PTH concentrations. Although the benefits of this treatment remain controversial, many investigators believe that PTH is a major uremic toxin that contributes to the progressive nature of CRF. Studies in dogs have shown that PTH concentrations are significantly increased in the setting of mild azotemia (serum creatinine concentrations as low as 1.5 to 2.5 mg/dl). Calcitriol treatment should be used only after hyperparathyroidism has been documented and the animal is well hydrated and is eating a phosphorus-reduced diet in conjunction with enteric phosphate binders. Serum phosphorus concentrations should be less than 6.0 mg/dl before and during calcitriol treatment, and the product of the calcium and phosphorus concentrations should be less than 70 mg/dl. Calcitriol may be given to animals with CRF that are hypercalcemic; however, both the serum calcium concentration and the product of the calcium

and phosphorus concentrations must be evaluated frequently to make sure they improve in response to treatment. In addition, calcium-containing enteric phosphate binders should be avoided if calcitriol is administered.

Calcitriol doses of 1.5 to 3.5 ng/kg and 1.5 ng/kg given orally once daily have been recommended for dogs and cats with CRF, respectively. The human formulation of calcitriol (Rocaltrol; Hoffmann-La Roche, Nutley, N.J.) comes in pharmacologic dose capsules and therefore is not suitable for dogs and cats. The proper calcitriol dose for dogs and cats should be formulated by compounding pharmacies. For follow-up, a serum chemistry profile should be obtained at 1 week, 1 month, and then monthly to ensure that hypercalcemia and hyperphosphatemia do not occur. Hypercalcemia caused by ultra-low-dose calcitriol is rare and should resolve within 4 days of the discontinuation of treatment. If hypercalcemia does not resolve after discontinuation, other potential causes (e.g., hypercalcemia of malignancy) should be investigated. If hyperphosphatemia develops during calcitriol treatment, further dietary phosphorus reduction or an increase in the dosage of enteric phosphate binders, or both, are necessary. Ideally, serum PTH concentrations should be measured before and at 1, 3, and 6 months after the start of calcitriol treatment to ensure that they have decreased and remain in the normal range. Intact-PTH assays should be used for measuring serum PTH concentrations, and specific instructions for sample handling should be obtained in advance from the laboratory (e.g., Animal Health Diagnostic Laboratory, Endocrine Diagnostic Section, B629 West Fee Hall, Michigan State University, East Lansing, MI 48824-1316).

Vomiting and anorexia are common in dogs and cats with CRF and can often result in decreased caloric intake and dehydration. Causes of the vomiting and anorexia include (1) stimulation of the chemoreceptor trigger zone by uremic toxins; (2) decreased excretion of gastrin, resulting in increased gastric acid secretion (serum gastrin concentrations in dogs and cats with renal failure may be as high as five and 20 times the normal concentrations, respectively); and (3) gastrointestinal tract irritation secondary to uremic vasculitis. Vomiting may be treated with trimethobenzamide or metoclopramide, which blocks the chemoreceptor trigger zone, or with chlorpromazine, which blocks the emetic center (see Tables 44-6 and 44-12 and Drugs Used in Dogs and Cats with Urinary Tract Disorders, p. 657). Metoclopramide also increases gastric motility and emptying without increasing gastric acid secretion and is the drug of choice for the management of vomiting associated with renal failure. Chlorpromazine ($\alpha$-adrenergic blocker) may cause hypotension and decreased renal blood flow and therefore should be used only if other antiemetics are ineffective. H$_2$-receptor blockers (e.g., ranitidine) have been shown to effectively decrease gastric acid secretion, which may attenuate vomiting in dogs and cats with CRF (see Table 44-12 and Drugs Used in Dogs and Cats with Urinary Tract Disorders). Oral ulcers, stomatitis, and glossitis may occur as a result of gastritis and vomiting or as a result of the effect of uremic toxins on mucous membranes. A Xylocaine viscous solution (0.5 to 1 ml PO), given before feeding in dogs, often lessens the pain associated with oral ulcerations, and this may encourage the animal to eat. If vomiting can be controlled but the animal still will not eat enough to meet its daily calorie requirements, a feeding tube may be indicated. Cats tend to tolerate gastrostomy tubes especially well, and they can remain in place for months. Esophagostomy and gastrostomy tubes not only facilitate provision of potentially unpalatable but appropriate calories but also provide a relatively stress-free route for fluid therapy.

The nonregenerative anemia observed in dogs and cats with CRF is the result of a combination of decreased erythropoietin production, shortened red blood cell survival, gastrointestinal tract blood loss, and the effects of uremic toxins such as PTH on erythropoiesis. Anabolic steroids may be of benefit to dogs and cats with CRF, because they promote red blood cell production and a positive nitrogen balance (see Table 44-12 and Drugs Used in Dogs and Cats with Urinary Tract Disorders, p. 657). These agents stimulate the differentiation of red blood cell precursors in the bone marrow, augment the renal activation of erythropoietin, and promote protein anabolism if caloric intake is adequate. In addition, increases in the red blood cell 2,3-diphosphoglycerate concentration stimulated by anabolic steroids facilitate the release of oxygen from hemoglobin to the tissues. However, several months of treatment with anabolic steroids is usually required before a response is observed, and the benefits are usually minimal. Short-term studies performed in uremic dogs treated with anabolic steroids have failed to show that they have any benefit in terms of increasing body weight, increasing the serum albumin concentration, and maintaining nitrogen balance and muscle mass. In contrast, studies assessing the effects of recombinant human erythropoietin ($_r$-HuEPO) treatment on anemia in dogs and cats with CRF have generally shown it to be successful. The cost of treatment for medium-sized and large dogs is high. Although not approved for use in dogs and cats, 100 units of $_r$-HuEPO (Epogen, Amgen, Thousand Oaks, Calif) per kilogram of body weight given subcutaneously three times weekly has been used successfully. The dose interval is lengthened once a target packed cell volume (PCV) is achieved (PCV of 30% to 35% in cats and 35% to 40% in dogs). This treatment, in addition to increasing the PCV, often results in increased appetite, weight gain, increased strength, and an improved sense of well-being. It should be noted, however, that there is a potential for antibodies to form in dogs and cats treated with $_r$-HuEPO. Most studies show that anti-$_r$-HuEPO antibodies will develop in approximately 30% to 40% of dogs and cats treated with $_r$-HuEPO. If antibodies are produced against $_r$-HuEPO, they may also react with endogenous erythropoietin, making the animal transfusion-dependent. In addition, oral iron supplementation may be necessary during $_r$-HuEPO treatment because of the rapid initiation of erythropoiesis and marginal depletion of iron stores that occur in animals with CRF. If canine and feline recombinant erythropoietin become available, our ability to treat the anemia of CRF will improve significantly.

Impaired immunity to infectious agents occurs in the uremic animal as a result of an altered inflammatory response and a defect in cellular immunity. Consequently the uremic animal is more susceptible to life-threatening infections. Indwelling urinary catheters should be used only if necessary, and an aseptic technique and closed collection systems are important. It is not recommended that prophylactic antibiotic treatment be instituted in conjunction with the placement of indwelling urinary catheters; urinary tract infections should be treated on the basis of culture and sensitivity results, and indwelling urinary catheters should be removed.

Caution should be taken to avoid using nephrotoxic antibiotics (e.g., gentamicin). Animals with CRF are particularly susceptible to adverse drug reactions. This is because many drugs and drug metabolites are excreted by the kidneys and therefore can accumulate in animals with decreased renal function and contribute to additional loss of nephrons. Package inserts should be studied to ascertain the route of drug excretion, potential toxicity, and the way to adjust dosage (increasing the dosing interval as opposed to decreasing the dose) in animals with CRF. Usually it is not necessary to adjust the drug dosage if the serum creatinine concentration is less than 2.5 mg/dl.

Stressful situations should be avoided if at all possible in dogs and cats with CRF, because stress is associated with the release of endogenous corticosteroids, which may result in endogenous protein catabolism. In addition, many dogs and cats with CRF are geriatric animals that respond better to outpatient treatment than to hospitalization. Follow-up examinations of these animals should be performed at least every 2 to 4 months. Body weight; a complete blood count; the serum urea nitrogen, creatinine, calcium, phosphorus, and total protein concentrations; and urinalysis should be assessed at each follow-up visit. The keeping of data flow charts facilitates monitoring the progress of these patients. Plots of the reciprocal of the serum creatinine concentration versus age or time may help demonstrate a progressive decline in renal function, or a positive response to therapy.

## Suggested Readings

Allen TA et al: A technique for estimating progression of chronic renal failure in the dog, *J Am Vet Med Assoc* 190:866, 1987.

Allen TA et al: Comparative aspects of nonoliguric acute renal failure, *Compend Contin Educ Pract Vet* 9:293, 1987.

Behrend EN et al: Effects of dietary protein conditioning on gentamicin pharmacokinetics in the dog, *J Vet Pharmacol Therap* 17:259, 1994.

Behrend EN et al: Hospital-acquired acute renal failure in dogs: 29 cases (1983-1992), *J Am Vet Med Assoc* 208:537, 1996.

Brown SA et al: Gentamicin-associated acute renal failure in the dog, *J Am Vet Med Assoc* 186:686, 1985.

Brown SA: Canine renal disease. In Wills J et al, editors: *The Waltham book of clinical nutrition of the dog & cat*, Oxford, 1994, Elsevier, p 963.

Brown SA: Reassessment of the use of calcitriol in chronic renal failure. In Kirk RW et al, editors: *Current veterinary therapy XII, small animal practice*, Philadelphia, 1995, WB Saunders.

Brown SA et al: Effects of the angiotensin-converting enzyme inhibitor benazepril in cats with induced renal insufficiency, *Am J Vet Res* 62:375, 2001.

Cowgill LD et al: Acute renal failure. In Ettinger SJ et al, editors: *Textbook of veterinary internal medicine,* ed 5, Philadelphia, 2000, WB Saunders, p 1615.

Finco DR et al: Effects of three diets on dogs with induced chronic renal failure, *Am J Vet Res* 46:646, 1985.

Finco DR et al: Effects of dietary phosphorus and protein in dogs with chronic renal failure, *Am J Vet Res* 53:2264, 1992.

Grauer GF et al: Effects of dietary protein conditioning on gentamicin-induced nephrotoxicosis in healthy male dogs, *Am J Vet Res* 55:90, 1994.

Grauer GF et al: Acute renal failure. In Ettinger SJ et al: editors: *Textbook of veterinary internal medicine,* ed 4, Philadelphia, 1995, WB Saunders, p 1720.

Grauer GF et al: Estimation of quantitative enzymuria in dogs with gentamicin-induced nephrotoxicosis using urine enzyme/creatinine ratios from spot urine samples, *J Vet Intern Med* 9:324, 1995.

Grauer GF et al: Effects of dietary n-3 fatty acid supplementation versus thromboxane synthetase inhibition on gentamicin-induced nephrotoxicosis in healthy male dogs, *Am J Vet Res* 57:948, 1996.

Pascoe PJ et al: Case-control study of the association between intraoperative administration of nafcillin and acute postoperative development of azotemia, *J Am Vet Med Assoc* 208:1043, 1996.

Polzin DJ et al: Chronic renal failure. In Ettinger SJ et al, editors: *Textbook of veterinary internal medicine,* ed 5, Philadelphia, 2000, WB Saunders, p 1634.

Rivers BJ et al: Evaluation of urine gamma glutamyl transpeptidase-to-creatinine ratio as a diagnostic tool in an experimental model of aminoglycoside-induced acute renal failure in the dog, *J Am Anim Hosp Assoc* 32:323, 1996.

Rivers BJ et al: Duplex Doppler estimation of resistive index in arcuate arteries of sedated, normal female dogs: implications for use in the diagnosis of renal failure, *J Am Anim Hosp Assoc* 33:69, 1997.

Thrall MA et al: Antifreeze poisoning. In Kirk RW et al, editors: *Current veterinary therapy XII,* Philadelphia, 1995, WB Saunders, p 232.

Vaden SL et al: Retrospective analysis of 106 dogs with acute renal failure, *J Vet Intern Med* 9:209, 1995.

# CHAPTER 45

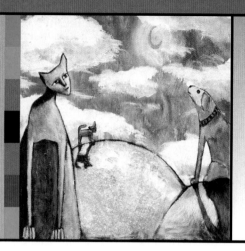

# Urinary Tract Infections

## CHAPTER OUTLINE

Etiology and pathogenesis, 624
Host defense mechanisms, 625
Complicated versus uncomplicated urinary tract
infections, 626
Relapses versus reinfections, 626
Clinical features, 626
Treatment, 627

Bacterial infections of the urinary tract occur more frequently in dogs than in cats. Although inflammation of the lower urinary tract is common in cats, bacterial infections are rare. Fewer than 2% of the cases of lower urinary tract inflammation (LUTI) in cats are caused by a primary urinary tract infection (UTI). Most of the UTIs in dogs involve bacterial inflammation of the lower urinary tract (bladder, urethra); however, the ascension of bacteria into the ureters and kidneys is a potential sequela of lower UTIs. Compared with the incidence of bacterial UTIs, mycoplasmal, chlamydial, viral, and fungal UTIs are rare in dogs. Most bacterial infections of the lower urinary tract respond quickly to appropriate antibiotic treatment; however, UTIs associated with defects in the host immune system (complicated UTIs) often fail to respond to antibiotic therapy, or the infection relapses shortly after antibiotic withdrawal.

## Etiology and Pathogenesis

The most common bacterial pathogens associated with UTIs in the dog include *Escherichia coli, Staphylococcus, Streptococcus, Enterococcus, Enterobacter, Proteus, Klebsiella,* and *Pseudomonas* organisms. *E. coli* is the most common isolate from canine and feline urine (Table 45-1). Although UTIs usually involve a single organism, as many as 20% to 30% may be mixed bacterial infections (i.e., two or more species). Most bacterial UTIs are thought to be caused by intestinal or cutaneous flora that ascend through the urethra to the bladder. Although many enteric organisms are anaerobes, the oxygen tension in urine probably inhibits the growth of strict anaerobic bacteria; therefore anaerobes rarely cause UTIs.

Bacterial virulence and the number of invading organisms are two major factors that determine whether a UTI becomes established (Table 45-2). The ability of bacteria to adhere to the epithelial surface of the urinary tract prevents bacterial washout during voiding and allows bacteria to proliferate between urine voidings. Infection of the urinary tract usually involves bacterial colonization of the genitalia, migration of the bacteria along the urethra, and adherence of the organisms to the uroepithelium. Uroepithelial adherence is facilitated by fimbriae, which are rigid, filamentous, proteinaceous appendages found on many gram-negative bacteria. Other factors that increase bacterial virulence include capsular K antigens, which interfere with opsonization and phagocytosis, and O antigens in endotoxin, which decrease smooth muscle contractility. The latter may stop ureteral peristalsis and facilitate the ascension of bacteria from the bladder to the kidney. *E. coli* isolates from dogs have a greater ability to produce colicins (resulting in increased vascular permeability), hemolysins (increasing their invasiveness through tissue damage), and β-lactamase (causing resistance to β-lactam antibiotics) and to ferment dulcitol (which is associated with resistance to phagocytosis), but they have a decreased ability to agglutinate red blood cells (RBCs; associated with uroepithelial adherence) compared with human *E. coli* isolates. Finally, cell wall–deficient bacterial variants may thrive in hypertonic environments such as the renal medulla and urine, where white blood cell (WBC) migration and phagocytosis may be compromised.

Bacterial resistance to antimicrobial drugs may result from inherent resistance, from mutation and selection, or from the transfer of resistance factors (R factors) between organisms through deoxyribonucleic acid (DNA) transfer. An entire bacterial population can acquire resistance by genetic transfer after only one dose of an antibiotic. The R factor phenomenon has been identified in gram-negative bacteria, including *E. coli, Enterobacter, Klebsiella,* and *Proteus.* R factor resistance to multiple drugs is common, and R factors are known to confer resistance to penicillins, cephalosporins, aminoglycosides, tetracyclines, chloramphenicol, sulfonamides, and trimethoprim.

Mycoplasmal organisms have also been associated with UTIs in dogs. Clinical signs of mycoplasmal cystitis may in-

TABLE 45-1

Approximate Percentages of Bacterial Isolates in Dogs With Urinary Tract Infections

| ISOLATES | PERCENTAGE OF TOTAL |
|---|---|
| *E. coli* | 45 |
| *Staphylococcus* spp. | 13 |
| *Proteus* spp. | 10 |
| *Enterococcus* | 8 |
| *Klebsiella* spp. | 7 |
| *Streptococcus* spp. | 6 |
| *Enterobacter* spp. | 3 |
| *Pseudomonas* spp. | 3 |
| Other organisms | 5 |

 TABLE 45-2

Factors Affecting Bacterial Virulence

Fimbriae—facilitate attachment to uroepithelium
Capsular K antigens—increase invasiveness and interfere with opsonization and phagocytosis
O antigens in endotoxin—decrease smooth muscle contractility
Cell wall–deficient bacterial variants—can exist in hypertonic environments (urine, renal medulla) where host defense mechanisms may be compromised
Colicins—increase vascular permeability
Hemolysins—increase invasiveness through tissue damage
β-Lactamase—causes resistance to β-lactam antibiotics
Dulcitol fermentation—causes resistance to phagocytosis
Erythrocyte agglutination—associated with uroepithelial adherence
Drug resistance
 Inherent resistance
 Mutation and selection
 Resistance factor transfer

 TABLE 45-3

Host Defense Mechanisms and Abnormalities That May Lead to Complicated Urinary Tract Infections

| HOST DEFENSES | ABNORMALITIES |
|---|---|
| **Normal Micturition** | |
| Normal urine volume | Urinary incontinence |
| Normal voiding frequency | Urine outflow tract obstruction |
| Small residual urine volume | Incomplete bladder emptying |
| **Anatomic Structures** | |
| Urethral high-pressure zone | Urethral anomalies |
| Urethral contraction and peristalsis | Urethrostomy surgery |
| Urethral length | Ectopic ureter |
| Vesicoureteral valvelike junction | Urachal diverticula |
| Ureteral contractions and peristalsis | Vesicoureteral reflux |
| | Indwelling urinary catheter |
| | Urinary incontinence |
| | Vaginal stricture |
| | Ureteral dilatation or hydroureter |
| **Mucosal Defense Barriers** | |
| Antibody and muco-protein production | Mucosal trauma |
| Nonpathogenic flora colonization | Urolithiasis |
| | Catheterization |
| | Immunoglobulin A deficiency |
| | Neoplasia |
| | Cyclophosphamide-induced damage |
| **Antimicrobial Properties of Urine** | |
| Hyperosmolality | Decreased urine concentration |
| High urea concentration | Glucosuria |
| Acidic pH | |
| **Systemic Immunocompetence** | |
| Cell-mediated immunity? | Immunosuppressive drug therapy |
| Humoral immunity | Hyperadrenocorticism |
| | Diabetes melitus |
| | Renal failure |
| | Neoplasia |

clude hematuria, pollakiuria, stranguria, incontinence, polydipsia-polyuria, and fever; however, some dogs with positive urine culture results are asymptomatic. Whether mycoplasmas are primary urinary tract pathogens remains unclear.

## Host Defense Mechanisms

The status of the host defense mechanisms appears to be the most important factor influencing the pathogenesis of UTI (Table 45-3). Normal voiding is an efficient natural defense mechanism against UTI. The mechanical washout that occurs as a result of complete voiding is responsible for removing more than 95% of nonadherent bacteria that gain entrance into the urinary bladder. Washout is enhanced by an increased urine production and frequency of voiding. Disorders that decrease the frequency of voiding or the volume of voided urine or that result in an increased urine residual volume may predispose animals to the development of UTIs. The normal urine residual volume for dogs and cats is less than 0.2 to 0.4 ml/kg.

Bacteria are normally present in increasing numbers from the midurethra to the distal urethra, but seldom do these organisms cause UTIs in normal dogs. The high-pressure zone in the midurethra and spontaneous urethral contractions help prevent the ascension of bacteria. Differences in epithelial morphology (decreased epithelial receptor sites) also help decrease the number of bacteria that can colonize the proximal and mid sections of the urethra. The length of the urethra and zinc-containing bacteriostatic/bactericidal prostatic secretions contribute to a lower incidence of UTIs in male dogs than in female dogs. In both genders the valvelike nature of the vesicoureteral junction confers protection against the ascension of bacteria to the kidneys.

The colonization of vulval and preputial luminal mucous membranes by nonpathogenic flora also serves to decrease colonization by uropathogens. Normal flora occupy most of the epithelial receptor sites, produce bacteriocins that interfere with uropathogen metabolism, and have a high affinity but low requirement for the essential nutrients required by uropathogens. In addition, mucosal secretions help prevent the adherence of uropathogens to epithelium; specifically, secretory immunoglobulins do so by coating pathogenic bacteria, and glycosaminoglycans do so by forming a protective barrier over the epithelial surface.

The antibacterial properties of urine constitute an important host defense mechanism against UTIs. Urine is frequently bacteriostatic and sometimes can be bactericidal, depending on its composition. The combination of a low pH and high concentrations of urea and weak organic acids in concentrated urine inhibits bacterial growth. The increased urine concentrating ability of cats compared with dogs is thought to be one of the reasons that normal cats have so few bacterial UTIs. Dilute urine formed in animals with polydipsic-polyuric disorders has fewer antibacterial properties than hypersthenuric urine does. For example, the incidence of bacterial UTI is higher in both dogs and cats with chronic renal failure (CFR).

## Complicated Versus Uncomplicated Urinary Tract Infections

Uncomplicated UTIs occur in the absence of underlying structural or functional abnormalities in the host defense mechanisms. They are easier to treat than complicated UTIs and are usually cleared soon after appropriate antibiotic treatment is initiated. Complicated UTIs are associated with defects in the host defense mechanisms (i.e., interference with normal micturition, anatomic defects, damage to mucosal barriers, alterations in urine volume or composition). It is usually not possible to eliminate the clinical and clinicopathologic signs of complicated UTIs with antibiotic treatment; signs either persist during antibiotic treatment or recur shortly after antibiotic withdrawal. Because of the relatively low prevalence of UTIs in male dogs compared with female dogs, any UTI in a male dog should be considered a complicated infection.

Abnormal micturition often results in incomplete voiding and the retention of urine, which allows more time for bacteria to multiply within the urinary tract. Bladder wall distention that may occur with urine retention will compress intramural vessels and thereby decrease the number of WBCs and other antimicrobial factors that may enter the bladder lumen. Damage to mucosal barriers (e.g., transitional cell carcinoma [TCC]) may also result in the development of a complicated UTI, depending on the extent of the lesion and whether uropathogens are concurrently introduced. Interestingly, bacterial inoculation of the urinary bladder in experimental animals usually fails to establish a UTI that lasts beyond 2 to 3 days, unless the uroepithelium is first damaged by a chemical or mechanical insult.

Anytime the urinary bladder is catheterized, bacteria are carried up the urethra to the bladder. If the catheter is inserted too far and damages the bladder mucosa, the chance of infection increases greatly. Anatomic defects may also allow the ascending migration of bacteria (e.g., indwelling urinary catheter, ectopic ureter) or may damage mucosal barriers (e.g., urolithiasis, neoplasia, urachal remnant, thickened bladder wall caused by chronic inflammation). Decreased urine volume may also be associated with a heightened risk for UTI because of decreased washout (although concentrated urine has greater antibacterial properties), and altered urine composition (glucosuria or the excretion of irritating substances such as cyclophosphamide metabolites that result in hematuria) can make the environment more receptive to bacterial growth. In addition to these local factors, systemic disorders, such as renal failure, hyperadrenocorticism, prolonged corticosteroid administration, neoplasia, and diabetes mellitus, can result in a complicated UTI.

## Relapses Versus Reinfections

Recurrences of clinical and clinicopathologic signs of UTI can be classified into two categories: relapses and reinfections. Relapses are infections caused by the same species of bacteria occurring within several weeks of the cessation of treatment. In this case the previous antibacterial treatment has failed to eliminate the organism. Relapses may result from the use of an improper antibiotic or dosage, the emergence of drug-resistant pathogens, or failure to eliminate factors that alter normal host defense mechanisms and allow the bacteria to persist (e.g., bacteria inside a urolith). UTIs in animals that relapse are frequently associated with a greater antimicrobial resistance than that observed in the original infection. Relapses in male dogs may result from chronic prostatic infections. Because of the blood-prostate barrier antibiotics must be lipid soluble and have an alkaline or neutral $pK_a$ (e.g., fluoroquinolones, trimethoprim-sulfa, chloramphenicol, carbenicillin) in order to gain access to the prostate. On the other hand, recurrent UTIs may also result from reinfection. In this case, the previous antibacterial treatment cleared the first infection, but the urinary tract has subsequently become infected with another bacterium. In most cases the interval between reinfections is longer than the interval between relapses (>2 weeks). The occurrence of reinfections often indicates that the factors that alter normal host defense mechanisms have not been eliminated. Alternatively, reinfections may be iatrogenic and occur as a result of follow-up catheterization. Reinfections with less invasive bacteria (*Pseudomonas aeruginosa, Klebsiella pneumoniae, Enterobacter cloacae*) generally indicate that the host's immune system is compromised.

## Clinical Features

Inflammation of the lower urinary tract often results in pollakiuria, stranguria or dysuria, and gross or microscopic hematuria. Urinalysis findings compatible with a lower UTI include bacteriuria, hematuria, pyuria, and increased numbers of transitional epithelial cells in the urine sediment. In addition, an increased urine protein concentration and alkaline urine may be observed. However, bacteria as well as other urine sediment abnormalities are not always observed during urine sediment examination in animals with a bacterial UTI, especially if the urine is hyposthenuric or isosthenuric. Therefore urine bacterial cultures should be performed to confirm the presence and type of bacteria. Similarly, research has shown that the testing of canine urine with commercially available dipstick leukocyte esterase assays is not reliable, and the false-negative rate can exceed 10% in the absence of a urine sediment examination. Some urine dipsticks also have a nitrate pad to detect nitrate-reducing bacteria, but this test has been shown to be inaccurate in dogs and cats as well.

Cystocentesis constitutes the best way to collect urine for urinalysis and bacterial culture, because it prevents urine from being contaminated by bacteria inhabiting the distal urethra, prepuce, or vulva. If urine collected by catheterization, voiding, or bladder expression is cultured, it is important to quantify the number of organisms per milliliter to differentiate a true infection from contamination (see Table 41-1). Bacterial antibiotic sensitivity testing should be performed to guide the selection of antibiotic treatment and, in cases of recurrent UTI, help differentiate relapses from reinfections. It is difficult to differentiate a lower UTI from upper tract involvement (as well as prostatitis), but this should be attempted to prevent renal damage in dogs and cats with pyelonephritis, which will require long-term antibiotic treatment and close monitoring (Table 45-4). Animals with acute bacterial pyelonephritis and prostatitis may manifest nonspecific systemic signs of lethargy, depression, anorexia, fever, and leukocytosis, which rarely occur in the setting of bacterial

infections of the bladder and urethra. However, these systemic signs are often not present in animals with chronic pyelonephritis and prostatitis. Bilateral pyelonephritis may result in renal failure and subsequent azotemia and the loss of urine concentrating ability. Cylindruria, especially WBC cellular casts, indicates the presence of renal disease and, if coupled with a significant bacteriuria, is highly suggestive of bacterial pyelonephritis. Several tests have been developed to differentiate upper and lower UTIs in people (see Table 45-4); however, these tests are difficult to perform and in some cases have not proved reliable in veterinary medicine.

## Treatment

It is important to try to identify those animals with immune system defects or disorders that may be treatable (e.g., diabetes mellitus, hyperadrenocorticism, chronic renal failure, urolithiasis, urachal remnants, excessive perivulvar skin folds or pyoderma, incontinence) and that predispose to the development of UTIs. Therefore a complete physical examination should be performed in all animals with signs of a UTI. Similarly, urinalysis and culture should be performed in all dogs and cats with suspected immune system defects. Although antibiotic treatment is the cornerstone of management, the status of host defense mechanisms is thought to be the single most important determinant of the outcome of treatment for a UTI. Antibiotic treatment should control the pathogenic bacterial growth for enough time to allow host defense mechanisms to prevent colonization of the urinary tract without the need for further antibiotic administration. Although it is advisable to evaluate the bacterial sensitivity to antimicrobial drugs, the treatment of acute, uncomplicated UTIs is often dictated by economic and time considerations. If bacterial sensitivity results are not available, the antibiotic should be chosen on the basis of bacterial identification or the Gram's staining characteristics of the bacteria (Fig. 45-1). Clinical experience at several veterinary teaching hospitals has shown that intelligent guesses may be made about bacterial susceptibility to antibiotics. In the absence of bacterial sensitivity testing, the following are the drugs of choice for the treatment of infection with the bacteria listed: *E. coli*, trimethoprim-sulfa or enrofloxacin; *Proteus*, amoxicillin; *Staphylococcus*, amoxicillin; *Streptococcus* spp., amoxicillin; *Enterobacter* spp., trimethoprim-sulfa or enrofloxacin; *Klebsiella* spp., first-generation cephalosporins or enrofloxacin; and *Pseudomonas* spp., tetracycline (Table 45-5). If the identity of the bacteria is unknown, treatment should be determined on the basis of the Gram's staining characteristics (i.e., ampicillin, amoxicillin, or amoxicillin–clavulanic acid for gram-positive bacteria and trimethoprim-sulfa or enrofloxacin for gram-negative bacteria).

The steps to follow in the management of a UTI are given in Table 45-6, and a flow diagram is shown in Fig. 45-1. The duration of therapy for a lower UTI must be individualized and should be based on the cessation of clinical signs and elimination of the abnormal urine sediment, as well as negative urine culture results. In general, uncomplicated lower UTIs should be treated for 2 to 3 weeks, whereas complicated

 TABLE 45-4

**Clinicopathologic Findings That Can Be Associated With Bacterial Pyelonephritis in Dogs and Cats**

Fever, leukocytosis, renal pain
Cellular casts in urine sediment
Renal failure (i.e., azotemia, inability to concentrate urine, polydipsia-polyuria)
Excretory urogram and ultrasonographic abnormalities (i.e., renal pelvis dilatation or asymmetric filling of diverticula, dilated ureters)
Bacteria in inflammatory lesions identified by renal histologic studies
Positive result from bacterial culture of ureteral urine obtained at cystoscopy (Stamey test)
Positive result from bacterial culture of urine obtained after bladder rinsing with sterile saline solution (Fairley test)
Positive result from bacterial culture of fluid aspirated from the renal pelvis (pyelocentesis) under ultrasound guidance

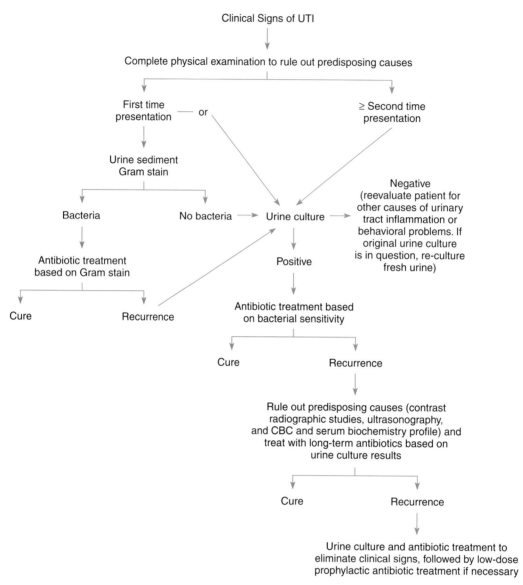

**FIG 45-1**
Flow diagram for management of urinary tract infections.

UTIs should be treated for a minimum of 4 weeks. Proper selection of antibiotic therapy can be verified after 3 to 5 days of therapy by determining whether the urine is sterile. The urine sediment, however, may still be abnormal at this time.

Reasons for a poor therapeutic response are listed in Table 45-7. Urine culture and sensitivity testing should always be done in animals with recurrent UTIs. In addition, attempts should be intensified to identify defects in the host's immune system. Double-contrast enhanced cystography and ultrasonography may be used to identify anatomic abnormalities, mucosal lesions of the bladder, or urolithiasis. In male dogs, semen and prostatic wash cytologic and culture studies, as well as ultrasonography, should be done to rule out or identify bacterial prostatitis. Excretory urographic, ultrasonographic, and renal biopsy findings may confirm the presence

of pyelonephritis; however, results of these studies may be normal in dogs and cats with chronic pyelonephritis. Finally, the possibility of otherwise asymptomatic hyperadrenocorticism causing the recurrent UTIs should be considered, especially in animals with infections associated with low numbers of WBCs and RBCs in the urine sediment.

Long-term (4 to 6 weeks) antibiotic treatment is required for patients with complicated UTIs, and careful follow-up examinations should be performed in such animals (see Table 45-6). When antibiotic treatment is used for this period of time, long-term antibiotic adverse effects should also be considered. Keratoconjunctivitis sicca and folate deficiency anemia may occur in association with long-term use of trimethoprim-sulfa (although they are rare), and nephrotoxicity is always a concern in animals receiving aminoglycosides, even for a short time.

TABLE 45-5

**Antimicrobial Agents to Which More Than 90% of Urinary Isolates Are Susceptible In Vitro at Concentrations Less Than One Fourth of the Expected Urinary Concentration**

| ORGANISM | ANTIMICROBIAL AGENTS |
| --- | --- |
| E. coli* | Trimethoprim-sulfa<br>Fluoroquinolone<br>Amoxicillin–clavulanic acid |
| Coagulase-positive<br>Staphylococcus spp. | Amoxicillin<br>Chloramphenicol<br>Trimethoprim-sulfa<br>Cephalosporins (first generation) |
| Proteus mirabilis | Amoxicillin<br>Fluoroquinolone<br>Cephalosporins (first, second,<br>third generations)<br>Amoxicillin–clavulanic acid |
| Klebsiella<br>pneumoniae* | Cephalosporins (first, second,<br>third generations)<br>Fluoroquinolone<br>Amoxicillin–clavulanic acid<br>Trimethoprim-sulfa |
| Streptococcus spp. | Amoxicillin<br>Amoxicillin–clavulanic acid<br>Chloramphenicol<br>Cephalosporins (first, second,<br>third generations) |
| Pseudomonas<br>aeruginosa | Tetracycline<br>Fluoroquinolone<br>Carbenicillin |
| Enterobacter spp.* | Trimethoprim-sulfa<br>Fluoroquinolone |
| Enterococcus spp. | Fluoroquinolone<br>Trimethoprim-sulfa<br>Chloramphenicol<br>Tetracyline |

*These bacteria are capable of major changes in their susceptibility to antibiotics and are therefore less predictable.

The prognosis for an animal with a complicated UTI as opposed to an uncomplicated UTI is always guarded. The single most important treatment for a complicated UTI is correction of the underlying defect in the host defense mechanisms. If predisposing factors cannot be identified or eliminated, relapses and reinfections are common. Low-dose (one third to one half of the conventional daily dose) antimicrobial treatment administered at bedtime may be recommended for animals with frequent infections associated with host defense mechanism problems that cannot be cured. This allows the drug to be present in the bladder overnight, supplementing the animal's defense mechanisms. Penicillins are recommended for the treatment of recurrences caused by gram-positive bacteria, whereas trimethoprim-sulfa or enrofloxacin is recommended for the treatment of

 TABLE 45-6

**Ideal Steps to Follow in the Management of Urinary Tract Infections in Dogs and Cats**

Diagnosis should be determined on the basis of history, urine sediment, and, ideally, urine culture and sensitivity findings.

Select an antimicrobial agent.

Reculture urine in 3 to 5 days to ascertain effectiveness of selected antimicrobial agent.

Examine urine sediment 3 to 4 days before discontinuing antibiotic treatment.

Repeat urinalysis and culture 10 to 14 days after cessation of antibiotic therapy.

Patients with recurrent urinary tract infections should undergo contrast-enhanced radiography, ultrasonography, a complete blood count, and serum biochemistry profile to determine whether they have underlying predisposing factors.

Frequent reinfections may need to be treated with prophylactic doses of antibiotics after the initial inflammation has been cleared up in response to standard-dose antibiotic treatment.

 TABLE 45-7

**Reasons for Poor Therapeutic Response in Dogs and Cats with Urinary Tract Infections**

Use of ineffective drugs or ineffective duration of therapy

Failure of owner to administer prescribed dose at proper intervals

Gastrointestinal tract disease or concurrent oral intake of food and drug resulting in decreased drug absorption

Impaired action of drugs, either because bacteria are not multiplying or because they are sequestered in an inaccessible site (e.g., prostate or uroliths)

Failure to recognize and eliminate predisposing causes

Presence of mixed bacterial infections in which only one of the pathogens is eradicated by antimicrobial therapy

Iatrogenic reinfection caused by catheterization

Development of drug resistance in bacteria

recurrences caused by gram-negative bacteria. It should be noted, however, that low-dose, long-term antibiotic treatment can predispose the animal to the development of a very resistant UTI.

Urinary acidification (ammonium chloride) has been advocated as adjunctive therapy for lower UTIs because acidic urine provides a less favorable environment for bacterial growth. However, the antimicrobial activity of acidic urine is inferior to that of antibiotics and should not be expected to eradicate infection; ammonium chloride should only be used in conjunction with other modes of therapy. Urinary acidification may also be an effective adjunctive therapy to adjust the urine pH and thereby optimize the efficacy of certain antibiotics (penicillin, ampicillin, carbenicillin, tetracycline, nitrofurantoin). Ammonium chloride (60 to 100 mg/kg) should be given orally twice daily to maintain a urine pH of less than 6.5. The use of ammonium chloride is not without risk, however, especially in male dogs, because oxalate, silicate, urate, and cystine are all less soluble in acidic urine and urolithiasis may result from excessive acidification.

Urinary antiseptics have also been advocated as adjunctive therapy in the control or prophylaxis of lower urinary tract disease. Although they are less effective than specific antimicrobial therapy in eradicating infections, they are probably more effective than urinary acidifiers. Methenamine mandelate is a cyclic hydrocarbon and is the most commonly used urinary tract antiseptic. The dose for dogs is 10 mg/kg PO every 6 hours. In an acidic environment (pH <6), methenamine hydrolyzes to form formaldehyde. It should be used in conjunction with ammonium chloride to enhance its effectiveness. Methylene blue (tetramethylthionine chloride) is a weak urinary antiseptic agent that used to be common in combination products designed to treat lower urinary tract inflammation. These products should be avoided in cats, however, because methylene blue has the potential to cause Heinz bodies and hemolytic anemia. Similarly, phenazopyridine, a urinary tract analgesic, should not be used in cats.

## Suggested Readings

Allen TA et al: Microbiologic evaluation of canine urine: direct microscopic examination and preservation of specimen quality for culture, *J Vet Med Assoc* 190:1289, 1987.

Fettman MJ: Evaluation of the usefulness of routine microscopy in canine urinalysis, *J Am Vet Med Assoc* 190:892, 1987.

Forrester SD et al: Retrospective evaluation of urinary tract infection in 42 dogs with hyperadrenocorticism or diabetes mellitus or both, *J Vet Intern Med* 13:557, 1999.

Hess RS et al: Concurrent disorders in dogs with diabetes mellitus: 221 cases (1993-1998), *J Am Vet Med Assoc* 217:1166, 2000.

Lees GE et al: Treatment of urinary tract infections in dogs and cats, *J Am Vet Med Assoc* 189:648, 1986.

Ling GV et al: Canine urinary tract infections: a comparison of in vitro antimicrobial susceptibility test results and response to oral therapy with ampicillin or with trimethoprim-sulfa, *J Am Vet Med Assoc* 185:277, 1984.

Ling GV: Bacterial infections of the urinary tract. In Ettinger SJ et al, editors: *Textbook of veterinary internal medicine,* Philadelphia, 2000, WB Saunders, p 1678.

Nolan LK et al: Comparison of virulence factors and antibiotic resistance profiles of *Escherichia coli* strains from humans and dogs with urinary tract infections, *J Vet Intern Med* 1:152, 1987.

Norris CR et al: Recurrent and persistent urinary tract infections in dogs: 383 cases (1969-1995), *J Am Anim Hosp Assoc* 36:484, 2000.

Oluch AO et al: Nonenteric *Escherichia coli* isolates from dogs: 674 cases (1990-1998), *J Am Vet Med Assoc* 218:381, 2001.

Osborne CA et al: Bacterial infections of the canine and feline urinary tract. In Osborne CA et al, editors: *Canine and feline nephrology and urology,* Philadelphia, 1995, WB Saunders, p 759.

Senior DF: Bacterial urinary tract infections: invasion, host defenses, and new approaches to prevention, *Comp Cont Educ Pract Vet* 7:334, 1985.

Senior DF: Serotype, hemolysin production, and adherence characteristics of strains of *Escherichia coli* causing urinary tract infection in dogs, *Am J Vet Res* 53:494, 1992.

Wilson RA et al: Strains of *Escherichia coli* associated with urogenital disease in dogs and cats, *Am J Vet Res* 49:743, 1988.

# CHAPTER 46

## Canine Urolithiasis

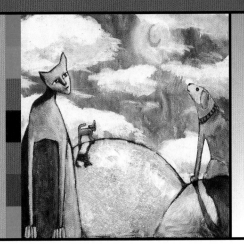

### CHAPTER OUTLINE

Etiology and pathogenesis, 631
Clinical features and diagnosis, 636
Treatment, 636
Reevaluation of the patient with urolithiasis, 641

Canine urine is a complex solution in which salts (e.g., calcium oxalate, magnesium ammonium phosphate) can remain in solution under conditions of supersaturation. However, supersaturated urine has a potential energy of precipitation, or the tendency to form solids from the dissolved salts. Crystalluria is a consequence of urine supersaturation, and uroliths may form if crystals aggregate and are not excreted. Uroliths may damage the uroepithelium and result in urinary tract inflammation (hematuria, pollakiuria, dysuria-stranguria). They may also predispose the animal to the development of a bacterial urinary tract infection (UTI). If uroliths lodge in the ureters or urethra, urine flow may be obstructed.

Most uroliths in dogs are found in the bladder or urethra; only about 5% are located in the kidneys or ureters. Uroliths are usually named according to their mineral content. Data collected at the College of Veterinary Medicine of the University of Minnesota have shown that approximately 50% of canine uroliths are struvite (magnesium ammonium phosphate), 33% are calcium oxalate, 8% are urate, 1% are silicate, 1% are cystine, and 7% are mixed (i.e., the urolith contains less than 70% of any one mineral type). Crystalline aggregates constitute approximately 95% of the urolith weight, and an organic matrix composed of protein and mucoprotein complexes may constitute as much as 5%. Factors associated with particular types of uroliths are summarized in Table 46-1.

### Etiology and Pathogenesis

Conditions that contribute to the crystallization of salts and the formation of uroliths include a sufficiently high concentration of salts in the urine, adequate time in the urinary tract (urinary retention of salts and crystals), a urine pH favorable for salts to crystallize, a nucleation center or nidus on which crystallization can occur, and decreased concentrations of crystallization inhibitors in the urine. The combination of a high dietary intake of minerals and protein and the ability of dogs to produce highly concentrated urine contributes to urine becoming supersaturated with salts. In some cases, decreased tubular resorption (e.g., calcium, cystine, uric acid) or an increased production secondary to bacterial infection (e.g., ammonium and phosphate ions) also contributes to urine becoming supersaturated.

Several theories exist concerning the pathogenesis of uroliths. In the precipitation-crystallization theory, the supersaturation of urine with salts is thought to be the primary factor responsible for initiating nidus formation and sustaining the growth of the urolith. Normal canine urine is supersaturated with several salts. However, the greater the concentration of salts in urine and the less often voiding occurs (e.g., decreased water intake), the greater the chance of urolith formation. Supersaturated urine has a potential energy of precipitation, or a driving force that favors crystal formation. The greater the magnitude of the supersaturation, the greater the potential for crystallization to occur. Conversely, undersaturated solutions have a potential energy of dissolution, such that previously formed crystals dissolve at a rate proportional to the degree of undersaturation.

In other theories of urolith formation, it is thought that substances in urine may promote or inhibit crystal formation. For example, in the matrix nucleation theory, an organic matrix substance in urine is thought to promote initial nidus formation. This matrix substance may be albumin, globulin, Tamm-Horsfall mucoprotein, or an immunologically unique hydroxyproline-deficient protein called matrix substance A. The proteinaceous matrix substance may promote crystallization by providing a surface where crystallization can occur and by binding crystals together, which may increase their urinary retention. In another theory, the crystallization inhibitor theory, the absence of a critical inhibitor of crystal formation is considered to be the primary factor that allows initial nidus formation. Examples of crystallization inhibitors are citrates, glycosaminoglycans, and pyrophosphates. Decreased concentrations of these substances in urine may facilitate

TABLE 46-1

Factors That Help Predict Urolith Composition

| UROLITH TYPE | RADIOGRAPHIC DENSITY (1.0-3.0 scale) | USUAL URINE pH | URINARY TRACT INFECTION | GENDER PREDISPOSITION | COMMONLY AFFECTED BREEDS | COMMON AFFECTED AGES (yr) | CLINICOPATHOLOGIC ABNORMALITIES |
|---|---|---|---|---|---|---|---|
| Magnesium ammonium phosphate (struvite) | 2.5 | Neutral to alkaline | Very common, especially urease-producing bacteria (e.g., *Staphylococcus, Proteus*) | Female (>80%) | Miniature Schnauzers, Bichon Frises, Cocker Spaniels, Miniature Poodles | 1-8 | Usually none |
| Calcium oxalate | 3.0 | Acidic to neutral | Rare | Male (>70%) | Miniature Schnauzers, Miniature Poodles, Yorkshire Terriers, Lhasa Apsos, Bichon Frises, Shih Tzus, Cairn Terriers | 5-12 | Occasional hypercalcemia |
| Urate | 1.0 | Acidic to neutral | Uncommon | Male (>90%) | Dalmatians, English Bulldogs, Miniature Schnauzers (PSS), Yorkshire Terriers (PSS) | 1-4 | Decreased serum urea, nitrogen, and albumin concentrations and abnormal preprandial and postprandial bile acid concentrations in dogs with PSS |
| Cystine | 1.5 | Acidic | Rare | Male (>95%) | Dachshunds, Basset Hounds, English Bulldogs, Yorkshire Terriers, Irish Terriers, Rottweilers, Chihauhaus, Mastiffs, Tibetan Spaniels | 1-7 | Usually none |
| Silicate | 2.5 | Acidic to neutral | Uncommon | Male (>95%) | German Shepherds, Golden Retrievers, Labrador Retrievers Old English Sheepdogs | 4-9 | Usually none |

*PSS,* Portosystemic shunt.

spontaneous crystallization and urolith growth. The extent to which promoters and inhibitors of crystallization are involved in urolith formation in dogs is unknown. In all cases, however, supersaturation of the urine with urolith constituents is essential for uroliths to form.

**Struvite uroliths.** Struvite or magnesium ammonium phosphate uroliths are the most common uroliths in dogs (Fig. 46-1). Uroliths that predominantly consist of struvite may also contain a small amount of calcium phosphate (hydroxyapatite) or calcium carbonate. A UTI is an important factor predisposing to the formation of struvite uroliths in dogs; *Staphylococcus* and *Proteus* organisms are commonly associated pathogens. These bacteria contain urease and are capable of splitting urea into ammonia and carbon dioxide. Hydroxyl and ammonium ions are formed by the hydrolysis of ammonia, which decreases hydrogen ion concentrations in urine, resulting in an alkaline urine and decreased struvite solubility. The hydrolysis of urea increases the urine concentrations of ammonium and phosphate (a result of the increased dissociation of phosphorus) ions, which augments urine supersaturation. High urine ammonia concentrations may also damage glycosaminoglycans that prevent bacteria

from adhering to the urinary mucosa. Bacterial cystitis also increases the amount of organic debris available as a crystallization surface. Because of their high association with UTIs, struvite uroliths are more common in female dogs (80% to 97% of uroliths in female dogs are struvite). Uroliths in dogs less than 1 year of age are usually struvite and are also frequently associated with a UTI.

The factors involved in the pathogenesis of struvite uroliths in sterile urine are not known; however, the struvite uroliths that form in cats usually do so in the absence of a UTI. A greater urine-concentrating ability, and therefore a greater degree of urine supersaturation, may be partially responsible for causing uroliths to form in cats and in those dogs without UTIs. Because most canine diets are rich in minerals and protein, the dog's urine frequently becomes supersaturated with magnesium, ammonium, and phosphate. In addition, a consistently high urine pH in the absence of a UTI (potentially caused by drugs, diet, or renal tubular disorders) may facilitate struvite urolith formation.

Struvite uroliths may occur in any breed; however, those commonly affected include Miniature Schnauzers, Miniature Poodles, Bichon Frises, and Cocker Spaniels. The high prevalence of struvite uroliths in Miniature Schnauzers and Miniature Poodles has led to the suggestion that there is a familial predisposition in these breeds (see Table 46-1). Uroliths larger than 10 mm in any dimension are likely to be struvite. In addition, struvite uroliths found in the urinary bladder are most likely to be smooth, blunt-edged or faceted, or pyramidal.

**Calcium oxalate uroliths.** Calcium oxalate uroliths in dogs are often the monohydrate (whewellite) form (see Figs. 41-3 and 46-2, *A*) rather than the dihydrate (weddellite) form (see Figs. 41-4 and 46-2, *B*). The factors involved in the pathogenesis of calcium oxalate urolithiasis in dogs are not completely understood but frequently involve increased concentrations of calcium in the urine. Hypercalciuria probably occurs most commonly in dogs postprandially and is associated with increased absorption of calcium from the gut. Another potential cause of hypercalciuria is the defective tubular resorption of calcium. Hypercalciuria may also occur secondary to overt hypercalcemia (e.g., that resulting from primary hyperparathyroidism, neoplasia, or vitamin D intoxication); however, this is thought to be an infrequent cause of calcium oxalate uroliths. Treatment with certain drugs (e.g., glucocorticoids, furosemide) as well as dietary supplementation with calcium or sodium chloride may also result in hypercalciuria. An association between hyperadrenocorticism and the development of calcium-containing uroliths has also been identified in dogs. Finally, decreased urine concentrations of glycosaminoglycans, Tamm-Horsfall protein, osteopontine, and/or citrate, which are calcium oxalate crystallization inhibitors, or defective urinary nephrocalcin or increased dietary intake of oxalate (e.g., vegetables, grass, vitamin C) may play a role in the pathogenesis of calcium oxalate urolithiasis in some dogs. The overall prevalence of calcium oxalate uroliths in dogs has increased significantly over the past 10 years and may be related to the increased use of urine-acidifying diets or other unidentified environmental factors.

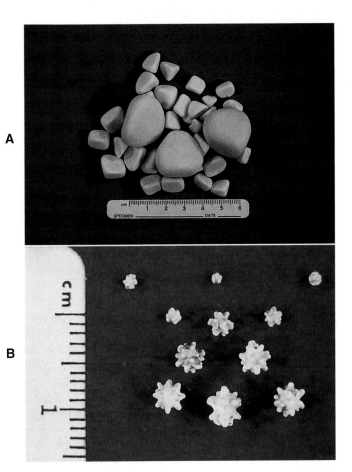

**FIG 46-1**
**A,** Typical appearance of struvite stones; however, struvite stones may also be jack-shaped, **B.** (**B** courtesy Dr. Howard Seim, Colorado State University.)

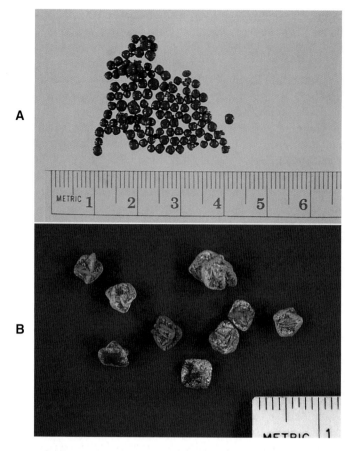

A

B

**FIG 46-2**
Typical appearance of monohydrate calcium oxalate stones, **A,** and dihydrate calcium oxalate stones, **B.**

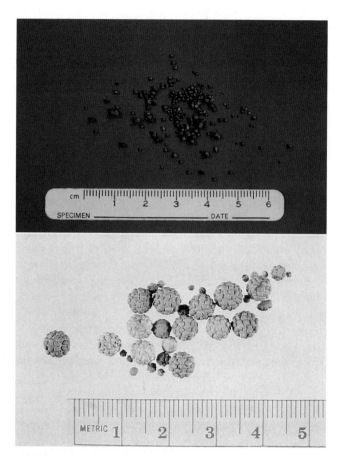

**FIG 46-3**
Appearance of ammonium urate stones from two different dogs.

Approximately 70% of calcium oxalate uroliths are found in male dogs, and Miniature and Standard Schnauzers, Miniature Poodles, Yorkshire Terriers, Lhasa Apsos, Bichon Frises, and Shih Tzus are the breeds commonly affected. Obesity also appears to increase the risk of calcium oxalate urolithiasis. The increased prevalence in male dogs may be related to an increase in the hepatic production of oxalate mediated by testosterone. Conversely, estrogens in female dogs may increase the urinary excretion of citrate. Calcium oxalate uroliths frequently occur in older dogs (mean age, 8 to 12 years), and a concurrent UTI appears to be rare. Calcium oxalate solubility is increased in urine with a pH above 6.5, whereas a urine pH of less than 6.5 favors calcium oxalate crystal formation.

**Urate uroliths.** Most urate uroliths are composed of ammonium acid urate; 100% uric acid and sodium urate uroliths are relatively rare (Fig. 46-3). Uric acid is derived from the metabolic degradation of endogenous purine ribonucleotides and dietary nucleic acids. It is hypothesized that the hepatic transport of uric acid is defective in Dalmatians and some English Bulldogs, because uric acid conversion to allantoin has been found to be decreased in them, even though hepatocyte uricase activities are often adequate. The decreased production of allantoin seen in these breeds

results in the increased urinary excretion of uric acid. Normally, allantoin, which is produced through the oxidation of uric acid by uricase, is the major metabolite generated during purine metabolism. In comparison with uric acid, allantoin is quite soluble in urine.

In addition to a decreased hepatic metabolism of uric acid, the proximal tubular resorption of uric acid appears to be decreased in Dalmatians. This increases the uric acid and sodium urate (the salt of uric acid) concentrations in urine. Although urinary uric acid excretion in Dalmatians is approximately 10 times that of other dogs, urate stones form in only a small percentage. For unknown reasons, male Dalmatians are at greater risk of having urate stones than are female Dalmatians. In a recently published study, the male/female ratio for urate stone–forming Dalmatians was reported to be 16.4:1 (Bartges and colleagues, 1994).

Another possible cause of urate stone formation is a decreased glycosaminoglycan concentration in the urine. Glycosaminoglycans in urine may combine with urate salts, resulting in an overall negative charge and reduced crystallization. Obviously, if the concentration in urine is decreased, the risk of urate stone formation may then increase. An additional possible cause of urate stone formation is an increase in the urinary excretion of both uric acid and ammonium ions

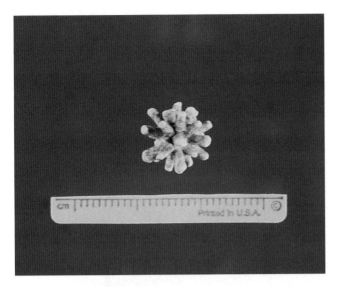

**FIG 46-4**
Typical appearance of a silicate stone.

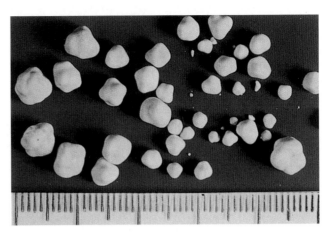

**FIG 46-5**
Typical appearance of cystine stones.

secondary to protein ingestion. Ammonia, which is produced by renal tubular cells from glutamine, diffuses into the tubular lumen and serves as a buffer for secreted hydrogen ions, thereby forming ammonium ions. Ammonium ions are relatively lipid insoluble and therefore become trapped within the tubular fluid.

Approximately 60% of urate uroliths occur in Dalmatians, and conversely, approximately 75% of the uroliths in Dalmatians are urate uroliths. In addition to Dalmatians, English Bulldogs have an increased incidence of urate uroliths. Ammonium acid urate stones may also form in any dog with hepatic insufficiency (e.g., hepatic cirrhosis, a portosystemic shunt [PSS]) as a result of increased renal excretion of ammonium urates. PSSs are common in Miniature Schnauzers, Yorkshire Terriers, and Pekingese dogs; therefore ammonium acid urate uroliths are more common in these breeds. UTIs, especially those with urease-producing bacteria, may facilitate ammonium acid urate crystallization by increasing urine ammonia concentrations. A UTI may also occur secondary to urolith-induced mucosal irritation. Uric acid crystallization is facilitated in acidic urine, whereas an alkaline urine appears to favor ammonium urate crystallization.

**Silicate uroliths.** Silicate uroliths were first reported in the United States in 1976 when crystallographic analysis of uroliths became available. Silicate uroliths frequently, but not always, have a jack shape (Fig. 46-4), although not all jackstones are silicates (ammonium urate and struvite uroliths may also be jack-shaped) (see Fig. 46-1, *B*). The factors responsible for the pathogenesis of silicate uroliths are unknown, but their formation is probably related to the dietary intake of silicates, silicic acid, or magnesium silicate. There appears to be a link between the formation of silicate uroliths and the consumption of large amounts of corn gluten or soybean hulls, which can be high in silicates. Many of the reported silicate uroliths in the United States have occurred in

male German Shepherd Dogs, Old English Sheepdogs, and Golden and Labrador Retrievers. Most silicate uroliths are diagnosed in dogs 6 to 8 years of age. Alkaline urine appears to increase silicate solubility, and secondary UTIs may occur as a result of mucosal irritation caused by these jack-shaped uroliths.

**Cystine uroliths.** Cystinuria, an inherited disorder of renal tubular transport, is thought to be the primary cause of cystine uroliths. The tubular resorptive defect involves cystine and, in some cases, other amino acids (tubular resorption of cysteine, the immediate precursor of cystine, glycine, ornithine, carnitine, arginine, and lysine, may also be decreased). Although the plasma cystine concentrations are normal in these dogs, the concentration of plasma methionine, a precursor of cystine, may be increased. Plasma cystine is freely filtered through the glomeruli and is actively resorbed by proximal tubular epithelial cells in normal dogs. Were it not for the relative insolubility of cystine in urine and the potential for uroliths to form, cystinuria would be of little consequence. Cystine is most soluble in alkaline solutions; therefore cystine stones usually form in acidic urine. Cystine uroliths do not form in all dogs with cystinuria; therefore cystinuria is a predisposing rather than a primary causative factor. Cystine uroliths (Fig. 46-5) are most frequently observed in male dogs, and Dachshunds are the breed principally affected, but Basset Hounds, Tibetan Spaniels, English Bulldogs, Yorkshire Terriers, Irish Terriers, Chihuahuas, Mastiffs, and Rottweilers also appear to be at increased risk for cystine urolithiasis.

For unknown reasons, cystine uroliths usually do not form in immature dogs; the average age at detection is 3 to 6 years. The incidence of cystine urolithiasis in dogs in the United Kingdom has been reported to be approximately 10 times that seen in dogs in the United States, probably reflecting the increased popularity of affected breeds in the United Kingdom. UTIs may occur secondarily; however, infection is not

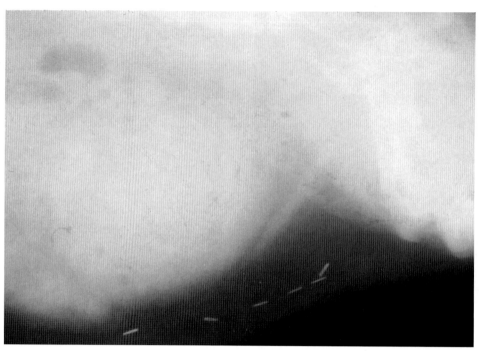

**FIG 46-6**
Radiograph of a male dog with an opaque urethral calculus at the caudal aspect of the os penis. Note the distended bladder associated with the obstructive uropathy and the staples from a previous cystotomy for urolith removal.

thought to play a primary role in the pathogenesis of cystine uroliths.

## Clinical Features and Diagnosis

The clinical features of urolithiasis depend on the number, type, and location of the stones in the urinary tract. Most uroliths are located in the urinary bladder; therefore clinical signs of cystitis (hematuria, pollakiuria, dysuria-stranguria) are frequently observed. Mucosal irritation is relatively severe in dogs with jack-shaped uroliths, as opposed to that seen in those with solitary, smooth stones. In male dogs, smaller uroliths may pass into the urethra, causing partial or complete obstruction with signs of bladder distention, dysuria-stranguria, and postrenal azotemia (depression, anorexia, vomiting). Uroliths frequently lodge in the male urethra at the caudal aspect of the os penis (Fig. 46-6). Occasionally the urinary bladder or urethra may rupture and result in an abdominal effusion or subcutaneous perineal fluid accumulation and postrenal azotemia. Animals with unilateral renal uroliths may be asymptomatic, or they may have hematuria and chronic pyelonephritis. Frequently, chronic renal failure develops in animals with bilateral renal uroliths, especially if pyelonephritis is also present. Dogs with ureteral uroliths may also be asymptomatic, or they may have hematuria and abdominal pain. Unilateral obstruction of a ureter often results in unilateral hydronephrosis without evidence of decreased renal function.

Canine urolithiasis is usually diagnosed on the basis of a combination of historical, physical examination, and radio-

graphic or ultrasonographic findings (Fig. 46-7). In male dogs with dysuria and stranguria caused by urethral stones, attempted passage of a urinary catheter will often be met with a "gritty feeling" of resistance. In this case, the diagnosis can usually be confirmed with retrograde positive-contrast–enhanced urethrography. In some cases, cystouroliths can be detected during abdominal palpation in dogs with signs of cystitis. Plain film radiographs and ultrasonography will usually confirm the presence of cystouroliths unless the stones are radiolucent or very small. Double-contrast–enhanced cystography is the most sensitive diagnostic tool for detecting cystouroliths. Finally, ultrasonography works well for confirming the presence of renoliths as well as hydronephrosis-hydroureter.

## Treatment

General principles for the treatment of urolithiasis include the relief of any urethral obstruction and decompression of the bladder if necessary. This can usually be accomplished by the passage of a small-bore catheter, cystocentesis, dislodgment of the urethral calculi by hydropulsion, or emergency urethrotomy. Fluid therapy should be initiated to restore water and electrolyte balance if postrenal azotemia exists. Hyperkalemia is a potentially life-threatening electrolyte disturbance that may occur in dogs and cats with postrenal azotemia caused by urethral obstruction or rupture of the urinary bladder or urethra. The serum potassium concentration as well as the blood urea nitrogen and creatinine concentrations should be measured in dogs and cats with a

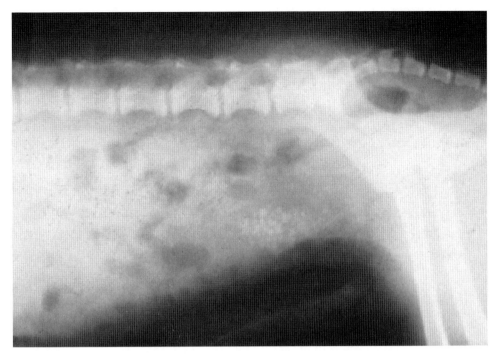

**FIG 46-7**
Typical appearance of radiopaque cystouroliths on plain film radiographs. (Courtesy Dr. Philip Steyn, Colorado State University, Fort Collins, Colo.)

suspected obstruction. Alternatively, bradycardia and electrocardiographic findings of flattened P waves, a prolonged PR interval, widened QRS complexes, and tall or spiked T waves are suggestive of hyperkalemia and indicate the need for aggressive treatment to lower the serum potassium concentration. Hyperkalemia should be promptly treated according to the regimen outlined in Table 46-2.

The medical dissolution of struvite, urate, and cystine uroliths has been shown to be effective (Table 46-3); however, the choice between the surgical removal of uroliths and medical dissolution is not always clear. Disadvantages of surgery include the need for anesthesia, the invasiveness of the procedure (potential surgical complications), the possibility of incomplete removal of uroliths, and the persistence of underlying causes. Inasmuch as the underlying cause is usually not eliminated, surgery typically does not lead to a decrease in the rate of urolith recurrence. Advantages of surgery include the fact that the urolith type can be definitively diagnosed, any concurrent or predisposing anatomic abnormalities (e.g., urachal remnants, urinary bladder polyps) can be corrected, and urinary bladder mucosal samples can be obtained for bacterial culture if the urine yields no growth on culture.

Medical treatment decreases the concentration of calculogenic salts in the urine, increases salt solubility in urine, and increases urine volume, which produces urine with a lower concentration of calculogenic salts. The major disadvantage of the medical treatment of urolithiasis is that considerable owner compliance is required for several weeks to months. The cost of medical dissolution is comparable to the cost of surgery, because multiple urinalyses, bacterial cultures, and

 TABLE 46-2

**Electrocardiographic Findings and Treatment Recommendations for Dogs and Cats With Hyperkalemia**

**ECG Findings**

1. Bradycardia
2. Flattened waves
3. Prolonged PR interval
4. Widened QRS complexes
5. Tall or spiked T waves
6. Arrhythmias

**Treatment Recommendations**

1. Fluid therapy with 0.9% saline solution
2. Slow IV bolus of regular insulin (0.25-0.5 U/kg), followed by 50% dextrose (4 ml/U of administered insulin), or
3. Slow IV bolus of sodium bicarbonate (1-2 mEq/kg), or
4. Slow IV bolus of 10% calcium gluconate (0.5-1.0 ml/kg while monitoring the ECG)

radiographs are frequently required for follow-up. Animals with urolith-induced obstructive uropathy cannot be treated medically, and some uroliths (calcium oxalate, calcium phosphate, silicate, and mixed-composition uroliths) do not respond to medical dissolution. In addition to the medical dissolution of uroliths, voiding urohydropropulsion or catheter urolith retrieval can be used to nonsurgically remove cystouroliths in some animals (see Lulich and colleagues, 1992,

## TABLE 46-3

**Treatment and Prevention of Urolithiasis in Dogs**

| UROLITH TYPE | TREATMENT OPTIONS | PREVENTION |
|---|---|---|
| Struvite | Surgical removal or dissolution:<br>Hill's s/d diet<br>Control infection<br>Urease inhibitor?<br>Keep urine pH <6.5, BUN <10 mg/dl, and urine specific gravity <1.020 | Hill's c/d diet<br>Monitor urine pH and urine sediment, and treat any infections quickly and appropriately |
| Calcium oxalate | Surgical removal | Hill's u/d diet? |
| Urate | Surgical removal or dissolution:<br>Hill's u/d diet<br>Allopurinol (7-10 mg/kg tid-sid PO)<br>Control infection | Potassium citrate?<br>Hill's u/d diet<br>Allopurinol if necessary |
| Silicate | Surgical removal | Hill's u/d diet<br>Prevent consumption of dirt and grass |
| Cystine | Surgical removal or dissolution:<br>Hill's u/d diet<br>N-(2-mercaptopropionyl)-glycine (15-20 mg/kg bid PO) | Hill's u/d diet<br>Thiol-containing drugs if necessary |

*BUN,* Blood urea nitrogen.

## TABLE 46-4

**Guidelines for Urohydropropulsion**

1. Assess urolith size and shape in relation to animal size:
   Uroliths must be smaller than the smallest urethral diameter.
   Smooth uroliths will pass more readily than those with irregular surfaces.
2. Sedation facilitates animal positioning. Consider analgesia and muscle relaxation.
3. General anesthesia may also be used.
4. Moderately distend the bladder with sterile saline solution administered through a urethral catheter (4-6 ml/kg of body weight), and assess bladder size by abdominal palpation.
5. Remove urethral catheter.
6. Position the animal so that its vertebral column is vertical.
7. Gently agitate the bladder using abdominal palpation to move uroliths into the trigone region.
8. Apply steady digital pressure to the bladder to express urine and uroliths.
9. Steps 4 through 8 can be repeated as necessary.
10. Assess complete urolith removal with follow-up radiographs or double-contrast-enhanced cystograms.

1993, for detailed instructions and Table 46-4). Lithotripsy, available at some referral centers, has also been used successfully to treat nephroliths and ureteroliths in dogs.

General preventive measures to be taken in addition to the surgical or medical management of uroliths include the induction of diuresis and the eradication of UTIs. Diuresis is important because it lowers the urine specific gravity and the urinary concentration of calculogenic salts. The addition of 0.5 to 1 g of salt (1 tsp = 3.5 g of NaCl) to the diet per day is often recommended; however, there are exceptions to this.

For example, Hill's Canine Prescription Diet s/d contains high levels of salt and should not be further supplemented. In addition, the preventive or dissolution treatment of calcium oxalate and cystine uroliths should not include increased dietary salt, because the resulting natriuresis may increase urine calcium and cystine excretion. In general, the maintenance of a urine specific gravity of less than 1.020 is ideal, and dogs should be allowed frequent opportunities to void. The urine sediment and pH should be monitored routinely, and UTIs should be treated promptly on the basis of bacterial culture and sensitivity results (see specific instructions in discussion of each type of urolith).

**Struvite uroliths.** Struvite uroliths can usually be dissolved by feeding the animal Hill's Canine Prescription Diet s/d. The protein, calcium, phosphorous, and magnesium content of the diet is markedly restricted; it has a high salt content; and it results in the production of acidic urine. The marked protein restriction in the diet reduces the hepatic production of urea and decreases urea concentrations in urine and the renal medulla. The result is decreased urea for bacterial urease, decreased medullary hypertonicity, and therefore decreased urine-concentrating ability. It takes an average of 8 to 10 weeks (range, 2 weeks to 7 months) for struvite uroliths to be dissolved this way. The rate at which uroliths dissolve is proportional to the surface area of the urolith exposed to the undersaturated urine. This diet cannot be fed routinely as a maintenance diet and should not be used in pregnant, lactating, or growing animals or after surgery, since wound healing may be compromised as a result of the restricted protein in the diet. In addition, because of its high salt content, the s/d diet should not be fed to dogs with congestive heart failure, hypertension, or nephrotic syndrome. In Miniature Schnauzers, the high fat content of s/d may exacerbate any lipid abnormalities and increase the risk of pancreatitis. The s/d diet should be fed for a minimum of 30 days after the calculi are no longer visible radiographically. It should be noted that the diet will not dissolve nonstruvite uroliths and it will not be effective if a UTI persists or the animal is fed anything in addition to the s/d diet. Lack of owner compliance with the dietary recommendations (i.e., instructions to feed s/d only) is indicated if the serum urea nitrogen concentrations remain greater than 10 mg/dl after the diet has been initiated.

In addition to decreasing the concentration of crystalloids in the urine, the elimination of any bacterial UTI is an essential part of the medical treatment of struvite urolithiasis. If infection is present at the start of treatment, antibiotics should be continued throughout the course of the medical dissolution treatment to destroy viable bacteria that may be liberated from the urolith as it dissolves. Antibiotics should be selected on the basis of urine culture and sensitivity findings; in cases of severe or persistent UTIs caused by urease-producing bacteria, the urease inhibitor acetohydroxamic acid (Lithostat; Mission Pharmacal, San Antonio, Tex) may be added to the treatment. At a dose of 12.5 mg/kg PO q12h, it may help dissolve struvite uroliths that are resistant to antibiotic and dietary treatment. Adjunctive treatment with urinary acidifiers in conjunction with the s/d diet is usually not recommended. The most common causes of alkaline urine during s/d diet treatment are a persistent bacterial infection and lack of dietary compliance. The medical treatment of sterile struvite uroliths is the same as that described in previous paragraphs, except that antibiotics and acetohydroxamic acid are not necessary. Sterile struvite uroliths usually dissolve more rapidly than do those associated with UTIs (range, 1 to 3 months).

Measures to prevent struvite urolith recurrence include preventing and controlling UTIs, maintaining an acidic urine, and decreasing the dietary intake of calculogenic salts. Hill's Canine Prescription Diet c/d is a good maintenance diet to prevent sterile struvite urolith recurrence, because the protein, magnesium, calcium, and phosphorous content is only moderately restricted and it produces an acidic urine. However, because the sodium content of the c/d diet is mildly restricted, 0.5 g of salt (approximately ⅛ tsp) should be supplemented daily to increase water consumption and urine production. In dogs with recurrent UTIs, predisposing abnormalities (e.g., urachal remnant, urinary bladder polyp) should be identified or ruled out with double-contrast–enhanced cystography or ultrasonography. Otherwise, silent hyperadrenocorticism may also result in recurrent UTI (see Chapter 45). Occasionally, long-term, lower-dose prophylactic antibiotic treatment may be necessary to prevent recurrent UTIs. Routine urinalyses should be performed every 2 to 4 months in asymptomatic animals and follow-up urine cultures performed in animals with clinical signs of lower urinary tract inflammation.

**Calcium oxalate uroliths.** A medical treatment for the dissolution of oxalate urolithiasis has not yet been developed. A moderate restriction of protein, calcium, oxalate, and sodium intake, with a normal intake of phosphorus, magnesium, and vitamins C and D, is recommended to prevent recurrence of calcium oxalate uroliths after surgical removal (Hills' Canine Prescription Diet u/d is recommended for this). Increased dietary sodium intake may result in an increase in the urinary excretion of calcium and therefore should be avoided. Potassium citrate, given by mouth, may help prevent recurrence of calcium oxalate uroliths, because citrate complexes with calcium, thereby forming a relatively soluble calcium citrate. In addition, it results in mild urine alkalinization, which increases the solubility of calcium oxalate. However, overzealous urine alkalinization may result in the formation of calcium phosphate uroliths, so this should be avoided. The recommended dose of potassium citrate is 40 to 75 mg/kg PO q12h. Thiazide diuretics have also been recommended to decrease the urinary excretion of calcium; hydrochlorothiazide (2 mg/kg PO q12h) has been shown to reduce urine calcium excretion in dogs. This effect was enhanced by combining the treatment with the u/d diet.

**Urate uroliths.** The medical dissolution of urate uroliths that are not associated with hepatic insufficiency (e.g., PSSs) should include a diet low in protein and nucleic acids, alkalinization of the urine, xanthine oxidase inhibition, and the elimination of UTIs. Hill's Canine Prescription Diet u/d has a reduced protein and purine content and produces alkaline urine; therefore it is recommended for the dissolution and prevention of urate uroliths. Similar to the s/d diet, the u/d diet decreases the hepatic formation of urea and hence renal medullary hypertonicity and the urine-concentrating ability. Inasmuch as the u/d diet has a restricted salt content, 0.5 to 1 g of salt (⅛ to ¼ tsp) may be supplemented on a daily basis to increase water consumption and urine production. In addition, allopurinol, a competitive inhibitor of the enzyme xanthine oxidase, which converts hypoxanthine to xanthine and xanthine to uric acid (Fig. 46-8), should be administered at a dose of 10 to 15 mg/kg PO q12h or once daily, and if necessary, sodium bicarbonate or potassium citrate should be administered orally to maintain a urine pH of 7.0. The dose of the urine alkalinizer has to be individualized for each animal. Potassium citrate is available in a wax matrix tablet (Urocit-K; Mission Pharmacal, San Antonio, Tex). Treatment can be started with a one-quarter tablet q8h and the dosage adjusted up or down based on the urine pH. Allopurinol metabolism does not appear to be influenced by dietary protein in dogs, and therefore the formation of xanthine calculi in dogs consuming a high protein diet and receiving allopurinol is not thought to be associated with altered allopurinol metabolism. It is unknown if the long-term use of allopurinol to prevent the recurrence of urate uroliths increases the risk of xanthine uroliths forming. The benefits of allopurinol may, however, outweigh the risks in animals that have had multiple episodes of urate urolithiasis. Just as in the management of struvite uroliths, any UTI should be appropriately treated, because urease-producing organisms will increase the urine ammonium ion concentration and potentiate ammonium urate crystal production.

In dogs with urate urolithiasis secondary to severe hepatic insufficiency, the underlying disorder should be corrected if possible. If hepatic function can be improved (e.g., surgical correction of a PSS) and the urine becomes undersaturated with ammonium and urate ions, uroliths may dissolve spontaneously. Even though spontaneous dissolution after surgical correction of a PSS is possible, it is usually recommended to perform a cystotomy for urolith removal at the time of PSS correction. In dogs with inoperable PSS, the u/d diet has decreased urine saturation with ammonium urate and reduced signs of hepatoencephalopathy.

**Silicate uroliths.** The medical dissolution of silicate uroliths is not yet feasible; however, recommended ways to decrease recurrence after surgical removal include a dietary change, increasing the urine volume, and urine alkalinization. Hill's Canine Prescription Diet u/d may be beneficial, because it contains low amounts of silicates and produces alkaline urine. Sodium chloride should be supplemented at a dose of 0.5 to 1 g/day (⅛ to ¼ tsp). In addition, in certain regions, soil may contain high concentrations of silicate; therefore the consumption of dirt and grass should be discouraged.

**Cystine uroliths.** Recommendations for the medical dissolution and prevention of cystine uroliths include a reduction in the dietary intake of protein and methionine, alkalinization of the urine, and the administration of thiol-containing drugs. Hill's Canine Prescription Diet u/d is appropriate, because it has a very low protein content, produces alkaline urine, and decreases the urine-concentrating ability. Urine pH should be maintained at approximately 7.5 with potassium citrate given orally if necessary. Treatment can be started with a one-quarter tablet q8h and the dosage adjusted up or down based on the urine pH. Sodium bicarbonate supplementation should be avoided, because the resulting natriuresis may enhance cystinuria. D-Penicillamine forms a disulfide compound with cysteine and therefore decreases the cystine content of the urine (Fig. 46-9). This disulfide compound is approximately 50 times more soluble than cystine in urine. D-Penicillamine may interfere with surgical wound healing, and treatment should not be initiated ear-

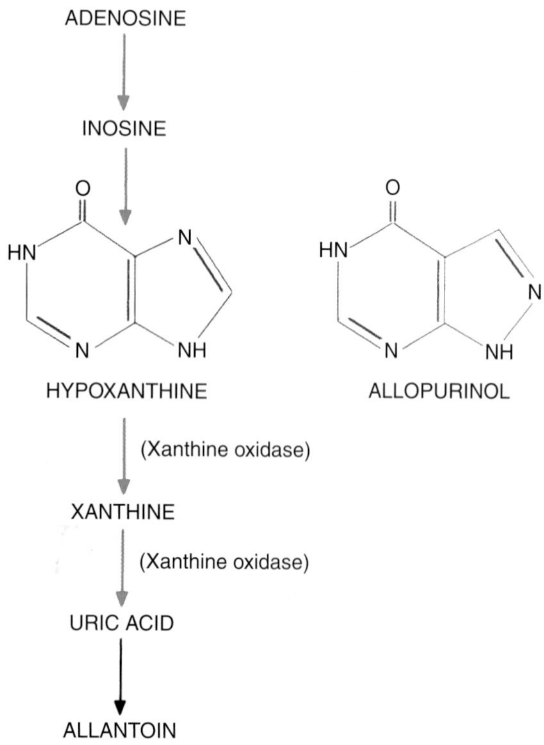

**FIG 46-8**
Metabolism of purine adenosine and a comparison of the structures of hypoxanthine and allopurinol.

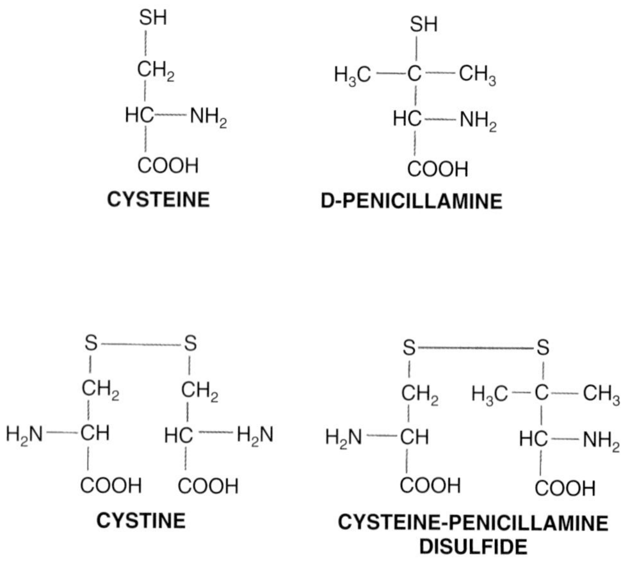

**FIG 46-9**
Structures of cystine, cysteine, D-penicillamine, and cysteine-penicillamine disulfide.

lier than 2 weeks after surgery. Other possible adverse effects of D-penicillamine include immune complex glomerulonephritis, fever, lymphadenopathy, and skin hypersensitivity. Another thiol-containing drug, N-(2-mercaptopropionyl)-glycine (MPG), increases the solubility of cystine in urine by means of a disulfide exchange reaction similar to that produced by D-penicillamine and may have fewer adverse effects. The dose of MPG that has been recommended for dogs for urate urolith dissolution is 15 to 20 mg/kg PO q12h. Thiol-containing drugs should be used along with Hill's Canine Prescription Diet u/d if necessary to prevent cystine urolith formation.

## REEVALUATION OF THE PATIENT WITH UROLITHIASIS

Whenever medical dissolution of uroliths is being attempted, the patient should be reexamined at least monthly. A complete urinalysis should be performed and abdominal radiographs or ultrasonography taken to assess urolith size. If urinalysis findings are suggestive of a UTI, bacterial culture and sensitivity testing should be performed and antibiotic treatment initiated or adjusted accordingly. If the urolith has not gotten smaller after 2 months of dissolution treatment, owner compliance, the control of infection, and urolith type should be reassessed and surgical removal considered.

Uroliths recur in up to 25% of dogs, and it is not uncommon for individual dogs to have three or more episodes of urolithiasis in their lifetime. The likelihood of recurrence appears to be greatest in dogs with metabolic uroliths (calcium oxalate, urate, and cystine uroliths) or a familial predisposition (e.g., Miniature Schnauzers with struvite uroliths). Therefore appropriate preventive measures and frequent reevaluations are important in such dogs.

### Suggested Readings

Aldrich J et al: Silica-containing urinary calculi in dogs (1981-1993), *J Vet Intern Med* 11:288, 1997.

Bartges JW et al: Prevalence of cystine and urate uroliths in Bulldogs and urate uroliths in Dalmatians, *J Am Vet Med Assoc* 204:1914, 1994.

Bartges JW et al: Influence of four diets on uric acid metabolism and endogenous acid production in healthy Beagles, *Am J Vet Res* 57:324, 1996.

Bartges JW et al: Bioavailability and pharmacokinetics of intravenously and orally administered allopurinol in healthy Beagles, *Am J Vet Res* 58:504, 1997.

Bartges JW et al: Influence of two diets on pharmacokinetic parameters of allopurinol and oxypurinol in healthy Beagles, *Am J Vet Res* 58:511, 1997.

Bartges JW et al: Ammonium urate uroliths in dogs with portosystemic shunts. In Bonagura JD, editor: *Current veterinary therapy XIII*, Philadelphia, 2000, WB Saunders, p 872.

Block G et al: Use of extracorporeal shock wave lithotripsy for treatment of nephrolithiasis and ureterolithiasis in five dogs, *J Am Vet Med Assoc* 208:531, 1996.

Hess RS et al: Association between hyperadrenocorticism and development of calcium-containing uroliths in dogs with urolithiasis, *J Am Vet Med Assoc* 212:1889, 1998.

Hoppe A et al: Cystinuria in the dog: clinical studies during 14 years of medical treatment, *J Vet Intern Med* 15:361, 2001.

Krawiec DR et al: Effect of acetohydroxamic acid on dissolution of canine struvite uroliths, *Am J Vet Res* 45:1266, 1984.

Ling GV et al: Xanthine-containing urinary calculi in dogs given allopurinol, *J Am Vet Med Assoc* 198:1935, 1991.

Ling GV et al: CVT update: management and prevention of urate urolithiasis. In Bonagura JD, editor: *Current veterinary therapy XII*, Philadelphia, 1995, WB Saunders, p 985.

Lulich JP et al: Evaluation of urine and serum metabolites in Miniature Schnauzers with calcium oxalate urolithiasis, *Am J Vet Res* 52:1583, 1991.

Lulich JP et al: Prevalence of calcium oxalate uroliths in Miniature Schnauzers, *Am J Vet Res* 52:1579, 1991.

Lulich JP et al: Catheter-assisted retrieval of urocystoliths from dogs and cats, *Am J Vet Med Assoc* 201:111, 1992.

Lulich JP et al: Nonsurgical removal of urocystoliths by voiding urohydropropulsion, *Am J Vet Med Assoc* 203:660, 1993.

Lulich JP et al: Canine calcium oxalate uroliths. In Bonagura JD, editor: *Current veterinary therapy XII*, Philadelphia, 1995, WB Saunders, p 992.

Lulich JP et al: Voiding urohydropropulsion: a nonsurgical technique for removal of urocystoliths. In Bonagura JD, editor: *Current veterinary therapy XII*, Philadelphia, 1995, WB Saunders, p 1003.

Lulich JP et al: Effects of hydrochlorothiazide and diet in dogs with calcium oxalate urolithiasis, *J Am Vet Med Assoc* 218:1583, 2001.

Osborne CA et al: Medical dissolution and prevention of cystine urolithiasis. In Kirk RW, editor: *Current veterinary therapy X*, Philadelphia, 1989, WB Saunders, p 1189.

Osborne CA et al: Canine and feline nephroliths. In Bonagura JD, editor: *Current veterinary therapy XII*, Philadelphia, 1995, WB Saunders, p 981.

Osborne CA et al: Canine and feline calcium phosphate urolithiasis. In Bonagura JD, editor: *Current veterinary therapy XII*, Philadelphia, 1995, WB Saunders, p 996.

Osborne CA et al: Canine and feline urolithiases: relationship of etiopathogenesis to treatment and prevention. In Osborne CA et al, editors: *Canine and feline nephrology and urology*, Philadelphia, 1995, Williams & Wilkins, p 798.

Sanderson SL et al: Evaluation of urinary carnitine and taurine excretion in 5 cystinuric dogs with carnitine and taurine deficiency, *J Vet Intern Med* 15:94, 2001.

Seaman R et al: Canine struvite urolithiasis, *Compend Contin Educ Pract Vet* 23:407, 2001.

Stevenson AR et al: Effects of dietary potassium citrate supplementation on urine pH and urinary relative supersaturation of calcium oxalate and struvite in healthy dogs, *Am J Vet Res* 61:430, 2000.

Weichselbaum RC et al: Evaluation of the morphologic characteristics and prevalence of canine urocystoliths from a regional urolith center, *Am J Vet Res* 59:379, 1998.

# CHAPTER 47

## Feline Lower Urinary Tract Inflammation

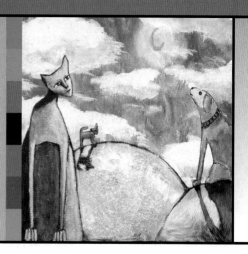

### CHAPTER OUTLINE

Etiology and pathogenesis, 642
Clinical features and diagnosis, 645
Management, 645

Feline lower urinary tract inflammation (FLUTI) is characterized by one or more of the following clinical signs: pollakiuria, hematuria, dysuria-stranguria, inappropriate urination, and partial or complete urethral obstruction. These clinical signs have historically been termed *feline urologic syndrome;* however, this syndrome is not a single disease entity. The definition of the syndrome has varied among studies and authors, and it is difficult to interpret the literature without a broader definition that includes all disorders associated with FLUTI.

FLUTI can be divided into two broad categories based on the presence or absence of struvite (magnesium ammonium phosphate) crystalluria and/or struvite uroliths (Fig. 47-1). Cats that have struvite-related disease may have overt urolithiasis, crystalluria without obstruction, or a urethral obstruction with struvite-containing mucous plugs. However, apparently normal cats can have struvite crystalluria, and mucous plugs without struvite crystals can cause urethral obstructions. Cats in the second group usually have urinary tract inflammation but no detectable struvite crystals or urolith formation. A small percentage (>2%) of young cats in either group may have primary bacterial urinary tract infections; bacterial urinary tract infections are more common in older cats with compromised host defense mechanisms (e.g., chronic renal failure). In most cats with FLUTI, the cause of the inflammation is unknown.

FLUTI has been reported to occur in 0.34% to 0.64% of all cats, and it is thought to be the reason for 4% to 10% of all feline admissions to veterinary hospitals. It appears to be equally prevalent in male and female cats; however, overweight cats are thought to be predisposed to cystitis. Indoor cats are also reported to be more predisposed to the syndrome than outdoor cats; however, because the urination habits of indoor cats are more closely observed than those of outdoor cats, this may be an artificial difference. Most feline lower urinary tract disorders occur in cats between 2 and 6 years of age, with an increased prevalence often observed in the winter and spring months. Between 30% and 70% of cats that have one episode of FLUTI will have a recurrence.

The reported mortality rates for cats with FLUTI range from 6% to 36%. Hyperkalemia and uremia are major causes of death in male cats with a urethral obstruction; however, many cats with recurrent FLUTI are euthanized because owners are unwilling to repeatedly finance the treatment, diagnostics, or hospitalization necessary to relieve urethral obstruction. Chronic renal disease or failure secondary to ascending pyelonephritis is a possible long-term sequela or complication of FLUTI, especially if there have been repeated urethral catheterizations.

### Etiology and Pathogenesis

FLUTI may occur in association with struvite uroliths, microcalculi, or crystals, which irritate the uroepithelium. As with canine urolithiasis, there must be a sufficiently high concentration of urolith-forming constituents in the urine, a favorable pH, and adequate time in the urinary tract for crystals to form.

Dietary factors, especially a high dietary intake of magnesium, are currently thought to play a role in the development of struvite crystals and uroliths. Diets with a high ash content have also been implicated in the past and are a major concern to cat owners; however, dietary ash consists of all noncombustible materials in the diet, including magnesium, calcium, phosphorus, sodium, and chloride. The magnesium content is related to the total ash content in dry and semimoist foods but not in canned foods. Despite owner concern, a high dietary ash content may be beneficial if it resulted from high salt content. In contrast, a low-ash diet may promote the development of crystalluria if the dietary magnesium content is high. Obesity has been linked to the struvite-associated FLUTI; however, obesity and struvite-induced inflammation may both be linked to excessive food, and therefore magnesium, consumption.

In general, the available energy density is lower in dry cat foods than in canned foods, and dry cat foods contain more

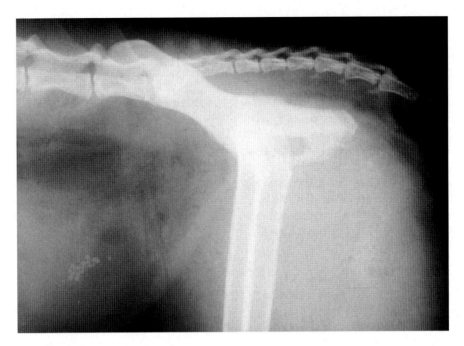

**FIG 47-1**
Radiographic appearance of struvite uroliths in the bladder and urethra of a cat.

magnesium per kilocalorie than do canned or semimoist foods. In addition, most dry cat foods have a high fiber content and are less digestible than canned or semimoist foods, resulting in an increased total intake of magnesium (most cats eat to meet their caloric needs). The consumption of dry food also results in a larger fecal volume and greater fecal water loss, which may decrease urine volume. A decreased urine volume in turn increases the concentration of magnesium and other calculogenic substances in the urine and increases the time these substances are present in the urinary tract.

Even more important than the urine magnesium concentrations in the pathogenesis of struvite crystalluria is the urine pH. Struvite is approximately 100 times more soluble at a urine pH of 6.4 than at a pH of 7.7. In fact, if dietary magnesium chloride is used to acidify the urine, the urine magnesium concentrations are relatively high but crystalluria and bladder inflammation do not occur. On the other hand, if magnesium oxide or magnesium sulfate is added to the diet, urine alkalinization, crystalluria, and inflammation usually occur rapidly. Many standard cat foods produce a postprandial increase in the urine pH of approximately 1 U, which lasts 3 to 5 hours. Cats fed standard foods ad libitum usually have less fluctuation in their urinary pH but may have a higher daily average urine pH than meal-fed cats.

Approximately 30% of the uroliths in cats consist either entirely or predominantly of struvite. Most struvite uroliths form in the urinary bladder of female cats between 1 and 2 years of age. In contrast to dogs, most feline struvite uroliths form in sterile urine. When a bacterial infection is present, the most common organism is a urease-producing *Staphylococcus* sp. Tamm-Horsfall mucoprotein, secreted by the renal tubules, is the major protein found in feline struvite

uroliths. It may also play a role in the pathogenesis of urethral plugs.

Urethral obstruction is more common in the male cat; the length and diameter of the urethra play a relevant role in this. Many obstructions are caused by mucous and struvite plugs that lodge in the penile urethra. Uroliths may lodge in any portion of the urethra, including sections proximal to fibrous connective tissue strictures resulting from previous injuries. Local inflammation that develops in response to urethral calculi or plugs may exacerbate the obstruction by causing urethral edema. Iatrogenic trauma created by urethral catheterization may also cause urethritis or inflammation of the periurethral tissue, leading to urethral compression.

Struvite-associated FLUTI may alter normal host defense mechanisms and allow bacteria to colonize the bladder or urethra. Complete voiding (bladder content washout) is a major host defense mechanism against bacterial infection. Therefore anatomic abnormalities or partial obstructions that may interfere with normal voiding can result in an increased urine residual volume. In addition, chronic inflammation of the urinary bladder with fibrosis and thickening of the bladder wall may cause decreased detrusor tone and incomplete voiding. Perhaps the most important factor predisposing to the development of bacterial cystitis in association with struvite-induced inflammation is urethral catheterization (especially placement of indwelling urinary catheters), combined with fluid therapy and the formation of dilute urine. A primary bacterial infection of the feline urinary tract, although rare in young cats compared with the incidence in dogs, may also cause the clinical signs observed in FLUTI. Bacterial cystitis-urethritis, viral cystitis, mycoplasmal or ureaplasmal cystitis, neoplasia, trauma, irritant cystitis-urethritis, urolithiasis, vesicourachal diverticuli, urethral strictures secondary to scar tissue, extraluminal inflammation and masses, and neurologic disorders can all cause or mimic FLUTI.

In addition to struvite uroliths, other types of uroliths, including calcium oxalate and urate stones, can cause signs of FLUTI. Calcium oxalate uroliths account for approximately 50% of feline uroliths, and urate uroliths constitute approximately 7%. Based on the findings from a recent study, Burmese, Persian, and Himalayan cats may be at higher risk for calcium oxalate urolithiasis (Thumchai and colleagues, 1996). Calcium oxalate uroliths are also more common in neutered male cats than in female cats, their prevalence is higher in older animals, and they occur more frequently in the kidneys than struvite uroliths do. Calcium oxalate uroliths are becoming more prevalent in cats, and this may be related to the widespread use of acidifying diets designed to prevent struvite-related FLUTI. Epidemiologic studies indicate that cats fed diets low in sodium or potassium or formulated to maximize urine acidity have an increased risk of developing calcium oxalate uroliths but a decreased risk of developing struvite uroliths. Another recent retrospective study identified the feeding of urine-acidifying diets, feeding a single brand of cat food, and maintaining cats in an indoor-only environment as factors associated with development of calcium oxalate urolithiasis (Kirk and colleagues, 1995). The increase in prevalence of calcium oxalate uroliths in cats may also correlate with the observation that cats are living longer lives than they were 10 to 15 years ago. Finally since the prevalence of calcium oxalate uroliths is also increasing in people and dogs, there may be unidentified environmental factors common to all three species influencing the development of these uroliths.

A decreased urine volume and decreased frequency of urination are also thought to facilitate the development of struvite-associated and non–struvite-associated FLUTI. Possible causes of a decreased urine volume and frequency of urination include a dirty or poorly available litter box; decreased physical activity as a result of cold weather, castration, obesity, illness, or confinement; and decreased water consumption because of water taste, availability, or temperature. Stress may also contribute to the development of the clinical signs of urinary tract disease. Although the role of stress is difficult to prove, it is often implicated; the history provided by owners frequently points to a recent association with boarding, cat shows, a new pet or baby in the home, a vacation, or cold or rainy weather.

From time to time, researchers have implicated viruses, including feline calicivirus, bovine herpesvirus 4, and feline syncytia-forming virus, in the pathogenesis of FLUTI. Recent findings of bovine herpesvirus 4 antibodies in cats and the detection of calicivirus-like particles in the crystalline-mucous urethral plugs of male cats have sparked renewed interest in the possibility of a viral component in the syndrome (Osborne and colleagues, 1999). Whether viruses play a major role remains to be determined.

In previous studies of cats with naturally occurring FLUTI, approximately 25% had vesicourachal diverticuli (Fig. 47-2) (Osborne and colleagues, 1999). These may be congenital or acquired; the acquired diverticuli are observed primarily in cats older than 1 year, with a mean age of 3.7 years. Male cats are twice as likely to acquire the abnormality as fe-

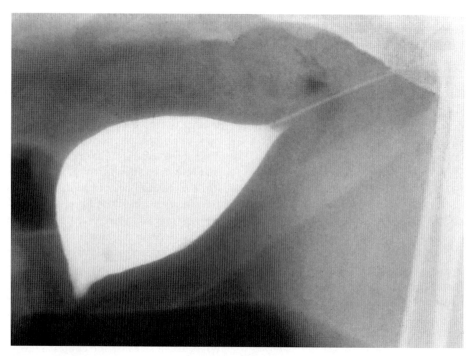

**FIG 47-2**
Positive-contrast–enhanced cystogram of a feline bladder showing a urachal remnant.

male cats, and increased intravesical pressure and bladder inflammation during urethral obstruction may play a major role in its pathogenesis. Although a urachal diverticulum may be an incidental finding in an asymptomatic cat, hematuria and dysuria are frequently noted clinical signs. Vesicourachal diverticuli are currently thought to develop secondary to FLUTI and increased intravesical pressure and are not thought to be a major initiating factor.

In large retrospective studies of cats with FLUTI conducted at the University of Minnesota (Kruger and colleagues, 1991) and The Ohio State University (Buffington and colleagues, 1997), a cause for the inflammation could not be found in 54% and 79% of the cats, respectively. Researchers at The Ohio State University have found numerous similarities between cats with idiopathic FLUTI and women with interstitial cystitis. These similarities include chronic irritative voiding patterns, sterile urine, a prominent bladder mucosal vascularity with spontaneous hemorrhages observed during cystoscopy, decreased mucosal production of glycosaminoglycan, and increased numbers of mast cells and sensory afferent neurons in bladder mucosal biopsy samples. The cause of interstitial cystitis in women is also unknown.

## Clinical Features and Diagnosis

The clinical signs of FLUTI depend on the component of the disease complex present (Table 47-1). Unobstructed cats usu-

TABLE 47-1

**Clinical Signs Associated With Lower Urinary Tract Inflammation in Cats**

### Cystitis-Urethritis

Hematuria
Pollakiuria
Dysuria-stranguria
Vocalizing during voiding
Licking at genitalia
Urination in inappropriate places

### Partial or Complete Urethral Obstruction

Inability to urinate, straining in the litter box
Hiding behavior
Vocalizing during voiding
Painful abdomen
Licking at genitalia
Congested penis extended from prepuce
Signs of postrenal azotemia
    Depression
    Weakness
    Anorexia
    Emesis
    Dehydration
    Hypothermia
    Acidosis and hyperventilation
    Electrolyte disturbances (hyperkalemia)
    Bradycardia

ally have pollakiuria, dysuria-stranguria, and microscopic or gross hematuria, and they urinate in inappropriate places, often in a bathtub or sink (also see Chapter 41). These clinical signs may be readily apparent in cats that live indoors but may be missed in cats that live primarily outdoors.

In male cats with urinary obstruction, the presenting signs depend on the duration of the obstruction. Within 6 to 24 hours, most obstructed cats will make frequent attempts to urinate, pace, vocalize, hide under beds or behind couches, lick their genitalia, and display anxiety. If the obstruction is not relieved within 36 to 48 hours, clinical signs characteristic of postrenal azotemia, including anorexia, vomiting, dehydration, depression, weakness, collapse, stupor, hypothermia, acidosis with hyperventilation, bradycardia, or sudden death may occur.

On physical examination, an unobstructed cat will be apparently healthy, except for a small, easily expressed bladder. The bladder wall may also be thickened. Abdominal palpation may be painful for the unobstructed cat; however, the obstructed cat always resents manipulation of the caudal area of the abdomen. The most relevant finding during a physical examination of the obstructed cat is a turgid, distended bladder that is difficult or impossible to express. Care should be exercised when manipulating the distended bladder, however, because the wall has been injured by the increased intravesical pressure and is susceptible to rupture. In the cat with a urethral obstruction, the penis may be congested and protrude from the prepuce. Occasionally a urethral plug is observed to extend from the urethral orifice; in some cases the cat may lick his penis until it becomes excoriated and bleeds.

The diagnosis of urethral obstruction is usually straightforward and is based on history and physical examination findings. In unobstructed cats with FLUTI, urinalysis usually reveals hematuria; if not, behavioral causes of abnormal urination should be considered (Table 47-2 and Fig. 47-3). Struvite-associated disease is likely in cats in which the initial urine pH is alkaline and struvite crystals are observed in the urine sediment. Radiography or ultrasonography and urine cultures should be employed to rule out or identify overt urolithiasis and a urinary tract infection in cats with suspected struvite-associated disease, especially if there is no response to a magnesium-restricted, acidifying diet (see Fig. 47-3 and Management section). In cats with FLUTI that have acidic urine, radiography or ultrasonography can help identify or rule out anatomic abnormalities (e.g., thickened bladder wall, polyps, tumors, non–struvite-associated urolithiasis). Cystoscopy is also a valuable tool in cats with FLUTI. Nonspecific cystoscopic findings include prominent mucosal vascularity and submucosal petechial hemorrhages. Radiography (plain and double-contrast–enhanced cystography), ultrasonography, or cystoscopy and urine culture should be performed in all cats with recurrent FLUTI.

## Management

**Unobstructed cats.** The nature of the treatment for FLUTI depends on the clinical signs at presentation (see Table 47-2 and Fig. 47-3). Unobstructed cats with idiopathic dysuria-

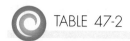

TABLE 47-2

## Diagnostic and Therapeutic Plan for Cats With Lower Urinary Tract Inflammation

1. Rule out urethral obstruction; relieve obstruction, if present.
2. Assess degree of hyperkalemia with an electrocardiogram; measure serum urea nitrogen, creatinine, and potassium concentrations; and initiate IV fluid therapy if cat is obstructed and depressed.
3. In both obstructed and unobstructed cats, obtain a urine sample by cystocentesis, if possible, for the evaluation of urine pH and urine sediment. Culture urine if there is evidence of a urinary tract infection (pyuria, bacteriuria).
4. Manage cats with suspected struvite-associated FLUTI using a diet containing less than 20 mEq of magnesium per 100 kCal, and acidify urine (between 6.2 and 6.4) with ammonium chloride or methionine, if necessary.

5. Obtain a urine sample in cats with non–struvite-associated FLUTI or in cats with struvite-associated FLUTI with persistent or recurring clinical signs:
   a. If there is no evidence of urinary tract infection, examine the bladder using radiography or ultrasonography or examine the bladder and urethra using contrast-enhanced radiography or cystoscopy.
   b. If there is evidence of urinary tract infection, perform bacterial culture and sensitivity testing and treat with an appropriate antibiotic. If signs persist or recur, examine the bladder using radiography or ultrasonography or examine the bladder and urethra with contrast-enhanced radiography or cystoscopy.
6. In cases of idiopathic FLUTI, try antiinflammatory treatment.

*FLUTI,* Feline lower urinary tract inflammation.

Clinical signs (dysuria/stranguria, hematuria, pollakiuria, inappropriate urination)

↓

Urinalysis

Normal
(rule out behavioral
and neurologic causes)

Abnormal
(most likely abnormality
is hematuria)

Alkaline pH
Struvite crystalluria

Acidic pH
No crystalluria

Dietary trial
(low Mg and urine
acidification)

(If bacteria
or pyruria present)

Quantative urine culture

No growth          Significant growth

Antibiotic trial

Response     No response/
recurrence

No response/
recurrence          Response

Survey and contrast radiographs or ultrasonography of urinary tract or cysto-urethroscopy

Specific findings (e.g.,
focal bladder wall thickening,
tumor, polyps, uroliths)

↓

Surgery/biopsy

Nonspecific findings
(e.g., generalized bladder
wall thickening, prominent
mucosal vascularity, spontaneous
submucosal petechial hemorrhages)
Try anti-inflammatory treatment
if urine is bacteriologically sterile

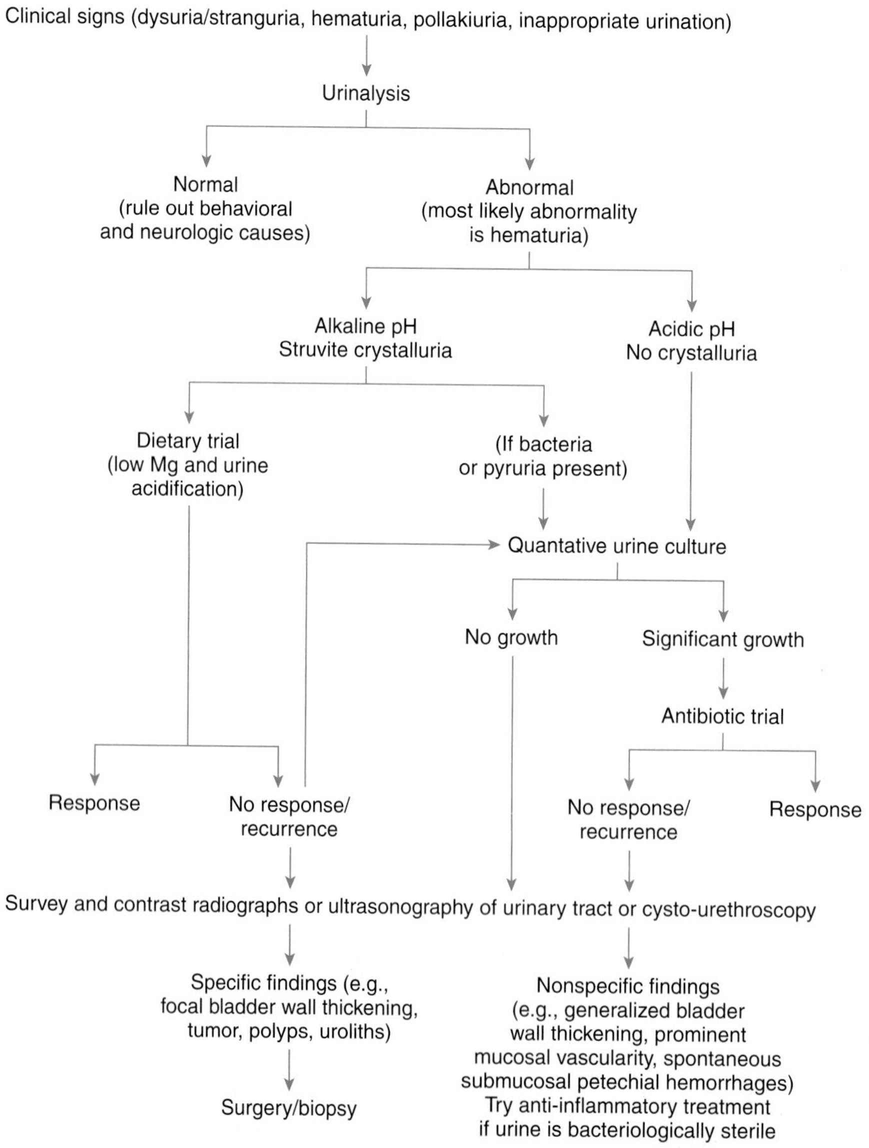

**FIG 47-3**
Diagnostic and therapeutic flow chart for unobstructed cats with lower urinary tract inflammation.

stranguria and hematuria will often become asymptomatic within 5 to 7 days of presentation, whether therapy is instituted or not. Many cats are treated with antibiotics, and if clinical signs abate, a cause-and-effect relationship is often established in the minds of the clinician and cat owner. The clinician should remember, however, that more than 95% of young cats with FLUTI have sterile urine and that the same results could be obtained by treating with numerous placebos.

If the initial urinalysis reveals an alkaline urine with struvite crystalluria, the cat should be fed a magnesium-restricted, acidifying diet that will maintain an average urine pH of less than 6.4. Urine culture and sensitivity tests should be performed if pyuria or bacteriuria is observed in the urine sediment, and appropriate antibiotics should be administered if urine cultures are positive. Cystocentesis is the ideal way to obtain urine for bacterial culture; if urine is obtained by any other method, a quantitative urine culture should be performed. Several sources of fresh water should be made available to the cat. The litter boxes should also be cleaned frequently and placed in convenient locations. The length of treatment with a struvite-prevention diet is controversial, but 2 months is a good initial trial. If struvite-associated FLUTI recurs after the initial treatment, a longer therapeutic trial is indicated. Lifetime feeding of a struvite-prevention diet to a cat that has had one or two episodes of struvite-associated FLUTI is usually not recommended.

Hill's Feline Prescription Diet s/d can be used to effectively dissolve struvite uroliths. It takes an average of 36 days for sterile struvite uroliths to dissolve, whereas struvite uroliths associated with urease-producing bacterial infections in cats take an average of 79 days to dissolve. Antibiotic treatment in cats with struvite urolithiasis and a concurrent bacterial urinary tract infection should be determined on the basis of urine culture and sensitivity results and continued throughout the period of dissolution. The diet should be fed for 30 days beyond the point when the uroliths are no longer visible in radiographs.

If struvite crystalluria and alkaline urine recur repeatedly, longer-term dietary therapy is warranted. Examples of diets that can be used to treat struvite-associated FLUTI as well as prevent recurrence include Hill's Feline Prescription Diet c/d (canned or dry), Science Diet Feline Maintenance (canned or dry), Iams pH/S, Purina UR–Formula Feline Diet, and Waltham Veterinarium Feline Control pHormula Diet. The composition of many over-the-counter cat foods is not constant; therefore it is difficult to make recommendations regarding their use. Ideally, the urine pH, measured 4 to 8 hours after feeding, should be maintained between 6.2 and 6.4. The prescription diets just mentioned are metabolized to form acid ions, which are excreted in the urine. If these diets cannot maintain an acidic urine, urinary acidifiers may be added to the treatment regimen. Ammonium chloride is the most effective urinary acidifier (800 mg/day, or approximately ¼ tsp, on food); however, diarrhea, vomiting, and anorexia are potential adverse effects. If the diarrhea persists after 7 to 10 days of use, methionine (500 mg q12h) may be substituted for the ammonium chloride. It is rare, however, for these prescription diets to not maintain an acidic urine in cats. A urease-producing bacterial infection and dietary indiscretion

should be identified or ruled out if alkaline urine is found to persist during dietary therapy. Excessive urine acidification may result in a chronic metabolic acidosis and in increases in serum calcium and phosphorous concentrations associated with chronic bone buffering, so this should be avoided. Hypokalemia and weakness develop in some cats with renal tubular disorders and a decreased ability to excrete hydrogen-fed acidifying diets.

In most cases of FLUTI, the urine is acidic and no struvite crystals are observed; therefore magnesium-restricted, acidifying diets are not recommended. A urine sample should be obtained by cystocentesis for urine culture, and plain abdominal radiography or ultrasonography, contrast-enhanced radiographic studies of the bladder and urethra, or cystoscopy should be performed to identify or rule out anatomic abnormalities if the urine is bacteriologically sterile (see Table 47-2 and Fig. 47-3). Numerous agents, including antibiotics, tranquilizers, anticholinergics, antispasmodics, and anti-inflammatory drugs (e.g., dimethylsulfoxide, glucocorticoids), have been recommended for the treatment of idiopathic cystitis in cats; however, no controlled studies have demonstrated the efficacy of any of these agents. More recently glycosaminoglycans, amitriptyline, and nonsteroidal antiinflammmatory drugs (NSAIDs) have been recommended for the treatment of idiopathic FLUTI, but again no controlled studies document the efficacy of these treatments in cats. Oxybutynin and propantheline are antispasmodic drugs that may alleviate pollakiuria in some cats. Keep in mind that in controlled studies, more than 70% of cats with idiopathic FLUTI have appeared to respond to placebo treatments (lactose, wheat flour). Just because we administer a drug and the patient appears to respond does not mean there is a cause-and-effect relationship.

**Obstructed cats.** In cats with a urethral obstruction, the relative urgency for relieving the obstruction depends on the physical status of the cat. Cats that are alert and not azotemic may be sedated for urethral catheterization without further diagnostic tests or treatment; however, in a depressed cat with urethral obstruction, the serum potassium concentration should be measured in-house or an electrocardiographic rhythm strip should be evaluated to assess the degree of hyperkalemia (see Table 46-2) and an intravenous (IV) catheter should be placed for the administration of normal (0.9%) saline solution before establishing urethral patency. If the electrocardiogram or blood tests confirm the presence of hyperkalemia, the cat should be treated aggressively to decrease serum potassium concentrations or counteract the effects of hyperkalemia on cardiac conduction (see Table 46-2).

The degree of restraint required for urethral catheterization depends on the cat's temperament and physical status. Physical restraint in a towel or cat bag, with or without the topical application of lidocaine, may be all that is required in a severely depressed cat. In cats requiring more restraint, ketamine HCl (1 to 2 mg/kg IV), an ultra–short-acting barbiturate (thiamylal sodium or thiopental sodium, 1 mg/kg IV titrated to effect), or propofol may be used to effect. Because ketamine is eliminated by the kidneys, low IV doses (10 to 20 mg total) are frequently adequate for restraint. The administration of additional doses of ketamine should be avoided in severely azotemic cats.

A urethral obstruction may be relieved in some cases by penile massage and gentle expression of the bladder. If this does not result in urine flow, palpation of the urethra per rectum may dislodge a urethral plug or calculus. Sterile isotonic saline solution, administered through well-lubricated catheters or cannulas, should be used to hydropulse urethral plugs into the bladder. A variety of cannulas and catheters may be used for this purpose; however, nonmetal catheters with smooth, open ends are preferred to prevent iatrogenic damage to the urethral mucosa. Use of a strict aseptic technique is essential to prevent bacterial urinary tract infections. If it proves difficult to catheterize the bladder, cystocentesis may be performed to decrease the intravesical pressure and allow for the urethral obstruction to be back-flushed into the bladder.

Questions frequently arise as to the appropriate indications for the placement of indwelling urinary catheters in male cats with obstructions that have just been relieved. These are (1) an inability to restore a normal urine stream, (2) an abundance of debris that cannot be extracted via repeated bladder lavage, (3) evidence of detrusor atony in cats that cannot be manually expressed four to six times per day, or (4) intensive care of critically ill animals in which urine formation is being monitored as a guide to fluid therapy requirements. When an indwelling urinary catheter is necessary, again, strict aseptic technique should be used during placement. A soft, red rubber feeding tube (3F to 5F) should be used; placing the feeding tube in the freezer for 30 minutes before use facilitates its passage. The catheter should be inserted only as far as the neck of the bladder; an ability to aspirate urine indicates proper placement of the catheter. A closed urine-collection system should be used, and the catheter should be sutured to the prepuce and left in place for as short a time as possible (2 to 3 days is the average). An Elizabethan collar or tape hobbles are needed to prevent the cat from chewing out the sutures and removing the catheter. Prophylactic antibiotic treatment is not recommended; however, the urine sediment should be examined daily for bacteria and white blood cells and the urine cultured if necessary. Secondary bacterial urinary tract infections are common in cats with indwelling urinary catheters receiving IV fluids to promote diuresis.

The degree of postrenal azotemia should be assessed by measuring the serum urea nitrogen, creatinine, and potassium concentrations. IV fluid therapy is indicated, especially in cats with azotemia. Maintenance therapy (approximately 60 to 70 ml/kg/day) and replacement therapy (percentage of dehydration × body weight [in kilograms] = liters to administer) should be administered IV over 24 hours. The subcutaneous administration of a balanced electrolyte solution is an acceptable mode of fluid therapy in some cats once the initial uremic crisis is under control. Measurement of the urine volume every 4 to 8 hours will facilitate the administration of correct replacement therapy. A large-volume, postobstructive diuresis may develop in some cats, and IV fluid replacement therapy is essential in these animals. Serum urea

nitrogen, creatinine, and serum electrolyte concentrations should be reassessed as needed, depending on the degree of azotemia and the response to treatment, to ensure the adequate recovery of renal function. Occasionally, hypokalemia occurs in a cat with a prolonged and severe diuresis. In addition, if severe hematuria persists, the hematocrit should be monitored once or twice daily.

Detrusor atony is fairly common in cats obstructed for more than 24 hours and is associated with bladder overdistention. If the bladder can be expressed four to six times per day, an indwelling catheter may not be necessary. If the bladder cannot be expressed at least four times per day, an indwelling catheter is indicated. Bethanechol (2.5 mg q8h PO) may be administered to stimulate detrusor contractility only after the finding of a wide urine stream or the placement of an indwelling urinary catheter has confirmed that the urethra is patent. Acepromazine and phenoxybenzamine can significantly lower intraurethral pressures in anesthetized, healthy, intact male cats, and therefore these compounds may also be helpful in the management of a functional urethral obstruction in cats with FLUTI.

Perineal urethrostomy is rarely required for the emergency relief of a urethral obstruction. If the obstruction cannot be relieved by medical means, the condition of uremic cats must be stabilized before surgery is performed. Repeated cystocentesis should be done to keep the bladder empty until hyperkalemia, acidosis, and uremia resolve. Elective perineal urethrostomies are occasionally advisable in male cats with recurrent obstructions to decrease the likelihood of death from postrenal azotemia. However, a perineal urethrostomy does not decrease the risk of recurrence of clinical signs of cystitis, and it has been documented that cats with cystitis that undergo perineal urethrostomies are more susceptible to bacterial urinary tract infections.

The dietary management of a previously obstructed cat with struvite crystalluria is similar to that of an unobstructed cat with struvite crystalluria and alkaline urine. Magnesium-restricted, acidifying diets should be fed to help prevent recurrences of lower urinary tract inflammation or obstruction.

Probably the most important aspect of long-term patient monitoring is ensuring that the owner recognizes both the significance and the clinical signs of urethral obstruction. Owners of male cats with urinary obstruction must be warned of the risks of reobstruction, especially during the first 24 to 48 hours after the relief of an obstruction or the removal of an indwelling urinary catheter. Allowing the owner to palpate the distended bladder during the initial examination is a good way to teach him or her how to differentiate between pollakiuria and dysuria-stranguria, and an obstruction. Any straining in the litter box should be cause for alarm in a male cat with a history of urethral obstruction, and careful observation for continued voiding of urine is essential for the early detection of a recurrence.

Follow-up urinalysis and urine culture should be performed 5 to 7 days after catheterization in all cats that have been catheterized to relieve a urethral obstruction. Because normal host defenses are bypassed when a catheter is introduced into the bladder, urinary tract infections are common after catheterization, especially if an indwelling urinary catheter has been used. A follow-up urinalysis and urine culture should also be performed in all cats receiving corticosteroids, because these may decrease immune system function (and decrease inflammation-related changes in the urine sediment) and predispose cats to the development of bacterial urinary tract infections. Ascending pyelonephritis is a significant concern in cats with any urinary tract infection, and it is a potential complication of FLUTI, especially if corticosteroids are used.

Periodic urinalyses to measure pH are beneficial in cats with struvite-associated disease being managed by diet to prevent recurrent episodes. The urine pH 4 to 8 hours after eating should be 6.4 or less. Yearly urinalysis and bacterial culture are especially important in cats with perineal urethrostomies, because the normal host defense mechanisms of the lower urethra have been surgically removed in these cats.

The prognosis for male cats with recurrent urethral obstruction is guarded, and perineal urethrostomy should be considered, especially if the second obstruction occurs during medical management designed to prevent recurrence. The prognosis for cats with recurrent, nonobstructed FLUTI is fair to good, inasmuch as this syndrome is rarely life-threatening. Pyelonephritis, renal urolithiasis, and chronic renal failure are potential sequelae of recurrent, nonobstructed FLUTI.

## Suggested Readings

Barsanti JA et al: The role of dimethyl sulfoxide and glucocorticoids in lower urinary tract diseases. In Bonagura JD, editor: *Current veterinary therapy XII,* Philadelphia, 1995, WB Saunders.

Bartges JW et al: Bacterial urinary tract infection in cats. In Bonagura JD, editor: *Current veterinary therapy XIII,* Philadelphia, 2000, WB Saunders, p 880.

Buffington CAT et al: Clinical evaluation of cats with nonobstructive urinary tract diseases, *J Am Vet Med Assoc* 210:46, 1997.

Buffington CAT et al: Feline interstitial cystitis, *J Am Vet Med Assoc* 215:682, 1999.

Buffington CAT et al: CVT update: idiopathic (interstitial) cystitis in cats. In Bonagura JD, editor: *Current veterinary therapy XIII,* Philadelphia, 2000, WB Saunders, p 894.

Kirk CA et al: Evaluation of factors associated with development of calcium oxalate urolithiasis in cats, *J Am Vet Med Assoc* 207:1429, 1995.

Kruger JM et al: Clinical evaluation of cats with lower urinary tract disease, *J Am Vet Med Assoc* 199:211, 1991.

Kruger JM et al: Nonobstructive idiopathic feline lower urinary tract disease: therapeutic rights and wrongs. In Bonagura JD, editor: *Current veterinary therapy XIII,* Philadelphia, 2000, WB Saunders, p 888.

Lekcharoensuk C et al: Association between dietary factors and calcium oxalate and magnesium ammonium phosphate urolithiasis in cats, *J Am Vet Med Assoc* 219:1228, 2001.

Lekcharoensuk C et al: Epidemiologic study of risk factors for lower urinary tract disease in cats, *J Am Vet Med Assoc* 218:1429, 2001.

Marks SL et al: Effects of acepromazine maleate and phenoxybenzamine on urethral pressure profiles of anesthetized, healthy, sexually intact male cats, *Am J Vet Res* 57:1497, 1996.

Osborne CA et al: Canine and feline nephroliths. In Bonagura JD, editor: *Current veterinary therapy XII,* Philadelphia, 1995, WB Saunders, p 981.

Osborne CA et al: Disorders of the feline lower urinary tract. In Osborne CA et al, editors: *Canine and feline nephrology and urology,* Philadelphia, 1995, Williams & Wilkins, p 625.

Osborne CA et al: Feline calcium oxalate uroliths. In Bonagura JD, editor: *Current veterinary therapy XII,* Philadelphia, 1995, WB Saunders, p 989.

Osborne CA et al: Disorders of the feline lower urinary tract. I. Etiology and pathophysiology, *Vet Clin North Am Small Anim Pract* 26:169, 1996.

Osborne CA et al: Disorders of the feline lower urinary tract. II. Diagnosis and therapy, *Vet Clin North Am Small Anim Pract* 26:423, 1996.

Osborne CA et al: Feline urologic syndrome, feline lower urinary tract disease, feline interstitial cystitis: what's in a name? *J Am Vet Med Assoc* 214:1470, 1999.

Selcer BA: Ultrasonographic findings in feline lower urinary tract diseases. In Bonagura JD, editor: *Current veterinary therapy XII,* Philadelphia, 1995, WB Saunders, p 1007.

Thumchai R et al: Epizootiologic evaluation of urolithiasis in cats: 3,498 cases (1982-1992), *J Am Vet Med Assoc* 208:547, 1996.

# CHAPTER 48

# Disorders of Micturition

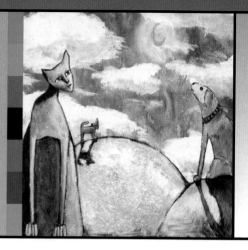

## CHAPTER OUTLINE

PHYSIOLOGY OF MICTURITION, 650
ETIOLOGY AND CLINICAL FEATURES OF DISORDERS
OF MICTURITION, 651
    Distended bladder, 651
    Small or normal-sized bladder, 652
    Geriatric incontinence, 653
DIAGNOSIS, 653
    Initial evaluation, 654
    Pharmacologic testing, 654
TREATMENT, 655
    Lower motor neuron disorders, 655
    Upper motor neuron disorders, 655
    Reflex dyssynergia, 655
    Functional urethral obstruction, 655
    Urethral sphincter mechanism incompetence, 656
    Detrusor hyperreflexia or instability, 656
    Congenital disorders, 656
    Anatomic urethral obstruction, 656
PROGNOSIS, 656

Micturition is the normal process of the passive storage and active voiding of urine. Disorders of micturition encompass problems with urine storage (incontinence) and bladder emptying (urine retention). Urinary incontinence is the inappropriate passage of urine during the storage phase of micturition. The most common forms of urinary incontinence are detrusor hyperreflexia or instability, and urethral sphincter mechanism incompetence (USMI). Urine retention can occur in patients with decreased detrusor muscle contractility or with increased urethral resistance. Armed with an understanding of bladder and urethral neuroanatomy, as well as the mechanism of action of the currently available drugs, clinicians are able to effectively control many disorders of micturition.

## PHYSIOLOGY OF MICTURITION

Micturition is controlled by a combination of autonomic and somatic innervation (Fig. 48-1). Parasympathetic innervation to the bladder is provided by the sensory and motor portions of the pelvic nerve that arises from sacral spinal cord segments S1 to S3. The sensory portion relays the sensation of bladder fullness as the stretch receptors associated with detrusor muscle fibers are activated. The motor portion of this parasympathetic innervation predominates during the voiding phase of micturition, with stimulation of the pelvic nerve resulting in the depolarization of pacemaker fibers throughout the detrusor muscle. The subsequent spread of excitation to adjoining muscle fibers through tight junctions of smooth muscle cells leads to contraction of the detrusor muscle.

The S1 to S3 spinal cord segments are also the source of the somatic innervation to the external urethral sphincter via the pudendal nerve. The external urethral sphincter is located predominantly in the midportion of the female urethra and in the membranous portion of the male urethra. Stimulation of the pudendal nerve causes the striated skeletal muscle of the external urethral sphincter to contract. This contraction is under conscious control; additional somatic functions under conscious control are relaxation of the pelvic musculature and initiation of an abdominal press, which facilitate bladder emptying. The pudendal nerve also has sensory and motor function to the perineal region, including the anal sphincter, vulva, and prepuce.

Sympathetic innervation to the bladder is provided by the hypogastric nerve and is composed of preganglionic fibers exiting spinal cord segments L1 to L4 and synapsing in the caudal mesenteric ganglion. β-Adrenergic fibers terminate in the detrusor muscle; stimulation of these fibers results in detrusor muscle relaxation, which facilitates urine storage. α-Adrenergic fibers innervate the smooth muscle fibers in the trigone and urethra; stimulation of these fibers causes contraction and formation of the functional internal urethral

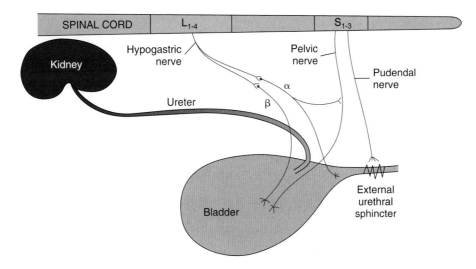

**FIG 48-1**
Autonomic and somatic innervation of the urinary bladder.

sphincter. α-Adrenergic receptors also have a modulating effect on the external urethral sphincter.

The normal storage phase of micturition is governed by sympathetic autonomic domination, which causes the detrusor muscle to relax as a result of α-adrenergic stimulation and the internal urethral sphincter to contract as a result of α-adrenergic stimulation. Voiding is also consciously inhibited by the contraction of striated urethral muscles distal to the bladder and involuntarily inhibited by a spinal reflex that tightens the external urethral sphincter when there is a sharp increase in intraabdominal pressure (e.g., during abdominal palpation or bladder expression, barking, coughing, sneezing, retching). Urinary incontinence occurs if the pressure in the bladder exceeds the pressure exerted by the urethral sphincters.

Stretch receptors in the bladder send impulses through the pelvic nerve and spinal cord pathways to the thalamus and cerebral cortex when the urinary bladder fills and intramural tension exceeds the threshold. Voluntary control of voiding is mediated by the cerebral cortex, pons (main micturition center), and the cerebellum through the reticulospinal tracts to the sacral nuclei. The voiding phase of micturition is characterized by parasympathetic activity. In this phase the detrusor muscle contracts and the sympathetic stimulation to the internal urethral sphincter is simultaneously inhibited. When the bladder is empty, the normal sympathetic domination resumes and the detrusor muscle relaxes to allow filling to occur. The normal residual volume of urine after complete voiding is approximately 0.2 to 0.4 ml/kg in both dogs and cats.

## ETIOLOGY AND CLINICAL FEATURES OF DISORDERS OF MICTURITION

Disorders of micturition can be divided into two major categories: those associated with a large or distended bladder and those associated with a small or normal-sized bladder (Table 48-1). Disorders associated with distended bladders include neurogenic disorders (upper [UMN] and lower [LMN] motor neuron disease, functional urethral obstruction, reflex dyssynergia) and anatomic obstructive disorders. Neurologic disorders may be caused by any condition that produces compression, damage, or degeneration of the spinal cord, pelvic nerve, or pudendal nerve. Overdistention of the bladder for a prolonged time may also cause a neurogenic incontinence by decreasing bladder detrusor muscle tone (a type of LMN disorder). Dysautonomia in dogs and cats, an autonomic polyganglionopathy, also produces an LMN incontinence that is associated with weak and ineffective detrusor activity. Disorders associated with a small or normal-sized bladder may be caused by detrusor hyperreflexia or instability (urethral sphincter mechanism incompetence [USMI]). Hormone-responsive incontinence is a type of USMI that occurs in middle-age to older, female, spayed dogs, probably because the decrease in estrogen concentration down-regulates the α-adrenergic receptors of the internal urethral sphincter. Finally, congenital abnormalities of the urinary system (e.g., ectopic ureters, vaginal strictures) can result in urinary incontinence associated with a small or normal-sized urinary bladder.

### DISTENDED BLADDER

If neurologic lesions or deficits are detected during neurologic examination, the status of the bladder helps localize the lesion and helps classify the injury as either a UMN lesion (above the fifth lumbar vertebral body) or an LMN lesion (at or below the fifth lumbar vertebral body). The most characteristic sign of an LMN lesion affecting the bladder is a distended bladder that is easily expressed. An LMN injury affecting the bladder causes both sphincter and detrusor hyporeflexia; if the lesion involves spinal cord segments S1 to S3, both perineal and bulbospongiosus reflexes of the pudendal nerve are absent.

UMN lesions affecting the bladder are characterized by a large, distended bladder that is difficult to express. Thoracolumbar spinal cord lesions causing paresis or paralysis are

TABLE 48-1

Disorders of Micturition

| DISORDER | CAUSES |
|---|---|
| **Distended Bladder** | |
| Neurogenic | |
|    Lower motor neuron disease | Lesion to S1 to S3 spinal cord segment (at or below fifth lumbar vertebral body), neoplasia, trauma, cauda equina syndrome |
| | Trauma to pelvic nerve, detrusor atony, canine and feline dysautonomia |
|    Upper motor neuron disease | Lesion cranial to S1 spinal cord segment (above fifth lumbar vertebral body), intervertebral disk protrusion, neoplasia, trauma, fibrocartilaginous infarct, meningitis |
| | Cerebral disease, cerebellar disease, brainstem disease |
| Reflex dyssynergia (detrusor-urethral dyssynergia) | Unknown |
| Functional urethral obstruction | Urethral muscular spasm, often associated with urethral inflammation or trauma |
| Anatomic outflow tract obstruction | Urethral stricture, neoplasia, cystic or urethral calculi, granulomatous urethritis, prostatic disease |
| **Small or Normal-Sized Bladder** | |
| Urethral sphincter mechanism incompetence | Deficient bladder/urethral support, hormone-responsive |
| Detrusor hyperreflexia or instability | Bladder irritation, urethral irritation |
| Congenital incontinence | Ectopic ureters, patent urachus, urethral fistula (rectal or vaginal), pseudohermaphroditism, vaginal strictures |

frequent causes of UMN bladder disorders. In an animal with a UMN lesion there is no voluntary control of micturition and the urethral sphincter shows reflex hyperexcitability, because the somatic efferents in the pudendal nerve are not inhibited, making it difficult to express the bladder. Even though this is a primary urine retention disorder, urinary incontinence occurs when the intravesical pressure exceeds the outflow resistance and urine leaks through the urethral sphincter. This is known as *paradoxic incontinence.*

Reflex dyssynergia, or detrusor-urethral dyssynergia, is seen primarily in larger-breed male dogs. The cause is usually difficult to determine but may include any of several neurologic lesions of the spinal cord or autonomic ganglia. Pathophysiologically, reflex dyssynergia results from the active contraction of the detrusor without relaxation of the internal or external urethral sphincters. Characteristic signs of reflex dyssynergia include normal or near-normal initiation of voiding, followed by a narrowed urine stream. Urine may be delivered in spurts, or flow may be completely disrupted and the dog will often strain to produce urine. After a while the dog will lower his leg and then often begins dribbling urine as he walks away. It is difficult to express urine from the bladder of a dog with reflex dyssynergia; however, urethral catheterization is usually easy. With reflex dyssynergia, increased outflow resistance occurs when the dog tries to initiate voiding. Recently, a type of functional urethral obstruction was described in three male dogs in which resting outflow resistance was increased (Lane, 2000). Prostatitis and a history of urethral calculi were associated with the func-

tional urethral obstruction in two cases, respectively; the third case was labeled as idiopathic.

Incontinence in an animal with a urinary outflow tract obstruction is called *paradoxic incontinence.* It occurs because, when intravesical pressure exceeds the pressure within the urethra, urine usually leaks past the obstruction before urethral or bladder rupture occurs. Clinical signs associated with a functional or anatomic urethral obstruction include dribbling of urine, straining to urinate without producing urine, restlessness, and abdominal pain. The most common causes of anatomic urethral obstruction are calculi and neoplasia in dogs, and struvite/mucous plugs in cats; however, urethral strictures and granulomatous urethritis can also create obstructions to urine flow. Any type of prostatic disease in dogs may produce an outflow tract obstruction. Older male dogs with benign prostatic hyperplasia may be evaluated because of stranguria and tenesmus; however, bacterial prostatitis, prostatic neoplasia, and prostatic abscesses are more likely causes of a urinary outflow tract obstruction.

## SMALL OR NORMAL-SIZED BLADDER

Causes of urinary incontinence associated with a small or normal-sized bladder include detrusor muscle hyperreflexia and/or instability, urethral sphincter mechanism incompetence (USMI), and congenital abnormalities. Recently, abnormal caudad bladder movement with the animal under anesthesia has been identified in bitches with USMI. This is thought to be due to deficient bladder and urethral support mechanism in these dogs. Estrogen and testosterone are believed to contribute to the integrity of urethral muscle tone by augmenting its responsiveness to α-adrenergic innervation. Thus middle-age to older, spayed, female dogs are prone to incontinence because of decreased estrogen concentrations. This incontinence is most pronounced when the animal is asleep or relaxed and often responds to estrogen replacement or α-adrenergic therapy. Less frequently, incontinence develops in male dogs after castration; the condition seems to occur most commonly in dogs castrated at an older age and often responds to α-adrenergic treatment or hormone replacement. Both processes are diagnosed on the basis of history, urinalysis (lack of evidence of lower urinary tract inflammation), physical examination findings, and the animal's response to therapy. Frequently, α-adrenergic treatment (e.g., phenylpropanolamine) may be combined with hormone replacement treatment in severe cases of USMI.

Detrusor muscle hyperreflexia and/or instability incontinence is the inability to control voiding owing to a strong urge to urinate. Inflammation of the bladder or urethra may trigger the voiding reflex by creating a sensation of bladder fullness. Clinical signs of this type of incontinence include pollakiuria, dysuria-stranguria, and, frequently, hematuria. A bacterial urinary tract infection is the most common cause in the dog, and sterile inflammation of the lower urinary tract is the most common cause in cats. Evidence of a urinary tract infection or inflammation revealed by urinalysis (e.g., bacteriuria, pyuria, or hematuria) initially supports the tentative diagnosis of urge or inflammatory incontinence. If clinical signs persist after appropriate treatment for the urinary tract inflammation has been initiated, further diagnostic studies, including ultrasonography, contrast-enhanced radiography, and cystoscopy, are indicated, because infiltrative disease of the bladder (e.g., neoplasia, chronic cystitis), polyps, uroliths, or urachal remnants can result in pollakiuria and stranguria. It should also be noted that detrusor hyperreflexia/instability may be a primary or idiopathic disorder that is not associated with bladder or urethral inflammation.

Urinary incontinence in a young animal may be associated with a variety of congenital defects of the urinary or genital systems. The most common defects are ectopic ureters and vaginal strictures, but patent urachus, urethrorectal and urethrovaginal fistulae, and female pseudohermaphroditism have also been associated with urinary incontinence. Ectopic ureters are most commonly observed in female dogs. Breeds in which the incidence of ectopic ureters is high include Siberian Huskies, Miniature and Toy Poodles, Labrador Retrievers, Fox Terriers, West Highland White Terriers, Collies, and Welsh Corgis. Ectopic ureters are rarely seen in cats, but the gender predisposition is reversed, with the prevalence higher in male than in female cats.

The most common clinical sign of ectopic ureters is constant dribbling of the urine, although dogs and cats with a unilateral ectopic ureter also may void normally. Because 70% of ectopic ureters in dogs terminate in the vagina, vaginoscopy may allow visualization of the opening of the ectopic ureter; however, the orifice may be difficult to see even if the vagina is fully distended with air. Intravenous urography and retrograde vaginourethrography are the diagnostic tests of choice for characterizing the defect. In contrast to the incontinence seen in animals with ectopic ureters, the incontinence associated with a vaginal stricture is often intermittent, occurring with changes in body position. Vaginal strictures can be diagnosed by digital vaginal examination, vaginoscopy, or contrast-enhanced vaginography.

## GERIATRIC INCONTINENCE

Incontinence may also be caused by cognitive disorders (CDs), decreased bladder capacity, or decreased mobility in geriatric animals. Polyuric-polydipsic disorders, such as chronic renal insufficiency or failure in geriatric animals, will also often exacerbate incontinence. Likewise, diuretic and corticosteroid use should be avoided, if possible, in incontinent animals because of their negative effects on urine-concentrating ability.

## *DIAGNOSIS*

Clinical features of disorders of micturition often help one discern the underlying problem. For example, if continuous urinary incontinence has been present from birth, the likely underlying problem is a congenital abnormality. Incontinence associated with hematuria, pollakiuria, and dysuria-stranguria usually indicates the presence of inflammation of the bladder or urethra or both. Inappropriate dribbling of urine during sleep or relaxation indicates USMI, and leakage of urine in female animals associated with postural changes may point to the pooling of urine behind a vaginal stricture. Dogs with pelvic bladders, which is a more caudal abdominal location in which the bladder neck is caudal to the pecten of the pubic bone (Fig. 48-2), can also have urethral sphincter incompetence that results in urinary incontinence. All these forms of incontinence are usually associated with a small or normal-sized bladder.

Dysuria and stranguria that occur in association with an abnormal or absent urine stream are typical of an obstructive uropathy. Urethral obstructions may be caused by anatomic (e.g., uroliths, tumors) or functional (e.g., reflex dyssynergia) problems. Urinary incontinence that occurs in association with trauma or pelvic surgery is usually neurogenic in origin (LMN disease); if paresis or paralysis is present, the lesion is usually above the fifth lumbar vertebral body and is a UMN lesion. Obstructive uropathies and UMN and LMN disorders result in large, distended bladders.

As noted earlier, incontinence in geriatric animals may be caused by CDs, a decreased bladder capacity, or decreased physical control. Physical problems in such animals, especially polyuric disorders and disabilities that impair mobility, should be identified and treated. Polyuria and polydipsia can trigger urge incontinence by placing continual stress on the bladder wall and urethral sphincter; however, in these cases the urine volume is large. A normally well-housebroken animal with polyuria and polydipsia may start urinating in the house if frequent access to the outdoors is not provided. If increased thirst and large urine volume are described by the

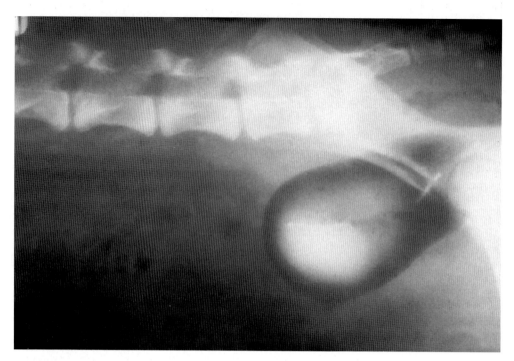

**FIG 48-2**
Double-contrast–enhanced cystogram showing a pelvic bladder in a 2-year-old spayed female Doberman Pinscher with urethral sphincter mechanism incompetence.

owner, appropriate diagnostic tests should be performed to identify conditions that cause polydipsia and polyuria (e.g., diabetes mellitus, pyometra, chronic renal insufficiency/ failure, hyperadrenocorticism, hypercalcemia).

Owners frequently mistake submissive urination, which may be a normal behavioral pattern of young dogs, with urinary incontinence. Other voiding patterns that are construed by some owners as incontinence are the urine marking used by male and occasionally female animals and inappropriate elimination behavior problems. The owner's description of the animal's voiding pattern may reveal a behavioral basis for the abnormal micturition, although a complete physical examination and a urinalysis should always be performed to identify or rule out a urinary tract disorder.

## INITIAL EVALUATION

The age of onset, sexual status of the animal, age at neutering, current medications, and history of trauma or previous urinary tract disorders are important anamnestic points to cover during the history-taking in an animal with any disorder of micturition. The physical examination should include evaluation of the perineum for evidence of urine scalding or staining. A thorough palpation of the bladder to assess its size and wall thickness and a rectal examination to assess anal tone, the prostate gland, the pelvic urethra, and the trigone region of the bladder should be performed in all cases. A digital vaginal examination is indicated, and vaginoscopy may be used to help identify congenital defects (e.g., vaginal strictures, ectopic ureters) in larger female dogs.

A neurologic examination should include evaluation of the perineal and bulbospongiosus reflexes. The perineal reflex causes the anal sphincter to contract and the tail to ventroflex in response to pinching the perineal skin. The bulbospongiosus reflex causes the anal sphincter to contract in response to gentle compression of the bulb of the penis or the vulva. Both these reflexes depend on an intact pudendal nerve (sensory and motor) and spinal cord segments S1 to S3. If both reflexes are normal, the pudendal reflex arc is intact. Because of their common origin, injury to the pudendal nerve may also affect the pelvic nerve.

Dogs should be walked outside so that the voiding posture and urine stream size and character can be observed. Immediately after the animal has attempted to void, the bladder should be palpated to determine the residual volume (normal residual volume is approximately 0.2 to 0.4 ml/kg). Catheterization is indicated to quantify the residual volume if a large bladder is palpable after voiding (in male dogs, however, behavioral urine marking can make assessment of residual urine volume difficult).

Urinalysis should be performed in all animals with urinary incontinence. If a urine culture is indicated, cystocentesis is the preferred method of collection; however, animals with a distended bladder should be catheterized instead to empty the bladder and to avoid the problem of urine leaking from the cystocentesis site.

## PHARMACOLOGIC TESTING

Frequently the diagnosis of disorders of micturition is based to some degree on the animal's response to pharmacologic testing or therapy. For example, detrusor hypocontractility should improve in response to a parasympathomimetic drug (e.g., bethanechol) and decreased urethral tone should respond to α-adrenergic agents (e.g., phenylpropanolamine) or to hormone replacement therapy. Increased urethral tone is treated with α-sympatholytics (e.g., phenoxybenzamine) and striated muscle relaxants (e.g., diazepam). Detrusor hypercontractility often responds to treatment of the underlying inflammatory process, such as bacterial cystitis or urolithiasis; however, smooth muscle antispasmodics (e.g., oxybutynin) and parasympatholytics (e.g., propantheline) may be useful in cases of severe inflammation.

## TREATMENT

### LOWER MOTOR NEURON DISORDERS

Animals with LMN diseases resulting from sacral spinal cord lesions or from dysautonomia require expression or strict aseptic catheterization of their bladder at least three times per day. Urinalysis or examination of the urine sediment should be performed weekly, and a urine bacterial culture should be performed if there is any evidence of a urinary tract infection. Care should be taken to prevent urine scalding by applying petroleum jelly to the perivulvar or peripreputial and abdominal skin. Bethanechol may be administered to increase detrusor contractility if the urethra is confirmed to be patent by bladder expression (see Drugs Used in Dogs and Cats with Urinary Tract Disorders, p. 657). Adverse effects of bethanechol include salivation, vomiting, diarrhea, or coliclike signs that indicate intestinal cramping. These signs are normally noticed within 1 hour of drug administration, and if they are observed, the dose of bethanechol should be decreased.

To manage detrusor atony the bladder must be expressed or urinary catheterization done intermittently to keep the bladder empty for a period of days to weeks. A closed urine-collection system should always be used with indwelling catheters. Urinalysis should be performed every 3 or 4 days and a urine bacterial culture and antibiotic sensitivity testing done if there is any evidence of urinary tract inflammation. Bethanechol may be administered to increase detrusor contractility but only after increased outflow resistance has been ruled out.

### UPPER MOTOR NEURON DISORDERS

The nature of the management of animals with a UMN lesion affecting the bladder depends on whether the animal has an autonomic bladder. A reflex or "autonomic" bladder often develops 5 to 10 days after a spinal cord injury, and it occurs because stretching of the bladder wall stimulates a local reflex arc that results in detrusor contraction. There is no cortical perception or voluntary control, and voiding is usually incomplete, resulting in a large urine residual volume. Treatment in an animal before an autonomic bladder develops should include aseptic catheterization three times per day. The use of corticosteroids for the treatment of neurologic disease may cause polyuria, necessitating more frequent catheterization to prevent overdistention of the bladder. Corticosteroids also predispose animals to urinary tract infections. During the initial stages of treatment, urinalysis or urine sediment examination should be performed every 3 or 4 days, and urine bacterial culture and antibiotic sensitivity testing should be performed if there is evidence of urinary tract inflammation (corticosteroids frequently mask signs of inflammation). Because these animals are usually in pain and reluctant to move, it is important to prevent urine scalding. The use of elevated racks or absorbent bedding is indicated, and petroleum jelly applied around the perineum or prepuce may minimize urine scalding.

After an autonomic bladder develops, the bladder should be palpated after urination to determine the residual urine volume. It may still be necessary to catheterize (express if possible) the bladder two or three times per day to minimize urine stasis. Urinalyses should continue to be done on a monthly schedule (weekly if the animal is receiving corticosteroids), and owners should be instructed to bring in a urine sample if a change in urine color or odor is noted. Nursing care to prevent urine scalding should be continued.

### REFLEX DYSSYNERGIA

Reflex dyssynergia often responds to pharmacologic management; however, a therapeutic response may not be seen for several days. Drugs commonly used include an α-blocker (e.g., prazosin or phenoxybenzamine), a somatic muscle relaxant (e.g., diazepam), and occasionally, bethanechol (see Drugs Used in Dogs and Cats with Urinary Tract Disorders at the end of this section). Intermittent urinary catheterization should be done as necessary to keep the bladder small and combat detrusor atony that may be caused by overdistention of the bladder.

Phenoxybenzamine has a slow onset of action, and the dose should be increased only at 3- to 4-day intervals. The urine stream should be evaluated to gauge drug effectiveness. If the stream is weak but continuous and of normal diameter, bethanechol may be used to increase detrusor contractility; however, it must not be used until the functional urethral obstruction has been relieved. If the urine stream is intermittent or narrowed, increased doses of diazepam or phenoxybenzamine or both are required (see Drugs Used in Dogs and Cats with Urinary Tract Disorders, p. 657). Because diazepam has a very short duration of action (approximately 1 to 2 hours when administered orally), administering it 30 minutes before walking the animal sometimes aids in the management of reflex dyssynergia. It may be several weeks before a correct combination of drugs is determined, however, and drug dosages may have to be modified over time. Periodic urinalyses are indicated to detect urinary tract inflammation or infection at an early stage.

Hypotension is the major adverse effect of phenoxybenzamine, and the dose should be decreased immediately if the animal shows any indication of lethargy, weakness, or disorientation. The dose should only be increased if a favorable response is not observed after 3 or 4 days; rapid dose changes should be avoided. Nausea is an adverse effect that can be minimized by administering the medication with a small meal. Glaucoma is a rare complication of phenoxybenzamine treatment in people; it is unknown if this occurs in dogs.

### FUNCTIONAL URETHRAL OBSTRUCTION

Nonneurogenic functional urethral obstruction, where resting as well as voiding urethral pressures are abnormally high, has been associated with prostatic disease; urinary tract infection; urethral muscular spasm; and urethral inflammation, hemorrhage, or edema in dogs and cats. Affected animals have clinical signs and histories similar to those in dogs with reflex dyssynergia. Resting urethral pressure profilometry is usually necessary to differentiate these two syndromes. When treatment of the underlying disorder fails to decrease the increased outflow resistance, α-blockers (e.g., prazosin or phenoxybenzamine) and skeletal muscle relaxants (e.g., diazepam) should be employed.

## URETHRAL SPHINCTER MECHANISM INCOMPETENCE

The treatment of urinary incontinence associated with decreased sphincter tone includes hormone replacement or α-adrenergic drugs or both (see Drugs Used in Dogs and Cats with Urinary Tract Disorders, p. 657). The usual induction therapy for estrogen-responsive incontinence consists of diethylstilbestrol (DES; 0.1 to 1.0 mg total PO q24h for 3 to 5 days). The frequency of administration is then decreased to the lowest possible one that will maintain continence. Some dogs can be successfully tapered to a very low maintenance schedule (e.g., 0.1 to 1.0 mg per dog every 7 to 10 days). Phenylpropanolamine (1.5 to 2.0 mg/kg PO q8h) may be used as an alternative drug or in addition to DES. Owners of dogs receiving phenylpropanolamine should be cautioned to observe their dog for hyperexcitability, panting, or anorexia and to decrease the dose if these signs develop. Although initially administered on a three times per day schedule, in some animals the dosing frequency of timed-release or precision-release phenylpropanolamine can be decreased to a once or twice daily schedule. Careful observation by the owner for recurrence of signs usually reveals when the dose needs to be increased. Dogs with increasing resistance to DES pose the greatest worry, because the development of estruslike signs and bone marrow toxicity are possible adverse effects of higher-dose DES therapy. Endocrine alopecia is another possible adverse effect. If DES-resistant dogs are not concurrently receiving phenylpropanolamine, a trial of it should be instituted before the DES dose exceeds recommended levels.

Urethral sphincter incompetence in neutered male dogs is best treated with α-adrenergic drugs. If testosterone is to be used, it should be parenterally administered, because most testosterone administered orally undergoes rapid hepatic degradation. Depository forms injected intramuscularly may be effective for 4 to 6 weeks. Male dogs receiving testosterone should have regular rectal examinations to evaluate prostate size. Testosterone should not be used in dogs that were previously neutered because of a testosterone-responsive disease (e.g., benign prostatic hypertrophy, perianal adenomas) or behavioral disorders (e.g., aggression).

## DETRUSOR HYPERREFLEXIA OR INSTABILITY

Smooth muscle relaxants and anticholinergics (e.g., dicyclomine, oxybutynin, propantheline bromide, imipramine, flavoxate) have been used to decrease inappropriate, involuntary detrusor contractions associated with lower urinary tract

inflammation, but their use should be reserved for those animals that do not respond to treatment of the primary disorder (e.g., antibiotics for bacterial urinary tract infections). Caution must be taken to avoid the use of phenazopyridine dyes commonly used as urinary analgesics in human patients (e.g., Azo-Gantrisin), because they have been associated with the development of Heinz body hemolysis and methemoglobinemia, especially in cats. Animals with chronic or recurrent cystitis require a thorough evaluation of the cause of the urinary tract infection (see Chapter 45). Antispasmodics may provide a small degree of relief; however, the identification and elimination of the underlying inflammatory disorder should be the priority. In cases where the detrusor hyperreflexia/instability is primary or idiopathic, anticholingeric agents may be beneficial.

## CONGENITAL DISORDERS

The correction of congenital defects depends on the nature and extent of the defect. For example, a patent urachus or urachal diverticulum is surgically correctable, as are many forms of ectopic ureters. However, urethral sphincter incompetence may occur in conjunction with an ectopic ureter, so that surgical reimplantation of the ureter does not guarantee continence. The use of α-adrenergic drugs after surgery increases the likelihood of success. Urethral pressure profilometry can be used to detect sphincter incompetence and measure the response to α-adrenergic drugs before surgery.

## ANATOMIC URETHRAL OBSTRUCTION

In animals with an anatomic urethral obstruction, the size and nature of the lesion can usually be determined by retrograde positive-contrast–enhanced urethrography. The prevention of renal damage secondary to urinary obstruction and the relief of urinary obstruction to prevent detrusor atony resulting from overdistention are the main priorities in dogs and cats with urine outflow tract obstructions. If the obstruction is created by a urethral urolith, retropulsion of the urolith into the bladder may be successful. If the urolith cannot be moved by retropulsion, a temporary or permanent perineal urethrostomy may be necessary.

In dogs with benign prostatic hyperplasia resulting in urethral obstruction, castration usually leads to a rapid decrease in the size of the prostate. The use of estrogens to decrease prostatic size is not recommended because of the potential for systemic adverse effects and squamous metaplasia of the prostate. Surgical drainage and marsupialization may be necessary to manage prostatic abscesses or prostatic cysts. In some cases of prostatic neoplasia, partial or complete prostatectomy may be beneficial; however, this surgery is difficult and frequently results in neurologic damage and urethral sphincter incompetence.

## *PROGNOSIS*

In general the prognosis for animals with neurogenic forms of urinary incontinence is poor. The long-term prognosis for animals with most types of spinal cord lesions is unfavorable, unless an intervertebral disk protrusion can be successfully decompressed or an extradural mass successfully removed or treated with chemotherapy or radiotherapy. Even if the spinal cord is decompressed, normal micturition may not completely return, because the central nervous system has a minimal capacity for regeneration. Damage to the pudendal nerve, pelvic nerve, or sacral nerve roots is associated with a more favorable prognosis, because peripheral nerves have a greater capacity to regenerate.

Long-term urinary care of paralyzed animals is necessary in most cases. Many owners can be taught to express the bladder, and some can learn to catheterize the urinary bladder. Although animals kept outdoors are easiest to manage, a modified diaper may be useful for indoor pets. Some owners cannot or will not deal with an incontinent animal; however, many owners will take the necessary steps to help their animal. Frequent urinalyses should be performed in these animals because of the high risk of urinary tract infections.

Most of the time, reflex dyssynergia responds to pharmacologic management, but occasionally the underlying disease worsens, making pharmacologic management ineffective. Drug doses should be reevaluated and increased if this happens, but this is not always successful. Diagnostic procedures such as myelography, an epidurography, computed tomography (CT), or magnetic resonance imaging (MRI) may be indicated in these refractory cases. Catheterization using aseptic techniques may be necessary for the long-term management of these animals.

Periodic urinalyses to identify or rule out urinary tract infections constitute an important aspect of follow-up care in an animal with any disorder of micturition. The frequency of the urinalyses depends on the nature of the disorder. Owners can be instructed to evaluate the color and odor of the urine and to bring in a urine sample immediately if they suspect an infection; however, routine monitoring is the cornerstone of the prevention of severe urinary tract infections.

In contrast to a dog with neurogenic urinary incontinence, the monitoring of a dog with USMI urinary incontinence requires less frequent urinalyses. The prognosis for animals with hormone-responsive urinary incontinence is usually excellent, although some dogs require multiple drugs for management.

Dogs treated for urge or inflammatory incontinence secondary to a urinary tract infection should undergo follow-up urinalysis or urine bacterial culture studies to confirm that the urinary tract infection has been eliminated. Long-term dietary management may help prevent recurrences in animals with urolithiasis- or struvite-associated feline lower urinary tract inflammation.

The prognosis for dogs and cats with trigonal or urethral neoplasia is usually poor. In most cases, urethral neoplasia is inoperable, because the clinical signs (dysuria, stranguria, hematuria, urethral obstruction) are usually not observed until the tumor is invasive. In contrast, most female dogs with granulomatous (chronic active) urethritis respond well to a combination of prednisolone, cyclophosphamide, and antibiotics.

## Suggested Readings

Adams WM et al: Radiographic and clinical features of pelvic bladder in the dog, *J Am Vet Med Assoc* 182:1212, 1983.

Arnold S et al: Urethral sphincter mechanism incompetence in male dogs. In Bonagura JD, editor: *Current veterinary therapy XIII*, Philadelphia, 2000, WB Saunders, p 896.

Atalan G et al: Ultrasonographic assessment of bladder neck mobility in continent bitches and bitches with urinary incontinence attributable to urethral sphincter mechanism incompetence, *Am J Vet Res* 53:673, 1998.

Holt PE: Feline urinary incontinence. In Bonagura JD, editor: *Current veterinary therapy XII*, Philadelphia, 1995, WB Saunders, p 1018.

Kyles AE et al: Vestibulovaginal stenosis in dogs: 18 cases (1987-1995), *J Am Vet Med Assoc* 209:1889, 1996.

Lane IF: Disorders of micturition. In Osborne CA et al, editors: *Canine and feline nephrology and urology*, Philadelphia, 1995, Williams & Wilkins, p 693.

Lane IF et al: Urinary incontinence and congenital urogenital anomalies in small animals. In Bonagura JD, editor: *Current veterinary therapy XII*, Philadelphia, 1995, WB Saunders, p 1022.

Lane IF et al: Functional urethral obstruction in 3 dogs: clinical and urethral pressure profile findings, *J Vet Intern Med* 14:43, 2000.

Lane IF: Urinary obstruction and functional urine retention. In Ettinger SJ et al, editors: *Textbook of veterinary internal medicine*, ed 5, Philadelphia, 2000a, WB Saunders, p 93.

Lane IF: Use of anticholinergic agents in lower urinary tract disease. In Bonagura JD, editor: *Current veterinary therapy XIII*, Philadelphia, 2000b, WB Saunders, p 899.

Lees GE: Incontinence, enuresis, dysuria, and nocturia. In Ettinger SJ et al, editors: *Textbook of veterinary internal medicine*, ed 5, Philadelphia, 2000, WB Saunders, p 89.

Moroff SD et al: Infiltrative urethral disease in female dogs: 41 cases (1980-1987), *J Am Vet Med Assoc* 199:247, 1991.

## Drugs Used in Dogs and Cats with Urinary Tract Disorders

| DRUG | TRADE NAME | ACTION | DOSE |
|---|---|---|---|
| Allopurinol | Zyloprim | Xanthine oxidase inhibitor | 10 mg/kg q8-24h PO (dog) |
| Aluminum carbonate, aluminum hydroxide | Basal gel, Amphojel | Enteric phosphate binders | 10-30 mg/kg q8h PO with or immediately after meals |
| Amitriptyline | Elavil | Anticholinergic effects, decreased histamine release from mast cells, increased bladder compliance | 5-10 mg q24h (evening) PO (cat) |

*Continued*

### Drugs Used in Dogs and Cats with Urinary Tract Disorders—cont'd

| DRUG | TRADE NAME | ACTION | DOSE |
|---|---|---|---|
| Amlodipine | Norvasc | Calcium antagonist | 2.5 mg q24h (dog); 0.625 mg q24h (cat) |
| Ammonium chloride | | Urinary acidifier | 100 mg/kg q12h PO (dog); 800 mg mixed with food daily (approximately ¼ tsp) (cat) |
| Aspirin | | Antiplatelet, antiinflammatory | 0.5-5 mg/kg q12h (dog); 0.5-5 mg/kg q24h (cat) |
| Azathioprine | Imuran | Immunosuppressant | 50 mg/m² PO q24h × 7 days, then q48h (dogs only) |
| Benazepril | Lotensin | Angiotensin-converting enzyme inhibitor | 0.25-0.5 mg/kg PO q24h |
| Bethanechol | Urecholine | Cholinergic (increases detrusor contractility) | 5-15 mg q8h PO (dog); 1.25-5 mg q8h PO (cat) |
| Chlorpromazine | Thorazine | Antiemetic | 0.25-0.5 mg/kg q6-8h IM, SQ, PO (after rehydration only) |
| Cimetidine | Tagamet | H₂ blocker | 2.5-5.0 mg/kg q12h PO, IV, IM |
| Cyclophosphamide | Cytoxan, Neosar | Immunosuppressant | 50 mg/m² PO q48h (dogs); 200-300 mg/m² PO q3wk (cats) |
| Cyclosporine | Neoral, Sandimmune | Immunosuppressant | 10 mg/kg q12-24h, adjust dose via monitoring |
| Diazepam | Valium | Skeletal muscle relaxant | 2-5 mg q8h PO |
| Dicyclomine | Bentyl, Bentylol | Antispasmodic, antimuscarinic | 10 mg PO q6-8h (dog) |
| Diethylstilbestrol (DES) | | Increased urethral sphincter tone | 0.1-1.0 mg q24h PO for 3-5 days and then same dose q3-7days (dog); 0.05-0.1 mg q24h PO q3-5days and then same dose q3-7days (cat) |
| 1,25-Dihydroxychole-calciferol, calcitriol | Rocaltrol | Active vitamin D₃, decreases parathyroid hormone | 1.5-3.5 ng/kg q24h PO |
| Dopamine | Intropin | Renal vasodilator | 2-10 µg/kg/min IV |
| Enalapril | Enacard | Angiotensin-converting enzyme inhibitor | 0.5 mg/kg q12-24h PO (dog); 0.25-0.5 mg/kg q12h PO (cat) |
| Ephedrine | | α-Adrenergic, increases urethral sphincter tone | 12.5-50 mg q8-12h PO (dog); 2-4 mg/kg q8-12h PO (cat) |
| Erythropoietin (r-Hu-EPO), epoetin alfa | Epogen | Stimulate erythrogenesis | 35-50 U/kg IV, SQ 3 times/wk or 400 U/kg IV, SQ weekly; adjust dose to PCV of 30%-35% |

*PCV,* Packed cell volume.

## Drugs Used in Dogs and Cats with Urinary Tract Disorders—cont'd

| DRUG | TRADE NAME | ACTION | DOSE |
|------|-----------|--------|------|
| Famotidine | Pepcid | $H_2$ blocker | 0.5 mg/kg IM, SQ, PO q12-24h |
| Flavoxate | Urispas | Muscle relaxant | 100-200 mg q6-8h |
| Furosemide | Lasix | Loop diuretic | 2-4 mg/kg q8-12h IV, PO |
| Hydralazine | Apresoline | Arterial vasodilator | 0.5-2.0 mg/kg q12h PO (dog); 2.5 mg q24h-q12h PO (cat) |
| Imipramine | Tofranil | Antimuscarinic, adrenergic agonist, muscle relaxant | 5-15 mg PO q12h (dog); 2.5-5 mg PO q12h (cat) |
| Lisinopril | Prinivil, Zestril | Angiotensin-converting enzyme inhibitor | 0.5 mg/kg PO q24h (dog) |
| Mannitol | Osmitrol | Osmotic diuretic | 0.5-1.0 g/kg as 20%-25% solution, slow IV bolus over 5-10 min |
| N-(2-mercaptopropionyl)-glycine | | Disulfide bond formation with cysteine | 10-15 mg/kg q12h PO (dog) |
| Metoclopramide | Reglan | Antiemetic | 0.2-0.5 mg/kg q8h PO, SQ |
| Nandrolone decanoate | Deca-Durabolin | Anabolic steroid | 1.0-1.5 mg/kg weekly IM (dog); 1.0 mg weekly IM (cat) |
| Oxybutynin | Ditropan | Direct antispasmodic effect on smooth muscle | 0.2-0.5 mg/kg q8-12h PO (dog) |
| D-Penicillamine | Cuprimine | Disulfide bond formation with cysteine | 10-15 mg/kg q12h PO (dog) |
| Phenoxybenzamine | Dibenzyline | α-Blocker, decreases urethral sphincter tone | 0.2-0.5 mg/kg q24h PO (dog); 0.5 mg/kg q24h PO (cat) |
| Phenylpropanolamine | Propagest | α-Adrenergic, increases urethral sphincter tone | 1.5-2.0 mg/kg q8-12h PO |
| Prazosin | Minipress | α-Blocker | 1 mg/15 kg PO q6-8h |
| Propantheline bromide | Pro-Banthine | Anticholinergic, decreases detrusor contractility | 0.25-0.5 mg/kg q8-12h PO |
| Racemethionine | Uroeze, Methio-Form | Urinary acidifier | 150-300 mg/kg/day PO (dog); 1.0-1.5 g/day PO (cat) |
| Ranitidine | Zantac | $H_2$ blocker | 2.0 mg/kg q8h PO, IV (dog); 2.5 mg/kg q12h IV, 3.5 mg/kg q12h PO (cat) |
| Testosterone cypionate | Andro-Cyp | Increased urethral sphincter tone | 1.0-2.2 mg/kg q30days IM (dog) |
| Trimethobenzamide | Tigan | Antiemetic | 3.0 mg/kg q8h PO, IM (dog) |

C H A P T E R **49**

# Disorders
# of the Hypothalamus
# and Pituitary Gland

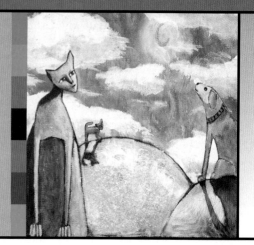

## CHAPTER OUTLINE

POLYURIA AND POLYDIPSIA, 660
DIABETES INSIPIDUS, 661
PRIMARY (PSYCHOGENIC) POLYDIPSIA, 667
ENDOCRINE ALOPECIA, 667
GROWTH HORMONE–RESPONSIVE DERMATOSIS
IN THE ADULT DOG, 670
FELINE ACROMEGALY, 673
PITUITARY DWARFISM, 677

## POLYURIA AND POLYDIPSIA

Water consumption and urine production are controlled by complex interactions among plasma osmolality and volume, the thirst center, the kidney, the pituitary gland, and the hypothalamus. Dysfunction in any of these areas results in the clinical signs of polyuria (PU) and polydipsia (PD). In dogs and cats, normal water intake varies from 20 to 70 ml/kg/day, and normal urine output varies between 20 and 45 ml/kg/day. PD and PU in the dog and cat have been defined as water consumption greater than 100 ml/kg/day and urine production greater than 50 ml/kg/day, respectively. It is possible, however, for thirst and urine production to be abnormal within the limits of these normal values in individual dogs and cats. PU and PD usually exist concurrently, and determining the primary component of the syndrome is one of the initial diagnostic considerations in an animal with PU/PD.

A variety of metabolic disturbances can cause PU/PD (see Table 41-5, p. 577). Primary polyuric disorders can be classified on the basis of the underlying pathophysiology into primary pituitary and nephrogenic diabetes insipidus; secondary nephrogenic diabetes insipidus, resulting from interference with the normal interaction of arginine vasopressin (AVP) and renal tubular AVP receptors, with the generation of intracellular cyclic adenosine monophosphate, or with renal tubular cell function or resulting from the loss of the renal medullary

interstitial concentration gradient; osmotic diuresis–induced PU and PD; and interference with the hypothalamic-pituitary secretion of AVP. Primary polydipsic disorders resulting from a defect in the thirst center have not been reported in dogs or cats, although an abnormal vasopressin response to hypertonic saline infusion has been reported in dogs with suspected primary polydipsia. A psychogenic or behavioral basis for compulsive water consumption does occur in dogs and is called *psychogenic polydipsia*. A complete discussion of the diagnostic approach to PU/PD is presented on p. 577. An index of suspicion for most of the endocrinopathies that cause PU/PD can be raised after a review of the history and physical examination findings, as well as a review of the initial database (i.e., complete blood count [CBC], serum biochemistry panel, and urinalysis). Specific tests may be necessary to confirm the diagnosis (Table 49-1). See the appropriate chapters in this section for a more complete discussion of the diagnosis and therapy of each of these endocrinopathies.

Occasionally the physical examination findings and initial database are normal in the dog or cat with PU and PD. Possible diagnoses in these dogs and cats then include diabetes insipidus, psychogenic water consumption, unusual hyperadrenocorticism, uncommon renal insufficiency without azotemia, and possibly mild hepatic insufficiency. Hyperadrenocorticism, renal insufficiency, and hepatic insufficiency should be ruled out before performing tests for diabetes insipidus or psychogenic polydipsia. Diagnostic tests to consider include tests of the pituitary-adrenocortical axis, liver function tests (e.g., measurement of preprandial and postprandial bile acid levels), determination of the urine protein/creatinine (P/C) ratio, abdominal ultrasonography, and, if indicated, renal biopsy.

Urine specific gravity varies widely among healthy dogs and, in some dogs, can range from 1.006 to greater than 1.040 within a 24-hour period. Wide fluctuations in urine specific gravity have not been reported in healthy cats. To assess the fluctuation in urine specific gravity in a dog or cat with suspected PU and PD, this author prefers to have the owner collect several urine samples at different times of the day for 2 to

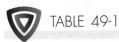 TABLE 49-1

Endocrine Disorders Causing Polyuria and Polydipsia in the Dog and Cat

| DISORDER | TESTS TO ESTABLISH THE DIAGNOSIS |
|---|---|
| Diabetes mellitus | Fasting blood glucose, urinalysis |
| Hyperadrenocorticism | ACTH stimulation test, low-dose dexamethasone suppression test |
| Hypoadrenocorticism | Blood electrolytes, ACTH stimulation test |
| Primary hyperparathyroidism | Blood calcium/phosphorus, serum PTH concentration, surgical exploration |
| Hyperthyroidism | Serum thyroxine concentration |
| Diabetes insipidus | Modified water deprivation test, response to dDAVP therapy |
|    Pituitary | |
|    Nephrogenic | |
| Acromegaly | Baseline growth hormone concentration, CT or MR scan |
| Primary hyperaldosteronism | Blood electrolytes, ACTH stimulation test–measure aldosterone |

*ACTH,* Adrenocorticotropic hormone; *PTH,* parathyroid hormone; *CT,* computed tomographic; *MR,* magnetic resonance.

 TABLE 49-2

Results of Urinalysis in Dogs with Selected Disorders Causing Polyuria and Polydipsia

| DISORDER | NO. OF DOGS | URINE SPECIFIC GRAVITY MEAN | URINE SPECIFIC GRAVITY RANGE | PROTEINURIA (%) | WBC (>5/HPF) (%) | BACTERIURIA (%) |
|---|---|---|---|---|---|---|
| Central diabetes insipidus | 20 | 1.005 | 1.001-1.012 | 5 | 0 | 0 |
| Psychogenic polydipsia | 18 | 1.011 | 1.003-1.023 | 0 | 0 | 0 |
| Hyperadrenocorticism | 20 | 1.012 | 1.001-1.027 | 48 | 0 | 12 |
| Renal insufficiency | 20 | 1.011 | 1.008-1.016 | 90 | 25 | 15 |
| Pyelonephritis | 20 | 1.019 | 1.007-1.045 | 70 | 75 | 80 |

*WBC,* White blood cells; *HPF,* high-power field.

3 days, storing the urine samples in the refrigerator until they can be brought to the veterinary hospital for determination of urine specific gravity. Critical evaluation of urine specific gravity measured from several urine samples obtained by the owner may provide clues to the underlying disorder (Table 49-2). For example, if the urine specific gravity is consistently in the isosthenuric range (1.008 to 1.015), renal insufficiency should be considered the primary differential diagnosis, especially if the blood urea nitrogen and serum creatinine concentration are high normal or increased (i.e., 25 mg/dl or more and 1.8 mg/dl or more, respectively). The presence of proteinuria, as determined by the urine P/C ratio, provides additional evidence for renal insufficiency. Isosthenuria is relatively common in dogs with hyperadrenocorticism, psychogenic water consumption, hepatic insufficiency, pyelonephritis, and partial diabetes insipidus with concurrent water restriction, but urine specific gravities above (e.g., pyelonephritis, psychogenic water consumption) or below (e.g., hyperadrenocorticism, partial diabetes insipidus) the isosthenuric range also occur with these disorders. If urine specific gravities less than 1.005 (i.e., hyposthenuric) are identified, renal insufficiency and pyelonephritis are ruled out and diabetes in-

sipidus, psychogenic water consumption, and hyperadrenocorticism should be considered.

The diagnosis of diabetes insipidus and psychogenic water consumption should be based on the results of the modified water deprivation test (see p. 663), the plasma osmolality, and the response to synthetic vasopressin therapy (see diagnosis of diabetes insipidus, below). Ideally, all realistic causes of secondary acquired nephrogenic diabetes insipidus should be ruled out before performing tests (especially the modified water deprivation test) for primary pituitary and nephrogenic diabetes insipidus and psychogenic polydipsia. Performing the recommended initial laboratory studies ensures that the veterinarian is pursuing a correct diagnosis and identifies the existence of concomitant medical problems.

## *DIABETES INSIPIDUS*

### Etiology

AVP plays a key role in the control of renal water resorption, urine production and concentration, and water balance. AVP is produced in the supraoptic and paraventricular nuclei of the hypothalamus, is stored in and secreted from the posterior pituitary gland, and interacts with distal tubular and collecting duct cells of the kidney to promote water resorption and the formation of concentrated urine. The defective synthesis or secretion of AVP or an inability of the renal tubules to respond to AVP causes diabetes insipidus.

**Central diabetes insipidus.** Central diabetes insipidus (CDI) is a polyuric syndrome that results from an insufficient secretion of AVP to concentrate the urine for water conservation. This deficiency may be absolute or partial. An absolute deficiency of AVP causes persistent hyposthenuria and severe diuresis. The urine specific gravity in dogs and cats with CDI usually remains hyposthenuric (i.e., 1.005 or less), even in those with severe dehydration. A partial deficiency of AVP, referred to as partial CDI, also causes persistent hyposthenuria and a marked diuresis as long as the dog or cat has unlimited access to water. During periods of water restriction, the urine specific gravity can increase into the isosthenuric range (i.e., 1.008 to 1.015), but typically the urine cannot be concentrated to more than 1.015 to 1.020 even when the animal is severely dehydrated. In any dog or cat with partial CDI, the maximum urine-concentrating ability during dehydration is inversely related to the severity of the deficiency in AVP secretion; that is, the more severe the AVP deficiency, the less concentrated the urine specific gravity during dehydration.

CDI may result from any condition that damages the neurohypophyseal system (Table 49-3). Idiopathic CDI is the most common form, appearing at any age, in any breed, and affecting animals of either sex. Necropsies performed in dogs and cats with idiopathic CDI usually fail to identify an underlying reason for the AVP deficiency. Although CDI is well documented in kittens and puppies, a hereditary form of CDI has not yet been documented. The most common identifiable causes of CDI in dogs and cats are head trauma (accidental or neurosurgical), neoplasia, and hypothalamic-pituitary malformations (e.g., cystic structures). Head trauma may cause a transient or permanent CDI, depending on the viability of the cells in the supraoptic and paraventricular nuclei. Trauma-induced transection of the pituitary stalk often results in a transient CDI, usually lasting 1 to 3 weeks.

Primary intracranial tumors that are associated with diabetes insipidus in dogs and cats include craniopharyngioma, pituitary chromophobe adenoma, and pituitary chromophobe adenocarcinoma. Metastatic tumors in the hypothalamus and pituitary can also cause CDI. Metastatic mammary carcinoma, lymphoma, malignant melanoma, and pancreatic carcinoma have been reported to cause CDI in dogs through their presence in the pituitary gland or hypothalamus. Metastatic neoplasia has not yet been reported to be a cause of CDI in cats.

**Nephrogenic diabetes insipidus.** Nephrogenic diabetes insipidus (NDI) is a polyuric disorder that results from an impaired responsiveness of the nephron to AVP. Plasma AVP concentrations are normal or increased in animals with this disorder. NDI is classified as either primary (familial) or secondary (acquired). Primary or familial NDI is a rare congenital disorder in dogs and cats, with only a few reports of congenital (primary) NDI in dogs in the literature. The etiology of primary NDI in dogs and cats in unknown. Familial NDI has been reported in a family of Huskies. Affected puppies possessed normal numbers of AVP receptors in the renal medulla, but the receptors had a tenfold-lower binding affinity for AVP compared with that in normal dogs. Affected dogs also showed antidiuretic responses to high doses of synthetic vasopressin (desmopressin [dDAVP]), consistent with their possessing AVP receptors with a lower binding affinity.

The most common form of diabetes insipidus is acquired secondary NDI. This form includes a variety of renal and metabolic disorders in which the renal tubules lose the ability to adequately respond to AVP (see p. 577). Most of these acquired forms are potentially reversible after elimination of the underlying illness.

## Clinical Features

**Signalment.** There is no apparent breed-, sex-, or age-related predilection for CDI. In one study, the age at the time of the diagnosis of CDI in dogs ranged from 7 weeks to 14 years, with a median of 5 years. Similarly, most cats with CDI are domestic short- and long-haired cats, although the disorder has also been documented in Persians and Abyssinians. The age at the time of diagnosis of CDI in cats ranged from 8 weeks to 6 years, with a mean of 1.5 years. Primary NDI has been identified only in puppies, kittens, and young adult dogs and cats less than 18 months of age. The clinical signs have been present since the owners acquired these pets.

**Clinical signs.** PU and PD are the hallmark signs of diabetes insipidus and are typically the only signs seen in dogs and cats with congenital and idiopathic CDI and in those with primary NDI. Affected animals may appear incontinent to their owners because of the frequency of urination and loss of normal housebroken behavior. Owners of cats with diabetes insipidus often complain of changing the kitty litter more frequently than expected. Additional clinical signs may

### TABLE 49-3

**Recognized Causes of Diabetes Insipidus in Dogs and Cats**

| CENTRAL DIABETES INSIPIDUS | NEPHROGENIC DIABETES INSIPIDUS |
|---|---|
| Idiopathic | Primary idiopathic |
| Traumatic | Primary familial (Huskies) |
| Neoplasia | Secondary acquired (see Table 41-5, p. 577) |
|    Craniopharyngioma | |
|    Chromophobe adenoma | |
|    Chromophobe adenocarcinoma | |
|    Metastasis | |
| Pituitary malformation | |
| Cysts | |
| Inflammation | |
| Familial (?) | |

be found in dogs and cats with secondary causes of diabetes insipidus. The most worrisome are neurologic signs, which may indicate the presence of an expanding hypothalamic or pituitary tumor in the dog or cat with diabetes insipidus that has not had head trauma.

**Physical examination.** The physical examination findings are usually unremarkable in animals with CDI, although some dogs and cats are thin, presumably because the pet's strong desire for water overrides its normal appetite. As long as access to water is not restricted, the animal's hydration status, mucous membrane color, and capillary refill time remain normal. The presence of neurologic abnormalities is variable in dogs and cats with either trauma-induced CDI or neoplastic destruction of the hypothalamus or pituitary gland. Physical examination reveals no perceptible neurologic alterations in many of these animals, whereas others show mild-to-severe neurologic signs, including stupor, disorientation, ataxia, circling, pacing, and convulsions. Severe hypernatremia may also cause neurologic signs in the traumatized dog or cat with undiagnosed CDI given inadequate fluid therapy (see p. 828). Persistent hypernatremia and hyposthenuria in a traumatized dog or cat should raise the clinical suspicion of diabetes insipidus.

## Diagnosis

In the dog or cat with suspected CDI or primary NDI, the diagnostic workup should initially rule out causes of acquired secondary NDI (see p. 577). Recommended initial diagnostic studies include a CBC, biochemistry panel, urinalysis with bacterial culture, abdominal ultrasonography or radiography, and an adrenocorticotropic hormone (ACTH) stimulation test. The results of these screening tests are usually normal in dogs and cats with CDI, primary NDI, and psychogenic water consumption, although a low-normal serum urea nitrogen concentration (5 to 10 mg/dl) may be found. Random urine specific gravity is usually less than 1.006, and is often as low as 1.001 if the dog or cat has unlimited access to water. The urine osmolality is less than 300 mOsm/kg. A urine specific gravity in the isosthenuric range (i.e., 1.008 to 1.012) does not rule out diabetes insipidus (Fig. 49-1), especially if the urine has been obtained after water is knowingly or inadvertently (e.g., a long car ride and wait in the veterinary office) withheld. The urine of dogs and cats with partial diabetes insipidus can be concentrated into the isosthenuric range if they are dehydrated. Erythrocytosis (packed cell volume of 50% to 60%), hyperproteinemia, hypernatremia, and azotemia may be found in animals if their access to water has been restricted.

Diagnostic tests to confirm and differentiate among CDI, primary NDI, and psychogenic water consumption include the modified water deprivation test, random plasma osmolality determination, and the response to AVP supplementation. The results of these tests can be interpreted only after the causes for acquired secondary NDI have been ruled out.

**Modified water deprivation test.** The modified water deprivation test is considered the best diagnostic test for differentiating among the primary causes of PU and PD. The technique, interpretation, contraindications, and complications of the test are described in Chapter 42 (see p. 587). The test consists of two phases. In phase I, the AVP secretory capabilities and renal distal and collecting tubule responsiveness to AVP are evaluated by assessing the effects of dehydration (i.e., water restriction until the animal loses 3% to 5% of its body weight) on urine specific gravity. The normal dog and cat, as well as those with psychogenic water consumption, should be able to concentrate urine to greater than 1.030

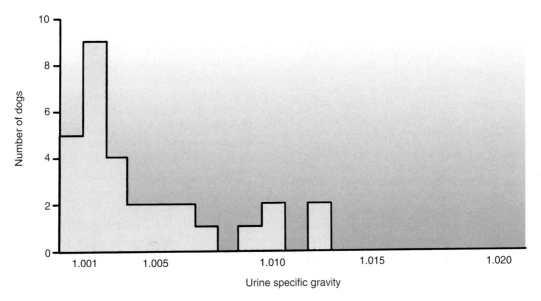

**FIG 49-1**
Urine specific gravity measured in 30 dogs with central diabetes insipidus at the time of initial presentation to the veterinarian. (From Feldman EC, Nelson RW: *Canine and feline endocrinology and reproduction*, ed 2, Philadelphia, 1996, WB Saunders.)

TABLE 49-4

Guidelines for Interpretation of the Water Deprivation Test

| | URINE SPECIFIC GRAVITY | | | TIME TO 5% DEHYDRATION | |
| DISORDER | INITIALLY | 5% DEHYDRATION | POST ADH | MEAN (hr) | RANGE (hr) |
|---|---|---|---|---|---|
| Central DI | | | | | |
|    Complete | <1.006 | <1.006 | >1.008 | 4 | 3-7 |
|    Partial | <1.006 | 1.008-1.020 | >1.015 | 8 | 6-11 |
| Primary nephrogenic DI | <1.006 | <1.006 | <1.006 | 5 | 3-9 |
| Primary polydipsia | 1.002-1.020 | >1.030 | NA | 13 | 8-20 |

*ADH,* Antidiuretic hormone; *DI,* diabetes insipidus; *NA,* not applicable.

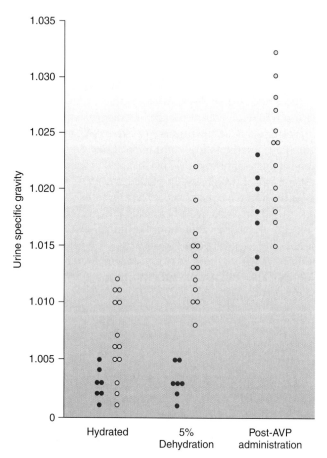

**FIG 49-2**
Urine specific gravity in 7 dogs with complete central diabetes insipidus (red circle) and 13 dogs with partial central diabetes insipidus (yellow circle) at the beginning (hydrated) end of phase I (5% hydrated) and end of phase II (post-AVP administration) of the modified water deprivation test. (From Feldman EC, Nelson RW: *Canine and feline endocrinology and reproduction,* ed 2, Philadelphia, 1996, WB Saunders.)

(1.035 in the cat) if dehydrated. Dogs and cats with partial and complete CDI and primary NDI have an impaired ability to concentrate urine in the face of dehydration (Table 49-4 and Fig. 49-2). The time required to attain 3% to 5% dehydration can sometimes be helpful in establishing the diag-

nosis. It often takes less than 6 hours for dogs and cats with complete CDI to attain 3% to 5% dehydration, whereas it often takes more than 8 to 10 hours for dogs and cats with partial CDI and especially those with psychogenic water consumption to attain 3% to 5% dehydration.

Phase II of the water deprivation test is indicated for dogs and cats that do not concentrate urine to greater than 1.030 during phase I of the test. Phase II determines the effect, if any, that exogenous AVP has on the renal tubular ability to concentrate urine in the face of dehydration (see Fig. 49-2). This phase differentiates impaired AVP secretion from impaired renal tubular responsiveness to AVP (see Table 49-4).

**Response to desmopressin (dDAVP).** An alternative approach to establishing the diagnosis is to evaluate the animal's response to trial therapy with dDAVP (desmopressin acetate, Aventis Pharmaceuticals, Parsippany, N.J.). One-half to one 0.1 mg or 0.2 mg dDAVP tablet is administered orally every 8 hours, or 1 to 4 drops of dDAVP nasal spray is administered from an eye dropper into the conjunctival sac every 12 hours for 5 to 7 days. Owners should notice a decrease in PU and PD by the end of the treatment period if the PU and PD are caused by CDI. Urine specific gravity should be measured on several urine samples collected by the owner on the last couple of days of trial therapy. An increase in urine specific gravity by 50% or more, compared with pretreatment specific gravities, supports the diagnosis of CDI, especially if the urine specific gravity exceeds 1.030. There should be only minimal improvement in dogs and cats with primary NDI, although a response may be observed with very high doses of dDAVP. Dogs and cats with psychogenic water consumption may exhibit a mild decline in urine output and water intake because the chronically low serum osmolality tends to depress AVP production.

This approach to diagnosis requires that all other causes of PU and PD, except CDI, primary NDI, and psychogenic PD, be previously ruled out. Tests for hyperadrenocorticism should always be evaluated before trial therapy with dDAVP is considered. Hyperadrenocorticism mimics partial CDI, in part because of suppression of vasopressin secretion with hyperadrenocorticism. Dogs with hyperadrenocorticism typically have a positive, albeit moderate, response to dDAVP treatment, which can result in a misdiagnosis of partial CDI

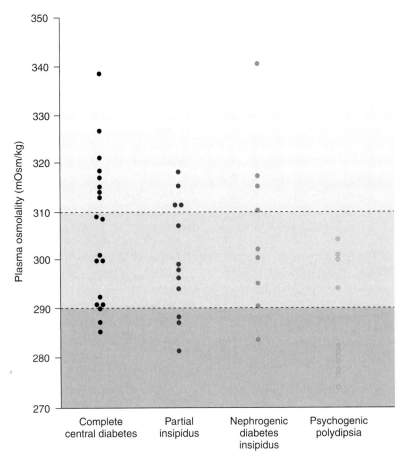

**FIG 49-3**
Random plasma osmolality in 19 dogs with complete central diabetes insipidus, 12 dogs with partial central diabetes insipidus, 9 dogs with primary nephrogenic diabetes insipidus, and 11 dogs with primary (psychogenic) polydipsia. Note the overlap in values between groups of dogs. *Dashed lines,* Upper and lower limits for normal plasma osmolality. (From Feldman EC, Nelson RW: *Canine and feline endocrinology and reproduction,* ed 2, Philadelphia, 1996, WB Saunders.)

as the cause of PU and PD. Unlike partial CDI, the beneficial response to dDAVP wanes over the ensuing weeks in dogs with hyperadrenocorticism.

The effect of dDAVP should not be critically evaluated until after 5 to 7 days of therapy, because renal medullary solute washout may prevent a dog or cat with CDI from forming concentrated urine in response to only one or two administrations. Although less time-consuming than the water deprivation test, the expense is often comparable, in part because of the cost of the dDAVP. In addition, the modified water deprivation test may still have to be performed if ambiguous results are obtained using this simpler approach.

**Random plasma osmolality.** Measurement of the random plasma osmolality may help in the diagnosis of primary or psychogenic PD. The plasma osmolality in normal dogs and cats is approximately 280 to 310 mOsm/kg. Diabetes insipidus is a primary polyuric disorder, with the compensatory PD preventing severe hyperosmolality, whereas psychogenic PD is a primary polydipsic disorder, with the compensatory PU preventing hyposmolality and water intoxication. In theory, the finding of high normal–to-high (i.e., 300 to 320 mOsm/kg)

random plasma osmolality in the dog or cat with unlimited access to water indicates the animal has diabetes insipidus, and the finding of low normal–to-low (i.e., 275 to 280 mOsm/kg) random plasma osmolality indicates the animal has psychogenic water consumption. Unfortunately, there is considerable overlap in the random plasma osmolality in animals with these disorders (Fig. 49-3). Based on our experience, a random plasma osmolality of less than 280 mOsm/kg obtained while the dog or cat has free access to water suggests the presence of psychogenic PD, whereas a plasma osmolality greater than 280 mOsm/kg is consistent with CDI, NDI, or psychogenic PD.

**Additional diagnostic tests.** Further diagnostic tests may be warranted when CDI or primary NDI is diagnosed in older dogs or cats. Pituitary or hypothalamic neoplasia should be considered in the older dog or cat in which CDI develops. A complete neurologic evaluation (e.g., cerebrospinal fluid evaluation, computed tomographic [CT] or magnetic resonance [MR] scan) may be warranted before idiopathic CDI is arbitrarily diagnosed, especially if the owner is willing to consider radiotherapy or chemotherapy should a tumor be identified. Similarly, a more complete evaluation of the kidney (e.g., abdominal ultrasound, renal biopsy) may be warranted in the older dog or cat tentatively considered to have primary NDI.

## Treatment

Therapeutic options for dogs and cats with diabetes insipidus are listed in Table 49-5. The synthetic analog of vasopressin, dDAVP, is the standard therapy for CDI. dDAVP has almost three times the antidiuretic action of AVP, with minimal-to-no vasopressor or oxytocic activity. The intranasal dDAVP

## TABLE 49-5

**Therapies Available for Polydipsic/Polyuric Dogs with Central Diabetes Insipidus, Nephrogenic Diabetes Insipidus, or Primary (Psychogenic) Polydipsia**

A. Central diabetes insipidus (severe)
  1. dDAVP (desmopressin acetate)
    a. Effective
    b. Expensive
    c. May require drops in conjunctival sac if oral form is ineffective
  2. LVP (lypressin [Diapid])
    a. Short duration of action; less potent than dDAVP
    b. Expensive
    c. Requires drops in nose or conjunctival sac
  3. No treatment—provide continuous source of water
B. Central diabetes insipidus (partial)
  1. dDAVP
  2. LVP
  3. Chlorpropamide
    a. 30%-70% effective
    b. Inexpensive
    c. Pill form
    d. Takes 1-2 weeks to obtain effect of drug
    e. May cause hypoglycemia
  4. Clofibrate—untested in veterinary medicine
  5. Thiazides
    a. Mildly effective
    b. Inexpensive
    c. Pill form
    d. Should be used with low-sodium diet
  6. Low-sodium diet
  7. No treatment—provide continuous source of water
C. Nephrogenic diabetes insipidus
  1. Thiazides—as above
  2. Low-sodium diet
  3. No treatment—provide continuous source of water
D. Primary (psychogenic) polydipsia
  1. Water restriction at times
  2. Water limitation
  3. Behavior modification
    a. Exercise
    b. Another pet
    c. Larger living environment

preparation (DDAVP nasal drops, 2.5 and 5.0 ml bottles containing 100 μg dDAVP/ml) is used most commonly for treating CDI in dogs and cats. Administration of medication to animals via the intranasal route is possible but not recommended. The dDAVP nasal preparation may be transferred to a sterile eye dropper bottle and drops placed into the conjunctival sac of the dog or cat. Although the solution is acidic, ocular irritation rarely occurs. One drop of dDAVP contains 1.5 to 4 μg of dDAVP, and a dosage of one to four drops administered once or twice daily appears sufficient to control signs of CDI in most animals.

Oral dDAVP (DDAVP tablets, 0.1 and 0.2 mg) can be used to treat CDI in dogs and presumably cats, although the response may be variable. The bioavailability of oral dDAVP is approximately 5% to 15% of the intranasal dose in humans. The initial oral dDAVP dose in dogs is 0.1 mg given three times a day. The dose is gradually increased to effect if unacceptable PU and PD persist 1 week after therapy is initiated. A decrease in frequency of administration to twice a day can be tried once clinical response has been documented. To date, dogs have required 0.1 to 0.2 mg of DDAVP two to three times a day to control polyuria and polydipsia. The use of oral dDAVP for treating CDI in cats has not been reported.

dDAVP for parenteral (SC) administration (dDAVP injection, 1 and 2 ml ampules containing 15 μg dDAVP/ml and 1 and 10 ml ampules containing 4 μg dDAVP/ml) can be used in lieu of eye drops or oral tablets. The initial parenteral dosage of dDAVP is 0.5 to 2 μg given subcutaneously once or twice daily. Because of cost differences between the parenteral and nasal preparations, the intranasal form of dDAVP, although not designed for parenteral use, has been given to dogs and cats by injection with no apparent adverse reactions. However, the intranasal form of dDAVP is not sterile, therefore the solution should be passed through a bacteriostatic filter before administration.

The maximal effect of dDAVP, regardless of the route of administration, occurs from 2 to 8 hours after administration, and the duration of action varies from 8 to 24 hours. Larger doses of dDAVP appear to both increase its antidiuretic effects and prolong its duration of action; however, expense becomes a limiting factor. The medication may be administered exclusively in the evening as insurance against nocturia.

Chlorpropamide, thiazide diuretics, and oral sodium chloride restriction have a limited efficacy in the treatment of NDI. dDAVP may control the clinical signs if administered in massive amounts (i.e., five to ten times the amount used for the treatment of CDI), but the drug's cost obviously detracts from the attractiveness of this therapeutic approach. Fortunately, therapy for CDI or NDI is not mandatory as long as the dog or cat has unlimited access to water and is housed in an environment that cannot be damaged by severe PU. A constant water supply is of paramount importance, because relatively short periods of water restriction can have catastrophic results (i.e., the development of hypernatremic, hypertonic dehydration and neurologic signs).

## Prognosis

Dogs and cats with idiopathic or congenital CDI usually become relatively asymptomatic in response to appropriate therapy, and with proper care these animals have an excellent life expectancy. Without therapy, these animals often lead acceptable lives as long as water is constantly provided and they are housed in an environment that cannot be damaged by severe PU. PU and PD frequently resolve in dogs and cats with trauma-induced CDI, often within 2 weeks of the traumatic incident. The prognosis in dogs and cats with hypothalamic and pituitary tumors is guarded to grave. Neurologic signs typically develop within 6 months after the diagnosis of CDI. Radiotherapy and chemotherapy using carmustine (BCNU) have been associated with improvement in some dogs with CDI and a pituitary or hypothalamic mass; however, the clinical response is variable and unpredictable.

The prognosis for animals with primary NDI is guarded to poor because of the limited therapeutic options and the generally poor response to therapy. The prognosis for animals with secondary NDI depends on the prognosis of the primary problem.

## PRIMARY (PSYCHOGENIC) POLYDIPSIA

Primary polydipsia is defined as a marked increase in water intake that cannot be explained as a compensatory mechanism for excessive fluid loss. In humans, primary polydipsia results from a defect in the thirst center or may be associated with mental illness. Primary dysfunction of the thirst center resulting in compulsive water consumption has not been reported in the dog or cat, although an abnormal vasopressin response to hypertonic saline infusion has been reported in dogs with suspected primary polydipsia. A psychogenic or behavioral basis for compulsive water consumption does occur in the dog but has not been reported in the cat. Psychogenic polydipsia may be induced by concurrent disease (e.g., hepatic insufficiency, hyperthyroidism) or may represent a learned behavior following a change in the pet's environment. Polyuria is compensatory to prevent overhydration.

Dogs, and presumably cats, with primary or psychogenic polydipsia have an intact hypothalamic-pituitary-renal axis for controlling fluid balance and variable severity of renal medullary solute washout. Because pituitary AVP secretion and renal tubular response to AVP are normal, these dogs can concentrate urine in excess of 1.030. Depending on the severity of renal medullary solute washout, it may take 12 to 24 hours of water deprivation to attain concentrated urine. Psychogenic polydipsia is diagnosed by exclusion of other causes of polyuria and polydipsia and by demonstrating that the dog or cat can concentrate urine to a specific gravity in excess of 1.030 during water deprivation.

Treatment is aimed at gradually limiting water intake to amounts in the high-normal range. The owner should determine the dog's approximate water intake per 24 hours when free-choice water is allowed, and this volume of water is then reduced by 10% per week until water volumes of 60 to 80 ml/kg/24 hours are reached. The total 24-hour volume of water should be divided into several aliquots, with the last aliquot given at bedtime. Oral salt (1 g/30 kg q12h) and/or oral sodium bicarbonate (0.6 g/30 kg q12h) may also be administered for 3 to 5 days in order to reestablish the renal medullary concentration gradient. For dogs that fail to respond to water restriction, the owner can consider changing the dog's environment or daily routine, such as initiating a daily exercise routine; bringing a second pet into the home; providing some distraction, such as a radio playing when the owners are not home; or moving the dog to an area with an increased amount of contact with humans.

## ENDOCRINE ALOPECIA

Endocrine alopecia is a common clinical problem in dogs and to a lesser extent in cats. It is typically bilaterally symmetrical, with the distribution pattern varying depending on the cause (Fig. 49-4). Hairs are easily epilated, and the skin is often thin and hypotonic; hyperpigmentation is common. Other dermatologic lesions such as scales, crusts, and papules are absent. Seborrhea and pyoderma may develop, depending on the underlying cause.

The potential causes of endocrine alopecia are listed in Table 49-6. The history and physical examination findings frequently provide clues to the underlying cause; if these are detected, appropriate diagnostic tests can then be done to confirm the diagnosis. If the history and physical examination fail to provide insight into the cause, the clinician should sequentially rule out the causes of endocrine alopecia, beginning with the most likely one.

In dogs the most common causes of endocrine alopecia are hypothyroidism and glucocorticoid excess (iatrogenic or spontaneous). Feline endocrine alopecia is perhaps the most

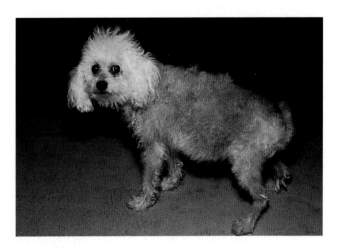

**FIG 49-4**
Endocrine alopecia in an 11-year-old male Miniature Poodle with pituitary-dependent hyperadrenocorticism.

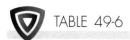

TABLE 49-6

Disorders Causing Endocrine Alopecia

| DISORDER | COMMON CLINICOPATHOLOGIC ABNORMALITIES | DIAGNOSTIC TESTS |
|---|---|---|
| Hypothyroidism | Hypercholesterolemia, mild nonregenerative anemia | Baseline $T_4$, free $T_4$, and TSH measurement |
| Hyperadrenocorticism | Stress leukogram, increased SAP, hypercholesterolemia, hyposthenuria, urinary tract infection | ACTH-stimulation test, low-dose dexamethasone suppression test, urine cortisol/creatinine ratio |
| Growth hormone deficiency pituitary dwarfism | None | Signalment, physical findings, growth hormone response test |
| Growth hormone–responsive dermatosis—adult dog | None | Growth hormone response test, response to growth hormone supplementation |
| Castration-responsive dermatosis | None | Response to castration |
| Hyperestrogenism | | |
|   Functional Sertoli cell tumor—male dog | None (bone marrow depression uncommon) | Physical findings, histopathologic findings, plasma estrogen and inhibin concentration |
|   Hyperestrogenism in intact female dog | None (bone marrow depression uncommon) | Abdominal ultrasonography, plasma estrogen concentration, response to ovariohysterectomy |
| Hypoestrogenism (?) | | |
|   Extrogen-responsive dermatosis of spayed female dogs | None | Response to estrogen therapy |
|   Feline endocrine alopecia | See below | See below |
| Hypoandrogenism (?) | | |
|   Testosterone-responsive dermatotsis—male dog | None | Response to testosterone therapy |
|   Feline endocrine alopecia | None | Response to combined estrogen-testosterone or progestin therapy |
| Telogen defluxion (effluvium) | None | History of recent pregnancy or diestrus |
| Diabetes mellitus | Hyperglycemia, glycosuria | Blood and urine glucose measurement |
| Adrenal sex hormone dermatosis | None | Sex hormones and precursors before and after ACTH stimulation |
| Progestin excess | None | Blood progesterone and 17-OH-progesterone concentration |

$T_4$, Tetraiodothyronine; *TSH*, thyroid-stimulating hormone; *SAP*, serum alkaline phosphatase; *ACTH*, adrenocorticotropic hormone.

common endocrine alopecia in cats. The diagnostic workup in both dogs and cats should begin with a CBC, serum biochemistry panel, and urinalysis. If the results of initial blood work are not helpful (e.g., normal) in dogs, definitive diagnostic tests for hypothyroidism (see p. 697) and hyperadrenocorticism (see p. 786) should be performed concurrently because of the suppressive effects of glucocorticoid excess on baseline thyroid hormone concentrations. Diagnosis becomes more difficult once hypothyroidism and hyperadrenocorticism have been ruled out. Growth hormone (GH)–responsive dermatosis, gonadal-dependent sex hormone imbalance, and adrenal-dependent sex hormone imbalance then constitute the primary differential diagnoses. Unfortunately, differentiating between these disorders is difficult, in part because the clinical and histologic abnormalities affecting the skin are similar for these disorders and tests to establish a definitive diagnosis for most of these disorders are lacking. Follicular dysplasia can cause a similar clinical picture and should also be considered.

**Growth hormone–responsive dermatosis.** Growth hormone deficiency in a juvenile dog is characterized by short stature and dermatologic problems, including retention of the puppy coat and subsequent development of endocrine alopecia, hyperpigmentation, and thin hypotonic skin (see Pituitary Dwarfism, p. 677). Similar dermatologic problems develop in an adult dog that develops GH deficiency, but the dog has a normal haircoat before hair loss begins (see Growth Hormone–Responsive Dermatosis, p. 670). Diagnosis of these disorders is based on the signalment, findings on physical examination, measurement of plasma GH or serum insulin-like growth factor-I (IGF-I) after the administration of a GH-secretagogue, and response to GH treatment.

**Gonadal-dependent sex hormone imbalance.** Endocrine alopecia can result from an excess or deficiency of one of the sex hormones, most notably estrogens and androgens, or may be responsive to treatment with one of the sex hormones (see Table 49-6). Dermatologic manifestations are

TABLE 49-7

Dermatohistopathologic Alterations Associated with Endocrinopathy-Induced Alopecia

| ABNORMALITY | SPECIFIC ENDOCRINE DISORDER |
| --- | --- |
| **Nonspecific Abnormalities Supporting an Endocrinopathy** | |
| Orthokeratotic hyperkeratosis | — |
| Follicular keratosis | — |
| Follicular dilation | — |
| Follicular atrophy | — |
| Predominance of telogen hair follicles | — |
| Sebaceous gland atrophy | — |
| Epidermal atrophy | — |
| Epidermal melanosis | — |
| Thin dermis | — |
| Dermal collagen atrophy | — |
| **Abnormalities Suggestive of a Specific Endocrine Disorder** | |
| Decreased amount and size of dermal elastin fibers | Hyposomatotropism |
| Excessive trichilemmal keratinization (flame follicles) | Growth hormone– and castration-responsive dermatosis |
| Vacuolated and/or hypertrophied arrector pilae muscles | Hypothyroidism |
| Increased dermal mucin content | Hypothyroidism |
| Thick dermis | Hypothyroidism |
| Comedones | Hyperadrenocorticism |
| Calcinosis cutis | Hyperadrenocorticism |
| Absence of arrector pilae muscles | Hyperadrenocorticism |

similar for most sex hormone–induced or sex hormone–responsive dermatoses and include endocrine alopecia that initially begins in the perineal, genital, and ventral abdominal regions and spreads cranially; dull, dry, easily epilated hair; failure of the haircoat to regrow after clipping; and variable presence of seborrhea and hyperpigmentation. Additional clinical findings are dependent on the underlying etiology. For example, additional clinical signs of hyperestrogenism may include gynecomastia, a pendulous prepuce, the attraction of other male dogs, squatting to urinate, and unilateral testicular atrophy (contralateral to the testicular tumor) in the male dog and vulvar enlargement and persistent proestrus, estrus, or anestrus in the bitch. Dermatologic signs of sex hormone–induced or sex hormone–responsive dermatosis can mimic GH-responsive dermatosis, creating a difficult diagnostic challenge for the veterinarian, especially when the alopecia occurs in a breed with a known predisposition for GH-responsive dermatosis (e.g., Pomeranians).

Diagnosis of sex hormone–induced or sex hormone–responsive dermatosis is based on the signalment, history, findings on physical examination, results of routine biochemical and hormonal tests used to rule out other causes of endocrine alopecia, and response to treatment. Histologic assessment of a skin biopsy specimen can be used to identify nonspecific endocrine-related alterations and support the diagnosis of endocrine alopecia (Table 49-7). There are no pathognomonic histologic changes for sex hormone–induced or sex hormone–responsive dermatoses. The identification of an increased plasma estrogen concentration would support

the presence of a functional Sertoli cell tumor in the dog and hyperestrogenism in the bitch (assuming that the bitch is not in proestrus or early estrus). Abdominal ultrasonography may identify ovarian cysts or neoplasia in the bitch with hyperestrogenism. The diagnosis in animals with most of these disorders, however, ultimately depends on the animal's response to therapy (Table 49-8). Because of potentially serious adverse reactions to therapy, the more common causes of endocrine alopecia should always be ruled out before one initiates treatment with one of the sex hormones (e.g., diethylstilbestrol, methyltestosterone). The haircoat should improve within 3 months of the start of therapy. If there is no improvement within this time, another diagnosis should be considered.

**Adrenal-dependent sex hormone imbalance.** Adrenal-dependent sex hormone imbalance may occur as a primary disorder or may occur in association with hyperadrenocorticism. Sex hormones and their precursors may be increased in dogs with pituitary-dependent hyperadrenocorticism, but the predominant clinical signs in these dogs result from hypercortisolism (e.g., polyuria, polydipsia). Sex hormones may also be increased in adrenal-dependent hyperadrenocorticism and may affect the dermatologic manifestations of the disease (e.g., alopecia of the flank, color change of the haircoat). Progesterone-secreting adrenocortical tumors have been described in cats. Clinical features in affected cats mimic hyperadrenocorticism, presumably because progesterone acts as a glucocorticoid agonist (see p. 812). An increase in baseline and/or post-ACTH plasma 17-hydroxyprogesterone has also been documented in dogs with clinical

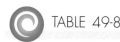

TABLE 49-8

Treatment for Sex Hormone–Induced or Sex Hormone–Responsive Endocrine Alopecia

| DISORDER | PRIMARY TREATMENT | POTENTIAL ADVERSE REACTIONS TO THERAPY |
|---|---|---|
| Sertoli cell neoplasia | Castration | None |
| Castration-responsive dermatosis | Castration | None |
| Hyperestrogenism in the intact female dog | Ovariohysterectomy | None |
| Estrogen-responsive dermatosis of spayed female dogs | Diethylstilbestrol, 0.1-1.0 mg PO q24h 3 weeks per month; once responds, 0.1-1 mg q4-7d | Aplastic anemia |
| Feline endocrine alopecia | Megestrol acetate, 2.5-5 mg/cat q48h until hair regrows; then 2.5-5 mg/cat q7-14d | Adrenocortical suppression, benign mammary hypertrophy, mammary neoplasia, pyometra (female cats); infertility (male cats); diabetes mellitus |
| Testosterone-responsive dermatosis | Methyltestosterone, 1 mg/kg (maximum, 30 mg) PO q48h until hair regrows, then q4-7d | Aggression, hepatopathy |
| Telogen defluxion (effluvium) | None | None |
| Adrenal sex hormone dermatosis | Growth hormone, castration, melatonin (see p. 669), mitotane | Diabetes mellitus, hypoadrenocorticism |

manifestations of hyperadrenocorticism but normal plasma cortisol concentrations following administration of ACTH or dexamethasone (see p. 812).

Congenital adrenal hyperplasia–like syndrome has clinical signs similar to those with GH-responsive dermatosis and has been identified in many breeds but especially in the Pomeranian, Chow Chow, Keeshond, and Samoyed. Both sexes are affected, but males are overrepresented. A partial deficiency of one of the adrenal enzymes, 11-hydroxylase, 21-hydroxylase, or 3-hydroxysteroid dehydrogenase, is believed to cause a partial deficiency of cortisol or aldosterone in affected dogs, which in turn promotes pituitary ACTH secretion, the development of adrenocortical hyperplasia, and increased adrenal sex hormone production. Elevations in progesterone and its precursors are common in affected dogs. Progesterone can have antiandrogenic activity, and the alopecia may be attributable to local hypoandrogenism; regrowth of hair occurs in some affected dogs with methyltestosterone treatment. Skin biopsies from affected dogs show the typical changes of endocrine alopecia (see Table 49-7) and may also show features of follicular dysplasia. Diagnosis requires evaluation of sex hormones and their precursors before and after ACTH administration. Currently, the only laboratory with well-established normal values for sex steroids is the Endocrinology Laboratory at the University of Tennessee, College of Veterinary Medicine, Knoxville, TN 37901-1071. Treatment has included castration, methyltestosterone (see Table 49-8), growth hormone (see p. 671), melatonin (3 to 6 mg q12-24h for 6 weeks), and o,p'DDD (mitotane) (induction dose: 15 to 25 mg/kg daily until post-ACTH plasma cortisol concentration is between 2 and 5 μg/dl, then initiate

maintenance therapy; see p. 792). Dogs with congenital adrenal hyperplasia–like syndrome are healthy aside from the alopecia, and many owners elect not to treat their dog because of the expense and/or risk of complications associated with methyltestosterone, GH or o,p'DDD treatment.

## GROWTH HORMONE–RESPONSIVE DERMATOSIS IN THE ADULT DOG

### Etiology

GH-responsive dermatosis is a poorly defined dermatologic disorder affecting adult dogs. It may represent an initially mild (partial?) but progressive form of congenital hyposomatotropism that is not severe enough to cause dwarfism but that, with time, results in dermatologic manifestations in young adult dogs. Alternatively, hyposomatotropism may be a disorder that is acquired after normal growth has occurred. Currently the etiology remains unknown. Baseline plasma GH concentrations in these dogs are low, and there is no increase in the plasma concentration after stimulation of the somatotrophs, suggesting a problem with somatotroph function. Given the strong breed-related predisposition for this disorder, genetics undoubtedly plays a role, at least in some breeds. The sex of animals may also play a role, given the predominance of this dermatosis in intact male dogs. The lesion does not appear to be progressive or to affect other endocrine functions of the pituitary.

Some dogs with the typical signalment and clinical signs of GH-responsive dermatosis respond to GH therapy despite having either normal or abnormal GH stimulation test results but normal baseline serum IGF-I concentrations. These findings indicate that true GH deficiency may not be present in some dogs (especially Chow Chows, Keeshonds, Pomeranians, and Samoyeds) with GH-responsive dermatosis, that other, as yet poorly characterized causes of endocrine dermatosis exist that mimic GH-responsive dermatosis (see discussion on endocrine alopecia), and that dogs that do not have hyposomatotropism may respond to GH therapy.

## Clinical Features

**Signalment.** Although many breeds have GH-responsive dermatosis, Chow Chows, Pomeranians, Toy and Miniature Poodles, Keeshonds, American Water Spaniels, and Samoyeds are overrepresented. Because the Chow Chow, Keeshond, Pomeranian, and Samoyed are overrepresented in congenital adrenal hyperplasia–like syndrome (see p. 670), any GH irregularity in these breeds may be coincidental or a secondary problem. There also seems to be a predilection for the disorder in male animals. Clinical signs usually develop in young animals (1 to 4 years of age), although the age at which an initial examination for the evaluation of related signs is performed by the veterinarian is reported to extend up to 11 years.

**Clinical signs.** Hyposomatotropism in the mature dog primarily affects hair growth and skin pigmentation. GH-responsive dermatosis is characterized by bilaterally symmetrical alopecia of the trunk, neck, pinnae, tail, and caudomedial thighs (Fig. 49-5). Alopecia frequently begins in areas of friction or wear (e.g., around the neck in the vicinity of the collar). Initially there is a gradual loss of guard (primary) hairs in affected areas, giving the haircoat a puppylike appearance. With time, undercoat (secondary) hairs are lost. Truncal primary hairs are then gradually lost, followed by secondary hairs. Complete truncal alopecia is uncommon. The head is not involved, and the legs are involved to a lesser extent than the trunk. Hair in affected areas is easily epilated, and the remaining haircoat is usually dry and lusterless. Hyperpigmentation develops in areas of alopecia. In chronic cases the skin becomes thin and hypotonic. These dogs are otherwise normal.

**Clinical pathology.** Routine clinical pathologic test results, including those of a CBC, serum biochemistry panel, and urinalysis, are normal in mature dogs with GH-responsive dermatosis.

**Dermatohistopathology.** Histologic assessment of a skin biopsy specimen may reveal the presence of nonspecific alterations found in endocrine skin diseases (see Table 49-7), decreased amounts and size of dermal elastin fibers, and flame follicles. Flame follicles are exaggerated forms of catagen follicles in which large spikes of fused keratin appear to protrude through the outer root sheath into the vitreous layer of the follicle. Flame follicles are seen with endocrine and developmental disorders, most notably GH-responsive dermatosis, castration-responsive dermatosis, postclipping alopecia, and the follicular dysplasia seen in Siberian Huskies. The tendency to form flame follicles may also be breed dependent; flame follicles may develop in dogs such as Chow Chows or Pomeranians as a result of other atrophic influences on the hair follicle (e.g., hyperestrogenism, hyperadrenocorticism).

## Diagnosis

GH-responsive dermatosis is diagnosed on the basis of the results of a GH-stimulation test (Table 49-9) and the animal's response to GH-replacement therapy. Baseline GH concentrations are similar in normal dogs and dogs with GH-responsive dermatosis. The clonidine-stimulation test is the most commonly used GH-stimulation test. In normal dogs the plasma GH concentration should exceed 10 ng/ml 15 to 30 minutes after the administration of the secretagogue and should remain less than 10 ng/ml (preferably undetectable) in dogs with suspected GH-deficiency syndrome. Hypothyroidism, hyperadrenocorticism, and possibly sex hormone imbalances suppress pituitary GH secretion and should be ruled out before the results of GH-stimulation tests are interpreted. Unfortunately, the means to measure GH in the dog is severely limited. As such, a tentative diagnosis is made based on the signalment, the history and physical examination findings, an absence of clinicopathologic alterations, the finding of appropriate dermatohistopathologic alterations on skin biopsy specimens, and the ruling out of more common causes of endocrine alopecia. If all of the findings support the existence of GH-responsive dermatosis, the animal's response to GH-replacement therapy can then be used to help establish the diagnosis.

## Treatment

Historically, treatment of GH-responsive dermatosis has involved the administration of GH. Unfortunately, an effective GH product is not readily available for use in dogs. Recombinant human GH is expensive, difficult to procure, and may induce antibody formation, which can interfere with effectiveness when administered to dogs. Recombinant bovine GH is designed for use in cows and is not suitable for dilution to concentrations suitable for use in dogs. Porcine GH is immunologically similar to canine GH, but its availability is unpredictable. If available, the recommended dose of porcine GH is 0.1 IU (0.05 mg/kg) given subcutaneously three times per week for 4 to 6 weeks. Hypersensitivity reactions (including angioedema), carbohydrate intolerance, and overt diabetes mellitus are the primary adverse reactions associated with GH injections. Frequent monitoring of urine for glucose and blood for the development of hyperglycemia (blood glucose >150 mg/dl) should be done, and GH therapy should be stopped if either develops. Regrowth of hair and thickening of the skin are used to assess the response to therapy. The haircoat should improve within 4 to 6 weeks of the start of therapy (Fig. 49-6). The hair that grows back consists primarily of lanugo hairs, with variable regrowth of primary or guard hairs. The duration of clinical remission in dogs with GH-responsive dermatosis that respond to GH treatment is variable but may last up to 3 years after therapy. A 1-week course of GH treatment should be given if dermatologic signs begin to recur.

Alternative treatments that have been reported to be effective include castration, melatonin, and o,p'DDD (see Endocrine

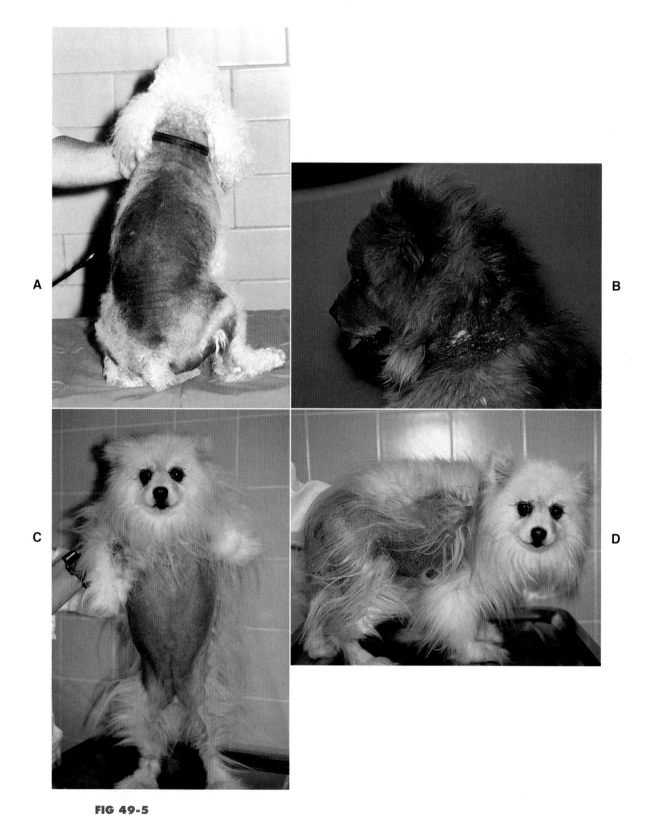

**FIG 49-5**
**A,** A 3-year-old Poodle with adult-onset growth hormone (GH)–responsive dermatosis. Note the symmetrical truncal alopecia and hyperpigmentation, with lesser involvement of the distal extremities and sparing of the head. **B,** A 2-year-old Chow Chow with adult-onset GH-responsive dermatosis. Note the alopecia and hyperpigmentation around the neck, probably related to the excessive epilation of hair caused by the dog's collar. **C** and **D,** A 6-year-old Pomeranian with adult-onset, GH-responsive dermatosis. Note the symmetrical truncal alopecia with lesser involvement of the extremities and sparing of the head. (**A** courtesy J.C. Blakemore, West Lafayette, Ind; **B** courtesy D. Serra, Wyoming, R.I.)

## TABLE 49-9

Growth Hormone–Stimulation Testing Protocols

| TEST | DESCRIPTION AND RESULTS |
|------|-------------------------|
| Xylazine-stimulation test* | |
|   Protocol | 100 µg/kg IV; plasma samples obtained before and at 15, 30, 45, and 60 minutes after administration of xylazine† |
|   Normal results | Plasma GH, >10 ng/ml 15 to 30 minutes after xylazine administration |
|   Adverse reactions | Sedation (common), bradycardia, hypotension, collapse, shock, seizures |
| Clonidine-stimulation test | |
|   Protocol | 10 µg/kg IV; plasma samples obtained before and at 15, 30, 45, and 60 minutes after administration of clonidine† |
|   Normal results | Plasma GH, >10 ng/ml 15 to 30 minutes after clonidine administration |
|   Adverse reactions | Sedation (common), bradycardia, hypotension, collapse, aggressive behavior |
| GHRH-stimulation test | |
|   Protocol | 1 µg/kg GHRH IV; plasma samples obtained before and at 10, 20, 30, 45, and 60 minutes after GHRH administration |
|   Normal results | Plasma GH, >10 ng/ml 15 to 30 minutes after GHRH administration |
|   Adverse reactions | None reported |

*Currently preferred GH-stimulation test.
†An abbreviated protocol in which plasma samples are obtained before and 20 and 30 minutes after stimulation can be done.
*GH,* Growth hormone; *GHRH,* growth hormone–releasing hormone.

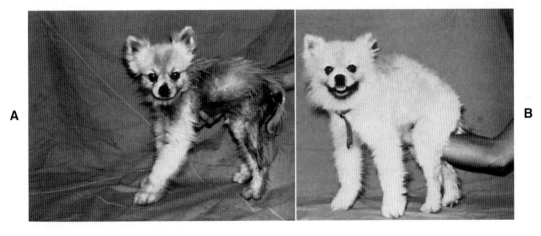

### FIG 49-6
**A,** A 6-year-old female Pomeranian with adult-onset, GH-responsive dermatosis. **B,** Same dog as in **A** 3 months after the start of exogenous porcine GH replacement therapy.

Alopecia, above). Response to treatments other than GH casts doubt on the role of GH in the development of this clinical syndrome and emphasizes the difficulty in separating GH-responsive, sex hormone–induced, and sex hormone–responsive endocrine alopecia. Spontaneous regrowth of hair has also occurred in some untreated dogs.

### Prognosis

The long-term prognosis is good, even in dogs not treated with GH. Most untreated dogs eventually lose most of their hair on the thorax and abdomen (the head and distal ex-

tremities are spared), and the skin turns black. The dogs are otherwise healthy.

## FELINE ACROMEGALY

### Etiology

Chronic excessive secretion of GH in adult cats results in acromegaly, a disease characterized by the overgrowth of connective tissue, bone, and viscera. In cats, acromegaly is caused by a functional adenoma of the somatotropic cells of the

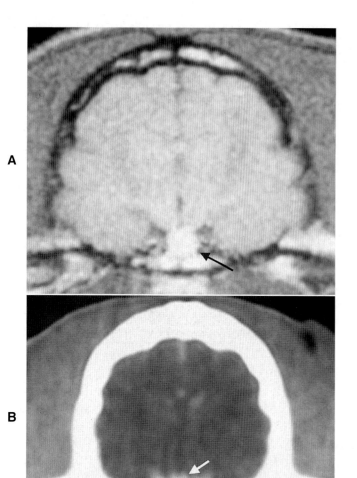

**FIG 49-7**

**A,** Magnetic resonance image of the pituitary region of a 5-year-old male, castrated domestic long-haired cat with insulin-resistant diabetes mellitus and acromegaly. A mass is evident in the hypothalamic-pituitary region *(arrow).* **B,** Computed tomographic scan of the pituitary region 1 year after completion of radiation therapy. The volume of the mass was decreased by approximately 65% compared with the volume prior to treatment. Insulin-requiring diabetes mellitus persisted, but insulin-resistance had resolved.

pituitary pars distalis (Fig. 49-7). In more than 90% of cats in which necropsies have been performed, the pituitary tumor has proved to be a macroadenoma that extends dorsally into or compresses the hypothalamus and thalamus. GH secretion by these tumors is increased, and presumably feedback control of the GH secretion is abnormal. Progestin-induced acromegaly has not been documented in the cat. Progestins, including megestrol acetate, do not appear to stimulate GH or IGF-I secretion in the cat. In contrast, acromegaly in the dog is seen most commonly after prolonged exposure to progestins, either exogenously administered (e.g., medroxyprogesterone acetate) or late in life fol-

lowing years of endogenous progesterone secretion during the diestrual phase of the estrous cycle in the intact bitch.

Chronic GH hypersecretion has both catabolic and anabolic effects. The anabolic effects are caused by increased concentrations of IGF-I. The growth-promoting effects of IGF-I result in the proliferation of bone, cartilage, and soft tissues and in organomegaly, most notably of the kidney and heart. These anabolic effects are responsible for producing the classic clinical manifestations of acromegaly (Table 49-10). The catabolic effects of GH are a direct result of the antiinsulin effects of GH on tissues. Excess GH causes insulin antagonism by inducing a postreceptor defect in glucose transport, which may lead to hyperinsulinism and the subsequent downregulation of insulin receptors. These abnormalities in the binding and action of insulin result in carbohydrate intolerance, hyperglycemia, and eventually insulin-resistant diabetes mellitus. Most but not all cats with acromegaly have diabetes mellitus at the time acromegaly is diagnosed, and most eventually develop severe insulin resistance.

## Clinical Features

Acromegaly typically occurs in older (mean age, 10 years; range, 8 to 14 years) male, domestic short-haired or long-haired cats. Clinical signs result from the catabolic, diabetogenic effects of GH, the anabolic actions of chronic IGF-I secretion by the liver, and growth of the pituitary macroadenoma (see Table 49-10). The earliest clinical signs are usually PU, PD, and polyphagia resulting from the concurrent diabetes mellitus. Polyphagia may also develop as a direct result of hypersomatotropism, independent of the diabetes mellitus, and can become quite intense. Weight loss varies and depends in part on whether the anabolic effects of IGF-I or the catabolic effects of hyperglycemia predominate. Most cats initially lose weight followed by a period of stabilization and then a slow, progressive gain in body weight as the anabolic effects of IGF-I begin to dominate the clinical picture. Severe insulin resistance eventually develops. In most cats, the clinician considers acromegaly only after he or she realizes that insulin therapy has been ineffective in establishing glycemic control of the diabetic state. Insulin dosages in cats with acromegaly frequently exceed 2 to 3 U/kg of body weight twice a day, with no apparent decline in the blood glucose concentration.

Clinical signs related to the anabolic actions of excess GH secretion (see Table 49-10) may be evident at the time diabetes mellitus is diagnosed. More commonly, however, they become apparent several months after the diabetes has been diagnosed, often in conjunction with the realization that hyperglycemia is difficult to control with exogenous insulin therapy. Because of the insidious onset and slowly progressive nature of the anabolic clinical signs, owners are often not aware of the subtle changes in the appearance of their cat until the clinical signs are quite obvious. Anabolic changes in acromegalic cats include an increase in body size, enlargement of the abdomen and head, development of prognathia inferior, and weight gain (Fig. 49-8). Weight gain in a cat with poorly regulated diabetes mellitus is an impor-

## TABLE 49-10

### Clinical Signs Associated with Acromegaly in Dogs and Cats

**Anabolic, IGF-I–Induced**

Respiratory
  Inspiratory stridor
  Transient apnea
  Panting
  Exercise intolerance
  Fatigue
Dermatologic
  Myxedema
  Excessive skin folds
  Hypertrichosis
Conformational
  Increased size
  Increased soft tissue in oropharyngeal/laryngeal area
Enlargement of:
  Abdomen
  Head
  Feet
  Viscera
Broad face
Prominent jowls
Prognathia inferior
Increased interdental space
Rapid toenail growth
Degenerative polyarthropathy

**Catabolic, GH-Induced**

Polyuria, polydipsia
Polyphagia

**Iatrogenic**

Progestins
  Mammary nodules
  Pyometra

**Neoplasia-Induced**

Lethargy, stupor
Adipsia
Anorexia
Temperature deregulation
Papilledema
Circling
Seizures
Pituitary dysfunction
  Hypogonadism
  Hypothyroidism
  Hypoadrenocorticism

*IGF-I,* Insulin-like growth factor-I; *GH,* growth hormone.

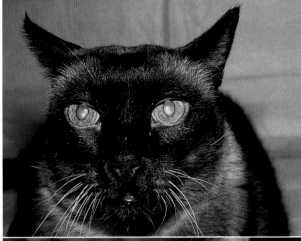
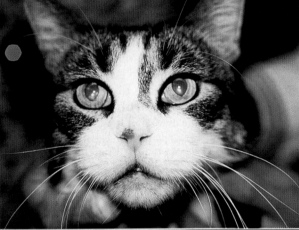
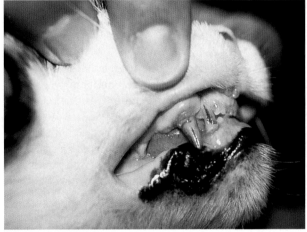

**FIG 49-8**
**A,** A 13-year-old male, castrated Siamese with insulin-resistant diabetes mellitus and acromegaly. The owners had noticed a gradual increase in the size of the cat's head. Note the broad face and mildly protruding mandible (prognathia inferior). **B** and **C,** An 8-year-old male, castrated domestic short-haired cat with insulin-resistant diabetes mellitus and acromegaly. Note the broad head, mildly protruding mandible, and prognathia inferior with displacement of the lower canine teeth. (From Feldman EC, Nelson RW: *Canine and feline endocrinology and reproduction,* ed 2, Philadelphia, 1996, WB Saunders.)

tant diagnostic clue to acromegaly. With time, organomegaly, especially of the heart, kidney, liver, and adrenal gland, develop. Diffuse thickening of soft tissues in the pharyngeal region can lead to extrathoracic upper airway obstruction and respiratory distress.

Neurologic signs may develop as a result of pituitary tumor growth and the resultant invasion and compression of the hypothalamus and thalamus. Signs include stupor, somnolence, adipsia, anorexia, temperature deregulation, circling, seizures, and changes in behavior. Blindness is not common, because the optic chiasm is located anterior to the pituitary gland. Papilledema may be evident during an ophthalmic examination. Peripheral neuropathy causing weakness, ataxia, and a plantigrade stance may develop as a result of poorly controlled diabetes mellitus. Other endocrine and metabolic abnormalities resulting from the compressive effects of the tumor on the pituitary are uncommon.

## Clinical Pathology

Concurrent, poorly controlled diabetes mellitus is responsible for causing most of the abnormalities identified on a serum biochemistry panel and urinalysis, including hyperglycemia, glycosuria, hypercholesterolemia, and a mild increase in the alanine transaminase and alkaline phosphatase activities. Ketonuria is an infrequent finding. Mild erythrocytosis, persistent mild hyperphosphatemia without concurrent azotemia, and persistent hyperproteinemia (total serum protein concentration of 8.2 to 9.7 mg/dl) with a normal pattern of distribution on protein electrophoretic studies may also be found. Renal failure is a potential sequela of acromegaly and, if present, will be associated with azotemia, isosthenuria, and proteinuria.

## Diagnosis

A definitive diagnosis of acromegaly requires the documentation of an increased baseline serum GH concentration. The baseline GH concentration in cats with acromegaly typically exceeds 10 ng/ml (normal concentration is less than 5 ng/ml). Unfortunately, a commercial GH assay is not available for cats, and it may take months before results are obtained when blood samples are submitted to research laboratories. Therefore the diagnosis is based on (1) the identification of conformational alterations (e.g., increased body size, large head, prognathia inferior, organomegaly) in a cat with insulin-resistant diabetes mellitus; (2) a persistent increase rather than decrease in the body weight of a cat with poorly controlled diabetes mellitus; and (3) the documentation of a pituitary mass by CT or MR scanning (see Fig. 49-7). It is usually necessary to administer a positive contrast agent to visualize a pituitary mass using CT or MR imaging. In addition, hyperadrenocorticism must be ruled out before a tentative diagnosis of acromegaly can be made.

Measurement of the serum IGF-I concentration can be used to provide further evidence for the diagnosis of acromegaly. Measurement of serum IGF-I is commercially available (e.g., Diagnostic Endocrinology Laboratory, College of Veterinary Medicine, Michigan State University, East Lansing, MI, 48909-7576). Serum IGF-I concentrations are considered to reflect overall GH secretion during the previous 24 hours. Concentrations are usually increased in acromegalic cats; however, serum IGF-I values may fall in the upper normal range in the early stages of the disease (Fig. 49-9). Repeat

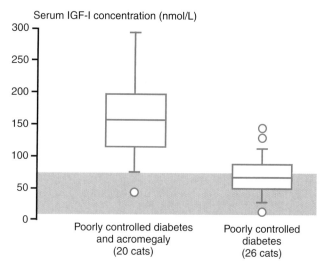

**FIG 49-9**
Box plots of serum concentrations of insulin-like growth factor-I (IGF-I) in 20 cats with poorly controlled diabetes caused by concurrent acromegaly and 26 cats with poorly controlled diabetes caused by another disorder. For each box plot, T-bars represent the main body of data, which in most instances is equal to the range. Each box represents the interquartile range (25th to 75th percentile). The horizontal bar in each box is the median. The solid circles represent outlying data points. Shaded area is the normal range.

measurements performed 3 to 4 months later will usually demonstrate an increase in serum IGF-I if acromegaly is present. The increase in serum IGF-I typically coincides with development and growth of the pituitary somatotropic adenoma. Measurement of serum IGF-I can be used as a screening test for acromegaly prior to performing a CT or MR scan. The clinical picture and severity of insulin resistance must always be taken into consideration when interpreting serum IGF-I results.

## Treatment

Radiotherapy is currently considered the best treatment option for acromegaly in cats. Unfortunately, the response to cobalt teletherapy is unpredictable and ranges from no response to a dramatic response, characterized by shrinkage of the tumor, elimination of hypersomatotropism, resolution of insulin resistance, and, in some cats, reversion to a subclinical diabetic state (see Fig. 49-7). Typically, the tumor size and the plasma growth hormone and serum IGF-I concentrations decrease and insulin responsiveness improves after cobalt teletherapy. However, hypersomatotropism usually recurs 6 to 18 months after treatment. Disadvantages of radiotherapy include limited availability, expense, the need for extended hospitalization, frequent anesthesia, and an unpredictable outcome.

The long-acting somatostatin analog Octreotide (Novartis Pharmaceuticals, East Hanover, N.J.) has been unsuccessful in lowering serum GH concentration or improving insulin sensitivity in the acromegalic cats in which it has been used.

Dosages used in cats have ranged from 10 to 200 μg/cat, given subcutaneously two to three times daily. The reason for its ineffectiveness in cats is not understood; it may be that the GH-secreting somatotroph adenomas of cats lack the somatostatin receptors for the somatostatin analogs.

Microsurgical transsphenoidal hypophysectomy has been shown to be effective for the treatment of feline pituitary-dependent hyperadrenocorticism, but use of this specialized surgical technique for the treatment of acromegaly has not been reported. Successful use of transsphenoidal cryotherapy of a pituitary tumor has been described in a cat with acromegaly.

## Prognosis

The short- and long-term prognosis for cats with tumor-induced acromegaly is guarded to good and poor, respectively. The survival time has ranged from 4 to 60 months (typically 1.5 to 3 years) from the time the diagnosis of acromegaly is established. The GH-secreting pituitary tumor usually grows slowly, and neurologic signs associated with an expanding tumor are uncommon until late in the disorder. Diabetes mellitus is difficult to control, even with the administration of large doses of insulin (20 units or more/injection) given twice daily. Administration of large doses of insulin should be avoided. The severity of insulin resistance fluctuates unpredictably in cats with acromegaly, and severe, life-threatening hypoglycemia may suddenly develop after months of insulin resistance and blood glucose concentrations in excess of 400 mg/dl. To prevent severe hypoglycemia, insulin doses should not exceed 12 to 15 units per injection. Most cats with acromegaly eventually die or are euthanized because of the development of severe congestive heart failure, renal failure, respiratory distress, the neurologic signs of an expanding pituitary tumor, or coma caused by severe hypoglycemia.

## *PITUITARY DWARFISM*

### Etiology

Pituitary dwarfism results from a congenital deficiency of GH. In dogs and probably cats, it is most commonly associated with pressure atrophy of the anterior lobe of the pituitary gland caused by cystic enlargement of the residual craniopharyngeal duct (i.e., Rathke's cleft) and with pituitary hypoplasia resulting from primary failure of differentiation of the craniopharyngeal ectoderm of Rathke's pouch into a normal anterior lobe. Pituitary dwarfism is encountered most often as a simple, autosomal recessive inherited abnormality in the German Shepherd Dog. A similar mode of inheritance has been reported in Carnelian Bear dogs. Inherited pituitary dwarfism may be due to isolated GH deficiency or may be part of a combined pituitary hormone deficiency. Concurrent deficiency in thyroid-stimulating hormone (TSH) and prolactin are most commonly identified in affected German Shepherd Dogs; ACTH secretion is preserved. Kooistra and colleagues (2000) hypothesize that the disorder is caused by a mutation in a developmental transcription factor that pre-

## TABLE 49-11

### Clinical Signs Associated with Pituitary Dwarfism

**Musculoskeletal**

Stunted growth
Thin skeleton, immature facial features
Square, chunky contour (adult)
Bone deformities
Delayed closure of growth plates
Delayed dental eruption

**Reproduction**

Testicular atrophy
Flaccid penile sheath
Failure to have estrous cycles

**Other Signs**

Mental dullness
Shrill, puppy-like bark
Signs of secondary hypothyroidism
Signs of secondary adrenal insufficiency (uncommon)

**Dermatologic**

Soft, wooly haircoat
Retention of lanugo hairs
Lack of guard hairs
Alopecia
   Bilaterally symmetrical
   Trunk, neck, proximal extremities
Hyperpigmentation of skin
Thin, fragile skin
Wrinkles
Scales
Comedones
Papules
Pyoderma
Seborrhea sicca

cludes effective expansion of a pituitary stem cell after the differentiation of the corticotropic cells that produce ACTH. Pituitary dwarfism resulting from a mutant GH or an insensitivity to GH owing to a lack of or defect in GH receptors (e.g., Laron-type dwarfism in human beings) has not been documented in dogs or cats.

### Clinical Features

**Signalment.** Pituitary dwarfism occurs primarily in German Shepherds, although pituitary dwarfism in other breeds, including the Weimaraner, Spitz, Toy Pinscher, and Carnelian Bear dog, has also been observed. Pituitary dwarfism has also been observed in cats. There does not appear to be a sex-related predilection.

**Clinical signs.** The most common clinical manifestations of pituitary dwarfism are a lack of growth (i.e., short stature), endocrine alopecia, and hyperpigmentation of the skin (Table 49-11). Affected animals are usually a normal size during the

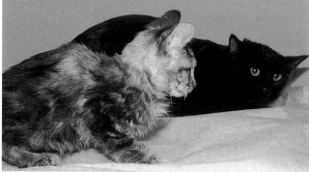

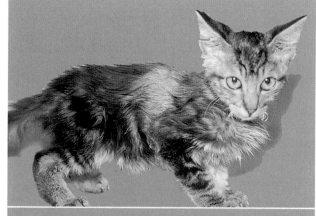

**FIG 49-10**
**A,** An 8-month-old male domestic short-haired cat with pituitary dwarfism The size of the pituitary dwarf cat was similar to that of an 8-week-old kitten. Note the normal body contour and juvenile appearance. **B,** Same cat as in **A** (foreground) with an age-matched normal cat (background) to illustrate the small stature and juvenile appearance of the pituitary dwarf. (From Feldman EC, Nelson RW: *Canine and feline endocrinology and reproduction,* ed 2, Philadelphia, 1996, WB Saunders.)

first 1 to 2 months of life, but after that grow more slowly than their littermates. By 3 to 4 months of age, affected dogs and cats are obviously runts of the litter and usually never attain full adult dimensions. Dwarfs with an isolated GH deficiency typically maintain a normal body contour and body proportions as they age (i.e., proportionate dwarfism), whereas dwarfs with combined deficiencies (most notably TSH) may acquire a square or chunky contour typically associated with congenital hypothyroidism (i.e., disproportionate dwarfism) (Fig. 49-10).

The most notable dermatologic sign is a retention of the lanugo or secondary hairs, with a concurrent lack of the primary or guard hairs. As a result the haircoat in a dwarf is initially soft and wooly. The lanugo hairs are easily epilated, and a bilateral symmetrical alopecia gradually develops. Initially, hair loss is confined to areas of wear, such as the neck (collar) and posterolateral aspects of the thighs (from sitting). Eventually the entire trunk, neck, and proximal limbs become alopecic, with primary hairs remaining only on the face and distal extremities. The skin is initially normal but becomes

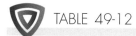

## TABLE 49-12

### Some Potential Causes of Small Stature in Dogs and Cats

| ENDOCRINE CAUSES | NONENDOCRINE CAUSES |
|---|---|
| Hyposomatotropism | Malnutrition |
| Hypothyroidism | Gastrointestinal tract disorders |
| Hyperadrenocorticism | |
| Hypoadrenocorticism | Maldigestion |
| Diabetes mellitus | Pancreatic exocrine insufficiency |
| | Malabsorption |
| | Heavy intestinal parasitism |
| | Hepatic disorders |
| |    Portosystemic vascular shunt |
| |    Glycogen storage disease |
| | Renal disease |
| | Cardiovascular disease, anomalies |
| | Skeletal dysplasia, chondrodystrophy |
| | Mucopolysaccharidoses |
| | Hydrocephalus |

hyperpigmented, thin, wrinkled, and scaly. Comedones, papules, and secondary pyoderma frequently develop in the adult dwarf. Secondary bacterial infections of the skin and respiratory tract are common long-term complications.

Hypogonadism may also develop, although normal reproductive function has been observed in some animals with pituitary dwarfism. In the male animal, testicular atrophy, azoospermia, and a flaccid penile sheath are typical; in the female, estrous activity ceases after the secretion of pituitary gonadotropins is impaired.

### Clinical Pathology

The results of a CBC, serum biochemical panel, and urinalysis are usually normal in animals with uncomplicated pituitary dwarfism. Hypophosphatemia may result from decreased renal tubular phosphorus resorption secondary to the GH deficiency. Mild hypoalbuminemia, anemia, and azotemia may develop as a result of decreases in anabolic processes stemming from GH and IGF-I deficiencies. Other clinicopathologic alterations may also be present, primarily as a result of concurrent hypothyroidism (see Chapter 51).

### Diagnosis

The signalment, history, and physical examination usually provide sufficient evidence for pituitary dwarfism to be included among the tentative diagnoses of short stature. Strong presumptive evidence can be obtained by ruling out other potential causes of small size (Table 49-12) after a thorough evaluation of the history and physical examination findings, the results of routine laboratory studies (i.e., CBC, fecal examinations, serum biochemical panel, urinalysis), and radiographic studies (Fig. 49-11). A definitive diagnosis of hypo-

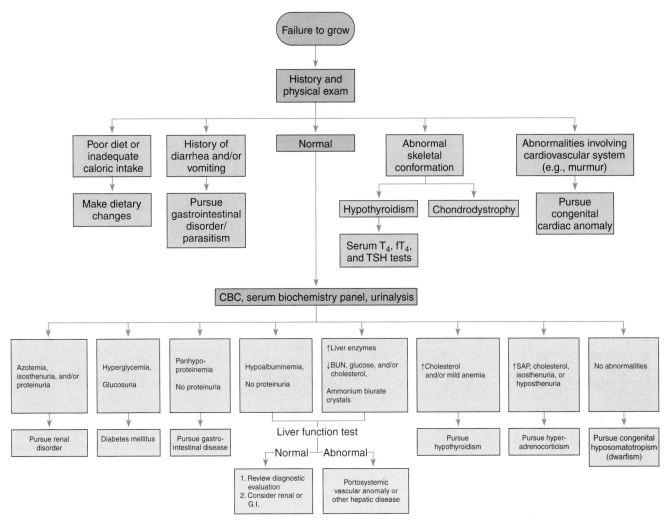

**FIG 49-11**
Diagnostic approach to the puppy or kitten that fails to grow. (From Feldman EC, Nelson RW: *Canine and feline endocrinology and reproduction,* ed 2, Philadelphia, 1996, WB Saunders.)

somatotropism should rely on an evaluation of somatotroph responsiveness to provocative testing (see Table 49-9). In most pituitary dwarfs, there is no increase in the plasma GH concentration after the administration of a GH secretagogue. A partial GH deficiency may be suspected whenever subnormal results are obtained. Baseline serum IGF-I concentrations are low in dogs with pituitary dwarfism, but breed size should be considered when evaluating test results.

## Treatment

The therapy for pituitary dwarfism relies on the administration of GH, as discussed on p. 671. Because of the synergistic influence of GH and thyroid hormone on growth processes, however, subnormal concentrations of thyroid hormone may diminish the effectiveness of GH therapy. Therefore dogs and cats with suspected panhypopituitarism should concurrently receive daily thyroid hormone supplementation, outlined in Chapter 51, and this should be continued for the rest of the animal's life.

A beneficial response in the skin and haircoat usually occurs within 6 to 8 weeks of the start of GH and thyroid hormone supplementation. The hair that grows back is primary lanugo or secondary hairs; the growth of primary or guard hairs is variable and may occur sporadically over the body. An increase in height is dependent on the status of the growth plates at the time treatment is initiated. A significant increase in height may occur if the growth plates are open, and minimal to no change in height will occur if the growth plates have closed or are about to close at the time treatment is initiated.

Improvement in clinical signs has been reported in two German Shepherd dwarfs treated with medroxyprogesterone acetate at 3- to 6-week intervals. Progestogens induce the expression of the GH gene in the mammary gland of dogs, resulting in GH secretion from foci of hyperplastic ductular epithelial cells and increased plasma concentrations of GH and IGF-I. Adverse reactions included pruritic pyoderma in both dogs, cystic endometrial hyperplasia with mucometra in the female dog, and signs of acromegaly in the male dog.

## Prognosis

The long-term prognosis for animals with pituitary dwarfism is poor. Most animals die by 3 to 5 years of age despite therapy. Death is usually a result of infections, degenerative diseases, or neurologic dysfunction.

## *Suggested Readings*

Feldman EC, Nelson RW: *Canine and feline endocrinology and reproduction,* ed 3, Philadelphia, 2004, WB Saunders.

DIABETES INSIPIDUS

Harb MF et al: Central diabetes insipidus in dogs: 20 cases (1986-1995), *J Am Vet Med Assoc* 209:1884, 1996.

Kraus KH: The use of desmopressin in diagnosis and treatment of diabetes insipidus in cats, *Comp Contin Educ Small Anim Pract* 9:752, 1987.

Luzius H et al: A low affinity vasopressin $V_2$-receptor in inherited nephrogenic diabetes insipidus, *J Recept Res* 12:351, 1992.

Nichols R: Clinical use of the vasopressin analogue DDAVP for the diagnosis and treatment of diabetes insipidus. In Bonagura JD, editor: *Kirk's current veterinary therapy XIII,* Philadelphia, 2000, WB Saunders, p 325.

van Vonderen IK et al: Intra- and interindividual variation in urine osmolality and urine specific gravity in healthy pet dogs of various ages, *J Vet Intern Med* 11:30, 1997.

van Vonderen IK et al: Disturbed vasopressin release in 4 dogs with so-called primary polydipsia, *J Vet Intern Med* 13:419, 1999.

ENDOCRINE ALOPECIA AND GROWTH HORMONE–RESPONSIVE DERMATOSIS

Ashley PF et al: Effect of oral melatonin administration on sex hormone, prolactin, and thyroid hormone concentrations in adult dogs, *J Am Vet Med Assoc* 215:1111, 1999.

Bell AG et al: Growth hormone responsive dermatosis in three dogs, *NZ Vet J* 41:195, 1993.

Paradis M: Melatonin therapy for canine alopecia. In Bonagura JD, editor: *Kirk's current veterinary therapy XIII,* Philadelphia, 2000, WB Saunders, p 546.

Schmeitzel LP et al: Hormonal abnormalities in Pomeranians with normal coat and in Pomeranians with growth hormone–responsive dermatosis, *J Am Vet Med Assoc* 197:1333, 1990.

Schmeitzel LP: Sex hormone–related and growth hormone–related alopecias, *Vet Clin North Am* 20:1579, 1990.

Schmeitzel LP et al: Congenital adrenal hyperplasia–like syndrome. In Bonagura JD et al, editors: *Kirk's current veterinary therapy XII,* Philadelphia, 1995, WB Saunders, p 600.

Scott DW et al, editors: *Muller and Kirk's small animal dermatology,* ed 6, Philadelphia, 2001, WB Saunders.

van Herpen H et al: Production of antibodies to biosynthetic human growth hormone in the dog, *Vet Rec* 134:171, 1994.

FELINE ACROMEGALY

Abrams-Ogg ACG et al: Acromegaly in the cat: diagnosis with magnetic resonance imaging and treatment by cryohypophysectomy, *Can Vet J* 34:682, 1993.

Goossens MMC et al: Cobalt 60 irradiation of pituitary gland tumors in three cats with acromegaly, *J Am Vet Med Assoc* 213:374, 1998.

Peterson ME et al: Acromegaly in fourteen cats, *J Vet Intern Med* 4:192, 1990.

PITUITARY DWARFISM

Kooistra HS et al: Progestin-induced growth hormone (GH) production in the treatment of dogs with congenital GH deficiency, *Domest Anim Endocrinol* 15:93, 1998.

Kooistra HS et al: Combined pituitary hormone deficiency in German Shepherd dogs with dwarfism, *Domest Anim Endocrinol* 19:177, 2000.

Rijnberk A et al: Disturbed release of growth hormone in mature dogs: a comparison with congenital growth hormone deficiency, *Vet Rec* 133:542, 1993.

## CHAPTER 50

# Disorders of the Parathyroid Gland

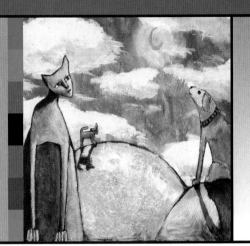

## CHAPTER OUTLINE

CLASSIFICATION OF HYPERPARATHYROIDISM, 681
PRIMARY HYPERPARATHYROIDISM, 681
PRIMARY HYPOPARATHYROIDISM, 686

## CLASSIFICATION OF HYPERPARATHYROIDISM

Hyperparathyroidism is a sustained increase in parathyroid hormone (PTH) secretion. Chief cells located within the parathyroid gland synthesize and secrete PTH—a peptide hormone that controls the minute-to-minute level of ionized calcium in the blood and extracellular fluids (ECFs). The major regulator of PTH secretion is the concentration of ionized calcium in the blood. Decreased serum ionized calcium increases PTH secretion, and vice versa. PTH stimulates calcium reabsorption and inhibits phosphate reabsorption by the kidney, stimulates synthesis of the active form of vitamin D in the kidney, and stimulates bone resorption. The net effect is to increase the serum ionized and total calcium concentration and decrease the serum phosphorus concentration.

Hyperparathyroidism can result from a normal physiologic response to decreased serum ionized calcium concentrations (renal or nutritional secondary hyperparathyroidism) or a pathologic condition resulting from the excessive synthesis and secretion of PTH by abnormal, autonomously functioning parathyroid chief cells (i.e., primary hyperparathyroidism [PHP]). In PHP, increased secretion of PTH is maintained regardless of the serum ionized calcium concentration.

Hypercalcemia and hypophosphatemia develop as a result of the physiologic actions of PTH. In renal secondary hyperparathyroidism, renal failure causes retention of phosphate and development of hyperphosphatemia. Hyperphosphatemia decreases serum ionized calcium concentration by the mass law effect ($[Ca] \times [Pi] = constant$). The decrease in serum ionized calcium, in turn, stimulates PTH secretion. The net effect is increased serum phosphate, normal-to-low serum ionized calcium, increased serum PTH concentration, and diffuse parathyroid gland hyperplasia. The etiogenesis of hyperparathyroidism is similar in nutritional secondary hyperparathyroidism, except the decrease in calcium results from feeding diets containing low calcium-to-phosphorus ratios, such as beef heart or liver. Dietary calcium deficiency or phosphorus excess decreases serum calcium concentration, inducing increased PTH secretion and parathyroid gland hyperplasia.

## PRIMARY HYPERPARATHYROIDISM

### Etiology

PHP is a disorder resulting from the excessive, relatively uncontrolled secretion of PTH by one or more abnormal parathyroid glands. It is an uncommon disorder in the dog and rare in the cat. Parathyroid adenoma is the most common histologic finding; parathyroid carcinoma and parathyroid adenomatous hyperplasia have also been described. Parathyroid adenomas are typically small, well-encapsulated, light brown to red tumors located in close apposition to the thyroid gland (Fig. 50-1). The remaining parathyroid glands are normal, atrophied, or not visible at surgery. Parathyroid carcinomas are rare in dogs and cats, and their biologic behavior is not well characterized. In our experience, carcinomas grossly appear similar to adenomas and the diagnosis has been based on the finding of certain histologic features (e.g., capsular or vascular invasion). Parathyroid hyperplasia is tentatively diagnosed if more than one parathyroid gland is found to be grossly and microscopically abnormal and renal and nutritional secondary hyperparathyroidism are ruled out. Histologically, affected glands contain multiple nodules less than 5 mm in diameter, as opposed to adenomas, which are defined as consisting of a single nodule typically greater than 5 mm in diameter.

The differentiation between hyperplasia and adenoma has important prognostic implications. That is, the surgical removal of a solitary parathyroid adenoma results in cure, assuming that at least one normal parathyroid gland remains to prevent hypoparathyroidism. However, the likelihood of persistent hyperparathyroidism is high in animals with parathyroid hyperplasia, unless all abnormal parathyroid tissue is

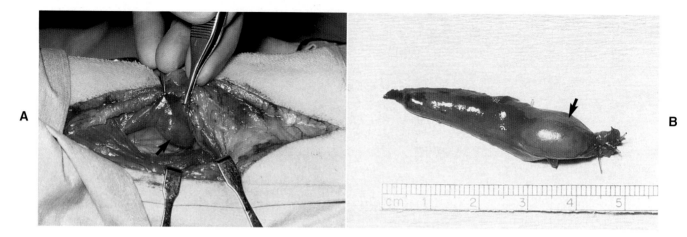

**FIG 50-1**
**A,** Surgical site in a 12-year-old dog with primary hyperparathyroidism (PHP). A parathyroid adenoma *(arrow)* can be seen in the thyroid lobe. **B,** Gross appearance of parathyroid adenoma *(arrow)* and thyroid lobe after removal from the dog in **A.**

TABLE 50-1

Biologic Actions of the Hormones that Affect Calcium and Phosphorus Metabolism

| HORMONE | BONE | KIDNEY | INTESTINE | NET EFFECT | |
|---|---|---|---|---|---|
| | | | | SERUM Ca | PO₄ |
| Parathyroid hormone | Increased bone resorption | ↑ Ca absorption<br>↑ PO₄ excretion | No direct effect | ↑ | ↓ |
| Calcitonin | Decreased bone resorption | ↓ Ca resorption<br>↓ PO₄ resorption | No direct effect | ↓ | ↓ |
| Vitamin D | Maintain Ca transport system | ↓Ca resorption | ↑ Ca absorption<br>↑ PO₄ absorption | ↑ | ↑ |

↑, Increased; ↓, decreased.

removed, and recurrence of hyperparathyroidism weeks to months after surgery is high. Often all four parathyroid glands must ultimately be removed to resolve the hyperparathyroid problem, which leads to the development of iatrogenic permanent hypoparathyroidism.

The clinical signs of PHP stem from the physiologic actions of excessive PTH secretion rather than from the space-occupying nature of the tumor. The physiologic actions of PTH ultimately cause hypercalcemia and hypophosphatemia (Table 50-1). Hyperphosphatemia may be found in some dogs with secondary renal failure induced by prolonged, severe hypercalcemia; a problem that is not common with PHP.

## Clinical Features

**Signalment.** PHP occurs in older dogs (mean age, 10 years; range, 4 to 16 years), and there is no sex-related predilection. A genetic predisposition is suspected in the Keeshond. Hereditary neonatal PHP, which is possibly inherited in an autosomal recessive fashion, has been reported in two German Shepherd puppies. Eight cats with hypercalcemia caused by PHP have also been described. Their mean age was approximately 12

years (range, 8 to 15 years), five were female, five were Siamese, and three were of mixed breed.

**Clinical signs.** Clinical signs of PHP are caused by hypercalcemia, which is the hallmark of this disorder. Clinical signs are absent in most dogs and cats with the mildest form of PHP, and hypercalcemia is discovered only after a serum biochemistry panel is performed, often for unrelated reasons. When clinical signs do develop, they initially tend to be nonspecific and insidious in onset. The clinical signs in dogs are typically renal, gastrointestinal, and neuromuscular in origin (Table 50-2). The most common clinical signs in cats with PHP are anorexia and lethargy.

**Physical examination.** The physical examination findings are usually normal, which is an important diagnostic finding when differentiating dogs with PHP from dogs with hypercalcemia of malignancy (see p. 836). Lethargy, generalized muscle atrophy, weakness, and cystic calculi (calcium phosphate or calcium oxalate, or both types) may be noted in some dogs with PHP. The severity of weakness is variable but usually subtle. A parathyroid adenoma is rarely identified by palpation of the ventral neck in dogs. If a mass is palpated,

TABLE 50-2

## Clinical Signs Associated with Primary Hyperparathyroidism in Dogs

Polyuria and polydipsia*
Listlessness*
Urinary incontinence*
Weakness, exercise intolerance*
Dysuria, pollakiuria, hematuria
Inappetence
Shivering
Muscle wasting
Vomiting
Constipation
Stiff gait

*Common sign.

the possibility of a carcinoma should be considered. In contrast to the rarity of palpable masses in dogs, cats with PHP can have palpable parathyroid masses that are typically located in the region of the thyroid gland. As such, a palpable mass in the ventral cervical region of the neck should raise suspicion for hyperthyroidism (common), as well as PHP (rare).

### Diagnosis

PHP should be suspected in a dog or cat with persistent hypercalcemia and normophosphatemia to hypophosphatemia. The serum calcium concentration is typically 12 to 15 mg/dl but can exceed 16 mg/dl. The serum ionized calcium concentration is typically 1.4 to 1.8 mmol/L but can exceed 2.0 mmol/L. The serum phosphorus concentration is typically less than 4 mg/dl, unless concurrent renal insufficiency is present. Although hypercalcemia in dogs and cats has several causes (Table 50-3), the primary differential diagnoses for hypercalcemia and hypophosphatemia are hypercalcemia of malignancy and PHP (see p. 836). The history, findings on physical examination, results of routine blood and urine tests, thoracic radiographs, abdominal and cervical ultrasound, and measurement of PTH and PTHrp will usually establish the diagnosis. For PHP, clinical signs are usually mild to absent, the physical examination is normal, and results of routine blood work, thoracic and abdominal radiography, and abdominal ultrasonography are unremarkable, except for the hypercalcemia and hypophosphatemia. Additional tests used to identify lymphoma as the cause of hypercalcemia (i.e., cytologic evaluations of bone marrow and lymph node aspirates and PTHrp concentrations) are normal in dogs with PHP. Ultrasonographic examination of the thyroparathyroid complex may reveal enlargement of one or more parathyroid glands. Most parathyroid adenomas measure 4 to 8 mm in diameter, although an occasional parathyroid adenoma will exceed 1 cm (Fig. 50-2). A urine specific gravity of less than 1.015 is common and a consequence of hypercalcemia interfering with the action of antidiuretic hormone and renal con-

centrating ability. Hematuria, pyuria, bacteriuria, and crystalluria may be identified if cystic calculi and secondary bacterial cystitis develop. Hypercalciuria, proximal renal tubular acidosis with impaired bicarbonate resorption, and the production of alkaline urine may predispose dogs to the development of cystic or renal calculi and bacterial cystitis. Uroliths are typically composed of calcium phosphate, calcium oxalate, or mixtures of the two salts. Prolonged (severe) hypercalcemia may cause progressive nephrocalcinosis, renal damage, and azotemia with a resultant increase in the serum urea nitrogen, creatinine, and phosphorus concentrations. Serum ionized calcium concentration will be increased in dogs with PHP-induced renal failure and normal or low in primary renal failure–induced hypercalcemia (see p. 836).

Measurement of serum PTH concentration helps confirm a diagnosis of PHP. Assays that measure the intact PTH molecule are recommended. Interpretation of the serum PTH concentration must be done in conjunction with the serum calcium concentration. If the parathyroid gland is functioning normally, the serum PTH concentration should be low or undetectable in the face of hypercalcemia because of the inhibitory effects of an increased serum calcium concentration on parathyroid gland function. Dogs with nonparathyroid-induced hypercalcemia should have low-to-undetectable serum PTH concentrations. A midnormal to increased serum PTH concentration is inappropriate in the face of hypercalcemia and indicative of an autonomously functioning parathyroid gland (Fig. 50-3). Increased serum PTH concentrations can be found in dogs with renal failure resulting from concurrent secondary renal hyperparathyroidism. Because of the influence of the kidney on circulating PTH concentration, it is essential that renal function be normal in the hypercalcemic dog for an evaluation of the serum PTH concentration to be meaningful. Alternatively, the serum PTH concentration should be evaluated in conjunction with the serum ionized calcium concentration. The latter is typically normal to low in animals with renal failure and increased in those with PHP, whereas the serum PTH concentration is increased in both disorders.

Surgical exploration of the neck is ultimately required to establish a diagnosis of PHP. If the signalment, history, and physical examination findings are consistent with PHP, a thorough diagnostic evaluation has failed to identify another cause for the hypercalcemia and the serum PTH concentration is inappropriately increased, compared with the corresponding serum calcium concentration; the likelihood of PHP is high and surgical exploration of the neck is warranted. Ultrasonographic evaluation of the thyroparathyroid complex adds further evidence for PHP and provides useful information before surgical exploration regarding the number and location of hyperfunctioning parathyroid glands.

### Treatment

Surgical removal of the abnormal parathyroid tissue is the treatment of choice. Bojrab (1998) and Fossum (2002) have adequately described the surgical techniques for the thyroparathyroid complex (see Suggested Readings). Ethanol injection or

TABLE 50-3

Causes of Hypercalcemia in Dogs and Cats

| DISORDER | TESTS TO HELP ESTABLISH THE DIAGNOSIS |
|---|---|
| Primary hyperparathyroidism | Serum PTH concentration, cervical ultrasound, surgery |
| Hypercalcemia of malignancy | Physical examination, thoracic and abdominal radiography, |
|   Humorally mediated: LSA, apocrine gland adeno-carcinoma, carcinoma (nasal, mammary gland, gastric, thyroid, pancreatic, pulmonary) |   abdominal ultrasonography, lymph node and bone marrow aspiration, serum PTHrp |
|   Locally osteolytic (multiple myeloma, LSA, squamous cell carcinoma, osteosarcoma, fibrosarcoma) | |
| Hypervitaminosis D | History, serum biochemistry panel, serum vitamin D concentration |
|   Cholecalciferol rodenticides, plants | |
|   Excessive supplementation | |
| Hypoadrenocorticism | Serum Na$^+$, K$^+$, ACTH stimulation tests |
| Renal failure | Serum biochemistry panel, urinalysis |
| Granulomatous disease (rare) | Thoracic radiography, fundic examination, cytologic studies of |
|   Systemic mycosis-Blastomycosis |   tracheal wash or intestinal biopsy specimens, serum fungal titers |
|   Schistosomiasis, FIP | |
| Nonmalignant skeletal disorder (rare) | Radiography of peripheral skeleton |
|   Osteomyelitis | |
|   Hypertrophic osteodystrophy | |
| Iatrogenic disorder (rare) | — |
|   Excessive calcium supplementation | |
|   Excessive oral phosphate binders | |
| Dehydration (mild hypercalcemia) | — |
| Factitious disorder | — |
|   Lipemia | |
|   Postprandial measurement | |
|   Young animal (<6 months) | |
| Laboratory error | — |
| Idiopathic (cats) | — |

*LSA,* Lymphosarcoma; *ACTH,* adrenocorticotropic hormone; *FIP,* feline infectious peritonitis.

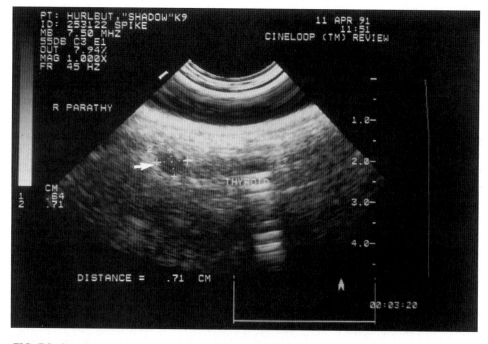

**FIG 50-2**
Ultrasound image of the right thyroid lobe of an 11-year-old German Shepherd with hypercalcemia. A mass is seen in the region of the parathyroid gland *(arrow).* Parathyroid adenoma was diagnosed histologically, after surgical removal of the mass.

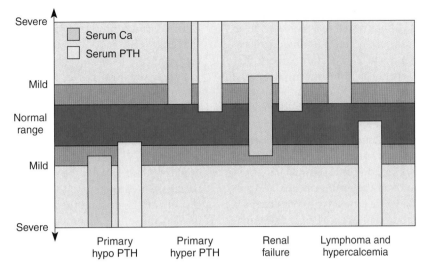

**FIG 50-3**
Ranges of the serum calcium and parathyroid hormone (PTH) concentrations in the more common disorders causing alterations in serum calcium concentration, parathyroid gland function, or both. *PTH,* Parathyroid hormone; *hypo PTH,* hypoparathyroidism; *hyper PTH,* hyperparathyroidism.

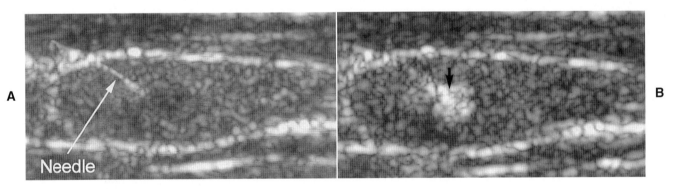

**FIG 50-4**
**A,** Ultrasound image of the left thyroid lobe of an 12-year-old Keeshond with hypercalcemia. A mass is in the region of the parathyroid gland *(arrow)* and a needle has been inserted into the mass using ultrasound guidance before heat ablation of the mass.
**B,** Heat is being administered to the mass, causing hyperechogenicity of the mass *(arrow).*

heat ablation of abnormal parathyroid tissue under ultrasound guidance is also an effective treatment for PHP (Fig. 50-4). Although surgery is avoided with these techniques, anesthesia is still required, development of posttreatment hypocalcemia is not avoided, and results are less consistent than with surgical removal of the abnormal parathyroid tissue.

During surgery, it is important to evaluate all four parathyroid glands before deciding on which gland, or glands, to remove. Almost all dogs and cats with PHP have a solitary, easily identified parathyroid adenoma (see Fig. 50-1). Enlargement of more than one parathyroid gland indicates the presence of either multiple adenomas or, more likely, parathyroid hyperplasia. If more than one enlarged gland is identified, this raises concern as to whether there is primary or sec-

ondary (i.e., renal or nutritional) hyperparathyroidism. However, a thorough presurgical evaluation tends to rule out the existence of secondary disease. If the clinician is convinced that primary disease is present, a decision to remove three, as opposed to four, glands should be made on the basis of the animal's clinical status and renal function, as well as on the ability of the owner to treat permanent hypoparathyroidism. If none of the parathyroid glands appear enlarged or if all appear small, the diagnosis of PHP must be questioned and hypercalcemia stemming from occult neoplasia or PTH production by a parathyroid tumor in an ectopic site (e.g., cranial mediastinum) or by a nonparathyroid tumor considered.

An attempt must be made to ensure that at least one parathyroid gland remains intact to maintain calcium homeostasis and prevent permanent hypocalcemia. Surgical removal of the parathyroid tumor results in a rapid decline in the circulating PTH concentration and the subsequent development of hypocalcemia 1 to 7 days after surgery. The higher the preoperative serum calcium concentration, the more chronic the hypercalcemic condition, or both, the more likely the dog or cat will become clinically hypocalcemic after removal of the abnormal parathyroid gland or glands. As a general rule, if the serum calcium concentration before surgery is less than 14 mg/dl or ionized calcium concentration is less than 1.6 mmol/L, the dog or cat should be kept in the hospital for 5 to 7 days and the serum calcium concentration monitored twice daily. Treatment for hypocalcemia is not initiated unless clinical signs of hypocalcemia develop or the serum calcium or ionized calcium concentration declines below 9 mg/dl and 0.9 mmol/L, respectively; whichever comes first. In most of these animals, the remaining parathyroid glands are capable of secreting adequate amounts of PTH to prevent severe hypocalcemia and the associated clinical signs, the hypocalcemia gradually resolves during the ensuing week, and postoperative calcium and vitamin D supplementation is not required.

Serum calcium or ionized calcium concentrations greater than 14 mg/dl and 1.6 mmol/L, respectively, in animals with PHP, suggest the existence of chronic hypercalcemia, marked atrophy of the remaining parathyroid glands, and a high probability for the development of signs of hypocalcemia (i.e., panting, nervousness, facial rubbing, muscle twitching, ataxia, seizures) after surgery. In these animals, vitamin D and calcium therapy should be started once a decrease in the serum calcium or ionized calcium concentration is documented to attempt to prevent hypocalcemia. A decrease in serum calcium is usually evident within 6 to 8 hours of surgery. In some animals with severe hypercalcemia (total calcium or ionized calcium >18 mg/dl and 2.0 mmol/L, respectively), vitamin D therapy can be initiated 24 to 36 hours before surgery because of the known delay in the onset of vitamin D's action.

Therapy for hypocalcemia includes the acute administration of calcium intravenously (IV) or subcutaneously (SC) to control immediate clinical signs and the long-term oral administration of calcium and vitamin D supplements to maintain low-normal blood calcium concentrations while the parathyroid gland atrophy resolves (see p. 688). The onset of action of vitamin D varies depending on the formulation of vitamin D that is administered. In general, 1,25-dihydroxyvitamin $D_3$ has the fastest onset of action, vitamin $D_2$ (ergocalciferol) has the slowest onset of action, and dihydrotachysterol falls in between (see Table 50-7). Some dogs, but more often cats, seem resistant to vitamin D given in tablet form but respond appropriately to the liquid form. (See p. 840 for details about the management of hypocalcemia.)

The goal of calcium and vitamin D therapy is to maintain the serum calcium concentration within the low to low-normal range (9 to 10 mg/dl). Maintaining the serum calcium concentration in the low normal range prevents the development of clinical signs of hypocalcemia, minimizes the risk of hypercalcemia, and stimulates a return of function in the re-

maining atrophied parathyroid glands. Once the parathyroid glands regain control of calcium homeostasis and the serum calcium concentration is stable in the dog or cat in the home environment, the calcium and vitamin D supplements can be gradually withdrawn over a period of 3 to 6 months. This gradual withdrawal allows time for the parathyroid glands to become fully functional and thereby prevents hypocalcemia.

Vitamin D therapy should be withdrawn first; this is done by gradually increasing the number of days between administrations. The dosing interval should be increased by 1 day every 2 to 3 weeks, after the serum calcium concentration has been measured and found to be 9 mg/dl or greater. Vitamin D therapy can be discontinued once the dog or cat is clinically normal, the serum calcium concentration is stable between 9 and 11 mg/dl, and the vitamin D dosing interval is every 7 days. The oral calcium supplementation can then be gradually reduced and discontinued over the ensuing month.

### Prognosis

The prognosis for animals with PHP depends on the severity of secondary changes induced by the hypercalcemia, specifically those affecting renal function, and on the ability to prevent severe hypocalcemia postoperatively. If serious renal damage has not occurred and severe hypocalcemia can be prevented postoperatively, the prognosis is excellent. Hypercalcemia may recur weeks to months after surgery in dogs and cats with PHP caused by parathyroid hyperplasia, if one or more parathyroid glands have been left in situ.

## PRIMARY HYPOPARATHYROIDISM

### Etiology

Primary hypoparathyroidism develops as a result of an absolute or relative deficiency in the secretion of PTH. This deficiency ultimately causes hypocalcemia and hyperphosphatemia because of a loss of PTH effects on bone, kidney, and intestine (see Table 50-1). The major signs of hypoparathyroidism are directly attributable to the decreased concentration of ionized calcium in the blood, which leads to increased neuromuscular activity.

Spontaneous primary hypoparathyroidism is rare in dogs and cats. Most cases are classified as idiopathic (i.e., there is no evidence of trauma, malignant or surgical destruction, or other obvious damage to the neck or parathyroid glands). The glands are difficult to locate visually and microscopically show evidence of atrophy. Histologic evaluation of the parathyroid gland often reveals a diffuse lymphocytic, plasmacytic infiltration and fibrous connective tissue, suggesting an underlying immune-mediated cause of the disorder.

Iatrogenic hypoparathyroidism after performance of bilateral thyroidectomy for the treatment of hyperthyroidism is common in cats. The parathyroid tissue in such animals may be excised or traumatized, or its blood supply may be interrupted during surgery. This form of hypoparathyroidism may be transient or permanent, depending on the viability of the parathyroid gland or glands saved at the time of surgery.

Only one viable parathyroid gland is needed to maintain a normal serum calcium concentration.

Transient hypoparathyroidism may develop secondary to severe magnesium depletion (serum magnesium concentration <1.2 mg/dl). Severe magnesium depletion may suppress PTH secretion without parathyroid destruction, increase end-organ resistance to PTH, and impair the synthesis of the active form of vitamin D (i.e., calcitriol). The end result is mild hypocalcemia and hyperphosphatemia. Magnesium repletion reverses the hypoparathyroidism. Serum magnesium concentrations in dogs and cats with spontaneous primary hypoparathyroidism usually have been normal when measured. The reader is referred to p. 843 for more information on magnesium.

## Clinical Features

**Signalment.** The age at which the clinical signs of hypoparathyroidism appear in dogs ranges from 6 weeks to 13 years, with a mean of 4.8 years. There may be a sex-related predisposition in female dogs. There is no apparent breed-related predisposition, although Toy Poodles, Miniature Schnauzers, Labrador Retriever, German Shepherd, and Terriers are commonly affected breeds. However, this increased prevalence may merely reflect the popularity of these breeds. Only a few cases of primary hypoparathyroidism in cats have been reported. To date, these cats have been young to middle-aged (6 months to 7 years), of several breeds, and usually male.

**Clinical signs.** The clinical signs and physical examination findings in dogs and cats with primary hypoparathyroidism are similar. The major clinical signs are directly attributable to hypocalcemia, most notably its effects on the neuromuscular system. Neuromuscular signs include nervousness, generalized seizures, focal muscle twitching, rear-limb cramping or tetany, ataxia, and weakness (Table 50-4). Additional signs include lethargy, inappetence, intense facial rubbing, and panting. The onset of clinical signs tends to be abrupt and severe and to occur more frequently during exercise, excitement, and stress. Clinical signs also tend to occur episodically. Episodes of clinical hypocalcemia are interspersed with relatively normal periods, lasting minutes to days. Interestingly, the hypocalcemia persists during these "normal" periods.

**Physical examination.** The most common physical examination findings are related to muscular tetany and include a stiff gait; muscle rigidity; a tense, splinted abdomen; and muscle fasciculations. Fever, panting, and nervousness, often to the point of interfering with the examination, are also common. Potential cardiac abnormalities include paroxysmal tachydysrhythmias, muffled heart sounds, and weak femoral pulses. Cataracts have been noted in a few dogs and in one cat with primary hypoparathyroidism. In dogs these cataracts were small, punctate-to-linear, white opacities that were randomly distributed in the anterior and posterior cortical subcapsular region of the lens; there was no loss of vision. The physical examination findings are occasionally normal, despite the previous history of neuromuscular disorders.

## Diagnosis

Primary hypoparathyroidism should be suspected in a dog or cat with persistent hypocalcemia, hyperphosphatemia, and normal renal function. The serum calcium concentration is usually less than 7 mg/dl, the serum ionized calcium is usually less than 0.8 mmol/L, and the serum phosphorus is usually greater than 6 mg/dl. Low serum calcium and high serum phosphorus concentrations can also be encountered during nutritional and renal secondary hyperparathyroidism, after phosphate-containing enema, and during tumor lysis syndrome. The diagnosis of primary hypoparathyroidism is established by identifying an undetectable serum PTH concentration in the face of severe hypocalcemia in a dog or cat in which other causes of hypocalcemia have been ruled out (Table 50-5). Most causes of hypocalcemia can be identified after evaluation of the history, findings on physical examination, and results of routine blood and urine tests and an abdominal ultrasound. The history and physical examination findings are essentially unremarkable in dogs and cats with primary hypoparathyroidism, other than those findings caused by hypocalcemia. The only relevant abnormalities identified on routine blood and urine tests is severe hypocalcemia and, in most dogs and cats, hyperphosphatemia. The serum total protein, albumin, urea nitrogen, creatinine, and magnesium concentrations are normal. Abdominal ultrasound is also normal.

Measurement of serum PTH concentration helps confirm a diagnosis of primary hypoparathyroidism. Blood for PTH determination should be obtained before the initiation of calcium and vitamin D therapy while the animal is still hypocalcemic. Assays that measure the intact PTH molecule are recommended. Interpretation of the serum PTH concentration must be done in conjunction with the serum calcium concentration. If the parathyroid gland is functioning normally, the serum PTH concentration should be increased in the face of hypocalcemia because of the stimulatory effects of a decreased serum ionized calcium concentration on parathyroid gland function. A low-to-undetectable serum PTH concentration in a hypocalcemic dog or cat is strongly suggestive of primary hypoparathyroidism (see Fig. 50-3). Dogs and cats

## TABLE 50-4

### Clinical Signs of Primary Hypoparathyroidism in Dogs

Nervousness
Generalized seizures
Rear leg cramping or pain
Focal muscle fasciculations, twitching
Ataxia, stiff gait
Facial rubbing (intense)
Aggressive behavior
Panting
Weakness
Inappetence
Listlessness, lethargy
Biting, licking paws (intense)

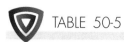

## TABLE 50-5

### Causes of Hypocalcemia in Dogs and Cats

| DISORDER | TESTS TO HELP ESTABLISH THE DIAGNOSIS |
|---|---|
| Primary hypoparathyroidism<br>    Idiopathic<br>    Post-thyroidectomy | History, serum PTH concentration, rule out other causes |
| Puerperal tetany | History |
| Renal failure<br>    Acute<br>    Chronic | Serum biochemistry panel, urinalysis |
| Ethylene glycol toxicity | History, urinalysis |
| Acute pancreatitis | Physical findings, serum lipase or amylase activities |
| Intestinal malabsorption syndromes | History, digestion or absorption tests, intestinal biopsy |
| Hypoproteinemia or hypoalbuminemia | Serum biochemistry panel |
| Hypomagnesemia | Serum total and ionized mg |
| Nutritional secondary hyperparathyroidism | Dietary history (history of what dog or cat eats) |
| Tumor lysis syndrome | History |
| Phosphate-containing enemas | History |
| Anticonvulsant medications | History |
| NaHCO₃ administration | History |
| Laboratory error | History |

## TABLE 50-6

### Injectable and Oral Calcium Preparations

| PREPARATION | DOSAGE FORM | APPROXIMATE CALCIUM CONTENT | DOSE |
|---|---|---|---|
| **Injectable (IV)** | | | |
| Calcium gluconate | 10% solution | 9.3 mg Ca/ml | 0.5-1.5 ml/kg (5-15 mg Ca/kg) |
| Calcium chloride | 10% solution | 27.2 mg Ca/ml | 0.25-0.75 ml/kg (5-15 mg Ca/kg) |
| **Oral** | | | |
| Calcium gluconate | 325, 500, 650, and 1000 mg tablets | 30, 45, 60, and 90 mg of Ca/tablet | 25 mg of Ca/kg q8-12h |
| Calcium lactate | 325 and 650 mg tablets | 42 and 85 mg of Ca/tablet | 25 mg of Ca/kg q8-12h |
| Calcium carbonate | 500, 650, and 1250 mg tablets | 200, 260, and 500 mg of Ca/tablet | 25 mg of Ca/kg q8-12h |
| Calcium carbonate/gluconate | 700 mg tablets | 250 mg of Ca/tablet | 25 mg of Ca/kg q8-12h |

with nonparathyroid-induced hypocalcemia should have normal or high serum PTH concentrations; the exception are those disorders causing severe hypomagnesemia.

### Treatment

The therapy for primary hypoparathyroidism involves the administration of vitamin D and calcium supplements (see p. 840). Therapy is typically divided into two phases: The first phase (i.e., acute therapy) should initially control hypocalcemic tetany and involves the slow administration of calcium gluconate IV (not calcium chloride), to effect (Table 50-6). Once the clinical signs of hypocalcemia are controlled, calcium gluconate should then be administered by continuous IV infusion or SC every 6 to 8 hours until the orally administered calcium and vitamin D therapy (i.e., second phase of therapy) becomes effective. The dose of calcium gluconate

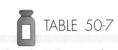 TABLE 50-7

Vitamin D Preparations

| PREPARATION | DOSAGE FORM | DOSE | TIME FOR MAXIMAL EFFECT | TIME FOR RELIEF OF TOXICITY |
|---|---|---|---|---|
| Vitamin D$_2$ (ergocalciferol) | Capsules: 25,000 U, 50,000 U<br>Syrup: 8000 U/ml*<br><br>IM injectable: 50,000 U/ml | Initial: 4000-6000 U/kg/day<br>Maintenance: 1000-2000 U/kg once daily to once every 7-14 days | 5-21 days | 1-18 weeks |
| Dihydrotachysterol | Tablets: 0.125 mg,* 0.2 mg, 0.4 mg<br><br>Capsules: 0.125 mg*<br>Oral solution: 0.25 mg/ml* | Initial: 0.02-0.03 mg/kg/day<br>Maintenance: 0.01-0.02 mg/kg/day every 24-48h | 1-7 days | 1-3 weeks |
| 1,25-Dihydroxy vitamin D$_3$ | Capsules: 0.25 µg | Initial: 0.02-0.03 µg/kg/day<br>Maintenance: 0.005-0.015 µg/kg/day | 1-4 days | 2-14 days |

*Dose form suitable for administration in cats.

administered SC is the same as that administered IV to control the tetany originally; calcium gluconate should be diluted at least 1:1 in saline before administration. During this period of parenteral calcium and oral calcium and vitamin D therapy, the serum calcium concentration should be measured twice daily and the dose or frequency of the calcium administered SC should be adjusted accordingly to control clinical signs and maintain the serum calcium concentration between 8 and 10 mg/dl. The SC calcium therapy should be gradually discontinued by increasing the interval between administrations once the serum calcium concentration remains greater than 8 mg/dl for 48 hours.

The second phase of therapy (i.e., maintenance therapy) should maintain the blood calcium concentration between 9 and 10 mg/dl through the daily administration of vitamin D and calcium (see Table 50-6; Table 50-7). These calcium concentrations are above the level at which there is a risk for clinical hypocalcemia and below the level at which hypercalciuria (risk of calculi formation) or severe hypercalcemia and hyperphosphatemia (risk of nephrocalcinosis and renal failure) may occur. Maintenance therapy should be initiated once the hypocalcemic tetany is controlled with IV and SC calcium therapy. Dogs and cats should ideally remain hospitalized until their serum calcium concentration remains between 9 and 10 mg/dl without parenteral support. Serum calcium concentrations should be monitored weekly, with the vitamin D dose adjusted to maintain a concentration of 9 to 10 mg/dl. The aim of therapy is to prevent hypocalcemic tetany and not induce hypercalcemia. Serum calcium concentrations of more than 10 mg/dl are unnecessary to prevent tetany and only increase the likelihood of unwanted hypercalcemia.

Once the serum calcium concentration has stabilized, attempts can be made to slowly taper the dose of oral calcium and then vitamin D to the lowest one that still maintains the

serum calcium concentration between 9 and 10 mg/dl. Vitamin D is critical for establishing and maintaining a normal blood calcium concentration. Most dogs and cats with primary hypoparathyroidism require permanent vitamin D therapy. The calcium supplement can often be gradually tapered over a period of 2 to 4 months and then stopped once the animal's serum calcium concentration is stable between 9 and 10 mg/dl. Calcium in the diet is often sufficient for maintaining the calcium needs of the animal. Supplementing the diet with calcium-rich foods (e.g., dairy products) helps ensure an adequate source of dietary calcium. Once the dog or cat's serum calcium concentration is stable and maintenance therapy has become established, reevaluation of the concentration every 3 to 4 months is advisable.

### Prognosis

The prognosis depends on the dedication of the owner. The prognosis is excellent if proper therapy is instituted and timely reevaluations are performed. Proper management requires close monitoring of the serum calcium concentration. The more frequent the rechecks, the better the chance of preventing extremes in the concentration and the better the chance of a normal life expectancy.

### Suggested Readings

Bojrab MJ: *Current techniques in small animal surgery,* ed 4, Philadelphia, 1998, William & Wilkins.

Feldman EC, Nelson RW: *Canine and feline endocrinology and reproduction,* ed 3, Philadelphia, 2004, WB Saunders.

Fossum TW: *Small animal surgery,* ed 2, St Louis, 2002, WB Saunders.

PRIMARY HYPERPARATHYROIDISM
Berger B et al: Primary hyperparathyroidism in dogs: 21 cases (1976-1986), *J Am Vet Med Assoc* 191:350, 1987.

DeVries SE et al: Primary parathyroid gland hyperplasia in dogs: six cases (1982-1991), *J Am Vet Med Assoc* 202:1132, 1993.

Kallet AJ et al: Primary hyperparathyroidism in cats: seven cases (1984-1989), *J Am Vet Med Assoc* 199:1767, 1991.

Long CD et al: Percutaneous ultrasound-guided chemical parathyroid ablation for treatment of primary hyperparathyroidism in dogs, *J Am Vet Med Assoc* 215:217, 1999.

Pollard RE et al: Percutaneous ultrasonographically guided radiofrequency heat ablation for treatment of primary hyperparathyroidism in dogs, *J Am Vet Med Assoc* 218:1106, 2001.

Reusch CE et al: Ultrasonography of the parathyroid glands as an aid in differentiation of acute and chronic renal failure in dogs, *J Am Vet Med Assoc* 217:1849, 2000.

Thompson KG et al: Primary hyperparathyroidism in German Shepherd Dogs: a disorder of probable genetic origin, *Vet Pathol* 21:370, 1984.

Torrance AG et al: Human-parathormone assay for use in dogs: validation, sample handling studies, and parathyroid function testing, *Am J Vet Res* 50:1123, 1989.

Wisner ER et al: High-resolution parathyroid sonography, *Vet Radiol Ultrasound* 38:462, 1997.

PRIMARY HYPOPARATHYROIDISM

Bruyette DS et al: Primary hypoparathyroidism in the dog: report of 15 cases and review of 13 previously reported cases, *J Vet Intern Med* 2:7, 1988.

Peterson ME et al: Idiopathic hypoparathyroidism in five cats, *J Vet Intern Med* 5:47, 1991.

## CHAPTER 51

# Disorders
# of the Thyroid Gland

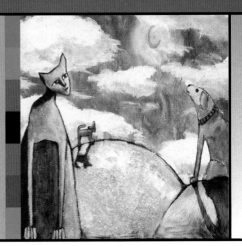

## CHAPTER OUTLINE

HYPOTHYROIDISM IN DOGS, 691
HYPOTHYROIDISM IN CATS, 709
HYPERTHYROIDISM IN CATS, 712
CANINE THYROID NEOPLASIA, 724

## HYPOTHYROIDISM IN DOGS

### Etiology

Structural or functional abnormalities of the thyroid gland can lead to deficient production of thyroid hormones. A convenient classification scheme for hypothyroidism has been devised that is based on the location of the problem within the hypothalamic-pituitary-thyroid gland complex (Fig. 51-1). Primary hypothyroidism is the most common form of this disorder in dogs; it results from problems within the thyroid gland, usually destruction of the thyroid gland (Table 51-1). The two most common histologic findings in this disorder are lymphocytic thyroiditis and idiopathic atrophy of the thyroid gland (Fig. 51-2). Lymphocytic thyroiditis is an immune-mediated disorder characterized by a diffuse infiltration of lymphocytes, plasma cells, and macrophages into the thyroid gland. The factors that trigger the development of lymphocytic thyroiditis are poorly understood, but genetic factors undoubtedly play a role.

Idiopathic atrophy of the thyroid gland is characterized by loss of the thyroid parenchyma. There is no inflammatory infiltrate, even in areas where small follicles or follicular remnants are present. The cause of idiopathic thyroid atrophy is not known, but it may be a primary degenerative disorder. It may also represent an end stage of autoimmune lymphocytic thyroiditis.

Secondary hypothyroidism results from failure of pituitary thyrotropic cells to develop (pituitary hypoplasia causing pituitary dwarfism; see p. 677) or from dysfunction within the pituitary thyrotropic cells causing impaired secretion of thyrotropin (thyroid-stimulating hormone [TSH]) and a "secondary" deficiency in thyroid hormone synthesis and secretion. Follicular atrophy gradually develops owing to the lack of

TSH. Secondary hypothyroidism could also follow the destruction of pituitary thyrotrophs (e.g., pituitary neoplasia [rare]) or the suppression of thyrotroph function by hormones or drugs (e.g., glucocorticoids [common]) (see Table 51-1).

Tertiary hypothyroidism is a deficiency in the secretion of thyrotropin-releasing hormone (TRH) by peptidergic neurons in the supraoptic and paraventricular nuclei of the hypothalamus. Lack of TRH secretion should cause a deficiency in TSH secretion and secondary follicular atrophy in the thyroid gland. Although several causes of this have been identified in people, it has not been reported in dogs and can be assumed to be rare.

Congenital defects in hormonogenesis have been documented in dogs but are rare. Documented causes of congenital primary hypothyroidism in dogs include deficient dietary iodine intake, dyshormonogenesis (i.e., an iodine organification defect), and thyroid dysgenesis. Secondary hypothyroidism resulting from an apparent deficiency of TSH has also been reported in a family of Giant Schnauzers and in a Boxer. Pedigree analysis showed that it may be inherited in an autosomal recessive fashion in the family of Giant Schnauzers. The development of an enlarged thyroid gland (i.e., goiter) depends on the etiology. If the hypothalamic-pituitary-thyroid gland axis is intact (e.g., as occurs with an iodine organification defect), goiter will develop, and if it is not intact (e.g., as occurs with pituitary TSH deficiency), goiter will not develop.

### Clinical Features

Clinical signs of the more common forms of primary hypothyroidism usually develop during middle age (i.e., 2 to 6 years). Clinical signs tend to develop at an earlier age in breeds at increased risk than in other breeds (Table 51-2). There is no apparent sex-related predilection.

Clinical signs are quite variable and depend in part on the age of the dog at the time a deficiency in thyroid hormone develops (Table 51-3). Clinical signs may also differ between breeds. For example, truncal alopecia may dominate in some breeds, whereas thinning of the haircoat dominates in other breeds. In adult dogs the most consistent clinical signs of hypothyroidism result from decreased cellular metabolism and

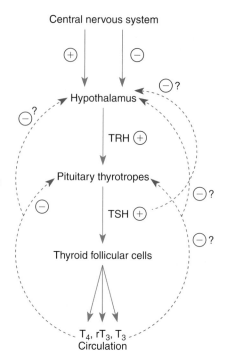

**FIG 51-1**
The hypothalamic-pituitary-thyroid gland axis. *TRH,*
Thyrotropin-releasing hormone; *TSH,* thyrotropin; *T₄,* thyroxine;
*T₃,* 3,5,3'-triiodothyronine; *rT₃,* 3,3',5'-triiodothyronine; +,
stimulation; −, inhibition.

 TABLE 51-1

## Potential Causes of Hypothyroidism in Dogs

**Primary Hypothyroidism**

Lymphocytic thyroiditis
Idiopathic atrophy
Neoplastic destruction
Iatrogenic causes
    Surgical removal
    Antithyroid medications
    Radioactive iodine treatment
    Drugs (e.g., sulfamethoxazole)

**Secondary Hypothyroidism**

Pituitary malformation
    Pituitary cyst
    Pituitary hypoplasia
Pituitary destruction
    Neoplasia
Pituitary thyrotropic cell suppression
    Naturally acquired hyperadrenocorticism
    Euthyroid sick syndrome
Iatrogenic causes
    Drug therapy, most notably glucocorticoids
    Radiation therapy
    Hypophysectomy

**Tertiary Hypothyroidism**

Congenital hypothalamic malformation(?)
Acquired destruction of hypothalamus(?)

**Congenital Hypothyroidism**

Thyroid gland dysgenesis (aplasia, hypoplasia, ectasia)
Dyshormonogenesis: iodine organification defect
Deficient dietary iodine intake

 TABLE 51-2

## Dog Breeds Reported to Have an Increased Prevalence of Thyroid Hormone Autoantibodies

| | |
|---|---|
| Pointer | Skye Terrier |
| English Pointer | Old English Sheepdog |
| German Wirehaired Pointer | Maltese |
| Boxer | Petit Basset Griffon |
| Kuvasz |   Vendeen |
| American Staffordshire Terrier | Beagle |
| American Pit Bull Terrier | Dalmatian |
| Giant Schnauzer | Rhodesian Ridgeback |
| Golden Retriever | Shetland Sheepdog |
| Chesapeake Bay Retriever | Siberian Husky |
| Brittany Spaniel | Borzoi |
| Australian Shepherd | Doberman Pinscher |
| Malamute | Cocker Spaniel |
| English Setter | |

From Nachreiner RF et al: Prevalence of serum thyroid hormone
autoantibodies in dogs with clinical signs of hypothyroidism, *J Am
Vet Med Assoc* 220:466, 2002.

its effects on the dog's mental status and activity. Most dogs
with hypothyroidism show some mental dullness, lethargy,
exercise intolerance or unwillingness to exercise, and a
propensity to gain weight without a corresponding increase
in appetite or food intake. These signs are often gradual in
onset, subtle, and not recognized by the owner until after thyroid hormone supplementation has been initiated. Additional
clinical signs of hypothyroidism typically involve the skin
and, less commonly, the neuromuscular system.

**Dermatologic signs.** Alterations in the skin and haircoat are the most common observable abnormalities in dogs
with hypothyroidism. The classic cutaneous signs include bi-

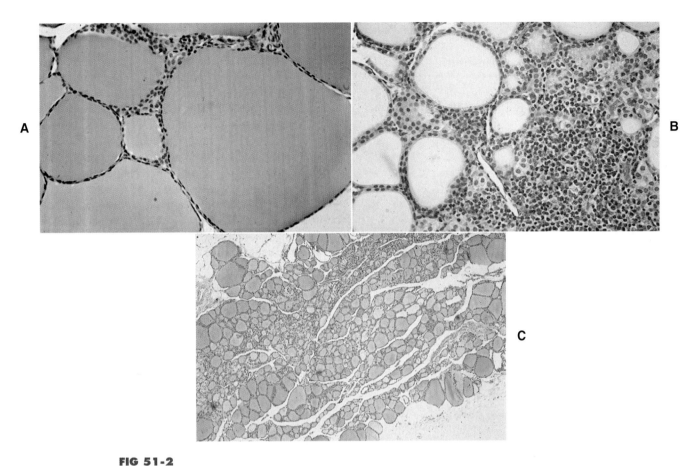

**FIG 51-2**
Histologic section of a thyroid gland from a healthy dog **(A),** from a dog with lymphocytic thyroiditis and hypothyroidism **(B),** and from a dog with idiopathic atrophy of the thyroid gland and hypothyroidism **(C).** Note the mononuclear cell infiltration, disruption of the normal architecture, and loss of colloid-containing follicles in **B** and the small size of the gland, decrease in follicular size and colloid content, and lack of a cellular infiltration in **C,** compared with **A.** (**A** and **B,** Hematoxylin and eosin stain; magnification ×250; **C,** hematoxylin and eosin stain; magnification ×40). (From Feldman EC, Nelson RW: *Canine and feline endocrinology and reproduction,* ed 2, Philadelphia, 1996, WB Saunders.)

laterally symmetric, nonpruritic truncal alopecia that tends to spare the head and extremities (Fig. 51-3). Alopecia may be local or generalized and symmetric or asymmetric; it may involve only the tail (i.e., "rat tail"); and it often initially starts over sites of wear. Although nonpruritic endocrine alopecia is not pathognomonic for hypothyroidism (see p. 667), hypothyroidism is certainly the most likely diagnosis in an affected dog with lethargy, weight gain, and no polyuria-polydipsia.

Seborrhea and pyoderma are also common signs of hypothyroidism. Depletion of thyroid hormone suppresses humoral immune reactions, impairs T-cell function, and reduces the number of circulating lymphocytes—defects that can be reversed by exogenous thyroid hormone therapy. All forms of seborrhea (i.e., sicca, oleosa, dermatitis) are possible. Seborrhea and pyoderma may be focal, multifocal, or generalized. Because both frequently result in pruritus, hypothyroid dogs with secondary pyoderma or seborrhea may initially be brought to the veterinarian because of a pruritic skin disorder.

The haircoat in dogs with hypothyroidism is often dull, dry, and easily epilated. Hair regrowth is slow. Hyperkerato-

sis leads to the development of scales and dandruff. Variable degrees of hyperpigmentation may also be noted. Chronic otitis externa has been noted in some dogs with hypothyroidism. In severe cases of hypothyroidism, acidic and neutral mucopolysaccharides may accumulate in the dermis, bind water, and cause skin to thicken. Referred to as *myxedema,* the condition causes the skin to thicken predominantly in the forehead and face of dogs, resulting in rounding of the temporal region of the forehead, puffiness and thickening of the facial skin folds, and, in conjunction with drooping of the upper eyelids, the development of a "tragic facial expression."

**Neuromuscular signs.** Neurologic signs may be the predominant problem in some dogs with hypothyroidism (see Table 51-3). Hypothyroidism-induced segmental demyelination and axonopathy may cause signs referable to the central or peripheral nervous system. Clinical signs referable to the central nervous system (CNS) may also appear after mucopolysaccharide accumulates in the perineurium and endoneurium or after cerebral atherosclerosis or severe hyperlipidemia develops, and include seizures, ataxia, and circling.

## TABLE 51-3

Clinical Manifestations of Hypothyroidism in Adult Dogs

**Metabolic**

Lethargy*
Mental dullness*
Inactivity*
Weight gain*
Cold intolerance

**Dermatologic**

Endocrine alopecia*
  Symmetric or asymmetric
  "Rat tail"
Dry, brittle haircoat
Hyperpigmentation
Seborrhea sicca or oleosa, or dermatitis*
Pyodermal*
Otitis externa
Myxedema

**Reproductive**

Persistent anestrus
Weak or silent estrus
Prolonged estrual bleeding
Inappropriate galactorrhea or gynecomastia
Testicular atrophy(?)
Loss of libido(?)

**Neuromuscular**

Weakness*
Knuckling
Ataxia
Circling
Vestibular signs
Facial nerve paralysis
Seizures
Laryngeal paralysis

**Ocular**

Corneal lipid deposits
Corneal ulceration
Uveitis

**Cardiovascular**

Decreased contractility
Bradycardia
Cardiac arrhythmias

**Gastrointestinal**

Esophageal hypomotility(?)
Diarrhea
Constipation

**Hematologic**

Anemia*
Hyperlipidemia*
Coagulopathy

**Behavioral Abnormalities(?)**

*Common.

These signs are often present in conjunction with vestibular signs (e.g., head tilt, positional vestibular strabismus) or facial nerve paralysis. Peripheral neuropathies include facial nerve paralysis, weakness, and knuckling or dragging of the feet, with excessive wear of the dorsal part of the toenail. Muscle wasting may also be evident, although myalgia is not common. Thyroxine-responsive unilateral forelimb lameness has also been observed in dogs. The relationship between hypothyroidism and laryngeal paralysis or esophageal hypomotility remains controversial, in part because it is difficult to prove a cause-and-effect relationship between these disorders and because treatment of hypothyroidism usually does not improve the clinical signs caused by laryngeal paralysis or esophageal hypomotility.

**Reproductive signs.** Historically, hypothyroidism was believed to cause lack of libido, testicular atrophy, and oligospermia to azoospermia in male dogs. However, work by Johnson and colleagues (1999) in Beagles failed to document any deleterious effect of experimentally induced hypothyroidism on any aspect of male reproductive function. Although other classic clinical signs and clinicopathologic abnormalities of hypothyroidism developed in dogs studied, libido, testicular size, and the total sperm count per ejaculate remained normal. These findings indicate that hypothyroidism may, at best, be an uncommon cause of reproductive dysfunction in male dogs, assuming that the Beagle is representative of other dog breeds.

Clinical experience has shown that hypothyroidism can cause prolonged interestrus intervals and failure to cycle in the bitch. Additional reproductive abnormalities include weak or silent estrous cycles, prolonged estrual bleeding (which may be caused by acquired problems in the coagulation system), and inappropriate galactorrhea and gynecomastia. An association between hypothyroidism and fetal resorption, abortion, and stillbirth has been suggested in the bitch; however, there is no published documentation of this association. Maternal hypothyroidism has also been suggested to result in the birth of weak puppies that die shortly after birth.

**Miscellaneous clinical signs.** Ocular, cardiovascular, gastrointestinal, and clotting abnormalities are uncommon clinical manifestations of hypothyroidism (see Table 51-3). More commonly, biochemical or functional abnormalities of these organ systems are identified in dogs exhibiting the more common clinical signs of hypothyroidism. Echocardiography may identify a decrease in cardiac contractility that is usually mild and asymptomatic but that may become relevant during a surgical procedure requiring prolonged anesthesia and aggressive fluid therapy.

A reduction in the activity of factor VIII–related antigen (von Willebrand factor) activity has been inconsistently documented in dogs with hypothyroidism, and the development of clinical signs of a bleeding disorder in hypothyroid dogs is uncommon. An evaluation of the coagulation cascade or von Willebrand factor activity is not indicated in dogs with untreated hypothyroidism unless there are concurrent bleeding problems. Thyroid hormone supplementation has a variable and sometimes deleterious effect on the blood concentration

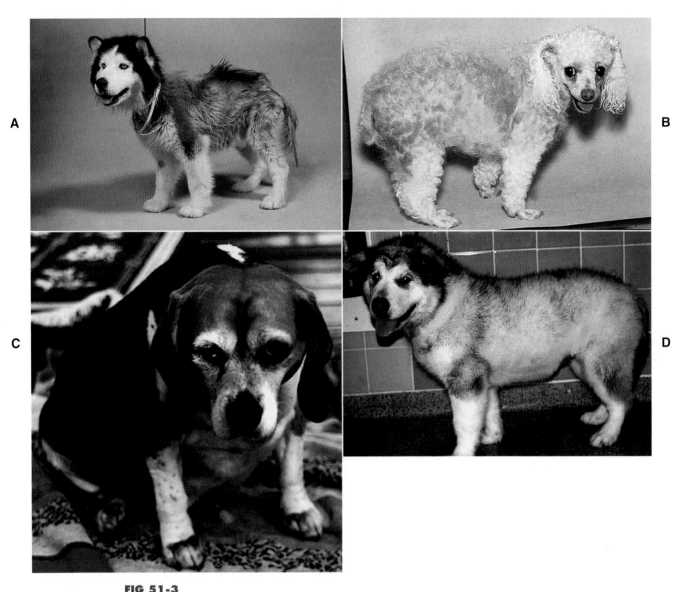

**FIG 51-3**
**A,** A 4-year-old male Malamute with hypothyroidism; a dry, lusterless haircoat; and thinning of the truncal hairs. **B,** A 6-year-old female spayed Poodle with hypothyroidism and endocrine alopecia. In both dogs, note the truncal distribution of the dermatologic problem with sparing of the head and extremities. **C,** An 8-year-old male castrated Beagle with hypothyroidism, obesity, and myxedema of the face. Note the "tragic facial expression" and "mental dullness" evident from the dog's facial expression. **D,** A 7-month-old female Malamute with congenital hypothyroidism. Note the retention of the puppy haircoat and small stature of the dog.

of von Willebrand factor in euthyroid dogs with von Willebrand's disease.

A cause-and-effect relationship between hypothyroidism and behavioral problems (e.g., aggression) has not been established in dogs. To date, most reports have been anecdotal and based on improvement in behavior following initiation of thyroid hormone treatment. An inverse relationship between development of aggression and serotonin activity in the CNS has been documented in several species, including dogs. Serotonin turnover and sympathetic activity in the CNS increase in rats made hypothyroid following surgical thyroidectomy, dopamine receptor sensitivity is affected by thy-

roid hormone in rats, and thyroid hormone potentiates the activity of tricyclic antidepressants in humans suffering from certain types of depression. These studies suggest that thyroid hormone may have an influence on the serotonin-dopamine pathway in the CNS, regardless of the functional status of the thyroid gland. The benefits, if any, of using thyroid hormone to treat behavioral disorders such as aggression in dogs remains to be clarified.

**Cretinism.** Hypothyroidism in puppies is termed *cretinism.* As the age of onset increases, the clinical appearance of animals with cretinism merges imperceptibly with that of adult hypothyroidism. Retarded growth and impaired mental

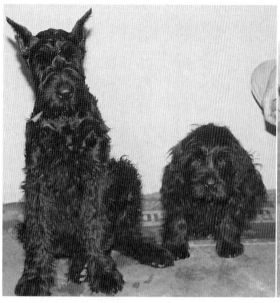

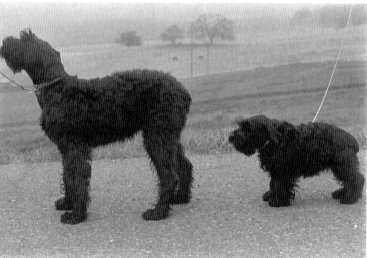

A

B

**FIG 51-4**
**A** and **B,** Eight-month-old female Giant Schnauzer littermates. The dog on the left is normal, whereas the smaller dog on the right has congenital hypothyroidism (cretinism). Note the small stature; disproportionate body size; large, broad head; wide, square trunk; and short limbs in the cretin. (From Feldman EC, Nelson RW: *Canine and feline endocrinology and reproduction,* ed 2, Philadelphia, 1996, WB Saunders.)

TABLE 51-4

### Clinical Signs of Cretinism

Disproportionate dwarfism
Short, broad skull
Shortened mandible
Enlarged cranium
Shortened limbs
Kyphosis
Mental dullness
Constipation
Inappetence
Gait abnormalities
Delayed dental eruption
Alopecia
Retention of puppy haircoat
Dry hair
Thick skin
Lethargy
Dyspnea
Goiter

development are the hallmarks of cretinism (Table 51-4). Dogs with cretinism have a disproportionate body size, with large, broad heads; thick, protruding tongues; wide, square trunks; and short limbs (Fig. 51-4). This is in contrast to the proportionate dwarfism caused by growth hormone deficiency. Cretins are mentally dull and lethargic and do not show the typical playfulness seen in normal puppies. Persistence of the puppy haircoat, alopecia, inappetence, delayed dental eruption, and goiter are additional signs. Differential diagnoses for failure to grow include endocrine (e.g., dwarfism) and nonendocrine causes (see Table 49-12 and Fig. 49-11). The presence of goiter is variable and dependent on the underlying etiology.

**Immunoendocrinopathy syndromes.** Because autoimmune mechanisms play an important role in the pathogenesis of lymphocytic thyroiditis, it is not surprising that lymphocytic thyroiditis may occur in conjunction with other immune-mediated endocrinopathies. Presumably, the immune-mediated attack is directed against antigens shared by the endocrine system. In human beings, autoimmune polyglandular syndrome type II (Schmidt's syndrome) is the most common of the immunoendocrinopathy syndromes, and it usually consists of primary adrenal insufficiency, autoimmune thyroid disease, and type 1 diabetes mellitus. Immunoendocrinopathy syndromes are uncommon in dogs and should be suspected in a dog found to have multiple endocrine gland failure. Hypothyroidism, hypoadrenocorticism, and, to a lesser extent, diabetes mellitus, hypoparathyroidism, and lymphocytic orchitis are recognized combined syndromes. In most affected dogs, each endocrinopathy is manifested separately, with additional disorders ensuing one by one after variable periods (weeks to months). Diagnostic tests and treatment are directed at each disorder as it is recognized, because it is not possible to reliably predict or prevent any of these problems. Immunosuppressive drug therapy is not indicated for animals with these syndromes,

Blood vessel

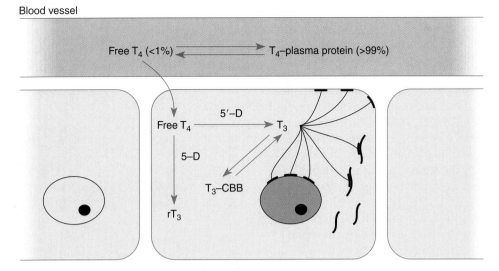

**FIG 51-5**
Intracellular metabolism of free $T_4$ to either $T_3$ or reverse $T_3$ by 5'- or 5-monodeiodinase, respectively. Intracellular $T_3$ formed from monodeiodination of free $T_4$ can interact with $T_3$ receptors on the cell membrane, mitochondria, or nucleus of the cell and stimulate the physiologic actions of thyroid hormone or bind to cytoplasmic binding proteins *(CBB)*. The latter form an intracellular storage pool for $T_3$. (From Feldman EC, Nelson RW: *Canine and feline endocrinology and reproduction*, ed 2, Philadelphia, 1996, WB Saunders.)

because the adverse effects of immunosuppressive therapy and the difficulty posed by suppression of the immune destruction of affected endocrine glands outweigh the potential benefits of such therapy.

## Clinical Pathology

The most consistent clinicopathologic findings in dogs with hypothyroidism are hypercholesterolemia and hypertriglyceridemia; the latter is identified as lipemia. Hypercholesterolemia is identified in approximately 75% of hypothyroid dogs, and the cholesterol concentration can exceed 1000 mg/dl. Although fasting hypercholesterolemia and hypertriglyceridemia can be associated with several other disorders (see p. 822), their presence in a dog with appropriate clinical signs is strong evidence for hypothyroidism.

A mild normocytic, normochromic, nonregenerative anemia (packed cell volume [PCV] of 28% to 35%) is a less consistent finding. Evaluation of red blood cell morphology may reveal an increase in the numbers of leptocytes (target cells), which develop as a result of increased erythrocyte membrane cholesterol loading. The white blood cell count is typically normal, and platelet counts are normal to increased.

A mild to moderate increase in lactate dehydrogenase, aspartate aminotransferase, alanine transaminase, alkaline phosphatase, and, rarely, creatine kinase activities may also be identified but are extremely inconsistent findings and may not be directly related to the hypothyroid state. Mild hypercalcemia may be found in some dogs with congenital hypothyroidism. Results of urinalysis are usually normal in dogs with hypothyroidism. Polyuria, hyposthenuria, and urinary tract infections are not typical of hypothyroidism.

## Dermatohistopathologic Findings

Skin biopsies are often performed in dogs with suspected endocrine alopecia, especially if screening diagnostic tests (including tests to assess thyroid gland function) have failed to identify the cause. Nonspecific histologic changes are associated with various endocrinopathies, including hypothyroidism (see Table 49-7); histologic alterations that are claimed to be specific to hypothyroidism may also be seen. A variable inflammatory cell infiltrate may be present if a secondary pyoderma has developed. The finding of "hypothyroid-specific" histopathologic alterations is an indication for further evaluation of thyroid gland function.

## Tests of Thyroid Gland Function

**Overview.** Function of the thyroid gland is typically assessed by measuring the baseline serum thyroid hormone concentrations. Several baseline thyroid hormone tests are available, including those that measure thyroxine ($T_4$), free $T_4$ ($fT_4$), 3,5,3'-triiodothyronine ($T_3$), free $T_3$ ($fT_3$), 3,3',5'-triiodothyronine (reverse $T_3$ [$rT_3$]), and endogenous TSH concentration. $T_4$ accounts for most of the thyroid hormone secreted by the thyroid gland, with only small quantities of $T_3$ and minor amounts of $rT_3$ released. Once it is secreted into the circulation, more than 99% of $T_4$ is bound to plasma proteins. The unbound, or free, $T_4$ is biologically active, exerts negative feedback inhibition on pituitary TSH secretion (see Fig. 51-1), and is capable of entering cells throughout the body (Fig. 51-5). Protein-bound $T_4$ acts as a reservoir and buffer to maintain a steady concentration of free hormone in the plasma, despite rapid alterations in the delivery of thyroid hormone to tissues. Within the cell, $fT_4$ is deiodinated to form either $T_3$ or $rT_3$, depending on the metabolic demands of the tissues at that particular time. $T_3$ is preferentially produced during normal metabolic states, whereas $rT_3$, which is biologically inactive, appears to be produced during periods of illness, starvation, or excessive endogenous catabolism. Intracellular $T_3$ binds to receptors on the mitochondria, nucleus, and plasma membrane and exerts its physiologic effects. $T_3$ is believed to be the primary hormone that induces physiologic effects, because of its greater biologic activity and volume of distribution compared with those of $T_4$, the preferential deiodination of $T_4$ to $T_3$ within the cell, and the presence of specific intracellular receptors for $T_3$.

All serum $T_4$, both protein bound and free, comes from the thyroid gland. Therefore tests that measure the serum total and $fT_4$ concentrations, in conjunction with the serum TSH concentration, are currently recommended for the assessment of thyroid gland function in dogs suspected of having hypothyroidism. In contrast, most $T_3$ and $rT_3$ is formed through the deiodination of $T_4$ in extrathyroidal sites, most notably the liver, kidney, and muscle. Serum $T_3$ concentration is a poor gauge of thyroid gland function because of its predominant location within cells and the minimal amount secreted by the thyroid gland in comparison with the amount of $T_4$ secreted (Fig. 51-6). Thus measurement of serum $T_3$, $fT_3$, and $rT_3$ concentration is not recommended for the assessment of thyroid gland function in dogs.

**Baseline serum $T_4$ concentration.** The baseline serum $T_4$ concentration is the sum of the protein-bound and free levels circulating in the blood. Measurement of the serum $T_4$ concentration can be used as the initial test for hypothyroidism or be part of a thyroid panel containing $T_4$, $fT_4$, TSH, and an antibody test for lymphocytic thyroiditis (Table 51-5).

Measurement of serum $T_4$ by radioimmunoassay (RIA) is more accurate than in-clinic ELISA methods (e.g., Snap $T_4$ Test; IDEX Laboratories). Theoretically, the interpretation of baseline serum $T_4$ concentration should be straightforward in that dogs with hypothyroidism should have low values as compared with the values in healthy dogs. Unfortunately, the serum $T_4$ concentration range in hypothyroid dogs overlaps with that in healthy dogs, and this overlap becomes more evident in euthyroid dogs with concurrent illness. The amount of residual thyroid gland function at the time the sample is obtained, the suppressive effects of extraneous factors on serum thyroid hormone concentrations, and the presence of circulating antithyroid hormone antibodies all affect the sensitivity and specificity of the serum $T_4$ concentration in the diagnosis of hypothyroidism.

An arbitrary serum $T_4$ value is not used to distinguish euthyroidism from hypothyroidism. Rather, the $T_4$ value should be evaluated in the context of the history, physical examination findings, and other clinicopathologic data. All of this information yields an index of suspicion for euthyroidism or hypothyroidism. As a clinician, it is difficult to judge the effect that extraneous factors, especially concurrent illness, have on the serum $T_4$ concentration. Because these variables can suppress a baseline serum $T_4$ concentration to less than 0.5 µg/dl

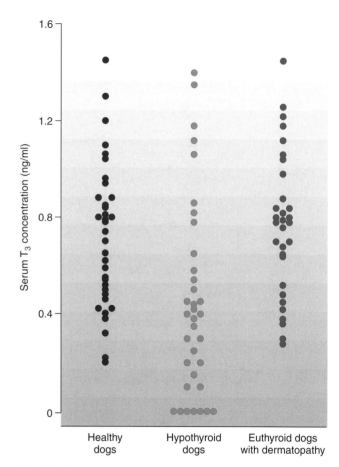

**FIG 51-6**
Baseline serum $T_3$ concentrations in 35 healthy dogs, 35 dogs with hypothyroidism, and 30 euthyroid dogs with concurrent dermatopathy. Note the overlap in serum $T_3$ concentrations among the three groups of dogs.

in a euthyroid dog and hypothyroid dogs rarely have a serum $T_4$ concentration greater than 1.5 µg/dl, the baseline serum $T_4$ concentration is used as a measure of euthyroidism. The higher the $T_4$ concentration, the more likely it is that the dog is euthyroid (Table 51-6). The one exception is the hypothyroid dog with circulating antithyroid hormone antibodies (see p. 700). Conversely, the lower the $T_4$ value, the more likely it is that the dog has hypothyroidism, assuming that the history, physical examination findings, and clinicopathologic data are also consistent with the disease. If the clinician's index of suspicion for hypothyroidism is not high but the serum $T_4$ concentration is low, then other factors such as euthyroid sick syndrome must also be considered (see p. 702).

**Baseline serum $fT_4$ concentrations.** Serum $fT_4$ is currently measured by one of two methods: RIA using kits designed for use in human beings and a modified equilibrium dialysis (MED) technique that uses a short dialysis step to separate $fT_4$ from protein-bound $T_4$, followed by RIA for $fT_4$. The MED technique (Nichols Institute, San Juan Capistrano, Calif) is the most accurate method for determining serum $fT_4$ concentrations and is the preferred $fT_4$ test for assessing

## TABLE 51-5

### Diagnostic Recommendations for Evaluating Thyroid Gland Function in Dogs

1. The decision to assess thyroid gland function should be based on results of the history, physical examination, and routine bloodwork (CBC, serum biochemistry panel, urinalysis).
2. Initial single screening tests include baseline serum $T_4$ and baseline serum free $T_4$ measured by modified equilibrium dialysis (MED).
   a. Treatment is indicated if the serum $T_4$ or free $T_4$ concentration is low and the initial evaluation of the dog strongly supports the diagnosis of hypothyroidism.
   b. Treatment is not indicated if the serum $T_4$ or free $T_4$ concentration is normal and the initial evaluation of the dog does not strongly support the diagnosis of hypothyroidism.
   c. Additional diagnostic tests (i.e., endogenous TSH, thyroglobulin autoantibody, or thyroid hormone autoantibody) are indicated if the serum $T_4$ concentration is normal but the initial evaluation of the dog strongly supports the diagnosis of hypothyroidism, or if the veterinarian is uncertain whether hypothyroidism exists after evaluation of the history, physical examination, routine bloodwork, and serum $T_4$ or free $T_4$ concentration.
3. Commonly used screening protocols using two diagnostic tests include baseline serum $T_4$ or baseline serum free $T_4$ measured by MED and serum TSH concentration.
   a. Treatment is indicated if the serum $T_4$ or free $T_4$ concentration is low and the initial evaluation of the dog strongly supports the diagnosis of hypothyroidism, regardless of the serum TSH test result.
   b. Treatment is not indicated if all of these tests are normal and the initial evaluation of the dog does not strongly support the diagnosis of hypothyroidism.
   c. Treatment is not indicated and the tests should be repeated in 8 to 12 weeks if the serum free $T_4$ concentration is normal and the serum TSH concentration is increased.
   d. Evaluation of serum thyroglobulin or a $T_4$ autoantibody test is indicated if serum $T_4$ concentration is normal, serum TSH concentration is increased, and the initial evaluation of the dog strongly supports the diagnosis of hypothyroidism.
4. Common components of a thyroid panel include serum $T_4$ concentration, serum $T_4$ concentration measured by MED, serum TSH concentration, and an antibody test for lymphocytic thyroiditis.
   a. Treatment is indicated if all of the tests for thyroid gland function are abnormal and the initial evaluation of the dog strongly supports the diagnosis of hypothyroidism, regardless of the thyroid hormone antibody test results.
   b. Treatment is not indicated if all of the tests for thyroid gland function are normal and the initial evaluation of the dog does not strongly support the diagnosis of hypothyroidism, regardless of the thyroid hormone antibody test results. Positive thyroid hormone antibody test results support the presence of lymphocytic thyroiditis and the need to monitor tests of thyroid gland function every 3 to 6 months.
   c. When discordant thyroid gland function test results are obtained, the decision to treat should be based on the initial evaluation of the dog, the clinician's index of suspicion for hypothyroidism, and a critical evaluation of each thyroid gland function test result. Serum free $T_4$ concentration by MED is the most accurate test of thyroid gland function.

Modified from the International Symposium on Canine Hypothyroidism, published in *Canine Practice*, vol 22, 1997.

---

thyroid gland function in dogs. Accuracy of the MED assay has been greater than 90% in all studies in which it has been critically evaluated, compared with an accuracy of 75% to 85% for serum $T_4$. In general, serum $fT_4$ values obtained by the MED technique that are greater than 1.5 ng/dl are consistent with euthyroidism, and values less than 1.0 ng/dl (especially those <0.5 ng/dl) are suggestive of hypothyroidism, assuming that the history, physical examination, and clinicopathologic abnormalities are also consistent with the disorder. Circulating antithyroid hormone antibodies do not affect the $fT_4$ results determined by the MED test. Serum $fT_4$ is not affected by the suppressive effects of concurrent illness as much as serum $T_4$, although severe illness can cause $fT_4$ concentrations to decrease below 0.5 ng/dl (see Concurrent Illness [Euthyroid Sick Syndrome], p. 702).

## TABLE 51-6

### Interpretation of Baseline Serum Thyroxine ($T_4$) and Free Thyroxine ($fT_4$) Concentration in Dogs with Suspected Hypothyroidism

| SERUM $T_4$ CONCENTRATION ($\mu g/dl$) | SERUM $fT_4$ CONCENTRATION (ng/dl) | PROBABILITY OF HYPOTHYROIDISM |
|---|---|---|
| >2.0 | >2.0 | Very unlikely |
| 1.5-2.0 | 1.5-2.0 | Unlikely |
| 1.0-1.5 | 0.8-1.5 | Unknown |
| 0.5-1.0 | 0.5-0.8 | Possible |
| <0.5 | <0.5 | Very likely* |

*Assuming that a severe systemic illness is not present.

**Baseline endogenous canine TSH concentration.**
Currently there are two validated canine TSH (cTSH) assays: a commercially available immunoradiometric assay manufactured by the Diagnostic Products Corporation (DPC, Los Angeles, Calif) and an in-house cTSH assay offered by the Endocrine Section, Animal Health Diagnostic Laboratory, College of Veterinary Medicine, Michigan State University, East Lansing. Unfortunately, serum cTSH concentrations measured in hypothyroid dogs overlap with those for euthyroid dogs with concurrent illness, and approximately 20% of hypothyroid dogs have normal cTSH concentrations (i.e., $<0.6$ ng/ml) (Fig. 51-7). In most studies the sensitivity and specificity of the cTSH assay have averaged approximately 80%.

The endogenous cTSH concentration should always be interpreted in conjunction with the serum $T_4$ or $fT_4$ concentrations measured in the same blood sample and should never be used as the sole test of thyroid gland function. Finding a low serum $T_4$ or $fT_4$ concentration and a high cTSH concentration in a blood sample obtained from a dog with appropriate history and physical examination findings supports the diagnosis of primary hypothyroidism, and finding normal serum $T_4$, $fT_4$, and cTSH concentrations rules out hypothyroidism. Any other combination of serum $T_4$, $fT_4$, and cTSH concentrations is difficult to interpret, but because of the high accuracy of the assay, reliance on $fT_4$ measured by MED technique is recommended. A normal serum $T_4$ or $fT_4$ concentration and an increased serum cTSH concentration are found in the early stages of primary hypothyroidism in humans. Although similar thyroid hormone and cTSH results have been identified in dogs, it is not known what percent of these dogs will progress to clinical hypothyroidism. Clinical signs of hypothyroidism are usually not evident in these dogs, in part because serum $T_4$ and $fT_4$ concentrations are in the normal range. Treatment with sodium levothyroxine is not indicated. Rather, assessment of thyroid gland function should be repeated in 2 to 4 months, especially if antibody tests for lymphocytic thyroiditis are positive. If progressive destruction of the thyroid gland is occurring, serum $T_4$ and $fT_4$ will gradually decrease and endogenous cTSH will increase with time, and clinical signs will eventually develop.

**TSH and TRH stimulation tests.** TSH and TRH stimulation tests evaluate the thyroid gland's responsiveness to exogenous TSH and TRH administration, respectively. The primary advantage of these tests is that they differentiate hypothyroidism from euthyroid sick syndrome (see p. 702) in dogs with low baseline thyroid hormone concentrations. Although the TSH stimulation test is preferred, TSH for injection is no longer available at a reasonable cost for use in dogs and cats. The TRH stimulation test is still available for use in dogs and cats, although TRH for injection is becoming difficult to obtain. This test is not commonly performed. Numerous different protocols for the TRH stimulation test have been recommended in the literature, which emphasizes the importance of following the procedure recommended by the specific laboratory performing the measurement. Adverse effects of TRH doses in excess of 0.1 mg/kg include increased salivation, urination, defecation, vomiting, miosis, tachycardia, and tachypnea. The lowest dose of TRH that maximally stimulates $T_4$ secretion without causing adverse reactions should be used in the TRH stimulation test. At our hospital, 0.2 mg of TRH per dog (regardless of dog size) is administered intravenously, and blood for the serum total $T_4$ determination is obtained before and 4 hours after TRH administration.

Using the TRH protocol just described, euthyroid dogs should have a post–TRH administration serum $T_4$ concentration of greater than 2 $\mu$g/dl. Alternatively, the post-TRH serum $T_4$ concentration should increase by at least 0.5 $\mu$g/dl above the baseline serum $T_4$ concentration in a euthyroid dog. In contrast, dogs with primary hypothyroidism should have a post-TRH serum $T_4$ concentration below the normal baseline serum $T_4$ concentration range (i.e., $<1.5$ $\mu$g/dl), and there should be a less than 0.5 $\mu$g/dl increase in the serum $T_4$ concentration after TRH administration (Fig. 51-8). Post-TRH serum $T_4$ concentrations between 1.5 and 2.0 $\mu$g/dl are nondiagnostic and may be found in the early stages of hypothyroidism or may represent suppression of thyroid gland function as a result of concurrent illness or drug therapy in an otherwise euthyroid dog.

**Tests for lymphocytic thyroiditis**
The finding of circulating thyroid hormone ($T_4$ and $T_3$) and thyroglobulin (Tg) autoantibodies is believed to correlate with the presence of lymphocytic thyroiditis. Tg autoantibodies occur in conjunction with $T_3$ and $T_4$ autoantibodies and are identified in dogs with lymphocytic thyroiditis who are not positive for $T_3$ and $T_4$ autoantibodies, implying that Tg autoantibody determination is a better screening test for lymphocytic thyroiditis than $T_3$ and $T_4$ autoantibodies. Presence of Tg autoantibodies implies pathology in the thyroid gland but provides no information about the severity or progressive nature of the inflammatory response or the extent of thyroid gland involvement; nor is this test an indicator of thyroid gland function. Tg autoantibodies should not be used alone in the diagnosis of hypothyroidism. Dogs with confirmed hypothyroidism can be negative and euthyroid dogs can be positive for Tg autoantibodies. Identification of Tg autoantibodies would support hypothyroidism caused by lymphocytic thyroiditis if the dog had clinical signs, physical findings, and thyroid hormone test results consistent with the disorder.

Tg autoantibodies may be used as a prebreeding screen for lymphocytic thyroiditis in valuable breeding dogs. Currently a positive Tg autoantibody test is considered suggestive of lymphocytic thyroiditis and supports retesting in several months, before breeding the dog. The value of serum Tg autoantibodies as a marker for eventual development of hypothyroidism remains to be clarified. A recent 1-year prospective study found that approximately 20% of 171 dogs with positive Tg autoantibody and normal $fT_4$ and cTSH test results developed changes in $fT_4$ and/or had cTSH test results consistent with hypothyroidism 1 year later; 15% reverted to a negative Tg autoantibody test with no change in $fT_4$ and cTSH test results, and 65% remained Tg autoantibody positive or had an inconclusive result with no change in $fT_4$ and cTSH test results 1 year later (Graham and colleagues, 2001).

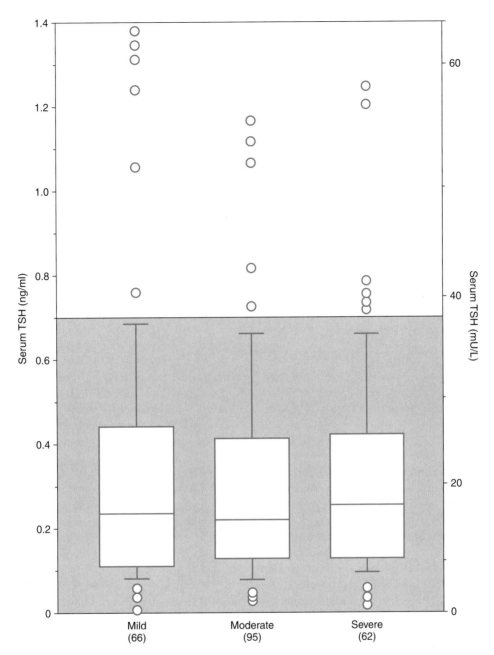

**FIG 51-7**
Box plots of serum concentrations of thyrotropin (TSH) concentrations in 223 dogs with nonthyroidal disease stratified according to severity of disease. For each box plot, T-bars represent the main body of data, which in most instances is equal to the range. Each box represents an interquartile range (25th to 75th percentile). The horizontal bar in each box is the median. Open circles represent outlying data points. Numbers in parentheses indicate the numbers of dogs in each group. Shaded area is the normal range. (From Kantrowitz LB et al: Serum total thyroxine, total triiodothyronine, free thyroxine, and thyrotropin concentrations in dogs with nonthyroidal disease, *J Am Vet Med Assoc* 219:765, 2001.)

Testing for serum $T_4$ autoantibodies is indicated in dogs with unusual serum $T_4$ values. $T_4$ autoantibodies may interfere with the RIAs used to measure serum $T_4$ concentrations, which thereby yield spurious and thus unreliable values. The type of interference depends on the separation system used in the RIA. Falsely low results are obtained if nonspecific sepa-

ration methods are used (e.g., ammonium sulfate, activated charcoal); falsely increased values are obtained if single-step separation systems utilizing antibody-coated tubes are used. Fortunately, spurious $T_4$ values resulting from clinically relevant concentrations of thyroid hormone antibody account for less than 1% of such results from commercial endocrine

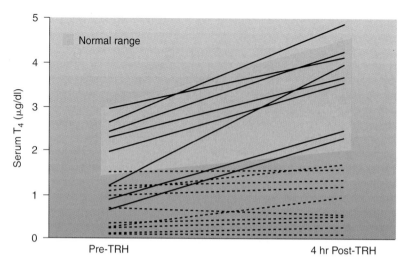

**FIG 51-8**
Results of a TRH stimulation test in 10 dogs with naturally developing hypothyroidism *(dotted lines)* and 8 euthyroid dogs with concurrent pyoderma *(solid lines)*. The dark gray region represents the reference range for pre– and post–TRH administration serum T$_4$ concentrations.

laboratories. Serum fT$_4$ measured by MED is not affected by T$_4$ autoantibodies and should be evaluated in lieu of serum T$_4$ in dogs suspected of having T$_4$ autoantibodies.

## Factors Affecting Thyroid Gland Function Tests

There are many factors that affect baseline thyroid hormone and endogenous cTSH concentrations (Table 51-7). Unfortunately, many of these factors decrease baseline thyroid hormone concentrations and may increase endogenous cTSH in euthyroid dogs, potentially causing misdiagnosis of hypothyroidism if the clinician accepts the results out of context. The most common factors that result in lower baseline thyroid hormone concentrations in euthyroid dogs are concurrent illness (i.e., euthyroid sick syndrome), drugs (especially glucocorticoids; see Table 51-7), and random fluctuations in thyroid hormone concentrations. Such random fluctuations in baseline serum T$_4$ concentrations occur in healthy dogs, euthyroid dogs with concurrent illness, and hypothyroid dogs, and in euthyroid dogs these fluctuations may result in a serum T$_4$ concentration below 1.0 µg/dl (Fig. 51-9). A diurnal pattern for thyroid hormone secretion has not been identified in dogs.

**Concurrent illness (euthyroid sick syndrome).** *Euthyroid sick syndrome* refers to suppression of serum thyroid hormone concentrations in euthyroid dogs in response to concurrent illness. A decrease in serum thyroid hormone concentrations may result from a decline in TSH secretion secondary to suppression of the hypothalamus or pituitary gland, from decreased synthesis of T$_4$, from decreased concentration or binding affinity of circulating binding proteins (e.g., thyroid binding globulin), from inhibition of the deiodination of T$_4$ to T$_3$, or any combination of these factors. The subsequent decrease in serum total T$_4$ and, in many cases, fT$_4$ concentrations is believed to represent a physiologic adapta-

tion by the body, with the purpose being to decrease cellular metabolism during periods of illness. It is not indicative of hypothyroidism, per se. Generally, the type and magnitude of most alterations in serum thyroid hormone concentrations are not unique to a specific disorder but reflect the severity of the illness or the catabolic state and appear to represent a continuum of changes. Systemic illness has more of an effect in lowering serum thyroid hormone concentrations than do, for example, dermatologic disorders. In addition, the more severe the systemic illness, the more suppressive the effect on the serum thyroid hormone concentration (Fig. 51-10).

Unfortunately, euthyroid dogs with concurrent illness can have serum T$_4$ concentrations that often fall between 0.5 and 1.0 µg/dl, and with severe illness (e.g., cardiomyopathy, severe anemia) these concentrations can be less than 0.5 µg/dl. Alterations in serum concentrations of fT$_4$ and cTSH are more variable and probably depend in part on the pathophysiologic mechanisms involved in the illness. In general, serum fT$_4$ concentrations tend to be decreased in dogs with concurrent illness but to a lesser extent than total T$_4$ concentrations. However, fT$_4$ concentrations can be less than 0.5 ng/dl if severe illness is present. cTSH concentrations may be normal or increased depending, in part, on the effect of the concurrent illness on fT$_4$ concentrations and on pituitary function. If pituitary function is suppressed, cTSH concentrations will be in the normal range or undetectable. If pituitary response to changes in fT4 concentration is not affected by the concurrent illness, cTSH concentrations will increase in response to a decrease in fT$_4$. Serum cTSH concentrations can easily exceed 1.0 ng/ml in dogs with euthyroid sick syndrome.

Treatment of euthyroid sick syndrome should be aimed at the concurrent illness. The serum thyroid hormone concentrations return to normal once the concurrent illness is eliminated. Treatment of euthyroid sick syndrome with sodium levothyroxine is not recommended.

TABLE 51-7

Variables That May Affect Baseline Serum Thyroid Hormone Function Test Results in Dogs

| FACTOR | EFFECT |
|---|---|
| Age | Inversely proportional effect |
|   Neonate (<3 mo) | Increased $T_4$ |
|   Aged (>6 yr) | Decreased $T_4$ |
| Body size | Inversely proportional effect |
|   Small (<10 kg) | Increased $T_4$ |
|   Large (>30 kg) | Decreased $T_4$ |
| Breed | |
|   Sight Hounds (e.g., Greyhound) | $T_4$ and free $T_4$ lower than normal range established for dogs; no difference for TSH |
| Gender | No effect |
| Time of day | No effect |
| Weight gain/obesity | Increased |
| Weight loss/fasting | Decreased $T_4$; no effect on free $T_4$ |
| Strenuous exercise | Increased $T_4$; decreased TSH; no effect on free $T_4$ |
| Estrus (estrogen) | No effect on $T_4$ |
| Pregnancy (progesterone) | Increased $T_4$ |
| Surgery/anesthesia | Decreased $T_4$ |
| Concurrent illness* | Decreased $T_4$ and free $T_4$; depending on illness, TSH may increase, decrease, or not change |
| Drugs | |
|   Carprofen | Decreased $T_4$, free $T_4$, and TSH |
|   Etodolac | No effect on $T_4$, free $T_4$, or TSH |
|   Glucocorticoids | Decreased $T_4$ and free $T_4$; decreased or no effect on TSH |
|   Furosemide | Decreased $T_4$ |
|   Methimazole | Decreased $T_4$ and free $T_4$; increased TSH |
|   Phenobarbital | Decreased $T_4$ and free $T_4$; delayed increase in TSH |
|   Phenylbutazone | Decreased $T_4$ |
|   Potassium bromide | No effect on $T_4$, free $T_4$, or TSH |
|   Progestagens | Decreased $T_4$ |
|   Propylthiouracil | Decreased $T_4$ and free $T_4$; increased TSH |
|   Sulfonamides | Decreased $T_4$ and free $T_4$; increased TSH |
|   Ipodate | Increased $T_4$; decreased $T_3$ |
| Dietary iodine intake | If excessive, decreased $T_4$ and free $T_4$; increased TSH |
| Thyroid hormone autoantibodies | Increased or decreased $T_4$; no effect on free $T_4$ or TSH |

*There is a direct correlation between the severity and systemic nature of the illness and suppression of the serum $T_4$ and free $T_4$ concentration.

## Diagnosis

The recommendations regarding the approach to the diagnosis of hypothyroidism, reached at an international symposium on canine hypothyroidism held at the University of California, Davis, in August 1996 (*Canine Practice*, Vol. 77, 1997), are given in Table 51-5.

Although measurement of serum $T_4$ concentration can be used as an initial screening test, evaluation of a thyroid panel that includes $T_4$, $fT_4$ measured by MED, cTSH, and Tg autoantibodies provides a more informative analysis of the pituitary-thyroid axis and thyroid gland function. Low serum $T_4$ and $fT_4$, and increased serum cTSH concentrations in a dog with appropriate clinical signs and clinicopathologic abnormalities strongly support the diagnosis of hypothyroidism. Concurrent presence of Tg autoantibodies suggests lymphocytic thyroiditis as the underlying etiology. Unfortu-

nately, discordant test results are common. When this occurs, the appropriateness of clinical signs, clinicopathologic abnormalities, and clinician index of suspicion become the most important parameters when determining whether to treat the dog with sodium levothyroxine. Serum $fT_4$ concentration measured by MED is the most accurate test of thyroid gland function and carries the highest priority when assessing thyroid gland function, followed by serum $T_4$ concentration. Results of cTSH concentration increase the likelihood of euthyroidism or hypothyroidism when these results are consistent with results of serum $fT_4$, but cTSH test results should not be used as the sole indicator of hypothyroidism. Low serum $fT_4$ and normal cTSH test results occur in approximately 20% of dogs with hypothyroidism, and high cTSH test results occur in euthyroid dogs with euthyroid sick syndrome. Normal serum $fT_4$ and high cTSH may suggest early compensated

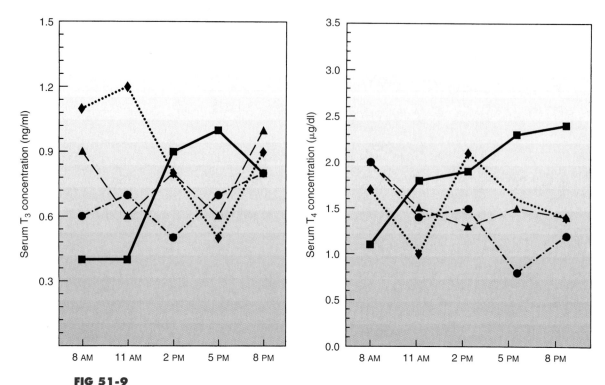

**FIG 51-9**

Sequential baseline serum $T_3$ and $T_4$ concentrations measured in blood samples obtained at 8 AM, 11 AM, 2 PM, 5 PM, and 8 PM in four healthy dogs. Note the random fluctuation in the serum $T_3$ and $T_4$ concentrations throughout the day and the occasional low value, which could result in a misdiagnosis of hypothyroidism. (From Feldman EC, Nelson RW: *Canine and feline endocrinology and reproduction,* ed 2, Philadelphia, 1996, WB Saunders.)

hypothyroidism, but one has to wonder why clinical signs would develop if serum $fT_4$ were normal. Positive Tg autoantibody findings merely suggest the possibility of lymphocytic thyroiditis; Tg autoantibody determination is not a thyroid function test. Positive results increase the suspicion for hypothyroidism if serum $T_4$ or $fT_4$ concentrations are low but have no bearing on the generation of clinical signs if serum $T_4$ and $fT_4$ concentrations are normal. When faced with discordant test results, the decision becomes one of initiating trial therapy with sodium levothyroxine or repeating the tests sometime in the future—a decision that I usually base on the appropriateness of clinical signs and results of the $fT_4$ measured by MED.

Admittedly, interpretation of serum $T_4$, $fT_4$, and cTSH concentrations is not always simple. Because of expense and the frustration of working with tests that can fail to be reliable, many veterinarians and some clients prefer trial therapy as a diagnostic test. Trial therapy should be done only when thyroid hormone supplementation does not pose a risk to the patient. Response to trial therapy with sodium levothyroxine is nonspecific. A dog that has a positive response to therapy either has hypothyroidism or "thyroid-responsive disease." Because of its anabolic nature, thyroid supplementation can create an effect in a dog without thyroid dysfunction, especially regarding quality of the haircoat. Therefore if a positive response to trial therapy is observed, thyroid supplementa-

tion should be gradually discontinued once clinical signs have resolved. If clinical signs recur, hypothyroidism is confirmed and the supplement should be reinitiated. If clinical signs do not recur, a "thyroid-responsive disorder" or a beneficial response to concurrent therapy (e.g., antibiotics, flea control) should be suspected.

**Diagnosis in a previously treated dog.** Occasionally a clinician wants to determine if a dog receiving thyroid hormone supplementation is in fact hypothyroid. The exogenous administration of thyroid hormone, either $T_4$ or $T_3$, will suppress pituitary TSH secretion and cause pituitary thyrotroph atrophy and subsequently thyroid gland atrophy in a healthy euthyroid dog. Serum $T_4$, $fT_4$, and cTSH concentrations are decreased or undetectable; the severity of the decrease is dependent on the severity of thyroid gland atrophy induced by the thyroid supplement. Serum $T_4$ and $fT_4$ results are often suggestive of hypothyroidism, even in a previously euthyroid dog, if testing is performed within a month of discontinuing treatment. Thyroid hormone supplementation must be discontinued and the pituitary-thyroid axis allowed to regain function before meaningful baseline serum $T_4$ concentrations can be obtained. The time between the discontinuation of thyroid hormone supplementation and the acquisition of meaningful results regarding thyroid gland function depends on the duration of treatment, the dose and frequency of administration of the thyroid hormone supplement, and indi-

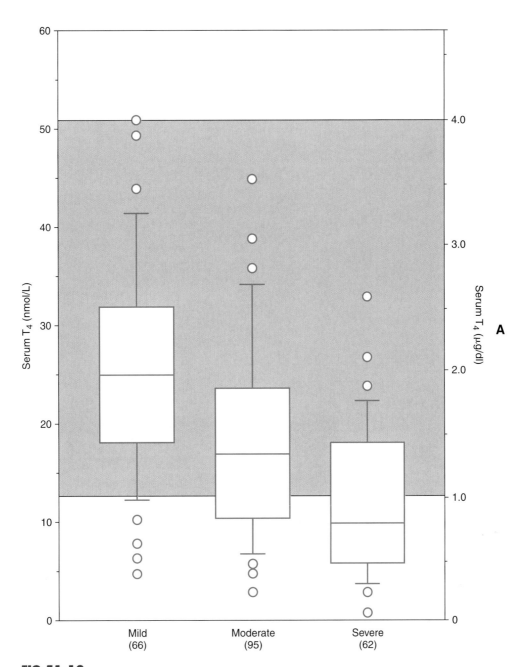

**FIG 51-10**
Box plots of serum total T$_4$ **(A)** and free T$_4$ **(B)** concentrations in 223 dogs with nonthyroidal disease stratified according to severity of disease. See Fig. 51-7 for explanation. (From Kantrowitz LB et al: Serum total thyroxine, total triiodothyronine, free thyroxine, and thyrotropin concentrations in dogs with nonthyroidal disease, *J Am Vet Med Assoc* 219:765, 2001.)

*Continued*

vidual variability. As a general rule, thyroid hormone supplements should be discontinued for a minimum of 4 weeks, but preferably 6 to 8 weeks, before thyroid gland function is critically assessed.

**Diagnosis in puppies.** A similar approach as discussed above is used to diagnose congenital hypothyroidism. However, serum cTSH concentrations are dependent on the etiology. cTSH concentrations will be increased in dogs with primary dysfunction of the thyroid gland (e.g., iodine organification defect) and an intact hypothalamic-pituitary-thyroid gland axis. However, cTSH concentrations will be within the normal range or undetectable in dogs with pituitary or hypothalamic dysfunction as the cause of the hypothyroidism. Results of a TRH stimulation test with measurement of cTSH and serum thyroid hormone concentrations may help localize the site of the problem.

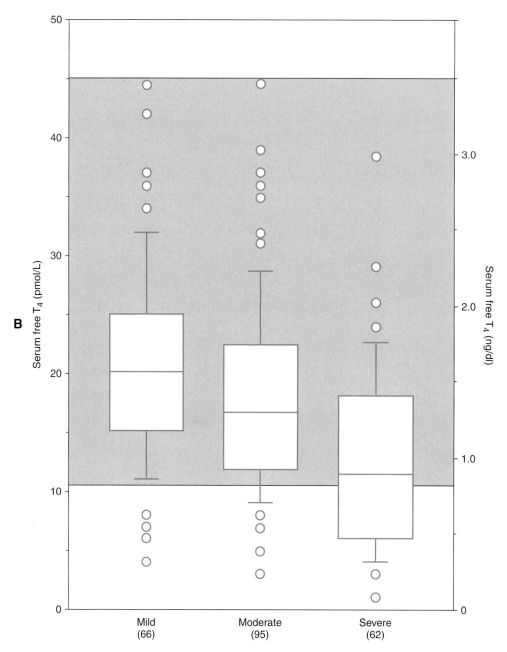

**FIG 51-10, cont'd**
Box plots of serum total T$_4$ **(A)** and free T$_4$ **(B)** concentrations in 223 dogs with nonthyroidal disease stratified according to severity of disease. See Fig. 51-7 for explanation. (From Kantrowitz LB et al: Serum total thyroxine, total triiodothyronine, free thyroxine, and thyrotropin concentrations in dogs with nonthyroidal disease, *J Am Vet Med Assoc* 219:765, 2001.)

## Treatment

### Initial therapy with sodium levothyroxine (synthetic T$_4$).

Synthetic levothyroxine is the treatment of choice for hypothyroidism. Its administration orally should result in normal serum concentrations of T$_4$, T$_3$, and cTSH, attesting to the fact that these products can be converted to the more metabolically active T$_3$ by peripheral tissues. A sodium levothyroxine product approved for use in dogs (e.g., Soloxine; King Pharmaceuticals, Bristol, Tenn) is recommended.

The initial dosage is 0.02 mg/kg body weight (0.1 mg/10 lb; maximum dose, 0.8 mg) every 12 hours. Because of variability in its absorption and metabolism, the dose and frequency may have to be adjusted before a satisfactory clinical response is observed; this variability is one reason for the monitoring of therapy in dogs.

**Response to sodium levothyroxine therapy.** Thyroid hormone supplementation should be continued for a minimum of 6 to 8 weeks before critically evaluating the effectiveness of treatment. With appropriate therapy, all of the clinical signs and clinicopathologic abnormalities associated with hypothyroidism are reversible. An increase in mental alertness and activity usually occurs initially and is seen within the first week of treatment; this is an important early indicator that the diagnosis of hypothyroidism was correct. Although some hair regrowth usually occurs within the first month in dogs with endocrine alopecia, it may take several months for complete regrowth and a marked reduction in hyperpigmentation of the skin to occur. Initially the haircoat may worsen as large amounts of hair in the telogen stage of the hair cycle are shed. Improvement in neurologic manifestations is usually evident within 1 to 2 weeks of initiating treatment; complete resolution of neurologic signs is unpredictable and may take 3 to 6 months of treatment before it occurs.

**Failure to respond to sodium levothyroxine therapy.** Problems with levothyroxine therapy should be suspected if clinical improvement is not seen within 8 weeks of the initiation of therapy. There are several possible reasons for a poor response to therapy (Table 51-8). An inappropriate diagnosis of hypothyroidism is the most obvious. Hyperadrenocorticism can be mistaken for hypothyroidism if other clinical signs (e.g., polyuria, polydipsia) commonly associated with hyperadrenocorticism are not present, because of the suppressive effects of cortisol on serum thyroid hormone concentrations (see p. 702). Failure to recognize the impact of concurrent illness on thyroid hormone test results is another common cause for misdiagnosing hypothyroidism. Concurrent disease (e.g., allergic skin disease, flea hypersensitivity) is common in dogs with hypothyroidism and may affect the clinical impression of response to sodium levothyroxine therapy if the disease is not recognized. Whenever a dog shows a poor response to levothyroxine therapy, the history, physical examination findings, and diagnostic test results that prompted the initiation of levothyroxine therapy should be critically reevaluated. A poor response to therapy may also be due to an inappropriate dose or frequency of administration of sodium levothyroxine, the use of some generic levothyroxine products, or poor intestinal absorption of the levothyroxine. The serum thyroid hormone concentrations should be monitored closely to identify these possibilities. Before measuring them, however, the clinician should investigate whether the poor response is a consequence of inadequate owner compliance in administering the hormone or the use of outdated preparations.

**Therapeutic monitoring.** Therapeutic monitoring includes evaluation of the clinical response to thyroid hormone supplementation and measurement of serum $T_4$ and cTSH concentrations before or after sodium levothyroxine administration, or both. These concentrations should be measured 4 to 8 weeks after initiating therapy, whenever signs of thyrotoxicosis develop, or if there has been minimal or no response to therapy. They should also be measured 2 to 4 weeks after an adjustment in levothyroxine therapy in dogs showing a poor response to treatment.

Serum $T_4$ and cTSH concentrations are typically evaluated 4 to 6 hours after the administration of levothyroxine in dogs

 **TABLE 51-8**

**Potential Reasons for Poor Clinical Response to Treatment with Sodium Levothyroxine (Synthetic $T_4$)**

Owner compliance problems
Use of inactivated or outdated product
Inappropriate sodium levothyroxine dose
Inappropriate frequency of administration
Low tablet strength*
Poor bioavailability (e.g., poor gastrointestinal tract absorption)
Inadequate time for clinical response to occur
Incorrect diagnosis of hypothyroidism

*Tablet strength refers to the actual amount of active drug in the tablet, as opposed to the stated amount.

receiving the medication twice daily and just before and 4 to 6 hours after administration in dogs receiving it once a day. This information allows the clinician to evaluate the dose, frequency of administration, and adequacy of intestinal absorption of sodium levothyroxine. Measurement of serum $fT_4$ by the MED technique can be done in lieu of measuring $T_4$ but is more expensive and probably does not offer additional information except in dogs with $T_4$ autoantibodies (see p. 700). The presence of thyroid hormone autoantibodies does not interfere with the physiologic actions of thyroid hormone supplements.

Post-dosing serum $T_4$ concentrations and recommendations for changes in therapy are given in Fig. 51-11. If the dose of the thyroid hormone supplement and the dosing schedule are appropriate, the serum $T_4$ concentrations should be in the upper half of or above the reference baseline range (i.e., 2.5 to 4.5 μg/dl) when measured 4 to 6 hours after thyroid hormone administration and cTSH concentration should be in the normal range (i.e., <0.6 ng/ml) in all blood samples evaluated. Post-dosing serum $T_4$ concentrations are frequently above the normal range. The finding of an increased postdosing serum $T_4$ concentration is therefore not an absolute indication to reduce the dose of sodium levothyroxine, especially if there are no clinical signs of thyrotoxicosis. However, a reduction in the dose is recommended whenever serum $T_4$ concentrations exceed 6.0 μg/dl.

**Thyrotoxicosis.** It is unusual for thyrotoxicosis to develop as a result of the excessive administration of sodium levothyroxine in the dog, owing to physiologic adaptations that impair gastrointestinal tract absorption and enhance clearance of thyroid hormone by the liver and kidneys. Nevertheless, thyrotoxicosis may develop in dogs receiving excessive amounts of sodium levothyroxine; in dogs in which the plasma half-life for levothyroxine is inherently prolonged, especially in those receiving levothyroxine twice daily; and in dogs with impaired metabolism of levothyroxine (e.g., concurrent renal or hepatic insufficiency). Rarely, thyrotoxicosis develops in a dog given minute amounts of sodium levothyroxine. The reason for this marked sensitivity to the hormone is not known.

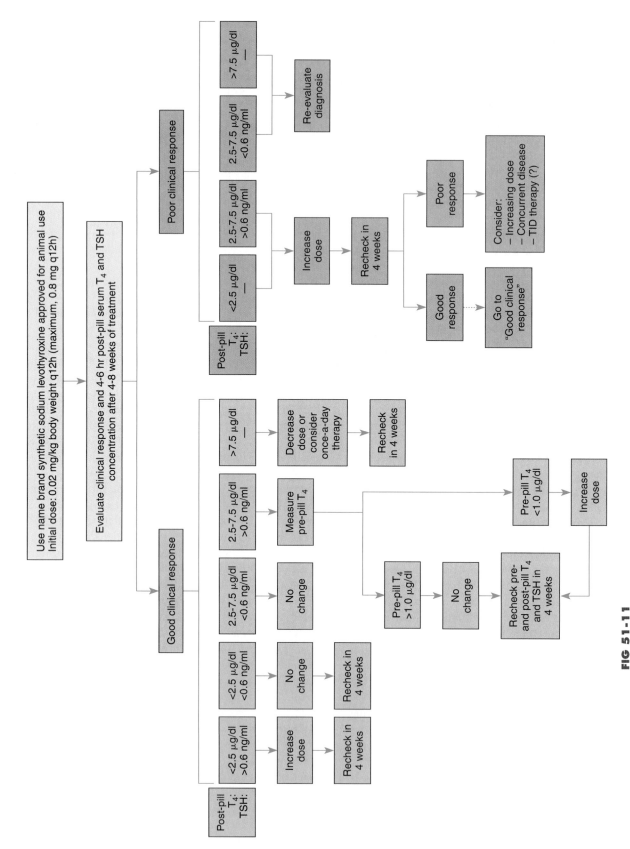

**FIG 51-11**
Initial therapeutic approach and monitoring recommendations for dogs with hypothyroidism.

Clinical signs of thyrotoxicosis include panting, nervousness, aggressive behavior, polyuria, polydipsia, polyphagia, and weight loss. The documentation of increased serum thyroid hormone concentrations supports the diagnosis. However, these concentrations can occasionally be within the normal range in a dog with signs of thyrotoxicosis, and they are commonly increased in dogs with no signs of thyrotoxicosis. Adjustments in the dose or frequency of administration of thyroid hormone medication, or both measures, are indicated if appropriate clinical signs develop in a dog receiving thyroid hormone supplements. Supplementation may have to be discontinued for a few days in such animals if the clinical signs are severe. Signs of thyrotoxicosis should resolve within 1 to 3 days if they are due to the thyroid medication and the adjustment in treatment has been appropriate. It is recommended that therapy be monitored 2 to 4 weeks after sodium levothyroxine treatment has been adjusted and the clinical signs have resolved.

### Prognosis

The prognosis for dogs with hypothyroidism depends on the underlying cause. The life expectancy of an adult dog with primary hypothyroidism that is receiving appropriate therapy should be normal. Most, if not all, of the clinical manifestations will resolve in response to thyroid hormone supplementation. The prognosis for puppies with hypothyroidism (i.e., cretinism) is guarded and depends on the severity of skeletal and joint abnormalities at the time treatment is initiated. Although many of the clinical signs resolve with therapy, musculoskeletal problems, especially degenerative osteoarthritis, may develop owing to abnormal bone and joint development. The prognosis for dogs with secondary hypothyroidism caused by malformation or destruction of the pituitary gland is guarded to poor. The life expectancy is shortened in dogs with congenital malformation of the pituitary gland (i.e., pituitary dwarfism), primarily because of the multiple problems that develop in early life (p. 677). Acquired secondary hypothyroidism is usually caused by destruction of the region by a space-occupying mass, which has the potential to expand into the brainstem.

## HYPOTHYROIDISM IN CATS

### Etiology

Iatrogenic hypothyroidism is the most common cause of hypothyroidism in cats and can result from bilateral thyroidectomy, radioactive iodine treatment, or an overdose of antithyroid drugs. Naturally acquired adult-onset primary hypothyroidism is rare; one cat with lymphocytic thyroiditis and clinical hypothyroidism has been described in the literature. Congenital primary hypothyroidism causing disproportionate dwarfism is recognized more frequently in cats than adult-onset hypothyroidism is. Reported causes of congenital hypothyroidism include a defect in thyroid hormone biosynthesis, most notably an iodine organification defect, and thyroid dysgenesis. Goiter is common in cats with defects in thyroid hormone biosynthesis because the hypothalamic-pituitary-thyroid gland axis remains intact. An inherited defect in iodine organification was documented in a family of Abyssinian cats with congenital hypothyroidism. The inbreeding of affected cats resulted in hypothyroidism in all offspring, whereas the breeding of affected cats with unrelated cats resulted in the birth of phenotypically normal kittens. These results indicate that the disease is inherited in an autosomal recessive fashion in this family of cats. Although rare, iodine deficiency has been reported to cause hypothyroidism in kittens fed a strict all-meat diet.

### Clinical Signs

Clinical signs of feline hypothyroidism are listed in Table 51-9. The most common are lethargy, inappetence, obesity, and seborrhea sicca. The lethargy and inappetence may become severe. Additional dermatologic signs may include a dry, lusterless, unkempt haircoat; easily epilated hair; poor regrowth of hair; and alopecia of the pinnae. Alopecia, if it develops, may be asymmetric or bilaterally symmetric, initially involving the lateral neck, thorax, and abdomen. Myxedema of the face resulting a "puffy" appearance has also been reported. Bradycardia and mild hypothermia may be additional physical examination findings.

The clinical signs of congenital hypothyroidism are similar to those in dogs (see p. 695). Affected kittens typically appear normal at birth, but a slowing of growth usually becomes evident by 6 to 8 weeks of age. Disproportionate dwarfism develops over the ensuing months, with large heads; short, broad necks; and short limbs developing in affected kittens (Fig. 51-12). Additional findings include lethargy, mental dullness, constipation, hypothermia, bradycardia, and

TABLE 51-9

**Clinical Manifestations of Feline Hypothyroidism**

| ADULT-ONSET HYPOTHYROIDISM | CONGENITAL HYPOTHYROIDISM |
|---|---|
| Lethargy | Disproportionate dwarfism |
| Inappetence | Failure to grow |
| Obesity | Large head |
| Dermatologic | Short, broad neck |
|   Seborrhea sicca | Short limbs |
|   Dry, lusterless haircoat | Lethargy |
|   Easily epilated hair | Mental dullness |
|   Poor regrowth of hair | Constipation |
|   Endocrine alopecia | Hypothermia |
|   Alopecia of pinnae | Bradycardia |
|   Thickened skin | Retention of kitten haircoat |
|   Myxedema of the face | Retention of deciduous teeth |
| Reproduction | |
|   Failure to cycle | |
|   Dystocia | |
| Bradycardia | |
| Mild hypothermia | |

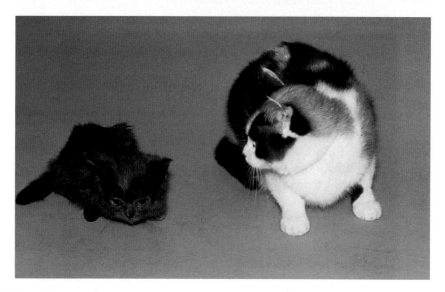

**FIG 51-12**
A 1-year-old domestic long-haired cat with pituitary dwarfism. A comparably aged cat is also present to illustrate the small size of the pituitary dwarf. Note the square, chunky contour of the head and the dull facial expression of the cat—findings that are suggestive of cretinism (see Fig. 49-10, p. 678, for comparison). The cat had concurrent growth hormone and thyroid hormone deficiency. (From Feldman EC, Nelson RW: *Canine and feline endocrinology and reproduction,* ed 2, Philadelphia, 1996, WB Saunders.)

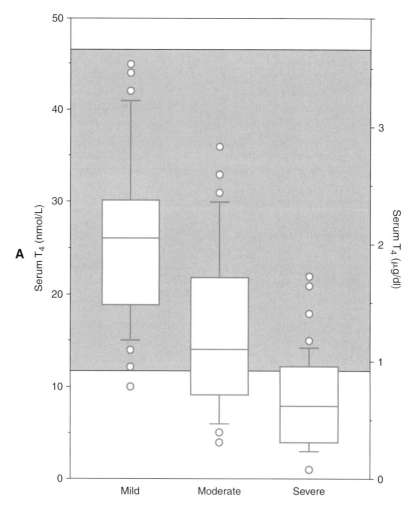

**FIG 51-13**
Box plots of serum total T$_4$ **(A)** and free T$_4$ **(B)** concentrations in 221 cats with nonthyroidal disease, grouped according to severity of illness. Of 221 cats with nonthyroidal illness, 65 had mild disease, 83 had moderate disease, and 73 had severe disease. See Fig. 51-7 for explanation. (From Peterson ME et al: Measurement of serum concentrations of free thyroxine, total thyroxine, and total triiodothyronine in cats with hyperthyroidism and cats with nonthyroidal disease, *J Am Vet Med Assoc* 218:529, 2001.)    *Continued*

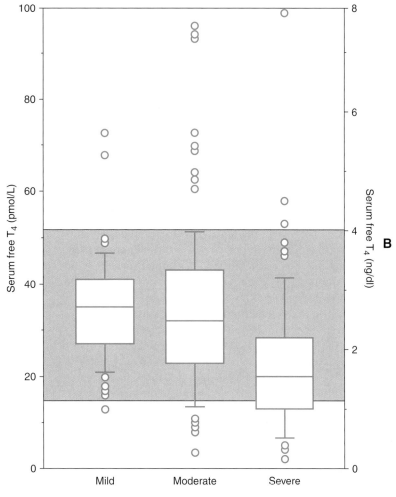

**FIG 51-13, cont'd**
For legend, see opposite page.

prolonged retention of deciduous teeth. The haircoat may consist mainly of an undercoat with primary guard hairs scattered thinly throughout.

## Diagnosis

The diagnosis of hypothyroidism in the cat should be based on a combination of history, clinical signs, physical examination findings, baseline serum $T_4$ or $fT_4$ concentrations, and, if indicated, the animal's response to exogenous TRH. The prevalence of hypercholesterolemia and normocytic, normochromic, nonregenerative anemia in adult cats with naturally acquired hypothyroidism is not known, but it is occasionally identified in cats with iatrogenic and congenital hypothyroidism. Therefore the initial screening blood tests for hypothyroidism in cats should include a complete blood count (CBC), measurement of the serum cholesterol concentration, and measurement of the baseline serum $T_4$ or $fT_4$ concentration. A normal serum $T_4$ or $fT_4$ concentration indicates that the cat is euthyroid. A low serum $T_4$ or $fT_4$ concentration in a cat that has undergone thyroidectomy or radioactive iodine treatment, or in a kitten with disproportion-

ate dwarfism, supports the diagnosis of hypothyroidism. The definitive diagnosis must then rely on the cat's response to trial therapy with sodium levothyroxine. Treatment with sodium levothyroxine is indicated for cats with iatrogenic hypothyroidism if they have appropriate clinical signs. Asymptomatic cats with a low serum $T_4$ or $fT_4$ concentration should not be treated until clinical signs become evident in the hope that additional time will allow atrophied or ectopic thyroid tissue to become functional.

Because naturally acquired primary hypothyroidism is rare, and because in our experience a low serum $T_4$ or $fT_4$ concentration in an adult cat is almost always caused by euthyroid sick syndrome (see p. 702; Fig. 51-13) or some other nonthyroidal factor, we are reluctant to diagnose hypothyroidism solely on the basis of the serum $T_4$ or $fT_4$ concentration in an adult cat that has not been previously treated for hyperthyroidism. A TRH (see p. 700) stimulation test should be performed to prove or disprove the diagnosis. The response to trial therapy with sodium levothyroxine is nonspecific and does not by itself establish or rule out the diagnosis. If trial therapy is attempted and a positive response is observed, thyroid supplementation should be gradually discontinued once the clinical signs have resolved. Hypothyroidism is likely if clinical signs recur after thyroid hormone treatment is discontinued and resolve after treatment is reinitiated.

## Treatment

Treatment of hypothyroidism in cats is similar to that used in dogs, which is described in detail on p. 706. Sodium levothyroxine is the recommended thyroid hormone supplement. The initial dosage for cats is 0.05 or 0.1 mg once or twice daily. A minimum of 4 to 8 weeks should elapse before the cat's clinical response to treatment is critically assessed. Subsequent reevaluations should include a history, physical examination, and measurement of serum $T_4$ concentrations (see Therapeutic Monitoring, p. 707). The goal of therapy is to eliminate the clinical signs of hypothyroidism but prevent signs of hyperthyroidism. This can usually be accomplished by maintaining the serum $T_4$ concentration between 1.0 and 2.5 mg/dl. The dose and frequency of sodium levothyroxine administration may have to be modified to attain these goals. If the serum thyroid hormone concentrations are normal after 4 to 8 weeks of treatment but there is no clinical response, the clinician should reassess the diagnosis.

## Prognosis

The prognosis for cats with hypothyroidism depends on the underlying cause and the age of the cat at the time clinical signs develop. The life expectancy of an adult cat with primary hypothyroidism that is receiving appropriate therapy should be normal. The prognosis for kittens with congenital hypothyroidism is guarded and depends on the severity of the skeletal changes at the time treatment is initiated. Although many of the clinical signs resolve with therapy, musculoskeletal problems may persist or develop owing to abnormal bone and joint development.

# HYPERTHYROIDISM IN CATS

## Etiology

Hyperthyroidism is a multisystemic disorder resulting from the excessive production and secretion of $T_4$ and $T_3$ by the thyroid gland and is almost always a result of chronic intrinsic disease in one or both thyroid lobes. One or more usually small, discrete thyroid masses are palpable in the ventral region of the neck in most cats with hyperthyroidism. Multinodular adenomatous goiter is the most common histologically observed thyroid lesion in thyrotoxic cats. Small, multifocal nodules are found throughout the gland in such cats; the lesions are histologically similar to the nodular hyperplasia seen in human beings. Less common are thyroid adenomas that cause the lobes to be enlarged and distorted; thyroid carcinoma accounts for less than 5% of clinical cases.

One or both thyroid lobes can be affected in thyrotoxic cats. Approximately 20% of hyperthyroid cats have unilateral thyroid lobe involvement (Fig. 51-14). The lobe causing the disease usually contains a solitary adenoma or adenomatous

hyperplasia. The nondiseased thyroid lobe is nonfunctioning and atrophied because of the suppressive effects of the hyperactive thyroid tissue on TSH secretion. More than 70% of hyperthyroid cats have bilateral involvement (Fig. 51-15). Of these cats, the thyroid lobes are symmetrically enlarged in 10% to 15% and asymmetrically enlarged in the remainder. Two distinct masses cannot always be appreciated on palpation, even if both lobes are large. Approximately 3% to 5% of thyrotoxic cats have hyperactive thyroid tissue in the anterior mediastinum, with or without a palpable mass in the neck (Fig. 51-16). It is not known whether this tissue represents ectopic thyroid tissue or one or more thyroid lobes that have gravitated down the neck as they got heavier and simply become trapped in the thorax. Functional thyroid carcinoma is the most likely diagnosis if more than two thyroid masses are present (see Fig. 51-16). Some of these cats initially have only one or two thyroid masses, emphasizing the importance of always histologically evaluating surgically removed tissue.

The pathogenesis of the adenomatous hyperplastic changes of the thyroid gland remains unclear. It has been postulated that immunologic, infectious, nutritional, environmental, or genetic factors may interact to cause pathologic changes. Epidemiologic studies have identified consumption of commercial canned cat foods as a risk factor for development of hyperthyroidism, suggesting that a goitrogenic compound (e.g., excess iodine, soy isoflavones) may be present in the diet. Environmental factors such as use of kitty litter may also be involved. The increase in the number of cats housed indoors and the corresponding change in quality of care and the types of cat food in the late 1960s and early 1970s followed by the "sudden" recognition of the disorder in the late 1970s supports a role for diet or the environment in the pathogenesis of hyperthyroidism. Recent studies have also identified overexpression of the *c-ras* oncogene in areas of nodular follicular hyperplasia in feline thyroid glands, suggesting that mutations in this oncogene may play a role in the pathogenesis of hyperthyroidism in cats (Merryman and colleagues, 1999). In the normal cell, activation of the *ras* protein leads to mitosis. Mutation of the *ras* oncogene produces mutated *ras* proteins that are not subject to the normal cellular feedback mechanisms that prevent uncontrolled mitosis. Altered expression of G proteins involved in the signal transduction pathway that stimulates growth and differentiation of thyroid cells may also play a role (Hammer and colleagues, 2000).

## Clinical Features

**Signalment.** Hyperthyroidism is the most common endocrinopathy affecting cats older than 8 years. The average age at the time of initial presentation to the veterinarian is 13 years, with a range of 4 to 20 years. Less than 5% of cats with this disorder are younger than 8 years. There is no sex-related predisposition; domestic short-haired and long-haired cats are the most frequently affected breeds. Siamese and Himalayans have a decreased risk for development of hyperthyroidism.

**Clinical signs.** Clinical signs are a result of the excessive secretion of thyroid hormone by the thyroid mass. Rarely, an

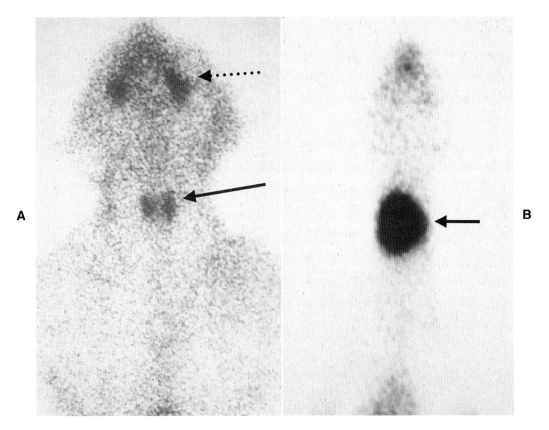

**FIG 51-14**
**A,** Sodium pertechnetate scan of the head, neck, and proximal thorax of a healthy cat. Note that the uptake of pertechnetate (i.e., darkness) is comparable between the two thyroid lobes *(solid arrow)* and the salivary glands *(broken arrow).* **B,** Sodium pertechnetate scan of the head, neck, and proximal thorax of a cat with hyperthyroidism caused by unilateral disease affecting the right thyroid lobe *(arrow).* Note the difference in uptake of pertechnetate between the hyperfunctioning thyroid lobe and the salivary glands.

owner will seek veterinary care because of an observed mass in the ventrocervical region of the neck. The classic clinical signs of hyperthyroidism are weight loss (which may progress to cachexia), polyphagia, and restlessness or hyperactivity. Additional clinical signs include haircoat changes (patchy alopecia, matted hair, no or excessive grooming behavior), polyuria, polydipsia, vomiting, and diarrhea (Table 51-10). Some cats show aggressive behavior that resolves in response to successful treatment of the hyperthyroid state. In some cats, lethargy, weakness, and anorexia are the dominant clinical features, in addition to weight loss. Because of the multisystemic effects of hyperthyroidism, the variable clinical signs, and its resemblance to many other diseases of the cat, hyperthyroidism should be suspected in any aged cat (i.e., older than 10 years) with medical problems.

**Physical examination.** Physical examination findings are listed in Table 51-10. A discrete thyroid mass is palpable in approximately 90% of cats with hyperthyroidism. However, the palpation of a cervical mass is not pathognomonic for hyperthyroidism, because some cats with palpable thyroids are clinically normal and because some cervical masses are not

thyroids. Because the thyroid lobes are loosely attached to the trachea, the increase in the weight of the gland resulting from adenomatous hyperplasia or neoplasia usually causes it to descend in the neck. The thyroid mass is commonly palpated in the region of the thoracic inlet. The abnormal thyroid lobe, or lobes, may even descend into the anterior mediastinum. This should be suspected in the hyperthyroid cat without a palpable thyroid mass, although a small, nonpalpable mass is also possible. It is frequently difficult to accurately assess unilateral or bilateral thyroid lobe involvement solely on the basis of palpation findings. A solitary mass is frequently palpated in cats with bilateral thyroid lobe involvement.

## Clinical Pathology

Results of a CBC are usually normal in hyperthyroid cats. The most common abnormalities are a mild increase in the PCV and mean corpuscular volume. Neutrophilia, lymphopenia, eosinopenia, or monocytopenia is identifed in less than 20% of hyperthyroid cats. Common serum biochemical abnormalities include an increase in serum activities of alanine aminotransferase, alkaline phosphatase, and

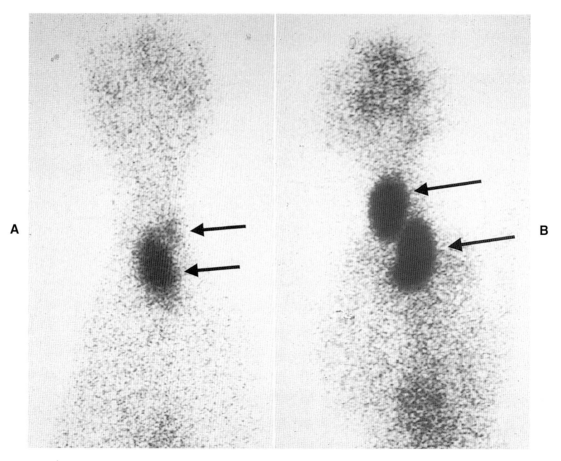

**FIG 51-15**
**A,** Sodium pertechnetate scan of the head, neck, and proximal thorax of a cat with hyperthyroidism caused by bilateral, asymmetric disease affecting both thyroid lobes *(arrows),* with the right lobe more severely involved. This is the most common form of the disease. **B,** Sodium pertechnetate scan of the head, neck, and proximal thorax of a cat with hyperthyroidism caused by bilateral, symmetric disease affecting both thyroid lobes *(arrows).* Hypocalcemia after bilateral thyroidectomy is a major concern.

aspartate aminotransferase; the increase is typically in the mild to moderate range (i.e., 100 to 400 IU/L). One or more of these liver enzymes are increased in approximately 90% of hyperthyroid cats. Additional evaluation of the liver should be considered if liver enzyme activities are greater than 500 IU/L (see Chapter 36). Increased serum urea nitrogen and creatinine concentrations are identified in approximately 30%, and hyperphosphatemia in 20%, of hyperthyroid cats at our clinic—findings that have important implications from the standpoint of the initial treatment implemented (see Renal Insufficiency, p. 716). The urine specific gravity ranges from 1.008 to greater than 1.050. Most hyperthyroid cats have urine specific gravities greater than 1.035. The documentation of a concentrated urine specific gravity is helpful in differentiating primary renal insufficiency from prerenal azotemia in cats with an increased blood urea nitrogen level. Urinalysis findings are also helpful in ruling out diabetes mellitus if the serum biochemistry panel reveals hyperglycemia.

## Common Concurrent Problems

**Thyrotoxic cardiomyopathy.** Hypertrophic and, less commonly, dilative thyrotoxic cardiomyopathy may develop in cats with hyperthyroidism. Cardiovascular abnormalities detectable during physical examination include tachycardia, a "pounding" heartbeat noted on palpation of the ventral thorax, and, less frequently, pulse deficits, gallop rhythms, cardiac murmur, and muffled heart sounds resulting from a pleural effusion. Electrocardiographic abnormalities include tachycardia, an increased R-wave amplitude in lead II, and, less commonly, a right bundle-branch block, a left anterior fascicular block, widened QRS complexes, and atrial and ventricular arrhythmias. Thoracic radiographs may reveal cardiomegaly, pulmonary edema, or a pleural effusion. Echocardiographic abnormalities identified in cats with hypertrophic thyrotoxic cardiomyopathy include left ventricular hypertrophy, thickening of the interventricular septum, left atrial and ventricular dilation, and myocardial hypercontractility. Those seen in cats with dilative thyrotoxic cardiomyopathy include

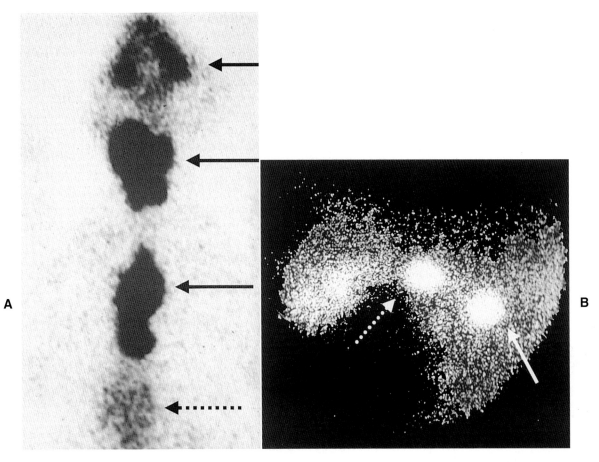

**FIG 51-16**
**A,** Sodium pertechnetate scan of the head, neck, and proximal thorax of a cat with hyperthyroidism caused by metastatic thyroid adenocarcinoma with multiple masses present in the head, neck, and anterior mediastinum *(arrows)*. **B,** Sodium pertechnetate scan of the head, neck, and proximal thorax of a cat with hyperthyroidism caused by two hyperfunctioning masses: one located in the neck *(broken arrow)* and one in the anterior mediastinum (i.e., ectopic site) *(solid arrow)*. $^{131}$I therapy is the treatment of choice for both forms of hyperthyroidism illustrated in this figure.

 TABLE 51-10

Clinical Signs and Physical Examination Findings in Cats with Hyperthyroidism

| CLINICAL SIGNS | PHYSICAL EXAMINATION FINDINGS |
|---|---|
| Weight loss* | Palpable thyroid* |
| Polyphagia* | Thin* |
| Unkempt haircoat, patchy alopecia* | Hyperactive, difficult to examine* |
| Polyuria-polydipsia* | Tachycardia* |
| Vomiting* | Hair loss, unkempt haircoat* |
| Nervous, hyperactive | Small kidneys |
| Diarrhea, "bulky" stools | Heart murmur |
| Decreased appetite | Easily stressed |
| Tremor | Dehydrated, cachectic appearance |
| Weakness | Premature beats |
| Dyspnea, panting | Gallop rhythm |
| Decreased activity, lethargy | Aggressive |
| Anorexia | Depressed, weak |
| | Ventral flexion of the neck |

*Common.

subnormal myocardial contractility and marked ventricular dilation. Either form of cardiomyopathy may result in the development of congestive heart failure. Hypertrophic thyrotoxic cardiomyopathy is usually reversible, after the hyperthyroid state is corrected, whereas dilative thyrotoxic cardiomyopathy is not.

**Renal insufficiency.** Hyperthyroidism and renal insufficiency are common diseases of older cats and often occur concurrently. Identification of small kidneys on physical examination or increased blood urea nitrogen and serum creatinine concentrations and urine specific gravity between 1.008 and 1.020 should raise suspicion for concurrent renal insufficiency in a cat with hyperthyroidism. Unfortunately, hyperthyroidism increases the glomerular filtration rate (GFR), renal plasma flow, and renal tubular resorptive and secretory capabilities in normal and compromised kidneys. The clinical and biochemical manifestations of renal failure may be masked in cats with both thyroid and renal disease whose renal perfusion is enhanced by the circulatory dynamics produced by hyperthyroidism. Renal perfusion and GFR may acutely decrease and azotemia or clinical signs of renal insufficiency become apparent or significantly worsen after treatment of the hyperthyroid state. Because it is not easy to determine what impact the hyperthyroid state is having on renal function, cats with hyperthyroidism should initially be given reversible therapy (i.e., oral antithyroid drugs) until the impact of establishing euthyroidism on renal function can be determined (see p. 721).

**Systemic hypertension.** Systemic hypertension is common in cats with hyperthyroidism and results from the effects of increased β-adrenergic activity on heart rate, myocardial contractility, systemic vasodilation, and activation of the renin-angiotensin-aldosterone system. Hypertension caused by hyperthyroidism is usually clinically silent. Retinal hemorrhages and retinal detachment are the most common clinical complications of systemic hypertension in hyperthyroid cats, but in general, ocular lesions are not commonly identified in cats with hyperthyroidism.

**Gastrointestinal tract disorders.** Gastrointestinal tract signs are common in cats with hyperthyroidism and include polyphagia, weight loss, anorexia, vomiting, diarrhea, increased frequency of defecation, and increased volume of feces. Intestinal hypermotility and malassimilation have been documented in some cats with hyperthyroidism and are responsible for producing some of the gastrointestinal tract signs. Inflammatory bowel disease is a common concurrent gastrointestinal tract disorder that should be considered in any hyperthyroid cat that has persistence of gastrointestinal signs following correction of the hyperthyroid state (see p. 447). Intestinal neoplasia, most notably lymphoma, is perhaps the most important differential diagnosis in cats seen because of polyphagia and weight loss (see p. 816). The abdomen should be carefully palpated in a search for thickening of the intestinal tract and mesenteric lymphadenopathy—findings that may be the only clues to an intestinal lymphoma. Abdominal ultrasonography may also provide clues to the possibility of lymphoma.

## Diagnosis

The diagnosis of hyperthyroidism is based on identification of appropriate clinical signs, palpation of a thyroid nodule, and documentation of an increased serum $T_4$ concentration. Increasing awareness of the disease in the 1980s and the incorporation of serum $T_4$ as a routine part of the feline biochemistry panel performed by commercial diagnostic laboratories in the late 1980s has created a diagnostic challenge for veterinarians as they try to differentiate healthy cats from cats with mild or occult hyperthyroidism. *Occult hyperthyroidism* refers to the condition in a cat with mild clinical signs, a palpable nodule in the ventral region of the neck, and a nondiagnostic serum $T_4$ concentration that falls within the upper half of the reference range (i.e., 2.5 to 3.5 μg/dl). Random fluctuations of serum $T_4$ concentration into the normal range in cats with mild hyperthyroidism or a decrease in serum $T_4$ as a consequence of concurrent nonthyroidal illness (see Fig. 51-13) account for the nondiagnostic serum $T_4$ test result. Additional diagnostic tests (e.g., serum $fT_4$ concentration, radionuclide thyroid scan) are often needed to establish the diagnosis of hyperthyroidism in cats with mild or occult disease.

**Baseline serum T₄ concentration.** Measurement of random baseline serum $T_4$ concentrations has been extremely reliable in differentiating hyperthyroid cats from those without thyroid disease (Fig. 51-17). An abnormally high serum $T_4$ concentration strongly supports the diagnosis of hyperthyroidism, especially if appropriate clinical signs are present, and a low serum $T_4$ concentration rules out hyperthyroidism, except in extremely uncommon situations where severe life-threatening nonthyroidal illness is present (Table 51-11). Serum $T_4$ concentrations that fall within the upper half of the normal range create a diagnostic dilemma, especially if clinical signs are suggestive of hyperthyroidism and a nodule is palpable in the ventral region of the neck. Cats with mild or occult hyperthyroidism and hyperthyroid cats with significant nonthyroidal illness (e.g., neoplasia, systemic infection, organ system failure; Fig. 51-18) can have "normal" serum $T_4$ concentrations. The diagnosis of hyperthyroidism should not be excluded on the basis of one "normal" test result, especially in a cat with appropriate clinical signs and a palpable mass in the neck. If the serum $T_4$ test result is not definitive, the recommendation is to measure serum $T_4$ and $fT_4$ using the MED technique in 1 to 2 weeks and to rule out nonthyroidal illness. If the diagnosis is still not established, the veterinarian should consider repeating the serum $T_4$ and $fT_4$ tests in 4 to 8 weeks, obtaining a radionuclide thyroid scan, or completing a $T_3$ suppression test. If available, a radionuclide thyroid scan is preferable over the $T_3$ suppression test for diagnosing hyperthyroidism in cats with nondiagnostic serum $T_4$ and $fT_4$ concentrations. The $T_3$ suppression test should be considered only in cats with persistently nondiagnostic serum $T_4$ and $fT_4$ concentrations and no access to radionuclide scanning facilities. It is important to remember that the thyroid nodule may also be nonfunctional and the clinical signs may be the result of another disease (see p. 816).

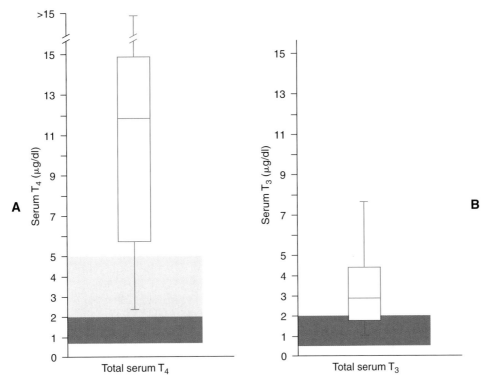

**FIG 51-17**
Mean and range of random total serum $T_4$ **(A)** and total serum $T_3$ **(B)** concentrations in hyperthyroid cats. Seventy-five percent of hyperthyroid cats have values within the box, and the balance is within the limitation bars above and below the box. Note that virtually all hyperthyroid cats have abnormal or "borderline" serum $T_4$ concentrations, whereas serum $T_3$ concentrations are less sensitive. The purple region represents the normal reference range, and the pink region represents the "borderline" or "nondiagnostic" range.

TABLE 51-11

Interpretation of Baseline Serum Thyroxine ($T_4$) Concentration in Cats with Suspected Hyperthyroidism

| SERUM $T_4$ CONCENTRATION ($\mu$g/dl) | PROBABILITY OF HYPERTHYROIDISM |
|---|---|
| >4.0 | Very likely |
| 3.0-4.0 | Possible |
| 2.5-3.0 | Unknown |
| 2.0-2.5 | Unlikely |
| <2.0 | Very unlikely* |

*Assuming that a severe systemic illness is not present.

**Serum free $T_4$ concentration.** Measurement of the baseline serum $fT_4$ concentration by the MED technique (see p. 698) is a more reliable means of assessing thyroid gland function than measurement of the serum total $T_4$ concentration, in part because nonthyroidal illness has more of a suppressive effect on serum total $T_4$ than on $fT_4$ (see Fig. 51-13) and

serum $fT_4$ is increased in many cats with occult hyperthyroidism and "normal" $T_4$ test results. Because of cost, measurement of $fT_4$ concentration by MED is often reserved for cats with suspected hyperthyroidism where $T_4$ values are borderline. Occasionally concurrent illness causes an increase in serum fT4 concentration in cats—an increase that can exceed the reference range (see Fig. 51-18). For this reason, serum fT4 concentration should always be interpreted in conjunction with total $T_4$ concentration measured from the same blood sample. An increased serum $fT_4$ concentration in conjunction with high-normal or increased serum $T_4$ concentration is supportive of hyperthyroidism. An increased serum $fT_4$ concentration in conjunction with a low-normal or low serum $T_4$ concentration is supportive of euthyroid sick syndrome rather than hyperthyroidism.

**$T_3$ suppression test.** The $T_3$ suppression test evaluates the responsiveness of pituitary TSH secretion to suppression by sodium liothyronine (synthetic $T_3$; Fig. 51-19). The administration of $T_3$ to normal cats should suppress pituitary TSH secretion, causing a subsequent decrease in the serum $T_4$ concentration. The serum $T_4$ concentration is a valid marker of thyroid gland function because exogenous $T_3$ cannot be converted to $T_4$. Cats with hyperthyroidism have autonomous secretion of

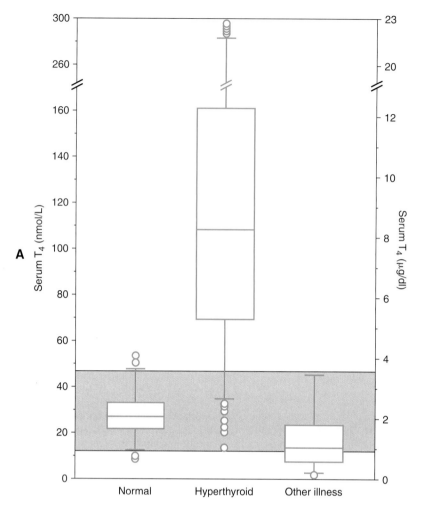

**FIG 51-18**
Box plots of serum total T$_4$ **(A)** and free T$_4$ **(B)** concentrations in 172 clinically normal cats, 917 cats with untreated hyperthyroidism, and 221 cats with nonthyroidal disease. See Fig. 51-7 for explanation. (From Peterson ME et al: Measurement of serum concentrations of free thyroxine, total thyroxine, and total triiodothyronine in cats with hyperthyroidism and cats with nonthyroidal disease, *J Am Vet Med Assoc* 218:529, 2001.)

thyroid hormone, independent of pituitary control. The administration of T$_3$ to hyperthyroid cats should therefore have little to no effect on the serum T$_4$ concentration, because pituitary TSH secretion has already been chronically suppressed. T$_3$ administration has no further suppressive effect. Results of the T$_3$ suppression test should allow cats with a normal pituitary-thyroid axis to be differentiated from those with autonomous thyroid hormone secretion and probable hyperthyroidism. Disadvantages of the test are the 3 days it takes to complete it, the need to rely on owners to administer the drug seven times, and the problem with getting cats to swallow the tablets.

To perform this test, serum is first obtained for determination of baseline serum T$_4$ and T$_3$ concentrations. The owner is then instructed to administer 25 mg of sodium liothyronine (synthetic T$_3$; Cytomel; JPI Jones, St. Louis) three times a day for 2 days, beginning the following morning. On the morning of day 3, a seventh 25-mg dose should be ad-

ministered and the cat returned to the hospital 2 to 4 hours later to obtain a second blood sample for measurement of the serum T$_4$ and T$_3$ concentrations.

Normal cats consistently have post-dosing serum T$_4$ concentrations of less than 1.5 µg/dl, whereas hyperthyroid cats have post-dosing T$_4$ concentrations of greater than 2.0 µg/dl. Values of 1.5 to 2.0 µg/dl should be considered nondiagnostic. The percentage decrease in the serum T$_4$ concentration is not as reliable a gauge as the absolute value, although suppression of more than 50% below the baseline value occurs in normal but not hyperthyroid cats. The serum T$_3$ concentrations are used to determine whether the owner has successfully administered the thyroid medication to the cat. Serum T$_3$ concentration measured in the post-pill blood sample should be increased compared with results obtained before initiating the test in all cats properly tested, regardless of the status of thyroid gland function. If the serum T$_4$ concentration fails to

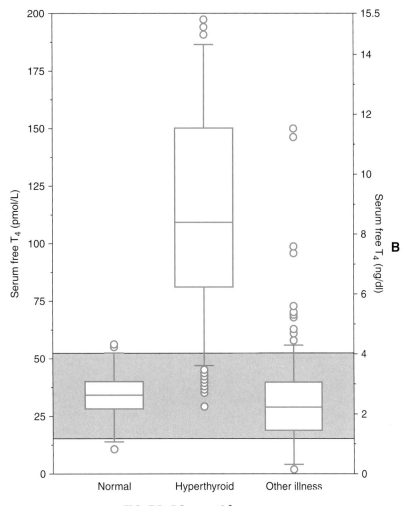

**FIG 51-18, cont'd**
For legend, see opposite page.

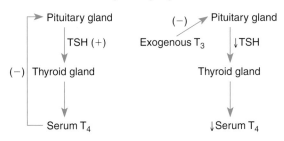

**Normal pituitary-thyroid axis**

**Hyperthyroidism**

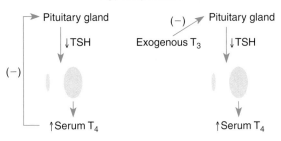

**FIG 51-19**
Effect of $T_3$ supplementation on the pituitary-thyroid axis in healthy cats and cats with hyperthyroidism. Suppression of pituitary TSH secretion by the $T_3$ supplement decreases serum $T_4$ concentration in healthy cats. In hyperthyroid cats the serum TSH concentration is already suppressed; the $T_3$ supplementation has no effect. The serum $T_4$ concentration remains increased.

TABLE 51-12

Indications, Contraindications, and Disadvantages of the Three Modes of Therapy for Hyperthyroidism in Cats

| THERAPY | INDICATIONS | RELATIVE CONTRAINDICATIONS | DISADVANTAGES |
|---------|-------------|---------------------------|---------------|
| Methimazole, propylthiouracil, carbimazole | Long-term therapy for all forms of hyperthyroidism; initial therapy to stabilize cat's condition and assess renal function before thyroidectomy or radioactive iodine | None | Daily therapy required; no effect on growth of tumor; mild adverse reactions common; severe reactions possible |
| Thyroidectomy | Unilateral lobe involvement; bilateral lobe involvement, asymmetric sizes | Ectopic thyroid lobe; metastatic carcinoma; bilateral, symmetric, large lobes (high risk of hypocalcemia); severe systemic signs; cardiac arrhythmias or failure; renal failure | Anesthetic risks; relapse of disease; postoperative complications, especially hypocalcemia |
| Radioactive iodine ($^{131}$I) | Therapy for all forms of hyperthyroidism; treatment of choice for ectopic thyroid lobe and thyroid carcinoma | None | Limited availability; prolonged hospitalization; potential for retreatment; hazardous to humans |

decline in a cat that does not show an increase in the serum $T_3$ concentration, problems with owner compliance should be considered and the test results not trusted.

**TRH stimulation test.** The intravenous (IV) administration of TRH will stimulate pituitary TSH secretion and cause a subsequent increase in the serum $T_4$ concentration in cats with a normal pituitary-thyroid axis. Pituitary TSH secretion is chronically suppressed in cats with hyperthyroidism; thus a single administration of TRH should not increase pituitary TSH secretion. Consequently, TRH administration in hyperthyroid cats should have little or no effect on the serum $T_4$ concentrations. For the TRH stimulation test in cats, blood is obtained for serum $T_4$ measurement before and 4 hours after the IV administration of TRH (0.1 mg/kg body weight). Disadvantages of the TRH stimulation test include its cost and the frequent occurrence of adverse effects, including salivation, vomiting, tachypnea, and defecation. These adverse effects usually begin immediately after TRH administration and may continue for as long as 4 hours. The TRH stimulation test is no longer recommended for identifying hyperthyroidism.

**Radionuclide thyroid scanning.** The thyroid scan is used as a diagnostic test in those cats with appropriate signs of hyperthyroidism but nondiagnostic serum $T_4$ concentrations; to identify ectopic thyroid tissue in cats with appropriate signs of hyperthyroidism and increased serum $T_4$ concentrations but no palpable thyroid nodule in the neck; and to help formulate the best treatment plan, especially by predicting the likelihood of success and the risk of hypocalcemia developing after thyroidectomy. Radioactive technetium 99m (pertechnetate) is used for routine imaging of the thyroid gland in cats. It has a short physical half-life (6 hours), is concentrated within functioning thyroid follicular cells, and reflects the trapping mechanism of the gland. Because antithyroid drugs do not affect the

trapping mechanism of the thyroid pump, pertechnetate still concentrates in the thyroid gland, even after complete blockade of thyroid hormone synthesis by antithyroid drugs. Salivary glands and the gastric mucosa also concentrate pertechnetate; it is excreted by the kidneys.

Scanning of the thyroid provides a picture of all functioning thyroid tissue and permits the delineation and localization of functioning as opposed to nonfunctioning areas of the thyroid. Fig. 51-14 shows the similarity between the size and shape of the thyroid lobes and similarity of radionuclide uptake by the thyroid and salivary glands in a normal cat. This 1:1 ratio of salivary gland to thyroid lobe uptake is the standard by which to judge the status of the thyroid. Findings in most hyperthyroid cats are markedly abnormal and usually easy to interpret (see Figs. 51-14 to 51-16).

### Treatment

Hyperthyroidism in cats can be managed by thyroidectomy, oral antithyroid medications, or radioactive iodine. All three modes of therapy are effective. Surgery and radioactive iodine treatments are used in the hope of providing a permanent cure for the disease; oral antithyroid drugs only "control" the hyperthyroidism and must be given daily to achieve and maintain their effect. The mode ultimately chosen depends on a number of factors, including the general health and age of the cat; the status of its renal function; the severity of any concurrent disease (e.g., thyrotoxic cardiomyopathy); the existence of adenomatous hyperplasia, adenoma, or carcinoma; unilateral versus bilateral lobe involvement; the size of the thyroid masses if bilateral disease is present; the availability of radioactive iodine; the surgical expertise of the clinician; the ease of administration of oral medications to the cat; and the owner's wishes (Table 51-12).

Hyperthyroid cats should be treated initially with the oral antithyroid drug methimazole to reverse the hyperthyroid-induced metabolic and cardiac derangements, decrease the anesthetic risk associated with thyroidectomy, and assess the impact of treatment on renal function. Hyperthyroidism may mask renal insufficiency in some cats because renal perfusion and GFR are enhanced by the circulatory dynamics of the hyperthyroid state (see p. 716). Azotemia may develop or worsen, and clinical signs of renal insufficiency may develop following treatment of the hyperthyroid state. Because it is not easy to determine what impact the hyperthyroid state is having on renal function, it is preferable to treat cats with reversible therapy (i.e., methimazole) until the impact of hyperthyroidism on renal function can be determined. If renal parameters remain static or improve following resolution of the hyperthyroidism with methimazole, a more permanent treatment for hyperthyroidism can be recommended. If significant azotemia or clinical signs of renal insufficiency develop during methimazole therapy, the treatment protocol for the antithyroid drug should be modified to attain the best possible control of both disorders, and treatment for renal insufficiency instituted. Maintaining a mild hyperthyroid state may be necessary to improve renal perfusion and GFR and avoid the uremia of renal failure.

**Antithyroid drugs.** Oral antithyroid drugs (e.g., methimazole, propylthiouracil, carbimazole) are inexpensive, readily available, relatively safe, and effective in the treatment of hyperthyroidism in cats. They inhibit the synthesis of thyroid hormone by blocking the incorporation of iodine into the tyrosyl groups in thyroglobulin and by preventing the coupling of these iodotyrosyl groups into $T_3$ and $T_4$, hence inhibiting the synthesis of thyroid hormone. Antithyroid drugs do not block the release of stored thyroid hormone into the circulation and do not have antitumor actions. Therapy can be initiated before pertechnetate scanning because, as already noted, these drugs do not interfere with the results of scanning. Indications for oral antithyroid drugs include (1) test treatment to normalize serum $T_4$ concentrations and assess the effect of resolving hyperthyroidism on renal function, (2) initial treatment to alleviate or eliminate any medical problems associated with the syndrome before thyroidectomy is performed or before the hospitalization required for radioactive iodine treatment, and (3) long-term treatment of hyperthyroidism.

Methimazole (Tapazole; Eli Lilly & Co., Indianapolis, Ind) is currently the antithyroid drug of choice because the incidence of adverse reactions associated with its use is lower than that associated with the use of propylthiouracil (Table 51-13). Adverse reactions are less likely to occur when the dosage of methimazole is started low (typically at subtherapeutic dose initially) and gradually increased to effect. The recommended initial dose of methimazole is 2.5 mg administered orally once a day for 2 weeks. If adverse reactions are not observed by the owner, if the physical examination reveals no new problems, if results of a CBC and platelet count are within reference limits, and if serum $T_4$ concentration is greater than 2 μg/dl after 2 weeks of therapy, the dose is increased to 2.5 mg twice daily and the same parameters evaluated 2 weeks later. The dosage should continue to be in-

TABLE 51-13

**Abnormalities Associated with Methimazole Therapy in 262 Cats with Hyperthyroidism**

| CLINICAL SIGNS AND PATHOLOGY | PERCENTAGE OF CATS | TIME TO DEVELOP (DAYS) MEAN | TIME TO DEVELOP (DAYS) RANGE |
|---|---|---|---|
| **Clinical Signs** | | | |
| Anorexia | 11 | 24 | 1-78 |
| Vomiting | 11 | 22 | 7-60 |
| Lethargy | 9 | 24 | 1-60 |
| Excoriations | 2 | 21 | 6-40 |
| Bleeding | 2 | 31 | 15-50 |
| **Clinical Pathology** | | | |
| Positive antinuclear antibody titer | 22 | 91 | 10-870 |
| Eosinophilia | 11 | 57 | 12-490 |
| Lymphocytosis | 7 | 25 | 14-90 |
| Leukopenia | 5 | 23 | 10-41 |
| Thrombocytopenia | 3 | 37 | 14-90 |
| Agranulocytosis | 2 | 62 | 26-95 |
| Hepatopathy | 2 | 39 | 15-60 |

Adapted from Peterson ME et al: Methimazole treatment of 262 cats with hyperthyroidism, *J Vet Intern Med* 2:150, 1988.

creased every 2 weeks by 2.5 mg/day increments until the serum $T_4$ concentration is between 1 and 2 μg/dl or adverse reactions develop. Serum $T_4$ concentrations decline into the reference range within 1 to 2 weeks once the cat is receiving an effective dose of methimazole; clinical improvement is usually noted by owners within 2 to 4 weeks once good control of serum $T_4$ concentration is achieved.

Rarely, cats are encountered that seem particularly resistant to methimazole, requiring as much as 20 mg/day. The most common cause for apparent resistance to methimazole is the inability of some owners to administer the drug to their cats. An alternative is the topical application of methimazole to the pinna of the ear. Custom veterinary pharmacies offer transdermal methimazole in a pluronic lecithin organogel (PLO), typically at a concentration of 5 mg of methimazole per 0.1 ml of gel. The gel is applied to the pinna of the ear using a tuberculin syringe and rubbed into the skin; the owner must wear gloves to avoid absorption of methimazole. The dosage and frequency of administration is as discussed with oral methimazole treatment. Bioavailability following a single administration is poor but variable (Hoffman and colleagues, 2002). However, transdermal methimazole in a PLO has been efficacious with chronic dosing in hyperthyroid cats; chronic dosing may enhance absorption secondary to changes in the stratum corneum that occur with chronic PLO administration.

Adverse reactions to methimazole typically occur within the first 4 to 8 weeks of therapy (see Table 51-13). The cat should be examined during the first 3 months of methimazole treatment and a CBC, platelet count, and assessment of kidney function performed every 2 weeks. After the initial 3 months of therapy, a CBC, platelet count, and serum biochemistry panel should be evaluated every 3 to 6 months. Using the dosing protocol described above, lethargy, vomiting, and anorexia occur in less than 10% of cats; these mild adverse reactions are usually transient and often resolve despite continued administration of the drug. Mild methimazole-induced hematologic changes occur in less than 10% of cats and include eosinophilia, lymphocytosis, and transient leukopenia. More worrisome but less common (<5% of cats) alterations include severe thrombocytopenia (platelet counts <75,000/mm$^3$), neutropenia (total white blood cell counts <2000/mm$^3$), and immune-mediated hemolytic anemia. Apparent hepatic toxicity or injury occurs in less than 2% of cats receiving methimazole, and this is characterized by clinical signs of liver disease (i.e., lethargy, anorexia, vomiting), icterus, and abnormalities in the serum alanine transaminase and alkaline phosphatase activities. Some cats test positively for antinuclear antibodies, but the importance of this finding is not known. If any of these serious complications develop, methimazole treatment should be discontinued and supportive care (e.g., IV fluids, blood transfusions, antibiotics) given. The adverse reactions typically resolve within a week of the discontinuation of methimazole treatment. It is common for these potentially life-threatening adverse reactions to recur, regardless of the antithyroid drug used; thus alternative therapy (i.e., surgery, radioactive iodine) is recommended.

Carbimazole (Neo-Mercazole; Roche) is an antithyroid drug that is converted to methimazole in vivo; it is an effective alternative treatment if methimazole is not available. In contrast to methimazole treatment, twice-daily treatment schedules may be inadequate during the initial weeks of administration; an initial dosage of 5 mg three times a day is recommended initially. Euthyroidism is typically attained within 2 weeks of the start of therapy. Long-term, twice-daily schedules are effective in controlling hyperthyroidism. Adverse reactions are similar to those seen in cats receiving methimazole, but they occur less frequently. Cats being treated with carbimazole should be monitored in the same manner as that suggested for cats receiving methimazole.

**Surgery.** Thyroidectomy is the treatment of choice unless the risk of anesthesia in the cat is unacceptable, its renal function is questionable, the likelihood of postoperative hypocalcemia is great, ectopic thyroid tissue is present in the thorax, or thyroid carcinoma with metastasis is suspected. If the animal is a poor anesthetic risk or renal insufficiency is suspected, methimazole can be administered orally for 1 to 2 months before performing surgery to reestablish euthyroidism, reverse the metabolic derangements associated with hyperthyroidism, reevaluate the effect of hyperthyroidism on GFR and renal function, and improve the likelihood of a successful outcome after thyroidectomy. Surgery should always be considered an elective procedure.

If possible, an ultrasound examination of the ventral neck or a pertechnetate scan should be performed before surgery to identify the location of the abnormal thyroid tissue, differentiate unilateral from bilateral lobe involvement, and pro-

vide some insight into the probability of hypocalcemia developing postoperatively (Fig. 51-20). Similar information can also be gained by direct visualization at the time of surgery. Normal thyroid glands are flat, smooth, and salmon colored. Adenomatous thyroid glands are variably enlarged, are often nodular or cystic, and vary in color from yellow to reddish brown. If a unilateral thyroid mass is present, the opposite thyroid lobe may be normal or atrophic. All grossly abnormal thyroid tissue should be removed.

There is a direct correlation between the size of the thyroid lobes, the inability to visualize the external parathyroid glands, and the risk of hypocalcemia. Care must be taken to preserve at least one, but preferably both, external parathyroid glands and their associated blood supply. Even in cats with unilateral disease, an attempt should be made to preserve the external parathyroid on the involved side because of the potential need to remove the other thyroid lobe in the future. A "subcapsular" thyroidectomy affords the best chance of retaining functional parathyroid glands. (See Suggested Readings for thyroidectomy procedures.) Abnormal, adenomatous thyroid cells may remain adhered to the capsule after

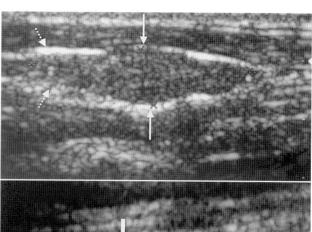

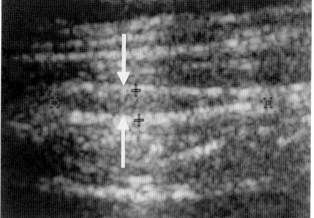

**FIG 51-20**

**A,** Ultrasound image of the right thyroid lobe of a 13-year-old domestic short-haired cat with hyperthyroidism. A mass is in the mid-region of the thyroid lobe *(solid arrows)*. **B,** Ultrasound image of the normal-appearing left thyroid lobe. Results of the ultrasound examination supported unilateral disease affecting the right thyroid lobe, which was confirmed with a sodium pertechnetate scan.

subcapsular thyroidectomy, and these "rest" cells may serve as the source for the redevelopment of hyperthyroidism 6 to 24 months later. If all four parathyroid glands are inadvertently removed, the two external parathyroid glands should be removed from their respective thyroid lobes, minced, and placed within the muscle belly of one of the sternohyoideus muscles by bluntly dissecting parallel to the muscle fibers. Hypoparathyroidism usually resolves within a month of surgery if revascularization of the parathyroid autotransplant occurs.

***Postoperative complications.*** The most worrisome complication is hypocalcemia (Table 51-14). The serum calcium concentration should be assessed at least once daily for 5 to 7 days if a bilateral thyroidectomy has been performed. Clinical signs of hypocalcemia typically develop within 72 hours of surgery, although signs may not develop for 5 to 7 days. These signs include lethargy, anorexia, reluctance to move, facial twitching (especially the ears), muscle tremors and cramping, tetany, and convulsions. If all four parathyroid glands are removed at surgery, appropriate calcium and vitamin D supplementation (see p. 688) should be initiated once the cat has recovered from anesthesia. If the parathyroid gland (or glands) has been spared, transient hypocalcemia may still develop and last for several days to weeks, probably as a result of disruption of blood flow to the parathyroid glands after surgical manipulation. In these cats, oral vitamin D and calcium therapy should be initiated only if clinical signs develop or if hypocalcemia becomes severe (i.e., a serum total calcium concentration <8 mg/dl; a serum ionized calcium concentration <0.8 mmol/L). A decline in the blood calcium concentration is not an absolute indication to begin therapy, however, because the remaining parathyroid glands may respond before clinical signs or severe hypocalcemia develops.

The persistence of apparent hypoparathyroidism is variable and difficult to predict. Parathyroid function may recover after days, weeks, or months of vitamin D and calcium supplementation. Whenever resolution of hypoparathyroidism is observed, it is assumed that reversible parathyroid damage occurred, accessory parathyroid tissue may be starting to compensate for glands damaged or removed at surgery, or the parathyroid autotransplant (if performed at surgery) has revascularized and become functional. It is also possible that calcium-regulating mechanisms are functioning in the absence of parathyroid hormone. Because it is difficult to predict the long-term requirement for vitamin D therapy in any cat, an attempt should be made to gradually wean all treated cats off medication while monitoring the serum calcium concentration. The tapering process can begin several weeks after vitamin D therapy is initiated and should extend over a period of at least 12 to 16 weeks. The goal is to maintain the serum calcium concentration within the low-normal range (8.5 to 9.5 mg/dl). If hypocalcemia recurs, therapy with vitamin D and calcium must be reinstituted.

Hypothyroidism may develop in some cats after bilateral thyroidectomy. The clinical signs, diagnosis, and treatment are discussed on p. 709. The decision to initiate sodium levothyroxine treatment should be based on the presence or absence of clinical signs, not on the serum $T_4$ concentration, per se. Serum $T_4$ concentrations commonly decrease following surgery, often to less than 0.5 μg/dl, but thyroid function returns in most cats before clinical signs become apparent. Thyroid hormone supplementation should be initiated in cats that develop clinical signs (i.e., lethargy, inappetence) in conjunction with a low serum $T_4$ concentration. Thyroid replacement therapy may not be needed long term in some of these cats, because they may recover some endogenous thyroid function. Therefore thyroid replacement therapy should be tapered slowly and then discontinued after 1 to 3 months to determine the continued need for treatment.

If clinical signs persist despite thyroidectomy, the serum $T_4$ concentration should be measured. If the serum $T_4$ concentration is low-normal or low (i.e., <2.0 μg/dl), another disorder should be suspected (see p. 816). If the serum $T_4$ concentration is high-normal or high (i.e., >3.0 μg/dl), ectopic abnormal thyroid tissue, metastatic thyroid carcinoma, or, if unilateral thyroidectomy was performed, abnormal tissue in the remaining thyroid lobe should be suspected. Ectopic thyroid tissue would most likely be in the mediastinum, cranial to the heart (see Fig. 51-16). Thyroid scanning must usually be done to identify ectopic or metastatic thyroid tissue. Alternatively, oral antithyroid drugs or radioactive iodine therapy can be considered. Clinical signs of hyperthyroidism may also recur months to years after thyroidectomy. The serum $T_4$ concentration should be monitored once or twice a year in all cats successfully treated with surgery.

**Radioactive iodine.** Iodine 131 (half-life, 8 days) is the radionuclide of choice for the treatment of functional thyroid tumors causing hyperthyroidism. [131]I administered intravenously or subcutaneously is concentrated within the thyroid, and the emitted radiation destroys surrounding functioning follicular cells without causing radiation damage to contiguous structures. The cells killed are those that are

TABLE 51-14

**Complications of Thyroidectomy in Cats with Hyperthyroidism**

Transient or permanent hypoparathyroidism causing
 hypocalcemia:
 Restlessness
 Irritability
 Abnormal behavior
 Muscle cramping, pain
 Muscle tremors, especially ears and face
 Tetany
 Convulsions
Laryngeal paralysis
Horner's syndrome
Hypothyroidism
Exacerbation of concurrent renal insufficiency
No amelioration of the hyperthyroidism

functioning. Atrophied normal cells are spared, preventing long-term hypothyroidism in most cats. Depending on the dose administered, more than 80% of treated cats become euthyroid within 3 months—most within 1 week—and more than 95% of treated cats are euthyroid at 6 months. Clinical signs and laboratory data consistent with hypothyroidism develop in approximately 2% of $^{131}$I-treated cats, 2% to 4% require a second $^{131}$I treatment, and hyperthyroidism recurs in 2% within 1 to 6 years of treatment. The only recognized adverse reaction is hypothyroidism, which typically develops in cats with bilateral, large, diffusely affected thyroid lobes. Hypothyroidism can be treated with 0.05 to 0.1 mg of sodium levothyroxine given orally once or twice daily. The duration of hospitalization following $^{131}$I administration varies depending on state regulations and the dosage of $^{131}$I administered. In our hospital, the average cat is treated with 2 to 4 mCi of $^{131}$I and requires 5 to 8 days of hospitalization after therapy until the radioactivity of the cat and its excretions reaches an acceptable level. Unfortunately, the limited availability of facilities that offer $^{131}$I treatment often precludes its use in many areas of the country. This form of treatment remains a valuable option for cats with bilateral, markedly enlarged thyroid lobes identified at surgery or by ultrasound or sodium pertechnetate scanning; for cats with a hyperfunctioning, nonaccessible ectopic thyroid mass; and for cats with metastatic or nonresectable thyroid carcinoma. Cats in these categories can be referred to facilities that offer $^{131}$I treatment.

## Prognosis

The prognosis for a hyperthyroid cat depends on its physical condition at the time of diagnosis; the presence and severity of concurrent disease, especially renal insufficiency; the histologic characteristics of the mass (i.e., hyperplasia or adenoma versus carcinoma); the selection of an appropriate therapy given the cat's clinical condition, the number of hyperfunctioning thyroid masses, and the location of thyroid masses; and the avoidance of adverse reactions associated with therapy. Any of the three major treatments can be successful if used under appropriate circumstances. Surgery and $^{131}$I therapy have the potential for cure, whereas clinical signs can be expected to resolve in response to any of the three forms of treatment. Hyperthyroid cats with adenomatous hyperplasia or adenoma can be maintained on methimazole for years, assuming adverse reactions related to the medication are avoided. Hyperthyroidism may recur months to years (or not at all) after thyroidectomy or $^{131}$I treatment. In one epidemiologic study, the median survival time was 25 months (range, 3 days to 8 years) in 231 hyperthyroid cats treated with $^{131}$I (Slater and colleagues, 2001). Renal-related problems and neoplasia were the most common health problems at the time of death.

## CANINE THYROID NEOPLASIA

### Etiology

Thyroid adenomas are usually small, nonfunctional masses that do not cause clinical signs and are found incidentally at necropsy. Exceptions are thyroid adenomas that are functional and cause hyperthyroidism or are unexpectedly identified during ultrasound examination of the ventral neck. In contrast, the more clinically common thyroid carcinomas are usually large, solid masses that cause clinical signs that can be recognized by owners and are easily palpated by veterinarians. Thyroid carcinomas frequently extend into the esophagus, trachea, cervical musculature, nerves, and thyroidal vessels. Distant metastasis to the lungs and retropharyngeal lymph nodes is common. Metastasis to other locations, including the liver, kidneys, heart base, bones, and spinal cord, is also possible. Because of the high prevalence of malignancy, all thyroid masses discovered antemortem in the dog should be assumed to be malignant until proven otherwise.

Most dogs with thyroid tumors are euthyroid or hypothyroid; approximately 10% of dogs have functional thyroid tumors that secrete excess thyroid hormone, causing hyperthyroidism. Clinical signs of hyperthyroidism may predominate in these dogs. Hyperthyroidism may be caused by functional thyroid adenomas and carcinomas. In contrast, adenomatous hyperplasia is the most common cause of hyperthyroidism in cats but has not been described in dogs.

## Clinical Features

**Signalment.** The average age at which the clinical signs of thyroid tumors appear in dogs is 10 years, with a range of 5 to 15 years. There is no sex-related predilection. Although any breed can be affected, Boxers, Beagles, and Golden Retrievers may be at an increased risk.

**Clinical signs.** Dogs with nonfunctional thyroid tumors are usually brought to veterinarians because the owner has seen or felt a mass in the dog's neck or because the mass is causing clinical signs. The most common reason for bringing the dog to the veterinarian is a mass in the ventral region of the neck (Fig. 51-21). Additional clinical signs (e.g., dyspnea, dysphagia) may develop as a result of the mass compressing on adjacent structures or as a result of metastasis (e.g., exercise intolerance, weight loss; Table 51-15). Clinical signs of hyperthyroidism occur in approximately 10% of dogs with thyroid tumors and are similar to those seen in cats (see p. 712).

**Physical examination.** Most thyroid tumors are found to be firm, asymmetric, lobulated, and nonpainful masses that are located close to the typical thyroid region in the neck. The mass is usually well embedded in surrounding tissue and not freely moveable. Additional physical examination findings may include dyspnea, cough, cachexia, lethargy, Horner's syndrome, and dehydration. A dry, lusterless haircoat is common, but alopecia is rare. Mandibular or cervical lymph nodes, or both, may be enlarged as a result of tumor spread or lymphatic obstruction. Dogs with functional thyroid tumors may be restless, thin, and panting, and auscultation of the heart frequently reveals tachycardia. Surprisingly, many dogs are found to be remarkably healthy on physical examination.

**Clinical pathology.** CBC, serum biochemistry panel, and urinalysis findings usually do not help establish the diagnosis. A mild normocytic, normochromic, nonregenerative anemia, hypercholesterolemia, and hypertriglyceridemia causing lipemia may be present in dogs with concurrent hypothyroidism. A mild increase in the blood urea nitrogen

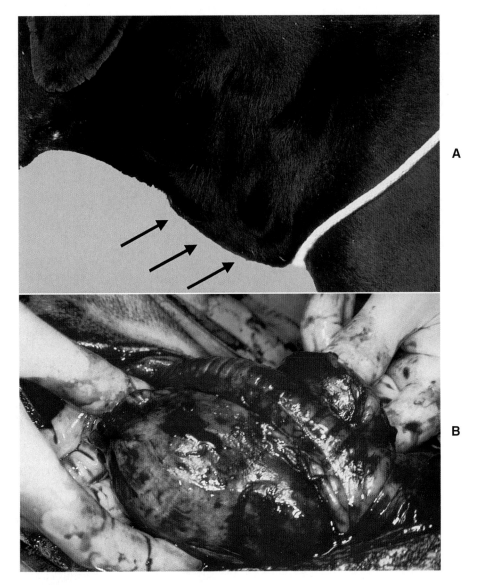

**FIG 51-21**
**A,** A 13-year-old male Labrador Retriever was presented to the veterinarian because the owner noticed a mass in the neck *(arrows)*. The mass was a thyroid adenocarcinoma.
**B,** Thyroid adenocarcinoma in an 11-year-old mixed-breed dog. Clinical signs included dysphagia, coughing, and a visible mass in the ventral region of the neck.

concentration and liver enzyme activities has been identified in less than 35% of dogs; however, the latter changes were not found to be indicative of hepatic metastasis. Hypercalcemia has also been noted in a few dogs.

**Serum thyroid hormone concentrations.** Baseline serum $T_4$ and $fT_4$ concentrations are increased and serum cTSH is undetectable in dogs with a functional thyroid tumor causing hyperthyroidism. However, most canine thyroid tumors are nonfunctional, and most of these dogs are found to be euthyroid when thyroid hormone concentrations are evaluated. At our hospital, approximately 25% of dogs with thyroid tumors are found to be hypothyroid secondary to the destruction of normal glandular tissue by an expanding nonfunctioning tumor.

**Diagnostic imaging.** Ultrasonography of the neck will confirm the presence of a mass, regardless of its size and

 TABLE 51-15

**Clinical Signs Caused by Thyroid Neoplasia in Dogs**

| NONFUNCTIONAL | FUNCTIONAL (HYPERTHYROID) |
| --- | --- |
| Swelling or mass in neck | Swelling or mass in neck |
| Dyspnea | Polyphagia and weight loss |
| Cough | Hyperactivity |
| Lethargy | Polyuria and polydipsia |
| Dysphagia | Panting |
| Regurgitation | Change in behavior |
| Anorexia | (aggression) |
| Weight loss | |
| Horner's syndrome | |
| Change in bark | |
| Facial edema | |

location; can distinguish among cavitary, cystic, and solid tumors; can identify the presence and severity of local tumor invasion; can identify the presence and location of metastatic sites in the cervical region; and improves the likelihood that representative tissue for cytologic or histologic evaluation is obtained during fine-needle aspiration or percutaneous biopsy of the mass (Fig. 51-22). Because pulmonary metastasis is common with thyroid carcinoma, thoracic radiographs should be included in the routine diagnostic evaluation of dogs with a suspected thyroid mass. In our hospital, approximately 50% of dogs with necropsy-confirmed pulmonary metastasis were identified by thoracic radiography. Cervical radiographs may identify a small mass that was suspected but not definitively identified on physical examination, may show the severity of the displacement of adjacent structures, and may identify local invasion of the mass into the larynx and trachea. Abdominal ultrasonography can be used to identify abdominal (most notably hepatic) metastatic lesions. Computed tomography and magnetic resonance imaging of the cervical region can define the extent of tumor invasion into surrounding structures (Fig. 51-23)—information that is valuable if surgery is being considered.

Thyroid scans using pertechnetate as the contrast agent (see p. 720) can be used to assess the size of the thyroid mass and the extent of invasion. If cells within metastatic sites retain the ability to trap iodine, those sites should also be visualized. Ectopic sites of thyroid tissue (neoplastic or normal) may also be seen. Pertechnetate scans do not provide information regarding thyroid function (i.e., euthyroid, hypothyroid, or hyperthyroid) or the benign versus malignant nature of the tumor.

## Diagnosis

For a definitive diagnosis to be rendered, a biopsy specimen must be obtained from the tumor and evaluated histologically. Unfortunately, canine thyroid tumors are highly vascular, and it is common for hemorrhage to occur after biopsy. Fine-needle aspiration using a 21- or 23-gauge needle and cytologic examination of the mass are recommended initially to confirm that the mass is of thyroid origin. Contamination of the aspirate with blood is very common, and differentiation between adenoma and carcinoma is difficult. Large-bore needle biopsy, surgical exploration, or ultrasound-guided biopsy is often required to confirm the diagnosis. Ultrasonography identifies solid areas of the mass for which biopsy is required and large blood vessels to be avoided. This procedure is preferred if the findings yielded by needle aspiration are inconclusive.

## Treatment

Treatment of thyroid tumors is dependent, in part, on the size of the mass, extent of invasion of surrounding soft tissues, functional status regarding secretion of thyroid hormone, and histologic diagnosis of adenoma versus carcinoma. All thyroid tumors should be considered malignant until proven otherwise. As such, surgical removal is the treatment of choice whenever possible, regardless of the functional status of the

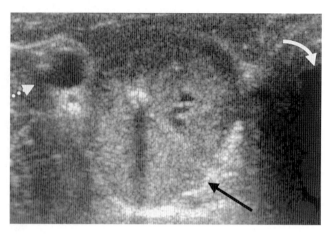

**FIG 51-22**
Ultrasound image of a mass in the region of the right thyroid lobe *(straight arrow)*, the carotid artery *(broken arrow)*, and the trachea *(curved arrow)* in an 11-year-old female spayed Labrador mix. A small region of mineralization causing a shadowing effect is evident within the mass. The mass was an unexpected finding during a routine physical examination. Thyroid adenocarcinoma was the histopathologic diagnosis following surgical removal of the mass.

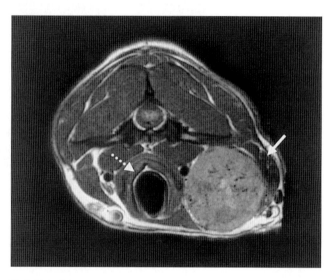

**FIG 51-23**
Magnetic resonance image of a right-sided thyroid mass *(solid arrow)* adjacent to the trachea *(broken arrow)* in a 10-year-old male castrated Golden Retriever that was presented for a swelling in the neck. The histopathologic diagnosis was thyroid C-cell carcinoma with vascular invasion. The affected region of the neck was treated with radiation following thyroidectomy.

tumor. Radiation therapy and chemotherapy are indicated following removal of a thyroid carcinoma, especially if surgical debulking was incomplete or metastasis is suspected (e.g., histologic identification of vascular invasion), and before surgical debulking of a large mass to improve the success of surgery while minimizing postoperative complications. Radioactive iodine and methimazole can be used to treat functional thyroid tumors causing hyperthyroidism, especially if surgery does not provide a cure.

**Surgery.** Surgical excision of thyroid adenomas and small, well-encapsulated, moveable thyroid carcinomas is likely to be curative. However, the potential for cure after surgical removal of most thyroid carcinomas depends on the size of the tumor, the amount of local tissue invasion, and the presence or absence of distant metastasis. Incomplete surgical excision is common because of the tendency for there to be significant local invasion of the tumor into surrounding tissue; incomplete excision should not be considered a surgical problem, however. Cobalt radiation or doxorubicin therapy should be considered after surgery, regardless of how successful the surgery appears to have been. There are two notable contraindications to surgery as the initial therapy. First are known distant metastatic lesions; biopsy of such masses should provide information that can be used to definitively confirm the presence of thyroid malignancy. Second are tumors thought to be too large, too vascular, or too invasive to warrant surgery and its complications. Cobalt irradiation or doxorubicin can be used to initially shrink the mass, followed by surgical removal weeks later.

The debulking of large tumors, even if distant metastatic lesions have been identified, may make the dog more comfortable, relieve dyspnea and dysphagia, and buy time for other therapies to work. However, extensive tumor invasion and aggressive attempts at surgical removal, especially of bilateral tumors, threaten the integrity of recurrent laryngeal nerves, parathyroid glands, and normal thyroid tissue. It is important to monitor serum calcium concentrations before and for 5 to 7 days after surgery if there is any chance that the parathyroid glands have been completely excised or damaged; vitamin D and calcium therapy should be initiated if any evidence of hypoparathyroidism is found (see p. 688). Serum $T_4$, $fT_4$, and cTSH concentrations should be assessed 1 to 3 weeks after surgery and, depending on clinical signs, replacement therapy implemented accordingly (see p. 706). (See Bojrab [1998] and Fossum [2002] for information on surgical techniques for the thyroparathyroid complex.)

**Chemotherapy.** Chemotherapy is indicated if total surgical removal is not successful, if distant metastatic lesions have been identified, or if the size of the primary tumor is such that local invasion or metastasis is likely, even though it cannot be identified with diagnostic tests. Whenever the thyroid mass exceeds approximately 4 cm in diameter, the probability of metastasis becomes extremely high. Doxorubicin given in a dosage of 30 mg/m² body surface area intravenously every 3 to 6 weeks is the historic treatment of choice. The response of canine thyroid tumors to doxorubicin is variable. In most dogs, doxorubicin prevents further growth of the tumor and may cause the tumor size to shrink, but it rarely causes total remission of the tumor. Combination chemotherapy with 5-fluorouracil, cyclophosphamide, and/or vincristine may enhance the effectiveness of doxorubicin. Cisplatin or carboplatin should be considered in dogs that fail to respond to or have recurrence of disease with doxorubicin therapy. The response to cisplatin has been reported to be similar to the response to doxorubicin, although several cisplatin-treated dogs were previously treated with doxorubicin (Fineman and colleagues, 1998). (See Chapters 79 and 80 for a discussion of the use of these chemotherapeutic agents.)

**Radioactive iodine.** Reports evaluating the effectiveness of ¹³¹I for the treatment of thyroid tumors in large groups of dogs have not appeared in the literature. On the basis of limited experience, ¹³¹I therapy appears to have limited efficacy in dogs with functional thyroid tumors. When given in large doses (i.e., 50 to 150 mCi), ¹³¹I may be effective in controlling the thyrotoxic state in dogs with hyperthyroidism caused by relatively small tumors but is only palliative for advanced functional thyroid carcinomas, even with multiple treatments. ¹³¹I therapy is ineffective in "cold" tumors (i.e., those that neither extract iodine from the circulation nor secrete thyroid hormone). It is recommended that kinetic studies using ¹³¹I be conducted before treatment, because most canine thyroid tumors and metastatic lesions do not adequately trap, concentrate, or retain the iodine. These factors limit the use of this therapy in dogs.

**Cobalt irradiation.** Cobalt teletherapy can be used for extensive or invasive tumors, for gross postoperative residual cancer, and when the tumor is unresectable. Cobalt teletherapy can be used alone or in conjunction with surgery or chemotherapy. In most dogs, cobalt irradiation is done after incomplete surgical excision of the thyroid tumor and in cases in which distant metastasis was not identified, and to shrink large, invasive, and nonresectable thyroid tumors. There is a slow regression rate of thyroid carcinoma following radiation therapy in dogs. In one study involving 25 dogs with unresectable differentiated thyroid carcinoma and no evidence of metastasis, the time to attain maximum tumor size reduction varied from 8 to 22 months and progression-free survival rates (defined as the time between completion of irradiation and detection of measurable local tumor recurrence or death from causes unrelated to tumor progression) were 80% at 1 year and 72% at 3 years (Theon and colleagues, 2000).

**Oral antithyroid drugs.** Oral antithyroid drugs are not recommended as a primary mode of therapy for hyperthyroidism in dogs because they are not cytotoxic. However, they can be used as palliative therapy to control the clinical signs of hyperthyroidism in untreated dogs or those in which hyperthyroidism recurs after surgery, ¹³¹I irradiation, or doxorubicin therapy. The therapeutic approach is similar to that used in hyperthyroid cats (see p. 721), beginning with 2.5 mg of methimazole administered twice a day, with subsequent increases in the dosage as needed to control clinical signs and maintain the serum $T_4$ concentration within the reference range.

### Prognosis

The prognosis is excellent after surgical resection of thyroid adenomas. The prognosis is good for those dogs that undergo surgical resection of small, well-encapsulated carcinomas. Unfortunately, most dogs have relatively large thyroid masses, which have frequently invaded surrounding tissues or metastasized at the time of diagnosis. In these dogs, aggressive therapy using multiple treatments can alleviate the clinical signs and in some cases dramatically reduce the tumor burden. The long-term prognosis, however, remains guarded to poor, with survival times typically ranging from 6 to 24 months, depending on the aggressiveness of treatment. Surgical debulking of the primary tumor often enhances long-term survival.

## Suggested Readings

Bojrab MJ: *Current techniques in small animal surgery,* ed 4, Philadelphia, 1998, William & Wilkins.

Feldman EC, Nelson RW: *Canine and feline endocrinology and reproduction,* ed 3, Philadelphia, 2004, WB Saunders.

Fossum TW: *Small animal surgery,* ed 2, St Louis, 2002, Mosby.

CANINE AND FELINE HYPOTHYROIDISM

Calvert CA et al: Thyroid-stimulating hormone stimulation tests in cardiomyopathic Doberman Pinschers: a retrospective study, *J Vet Intern Med* 12:343, 1998.

Gaskill CL et al: Effects of phenobarbital treatment on serum thyroxine and thyroid-stimulating hormone concentrations in epileptic dogs, *J Am Vet Med Assoc* 215:489, 1999.

Graham PA et al: A 12-month prospective study of 234 thyroglobulin antibody positive dogs which had no laboratory evidence of thyroid dysfunction, *J Vet Intern Med* 15:298, 2001.

Greco DS et al: Congenital hypothyroid dwarfism in a family of Giant Schnauzers, *J Vet Intern Med* 5:57, 1991.

Jaggy A et al: Neurological manifestations of hypothyroidism: a retrospective study of 29 dogs, *J Vet Intern Med* 8:328, 1994.

Johnson C et al: Effect of [131]I-induced hypothyroidism on indices of reproductive function in adult male dogs, *J Vet Intern Med* 13:104, 1999.

Jones BR et al: Preliminary studies on congenital hypothyroidism in a family of Abyssinian cats, *Vet Rec* 131:145, 1992.

Kantrowitz LB et al: Serum total thyroxine, total triiodothyronine, free thyroxine, and thyrotropin concentrations in epileptic dogs treated with anticonvulsants, *J Am Vet Med Assoc* 214:1804, 1999.

Kantrowitz LB et al: Serum total thyroxine, total triiodothyronine, free thyroxine, and thyrotropin concentrations in dogs with nonthyroidal disease, *J Am Vet Med Assoc* 219:765, 2001.

Nachreiner RF et al: Radioimmunoassay monitoring of thyroid hormone concentrations in dogs on thyroid replacement therapy: 2,674 cases (1985-1987), *J Am Vet Med Assoc* 201:623, 1992.

Nachreiner RF et al: Prevalence of autoantibodies to thyroglobulin in dogs with nonthyroidal illness, *Am J Vet Res* 59:951, 1998.

Nachreiner RF et al: Prevalence of serum thyroid hormone autoantibodies in dogs with clinical signs of hypothyroidism, *J Am Vet Med Assoc* 220:466, 2002.

Panciera DL: Hypothyroidism in dogs: 66 cases (1987-1992), *J Am Vet Med Assoc* 204:761, 1994.

Panciera DL et al: Plasma von Willebrand factor antigen concentration and buccal mucosal bleeding time in dogs with experimental hypothyroidism, *J Vet Intern Med* 10:60, 1996.

Peterson ME et al: Measurement of serum total thyroxine, triiodothyronine, free thyroxine, and thyrotropin concentrations for diagnosis of hypothyroidism in dogs, *J Am Vet Med Assoc* 211:1396, 1997.

Rand JS et al: Spontaneous adult-onset hypothyroidism in a cat, *J Vet Intern Med* 7:272, 1993.

Scott-Moncrieff JCR et al: Comparison of serum concentrations of thyroid-stimulating hormone in healthy dogs, hypothyroid dogs, and euthyroid dogs with concurrent disease, *J Am Vet Med Assoc* 212:387, 1998.

FELINE HYPERTHYROIDISM

Adams WH et al: Changes in renal function in cats following treatment of hyperthyroidism using [131]I, *Vet Radiol Ultrasound* 38:231, 1997.

Adams WH et al: Investigation of the effects of hyperthyroidism on renal function in the cat, *Can Vet Res* 61:53, 1997.

Becker TJ et al: Effects of methimazole on renal function in cats with hyperthyroidism, *J Am Anim Hosp Assoc* 36:215, 2000.

Court MH et al: Identification and concentration of soy isoflavones in commercial cat foods, *Am J Vet Res* 63:181, 2002.

Graves TK et al: Changes in renal function associated with treatment of hyperthyroidism in cats, *Am J Vet Res* 55:1745, 1994.

Hammer KB et al: Altered expression of G proteins in thyroid gland adenomas obtained from hyperthyroid cells, *Am J Vet Res* 61:874, 2000.

Hoffman SB et al: Bioavailability of transdermal methimazole in a pluronic lecithin organogel (PLO) in healthy cats, *J Vet Intern Med* 16:359, 2002.

Kass PH et al: Evaluation of environmental, nutritional, and host factors in cats with hyperthyroidism, *J Vet Intern Med* 13:323, 1999.

Martin KM et al: Evaluation of dietary and environmental risk factors for hyperthyroidism in cats, *J Am Vet Med Assoc* 217:853, 2000.

Merryman JI et al: Overexpression of c-ras in hyperplasia and adenomas of the feline thyroid gland: an immunohistochemical analysis of 34 cases, *Vet Pathol* 36:117, 1999.

Padgett SL et al: Efficacy of parathyroid gland autotransplantation in maintaining serum calcium concentrations after bilateral thyroparathyroidectomy in cats, *J Am Anim Hosp Assoc* 34:219, 1998.

Peterson ME et al: Radioiodine treatment of 524 cats with hyperthyroidism, *J Am Vet Med Assoc* 207:1422, 1995.

Peterson ME et al: Measurement of serum concentrations of free thyroxine, total thyroxine, and total triiodothyronine in cats with hyperthyroidism and cats with nonthyroidal disease, *J Am Vet Med Assoc* 218:529, 2001.

Slater MR et al: Long-term health and predictors of survival for hyperthyroid cats treated with iodine-131, *J Vet Intern Med* 15:47, 2001.

van der Woerdt, Peterson ME: Prevalence of ocular abnormalities in cats with hyperthyroidism, *J Vet Intern Med* 14:202, 2000.

CANINE THYROID NEOPLASIA

Adams WH et al: Treatment of differentiated thyroid carcinoma in 7 dogs utilizing [131]I, *Vet Radiol Ultrasound* 36:417, 1995.

Brearley MJ et al: Hypofractional radiation therapy for invasive thyroid carcinoma in dogs: a retrospective analysis of survival, *J Small Anim Pract* 40:206, 1999.

Fineman LS et al: Cisplatin chemotherapy for treatment of thyroid carcinoma in dogs: 13 cases, *J Am Anim Hosp Assoc* 34:109, 1998.

Jeglum KA et al: Chemotherapy of canine thyroid carcinoma, *Compend Contin Educ Pract Vet* 5:96, 1983.

Klein MK et al: Treatment of thyroid carcinoma in dogs by surgical resection alone: 20 cases (1981-1989), *J Am Vet Med Assoc* 206:1007, 1995.

Marks SL et al: [99m]Tc-pertechnetate imaging of thyroid tumors in dogs: 29 cases (1980-1992), *J Am Vet Med Assoc* 204:756, 1994.

Theon AP et al: Prognostic factors and patterns of treatment failure in dogs with unresectable differentiated thyroid carcinomas treated with megavoltage irradiation, *J Am Vet Med Assoc* 216:1775, 2000.

# 52

# Disorders of the Endocrine Pancreas

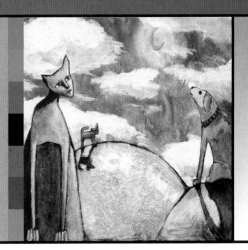

## CHAPTER OUTLINE

HYPERGLYCEMIA, 729
HYPOGLYCEMIA, 729
DIABETES MELLITUS IN DOGS, 731
DIABETES MELLITUS IN CATS, 749
DIABETIC KETOACIDOSIS, 762
INSULIN-SECRETING β-CELL NEOPLASIA, 769
GASTRINOMA: ZOLLINGER-ELLISON
SYNDROME, 775

## HYPERGLYCEMIA

### Etiology

Hyperglycemia is present if the blood glucose concentration is greater than 130 mg/dl, although clinical signs of hyperglycemia do not develop until the renal tubular threshold for the resorption of glucose is exceeded. In dogs this typically occurs whenever the blood glucose concentration exceeds 180 to 220 mg/dl. The threshold for glucose resorption appears more variable in cats, ranging from 200 to 280 mg/dl. Glycosuria causes an osmotic diuresis, which in turn causes polyuria and polydipsia, the hallmark clinical signs of severe hyperglycemia (>180 mg/dl in dogs and >200 to 280 mg/dl in cats). The most common cause of hyperglycemia and glycosuria is diabetes mellitus. Severe hyperglycemia without glycosuria also occurs commonly in cats with stress-induced hyperglycemia, presumably resulting from the secretion of catecholamines and possibly lactate (see p. 759). Transient glycosuria (typically <1% on urine glucose test strips) may occur in some cats with severe or prolonged stress-induced hyperglycemia.

### Clinical Features

Hyperglycemia of between 130 and 180 mg/dl (possibly as high as 280 mg/dl in cats) is clinically silent and is often an unsuspected finding encountered during clinical pathologic testing. If a dog or cat with mild hyperglycemia (<180 mg/dl) and no glycosuria is seen because of polyuria and polydipsia, a disorder other than overt diabetes mellitus should be suspected. Mild hyperglycemia can occur in some dogs and cats up to 2

hours after the consumption of diets containing increased quantities of monosaccharides and disaccharides or propylene glycol or during the intravenous (IV) administration of total parenteral nutrition fluids, in "stressed" cats (and rarely dogs), in animals in the early stages of diabetes mellitus, and in animals with disorders and drugs causing insulin resistance (Table 52-1). A diagnostic evaluation for disorders causing insulin resistance is indicated if mild hyperglycemia is found to persist in a fasted, unstressed dog or cat, especially if the blood glucose concentration is increasing over time (see p. 747).

## HYPOGLYCEMIA

### Etiology

Hypoglycemia is present if the blood glucose concentration is less than 60 mg/dl. It typically results from the excessive use of glucose by normal cells (e.g., during periods of hyperinsulinism) or neoplastic cells, impaired hepatic gluconeogenesis and glycogenolysis (e.g., portal shunt, hepatic cirrhosis), a deficiency in diabetogenic hormones (e.g., hypocortisolism), an inadequate dietary intake of glucose and other substrates required for hepatic gluconeogenesis (e.g., starvation), or a combination of these mechanisms (e.g., sepsis; Table 52-2). Iatrogenic hypoglycemia is a common problem resulting from overzealous insulin administration in diabetic dogs and cats.

Prolonged storage of blood before separation of serum or plasma causes the glucose concentration to decrease at a rate of approximately 7 mg/dl/hr. Glycolysis by red and white blood cells becomes even more apparent in dogs and cats with erythrocytosis, leukocytosis, or sepsis. Therefore whole blood obtained for the measurement of the glucose concentration should be separated soon after collection (within 1 hour) and the serum or plasma refrigerated or frozen until the assay is performed, to minimize artifactual lowering of the blood glucose concentration. Glucose determinations from separated and refrigerated plasma or serum are reliable for as long as 48 hours after the separation and refrigeration of the specimen. Alternatively, plasma can be collected in sodium fluoride tubes. Unfortunately, hemolysis is common in blood collected in sodium fluoride–treated tubes, which

TABLE 52-1

Causes of Hyperglycemia in Dogs and Cats

Diabetes mellitus*
"Stress" (cat)*
Postprandial effects (diets containing monosaccharides,
    disaccharides, and propylene glycol)
Hyperadrenocorticism*
Acromegaly (cat)
Diestrus (bitch)
Pheochromocytoma (dog)
Pancreatitis
Exocrine pancreatic neoplasia
Renal insufficiency
Drug therapy*
    Glucocorticoids
    Progestagens
    Megestrol acetate
    Thiazide diuretics
Dextrose-containing fluids*
Parenteral nutrition*
Head trauma

*Common cause.

 TABLE 52-2

Causes of Hypoglycemia in Dogs and Cats

β-Cell tumor (insulinoma)
Extrapancreatic neoplasia
    Hepatocellular carcinoma, hepatoma
    Leiomyosarcoma, leiomyoma
    Hemangiosarcoma
    Carcinoma (mammary, salivary, pulmonary)
    Leukemia
    Plasmacytoma
    Melanoma
Hepatic insufficiency*
    Portal caval shunts
    Chronic fibrosis, cirrhosis
Sepsis*
Hypoadrenocorticism
Hypopituitarism
Idiopathic hypoglycemia*
    Neonatal hypoglycemia
    Juvenile hypoglycemia (especially toy breeds)
    Hunting dog hypoglycemia
Renal failure
Exocrine pancreatic neoplasia
Hepatic enzyme deficiencies
    Von Gierke's disease (type I glycogen storage disease)
    Cori's disease (type III glycogen storage disease)
Severe polycythemia
Prolonged starvation
Prolonged sample storage*
Iatrogenic*
    Insulin therapy
    Sulfonylurea therapy
    Ethanol ingestion
    Ethylene glycol ingestion
Artifact
    Portable blood glucose–monitoring devices
    Laboratory error

*Common cause.

can result in slight decrements in glucose values owing to methodologic problems in laboratory determinations. Blood glucose values determined by many portable home blood glucose–monitoring devices are typically lower than actual glucose values determined by bench-top methodologies (i.e., glucose oxidase and hexokinase methods), and this may result in an incorrect diagnosis of hypoglycemia (see p. 739). Finally, a laboratory error may also result in an incorrect value. Therefore it is wise to confirm hypoglycemia by determining the blood glucose concentration from a second blood sample and using bench-top methodology before embarking on a search for the cause of hypoglycemia.

## Clinical Features

Clinical signs of hypoglycemia usually develop if the blood glucose concentration is less than 45 mg/dl, although this can be quite variable. The development of clinical signs depends on the nadir of the blood glucose concentration, the rate of decline in the concentration, and the duration of hypoglycemia. Clinical signs are a result of neuroglycopenia and hypoglycemia-induced stimulation of the sympathoadrenal nervous system. Neuroglycopenic signs include seizures, weakness, collapse, ataxia, and, less commonly, lethargy, blindness, bizarre behavior, and coma. Signs of increased secretion of catecholamines include restlessness, nervousness, hunger, and muscle fasciculations.

Depending on the cause, the signs of hypoglycemia may be persistent or intermittent. The hallmark clinical sign of hypoglycemia (i.e., seizures) tends to be intermittent, regardless of the cause. Dogs and cats usually recover from hypoglycemic seizures within 30 seconds to 5 minutes as a result of the activation of counterregulatory mechanisms (e.g., secre-

tion of catecholamines and glucagon) that block the effects of insulin, stimulate hepatic glucose secretion, and promote an increase in the blood glucose concentration.

## Diagnostic Approach

Hypoglycemia should always be confirmed before beginning diagnostic studies to identify the cause. Careful evaluation of the animal's history, physical examination findings, and results of routine blood tests (i.e., complete blood count [CBC], serum biochemistry panel, urinalysis) usually provide clues to the underlying cause. Hypoglycemia in the puppy or kitten is usually caused by idiopathic hypoglycemia, starvation, liver insufficiency (i.e., portal shunt), or sepsis. In young adult dogs or cats, hypoglycemia is usually caused by liver insufficiency, hypoadrenocorticism, or sepsis. In older dogs or cats, liver insufficiency, β-cell neoplasia, extrapancreatic neoplasia, hypoadrenocorticism, and sepsis are the most common causes.

Hypoglycemia tends to be mild (>45 mg/dl) and is often an incidental finding in dogs and cats with hypoadrenocorticism or liver insufficiency. Additional clinical pathologic alterations are usually present (e.g., hyponatremia and hyperkalemia in animals with Addison's disease or increased alanine aminotransferase activity, hypocholesterolemia, hypoalbuminemia, and a low blood urea nitrogen [BUN] concentration in animals with liver insufficiency). An adrenocorticotropic hormone (ACTH) stimulation test or liver function test (i.e., preprandial and postprandial bile acids) may be required to confirm the diagnosis. Severe hypoglycemia (<40 mg/dl) may develop in neonates and juvenile kittens and puppies (especially toy breeds) and in animals with sepsis, β-cell neoplasia, and extrapancreatic neoplasia, most notably hepatic adenocarcinoma and leiomyosarcoma. Sepsis is readily identified based on physical examination findings and abnormal CBC findings and includes a neutrophilic leukocytosis (typically >30,000/μl), a shift toward immaturity, and signs of toxicity. Extrapancreatic neoplasia can usually be identified based on the physical examination, abdominal or thoracic radiography, and abdominal ultrasonography findings. Dogs with β-cell neoplasia typically have normal physical examination findings and no abnormalities other than hypoglycemia shown by other diagnostic tests. Measurement of the baseline serum insulin concentration when the blood glucose is less than 60 mg/dl (preferably <50 mg/dl) is necessary to confirm the diagnosis of a β-cell tumor (see p. 770).

## Treatment

Whenever possible, therapy should always be directed at eliminating the underlying cause of the hypoglycemia. If the disorder cannot be eliminated and the clinical signs of hypoglycemia persist, long-term symptomatic therapy designed to increase the blood glucose concentration may be necessary to minimize clinical signs (see Table 52-19). Such therapy is usually required for animals with metastatic β-cell or extrapancreatic neoplasia.

Symptomatic therapy for animals with severe hypoglycemia of acute onset relies on the administration of glucose. If the dog or cat is having a hypoglycemic seizure at home, the owner should rub or pour a sugar mixture (e.g., Karo syrup) on the pet's buccal mucosa. Most dogs and cats respond within 1 to 2 minutes. Never have owners place fingers in or pour the sugar solution down the pet's mouth. Once the dog or cat is sternal and cognizant of its surroundings, it should be fed a small meal and brought to the veterinarian.

If collapse, seizures, or coma develops in the hospital, a blood sample should be obtained to measure the glucose concentration and other variables before reversing the signs with the IV administration of 50% dextrose. Dextrose should be administered in small amounts slowly rather than in large boluses rapidly. Commonly, 2 to 15 ml of 50% dextrose is required to alleviate the signs. Dogs and cats with hypoglycemia usually respond to glucose administration within 2 minutes.

Aggressive glucose therapy should be done with caution in dogs with β-cell neoplasia to minimize the degree of re-bound hypoglycemia. A continuous IV infusion of 2.5% to 5% dextrose in water or glucagon (see p. 772) may be required for several hours to days to prevent the recurrence of severe hypoglycemia until other therapy effectively maintains an adequate blood glucose concentration.

## Prognosis

In most dogs and cats, clinical signs of hypoglycemia can be controlled with glucose administration. Recurrence of hypoglycemia is dependent on the ability to correct the underlying etiology. Occasionally, a dog or cat with severe central nervous system (CNS) signs (e.g., blindness, coma) caused by hypoglycemia does not respond to initial glucose therapy. Irreversible cerebral lesions may result from prolonged severe hypoglycemia and the resultant cerebral hypoxia. The prognosis in these animals is guarded to poor. Therapy is directed at providing a continuous supply of glucose by administering a 2.5% to 5% solution IV or increasing hepatic gluconeogenesis with a constant rate infusion of glucagon. Seizure activity is controlled with diazepam or a stronger anticonvulsant medication. Glucocorticoids and mannitol may be necessary to combat cerebral edema.

# DIABETES MELLITUS IN DOGS

## Etiology

Virtually all dogs with diabetes have insulin-dependent diabetes mellitus (IDDM) at the time of diagnosis. IDDM is characterized by hypoinsulinemia, essentially no increase in the endogenous serum insulin concentration after the administration of an insulin secretagogue (e.g., glucose or glucagon) at any time after the diagnosis of the disease, failure to establish glycemic control in response to diet or treatment with oral hypoglycemic drugs, or both, and an absolute need for exogenous insulin to maintain glycemic control. The cause of diabetes mellitus has been poorly characterized in dogs but is undoubtedly multifactorial. A genetic predisposition, infection, insulin-antagonistic diseases and drugs, obesity, immune-mediated insulitis, and pancreatitis have been identified as inciting factors in the development of IDDM. The end result is a loss of β-cell function, hypoinsulinemia, impaired transport of circulating glucose into most cells, and accelerated hepatic gluconeogenesis and glycogenolysis. The subsequent development of hyperglycemia and glycosuria causes polyuria, polydipsia, polyphagia, and weight loss. Ketoacidosis develops as the production of ketone bodies increases to compensate for the underutilization of blood glucose (see p. 762). Loss of β-cell function is irreversible in dogs with IDDM, and lifelong insulin therapy is mandatory to maintain glycemic control of the diabetic state.

Unlike cats, a transient or reversible form of diabetes mellitus is uncommon in dogs. The most common scenario for transient diabetes mellitus in dogs is correction of insulin antagonism after ovariohysterectomy in a bitch in diestrus. Progesterone stimulates secretion of growth hormone in the bitch. Ovariohysterectomy removes the source of progesterone, plasma growth hormone concentration declines, and insulin antagonism resolves. If an adequate population of functional β cells are still present in the pancreas, hyperglycemia may resolve without the need for insulin treatment. These dogs have a significant reduction in β-cell numbers (i.e., subclinical diabetes), compared with healthy dogs, before the development of hyperglycemia during diestrus and are prone to redevelopment of hyperglycemia and diabetes mellitus if insulin antagonism recurs for any reason after ovariohysterectomy. Although uncommon, a similar situation can occur in dogs with subclinical diabetes treated with insulin-antagonistic drugs (e.g., glucocorticoids) or in the very early stages of an insulin-antagonistic disorder (e.g., hyperadrenocorticism). Failure to quickly correct the insulin antagonism will result in IDDM and the lifelong requirement for insulin treatment to control the hyperglycemia.

A honeymoon period occurs in some dogs with newly diagnosed IDDM. It is characterized by excellent glycemic control in response to small doses of insulin (<0.2 U/kg/injection), presumably because of the presence of residual β-cell function. However, glycemic control becomes more difficult and insulin doses usually increase within 3 to 6 months of starting treatment as residual functioning β cells are destroyed and endogenous insulin secretion declines. It is very uncommon for non–insulin-dependent diabetes mellitus (NIDDM) to be recognized clinically in dogs, despite the documentation of obesity-induced carbohydrate intolerance in dogs and the identification of residual β-cell function in some diabetic dogs. A juvenile form of canine diabetes mellitus that closely resembles human maturity-onset diabetes of the young, a subclassification of NIDDM, has been described but is rare. The clinical characteristics of juvenile canine NIDDM resemble those of IDDM in dogs with residual β-cell function, with the result that dogs with either condition are treated with insulin to manage the hyperglycemia.

## Clinical Features

**Signalment.** Most dogs are 4 to 14 years old at the time diabetes mellitus is diagnosed, with a peak prevalence at 7 to 9 years of age. Juvenile-onset diabetes occurs in dogs less than 1 year of age and is uncommon. Female dogs are affected about twice as frequently as male dogs. Genetic predispositions to the development of diabetes have been indicated by the finding of familial associations in dogs and by pedigree analysis of Keeshonds. An epidemiologic study performed by Guptill and colleagues (1999) identified the Australian, Fox, Cairn, and Yorkshire Terrier, Standard and Miniature Schnauzer, Bichon Frise, Spitz, Miniature and Toy Poodle, Samoyed, and Lhasa Apso as breeds at increased risk for development of diabetes mellitus, and the German Shepherd, Collie, Shetland Sheepdog, Golden Retriever, Cocker Spaniel, Australian Shepherd, Labrador Retriever, Boston Terrier, and Rottweiler as breeds at decreased risk for development of diabetes mellitus.

**History.** The history in virtually all diabetic dogs includes the classic signs polydipsia, polyuria, polyphagia, and weight loss. Polyuria and polydipsia do not develop until hyperglycemia results in glycosuria. Occasionally, an owner brings

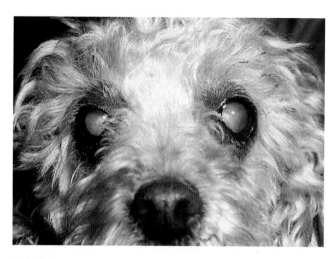

**FIG 52-1**
Bilateral cataracts causing blindness in a diabetic dog. (From Feldman EC, Nelson RW: *Canine and feline endocrinology and reproduction,* ed 2, Philadelphia, 1996, WB Saunders.)

in a dog because of sudden blindness caused by cataract formation (Fig. 52-1). The classic signs of diabetes mellitus may have gone unnoticed or been considered irrelevant by the owner. If the clinical signs associated with uncomplicated diabetes are not observed by the owner and impaired vision caused by cataracts does not develop, a diabetic dog is at risk for the development of systemic signs of illness as progressive ketonemia and metabolic acidosis develop (see p. 762). The time sequence from the onset of initial clinical signs to the development of diabetic ketoacidosis (DKA) is unpredictable, ranging from days to weeks.

**Physical examination.** The physical examination findings depend on whether DKA is present and its severity, on the duration of diabetes before its diagnosis, and on the nature of any other concurrent disorder. The nonketotic diabetic dog has no classic physical examination findings. Many diabetic dogs are obese but are otherwise in good physical condition. Dogs with prolonged untreated diabetes may have lost weight but are rarely emaciated unless concurrent disease (e.g., pancreatic exocrine insufficiency) is present. The haircoat may be sparse, the hairs dry, brittle and lusterless, and scales from hyperkeratosis may be present. Diabetes-induced hepatic lipidosis may cause hepatomegaly. Lenticular changes consistent with cataract formation are another common clinical finding in diabetic dogs. Additional abnormalities may be identified in the ketoacidotic diabetic dog (see p. 763).

## Diagnosis

For diabetes mellitus to be diagnosed, the dog must show the appropriate clinical signs (i.e., polyuria, polydipsia, polyphagia, weight loss) and a persistent fasting hyperglycemia and glycosuria must be documented. Measurement of the blood glucose concentration using a portable blood glucose–monitoring device (see p. 739) and testing for the presence of glycosuria using urine reagent test strips (e.g., KetoDiastix; Ames Division, Miles Laboratories Inc., Elkhart, Ind) allows the rapid confirmation of diabetes mellitus. The concurrent documentation of ketonuria establishes a diagnosis of DKA.

It is important to document both persistent hyperglycemia and glycosuria to establish a diagnosis of diabetes mellitus, because hyperglycemia differentiates diabetes mellitus from primary renal glycosuria, whereas glycosuria differentiates diabetes mellitus from other causes of hyperglycemia (see Table 52-1), most notably epinephrine-induced stress hyperglycemia that may develop around the time of blood sampling. Stress-induced hyperglycemia is a common problem in cats and occasionally occurs in dogs, especially those that are very excited, hyperactive, or aggressive. The reader is referred to p. 759 for more information on stress-induced hyperglycemia.

A thorough evaluation of the dog's overall health is recommended once the diagnosis of diabetes mellitus has been established to identify any disease that may be causing or contributing to the carbohydrate intolerance (e.g., hyperadrenocorticism), that may result from the carbohydrate intolerance (e.g., bacterial cystitis), or that may mandate a modification of therapy (e.g., pancreatitis). The minimum laboratory evaluation should include a CBC, serum biochemical panel, measurement of serum trypsinlike immunoreactivity, and urinalysis with bacterial culture. Serum progesterone concentration should be determined if diabetes mellitus is diagnosed in an intact bitch, regardless of her cycling history. If available, abdominal ultrasound is indicated to assess for pancreatitis, adrenomegaly, pyometritis in an intact bitch, and abnormalities affecting the liver and urinary tract (e.g., changes consistent with pyelonephritis or cystitis). Measurement of the baseline serum insulin concentration or an insulin response test is not routinely done. Additional tests may be warranted after obtaining the history, performing the physical examination, or identifying ketoacidosis. Potential clinical pathologic abnormalities are listed in Table 52-3.

## Treatment

The primary goal of therapy is elimination of the owner-observed signs occurring secondary to hyperglycemia and glycosuria. A persistence of clinical signs and the development of chronic complications (Table 52-4) are directly correlated with the severity and duration of hyperglycemia. Limiting blood glucose concentration fluctuations and maintaining nearly normal glycemia will help minimize the severity of clinical signs and prevent the complications of poorly controlled diabetes. In the diabetic dog, this can be accomplished through proper insulin therapy, diet, exercise, and the prevention or control of concurrent inflammatory, infectious, neoplastic, and hormonal disorders.

Although it is worthwhile attempting to normalize the blood glucose concentration, the veterinarian must also guard against the development of hypoglycemia, a serious and potentially fatal complication of therapy. Hypoglycemia is most apt to occur as the result of overzealous insulin therapy. The veterinarian must balance the benefits of tight glucose control obtainable with aggressive insulin therapy against the risk of hypoglycemia.

## TABLE 52-3

### Clinicopathologic Abnormalities Commonly Found in Dogs and Cats with Uncomplicated Diabetes Mellitus

**Complete Blood Count**

Typically normal
Neutrophilic leukocytosis, toxic neutrophils if pancreatitis or infection present

**Biochemistry Panel**

Hyperglycemia
Hypercholesterolemia
Hypertriglyceridemia (lipemia)
Increased alanine aminotransferase activity (typically <500 IU/L)
Increased alkaline phosphatase activity (typically <500 IU/L)

**Urinalysis**

Urine specific gravity typically >1.025
Glycosuria
Variable ketonuria
Proteinuria
Bacteriuria

**Ancillary Tests**

Hyperlipasemia if pancreatitis present
Hyperamylasemia if pancreatitis present
Serum trypsinlike immunoreactivity usually normal
Low with pancreatic exocrine insufficiency
High with acute pancreatitis
Normal to high with chronic pancreatitis
Variable serum baseline insulin concentration
  IDDM: low, normal
  NIDDM: low, normal, increased
  Insulin resistance induced: low, normal, increased

*IDDM,* Insulin-dependent diabetes mellitus; *NIDDM,* non–insulin-dependent diabetes mellitus.

**Initial insulin therapy.** Intermediate-acting insulin (i.e., Lente, NPH) is the initial insulin of choice for establishing control of glycemia in diabetic dogs (Table 52-5). Recombinant human-source insulin should be used to avoid problems with insulin effectiveness presumably caused by circulating insulin antibodies (see p. 746). Insulin therapy is begun with Lente or NPH insulin of recombinant human origin at an approximate dose of 0.25 U/kg twice a day. Because greater than 90% of diabetic dogs require recombinant human Lente or NPH insulin twice a day, the preference is to start with twice-a-day insulin therapy. Establishing control of glycemia is easier and problems with hypoglycemia and the Somogyi effect (see p. 744) are less likely when twice daily insulin therapy is initiated while the insulin dose is low (i.e., at the time insulin treatment is initiated). Glycemic regulation is more problematic and development of hypoglycemia and the Somogyi effect more likely when poorly controlled diabetic

### TABLE 52-4

Complications of Diabetes Mellitus in Dogs and Cats

| COMMON | UNCOMMON |
|---|---|
| Iatrogenic hypoglycemia | Peripheral neuropathy (dog) |
| Persistent polyuria, polydipsia, weight loss | Glomerulonephropathy, glomerulosclerosis |
| Cataracts (dog) | Retinopathy |
| Bacterial infections, especially in the urinary tract | Exocrine pancreatic insufficiency |
| Pancreatitis | Gastric paresis |
| Ketoacidosis | Diabetic diarrhea |
| Hepatic lipidosis | Diabetic dermatopathy (dog) (i.e., superficial necrolytic dermatitis) |
| Peripheral neuropathy (cat) | |

### TABLE 52-5

Properties of Recombinant Human Insulin Preparations Used in Dogs and Cats*

| TYPE OF INSULIN | ROUTE OF ADMINISTRATION | ONSET OF EFFECT | TIME OF MAXIMUM EFFECT (HR) | | DURATION OF EFFECT (HR) | |
|---|---|---|---|---|---|---|
| | | | DOG | CAT | DOG | CAT |
| Regular crystalline | IV | Immediate | ½-2 | ½-2 | 1-4 | 1-4 |
| | IM | 10-30 min | 1-4 | 1-4 | 3-8 | 3-8 |
| | SC | 10-30 min | 1-5 | 1-5 | 4-10 | 4-10 |
| NPH (isophane) | SC | ½-2 hr | 2-10 | 2-8 | 6-18 | 4-12 |
| Lente† | SC | ½-2 hr | 2-10 | 2-10 | 8-20 | 6-18 |
| Ultralente | SC | ½-8 hr | 4-16 | 4-16 | 6-24 | 6-24 |

*Purified pork insulin has similar properties; beef/pork insulin mixtures are less potent and may have a longer duration of action than recombinant human insulins.
†Initial insulin of choice for the diabetic dog and cat. Beef/pork PZI is also a good initial insulin for the diabetic cat.

dogs receiving a high dose of insulin once daily are switched to insulin twice a day but the dose per injection is arbitrarily chosen.

**Dietary therapy.** Adjustments in diet and feeding practices should be directed at correcting or preventing obesity, maintaining consistency in the timing and caloric content of the meals, and furnishing a diet that helps minimize the postprandial increase in blood glucose concentration (Table 52-6). Diets containing increased fiber content are beneficial for treating obesity and improving control of glycemia in diabetics.

Several mechanisms have been proposed to explain the fiber-induced slowing of intestinal glucose absorption and the corresponding improvement in glycemic control of the diabetic dog. These include a delay in the gastric emptying of nutrients; a delay in the intestinal absorption of nutrients, most likely resulting from an effect on the diffusion of glucose toward the brush border of the intestine; and a fiber-induced effect on the release of regulatory gastrointestinal tract hormones into the circulation. The improvement in glycemic control depends in part on the type of fiber consumed. The two basic types of fiber are differentiated by their solubility in water: (1) insoluble fiber (e.g., lignin, cellulose) and (2) soluble fiber (e.g., gums, pectins). In most studies the consumption of soluble fiber has been found to be more effective in improving glycemic control than the consumption of insoluble fiber. However, studies in diabetic dogs have documented glycemic improvement in response to the consumption of diets containing increased amounts of insoluble fiber (Fig. 52-2). Most commercial high-fiber diets predominantly contain insoluble fiber, although diets containing mixtures of soluble and insoluble fiber are becoming available (Table 52-7). The amount of fiber varies considerably among products, ranging from 3% to 25% of dry matter (normal diets contain <2% fiber on a dry matter basis). In general, diets containing 12% or more insoluble fiber or 8% or more of a mixture of soluble and insoluble fiber are most likely to be effective in improving glycemic control in diabetic dogs.

The dog's susceptibility to the complications of high-fiber diets, its body weight and condition, and the presence of a concurrent disease (e.g., pancreatitis, renal failure) in which

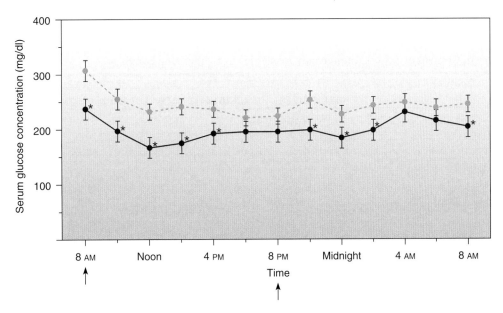

**FIG 52-2**

Mean (± standard error of the mean) serum concentration of glucose in 11 dogs with naturally occurring diabetes mellitus fed high-insoluble fiber (i.e., cellulose) *(red)* and low-fiber *(blue)* diet. ↑, Insulin administration and consumption of half of daily caloric intake; *p <0.05, compared with low-fiber diet. (From Nelson RW et al: Effect of dietary insoluble fiber on glycemic control in dogs with naturally-occurring diabetes mellitus, *J Am Vet Med Assoc* 212:280, 1998.)

 TABLE 52-6

**Recommendations for Dietary Treatment of Diabetes Mellitus in Dogs**

| | |
|---|---|
| I. Dietary composition<br>  Increased fiber content (see Table 52-7)<br>  Increased digestible carbohydrate content<br>    (45%-60% ME)<br>  Decreased fat content (<25% ME)<br>  Adequate protein content (15%-30% ME)<br>II. Feed canned and/or dry kibble foods; avoid diet<br>  containing monosaccharides, disaccharides, and pro-<br>  pylene glycol<br>III. Caloric intake and obesity<br>  Average daily caloric intake in geriatric pet:<br>    40-60 kcal/kg<br>  Adjust daily caloric intake on individual basis | Eliminate obesity, if present by:<br>  Increasing daily exercise<br>  Decreasing daily caloric intake<br>  Feeding low-calorie-dense, low-fat, high-fiber<br>    (preferred in diabetics) or low-calorie-dense, low-<br>    fat, low-fiber diet designed for weight loss<br>  Eliminating treats<br>IV. Feeding schedule<br>  Maintain consistent caloric content of the meals<br>  Maintain consistent timing of feeding<br>  Feed within time frame of insulin action<br>  Feed one-half the total daily caloric intake at time of<br>    each insulin injection<br>  Let "nibbler" dogs continue to nibble throughout day<br>    and night |

*ME,* Metabolizable energy.

diet is an important aspect of therapy ultimately dictate which, if any, fiber diet is fed. Common clinical complications of high insoluble fiber diets include excessive frequency of defecation; constipation and obstipation; hypoglycemia 1 to 2 weeks after the increase in fiber content of the diet; and refusal to eat the diet. Complications of soluble fiber-containing diets include soft-to-watery stools; excessive flatulence; hypoglycemia 1 to

2 weeks after the increase in fiber content of the diet; and refusal to eat the diet. If firm stools or constipation become a problem with high insoluble fiber diets, a mixture of insoluble and soluble fiber diets can be fed or soluble fiber (e.g., sugar-free Metamucil, canned pumpkin) can be added to the diet to soften the stool. Alternatively, if soft or watery diarrhea or flatulence become a problem with soluble fiber-

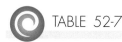

TABLE 52-7

**Approximate Nutrient Content of Some Commercially Available High-Fiber Dog Foods**

| | CRUDE FIBER* | CARBOHYDRATE† | FAT† | PROTEIN† | CALORIES‡ (CAN/CUP) |
|---|---|---|---|---|---|
| **Prescription Diet r/d** | | | | | |
| Canned | 26 | 45 | 22 | 33 | 249 |
| Dry | 24 | 49 | 21 | 30 | 205 |
| **Prescription Diet w/d** | | | | | |
| Canned | 14 | 54 | 29 | 16 | 390 |
| Dry | 17 | 62 | 19 | 19 | 226 |
| **Purina OM** | | | | | |
| Canned | 19 | 17 | 28 | 55 | 189 |
| Dry | 11 | 47 | 16 | 37 | 276 |
| **Science Diet Light** | | | | | |
| Canned | 10 | 58 | 24 | 18 | 364 |
| Dry | 14 | 62 | 18 | 20 | 295 |
| **Purina DCO** | | | | | |
| Dry | 8 | 45 | 32 | 24 | 320 |
| **Waltham Glucomodulation Control Diet** | | | | | |
| Canned | 10 | 55 | 11 | 34 | 339 |
| Dry | 5 | 62 | 10 | 28 | 316 |
| **Iams Eukanuba Optimum Weight Control** | | | | | |
| Dry | 3 | 52 | 19 | 29 | 253 |

*Expressed as a percentage of the diet dry matter.
†Expressed as percent metabolizable energy derived from carbohydrate, fat, or protein.
‡Expressed as kilocalories of metabolizable energy per can (15 oz) or for the dry diets per standard (8 oz volume) measuring cup full.

containing diets, an insoluble fiber diet can be added and the quantity of the soluble fiber diet decreased. If palatability is a problem initially, the animal can be gradually switched from its regular diet to a diet containing small amounts of fiber, after which diets containing more fiber are provided. Refusal to consume high-fiber diets months after their initiation is usually a result of boredom with the food. Periodic changes in the types of high-fiber diets and mixtures of diets have been helpful in alleviating this problem.

Diets containing an increased amount of fiber should not be fed to thin or emaciated diabetic dogs because high-fiber diets have a low caloric density, which can interfere with weight gain and may result in further weight loss. For thin diabetic dogs to gain weight, usually glycemic control must be reestablished through insulin therapy and the feeding of a higher-calorie-dense, lower-fiber diet designed for maintenance. Once a normal body weight has been attained, a diet containing more fiber can be gradually substituted for the prior diet.

**Exercise.** Exercise plays an important role in maintaining glycemic control in the diabetic dog by helping promote weight loss and by eliminating the insulin resistance induced by obesity. Exercise also has a glucose-lowering effect by increasing the mobilization of insulin from its injection site, presumably resulting from increased blood and lymph flow, by increasing blood flow (and therefore insulin delivery) to exercising muscles, and by stimulating glucose transporters in muscle cells. The daily routine for diabetic dogs should include exercise, preferably at the same time each day. Strenuous and sporadic exercise can cause severe hypoglycemia and should be avoided. The insulin dose should be decreased in dogs subjected to sporadic strenuous exercise (e.g., hunting dogs during hunting season) on those days of anticipated increased exercise. The reduction in insulin dose required to prevent hypoglycemia is variable and determined by trial and error. Reducing the insulin dose by 50% initially is recommended with further adjustments based on the occurrence of symptomatic hypoglycemia and the severity of polyuria and polydipsia that develops during the ensuing 24 to 48 hours. In addition, owners must be aware of the signs of hypoglycemia and have a source of glucose (e.g., Karo syrup, candy, food) readily available to give their dog should any of these signs develop.

**Acarbose.** Acarbose is a complex oligosaccharide of microbial origin that competitively inhibits pancreatic α-amylase and α-glucosidases (i.e., glucoamylase, sucrase, maltase, isomaltase) in the brush border of the small intestinal mucosa. Inhibition of these enzymes delays digestion of complex carbohydrates and disaccharides to monosaccharides. This inhibition delays absorption of glucose from the intestinal tract and decreases postprandial blood glucose concentrations. Acarbose is beneficial in improving control of glycemia in some dogs with IDDM. The high prevalence of adverse effects (e.g., diarrhea, weight loss) resulting from carbohydrate malassimilation and the expense of the drug limit its usefulness. Acarbose is reserved for treating poorly controlled diabetic dogs where the cause for poor control of glycemia cannot be identified and insulin treatment, by itself, is ineffective in preventing clinical signs of diabetes. The initial dose should be kept low (i.e., 12.5 to 25 mg/dog at each meal) and always administered at the time of feeding. A stepwise increase to 50 mg/dog and, in large dogs (i.e., >25 kg), a further increase to 100 mg/dog can be considered in dogs that fail to show improvement in control of glycemia after 2 weeks at lower doses.

**Identification and control of concurrent problems.** Concurrent disease and insulin-antagonistic drugs can interfere with tissue responsiveness to insulin. Tissue responsiveness to insulin may be impaired as a result of decreased number of insulin receptors at the surface of the cell membrane, alterations in insulin receptor binding affinity, or impairment in one of several postreceptor steps responsible for activation of glucose transport systems. Loss of tissue responsiveness results in insulin resistance, and the severity of insulin resistance depends, in part, on the underlying etiology (see p. 747). Insulin resistance may be mild and easily overcome by increasing the dose of insulin or may be severe, causing marked hyperglycemia regardless of the type and dose of insulin administered. Some causes of insulin resistance are readily apparent at the time diabetes is diagnosed, such as obesity and the administration of insulin-antagonistic drugs (e.g., glucocorticoids, megestrol acetate). Other causes of insulin resistance are not readily apparent and require an extensive diagnostic evaluation to be identified. In general, any concurrent inflammatory, infectious, hormonal, or neoplastic disorder can cause insulin resistance and interfere with the effectiveness of insulin therapy. Identification and treatment of concurrent disease plays an integral role in the successful management of the diabetic dog. A thorough history, physical examination, and complete diagnostic evaluation are imperative in the newly diagnosed diabetic dog (see Diagnosis, p. 732).

**Initial adjustments in insulin therapy.** Diabetic dogs require several days to equilibrate to changes in insulin dose or preparation. Therefore newly diagnosed diabetic dogs are typically hospitalized for no more than 24 to 48 hours to finish the diagnostic evaluation of the patient and to begin insulin therapy. During hospitalization, blood glucose concentrations are typically determined at the time insulin is administered and at 11 AM, 2 PM, and 5 PM. The intent is to identify hypoglycemia (i.e., blood glucose <80 mg/dl) in those dogs that are unusually sensitive to the actions of insulin. If hypoglycemia occurs, the insulin dose is decreased before sending the dog home. The insulin dose is not adjusted in those dogs that remain hyperglycemic during these first few days of insulin therapy. The objective during this first visit is *not* to establish perfect glycemic control before sending the dog home. Rather, the objective is to begin to reverse the metabolic derangements induced by the disease, allow the patient to equilibrate to the insulin and change in diet, teach the owner how to administer insulin, and give the owner a few

days to become accustomed to treating the diabetic dog at home. Adjustments in insulin therapy are made on subsequent evaluations, once the owner and pet have become accustomed to the treatment regimen.

Diabetic dogs are typically evaluated once weekly until an effective insulin treatment protocol is identified. The owner is informed at the time insulin therapy is initiated that it will take approximately 1 month to establish a satisfactory insulin treatment protocol, assuming unidentified insulin-antagonistic disease is not present. The goals of therapy are also explained to the owner. During this month, changes in insulin dose, type, and frequency of insulin administration are common and should be anticipated by the owner. At each evaluation, the owner's subjective opinion of water intake, urine output, and overall health of the pet is discussed; a complete physical examination is performed; change in body weight noted; and serial blood glucose measurements between 7 and 9 AM and 4 and 6 PM are assessed. Adjustments in insulin therapy are based on this information, the pet is sent home, and an appointment is scheduled for the next week to reevaluate the response to any change in therapy. Glycemic control is attained when clinical signs of diabetes have resolved, the pet is healthy and interactive in the home, its body weight is stable, the owner is satisfied with the progress of therapy, and, if possible, the blood glucose concentrations range between 100 and 250 mg/dl throughout the day.

The insulin dose required to maintain glycemic control typically changes (increase or decrease) with time. Initially, a fixed dose of insulin is administered at home and changes are made only after the owner consults with the veterinarian. As the insulin dose range required to maintain glycemic control becomes apparent and as confidence is gained in the owner's ability to recognize signs of hypo- and hyperglycemia, the owner is eventually allowed to make *slight* adjustments in the insulin dose at home based on clinical observations of the pet's well-being. However, the owner is instructed to stay within the agreed upon insulin dose range. If the insulin dose is at the upper or lower end of the established range and the pet is still symptomatic, the owner is instructed to call the veterinarian before making further adjustments in the insulin dose.

## Techniques for Monitoring Diabetic Control

The basic objective of insulin therapy is to eliminate the clinical signs of diabetes mellitus while avoiding the common complications associated with the disease. Common complications in dogs include blindness caused by cataract formation, weight loss, hypoglycemia, recurring ketosis, and poor control of glycemia secondary to concurrent infection, inflammation, neoplasia, or hormonal disorders. The devastating chronic complications of human diabetes (e.g., nephropathy, vasculopathy, coronary artery disease) require several decades to develop and are uncommon in diabetic dogs.

As such, the need to establish nearly normal blood glucose concentrations is not necessary in diabetic dogs. Most owners are happy and most dogs are healthy and relatively asymptomatic if most blood glucose concentrations are kept between 100 mg/dl and 250 mg/dl.

**History and physical examination.** The most important initial parameters to assess when evaluating control of glycemia are the owner's subjective opinion of severity of clinical signs and overall health of the pet, findings on physical examination, and stability of body weight. If the owner is happy with results of treatment, the physical examination is supportive of good glycemic control, and the body weight is stable, the diabetic dog is usually adequately controlled. The preference is to talk to the owner and perform the physical examination of the dog at the beginning of the day (between 7:30 and 9:00 AM), before or within 1 hour of insulin administration, and to obtain blood for determination of glucose and serum fructosamine concentration (see following) at that time. In most well-regulated diabetic dogs, the blood glucose concentration measured between 7:30 and 9:00 AM and before or within 1 hour of insulin administration will be between 150 and 250 mg/dl. An early-morning blood glucose concentration less than 150 mg/dl in a presumably well-controlled diabetic dog raises concern for development of hypoglycemia several hours after insulin administration that is either asymptomatic or has clinical signs that are not recognized by the owner. Measurement of serum fructosamine concentration is indicated in this situation; identification of a low serum fructosamine concentration (<350 μmol/L) suggests periods of hypoglycemia and a need to reduce the insulin dose. Poor control of glycemia should be suspected and additional diagnostics (i.e., serial blood glucose curve, serum fructosamine concentration, tests for concurrent disorders) or a change in insulin therapy considered if the owner reports clinical signs (i.e., polyuria, polydipsia, lethargy, signs of hypoglycemia), the physical examination identifies problems consistent with poor control of glycemia (e.g., thin or emaciated, poor haircoat), the dog is losing weight, or the blood glucose concentration measured in the early morning is greater than 300 mg/dl.

**Serum fructosamine concentration.** Documenting an increased blood glucose concentration does not, *by itself,* confirm poor control of glycemia. Stress or excitement can cause marked hyperglycemia that does not reflect the patient's responsiveness to insulin and can lead to the erroneous belief that the diabetic dog is poorly controlled (see p. 759). If a discrepancy exists between the history, physical examination findings, and blood glucose concentration or the dog is fractious, aggressive, excited, or scared and the blood glucose concentration is known to be unreliable, measurement of serum fructosamine concentration should be done to further evaluate status of glycemic control. Fructosamines are glycated proteins found in blood that are used to monitor glycemic control. Fructosamines result from an irreversible, nonenzymatic, insulin-independent binding of glucose to serum proteins. The extent of glycosylation of serum proteins is directly related to the blood glucose concentration; the higher the average blood glucose concentration during the preceding 2 to 3 weeks, the higher the serum fructosamine concentration, and vice versa. Serum fructosamine concentration is not affected by acute increases in the blood glucose concentration, as occurs with stress or excitement-induced hyperglycemia. Serum fructosamine concentrations can be measured during the routine evaluation of glycemic control performed every 3 to 6 months; to clarify the effect of stress or excitement on blood glucose concentrations; to clarify discrepancies between the history, physical examination findings, and serial blood glucose concentrations; and to assess the effectiveness of changes in insulin therapy (see p. 741).

In our laboratory the normal reference range for serum fructosamine is 225 to 375 μmol/L; a range determined in healthy dogs with persistently normal blood glucose concentrations. Interpretation of serum fructosamine in a diabetic dog must take into consideration the fact that hyperglycemia is common, even in well-controlled diabetic dogs (Table 52-8).

 TABLE 52-8

Sample Handling, Methodology, and Normal Values for Serum Fructosamine Concentrations Measured in the Laboratory

| | **FRUCTOSAMINE** |
|---|---|
| Blood sample | 1-2 ml serum |
| Sample handling | Freeze until assayed |
| Methodology | Automated colorimetric assay using nitroblue tetrazolium chloride |
| Factors affecting results | Hypoalbuminemia (decreased), hyperlipidemia (mild decrease—dogs), azotemia (mild decrease—dogs), storage at room temperature (decreased) |
| Normal range | 225-375 μmol/L |
| **Interpretation in Diabetics:** | |
| Excellent control | 350-400 μmol/L |
| Good control | 400-450 μmol/L |
| Fair control | 450-500 μmol/L |
| Poor control | >500 μmol/L |
| Prolonged hypoglycemia | <300 μmol/L |

Most owners are happy with the pet's response to insulin treatment if serum fructosamine concentrations can be kept between 350 and 450 μmol/L. Values greater than 500 μmol/L suggest inadequate control of the diabetic state and values greater than 600 μmol/L indicate serious lack of glycemic control. Serum fructosamine concentrations in the lower half of the normal reference range (<300 μmol/L) or below the normal reference range should raise concern for significant periods of hypoglycemia in the diabetic dog. The Somogyi phenomenon (i.e., glucose counterregulation) should be suspected if clinical signs (i.e., polyuria, polydipsia, polyphagia, weight loss) are present in a diabetic dog with a serum fructosamine concentration less than 400 μmol/L. Increased serum fructosamine concentrations (>500 μmol/L) suggest poor control of glycemia and a need for insulin adjustments; however, increased serum fructosamine concentrations do not identify the underlying problem.

**Urine glucose monitoring.** Occasional monitoring of urine for glycosuria and ketonuria is helpful in those diabetic dogs that have problems with recurring ketosis or hypoglycemia to determine whether ketonuria or persistent negative glycosuria is present, respectively. The owner is instructed not to adjust daily insulin doses based on morning urine glucose measurements in diabetic dogs, except to decrease the insulin dose in dogs with recurring hypoglycemia and persistent negative glycosuria. The vast majority of diabetic dogs develop complications as a result of owners being misled by morning urine glucose concentrations. A weekend evaluation of multiple urine samples that have been obtained throughout the day and early evening is recommended. The well-controlled diabetic pet should have urine that is free of glucose for most of each 24-hour period. Persistent glycosuria throughout the day and night suggests a problem that may require evaluation via in-hospital or at home blood glucose determinations.

**Serial blood glucose curve.** If an adjustment in insulin therapy is deemed necessary after reviewing the history, physical examination, changes in body weight, and serum fructosamine concentration, then a serial blood glucose curve should be generated to provide guidance in making the adjustment unless blood glucose measurements are unreliable because of stress, aggression, or excitement (see p. 759). Evaluation of a serial blood glucose curve is mandatory during the initial regulation of the diabetic patient, is periodically of value to assess glycemic control despite the fact that a dog may appear to be doing well in the home environment, and is necessary to reestablish glycemic control in the patient in which clinical manifestations of hyperglycemia or hypoglycemia have developed.

***Protocol for generating the serial blood glucose curve in the hospital.*** When assessing glycemic control, the insulin and feeding schedule used by the owner should be followed and blood should be obtained every 1 to 2 hours throughout the day for glucose determination. The owner should feed the pet at home, not at the hospital. If insulin is usually given within 1 hour before the pet's presentation to the clinic, the owner administers insulin (using his or her own insulin and syringe) in the hospital *after* initial blood glucose is obtained. A veterinary technician should closely evaluate the entire insulin administration procedure. If the owner usually administers insulin before 6 AM, the owner should give the insulin at 6 AM and bring the pet to the hospital at the first appointment of the day. It is more important to maintain the pet's daily routine than to risk inaccurate blood glucose results caused by inappetence in the hospital or insulin administration at an unusual time. The exception are those instances where the clinician wants to evaluate owner administration technique of insulin rather than physiologic saline.

Blood glucose concentrations are typically determined by either an in-house bench-top method or hand held portable blood glucose-monitoring device. Blood glucose values determined by many portable blood glucose-monitoring devices are typically lower than actual glucose values determined by bench-top methodologies (i.e., glucose oxidase and hexokinase methods; Fig. 52-3). This may result in an incorrect diagnosis of hypoglycemia or the misperception that glycemic control is better than it actually is. Failure to consider this "error" could result in insulin underdosing and the potential for persistence of clinical signs despite "acceptable" blood glucose results.

By evaluating serial blood glucose measurements every 1 to 2 hours throughout the day, the clinician will be able to determine if the insulin is effective and to identify the glucose nadir, time of peak insulin effect, duration of insulin effect, and severity of fluctuation in blood glucose concentrations in that particular diabetic dog. Obtaining only 1 or 2 blood glucose concentrations has not been reliable for evaluating the effect of a given insulin dose (Fig. 52-4).

The *ideal* goal of insulin therapy in diabetic dogs is to maintain the blood glucose concentration between 100 mg/dl and 250 mg/dl throughout the day and night. These goals can be very difficult, and in some diabetic dogs, impossible to attain. The ultimate decision on whether to adjust insulin therapy must always take into consideration the owner's perception of how the pet is doing at home, findings on physical examination, changes in body weight, serum fructosamine concentrations, and results of serial blood glucose measurements. Many diabetic dogs do well despite blood glucose concentrations consistently in the high 100s to low 300s.

***Protocol for generating the serial blood glucose curve at home.*** Hyperglycemia induced by stress, aggression, or excitement is the single biggest problem affecting accuracy of the serial blood glucose curve, especially in cats. Stress can override the glucose-lowering effect of the insulin injection, causing high blood glucose concentrations despite the presence of adequate amounts of insulin in the circulation and leading to a spiraling path of insulin overdosing, hypoglycemia, Somogyi phenomenon, and poor control of glycemia. The biggest factors inducing stress hyperglycemia are hospitalization and multiple venipunctures. An alternative to hospital-generated blood glucose curves is to have the owner generate

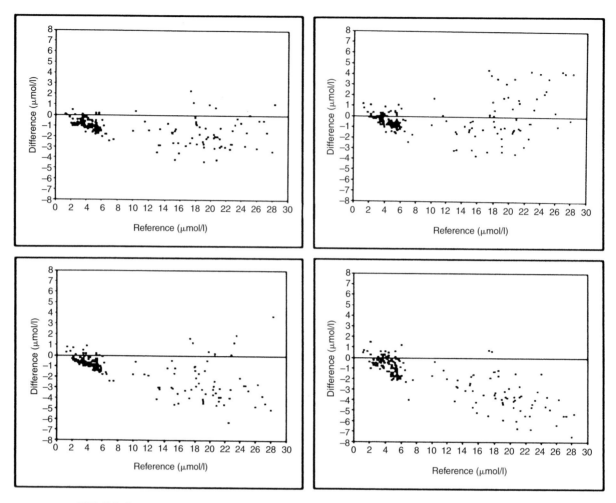

**FIG 52-3**
Scatterplots of the difference between blood glucose concentration obtained with four portable blood glucose meters and concentration obtained with a reference method versus concentration obtained with the reference method for blood samples from 170 dogs. (From Wess G et al: Evaluation of five portable blood glucose meters for use in dogs, *J Am Vet Med Assoc* 216:203, 2000.)

the blood glucose curve at home using the ear or lip prick technique and a portable home glucose-monitoring device that allows the owner to touch the drop of blood on the ear or lip with the end of the glucose test strip. This technique is usually reserved for diabetic dogs in which the reliability of blood glucose results generated in the veterinary hospital are questionable. The reader is referred to p. 758 for more information on monitoring blood glucose concentrations at home.

***Interpreting the serial blood glucose curve.*** Results of the blood glucose curve will allow the veterinarian to assess the effectiveness of the administered insulin to lower the blood glucose concentration and to determine the glucose nadir and duration of insulin effect (Fig. 52-5). Ideally, all blood glucose concentrations should range between 100 and 250 mg/dl during the time period between insulin injections. Typically, the highest blood glucose concentrations occur at the time of each insulin injection, but this does not always

occur. If the blood glucose nadir is greater than 150 mg/dl, the insulin dose may need to be increased, and if the nadir is less than 80 mg/dl, the insulin dose should be decreased.

Duration of insulin effect can be assessed if the glucose nadir is greater than 80 mg/dl and there has not been a rapid decrease in the blood glucose concentration after insulin administration. Assessment of duration of insulin effect may not be valid when the blood glucose decreases to less than 80 mg/dl or decreases rapidly because of the potential induction of the Somogyi phenomenon, which can falsely decrease the apparent duration of insulin effect (see p. 744). The duration of effect is roughly defined as the time from the insulin injection through the lowest glucose level and until the blood glucose concentration exceeds 200 to 250 mg/dl. Duration of effect of Lente and NPH insulin is 10 to 14 hours in approximately 90% of diabetic dogs, necessitating twice daily insulin treatment. Dogs are usually symptomatic for diabetes if the

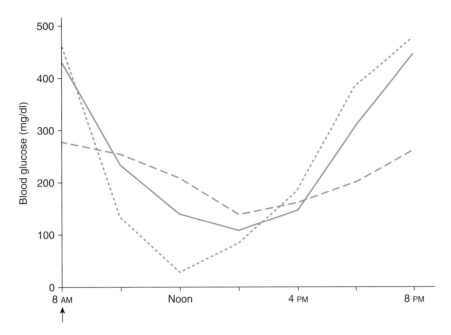

**FIG 52-4**
Blood glucose concentration curve in a Dachshund receiving 0.8 U of recombinant human Lente insulin per kilogram of body weight twice a day *(solid line),* a Miniature Poodle receiving 0.6 U of recombinant human Lente insulin per kilogram of body weight twice a day *(dashed line),* and a Terrier-mix receiving 1.1 U of recombinant human Lente insulin per kilogram of body weight twice a day *(dotted line).* Insulin and food was given at 8 AM for each dog. Interpretation of the blood glucose curves suggest short duration of insulin effect in the Dachshund, insulin underdosing in the Miniature Poodle, and the Somogyi effect in the Terrier-mix. The blood glucose concentrations were similar in all dogs at 2 and 4 PM; the glucose results at these times do not establish the diagnosis in any of the dogs.

duration of insulin effect is less than 10 hours (see p. 746) and may develop hypoglycemia or the Somogyi phenomenon if the duration of insulin effect is greater than 14 hours and the insulin is being administered twice a day (Fig. 52-6).

***Problems with serial blood glucose curves.*** The results of serial blood glucose determinations can be affected by many variables, including stress, excitement, inappetence, and the prolonged insulin-antagonistic effects of the diabetogenic hormones (i.e., glucagon, catecholamines, cortisol, growth hormone). Hyperglycemia induced by stress, excitement, or aggressive behavior should be considered whenever results of a serial blood glucose curve suggest insulin ineffectiveness, especially when the history, physical examination, and body weight suggest good glycemic control (Fig. 52-7; see p. 743).

Finicky diabetic dogs frequently refuse to eat in the veterinary hospital. Unfortunately, inappetence can profoundly alter the results of a serial blood glucose curve (see Fig. 52-7). To counter the effects of inappetence, the owner should feed the finicky dog before presenting the animal to the hospital. Blood samples can then be obtained until the next scheduled meal. The information gained in this manner will more reliably reflect what is happening at home.

The reproducibility of serial blood glucose curves varies from patient to patient. In some dogs, results of serial blood glucose curves may vary dramatically from day to day or month to month, depending, in part, on the actual amount of insulin administered and absorbed from the subcutaneous (SC) site of deposition and the interaction between insulin, diet, exercise, stress, and counterregulatory hormone secretion. In other dogs, serial blood glucose curves are reasonably consistent from day to day and month to month. Generally, information gained from a prior serial blood glucose curve should never be assumed to be reproducible on subsequent curves, especially if several weeks to months have passed or the dog has developed recurrence of clinical signs.

Despite these problems, serial blood glucose curves are valuable in assessing glycemic control. These curves provide guidelines for making rational adjustments in insulin therapy. The clinician, however, must also consider the owner's perceptions of the pet's health, physical examination findings, changes in body weight, and, if available, serum fructosamine concentrations when assessing the effectiveness of insulin therapy.

***Role of serum fructosamine in aggressive, excitable, or stressed dogs.*** Serial blood glucose curves are unreliable in aggressive, excitable, or stressed dogs because of problems related to stress-induced hyperglycemia. In these dogs the clinician must make an educated guess as to where the problem lies (e.g., wrong type of insulin, low dose), make

**Guidelines for Interpreting Serial
Blood Glucose Curve**

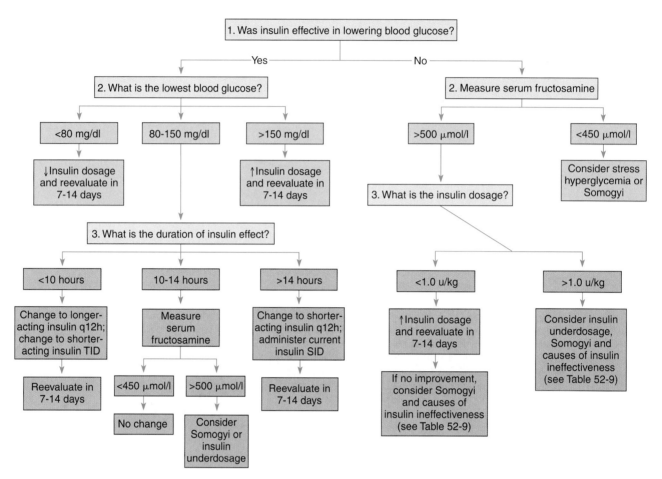

**FIG 52-5**
Algorithm for interpreting results of a blood glucose concentration curve.

an adjustment in therapy, and rely on changes in serum fructosamine to assess the benefit of the change in treatment. The reader is referred to p. 758 for more information on use of serum fructosamine in diabetic pets with stress-induced hyperglycemia.

## Insulin Therapy During Surgery

Generally, surgery should be delayed in diabetic dogs until the animal's clinical condition is stable and the diabetic state is controlled with insulin. The exception are those situations in which surgery is required to eliminate insulin resistance (e.g., ovariohysterectomy in a diestrus bitch) or to save the animal's life. The surgery itself does not pose a greater risk in a stable diabetic animal than in a nondiabetic animal. The concern is the interplay between insulin therapy and the lack of food intake during the perioperative period. The stress of anesthesia and surgery also cause the release of diabetogenic hormones, which in turn promote ketogenesis. Insulin must be administered during the perioperative period to prevent severe hyperglycemia and minimize ketone formation. To compensate for the lack of food intake and prevent hypoglycemia, the amount

of insulin administered during the perioperative period is decreased and IV dextrose is administered, when needed. To correct marked hyperglycemia (>300 mg/dl blood glucose concentration), regular crystalline insulin is administered intramuscularly (IM) or by continuous IV infusion.

The following protocol is used during the perioperative period in dogs and cats undergoing surgery. The day before surgery the animal is given its normal dose of insulin and fed as usual. Food is withheld after 10 PM. On the morning of the procedure, the blood glucose concentration is measured before the animal is given insulin. If the blood glucose concentration is less than 100 mg/dl, insulin is not given and an IV infusion of 2.5% to 5% dextrose is initiated. If the blood glucose concentration is between 100 and 200 mg/dl, one quarter of the animal's usual morning dose of insulin is given and an IV infusion of dextrose is initiated. If the blood glucose concentration is more than 200 mg/dl, one half of the usual morning dose of insulin is given but the IV dextrose infusion is withheld until the blood glucose concentration is less than 150 mg/dl. In all three situations the blood glucose concentration is measured every 30 to 60 minutes during the surgical

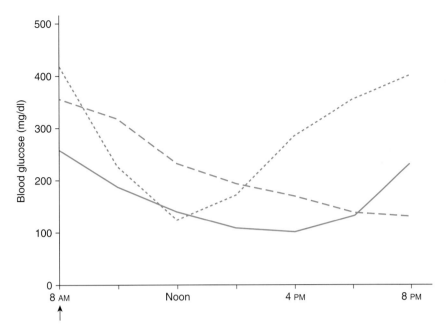

**FIG 52-6**
Blood glucose concentration curves obtained from three diabetic dogs treated with recombinant human Lente insulin twice a day, illustrating a difference between dogs in the duration of insulin effect. The insulin is effective in lowering the blood glucose concentration in all dogs, and the blood glucose nadir is between 100 and 175 mg/dl for the dogs. However, the duration of insulin effect is approximately 12 hours *(solid line)* in one dog with good control of glycemia (ideal duration of effect), approximately 8 hours *(dotted line)* in one dog with persistently poor control of glycemia (short duration of effect), and greater than 12 hours *(dashed line)* in one dog with a history of good days and bad days of glycemic control (prolonged duration of effect); a history suggestive of the Somogyi phenomenon (see Fig. 52-8).

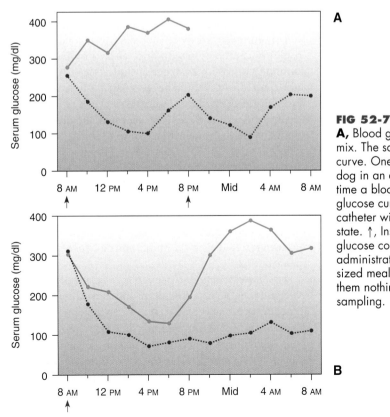

**FIG 52-7**
**A,** Blood glucose concentration curves in a fractious Terrier-mix. The same dose of NPH insulin was given for each curve. One glucose curve *(blue line)* was obtained with the dog in an agitated state requiring physical restraint each time a blood specimen was obtained; blood for the other glucose curve *(red line)* was obtained through a jugular catheter with minimal-to-no restraint and the dog in a quiet state. ↑, Insulin administration and food. **B,** Mean blood glucose concentrations in eight diabetic dogs after the administration of NPH insulin (↑) and the feeding of equal-sized meals at 8 AM and 6 PM *(blue line)* or after feeding them nothing *(red line)* during the 24 hours of blood sampling.

procedure. The goal is to maintain the blood glucose concentration between 150 and 250 mg/dl during the perioperative period. A 2.5% to 5% dextrose infusion is administered IV, and regular crystalline insulin is administered intermittently as needed to eliminate or prevent hypoglycemia and severe hyperglycemia, respectively. When the blood glucose concentration exceeds 300 mg/dl, the dextrose infusion should be discontinued and the blood glucose concentration evaluated 30 and 60 minutes later. If the blood glucose concentration remains greater than 300 mg/dl, regular crystalline insulin is administered IM at approximately 20% of the dose of long-acting insulin being used at home. Subsequent doses of regular crystalline insulin should be given no more frequently than every 4 hours, and the dose should be adjusted based on the effect of the first insulin injection on the blood glucose concentrations.

On the day after surgery the diabetic dog or cat can usually be returned to the routine schedule of insulin administration and feeding. An animal that is not eating can be maintained with IV dextrose infusions and regular crystalline insulin injections given SC every 6 to 8 hours. Once the animal is eating regularly, it can be returned to its normal insulin and feeding schedule.

### Complications of insulin therapy

**Hypoglycemia.** Hypoglycemia is a common complication of insulin therapy. Signs of hypoglycemia are most apt to occur after sudden large increases in the insulin dose, with excessive overlap of insulin action in dogs receiving insulin twice a day, and after prolonged inappetence. In these situations, severe hypoglycemia may occur before the diabetogenic hormones (i.e., glucagon, catecholamines, cortisol, growth hormone) are able to compensate for and reverse low blood glucose concentrations. In many diabetic dogs, signs of hypoglycemia are not apparent to owners and hypoglycemia is identified during evaluation of a serial blood glucose curve or serum fructosamine concentration. Clinical signs and treatment of hypoglycemia are discussed on p. 729. If clinical signs of hypoglycemia have occurred, insulin therapy should be stopped until hyperglycemia and glycosuria recur. The adjustment in the subsequent insulin dose is somewhat arbitrary; as a general rule of thumb, the insulin dose initially should be decreased 25% to 50% and subsequent adjustments in the dose based on clinical response and results of blood glucose measurements.

**Recurrence of clinical signs.** Recurrence or persistence of clinical signs is perhaps the most common "complication" of insulin therapy in diabetic dogs. This is usually caused by problems with owner technique in administering insulin; problems with insulin therapy relating to the insulin type, dose, species, or frequency of administration; or problems with responsiveness to insulin caused by concurrent inflammatory, infectious, neoplastic, or hormonal disorders (i.e., insulin resistance).

*Problems with owner administration and insulin action.* Insulin ineffectiveness will result in recurrence or persistence of clinical signs. Insulin ineffectiveness may be caused by problems related to insulin activity or administration technique. Failure to administer an appropriate dose of biologically active insulin can mimic insulin resistance because of unrecognized insulin underdosing. Insulin underdosing can result from administration of biologically inactive insulin (e.g., outdated, overheated, mixed by shaking), administration of diluted insulin, use of inappropriate insulin syringes for the concentration of insulin (e.g., U100 syringe with U40 insulin), or problems with insulin administration technique (e.g., misunderstanding how to read the insulin syringe, inappropriate injection technique). These problems are identified by evaluating the owner's insulin administration technique and by administering new, undiluted insulin and measuring several blood glucose concentrations throughout the day.

*Problems with insulin treatment regimen.* The most common problems causing poor control of glycemia in this category include insulin underdosing, the Somogyi phenomenon, short duration of effect of Lente and NPH insulin, and once-a-day insulin administration. The insulin treatment regimen should be critically evaluated for possible problems in these areas and appropriate changes made to try to improve insulin effectiveness, especially if the history and physical examination do not suggest a concurrent disorder causing insulin resistance.

*Diluted insulin.* Diluted insulin should be replaced with full-strength insulin. In some dogs insufficient amounts of insulin are administered when diluted insulin is used, despite appropriate dilution and insulin administration techniques. These inadequacies are corrected when full-strength insulin is used. Small insulin syringes (e.g., U100, 0.3 ml) should be used with full-strength U100 insulin for dogs receiving small amounts of insulin.

*Insulin underdosing.* Control of glycemia can be established in most dogs using less than 1.0 U of insulin/kg of body weight administered twice each day. An inadequate dose of insulin in conjunction with once-a-day insulin therapy is a common cause for persistence of clinical signs. In general, insulin underdosing should be considered if the insulin dose is less than 1.0 U/kg and the animal is receiving insulin twice a day. If insulin underdosing is suspected, the dose of insulin should be gradually increased by 1 to 5 U/injection (depending on the size of the dog) per week. The effectiveness of the change in therapy should be evaluated by client perception of clinical response and measurement of serum fructosamine or serial blood glucose concentrations. Other causes for insulin ineffectiveness and resistance should be considered once the insulin dose exceeds 1.0 U/kg/injection, the insulin is being administered every 12 hours, and control of glycemia remains poor.

*Insulin overdosing and glucose counterregulation (Somogyi phenomenon).* A high dose of insulin may cause overt hypoglycemia or induce glucose counterregulation (i.e., Somogyi phenomenon) and transient insulin resistance. The Somogyi phenomenon results from a normal physiologic response to impending hypoglycemia induced by excessive insulin. When the blood glucose concentration declines to less than 65 mg/dl or when the blood glucose concentration decreases rapidly regardless of the glucose nadir, direct hypoglycemia-induced stimulation of hepatic glycogenolysis and secretion of diabetogenic hormones, most notably epinephrine and glucagon, increase the blood glucose concentration, minimize signs of hypoglycemia, and cause marked hyperglycemia within 12 hours of glucose counterregulation. Clinical signs of hypoglycemia are typically mild or not recognized by the owner; clinical signs caused by hyperglycemia tend to dominate the clinical picture. Diagnosis of insulin-induced hyperglycemia requires demonstration of hypoglycemia (<65 mg/dl) that reverts to hyperglycemia (>300 mg/dl) after insulin administration. If the duration of insulin effect is greater than 12 hours, hypoglycemia often occurs at night after the evening dose of insulin and the serum glucose concentration is typically greater than 300 mg/dl the next morning (Fig. 52-8). Serum fructosamine concentrations are unpredictable in dogs with the Somogyi phenomenon, ranging from 300 to greater than 600 μmol/l. Values below 400 μmol/l in diabetic dogs with suspected poor control of glycemia suggest the Somogyi

phenomenon. High serum fructosamine values identify poor control of glycemia but are not helpful in identifying the cause. The Somogyi phenomenon should be included in the list of causes for high serum fructosamine concentrations.

Therapy involves reducing the insulin dose. If the diabetic dog is receiving an "acceptable" dose of insulin (<1.0 U/kg/injection), the insulin dose should be decreased 10% to 25%. If the insulin dose exceeds these amounts, glycemic regulation should be started over again using an initial dose of 0.25 U/kg given twice daily. Evaluation of glycemic control should be done 5 to 7 days after initiating the new dose of insulin and further adjustments in the insulin dose made accordingly.

Secretion of diabetogenic hormones during the Somogyi phenomenon may induce insulin resistance, which can last 24 to 72 hours after the hypoglycemic episode. This is a common cause of poor control of glycemia in diabetic cats. The reader is referred to p. 761 for more information on insulin resistance induced by the Somogyi phenomenon.

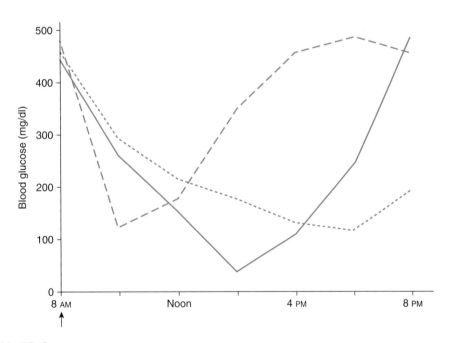

**FIG 52-8**

Blood glucose concentration curves obtained from three poorly controlled diabetic dogs treated with recombinant human Lente insulin twice a day, illustrating the typical blood glucose curves suggestive of the Somogyi phenomenon. In one dog *(solid line)*, the glucose nadir is less than 80 mg/dl and is followed by a rapid increase in the blood glucose concentration. In one dog *(dashed line)* a rapid decrease in the blood glucose concentration occurs within 2 hours of insulin administration and is followed by a rapid increase in the blood glucose concentration; the rapid decrease in blood glucose stimulates glucose counterregulation, despite maintaining the blood glucose nadir above 80 mg/dl. In one dog *(dotted line)* the blood glucose curve is not suggestive of the Somogyi phenomenon, per se. However, the insulin injection causes the blood glucose to decrease by approximately 300 mg/dl during the day, and the blood glucose concentration at the time of the evening insulin injection is considerably lower than the 8 AM blood glucose concentration. If a similar decrease in the blood glucose occurs with the evening insulin injection, hypoglycemia and the Somogyi phenomenon would occur at night and would explain the high blood glucose concentration in the morning and the poor control of the diabetic state.

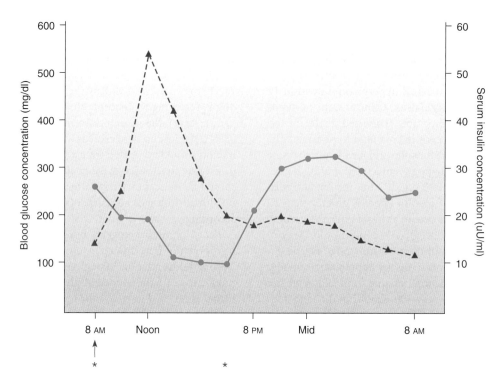

**FIG 52-9**
Mean blood glucose *(blue line)* and serum insulin *(red line)* concentrations in eight dogs with diabetes mellitus treated with a beef-pork source NPH insulin subcutaneously (SC) once daily. The duration of NPH effect is too short, resulting in prolonged periods of hyperglycemia beginning shortly after the evening meal. ↑, Insulin injection; *, equal-sized meals consumed.

*Short duration of insulin effect.* For most dogs, the duration of effect of recombinant human-source Lente and NPH insulin is 10 to 14 hours and twice-a-day insulin administration is effective in controlling blood glucose concentrations (Fig. 52-9). However, in some diabetic dogs, the duration of effect of Lente and NPH insulin is less than 10 hours; a duration that is too short to prevent periods of hyperglycemia and persistence of clinical signs. A diagnosis of short duration of insulin effect is made by demonstrating recurrence of hyperglycemia (>250 mg/dl) within 6 to 10 hours of the insulin injection, while the lowest blood glucose concentration is maintained above 80 mg/dl (see Fig. 52-6). Treatment involves changing to longer-acting insulin (e.g., switching to Ultralente insulin; Fig. 52-10) or increasing the frequency of insulin administration (e.g., initiating q8h therapy). PZI insulin of beef/pork source should not be used in dogs because of potential problems with insulin antibodies (see following).

*Prolonged duration of insulin effect.* In some diabetic dogs the duration of effect of Lente and NPH insulin is greater than 12 hours and twice-a-day insulin administration creates problems with hypoglycemia and the Somogyi phenomenon. In these dogs, the glucose nadir after the morning administration of insulin typically occurs near the time of the evening insulin administration, and the morning blood glucose concentration is usually greater than 300 mg/dl (see Fig. 52-6). The effectiveness of insulin in lowering the blood glucose concentration is variable from day to day, presumably because of varying concentrations of diabetogenic hormones, the secretion of which was induced by prior hypoglycemia. Serum fructosamine concentrations are variable but usually greater than 500 μmol/L. An effective treatment depends, in part, on the duration of effect of the insulin. A 24-hour blood glucose curve should be generated after administration of insulin once in the morning and feeding the dog at the normal times of the day. This will allow the clinician to estimate the duration of effect of the insulin. If the duration of effect is less than 16 hours, a shorter-acting insulin given twice a day or a lower dose of the same insulin given in the evening, compared with the morning insulin dose, can be tried (see Fig. 52-10). If the duration of effect is 16 hours or longer, switching to a longer-acting insulin administered once a day or administering NPH or Lente insulin in the morning and regular insulin at bedtime (i.e., 16 to 18 hours after the morning insulin injection) can be tried.

*Inadequate insulin absorption.* Slow or inadequate absorption of insulin deposited SC is an uncommon problem in diabetic dogs treated with NPH or Lente insulin. The reader is referred to p. 762 for information on inadequate insulin absorption.

*Circulating insulin-binding antibodies.* The amino acid sequence of canine, porcine, and recombinant human insulin are similar, suggesting that recombinant human insulin should not be strongly antigenic when administered to diabetic dogs. Studies using an ELISA to detect insulin antibod-

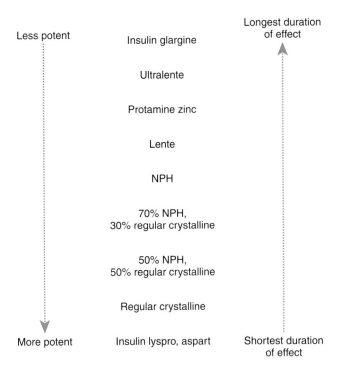

**FIG 52-10**
Categorization of types of commercial insulin based on the potency and duration of effect. An inverse relationship exists between the potency and duration of effect.

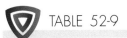 TABLE 52-9

**Recognized Causes of Insulin Ineffectiveness or Insulin Resistance in Diabetic Dogs and Cats**

| CAUSED BY INSULIN THERAPY | CAUSED BY CONCURRENT DISORDER |
|---|---|
| Inactive insulin | Diabetogenic drugs |
| Diluted insulin | Hyperadrenocorticism |
| Improper administration technique | Diestrus (bitch) |
| Inadequate dose | Acromegaly (cat) |
| Somogyi effect | Infection, especially of oral cavity and urinary tract |
| Inadequate frequency of insulin administration | Hypothyroidism (dog) |
| Impaired insulin absorption, especially Ultralente insulin | Hyperthyroidism (cat) |
| Anti-insulin antibody excess | Renal insufficiency |
| | Liver insufficiency |
| | Cardiac insufficiency |
| | Glucagonoma (dog) |
| | Pheochromocytoma |
| | Chronic inflammation, especially pancreatitis |
| | Pancreatic exocrine insufficiency |
| | Severe obesity |
| | Hyperlipidemia |
| | Neoplasia |

ies in serum of insulin-treated diabetic dogs identified serum insulin antibodies in approximately 5% of dogs treated with recombinant human insulin. In contrast, the amino acid sequence of canine and beef insulin differ and serum insulin antibodies were identified in approximately 45% of dogs treated with beef/pork-source insulin (which is 90% beef insulin). Presence of serum insulin antibodies in these dogs was associated with erratic and often poor control of glycemia, an inability to maintain control of glycemia for extended periods of time, frequent adjustments in insulin dose, and occasional development of severe insulin resistance (i.e., blood glucose concentrations consistently >400 mg/dl). Erratic fluctuations in the blood glucose concentration has been described in diabetic humans with insulin antibodies and results from changes in circulating free-insulin concentration as antibody-binding affinity for insulin changes. Dogs treated with recombinant human insulin consistently had more stable control of glycemia for extended periods of time. Interestingly, ELISA titers reverted to negative and glycemic control improved by 4 to 6 weeks after changing from beef/pork to human recombinant insulin in insulin-antibody positive dogs. Recombinant human-source insulin should be used in diabetic dogs to avoid problems with insulin effectiveness presumably caused by circulating insulin antibodies.

*Allergic reactions to insulin.* Significant reactions to insulin occur in up to 5% of human diabetics treated with insulin and include erythema, pruritus, and induration at the injection site and, uncommonly, systemic manifestations characterized by urticaria, angioneurotic edema or frank anaphy-

laxis. Atrophy or hypertrophy of SC tissue (i.e., lipoatrophy, lipodystrophy) may also occur at the insulin injection site. Many humans with insulin allergy have histories of sensitivity to other drugs as well. Allergic reactions to insulin have been poorly documented in diabetic dogs and cats. Pain on injection of insulin is usually caused by inappropriate injection technique or site of injection and not an adverse reaction to insulin, per se. Chronic injection of insulin in the same area of the body may cause thickening of the skin and SC tissues and may be caused by an immune reaction to insulin or some other protein (e.g., protamine) in the insulin bottle. Thickening of the skin and SC tissues may impair insulin absorption, resulting in recurrence of clinical signs of diabetes. Rotation of the injection site will help prevent this problem. Rarely, diabetic dogs and cats will develop focal SC edema and swelling at the site of insulin injection. Insulin allergy is suspected in these animals. Treatment includes switching to a less antigenic insulin (recombinant human insulin for dogs, beef insulin for cats) and to a more purified insulin preparation (e.g., regular crystalline insulin) in the hopes of minimizing a potential immune reaction to the species of insulin or some contaminant in the insulin preparation. Systemic allergic reactions to insulin in dogs or cats have yet to be identified.

*Concurrent disorders causing insulin resistance.* Many disorders can interfere with insulin action (Table 52-9). The most common concurrent disorders interfering with insulin effectiveness in dogs include diabetogenic drugs (i.e., glucocorticoids), severe obesity, hyperadrenocorticism, diestrus, chronic pancreatitis, renal insufficiency, oral and urinary tract infections, hyperlipidemia, and insulin antibodies in dogs receiving beef insulin. Obtaining a complete history and performing a thorough physical examination is the most important step in identifying these concurrent disorders. Abnormalities identified on a thorough physical examination may suggest a concurrent insulin-antagonistic disorder or infectious process, which will give the clinician direction in the diagnostic evaluation of the patient. If the history and physical examination are unremarkable, a CBC, serum biochemical analysis, serum progesterone concentration (intact female dog), abdominal ultrasound, and urinalysis with bacterial culture should be obtained to further screen for concurrent illness. Additional tests will be dependent on the results of the initial screening tests (Table 52-10).

## Chronic Complications of Diabetes Mellitus

Complications resulting from the diabetes (e.g., cataracts) or the therapy (e.g., insulin-induced hypoglycemia) are common in diabetic dogs (see Table 52-4). The most common complications in the dog are blindness and anterior uveitis

 TABLE 52-10

**Diagnostic Tests to Consider for the Evaluation of Insulin Resistance in Diabetic Dogs and Cats**

CBC, serum biochemistry panel, urinalysis
Bacterial culture of the urine
Serum lipase and amylase activities (pancreatitis)
Serum trypsin-like immunoreactivity (exocrine pancreatic insufficiency, pancreatitis)
Adrenocortical function tests
   ACTH stimulation test (spontaneous or iatrogenic hyperadrenocorticism)
   Low-dose dexamethasone suppression test (spontaneous hyperadrenocorticism)
Thyroid function tests
   Baseline serum total and free thyroxine (hypothyroidism or hyperthyroidism)
   Endogenous TSH (hypothyroidism)
   Thyroid-stimulating hormone stimulation test (hypothyroidism)
   Thyroid-releasing hormone stimulation test (hypothyroidism or hyperthyroidism)
   Triiodothyronine suppression test (hyperthyroidism)
Serum progesterone concentration (diestrus in intact female dog)
Plasma growth hormone or serum insulin-like growth factor I concentration (acromegaly)
Serum insulin concentration 24 hours after discontinuation of insulin therapy (insulin antibodies)
Serum triglyceride concentration (hyperlipidemia)
Abdominal ultrasonography (adrenomegaly, adrenal mass, pancreatitis, pancreatic mass)
Thoracic radiography (cardiomegaly, neoplasia)
Computed tomography or magnetic resonance imaging (pituitary mass)

resulting from cataract formation; chronic pancreatitis; recurring infections of the urinary tract, respiratory system, and skin; hypoglycemia; and ketoacidosis.

***Cataracts.*** Cataract formation is the most common and one of the most important long-term complications of diabetes mellitus in the dog. Cataracts are highly prevalent in diabetic dogs because many of these animals have significant hyperglycemia despite insulin therapy. Diabetic cataract formation is thought to be related to altered osmotic relationships in the lens, which develop secondary to an accumulation of sorbitol and fructose resulting from the metabolism of glucose via the sorbitol pathway in the lens.

The cell membrane is not freely permeable to sorbitol and fructose, and these substances act as potent hydrophilic agents, causing an influx of water into the lens, leading to swelling and rupture of the lens fibers and hence to the development of cataracts. Cataract formation is an irreversible process once it begins, and it can occur quite rapidly. Diabetic dogs that are poorly controlled and have problems with wide fluctuations in the blood glucose concentration seem especially at risk for rapid development of cataracts. Good glycemic control and minimal fluctuation in the blood glucose concentration decrease the risk of cataract formation. Once blindness occurs as a result of cataract formation, the need for stringent blood glucose control is reduced. Hyperglycemia-induced cataracts do not develop in cats. The reason for this is not known, but it may be related to the decreased permeability of the lens to glucose, compared with that in dogs, or to differences in the metabolism of glucose within the lens.

Blindness may be eliminated by removing the abnormal lens. Vision is restored in approximately 75% to 80% of diabetic dogs that undergo cataract removal. Factors that affect the success of surgery include the degree of glycemic control, the presence of retinal disease, and the presence of lens-induced uveitis. Ideally, glycemic control should be the best possible before surgery, and retinal function should be normal. Acquired retinal degeneration affecting vision is more of a concern in older diabetic dogs than is diabetic retinopathy. Fortunately, acquired retinal degeneration is unlikely in an older diabetic dog with vision immediately before cataract formation. If available, electroretinography should be performed before surgery to evaluate retinal function.

***Lens-induced uveitis.*** Uveitis that occurs in association with a resorbing, hypermature cataract may decrease the success of cataract surgery and must be controlled before surgery. The treatment of lens-induced uveitis focuses on decreasing the inflammation and preventing further intraocular damage. Topical ophthalmic corticosteroids are the most commonly used drug for the control of ocular inflammation. However, the systemic absorption of topically applied corticosteroids may induce insulin resistance. An alternative is to topically apply nonsteroidal antiinflammatory agents (e.g., 0.03% flurbiprofen [Ocufen; Allergan Pharmaceuticals, Irvine, Calif]). Although not as potent as corticosteroids, nonsteroidal antiinflammatory drugs do not interfere with glycemic control.

## Prognosis

The prognosis is dependent on the presence and reversibility of concurrent diseases, ease of regulation of the diabetic state with insulin, and owner commitment toward treating the disease. The mean survival time in diabetic dogs is approximately 3 years from time of diagnosis. This survival time is somewhat skewed, because dogs are usually 8 to 12 years old at the time of diagnosis and a relatively high mortality rate exists during the first 6 months because of concurrent life-threatening or uncontrollable disease (e.g., ketoacidosis, acute pancreatitis, renal failure). Diabetic dogs that survive the first 6 months can easily live longer than 5 years with the disease.

## DIABETES MELLITUS IN CATS

### Etiology

The most commonly recognized form of diabetes mellitus in the cat is IDDM. Cats with IDDM fail to respond to diet and oral hypoglycemic drugs and must be treated with exogenous insulin to obtain control of glycemia and prevent ketoacidosis. Common histologic abnormalities in cats with IDDM include islet-specific amyloidosis, β-cell vacuolation and degeneration, and chronic pancreatitis (Fig. 52-11). Still other diabetic cats do not have amyloidosis, inflammation, or degeneration of their pancreatic islets; instead immunohistochemical evaluation shows a reduction in the number of pancreatic islets

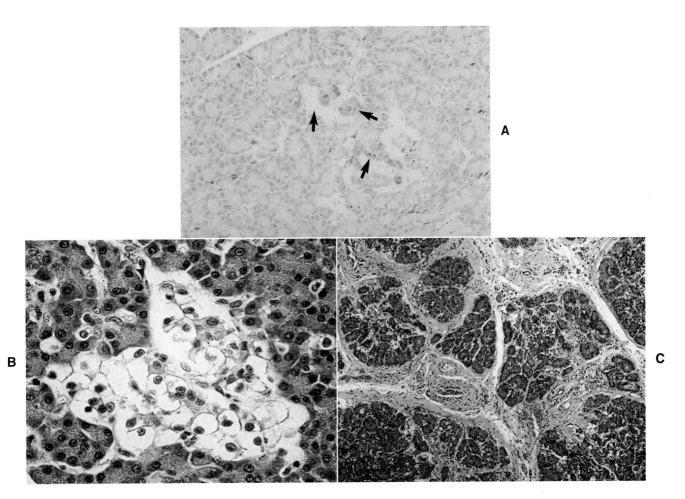

**FIG 52-11**
**A,** Severe islet amyloidosis *(straight arrow)* in a cat with initial NIDDM that progressed to insulin-dependent diabetes mellitus (IDDM). A pancreatic biopsy specimen was obtained while the animal was in the IDDM state. Residual β cells containing insulin *(curved arrows)* are also present. (Immunoperoxidase stain, X100.) **B,** Severe vacuolar degeneration of islet cells. Pancreatic tissue was evaluated at necropsy 28 months after diabetes was diagnosed and 20 months after cat progressed from NIDDM to IDDM, requiring insulin to control blood glucose concentrations. The cat died from metastatic exocrine pancreatic adenocarcinoma. (H&E, X500.) **C,** Severe chronic pancreatitis with fibrosis in a diabetic cat with IDDM. The cat was euthanized because of persistent problems with lethargy, inappetence, and poorly controlled diabetes mellitus. (H&E, X100.) (**A** from Feldman EC, Nelson RW: *Canine and feline endocrinology and reproduction,* ed 2, Philadelphia, 1996, WB Saunders.)

or insulin-containing β cells, or both. The lymphocytic infiltration of islets, in conjunction with islet amyloidosis and vacuolation, has also been observed in a few diabetic cats and suggests the possibility of an immune-mediated insulitis. However, this histologic finding is very uncommon; the role of immune destruction and genetic factors in the development of IDDM in cats remains to be determined.

NIDDM is diagnosed in approximately 30% of diabetic cats at our hospital. The etiopathogenesis of NIDDM is undoubtedly multifactorial. Islet-specific amyloid deposition in the islets represents a potential causative factor in cats. Amyloid is a common albeit not the only pathologic finding in the islets of diabetic cats. Amyloid results from aggregation of a specific islet polypeptide called *amylin*. Amylin is produced by the β cells and cosecreted with insulin. The physiologic actions of amylin include increased satiety, decreased gastric emptying, and decreased glucagon secretion. Stimulants of insulin secretion also stimulate the secretion of amylin. Excessive secretion of amylin results in aggregation and deposition of amylin in the islets as amyloid (see Fig. 52-11). Amyloid is toxic to islet cells. If deposition of amyloid is progressive (e.g., persistent insulin resistant states), islet cell destruction progresses and eventually leads to diabetes mellitus. Total destruction of the islets results in IDDM; partial destruction may lead to NIDDM.

The presence and severity of concurrent insulin resistance is an important variable that influences the clinical impact of partial destruction of the pancreatic islets. Tissue sensitivity to insulin is dependent on an appropriate number of insulin receptors on the cell membrane, normal binding affinity of insulin receptors for insulin, and normal stimulation of postreceptor processes responsible for insulin action in the cell. Problems in any of these areas results in insulin resistance. Type II diabetes mellitus in humans results from a primary, probably genetic, problem with insulin sensitivity of tissues combined with impaired responsiveness of β cells to stimulants of insulin secretion (e.g., glucose, fatty acids). To date, no evidence indicates that diabetes in cats results from a primary defect in insulin sensitivity. However, secondary insulin resistance caused by concurrent obesity, disease, or drugs does play a role in development of diabetes in cats. Examples of diseases include chronic pancreatitis and other chronic inflammatory diseases, infection, and insulin-resistant disease like hyperthyroidism, hyperadrenocorticism, and acromegaly. Cats with partial destruction of islets have impaired ability to secrete insulin in response to increased demand, such as occurs during insulin resistance. The more severe the insulin resistance, the more likely cats with partial destruction of islets will develop hyperglycemia, and vice versa.

Persistent hyperglycemia can, in turn, suppress function of remaining β cells present in the islets, causing hypoinsulinemia and worsening hyperglycemia. Suppression of β-cell function is initially reversible if hyperglycemia is improved (referred to as *glucose desensitization*), but chronic exposure to hyperglycemia eventually results in permanent suppression of β-cell function (i.e., glucose toxicity). Identification

and correction of concurrent problems that affect insulin sensitivity is critical to the successful treatment of diabetes in cats.

Clinicians usually classify diabetic cats as either IDDM or NIDDM, based on their need for insulin treatment. This can be confusing because some diabetic cats can initially appear to have NIDDM that progresses to IDDM, or the cat's condition flips back and forth between IDDM and NIDDM as severity of insulin resistance and impairment of β-cell function waxes and wanes. Apparent changes in the diabetic state (i.e., IDDM, NIDDM) are understandable when one realizes that islet pathology may be mild to severe and progressive or static; that the ability of the pancreas to secrete insulin depends on the severity of islet pathology and can decrease with time; that responsiveness of tissues to insulin varies, often in conjunction with the presence or absence of concurrent inflammatory, infectious, neoplastic, or hormonal disorders; and that all these variables affect the cat's need for insulin, insulin dose, and ease of diabetic regulation.

Approximately 20% of diabetic cats become "transiently diabetic" usually within 4 to 6 weeks of establishing the diagnosis of diabetes and initiating treatment. In these cats, hyperglycemia, glycosuria, and clinical signs of diabetes resolve and insulin treatment can be discontinued. Some diabetic cats may never require insulin treatment once the initial bout of clinical diabetes mellitus has dissipated, whereas others become permanently insulin dependent weeks to months after the resolution of a prior diabetic state. Based on findings from a recent evaluation of a group of cats with transient diabetes mellitus, cats with transient diabetes are theoretically in a subclinical diabetic state that becomes clinical when the pancreas is stressed by exposure to a concurrent insulin-antagonistic drug or disease, most notably glucocorticoids, megestrol acetate, and chronic pancreatitis (Fig. 52-12). Unlike healthy cats, those with transient diabetes mellitus have some abnormality of the islets that impairs their ability to compensate for concurrent insulin resistance and results in carbohydrate intolerance. Insulin secretion by β cells becomes reversibly suppressed, most likely stemming from a worsening carbohydrate intolerance. Chronic hyperglycemia impairs insulin secretion by β cells and induces peripheral insulin resistance by promoting the down-regulation of glucose transport systems and causing a defect in posttransport insulin action; this phenomenon is referred to as glucose toxicity. β cells have an impaired response to stimulation by insulin secretagogues, thereby mimicking IDDM. The effects of glucose toxicity are potentially reversible upon correction of the hyperglycemic state. The clinician makes a correct diagnosis of IDDM. However, insulin therapy and the treatment of insulin-antagonistic disorders lower the blood glucose concentration and reduce insulin resistance; β-cell function improves, insulin secretion returns, and an apparent IDDM state resolves. The future requirement for insulin treatment depends on the underlying abnormality in the islets. If it is progressive (e.g., amyloidosis), eventually enough β cells will be destroyed and IDDM will develop.

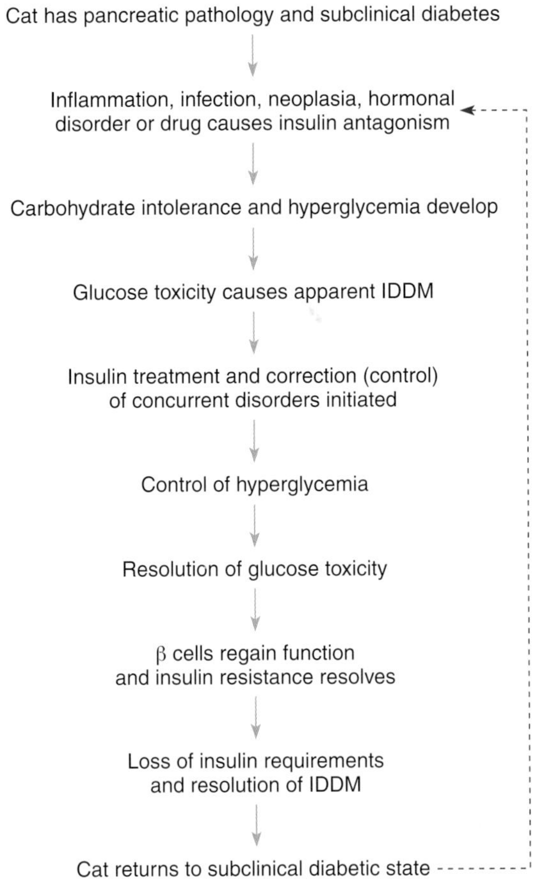

Cat has pancreatic pathology and subclinical diabetes

↓

Inflammation, infection, neoplasia, hormonal disorder or drug causes insulin antagonism

↓

Carbohydrate intolerance and hyperglycemia develop

↓

Glucose toxicity causes apparent IDDM

↓

Insulin treatment and correction (control) of concurrent disorders initiated

↓

Control of hyperglycemia

↓

Resolution of glucose toxicity

↓

β cells regain function and insulin resistance resolves

↓

Loss of insulin requirements and resolution of IDDM

↓

Cat returns to subclinical diabetic state - - - - - - - -

**FIG 52-12**
Sequence of events in the development and resolution of an insulin-requiring diabetic episode in cats with transient diabetes. (From Feldman EC, Nelson RW: *Canine and feline endocrinology and reproduction,* ed 2, Philadelphia, 1996, WB Saunders.)

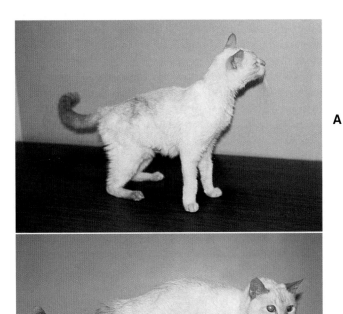

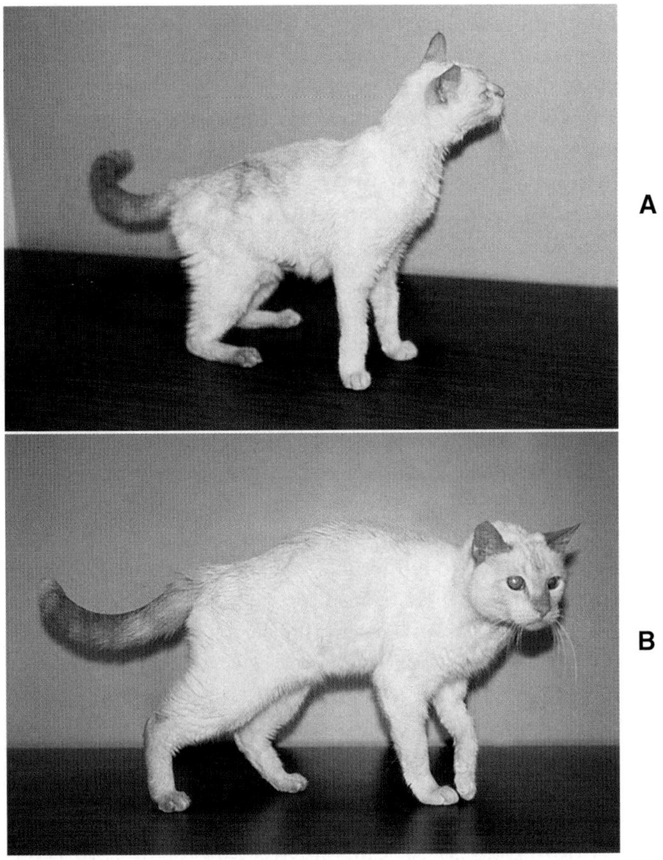

**FIG 52-13**
**A,** Plantigrade posture in a cat with diabetes mellitus and exocrine pancreatic insufficiency. **B,** Resolution of hind limb weakness and plantigrade posture after improving glycemic control by adjusting insulin therapy and initiating pancreatic enzyme replacement therapy.

## Clinical Features

**Signalment.** Although diabetes mellitus may be diagnosed in cats of any age, most diabetic cats are more than 9 years old (mean, 10 years) at the time of diagnosis. Diabetes mellitus occurs predominantly in neutered male cats; no apparent breed predisposition has been discovered, although Burmese cats may be overrepresented in Australia.

**History.** The history in virtually all diabetic animals includes the classic signs polydipsia, polyuria, polyphagia, and weight loss. A common complaint of cat owners is the constant need to change the litter and in increase in the size of the "kitty litter clumps." Additional clinical signs include lethargy; decreased interaction with family members; lack of grooming behavior and development of a dry, lusterless, unkept or matted haircoat; and decreased jumping ability, rear limb weakness, or development of a plantigrade posture (Fig. 52-13). If the clinical signs associated with uncomplicated diabetes are not observed by the owner, a diabetic cat may be at risk for development of systemic signs of illness as progressive ketonemia and metabolic acidosis develop (see p. 762). The time sequence from the onset of initial clinical signs to the development of DKA is unpredictable.

**Physical examination.** The physical examination findings depend on whether DKA is present and its severity and on the nature of any other concurrent disorder. The nonketotic diabetic cat has no classic physical examination findings. Many diabetic cats are obese but are otherwise in good physical condition. Cats with prolonged untreated diabetes may have lost weight but are rarely emaciated unless concurrent disease (e.g., hyperthyroidism) is present. Newly diagnosed and poorly controlled diabetic cats often stop grooming and develop a dry, lusterless haircoat. Diabetes-induced hepatic lipidosis may cause hepatomegaly. Impaired ability to jump, weakness in the rear limbs, ataxia, or a plantigrade posture (i.e., the hocks touch the ground when the cat walks) may be evident if the cat has developed diabetic neuropathy. Distal muscles of the rear limbs may feel hard on digital palpation, and cats may object to palpation or manipulation of the rear limbs, presumably because of pain associated with the neuropathy. Additional abnormalities may be identified in the ketoacidotic diabetic cat (see p. 763).

## Diagnosis

Establishing the diagnosis of diabetes mellitus is similar for cats and dogs and is based on identification of appropriate clinical signs, hyperglycemia, and glycosuria (see p. 732). Transient, stress-induced hyperglycemia is a common problem in cats and can cause the blood glucose concentration to increase above 300 mg/dl (see p. 759). Unfortunately, stress is a subjective state that cannot be accurately measured, is not always easily recognized, and may evoke inconsistent responses among individual cats. Glycosuria usually does not develop in cats with stress hyperglycemia, because the transient increase in the blood glucose concentration prevents glucose from accumulating in urine to a detectable concentration. For this reason, persistent hyperglycemia and glycosuria should always be documented when establishing a diagnosis of diabetes mellitus in cats. If the clinician is in doubt, the "stressed" cat can be sent home with instructions for the owner to monitor the urine glucose concentration with the cat in the nonstressed home environment. Alternatively, a serum fructosamine concentration can be measured (see p. 738). Documenting an increase in the serum fructosamine concentration supports the presence of sustained hyperglycemia; however, a serum fructosamine concentration in the upper range of normal can occur in symptomatic diabetic cats if the diabetes developed shortly before presentation of the cat to the veterinarian.

Clinical signs do not develop until hyperglycemia causes glycosuria and are the same regardless of the functional status of pancreatic islets. Information used to establish the diagnosis of diabetes mellitus does not provide information on the status of pancreatic islet health, presence of glucose toxicity, ability of the cat to secrete insulin, or the severity and reversibility of concurrent insulin resistance. Identification of a serum insulin concentration greater than 15 µU/ml in a newly diagnosed, untreated diabetic cat supports the presence of functional β cells and partial destruction of the islets; however, low or undetectable serum insulin concentrations do not rule out partial islet cell loss because of the suppressive effects of glucose toxicity on circulating insulin concentrations.

Simply establishing the diagnosis of diabetes does not provide the whole picture; a thorough evaluation for concurrent disorders that may affect insulin sensitivity of tissues and evaluation of response to treatment are also important pieces of the puzzle when trying to determine if the diabetic cat has IDDM, NIDDM, or transient diabetes mellitus. The minimum laboratory evaluation in any diabetic cat should include a CBC, serum biochemical panel, serum thyroxine concentration, and urinalysis with bacterial culture. If available, abdominal ultrasound should also be a routine part of the diagnostic evaluation because of the high prevalence of chronic pancreatitis in diabetic cats. Measurement of the baseline serum insulin concentration or an insulin response test is not routinely done in cats because of the problems encountered with glucose toxicity. Additional tests may be warranted after obtaining the history, performing the physical examination, or identifying ketoacidosis. See Table 52-3 for a list of potential clinical pathologic abnormalities.

## Treatment

The significant incidence of NIDDM in cats raises interesting questions concerning the need for insulin treatment. Glycemic control can be maintained in some diabetic cats with dietary changes, oral hypoglycemic drugs, and control of current diseases.

Obviously it would be advantageous to be able to prospectively differentiate IDDM from NIDDM by assessing β-cell function. Unfortunately, measurement of baseline serum insulin concentration or serum insulin concentrations after administration of an insulin secretagogue have not been consistent aids in differentiating IDDM and NIDDM in the cat (see Diagnosis). The ultimate differentiation between IDDM and NIDDM is often made retrospectively, after the clinician has had several weeks to assess the response of the cat to therapy and to determine the cat's need for insulin. The initial decision between insulin treatment versus oral hypoglycemic drugs is based on the severity of clinical signs, presence or absence of ketoacidosis, general health of the cat, and owner wishes.

**Initial insulin therapy.** Diabetic cats are notoriously unpredictable in their response to exogenous insulin. No single type of insulin is routinely effective in maintaining control of glycemia, even with twice-a-day administration. Since the loss of PZI insulin a decade ago, NPH, Lente, and Ultralente insulin have all been used to treat diabetic cats. Ultralente insulin is the longest-acting but least potent of the commonly used commercial insulins (see Fig. 52-10). Although considered a long-acting insulin, Ultralente has to be administered twice a day in most diabetic cats, and absorption of Ultralente insulin is inadequate for controlling glycemia in approximately 25% of cats. Lente and NPH insulin are more potent insulin preparations that are more consistently and rapidly absorbed after SC administration than Ultralente insulin. Unfortunately, the duration of effect of Lente and especially NPH insulin can be considerably shorter than 12 hours in some diabetic cats, resulting in inadequate control of glycemia despite twice-a-day administration (see Table 52-5). It is not possible to predict which type of insulin will work best in individual diabetic cats. The initial insulin of choice ultimately is based on personal preference and experiences. Currently, Lente of recombinant human origin is initially used at a dose of 1 to 2 U per cat administered twice daily. The prevalence of insulin antibodies causing problems with control of glycemia is uncommon in cats treated with recombinant human insulin (see p. 762).

Recently, production of PZI of beef/pork origin was begun by an animal health pharmaceutical company (IDEXX Pharmaceuticals, Inc., Westbrook, Me) using the same methods as the original manufacturer. PZI is a longer-acting insulin that is more consistently absorbed than Ultralente insulin and has a more acceptable duration of effect than NPH insulin. However, the timing of the glucose nadir is quite variable and occurs within 9 hours of PZI administration in greater than 80% of treated diabetic cats. Routinely, PZI is administered twice a day. In a recent study, PZI was very effective in significantly improving control of glycemia in poorly controlled diabetic cats previously treated with Ultralente or NPH insulin (Nelson and colleagues, 2001). Comparison of efficacy between PZI and Lente has not been reported.

Glargine (Lantus, Aventis Pharmaceuticals, Bridgewater, N.J.) is an insulin analog that has a prolonged duration of action after SC administration in human diabetic patients. It was designed to provide a sustained mild increase in serum insulin concentration to control hepatic glucose production. Preliminary studies in healthy cats suggest that the duration of effect of glargine and PZI are similar. Initial clinical impressions are that glargine may be effective in improving control of glycemia in cats in which lente and PZI insulin have too short of a duration of effect and are unable to control the diabetic state.

**Dietary therapy.** The general principles for dietary therapy are discussed on p. 734 (Table 52-11). Obesity, feeding practices, and content of the diet warrant discussion in diabetic cats. Obesity is common in diabetic cats and results from excessive caloric intake typically caused by free-choice feeding of dry cat food. Obesity causes reversible insulin resistance that resolves as obesity is corrected. Control of glycemia often improves, and some diabetic cats may revert to a subclinical diabetic state after weight reduction. Correction of obesity is

TABLE 52-11

**Recommendations for Dietary Treatment of Diabetes Mellitus in Cats**

I. Dietary composition (see Table 52-12)
   Option 1—Moderate carbohydrate and fat, high fiber content
   Option 2—High protein, low carbohydrate, low fiber content
   Option 3—High fat, low carbohydrate, low fiber content
   Diet options can be used interchangeably
   Which diet composition improves glycemic control the most is unpredictable
II. Feed canned and/or dry kibble foods; avoid diets containing monosaccharides, disaccharides, propylene glycol
III. Caloric intake and obesity
   Average daily caloric intake in geriatric pet: 40-60 kcal/kg
   Adjust daily caloric intake on individual basis
   Eliminate obesity, if present, by:
      Decreasing daily caloric intake
      Feeding diets designed for weight loss
IV. Feeding schedule
   Maintain consistent caloric content of meals
   Maintain consistent timing of feeding
   Feed within time frame of insulin action
   Feed one-half the total daily caloric intake at time of each insulin injection
   Let "nibbler" cats continue to nibble throughout day and night

*DM,* Dry matter; *ME,* metabolizable energy.

difficult in cats because it requires restriction of daily caloric intake without a corresponding increase in caloric expenditure (i.e., exercise). The reader is referred to Chapter 54 for more information on correction of obesity in cats.

The eating habits of cats vary considerably, from those cats that eat everything at the time it is offered to those that graze throughout the day and night. The primary goal of dietary therapy is to minimize the impact of a meal on postprandial blood glucose concentrations. Consuming the same amount of calories in multiple small amounts throughout a 12-hour period should have less impact than consuming the calories at a single large meal. Half of the cat's total daily caloric intake should be offered at the time of each insulin injection and remain available to the cat to consume when it wishes. Attempts to force a "grazing" cat to eat the entire meal at one time usually fail and are not warranted as long as the cat has access to the food during the ensuing 12 hours. A similar approach is taken for diabetic dogs that are finicky eaters.

During the past decade, high-fiber, moderately fat-restricted diets have been recommended for diabetic cats based on studies that documented a significant improvement in glycemic control when diabetic cats consumed a canned insoluble-fiber (i.e., cellulose) diet containing 12% insoluble fiber on a dry-matter basis, compared with a canned low-fiber diet (Fig. 52-14). As with diabetic dogs, when diabetic cats are fed diets containing large amounts of insoluble fiber, they show increased frequency of defecation, inappetence caused by poor palatability, constipation, and obstipation. Recently, dietary recommendations for diabetic cats have come under scrutiny. Cats are carnivores and have higher dietary protein requirements than omnivores, such as humans and dogs. Hepatic glucokinase and hexokinase activity is lower in cats, compared with that for carnivores with omnivorous dietary habits, and may predispose the diabetic cat to developing higher postprandial blood glucose concentrations after consumption of diets containing a high carbohydrate load, and vice versa. Two carbohydrate-restricted diets that have been recommended for diabetic cats are Purina DM (Ralston Purina Co., St. Louis) and Science Diet Feline Growth (Hill's Pet Products, Topeka, Kan). Purina DM is a high-protein, low-carbohydrate, low-fiber diet, and Science Diet Growth is a high-fat, low-carbohydrate, low-fiber diet (Table 52-12). Preliminary studies suggest that these diets may be as effective in improving glycemic control as diets moderate in protein, fat, and digestible carbohydrate content and high in fiber. All of these diets have one central theme: carbohydrate restriction, either by decreasing intake or slowing absorption using fiber. The diets listed in Table 54-12 provide the veterinarian with dietary choices for the management of diabetes in cats, especially when palatability issues develop or poor control of glycemia persists despite adjustments in insulin therapy.

**Identification and control of concurrent problems.** In general, any concurrent inflammatory, infectious, hormonal, or neoplastic disorder can cause insulin resistance and interfere with the effectiveness of insulin therapy (see p. 762). Identification and treatment of concurrent disease plays an integral role in the successful management of the diabetic cat.

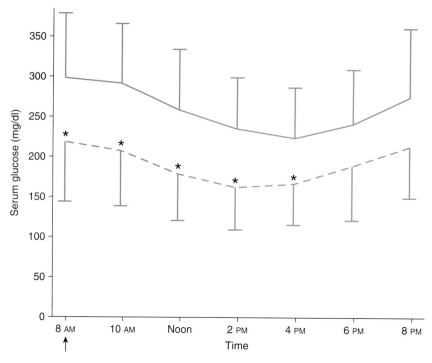

**FIG 52-14**

Mean (± SD) serum concentration of glucose in samples obtained from sixteen cats with naturally acquired diabetes mellitus before feeding (8 AM) and obtained for 12 hours after insulin administration and concurrent consumption of a meal high in insoluble fiber (------------) or low in fiber (————) *(arrow)*. Mean serum concentration of glucose is the mean of all corresponding serum glucose values obtained during the 12-hour blood glucose-sampling period for each cat at 6, 12, 18, and 24 weeks after initiation of each diet. *, Values differ significantly (P <0.05) from those for the low-fiber diet. (From Nelson RW et al: Effect of dietary insoluble fiber on control of glycemia in cats with naturally acquired diabetes mellitus, *J Am Vet Med Assoc* 216:1082, 2000.)

 TABLE 52-12

**Approximate Nutrient Content of Some Commercially Available Diets Used for the Treatment of Diabetes Mellitus in Cats**

| | CRUDE FIBER* | CARBOHYDRATES† | FAT† | PROTEIN† | CALORIES‡ (CAN/CUP) |
|---|---|---|---|---|---|
| Prescription Diet w/d | | | | | |
|   Canned | 13 | 22 | 39 | 39 | 148 |
|   Dry | 9 | 37 | 23 | 40 | 246 |
| Purina DM | | | | | |
|   Canned | 4 | 7 | 44 | 49 | 194 |
|   Dry | 1 | 11 | 37 | 52 | 592 |
| Science Diet Feline Growth | | | | | |
|   Canned | 1 | 7 | 60 | 33 | 230 |
|   Dry | 1 | 21 | 50 | 29 | 510 |

*Expressed as a percentage of the diet dry matter.
†Expressed as percent metabolizable energy derived from carbohydrate, fat, or protein.
‡Expressed as kilocalories of metabolizable energy per can (5.5 oz) or for the dry diets per standard (8 oz volume) measuring cup full.

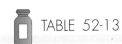

TABLE 52-13

Indications, Efficacy, and Adverse Effects of Oral Hypoglycemic Drugs in Diabetic Cats and Dogs

| DRUG CLASSIFICATION | MECHANISM OF ACTION | INDICATIONS | EFFICACY | ADVERSE EFFECTS | PREVALENCE OF ADVERSE EFFECTS |
|---|---|---|---|---|---|
| Sulfonylureas (e.g., glipizide, glyburide) | Stimulate insulin secretion | Cats with NIDDM Not indicated in dogs | Cats: ~25% respond | Cats: vomiting, icterus, increased liver enzymes, hypoglycemia | <15% of treated cats |
| Meglitinides (e.g., rapaglinide) | Stimulate insulin secretion | Possibly cats with NIDDM | Unknown | Unknown | Unknown |
| Biguanides (e.g., metformin) | Insulin sensitizer | Possibly cats with NIDDM | Cats: <25% respond Dogs: unknown | Cats: inappetence, vomiting, weight loss Dogs: unknown | Cats: common at doses >75 mg/cat Dogs: unknown |
| Thiazolidinediones (e.g., rosiglitazone pioglitazone) | Insulin sensitizer | Unknown | Unknown | Unknown | Unknown |
| α-Glucosidase inhibitors (e.g., acarbose) | Slows intestinal glucose absorption | Adjunct treatment in dogs and possibly cats | Cats: unknown Dogs: dose dependent | Cats: unknown Dogs: diarrhea, weight loss | Cats: unknown Dogs: 35% of treated dogs |

A thorough history, physical examination, and complete diagnostic evaluation (including CBC, serum biochemistry panel, serum $T_4$, urinalysis, and abdominal ultrasound) are imperative in any newly diagnosed diabetic cat.

**Oral hypoglycemic drugs.** Oral hypoglycemic drugs are primarily used for the treatment of NIDDM; a form of diabetes that is very uncommon in dogs but common in cats (see Etiology, p. 749). In the United States, five classes of oral hypoglycemic drugs are approved for the treatment of NIDDM in human beings: (1) sulfonylureas, (2) meglitinides, (3) biguanides, (4) thiazolidinediones, and (5) α-glucosidase inhibitors (Table 52-13). These drugs work by stimulating pancreatic insulin secretion, enhancing tissue sensitivity to insulin or slowing postprandial intestinal glucose absorption. In addition, chromium and vanadium are trace minerals that may also enhance tissue sensitivity to insulin. Sulfonylureas have been the most extensively evaluated of the oral hypoglycemic drugs in diabetic cats.

**Sulfonylureas.** Sulfonylurea drugs (e.g., glipizide, glyburide) are the most commonly used oral hypoglycemic drugs for the treatment of diabetes mellitus in cats. The primary effect of sulfonylureas is the direct stimulation of insulin secretion by the β cells of the pancreas (Fig. 52-15). Some endogenous pancreatic insulin secretory capacity must exist for sulfonylureas to be effective in improving glycemic control. The sulfonylurea drug glipizide (Glucotrol; Pfizer Inc., New York) has been used successfully as an alternative to insulin therapy in healthy, newly diagnosed diabetic cats. Clinical response is variable, ranging from excellent (i.e., blood glucose concentrations decreasing to <200 mg/dl) to partial response (i.e., clinical improvement but failure to resolve hyperglycemia) to no response. Presumably the population of functioning β cells varies from none (severe IDDM) to near normal (mild NIDDM) in treated cats, resulting in a response range from none to excellent. Cats with a partial response to glipizide have some functioning β cells but not enough to decrease the blood glucose concentration to less than 200 mg/dl. These cats may have severe NIDDM or the early stages of IDDM. Glipizide treatment has been found effective in improving clinical signs and severity of hyperglycemia in approximately 30% of diabetic cats.

Glipizide is initially administered at a dose of 2.5 mg per os two times a day in conjunction with a meal to those diabetic cats which are nonketotic and relatively healthy on physical examination (Fig. 52-16). Each cat is examined weekly during the first month of glipizide therapy. A history, complete physical examination, body weight, urine glucose/ketone measurement, and blood glucose concentration are evaluated at each examination. If adverse reactions (Table 52-14) have not occurred after 2 weeks of treatment, the glipizide dose is increased to 5.0 mg two times per day. Therapy is continued as long as the cat is stable. If euglycemia or hypoglycemia develop, glipizide dose may be tapered down or discontinued and blood glucose concentrations reevaluated 1 week later to assess the need for the drug. If hyperglycemia recurs, the dose is increased or glipizide is reinitiated, with a reduction in dose in those cats previously developing hypoglycemia. Glipizide is discontinued and insulin therapy initiated if clinical signs continue to worsen, the cat becomes ill or develops ketoacidosis or peripheral neuropathy, blood glucose concentrations remain greater than 300 mg/dl after 1 to 2 months of therapy, or the owners become dissatisfied with the treatment. In some cats, glipizide becomes ineffective weeks to months later, and exogenous insulin is ultimately required to control the diabetic state. Presumably the need to be switched from glipizide to insulin treatment results from the progression of the underlying pathophysiologic condition (e.g., islet-specific amyloid deposition). The more rapid the progression, the shorter the beneficial response to glipizide.

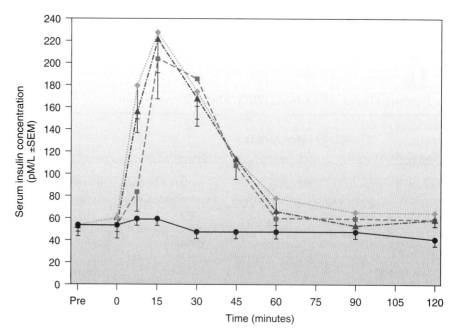

**FIG 52-15**
Mean serum insulin concentrations after oral administration of a placebo and three doses of glipizide (2.5, 5, and 10 mg) to 10 healthy cats. Placebo *(red)*; 2.5 mg glipizide *(green)*; 5 mg glipizide *(pink)*; 10 mg glipizide *(blue)*. (From Miller AB et al: Effect of glipizide on serum insulin and glucose concentrations in healthy cats, *Res Vet Sci* 52:177, 1992.)

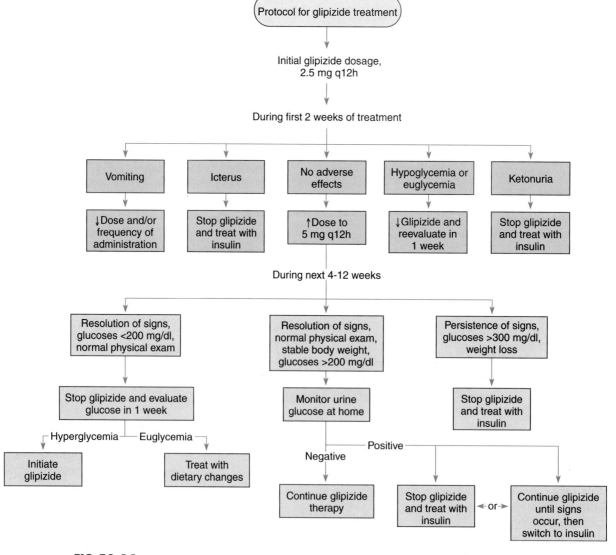

**FIG 52-16**
Algorithm for treating diabetic cats with the oral sulfonylurea drug, glipizide. (From Feldman EC, Nelson RW: *Canine and feline endocrinology and reproduction*, ed 2, Philadelphia, 1996, WB Saunders.)

TABLE 52-14

**Adverse Reactions to Glipizide Treatment in Diabetic Cats**

| ADVERSE REACTION | RECOMMENDATION |
|---|---|
| Vomiting within 1 hour of administration | Vomiting usually subsides after 2 to 5 days of glipizide therapy; decrease dose or frequency of administration if vomiting is severe; discontinue if vomiting persists >1 week |
| Increased serum hepatic enzyme activities | Continue treatment and monitor enzymes every 1 to 2 weeks initially; discontinue glipizide if cat becomes ill (lethargy, inappetence, vomiting) or the alanine transferase activity exceeds 500 IU/L |
| Icterus | Discontinue glipizide treatment; reinstitute glipizide treatment at lower dose and frequency of administration once icterus resolves (usually within 2 weeks); discontinue treatment permanently if icterus recurs |
| Hypoglycemia | Discontinue glipizide treatment; recheck blood glucose concentration in 1 week; reinstitute glipizide therapy at lower dose or frequency of administration if hyperglycemia recurs |

Glyburide (Micronase; Pharmacia and Upjohn Company, Kalamazoo, Mich) is another sulfonylurea with similar actions as glipizide. Glyburide has a longer duration of action than glipizide and is usually administered once a day, versus twice a day for glipizide. Most studies in human diabetics have reported similar responses in comparisons of glyburide and glipizide. In countries where glipizide is not available, treatment with glyburide should be considered at an initial dose of 0.625 mg (one-half of 1.25 mg tablet) per cat once daily. Response to therapy and adverse reactions to glyburide are similar to those described for glipizide.

**Biguanides.** The most commonly used drug in this class of oral hypoglycemic agents is metformin (Glucophage; Bristol-Myers Squibb, Princeton, N.J.). Metformin has no direct effect on β-cell function but improves glycemic control in an insulin-dependent manner primarily by enhancing the sensitivity of both hepatic and peripheral tissues to insulin. Metformin inhibits hepatic gluconeogenesis and glycogenolysis and increases muscle glucose metabolism by enhancing muscle insulin sensitivity. The net effect of these actions is to lower blood glucose concentrations without causing hypoglycemia. Studies in cats have shown that plasma metformin concentrations fall within the therapeutic range for humans at doses of 25 to 50 mg/cat, and plasma metformin concentrations are near baseline 12 hours after metformin administration. Unfortunately, inappetence and vomiting are common adverse effects when diabetic cats are treated with 25 to 50 mg of metformin twice a day, and clinical response to metformin treatment has been discouraging.

**Thiazoledinediones.** Thiazoledinediones are a new class of antidiabetic drugs that increase the sensitivity of target tissues to the action of insulin without directly stimulating insulin secretion from pancreatic β cells. Thiazoledinediones enhance insulin sensitivity in hepatic, muscle, and adipose tissue, thereby inhibiting hepatic glucose production, stimulating muscle glucose metabolism, and reducing circulating free fatty acid (FFA) concentrations. Pioglitazone (Actos; Takeda Pharmaceuticals America, Lincolnshire, Ill) and rosiglitazone (Avandia; Bristol-Myers Squibb Co., Princeton, N.J.) are used as monotherapy and in combination with sul-

fonylureas, metformin, and insulin in diabetic humans. Currently no published reports exist on the use of thiazoledinediones for treating diabetes in cats or dogs.

**Vanadium.** Vanadium is a ubiquitous trace element that exerts insulin-like effects in vitro. The mechanism of action is not known but research suggests that vanadium acts at a postreceptor site to stimulate glucose metabolism. Vanadium does not increase serum insulin concentrations. Unpublished studies in cats suggest that vanadium may be effective in improving control of glycemia in cats in the early stages of NIDDM. The dose is 0.2 mg of vanadium/kg/day administered once a day in food or water. Adverse effects in cats include anorexia and vomiting. Long-term toxicity is related to the accumulation of the metal in organs such as the liver and kidneys, as well as in bone. Acute renal failure has been reported in 1 cat treated with vanadium for 1 year; the renal failure was reversible after discontinuation of vanadium treatment.

**Chromium.** Chromium is an ubiquitous trace element that exerts insulin-like effects in vitro. The exact mechanism of action is not known, but the overall effect of chromium is to increase insulin sensitivity, presumably through a postreceptor mechanism of action. Chromium does not increase serum insulin concentrations. Chromium is an essential cofactor for insulin function, and chromium deficiency results in insulin resistance. The effect of chromium tripicolinate supplementation on glucose tolerance has been controversial in cats, ranging from no effect in obese and nonobese healthy cats to a small but significant dose-dependent improvement in glucose tolerance in nonobese healthy cats. Oral chromium tripicolinate supplementation did not improve glycemic control in a group of dogs with IDDM. The effect of oral chromium tripicolinate supplementation in diabetic cats has not been reported.

**Acarbose.** Acarbose competitively inhibits pancreatic α-amylase and α-glucosidases in the brush border of the small intestinal mucosa, which delays digestion of complex carbohydrates and disaccharides and slows absorption of glucose from the intestinal tract (see p. 736). Feeding carbohydrate-restricted diets (see Table 52-12) is recommended in lieu of acarbose treatment in diabetic cats.

**Initial adjustments in insulin therapy.** The approach to initially adjusting insulin therapy is similar for the diabetic dog and cat (see p. 737). Most owners of diabetic cats are happy with the response to insulin treatment if the blood glucose concentrations range between 100 and 300 mg/dl throughout the day. Diabetic cats can have problems with insulin-induced hyperglycemia (Somogyi phenomenon, p. 761) at relatively small doses of insulin (2 to 3 U/injection). As such, the preference is to have the owner administer a fixed dose of insulin once control of glycemia is attained and discourage owners from adjusting the insulin dose at home without first consulting their veterinarian.

## Techniques for Monitoring Diabetic Control

The techniques for monitoring diabetic control have been discussed on p. 737. One important factor that affects monitoring of diabetic cats is the propensity to develop stress-induced hyperglycemia caused by frequent visits to the veterinary hospital for blood samplings (see p. 759). Once stress-induced hyperglycemia develops, it is a perpetual problem and blood glucose measurements can no longer be considered accurate. Veterinarians must remain wary of stress hyperglycemia in diabetic cats and should take steps to avoid its development. Micromanaging diabetic cats should be avoided, and serial blood glucose curves should only be done when the clinician perceives a need to change insulin therapy. The determination of good versus poor control of glycemia should be based on the owner's subjective opinion of the presence and severity of clinical signs and the overall health of the pet, ability of the cat to jump, its grooming behavior, findings on physical examination, and stability of body weight. Generation of a serial blood glucose curve should be reserved for newly diagnosed and poorly controlled diabetic cats unless stress-induced hyperglycemia is suspected. If suspected, a switch from reliance on serial blood glucose curves generated in the veterinary hospital to reliance on blood glucose results generated by the owner in the less stressful home environment (e.g., the ear prick technique) or evaluation of sequential serum fructosamine concentrations should be done, in addition to the history and physical examination findings.

***Protocol for generating the serial blood glucose curve at home.*** An alternative to hospital-generated blood glucose curves is to have the owner generate the blood glucose curve at home using the ear prick technique and a portable home blood glucose–monitoring device that allows the owner to touch the drop of blood on the ear with the end of the glucose test strip (Fig. 52-17). Several Internet web sites provide detailed explanations of the ear prick technique and supply information on owners' experiences with the technique, as well as with different portable blood glucose home monitors. At the time diabetes is diagnosed, a web address is given to the clients, and they are asked to visit the site to see whether they would be interested in monitoring blood glucose concentrations at home. Time is spent teaching the technique to those individuals willing to give it a try, and advice is given on how often to perform a blood glucose curve (ideally no more frequently than 1 day every 2 to 4 weeks), and how

often to measure the blood glucose concentration on the day of the curve (typically at the time of insulin administration and 3, 6, 9, and 12 hours later). Use of the ear prick technique in cats has produced very good results. Stress has been significantly reduced, and accuracy of the blood glucose measurements has improved immensely. The biggest problem has been overzealous owners who start monitoring blood glucose concentrations too frequently. A similar approach can be used in diabetic dogs, using either the ear or lip prick technique. However, home glucose monitoring is not encouraged in dogs as much as cats, primarily because stress-induced hyperglycemia is not as big of a problem in diabetic dogs.

***Role of serum fructosamine in stressed diabetic cats.*** Use of serum fructosamine concentrations for assessing control of glycemia has been discussed on p. 738. Serum fructosamine concentrations are not affected by acute transient increases in blood glucose concentration. Unlike blood glucose measurements, evaluation of serum fructosamine concentration in fractious or stressed diabetic cats provides reliable objective information on the status of glycemic control during the previous 2 to 3 weeks. In fractious or stressed cats, the clinician must make an educated guess as to where the problem lies (e.g., wrong type of insulin, low insulin dose), make an adjustment in therapy, and rely on changes in serum fructosamine to assess the benefit of the change in treatment. Because serum proteins have a relatively short half-life, serum fructosamine concentration changes relatively quickly (i.e., 2 to 3 weeks) in response to a change in glycemic control. This short period for change in serum fructosamine concentration is advantageous for detecting improvement or deterioration of glycemic control quickly in fractious, stressed, or scared cats in which blood glucose concentrations are unreliable. As such, serum fructosamine concentrations can be measured before and 2 to 3 weeks after changing insulin therapy to assess the effectiveness of the change. If changes in insulin therapy are appropriate, a decrease in serum fructosamine concentration should occur. If the serum fructosamine concentration is the same or has increased, the change was ineffective in improving glycemic control, another change in therapy based on an educated guess should be done, and the serum fructosamine measured again 2 to 3 weeks later.

## Insulin Therapy During Surgery

The approach to managing the diabetic cat and dog during surgery is similar and has been discussed on p. 742.

## Complications of Insulin Therapy

Complications of insulin therapy are similar for diabetic dogs and cats and have been discussed on p. 744. Complications of insulin therapy result in poor control of glycemia. Poor control is defined as an inability to meet the goals for treating diabetes (i.e., resolving clinical signs, maintaining a healthy pet, avoiding complications caused by diabetes and its treatment). In diabetic cats, poor control is characterized by persistence or recurrence of polyuria, polydipsia, and polyphagia; lethargy and decreased interaction with family members; progressive weight loss leading to a thin or emaciated body

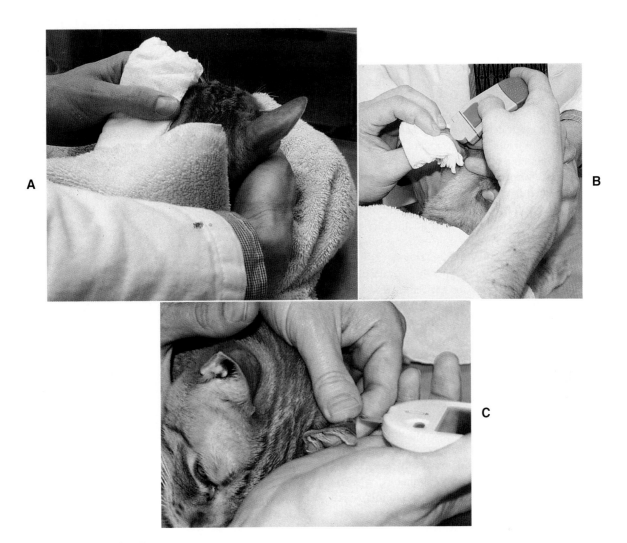

**FIG 52-17**
Ear prick technique for measuring blood glucose concentration. **A,** A hot washcloth is applied to the pinna for 2 to 3 minutes to increase circulation to the ear. **B,** A spot is identified on the periphery of the outer side of the pinna, a small coating of petrolatum jelly is applied, and the spot is pricked with the lancet device supplied with the portable blood glucose meter. Gauze should be placed between the pinna and the digit holding the pinna to prevent pricking the finger if the blade of the lancet accidentally passes through the pinna. Petrolatum jelly is applied to help the blood form into a ball on the pinna as it seeps from the site that is lanced. **C,** Digital pressure is applied in the area of the lanced skin to promote bleeding. The glucose test strip is touched to the drop of capillary blood that forms and is removed once enough blood has been drawn into the test strip to activate the meter.

condition (the exception is acromegaly); lack of grooming behavior leading to a poor, unkempt haircoat; and peripheral neuropathy causing weakness, inability to jump, a plantigrade stance, and ataxia. Poor control usually results from one of two basic problems: (1) an inability to resolve hyperglycemia and (2) an inability to avoid hypoglycemia. The most common complications of insulin therapy in the diabetic cat are recurring hypoglycemia, insulin overdose causing the Somogyi phenomenon, incorrect assessment of glycemic control caused by stress-induced hyperglycemia, inadequate absorption of longer-acting insulins, short duration of effect of intermediate-acting insulins, and insulin resistance caused by concurrent inflammatory and hormonal disorders, most notably

chronic pancreatitis. Although the etiologies, clinical presentations, diagnostic approach, and treatment are different for these basic problems, the end result is the same—a frustrated, unhappy owner and a symptomatic diabetic cat.

***Stress hyperglycemia.*** Transient hyperglycemia is a well-recognized problem in fractious, scared, or otherwise stressed cats. Hyperglycemia develops as a result of increased catecholamines and, in struggling cats, lactate concentrations. Blood glucose concentrations typically exceeded 200 mg/dl in these cats and values in excess of 300 mg/dl are common. Diabetes mellitus may be inadvertently diagnosed in these cats if the diagnosis is based solely on the blood glucose concentration. Because stress hyperglycemia is transient, clinical signs caused by hyperglycemia do not occur and urine testing for glucose is usually negative; findings that are inconsistent with a diagnosis of diabetes mellitus.

Stress hyperglycemia can significantly increase blood glucose concentrations in diabetic cats despite the administration of insulin (an effect that has serious consequences on the clinician's ability to accurately judge the effectiveness of the insulin injection). Unfortunately the frequent blood samples required for the generation of a serial blood glucose curve can become very stressful, especially if serial blood glucose curves are performed frequently, as occurs during the initial month of treatment in newly diagnosed diabetic cats and in poorly regulated diabetic cats. Most diabetic cats do not tolerate frequent venipunctures and eventually develop a change in temperament, typically toward aggression, and stress hyperglycemia. Induction of stress hyperglycemia is variable but usually starts during a venipuncture procedure and begins earlier and earlier on subsequent visits to the veterinarian, until eventually stress hyperglycemia is induced by hospitalization and ultimately by the car ride to the veterinary hospital. Blood glucose concentrations can remain greater than 400 mg/dl throughout the day when stress hyperglycemia develops before the first venipuncture of the day, despite administration of insulin. Failure to recognize the effect of stress on blood glucose results may lead to the erroneous perception that the diabetic cat is poorly controlled. Insulin therapy is invariably adjusted, often by increasing the insulin dose, and another blood glucose curve recommended 1 to 2 weeks later. A vicious cycle ensues, which eventually culminates in the Somogyi phenomenon, clinically apparent hypoglycemia, or referral for evaluation of insulin resistance.

Failure to identify the presence of stress hyperglycemia and its impact on interpretation of blood glucose measurements is one of the most important reasons for misinterpreting the status of glycemic control in diabetic cats.

Stress hyperglycemia should be suspected if the cat is visibly upset, aggressive or struggles during restraint and the venipuncture process. However, stress hyperglycemia can also be present in diabetic cats that are easily removed from the cage and do not resist the blood-sampling procedure. These cats are scared, but rather than become aggressive they remain crouched in the back of the cage, often have dilated pupils, and usually are flaccid when handled. Stress hyperglycemia should also be suspected if a disparity exists between assessment of glycemic control based on results of the history, physical examination, and stability of body weight; assessment of glycemic control based on results of blood glucose measurements; or when the initial blood glucose concentration measured in the morning is in an acceptable range (i.e., 150 to 250 mg/dl) but subsequent blood glucose concentrations increase steadily throughout the day (Fig. 52-18). Once stress hyperglycemia develops, it is a perpetual problem and blood glucose measurements can no longer be considered accurate. If stress hyperglycemia is suspected, a switch from reliance on serial blood glucose curves generated in the veterinary hospital to reliance on blood glucose results generated by the owner in the less stressful home environment (see p. 758) or evaluation of sequential serum fruc-

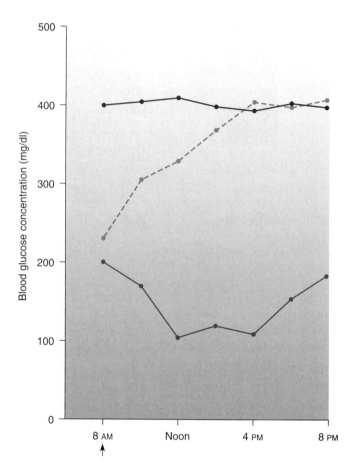

**FIG 52-18**

Blood glucose concentration curves in a 5.3-kg male cat receiving 2 U of recombinant human Ultralente insulin *(pink line)* 2 weeks after the initiation of insulin therapy, 2 U of recombinant human Ultralente insulin *(blue line)* 2 months later, and 6 U of recombinant human Ultralente insulin *(red line)* 4 months later. The insulin dose had been gradually increased based on the blood glucose concentration curves. The owner reported minimal clinical signs regardless of the insulin dose; at the 4-month recheck the cat had maintained its body weight and had a blood glycosylated hemoglobin concentration of 2.2%. The cat became progressively more fractious during each hospitalization, supporting the existence of stress-induced hyperglycemia as the reason for the discrepancy between the blood glucose values and other parameters used to evaluate glycemic control. ↑, Subcutaneous (SC) insulin injection and food. (From Feldman EC, Nelson RW: *Canine and feline endocrinology and reproduction,* ed 2, Philadelphia, 1996, WB Saunders.)

tosamine concentrations (see p. 758) should be done, in addition to the history and physical examination findings.

***Hypoglycemia.*** Hypoglycemia is a common complication of insulin therapy and has been discussed on p. 744. In diabetic cats, symptomatic hypoglycemia is most apt to occur after sudden large increases in the insulin dose, after sudden improvement in concurrent insulin resistance, with excessive overlap of insulin action in cats receiving insulin twice a day, after prolonged inappetence, and in insulin-treated cats that have reverted to a non–insulin-dependent state. In these situations, severe hypoglycemia may occur before the diabetogenic hormones (i.e., glucagon, cortisol, epinephrine, growth hormone) are able to compensate for and reverse low blood glucose concentrations. The initial treatment approach for hypoglycemia is to discontinue insulin until hyperglycemia recurs and then reduce the ensuing insulin dose 25% to 50%. If hypoglycemia remains a reoccurring problem despite reductions in the insulin dose, excessive overlap in insulin action or reversion to a non–insulin-dependent diabetic state should be considered. Excessive overlap in insulin action causing hypoglycemia is an uncommon problem in cats, occurring in less than 10% of diabetic cats treated with insulin. Excessive overlap of insulin action results from twice-a-day administration of a type of insulin with a duration of effect that is considerably longer than 12 hours (a problem that is associated with twice-a-day administration of Ultralente and PZI but usually not NPH or Lente insulin). Indications of excessive overlap include a glucose nadir that occurs 10 hours or later after insulin administration or gradually decreasing blood glucose concentrations measured at the time of sequential insulin injections (see Fig. 52-6). If excessive overlap of insulin action is suspected, a decrease in frequency of insulin administration to once a day or a switch to a shorter-acting insulin (e.g., Lente, NPH) administered twice a day can be tried.

Reversion to a non–insulin-dependent diabetic state should be suspected if hypoglycemia remains a persistent problem despite administration of small doses of insulin (i.e., 1 U or less per injection) and administration of insulin once a day, if blood glucose concentrations are consistently below 150 mg/dl before insulin administration, if serum fructosamine concentration is less than 350 μmol/L (reference range: 250 to 375 μmol/L), or if urine glucose test strips are consistently negative. Maintaining blood glucose concentrations below 150 mg/dl is very difficult to do with once- or twice-a-day injections of intermediate or long-acting insulin. All of the scenarios listed previously suggest the presence of endogenously derived circulating insulin, the existence of partial not complete destruction of the pancreatic islets, and probably the presence of glucose toxicity at the time diabetes was initially diagnosed (see p. 750). Correction of concurrent disorders identified around the time diabetes was diagnosed may have also improved insulin sensitivity of tissues. Insulin therapy should be discontinued and diet modified to help minimize recurrence of hyperglycemia (see Dietary Therapy, p. 753). Treatment with the oral sulfonylurea drug, glipizide, should also be considered (see Sulfonylureas, p. 755).

**Recurrence of clinical signs.** Recurrence or persistence of clinical signs is a common complication of insulin therapy in diabetic cats. This usually is caused by problems with insulin overdosing and the Somogyi phenomenon, short duration of insulin effect, poor absorption of long-acting insulins, or problems with responsiveness to insulin caused by concurrent insulin resistance.

*Insulin overdosing and glucose counterregulation (Somogyi phenomenon).* The Somogyi phenomenon is discussed on p. 744. A similar phenomenon, characterized by wide fluctuations in blood glucose concentration after which there are several days of persistent hyperglycemia, is recognized clinically in diabetic cats. However, the exact role of the counterregulatory hormones remains to be clarified. Insulin overdose inducing glucose counterregulation is one of the most common causes of insulin resistance and poor glycemic control in cats. It can be induced with insulin doses of 2 to 3 U per injection and can result in cats receiving 10 to 15 U of insulin per injection as veterinarians react to the persistence of clinical signs and increased blood glucose and serum fructosamine concentrations. A cyclic history of 1 or 2 days of good glycemic control after which there are several days of poor control should raise suspicion for insulin resistance caused by glucose counterregulation. Serum fructosamine concentrations are unpredictable but are usually increased (>500 μmol/L); these results confirm poor glycemic control but do not identify the underlying cause. Establishing the diagnosis may require several days of hospitalization and serial blood glucose curves; an approach that eventually leads to problems with stress-induced hyperglycemia. An alternative approach is to arbitrarily reduce the insulin dose 1 to 3 U and have the owner evaluate the cat's clinical response over the ensuing 2 to 5 days. If clinical signs of diabetes worsen after a reduction in the insulin dose, another cause for the insulin resistance should be pursued. However, if the owner reports no change or improvement in clinical signs, continued gradual reduction of the insulin dose should be pursued. Alternatively, glycemic regulation of the diabetic cat could be started over, using an insulin dose of 1 U/cat given twice daily.

*Insulin underdosing.* Control of glycemia can be established in most diabetic cats using 1 U or less of insulin/kg of body weight administered twice each day. An inadequate dose of insulin in conjunction with once-a-day insulin therapy is a common cause for persistence of clinical signs. In general, insulin underdosing should be considered if the insulin dose is less than 1 U/kg/injection and the cat is receiving insulin twice a day. If insulin underdosing is suspected, the dose of insulin should be gradually increased by 0.5 to 1 U/injection per week. The effectiveness of the change in therapy should be evaluated by client perception of clinical response and measurement of serum fructosamine or serial blood glucose concentrations. Other causes for insulin ineffectiveness and resistance should be ruled out before considering increasing the insulin dose above 1 U/kg/injection (most notably the Somogyi phenomenon and chronic pancreatitis).

*Short duration of insulin effect.* Short duration of insulin effect (<10 hours) is a common problem in diabetic cats despite twice-a-day insulin administration. Short duration of effect is most common with NPH and, to a lesser extent, Lente insulin. In some diabetic cats, duration of effect of NPH and Lente insulin is only 6 hours (see Table 52-5). As a result, hyperglycemia (>250 mg/dl) occurs for several hours each day, and owners of these pets usually mention continuing problems with polyuria and polydipsia, weight loss, or the development of weakness caused by development of peripheral neuropathy. A diagnosis of short duration of insulin effect is made by demonstrating hyperglycemia (>250 mg/dl) within 6 to 10 hours of the insulin injection, while the lowest blood glucose concentration is maintained above 80 mg/dl (see Fig. 52-6). Treatment involves changing the type of insulin (e.g., switching to Ultralente or PZI insulin) or the frequency of insulin administration (e.g., initiating q8h therapy).

*Prolonged duration of insulin effect.* Prolonged duration of insulin effect has been discussed on p. 746. In diabetic cats, problems with prolonged duration of insulin effect are most common with twice-a-day administration of PZI and, to a lesser extent, Ultralente insulin.

*Inadequate insulin absorption.* Slow or inadequate absorption of SC deposited insulin is most commonly observed in diabetic cats receiving Ultralente insulin, a long-acting insulin that has a slow onset and prolonged duration of effect. In approximately 25% of cats evaluated at our hospital, Ultralente insulin is absorbed from the SC site of deposition too slowly for it to be effective in maintaining acceptable glycemic control. In these cats the blood glucose concentration may not decrease until 6 to 10 hours after the injection or, more commonly, it decreases minimally despite insulin doses of 8 to 12 U/cat given every 12 hours. As a consequence, the blood glucose concentration remains greater than 300 mg/dl for most of the day. A similar problem may become apparent with glargine insulin as clinical experiences with this newer long-acting insulin analog increase. Switching from Ultralente to Lente or PZI insulin given twice a day has resulted in success in these cats. When switching type of insulin, the insulin dose is decreased (usually to amounts initially used to regulate the diabetic cat) to avoid hypoglycemia. The duration of effect of the insulin becomes shorter as the potency of the insulin increases, which may create problems with short duration of insulin effect (see Fig. 52-10).

*Circulating insulin-binding antibodies.* The amino acid sequence of feline and beef insulin are similar, but differences exist between feline and pork insulin and human insulin. Studies using an ELISA to detect insulin antibodies in serum of insulin-treated diabetic cats identified an approximately equal frequency of positive serum insulin antibody titers in diabetic cats treated with beef insulin, compared with recombinant human insulin. However, titers were weakly positive in most cats, prevalence of persistent titers was low, and presence of serum insulin antibodies did not appear to affect control of glycemia. These results suggest that the prevalence of insulin antibodies causing problems with control of glycemia similar to those identified in dogs (see p. 746) is uncommon in cats treated with recombinant human insulin. Overt insulin resistance caused by insulin antibody formation occurs in less than 5% of cats treated with recombinant human insulin.

*Concurrent disorders causing insulin resistance.* Many disorders can interfere with insulin action (see Table 52-9). The most common concurrent disorders interfering with insulin effectiveness in cats include severe obesity, chronic pancreatitis, renal insufficiency, hyperthyroidism, oral infections, acromegaly, and hyperadrenocorticism. Obtaining a complete history and performing a thorough physical examination is the most important step in identifying these concurrent disorders. Abnormalities identified on a thorough physical examination may suggest a concurrent insulin-antagonistic disorder or infectious process, which will give the clinician direction in the diagnostic evaluation of the patient. If the

history and physical examination are unremarkable, a CBC, serum biochemical analysis, serum thyroxine concentration, abdominal ultrasound, and urinalysis with bacterial culture should be obtained to further screen for concurrent illness. Additional tests will be dependent on the results of the initial screening tests (see Table 52-10).

## Chronic Complications of Diabetes Mellitus

Complications resulting from the diabetes (e.g., peripheral neuropathy) or the therapy (e.g., insulin-induced hypoglycemia) are common in diabetic cats (see Table 52-4). The most common complications in the cat are hypoglycemia, chronic pancreatitis, weight loss, poor grooming behavior causing a dry, lusterless and unkempt haircoat, and peripheral neuropathy of the hind limbs, causing weakness, inability to jump, a plantigrade stance, and ataxia. Diabetic cats are also at risk for ketoacidosis.

***Diabetic neuropathy.*** Diabetic neuropathy is one of the most common chronic complications of diabetes in cats, with a prevalence of approximately 10%. Clinical signs of a coexistent neuropathy in the diabetic cat include weakness, impaired ability to jump, knuckling, a plantigrade posture with the cat's hocks touching the ground when it walks (see Fig. 52-13), muscle atrophy, depressed limb reflexes, and deficits in postural reaction testing. Clinical signs may progress to include the thoracic limbs. Abnormalities on electrophysiologic testing are consistent with demyelination at all levels of the motor and sensory peripheral nerves and include abnormal spontaneous activity on electromyography and variably decreased motor nerve conduction velocities. The cause of diabetic neuropathy is not known, and no specific therapy for it exists. Aggressive glucoregulation with insulin may improve nerve conduction and reverse the posterior weakness and plantigrade posture (see Fig. 52-13). However, the response to therapy is variable. Generally the longer the neuropathy has been present and the more severe the neuropathy, the less likely improving glycemic control will reverse the clinical signs of neuropathy.

## Prognosis

The prognosis for diabetic cats and dogs is similar (see p. 749). The mean survival time in diabetic cats is approximately 3 years from time of diagnosis. However, this survival time is skewed because cats are usually 8 to 12 years old at the time of diagnosis and a high mortality rate exists during the first 6 months because of concurrent life-threatening or uncontrollable disease (e.g., ketoacidosis, acute pancreatitis, renal failure, hyperadrenocorticism). Diabetic cats that survive the first 6 months can easily live longer than 5 years with the disease.

## DIABETIC KETOACIDOSIS

### Etiology

The etiopathogenesis of ketoacidosis in diabetes mellitus is complex and is usually affected by concurrent clinical disorders. Virtually all dogs and cats with DKA have a relative or absolute deficiency of insulin. DKA develops in some diabetic dogs and cats even though they receive daily injections of insulin, and their circulating insulin concentrations may even be increased. A "relative" insulin deficiency is present in these animals. Presumably because of an increase in the circulating levels of diabetogenic hormones (i.e., epinephrine, glucagon, cortisol, growth hormone) and an altered metabolic milieu (e.g., increased levels of plasma FFAs and amino acids, metabolic acidosis), these dogs and cats have insulin resistance. To maintain normal glucose homeostasis there must be a balance between the body's sensitivity to insulin and the amount of insulin secreted by the β cell or injected exogenously. With the development of insulin resistance, the need for insulin may exceed the daily injected insulin dose, and this predisposes the animal to DKA.

Circulating levels of diabetogenic hormones are increased in human beings with DKA and presumably in dogs and cats as well. The body increases its production of diabetogenic hormones in response to a wide variety of stress situations. This response is usually beneficial. In the setting of DKA, however, the net effect of these hormonal disturbances is an accentuation of insulin deficiency through the development of insulin resistance; a stimulation of lipolysis, leading to ketogenesis; and the development of gluconeogenesis, which worsens hyperglycemia.

It is rare for the dog or cat with DKA not to have some coexisting disorder, such as pancreatitis, infection, or renal insufficiency. These disorders have the potential to cause an increase in diabetogenic hormone secretion. It is critically important that disorders that coexist with DKA be recognized and treated for DKA to be successfully managed.

Insulin deficiency and insulin resistance, together with increased circulating concentrations of diabetogenic hormones, play a critical role in the stimulation of ketogenesis. For the synthesis of ketone bodies (i.e., acetoacetic acid, β-hydroxybutyric acid, acetone) to be enhanced, there must be two major alterations in intermediary metabolism: (1) enhanced mobilization of FFAs from triglycerides stored in adipose tissue and (2) a shift in hepatic metabolism from fat synthesis to fat oxidation and ketogenesis. Insulin is a powerful inhibitor of lipolysis and FFA oxidation. A relative or absolute deficiency of insulin "allows" lipolysis to increase, thus increasing the availability of FFAs to the liver and in turn promoting ketogenesis. As ketones continue to accumulate in the blood, the body's buffering system becomes overwhelmed, causing metabolic acidosis to worsen. As ketones accumulate in the extracellular space, the amount eventually surpasses the renal tubular threshold for complete resorption and they spill into the urine, contributing to the osmotic diuresis caused by glycosuria and enhancing the excretion of solutes (e.g., sodium, potassium, magnesium). Insulin deficiency per se also contributes to the excessive renal losses of water and electrolytes. The result of this is an excessive loss of electrolytes and water, leading to volume contraction, an underperfusion of tissues, and the development of prerenal azotemia. The rise in the blood glucose concentration raises the plasma osmolality, and the resulting osmotic diuresis further aggravates the rise in plasma osmolality by causing water losses in excess of the salt loss. The increase in plasma osmolality causes water to be shifted out of cells, leading to cellular dehydra-

tion. The severe metabolic consequences of DKA, which include severe acidosis, hyperosmolality, obligatory osmotic diuresis, dehydration, and electrolyte derangements, can become life threatening.

## Clinical Features

DKA is a serious complication of diabetes mellitus that occurs most commonly in dogs and cats with diabetes that has gone undiagnosed. Less commonly, DKA develops in an insulin-treated diabetic dog or cat that is receiving an inadequate dose of insulin, often occurring in conjunction with an infectious, inflammatory, or insulin-resistant hormonal disorder. Because of the close association between DKA and newly diagnosed diabetes mellitus, the signalment of DKA in dogs and cats is similar to that of nonketotic diabetics (see p. 732 and p. 751).

The history and physical examination findings are variable, in part because of the progressive nature of the disorder and the variable time between the onset of DKA and owner recognition of a problem. The classic clinical signs of uncomplicated diabetes (i.e., polyuria, polydipsia, polyphagia, weight loss) develop initially but are either unnoticed or considered insignificant by the owner. Systemic signs (e.g., lethargy, anorexia, vomiting) ensue as ketonemia and metabolic acidosis develop and worsen, with the severity of these signs directly related to the severity of the metabolic acidosis and the nature of concurrent disorders (e.g., pancreatitis, infection) that are often present. The time interval from the onset of the initial clinical signs of diabetes to the development of systemic signs of DKA is unpredictable and ranges from a few days to longer than 6 months. Once ketoacidosis begins to develop, however, severe illness usually becomes evident within 7 days.

Common physical examination findings include dehydration, depression, weakness, tachypnea, vomiting, and sometimes a strong odor of acetone on the breath. Slow, deep breathing (i.e., Kussmaul's respiration) may be observed in animals with severe metabolic acidosis. Gastrointestinal tract signs such as vomiting, abdominal pain, and distention are common in animals with DKA, in part because of the common concurrent occurrence of acute and chronic pancreatitis in diabetic dogs and cats. Other intraabdominal disorders should also be considered and diagnostic tests (e.g., abdominal ultrasound) performed to help identify the cause of the gastrointestinal signs.

## Diagnosis

For diabetes mellitus to be diagnosed, the animal must show the appropriate clinical signs (i.e., polyuria, polydipsia, polyphagia, weight loss) and persistent fasting hyperglycemia and glucosuria must be documented. The concurrent documentation of ketonuria with reagent test strips that measure acetoacetic acid (KetoDiastix; Ames Division, Miles Laboratories, Elkhart, Ind) establishes the diagnosis of diabetic ketosis (DK) and documentation of metabolic acidosis establishes the diagnosis of DKA. If ketonuria is not present but DKA is suspected, the serum or urine can be tested for acetone using Acetest tablets (Ames Division, Miles Laboratories, Elkhart, Ind). β-hydroxybutyrate and acetone are derived from acetoacetic acid, and commonly used urine reagent strips do not detect β-hydroxybutyrate or acetone. However, it is extremely uncommon for DKA to develop without an excess of acetoacetic acid.

## Treatment of "Healthy" Dogs or Cats with DK or DKA

If systemic signs of illness are absent or mild, serious abnormalities are not readily identifiable on physical examination, and metabolic acidosis is mild (i.e., total venous carbon dioxide [$CO_2$] or arterial bicarbonate concentration >16 mEq/L), short-acting regular crystalline insulin can be administered SC three times daily until the ketonuria resolves. The insulin dose should be adjusted based on blood glucose concentrations. To minimize hypoglycemia, the dog or cat should be fed one third of its daily caloric intake at the time of each insulin injection. The blood glucose and urine ketone concentrations, as well as the animal's clinical status, should also be monitored. A decrease in blood glucose concentrations implies a decrease in ketone production. This, in combination with metabolism of ketones and loss of ketones in urine, will usually result in correction of ketosis within 48 to 96 hours of initiating aggressive insulin therapy. Prolonged ketonuria is suggestive of a significant concurrent illness or inadequate blood insulin concentrations to suppress lipolysis and ketogenesis. Once the ketosis has resolved and the dog's or cat's condition is stable (it is eating and drinking), insulin therapy may be initiated using the longer-acting insulin preparations (see p. 733 and p. 752).

## Treatment of Sick Dogs or Cats with DKA

Aggressive therapy is called for if the dog or cat has systemic signs of illness (e.g., lethargy, anorexia, vomiting); physical examination reveals dehydration, depression, weakness, or Kussmaul's respiration, or a combination of these; the blood glucose concentration is more than 500 mg/dl; or metabolic acidosis is shown to be severe by the finding of a total venous $CO_2$ or arterial bicarbonate concentration of less than 12 mEq/L. The five goals of treatment of a severely ill ketoacidotic, diabetic pet are (1) to provide adequate amounts of insulin to suppress lipolysis, ketogenesis, and hepatic gluconeogenesis; (2) to restore water and electrolyte losses; (3) to correct acidosis; (4) to identify the factors precipitating the present illness; and (5) to provide a carbohydrate substrate (i.e., dextrose) when necessary to allow continued administration of insulin without causing hypoglycemia (Table 52-15). Proper therapy does not imply forcing as rapid a return to a normal state as possible. Because osmotic and biochemical problems can arise as a result of overly aggressive therapy, as well as from the disease itself, rapid changes in various vital parameters can be as harmful as, or more harmful than, no change. If all abnormal parameters can be slowly returned toward normal (i.e., over a period of 36 to 48 hours), therapy is more likely to be successful.

To aid in the formulation of a treatment protocol, a collection of critically important studies should be performed in the ill ketoacidotic diabetic. The minimum required tests include urinalysis, hematocrit, measurement of the total plasma protein concentration, measurement of the blood glucose concentration, a venous total $CO_2$ or arterial acid-base evaluation, measurement of the BUN or serum creatinine concentration, and measurement of serum electrolytes (i.e., $Na^+$, $K^+$, $Ca^{2+}$, $PO4^{-2}$). Abnormalities frequently associated with DKA are listed in Table 52-16. Additional information, such as that provided by radiographs, abdominal ultrasound, or additional laboratory studies, are usually needed to identify underlying concurrent disorders (see Table 52-10).

**Fluid therapy.** It is important to replace fluid deficiencies and maintain normal fluid balance to ensure adequate cardiac output, blood pressure, and blood flow to all tissues. It is especially critical to improve renal blood flow. The type of parenteral fluid initially used depends on the animal's electrolyte status, blood glucose concentration, and osmolality. With rare exceptions, all dogs and cats with DKA have severe deficits in total body sodium content, regardless of the measured serum concentration. Unless serum electrolyte concentrations dictate otherwise, the initial IV fluid of choice is 0.9% (normal) sodium chloride, supplemented with potassium as appropriate (see Tables 55-2 and 55-4). Most dogs and cats with severe DKA usually are sodium depleted and therefore not suffering from dramatic hyperosmolality, despite potentially remarkable elevations in both the blood glucose and BUN concentrations. Hypotonic fluids must be used with caution in the dog or cat with DKA. Animals rarely die of hypertonicity, but they may die from the effects of volume contraction caused by the infusion of too much free water (i.e., hypotonic fluids). Appropriate fluid and insulin therapy readily corrects hyperosmolality during the initial 24 to 36 hours of treatment.

The initial volume and rate of fluid administration are determined by assessing the degree of shock, the dehydration deficit, the animal's maintenance requirements, the plasma protein concentration, and the presence or absence of cardiac disease. The typical dog or cat with DKA is 6% to 12% dehydrated. Fluid administration should be directed at gradually replacing all deficits over a period of 24 to 48 hours. Rapid replacement of fluids is rarely indicated, except if the dog or cat is in shock. Once the animal is out of this critical phase, the rate of fluid replacement should be decreased in an effort to correct the fluid imbalance in a slow but steady manner. A fluid rate of 1.5 to 2 times the maintenance rate (i.e., 60 to 100 ml/kg/24 hr) is typically chosen initially, with subsequent adjustments made based on frequent assessment of the animal's hydration status and urine output, the severity of azotemia, and the persistence of vomiting and diarrhea.

**Potassium supplementation.** Most dogs and cats with DKA initially have normal or decreased serum potassium concentrations. However, individual animals may have low, normal, or high potassium concentrations, depending on the duration of illness, the animal's renal function, and the animal's previous nutrition status. During therapy for DKA the serum potassium concentration decreases as a result of rehy-

## TABLE 52-15

Initial Management of Dogs or Cats with Severe Diabetic Ketoacidosis

### Fluid Therapy

Type: 0.9% saline solution.

Rate: 60 to 100 ml/kg/24 hr initially; adjust based on hydration status, urine output, persistence of fluid losses.

Potassium supplement: based on serum $K^+$ concentration (Table 55-2, p. 829); if unknown, initially add 40 mEq KCl to each liter of fluids.

Phosphate supplement: administer if serum phosphorus concentration <1.5 mg/dl, initial IV infusion rate is 0.01-0.03 mmol/kg/hr in calcium-free fluids (e.g., 0.9% saline).

Dextrose supplement: not indicated until blood glucose concentration is less than 250 mg/dl, then begin 5% dextrose infusion.

### Bicarbonate Therapy

Indication: administer if plasma bicarbonate concentration is less than 12 mEq/L or total venous $CO_2$ concentration is less than 12 mmol/L; if not known, do not administer unless animal is severely ill and then only once.

Amount: mEq $HCO_3^-$ = body weight (kg) × 0.4 × (12 − animal's $HCO_3^-$) × 0.5; if animal's $HCO_3^-$ or total $CO_2$ concentration is unknown, use 10 in place of (12 − animal's $HCO_3^-$).

Administration: add to IV fluids and give over 6 hours; do not give as bolus infusion.

Retreatment: only if plasma bicarbonate concentration remains less than 12 mEq/L after 6 hours of therapy.

### Insulin Therapy

Type: regular crystalline insulin.

Administration technique: *Intermittent M technique:* initial dose, 0.2 U/kg IM; then 0.1 U/kg IM hourly until blood glucose concentration is less than 250 mg/dl, then switch to SC regular insulin q6-8h. *Low-dose infusion technique:* initial rate, 0.05 to 0.1 U/kg/hr diluted in 0.9% NaCl and administered via infusion or syringe pump in a line separate from that used for fluid therapy; adjust infusion rate based on hourly blood glucose measurements, switch to SC regular insulin q6-8h once blood glucose concentration is less than 250 mg/dl.

Goal: gradual decline in blood glucose concentration, preferably around 75 mg/dl/hr until concentration is less than 250 mg/dl.

### Ancillary Therapy

Concurrent pancreatitis is common in DKA; nothing per os and aggressive fluid therapy usually indicated.

Concurrent infections are common in DKA; use of broad-spectrum, parenteral antibiotics usually indicated.

Additional therapy may be needed, depending on the nature of concurrent disorders.

### Patient Monitoring

Blood glucose measurement every 1 to 2 hours initially; adjust insulin therapy and begin dextrose infusion when decreases below 250 mg/dl.

Hydration status, respiration, pulse every 2 to 4 hours; adjust fluids accordingly.

Serum electrolyte and total venous $CO_2$ concentrations every 6 to 12 hours; adjust fluid and bicarbonate therapy accordingly.

Urine output, glycosuria, ketonuria every 2 to 4 hours; adjust fluid therapy accordingly.

Body weight, packed cell volume, temperature, and blood pressure daily.

Additional monitoring, depending on concurrent disease.

## TABLE 52-16

Common Clinicopathologic Abnormalities Identified in Dogs and Cats with Diabetic Ketoacidosis

| | |
|---|---|
| Neutrophilic leukocytosis, signs of toxicity if septic | Hypokalemia |
| Hemoconcentration | Metabolic acidosis (decreased total carbon dioxide concentration) |
| Hyperglycemia | Hyperlipasemia |
| Hypercholesterolemia, lipemia | Hyperamylasemia |
| Increased alkaline phosphatase activity | Hyperosmolality |
| Increased alanine aminotransferase activity | Glycosuria |
| Increased BUN and serum creatinine concentrations | Ketonuria |
| Hyponatremia | Urinary tract infection |
| Hypochloremia | |

dration (i.e., dilution), the correction of acidemia (i.e., shift of hydrogen ions out of cells in exchange for potassium; Fig. 52-19), the insulin-mediated cellular uptake of potassium (with glucose), and continued urinary losses. Severe hypokalemia is the most common complication that develops during the initial 24 to 36 hours of treatment of DKA. Dogs and cats with hypokalemia require aggressive potassium replacement therapy to replace deficits and prevent worsening, life-threatening hypokalemia after the initiation of insulin therapy. Normal saline solution does not contain potassium, and Ringer's solution contains 4 mEq of potassium per liter; thus these fluids must be supplemented, especially with initially low or normal serum potassium concentrations. The exception to this are animals with hyperkalemia associated with oliguric renal failure. Potassium supplementation should initially be withheld in these dogs and cats until glomerular filtration is restored, urine production increases, and the hyperkalemia is resolving.

Ideally the amount of potassium required should be determined based on an actually measured serum potassium concentration. If this is not available, 40 mEq of potassium should initially be added to each liter of IV fluids (36 mEq added to Ringer's solution). Fifty percent of the potassium added should be in the form of potassium chloride and 50% in the form of potassium phosphate to help prevent hypophosphatemia after the initiation of insulin therapy (see Phosphate Supplementation, below). Subsequent adjustments in potassium supplementation should be based on the serum potassium concentration measured preferably every 6 to 8 hours until the dog's or cat's condition is stable and serum electrolyte concentrations are in the normal range.

***Phosphate supplementation.*** Phosphate shifts between the intracellular and extracellular compartment in a manner similar to potassium. The metabolic acidosis of DKA causes phosphorus to shift from the intracellular to the extracellular compartment (see Fig. 52-19).

Consequently, hypophosphatemia may not be identified at the time the animal is first seen, even though total body phosphorus content may be severely deficient because of excess renal losses. With the initiation of insulin therapy and correction of metabolic acidosis, there may be a marked shift of phosphorus from the extracellular into the intracellular compartment, causing potentially severe hypophosphatemia (<1.5 mg/dl) to occur within 12 to 24 hours. Hemolytic anemia is the most common problem caused by severe hypophosphatemia and can be life-threatening if it goes unrecognized and untreated. Weakness, ataxia, and seizures may also be observed. Severe hypophosphatemia may be clinically silent in many animals.

Phosphate therapy is called for if clinical signs or hemolysis is identified or if the serum phosphorus concentration is less than 1.5 mg/dl. IV fluids are routinely supplemented with phosphorus to prevent the development of severe hypophosphatemia during therapy for severe DKA. The dose of phosphate recommended for dogs is 0.01 to 0.03 mmol/kg/hr, preferably administered in calcium-free IV fluids (e.g., 0.9% sodium chloride). An alternative approach is to determine the amount of potassium supplementation required in the dog or cat and then provide 75% in the form of potassium chloride and 25% in the form of potassium phosphate. This mixture is continued until serum electrolyte concentrations have stabilized in the normal range and metabolic acidosis has resolved or hyperphosphatemia develops. Adverse effects stemming from overzealous phosphate administration include iatrogenic hypocalcemia and its associated neuromuscular signs, hypernatremia, hypotension, and metastatic calcifica-

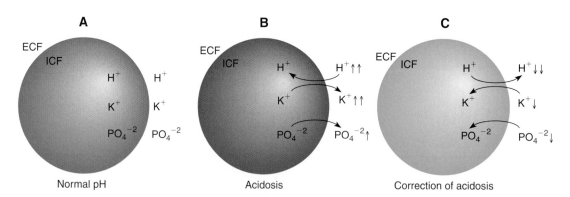

**FIG 52-19**
Redistribution of extracellular (ECF) and intracellular (ICF) hydrogen, potassium, and phosphate ions in response to a decrease in ECF pH (i.e., acidosis) and increase in ECF osmolality and subsequent correction of acidosis and hyperosmolality with fluid, insulin, and bicarbonate therapy. **A,** Normal ECF pH. **B,** Increase in ECF hydrogen ion concentration and osmolality, causing hydrogen ions to move into cells and water, potassium and phosphate to move out of cells. **C,** ECF hydrogen ion concentration decreases during correction of acidosis, causing hydrogen ions to move out of cells. Insulin treatment causes intracellular translocation of potassium and phosphate ions, decreasing ECF potassium and phosphate concentrations. (Feldman EC, Nelson RW: *Canine and feline endocrinology and reproduction,* ed 2, Philadelphia, 1996, WB Saunders.)

tion. Phosphorus supplementation is contraindicated in dogs and cats with hypercalcemia, hyperphosphatemia, oliguria, or suspected tissue necrosis.

***Bicarbonate therapy.*** The clinical presentation of the dog or cat, in conjunction with the plasma bicarbonate or total venous $CO_2$ concentration, should be used to determine the need for bicarbonate therapy. Bicarbonate supplementation is not recommended if the plasma bicarbonate (or total venous $CO_2$) concentration is 12 mEq/L or greater, especially if the animal is alert. An alert dog or cat probably has a normal or nearly normal pH in the cerebrospinal fluid (CSF). The acidosis in these animals is corrected through insulin and fluid therapy. An improvement in renal perfusion enhances the urinary loss of ketoacids, and insulin therapy markedly diminishes the production of ketoacids. Acetoacetate and β-hydroxybutyrate are also metabolically usable anions, and 1 mEq of bicarbonate is generated from each 1 mEq of ketoacid metabolized.

When the plasma bicarbonate concentration is 11 mEq/L or less (total venous $CO_2$ concentration is <12 mEq/L), bicarbonate therapy should be initiated. Many of these animals have severe depression that may be a result of concurrent severe CNS acidosis. These are difficult dogs and cats to treat, and the only safe therapeutic protocol involves correcting the metabolic acidosis slowly in the peripheral circulation by means of IV fluid supplementation, thereby avoiding major alterations in the pH of the CSF. As such, only a portion of the bicarbonate deficit is given initially over a 6-hour period.

The bicarbonate deficit (i.e., the milliequivalents of bicarbonate initially needed to correct acidosis to the critical level of 12 mEq/L over a period of 6 hours) is calculated by the following formula:

$$\text{mEq bicarbonate} = \text{body weight (kg)} \times 0.4 \times (12 - \text{animal's bicarbonate}) \times 0.5$$

If the serum bicarbonate concentration is not known, the following formula should be used:

$$\text{mEq bicarbonate} = \text{body weight (kg)} \times 2$$

The difference between the animal's serum bicarbonate concentration and the critical value of 12 mEq/L represents the treatable base deficit in DKA. If the animal's serum bicarbonate concentration is not known, the number 10 should be used for the treatable base deficit. The factor 0.4 corrects for the extracellular fluid (ECF) space in which bicarbonate is distributed (40% of body weight). The factor 0.5 provides one half of the required dose of bicarbonate in the IV infusion. In this manner, a conservative dose is given over a 6-hour period. Bicarbonate should not be given by bolus infusion nor should the metabolic acidosis be rapidly corrected. After 6 hours of therapy, the acid-base status should be reevaluated and a new dose calculated. Further bicarbonate supplementation is not needed once the plasma bicarbonate level is greater than 12 mEq/L.

***Magnesium supplementation.*** Hypomagnesemia is common in dogs and cats with DKA, often worsens during the initial treatment of DKA, but resolves without treatment as the DKA resolves. Clinical signs of hypomagnesemia do not usually occur until the serum total magnesium concentration is less than 1.0 mg/dl; even at these low levels many dogs and cats remain asymptomatic. Treatment with magnesium is usually not indicated unless problems with persistent lethargy, anorexia, weakness, or refractory hypokalemia are encountered (see p. 843).

**Insulin therapy.** Resolution of ketoacidosis can only be achieved through insulin therapy. As such, insulin therapy should be initiated within 1 to 4 hours of establishing the diagnosis of DKA; the more severe the hypokalemia, the longer the delay before starting insulin. If hypokalemia or hypophosphatemia are a concern, the initial insulin dose can be reduced to slow the intracellular shift of these electrolytes while still increasing blood insulin concentrations and decreasing lipolysis and generation of FFAs. Insulin therapy may not be as effective if a concurrent insulin-antagonistic disease is present, and it may be necessary to eliminate the disease while the animal is still ill to improve insulin effectiveness and resolve the ketoacidosis. Regardless, insulin therapy is still indicated. The amount of insulin needed by an individual animal is difficult to predict. Therefore an insulin with a rapid onset of action and a brief duration of effect would be ideal for making rapid adjustments in the dose and frequency of administration to meet the needs of that particular dog or cat. Rapid-acting regular crystalline insulin meets these criteria and is recommended for the treatment of DKA.

Insulin protocols for the treatment of DKA include the intermittent IM technique; the continuous low-dose IV infusion technique; and the initial IM then intermittent SC technique. All three routes (i.e., IV, IM, SC) of insulin administration are effective in decreasing plasma glucose and ketone concentrations. The successful management of DKA does not depend on the route of insulin administration. Rather, it depends on the proper treatment of each disorder associated with DKA.

***Intermittent intramuscular regimen.*** Dogs and cats with severe DKA should receive an initial regular crystalline insulin loading dose of 0.2 U/kg, after which a dose of 0.1 U/kg is given every hour. The insulin should be administered into the muscles of the rear legs to ensure that the injections go into muscle and not into fat or SC tissue. Diluting regular insulin 1:10 with sterile saline solution or special diluents available from the insulin manufacturer and using 0.3 ml U100 insulin syringes are helpful when administering small doses of insulin. The blood glucose concentration should be measured every hour using a portable blood glucose-monitoring device and the insulin dose adjusted accordingly. The goal of initial insulin therapy is to slowly lower the blood glucose concentration to the range of 200 to 250 mg/dl, preferably over a 6- to 10-hour period. An hourly decline of 50 to 100 mg/dl in the blood glucose concentration is ideal. This produces a steady, moderate decline and avoids large shifts in osmolality. A declining blood glucose concentration also ensures that lipolysis and the supply of FFAs for ketone production have been effectively turned off. However, glucose concentrations decrease much more rapidly than do ketone levels. In general, hyperglycemia is corrected in 4 to 8 hours, but ketosis takes 12 to 48 hours to resolve.

Once the initial hourly insulin therapy brings the blood glucose concentration below 250 mg/dl, the hourly administration of regular insulin should be discontinued and regular insulin given every 4 to 6 hours IM or, if the animal's hydration status is good, every 6 to 8 hours SC. The initial dose is usually 0.1 to 0.4 U/kg, with subsequent adjustments made based on the blood glucose concentrations. In addition, at this point the IV infusion solution should have enough 50% dextrose added to create a 5% dextrose solution (i.e., 100 ml of 50% dextrose added to each liter of fluids). The blood glucose concentration should be maintained between 150 and 300 mg/dl until the animal's condition is stable and the animal is eating. Usually a 5% dextrose solution is adequate for maintaining the desired blood glucose concentration. The insulin dose can be lowered or raised accordingly if the concentration decreases below 150 mg/dl or increases above 300 mg/dl. Dextrose helps minimize problems with hypoglycemia and allows insulin to be administered on schedule. Delaying the administration of insulin delays correction of the ketoacidotic state.

Longer-acting insulins (e.g., NPH, Lente, PZI) should not be administered until the dog or cat's condition is stable and the animal is eating, not vomiting, maintaining a fluid balance without any IV infusions, and no longer acidotic, azotemic, or electrolyte deficient. The initial dose of these longer-acting insulins is similar to the regular insulin dose that was being given just before the switch to the longer-acting insulins. Subsequent adjustments in the longer-acting insulin dose should be made based on clinical response and results of blood glucose and serum fructosamine concentrations, as described on p. 737 and p. 758.

***Constant low-dose insulin infusion technique.*** A constant IV infusion of regular crystalline insulin is also effective in decreasing blood glucose concentrations. The decision to use the intermittent IM technique as opposed to a constant IV insulin infusion is made primarily based on clinician preference and the availability of technical support and infusion pumps. The initial rate of regular crystalline insulin infusion is 0.05 to 0.1 U/kg/hr, and the infusion is given in an IV line separate from that used for fluid therapy. An infusion or syringe pump should be used to ensure a constant rate of insulin infusion. Insulin infusions administered using pediatric drip sets may not infuse insulin at a constant rate, and this may go unnoticed if it is not possible to frequently monitor the blood glucose concentration. The goal of therapy is identical to that described for the intermittent IM technique, that is, to provide a continuous source of insulin at a dose that will cause a gradual decline in the blood glucose concentration. This goal is best attained through the use of infusion or syringe pumps.

Regular crystalline insulin needs to be diluted before it is administered, simply because of the small amounts of insulin being infused into the animal. If a syringe pump is used, regular crystalline insulin can be diluted with sterile saline solution or a specific diluting solution available from the insulin

manufacturer. Assuming that U100 regular crystalline insulin is being used, the insulin should be diluted 1 to 10 to 1 to 100, depending on the size of the dog or cat. If an infusion pump is used, regular crystalline insulin can be added to 250 ml of 0.9% saline or Ringer's solution. Because insulin adheres to glass and plastic surfaces, approximately 50 ml of the insulin-containing fluid should be run through the drip set before it is administered to the animal.

The infusion rate is adjusted based on the hourly measured blood glucose concentration; an hourly decline of 50 to 100 mg/dl in the blood glucose concentration is ideal. Once the concentration approaches 250 mg/dl, the insulin infusion can be discontinued and regular insulin given every 4 to 6 hours IM or, if the animal's hydration status is good, every 6 to 8 hours SC, as described for the intermittent IM protocol. Alternatively, the insulin infusion can be continued (at a decreased rate to prevent hypoglycemia) until the insulin preparation is exchanged for a longer-acting product. Dextrose should be added to the IV fluids once the blood glucose concentration decreases below 250 mg/dl, as discussed in the section on the intermittent IM insulin technique.

***High-dose IM then intermittent SC technique.*** Although a high-dose IM then intermittent SC insulin technique has been used successfully for years, using the intermittent IM and constant IV insulin techniques are now recommended. Although the high-dose IM technique is less labor intensive than the other techniques of insulin administration, it can cause the blood glucose concentration to decrease rapidly, thereby increasing the risk of hypoglycemia, hypokalemia, and hypophosphatemia. The initial regular crystalline insulin dose is 0.25 to 0.5 U/kg, given IM every 4 hours. Usually insulin is administered IM only once or twice. Once the animal is rehydrated, insulin is administered SC every 6 to 8 hours. SC administration is not recommended initially because of problems with insulin absorption from SC sites of deposition in a dehydrated dog or cat. The dose of IM or SC insulin is adjusted according to the blood glucose concentrations, which initially should be measured hourly. Dextrose should be added to the IV fluids once the blood glucose concentration decreases below 250 mg/dl, as discussed in the section on the intermittent IM insulin technique.

**Concurrent illness.** Therapy for DKA frequently involves the management of concurrent, often serious illness. Common concurrent illnesses in dogs and cats with DKA include bacterial infection, pancreatitis, congestive heart failure, renal failure, and insulin-antagonistic disorders, most notably hyperadrenocorticism, hyperthyroidism, and diestrus. It may be necessary in such animals to modify the therapy for DKA (e.g., fluid therapy in animals with concurrent heart failure) or implement additional therapy (e.g., antibiotics), depending on the nature of the concurrent illness. Insulin therapy, however, should never be delayed or discontinued. Resolution of the ketoacidosis can only be achieved through insulin therapy. If nothing is to be given per os, insulin therapy should be continued and the blood glucose concentration maintained with IV dextrose infusions. If a concurrent insulin-antagonistic disease is present, it may be necessary to eliminate the disease while the animal is still ill to improve insulin effectiveness and resolve the ketoacidosis.

**Complications of therapy for DKA.** Complications caused by therapy for DKA are common and usually result from overly aggressive treatment, inadequate monitoring of the animal's condition, and failure to reevaluate biochemical parameters in a timely manner. DKA is a complex disorder that is associated with a high mortality rate if improperly managed. To minimize the risk of therapeutic complications and improve the chances of a successful response to therapy, all abnormal parameters should be slowly returned toward normal (over a period of 24 to 48 hours), the physical and mental status of the animal must be evaluated frequently (at least three to four times daily), and biochemical parameters (e.g., blood glucose, serum electrolyte, blood gas values) must be evaluated in a timely fashion. During the initial 24 hours the blood glucose concentrations should be measured every 1 to 2 hours and the serum electrolyte and blood gas values measured every 6 to 8 hours. Fluid, insulin, and bicarbonate therapy typically must be modified three or four times during the initial 24 hours of therapy.

Failure to recognize changes in the status of the animal with DKA and to respond accordingly will invariably lead to the development of potentially serious complications. The more common complications are hypoglycemia, CNS signs secondary to cerebral edema, severe hypokalemia, severe hypernatremia and hyperchloremia, and hemolytic anemia resulting from hypophosphatemia.

## Prognosis

DKA remains one of the most difficult metabolic therapeutic challenges in veterinary medicine. Despite all precautions and diligent therapy, a fatal outcome cannot be avoided in some cases. Approximately 30% of cats and dogs with severe DKA die or are euthanized during the initial hospitalization. Death is usually the result of a severe underlying illness (e.g., oliguric renal failure, necrotizing pancreatitis), severe metabolic acidosis (i.e., arterial blood pH of <7), or complications (e.g., cerebral edema, hypokalemia) that develop during therapy. Nevertheless, if logical therapy is implemented and animals are monitored carefully, the goal of therapy for DKA (i.e., achieving a healthy diabetic dog or cat) is attainable.

## INSULIN-SECRETING β-CELL NEOPLASIA

### Etiology

Functional tumors arising from the β cells of the pancreatic islets are malignant tumors that secrete insulin independent of the typically suppressive effects of hypoglycemia. β-cell tumors, however, are not completely autonomous and respond to provocative stimuli (e.g., glucose) by secreting insulin, often in excessive amounts. Immunohistochemical analysis of β-cell tumors has revealed a high incidence of multihormonal production, including pancreatic polypeptide, somatostatin, glucagon, serotonin, and gastrin. However, insulin has been the most common product demonstrated

within the neoplastic cells, and the clinical signs in such animals are primarily those that result from a hyperinsulinemia-induced hypoglycemia.

β-Cell tumors are uncommon in dogs and rare in cats. The malignant potential of β-cell tumors is often underestimated in the dog. Virtually all such tumors in dogs are malignant and most animals have microscopic or grossly visible metastatic lesions at the time of surgery. The most common metastatic sites are the lymphatics and lymph nodes (i.e., duodenal, mesenteric, hepatic, splenic), liver, and peripancreatic mesentery and omentum. Pulmonary metastasis is rare. In most dogs, hypoglycemia recurs weeks to months after surgical excision of the tumor. The high prevalence of metastatic lesions at the time afflicted dogs are initially examined results, in part, from the typically protracted time it takes for clinical signs to develop and the interval between the time an owner initially observes signs and seeks assistance from a veterinarian. Most dogs are symptomatic for 1 to 6 months before being brought to a veterinarian.

## Clinical Features

**Signalment.** Insulin-secreting tumors typically occur in middle-aged or older dogs. The mean age at the time of diagnosis of an insulin-secreting tumor in 77 dogs in our series was 9.5 years, with a median age of 10 years and an age range of 3 to 14 years. No sex-related predilection is seen. Insulin-secreting tumors are diagnosed in a wide variety of breeds but are most commonly diagnosed in large breeds of dogs such as the German Shepherd, Labrador Retriever, Golden Retriever, and Irish Setter.

**Clinical signs.** The clinical signs of an insulin-secreting tumor typically are caused by neuroglycopenia (i.e., hypoglycemia) and an increase in circulating catecholamine concentrations and include seizures, weakness, collapse, ataxia, muscle fasciculations, and bizarre behavior (Table 52-17). The severity of the clinical signs depends on the duration and severity of the hypoglycemia. Dogs with chronic fasting

 TABLE 52-17

**Clinical Signs Associated with Insulin-Secreting Tumors in Dogs**

| |
| --- |
| Seizures* |
| Weakness* |
| Collapse |
| Ataxia |
| Polyphagia |
| Weight gain |
| Muscle fasciculations |
| Posterior weakness (neuropathy) |
| Lethargy |
| Nervousness |
| Bizarre behavior |

*Common clinical signs.

hypoglycemia or with recurring episodes appear to tolerate low blood glucose concentrations (20 to 30 mg/dl) for prolonged periods without clinical signs, and only small additional changes in the blood glucose concentration are then required to produce symptomatic episodes. As such, fasting, excitement, exercise, and eating may trigger the development of clinical signs. Because of the compensatory counterregulatory mechanisms that are designed to increase the blood glucose concentration when hypoglycemia develops, clinical signs tend to be episodic and are generally observed for only a few seconds to minutes. If these counterregulatory mechanisms are inadequate, seizures typically occur as the blood glucose concentration continues to decrease. The seizures are often self-limiting, lasting from 30 seconds to 5 minutes, and may stimulate further catecholamine secretion and the activation of other counterregulatory mechanisms that increase the blood glucose concentration above critical levels.

**Physical examination.** Physical examination findings in animals with β-cell tumors are surprisingly unremarkable; dogs are usually free of visible or palpable abnormalities. Weight gain is evident in some dogs and is probably a result of the potent anabolic effects of insulin. Peripheral neuropathies have been observed in dogs with insulin-secreting tumors, which may be responsible for producing alterations detected during physical examination, including weakness of the rear limbs, proprioception deficits, depressed reflexes, and muscle atrophy. The pathogenesis of the polyneuropathy is not known. Proposed theories include metabolic derangements of the nerves induced by hyperinsulinemia or an immune-mediated reaction resulting from the sharing of antigens between the tumor and nerves.

**Clinical pathology.** Results of the CBC and urinalysis in dogs with an insulin-secreting tumor are usually normal. The only consistent abnormality identified in serum biochemistry profiles is hypoglycemia, which is typically 30 to 50 mg/dl. Dogs with insulin-secreting tumors may occasionally have a blood glucose concentration of 60 to 80 mg/dl revealed during random testing. Such a finding does not rule out hypoglycemia as a cause of episodic weakness or seizure activity. Fasting with hourly evaluations of the blood glucose concentration should be carried out in dogs with suspected hypoglycemia. A fast of 8 hours or less is usually successful in demonstrating hypoglycemia in dogs with insulin-secreting tumors. The remainder of the serum biochemistry profile is usually normal. Hypoalbuminemia, hypophosphatemia, hypokalemia, and increased alkaline phosphatase and alanine aminotransferase activities have been reported. However, these findings are considered nonspecific and not helpful in arriving at a definite diagnosis. A correlation between increased liver enzyme activities and obvious metastasis of β-cell tumors to the liver has not been established.

## Diagnosis

The diagnosis of an insulin-secreting tumor requires an initial confirmation of hypoglycemia, after which inappropriate insulin secretion is documented and a pancreatic mass is identified using ultrasonography or exploratory celiotomy.

Considering the potential differential diagnoses for hypoglycemia (see Table 52-2), a tentative diagnosis of insulin-secreting neoplasia can often be made based on the history, physical examination findings, and an absence of abnormalities other than hypoglycemia shown by routine blood tests. Abdominal ultrasonography can be used to identify a mass in the region of the pancreas and to look for evidence of potential metastatic disease in the liver and surrounding structures (Fig. 52-20). Because of the smallness of most insulin-secreting tumors, abdominal ultrasonographic findings are often interpreted as normal, although a pancreatic mass or metastatic lesion can be found at surgery. Therefore a normal abdominal ultrasonographic finding does not rule out the diagnosis of an insulin-secreting tumor. Thoracic radiographs are of minimal value in documenting metastatic disease, primarily because identifiable metastatic nodules in the lung occur late in the disease.

The diagnosis of an insulin-secreting tumor is established by evaluating the blood insulin concentration at a time when hypoglycemia is present. Hypoglycemia suppresses insulin secretion in normal animals, with the degree of suppression directly related to its severity. Hypoglycemia fails to have this same suppressive effect on insulin secretion if the insulin is synthesized and secreted from autonomous neoplastic cells, because tumor cells that produce and secrete insulin are less responsive to hypoglycemia than are normal β cells. Invariably the dog with an insulin-secreting tumor will have inappropriate excesses in its insulin concentration relative to that needed for a particular blood glucose concentration. The relative excess of insulin is easiest to recognize when the blood glucose concentration is low, preferably less than 50 mg/dl. If the blood glucose concentration is low and the insulin concentration is in the upper half of the normal range or increased, this indicates that the animal has a relative or absolute excess of insulin that can be explained by the presence of an insulin-secreting tumor that is insensitive to hypoglycemia.

Most dogs with insulin-secreting neoplasia are persistently hypoglycemic. If the blood glucose concentration is less than 60 mg/dl (preferably <50 mg/dl), serum should be submitted to a commercial veterinary endocrine laboratory for determination of the glucose and insulin concentration. If the dog is euglycemic, a 4- to 12-hour fast may be necessary to induce hypoglycemia. Blood glucose concentrations should be evaluated hourly during the fast. Portable home blood glucose–monitoring devices are typically used to monitor blood glucose concentration in most veterinary hospitals. Because blood glucose results obtained from most of these devices are erroneously low, a blood sample for submission to a commercial laboratory for glucose and insulin determinations should not be obtained until the blood glucose measured on these devices is approximately 40 mg/dl or less. The dog can then be fed several small meals over the next 1 to 3 hours to prevent marked fluctuations in the blood glucose concentration and a potential postprandial reactive hypoglycemia.

Serum insulin concentrations must be evaluated simultaneously in relation to the blood glucose concentration. The serum insulin and glucose concentrations in the healthy

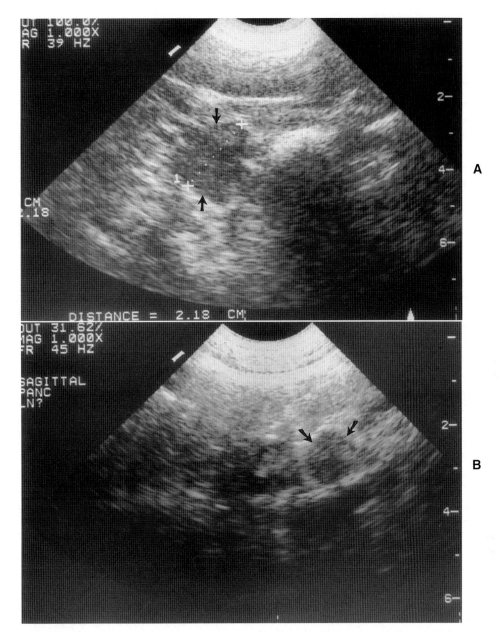

**FIG 52-20**
Ultrasonogram of the pancreas showing an islet β-cell tumor *(arrows)* in a 13-year-old
Borzoi **(A)** and of the peripancreatic tissue showing a metastatic β-cell tumor *(arrows)* in a
5-year-old Golden Retriever **(B).** (From Feldman EC, Nelson RW: *Canine and feline endocrinology and reproduction,* ed 2, Philadelphia, 1996, WB Saunders.)

fasted dog are usually between 5 and 20 μU/ml and 70 and
110 mg/dl, respectively. The finding of a serum insulin concentration that exceeds 20 μU/ml in a dog with a corresponding blood glucose concentration of less than 60 mg/dl
(preferably <50 mg/dl) in combination with appropriate
clinical signs and clinicopathologic findings strongly supports
the diagnosis of an insulin-secreting tumor. An insulin-
secreting tumor is also possible if the serum insulin concentration is in the high-normal range (10 to 20 μU/ml). Insulin
values in the low-normal range (5 to 10 μU/ml) may be
found in animals with other causes of hypoglycemia and

those with insulin-secreting tumors. Careful assessment of
the history, physical examination findings, clinical pathologic
and abdominal ultrasonographic findings, and, possibly, repeated serum glucose and insulin measurements can usually
identify the cause of the hypoglycemia.

Any serum insulin concentration that is below the normal
range (typically <5 μU/ml) is consistent with insulinopenia
and does not indicate the presence of an insulin-secreting tumor. Confidence in identifying inappropriate hyperinsulinemia is dependent on the severity of the hypoglycemia; the
lower the blood glucose concentration, the more confident

the clinician can be in identifying inappropriate hyperinsulinemia, especially when the serum insulin concentration falls in the normal range.

## Treatment

**Surgical treatment.** Surgical exploration appears to be the best diagnostic, therapeutic, and prognostic tool in dogs with insulin-secreting tumors. Surgery offers a chance to cure dogs with a resectable solitary mass. In dogs with nonresectable tumors or with obvious metastatic lesions, the removal or "debulking" of as much abnormal tissue as possible has frequently resulted in the remission, or at least alleviation, of clinical signs and an improved response to medical therapy lasting for weeks to months. Survival time is also longer in dogs undergoing surgical exploration and tumor debulking after which medical therapy is provided, compared with dogs only treated medically. Despite these benefits, surgery remains a relatively aggressive mode of diagnosis and treatment, in part because of the high prevalence of metastatic disease and the older age of many dogs at the time β-cell neoplasia is diagnosed. As a general rule, the authors of this text are less aggressive about recommending surgery in aged dogs (i.e., 12 years and older), dogs with metastatic disease identified by ultrasonography, and dogs with concurrent disease that enhances the anesthetic risk. (See Suggested Readings for detailed information on surgical techniques.)

Until surgery is performed, the dog with an insulin-secreting tumor must be protected from episodes of severe hypoglycemia. This can usually be accomplished through the frequent feeding of small meals and administration of glucocorticoid therapy (Table 52-18). A continuous IV infusion of a balanced electrolyte solution containing 2.5% to 5% dextrose before, during, and immediately after surgery is important. Although this does not restore euglycemia, these solutions provide a substrate for adequate CNS function, thereby preventing CNS signs in most dogs and cats. The IV dextrose infusion can be initiated the evening before surgery, at the time food and water are withheld, and continued throughout the perioperative period. Initiating fluid therapy before surgery also helps ensure adequate circulation to the pancreas, thereby minimizing the risk of postoperative pancreatitis. The goal of the dextrose infusion is to avoid clinical signs of hypoglycemia and maintain the blood glucose concentration at greater than 35 mg/dl.

If dextrose infusion is ineffective in preventing severe hypoglycemia during the perioperative period, a constant rate infusion of glucagon should be considered. Glucagon is a potent stimulant of hepatic gluconeogenesis and is effective in maintaining normal blood glucose concentrations in dogs with β-cell neoplasia when administered by constant-rate infusion. Lyophilized glucagon USP (1 mg) is reconstituted with the diluent provided by the manufacturer (Eli Lilly, Indianapolis, Ind), and the solution is added to 1 L of 0.9% saline, making a 1 μg/ml solution that can be administered by syringe pump. The initial dose is 5 to 10 ng/kg of body weight/min. The dose is adjusted, as needed, to maintain the blood glucose concentration within the normal range. When discontinuing glucagon, the dose should be gradually decreased over 1 to 2 days.

## TABLE 52-18

Long-Term Medical Therapy for Dogs with β-Cell Neoplasia

### Standard Treatments

1. Dietary therapy
   a. Feed canned or dry food in three to six small meals daily
   b. Avoid foods containing monosaccharides, disaccharides, or propylene glycol
2. Limit exercise
3. Glucocorticoid therapy
   a. Prednisone, 0.5 mg/kg divided q12h initially
   b. Gradually increase dose and frequency of administration, as needed
   c. Goal to control clinical signs, not to reestablish euglycemia
   d. Consider alternative treatments if signs of iatrogenic hypercortisolism become severe or glucocorticoids become ineffective

### Additional Treatments

1. Diazoxide therapy
   a. Continue standard treatment; reduce glucocorticoid dose to minimize adverse signs
   b. Diazoxide, 5 mg/kg q12h initially
   c. Gradually increase dose as needed, not to exceed 60 mg/kg/day
   d. Goal to control clinical signs, not to reestablish euglycemia
2. Somatostatin therapy
   a. Continue standard treatment; reduce glucocorticoid dose to minimize adverse signs
   b. Octreotide (Novartis Pharmaceuticals), 10 to 40 g/dog SC q8-12h
3. Streptozotocin therapy
   a. Continue standard treatment; reduce glucocorticoid dose to minimize adverse signs
   b. 0.9% saline diuresis for 3 hours, then streptozotocin, 500 mg/m², in 0.9% saline and administered IV over 2 hours, then 0.9% saline diuresis for 2 additional hours
   c. Administer antiemetics immediately after streptozotocin administration to minimize vomiting
   d. Repeat treatment every 3 weeks until hypoglycemia resolves or adverse reactions develop (e.g., pancreatitis, renal failure)

Most dogs with insulin-secreting tumors have masses that can be easily seen by the surgeon inspecting the pancreas. In a minority of dogs, the tumor is not visible but can be palpated during gentle but thorough digital examination of the pancreas. Multiple pancreatic masses may also occur. No predisposition for tumor location within the pancreas is seen (Fig. 52-21), and there appears to be little correlation between tumor size or shape and its malignant potential. A complete inspection of the abdominal contents is imperative to identify unsuspected abnormalities and sites of metastatic lesions. The

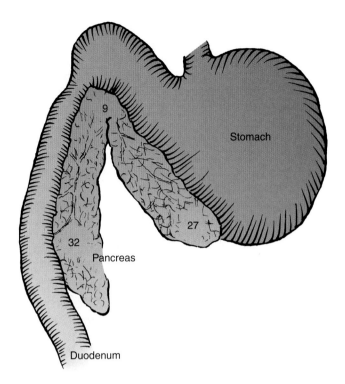

**FIG 52-21**
Tumor location in 68 dogs with islet β-cell tumors. (From Feldman EC, Nelson RW: *Canine and feline endocrinology and reproduction,* ed 2, Philadelphia, 1996, WB Saunders.)

most common sites of tumor spread include the lymphatics and lymph nodes (i.e., duodenal, mesenteric, hepatic, splenic), liver, and peripancreatic mesentery and omentum. It is common to fail to identify metastatic disease during surgery. A solitary pancreatic mass is commonly removed in toto with the belief that the dog has been "cured," only to have clinical signs of hyperinsulinism recur months later. As discussed previously, removing or debulking as much abnormal tissue as possible may result in the remission or alleviation of clinical signs, an improvement in the animal's response to medical treatment, and an increase in survival time.

The most common postoperative complications are pancreatitis, hyperglycemia, and hypoglycemia. The development of these complications is directly related to the expertise of the surgeon in the handling of the pancreas and excision of these tumors, the location of the tumor in the pancreas (i.e., peripheral lobe versus central region), the presence or absence of functional metastatic lesions, and the adequacy of fluid therapy during the perioperative period. The IV administration of polyionic fluids with 2.5% to 5% dextrose (60 to 100 ml/kg/24 hr) and nothing by mouth just before, during, and for 24 to 48 hours after surgery, followed by appropriate dietary therapy (see p. 558) during the ensuing week, is helpful in minimizing the risk of pancreatitis.

Occasionally, transient diabetes mellitus develops in dogs after the surgical removal of an insulin-secreting tumor; unfortunately, this is not an indication of cure. It is believed to result from inadequate insulin secretion by atrophied normal β cells. Removal of all, or most, of the neoplastic cells acutely

deprives the animal of insulin. Until the atrophied normal cells regain their secretory abilities, the animal will be hypoinsulinemic and may require exogenous insulin injections to maintain euglycemia. Insulin therapy is initiated postoperatively only if hyperglycemia and glucosuria persist for longer than 2 or 3 days beyond the time that all dextrose-containing IV fluids have been discontinued. Initial insulin therapy should be conservative, that is, 0.25 U of NPH or Lente insulin per kilogram of body weight given once daily. Subsequent adjustments in insulin therapy should be made based on clinical response and blood glucose and serum fructosamine determinations (see p. 737). The need for insulin treatment is usually transient, lasting from a few days to several months. Rarely, a dog will remain diabetic for more than 1 year. Owner evaluation of the pet's urine glucose level is helpful in identifying when insulin therapy is no longer needed. Failure to identify glucose in the urine in conjunction with the disappearance of polyuria-polydipsia is an indication to discontinue insulin therapy. If hyperglycemia and glucosuria recur, insulin therapy can be reinstituted but at a lower dose.

Dogs that remain hypoglycemic after surgical removal of an insulin-secreting tumor are assumed to have functional metastatic lesions. Medical therapy should be initiated in those dogs with persistent postoperative hypoglycemia. The IV infusion of 2.5% to 5% dextrose should be continued during the initial 48 to 72 hours after surgery. Additional therapy may be needed if hypoglycemic seizures occur (Table 52-19). The goal is to prevent clinical signs of hypoglycemia, not to reestablish a normal blood glucose concentration.

**Medical treatment for chronic hypoglycemia.** Medical measures for the management of chronic hypoglycemia should be initiated if an exploratory celiotomy is not performed or if the development of metastatic or inoperable neoplasia results in the recurrence of clinical signs. The goals of long-term therapy are to reduce the frequency and severity of clinical signs and to prevent an acute hypoglycemic crisis, not to establish euglycemia, per se. Medical therapy currently consists of nonspecific antihormonal therapy. This therapy is palliative and should minimize hypoglycemia by increasing the absorption of glucose from the intestinal tract; increasing hepatic gluconeogenesis and glycogenolysis; or inhibiting the synthesis, secretion, or peripheral cellular actions of insulin (see Table 52-18).

**Frequent feedings.** Dogs with insulin-secreting tumors have a persistent absolute or relative excess of circulating insulin. If a constant source of calories is provided as a substrate for this insulin, hypoglycemic episodes can be reduced in frequency or prevented. Diets that are high in fat, complex carbohydrates, and fiber will delay gastric emptying and slow intestinal glucose absorption, helping to minimize the increase in the portal blood glucose concentration and the stimulation of pancreatic insulin secretion. Simple sugars are rapidly absorbed, have a potent stimulatory effect on insulin secretion by neoplastic β cells and therefore should be avoided in the animal's diet. If dog food is used, a combination of canned and dry food, fed in three to six small meals daily, is recommended. Daily caloric intake should be controlled because

TABLE 52-19

**Medical Therapy for Hypoglycemia Seizures Caused by an Insulin-Secreting β-Cell Tumor**

**Seizures at Home**

Step 1. Rub or pour sugar solution on pet's gums
Step 2. Once pet is sternal, feed a small meal
Step 3. Call the veterinarian

**Seizures in Hospital**

Step 1. Administer 1 to 5 ml of 50% dextrose IV *slowly* over 10 minutes
Step 2. Once animal is sternal, feed a small meal
Step 3. Initiate long-term medical therapy (see Table 52-18)

**Intractable Seizures in Hospital**

Step 1. Administer 2.5% to 5% dextrose in water IV at 1.5 to 2 times maintenance fluid rate
Step 2. Add 0.5 to 1 mg of dexamethasone/kg to IV fluids and administer over 6 hours; repeat every 12 to 24 hours, as necessary
Step 3. Administer glucagon USP (Eli Lilly Co.) IV by constant rate infusion at an initial dose of 5 to 10 ng/kg/min (see page 772)
Step 4. Somatostatin analog (Octreotide, Novartis Pharmaceuticals), 20 to 40 μg SC q8-12h
Step 5. If above fails, anesthetize animal with pentobarbital for 4 to 8 hours while continuing above therapy; consider surgery to debulk functional tumor

hyperinsulinemia promotes obesity. Exercise should be limited to short walks on a leash.

***Glucocorticoid therapy.*** Glucocorticoid therapy should be initiated when dietary manipulations are no longer effective in preventing the signs of hypoglycemia. Glucocorticoids antagonize the effects of insulin at the cellular level, stimulate hepatic glycogenolysis, and indirectly provide the necessary substrates for hepatic gluconeogenesis. Prednisone is the glucocorticoid most often used and is given at an initial dose of 0.5 mg/kg/day in divided doses twice a day. If this controls the signs of hypoglycemia, the medication is continued without dose adjustment. If signs persist or recur, the dose of prednisone should be gradually increased until signs of hypoglycemia abate or signs of iatrogenic hypercortisolism develop (see p. 780). If evidence of hypercortisolism appears, the dose of prednisone should be reduced (therapy should not be stopped) and additional therapy considered.

***Diazoxide therapy.*** Diazoxide (Proglycem; Baker Norton Pharmaceuticals, Miami, Fla) is a benzothiadiazide diuretic that inhibits insulin secretion, stimulates hepatic gluconeogenesis and glycogenolysis, and inhibits tissue use of glucose. The net effect of this is that hyperglycemia develops. Unfortunately, diazoxide is difficult to procure and is expen-

sive. The initial dose is 10 mg/kg, divided into two doses daily. The dose may gradually be increased as needed to control the signs of hypoglycemia but should not exceed 60 mg/kg/day. The most common adverse reactions to diazoxide are anorexia and vomiting. Administering the agent with a meal or decreasing the dose, at least temporarily, is usually effective in controlling adverse gastrointestinal signs.

***Octreotide therapy.*** Octreotide (Sandostatin; Novartis Pharmaceuticals, East Hanover, N.J.) is an analog of somatostatin that inhibits the synthesis and secretion of insulin by normal and neoplastic β cells. The responsiveness of insulin-secreting tumors to the suppressive effects of octreotide is variable, being dependent on the presence of membrane receptors for somatostatin on the tumor cells. Octreotide is beneficial in alleviating hypoglycemia in approximately 40% to 50% of treated dogs. Unfortunately some of these dogs become refractory to octreotide treatment. Nevertheless, octreotide at a dose of 10 to 40 μg/dog SC twice a day to three times a day is well tolerated and can be considered for managing chronic hypoglycemia in dogs with insulin-secreting neoplasia. Adverse reactions have not been seen at these doses.

***Streptozotocin therapy.*** Streptozotocin is a naturally occurring nitrosourea that selectively destroys pancreatic β cells. Streptozotocin has been effective in reducing tumor size and improving clinical signs of hyperinsulinism in humans with advanced β-cell carcinoma and has been used to treat β-cell tumors in dogs. The treatment protocol involves a 0.9% saline diuresis for 7 hours with streptozotocin (500 mg/m²) administered over a 2-hour period beginning 3 hours after initiating the diuresis. Antiemetics are administered immediately after streptozotocin administration to minimize vomiting. Streptozotocin treatment is repeated every 3 weeks. Efficacy in controlling clinical signs of hypoglycemia and prolonging survival time has been variable. Adverse reactions of streptozotocin treatment include vomiting, pancreatitis, diabetes mellitus, and renal failure. Renal failure is less likely when the drug is administered during fluid diuresis as described previously. The reader is referred to the article by Moore and colleagues listed in the recommended readings for more information on using streptozotocin for treating β-cell neoplasia in dogs.

**Prognosis**

Owing to the extremely high likelihood of malignancy in any dog with an insulin-secreting tumor, the long-term prognosis is guarded to poor at best. Survival time is dependent, in part, on the willingness of the owner to treat the disease. Tobin and colleagues (1999) reported a median survival time after diagnosis of only 74 days (range, 8 to 508 days) in dogs treated medically, compared with 381 days (range, 20 to 1758 days) in dogs that initially underwent surgery. The extent to which surgery can alter the prognosis depends on the clinical stage of the disease, most notably the extent of metastatic lesions. Approximately 10% to 15% of dogs undergoing surgery for an insulin-secreting tumor die or are euthanized at the time of or within 1 month of surgery because of severe metastatic disease, uncontrollable postoperative hypoglycemia, or complications related to pancreatitis. An additional 20% to 25% of dogs die or are euthanized within 6 months of surgery because of severe metastatic disease and recurrence of clinical hypoglycemia. The remaining 60% to 70% live beyond 6 months postoperatively, many beyond 1 year after surgery, before uncontrollable hypoglycemia develops, resulting in death or necessitating euthanasia. Additional surgery to debulk metastatic lesions may improve the animal's responsiveness to medical therapy and prolong the survival time in some dogs that become nonresponsive to medical treatment after the initial surgery.

## GASTRINOMA: ZOLLINGER-ELLISON SYNDROME

Gastrinoma is a malignant, gastrin-secreting tumor that is almost always found in the pancreas of dogs and cats. Sites of metastasis include the liver, adjacent lymph nodes, spleen, and mesentery. The clinical syndrome results from the excess secretion of gastrin by the tumor. The main actions of gastrin are stimulation of gastric acid secretion and parietal cell growth. The resultant hypergastrinemia induces the excessive gastric secretion of hydrochloric acid, which is responsible for causing esophageal, gastric, and duodenal ulcers to form; disrupting intestinal digestive, and absorptive functions; and producing the clinical signs.

### Clinical Features

Dogs and cats with confirmed gastrinomas are usually 3 to 12 years old. There does not appear to be a sex- or breed-related predisposition, although the number of reported confirmed cases is too small to allow definite conclusions to be drawn in this regard.

The most consistent clinical signs are vomiting, weight loss, anorexia, and diarrhea (Table 52-20). These signs can be attributed to the hypergastrinemia and the excessive secretion of gastric hydrochloric acid. Gastric hyperacidity results in ulcer formation, most commonly in the stomach and duodenum. Ulcerations, in turn, may cause vomiting, hematemesis, hematochezia, melena, inappetence, weight loss, depression, and abdominal pain. The esophageal reflux of acidic gastric contents may lead to the development of esophagitis and ulceration, with worsening inappetence, regurgitation, and weight loss. Diarrhea with malabsorption and steatorrhea may develop after acidification of the intestinal contents, with the subsequent inactivation of lipase, precipitation of bile salts, interference with chylomicron formation, and damage to intestinal mucosal cells.

The physical examination findings in such animals can vary from being relatively unremarkable to extremely severe. Animals with a gastrinoma may be lethargic, thin to emaciated, febrile, dehydrated, and in shock. Mucous membranes may appear pale as a result of anemia caused by bleeding ulcers. A compensatory tachycardia and abdominal tenderness elicited by palpation may also be present. One cat with gastrinoma had a palpable abdominal mass at the time of presentation.

### TABLE 52-20

**Clinical Signs of Gastrinoma and the Zollinger-Ellison Syndrome in Dogs and Cats**

Vomiting*
Anorexia*
Lethargy, depression*
Diarrhea*
Weight loss*
Melena
Hematemesis
Fever
Polydipsia
Abdominal pain
Hematochezia

*Common clinical signs.

Potential abnormal CBC findings include a regenerative anemia, hypoproteinemia, and neutrophilic leukocytosis, presumably caused by gastrointestinal tract inflammation and blood loss. Abnormalities in the serum biochemistry panel include hypoproteinemia, hypoalbuminemia, hypocalcemia, and mild increases in serum alanine aminotransferase and alkaline phosphatase activities. Hypochloremia, hypokalemia, and metabolic alkalosis may develop in those dogs and cats that vomit frequently. Hyperglycemia and hypoglycemia have been noted in a few cases; the etiology of this is unknown but it may be related to the tumor-associated secretion of other hormones (e.g., ACTH, insulin). Urinalysis findings are usually unremarkable. Sudan staining of a fecal sample may reveal steatorrhea resulting from both lipid and fatty acid accumulation; a positive occult blood reaction or overt melena is usually also present.

Survey abdominal radiograph findings are usually normal. If an ulcer has perforated through the serosal surface, radiographic signs consistent with peritonitis may be present. Contrast-enhanced radiographic studies may show gastric or duodenal ulcers; thickening of the gastric rugal folds, pyloric antrum, or intestine; and the rapid intestinal transit of barium. In an animal with concurrent severe esophagitis, a secondary megaesophagus or aberrant, nonperistaltic esophageal motility may be shown fluoroscopically. Ultrasonographic evaluation of the gastrointestinal tract may confirm some of the changes identified on abdominal radiographs (e.g., gastric and intestinal thickening) and may identify a pancreatic mass or its metastasis. However, gastrinomas vary tremendously in size and may not be detected with ultrasound.

Gastroduodenoscopy in a dog or cat with gastrinoma may reveal severe esophagitis and ulceration, especially near the cardia. Gastric rugal folds may be thickened and persist despite insufflation of the gastric lumen with air. Gastric and duodenal hyperemia, erosions, or ulceration is often visible. Histologic evaluation of esophageal, gastric, and duodenal biopsy specimens obtained during endoscopy may be relatively normal or may reveal variable degrees of inflammation consisting of infiltrates of immunocytes and neutrophils, gastric mucosal hypertrophy, fibrosis, and loss of the mucosal barrier.

## Diagnosis

Gastrinoma should be included among the differential diagnoses for any dog or cat with melena or hematemesis or in which severe gastric and duodenal ulceration is identified by gastroduodenoscopy. Unless a pancreatic mass is identified by ultrasonography, most dogs and cats with gastrinoma will inadvertently be diagnosed with severe inflammatory bowel disease, gastroduodenal erosions, and ulcers, and they will be treated with inhibitors of gastric acid secretion, mucosal protectants, antibiotics, and changes in diet. The probability of gastrinoma increases if ultrasonography reveals a pancreatic mass, the dog or cat does not respond to medical therapy directed at nonspecific inflammation and ulceration of the gastrointestinal tract, or clinical signs and gastrointestinal tract ulceration recur after antiulcer therapy is discontinued. For a definitive diagnosis of gastrinoma to be rendered, histologic and immunocytochemic evaluation of a pancreatic mass excised at surgery must be performed. The finding of increased basal serum gastrin concentrations is helpful in increasing the suspicion of gastrinoma in dogs and cats. Unfortunately, few commercial endocrine laboratories offer a gastrin assay validated for use in the dog and cat. In addition, experience with provocative stimulation tests (e.g., secretin stimulation test, calcium challenge test) is limited in dogs and cats, acid secretory studies are cumbersome, and none of these tests are specific for gastrinoma. For this reason, exploratory surgery, paying special attention to the pancreas and peripancreatic region, is perhaps the most cost-effective way to diagnose (and treat) gastrinoma in dogs and cats.

## Treatment

The treatment of gastrinoma should be directed at surgical excision of the tumor and control of gastric acid hypersecretion. Gastrointestinal tract ulceration is common and can usually be successfully managed by reducing gastric hyperacidity through the administration of $H_2$-receptor antagonists (e.g., ranitidine, famotidine), proton pump inhibitors (e.g., omeprazole), gastrointestinal tract protectants (e.g., sucralfate), or prostaglandin $E_1$ analogs (e.g., misoprostol). The reader is referred to Chapter 30 for more information on these gastrointestinal tract drugs. Surgical resection of an ulcer may be required, especially if the ulcer has perforated the bowel. Surgical resection of the tumor is necessary to obtain a cure, although metastasis to the liver, regional lymph nodes, and mesentery is common. Nevertheless, surgery is the best way to both establish the diagnosis and possibly cure those few animals with solitary, nonmetastatic gastrinomas. Even if metastatic disease is present, tumor debulking may enhance the success of medical therapy.

## Prognosis

Gastrinomas in dogs and cats are malignant tumors, and the long-term prognosis in such animals is poor. Evidence of metastases was present in 76% of reported dogs and cats at the time gastrinoma was diagnosed. Dogs and cats treated surgically, medically, or both survived for 1 week to 18 months (mean, 4.8 months). However, the short-term prognosis has improved in recent years as drugs have come available that can reduce gastric hyperacidity (e.g., ranitidine, famotidine) and that can protect and promote healing of the ulcers (e.g., sucralfate, misoprostol).

## Suggested Readings

Bojrab MJ: *Current techniques in small animal surgery,* ed 4, Philadelphia, 1998, William & Wilkins.

Feldman EC, Nelson RW: *Canine and feline endocrinology and reproduction,* ed 3, Philadelphia, 2004, WB Saunders.

Fossum TW: *Small animal surgery,* ed 2, St Louis, 2002, WB Saunders.

DIABETES MELLITUS

Appleton DJ et al: Dietary chromium tripicolinate supplementation reduces glucose concentrations and improves glucose tolerance in normal-weight cats, *J Feline Med Surg* 4:13, 2002.

Briggs C et al: Reliability of history and physical examination findings for assessing control of glycemia in dogs with diabetes mellitus: 53 cases (1995-1998), *J Am Vet Med Assoc* 217:48, 2000.

Cohn LA et al: Effects of chromium supplementation on glucose tolerance in obese and nonobese cats, *Am J Vet Res* 60:1360, 1999.

Cohn LA et al: Assessment of five portable blood glucose meters, a point-of-care analyzer, and color test strips for measuring blood glucose concentration in dogs, *J Am Vet Med Assoc* 216:198, 2000.

Elliott DA et al: Comparison of serum fructosamine and blood glycosylated hemoglobin concentrations for assessment of glycemic control in cats with diabetes mellitus, *J Am Vet Med Assoc* 214:1794, 1999.

Feldman EC et al: Intensive 50-week evaluation of glipizide administration in 50 cats with previously untreated diabetes mellitus, *J Am Vet Med Assoc* 210:772, 1997.

Goossens M et al: Response to insulin treatment and survival in diabetic cats: 104 cases (1985-1995), *J Vet Intern Med* 12:1, 1998.

Guptill L et al: Is canine diabetes on the increase? In *Recent advances in clinical management of diabetes mellitus,* Dayton, Ohio, 1999, Iams Co, p 24.

Hess RS et al: Effect of insulin dosage on glycemic response in dogs with diabetes mellitus: 221 cases (1993-1998), *J Am Vet Med Assoc* 216:217, 2000.

Nelson RW: Oral medications for treating diabetes mellitus in dogs and cats, *J Sm Anim Pract* 41:486, 2000.

Nelson RW et al: Effect of dietary insoluble fiber on control of glycemia in dogs with naturally acquired diabetes mellitus, *J Am Vet Med Assoc* 212:380, 1998.

Nelson RW et al: Transient clinical diabetes mellitus in cats: 10 cases (1989-1991), *J Vet Intern Med* 13:28, 1998.

Nelson RW et al: Effect of dietary insoluble fiber on control of glycemia in cats with naturally acquired diabetes mellitus, *J Am Vet Med Assoc* 216:1082, 2000.

Nelson RW et al: Effect of the α-glucosidase inhibitor acarbose on control of glycemia in dogs with naturally acquired diabetes mellitus, *J Am Vet Med Assoc* 216:1265, 2000.

Nelson RW et al: Efficacy of protamine zinc insulin for treatment of diabetes mellitus in cats, *J Am Vet Med Assoc* 218:38, 2001.

Panciera DL et al: Epizootiologic patterns of diabetes mellitus in cats: 333 cases (1980-1986), *J Am Vet Med Assoc* 197:1504, 1990.

Schachter S et al: Oral chromium picolinate and control of glycemia in insulin-treated diabetic dogs, *J Vet Intern Med* 15:379, 2001.

Wess G et al: Assessment of five portable blood glucose meters for use in cats, *Am J Vet Res* 61:1587, 2000.

Wess G et al: Capillary blood sampling from the ear of dogs and cats and use of portable meters to measure glucose concentration, *J Sm Anim Pract* 41:60, 2000.

DIABETIC KETOACIDOSIS

Bruskiewicz KA et al: Diabetic ketosis and ketoacidosis in cats: 42 cases (1980-1995), *J Am Vet Med Assoc* 211:188, 1997.

Crenshaw KL et al: Pretreatment clinical and laboratory evaluation of cats with diabetes mellitus: 104 cases (1992-1994), *J Am Vet Med Assoc* 209:943, 1996.

Macintire DK: Treatment of diabetic ketoacidosis in dogs by continuous low-dose intravenous infusion of insulin, *J Am Vet Med Assoc* 202:1266, 1993.

Norris CR et al: Serum total and ionized magnesium concentrations and urinary fractional excretion of magnesium in cats with diabetes mellitus and diabetic ketoacidosis, *J Am Vet Med Assoc* 215:1455, 1999.

INSULIN-SECRETING ISLET CELL NEOPLASIA

Fischer JR et al: Glucagon constant-rate infusion: a novel strategy for the management of hyperinsulinemic-hypoglycemic crisis in the dog, *J Am Anim Hosp Assoc* 36:27, 2000.

Moore AS et al: A diuresis protocol for administration of streptozotocin to dogs with pancreatic islet cell tumors, *J Am Vet Med Assoc* 221:811, 2002.

Tobin RL et al: Outcome of surgical versus medical treatment of dogs with beta-cell neoplasia: 39 cases (1990-1997), *J Am Vet Med Assoc* 215:226, 1999.

GASTRINOMA

Green RA et al: Gastrinoma: a retrospective study of four cases (1985-1995), *J Am Anim Hosp Assoc* 33:524, 1997.

Simpson KW: Gastrinoma in dogs. In Bonagura JD, editor: *Kirk's current veterinary therapy XIII*, Philadelphia, 2002, WB Saunders, p 617.

Zerbe CA et al: Gastrointestinal endocrine disease. In Ettinger SJ et al, editors: *Textbook of veterinary internal medicine*, ed 5, Philadelphia, 2000, WB Saunders, p 1500.

# CHAPTER 53

# Disorders of the Adrenal Gland

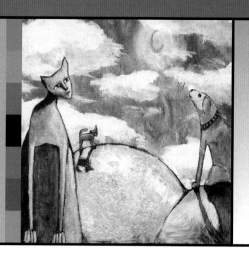

## CHAPTER OUTLINE

HYPERADRENOCORTICISM IN DOGS, 778
HYPERADRENOCORTICISM IN CATS, 798
HYPOADRENOCORTICISM, 804
PHEOCHROMOCYTOMA, 809
INCIDENTAL ADRENAL MASS, 812

## HYPERADRENOCORTICISM IN DOGS

### Etiology

Hyperadrenocorticism (Cushing's disease) is classified as pituitary dependent, adrenocortical dependent, or iatrogenic (i.e., resulting from excessive administration of glucocorticoids by the veterinarian or owner).

**Pituitary-dependent hyperadrenocorticism.** Pituitary-dependent hyperadrenocorticism (PDH) is the most common cause of spontaneous hyperadrenocorticism, accounting for approximately 80% to 85% of cases. A functional adrenocorticotropic hormone (ACTH)–secreting pituitary tumor is found at necropsy in approximately 85% of dogs with PDH. Adenoma of the pars distalis is the most common histologic finding, with a smaller percentage (approximately 20%) of dogs diagnosed with adenoma of the pars intermedia and a few dogs diagnosed with functional pituitary carcinoma. Approximately 50% of dogs with PDH have pituitary tumors less than 3 mm in diameter, and most of the remaining dogs, specifically those without central nervous system (CNS) signs, have tumors 3 to 10 mm in diameter at the time PDH is diagnosed. A small percentage of dogs (approximately 10% to 20%) have large pituitary tumors (i.e., macrotumors exceeding 10 mm in diameter) at the time PDH is diagnosed. These tumors have the potential to compress or invade adjacent structures and cause neurologic signs as they expand dorsally into the hypothalamus and thalamus (Fig. 53-1).

Diffuse hyperplasia of corticotroph cells has been noted in a small percentage (<15%) of dogs with PDH. It is believed to result from excessive stimulation of the anterior pituitary by corticotropin-releasing hormone (CRH), presumably as a result of a hypothalamic disorder or other CNS derangement. The etiology of hyperplasia of pituitary corticotrophs is unknown.

The primary derangement in dogs with PDH is an excessive secretion of ACTH, which causes bilateral adrenocortical hyperplasia and excess cortisol secretion to occur (Fig. 53-2). Normal feedback inhibition of ACTH secretion by physiologic levels of glucocorticoids is missing. Thus the excessive ACTH secretion persists despite increased adrenocortical secretion of cortisol. The episodic secretion of ACTH and cortisol results in fluctuating plasma concentrations that may at times be within the normal or reference range for most laboratories.

**Adrenocortical tumors.** Adrenocortical tumors (ATs) account for the remaining 15% to 20% of cases of spontaneous hyperadrenocorticism in dogs. Adrenocortical adenoma and carcinoma occur with equal frequency. There are no consistent clinical or biochemical features that help to distinguish dogs with functional adrenal adenomas from those with adrenal carcinomas. The only somewhat consistent characteristic is that carcinomas tend to appear larger than adenomas on abdominal ultrasound studies. Adrenocortical carcinomas may invade local structures (e.g., kidney, liver, vena cava) or metastasize hematogenously to the liver and lung.

Bilateral ATs can occur in dogs but are rare. A nonfunctional AT or an AT causing hyperadrenocorticism and a pheochromocytoma in the contralateral gland is a more common cause of bilateral adrenal masses in dogs. Macronodular hyperplasia of the adrenals has also been identified in dogs. The adrenals in such animals are usually grossly enlarged, with multiple nodules of varying sizes within the adrenal cortex. The exact pathogenesis of this latter syndrome is unclear, although most cases in dogs are presumed to represent an anatomic variant of PDH. Increased plasma 17-OH-progesterone concentrations have also been documented in dogs with an adrenal mass and clinical manifestations of hyperadrenocorticism, but normal plasma cortisol concentrations following administration of ACTH or dexamethasone (see p. 812).

ATs are autonomous and functional and randomly secrete excessive amounts of cortisol independently of pituitary control. The cortisol produced by these tumors suppresses hypothalamic CRH and circulating plasma ACTH concentrations,

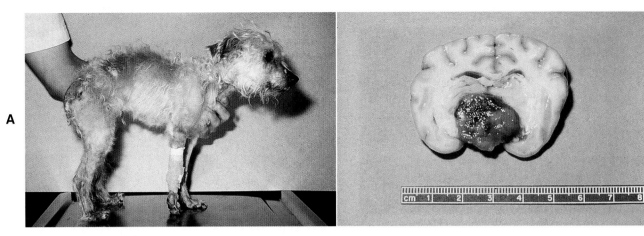

**FIG 53-1**
**A,** A 10-year-old male castrated mixed-breed dog with pituitary-dependent hyperadrenocorticism. Initial clinical signs of polyuria, polydipsia, and endocrine alopecia progressed to severe stupor, anorexia, adipsia, weight loss, and loss of body temperature regulation. **B,** Cross-section of the brain from the dog in **A** showing a pituitary macroadenoma that is severely compressing the surrounding brain structures.

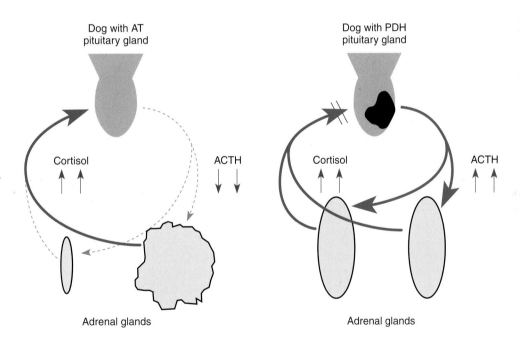

**FIG 53-2**
The pituitary-adrenocortical axis in dogs with a functioning adrenocortical tumor (AT; *left*) and in dogs with pituitary-dependent hyperadrenocorticism (PDH; *right*). Excess cortisol secretion from an AT causes pituitary suppression, decreased plasma ACTH concentration, and atrophy of the contralateral adrenal gland. Dogs with PDH have excess ACTH secretion, usually from a functional pituitary adenoma, which causes bilateral adrenomegaly and excess plasma cortisol concentrations.

causing cortical atrophy of the uninvolved adrenal and atrophy of all normal cells in the involved adrenal (see Fig. 53-2). This atrophy creates asymmetry in the size of the adrenal gland, which can be identified by abdominal ultrasonography. Most, if not all, of these tumors appear to retain ACTH receptors in that they respond to the administration of exogenous hormone. ATs are typically unresponsive to manip-

ulation of the hypothalamic-pituitary axis with pharmacologic agents such as dexamethasone.

**Iatrogenic hyperadrenocorticism.** Iatrogenic hyperadrenocorticism typically results from the excessive administration of glucocorticoids to control allergic or immune-mediated disorders. It can also develop as a result of the administration of eye, ear, or skin medications containing glucocorticoids, especially in small dogs (weight <10 kg) receiving them long term. Because the hypothalamic-pituitary-adrenocortical axis is normal, the prolonged excessive administration of glucocorticoids suppresses hypothalamic CRH and circulating plasma ACTH concentrations, causing bilateral adrenocortical atrophy. In these animals, ACTH stimulation test results are consistent with spontaneous hypoadrenocorticism despite clinical signs of hyperadrenocorticism.

## Clinical Features

**Signalment.** Hyperadrenocorticism typically develops in dogs 6 years of age and older (median age, 10 years) but has been documented in dogs as young as 1 year. There is no apparent sex-related predisposition, although AT appears to be diagnosed more commonly in female dogs than in male dogs. PDH and ATs have been diagnosed in numerous breeds. All Poodle breeds, Dachshunds, various Terrier breeds, German Shepherd Dogs, Beagles, and Labrador Retrievers are commonly represented among the breeds of dogs afflicted with hyperadrenocorticism. Boxers and Boston Terriers have also been mentioned to be at increased risk for PDH. PDH tends to occur more frequently in smaller dogs; 75% of dogs with PDH weigh less than 20 kg. Approximately 45% to 50% of dogs with functional ATs weigh more than 20 kg.

**Clinical signs.** The most common clinical signs in dogs with hyperadrenocorticism are polyuria-polydipsia, polyphagia, panting, abdominal enlargement, endocrine alopecia, mild muscle weakness, and lethargy (Fig. 53-3; Table 53-1). Not all dogs with hyperadrenocorticism exhibit the same signs; most dogs exhibit several, but not all, of these problems. The more signs evident in the history, the greater the index of suspicion for hyperadrenocorticism. Additional physical examination findings (see Table 53-1) help establish the diagnosis. In those dogs with multiple signs and physical examination findings consistent with the disorder, the diagnosis of hyperadrenocorticism is established in the examination room, and tests of the pituitary-adrenocortical axis are performed to confirm the diagnosis before initiating therapy.

Dogs are occasionally seen because of isolated polyuria-polydipsia, bilaterally symmetric endocrine alopecia, or, less commonly, panting. In dogs showing these signs there may be no other historic or physical examination findings consistent with hyperadrenocorticism. Although the diagnosis of hyperadrenocorticism is not readily apparent in these animals, it will eventually be identified, because it is a differential diagnosis for polyuria-polydipsia (see p. 660), endocrine alopecia (see p. 667), and panting. Similarly, hyperadrenocorticism causes insulin resistance and can lead to the development of diabetes mellitus. Clinical signs (other than polyuria and polydipsia) and physical examination findings suggestive of hyperadrenocorticism are often missing in diabetic dogs with concurrent hyperadrenocorticism. A clinical suspicion for hyperadrenocorticism develops after critical evaluation of routine blood test results (e.g., increased serum alkaline phosphatase [SAP] activity, isosthenuric urine) or after resistance to insulin treatment is identified.

 TABLE 53-1

**Clinical Signs and Physical Examination Findings in Dogs with Hyperadrenocorticism**

| CLINICAL SIGNS | PHYSICAL EXAMINATION FINDINGS |
|---|---|
| Polyuria, polydipsia | Endocrine alopecia |
| Polyphagia | Epidermal atrophy |
| Panting | Comedones |
| Abdominal enlargement | Calcinosis cutis |
| Endocrine alopecia | Hyperpigmentation |
| Weakness | Abdominal enlargement |
| Lethargy | Hepatomegaly |
| Calcinosis cutis | Muscle wasting |
| Hyperpigmentation | Bruising |
| Neurologic signs (PMA) | Testicular atrophy |
|   Stupor | Neurologic signs (PMA) |
|   Ataxia | Dyspnea (pulmonary |
|   Circling |   thromboemboli) |
|   Aimless wandering | |
|   Pacing | |
|   Behavioral alterations | |
| Respiratory distress-dyspnea (pulmonary thromboemboli) | |

*PMA,* Pituitary macroadenoma.

***Pituitary macrotumor syndrome.*** Neurologic signs may develop in dogs with PDH as a result of the pituitary tumor growing or expanding into the hypothalamus and thalamus (see Fig. 53-1). Neurologic signs typically develop 6 months or more after PDH has been diagnosed and appropriate medical therapy initiated. However, in approximately 10% to 20% of dogs with PDH, neurologic signs are present at the time the diagnosis of PDH is established or shortly afterward and may constitute the primary clinical manifestation of the disease. The most common neurologic sign is a dull, listless attitude (i.e., stupor). Additional signs of pituitary macroadenoma include inappetence, aimless wandering, pacing, ataxia, head pressing, circling, and behavioral alterations. In the event of severe compression of the hypothalamus, abnormalities related to dysfunction of the autonomic nervous system develop, including adipsia, loss of temperature regulation, erratic heart rate, and inability to be roused from a "sleeplike" state. For a definitive diagnosis to be rendered, a pituitary macrotumor must be identified using computed tomography (CT) or magnetic resonance imaging (MRI) (Fig. 53-4). There are no biochemical or endocrine test results that reliably correlate with the size of the pituitary tumor.

**Medical complications—pulmonary thromboembolism.** Several medical complications can develop secondary to prolonged steroid excess (Table 53-2). Perhaps the most worrisome is pulmonary thromboembolism (PTE), which is most commonly seen in dogs that have recently un-

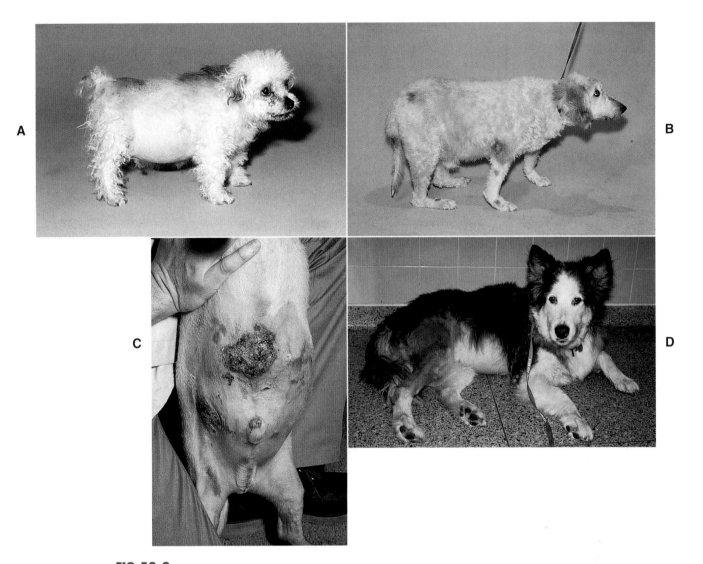

**FIG 53-3**
**A,** A 1-year-old male Miniature Poodle with pituitary-dependent hyperadrenocorticism (PDH). Note the truncal distribution of the endocrine alopecia with the pot-bellied appearance. **B,** A 9-year-old male castrated mixed-breed dog with PDH. Note the severe laxity of the ligaments, resulting in hyperextension of the carpal ligaments and ambulation on the hocks. A "rat tail" has also developed and is a finding also associated with hypothyroidism. **C,** An 8-year-old male castrated Chihuahua with PDH. Note the pot-bellied appearance and severe calcinosis cutis. **D,** A 7-year-old male castrated Malamute with PDH. Note the absence of hair growth on the right rear leg 1.5 years after the leg was shaved. The primary owner complaints at presentation were absence of hair growth, weakness, and recent onset of excessive panting.

dergone medical treatment for PDH or adrenalectomy for AT. There is no apparent correlation between the control of hyperadrenocorticism and the development of thromboemboli. Factors predisposing to the development of PTE in dogs with hyperadrenocorticism include inhibition of fibrinolysis (corticosteroids stimulate the release of plasminogen activator inhibitors), systemic hypertension, protein-losing glomerulonephropathy, decreased serum antithrombin III concentrations, increased concentrations of several coagulation factors, and an increased hematocrit value—factors that are common

complications of hyperadrenocorticism in dogs. Common clinical signs of PTE include acute respiratory distress, orthopnea, and, less commonly, a jugular pulse. Thoracic radiographs may reveal no abnormalities, or they may show hypoperfusion, alveolar pulmonary infiltrates, or a pleural effusion. There may be an increased diameter and blunting of the pulmonary arteries, absence of perfusion of the obstructed pulmonary vasculature, and overperfusion of the unobstructed pulmonary vasculature. Normal thoracic radiograph findings in a dyspneic dog that does not have a large

**FIG 53-4**
**A,** Post–gadolinium administration MRI scan of a 9-year-old male castrated German Shepherd Dog with pituitary-dependent hyperadrenocorticism (PDH) and a pituitary mass *(arrow).* There were no neurologic signs present at the time the MRI scan was performed.
**B,** Post–gadolinium administration MRI scan of an 8-year-old Boston Terrier with PDH, a large pituitary mass invading the brainstem, and signs of disorientation, ataxia, and circling. (From Feldman EC, Nelson RW: *Canine and feline endocrinology and reproduction,* ed 2, Philadelphia, 1996, WB Saunders.)

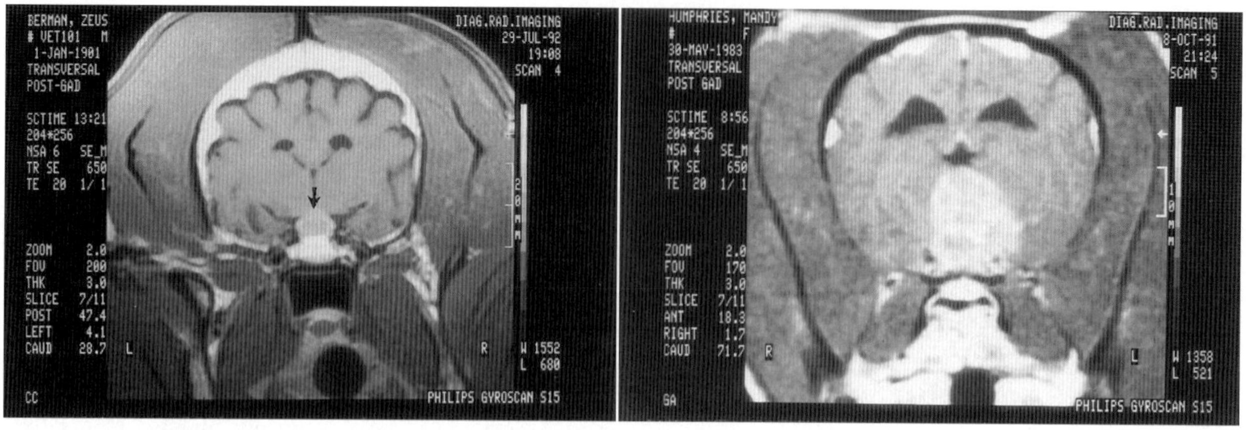

 TABLE 53-2

**Medical Complications Associated with Hyperadrenocorticism in Dogs**

Systemic hypertension
Pyelonephritis
Cystic calculi (calcium phosphate, oxalate)
Glomerulonephropathy, proteinuria
Congestive heart failure
Pancreatitis
Diabetes mellitus
Pulmonary thromboembolism
Pituitary macrotumor syndrome

TABLE 53-3

**Clinicopathologic Abnormalities Commonly Identified in Dogs with Hyperadrenocorticism**

Neutrophilic leukocytosis
Eosinopenia
Lymphopenia
Mild erythrocytosis
Increased alkaline phosphatase activity
Increased alanine aminotransferase activity
Hypercholesterolemia
Lipemia
Hyperglycemia
Hyposthenuria, isosthenuria
Urinary tract infection
Proteinuria

airway obstruction suggests a diagnosis of PTE. Arterial blood gas analysis typically reveals a decrease in the partial pressures of arterial oxygen and carbon dioxide, and mild metabolic acidosis. Thrombosis may be confirmed by angiography of the lungs or by radionuclear lung scanning. Therapy consists of general supportive care, oxygen, anticoagulants, and time (see p. 310). The prognosis for animals with PTE is guarded to grave. If animals do recover, it typically takes 5 to 10 days before they can be safely removed from oxygen support.

## Diagnosis

A thorough evaluation should be done in any dog suspected of having hyperadrenocorticism and should include a complete blood count (CBC), serum biochemistry panel, urinalysis with bacterial culture, and, if available, abdominal ultrasonography. Results of these tests will help increase or decrease the index of suspicion for hyperadrenocorticism, identify common concurrent problems (e.g., urinary tract in-

fection), and, in the case of ultrasonography, provide valuable information for localizing the cause of the disorder (i.e., PDH versus AT). Endocrine studies required to confirm the diagnosis and, if necessary, localize the cause of the disorder can then be performed.

**Clinical pathology.** Common clinicopathologic alterations caused by hyperadrenocorticism are listed in Table 53-3. An increase in SAP activity and cholesterol concentration are the most reliable indicators of hyperadrenocorticism; SAP and cholesterol are increased in approximately 95% and 75% of dogs with hyperadrenocorticism, respectively. Approximately 85% of dogs with hyperadrenocorticism have SAP activities that exceed 150 IU/L; values in excess of 1000 IU/L are common, and values in excess of 10,000 IU/L are occasionally identified. However, there is no correlation between the magnitude of increase in serum SAP activity and the severity of hyperadrenocorticism, response to therapy, or prognosis. There is also no correlation between the magnitude of increase in serum SAP activity and hepatocellular death or hepatic failure. The SAP activity can be normal in some dogs with hyperadrenocorticism, and an increase in the SAP activity by itself is not diagnostic for hyperadrenocorticism. Similarly, an increase in the activity of the steroid-induced isoenzyme of alkaline phosphatase (SIAP) is not a finding specific to hyperadrenocorticism or exogenous glucocorticoid administration; an increase in SIAP activity occurs commonly in the setting of numerous other disorders, including diabetes mellitus, primary hepatopathies, pancreatitis, congestive heart failure, and neoplasia, as well as in dogs receiving certain drugs (e.g., anticonvulsants). However, the serum SIAP activity is a sensitive test for hyperadrenocorticism: a finding of no SIAP in the serum may be of diagnostic value in ruling out hyperadrenocorticism. The serum bilirubin concentration is normal in dogs with hyperadrenocorticism and steroid hepatopathy; the finding of hyperbilirubinemia on a serum biochemistry panel suggests the existence of intrahepatic or posthepatic cholestasis or hemolysis (see p. 476). Preprandial and postprandial bile acid concentrations may be mildly increased in dogs with hyperadrenocorticism.

The urine specific gravity is typically less than 1.015 in dogs with hyperadrenocorticism that have free access to water; 85% of affected dogs seen at our hospital have urine specific gravities in this range. A finding of isosthenuria or hyposthenuria helps confirm polydipsia and polyuria and is further evidence in support of the diagnosis of hyperadrenocorticism. Water-deprived hyperadrenal dogs maintain the ability to concentrate urine, although usually the concentrating ability remains less than normal. As such, the urine specific gravity may exceed 1.025 if urine is obtained after water has been withheld from the dog (e.g., long car ride, hospitalization without water).

Possible additional urinalysis findings include glycosuria if there is concurrent undiagnosed diabetes mellitus, proteinuria, and alterations consistent with a urinary tract infection. Proteinuria is identified in approximately 45% of dogs with untreated hyperadrenocorticism. Proteinuria may be caused by glucocorticoid-induced systemic and glomerular hypertension, glomerulonephritis, or glomerulosclerosis. Urine protein/creatinine ratios are usually less than 4, although values in excess of 8 have been identified. Proteinuria decreases and often resolves in response to treatment of hyperadrenocorticism. Urinary tract infection is a common sequela of hyperadrenocorticism, occurring in approximately 50% of affected dogs. Hyposthenuria and the antiinflammatory effects of glucocorticoids commonly interfere with the identification of bacteria or inflammatory cells in the urine. Whenever hyperadrenocorticism is suspected, antepubic cystocentesis with bacterial culture and antibiotic sensitivity testing is strongly recommended, regardless of the urinalysis findings.

**Diagnostic imaging.** Abnormalities identified by thoracic and abdominal radiography and by abdominal ultrasonography are listed in Table 53-4. The most consistent radiographic findings in dogs with hyperadrenocorticism are enhanced ab-

 TABLE 53-4

**Abnormalities Identified by Abdominal and Thoracic Radiography in Dogs with Hyperadrenocorticism**

| ABDOMINAL RADIOGRAPHS | THORACIC RADIOGRAPHS |
|---|---|
| Excellent abdominal detail* | Calcification of trachea and bronchi* |
| Hepatomegaly* | Osteoporosis of vertebrae |
| Distention of urinary bladder* | Pulmonary metastasis from adrenocortical carcinoma |
| Cystic calculi | Pulmonary thromboembolism |
| Adrenal mass | Hypovascular lung fields |
| Calcified adrenal gland | Alveolar infiltrates |
| Dystrophic calcification of soft tissues, calcinosis cutis | Enlarged right pulmonary artery |
| Osteoporosis of vertebrae | Right-sided cardiomegaly |
|  | Pleural effusion |

*Common findings.

dominal contrast secondary to increased fat distribution in the abdomen; hepatomegaly caused by steroid hepatopathy; an enlarged urinary bladder secondary to the polyuric state; and dystrophic calcification of the trachea, bronchi, and occasionally the skin and abdominal blood vessels. The most important but least common abdominal radiograph finding is a soft-tissue mass or calcification in the area of an adrenal gland (Fig. 53-5). These findings are suggestive of an adrenal tumor. The larger the soft-tissue mass, the more likely it is that the tumor is a carcinoma. Approximately 50% of ATs are calcified, which allows them to be visualized radiographically; the frequency of calcification of an adrenal tumor is equally distributed between adenoma and carcinoma. Metastasis of an adrenocortical carcinoma to the pulmonary parenchyma is occasionally evident on thoracic radiographs.

Abdominal ultrasonography plays an integral role in the diagnostic evaluation of dogs suspected of having hyperadrenocorticism. It is used to search for any unexpected abnormalities in the abdomen (e.g., cystic calculi, masses) and to evaluate the size and shape of the adrenals (Fig. 53-6). The finding of bilaterally normal-sized or large adrenals (defined as having a maximum width >0.75 cm) visualized in a dog otherwise diagnosed as having hyperadrenocorticism is considered evidence for adrenal hyperplasia caused by PDH. The adrenal glands in dogs with PDH are similar but not exactly the same in size and shape; should have smooth, not irregular borders; can exceed 2 cm in maximum width; may have a bulbous cranial or caudal pole; and do not invade surrounding blood vessels or organs (see Fig. 53-6). An AT is typically identified as an adrenal mass (Fig. 53-7). Size is quite variable, ranging from 1.5 to greater than 8 cm in maximum width. Small adrenal masses (i.e., <3 cm in maximum width) often maintain a smooth contour and may distort only a portion of the adrenal gland; one or both poles of the adrenal gland may

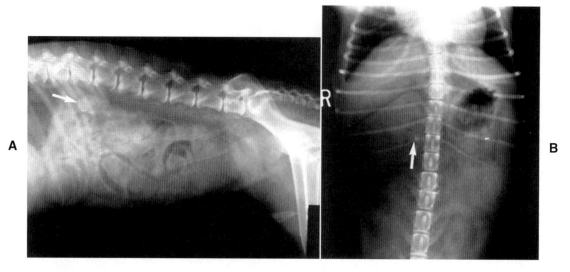

**FIG 53-5**
**A,** Lateral radiograph from a dog with adrenal-dependent hyperadrenocorticism showing a calcified adrenal mass cranial to the kidney *(arrow)*. **B,** Ventrodorsal radiograph from a dog with adrenal-dependent hyperadrenocorticism showing a calcified adrenal mass craniomedial to the kidney and lateral to the spine *(arrow)*. Compression of the abdomen in the region of the adrenal gland with a paddle has enhanced radiographic contrast, allowing better visualization of the adrenal mass.

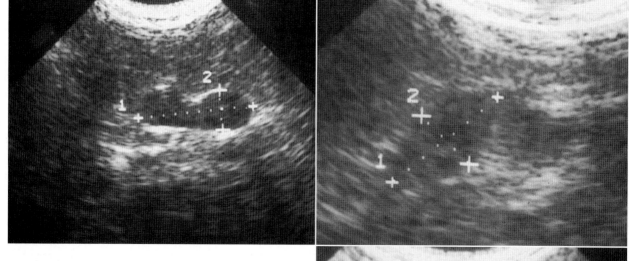

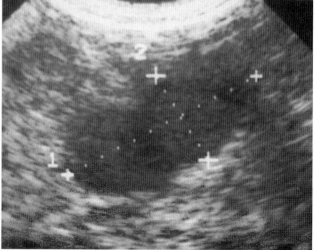

**FIG 53-6**
Ultrasound images of the adrenal gland in three dogs with pituitary-dependent hyperadrenocorticism (PDH) illustrating the differences in size and shape of the adrenal gland that can occur with PDH. **A,** The adrenal gland in this dog has maintained the typical kidney bean shape often identified in normal dogs. However, the maximum diameter of the gland was enlarged at 0.85 cm. The contralateral adrenal gland was similar in size and shape. **B,** The adrenal gland in this dog is uniformly thickened and appears plump rather than kidney bean shaped. The maximum diameter of the gland was 1.2 cm. The contralateral adrenal gland was similar in size and shape. **C,** Although the adrenal gland has maintained some semblance of a kidney bean shape in this dog, the gland has undergone marked enlargement, with a maximum diameter of 2.4 cm. The contralateral adrenal gland was similar in size and shape.

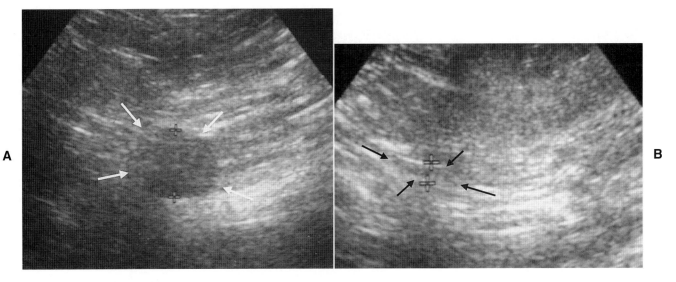

**FIG 53-7**
Ultrasound images of the adrenal glands in an 11-year-old male castrated Golden Retriever with adrenal-dependent hyperadrenocorticism. **A,** Cortisol-secreting tumor affecting the right adrenal gland *(arrows)*. The maximum diameter of the adrenal mass was 1.6 cm. **B,** The left adrenal gland has undergone marked atrophy *(arrows and crosses)* as a result of suppression of pituitary ACTH secretion following negative feedback inhibition caused by the adrenocortical tumor. The maximum diameter of the left adrenal gland was less than 0.2 cm.

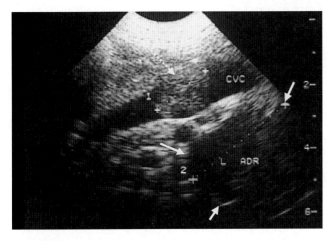

**FIG 53-8**
Ultrasound image of a mass affecting the left adrenal gland *(solid arrows)* and extending into the lumen of the caudal vena cava (CVC; *broken arrow*) in a 14-year-old male Standard Poodle. The maximum width of the adrenal mass was 1.8 cm. The histopathologic diagnosis was pheochromocytoma.

still appear normal. With large adrenal masses (typically >3 cm in maximum width), the adrenal gland usually becomes distorted and unrecognizable, the contour of the gland becomes irregular, and invasion into surrounding blood vessels and compression of adjacent organs may occur (Fig. 53-8). These changes suggest adrenocortical carcinoma. Identification of calcification within the mass does not differentiate adenoma from carcinoma. Generally, the larger the mass, the more likely it is to be carcinoma. The contralateral unaffected

adrenal should be small or undetectable (maximum width typically <0.3 cm) as a result of AT-induced adrenocortical atrophy (see Fig. 53-7); asymmetry in the size of the adrenals is evident on ultrasound studies (see Fig. 53-2). Identification of an adrenal mass and a normal to large contralateral adrenal gland in a dog with clinical signs supportive of hyperadrenocorticism suggests the presence of PDH and an incidental adrenal mass (Fig. 53-9; see Incidental Adrenal Mass, p. 812). The right adrenal gland is normally more difficult to identify, and this must be considered when interpreting ultrasonograms. If an adrenal mass is identified, ultrasonography can be used to search for metastasis in the liver or other organ systems, for tumor invasion of the vena cava or other structures, and for compression of adjacent tissues by the tumor. The finding of normal-sized adrenal glands in a dog with confirmed hyperadrenocorticism is most consistent with a diagnosis of PDH. Failure to identify either adrenal is considered an inconclusive finding, and in this event, ultrasonography should be repeated when the dog is calmer, intestinal gas has had a chance to pass, or a more experienced ultrasonographer is available.

Identification of bilateral adrenomegaly with the appearance of multiple nodules of varying size is suggestive of macronodular hyperplasia (Fig. 53-10). Bilateral adrenal macronodular hyperplasia is believed to represent an anatomic variant of PDH.

CT and MRI can be used to assess the size and symmetry of the adrenal glands and to evaluate the pituitary gland for a macroadenoma. Contrast enhancement using an iodinated contrast agent (CT) or gadolinium (MRI) given by continuous intravenous (IV) infusion during the imaging procedure aids in the identification of a pituitary macroadenoma and the

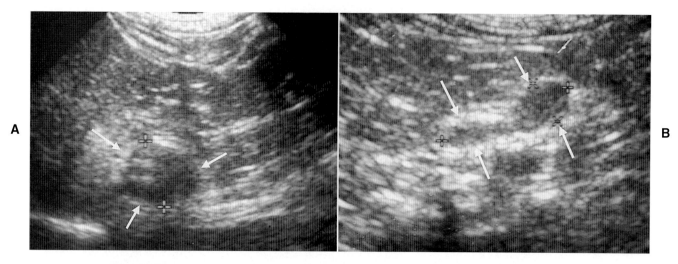

**FIG 53-9**
Ultrasound images of the adrenal glands in a 10-year-old female spayed Bichon Frise presented for acute onset of vomiting. **A,** An unexpected mass involving the right adrenal gland, measuring 1.4 cm in maximum diameter, was identified *(arrows)*. **B,** The left adrenal gland was normal in size and shape *(arrows)*; the maximum diameter was 0.6 cm. The normal-sized left adrenal gland suggests that the right adrenal mass is either a pheochromocytoma or is nonfunctional. Results of routine blood work and tests for hyperadrenocorticism were normal.

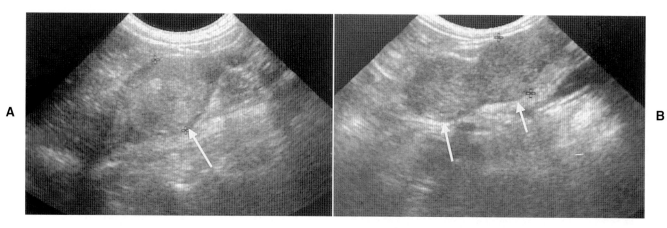

**FIG 53-10**
Ultrasound images of the adrenal glands *(arrows)* in an 11-year-old female spayed Shih Tzu. The right adrenal gland **(A)** measured 1.8 cm in maximum diameter and had a nodular echogenic pattern. In contrast, the left adrenal gland **(B)** had a large nodule located in each pole of the gland; each measured approximately 1.4 cm in maximum diameter. Tests of the pituitary-adrenocortical axis were diagnostic for pituitary-dependent hyperadrenocorticism; this finding, in conjunction with the findings on ultrasound, suggests macronodular hyperplasia of the adrenal glands.

adrenal glands during CT and MRI examination, respectively (see Fig. 53-4). The primary indication for CT or MRI is to confirm the presence of a visible pituitary tumor in a dog with clinical signs suggestive of macrotumor (see Pituitary Macrotumor Syndrome, p. 780) or in dogs diagnosed with PDH in which the owner is willing to consider radiation treatment should a pituitary mass be identified (see Radiation Therapy, p. 797). MRI is superior to CT in detecting small pituitary tumors; in detecting associated tumor features such as edema, cysts, hemorrhage, and necrosis; and in imaging the adrenal glands.

## Tests of the pituitary-adrenocortical axis

The clinical signs, physical examination findings, and clinicopathologic alterations usually establish a presumptive diagnosis of hyperadrenocorticism, and results of abdominal ultrasonography provide valuable information regarding the probable location of the lesion (i.e., pituitary gland versus adrenal cortex). Confirmation of the diagnosis and establishment of the cause require the performance of specific diagnostic tests of the pituitary-adrenocortical axis (Table 53-5). Tests to establish the diagnosis of hyperadrenocorticism

TABLE 53-5

## Diagnostic Tests to Assess the Pituitary-Adrenocorticol Axis in Dogs

| TEST | PURPOSE | PROTOCOL | RESULTS | INTERPRETATION |
|---|---|---|---|---|
| Endogenous ACTH | Differentiate PDH from AT | Plasma sample obtained between 8 and 10 AM; Special handling required | <10 pg/ml<br>10-45 pg/ml<br>>45 pg/ml | AT<br>Nondiagnostic<br>PDH |
| ACTH stimulation | Diagnose Cushing's syndrome | 2.2 IU of ACTH gel*/kg IM; plasma pre- and 2 hr post-ACTH *or* 0.25 mg of synthetic ACTH*/dog IM; plasma pre- and 1 hr post-ACTH | *Post-ACTH cortisol concentration:*<br>>24 μg/dl<br>19-24 μg/dl<br>8-18 μg/dl<br><8 μg/dl | Strongly suggestive†<br>Suggestive‡<br>Normal<br>Iatrogenic Cushing's syndrome |
| Low-dose dexamethasone suppression test | Diagnose Cushing's syndrome and differentiate PDH from AT | 0.01 mg dexamethasone/kg IV; plasma pre- and 4 and 8 hr post-dexamethasone | *4 hr post-dexamethasone:* / *8 hr post-dexamethasone:*<br>— / <1.4 μg/dl<br><1.4 μg/dl / >1.4 μg/dl<br><50% of pre-value / >1.4 μg/dl<br>— / >1.4 μg/dl and <50% of pre-value<br>>1.4 μg/dl / >1.4 mg/dl | Normal<br>PDH<br>PDH<br>PDH<br>PDH or AT |
| Combination dexamethasone suppression and ACTH stimulation test | Diagnose Cushing's syndrome | 0.1 mg of dexamethasone/kg IV; plasma pre- and 2 hr post-dexamethasone; then 2.2 IU of ACTH gel/kg or 0.25 mg of synthetic ACTH/dog IM; plasma 1 and 2 hr (ACTH gel) or 30 and 60 min (synthetic ACTH) post-ACTH | >1.4 μg/dl 4 hr post-dexamethasone and >50% of pre-value / *Post-ACTH*<br><1.5 μg/dl / 8-18 μg/dl<br>>1.5 μg/dl / 8-20 μg/dl<br>>1.5 μg/dl / >20 μg/dl<br>>1.5 μg/dl / >20 μg/dl<br><1.5 μg/dl / <8 μg/dl | Normal<br>Suggestive<br>Strongly suggestive<br>Suggestive<br>Iatrogenic Cushing's syndrome |
| High-dose dexamethasone suppression test | Differentiate PDH from AT | 0.1 mg of dexamethasone/kg IV; plasma pre- and 8 hr post-dexamethasone | *Post-dexamethasone cortisol concentration:*<br><50% of pre-value<br><1.4 μg/dl<br>≥50% of pre-value | PDH<br>PDH<br>PDH or AT |

*PDH*, Pituitary-dependent hyperadrenocorticism; *AT*, adrenocortical tumor.

*ACTH gel: Cortigel; Savage Laboratories; synthetic ACTH: Cortrosyn; Organon Pharmaceuticals.

†Strongly suggestive of hyperadrenocorticism.

‡Suggestive of hyperadrenocorticism.

include the ACTH stimulation test, the low-dose dexamethasone suppression (LDDS) test, and the combination dexamethasone suppression and ACTH stimulation test (V test). A baseline morning plasma cortisol measurement by itself is of no value in the diagnosis of hyperadrenocorticism. Similarly, a normal urine cortisol/creatinine ratio determined from a random free-catch urine specimen obtained in the home environment rules out hyperadrenocorticism, but an increased ratio cannot serve as the basis for a diagnosis of hyperadrenocorticism. Dogs with concurrent illness but without hyperadrenocorticism also commonly have increased urine cortisol/creatinine ratios (Fig. 53-11).

Once a diagnosis of hyperadrenocorticism is established, discriminatory testing may be warranted to identify the cause (i.e., PDH versus AT), to identify the most appropriate therapy, and to more accurately determine the prognosis. Discriminatory tests include the LDDS test, the high-dose dex-

amethasone suppression (HDDS) test, and the baseline plasma endogenous ACTH concentration. The need to perform discriminatory testing depends in part on the abdominal ultrasound findings and the owner's willingness to consider adrenalectomy should an AT be identified. Medical therapy for PDH should be initiated if the abdominal ultrasound results are inconclusive or the owner is not willing to consider surgery. The probability of a dog with hyperadrenocorticism having PDH is 80% to 85%, regardless of whether discriminatory tests are performed. This probability can be further enhanced by assessing abdominal ultrasound studies.

The tests most commonly used to diagnose hyperadrenocorticism and to differentiate PDH from AT at our hospital are the ACTH stimulation test, the LDDS test, and abdominal ultrasonography. The urine cortisol/creatinine ratio can be determined as part of the initial screen for hyperadrenocorticism; however, more commonly, it is used to further rule out

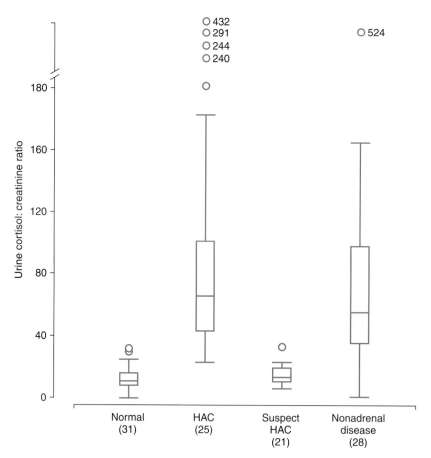

**FIG 53-11**

Box plots of the urine cortisol/creatinine ratios found in normal dogs, dogs with hyperadrenocorticism (HAC), dogs in which hyperadrenocorticism was initially suspected but that did not have the disease (suspect HAC), and dogs with a variety of severe, nonadrenal diseases. For each box plot, T-bars represent the main body of data, which in most instances are equal to the range. Each box represents an interquartile range (25th to 75th percentile). The horizontal bar in each box is the median. Open circles represent outlying data points. Numbers in parentheses indicate the numbers of dogs in each group. (From Smiley LE et al: Evaluation of a urine cortisol:creatinine ratio as a screening test for hyperadrenocorticism in dogs, *J Vet Intern Med* 7:163, 1993.)

hyperadrenocorticism if results of the previously named tests are normal or inconclusive and the dog has ambiguous clinical signs. An endogenous ACTH concentration is typically evaluated when findings on abdominal ultrasound are inconsistent with results of tests of the pituitary-adrenocortical axis (e.g., adrenal mass identified on ultrasound but test results suggestive of PDH) or results of abdominal ultrasound are confusing (e.g., bilateral adrenal masses or unilateral adrenal mass with normal-sized contralateral adrenal gland). The HDDS test is indicated only if abdominal ultrasound is not available and results of the LDDS test fail to confirm PDH.

None of the diagnostic tests for hyperadrenocorticism are foolproof. Results of all can be normal in a dog with hyperadrenocorticism and abnormal in a dog with nonadrenal disease. When the results are unexpected or questionable, another diagnostic test can be performed or the same diagnostic test repeated, preferably after waiting a month or two. Occasionally, results of different diagnostic tests performed in the same animal are contradictory. The decision to perform discriminatory tests or to initiate therapy should depend on the clinician's index of suspicion for the disorder. The history and physical examination findings, in conjunction with the results of routine blood tests and tests of the pituitary-adrenocortical axis, should all be considered when one is attempting to establish a diagnosis of hyperadrenocorticism. If there is doubt or uncertainty about the diagnosis, therapy for hyperadrenocorticism should be withheld and the dog reevaluated 1 to 3 months later.

**Urine cortisol/creatinine ratio.** The 24-hour urinary free cortisol excretion is increased in dogs with hyperadrenocorticism compared with that in healthy dogs; excretion is measured by routine cortisol radioimmunoassay technique on unextracted urine. The urine cortisol/creatinine ratio determined from a random urine sample is also significantly increased in dogs with spontaneous hyperadrenocorticism compared with that in healthy dogs. Unfortunately, the ratio is also increased in dogs with nonadrenal illness and in dogs with clinical signs consistent with hyperadrenocorticism but with a normal pituitary-adrenocortical axis (see Fig. 53-11). In one study in which sick dogs without hyperadrenocorticism were compared with dogs with hyperadrenocorticism, the specificity of the urine cortisol/creatinine ratio was only 20%. Thus a normal urine cortisol/creatinine ratio rules out hyperadrenocorticism and can be used as a screening test for normalcy; however, an increased urine cortisol/creatinine ratio is not diagnostic of spontaneous hyperadrenocorticism. Ideally, the urine cortisol/creatinine ratio should be determined from free-catch urine samples obtained by the owner in the nonstressful home environment. The stress associated with driving the dog to the veterinary hospital and having the dog undergo a physical examination before collecting urine can increase the test values.

**ACTH stimulation test.** The ACTH stimulation test is a relatively reliable, simple, and safe screening test in the diagnostic evaluation of dogs with hyperadrenocorticism, and if it is performed before the initiation of treatment, it can provide

information that can be used for posttreatment comparisons. The accuracy of the ACTH stimulation test for identifying hyperadrenocorticism is approximately 80%. Approximately 20% of dogs with hyperadrenocorticism have normal test results. If hyperadrenocorticism is suspected, the diagnosis should not be excluded because of normal ACTH stimulation test results. ACTH stimulation test results do not distinguish between PDH and AT, nor do they reliably distinguish between dogs with adrenal adenoma and those with adrenal carcinoma. The ACTH stimulation test is the only test that readily identifies iatrogenic hyperadrenocorticism.

The protocol for the ACTH stimulation test is given in Table 53-5. We use four ranges of values in the interpretation of the ACTH stimulation test (Fig. 53-12). At our laboratory, post–ACTH administration plasma cortisol values between 6 and 17 µg/dl are within the normal reference range; values of 5 µg/dl and below are suggestive of iatrogenic hyperadrenocorticism or spontaneous hypoadrenocorticism; values

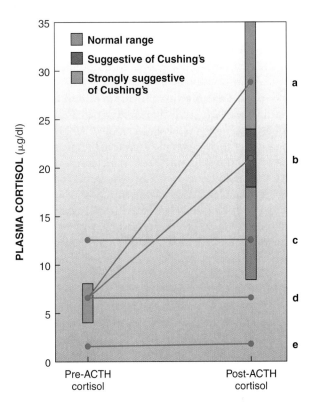

**FIG 53-12**
Interpretation of the ACTH stimulation test in dogs. Most dogs with Cushing's syndrome have an increased post–ACTH administration cortisol concentration *(line a)*. Post-ACTH cortisol values that fall into the "gray zone" *(line b)* could be consistent with Cushing's syndrome or result from the effects of concurrent illness or chronic stress. Less commonly, post-ACTH cortisol values fall into the normal range in dogs with Cushing's syndrome. The absence of a response to ACTH stimulation is suggestive of adrenocortical neoplasia *(lines c and d)* or iatrogenic hyperadrenocorticism *(lines d and e)*. History and physical examination findings should differentiate between these possibilities.

between 18 and 24 µg/dl are considered borderline for spontaneous hyperadrenocorticism; and values greater than 24 µg/dl are consistent with naturally occurring hyperadrenocorticism. An increased post–ACTH administration plasma cortisol value, especially one between 18 and 24 µg/dl, does not by itself confirm a diagnosis of hyperadrenocorticism, especially if the clinical features and clinicopathologic data are not consistent with the diagnosis. Some dogs that do not have hyperadrenocorticism have abnormal ACTH stimulation test results. Some of these dogs undoubtedly represent the extremes of normal; chronic stress (e.g., chronic severe illness), causing adrenocortical hyperplasia and adrenal hyperresponsiveness to ACTH, probably plays a role in the test results of other dogs.

If the post-ACTH plasma cortisol concentration does not increase above the preadministration value, this indicates a diagnosis of iatrogenic hyperadrenocorticism or spontaneous hypoadrenocorticism, especially if the cortisol values are below the normal baseline range (i.e., <5 µg/dl; see Fig. 53-12). A history of recent glucocorticoid administration and the clinical presentation of the dog can help differentiate iatrogenic hyperadrenocorticism from spontaneous hypoadrenocorticism. In rare instances a dog with AT will exhibit a minimal cortisol response to ACTH; however, its pre– and post–ACTH administration plasma cortisol values are within or above the reference range.

**Low-dose dexamethasone suppression test.** In the normal dog, relatively small doses of dexamethasone given intravenously can inhibit pituitary secretion of ACTH, causing a prolonged (i.e., up to 24 hours) decline in the circulating cortisol concentration (Fig. 53-13). Dexamethasone is used because it does not interfere with the radioimmunoassays used to measure the blood cortisol concentration. The abnormal pituitary in dogs with PDH is somewhat resistant to the negative feedback action of dexamethasone, and the metabolic clearance of dexamethasone may be abnormally accelerated as well. The administration of a small dose of dexamethasone to a dog with PDH soon causes the plasma cortisol concentration to be variably suppressed; however, it is no longer suppressed by 8 hours after dexamethasone administration. As such, the pituitary tumor is relatively resistant to the effects of dexamethasone compared with the response seen in normal dogs. Dogs with functioning ATs secrete cortisol autonomously, which suppresses endogenous ACTH secretion. Thus these tumors function independently of ACTH control. Dexamethasone does not affect the plasma cortisol concentration, regardless of the dose or time of blood sampling, in dogs with AT, because pituitary corticotrophs are already suppressed and blood ACTH concentration is undetectable.

The LDDS test is a reliable diagnostic test for differentiating normal dogs from those with hyperadrenocorticism. The accuracy of the LDDS is approximately 85%. This test has historically been used both as the initial diagnostic test to confirm spontaneous hyperadrenocorticism and as a "second opinion" test if the results of the ACTH stimulation test are unexpected. It does not identify iatrogenic hyperadrenocorticism, nor is it used to assess a dog's response to mitotane or ketoconazole therapy. A normal or inconclusive LDDS test

result does not by itself rule out hyperadrenocorticism. If hyperadrenocorticism is suspected, additional tests of the pituitary-adrenocortical axis should be performed. Similarly, an abnormal LDDS test result does not by itself confirm hyperadrenocorticism. Results of the LDDS test may be affected by concurrently administered anticonvulsant drugs, stress (e.g., bathing, concurrently performed diagnostic tests), exogenous glucocorticoids, and nonadrenal disease; the more severe the nonadrenal disease, the more likely it is that the LDDS test results will be falsely positive. When the LDDS test is being performed, it is important that all stresses be kept to a minimum; other procedures should not be performed until the test is completed; and the effect of the clinical problems should be considered when interpreting results.

The protocol for the LDDS test and the interpretation of the results are described in Table 53-5. One may use either dexamethasone sodium phosphate or dexamethasone in polyethylene glycol. The 8-hour post–dexamethasone administration plasma cortisol concentration is used to confirm hyperadrenocorticism. Normal dogs have plasma cortisol values of less than 1.0 µg/dl, whereas dogs with PDH and AT have plasma cortisol concentrations of 1.4 µg/dl or more 8 hours after dexamethasone administration. Cortisol concentrations of between 1.0 and 1.4 µg/dl are nondiagnostic and do not confirm or rule out the diagnosis. If results are in the nondiagnostic range, the clinician must rely on other information, including other tests of the pituitary-adrenocortical axis, to determine whether hyperadrenocorticism is the correct diagnosis.

If the 8-hour post–dexamethasone administration cortisol value supports a diagnosis of hyperadrenocorticism, the 4-hour post–dexamethasone administration plasma cortisol value may be of value in distinguishing between PDH and AT. Low doses of dexamethasone suppress pituitary ACTH secretion and plasma cortisol concentrations in approximately 60% of dogs with PDH during the initial 2 to 6 hours of the test. Suppression does not occur in dogs with AT, nor does it occur in approximately 40% of dogs with PDH. Suppression is defined as (1) a 4-hour post-dexamethasone plasma cortisol concentration of less than 1.4 µg/dl, (2) a 4-hour post-dexamethasone plasma cortisol concentration that is less than 50% of the baseline concentration, and (3) an 8-hour post-dexamethasone plasma cortisol concentration that is less than 50% of the baseline concentration. Any dog with hyperadrenocorticism that shows one or more of these three plasma cortisol concentrations most likely has PDH. If none of these three plasma cortisol concentrations occurs, then results of the LDDS test are consistent with a lack of suppression. Lack of suppression is considered a nonspecific result in that it is consistent with a diagnosis of hyperadrenocorticism but not informative in terms of whether it is pituitary or adrenal in origin. Differentiation between PDH and AT must rely on results of abdominal ultrasound, the HDDS test, or plasma endogenous ACTH concentration.

**Combined dexamethasone suppression and ACTH stimulation test.** The V test is an initial screening test for hyperadrenocorticism. It does not reliably differentiate PDH from AT and should not be used for this purpose. The proto-

**NORMAL DOG OR CAT**

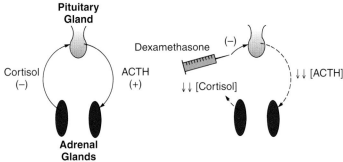

**PITUITARY-DEPENDENT HYPERADRENOCORTICISM**

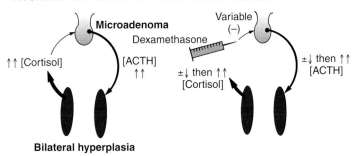

**ADRENOCORTICAL NEOPLASIA**

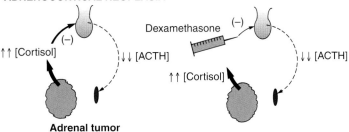

**FIG 53-13**

Effects of dexamethasone administration on the pituitary-adrenocortical axis in healthy dogs or cats and in dogs or cats with either pituitary-dependent hyperadrenocorticism (PDH) or adrenocortical neoplasia. In PDH, dexamethasone may initially suppress pituitary ACTH secretion, but the suppression is short-lived. The plasma cortisol concentrations initially decline but increase above normal within 2 to 6 hours of dexamethasone administration. In adrenocortical neoplasia, pituitary ACTH secretion is already suppressed; thus dexamethasone has no effect.

col for the V test is described in Table 53-5. Ideally, dogs with hyperadrenocorticism should not show suppression of the plasma cortisol concentration after the administration of dexamethasone and should show an exaggerated response to ACTH administration. Some dogs with hyperadrenocorticism, however, show suppression after dexamethasone administration or show a normal response to ACTH stimulation. Because of this, the post-dexamethasone and post-ACTH plasma cortisol concentrations should be interpreted independently of each other. When one "arm" of the V test indicates a diagnosis of hyperadrenocorticism but the other is normal, an additional screening test, preferably the LDDS test, should be performed to verify the diagnosis.

**High-dose dexamethasone suppression test.** Adrenocortical tumors function independently of pituitary ACTH; therefore regardless of the dose, dexamethasone should never suppress the plasma cortisol concentration if the source of the cortisol is an AT. In contrast, dexamethasone-induced suppression of ACTH secretion from a pituitary tumor is variable and may depend on the dexamethasone dose. The administration of larger and larger doses of dexamethasone should eventually suppress pituitary ACTH secretion in most dogs with PDH. The protocol for the HDDS test is similar to that for the LDDS test, except that a higher dose (i.e., 0.1 mg/kg body weight) of dexamethasone is used in an attempt to suppress pituitary ACTH secretion in dogs with PDH (see Table 53-5). Obtaining a 4-hour post-dexamethasone blood sample is optional; in our experience, this has been informative in only 2% of dogs tested with both the LDDS and HDDS tests. Suppression is defined as a 4-hour or 8-hour post-dexamethasone plasma cortisol concentration of less than 1.4 µg/dl and a 4-hour or 8-hour post-dexamethasone plasma cortisol concentration that is less than 50% of the baseline concentration. Any dog with hyperadrenocorticism that shows one or more of these four plasma cortisol concentrations most likely has PDH. Approximately 75% of dogs with PDH show at least one of the four. If an animal shows none of the four concentrations, this is consistent with a lack of suppression. Approximately 25% of dogs with PDH and essentially 100% of dogs with ATs do not show suppression. Higher doses of dexamethasone (e.g., 1.0 mg/kg) could be administered in an attempt to suppress pituitary ACTH secretion in dogs with dexamethasone-resistant PDH. However, the percentage of dogs with PDH that show suppression at higher doses of dexamethasone is similar to that observed for the 0.1 mg/kg protocol.

**Endogenous ACTH concentration.** Determination of a baseline plasma ACTH concentration is not used to diagnose hyperadrenocorticism, because many of the concentrations in dogs with hyperadrenocorticism are within the normal reference range (i.e., 10 to 110 pg/ml). However, determination of a single baseline plasma ACTH concentration may aid in distinguishing dogs with ATs from those with PDH once the diagnosis of hyperadrenocorticism is established. Adrenocortical tumors and iatrogenic hyperadrenocorticism should suppress ACTH secretion, and PDH is the result of excessive ACTH secretion (see Fig. 53-2). Approximately 60% of dogs with ATs causing hyperadrenocorticism have undetectable plasma ACTH concentrations, whereas 85% to 90% of dogs with PDH have plasma ACTH concentrations greater than 45 pg/ml and 35% have ACTH concentrations greater than 100 pg/ml. ACTH concentrations of 10 to 45 pg/ml are nondiagnostic. The final therapeutic plan is determined by abdominal ultrasound findings, the 4-hour post–low-dose dexamethasone cortisol concentration, and, if necessary, the post–high-dose dexamethasone plasma cortisol concentration. Several commercial veterinary endocrine laboratories now perform endogenous ACTH assays for dogs. The laboratory should be contacted for information on sample collection and handling; results should be interpreted on the basis of the reference range established for the laboratory being used.

## Medical Treatment of Pituitary-Dependent Hyperadrenocorticism

### Mitotane

Chemotherapy using mitotane (o,p'-DDD; Lysodren; Bristol Myers Oncology) is the most commonly used treatment for PDH. Mitotane also offers a viable alternative to adrenalectomy for treatment of AT, especially in aged dogs or dogs with worrisome concurrent disease. Although ATs are considered more resistant to the adrenocorticolytic effects of mitotane than normal or hyperplastic adrenal cortices, results

of mitotane treatment in some dogs with AT have been excellent. There are two treatment protocols for mitotane: the traditional approach, in which the goal is to control the hyperadrenal state without causing clinical signs of hypoadrenocorticism, and medical adrenalectomy, in which the goal is to destroy the adrenal cortex and convert from hyperadrenocorticism to hypoadrenocorticism. We prefer the traditional approach initially and consider medical adrenalectomy only in those dogs that fail to respond to the traditional approach or who become nonresponsive to mitotane after months or years of maintenance therapy. For the traditional approach there are two phases of mitotane therapy: an initial induction phase designed to gain control of the disorder and a lifelong maintenance phase designed to prevent recurrence of the signs of the disease.

***Induction phase of therapy.*** Before beginning induction therapy, the owner should determine the dog's water consumption during several 24-hour periods in the home environment. Normal dogs drink less than 100 ml/kg/24 hr (average, 60 ml/kg/24 hr), whereas dogs with polydipsia resulting from hyperadrenocorticism usually drink more than 100 ml/kg/24 hr. Once the daily quantity of water consumption has been established, therapy may be initiated at home, with the owner administering mitotane at a dosage of 40 to 50 mg/kg/day, divided into two doses. The total daily dose of mitotane is reduced to 25 to 35 mg/kg in dogs without polydipsia or with concurrent diabetes mellitus. Gastrointestinal absorption of mitotane is enhanced in the presence of fat. Mitotane is more effective when each dose is ground up, mixed with a small amount of vegetable oil, and administered with food.

Hyperadrenocorticism can be successfully treated with or without the concurrent administration of glucocorticoids. Glucocorticoid administration during induction therapy is a matter of personal preference. Advocates of the administration of low doses (0.25 mg/kg q24h) of prednisone during induction therapy believe that it may minimize or prevent adverse reactions caused by mitotane-induced hypocortisolism, without interfering with the resolution of the clinical signs of hyperadrenocorticism. Opponents of the routine administration of glucocorticoids during induction therapy rely on resolution of the polyphagia, polyuria, and polydipsia to identify control of hyperadrenocorticism; these are clinical signs that may persist because of concurrent glucocorticoid administration. Lethargy, inappetence, and vomiting are signs of mitotane overdosing—markers of overdosing that may not become apparent until later in the course of treatment because of concurrent glucocorticoid administration. Regardless of whether or not glucocorticoids are used during induction therapy, they should always be dispensed before beginning induction therapy, so that the owner has glucocorticoids on hand should adverse reactions to mitotane develop. Regardless of whether or not glucocorticoids are used, a thorough client understanding of the disorder and the potential problems with mitotane therapy plus close client-clinician communication during induction therapy are still the most important means of preventing complications.

***Monitoring induction therapy.*** The induction phase of mitotane treatment is typically done with the dog in the home environment. Owner awareness of the dog's activity, mental awareness, appetite, water consumption, and overall well-being is imperative for success without development of severe hypoadrenocorticism during induction. Owners are instructed to stop mitotane treatment and contact their veterinarian if lethargy, inappetance, vomiting, weakness, decreased water intake, or any change in the dog that does not seem right is observed. The usual amount of food offered to the dog can be decreased by approximately 25% during the induction phase to ensure that the dog remains hungry. The veterinarian should be contacted if there is any reduction in the dog's desire to eat. The veterinarian or a technician should call the owner every day, beginning with the second day of therapy, to check on the health of the animal and the possible development of signs related to hypocortisolism (i.e., lethargy, inappetence, vomiting). The induction phase of therapy is usually complete once any reduction in appetite is noted or once the daily water consumption decreases into the normal range (i.e., 80 ml/kg or less). Control is confirmed by the results of the ACTH stimulation test. An ACTH stimulation test should be performed 5 to 7 days after the start of induction therapy. Dogs that have responded clinically to the medication (or if the owner is not certain about response) should have further therapy withheld until results of the ACTH stimulation test are known. Dogs that have not yet responded clinically should have an ACTH stimulation test performed but should also remain on daily mitotane therapy pending results of the ACTH stimulation test.

The goal of therapy is to achieve an ACTH stimulation test result that is suggestive of hypoadrenocorticism (i.e., a post-ACTH plasma cortisol concentration of 2 to 5 μg/dl). A dog that shows a normal or exaggerated response to ACTH before therapy and a normal response (i.e., post-ACTH plasma cortisol concentration 6 to 17 μg/dl) after the initial phase of therapy usually remains clinically hyperadrenal. In these dogs, daily mitotane therapy and weekly ACTH stimulation tests should be continued until a post-ACTH plasma cortisol concentration falls within the desired range or signs of hypocortisolism develop. Maintenance therapy (see Maintenance Therapy) is initiated if the post-ACTH plasma cortisol concentration is less than 5 μg/dl and the dog appears healthy. The maintenance dose of mitotane is decreased from 50 mg/kg to 25 mg/kg, given orally, if the post-ACTH plasma cortisol concentration is less than 2 μg/dl and the dog appears healthy. Mitotane treatment is discontinued and prednisone treatment initiated if the post-ACTH plasma cortisol concentration is less than 2 μg/dl and the dog is systemically ill (i.e., lethargy, inappetence, vomiting; see Adverse Reactions to Mitotane Treatment).

In most dogs, clinical signs resolve and a post-ACTH plasma cortisol concentration of less than 5 μg/dl is achieved within 5 to 10 days of the start of the daily administration of mitotane at a dosage of 40 to 50 mg/kg. A small number of dogs, however, respond in less than 5 days, whereas an equally small number of dogs show minimal improvement after 20 to 30 consecutive days of therapy. Factors that can affect an animal's sensitivity to mitotane include the dose, gastrointestinal tract absorption, the rate of metabolism, and the cause of the hyperadrenocorticism. The dose of mitotane inversely correlates with the time it takes to attain a beneficial response. The greater the daily dose, the less time it takes to attain a response. The absorption of mitotane is improved if it is given with food, especially a fatty meal, and if the tablet is crushed, mixed with a small amount of vegetable oil, and mixed with food. The administration of mitotane to a fasted dog could result in decreased mitotane absorption and prolong induction therapy.

The method of disposition of mitotane in dogs is unknown. In people the hepatic microsomal enzyme system contributes to mitotane's biotransformation. The concurrent administration of drugs (e.g., phenobarbital) that stimulate hepatic microsomal drug-metabolizing enzymes could accelerate the biotransformation of mitotane and decrease its serum concentration. This phenomenon has been suspected in some hyperadrenal dogs insensitive to the effects of mitotane. Mitotane may also enhance its own degradation through the induction of hepatic microsomal enzyme synthesis.

The cause of hyperadrenocorticism can also affect an animal's sensitivity to mitotane. Typically, dogs with AT are more resistant to the adrenocorticolytic effects of mitotane than dogs with PDH. If tests to differentiate PDH from AT were not performed, those dogs that are shown to be resistant to therapy, defined as little or no reduction in the post-ACTH plasma cortisol concentration after 20 or more days of therapy, should undergo further evaluation (i.e., abdominal ultrasound) to determine whether an AT is an explanation for the resistance. Rarely, dogs with PDH require more than 30 consecutive days of mitotane therapy before the desired response is seen.

***Management of concurrent diabetes mellitus.*** Hyperadrenocorticism and diabetes mellitus are common concurrent diseases in dogs. Presumably, hyperadrenocorticism develops initially and subclinical diabetes mellitus becomes clinically apparent as a result of the insulin resistance caused by the hyperadrenal state. For most of these dogs, glycemic control remains poor despite insulin therapy, and good glycemic control is generally not possible until the hyperadrenocorticism is controlled. Occasionally, diabetic dogs presumably in the early stages of hyperadrenocorticism (often identified while pursuing the cause for an increased SAP) will be responsive to insulin and have good control of glycemia. Since the diabetes is well controlled, the decision to treat or not treat the hyperadrenocorticism in these dogs should be based on other factors (e.g., presence of additional clinical signs or physical examination findings; veterinarian's index of suspicion for the disease). A wait-and-see approach should be taken if there is not strong evidence for hyperadrenocorticism in these dogs. Poor control of the diabetic state will eventually occur if hyperadrenocorticism is present.

The initial focus should be on treating the hyperadrenal state in a poorly controlled diabetic dog diagnosed with hyperadrenocorticism. Insulin therapy is indicated during induction therapy; however, aggressive efforts to maintain the blood glucose concentration below 250 mg/dl should not be attempted. Rather, a conservative dose (0.5 to 1.0 U/kg) of intermediate-acting insulin (i.e., Lente or NPH) is administered twice a day to prevent ketoacidosis and severe hyperglycemia (blood glucose level >500 mg/dl). Monitoring induction therapy in the hyperadrenal dog with concurrent diabetes mellitus is similar to that used for the hyperadrenal dog (see Monitoring Induction Therapy) with one exception. Monitoring water consumption is not reliable when concurrent diabetes mellitus is present, since both diseases cause polyuria and polydipsia, and since polyuria and polydipsia may persist if poor control of glycemia persists despite attaining control of hyperadrenocorticism. Regardless, as control of the hyperadrenocorticism is achieved, insulin antagonism caused by the hyperadrenocorticism resolves and tissue sensitivity to insulin improves. To help prevent hypoglycemic reactions, owners are asked to test urine for the presence of glucose, preferably two or three times each day. Any urine sample found to be negative for glucose should be followed by a 10% to 20% reduction in the insulin dose. Mitotane therapy should be discontinued and an ACTH stimulation test performed if the urine continues to test negative for glucose. Critical assessment of glycemic control and adjustments in insulin therapy, if indicated, should be initiated once hyperadrenocorticism is controlled and maintenance therapy initiated (see p. 737).

***Maintenance therapy.*** Mitotane must continue to be administered periodically to prevent the recurrence of clinical signs. The maintenance phase of mitotane therapy should be initiated once a hypoadrenal response to ACTH is obtained. The maintenance dose is based on the weekly amount of mitotane administered, regardless of whether the weekly dose is given once per week or divided into multiple doses and given on several days. Adverse reactions caused by sensitivity to the drug (see Adverse Reactions to Mitotane Treatment) are less likely to occur when the weekly dose is divided and given on several days of the week. The typical initial weekly maintenance dosage of mitotane is 50 mg/kg orally, divided into two or three doses and administered on 2 or 3 days of each week (e.g., Monday and Thursday or Monday, Wednesday, and Friday). This is an arbitrary starting dose, and subsequent adjustments are made on the basis of the results of ACTH stimulation tests; the first test is performed 3 to 4 weeks after the start of maintenance therapy. The goal of maintenance therapy is to maintain the post-ACTH plasma cortisol concentration between 2 and 5 µg/dl in an otherwise healthy dog. The dose and frequency of administration of mitotane are adjusted, as needed, to maintain a hypoadrenal response to ACTH administration. If the post-ACTH cortisol concentration is between 2 and 5 µg/dl, a change in treatment is not indicated and the ACTH stimulation test should be repeated in 6 to 8 weeks. If the post-ACTH plasma cortisol concentration is greater than 5 to 6 µg/dl, the amount per administration or the frequency of administration is increased; if the post-ACTH plasma cortisol concentration is less than 2 µg/dl, the mitotane dose or frequency of administration is

decreased; mitotane therapy is temporarily discontinued if clinical signs of hypoadrenocorticism are present (see Adverse Reaction to Mitotane Treatment). An ACTH stimulation test is performed 3 to 4 weeks after changing the dose or frequency of administration of mitotane. Once the post-ACTH plasma cortisol concentration is stable and in the range of 2 to 5 µg/dl, the ACTH stimulation test should be repeated every 3 to 6 months thereafter unless clinical signs of hyperadrenocorticism or hypoadrenocorticism develop. With time (i.e., months to years), the dose and frequency of administration of mitotane must usually be increased to maintain this goal. Periodic ACTH stimulation testing will identify an increase in the post-ACTH plasma cortisol concentration above 5 µg/dl, allowing the clinician to adjust the mitotane treatment protocol before clinical signs of hyperadrenocorticism develop and another round of induction therapy is needed.

It is common for the clinical signs of hyperadrenocorticism to recur during the maintenance phase of mitotane therapy. In most dogs the maintenance dose of mitotane is either initially inadequate or becomes inadequate as the compensatory sustained increase in plasma ACTH concentration offsets the adrenocorticolytic effects of mitotane. In some dogs this can ultimately necessitate daily mitotane administration, sometimes with poor control of the disorder. Poor gastrointestinal tract absorption, rapid metabolism of the drug, and markedly increased plasma ACTH concentrations may, in part, cause the insensitivity to mitotane. Increasing the fat content of the meal or mixing mitotane with corn or peanut oil before administration may improve the dog's responsiveness to the drug. The relationship between mitotane insensitivity and the origin of the PDH (i.e., the pars distalis versus the pars intermedia) or the development of a macroadenoma is not known. Alternative therapy (i.e., medical adrenalectomy using mitotane, ketoconazole, trilostane) should be considered for those dogs that become insensitive to mitotane.

***Adverse reactions to mitotane treatment.*** Adverse reactions result from sensitivity to the drug or from excessive administration and the subsequent development of glucocorticoid and, if severe, mineralocorticoid deficiency (Table 53-6). The most common reactions to mitotane are gastric irritation and vomiting occurring shortly after its administration. If the gastric upset is the result of drug sensitivity and not hypoadrenocorticism, dividing the dose further or increasing the interval between administrations, or both, can help minimize vomiting. In some dogs it may be necessary to discontinue the medication for a few days. It may be necessary to perform an ACTH stimulation test to differentiate drug sensitivity from the completion of therapy.

The excessive administration of mitotane results in clinical signs of hypocortisolism, including weakness, lethargy, anorexia, vomiting, and diarrhea. If these signs develop, glucocorticoid therapy is warranted. Clinical improvement is usually seen within hours of the administration of prednisone (0.25 to 0.5 mg/kg PO). If the dog responds, the initial dosage of glucocorticoids should be continued for 3 to 5 days and then gradually decreased and stopped over the ensuing 1 to 2 weeks. Mitotane therapy should be stopped until the dog

## TABLE 53-6

### Adverse Effects of Mitotane in Dogs

**Direct Effect***

Lethargy
Inappetence
Vomiting
Neurologic signs
  Ataxia
  Circling
  Stupor
  Apparent blindness

**Promote Growth of PMA(?)**

Stupor
Disorientation
Circling
Ataxia
Aimless wandering
Pacing
Behavioral alterations

**Secondary to Overdosage***

Hypocortisolism
  Lethargy
  Anorexia
  Vomiting
  Diarrhea
  Weakness
Hypoaldosteronism (hyperkalemia, hyponatremia)
  Lethargy
  Weakness
  Cardiac disturbances
  Hypovolemia
  Hypotension

*PMA,* Pituitary macroadenoma.
*ACTH stimulation test, serum electrolyte concentration, response to discontinuation of mitotane, and response to glucocorticoid therapy are used to differentiate these categories of adverse reactions.

is normal when it is not receiving glucocorticoids. An ACTH stimulation test performed once the dog is healthy and not receiving glucocorticoids can help determine when to start mitotane treatment. Ideally, mitotane treatment should be started when the post-ACTH plasma cortisol concentration approaches 2 μg/dl. The weekly dose of mitotane should be reduced when therapy is reinitiated, and an ACTH stimulation test repeated 3 to 4 weeks later for comparison with results obtained before reinitiating mitotane therapy.

The excessive administration of mitotane can ultimately cause hypoaldosteronism. Mineralocorticoid deficiency should therefore be considered in any dog with signs of hypocortisolism that does not respond to glucocorticoid therapy. The finding of hyponatremia and hyperkalemia supports a diagnosis of hypoaldosteronism, and mineralocorticoid therapy is indicated in such dogs (see p. 807). An ACTH stimulation test, with measurement of the plasma aldosterone concentra-

tion, is performed to confirm the diagnosis. Hypoaldosteronism can develop quite quickly (i.e., within days of the start of mitotane therapy) in some dogs. Hypoaldosteronism can resolve and hyperadrenocorticism recur spontaneously, but this is unpredictable. Some dogs remain mineralocorticoid deficient for the remainder of their lives.

Mitotane may induce the development of neurologic signs, including stupor, head pressing, pacing, circling, seizures, ataxia, and blindness. Neurologic signs are usually transient, typically last 24 to 48 hours after mitotane administration, and usually occur in dogs that have been receiving the drug for more than 6 months. The primary differential diagnoses in such animals are pituitary macrotumor syndrome (see p. 780), hypoadrenocorticism, and thromboemboli. Adjustments in the dose or frequency of mitotane administration or temporary discontinuation of the therapy may alleviate the neurologic signs. An alternative mode of therapy should be considered if neurologic signs persist (see following discussion).

**Medical adrenalectomy using mitotane.** An alternative to the traditional mitotane treatment protocol is to intentionally cause complete destruction of the adrenal cortices by administering an excessive amount of mitotane. In theory, therapy for the ensuing adrenocortical insufficiency would then be necessary for the life of the dog. The protocol consists of administering mitotane at a dosage of 75 to 100 mg/kg daily for 25 consecutive days, given in three or four doses per day, with food, to minimize neurologic complications and ensure good intestinal absorption of the drug. Lifelong prednisone (0.1 to 0.5 mg/kg q12h initially) and mineralocorticoid (see p. 808) therapy is begun at the start of mitotane administration. The prednisone dose is tapered after completion of the 25-day protocol. Unfortunately, relapse with signs of hyperadrenocorticism occurs within the first year alone in approximately 33% of dogs so treated, indicating the need for periodic ACTH stimulation testing similar to that done in animals treated with the traditional mode of therapy. In addition, this treatment can be considerably more expensive than long-term treatment with mitotane because of the expense of treating addisonian dogs. For these reasons, we reserve this treatment for dogs that show a poor response to the traditional form of treatment.

### Ketoconazole

Ketoconazole (Nizoral; Janssen Pharmaceutical), with its low prevalence of toxicity, ability to reversibly inhibit adrenal steroidogenesis, and negligible effects on mineralocorticoid production, is an alternative to mitotane for the medical management of canine hyperadrenocorticism. Ketoconazole affects steroid biosynthesis by interacting with the imidazole ring and the cytochrome P-450 component of various mammalian steroidogenic enzyme systems. This agent can be used for stabilization of hyperadrenal dogs before adrenalectomy and as primary therapy in very small dogs (weight <5 kg), in which dosing of mitotane is problematic. It has also been used for medical management of dogs with malignant adrenocortical tumors in which surgical intervention is not an option but palliative therapy is desired; as "test" therapy for 4 to 8 weeks to obtain evidence for or against a diagnosis of hyperadreno-corticism in dogs with vague test results; and in dogs that cannot be treated with mitotane because of sensitivity to the drug.

Dogs seem to tolerate ketoconazole better when the dose is gradually increased over time. In addition, because this drug is an enzyme blocker, twice-daily administration has been necessary for the long-term management of these animals. The initial dosage of ketoconazole is 5 mg/kg twice a day, given for 7 days. If no problems with appetite or icterus are noted, the dose is increased to 10 mg/kg twice a day, given for 14 days. An ACTH stimulation test should be performed after 10 to 14 days of therapy at the higher dose and while the dog is still receiving ketoconazole. The goals of therapy are the same as those of mitotane therapy: the lack of an adreno-cortical response to ACTH and clinical improvement without illness developing. If a hypoadrenal response to ACTH (i.e., post-ACTH plasma cortisol concentration of between 2 and 5 μg/dl) is not obtained with a dosage of 10 mg/kg twice a day, then the dose should be increased to 15 mg/kg twice a day. Approximately half of the dogs that respond to keto-conazole require 15 mg/kg twice a day to maintain control of the hyperadrenocorticism. Approximately 20% to 25% of dogs do not respond to the drug as a result of poor intestinal absorption. Adverse reactions are primarily a result of hypocortisolism. The dose should be reduced or therapy discontinued if anorexia, depression, vomiting, or diarrhea is observed. Glucocorticoid treatment may be required if an overdose is suspected. Rechecks, including an ACTH stimulation test, every 3 to 6 months are recommended.

### Trilostane

Trilostane (Modrenal; Wanskerne) is a competitive inhibitor of 3-β-hydroxysteroid dehydrogenase, which mediates the conversion of pregnenolone to progesterone in the adrenal gland; the net effect is inhibition of cortisol production. Preliminary studies suggest that trilostane is effective in controlling clinical signs of hyperadrenocorticism in dogs for prolonged periods of time (>1 year) and may be a viable option for treatment of PDH in dogs, especially in those dogs in which mitotane is ineffective or in dogs that cannot tolerate mitotane because of drug sensitivity. Trilostane is currently available as 60- and 120-mg capsules. The recommended dosage is 60, 120, and 240 mg of trilostane orally once a day for dogs weighing 5 to 20 kg, 20 to 40 kg, and 40 to 60 kg, respectively. An ACTH stimulation test should be performed 10 to 14 days after initiating treatment and 4 to 6 hours after trilostane administration. The goals of therapy are the same as those of mitotane therapy: the lack of an adrenocortical response to ACTH and clinical improvement without illness developing. If a hypoadrenal response to ACTH (i.e., post-ACTH plasma cortisol concentration of between 2 and 5 μg/dl) is not obtained, the dosage should be increased by 60 mg increments, as necessary, until the goals of therapy are attained. If a hypoadrenal response is obtained but the dog still has clinical signs, twice-a-day therapy should be considered. An ACTH stimulation test should be done every 3 to 4 months once control of the hyperadrenal state is attained. Adverse effects are uncommon and include lethargy, vomiting,

and electrolyte shifts compatible with hypoadrenocorticism. A serum biochemistry panel and electrolytes should be monitored at the same time as the ACTH stimulation test. Trilostane is currently not available in the United States and is very expensive.

### L-Deprenyl

L-Deprenyl (Eldepryl; Somerset Pharmaceuticals) is approved for use in humans with Parkinson's disease, and recently selegiline hydrochloride, or L-Deprenyl (Anipryl; Deprenyl Animal Health), has been approved for treating PDH in dogs. It acts as an irreversible inhibitor of the enzyme monoamine oxidase type B, thereby promoting normalization of the dopamine level in people with Parkinson's disease. It is hypothesized by those who believe in this drug's effectiveness that the pituitary ACTH concentration is controlled in part by a negative feedback mechanism mediated by dopamine and that PDH may be caused by a loss of this negative suppression of ACTH, leading to the excess synthesis and secretion of the hormone. L-Deprenyl inhibits dopamine metabolism and increases hypothalamic and pituitary concentrations of dopamine, which in turn inhibits CRH and ACTH secretion and controls hypercortisolism and the associated clinical signs. Studies that have critically evaluated the efficacy of L-Deprenyl suggest efficacy in 20% to 30% of dogs with PDH. Interestingly, PDH originates from the pars intermedia and pars distalis in approximately 20% and 80% of affected dogs, respectively. Corticotrophs in the pars intermedia are under neurotransmitter control (dopamine), whereas corticotrophs in the pars distalis are controlled by CRH from the hypothalamus. Concentrations of an endogenous amphetamine, phenylethylamine, increase in the brain in dogs treated with L-Deprenyl, which may improve the dog's level of activity and its interactions with family members independent of any improvement in the hyperadrenal state. The current dosage recommendation for L-Deprenyl is 1 mg/kg once daily initially, with an increase to 2 mg/kg once daily if there is no response after 2 months. An alternative treatment should be considered if the dog fails to respond after 3 months of therapy, or earlier if clinical signs worsen or the physical condition of the dog deteriorates.

### Adrenalectomy

Adrenalectomy is the treatment of choice for an AT unless metastatic lesions or invasion of surrounding organs or blood vessels is identified during the preoperative evaluation, the dog is considered a poor anesthetic risk because it has a concurrent disease (e.g., heart failure) or is debilitated as a result of its hyperadrenal state, or the probability of perioperative thromboembolism is considered high because of systemic hypertension, an increased urine protein/creatinine ratio, or a decreased serum antithrombin III concentration. The probability of successful adrenalectomy is lower and the likelihood of perioperative complications is greater the larger the adrenal mass; removal of an adrenal mass that has a diameter in excess of 6 cm can be difficult even when the surgery is performed by an experienced surgeon. The probability that the adrenal mass is a carcinoma and that metastasis has occurred also is greater the larger the adrenal mass, regardless of findings during the preoperative evaluation. Treatment with mitotane or ketoconazole offers a viable alternative to adrenalectomy, especially for aged dogs or dogs at increased risk for anesthetic, surgical, or postsurgical problems. (See Suggested Readings for detailed information on surgical techniques.)

Glucocorticoid therapy is not indicated before adrenalectomy, because it may worsen hypertension, cause overhydration, and increase the risk of thromboembolic episodes. Beginning with anesthesia, fluids (e.g., lactated Ringer's solution) should be administered intravenously at a surgical maintenance rate. Acute hypocortisolism uniformly occurs after adrenalectomy. Therefore once the adrenal tumor is identified by the surgeon, dexamethasone (0.1 to 0.2 mg/kg) should be placed in the IV infusion bottle. This dose should be given over a 6-hour period. A tapering dose (e.g., decreasing the dose by 0.02 mg/kg/24 hr) of dexamethasone should continue to be administered intravenously at 12-hour intervals until the dog can be safely given oral medication without the danger of vomiting (typically 48 to 72 hours postoperatively). At that point, the glucocorticoid supplement should be switched to oral prednisone (0.25 to 0.5 mg/kg q12h initially). Once the dog is eating and drinking on its own, the frequency of prednisone administration should be decreased to once a day and given in the morning. The prednisone dosage is then gradually reduced during the ensuing 3 to 4 months. If a unilateral adrenalectomy has been performed, prednisone supplementation can eventually be discontinued once the contralateral normal adrenocortical tissue becomes functional. The condition in dogs that undergo bilateral adrenalectomy remains stable in response to prednisone at a dosage of 0.1 to 0.2 mg/kg administered once or twice daily.

Serum electrolyte concentrations should be closely monitored postoperatively. Serum sodium concentrations of less than 138 mEq/L or serum potassium concentrations of greater than 5.5 mEq/L develop in 30% to 40% of dogs in the 24- to 48-hour period after surgery. In most, these electrolyte abnormalities resolve in a day or two as exogenous steroid doses are reduced and the dog begins to eat. Mineralocorticoid treatment (see p. 807) is recommended if these abnormalities persist for longer than 48 hours or if they become more severe. An injection of desoxycorticosterone pivalate (DOCP; Percorten-V; Novartis Pharmaceuticals) is recommended, with measurement of serum electrolytes performed 14 and 25 days after the injection. If the dog is healthy and serum electrolytes are normal on day 25, the dog should be reevaluated 5 and 10 days later. If serum electrolytes are still normal on these days, additional DOCP treatment is not needed. If hyponatremia or hyperkalemia is identified on day 25, another injection of DOCP should be administered but the dosage reduced 50%; serum electrolytes are evaluated 25 days later, and if DOCP is still needed, the dosage is reduced by another 25% at the third injection. It would be rare for a dog to need more than two or three injections. Fludrocortisone acetate therapy, given orally, can be used in lieu of DOCP, although fludrocortisone acetate is not as effective as DOCP for correcting hyponatremia and hyperkalemia. Fludrocortisone acetate can usually be slowly tapered and then

discontinued after 14 to 21 days, to be given again only if hyperkalemia or hyponatremia recurs.

### Radiation therapy

Approximately 50% of dogs have a pituitary mass identified on CT or MRI at the time PDH is diagnosed. In approximately 50% of these dogs, the pituitary mass grows over the ensuing 1 to 2 years, eventually causing pituitary macrotumor syndrome (see p. 780). Pituitary macroadenoma is tentatively diagnosed by ruling out other causes of the neurologic disturbances and is confirmed by CT or MRI findings (see Fig. 53-4). Development of neurologic signs from a pituitary macrotumor is a common reason for owners to request euthanasia of dogs with PDH. Irradiation has successfully reduced the tumor size and lessened or eliminated neurologic signs in dogs with pituitary macrotumor syndrome (Fig. 53-14). However, a reduction in the secretory nature of pituitary tumors is variable; as a result, mitotane or an alternative form of medical therapy is usually necessary, in addition to pituitary irradiation. The primary mode of radiation treatment is cobalt 60 photon irradiation or linear accelerator photon irradiation. Treatment usually involves the delivery of a predetermined total dose of radiation given in fractions over a period of several weeks. Currently a total dose of 48 Gy, given in 4 Gy doses 3 to 5 days per week for 3 to 4 weeks, is typically administered to hyperadrenal dogs with pituitary macroadenoma at our hospital.

Prognostic factors that affect survival time after radiation therapy include the severity of neurologic signs and the relative size of the tumor. Generally, dogs with subtle or mild neurologic clinical signs and the smallest tumors show the best response to treatment. Theon and colleague (1998) found a mean survival time following radiation of 25 months in dogs with mild neurologic signs, 17 months in dogs with severe neurologic signs, and only 5 months in untreated dogs with neurologic signs. Because of the high prevalence of a pituitary mass at the time PDH is diagnosed and the potential for future growth and development of neurologic signs, examination of the pituitary gland using CT or MRI and radiation therapy if a mass is identified should be discussed with the owner at the time PDH is diagnosed. The goal of radiation therapy is to shrink the mass and prevent development of macrotumor syndrome; mitotane therapy may still be needed to control clinical signs of hyperadrenocorticism.

### Prognosis

The average life expectancy in dogs with adrenal-dependent hyperadrenocorticism that survive the initial postadrenalectomy month is approximately 36 months. Dogs with adrenocortical adenoma and adrenocortical adenocarcinoma that has not metastasized (uncommon) have a good prognosis, whereas dogs with metastatic adrenocortical adenocarcinoma (common) have a poor prognosis, with these dogs typically succumbing to the disease within a year of diagnosis. Although clinical signs can be controlled with ketoconazole and mitotane, death ultimately results from the debilitating effects of the tumor, complications of hyperadrenocorticism (e.g., pulmonary thromboembolism), or other geriatric disorders (e.g., renal insufficiency, congestive heart failure).

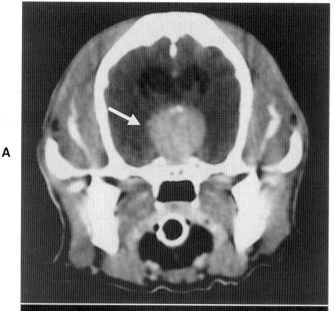

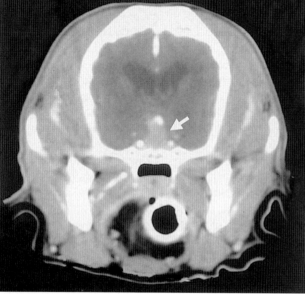

**FIG 53-14**

**A,** CT image of the pituitary region of a 9-year-old, female spayed Cocker Spaniel with pituitary-dependent hyperadrenocorticism (PDH). The PDH had been treated with mitotane for 2 years, at which time the dog developed lethargy, inappetance, and weight loss. A large mass measuring approximately 2.0 cm in diameter is evident in the hypothalamic-pituitary region *(arrow)*. **B,** CT image of the pituitary region 18 months after completion of radiation therapy. The volume of the mass decreased by approximately 75%, compared with the volume before treatment. Clinical signs related to the pituitary macrotumor resolved, and mitotane treatment was discontinued following radiation treatment.

The prognosis for dogs with PDH depends in part on the age and overall health of the dog and on the owner's commitment to therapy. The mean life span of affected dogs after diagnosis of PDH is approximately 30 months. Younger dogs may live considerably longer (i.e., 4 years or longer). Many dogs ultimately die or are euthanized because of complications related to hyperadrenocorticism (e.g., pituitary macrotumor syndrome, thromboembolism, infection) or other geriatric disorders.

## HYPERADRENOCORTICISM IN CATS

Hyperadrenocorticism is uncommon in cats. Although many of the clinical characteristics of feline hyperadrenocorticism are similar to those seen in dogs, there are some important differences that should be emphasized. Most notable is the very strong association with diabetes mellitus; the progressive, relentless weight loss leading to cachexia; and dermal and epidermal atrophy leading to extremely fragile, thin, easily torn and ulcerated skin (i.e., feline fragile skin syndrome) in cats with hyperadrenocorticism. Establishing the diagnosis is difficult, and effective medical treatment for hyperadrenocorticism in cats has yet to be identified.

### Etiology

Hyperadrenocorticism in cats is classified as either pituitary dependent (PDH) or adrenocortical dependent (i.e., neoplasia [AT]). Iatrogenic hyperadrenocorticism is uncommon in cats, and typically it takes months of prednisone administration before clinical signs occur. Cats with PDH have been found to have a pituitary microadenoma, macroadenoma, or carcinoma at necropsy. Interestingly, the prevalences of PDH and AT in cats with hyperadrenocorticism are comparable to those observed in dogs. Approximately 75% of cats with hyperadrenocorticism have PDH, and 25% have AT, with 50% of the ATs being adenomas and 50% adenocarcinomas.

### Clinical Features

**Clinical signs and physical examination findings.** Hyperadrenocorticism is a disease of older (average age, 10 years), mixed-breed cats. There is a strong correlation between hyperadrenocorticism and diabetes mellitus. Carbohydrate intolerance has been present in all cats with hyperadrenocorticism, and insulin-resistant diabetes mellitus has been present in many of these cats. The most common initial clinical signs of feline hyperadrenocorticism (i.e., polyuria, polydipsia, polyphagia) are more likely caused by the diabetes than by the hyperadrenocorticism. Consistent with this is the low prevalence of polyuria and polydipsia in cats receiving exogenous glucocorticoids and the common finding of a urine specific gravity of more than 1.030 in cats with spontaneous hyperadrenocorticism. Other clinical signs and physical examination findings are not as frequently observed in cats as in dogs and tend to be very subtle in the early stages of the disease (Table 53-7; Fig. 53-15). In the early stages, hyperadrenocorticism is typically suspected when the clinician begins to rule out causes of insulin ineffectiveness in a cat with diabetes mellitus (see p. 761). Establishing a definitive diagnosis is difficult when clinical signs of hyperadrenocorticism are mild, because tests of the pituitary-adrenocortical axis are usually inconclusive. As such, clinicians inadvertently pursue other causes for

TABLE 53-7

Clinical Features of Hyperadrenocorticism in Cats

| Clinical Signs | Clinical Signs—cont'd |
|---|---|
| Polyuria, polydipsia* | Weight loss* |
| Polyphagia* | Drooping of pinna |
| Patchy alopecia* | **Additional Physical Findings** |
| Unkempt haircoat* | "Pot-bellied" appearance* |
| Symmetric alopecia | Hepatomegaly* |
| Lethargy | Muscle wasting* |
| Thin, easily torn skin (feline fragile skin syndrome)* | Skin infections |

*Common.

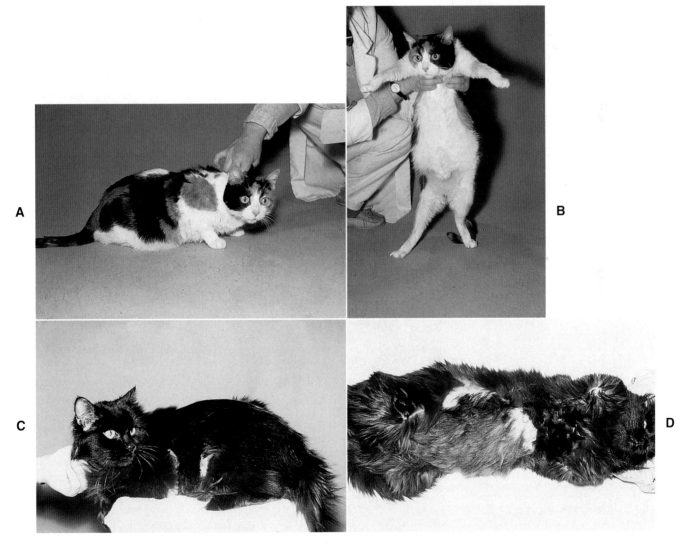

**FIG 53-15**
**A** and **B,** A 9-year-old cat with pituitary-dependent hyperadrenocorticism and insulin-resistant diabetes mellitus. Note the relatively normal physical appearance of the cat in its normal posture **(A).** Abdominal enlargement and inguinal alopecia are evident on physical examination **(B). C** and **D,** An 11-year-old cat with adrenal hyperadrenocorticism caused by bilateral adrenocortical adenomas and insulin-resistant diabetes mellitus. Note the relatively normal appearance of the cat and the patchy alopecia and thin haircoat affecting the ventral abdomen and rear legs.

poor control of the diabetic state. With time, hyperadreno-corticism becomes more apparent as affected cats become progressively more debilitated despite administration of high dosages of potent insulin, weight loss leads to severe cachexia, and dermal and epidermal atrophy result in extremely fragile, thin, easily torn, and ulcerated skin (i.e., feline fragile skin syndrome; Fig. 53-16). Dermal and epidermal lesions often occur when the cat is groomed or when the cat is handled during the physical examination. Insulin resistance is usually quite severe by the time cachexia and feline fragile skin syndrome develop. The primary differential diagnosis for insulin resistance, cachexia, and feline fragile skin syndrome is hyper-progesteronemia, as occurs with progesterone-secreting adrenal tumors (see p. 812).

**Clinical pathology.** The classic clinicopathologic alterations seen in dogs with hyperadrenocorticism are infrequently found in cats. The most frequently observed abnormalities in cats are hyperglycemia, glycosuria, hypercholesterolemia, and a mild increase in alanine aminotransferase activity. These alterations can be explained by the concurrent, poorly regulated diabetes mellitus. A stress leukogram, increase in SAP activity, and isosthenuric-hyposthenuric urine are not common clinicopathologic manifestations of feline hyperadrenocorticism. An inability to document histologic

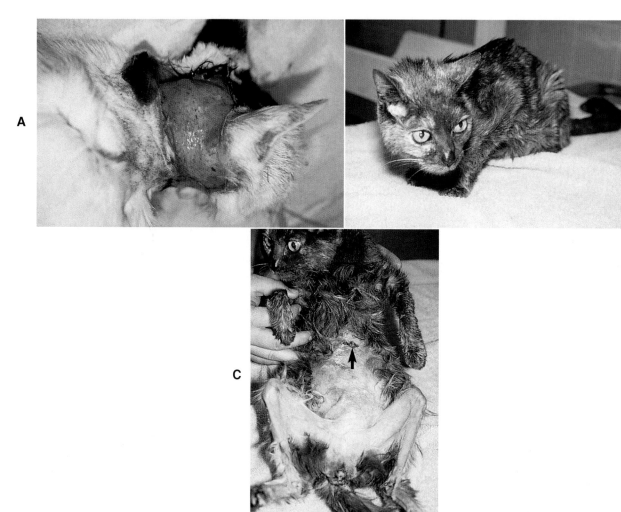

**FIG 53-16**
**A,** A 15-year-old cat with pituitary-dependent hyperadrenocorticism, insulin-resistant diabetes mellitus, and feline fragile skin syndrome. Note the torn skin over the back of the neck that occurred while restraining the cat during a physical examination. **B** and **C,** A 12-year-old cat with hyperadrenocorticism and severe insulin-resistant diabetes mellitus. This cat weighed 2.2 kg and was receiving 25 units of regular insulin three times a day with no glucose-lowering effect. Note the emaciated appearance, presumably resulting from protracted poor glycemic control, alopecia, severe dermal and epidermal atrophy, and lesions resulting from easily torn skin *(arrow)*. The dermatologic alterations resemble those seen in feline fragile skin syndrome, for which hyperadrenocorticism is a differential diagnosis.

changes in the liver consistent with steroid-induced hepatopathy, an absence of the steroid-induced alkaline phosphatase isoenzyme activity, and the relatively short half-life of SAP activity in cats may account for the absence of an observed increase in SAP activity. Urine abnormalities associated with canine hyperadrenocorticism (proteinuria, pyuria, bacteriuria) are not common in cats with hyperadrenocorticism.

## Tests of the Pituitary-Adrenocortical Axis

Although the tests used to diagnose hyperadrenocorticism in cats and dogs are similar (see p. 786), there are some important differences in the testing protocol and in the interpretation of results (Table 53-8). We rely most heavily on the urine cortisol/creatinine ratio, dexamethasone suppression test, and abdominal ultrasonography to establish the diagnosis of hyperadrenocorticism in cats. The ACTH stimulation test is not a very good test for diagnosing hyperadrenocorticism in cats. In our experience, the sensitivity of the ACTH stimulation test is less than 50% in cats. We also rely more heavily on results of abdominal ultrasound than on endogenous ACTH concentration to differentiate PDH from AT.

**Urine cortisol/creatinine ratio.** The theory behind and the specifics regarding the urine cortisol/creatinine ratio in cats are similar to those in dogs and are discussed on p. 789. In our laboratory, the normal urine cortisol/creatinine ratio is less than $1.5 \times 10^{-5}$; this value may vary among laboratories. We often use the urine cortisol/creatinine ratio as the initial screening test for hyperadrenocorticism in cats unless clinical signs strongly suggest the presence of hyperadrenocorticism. A normal urine cortisol/creatinine ratio is a strong finding against the diagnosis; an increased ratio does not establish the diagnosis, by itself, but supports performing the dexamethasone suppression test.

**Dexamethasone suppression test.** The duration of the suppressive effects of intravenously administered dexamethasone on plasma cortisol concentrations is more variable in cats than in dogs; approximately 20% of normal cats "escape" the suppressive effects of dexamethasone, and their cortisol concentrations fall outside the normal 8-hour post-dexamethasone reference range (i.e., 8-hour post-dexamethasone plasma cortisol concentration $>1.4$ μg/dl). This escape phenomenon is more likely to occur in cats receiving lower doses of dexamethasone. Because of potential misinterpretation caused by the escape phenomenon and the fragile state of many diabetic hyperadrenal cats, we typically use only one dexamethasone suppression test protocol (0.1 mg/kg dexamethasone IV; blood

 TABLE 53-8

Diagnostic Tests to Assess the Pituitary-Adrenocortical Axis in Cats

| TEST | PURPOSE | PROTOCOL | RESULTS | INTERPRETATION |
|---|---|---|---|---|
| Endogenous ACTH | Identify PDH | Plasma sample obtained between 8 and 10 AM; special handling required | >45 pg/ml<br><45 pg/ml | PDH<br>Nondiagnostic |
| ACTH stimulation | Diagnose Cushing's syndrome | 2.2 IU of ACTH gel*/kg IM; plasma pre- and 1 and 2 hr post-ACTH<br>or<br>0.125 mg of synthetic ACTH*/cat IM; plasma pre- and 30 and 60 min post-ACTH | *Post-ACTH cortisol concentration:*<br>>15 μg/dl<br>12-15 μg/dl<br>6-12 μg/dl<br><br><6 μg/dl | Strongly suggestive†<br>Suggestive‡<br>Normal<br><br>Iatrogenic Cushing's syndrome |
| Dexamethasone suppression test | Diagnose Cushing's syndrome | 0.1 mg of dexamethasone/kg IV; plasma pre- and 4, 6, and 8 hr post-dexamethasone | *Post-dexamethasone:*<br>8 hr:<br><1.0 μg/dl<br>1.0-1.4 μg/dl<br><1.4 μg/dl and 4 or 6 hr<br><1.4 μg/dl<br>>1.4 μg/dl and 4 and 6 hr<br>>1.4 μg/dl | <br><br>Normal<br>Nondiagnostic<br>Suggestive<br><br><br>Strongly suggestive |

*ACTH,* Adrenocorticotropic hormone; *PDH,* pituitary-dependent hyperadrenocorticism.
*ACTH gel: Cortigel, Savage Laboratories; Synthetic ACTH: Cortrosyn, Organon Pharmaceuticals.
†Strongly suggestive of hyperadrenocorticism.
‡Suggestive of hyperadrenocorticism.

obtained before and 4, 6, and 8 hours after dexamethasone administration) when evaluating the pituitary-adrenocortical axis in cats. An 8-hour post-dexamethasone plasma cortisol concentration of less than 1.0 μg/dl is suggestive of a normal pituitary-adrenocortical axis, values between 1.0 and 1.4 μg/dl are inconclusive, and values greater than 1.4 μg/dl are supportive of the diagnosis of hyperadrenocorticism. The higher the 8-hour post-dexamethsone plasma cortisol concentration above 1.4 μg/dl, the more supportive the test is for the diagnosis of hyperadrenocorticism. Similarly, plasma cortisol concentrations greater than 1.4 μg/dl at the 4- and 6-hour post-dexamethasone blood sampling times add further credence for the diagnosis of hyperadrenocorticism (Fig. 53-17). Whenever either or both the 4- and 6-hour post-dexamethasone cortisol values are less than 1.4 μg/dl (especially <1.0 μg/dl), the test results should be considered consistent with, but not definitively diagnostic of, hyperadrenocorticism and the clinician must rely on the clinical signs, physical examination findings, and results of other diagnostic tests to help establish the diagnosis. Results of the dexamethasone suppression test should never constitute the sole evidence for hyperadrenocorticism in cats.

**ACTH stimulation test.** The peak increase in the post–ACTH administration plasma cortisol concentration occurs earlier in cats than in dogs, with the plasma cortisol concentrations possibly approaching baseline values by 1 or 2 hours after the administration of synthetic or porcine ACTH, respectively. Whenever porcine ACTH gel is used, blood samples for the cortisol determination should be obtained 1 and 2 hours after its administration. Whenever synthetic ACTH is used, blood samples should be obtained 30 minutes and 1 hour after its administration. In our laboratory, a post-ACTH cortisol concentration of 12 μg/dl or less is normal, one between 12 and 15 μg/dl is borderline, one between 15 and 18 μg/dl is suggestive, and one greater than 18 μg/dl is con-

sistent with the diagnosis of hyperadrenocorticism. It is important that the endocrine laboratory have established reference values for cats. The sensitivity of the ACTH stimulation test in identifying hyperadrenocorticism is lower in cats than in dogs. In our experience, less than 50% of cats with hyperadrenocorticism confirmed at necropsy have abnormal ACTH stimulation test results consistent with the disease.

**Endogenous plasma ACTH concentration.** The endogenous plasma ACTH concentration test is discussed on p. 792. The normal range for baseline plasma ACTH concentrations in cats is undetectable to 110 pg/ml. The finding of an increased endogenous plasma ACTH concentration (i.e., >45 pg/ml) supports the diagnosis of PDH; values of less than 45 pg/ml are nondiagnostic. Values of less than 10 pg/ml are found in normal cats and cats with AT.

### Diagnostic Imaging

Abdominal ultrasonography is used to identify adrenal masses and to clarify the clinician's index of suspicion for PDH. The interpretation of results of adrenal imaging in cats is similar to that in dogs (see p. 783). Generally, however, the adrenal glands are more difficult to visualize in cats than in dogs. Failure to identify the adrenals represents an inconclusive finding, but it is considered more indicative of normal adrenals than of PDH. The maximum width of the adrenal gland in healthy cats is typically less than 0.5 cm. Adrenomegaly should be suspected when the maximum width is greater than 0.5 cm; a maximum width greater than 0.8 cm is strongly suggestive of adrenomegaly. The finding of easily visualized, bilaterally large adrenals in a cat with appropriate clinical signs, physical examination findings, and abnormal pituitary-adrenocortical axis test results is considered strong evidence for adrenal hyperplasia caused by PDH.

CT and MRI can be used to look for pituitary macroade-

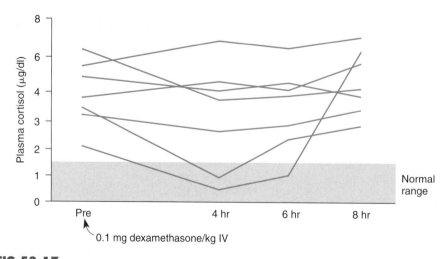

**FIG 53-17**

Dexamethasone suppression test results in seven cats with histologically confirmed hyperadrenocorticism. Blood for the cortisol determination was drawn before and 4, 6, and 8 hours after the IV administration of 0.1 mg of dexamethasone/kg body weight. In most cats the plasma cortisol concentration remained more than 1.4 μg/dl throughout the test—results that are very consistent with a diagnosis of hyperadrenocorticism.

noma (see p. 780). The primary differential diagnosis in cats with pituitary macroadenoma is acromegaly (see p. 673). Hyperadrenocorticism and acromegaly both cause insulin-resistant diabetes mellitus; however, additional clinical signs differ dramatically between these two disorders. Hyperadrenocorticism is a debilitating disease that results in progressive weight loss leading to cachexia, and dermal and epidermal atrophy leading to extremely fragile, thin, easily torn and ulcerated skin (i.e., feline fragile skin syndrome). In contrast, conformational changes caused by the anabolic actions of chronic insulin-like growth factor-I (IGF-I) secretion dominate the clinical picture in acromegaly. Conformational changes include an increase in body size, enlargement of the abdomen and head, prognathia inferior, and weight gain despite poorly regulated diabetes mellitus.

## Diagnosis

Hyperadrenocorticism is an elusive diagnosis in cats, in part because the clinical signs are often vague and easily attributed to concurrent diabetes mellitus until late in the disease and because none of the diagnostic tests used to establish the diagnosis in dogs are reliable in cats. The disease is suspected if the appropriate clinical signs, physical examination findings, clinicopathologic alterations, and abdominal ultrasound findings are noted. Abdominal ultrasonography may also provide information regarding the probable location of the lesion. The index of suspicion is further heightened if the urine cortisol/creatinine ratio and the results of the dexamethasone suppression test are abnormal. Ideally, all diagnostic tests performed in the assessment of a cat with suspected hyperadrenocorticism should be abnormal when the diagnosis of hyperadrenocorticism is being established; discordant test results raise doubt regarding the diagnosis. False-positive and false-negative results occur with all of the diagnostic tests used to assess the pituitary-adrenocortical axis. Normal results of the ACTH stimulation test are common in cats with hyperadrenocorticism. A normal urine cortisol/creatinine ratio and normal dexamethasone suppression test results are inconsistent with a diagnosis of hyperadrenocorticism; however, abnormal results of these tests do not, by themselves, confirm the diagnosis. Ultimately, hyperadrenocorticism is diagnosed on the basis of the clinical signs, physical examination, and abdominal ultrasonography findings; results of clinicopathologic and pituitary-adrenocortical axis tests; and the clinician's index of suspicion for the disease.

## Treatment

Treatment of hyperadrenocorticism is problematic in cats. Adrenalectomy is the treatment of choice for an adrenal mass. Unfortunately, a reliable medical treatment for PDH has not been identified in cats. Untreated hyperadrenal cats die as a result of the deleterious effects of chronic hypercortisolism and insulin-resistant diabetes mellitus on the skin (i.e., fragility) and on immune and cardiovascular function, and as a result of progressive weight loss leading to severe cachexia. Because treatment is indicated after hyperadrenocorticism has been diagnosed, the most viable option for PDH is bilateral

adrenalectomy. Medical treatment with metyrapone or aminoglutethemide (see below) is usually necessary for 4 to 6 weeks before adrenalectomy to reverse the catabolic state of the cat, improve skin fragility and wound healing, and decrease the potential for perioperative complications. Unfortunately, the suppressive effects of metyrapone and possibly aminoglutethemide on cortisol secretion by the adrenal cortex is short-lived; the hyperadrenal state typically recurs within 4 to 8 weeks of initiating treatment.

The surgical approach and medical management during and after surgery is similar to that used in dogs (see p. 796). After bilateral adrenalectomy, most cats remain in stable condition in response to fludrocortisone acetate (Florinef, 0.05 mg/cat PO q12h initially; ER Squibb & Sons) or injectable desoxycorticosterone pivalate (DOCP, 2.2 mg/kg IM every 25 days initially; Percoten-V; Novartis Pharmaceuticals), and prednisone (1.0 to 2.5 mg once daily). Subsequent adjustments in the dose of fludrocortisone acetate or DOCP should be based on periodically measured serum electrolyte concentrations (see p. 808). Insulin therapy can be discontinued in approximately 50% of cats once hyperadrenocorticism is eliminated, and diabetes is easier to control using less insulin in the remaining cats.

Medical therapy can be tried if the owner is unwilling to consider surgery or if metastatic lesions are identified. Consistently effective medical therapy remains to be identified. Although our numbers are small, we have had limited to no success with mitotane, despite its documented adrenocorticolytic effects in normal cats. We have also had limited to no success with ketoconazole. Metyrapone (Metopirone, 65 mg/kg PO q12h; Ciba-Geigy Pharmaceuticals), an 11-β-hydroxylase inhibitor, has been successful in controlling clinical signs of hyperadrenocorticism in a few cats, but the drug-induced blockade of cortisol synthesis and secretion can be overridden by increasing concentrations of circulating ACTH; the latter occurs in response to decreased cortisol secretion by the adrenal glands. Clinical signs may recur as early as 1 month after the start of metyrapone therapy. Metyrapone can be useful in stabilizing the cat's condition before adrenalectomy; however, this drug is not consistently available and can cause gastrointestinal problems (vomiting, diarrhea) in some cats. Aminoglutethimide (Cytadren, 30 mg/cat PO q12h; Ciba-Geigy Pharmaceuticals) inhibits the conversion of cholesterol to pregnenolone, thereby reducing cortisol hypersecretion. Aminoglutethimide has been used successfully in controlling clinical signs of hyperadrenocorticism and hyperprogesteronemia in cats with progesterone-secreting tumors (Fig. 53-18; see also p. 812). Aminoglutethimide is useful in stabilizing the cat's condition before adrenalectomy and appears to maintain its efficacy for a more prolonged period of time (i.e., months) compared with metyrapone. Cobalt irradiation may be tried in cats with pituitary macrotumor, although clinical signs of hypercortisolemia may persist despite shrinkage of the tumor.

## Prognosis

The prognosis in cats with hyperadrenocorticism is guarded to poor. Unilateral (AT) or bilateral (PDH) adrenalectomy

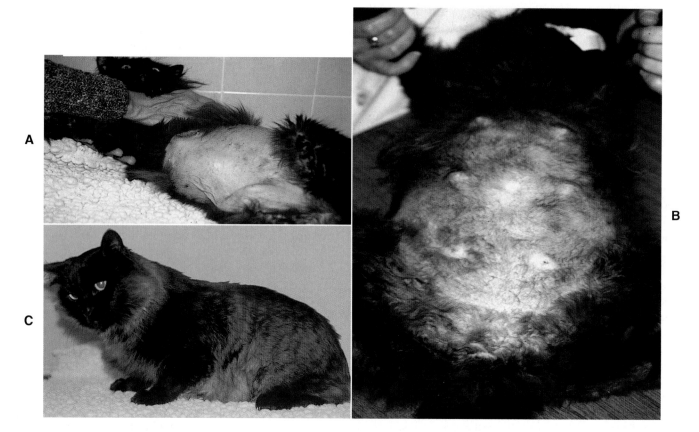

**FIG 53-18**
**A,** A 9-year-old male castrated domestic long-haired cat with a 2-year history of poorly controlled diabetes mellitus, failure of hair to regrow following clipping 1 year before presentation, and recent development of feline fragile skin syndrome. Diagnostic evaluation revealed an adrenocortical tumor, increased serum progesterone concentration, and suppression of the pituitary-adrenocortical axis on ACTH stimulation and dexamethasone suppression testing. A progesterone-secreting adrenocortical tumor was suspected. **B,** Five weeks after initiating treatment with aminoglutethemide. Feline fragile skin syndrome was resolving, hair was growing, and gynecomastia had developed. The serum progesterone concentration had decreased from a pretreatment value of 4.7 ng/ml to less than 1 ng/ml. **C,** Four months after adrenalectomy. Insulin-requiring diabetes mellitus had resolved.

has the potential for excellent success; however, success is dependent, in part, on correction of the debilitated state and skin fragility with medical treatment before surgery, involvement of a surgeon with expertise in adrenal surgery, avoidance of perioperative complications, and owner commitment to managing the iatrogenic adrenal insufficiency following bilateral adrenalectomy. Periodic evaluation of serum electrolytes and review of the treatment protocol is important. An addisonian crisis has occurred months after surgery in several of the cats treated in our clinic and was believed to be responsible for the death of some.

## HYPOADRENOCORTICISM

### Etiology

Hypoadrenocorticism is classified as either primary or secondary adrenocortical insufficiency. Primary adrenocortical insufficiency is the most common form and involves a defi-

ciency of both mineralocorticoid and glucocorticoid secretion. The etiology is usually classified as idiopathic because the cause of the disease is not obvious, and necropsies are usually done years after the diagnosis is established, at which time idiopathic atrophy of all layers of the adrenal cortex is the most frequent histopathologic finding. It is likely that immune-mediated destruction of the adrenal cortices occurs in most dogs and cats with idiopathic adrenal insufficiency; lymphocytes, plasma cells, and fibrosis are common findings in animals that undergo necropsy near the time of diagnosis. Bilateral destruction of the adrenal cortex by neoplasia (e.g., lymphoma), granulomatous disease, or arterial thrombosis can also cause primary adrenocortical insufficiency. For clinical signs to develop, it is believed that at least 90% of the adrenal cortices must be destroyed. The zones of the adrenal cortices are usually damaged at about the same rate, with aldosterone and glucocorticoid deficiency typically occurring in tandem. The rate of destruction is variable but progressive, ultimately leading to complete loss of adrenocortical function. Dogs typically have complete loss of adrenocortical function at the time Addison's disease is diagnosed. A partial deficiency syndrome characterized by inadequate adrenal reserve may occur initially, with clinical signs manifested only during times of stress (e.g., boarding, travel, surgery). As destruction of the adrenal glands progresses, hormone secretion becomes inadequate even under nonstressful conditions and a true metabolic crisis occurs without any obvious inciting event.

Mineralocorticoids (i.e., aldosterone) control sodium, potassium, and water homeostasis. In the setting of primary adrenocortical insufficiency, a loss of aldosterone secretion results in impaired renal conservation of sodium and chloride and the excretion of potassium, leading to the development of hyponatremia, hypochloremia, and hyperkalemia. The inability to retain sodium and chloride causes the extracellular fluid volume to be reduced, and this leads to the progressive development of hypovolemia, hypotension, a reduced cardiac output, and decreased perfusion of the kidneys and other tissues. Hyperkalemia has a deleterious effect on cardiac function, causing decreased myocardial excitability, an increased myocardial refractory period, and slowed conduction. A concurrent glucocorticoid deficiency typically results in gastrointestinal tract signs (anorexia, vomiting, weight loss) and changes in mental status (lethargy). One of the hallmark signs of hypocortisolism is impaired tolerance to stress, and clinical signs often become more pronounced when the animal is placed in stressful situations.

Secondary adrenocortical insufficiency involves only a deficiency of glucocorticoid secretion. Mineralocorticoid secretion, and thus serum electrolyte concentrations, are normal. The clinical signs result from the glucocorticoid deficiency. Secondary adrenocortical insufficiency is caused by the reduced secretion of pituitary ACTH. Destructive lesions (e.g., neoplasia, inflammation) in the pituitary gland or hypothalamus and the long-term administration of exogenous glucocorticoids or megestrol acetate (cats) are the most common causes of secondary adrenal insufficiency. Adrenocortical atrophy may develop after the injectable, oral, or topical administration of corticosteroids. Adrenal function usually returns within 2 to 4 weeks of the discontinuation of the administered medication unless long-acting depot forms of glucocorticoids are used. Naturally occurring, isolated hypoaldosteronism has not been described in dogs or cats.

## Clinical Features

**Signalment.** Hypoadrenocorticism is typically a disease of young to middle-aged (mean age, 4 years; age range, 2 months to 12 years) female dogs. There are no significant breed-related predilections, although genetics probably plays a role in the development of adrenal insufficiency in Standard Poodles and Portuguese Water Spaniels. Hypoadrenocorticism is rare in cats. There is no apparent sex-related predisposition in cats, although it also tends to occur in young to middle-aged cats (average age, 6 years). Hypoadrenocorticism can, however, occur in aged dogs and cats as well.

**Clinical signs and physical examination findings.** The clinical signs and physical examination findings in ani-

 TABLE 53-9

**Clinical Signs Caused by Hypoadrenocorticism in Dogs and Cats**

| DOGS | CATS |
|---|---|
| Lethargy* | Lethargy* |
| Anorexia* | Anorexia* |
| Vomiting* | Weight loss* |
| Weakness* | Vomiting |
| Diarrhea | Polyuria, polydipsia |
| Weight loss | |
| Shivering | |
| Polyuria, polydipsia | |
| Abdominal pain | |

*Common.

mals with hypoadrenocorticism result from a deficiency in glucocorticoid or mineralocorticoid secretion, or both (Table 53-9). The most common clinical manifestations are related to alterations in the gastrointestinal tract and mental status and include lethargy, anorexia, vomiting, and weight loss. Weakness is also a common owner complaint. Additional physical examination findings may include dehydration, bradycardia, weak femoral pulses, and abdominal pain. Hyperkalemia and hypoadrenocorticism should be suspected in an animal with bradycardia and signs consistent with hypovolemia. Bradycardia by itself, however, is not pathognomonic for hypoadrenocorticism, especially in an otherwise healthy dog. Similarly, dogs with hypoadrenocorticism can have normal heart rates. Polyuria and polydipsia are rarely presenting signs, although they may surface during the taking of a complete history.

Clinical signs are often vague and easily ascribed to more common disorders involving the gastrointestinal and urinary tracts. Observant owners may occasionally describe an illness with a waxing-waning or episodic course; however, this bit of historic information is the exception rather than the rule. Most dogs with hypoadrenocorticism are first seen because of progressive problems that vary in severity, depending on the degree of stress and the adrenocortical reserve.

If hyponatremia and hyperkalemia become severe, the resultant hypovolemia, prerenal azotemia, and cardiac arrhythmias may result in an addisonian crisis. The clinical manifestations are as previously described; the only difference is in the severity of signs. In severe cases the animal may be presented in shock and be moribund. An addisonian crisis must be differentiated from other life-threatening disorders, such as diabetic ketoacidosis, necrotizing pancreatitis, and septic peritonitis.

**Clinical pathology.** There are several abnormalities that may be identified on a CBC, serum biochemistry panel, and urinalysis (Table 53-10). Hyperkalemia, hyponatremia, and hypochloremia are the classic electrolyte alterations in animals with adrenal insufficiency and are perhaps the most important evidence ultimately used to establish a diagnosis of hypoadrenocorticism. Serum sodium concentrations vary

TABLE 53-10

Clinicopathologic Abnormalities Associated with Primary Hypoadrenocorticism in Dogs and Cats

**Hemogram**

Nonregenerative anemia
± Neutrophilic leukocytosis
± Mild neutropenia
± Eosinophilia
± Lymphocytosis

**Biochemistry Panel**

Hyperkalemia
Hyponatremia
Hypochloremia
Prerenal azotemia
Hyperphosphatemia
± Hypercalcemia
± Hypoglycemia
Metabolic acidosis (low total $CO_2$, $HCO_3^-$)

**Urinalysis**

Isosthenuria to hypersthenuria

---

from normal to as low as 105 mEq/L (mean, 128 mEq/L), and serum potassium concentrations vary from normal to greater than 10 mEq/L (mean, 7.2 mEq/L). The sodium/potassium ratio reflects changes in these electrolyte concentrations in serum and has been frequently used as a diagnostic tool to identify adrenal insufficiency. The normal ratio varies between 27:1 and 40:1. Values are often less than 27 and may be less than 20 in animals with primary adrenal insufficiency.

Electrolyte alterations, by themselves, can be misleading. Normal serum electrolyte concentrations do not rule out adrenal insufficiency. Electrolyte abnormalities may not be evident in the early stages of the disorder when clinical signs result from glucocorticoid deficiency and do not develop with secondary adrenal insufficiency caused by pituitary failure. Alternatively, other disorders can cause alterations in the serum electrolyte concentrations that mimic those seen in the setting of adrenal insufficiency, most notably disorders involving the hepatic, gastrointestinal, and urinary systems (see Tables 55-3 and 55-5). For most disorders a thorough history and physical examination, together with a critical evaluation of the CBC results, serum biochemistry profile, and urinalysis findings, allow the clinician to prioritize the potential differential diagnoses. The most challenging aspect of diagnosis is the differentiation between acute renal failure and primary adrenal insufficiency. The azotemia of adrenal insufficiency occurs secondary to reduced renal perfusion and an associated decrease in the glomerular filtration rate after the onset of hypovolemia and hypotension. A compensatory increase in the urine specific gravity (i.e., >1.030) allows prerenal azotemia to be differentiated from primary renal azotemia, and therefore adrenal insufficiency to be differentiated from acute renal failure, respectively.

Unfortunately, many hypoadrenal dogs and cats have an impaired ability to concentrate urine because of chronic urinary sodium loss, depletion of the renal medullary sodium content, loss of the normal medullary concentration gradient, and impaired water resorption by the renal collecting tubules. As a result, some hypoadrenal dogs and cats with prerenal azotemia have urine specific gravities in the isosthenuric range (i.e., 1.007 to 1.015). Fortunately, the initial therapy for acute renal failure and adrenal insufficiency is similar. Ultimately, the differentiation between these two disorders must rely on testing of the pituitary-adrenocortical axis and the animal's response to initial fluid and other supportive therapy.

**Electrocardiography.** Hyperkalemia causes cardiac conduction to be depressed and causes characteristic alterations on an electrocardiogram (ECG) (see Table 55-6). The severity of the ECG abnormalities correlates with the severity of the hyperkalemia. As a result, the ECG can be used as a diagnostic tool to identify and estimate the severity of hyperkalemia and as a therapeutic tool to monitor changes in the blood potassium concentration during therapy.

**Diagnostic imaging.** Hypoadrenal dogs and cats with severe hypovolemia often have microcardia, a descending aortic arch that is flattened and has a decreased diameter, and a narrow caudal vena cava, as seen on lateral thoracic radiographs. These findings are a crude means of evaluating the degree of hypovolemia and hypotension. Rarely, concurrent generalized megaesophagus may also be evident and may resolve in response to treatment for the hypoadrenocorticism. Abdominal ultrasonography may reveal small adrenal glands (i.e., maximum width <0.3 cm), a finding suggestive of adrenocortical atrophy. However, finding normal-sized adrenal glands does not rule out hypoadrenocorticism.

### Diagnosis

Hypoadrenocorticism is often tentatively diagnosed on the basis of the history, physical examination findings, clinicopathologic findings, and, in the case of primary adrenal insufficiency, the identification of appropriate electrolyte abnormalities. An ACTH stimulation test must be performed for the diagnosis to be confirmed (see Table 53-5). Baseline plasma cortisol concentrations and urine cortisol/creatinine ratios are not reliable ways to confirm the diagnosis. One major criterion is used in confirming the diagnosis of adrenal insufficiency: an abnormally decreased post-ACTH plasma cortisol concentration (i.e., post-ACTH plasma cortisol concentration <2 μg/dl; see Fig. 53-12). The finding of a normal plasma cortisol concentration (i.e., >5 μg/dl) after ACTH stimulation rules out adrenal insufficiency. Post-ACTH plasma cortisol values between 2 and 5 μg/dl are inconclusive.

Results of the ACTH stimulation test do not distinguish dogs and cats with naturally occurring primary adrenal insufficiency from those with secondary insufficiency resulting from pituitary failure, those with secondary insufficiency resulting from prolonged iatrogenic corticosteroid administra-

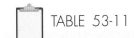 TABLE 53-11

Differentiation of Primary Versus Secondary Hypoadrenocorticism

|  | PRIMARY HYPOADRENOCORTICISM | SECONDARY HYPOADRENOCORTICISM |
|---|---|---|
| Serum electrolytes | Hyperkalemia Hyponatremia | Normal |
| ACTH stimulation test | | |
| Post-ACTH cortisol | Decreased | Decreased |
| Post-ACTH aldosterone | Decreased | Normal |
| Endogenous ACTH | Increased | Decreased |

tion, or dogs with primary adrenocortical destruction caused by mitotane overdosing. Concurrent abnormal serum electrolyte concentrations would imply the existence of primary adrenal insufficiency and the need for mineralocorticoid and glucocorticoid replacement therapy. Normal serum electrolyte concentrations do not differentiate early primary from secondary adrenal insufficiency. If secondary adrenal insufficiency can be documented, only glucocorticoid replacement therapy is indicated. Primary and secondary adrenal insufficiency can be differentiated prospectively by periodically measuring the serum electrolyte concentrations, by measuring the baseline endogenous ACTH concentration ($>100$ pg/ml in primary hypoadrenocorticism and $<45$ pg/ml in secondary hypoadrenocorticism), or by measuring plasma aldosterone concentrations during the ACTH stimulation test (Table 53-11). In theory, measurement of the blood aldosterone concentration should be of value when one is attempting to distinguish dogs with primary adrenal disease from those with secondary adrenal atrophy caused by a pituitary deficiency. Unfortunately, in our experience, there is no clear demarcation in blood aldosterone concentrations between these groups of dogs. After ACTH administration, the mean blood aldosterone concentration was found to be 306 pg/ml (range, 146 to 519 pg/ml) in 32 healthy dogs, 13 pg/ml (range, 0.1 to 91 pg/ml) in 15 dogs with naturally occurring primary hypoadrenocorticism, and 28 and 41 pg/ml in 2 dogs with secondary hypoadrenocorticism.

## Treatment

The aggressiveness of therapy depends in part on the clinical status of the animal and on the nature of the insufficiency (i.e., glucocorticoid or mineralocorticoid, or both). Many dogs and cats with primary adrenal insufficiency are presented in varying stages of an acute addisonian crisis, requiring immediate, aggressive therapy. In contrast, dogs and cats with secondary insufficiency often have a chronic course that poses more of a diagnostic than a therapeutic challenge.

### Therapy for acute addisonian crisis

An acute addisonian crisis implies both a mineralocorticoid and glucocorticoid deficiency. The treatment of acute primary adrenal insufficiency is directed toward eliminating

 TABLE 53-12

Initial Treatment for Acute Addisonian Crisis

**Fluid Therapy**

Type: 0.9% saline solution
Rate: 30 to 80 ml/kg IV initially
Potassium supplementation: contraindicated
Dextrose: 5% dextrose infusion (100 ml, 50% dextrose/L IV fluids)

**Glucocorticoid Therapy**

Hydrocortisone hemisuccinate or hydrocortisone phosphate,* 2 to 4 mg/kg IV, or prednisolone sodium succinate,* 4 to 20 mg/kg IV, then dexamethasone sodium phosphate, 0.05 to 0.1 mg/kg in IV fluids q12h; alternatively, dexamethasone sodium phosphate, 0.1 to 2 mg/kg IV, then 0.05 to 0.1 mg/kg in IV fluids q12h†

**Mineralocorticoid Therapy**

Desoxycorticosterone pivalate (DOCP; Percoten-V; Novartis), 2.2 mg/kg IM q25d initially

**Bicarbonate Therapy**

Indicated if $HCO_3^-$ <12 mEq/L or total venous $CO_2^-$ <12 mmol/L or animal is severely ill; mEq $HCO_3^-$ = body weight (kg) × 0.5 × base deficit (mEq/L); if base deficit unknown, use 10 mEq/L; add one quarter of calculated $HCO_3^-$ dose to IV fluids and administer over 6 hours; repeat only if plasma $HCO_3^-$ remains <12 mEq/L

*Hydrocortisone and prednisolone are assayed by most cortisol radioimmunoassays, interfering with interpretation of the ACTH stimulation test result.
†Higher doses of glucocorticoids may be required if the dog or cat is in shock.

the hypotension, hypovolemia, electrolyte imbalances, and metabolic acidosis; improving vascular integrity; and providing an immediate source of glucocorticoids (Table 53-12). Because death resulting from hypoadrenocorticism is often attributed to vascular collapse and shock, rapid correction of the hypovolemia is the first and most important therapeutic priority. Physiologic saline solution is the IV fluid of choice because it aids in correcting hypovolemia, hyponatremia, and hypochloremia. Hyperkalemia is reduced by simple dilution and by improved renal perfusion. Potassium-containing fluids (see Table 55-4) are relatively contraindicated but should be used in lieu of not giving IV fluids at all.

If hypoglycemia is suspected or known to be present, 50% dextrose should be added to the IV fluid to produce a 5% dextrose solution (i.e., 100 ml of 50% dextrose per liter of fluids). The addition of dextrose to isotonic solutions produces a hypertonic solution that should ideally be administered through a central vein, rather than through the smaller cephalic or saphenous vein, to minimize phlebitis.

Dogs and cats with acute adrenal insufficiency usually have a mild metabolic acidosis, which does not require therapy. Fluid therapy alone corrects the mild acidosis as the hypovolemia lessens and tissue perfusion and the glomerular filtration rate improve. If the total venous carbon dioxide or the serum bicarbonate concentration is less than 12 mmol/L or 12 mEq/L, respectively, conservative bicarbonate therapy is indicated. In a severely ill animal whose laboratory results are not yet known, a base deficit of 10 mEq/L can be assumed to be present. The milliequivalents of bicarbonate needed to correct the acidosis can be determined from the following equation:

Bicarbonate deficit (mEq/L) =
$$\text{Body weight (kg)} \times 0.5 \times \text{Base deficit (mEq/L)}$$

One fourth of the calculated bicarbonate dose should be administered in the IV fluids during the initial 6 to 8 hours of therapy. The acid-base status of the animal should be reassessed at the end of this time. Rarely, a dog or cat may require additional parenterally administered sodium bicarbonate.

Sodium bicarbonate therapy helps correct the metabolic acidosis and also decreases the serum potassium concentration. The intracellular movement of potassium ions after bicarbonate administration, in conjunction with the dilutional effects of saline fluid therapy and improved renal perfusion, is quite effective in lowering the serum potassium concentration and returning any ECG abnormalities toward normal. Additional therapy to rapidly correct life-threatening hyperkalemia is rarely needed (see Table 55-7).

Glucocorticoid and mineralocorticoid therapy is also indicated in the initial management of an acute addisonian crisis. Initially, a rapid-acting, water-soluble glucocorticoid (e.g., hydrocortisone hemisuccinate or hydrocortisone phosphate, 2 to 4 mg/kg IV; prednisolone sodium succinate, 4 to 20 mg/kg IV) should be administered. An ACTH stimulation test should be completed before administering hydrocortisone or prednisone, because these glucocorticoids are measured by the cortisol assay, causing falsely increased cortisol results. IV infusion of saline is sufficient therapy during the initial 1 or 2 hours while the ACTH stimulation test is being completed. After the initial administration of a rapid-acting glucocorticoid (i.e., hydrocortisone, prednisolone sodium succinate), we usually treat dogs and cats with dexamethasone sodium

phosphate at an initial dose of 0.05 to 0.1 mg/kg in the IV solution twice a day. IV dexamethasone treatment should be continued until oral medication can be safely given.

Currently available mineralocorticoid supplements include desoxycorticosterone pivalate (DOCP; Percorten-V; Novartis Pharmaceuticals) and fludrocortisone acetate (Florinef). Both are intended for the long-term maintenance therapy of primary adrenal insufficiency. Injectable DOCP is the preferred mineralocorticoid for the treatment of a sick dog or cat suspected of having adrenal insufficiency. The drug is usually administered at a dose of 2.2 mg/kg, either intramuscularly or subcutaneously, every 25 days initially. In an animal in an emergency hypoadrenal crisis, we administer the drug intramuscularly. The IV administration of saline solution and the intramuscular (IM) administration of DOCP correct electrolyte abnormalities in most hypoadrenal animals within 6 to 24 hours. There are no adverse reactions to a single injection of DOCP administered to dogs subsequently shown to have normal adrenocortical function. Atrial natriuretic peptide provides natural protection against hypernatremia. Fludrocortisone acetate is also an effective treatment. However, it is available only in tablet form, and most dogs and cats are too ill to receive oral therapy initially.

Most dogs and cats with acute adrenal insufficiency show dramatic clinical and biochemical improvement within 24 to 48 hours of the start of appropriate fluid and glucocorticoid therapy. Over the ensuing 2 to 4 days the animal should be gradually switched from IV fluids to the oral intake of water and food. In addition, maintenance mineralocorticoid and glucocorticoid therapy should be initiated. If the animal fails to make this transition smoothly, persistent electrolyte imbalance, insufficient glucocorticoid supplementation, a concurrent endocrinopathy (e.g., hypothyroidism), or concurrent illness (most notably renal damage resulting from poor perfusion and hypoxia caused by adrenal insufficiency) should be suspected.

### Maintenance therapy for primary adrenal insufficiency

Maintenance therapy can be initiated once the dog or cat is in stable condition in response to parenteral medication. Mineralocorticoids and usually glucocorticoids are required for maintenance of the dog or cat with primary adrenal insufficiency. The preferred mineralocorticoid supplementation is injectable DOCP, which slowly releases the hormone at a rate of 1 mg/day/25 mg suspension. The initial dosage is 2.2 mg/kg body weight, given intramuscularly or subcutaneously every 25 days. Subsequent adjustments are made on the basis of serum electrolyte concentrations, which are initially measured 12 and 25 days after each of the first two or three DOCP injections. If the dog or cat has hyponatremia or hyperkalemia, or both, on day 12, the next dose should be increased by approximately 10%. If the day 12 electrolyte profile is normal but the day 25 profile is abnormal, the interval between injections should be decreased by 48 hours. DOCP is very effective in normalizing serum electrolyte concentrations, and adverse reactions, such as those associated with fludrocortisone (see p. 809), are not observed. Most dogs (and presumably cats) receiving DOCP also require a low dose of glucocorticoids (prednisone, 0.22 mg/kg q12h initially). Drawbacks to DOCP are problems with availability and the inconvenience and expense associated with the need to make monthly visits to the veterinarian for the injection. To minimize the inconvenience and expense, the owner is routinely taught to give the injection subcutaneously in the home environment. Every third or fourth treatment, we have the owner bring the dog into the clinic for a complete physical examination, measurement of the serum electrolyte concentrations, and administration of the DOCP to ensure that problems with the administration of DOCP have not developed. The expense can also be reduced by decreasing the dosage and giving DOCP every 21 days.

Fludrocortisone acetate (Florinef) is another commonly used mineralocorticoid supplement. The initial dose is 0.02 mg/kg/day, divided into two doses, which is administered orally. Subsequent adjustments in the dose are determined on the basis of serum electrolyte concentrations, which are initially assessed every 1 to 2 weeks. The goal is to reestablish normal serum sodium and potassium concentrations. The dose of fludrocortisone acetate must typically be increased during the first 6 to 18 months of therapy. This increasing need may reflect the continuing destruction of the adrenal cortices. After this time, the dose usually plateaus and remains relatively stable.

The major drawbacks to oral therapy with fludrocortisone acetate have been the wide range in the doses required to control the serum electrolyte concentrations; the development of polyuria, polydipsia, and incontinence seen in some dogs (presumably caused by the potent glucocorticoid activity of this drug); resistance to the effects of the drug observed in some animals; and persistent mild hyperkalemia and hyponatremia, also observed in some animals. Ineffectiveness of fludrocortisone acetate should be suspected when owners report that their pet is "just not right" and hyponatremia and hyperkalemia persist despite high dosages of the mineralocorticoid supplement The concurrent administration of hydrocortisone hemisuccinate or oral salt may help alleviate the electrolyte derangements in dogs and cats in which fludrocortisone acetate, by itself, is not completely effective. Alternatively, switching to DOCP should be considered.

Glucocorticoid supplementation is initially indicated for all dogs and cats with primary adrenal insufficiency. Prednisone is given at an initial dose of 0.22 mg/kg twice a day. Over the ensuing 1 to 2 months, the dose of prednisone should gradually be reduced to the lowest amount given once a day that still prevents the signs of hypocortisolism (i.e., inappetence, vomiting, diarrhea). Approximately 50% of dogs receiving fludrocortisone ultimately do not require glucocorticoid medication, except during times of stress (e.g., boarding); if DOCP is used, the requirement for daily glucocorticoid replacement increases. All owners should have glucocorticoids available to administer to their dogs and cats in times of stress. Veterinarians should also be aware of the increased glucocorticoid requirements of hypoadrenal dogs and cats undergoing surgery or during times of illness with a non–adrenal-related disease. The glucocorticoid dose being administered should be doubled on days when increased stress is anticipated.

The most common reason for persistence of clinical signs despite appropriate treatment is inadequate glucocorticoid supplementation. When healthy and in a nonstressed environment, dogs and cats with adrenal insufficiency typically require small amounts of prednisone, if any. However, when stressed or ill, these same animals may require large amounts of prednisone (i.e., 0.5 to 1.0 mg/kg) given twice a day. Failure to provide adequate amounts of prednisone can lead to persistent and worsening lethargy, inappetance, and vomiting. The amount of prednisone required to offset the deleterious effects of stress and illness is variable and unpredictable. As such, it is always better to err on the high end of the dosage range and then gradually decrease the dosage over the ensuing 1 or 2 weeks.

### Therapy for secondary adrenal insufficiency

Therapy for secondary adrenal insufficiency involves the administration of glucocorticoids as previously described. The exception is secondary adrenal insufficiency induced by the overzealous administration of glucocorticoids or megestrol acetate, in which case therapy revolves around a gradual reduction in the dose and frequency of administration, with eventual discontinuation of the medication. Dogs and cats with secondary adrenal insufficiency should not have mineralocorticoid deficiency. The periodic measurement of serum electrolytes is advisable because primary adrenal insufficiency ultimately develops in some dogs and cats believed to have secondary adrenal insufficiency.

## Prognosis

The prognosis in dogs and cats with adrenal insufficiency is usually excellent. The most important factor in determining an animal's long-term response to therapy is owner education. If there is good client-veterinarian communication, if frequent rechecks are performed, and if owners are conscientious about carrying out therapy, dogs and cats with adrenal insufficiency can have a "normal" life expectancy.

## PHEOCHROMOCYTOMA

### Etiology

Pheochromocytoma is a catecholamine-producing tumor derived from the chromaffin cells of the adrenal medulla. Adrenal pheochromocytomas are diagnosed uncommonly in dogs and only rarely in cats and are often an incidental finding at necropsy. Pheochromocytomas are usually solitary, slow-growing tumors ranging in size from nodules of less than 0.5 cm in diameter to masses greater than 10 cm in diameter. Pheochromocytomas of both adrenal glands have also been reported. Pheochromocytoma should be considered a malignant tumor in dogs. It is common for the tumor to invade or extend into the lumen of the adjacent vena cava or entrap and compress the caudal vena cava, or both (see Fig. 53-8). Mural invasion or luminal narrowing of the aorta, renal vessels, adrenal vessels, and hepatic veins may also occur. Distant sites of metastasis include the liver, lung, regional lymph nodes, spleen, heart, kidney, bone, pancreas, and CNS. Extraadrenal pheochromocytomas (i.e., paragangliomas) have been reported but are rare in dogs and cats.

## Clinical Features

Pheochromocytomas occur most commonly in older dogs and cats (mean age, 11 years). There is no apparent sex- or breed-related predisposition.

Clinical signs and physical examination findings develop as a result of the space-occupying nature of the tumor and its metastatic lesions or as a result of the excessive secretion of catecholamines (Table 53-13). The most common clinical signs are generalized weakness and episodic collapse. The most common abnormalities identified during physical examination involve the respiratory (i.e., tachypnea, excessive panting), cardiovascular (i.e., tachycardia, cardiac arrhythmias, weak femoral pulses), and musculoskeletal (i.e., weakness, muscle wasting) systems. Excess catecholamine secretion may also cause potentially life-threatening systemic hypertension. Catecholamine secretion is sporadic and unpredictable. As such, clinical manifestations and systemic hypertension tend to be paroxysmal and are usually not evident at the time the dog is examined. Because clinical signs and physical examination findings are often vague, nonspecific, and easily associated with other disorders, pheochromocytoma is often not considered a possible differential diagnosis until an adrenal mass is identified with abdominal ultrasound (see Incidental Adrenal Mass, p. 812). Pheochromocytoma may also be an unexpected or incidental finding at necropsy; may result in sudden collapse and death from a sudden, massive, and sustained release of catecholamines by the tumor; or may cause periodic clinical signs (e.g., collapsing episodes, tachypnea, pounding heart rate), which strongly suggest pheochromocytoma at the time of initial examination. The size of a pheochromocytoma may also correlate with the presence or absence and severity of the clinical signs. Small, well-demarcated pheochromocytomas, often causing minimal enlargement of the adrenal gland, are more commonly identified as incidental findings during abdominal ultrasound or at necropsy, whereas pheochromocytomas that distort the adrenal gland and compress or invade surrounding structures often cause recognizable clinical signs that enhance the likelihood of antemortem diagnosis.

## Diagnosis

A diagnosis of pheochromocytoma requires a high index of suspicion on the part of the clinician. No consistent abnormalities in the CBC, serum biochemical panel, or urinalysis findings are seen that would raise suspicion of pheochromocytoma. A history of acute or episodic collapse, the identification of appropriate respiratory and cardiac abnormalities during physical examination, the documentation of systemic hypertension (particularly if it is paroxysmal), and identification of an adrenal mass by abdominal ultrasonography are most helpful in establishing a tentative diagnosis of pheo-

 TABLE 53-13

**Clinical Signs and Physical Examination Findings Associated with Pheochromocytomas in Dogs**

| CLINICAL SIGNS | PHYSICAL EXAMINATION FINDINGS |
|---|---|
| Intermittent weakness* | No identifiable abnormalities |
| Intermittent collapsing episodes* | Panting, tachypnea* |
| Intermittent panting* | Weakness* |
| Intermittent tachypnea* | Tachycardia* |
| Lethargy | Cardiac arrhythmias |
| Inappetence | Weak pulses |
| Vomiting | Pale mucous membranes |
| Diarrhea | Muscle wasting |
| Weight loss | Lethargy |
| Polyuria, polydipsia | Abdominal pain |
| Abdominal distention | Hemorrhage (nasal, surgery site) |
| Rear limb edema | Ascites |
| | Palpable abdominal mass |
| | Rear limb edema |

*Common signs and physical examination findings.

chromocytoma. Documentation of hypertension in the non-azotemic dog with an adrenal mass and normal adrenocortical function would be consistent with various disorders, including pheochromocytoma. Unfortunately, catecholamine secretion by the tumor, and thus systemic hypertension, tends to be episodic. Failure to document systemic hypertension in a dog with appropriate clinical signs does not rule out a diagnosis of pheochromocytoma.

The ultrasound identification of adrenomegaly (i.e., adrenal mass) with a normal-sized contralateral adrenal gland is further evidence of a pheochromocytoma. In dogs and cats with systemic hypertension, abdominal ultrasound assessment of adrenal size is perhaps the best screening test for pheochromocytoma, keeping in mind that a normal-sized adrenal gland does not rule out the diagnosis. Ultrasonography may also provide information regarding metastatic or local invasion of the mass into surrounding structures, such as the caudal vena cava. Other possibilities must be considered if an adrenal mass is identified, most notably an AT causing hyperadrenocorticism or a nonfunctional adrenal mass (Table 53-14). A pheochromocytoma and an AT can also occur simultaneously, which can pose a difficult diagnostic and therapeutic challenge. Many of the clinical signs (e.g., panting, weakness) and blood pressure alterations seen in dogs with hyperadrenocorticism (common) are similar to those seen in dogs with pheochromocytoma (uncommon). Therefore it is important to rule out hyperadrenocorticism through the performance of appropriate hormonal tests (see p. 786) before focusing on pheochromocytoma in a dog with an adrenal mass. Measurement of urinary catecholamine concentrations or their metabolites can strengthen the tentative diagnosis of pheochromocytoma. Unfortunately, these tests

TABLE 53-14

## Adrenal Tumors Reported in Dogs and Cats

|  | HORMONE SECRETED | SPECIES | CLINICAL SYNDROME | TESTS TO ESTABLISH DIAGNOSIS |
|---|---|---|---|---|
| Nonfunctional adrenal tumor | None | Dog*, cat | — | Diagnosis by exclusion<br>Histopathology |
| Functional adreno-cortical tumor | Cortisol | Dog*, cat | Hyperadrenocorticism<br>Cushing's syndrome | ACTH stimulation test—measure cortisol<br>Low dose dexamethasone suppression test |
|  | Aldosterone | Cat*, dog | Hyperaldosteronism<br>Conn's syndrome | Serum K/Na<br>ACTH stimulation—measure aldosterone |
|  | Progesterone | Cat*, dog | Mimics hyperadrenocorticism | Serum progesterone |
|  | Steroid hormone precursors<br>17-OH progesterone | Dog | Mimics hyperadrenocorticism | ACTH stimulation test—measure steroid hormone precursors |
|  | Deoxycorticosterone | Dog | Mimics hyperaldosteronism | ACTH stimulation test—measure steroid hormone precursors |
| Functional adreno-medullary tumor | Epinephrine | Dog*, cat | Pheochromocytoma | Diagnosis by exclusion<br>Histopathology |

*Species most commonly affected.

are not commonly performed in dogs and cats. As a result, the antemortem definitive diagnosis of pheochromocytoma in a dog or cat ultimately relies on the findings yielded by histologic evaluation of the surgically excised adrenal mass.

## Treatment

A period of medical therapy to reverse the effects of excessive adrenergic stimulation, followed by surgical removal of the tumor, is the treatment of choice for pheochromocytoma. The success of chemotherapy and radiation therapy in humans with pheochromocytoma has been limited, and results of the treatment of malignant pheochromocytoma with chemotherapy or radiation therapy in dogs or cats have not been reported. Mitotane is ineffective for treating tumors arising from the adrenal medulla. Long-term medical therapy is primarily designed to control excessive catecholamine secretion rather than lessen the risk of local invasion or metastasis of the tumor to other organs.

Potentially life-threatening complications are common, especially during the induction of anesthesia and manipulation of the tumor during surgery. The most worrisome complications include episodes of acute, severe hypertension (systolic arterial blood pressure >300 mm Hg), episodes of severe tachycardia (heart rate >250 beats/min) and arrhythmias, and hemorrhage. Preoperative α-adrenergic blockade is indicated to prevent severe clinical manifestations of hypertension in the preoperative period, to reverse the hypovolemia that is frequently present, and to promote a smooth anesthetic induction. Phenoxybenzamine (Dibenzyline; SmithKline Beecham)

is the drug of choice for α-adrenergic blockade. The initial dosage is 0.25 mg/kg given orally twice a day. Therapy is judged to be efficacious if the clinical signs are reduced and blood pressure is stabilized; an increase in the dose should be considered if clinical signs do not improve after 2 weeks of treatment. Currently we administer phenoxybenzamine for a minimum of 2 weeks before surgical excision of a pheochromocytoma. Complications may still occur despite prior treatment with α-adrenergic–blocking drugs. (See Suggested Readings for more information on the perioperative and surgical management of dogs with a pheochromocytoma.)

Long-term medical management is designed to control excessive catecholamine secretion. The α-adrenergic–blocking drug phenoxybenzamine (0.25 mg/kg PO q12h initially) is used to prevent severe clinical manifestations of hypertension. Propranolol may also be necessary to control tachycardia and cardiac arrhythmias. However, propranolol should never be administered without prior α-adrenergic blockade, because otherwise severe hypertension could develop.

## Prognosis

The prognosis depends in part on whether there is concurrent disease and the nature of the disease, if present; the size of the adrenal mass; whether metastasis and local invasion of the tumor have occurred; and whether perioperative complications are averted. Surgically excisable tumors carry a guarded to good prognosis. Pretreatment with an α-adrenergic blocking drug for several weeks before surgery and involvement of an experienced anesthesiologist and surgeon with expertise in adrenal surgery help minimize potentially serious perioperative complications associated with anesthesia and digital manipulation of the tumor. Medically treated dogs can live longer than a year from the time of diagnosis if the tumor is relatively small (<3 cm diameter), vascular invasion is not present, and treatment with an α-adrenergic blocking drug is effective in minimizing the deleterious effects of periodic catecholamine secretion by the tumor.

## INCIDENTAL ADRENAL MASS

During the past decade, ultrasound has become a routine diagnostic tool for the evaluation of soft-tissue structures in the abdominal cavity. One consequence of abdominal ultrasound is the unexpected finding of a seemingly incidental adrenal mass. The clinical relevance of an incidentally discovered adrenal mass is related to its malignant potential and functional status. An adrenal mass should be considered neoplastic until proven otherwise. Adrenalectomy is the treatment of choice if the mass is malignant and has not spread, but adrenalectomy may not be indicated if the mass is benign, small, and hormonally inactive. Unfortunately, it is not easy to determine if an adrenal mass is malignant or benign before surgical removal and histopathologic evaluation. Guidelines to suggest malignancy include the size of the mass, invasion of the mass into surrounding organs and blood vessels, and identification of additional mass lesions with abdominal ultrasound and thoracic radiographs. The bigger the mass, the more likely it is to be malignant and the more likely it is that metastasis has occurred, regardless of findings on abdominal ultrasound and thoracic radiographs. Cytologic evaluation of specimens obtained by ultrasound-guided fine-needle aspiration of the adrenal mass may provide guidance regarding malignancy and the origin of the mass (i.e., adrenal cortex versus medulla).

An adrenal tumor may be functional (i.e., producing and secreting a hormone) or nonfunctional. Excess secretion of cortisol, catecholamines, aldosterone, progesterone, and steroid hormone precursors have been documented in dogs and cats (see Table 53-14). The most common functional adrenal tumors secrete cortisol (i.e., adrenal-dependent hyperadrenocorticism; see p. 778) or catecholamines (i.e., pheochromocytoma; see p. 809). Aldosterone-secreting adrenal tumors causing primary hyperaldosteronism (Conn's syndrome) are rare in dogs and cats. Excessive secretion of aldosterone causes sodium retention and potassium depletion. The classic clinical manifestations of primary hyperaldosteronism are lethargy, weakness, mild hypernatremia, severe hypokalemia (<3.0 mEq/L), and systemic hypertension. The contralateral adrenal gland should be normal in size and shape on abdominal ultrasound. Documentation of increased plasma aldosterone concentrations before and after ACTH administration is used to confirm the diagnosis.

Although a functional tumor arising from the zona reticularis of the adrenal cortex could secrete excessive amounts of estrogen, progesterone, or testosterone, to date, only progesterone-secreting ATs have been documented, most notably in cats. Excessive progesterone secretion in affected cats caused diabetes mellitus and feline fragile skin syndrome, which was characterized by progressively worsening dermal and epidermal atrophy, patchy endocrine alopecia, and easily torn skin (see Fig. 53-18). The clinical features mimicked feline hyperadrenocorticism, which is the primary differential diagnosis. Results of tests of the pituitary-adrenocortical axis are normal to suppressed in cats with progesterone-secreting adrenal tumors, and the contralateral adrenal gland is normal in size and shape on abdominal ultrasound. Diagnosis requires documenting an increased plasma progesterone concentration.

Functional tumors producing excessive amounts of an intermediary in the biosynthetic pathway of adrenocortical steroids are rare in dogs and cats. A deoxycorticosterone-secreting adrenocortical carcinoma has been documented in a dog. Deoxycorticosterone is a precursor of aldosterone, has mineralocorticoid activity, and acts on the same receptors as does aldosterone. The major clinical features in this dog were weakness, marked hypokalemia, and systemic hypertension. Increased plasma deoxycorticosterone and nondetectable plasma aldosterone concentrations were documented in the dog.

Adrenal tumors secreting 17-OH-progesterone and progesterone have also been documented in dogs. 17-OH-progesterone is a precursor of cortisol. Affected dogs had clinical signs and physical examination findings suggestive of hyperadrenocorticism, results of tests to assess the pituitary-adrenocortical axis were normal or suppressed, and pre– and post–ACTH stimulation plasma 17-OH-progesterone concentrations were increased.

A thorough review of the clinical signs, physical examination findings, results of routine blood and urine tests, and performance of appropriate hormonal tests should be done to determine the functional status of an incidental adrenal mass. A urine cortisol/creatinine ratio, an ACTH stimulation test, and an LDDS test are used to rule out hyperadrenocorticism. If weakness and severe hypokalemia are present, plasma aldosterone concentrations can be measured in addition to plasma cortisol concentrations during the ACTH stimulation test. We do not routinely perform specific hormonal tests to identify pheochromocytoma. If hormonal tests for hyperadrenocorticism and serum electrolyte concentrations are normal and clinical signs suggestive of pheochromocytoma are present, we assume that the adrenal mass is a pheochromocytoma and begin treatment with an α-adrenergic antagonist (see p. 811). If hormonal tests for hyperadrenocorticism and serum electrolyte concentrations are normal, clinical signs suggestive of pheochromocytoma are not present, and adrenalectomy is planned, we still assume that the adrenal mass is a pheochromocytoma and begin phenoxybenzamine treatment before adrenalectomy.

Adrenalectomy may or may not be indicated if hormonal tests for hyperadrenocorticism and serum electrolyte concentrations are normal and clinical signs and systemic hypertension suggestive of pheochromocytoma are not present.

In theory, adrenalectomy offers the best chance for long-term survival of the dog or cat, assuming that the mass is a malignant tumor. However, when considering adrenalectomy, the clinician should also consider the age of the dog or cat, the severity of concurrent illness, the size and invasive nature of the mass, and the probability for metastasis. Surgery is generally not indicated in old dogs and cats, especially if concurrent illness raises the anesthetic risk to an unacceptable level, when metastasis has been identified, or if serious complications are likely because of the size or invasive nature of the mass. In addition, adrenalectomy may not be indicated when the mass is small (<3 cm diameter) and nonfunctional and the dog or cat is healthy. An alternative approach in these cases is to determine the rate of growth of the mass by repeating abdominal ultrasound initially at 2, 4, and 6 months. If the adrenal mass does not change in size, the time between ultrasound evaluations can be increased to every 4 to 6 months. However, if the adrenal mass is increasing in size, adrenalectomy should be considered.

## *Suggested Readings*

Bojrab MJ: *Current techniques in small animal surgery,* ed 4, Philadelphia, 1998, William & Wilkins.

Feldman EC, Nelson RW: *Canine and feline endocrinology and reproduction,* ed 3, Philadelphia, 2004, WB Saunders.

Fossum TW: *Small animal surgery,* ed 2, St Louis, 2002, Mosby.

#### HYPERADRENOCORTICISM IN DOGS

Barthez PY et al: Ultrasonographic evaluation of the adrenal glands in dogs, *J Am Vet Med Assoc* 207:1180, 1995.

Bertoy EH et al: One-year follow-up evaluation of magnetic resonance imaging of the brain in dogs with pituitary-dependent hyperadrenocorticism, *J Am Vet Med Assoc* 208:1268, 1996.

Feldman EC et al: Use of low- and high-dose dexamethasone tests for distinguishing pituitary-dependent from adrenal tumor hyperadrenocorticism in dogs, *J Am Vet Med Assoc* 209:772, 1996.

Hoerauf A et al: Ultrasonographic characteristics of both adrenal glands in 15 dogs with functional adrenocortical tumors, *J Am Anim Hosp Assoc* 35:193, 1999.

Huang H et al: Iatrogenic hyperadrenocorticism in 28 dogs, *J Am Anim Hosp Assoc* 35:200, 1999.

Kaplan AJ et al: Effects of disease on the results of diagnostic tests for use in detecting hyperadrenocorticism in dogs, *J Am Vet Med Assoc* 207:445, 1995.

Kintzer PP et al: Treatment and long-term follow-up of 205 dogs with hyperadrenocorticism, *J Vet Intern Med* 11:43, 1997.

Meij BP et al: Results of transsphenoidal hypophysectomy in 52 dogs with pituitary-dependent hyperadrenocorticism, *Vet Surg* 27:246, 1998.

Reusch CE et al: The efficacy of L-deprenyl in dogs with pituitary-dependent hyperadrenocorticism, *J Vet Intern Med* 13:291, 1999.

Ruckstuhl NS et al: Results of clinical examinations, laboratory tests, and ultrasonography in dogs with pituitary-dependent hyperadrenocorticism treated with trilostane, *Am J Vet Res* 63:506, 2002.

Theon AP et al: Megavoltage irradiation of pituitary macrotumors in dogs with neurologic signs, *J Am Vet Med Assoc* 213:225, 1998.

Van Sluijs FJ et al: Results of adrenalectomy in 36 dogs with hyperadrenocorticism caused by adrenocortical tumor, *Vet Q* 17:113, 1995.

Zimmer C et al: Ultrasonographic examination of the adrenal gland and evaluation of the hypophyseal-adrenal axis in 20 cats, *J Small Anim Pract* 41:156, 2000.

#### HYPERADRENOCORTICISM IN CATS

Duesberg CA et al: Adrenalectomy for treatment of hyperadrenocorticism in cats: 10 cases (1988-1992), *J Am Vet Med Assoc* 207:1066, 1995.

Meij BP et al: Transsphenoidal hypophysectomy for treatment of pituitary-dependent hyperadrenocorticism in 7 cats, *Vet Surg* 30:72, 2001.

#### HYPOADRENOCORTICISM

Lifton SJ et al: Glucocorticoid deficient hypoadrenocorticism in dogs: 18 cases (1986-1995), *J Am Vet Med Assoc* 209:2076, 1996.

Lynn RC et al: Efficacy of microcrystalline desoxycorticosterone pivalate for treatment of hypoadrenocorticism in dogs, *J Am Vet Med Assoc* 202:392, 1993.

Peterson ME et al: Pretreatment clinical and laboratory findings in dogs with hypoadrenocorticism: 225 cases (1979-1993), *J Am Vet Med Assoc* 208:85, 1996.

#### PHEOCHROMOCYTOMA

Gilson SD et al: Pheochromocytoma in 50 dogs, *J Vet Intern Med* 8:228, 1994.

Von Dehn BJ et al: Pheochromocytoma and hyperadrenocorticism in dogs: six cases (1982-1992), *J Am Vet Med Assoc* 207:322, 1995.

#### INCIDENTAL ADRENAL MASS

Rossmeisl JH et al: Hyperadrenocorticism and hyperprogesteronemia in a cat with an adrenocortical adenocarcinoma, *J Am Anim Hosp Assoc* 36:512, 2000.

Syme HM et al: Hyperadrenocorticism associated with excessive sex hormone production by an adrenocortical tumor in two dogs, *J Am Vet Med Assoc* 219:1725, 2001.

## Drugs Used in Endocrine Disorders

| GENERIC NAME (TRADE NAME) | PURPOSE | RECOMMENDED DOSE | |
|---|---|---|---|
| | | **DOG** | **CAT** |
| Acarbose (Precose) | Treat canine diabetes mellitus | 12.5-25 mg/dog PO initially and given with meal | Not applicable |
| Aminoglutethimide (Cytadren) | Treat feline hyperadrenocorticism | Not applicable | 30 mg/cat PO q12h |

*Continued*

## Drugs Used in Endocrine Disorders—cont'd

| GENERIC NAME (TRADE NAME) | PURPOSE | RECOMMENDED DOSE | |
| --- | --- | --- | --- |
| | | DOG | CAT |
| Calcium-injectable and oral preps | Treat hypocalcemia, hypoparathyroidism | See Table 50-6, p. 688 | See Table 50-6, p. 688 |
| Carbimazole (Neo-Mercazole) | Treat feline hyperthyroidism | Not applicable | 5 mg PO q8h initially |
| Chlorothiazide (Diuril) | Treat central/renal diabetes insipidus | 20-40 mg/kg PO q12h | 20-40 mg/kg PO |
| Chlorpropamide (Diabinese) | Treat partial central diabetes insipidus | 5-20 mg/kg PO q12h | Unknown |
| Desmopressin (DDAVP) | Treat central diabetes insipidus | 1-4 drops of nasal spray in eye q12-48h; 0.1 mg tablets PO q8h | 1-4 drops of nasal spray in eye q12-48h; 0.1 mg tablets/q8-12h |
| Desoxycorticosterone pivalate (DOCP; Percorten-V) | Treat hypoadrenocorticism | 2.2 mg/kg IM or SC q25d | 2.2 mg/kg IM or SC q25d |
| Dexamethasone sodium phosphate | Treat acute Addisonian crisis | 0.05-0.1 mg/kg in fluids q12h | 0.05-0.1 mg/kg in fluids q12h |
| Diazoxide (Proglycem) | Supportive treatment for β cell tumor | 5 mg/kg PO q12h initially; increase as needed | Unknown |
| Diethylstilbesterol | Treat estrogen-responsive dermatosis of spayed female dogs | 0.1-1.0 mg PO q24h 3 wk/mo; once dog responds, 0.1-1 mg q4-7d | Not applicable |
| Doxorubicin (Adriamycin) | Treat canine thyroid neoplasia | 30 mg/m² BSA IV q3-6wk | Not applicable |
| Fludrocortisone acetate (Florinef) | Treat hypoadrenocorticism | 0.01 mg/kg PO q12h initially | 0.05-0.1 mg/cat PO q12h |
| Glipizide (Glucotrol) | Treat feline NIDDM | Not applicable | 2.5-5 mg/cat PO q12h |
| Glucagon USP | Treat hypoglycemia caused by beta cell neoplasia | 5-10 ng/kg/min as continuous IV infusion; adjust dose to effect | Unknown |
| Glyburide (Diabeta, Micronase) | Treat feline NIDDM | Not applicable | 0.625-1.25 mg/cat PO q24h |
| Growth hormone—porcine origin | Treat growth hormone–responsive dermatosis Treat pituitary dwarfism | 0.1 IU/kg SC 3 times/wk for 4 to 6 wk | Unknown |
| Hydrocortisone sodium succinate (Solu-Cortef) | Treat acute Addisonian crisis | 2-4 mg/kg IV, then administer dexamethasone in IV fluids | 2-4 mg/kg IV, then administer dexamethasone in IV fluids |
| Insulin | Treat diabetic ketoacidosis Treat diabetes mellitus | See Table 52-15, p. 765 See Table 52-5, p. 734, and p. 733 of text | See Table 52-15, p. 765 See Table 52-5, p. 734, and p. 752 of text |
| | Supportive treatment for hyperkalemia | See Table 55-7, p. 834 | See Table 55-7, p. 834 |
| Ketoconazole (Nizoral) | Treat hyperadrenocorticism | 10-15 mg/kg PO q12h | 10-15 mg/kg PO q12h |
| L-Deprenyl (Eldepryl) | Treat canine hyperadrenocorticism | 1 mg/kg PO q24h initially | Not applicable |

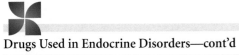

Drugs Used in Endocrine Disorders—cont'd

| GENERIC NAME (TRADE NAME) | PURPOSE | RECOMMENDED DOSE | |
|---|---|---|---|
| | | DOG | CAT |
| Megestrol acetate (Ovaban) | Treat feline endocrine alopecia | Not applicable | 2.5-5 mg/cat PO q48h; once cat responds, then q7-14d |
| Melatonin | Treat congenital adrenal hyperplasia-like syndrome | 3-6 mg PO q12-24h | Not applicable |
| Metformin (Glucophage) | Treat feline NIDDM | Not applicabl | 10-25 mg/cat PO q12-24h |
| Methimazole (Tapazole) | Treat hyperthyroidism | 2.5 mg/kg PO q12h initially; increase q2-4wk to effect | 2.5 mg/cat PO q24h initially; increase q2-4wk to effect |
| Methyltestosterone | Treat testosterone-responsive dermatosis | 1 mg/kg (max, 30 mg) PO q48h; once dog responds, then q4-7d | Not applicable |
| Metyrapone (Metopirone) | Treat feline hyperadrenocorticism | Not applicable | 65 mg/kg PO q12h |
| Mitotane (o,p'DDD; Lysodren) | Treat canine hyperadrenocorticism | Induction: 12-25 mg/kg PO q12h to effect  Maintenance: 25-50 mg/kg PO once weekly initially | Not applicable |
| Phenoxybenzamine (Dibenzyline) | Supportive treatment for pheochromocytoma | 0.25 mg/kg PO q12h initially | Unknown |
| Prednisone | Chronic treatment of hypoadrenocorticism | 0.2-0.5 mg/kg PO q12h initially | 2.5-5.0 mg/cat PO q12-24h initially |
| | Supportive treatment for β cell tumor | 0.25 mg/kg PO q12h initially; increase as needed | 0.25 mg/kg PO q12h initially; increase as needed |
| Prednisolone sodium succinate (Solu-Delta-Cortef) | Treat acute Addisonian crisis | 4-20 mg/kg IV, then administer dexamethasone in IV fluids | 4-20 mg/kg IV, then administer dexamethasone in IV fluids |
| Propylthiouracil (PTU) | Treat hyperthyroidism | 50 mg/dog PO q8-12h | 50 mg/cat PO q8-12h |
| Sodium levothyroxine-synthetic T$_4$ | Treat hypothyroidism | 0.02 mg/kg PO q12h initially | 0.05-0.1 mg/cat PO q12-24h |
| Sodium liothyronine-synthetic T$_3$ | Treat hypothyroidism | 4-6 μg/kg PO q8h initially | 25 μg/cat PO q8-12h |
| Somatostatin (Sandostatin, Octreotide) | Supportive treatment for β cell tumor | 10-40 μg/dog SC q8-12h | Unknown |
| Streptozotocin | Treat canine β cell tumor | 500 mg/m$^2$ BSA IV during saline diuresis q3wk; see Table 52-18 and p. 774 | Not applicable |
| Trilostane (Modrenal) | Treat hyperadrenocorticism | If dog weighs: 5-20 kg, give 60 mg PO q24h  20-40 kg, give 120 mg PO q24h | See Table 50-7, p. 689 |
| Vitamin D preparations | Treat hypoparathyroidism | See Table 50-7, p. 689 | See Table 50-7, p. 689 |

CHAPTER 54

# Disorders of Metabolism

Denise A. Elliott

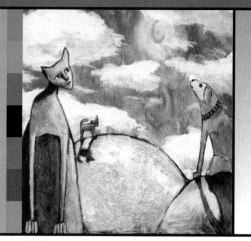

## CHAPTER OUTLINE

POLYPHAGIA WITH WEIGHT LOSS, 816
OBESITY, 817
HYPERLIPIDEMIA, 822

## POLYPHAGIA WITH WEIGHT LOSS

In most dogs and cats, polyphagia is usually accompanied by weight gain, and weight loss is accompanied by partial or complete anorexia. In some, however, polyphagia with concurrent weight loss is the presenting owner complaint. The most common cause of polyphagia and weight loss is inadequate caloric intake (Table 54-1). Daily caloric needs may not be met if inadequate quantities of food are being fed or if the diet is not balanced or is of poor quality. Alternatively, the owner may not recognize changes in nutritional needs (e.g., during pregnancy and lactation and at times of strenuous exercise, such as during hunting season) and may continue to feed the animal at previously adequate caloric levels.

Endocrinopathies and gastrointestinal tract disorders also cause polyphagia and weight loss in some dogs and cats (see Table 54-1) as a result of an increase in basal metabolism (hyperthyroidism), inadequate assimilation of dietary nutrients (gastrointestinal tract disorders), or inappropriate use of nutrients (diabetes mellitus). Gastrointestinal tract disorders include parasitism, pancreatic exocrine insufficiency, infiltrative bowel disorders, lymphangiectasia, and neoplasia, most notably lymphoma. In most of these disorders, the history and physical findings usually provide valuable clues to the diagnosis. For example, polyuria and polydipsia are common signs in diabetes mellitus. A thyroid nodule is usually palpable in dogs and cats with hyperthyroidism. Bulky, voluminous stools are noted in animals with pancreatic exocrine insufficiency. Diarrhea and vomiting may occur in animals with gastrointestinal tract disorders, and palpation of the abdomen may reveal abnormal loops of intestine and mesenteric lymph-adenopathy. The last condition may be discernible in animals with any of the infiltrative diseases but is especially noticeable in those with gastrointestinal tract lymphoma, eosinophilic enteritis, or histoplasmosis.

In addition to routine questions posed to the owner, the clinician should assess the type of diet, daily caloric intake, feeding routines, and competition for food from other dogs or cats. Daily caloric requirements in dogs and cats are quite variable and depend on numerous factors, such as the age of the animal and the amount of daily physical activity. Approximate daily caloric requirements in dogs and cats are 60 to 85 kcal of metabolizable energy (ME) per kilogram of body weight, with greater daily caloric requirements in younger dogs and cats and in smaller breeds of dogs. However, the daily caloric requirements in any individual dog or cat may vary by as much as 50% more or less than this average. The daily caloric intake can be estimated by dividing the number of calories currently being fed by the body weight of the dog or cat. The approximate caloric content of commercial dry dog and cat food is 300 kcal/cup (0.25 L), that of commercial canned dog food is 500 kcal/14 oz (400 g) can, and that of commercial canned cat food is 200 kcal/6 oz (170 g) can.

A complete blood count, serum biochemistry panel, measurement of baseline thyroxine concentration, urinalysis, and fecal examination for parasites should be done if the history and physical findings are unremarkable. Results of these tests usually help identify additional specific diagnostic tests that may be required to establish a definitive diagnosis (see Table 54-1). Inadequate nutrition should be suspected if the initial blood test results are unremarkable. Changes in the type of diet, daily caloric intake, and feeding routine should be made to ensure that the animal has an adequate caloric intake of a palatable and nutritionally complete diet. The animal's body weight should be determined 2 and 4 weeks after the start of an appropriate diet. The resolution of signs and weight gain confirm the diagnosis. Failure to gain weight indicates problems with owner compliance or the presence of occult disease, most likely disease involving the gastrointestinal tract.

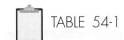

TABLE 54-1

Differential Diagnosis for Polyphagia and Weight Loss

| ETIOLOGY | DEFINITIVE DIAGNOSTIC TESTS |
| --- | --- |
| Inadequate nutrition | Response to diet change |
| Hyperthyroidism | Baseline $T_4$ and free $T_4$ concentration |
| Diabetes mellitus | Blood glucose concentration and urinalysis |
| Gastrointestinal disease | |
| Parasitism | Fecal examination, trial therapy |
| Infiltrative bowel disease: plasmacytic, lymphocytic, eosinophilic lymphosarcoma | Intestinal biopsy |
| Histoplasmosis | Intestinal biopsy, serology |
| Lymphangiectasia | Intestinal biopsy |
| Pancreatic exocrine insufficiency | Serum trypsinlike immunoreactivity, response to therapy |
| Protein-losing nephropathy | Urinalysis, urine protein/creatine ratio |
| Hypothalamic mass | Computed tomography |
| | Magnetic resonance imaging |

## OBESITY

Obesity is a clinical syndrome that involves the excess accumulation of body fat. Obesity is considered the most common form of malnutrition in small animal practice. Indeed, surveys suggest that 25% to 40% of cats and dogs presented to veterinary clinics are obese. The significance of obesity pertains to its role in the pathogenesis of a variety of diseases and to its ability to exacerbate preexisting disease. Obesity has been associated with an increased incidence of arthritis, diabetes mellitus, hepatic lipidosis, feline lower urinary tract disease (FLUTD), urine incontinence in spayed bitches, constipation, dermatitis, cardiovascular problems, respiratory problems, and increased anesthetic and surgical risk (Table 54-2). In addition, Scarlett and colleague (1998) found a threefold increase in risk of death in obese middle-aged cats when compared to the risk in lean middle-aged cats.

### Etiology

Obesity develops when energy intake consistently exceeds daily energy expenditure. There are numerous environmental and social factors that contribute to the formation of obesity (Table 54-3). These include decreased daily exercise as a result of confinement to the house and overfeeding of the pet by the client. Owners may overfeed their pet because a good appetite is a sign of good health, they may use food as a palliative agent when they leave the pet on its own, they may replace exercise with food, and they often indulge begging behavior because it is regarded as "cute." There is also a tendency to feed the same amount of food each day despite changes in energy requirements and the energy density of the diet. Daily energy requirements vary according to the environmental temperature, the life stage of the pet (i.e., growth, pregnancy, lactation, adult maintenance, old age), and the activity level of the pet. Therefore it is necessary to adjust the amount of food fed according to these factors.

TABLE 54-2

Potential Adverse Effects of Obesity

Problems with ambulation—aggravation of joint disease, intervertebral disk disease
Problems with respiration—impaired lung compliance, pickwickian syndrome
Cardiovascular disease and systemic hypertension
Exercise intolerance
Carbohydrate intolerance—predisposition for diabetes mellitus
Hyperlipidemia
Hepatic lipidosis
Predisposition for pancreatitis
Problems with constipation
Predisposition for feline lower urinary tract disease
Predisposition for urinary incontinence in spayed female dogs
Predisposition for reproductive problems—dystocia
Predisposition for dermatologic problems—seborrhea, pyoderma
Increased surgical and anesthetic risk
Increased susceptibility to infectious diseases(?)

Feeding errors also arise when an owner purchases a different type of food that has a higher energy density and continues to feed the same volume of food on a daily basis. Overfeeding may also arise if the feeding guidelines provided by pet food manufacturers are incorrect. In some situations, owners are simply not aware that they are overfeeding their pet. Ad libitum feeding may also predispose to overeating, particularly if the pet is bored and inactive. Likewise, highly palatable diets encourage overconsumption. Snacks and treats are a significant silent contributor to excess daily caloric intake.

TABLE 54-3

## Causes of Obesity in Cats and Dogs

**Primary Obesity**

Excess caloric intake
    Inappropriate feeding practices
    Inadequate feeding guidelines
    Ad libitum feeding
Reduced energy expenditure
Genetic predisposition
Obese owner

**Secondary Obesity**

Hypothyroidism
Hyperadrenocorticism
Hyperinsulinism
Acromegaly
Hypopituitarism
Hypothalamic dysfunction
Drugs
    Glucocorticoids
    Progestagens
    Phenobarbital
    Primidone

 TABLE 54-4

## Body Condition Scoring (BCS) System for Cats and Dogs Using a 5-Point System

| | |
|---|---|
| Thin (BCS 1/5) | Underweight; no obvious body fat |
| Lean (BCS 2/5) | Skeletal structure visible; little body fat |
| Optimum (BCS 3/5) | Rib cage easily palpable but not showing; moderate amount of body fat |
| Overweight (BCS 4/5) | Rib cage barely palpable; body weight more than normal |
| Obese (BCS 5/5) | Rib cage not palpable; large amount of body fat; physical impairment due to excess body fat |

Obese owners are an additional risk factor for obesity in pets. Lack of exercise by the owner may contribute to lack of exercise in the pet, and the consumption of high-fat foods by the owner may increase the likelihood that these scraps are fed to the pet. In addition, it is likely that obese owners simply do not recognize obesity as a problem in their pet.

There are genetic differences between animals such that some animals have significantly lower energy requirements and simply require fewer calories per day to maintain their ideal body weight. These genetic differences may be reflected by the increased propensity of certain dog breeds to gain weight. Breeds commonly recognized at risk for obesity include the Labrador Retriever, Golden Retriever, Cocker Spaniel, Collie, Dachshund, Cairn Terrier, Shetland Sheepdog, Beagle, Cavalier King Charles Spaniel, and Basset Hound. Neutering has been associated with an increased risk of obesity. It has been suggested that hormonal alterations secondary to neutering may alter energy expenditure and the regulation of food intake. Obesity has been reported to be more common in female neutered dogs and male neutered cats.

Obesity is less likely to result from a disease process or drug. Indeed, it has been suggested that less than 5% of obesity is due to a disease or drug. Endocrine abnormalities associated with obesity include hypothyroidism, hyperadrenocorticism, hyperinsulinism, and acromegaly. Drugs such as progestagens and corticosteroids have been associated with the development of obesity.

### Diagnosis

Obesity is defined as a "pathological condition characterized by an accumulation of fat much in excess of that required for optimal body function" (Mayer, 1973). However, what is an excess amount of body fat, and what is an acceptable amount? To answer these questions, we need to accurately determine the amount of body fat. Body fat can be assessed by techniques including morphometric measurements, dilutional techniques, bioelectrical impedance analysis, dual energy x-ray absorptiometry, densitometry, computed tomography, magnetic resonance imaging, determination of total body electrical conductivity, determination of total body potassium, and neutron activation analysis. Although numerous methods exist to determine body fat, measurement of body weight, body condition scoring (BCS), and morphometric measurements remain the most clinically useful techniques in small animal practice.

Measurement of body weight is the simplest technique available and should be included in the examination of every animal. Body weight provides a rough measure of total body energy stores, and changes in weight parallel energy and protein balance.

BCS provides a quick and simple subjective assessment of the animal's body condition. The two most commonly used scoring systems in small animal practice are a 5-point system where a BCS of 3 is considered ideal and a 9-point system where a BCS of 5 is considered ideal. Likewise, pets can be classified as being thin, lean, optimum weight, overweight, or obese (Table 54-4). The technique of BCS does depend on operator interpretation and does not provide any precise quantitative information concerning alteration in fat-free or lean body mass relative to fat mass.

Height and circumferential measurements of the abdomen, hip, thigh, and upper arm are commonly used to estimate the percent body fat in humans. Circumferential measurements have also been developed to estimate the percent body fat in cats. The Feline Body Mass Index (FBMI) is determined by measuring the rib cage circumference at the level of the ninth cranial rib and determining the leg index measurement (LIM), which is the distance from the patella to the calcanealtuber (Fig. 54-1, *A* and *B*). The percent body fat can be calculated as $1.5 - 9$ (rib cage measurement minus LIM) or determined by consulting a reference chart (Fig. 54-2). Cats with more than 30% body fat are candidates for a weight loss program. The FBMI is a very simple, yet objective tool for determining the body fat content of the cat. In addition, it

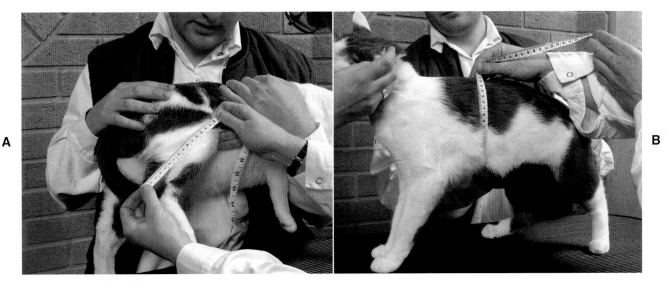

**FIG 54-1**
**A,** Length of the lower leg (LIM) from the middle of the patella. **B,** Measurement of the rib cage circumference.

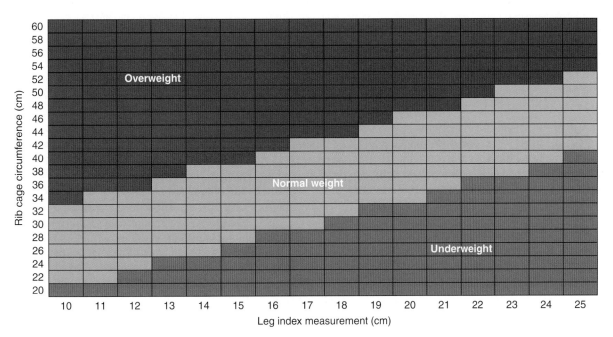

**FIG 54-2**
Feline Body Mass Index (FBMI).

is particularly valuable for convincing clients that their cat is indeed overweight and in need of weight loss. Pelvic circumference in relation to the distance from hock to stifle has been shown to predict body fat in dogs.

### Treatment

Once it has been determined that a pet is overweight or obese, a thorough dietary history should be obtained to calculate the daily caloric intake of the pet. Information that should be gathered includes the following:

- The name, manufacturer, and type (i.e., canned versus dry) of the current diet

- The amount of the diet that is fed each day (cans versus cups [250 g] of food)
- The method of feeding (ad libitum versus meal fed)
- The person responsible for feeding the pet
- Additional persons who may feed the pet (especially children, elderly parents, or friendly neighbors)
- The number and type of snacks or human foods given each day
- The potential access to foods for other pets

The pet's current body weight should be recorded, and the final ideal body weight of the pet should be calculated. The ideal body weight of the pet can be estimated either by

TABLE 54-5

Level of Key Nutrients in Selected Commercial Diets Suitable for Weight Loss in Dogs*

| | TYPE | PROTEIN (g/1000 kcal) | FAT (g/1000 kcal) | FIBER (g/1000 kcal) | ME (kcal/can/cup) |
|---|---|---|---|---|---|
| WALTHAM Canine Veterinary Diet Calorie Control | Dry | 80 | 29 | 9 | 226/cup |
| WALTHAM Canine Veterinary Diet Calorie Control in Gel | Can | 132 | 73 | 8 | 212/12.7 oz |
| Purina Veterinary Diets OM Overweight Management | Dry | 104 | 22 | 35 | 276/cup |
| Purina Veterinary Diets OM Overweight Management | Can | 178 | 34 | 77 | 189/12.5 oz |
| Hill's Prescription Diet Canine r/d | Dry | 84 | 29 | 77 | 205/cup |
| Hill's Prescription Diet Canine r/d | Can | 85 | 28 | 73 | 292/14.25 oz |
| Eukanuba Veterinary Diets Nutritional Weight Loss Formula Restricted-Calorie | Dry | 63 | 19 | 5 | 238/cup |

*ME*, Metabolizable energy.
*Information obtained from manufacturers' published information.

reviewing the medical record for the body weight when the pet was in an ideal body condition or by using breed-specific body weight charts. The optimum body weight for cats is generally between 3.5 and 5 kg. It is very important to set realistic and obtainable goals for weight loss in order to maintain client compliance. If the ideal body weight is below 15% of the current body weight, then it is crucial to use a stepwise process to gradually achieve the ideal body weight. The pet's initial goal should be set at a 15% body weight loss. Once this goal has been achieved, a new target body weight can be selected until the pet has reached the ideal body weight.

There are several valid reasons for using a stepwise approach. The pet's daily caloric intake will be determined on the basis of the target body weight. If the target weight is extremely low, then the total daily caloric intake will be low. Consequently, the pet will receive a very small allowance of food, which is most likely to encourage begging behavior and garbage scavenging. These undesirable behaviors will jeopardize owner compliance. In addition, the pet will lose weight rapidly. Extremely rapid weight loss is considered unhealthy and has been associated with a greater loss of lean body mass compared with fat mass. Furthermore, rapid weight loss is most likely to result in a rebound weight gain effect following cessation of the program.

To achieve a 15% body weight loss, cats can be fed 30 × [initial body weight (kg)] kcal per day and dogs can be fed 55 × [initial body weight (kg)$^{0.75}$] kcal per day. When fed at this level, cats will achieve a 15% body weight loss in 18 weeks, and dogs will achieve a 15% body weight loss in 12 weeks. The calculated amount of calories to achieve a 15% body weight loss should be compared with the current daily caloric intake obtained from the dietary history. Most pets will be consuming more calories than required for a 15%

body weight loss. However, if the amount of calories to achieve weight loss is actually less than the current daily caloric intake, then the dietary history should be reevaluated to search for additional calories. If no additional daily calories are identified, then the daily caloric intake of the pet should be reduced by 15% to 20%.

Once the daily caloric requirement to achieve a 15% body weight loss has been calculated, consideration should be given to the type of diet to feed. There are essentially two main dietary options: either feed a reduced amount of the regular maintenance diet or feed a diet that has been specifically formulated for weight reduction. It is not advisable to feed less of the regular diet, because this was the diet that resulted in the problem in the first place. More important, feeding a maintenance diet increases the risk of nutrient deficiency and unhealthy weight loss. Canine and feline maintenance diets are formulated according to energy intake. This means that if a dog or cat eats its daily energy requirement, it will automatically consume the required amounts of additional essential nutrients, such as amino acids, vitamins, minerals, and essential fatty acids. By feeding less of the maintenance diet, one is not only reducing the amount of energy but is also reducing the amount of protein, vitamins, minerals, and essential fatty acids and thereby risking malnutrition. Conversely, diets that have been specifically formulated for weight reduction have been formulated such that they contain more essential nutrients relative to the energy content of the diet. This means that the pet will receive the required amounts of nutrients such as proteins, vitamins, minerals, and essential fatty acids even though the pet is ingesting less energy.

Diets formulated specifically for weight reduction vary according to the fiber and protein content (Tables 54-5 and

TABLE 54-6

Level of Key Nutrients in Selected Commercial Diets Suitable for Weight Loss in Cats*

| | TYPE | PROTEIN (g/1000 kcal) | FAT (g/1000 kcal) | FIBER (g/1000 kcal) | ME (kcal/can/cup) |
|---|---|---|---|---|---|
| WALTHAM Feline Veterinary Diet Calorie Control | Dry | 128 | 28 | 13 | 208/8 oz |
| WALTHAM Feline Veterinary Diet Calorie Control in Gel | Can | 149 | 68 | 7 | 99/5.8 oz |
| Purina Veterinary Diets OM Overweight Management | Dry | 112 | 25 | 24 | 326/8 oz |
| Purina Veterinary Diets OM Overweight Management | Can | 113 | 37 | 26 | 150/5.5 oz |
| Hill's Prescription Diet Feline r/d | Dry | 114 | 29 | 44 | 263/cup |
| Hill's Prescription Diet Feline r/d | Can | 114 | 28 | 55 | 116/5.5 oz |
| Eukanuba Veterinary Diets Nutritional Weight Loss Formula Restricted-Calorie | Dry | 83 | 24 | 5 | 298/cup |

*ME*, Metabolizable energy.
*Information obtained from manufacturers' published information.

54-6). Traditionally, high-fiber diets have been suggested for weight loss. Fiber is used as a bulking agent to provide a satiating effect. However, recent research has suggested that fiber does not increase satiety. Rather, a high amount of fiber reduces the digestibility of the diet, increases the amount of fecal material, and increases the amount of water lost into the feces. Increases in fecal volume may not necessarily present a problem to owners of cats and small dogs; however, a fourfold increase in fecal volume is a substantial problem for owners of large-breed dogs. An increase in fecal water loss reduces the amount of water available to dilute urine. The higher urine specific gravity may predispose susceptible cats to the development of lower urinary tract disease. Furthermore, high-fiber diets are not palatable. If the pet will not eat the diet, client compliance will be reduced. In addition, inappetence in cats increases the risk of developing hepatic lipidosis.

High-protein diets have been reported to increase the proportion of fat loss while preserving or, indeed, increasing the lean body mass. The lean body mass is the most metabolically active portion of the body and includes skeletal muscle tissues. Preservation of lean body mass in humans has been shown to facilitate successful long-term maintenance of the ideal body weight once weight loss has been achieved.

Carnitine is an amino acid that is vital for energy metabolism. Carnitine facilitates the movement of long-chain fatty acids across the mitochondrial membrane, where they are used for energy production. Carnitine supplementation has been suggested to facilitate weight loss. However, a recent study evaluating the effect of carnitine supplementation on body weight loss failed to demonstrate any benefits (Center and colleagues, 2000). Cats that received carnitine supplementation lost the same percentage of body weight

in the same period of time as cats that did not receive carnitine supplementation. In addition, neither group of cats developed hepatic lipidosis.

Once the daily caloric intake has been calculated and the appropriate weight reduction diet chosen, the method of feeding should be determined. Ideally, the pet should be meal fed rather than ad libitum fed. The number of feedings per day can be selected to suit the client's schedule, but two to four meals per day is adequate. One member of the household should be selected to feed the pet. This will reduce inadvertent overfeeding by additional family members. The owner should be instructed to eliminate treats completely. If this is met with resistance, the owner should be instructed to limit the number of treats to less than 10% of the daily caloric intake. Ideally, low-calorie treats should be selected. Ice cubes are a valuable energy-free treat that many dogs enjoy. It is also important to modify the behavior of the owner such that the pet should not be allowed in the kitchen or dining room during meal preparation or eating. This will reduce the likelihood that the client will give the pet human snacks, which are generally high in calories. In addition, the client should inform and enlist the support of both family members and neighbors so that they do not unknowingly give the pet additional calories. In some cases it may be useful for the client to use a food diary to record the amount of food and snacks fed each day. For other clients this technique is often met with resistance and should not be considered.

Multicat households in which one cat is obese and the remainder are of normal body weight or are lean can present some management problems. Ideally, cats should be fed in separate rooms, but this is not always possible. In general, fat cats cannot jump. Hence, it may be useful to place the healthy cats' food on an elevated bench so that the healthy cats can jump up to consume their meals. Alternatively, a large cardboard box can be obtained. A small cat hole is cut into the box that will allow the cats with a normal body weight to fit but restricts the entry of the fat cat. The normal-weight cats are then fed in the box.

In addition to reducing the daily caloric intake, every effort should be made to increase the daily energy expenditure by encouraging exercise. Toys that the cat or dog can chase and play with should be encouraged. Laser pointers are particularly useful for encouraging play for cats. Ideally, dogs should receive two 20-minute walks per day. Swimming is an equally effective exercise, particularly for dogs with osteoarthritis. Providing the client with written instructions for weight loss will typically improve both compliance and success. Photographing the pet before institution of the weight reduction program will help clients to see the effects of the weight loss on their pet. Institution of reward boards or incentive programs will also increase compliance with the weight reduction program.

Pets on weight reduction programs should be reevaluated every 2 weeks. The body weight, BCS, and/or FBMI should be recorded. The dietary history should be reviewed. Ideally, cats should achieve about a 1% body weight loss per week. More rapid weight loss in cats increases the risk of hepatic lipidosis. Dogs should achieve a 1% to 2% body weight loss per week. If the rate of weight loss exceeds a 2% body weight loss per week, then the amount of calories fed to the pet should be increased by 10% to 15%. If there has not been any weight loss, the dietary history should be reevaluated for additional calories. If none are found, then the daily caloric intake should be further reduced by 10% to 15%.

Once the ideal body weight of the pet has been achieved, then the daily caloric intake can be adjusted to maintain optimal body weight. The diet can be altered to one formulated for weight maintenance or a "light" diet. The pet should be reevaluated every 2 to 3 months following weight loss to ensure that weight management is maintained and that the pet is not gaining weight on the new diet.

### Prevention

The key to obesity management is prevention. Energy requirements decrease when the animal is spayed or castrated. Therefore prevention should begin at the time that the pet is neutered. Owners should be counseled about the risk factors of obesity (male neutered cats; female neutered dogs; inactive, indoor lifestyle; inappropriate feeding practices) and the consequences of obesity (e.g., increased incidence of FLUTD, diabetes mellitus, arthritis). It is important that owners be instructed on both how to feed their pet and how to regularly determine the pet's body condition such that they can maintain the ideal body condition of their pet. Weight education should be reinforced at each annual health examination.

## HYPERLIPIDEMIA

Hyperlipidemia is defined as an increased concentration of triglycerides (hypertriglyceridemia), cholesterol (hypercho-

lesterolemia), or both, in the blood. In the fasted state, hyperlipidemia is an abnormal finding that represents either accelerated production or delayed degradation of lipoproteins. The lipoproteins function as a carrier system to transport insoluble triglycerides and cholesterol through the blood. Lipoproteins consist of a triglyceride and cholesterol ester core surrounded by a surface layer of cholesterol, phospholipid, and apolipoproteins. The apolipoproteins (A, B, C, and E) are responsible for the structure of the lipoprotein particle, for binding of the particle to cell surface receptors, and for the activation of enzymes. There are four major classes of lipoproteins. Each class differs in its lipid and apoprotein content and physicochemical characteristics, including size, density, and electrophoretic mobility. Lipoproteins are categorized according to their buoyant density on ultracentrifugation as chylomicrons, very-low-density lipoproteins (VLDLs), low-density lipoproteins (LDLs), or high-density lipoproteins (HDLs). The buoyant density is inversely proportional to the triglyceride content such that the chylomicrons are composed largely of triglyceride, whereas HDLs have virtually no triglyceride content. The classification system is somewhat arbitrary, and it should be appreciated that there is significant structural and functional heterogeneity within the classes. In addition, the system is a dynamic one, with one class producing another during its metabolism. Chylomicrons and VLDLs are primarily involved in triglyceride metabolism, whereas HDLs and LDLs are primarily involved in cholesterol metabolism.

### Pathophysiology

Following digestion and absorption, dietary cholesterol and triglyceride are packaged by the enterocyte into chylomicron particles. The chylomicron particles are secreted into the mesenteric lymph, through which they ultimately reach the systemic circulation. As the chylomicrons pass through the adipose and muscle tissue, they are exposed to lipoprotein lipase, an enzyme that is present on the surface of the capillary endothelial cells. Following activation by apoprotein C-II, lipoprotein lipase hydrolyzes the triglyceride from the core of the lipoprotein to free fatty acids and glycerol. The free fatty acids diffuse into the adjacent tissue and are either resynthesized into triglycerides and stored (adipocytes) or used for energy by the cell (myocytes and other cells). The activity of lipoprotein lipase is influenced by several factors, including heparin, insulin, glucagon, and thyroid hormone. Depletion of the triglyceride component of the chylomicron alters the surface such that the chylomicron is converted into a chylomicron remnant. The remnant particle is rapidly recognized by specific hepatic receptors and removed from the circulation. Within the hepatocyte, the contents of the chylomicron remnant are degraded and utilized. Chylomicrons are present in plasma 30 minutes to 2 hours following a fat-containing meal, and hydrolysis is normally complete within 6 to 10 hours.

The liver transforms excess free fatty acids that are not directly oxidized for energy into triglycerides. The free fatty acids may originate from residual dietary triglyceride present in chylomicron remnant particles, from endogenous production secondary to surplus dietary carbohydrate, and from excessive endogenous mobilization of free fatty acids. Free fatty acids can be mobilized from adipose tissue by the activation of the intracellular enzyme hormone-sensitive lipase (HSL). HSL hydrolyses stored triglycerides into free fatty acids and glycerol. Stimulators of HSL include epinephrine, norepinephrine, adrenocorticotropic hormone (ACTH), corticosteroids, growth hormone, and thyroid hormone. In addition, HSL is activated by insulin deficiency. Activation of HSL is a normal physiologic response to provide the body with energy during periods of fasting. In addition, HSL can be inappropriately activated in several pathologic conditions associated with an altered metabolic state.

The triglycerides produced by the hepatocyte are packaged into VLDL particles and subsequently secreted into the bloodstream. VLDL particles are produced continuously by the liver and, in the fasting state, are the main carriers of triglycerides. In addition, VLDL particles are used to export cholesterol from the liver and therefore contain a significant proportion of cholesterol. Analogous to chylomicron metabolism, endothelial lipoprotein lipase hydrolyzes the triglyceride portion of the VLDL particle into free fatty acids and glycerol. The free fatty acids can either be oxidized for energy or reconstituted into triglycerides and stored. Removal of the triglyceride core converts the VLDL particle into a remnant particle, which may be removed and catabolized by the liver. Alternatively, a second endothelial lipase, hepatic lipase, can further remove any residual triglyceride and convert the VLDL remnant particle into an LDL particle.

The LDL particle is a cholesterol and phospholipid–rich entity that functions to transport cholesterol to tissues, where it may be used for membrane synthesis or steroid hormone production. Ultimately, the LDL particle can bind to LDL receptors and is removed by the liver. In addition to VLDL particles, the liver also secretes nascent HDL particles into the circulation. HDL particles act to scavenge excess unesterified cholesterol from the cells and other lipoproteins and return it to the liver for excretion into bile. This process is often referred to as *reverse cholesterol transport.*

Hypertriglyceridemia can develop secondary to increased chylomicron production (excessive dietary intake of lipid), ineffective clearance of the chylomicron particle, increased VLDL production (excessive dietary intake of lipid and/or carbohydrate, excessive endogenous production or mobilization of lipids), and ineffective clearance of the VLDL particle. Hypercholesterolemia can arise from increased production of the LDL precursor particle (VLDL) or as a result of reduced clearance of the LDL or HDL particle.

## Classification

Postprandial hyperlipidemia is the most common cause of hyperlipidemia in the dog and cat. This is a normal physiologic manifestation that is due to the production of triglyceride-rich chylomicrons and usually resolves within 2 to 10 hours. Pathologic abnormalities in plasma lipids and lipoproteins

may be of genetic or familial origin (primary) or arise as a consequence of disease (Table 54-7).

Primary hypertriglyceridemias include the idiopathic hyperlipidemia of Miniature Schnauzers and hyperchylomicronemia of cats. Idiopathic hyperlipidemia of Miniature Schnauzers is characterized by severe hypertriglyceridemia due to excessive VLDL particles with or without concurrent hyperchylomicronemia, and by mild hypercholesterolemia. The exact mechanism and genetics have not been fully elucidated. Feline familial hyperlipidemia is characterized as a fasting hyperchylomicronemia with a slight increase in VLDL particles. The defect is due to the production of an inactive form of lipoprotein lipase. Idiopathic hyperchylomicronemia has also been observed in dogs. Similar to the situation with the cat, the disease in the dog is characterized by hypertriglyceridemia, hyperchylomicronemia, and normal serum cholesterol concentrations. Idiopathic hypercholesterolemia is rare but has been reported in Doberman Pinschers and Rottweilers. Lipid derangements consist of hypercholesterolemia due to an increased serum LDL concentration. The etiology of this disorder is unknown.

Diseases associated with secondary hyperlipidemia include endocrine disorders (hypothyroidism, diabetes mellitus, hyperadrenocorticism), nephrotic syndrome, and pancreatitis. Hypothyroidism is the most common cause of hypercholesterolemia in the dog. Hyperlipidemia secondary to hypothyroidism can be attributed to both a decrease in lipid synthesis and degradation (lipid degradation is more severely affected). Decreased lipoprotein lipase activity contributes to the impaired removal of triglyceride-rich lipoproteins. In addition, thyroid hormone deficiency reduces the biliary excretion of cholesterol. The resultant increase in intrahepatic cholesterol concentration down-regulates the hepatic LDL

 TABLE 54-7

**Causes of Hyperlipidemia in Dogs and Cats**

Postprandial hyperlipidemia
Primary hyperlipidemia
   Idiopathic hyperlipoproteinemia (Miniature Schnauzers)
   Idiopathic hyperchylomicronemia (cat)
   Lipoprotein lipase deficiency (cat)
   Idiopathic hypercholesterolemia
Secondary hyperlipidemia
   Hypothyroidism
   Diabetes mellitus
   Hyperadrenocorticism
   Pancreatitis
   Cholestasis
   Hepatic insufficiency
   Nephrotic syndrome
   Drug-induced hyperlipidemia
      Glucocorticoids
      Megestrol acetate (cat)

receptor, which increases the concentration of the circulating LDL and HDL cholesterol–rich particles.

Insulin deficiency (diabetes mellitus) reduces the production of lipoprotein lipase, which contributes to decreased clearance of triglyceride-rich lipoproteins. Furthermore, insulin deficiency activates HSL, causing the release of large quantities of free fatty acids into the blood. These free fatty acids are ultimately converted by the liver into triglycerides, packaged into VLDL particles, and secreted back into the circulation. Therefore the hypertriglyceridemia seen with diabetes mellitus is attributed to both a reduction of lipoprotein lipase and increased production and decreased clearance of VLDL particles. Insulin deficiency increases the synthesis of cholesterol in the liver. The increased intrahepatic cholesterol concentration down-regulates the hepatocyte LDL receptor, consequently reducing the clearance of circulating LDL and HDL particles, causing hypercholesterolemia.

The mechanism of hypertriglyceridemia associated with hyperadrenocorticism is probably due to stimulation of HSL with release of free fatty acids into the circulation. Similar to the situation with diabetes mellitus, excess free fatty acids are converted into VLDL particles. In addition, glucocorticoids inhibit lipoprotein lipase activity, thereby reducing the clearance of triglyceride-rich lipoproteins.

## Clinical Features

Waxing-and-waning vomiting, diarrhea, and abdominal discomfort are the most common clinical presentations associated with hypertriglyceridemia (Table 54-8). Severe hypertriglyceridemia (levels exceeding 1000 mg/dl) has been associated with pancreatitis, lipemia retinalis, seizures, cutaneous xanthomas, peripheral nerve paralysis, and behavioral changes. Cutaneous xanthomas, which represent lipid-laden macrophages and foam cells, are the most common manifestation of hypertriglyceridemia in the cat. Severe hypercholesterolemia has been associated with arcus lipoides corneae, lipemia retinalis, and atherosclerosis.

In addition to the clinical manifestations, hypertriglyceridemia may also interfere with the results of several routine biochemical tests (Table 54-9). The degree of interference depends on the specific assay used by the laboratory, the species (canine versus feline), and the severity of the hypertriglyceridemia. In addition, hyperlipidemia may also cause hemolysis, which in turn can interfere with the results of some biochemical assays. Alternatively, hyperbilirubinemia may cause the cholesterol concentration to be falsely lower. These potential alterations in biochemical data must be considered when interpreting results in animals with hyperlipidemia. Fortunately, many laboratories will attempt to clear the hypertriglyceridemia by ultracentrifugation before performing the biochemical assays.

## Diagnosis

The presence of lipemic serum suggests that the animal is hypertriglyceridemic. *Lactescence* refers to the opaque and milk-like appearance of plasma samples that occurs when the elevation of the triglyceride level is sufficient. Animals with

## TABLE 54-8

**Clinical Signs and Potential Consequences of Hypertriglyceridemia and Hypercholesterolemia**

| CLINICAL SIGNS | CONSEQUENCES |
|---|---|
| Seizures | Hypertriglyceridemia |
| Blindness | Seizures |
| Abdominal pain | Pancreatitis |
| Anorexia | Lipid-laden aqueous humor: |
| Vomiting | uveitis, blindness |
| Diarrhea | Lipemia retinalis |
| Behavioral changes | Xanthomas |
| Lipemia retinalis | |
| Uveitis | |
| Xanthoma formation | |
| Peripheral neuropathy | Hypercholesterolemia |
| Horner's syndrome | Corneal arcus lipoides |
| Tibial nerve paralysis | Lipemia retinalis |
| Radial nerve paralysis | Atherosclerosis |

lactescent serum typically have triglyceride concentrations that exceed 1000 mg/dl. Conversely, animals that are purely hypercholesterolemic do not exhibit lipemic or lactescent serum, since the cholesterol-rich LDL and HDL particles are too small to refract light. Blood samples to confirm hyperlipidemia should be obtained following a 12- to 18-hour fast. A serum sample rather than whole blood or plasma should be submitted for assessment. The sample can be refrigerated or frozen for several days without affecting the assays. When assessing the sample for hypertriglyceridemia, the laboratory should not clear the sample before determination of the triglyceride concentration. Clearing lipemic samples by centrifugation removes chylomicrons, which will artificially lower the triglyceride result. Reference ranges for serum triglyceride concentration are typically 50 to 150 mg/dl for the adult dog and 20 to 110 mg/dl for the adult cat. Reference ranges for serum cholesterol concentration are typically 125 to 300 mg/dl for the adult dog and 95 to 130 mg/dl for the adult cat.

The chylomicron test can be helpful to delineate whether the lipemia is predominantly a chylomicron or a VLDL defect. The test is performed by refrigerating a plasma sample for 12 hours. Chylomicrons are less dense than the other particles and hence will float to the top of the sample to form an opaque cream layer over a clear infranatant of serum. If the hypertriglyceridemia is due to excess VLDL particles, the plasma sample will remain turbid. Formation of a cream layer over a cloudy serum layer suggests both excess chylomicrons and VLDL particles.

Lipoprotein electrophoresis can be used to distinguish the lipoproteins, and ultracentrifugation can provide a quantitative measurement of each of the lipoprotein classes. However, both of these procedures are time consuming and are not routinely available for clinical application. The activity of lipoprotein lipase can be assessed by the heparin release test. Serum samples for the determination of triglyceride concentrations

TABLE 54-9

**Effect of Lipemia on Clinical Chemistry Analytes in Canine and Feline Sera***

| FALSE INCREASE IN VALUES | | FALSE DECREASE IN VALUES | |
|---|---|---|---|
| **CANINE SERA** | **FELINE SERA** | **CANINE SERA** | **FELINE SERA** |
| Total bilirubin | Total bilirubin | Creatinine | Creatinine |
| Conjugated bilirubin | Conjugated bilirubin | Total $CO_2$ | Total $CO_2$ |
| Phosphorus | Phosphorus | Cholesterol | Alanine aminotransferase |
| Alkaline phosphatase† | Alkaline phosphatase† | Urea nitrogen | |
| Glucose† | Glucose† | | |
| Total protein‡ | Total protein‡ | | |
| Lipase | | | |
| Alanine aminotransferase | | | |

Adapted from Jacobs RM et al: Effects of bilirubinemia, hemolysis and lipemia on clinical chemistry analytes in bovine, canine, equine and feline sera, *Can Vet J* 33:605, 1992.
*Analytes were measured using Coulter DACOS (Coulter Diagnostics, Hialeah, Fla).
†Interference occurs only at very high concentrations of lipid.
‡When measured using a refractometer.

 TABLE 54-10

**Level of Key Nutrients in Selected Commercial Diets Used for the Management of Canine Hypertriglyceridemia***

| | TYPE | FAT (g/1000 kcal) | PROTEIN (g/1000 kcal) | ME (kcal/can/cup) |
|---|---|---|---|---|
| WALTHAM Canine Veterinary Diet Low Fat | Dry | 20.58 | 66.06 | 274/cup |
| WALTHAM Canine Veterinary Diet Low Fat | Can | 19.9 | 92.45 | 377/13.6 oz |
| Purina Veterinary Diets En GastroENteric | Dry | 27.8 | 61.5 | 397/cup |
| Purina Veterinary Diets En GastroENteric | Can | 34.1 | 75.9 | 424/12.5 oz |
| Hill's Prescription Diet Canine w/d | Dry | 27 | 58 | 226/cup |
| Hill's Prescription Diet Canine w/d | Can | 38 | 53 | 372/14.75 oz |
| Eukanuba Veterinary Diets Nutritional Weight Loss Formula Restricted-Calorie | Dry | 19 | 63 | 238/cup |

*ME*, Metabolizable energy.
*Information obtained from manufacturers' published information.

(and, if possible, lipoprotein concentrations) are obtained before and 15 minutes following the intravenous administration of heparin (90 IU/kg body weight in dogs; 40 IU/kg body weight in cats). Heparin causes the release of lipoprotein lipase from the endothelium and stimulates the hydrolysis of triglycerides. A defect in lipoprotein lipase is suspected if there is no difference between the serum triglyceride concentrations before and after the administration of heparin.

**Treatment**

Before therapy is recommended, every attempt should be made to determine whether the hyperlipidemia is primary or secondary to an underlying disease process. Hyperlipidemia secondary to an underlying disorder will typically resolve or improve with correction of the metabolic disturbance. Therefore each animal requires a full history, physical examination, complete blood count, serum biochemistry panel, serum lipase and thyroxine concentrations, and urinalysis. The results of the initial diagnostic evaluation may indicate the need for additional diagnostic tests such as abdominal ultrasound and evaluation of an ACTH stimulation test. A recommendation to treat hyperlipidemia involves a lifelong commitment by the owner and must therefore not be undertaken lightly. In general, severe hypertriglyceridemia (levels exceeding 1000 mg/dl) mandates treatment. In this circumstance, catabolic mechanisms can be assumed to be overwhelmed, and the triglyceride level is very sensitive to a small increase from the intestine or liver. The triglyceride levels must be decreased to prevent possible complications, including pancreatitis. In other situations the recommendations will be influenced by additional variables, including the underlying disease process. A realistic goal of therapy is to reduce the triglyceride concentration to less than 400 mg/dl.

Chylomicrons are produced from dietary fat. Therefore restriction of dietary fat is the cornerstone of therapy for hypertriglyceridemia. The dietary history should be reviewed, and the diet altered to one that contains less than 20% fat on an ME basis (Table 54-10). Nutritional management of hypertriglyceridemia in cats is more difficult because of the limited availability of low-fat diets (Table 54-11). Treats should be restricted to 5% of the daily caloric intake and changed to low-fat commercial varieties. Carrots or brown rice crackers are useful alternatives. In addition to the provision of a low-fat diet, the absolute caloric intake should be evaluated. If the animal is overweight, caloric restriction is indicated and beneficial, since it decreases the production of VLDL particles from excess dietary energy. The plasma triglyceride concentration should be reevaluated after 4 weeks of a low-fat diet. If the reduction in triglyceride concentration is less than ideal, the dietary history should be reevaluated to ensure that there are no extra fat calories from treats, no access to other pet foods, and no additional family members or neighbors who are inadvertently providing the animal with dietary fat. In addition, the medical record should be reviewed to ensure the exclusion of underlying disorders that would contribute to hypertriglyceridemia. If the low-fat commercial products are not able to control the hypertriglyceridemia, then a complete and balanced ultra-low-fat (10% to 12% ME) home-prepared diet can be formulated specifically for the animal by a veterinary clinical nutritionist. Diets rich in omega-3 fatty acids have been suggested to improve hypertriglyceridemia in humans by decreasing the production of VLDL particles. In addition, fish oils are poor substrates for triglyceride-synthesizing enzymes, and their use leads to the formation of triglyceride-poor VLDL particles. Some authors have recommended menhaden fish oil in the amount of 200 mg/kg body weight/day to assist in the management of hypertriglyceridemia in dogs.

Treatment with drugs, all of which have the potential for toxicity, should be undertaken with particular care. In general, drugs should not be used in animals whose serum triglyceride concentration is less than 500 mg/dl. Several classes of drugs are used to treat hypertriglyceridemia in humans; however, there are few reports of their use in cats and dogs. Until there are further studies evaluating the dose, effect, and toxicity, drug therapy is indicated only in those animals that have clinical signs associated with severe elevations in triglyceride concentrations that cannot be ameliorated by dietary therapy.

Niacin (100 mg/day in dogs) reduces serum triglyceride concentrations by decreasing fatty acid release from adipocytes and reducing the production of VLDL particles. Adverse effects are frequent and include vomiting, diarrhea, erythema, pruritus, and abnormalities in liver function tests. Fibric acid derivatives (clofibrate, bezafibrate, gemfibrozil, ciprofibrate, fenofibrate) lower plasma triglyceride concentrations by stimulating lipoprotein lipase activity, in addition to reducing the free fatty acid concentration, which decreases the substrate for VLDL synthesis. In humans, the fibrates generally lower plasma triglyceride concentrations by 20% to 40%. Gemfibrozil has been used in the dog (200 mg/day) and cat (10 mg/kg q12h). Reported adverse effects include abdominal pain, vomiting, diarrhea, and abnormal liver function tests. The statins (lovastatin, simvastatin, pravastatin, fluvastatin, cerivastatin, atorvastatin) are hydroxymethyl-glutaryl coenzyme A (HMG-CoA) reductase inhibitors and therefore primarily suppress cholesterol metabolism. As a consequence of lower intracellular cholesterol concentrations, the hepatic LDL receptor is upregulated, thereby increasing the removal and clearance of LDL (VLDL remnant particles) from the circulation. In addition, the statins decrease hepatic production of VLDL. In humans the statins can lower triglyceride concentrations by 10% to 15%. Adverse effects include lethargy, diarrhea, muscle pain, and hepatotoxicity.

Hypercholesterolemia is most likely associated with the presence of an underlying disease and generally resolves with control of the altered metabolic state. Unlike the situation with humans, hypercholesterolemia rarely poses a health risk to the dog or cat. Specific therapy is indicated only for those animals with a prolonged marked increase in the serum cholesterol concentration (i.e., more than 800 mg/dl) that may be associated with the development of atherosclerosis. Nutritional therapy with low-fat diets is the initial treatment of choice for severe hypercholesterolemia. The addition of soluble fiber to the diet may also help to reduce plasma cholesterol concentrations by as much as 10%. Soluble fiber inter-

## TABLE 54-11

### Level of Key Nutrients in Selected Commercial Diets Used for the Management of Feline Hypertriglyceridemia*

| | TYPE | FAT (g/1000 kcal) | PROTEIN (g/1000 kcal) | ME (kcal/can/cup) |
|---|---|---|---|---|
| WALTHAM Feline Veterinary Diet Calorie Control | Dry | 28 | 128 | 208/8 oz |
| Purina Veterinary Diets OM Overweight Management | Dry | 25 | 112 | 326/8 oz |
| Hill's Prescription Diet Feline r/d | Dry | 29 | 114 | 263/cup |
| Hill's Prescription Diet Feline r/d | Can | 28 | 114 | 116/5.5 oz |
| Eukanuba Veterinary Diets Nutritional Weight Loss Formula Restricted-Calorie | Dry | 24 | 83 | 298/cup |

*ME,* Metabolizable energy.
*Information obtained from manufacturers' published information.

feres with the enteric reabsorption of bile acids. Consequently, the liver uses cholesterol to increase the synthesis of bile acids.

Pharmacologic agents that can be considered for the management of severe hypercholesterolemia include bile acid sequestrates, HMG-CoA reductase inhibitors, and probucol. Bile acid sequestrates are ion exchange resins that interrupt the enterohepatic circulation of bile acids. Decreased reabsorption of bile acids stimulates the liver to synthesize bile acids, utilizing intrahepatic cholesterol. Depletion of intrahepatic cholesterol stores stimulates the hepatic LDL receptor to increase the removal of LDL and HDL particles from the circulation. Cholestyramine (1 to 2 g PO q12h) is effective for lowering cholesterol concentrations; however, its use has been associated with constipation, it interferes with the absorption of several oral medications, and it may increase hepatic VLDL synthesis, resulting in an increase in plasma triglyceride concentrations. HMG-CoA reductase is the rate-limiting enzyme for cholesterol synthesis. The HMG-CoA reductase inhibitors (lovastatin, simvastatin, pravastatin, fluvastatin, cerivastatin, and atorvastatin) are the most potent cholesterol-lowering agents and in humans may reduce cholesterol concentrations by 20% to 40%. Lovastatin (10 to 20 mg PO q24h) may be tried in dogs with persistent, severe idiopathic hypercholesterolemia that does not respond to diet alone. Potential adverse effects include lethargy, diarrhea, muscle pain, and hepatotoxicity. Lovastatin should not be administered to dogs with hepatic disease. Probucol is a cholesterol-lowering agent whose mechanism of action is not completely clear. Probucol is not widely recommended for the management of hypercholesterolemia, since its effect on lowering cholesterol concentrations is variable and it has been associated with the development of arrhythmias.

## Suggested Readings

### OBESITY

Burkholder WJ: *Body composition of dogs determined by carcass composition analysis, deuterium oxide dilution, subjective and objective morphometry and bioelectrical impedance,* Blacksburg, 1994, Virginia Polytechnic Institute and State University.

Burkholder WJ et al: Foods and techniques for managing obesity in companion animals, *J Am Vet Med Assoc* 212:658, 1998.

Butterwick R et al: A study of obese cats on a calorie-controlled weight reduction programme, *Vet Rec* 134:372, 1994.

Butterwick R et al: Changes in the body composition of cats during weight reduction by controlled dietary energy restriction, *Vet Rec* 138:354, 1996.

Butterwick R et al: Effect of amount and type of dietary fiber on food intake in energy-restricted dogs, *Am J Vet Res* 58:272, 1997.

Center SA et al: The clinical and metabolic effects of rapid weight loss in obese pet cats and the influence of supplemental oral L-carnitine, *J Vet Intern Med* 14:598, 2000.

Edney AT et al: Study of obesity in dogs visiting veterinary practices in the United Kingdom, *Vet Rec* 188:391, 1986.

Hawthorne AJ et al: Predicting the body composition of cats: development of a zoometric measurement for estimation of percentage body fat in cats, *J Vet Intern Med* 14:365, 2000.

Mason E: Obesity in pet dogs, *Vet Rec* 86:612, 1970.

Mayer J: Obesity. In Goodhart R et al, editors: *Modern nutrition in health and disease,* Philadelphia, 1973, Lea & Febiger.

Scarlett JM et al: Overweight cats—prevalence and risk factors, *Int J Obes* 18(1):S22, 1994.

Scarlett JM et al: Associations between body condition and disease in cats, *J Am Vet Med Assoc* 212:1725, 1998.

Sloth C: Practical management of obesity in dogs and cats, *J Small Anim Pract* 33:178, 1992.

### HYPERLIPIDEMIA

Barrie J et al: Quantitative analysis of canine plasma lipoproteins, *J Small Anim Pract* 34:226, 1993.

Bauer JE: Evaluation and dietary considerations in idiopathic hyperlipidemia in dogs, *J Am Vet Med Assoc* 206:1684, 1995.

Bhatnagar D: Lipid-lowering drugs in the management of hyperlipidaemia, *Pharmacol Ther* 79:205, 1998.

Jacobs RM et al: Effects of bilirubinemia, hemolysis, and lipemia on clinical chemistry analytes in bovine, canine, equine, and feline sera, *Can Vet J* 33:605, 1992.

Jones BR: Inherited hyperchylomicronaemia in the cat, *J Small Anim Pract* 34:493, 1993.

Jones BR et al: Peripheral neuropathy in cats with inherited primary hyperchylomicronaemia, *Vet Rec* 119:268, 1986.

Watson TDG et al: Lipoprotein metabolism and hyperlipidaemia in the dog and cat: a review, *J Small Anim Pract* 34:479, 1993.

Whitney MS et al: Ultracentrifugal and electrophoretic characteristics of the plasma lipoproteins of miniature schnauzer dogs with idiopathic hyperlipoproteinemia, *J Vet Intern Med* 7:253, 1996.

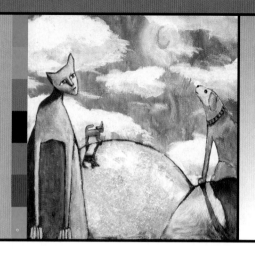

# CHAPTER 55

# Electrolyte Imbalances

Richard W. Nelson

## CHAPTER OUTLINE

HYPERNATREMIA, 828
HYPONATREMIA, 830
HYPERKALEMIA, 832
HYPOKALEMIA, 834
HYPERCALCEMIA, 836
HYPOCALCEMIA, 840
HYPERPHOSPHATEMIA, 841
HYPOPHOSPHATEMIA, 842
HYPERMAGNESEMIA, 843
HYPOMAGNESEMIA, 843

## HYPERNATREMIA

### Etiology

Hypernatremia exists if the serum sodium concentration exceeds 160 mEq/L, although reference ranges may vary between laboratories. It most commonly develops after water loss exceeds sodium loss (Table 55-1). The water loss may be pure (i.e., not accompanied by a loss of electrolytes, such as occurs with diabetes insipidus) or it may be hypotonic (i.e., loss of both water and sodium but with the water loss predominating, such as occurs with gastrointestinal fluid loss and renal failure). Insufficient water intake or an abnormal thirst mechanism are usually facets of an excessive water loss. Rarely, hypernatremia may occur in animals with hypodipsia caused by neurologic disease, an abnormal thirst mechanism, or defective osmoregulation of vasopressin release.

Less commonly, hypernatremia develops after sodium retention, such as occurs with iatrogenic sodium overload or primary hyperaldosteronism. Primary hyperaldosteronism is caused by an aldosterone-secreting adrenal tumor or idiopathic bilateral adrenal hyperplasia but is rare in dogs and cats. Increased serum aldosterone concentrations cause variable hypernatremia, hypokalemia, and systemic hypertension.

### Clinical Features

Clinical signs of hypernatremia are central nervous system (CNS) in origin and include lethargy, weakness, muscle fasciculations, disorientation, behavior changes, ataxia, seizures, stupor, and coma. Clinical signs typically become apparent when the plasma osmolality exceeds 350 mOsm/kg (serum sodium concentration of greater than 170 mEq/L). Clinical signs are caused by neuronal dehydration. Hypernatremia and hyperosmolality cause fluid to shift from the intracellular to the extracellular space. As the brain shrinks, meningeal vessels are damaged and torn, causing hemorrhage, hematoma, venous thrombosis, infarction of cerebral vessels, and ischemia. This gradient flow of water from the intracellular to the extracellular compartment often maintains adequate skin turgor and gives a false impression of hydration, even though there has been a detrimental loss of fluid from the animal.

The severity of clinical signs is related to the absolute increase in serum sodium concentration and especially the rapidity of onset of hypernatremia and hyperosmolality. Clinical signs usually do not develop until the serum sodium concentration approaches 170 mEq/L. If hypernatremia is rapid in onset, clinical signs may develop at a lower sodium concentration, and vice versa. With a gradual increase in the serum sodium concentration, the cells in the CNS can produce osmotically active solutes (idiogenic osmoles) intracellularly to reestablish osmotic equilibration between the extracellular and intracellular compartments, thereby minimizing cell shrinkage.

### Diagnosis

Measurement of the serum sodium concentration identifies hypernatremia. Once identified, the underlying cause should be sought. Careful evaluation of the history, physical examination findings, and results of routine clinical pathologic tests (i.e., complete blood count [CBC], serum biochemistry panel, urinalysis) usually yields clues to the cause. Evaluation of the urine specific gravity is especially helpful. Hypernatremia and hyperosmolality stimulate the release of vasopressin, resulting in hypersthenuria. A urine specific gravity of less than 1.008 in a dog or cat with hypernatremia is consistent with central or nephrogenic diabetes insipidus. A urine specific gravity of more than 1.030 in a dog and 1.035 in a cat implies a normal vasopressin–renal tubular axis and indicates the existence of sodium retention, primary hypodipsia-

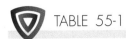

## TABLE 55-1

Causes of Hypernatremia in Dogs and Cats

**Caused by Pure Water Loss**

Central diabetes insipidus*
Nephrogenic diabetes insipidus*
Hypodipsia-adipsia*
   Neurologic disease
   Abnormal thirst mechanism
   Defective osmoregulation of vasopressin release
Inadequate access to water
High environmental temperature (heat stroke)
Fever

**Hypotonic Fluid Loss**

Gastrointestinal fluid loss*
   Vomiting
   Diarrhea
Chronic renal failure*
Polyuric acute renal failure*
Osmotic diuresis
   Diabetes mellitus
   Mannitol infusion
Diuretic administration
Postobstructive diuresis
Cutaneous burns
Third-space loss
   Pancreatitis
   Peritonitis

**Excess Sodium Retention**

Primary hyperaldosteronism
Iatrogenic
   Salt poisoning
   Hypertonic saline infusion
   Sodium bicarbonate therapy
   Parenteral nutrition*

Modified from DiBartola SP: Disorders of sodium and water: hypernatremia and hyponatremia. In DiBartola SP, editor: *Fluid therapy in small animal practice,* ed 2, Philadelphia, 2000, WB Saunders, p 53.
*Common causes.

adipsia, or gastrointestinal or insensible water loss. A urine specific gravity of between 1.008 and 1.030 (dog) or of 1.035 (cat) indicates the presence of partial vasopressin deficiency or an impaired renal tubular response to vasopressin, most likely secondary to a primary renal disorder.

## Treatment

The goal in treating hypernatremia is to restore the extracellular fluid (ECF) volume to normal and correct water deficits at a fluid rate that avoids significant complications and to identify and correct the underlying cause of the hypernatremia. The initial priority is to restore ECF volume to normal. In animals with modest volume contraction (e.g., tachycardia, dry mucous membranes, slow skin turgor), fluid

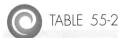

## TABLE 55-2

Guidelines for Potassium Supplementation in IV Fluids

| SERUM K+ (mEq/L) | K+ SUPPLEMENT/LITER OF FLUIDS* |
|---|---|
| >3.5 | 20 |
| 3.0-3.5 | 30 |
| 2.5-3.0 | 40 |
| 2.0-2.5 | 60 |
| <2.0 | 80 |

*Total hourly potassium administration should not exceed 0.5 mEq/kg body weight.

deficits should be corrected with 0.45% saline supplemented with an appropriate amount of potassium (Table 55-2). With severe dehydration, 0.9% saline solution or plasma should be used to expand vascular volume. In replacing deficits, rapid administration of fluids is contraindicated unless there are signs of significant hypovolemia. Any fluid should be administered in a volume only large enough to correct hypovolemia. Worsening neurologic status or sudden onset of seizures during fluid therapy is generally indicative of cerebral edema and the need for hypertonic saline solution or mannitol therapy. Once ECF deficits have been replaced, the serum sodium ($Na^+$) concentration should be reevaluated and water deficits corrected if hypernatremia persists. An approximation of the water deficit in liters may be calculated using the formula:

$$0.6 \times \text{Body weight (kg)} \times [1 - (\text{serum } Na^+_{desired}/\text{serum } Na^+_{present})]$$

Because the brain adjusts to hypertonicity by increasing the intracellular solute content via the accumulation of "idiogenic osmoles," the rapid repletion of body water with ECF dilution causes translocation of water into cells and can cause cerebral edema. If slower water repletion is undertaken, brain cells lose the accumulated intracellular solutes and osmotic equilibration can occur without cell swelling.

Half-strength (0.45%) saline solution with 2.5% dextrose or a 5% dextrose in water (D5W) solution is used to correct the water deficit in hypernatremic animals. Half-strength saline solution with 2.5% dextrose is the initial fluid used in hypernatremic animals with no signs of dehydration, and it should also be used in dehydrated animals with persistent hypernatremia after the correction of fluid deficits. D5W solution can be substituted for 0.45% saline solution with 2.5% dextrose if the hypernatremia does not abate after 12 to 24 hours of fluid therapy.

Oral fluid administration is preferable for correcting water deficits, with fluid administered intravenously (IV) if oral administration is not possible. The water deficit should be replaced slowly. Approximately 50% of the water deficit should be corrected in the first 24 hours, with the remainder corrected over the ensuing 24 to 48 hours. The serum sodium concentration should decline slowly, preferably at a rate of less than 1 mEq/L/hr. A gradual reduction in the serum sodium concentration minimizes the fluid shift from the extracellular to the intracellular compartment, thereby minimizing neuronal cell swelling and cerebral edema and increasing intracranial pressure. A deterioration in CNS status after the start of fluid therapy indicates the presence of cerebral edema and the immediate need to reduce the rate of fluid administration. Frequent monitoring of serum electrolyte concentrations, with appropriate adjustments in the type of fluid administered and rate of fluid administration, is important in the successful management of hypernatremia.

On rare occasions, a hypernatremic animal presents with an increase in the extracellular fluid volume. Such animals are difficult to treat. The goal is to lower the serum sodium concentration without exacerbating an increase in the ECF volume and causing pulmonary congestion and edema. To slowly correct hypernatremia in these animals, loop diuretics (e.g., furosemide, 1 to 2 mg/kg PO or IV q8-12h) are administered to promote sodium loss in the urine, and this in done in conjunction with the judicious administration of D5W.

## HYPONATREMIA

### Etiology

Hyponatremia is present if the serum sodium concentration is less than 140 mEq/L, although reference ranges may vary between laboratories. It can result from excessive sodium loss, primarily through the kidney, or from increased water conservation, or both. The latter condition may be an appropriate response to a reduction in the ECF volume or may be inappropriate (e.g., syndrome of inappropriate antidiuretic hormone secretion). In most cases, hyponatremia results from abnormalities in water balance (principally a defect in renal water excretion) rather than from abnormalities in sodium balance. Causes of hyponatremia in dogs and cats are listed in Table 55-3.

Hyponatremia must be differentiated from pseudohyponatremia, which is a decrease in the serum sodium concentration as a result of laboratory methodology in the presence of normal plasma osmolality. Pseudohyponatremia occurs in the presence of hyperlipidemia or severe hyperproteinemia. An increase in the concentration of triglycerides or proteins in plasma reduces the sodium concentration in the total plasma volume, but the sodium concentration in plasma water remains the same. Methods that measure the amount of sodium in a specific volume of plasma (e.g., flame photometry) result in falsely low sodium values, whereas methodologies that determine the sodium concentration in the aqueous phase of plasma (e.g., direct potentiometry using ion-selective electrodes) yield an accurate sodium value. Pseudohyponatremia can usually be identified if the method used to measure the sodium concentration is known, a blood sample is examined for the presence of gross lipemia, and a CBC and serum biochemistry panel are performed.

Hyponatremia may also occur after there is an increase in the concentration of osmotically active solutes (e.g., glucose,

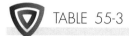

## TABLE 55-3

### Causes of Hyponatremia in Dogs and Cats

**With Normal Plasma Osmolality**

Hyperlipidemia
Hyperproteinemia

**With High Plasma Osmolality**

Hyperglycemia*
Mannitol infusion

**With Low Plasma Osmolality**

And hypervolemia
    Advanced liver failure*
    Advanced renal failure*
    Nephrotic syndrome*
    Congestive heart failure
And normovolemia
    Primary polydipsia
    Inappropriate antidiuretic hormone (ADH) secretion (SIADH)
    Myxedema coma of hypothyroidism
    Iatrogenic
        Hypotonic fluid administration
        Antidiuretic drugs (e.g., barbiturates, β-adrenergics)
And hypovolemia
    Hypoadrenocorticism*
    Gastrointestinal fluid loss*
    Third-space loss
        Pleural effusions (e.g., chylothorax)
        Peritoneal effusions
        Pancreatitis
    Cutaneous burns
    Diuretic administration

Modified from DiBartola SP: Disorders of sodium and water: hypernatremia and hyponatremia. In DiBartola SP, editor: *Fluid therapy in small animal practice*, ed 2, Philadelphia, 2000, WB Saunders, p 60.
*Common causes.

mannitol) in the ECF. An increase in the concentration of osmotically active solutes in the ECF causes a fluid shift from the intracellular to the extracellular compartment and a corresponding decrease in the serum sodium concentration. For example, the serum sodium concentration decreases 1.3 to 1.6 mEq/L for every 100 mg/dl increase in the serum glucose concentration. Estimation of the plasma osmolality is helpful in differentiating the cause of hyponatremia. Hyponatremia is usually associated with hyposmolality (less than 290 mOsm/kg), whereas pseudohyponatremia is associated with normal plasma osmolality, and hyponatremia caused by an increase in osmotically active solutes in the ECF is associated with hyperosmolality. Plasma osmolality can be estimated using the following formula:

$$\text{Plasma osmolality (mOsm/kg)} = (2 \times \text{Na [mEq/L]}) + \frac{\text{Glucose (mg/dl)}}{18} + \frac{\text{Urea nitrogen (mg/dl)}}{2.8}$$

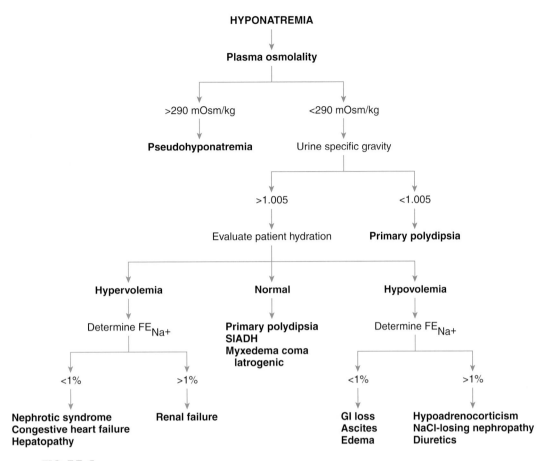

**HYPONATREMIA**
↓
**Plasma osmolality**

>290 mOsm/kg → **Pseudohyponatremia**

<290 mOsm/kg → Urine specific gravity

>1.005 → Evaluate patient hydration

<1.005 → **Primary polydipsia**

Evaluate patient hydration branches:
**Hypervolemia** | **Normal** | **Hypovolemia**

Hypervolemia → Determine $FE_{Na+}$
- <1% → **Nephrotic syndrome / Congestive heart failure / Hepatopathy**
- >1% → **Renal failure**

Normal → **Primary polydipsia / SIADH / Myxedema coma / Iatrogenic**

Hypovolemia → Determine $FE_{Na+}$
- <1% → **GI loss / Ascites / Edema**
- >1% → **Hypoadrenocorticism / NaCl-losing nephropathy / Diuretics**

**FIG 55-1**
Diagnostic approach to hyponatremia. *FE*$_{Na}$, Fractional excretion of sodium. (Adapted from DiBartola SP: Hyponatremia, *Vet Clin North Am* 19:215, 1989.)

Normal plasma osmolality in dogs and cats is approximately 280 to 310 mOsm/kg.

## Clinical Features

Clinical signs of hyponatremia include lethargy, anorexia, vomiting, weakness, muscle fasciculations, disorientation, seizures, and coma. CNS signs are the most worrisome and develop as changes in plasma osmolality cause fluid to shift from the extracellular to the intracellular space, resulting in neuronal swelling and lysis. The onset and severity of clinical signs depend on the rapidity with which the hyponatremia develops, as well as on the degree of hyponatremia. The more chronic the hyponatremia and the more slowly it develops, the more capable the brain is of compensating for changes in osmolality through the loss of potassium and organic osmolytes from cells. Clinical signs develop when the decrease in plasma osmolality occurs faster than the brain's defense mechanisms can counter the influx of water into the neurons.

## Diagnosis

Hyponatremia is readily evident from measurement of serum electrolyte concentrations. However, hyponatremia must be differentiated from pseudohyponatremia (see prior discussion). Hyponatremia is not a diagnosis per se but rather a manifestation of an underlying disorder. As such, a diagnos-

tic evaluation to identify the cause, as well as appropriate therapy to correct the hyponatremia, should be initiated. In most dogs and cats the cause of hyponatremia is readily apparent after evaluation of the history, physical examination findings, CBC, serum biochemistry panel, and urinalysis findings, but further diagnostic tests may be necessary. Careful assessment of the urine specific gravity, the hydration status of the animal, and, if necessary, the fractional excretion of sodium ($FE_{Na}$) help localize the problem (Fig. 55-1). The $FE_{Na}$ can be determined by first measuring the urine ($U_{Na}$) and plasma ($P_{Na}$) sodium and urine ($U_{Cr}$) and plasma ($P_{Cr}$) creatinine concentrations and then applying the following formula:

$$FE_{Na} = (U_{Na}/P_{Na}) \times (P_{Cr}/U_{Cr}) \times 100$$

## Treatment

The goals of therapy are to treat the underlying disease and, if necessary, to increase the serum sodium concentration and plasma osmolality. The goal of treatment directed at the hyponatremia is to correct body water osmolality and restore cell volume to normal by raising the ratio of sodium to water in extracellular fluid using IV fluid therapy, water restriction, or both. The increase in extracellular fluid osmolality draws water from cells and therefore reduces their volume. The

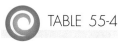

TABLE 55-4

Parenteral Fluid Solutions

| SOLUTION | ELECTROLYTE CONCENTRATION (mEq/L) | | | BUFFER (mEq/L) | OSMOLALITY (mOsm/L) | CALORIES (kcal/L) |
|---|---|---|---|---|---|---|
| | Na | K | Cl | | | |
| **Electrolyte Replacement Solutions** | | | | | | |
| Lactated Ringer's | 130 | 4 | 109 | Lactate 25 | 273 | 9 |
| Ringer's | 147 | 4 | 156 | — | 310 | — |
| Normal saline | 154 | — | 154 | — | 308 | — |
| Normosol R | 140 | 5 | 98 | Acetate 27 | 295 | 18 |
| **Maintenance Solutions** | | | | | | |
| 2½% Dextrose/0.45% saline | 77 | — | 77 | — | 280 | 85 |
| 2½% Dextrose/½ strength LRS | 65 | 2 | 54 | Lactate 14 | 263 | 89 |
| Normosol M | 40 | 13 | 40 | Acetate 16 | 112 | — |
| Normosol M in 5% dextrose | 40 | 13 | 40 | Acetate 16 | 363 | 175 |
| **Colloidal Solutions** | | | | | | |
| Dextran 70 (6% w/v in 0.9% saline) | 154 | — | 154 | | 300-303 | — |
| Hetastarch (6% in 0.9% saline) | 154 | — | 154 | — | — | — |
| Plasma (average values, dog) | 145 | 4 | 108 | 20 | 300 | — |
| **Other** | | | | | | |
| 5% Dextrose in water | — | — | — | — | 252 | 170 |

Adapted from Senior DF: Fluid therapy, electrolyte, and acid-base control. In Ettinger SJ, editor: *Textbook of veterinary internal medicine,* ed 3, Philadelphia, 1989, WB Saunders Co, p 429.
*Na,* Sodium; *K,* potassium; *Cl,* chloride; *LRS,* lactated Ringer's solution.

approach to treatment and the type of fluid used depend on the underlying etiology, the severity of the hyponatremia, and the presence or absence of clinical signs (Table 55-4). Chronic hyponatremia in an asymptomatic animal is best treated conservatively. Lactated Ringer's or Ringer's solution can be used for mild hyponatremia (serum sodium concentration of more than 135 mEq/L) and physiologic saline solution for more severe hyponatremia (serum sodium concentration of less than 135 mEq/L). Physiologic saline solution is typically used in symptomatic animals with severe hyponatremia. Hypertonic saline solutions (i.e., 3% NaCl) may be considered for the treatment of severe hyponatremia (serum sodium concentration of less than 120 mEq/L); however, this fluid should be used with caution and only if severe neurologic signs are present.

Fluid and electrolyte balance should gradually be restored over 24 to 48 hours, with periodic assessment of serum electrolyte concentrations. The more acute and severe the hyponatremia, the more slowly the serum sodium concentration should be corrected. A rapid increase in the serum sodium concentration to levels greater than 125 mEq/L is potentially dangerous and should be avoided in animals with acute, severe hyponatremia (serum sodium concentration of less than 120 mEq/L) and neurologic signs. For these animals, the serum sodium concentration should be gradually increased to

125 mEq/L or higher over 6 to 8 hours. Because loss of brain solute represents one of the compensatory mechanisms for preserving brain cell volume during dilutional states, an increase in serum sodium concentration toward normal is relatively hypertonic to brain cells that are partially depleted of solute as a result of hyponatremia. Consequently, raising the serum sodium concentration rapidly to greater than 125 mEq/L can cause CNS damage. Dietary sodium restriction (e.g., Prescription Diet h/d, Hill's Pet Products) and diuretic therapy should be considered in edematous animals.

## HYPERKALEMIA

### Etiology

Hyperkalemia is present if the serum potassium concentration exceeds 5.5 mEq/L, although reference ranges may vary between laboratories. Hyperkalemia can develop after an increased potassium intake (uncommon), after a compartmental shift in potassium from the intracellular to extracellular space (uncommon), or as a result of impaired potassium excretion in the urine (common; Table 55-5). Impaired urinary excretion of potassium is usually caused by renal dysfunction or hypoadrenocorticism. Iatrogenic-induced hyperkalemia is

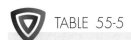 TABLE 55-5

## Causes of Hyperkalemia in Dogs and Cats

**Transcellular Shifts (ICF to ECF)**

Metabolic and respiratory acidosis
Insulin deficiency—DKA
Acute tumor lysis syndrome
Reperfusion post thrombus dissolution
Drugs—β-blockers (e.g., propranolol)

**Decreased Urinary Excretion**

Hypoadrenocorticism*
Acute oliguric-anuric renal failure*
End-stage chronic renal failure
Urethral obstruction*
Ruptured bladder—uroabdomen*
Selected gastroenteritis (e.g., trichuriasis, salmonellosis)
Chylothorax with repeated pleural fluid drainage
Hyporeninemic hypoaldosteronism

**Iatrogenic**

Excessive administration of potassium-containing fluids*
Potassium-sparing diuretics
Angiotensin-converting enzyme inhibitors (e.g., captopril)
Prostaglandin inhibitors (e.g., indomethacin)
Digitalis
α-Adrenergic agonists (e.g., phenylpropanolamine)

**Pseudohyperkalemia**

Hemolysis (Akita)
Thrombocytosis ($>10^6/mm^3$)
Leukocytosis ($>10^5/mm^3$)
Hypernatremia (dry reagent methods)

Modified from DiBartola SP et al: Disorders of potassium: hypokalemia and hyperkalemia. In DiBartola SP, editor: *Fluid therapy in small animal practice*, ed 2, Philadelphia, 2000, WB Saunders, p 100.
*ICF*, Intracellular fluid; *ECF*, extracellular fluid; *DKA*, diabetic ketoacidosis.
*Common causes.

 TABLE 55-6

## Electrocardiographic Alterations Associated with Hypokalemia and Hyperkalemia in Dogs and Cats

**Hypokalemia**

Depressed T-wave amplitude
Depressed ST segment
Prolonged QT interval
Prominent U wave
Arrhythmias
    Supraventricular
    Ventricular

**Hyperkalemia**

Serum potassium: 5.6-6.5 mEq/L
    Bradycardia
    Tall, narrow T waves
Serum potassium: 6.6-7.5 mEq/L
    Decreased R-wave amplitude
    Prolonged QRS interval
Serum potassium: 7.0-:8.5 mEq/L
    Decreased P-wave amplitude
    Prolonged P-R interval
Serum potassium: >8.5 mEq/L
    Invisible P wave
    Deviation of ST segment
    Complete heart block
    Ventricular arrhythmias
    Cardiac arrest

also common in dogs and cats. *Pseudohyperkalemia* refers to an increase in potassium in vitro and can occur in the setting of severe hypernatremia (if dry reagent methodologies are used), leukocytosis (white blood cell count of more than $100,000/mm^3$), thrombocytosis (more than $1 \times 10^6/mm^3$); if the blood specimen has been obtained from fluid lines or catheters contaminated with potassium-containing fluids; and in the setting of hemolysis in the Akita breed of dogs and in English Springer Spaniel dogs with phosphofructokinase deficiency.

## Clinical Features

The clinical manifestations of hyperkalemia reflect changes in cell membrane excitability and the magnitude and rapidity of onset of hyperkalemia. Mild-to-moderate hyperkalemia (serum potassium concentration of less than 6.5 mEq/L) is typically asymptomatic. Generalized skeletal muscle weakness develops as the hyperkalemia worsens. Weakness occurs after a hyperkalemia-induced decrease in the resting cell membrane potential to the level of the threshold potential, thereby impairing repolarization and subsequent cell excitation. The most prominent manifestations of hyperkalemia are cardiac in nature. Hyperkalemia causes decreased myocardial excitability, an increased myocardial refractory period, and slowed conduction; effects that may cause potentially life-threatening cardiac rhythm disturbances (Table 55-6).

## Diagnosis

Measurement of the serum potassium concentration or electrocardiography can identify hyperkalemia. Once identified, a careful review of the history, physical findings, CBC, serum biochemistry panel, and urinalysis usually yields clues to the cause. The most common causes for hyperkalemia in the dog and cat are iatrogenic, most notably excessive potassium administration in IV fluids; renal dysfunction, especially acute oliguric-anuric renal failure, urethral obstruction (tomcats), and rupture within the urinary system leading to uroabdomen; and hypoadrenocorticism. It can be a diagnostic challenge to differentiate renal dysfunction from hypoadrenocorticism, because both disorders can manifest a similar clinical picture. An adrenocorticotropic hormone (ACTH)

TABLE 55-7

Potential Therapies for the Management of Hyperkalemia in the Dog and Cat

| SOLUTION | DOSAGE | ROUTE OF ADMINISTRATION | DURATION OF EFFECT |
|---|---|---|---|
| Physiologic saline | ≥60-100 ml/kg/day | IV | Hours |
| Dextrose | 5%-10% in IV fluids *or* | IV, continuous | Hours |
| | 1-2 ml/kg 50% dextrose | IV, slow bolus | Hours |
| Regular insulin and dextrose | 0.5-1.0 U/kg in parenteral fluids plus | IV | Hours |
| | 2 g dextrose/U insulin administered | IV | |
| | | Monitor blood glucose | |
| Sodium bicarbonate | 1-2 mEq/kg | IV, slow bolus | Hours |
| 10% Calcium gluconate | 2-10 ml | IV, slow infusion | 30-60 min. |
| | | Monitor heart | |

stimulation test is needed to confirm hypoadrenocorticism (see p. 806). Measurement of the serum aldosterone concentration before and after ACTH administration should be considered, especially if plasma cortisol concentrations are normal and another cause for hyperkalemia cannot be identified. Small rents in the urinary bladder can be difficult to identify, and frequently contrast-enhanced radiographic studies or surgical exploration is necessary to confirm their presence.

### Treatment

For most animals, therapy for hyperkalemia is directed at treating the underlying cause. Symptomatic therapy for hyperkalemia should be initiated if the serum potassium concentration is greater than 7 mEq/L or if pronounced cardiac toxicity (i.e., complete heart block, premature ventricular contractions, arrhythmias) is identified on an electrocardiogram (ECG) (Table 55-7). The rapid institution of therapy in animals with marked hyperkalemia may be lifesaving. The goal of symptomatic therapy is to reverse the cardiotoxic effects of hyperkalemia and, if possible, reestablish normokalemia. Asymptomatic animals with normal urine output and chronic hyperkalemia of less than 7 mEq/L may not require immediate treatment, but a search for the underlying cause should be initiated.

IV fluid administration in amounts designed to correct fluid deficits and cause volume expansion rehydrates the animal, improves renal perfusion and potassium excretion, and dilutes the blood potassium concentration. Physiologic saline solution is the fluid of choice for this purpose. Potassium-containing fluids (e.g., lactated Ringer's solution) can be used if physiologic saline solution is not available, because the low potassium concentration in these fluids (see Table 55-4) in relation to that in blood will still have a dilutional effect on the blood potassium concentration. Dextrose can be added to the fluids to make a 5% to 10% dextrose-containing solution. Dextrose stimulates insulin secretion, which in turn promotes the movement of glucose and potassium from the

extracellular to the intracellular space. Fluids containing more than 5% dextrose should be given into a central vein to minimize the risk of phlebitis.

Rarely, additional therapy may be required to block the cardiotoxic effects of hyperkalemia (see Table 55-7). Sodium bicarbonate and regular insulin given with dextrose act to shift potassium from the extracellular to the intracellular space. IV calcium infusions block the effects of hyperkalemia on cell membranes but do not lower the blood potassium concentration. These therapies constitute aggressive, short-term, lifesaving measures that can reestablish normal cardiac conduction while one waits for more conventional therapy (i.e., fluids) to become effective.

## HYPOKALEMIA

### Etiology

Hypokalemia is present when the serum potassium concentration is less than 3.5 to 4.0 mEq/L, although reference ranges may vary between laboratories. Hypokalemia can develop after decreased dietary potassium intake (uncommon), translocation of potassium from the extracellular fluid to the intracellular fluid (common), or increased potassium loss in urine or gastrointestinal secretions (common) (Table 55-8). Iatrogenic hypokalemia is also common in dogs and cats. Pseudohypokalemia is uncommon and depends on the method used to measure the serum potassium concentration. Hyperlipidemia, hyperproteinemia (more than 10 g/dl), hyperglycemia (more than 750 mg/dl), and azotemia (urea nitrogen concentration of more than 115 mg/dl) can potentially cause pseudohypokalemia.

### Clinical Features

Most dogs and cats with mild-to-moderate hypokalemia (i.e., 3.0 to 4.0 mEq/L) are asymptomatic. Clinically severe hypokalemia primarily affects the neuromuscular and cardiovascular systems, owing to the hypokalemia-induced initial

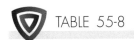

## TABLE 55-8

### Causes of Hypokalemia in Dogs and Cats

**Transcellular Shifts (ECF to ICF)**

Metabolic alkalosis
Diabetic ketoacidosis*
Hypokalemic periodic paralysis (Burmese cats)

**Increased Loss**

Gastrointestinal fluid loss*
Chronic renal failure, especially in cats*
Diet-induced hypokalemic nephropathy in cats
Distal (type I) renal tubular acidosis
Proximal (type II) renal tubular acidosis after sodium
    bicarbonate treatment
Postobstructive diuresis
Primary hyperaldosteronism
Secondary hyperaldosteronism*
    Liver insufficiency
    Congestive heart failure
    Nephrotic syndrome
Hyperthyroidism
Hypomagnesemia

**Iatrogenic***

Postassium-free fluid administration (e.g., 0.9% NaCl)
Parenteral nutritional solutions
Insulin and glucose-containing fluid administration
Sodium bicarbonate therapy
Loop (e.g., furosemide) and thiazide diuretics
Low dietary intake

**Pseudohypokalemia**

Hyperlipidemia (dry reagent methods; flame photometry)
Hyperproteinemia (dry reagent methods; flame
    photometry)
Hyperglycemia (dry reagent methods)
Azotemia (dry reagent methods)

Modified from DiBartola SP et al: Disorders of potassium: hypokalemia and hyperkalemia. In DiBartola SP, editor: *Fluid therapy in small animal practice,* ed 2, Philadelphia, 2000, WB Saunders, p 93.
*ECF,* Extracellular fluid; *ICF,* intracellular fluid; *NaCl,* sodium chloride.
*Common causes.

hyperpolarization followed by hypopolarization of cell membranes. The most common clinical sign of hypokalemia is generalized skeletal muscle weakness. In cats, ventroflexion of the neck (see Fig. 74-4, p. 1066), forelimb hypermetria, and a broad-based hindlimb stance may be observed. The timing of the onset of hypokalemia-induced weakness is extremely variable among animals. Cats seem more susceptible to the deleterious effects of hypokalemia than dogs do. In dogs, signs may not be evident until the serum potassium concentration is less than 2.5 mEq/L, whereas in cats signs can be seen when the serum potassium concentration is between 3 and 3.5 mEq/L.

Cardiac consequences of hypokalemia include decreased myocardial contractility, decreased cardiac output, and disturbances in cardiac rhythm. Cardiac disturbances assume a variable clinical expression, often evidenced only by ECG (see Table 55-6). Other metabolic effects of hypokalemia include hypokalemic nephropathy, which is characterized by chronic tubulointerstitial nephritis, impaired renal function, and azotemia and manifested clinically as polyuria, polydipsia, and impaired urine concentrating capability; hypokalemic polymyopathy, which is characterized by increased serum creatine kinase activity and electromyographic abnormalities; and paralytic ileus, manifested clinically as abdominal distention, anorexia, vomiting, and constipation. Hypokalemic nephropathy and polymyopathy are most notable in cats.

### Diagnosis

Measurement of the serum potassium concentration identifies hypokalemia. Once identified, a careful review of the history, physical findings, CBC, serum biochemistry panel, and urinalysis findings usually provides clues to the cause (see Table 55-8). If after review of this information the cause is not readily apparent, other, less likely causes for hypokalemia should be considered, such as renal tubular acidosis or another renal potassium-wasting disorder, primary hyperaldosteronism, and hypomagnesemia. To help differentiate renal and nonrenal sources of potassium loss, it may be necessary to determine the fractional excretion of potassium determined on the basis of a single urine and serum potassium and creatinine concentration or determine 24-hour urine potassium excretion (see p. 584).

### Treatment

Therapy is indicated if the serum potassium concentration is less than 3 mEq/L, if clinical signs related to hypokalemia are present, or if a serum potassium loss is anticipated (e.g., insulin therapy in diabetic ketoacidosis [DKA]) and the animal's ability to compensate for the loss is impaired. The goal of therapy is to reestablish and maintain normokalemia without inducing hyperkalemia.

Potassium supplements should be given orally whenever possible. Oral potassium supplements come in the form of elixirs, wax-matrix tablets, and microencapsulated slow-release formulations. Problems with oral preparations include poor palatability, which can be minimized by mixing them with food, and gastrointestinal tract irritation, which may cause vomiting, diarrhea, and melena. Two products that are well accepted by most dogs and cats and that have minimal gastrointestinal tract side effects are potassium gluconate elixir (Kaon Elixir, Adria Laboratories, Columbus, Ohio) and potassium gluconate prepared in a palatable protein base (Tumil-K, King Animal Health, St. Louis). The recommended dose for these products is 2.2 mEq of potassium per 100 calories of required energy intake per day or 2 mEq of potassium per 4.5 kg of body weight twice a day. Subsequent adjustments in dosage are made on the basis of clinical response and serum potassium concentrations. Bananas are also a good source of potassium.

Twenty inches (50 cm) of banana contains approximately 20 mEq of potassium.

Parenteral potassium supplementation is indicated if oral administration is not possible (e.g., vomiting, anorexia). Potassium chloride is the compound most commonly used, in part to help promote chloride as well as potassium repletion. Administration of potassium phosphate in addition to potassium chloride is indicated in dogs and cats with DKA to help prevent the onset of hypophosphatemia (see p. 766). IV administration is preferred, although potassium chloride can be given subcutaneously as long as the concentration of potassium does not exceed 30 mEq/L.

The initial amount of potassium added to fluids depends on the animal's serum potassium concentration (see Table 55-2) and the amount of potassium already present in the fluids (see Table 55-4). In dogs and cats with normal renal function, the maintenance amount of potassium supplementation is approximately 20 mEq/L of fluids when the fluid rate is 40 ml/kg/24 hr or 0.5 mEq/kg/day. The rate of IV potassium administration should not exceed 0.5 mEq/kg/hr. Subsequent adjustments in potassium therapy are based on the serum potassium concentration measured once or twice a day. An ECG, by showing alterations associated with hypokalemia and hyperkalemia, can also be used as a crude index of serum potassium concentration (see Table 55-6).

It is difficult to estimate the amount of potassium required to reestablish normal potassium balance based on the serum potassium concentration because potassium is primarily an intracellular cation. As such, serial measurement of the serum potassium concentration is important during treatment and should initially be done every 6 to 8 hours if potassium is being administered intravenously. Adjustments in potassium therapy should be made accordingly, with the goal of establishing a normal serum potassium concentration and then maintaining the serum potassium concentration in the normal range as treatment is withdrawn. Clinical signs of hypokalemia usually resolve within 1 to 5 days after correction of hypokalemia. Depending on the underlying cause, long-term oral potassium supplementation may be required to prevent the recurrence of hypokalemia.

## HYPERCALCEMIA

### Identification

Hypercalcemia is present if the serum calcium concentration is greater than 12 mg/dl or the serum ionized calcium concentration is greater than 1.45 mmol/L, although reference ranges may vary between laboratories. The serum total and ionized calcium concentration is higher in puppies than in adult dogs. A mild increase in the serum total calcium (i.e., less than 13 mg/dl), ionized calcium (i.e., less than 1.55 mmol/L), and phosphorus (i.e., less than 10 mg/dl) concentrations in a clinically healthy puppy, together with an increase in the serum alkaline phosphatase activity and normal urea nitrogen and creatinine concentrations,

should be considered normal. The serum total calcium concentration does not fluctuate with age in cats, but the serum ionized calcium concentration may be higher (less than 0.1 mmol/L) in cats less than 2 years of age compared with results in older cats.

The serum albumin and total protein concentrations should be measured when determining the total serum calcium concentration in the dog. Most automated and in-house serum chemistry analyzers measure the total serum calcium concentration, which consists of biologically active, ionized calcium (50%), protein-bound calcium (40%), and calcium complexes (10%). A drawback to this is that alterations in the plasma protein concentration may alter the total serum calcium concentration, yet the ionized calcium levels remain normal. Simple quantitative changes in the albumin and total plasma proteins do not cause hypocalcemia or hypercalcemia in dogs, even though the total serum calcium levels may "appear" low or high on the biochemistry panel. The following formulas can be used to determine the corrected total serum calcium concentration:

$$\text{Corrected calcium (mg/dl)} = \text{Serum calcium (mg/dl)} - \text{Serum albumin (g/dl)} + 3.5$$

or

$$\text{Corrected calcium (mg/dl)} = \text{Serum calcium (mg/dl)} - (0.4 \times \text{Serum total protein [g/dl]}) + 3.3$$

The formula based on albumin is preferred because of the stronger relationship between serum albumin and total calcium concentrations. The formulas should not be used in dogs less than 24 weeks of age, because high values may be obtained, nor should they be used in cats, because there is no linear relationship between serum total calcium and serum albumin and total protein concentrations in cats. These formulas yield a rough estimate of the corrected total serum calcium concentration and were developed without verification by serum ionized calcium measurements. Unfortunately, in one study by Mischke and colleagues (1996), correction of the total serum calcium concentration for albumin did not improve the correlation between the serum total and ionized calcium concentrations, suggesting that corrected total serum calcium concentrations may not be reliable indicators of calcium homeostasis.

Alternatively, the biologically active, ionized fraction of calcium can be determined directly, which bypasses the influence of plasma proteins on the total serum calcium concentration. Samples must be specially handled, specialized instrumentation must be used, and the sample pH must be adjusted (ionized calcium decreases as pH increases) to ensure the accuracy of this method.

### Etiology

Hypercalcemia is uncommon in dogs and cats. Persistent hypercalcemia usually results from increased calcium resorption from bone or kidney or increased calcium absorption from the gastrointestinal tract. Humoral hypercalcemia of malignancy (HHM) is the most common cause of hypercalcemia and occurs when the tumor produces substances that promote osteoclastic activity and renal calcium reabsorption. These substances include parathyroid hormone (PTH); parathyroid hormone–related peptide (PTHrP); 1,25-dihydroxyvitamin D; cytokines, such as interleukin-1 and tumor necrosis factor; prostaglandins; and humoral factors that stimulate renal 1-α-hydroxylase. Rarely, tumors induce hypercalcemia by local osteolytic activity after they metastasize to bone. Less commonly, hypercalcemia develops from impaired loss of calcium from the serum (e.g., reduced glomerular filtration) or reduced plasma volume (e.g., dehydration).

The list of differential diagnoses for hypercalcemia is relatively short in dogs and cats (see Table 50-3). In the dog, HHM (especially lymphoma), hypoadrenocorticism, chronic renal failure, hypervitaminosis D, and primary hyperparathyroidism are the most common diagnoses. In the cat, hypercalcemia of malignancy (especially lymphoma and squamous cell carcinoma), chronic renal failure, primary hyperparathyroidism, and idiopathic hypercalcemia are the most common diagnoses. Calcium oxalate urolithiasis and consumption of acidifying diets are commonly identified in cats with hypercalcemia, but their role, if any, in causing the disorder is unknown.

Hypercalcemia can develop in dogs and cats with chronic and, less commonly, acute renal failure. The pathogenesis of hypercalcemia associated with renal failure is complicated. The development of autonomously functioning parathyroid glands or an alteration of the set point for PTH secretion after the prolonged stimulation of renal secondary hyperparathyroidism (see p. 619), decreased PTH degradation by renal tubular cells, increased PTH-mediated intestinal absorption of calcium, increased PTH-mediated bone resorption, decreased renal excretion of calcium, and increased protein-bound or complexed fractions of calcium are believed to contribute to the hypercalcemia of renal failure. Prolonged hypercalcemia, especially in conjunction with concurrent high-normal to increased serum phosphorus concentration, can also cause renal insufficiency and azotemia. Determining whether the renal failure is primary or secondary in a dog with hypercalcemia, hyperphosphatemia, and azotemia poses an interesting diagnostic challenge (see Diagnosis).

## Clinical Features

Although all tissues can be affected by hypercalcemia, the neuromuscular, gastrointestinal, renal and cardiac systems are the most important clinically. Secondary nephrogenic diabetes insipidus, loss of the renal concentration gradient, and metastatic mineralization of the kidney cause polyuria and polydipsia. Decreased excitability of the central and peripheral nervous systems occurring in conjunction with decreased excitability of gastrointestinal smooth muscle cause lethargy, anorexia, vomiting, constipation, weakness and, rarely, seizures. In rare instances, cardiac arrhythmias may develop in animals with severe hypercalcemia (i.e., more than 18 mg/dl). Prolongation of the PR interval and shortening of the QT interval may be found on ECGs recorded in animals with milder hypercalcemia.

Clinical signs are often absent with mild increases in the serum calcium concentration, and hypercalcemia is discovered only after a serum biochemistry panel is performed, often for unrelated reasons. When clinical signs do develop, they initially tend to be insidious in onset. The severity of clinical signs depends in part on the severity, rate of onset, and duration of the hypercalcemia. Clinical signs become more severe as the magnitude of the hypercalcemia increases, regardless of the rate of onset or duration. Clinical signs are usually mild with serum calcium concentrations less than 14 mg/dl, are readily apparent with concentrations greater than 14 mg/dl, and become potentially life-threatening (i.e., cardiac arrhythmias) when the serum calcium concentration exceeds 18 to 20 mg/dl. Clinical signs resulting from the development of calcium uroliths may also occur.

## Diagnosis

Hypercalcemia should always be reconfirmed, preferably from a nonlipemic blood sample obtained from the dog or cat following a 12-hour fast, before embarking on an extensive diagnostic evaluation. Results of a CBC, serum biochemistry panel, and urinalysis, in conjunction with the history and physical examination findings, often provide clues to the diagnosis (see Table 50-3). Special attention should be paid to the serum electrolytes and renal parameters. Hypoadrenocorticism-induced hypercalcemia occurs in conjunction with mineralocorticoid deficiency; hyponatremia, hyperkalemia, and prerenal azotemia should be present. The serum phosphorus concentration is in the lower half of the normal range or low with HHM and primary hyperparathyroidism (Fig. 55-2). If the serum phosphorus concentration is increased and renal function is normal, hypervitaminosis D and bone osteolysis from metastatic or primary bone neoplasia are the primary differentials.

Determining whether renal failure is primary or secondary to hypercalcemia caused by another disorder when hyperphosphatemia and hypercalcemia coexist with azotemia can be difficult. Chronic and, less commonly, acute renal failure can cause hypercalcemia. Alternatively, disorders that cause persistent hypercalcemia with a concurrent high-normal to increased serum phosphorus concentration can cause progressive mineralization of the kidney and eventual renal failure. Measurement of the serum ionized calcium concentration may help identify dogs and cats with renal failure–induced hypercalcemia; serum ionized calcium concentrations are typically normal or decreased in renal failure and increased in hypercalcemia caused by other disorders.

Hypercalcemia of malignancy and primary hyperparathyroidism are the primary differentials when hypercalcemia and normal-to-low serum phosphorus concentrations are identified. The most common malignancy is lymphoma. A careful review of the history and physical examination findings may provide clues to the diagnosis. Systemic signs of illness suggest hypercalcemia of malignancy. Dogs and cats with primary hyperparathyroidism are usually healthy, and clinical

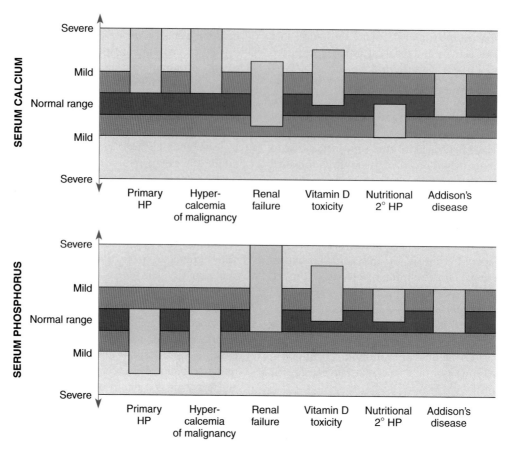

**FIG 55-2**

The range in serum calcium and phosphorus concentrations for the more common causes of hypercalcemia and/or hyperparathyroidism in the dog. *HP,* Hyperparathyroidism; *2° HP,* secondary hyperparathyroidism. (From Feldman EC, Nelson RW: *Canine and feline endocrinology and reproduction,* ed 2, Philadelphia, 1996, WB Saunders.)

signs are mild. The appendicular skeleton, peripheral lymph nodes, abdominal cavity, and rectum should be carefully palpated for masses, lymphadenopathy, hepatomegaly, splenomegaly, or pain on digital palpation of the long bones. Diagnostic tests that are helpful in identifying the underlying malignancy include thoracic and abdominal radiographs; abdominal ultrasound; cytologic evaluation of aspirates of the liver, spleen, lymph nodes, and bone marrow; determination of the serum ionized calcium, PTH, and PTHrP concentrations; and cervical ultrasound.

Sternal and hilar lymphadenopathy is common with lymphoma-induced hypercalcemia and can be readily identified with thoracic radiographs. Radiographs of the thorax and abdomen can also be used to evaluate bones; discrete lytic lesions in the vertebrae or long bones suggest multiple myeloma. Hyperproteinemia, proteinuria, and plasma cell infiltration in the bone marrow suggest multiple myeloma. Cytologic evaluation of peripheral lymph node, bone marrow, and splenic aspirates can be helpful in identifying lymphoma; involvement of the peripheral lymph nodes or spleen by lymphoma can be present without causing their enlargement. Ideally the largest

lymph node should be evaluated. Normal lymph node, bone marrow, and splenic aspirates do not rule out lymphoma.

Measurement of the serum ionized calcium, PTH, and PTHrP levels from the same blood sample is helpful in differentiating primary hyperparathyroidism from HHM. Excessive secretion of biologically active PTHrP plays a central role in the pathogenesis of hypercalcemia in most forms of HHM. An increased serum ionized calcium concentration, a detectable serum PTHrP concentration, and a nondetectable serum PTH concentration are diagnostic for HHM. Lymphoma is the most common cause of detectable PTHrP concentrations, but other tumors, including apocrine gland adenocarcinoma and various carcinomas (e.g., mammary gland, squamous cell, bronchogenic), can also cause hypercalcemia by this mechanism. In contrast, an increased serum ionized calcium concentration, a normal-to-increased serum PTH concentration, and a nondetectable PTHrP concentration are diagnostic of primary hyperparathyroidism. Ultrasonographic examination of the thyroparathyroid complex may reveal enlargement of one or more parathyroid glands. Most parathyroid adenomas measure 4 to 8 mm in diameter, although an occasional parathyroid adenoma will exceed 1 cm. In contrast, the parathyroid glands will be small or undetectable with hypercalcemia of malignancy.

Evaluation of the change in the serum calcium concentration following L-asparaginase administration should be considered for the animal with hypercalcemia of undetermined etiology to rule out occult lymphoma. For the L-asparaginase trial, 20,000 IU/m² of the drug is administered intravenously, and the serum calcium concentration is measured prior to and every 12 hours after administration for as long as 72 hours. A decline in the serum calcium level, usually into the normal range, is strongly suggestive of occult lymphoma. Hypersensitivity reactions are the most common adverse effect associated with L-asparaginase administration; pretreatment with an antihistamine is recommended.

Idiopathic hypercalcemia is an increasingly common diagnosis in young and middle-aged cats. Hypercalcemia is usually mild (less than 13 mg/dl) and asymptomatic. The serum phosphorus concentration and renal parameters are normal. The etiology is unknown. The results of a complete diagnostic evaluation as described above are unremarkable. Serum PTH concentrations are in the normal range or low; primary hyperparathyroidism has not been confirmed in any of these cats. Nephrocalcinosis and urolithiasis may develop, presumably secondary to increased urinary calcium excretion. Effective treatment has not been identified. Serum calcium concentrations have decreased in some cats following a dietary change to a high-fiber diet or after prednisone treatment was initiated, but the response has been unpredictable.

## Treatment

Medical therapy should be directed at eradicating the underlying cause of the hypercalcemia. Supportive therapy to decrease the serum calcium concentration to less toxic levels is indicated if clinical signs are severe, if the serum calcium concentration is greater than 16 mg/dl, if the calcium × phosphorus product is greater than 60 to 70 (implying metastatic mineralization of soft tissues), or if azotemia is present. In dogs and cats, correction of fluid deficits, saline diuresis, diuretic therapy with furosemide, and corticosteroids are the most commonly used modes of therapy (Table 55-9). Prerenal azotemia is common in dogs with hypercalcemia secondary to water restriction imposed by owners concerned about the polyuria and polydipsia. As such, diuretics should never be administered before volume replenishment is completed.

The supportive therapy implemented should not interfere with attempts to establish a definitive diagnosis. As a general rule, saline diuresis followed by diuretic therapy can be initiated without compromising the results of diagnostic tests. Because of the high incidence of lymphoma in animals with hypercalcemia, glucocorticoids should not be administered unless the cause of the hypercalcemia has been identified. Calcitonin may be useful in the treatment of animals with severe hypercalcemia and could be used in lieu of prednisone for treating hypercalcemia in animals without a definitive diagnosis. Calcitonin inhibits osteoclast activity and salmon

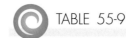

**TABLE 55-9**

**Nonspecific Therapy for Control of Hypercalcemia**

**Acute Therapy**

1. Correct fluid deficits
2. Physiologic saline diuresis, 60-180 mg/kg/day IV
3. Furosemide, 2-4 mg/kg IV, IM, PO q8-12h
4. Once diagnosis has been established: prednisone, 1-2 mg/kg q12h

**Additional therapy if above fails**

1. Sodium bicarbonate, 1-4 mEq/kg given in IV fluids
2. Salmon calcitonin, 4 U/kg IV then 4-8 U/kg SC q12-24h
3. Peritoneal dialysis/hemodialysis

**Long-Term Therapy**

1. Furosemide (see above)
2. Prednisone (see above)
3. Low-calcium diet: prescription diet k/d, u/d, s/d
4. Intestinal phosphate binders if hyperphosphatemia present (see p. 619)
5. Bisphosphonates (etidronate, 10-40 mg/kg PO divided q8-12h)

calcitonin has been used in combination with other therapies to treat hypercalcemia in dogs with cholecalciferol rodenticide toxicosis. Although calcitonin may rapidly decrease the magnitude of the hypercalcemia, its effect may be short-lived (hours), and resistance often develops within a few days, presumably because of downregulation of calcitonin receptors. The transitory effect of calcitonin has limited its usefulness for treating hypercalcemia.

The duration of therapy depends on the reversibility of the underlying cause. If prolonged supportive therapy is required (e.g., in an animal with cholecalciferol-containing rodenticide toxicity or nontreatable malignancy), furosemide, corticosteroids, and a low-calcium diet (e.g., prescription diets u/d and s/d canned, Hill's Pet Products, Topeka, Kan) can be used to help control the hypercalcemia. Non-calcium-containing intestinal phosphorus binders (e.g., aluminum hydroxide) should be administered if hyperphosphatemia is present. The dosage should be adjusted on the basis of serial serum phosphorus determinations. Oral bisphosphonate therapy (e.g., etidronate [Didronel, Proctor and Gamble Pharmaceuticals, Cincinatti, Ohio], 10 to 40 mg/kg orally divided q8-12h) has had some effectiveness in reducing hypercalcemia caused by lymphoma, myeloma, primary hyperparathyroidism, and hypervitaminosis D in dogs. Bisphosphonates decrease osteoclast activity and function and are generally used for maintenance treatment of hypercalcemia in humans. Bisphosphonate treatment has been associated with the development of renal impairment in humans and acute renal failure in animals.

# HYPOCALCEMIA

## Etiology

Hypocalcemia is present if the serum total calcium concentration is less than 9 mg/dl in adult dogs and cats and less than 7 mg/dl in dogs and cats less than 6 months of age or if the serum ionized calcium concentration is less than 1.0 mmol/L, although reference ranges may vary between laboratories. Hypocalcemia develops after increased calcium loss in milk (e.g., puerperal tetany), decreased calcium resorption from bone or kidney (e.g., primary hypoparathyroidism), decreased calcium absorption from the gastrointestinal tract (e.g., malassimilation syndromes), or increased precipitation-chelation of serum calcium (e.g., ethylene glycol toxicity, acute pancreatitis). The acute onset of hyperphosphatemia (see p. 841) can also cause hypocalcemia. The most common causes of hypocalcemia in dogs and cats are puerperal tetany, acute and chronic renal failure, malassimilation syndromes, and primary hypoparathyroidism (especially after thyroidectomy in hyperthyroid cats; see Table 50-5). Hypocalcemia is present in animals in hypoalbuminemic states; however, the ionized fraction of calcium is assumed to be normal. The serum calcium concentration should be adjusted proportionate to a low serum total protein or albumin concentration before rendering a diagnosis of hypocalcemia (see p. 836). However, the association between the total serum calcium concentration and the serum albumin or protein concentration is weak, and serum ionized calcium concentrations can be decreased despite a "corrected" serum total calcium concentration that is in the normal range.

## Clinical Features

Animals with hypocalcemia range from being asymptomatic to showing severe neuromuscular dysfunction. Serum total calcium concentrations between 7.5 and 9 mg/dl are often clinically silent; clinical signs usually occur if values are less than 7 mg/dl. The presence and severity of signs depend on the magnitude, rapidity of onset, and duration of hypocalcemia.

The most common clinical signs are directly attributable to a hypocalcemia-induced increase in neuronal excitability and include nervousness, behavioral changes, focal muscle twitching (especially ear and facial muscles), muscle cramping, stiff gait, tetany, and seizures. The seizures are not usually associated with loss of consciousness or urinary incontinence. Early indicators of hypocalcemia, especially in cats, include lethargy, anorexia, intense facial rubbing, and panting. Exercise, excitement, and stress may induce or worsen clinical signs. Additional physical examination findings may include fever, a "splinted" abdomen, cardiac abnormalities (weak femoral pulses, muffled heart sounds, tachyarrhythmias), and cataracts.

## Diagnosis

Hypocalcemia should be confirmed before initiating diagnostic tests to identify the cause. The list of differential diagnoses for hypocalcemia is relatively short, and the history, physical examination findings, CBC, serum biochemistry panel, serum lipase concentration, and urinalysis usually provide the clues necessary to establish the diagnosis (see Table 50-5). Primary hypoparathyroidism is the most likely diagnosis in the nonazotemic, nonlactating dog or cat with clinical signs of hypocalcemia (see p. 686). The finding of a low or nondetectable baseline serum PTH concentration confirms this diagnosis.

## Treatment

Therapy should be directed at eradicating the underlying cause of the hypocalcemia. Vitamin D or calcium therapy, or both, are indicated if clinical signs of hypocalcemia are present, if the serum calcium concentration is less than 7.5 mg/dl, or if the serum ionized calcium concentration is less than 0.8 mmol/L. If hypocalcemic tetany is present, calcium should be administered intravenously slowly to effect (see Table 50-6). Calcium gluconate is the preferred agent because it is not caustic if administered outside of the vein, unlike calcium chloride. Auscultation and ECG monitoring is advisable during calcium administration; if bradycardia or shortening of the QT interval occurs, the IV infusion should be stopped briefly. Calcium-rich fluids should be infused with caution in dogs or cats with hyperphosphatemia, because they can increase the probability of metastatic calcification of soft tissues, most notably in the kidney.

Once signs of hypocalcemic tetany have been controlled with IV calcium, subcutaneous or oral calcium and oral vitamin D supplementation may be needed to prevent the recurrence of clinical signs. If the cause of hypocalcemia is readily reversible and the hypocalcemia is anticipated to be short-lived (e.g., weaning puppies from bitch with puerperal tetany), an injection of calcium gluconate subcutaneously may be all that is necessary to prevent the recurrence of clinical signs. One can determine the dose of IV calcium gluconate required to control tetany originally, and this dose can then be administered subcutaneously after the calcium gluconate has been diluted in an equal volume of saline solution. Calcium chloride should not be administered subcutaneously. In animals with disorders causing prolonged hypocalcemia (e.g., primary hypoparathyroidism), the IV dose of calcium gluconate initially needed to control tetany can be injected subcutaneously every 6 to 8 hours until oral vitamin D and calcium supplements become effective in maintaining normocalcemia. Calcium gluconate should be diluted at least 1:1 before subcutaneous administration, and calcium chloride should not be used because it is highly irritating to tissues. Alternatively, calcium gluconate can be administered by continuous IV infusion at an initial dosage of 60 to 90 mg of elemental calcium/kg/day. Ten milliliters of 10% calcium gluconate provides 93 mg of elemental calcium. Calcium salts should not be added to fluids that contain lactate, acetate, bicarbonate, or phosphates, because calcium salt precipitates can result. The serum calcium concentration should be measured daily and subcutaneous or IV calcium therapy gradually decreased and then discontinued once the serum total calcium concentration is consistently greater than 8 mg/dl or the serum ionized calcium concentration is greater than 0.9 mmol/L.

Long-term maintenance therapy may be necessary to control hypocalcemia. It is most commonly required for the control of idiopathic hypoparathyroidism and hypoparathyroidism occurring after bilateral thyroidectomy in cats with hyperthyroidism. Oral vitamin D administration is the primary mode of treatment for the management of chronic hypocalcemia (see Table 50-7). Vitamin D works by stimulating intestinal calcium and phosphorus absorption and, together with parathyroid hormone, by mobilizing calcium and phosphorus from bone. Oral calcium supplements are needed early in maintenance therapy in addition to vitamin D (see Table 50-6).

The aim of maintenance therapy is to keep the serum calcium concentration between 9 and 10 mg/dl, which controls clinical signs, lessens the risk of hypercalcemia, and provides some stimulus for remaining or ectopic parathyroid tissue to become functional. The serum calcium concentration should be monitored closely (initially every 24 to 48 hours) and adjustments in therapy made accordingly. Vitamin D therapy is required permanently in animals with idiopathic hypoparathyroidism and in animals that have undergone total parathyroidectomy. Vitamin D therapy can usually be tapered and discontinued if there is only partial or transient parathyroid damage. Regardless, calcium supplementation often may be tapered and stopped. The reader is referred to Chapter 50 for more information on the treatment of hypocalcemia.

## HYPERPHOSPHATEMIA

### Etiology

Hyperphosphatemia is present when the serum phosphorus concentration is greater than 6.5 mg/dl in the adult dog and cat, although reference ranges may vary between laboratories. Dogs (especially large and giant breeds) and cats under 6 months of age normally have higher serum phosphorus concentrations (dog, 3.9 to 9 mg/dl; cat, 3.9 to 8.1 mg/dl) than their adult counterparts. Hyperphosphatemia can result from increased intestinal phosphorus absorption, decreased phosphorus excretion in the urine, or shift in phosphorus from the intracellular to the extracellular compartment. Translocation of phosphorus between the intracellular and extracellular compartment is similar to that of potassium. The most common cause of hyperphosphatemia in dogs and cats is decreased renal excretion secondary to renal failure (Table 55-10).

### Clinical Features

Hyperphosphatemia is a marker of underlying disease. By itself, hyperphosphatemia usually does not cause clinical signs. An acute increase in serum phosphorus may cause hypocalcemia and its associated neuromuscular signs (see p. 840). Sustained hyperphosphatemia can cause secondary hyperparathyroidism, fibrous osteodystrophy, and metastatic calcification in extraosseous sites. Fortunately, most causes of

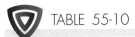

TABLE 55-10

### Causes of Hyperphosphatemia in Dogs and Cats

**Physiologic**

Young growing animal*

**Increased Input**

Hypervitaminosis D*
  Excess supplementation
  Cholecalciferol rodenticides
Jasmine toxicity
Excess dietary intake
Osteolytic bone lesions (neoplasia)

**Decreased Loss**

Acute or chronic renal failure*
Prerenal and postrenal azotemia*
Primary hypoparathyroidism*
Hyperthyroidism
Acromegaly

**Transcellular Shifts (ICF to ECF)**

Metabolic acidosis
Tumor cell lysis syndrome
Tissue trauma or rhabdomyolysis
Hemolysis

**Iatrogenic**

IV phosphorus administration
Phosphate-containing enemas
Anabolic steroids
Diuretics—furosemide and hydrochlorothiazides
Minocycline

**Laboratory Error**

Lipemia
Hyperproteinemia

Modified from Willard MD et al: Disorders of phosphorus: hypophosphatemia and hyperphosphatemia. In DiBartola SP, editor: *Fluid therapy in small animal practice*, ed 2, Philadelphia, 2000, WB Saunders, p 169.
*ICF*, Intracellular fluid; *ECF*, extracellular fluid.
*Common causes.

hyperphosphatemia cause a decrease in serum calcium concentration so that the calcium-phosphorus solubility product ($[Ca] \times [Pi]$) remains less than 60. The risk of soft tissue mineralization increases when the $[Ca] \times [Pi]$ solubility product exceeds 60 to 70. Chronic renal failure is the most common cause of sustained hyperphosphatemia and an increase in the solubility product above 60 to 70.

### Treatment

Hyperphosphatemia usually resolves with correction of the underlying disease. In dogs and cats with renal failure, hyperphosphatemia can initially be lowered with aggressive fluid therapy. Low-phosphorus diets and orally administered phosphate binders are the most effective way to treat sustained hyperphosphatemia caused by renal failure (see p. 619).

## HYPOPHOSPHATEMIA

### Etiology

Hypophosphatemia is present when the serum phosphorus concentration is less than 3 mg/dl in the dog and cat, although reference ranges may vary between laboratories. However, hypophosphatemia is usually not clinically worrisome until the serum phosphorus concentration is less than 1.5 to 2 mg/dl. Hypophosphatemia results from decreased phosphorus absorption in the intestinal tract, increased urinary phosphorus excretion, or a shift from the extracellular to the intracellular compartment. The most common cause of clinically significant hypophosphatemia in the dog and cat occurs within the first 24 hours of therapy for DKA, when there is a shift of potassium and phosphorus from the extracellular to the intracellular compartment (Table 55-11). Translocation of phosphorus between the intracellular and extracellular compartments is similar to that seen with potassium. Factors that promote a shift of potassium into the intracellular compartment (e.g., alkalosis, insulin, glucose infusion) promote a similar shift in phosphorus. During therapy for DKA, the serum phosphorus concentration can decline to severe levels (i.e., less than 1 mg/dl) as a result of the dilutional

## TABLE 55-11

### Causes of Hypophosphatemia in Dogs and Cats

**Decreased Intestinal Absorption**

Phosphate-binding antacids*
Vitamin D deficiency
Decreased dietary intake (?)
Malabsorption, steatorrhea (?)

**Increased Urinary Excretion**

Primary hyperparathyroidism*
Hypercalcemia of malignancy*
Diabetic ketoacidosis (DKA)*
Renal tubular disorders (Fanconi syndrome)
Proximally acting diuretics
Eclampsia

**Transcellular Shifts**

Insulin administration, especially for DKA*
Respiratory and metabolic alkalosis
Sodium bicarbonate administration*
Parenteral glucose administration*
Parenteral nutritional solutions
Hypothermia

Modified from Willard MD et al: Disorders of phosphorus: hypophosphatemia and hyperphosphatemia. In DiBartola SP, editor: *Fluid therapy in small animal practice*, ed 2, Philadelphia, 2000, WB Saunders, p 165.
*Common causes.

effects of fluid therapy and the intracellular shift of phosphorus following the initiation of insulin and bicarbonate therapy. Interestingly, the initial serum phosphorus concentration is usually normal or only mildly decreased, because the metabolic acidosis of DKA results in a shift of phosphorus from the intracellular to the extracellular compartment.

### Clinical Features

Clinical signs may develop when the serum phosphorus concentration is less than 1.5 mg/dl, although signs are quite variable, and severe hypophosphatemia is clinically silent in many animals. Hypophosphatemia primarily affects the hematologic and neuromuscular systems in the dog and cat. Hemolytic anemia is the most common sequela to hypophosphatemia. Hypophosphatemia decreases the erythrocyte concentration of ATP, which increases erythrocyte fragility, leading to hemolysis. Hemolysis is usually not identified until the serum phosphorus concentration is 1 mg/dl or less. Hemolytic anemia can be life-threatening if not recognized and treated. Neuromuscular signs include weakness, ataxia, and seizures, as well as anorexia and vomiting secondary to intestinal ileus.

### Treatment

For most dogs and cats, hypophosphatemia resolves after correction of the underlying cause. Phosphate therapy is probably not indicated for asymptomatic animals in which the serum phosphorus concentration is greater than 1.5 mg/dl and is unlikely to decrease further. Phosphate therapy is indicated if clinical signs or hemolysis are identified or if the serum phosphorus concentration is less than 1.5 mg/dl, especially if a further decrease is possible. It should also be considered during the initial 24 hours of therapy for DKA to help prevent the development of severe hypophosphatemia, especially if the serum phosphorus concentration is below the reference range at the time DKA is diagnosed. Phosphate supplementation is not indicated in dogs and cats with hypercalcemia, hyperphosphatemia, oliguric renal failure, or suspected tissue necrosis.

The goal of therapy is to maintain the serum phosphorus concentration greater than 2 mg/dl without causing hyperphosphatemia. Oral phosphate supplementation is preferred, using a buffered laxative (e.g., Phospho-Soda), balanced commercial diets, or milk. Intravenous phosphate supplementation is usually required to correct severe hypophosphatemia, especially with DKA. Potassium phosphate solutions are typically used. If potassium supplementation is contraindicated, sodium phosphate solutions can be substituted. Potassium and sodium phosphate solutions contain 3 mmol of phosphate per milliliter and either 4.4 mEq of potassium or 4 mEq of sodium per milliliter. The initial dosage of phosphate is 0.01 to 0.03 mmol/kg/hr, preferably administered by constant rate infusion in calcium-free intravenous fluids (i.e., 0.9% sodium chloride, D5W). Alternatively, the amount of potassium supplementation required in the animal can be determined and then provided with half potassium chloride and half potassium phosphate. Adverse effects from overzealous phosphate administration include iatrogenic hypocalcemia and its associated neuromuscular signs (see p. 840), hypernatremia, hypotension, and calcification of soft tissues. Because the dose of phosphate necessary to replete an animal and the animal's response to therapy cannot be predicted, it is important to initially monitor the serum phosphorus concentration every 6 to 8 hours and adjust the phosphate infusion accordingly.

## HYPERMAGNESEMIA

### Etiology

Hypermagnesemia is present if the serum magnesium concentration is greater than 2.5 mg/dl, although reference ranges may vary between laboratories. It is an uncommon clinical problem, owing to the remarkable ability of the kidney to efficiently eliminate excessive magnesium. Hypermagnesemia occurs in dogs and cats with renal insufficiency and failure or occurs iatrogenically after an excessive magnesium intake (e.g., IV administration, antacids, laxatives). Because excess magnesium is rapidly excreted by the healthy kidney, iatrogenic hypermagnesemia usually occurs in animals with renal insufficiency. Hypermagnesemia has also been reported in cats with thoracic neoplasia and pleural effusion, although the mechanism involved with the development of hypermagnesemia in these cats is unknown.

### Clinical Features

Clinical manifestations of hypermagnesemia include lethargy, weakness, and hypotension. Loss of deep tendon reflexes and ECG changes, consisting of prolonged PR intervals, widening QRS complexes, and heart block, occur at higher serum magnesium concentrations. Serious complications, including respiratory depression, apnea, coma, and cardiac arrest, occur in humans when serum magnesium concentrations exceed 10 mg/dl. At these high levels, magnesium acts as a nonspecific calcium-channel blocker.

### Diagnosis

Measurement of the serum magnesium concentration identifies hypermagnesemia. Unlike magnesium depletion, serum concentrations cannot be normal if there is an increase in magnesium stores (see Hypomagnesemia, below). A correlation between increased serum magnesium concentrations and the severity of total body excess has not been reported.

### Treatment

Treatment begins with the discontinuation of all exogenous sources of magnesium. Additional treatment that is implemented depends on the severity of the hypermagnesemia, the clinical presentation, and the status of renal function. Most dogs and cats with healthy kidneys only require supportive care and observation. Treatment aimed at improving renal function is indicated in animals with concurrent renal insufficiency (see Chapter 44). Dogs and cats with cardiac conduction disturbances, heart block, or hypotension should be treated with IV infusions of calcium (see Table 50-6) until cardiac function normalizes. Magnesium-free crystalloid fluids and furosemide can be administered to accelerate renal magnesium excretion.

## HYPOMAGNESEMIA

### Etiology

Hypomagnesemia is present if the serum magnesium concentration is less than 1.5 mg/dl, although reference ranges may vary between laboratories. It results from decreased oral intake or gastrointestinal tract absorption of magnesium (e.g., small intestinal disease causing malabsorption), increased gastrointestinal tract loss (e.g., protracted vomiting, diarrhea), increased urinary magnesium excretion (e.g., interstitial nephritis, diuretics), or a shift of the cation from the extracellular to the intracellular compartment. The most common causes of clinically significant hypomagnesemia in dogs and cats include disorders causing small intestinal malassimilation, renal disorders associated with a high urine output, the osmotic diuresis of DKA, and the shift of potassium, phosphorus, and magnesium from the extracellular to the intracellular compartment that occurs within the first 24 hours of therapy for DKA (Table 55-12). Magnesium is predominately an intracellular cation. The nature of the translocation of magnesium between the intracellular and the extracellular compartments is similar to that of potassium in that factors that promote a shift of potassium into the intracellular compartment (e.g., alkalosis, insulin, glucose infusion) promote a similar shift in magnesium. During therapy for DKA, the serum magnesium concentration can decline to severely low levels (i.e., less than 1 mg/dl) as a result of the dilutional effects of fluid therapy and the intracellular shift of magnesium after the initiation of insulin and bicarbonate therapy.

### Clinical Features

Hypomagnesemia is reported to be the most common electrolyte disorder in critically ill dogs and cats, and magnesium deficiency may predispose animals to a variety of cardiovascular, neuromuscular, and metabolic complications. Clinical signs of hypomagnesemia do not usually occur until the serum magnesium concentration is less than 1.0 mg/dl, and even at these low levels, many animals remain asymptomatic. A magnesium deficiency can result in several nonspecific clinical signs, including lethargy, anorexia, muscle weakness (including dysphagia and dyspnea), muscle fasciculations, seizures, ataxia, and coma. Concurrent hypokalemia, hyponatremia, and hypocalcemia occur in animals with hypomagnesemia, although the prevalence of these electrolyte abnormalities may differ between species. These electrolyte abnormalities may also contribute to the development of clinical signs. Magnesium is a cofactor for all enzyme reactions that involve ATP, most notably the sodium-potassium ATPase pump. Deficiencies in magnesium can lead to potassium wastage from the body, and the resultant hypokalemia

## TABLE 55-12

**Causes of Hypomagnesemia and Magnesium Depletion in Dogs and Cats**

### Gastrointestinal Causes

Inadequate intake
Chronic diarrhea and vomiting*
Malabsorption syndromes
Acute pancreatitis
Cholestatic liver disease
Nasogastric suction

### Renal Causes

Glomerulonephritis
Acute tubular necrosis
Postobstructive diuresis
Drug-induced tubular injury (e.g., aminoglycosides, cisplatin)
Prolonged IV fluid therapy*
Diuretics*
Digitalis administration
Hypercalcemia
Hypokalemia

### Endocrine Causes

Diabetic ketoacidosis*
Hyperthyroidism
Primary hyperparathyroidism
Primary hyperaldosteronism

### Miscellaneous Causes

Acute administration of insulin, glucose, or amino acids
Sepsis
Hypothermia
Massive blood transfusion
Peritoneal dialysis, hemodialysis
Total parenteral nutrition

*Common causes.

may be refractory to appropriate potassium replacement therapy. Magnesium deficiency inhibits PTH secretion from the parathyroid gland, resulting in hypocalcemia. Magnesium deficiency causes the resting membrane potential of myocardial cells to be decreased and leads to increased Purkinje fiber excitability, with the consequent generation of arrhythmias. ECG changes include a prolonged PR interval, widened QRS complex, depressed ST segment, and peaked T waves. Cardiac arrhythmias associated with magnesium deficiency include atrial fibrillation, supraventricular tachycardia, ventricular tachycardia, and ventricular fibrillation. Hypomagnesemia also predisposes animals to digitalis-induced arrhythmias.

## Diagnosis

Serum magnesium is an infrequently measured electrolyte in dogs and cats. Measurement is indicated in those dogs and cats with disorders and predisposing factors that are associated with hypomagnesemia (see Table 55-12). Assessing an animal's magnesium status is problematic, however, because there is no simple, rapid, and accurate laboratory test to gauge the total body magnesium status. Approximately 1% of total body magnesium is present in serum; as a result, serum magnesium concentrations do not always reflect the total body magnesium status. A normal serum magnesium concentration may exist despite an intracellular magnesium deficiency. However, a low serum magnesium concentration does support the presence of a total body magnesium deficiency. Magnesium exists in three distinct forms in serum: an ionized fraction, an anion-complexed fraction, and a protein-bound fraction. A serum ionized magnesium concentration determined using an ion-selective electrode more accurately assesses total body magnesium content than measurement of serum total magnesium and is recommended. Alternative methods of evaluating an animal's magnesium status include determining the ultrafilterable magnesium and the mononuclear blood cell magnesium content; however, these techniques are primarily used in research settings.

## Treatment

The amount of magnesium replaced and the route of administration depend on the severity of hypomagnesemia and the animal's clinical condition. To date there are no clinical studies that have yielded guidelines for magnesium replacement in dogs and cats; currently it is determined empirically. Mild hypomagnesemia may resolve in response to treatment of the underlying disease, the administration of magnesium-containing fluids, or the correction of hypophosphatemia, if present. Dogs receiving long-term diuretic and digoxin therapy may benefit from oral magnesium supplementation or the administration of potassium (and magnesium)-sparing diuretics. Supplementation is indicated if serum magnesium concentrations are less than 1.0 mg/dl, if clinical signs of hypomagnesemia are present, or if refractory hypokalemia or hypocalcemia is present. Renal function must be assessed before the administration of magnesium; the magnesium dose should be reduced by 50% to 75% in azotemic animals, and the serum magnesium concentrations must be monitored frequently to eliminate the risk of hypermagnesemia. The use of magnesium with digitalis cardioglycosides may cause serious conduction disturbances.

Oxide and hydroxide salts of magnesium (1 to 2 mEq/kg/day) are available for oral therapy. The primary adverse reaction is diarrhea. Parenteral solutions of magnesium sulfate (8.13 mEq of magnesium per gram) and magnesium chloride (9.25 mEq of magnesium per gram) salts are available; the IV dose is 0.75 to 1 mEq/kg/day, administered by continuous-rate infusion in 5% dextrose in water. For the treatment of life-threatening ventricular arrhythmias, a dose of 0.15 to 0.3 mEq/kg of magnesium is administered intravenously over 5 to 15 minutes. The magnesium solution should be diluted to 20% or less in D5W. Magnesium is incompatible with solutions containing sodium bicarbonate, calcium, hydrocortisone, and dobutamine hydrochloride. Serum magnesium, calcium, and potassium concentrations should be monitored daily. The goal of magnesium therapy is the resolution of clinical signs or refractory hypokalemia and hypocalcemia. The parenteral administration of magnesium sulfate may cause significant hypocalcemia such that calcium infusion may be necessary. Other adverse effects of magnesium therapy include hypotension, atrioventricular and bundle-branch blocks, and in the event of overdose, respiratory depression and cardiac arrest. Overdoses are treated with calcium gluconate (10 to 50 mg/kg IV).

## Suggested Readings

Bissett SA et al: Hyponatremia and hyperkalemia associated with peritoneal effusion in four cats, *J Am Vet Med Assoc* 218:1590, 2001.

Deniz A et al: Ionized calcium and total calcium in the cat, *Berl Munch Teirarztl Wochenschr* 108:105, 1995.

DiBartola SP, editor: *Fluid therapy in small animal practice,* ed 2, Philadelphia, 2000, WB Saunders.

Feldman EC et al: *Canine and feline endocrinology and reproduction,* ed 3, Philadelphia, 2003, WB Saunders.

Khanna C et al: Hypomagnesemia in 188 dogs: a hospital population–based prevalence study, *J Vet Intern Med* 12:304, 1998.

Kimmel SE et al: Hypomagnesemia and hypocalcemia associated with protein-losing enteropathy in Yorkshire Terriers: five cases (1992-1998), *J Am Vet Med Assoc* 217:703, 2000.

Kimmel SE et al: Incidence and prognostic value of low plasma ionized calcium concentration in cats with acute pancreatitis: 46 cases (1996-1998), *J Am Vet Med Assoc* 219:1105, 2001.

Machado CE et al: Safety of pamidronate in patients with renal failure and hypercalcemia, *Clin Nephrol* 45:175, 1996.

Mann FA et al: Ionized and total magnesium concentrations in blood from dogs with naturally acquired parvoviral enteritis, *J Am Vet Med Assoc* 212:1398, 1998.

Martin LG et al: Magnesium in the 1990s: implications for veterinary critical care, *J Vet Emer Crit Care* 3:105, 1993.

Martin LG et al: Abnormalities of serum magnesium in critically ill dogs: incidence and implications, *J Vet Emer Crit Care* 4:15, 1994.

Midkiff AM et al: Idiopathic hypercalcemia in cats, *J Vet Intern Med* 14:619, 2000.

Mischke R et al: The effect of the albumin concentration on the relation between the concentration of ionized calcium and total calcium in the blood of dogs, *Dtsch Tierarztl Wochenschr* 103:199, 1996.

Norris CR et al: Serum total and ionized magnesium concentrations and urinary fractional excretion of magnesium in cats with diabetes mellitus and diabetic ketoacidosis, *J Am Vet Med Assoc* 215:1455, 1999.

Savary KCM et al: Hypercalcemia in cats: a retrospective study of 71 cases (1991-1997), *J Vet Intern Med* 14:184, 2000.

Toll J et al: Prevalence and incidence of serum magnesium abnormalities in hospitalized cats, *J Vet Intern Med* 16:217, 2002.

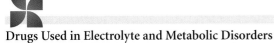

## Drugs Used in Electrolyte and Metabolic Disorders

| GENERIC NAME (TRADE NAME) | PURPOSE | RECOMMENDED DOSE | |
|---|---|---|---|
| | | **DOG** | **CAT** |
| Calcitonin—salmon (Calcimar) | Treat hypercalcemia | 4 U/kg IV, then 4-8 U/kg q12-24h | Unknown |
| Calcium—injectable and oral preparations | Treat hypocalcemia | See Table 50-6, p. 688 | See Table 50-6 |
| Calcium gluconate-10% | Treat hyperkalemia | 2-10 ml IV, slow infusion; 0.5-1.0 ml/kg, slow IV infusion | 2-10 ml IV, slow infusion |
| Cholestyramine (Questran) | Treat idiopathic hypercholesterolemia | 1-2 g PO q12h | Unknown |
| Clofibrate (Atromid-S) | Treat idiopathic hypertriglyceridemia | 500 mg PO q12h | Unknown |
| Etidronate disodium (Didronel) | Treat hypercalcemia | 10-40 mg/kg PO divided q8-12h | 10-40 mg/kg PO divided q8-12h |
| Furosemide (Lasix) | Treat hypercalcemia and hypermagnesemia | 2-4 mg/kg PO, IV q8-12h | 2-4 mg/kg PO, IV q8-12h |
| Gemfibrozil (Lopid) | Treat idiopathic hypertriglyceridemia | 200 mg PO q24h | 10 mg/kg PO q12h |
| Insulin—regular crystalline | Treat hyperkalemia | 0.5-1.0 U/kg plus 2 g dextrose/U of insulin in parenteral fluids IV | 0.5-1.0 U/kg plus 2 g dextrose/U of insulin in parenteral fluids IV |
| Lovastatin (Mevacor) | Treat idiopathic hypercholesterolemia | 10-20 mg PO q24h | Unknown |
| Magnesium—injectable and oral preparations | Treat hypomagnesemia | See p. 844 | See p. 844 |
| Marine-life oil supplements | Treat idiopathic hypertriglyceridemia | 10-30 mg/kg PO q24h | 10-30 mg/kg PO q24h |

*Continued*

Drugs Used in Electrolyte and Metabolic Disorders—cont'd

| GENERIC NAME (TRADE NAME) | PURPOSE | RECOMMENDED DOSE | |
|---|---|---|---|
| | | DOG | CAT |
| Niacin | Treat idiopathic hypertriglyceridemia | 100 mg PO q24h | Unknown |
| Potassium gluconate (Kaon Elixir, Tumil-K) | Treat hypokalemia | 2.2 mEq L/100 kcal food consumed *or* 2 mEq K/ 4.5 kg PO q12h | 2.2 mEq L/100 kcal food consumed *or* 2 mEq K/ 4.54 PO q12h |
| Prednisone | Treat hypercalcemia | 1-2 mg/kg PO q12h | 1-2 mg/kg PO q12h |
| Sodium bicarbonate | Treat hyperkalemia | 1-2 mEq/kg IV, slow bolus | 1-2 mEq/kg IV, slow bolus |
| Vitamin D preparations | Treat hypocalcemia | See Table 50-7, p. 689 | See Table 50-7 |

# CHAPTER 56

## Disorders of the Estrous Cycle

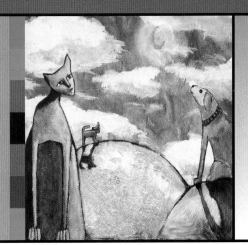

### CHAPTER OUTLINE

NORMAL ESTROUS CYCLE, 847
    The bitch, 847
    The queen, 851
DIAGNOSTIC TESTS FOR THE FEMALE
REPRODUCTIVE TRACT, 853
    Vaginal cytology, 853
    Vaginoscopy, 853
    Vaginal bacterial cultures, 854
    Virology, 854
    Assessment of reproductive hormones, 855
    Radiology and ultrasonography, 858
    Karyotyping, 858
    Laparoscopy and celiotomy, 858
FEMALE INFERTILITY, 859
    Failure to cycle, 860
    Prolonged interestrous interval, 862
    Short interestrous interval, 862
    Abnormal proestrus and estrus, 863
    Prolonged estrus, 863
    Short estrus, 864
    Normal cycles, 864
ESTRUS SUPPRESSION AND POPULATION
CONTROL, 865
    Megestrol acetate, 866
    Androgens, 867
    GnRH agonists, 867
OVARIAN REMNANT SYNDROME, 867
ESTRUS INDUCTION, 868
    The queen, 868
    The bitch, 868
INDUCTION OF OVULATION, 869
    The queen, 869
    The bitch, 869

## NORMAL ESTROUS CYCLE

### THE BITCH

The average age at the time of puberty in bitches is 9 to 10 months, and the range is 6 to 24 months of age. The interval from the beginning of one cycle to the beginning of the next, or the interestrous interval, varies from 4 to 12 months and averages 7 months. The interestrous interval is extremely variable within bitches, more so than it is among bitches. Because of this variability, the past interestrous interval cannot be used to accurately predict the next cycle in an individual bitch. Although a few bitches are very consistent, in most there is more than a month's variation from cycle to cycle. The interestrous interval is not influenced by pregnancy or the photoperiod, although breeds such as the Basenji cycle only once each year, indicating a possible effect of the photoperiod in some individuals. The estrous cycle in the bitch is divided into four components: proestrus, estrus, diestrus, and anestrus. Proestrus and estrus together are often referred to as *heat* or *season*. Together they constitute the follicular phase of the reproductive cycle.

#### Proestrus

Proestrus is considered to begin when vulvar swelling and a sanguineous discharge are first observed. It ends when the bitch allows copulation. Proestrus is characterized by increasing serum concentrations of estradiol that cause vulvar swelling, vaginal edema and cornification, and uterine bleeding that is recognized by a serosanguineous vulvar discharge. The average duration of proestrus is 9 days, and the range is 3 to 17 days. Attractiveness to males and receptivity to them gradually increase throughout proestrus.

The factor, or factors, responsible for initiating proestrus and the start of each new estrous cycle in bitches have not been completely elucidated. Sporadic bursts of luteinizing hormone (LH) secretion and fluctuations of follicle-stimulating hormone (FSH) secretion from the pituitary occur throughout anestrus and are often similar in magnitude to the periovulatory peak. From early anestrous onward there is an increase in FSH secretion without a concomitant increase in LH, until the end of anestrus, when there is an increase in LH pulse frequency and amplitude. In addition to the change in FSH and LH pulsatility, the termination of anestrus may also depend on increased ovarian responsiveness to the gonadotropins. Regardless of the initiating factors, ovarian follicles develop and mature and secrete 17-β-estradiol during proestrus (Fig. 56-1). The plasma estradiol concentrations

gradually increase from average anestrual concentrations of less than 15 pg/ml to peak concentrations of greater than 50 pg/ml 1 or 2 days before the LH surge. The estradiol concentrations then decline rapidly during the 1 to 2 days before the LH surge and the onset of estrus.

Estrogen causes the vaginal epithelial cells to proliferate and mature (*cornification*). The degree of estrogenic influence and therefore the stage of the estrous cycle with respect to the serum estrogen concentration can be monitored by vaginal cytology (Fig. 56-2). During early proestrus, parabasal and intermediate vaginal epithelial cells are the predominant cells

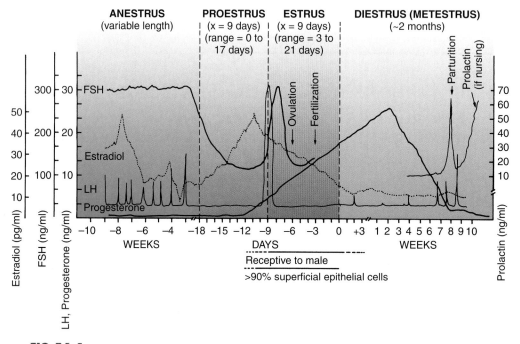

**FIG 56-1**
The canine estrous cycle. (From Morrow DA, editor: *Current therapy in theriogenology,* ed 2, Philadelphia, 1986, WB Saunders.)

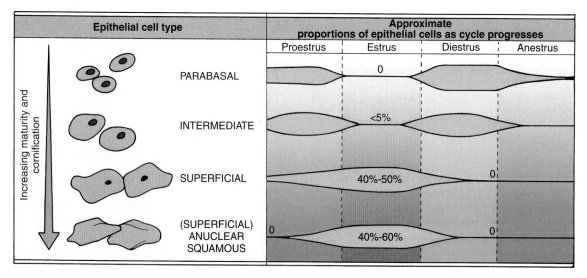

**FIG 56-2**
Cytologic changes of vaginal epithelial cells.

(more than 80%). As proestrus progresses, the population of exfoliated cells gradually matures; parabasal cells disappear as superficial cells increase in number. By late proestrus, superficial and anuclear squamous cells account for 70% to 80% of the epithelial cells. Red blood cells (RBCs) are present throughout proestrus. White blood cells (WBCs) decrease in number. Extracellular bacteria may be present throughout proestrus and estrus.

## Estrus

Behavioral estrus is characterized by acceptance of mating. The bitch's feet are firmly planted to allow the male to mount, hence the term *standing heat.* The tail is deviated to the side to allow intromission; this behavior has been referred to as "flagging." Stroking the perineum may occasionally elicit flagging, which would be an indication that the bitch is in estrus. The average duration of estrus is 9 days, and the range is 3 to 21 days. The swollen vulva is less turgid than during proestrus. The vulvar discharge of estrus is usually less bloody than that of proestrus, but normal bitches often have a sanguineous discharge throughout proestrus and estrus. Therefore changes in the gross appearance of the discharge are not reliable indicators of the transition from proestrus to estrus.

Coincident with the decline in the serum estradiol concentration, canine ovarian follicular cells begin to luteinize and secrete progesterone. The serum progesterone concentration increases above anestrual concentrations of less than 1 ng/ml (approximately 3 nmol/L) just before the LH surge. The decline in the serum estrogen concentration and the increase in the serum progesterone concentration in late proestrus are believed to be responsible for initiating the change in behavior associated with the onset of estrus, and for inducing the preovulatory surge in FSH and LH secretion (see Fig. 56-1). The LH surge in turn initiates ovulation and the subsequent formation of corpora lutea. Although the onset of behavioral estrus usually occurs within a day or two of the LH surge, behavioral estrus may occur as early as 4 days before or as late as 6 days after the LH surge.

In most bitches, ovulation occurs within 48 hours of the LH surge (the range is 0 to 96 hours). Primary oocytes are ovulated and take another 2 to 3 days to mature before fertilization can occur. Mature oocytes apparently have a fertile life of 2 to 3 days. The time during which mature oocytes are available for fertilization has been referred to as the *fertile period.* Freshly ejaculated canine sperm remains capable of fertilization in the female tract for 3 to 4 days and occasionally for as long as 6 days.

Vaginal cytologic specimens obtained during estrus are characterized by a predominance of superficial cells, an absence of neutrophils, and a clear background. During estrus, 90% or more of the epithelial cells are superficial and anuclear squamous cells. WBCs are normally absent during estrus. RBCs and extracellular bacteria are often present.

## Breeding Management

Because of the importance of territorial and social dominance to canine reproduction (see p. 907), the usual practice is to take the bitch to the stud for breeding. To optimize conception rates and litter size, viable sperm that are capable of fertilization and mature oocytes that are capable of being fertilized must be present simultaneously. This can be accomplished by a number of different strategies. A common practice is to begin breeding on a predetermined day of the cycle and to breed every other day for as long as behavioral estrus lasts, or for at least two breedings. Often day 10 to day 12 after the onset of proestrus is chosen. Because the average length of proestrus is 9 days, bitches experiencing an "average" cycle would be in estrus at that time. Because the LH surge usually occurs close to the onset of behavioral estrus, because ovulation usually occurs 2 days after the LH surge, because ova would be fertilizable 2 days later, and because freshly ejaculated semen is capable of fertilization for 4 days, this method of breeding management is often successful. As with other management schemes, multiple inseminations once every 1 to 3 days enhance conception rates and litter size. Breeding every other day is certainly acceptable but probably unnecessary for animals with normal fertility, providing that at least two breedings are done during the fertile period.

The management scheme of breeding on a predetermined day of the cycle is often modified according to the behavior of the bitch and occasionally according to the behavior of the stud. Bitches not in estrus will not allow copulation. Putting the breeding pair together for supervised periods (15 to 60 minutes) and observing their behavior, a practice called *teasing,* before the anticipated onset of estrus will enable the manager to identify the first day of behavioral estrus; thereafter, breeding can be done several times throughout estrus. Certain males will occasionally show distinctly greater interest in breeding on a particular day during estrus than on other days of that cycle. Some kennel managers believe that such behavior in a male signals the optimal time for insemination and cite excellent conception rates and large litters from these males as validation of their belief.

Vaginal cytology is a very useful adjunct to these management schemes, especially in instances in which the female does not exhibit strong behavioral estrus or in which the breeding pair is separated geographically, necessitating transportation of the animals or the semen. The changes in the exfoliated cells reflect the effects of estrogen on the vaginal epithelium. Under the influence of estrogen, the vaginal epithelium changes in thickness from a thin layer of stratified squamous cells without cornification to many cell layers in depth with prominent cornification and rete pegging. The epithelial cells exfoliate easily. Vaginal cytology therefore can be used as a bioassay for estrogen to monitor the follicular phase of the ovarian cycle. As the cytologic changes in proestrus approach those characteristic of estrus, the animal, or the semen, should be shipped to ensure safe arrival for insemination during the fertile period. Females that do not show normal behavioral estrus during the time that the findings of exfoliative vaginal cytology are consistent with estrus (i.e., greater than 90% superficial cells) could be bred using artificial insemination.

The success of these management methods is predicated on the assumptions that ovulation will occur some time during behavioral and cytologic estrus, and multiple inseminations will ensure that viable sperm, capable of fertilization, are present whenever ovulation and oocyte maturation actually do occur. If the LH surge could be identified and used in conjunction with the other management tools, this would greatly enhance the certainty that insemination was performed during the optimal fertile period. This is especially true in situations in which gamete viability is less than optimal, such as when thawed frozen semen is used (see p. 942). The success of breeding dogs in which fertility is suboptimal and the success of breeding with thawed frozen semen have been greatly improved by breeding according to the LH surge, a practice that has been referred to as *ovulation timing.* The LH surge can be identified by measuring serum LH concentrations on a daily basis or by identifying the preovulatory increase in the serum concentrations of progesterone that coincides with the LH surge in bitches. Inseminations should be done 4 to 6 days after the LH surge. Interpretation of LH and progesterone results is discussed in greater detail in the section on the assessment of reproductive hormones (see p. 855).

Unlike the situation with queens, breeding a bitch several times during the same day appears to offer no advantage over breeding a single time on a given day. The day of insemination with respect to the occurrence of ovulation is more important than the number of inseminations per day. As the time between insemination and the fertile period lengthens, both litter size and conception rates decrease. Inseminations during proestrus or diestrus are rarely successful. Conception rates and litter size are also affected by maternal age. Conception rates, litter size, and neonatal survival are greatest for Beagle bitches between 2 and 3.5 years of age. After 5 years of age the conception rate and litter size decline, and neonatal mortality begins to increase. Similarly, in Labrador Retriever, Golden Retriever, and German Shepherd bitches studied from 1 to 10 years of age, it was found that the number of pups born declines when bitches are 7 years of age or older. Litter size differs among breeds, with the bitches of smaller breeds tending to have fewer pups per litter because they tend to ovulate fewer ova.

### Diestrus

Diestrus begins with the bitch's refusal to mate. There are no external signs to mark the onset of diestrus other than the cessation of the signs of estrus. Diestrus represents the luteal phase of the cycle. The luteal secretion of progesterone depends on pituitary LH and prolactin. The serum progesterone concentration increases rapidly during the first 2 weeks after the LH surge and ovulation (see Fig. 56-1). It peaks at 15 to 80 ng/ml (approximately 47 to 250 nmol/L) by 15 to 30 days after ovulation. The plasma progesterone concentration remains elevated but gradually declines during the next 2 months regardless of whether pregnancy occurs. In pregnant bitches there is a rapid prepartum drop in the progesterone concentration to less than 2 ng/ml (approximately 6.4 nmol/L). This occurs approximately 64 days after the LH surge and approx-

imately 24 hours before the onset of parturition. The decline in the progesterone concentration may be more gradual in nonpregnant bitches and may not reach basal levels of 0.2 to 0.5 ng/ml (approximately 0.6 to 1.6 nmol/L) for 90 days. Specific luteotropic or luteolytic factors produced by the canine uterus or placenta that regulate ovarian function have yet to be identified. Although LH and prolactin are luteotropic, the canine corpus luteum appears to be unaffected by pregnancy. Instead, luteal regression appears to occur after a predetermined life span irrespective of the continuing availability of LH.

The beginning of diestrus is marked by an abrupt change in vaginal cytology. Diestrus is characterized by a sudden reduction in the number of superficial cells and the reappearance of intermediate cells, neutrophils, and background debris (see Fig. 56-2). On the first day of cytologic diestrus, parabasal and intermediate cells outnumber the superficial and anuclear squamous cells. Sheets of intermediate cells are also often observed. WBCs return in high numbers during the first day or two of diestrus. RBCs and bacteria disappear. The initial dramatic change in cytologic appearance is followed by a gradual change to the anestrual cytologic appearance (i.e., a predominance of parabasal cells). On the basis of the examination of only a single cytologic specimen, early proestrus to midproestrus cannot be distinguished from diestrus. The transition from proestrus, through estrus, and into diestrus is usually adequately monitored by cytologic studies done every other day. Parturition or signs of false pregnancy (see p. 886) are the only clinical evidence of the end of diestrus. Endocrinologically, diestrus ends when the serum progesterone concentrations decline to less than 1 ng/ml (approximately 3 nmol/L).

### Anestrus

Anestrus follows diestrus and ends with the onset of proestrus of the next cycle. The interval from the end of diestrus, as defined by basal serum progesterone concentrations, to the onset of proestrus is quite variable but averages 4.5 months. Because there are no external signs associated with anestrus, this phase of the cycle has been described erroneously as a period of sexual quiescence. In fact, the pituitary-ovarian axis and the uterus are active during anestrus. Pulsatile fluctuations in the pituitary hormones LH and FSH and in ovarian estrogen secretion have been identified. During anestrus, the endometrium sloughs. The size and activity of the endometrial glands and the thickness of the myometrium and endometrium all decrease, although not to the parameters seen in prepubertal bitches. Endometrial repair continues for about 120 days after nonpregnant cycles and for slightly longer (150 days) after a pregnant cycle. The vaginal cytology of anestrus is quite acellular; it contains primarily parabasal cells and small intermediate epithelial cells. The duration of anestrus per se is rarely determined in clinical practice because anestrus has no external indicators. Rather, the interestrous interval, the onset of proestrus of one cycle to the onset of proestrus of the next cycle, is usually described.

Given the extreme variations in the durations of proestrus and estrus, the lack of correlation between the first day of behavioral estrus and the LH surge, the variable interval from the LH peak to ovulation, the need for oocyte maturation after ovulation, and the fertilizable life spans of mature oocytes and sperm, it is readily apparent that events of the canine reproductive cycle cannot be adequately predicted or monitored solely on the basis of the number of days from the onset of proestrus, the physical and behavioral changes in the bitch, or the number of days since breeding.

## THE QUEEN

Female cats are seasonally polyestrous. Cyclicity is controlled by the photoperiod, which must be approximately 12 to 14 hours of light with an intensity of 50 footcandles. Therefore cats exposed to natural light usually cease cycling during winter months, whereas cats maintained under artificial light often cycle throughout the year. It has been shown that maintaining 14:10 to 16:8 hour light:dark schedules maximizes the number of cycling queens in the colony. In the presence of adequate light, sexual maturity and the first estrous cycle normally occur at 6 to 9 months of age, with a range of 5 to 12 months. Unlike bitches, which ovulate spontaneously, queens are induced to ovulate by coital stimulation of the vagina. In addition to coitally induced ovulation, many domestic cats have cycles in which spontaneous ovulation occurs.

The follicular phase of the cycle is characterized by increasing serum concentrations of 17-β-estradiol associated with the onset of proestrus and estrus. Because there is negligible vulvar swelling or discharge in queens compared to bitches, proestrus and estrus are usually recognized by behavioral changes. Proestrus is characterized by increasingly affectionate behavior, rubbing, treading with the rear feet, vocalization, and decreasing hostility toward the male. Proestrus may be so short as to be unrecognized, but more typically it lasts 1 to 2 days.

Estrus is characterized by increased vocalization, lordosis, holding the tail to one side, and allowing copulation. This characteristic estrual posture can sometimes be stimulated by stroking the perineum (Fig. 56-3). The cytologic appearance of exfoliated vaginal epithelial cells (see Fig. 56-2) during the estrous cycle is similar to that of bitches, except that RBCs are much less common. The duration of estrus among queens is quite variable but is usually about 6 days. It is not influenced by copulation. Anovulatory cycles occur every 2 to 3 weeks as long as light is adequate.

Ovulation occurs as a result of a neuroendocrine reflex that is initiated by the mechanical stimulation of sensory receptors in the vagina and cervix. This sensory input causes a surge of LH to be released from the pituitary gland (Fig. 56-4), which in turn causes ovulation. The intensity of the copulatory stimulation necessary to induce the LH surge is unknown but varies among queens. The frequency of coital stimulation is apparently the single most important determinant of ovulation in cats. A single copulation

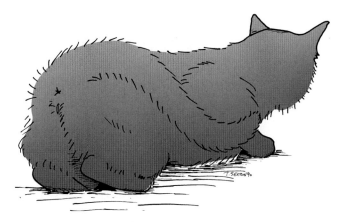

**FIG 56-3**
Estrual posture of the queen.

induces the LH surge necessary for ovulation in approximately 50% of cats, whereas more than 90% of normal domestic shorthair cats ovulate if bred three times daily for the first 3 days of estrus. The day of estrus on which mating occurs and the duration of estrus have no apparent effect on ovulation. Once the LH surge occurs, hormonal responses to additional copulatory stimuli are diminished. Ovulation occurs approximately 48 hours after the LH surge. Although cats continue to be referred to as *induced ovulators,* several investigators have shown that 35% to 60% of colony cats ovulate spontaneously, in the absence of coital stimulation or direct physical contact of any kind with other cats.

After intromission and ejaculation, the queen emits a characteristic "scream" that signals to the male to dismount. Because cats often prefer seclusion, breeding may not be witnessed by the owner. The queen's scream may be the only evidence that mating has occurred. The queen then begins frenzied rolling and grooms her perineum for several minutes and aggressively rebuffs the male. When this "after reaction" subsides, the queen allows another mating. Mating frequency is greatest during the first 2 hours (average of five copulations per hour), after which the frequency decreases to somewhat less than one copulation per hour for the next 3 days.

To ensure adequate copulatory stimulation to induce ovulation and to ensure the presence of adequate numbers of viable sperm at the time of ovulation, three breedings per day for the first 3 days of estrus are recommended. Because of the territorial nature of cats, especially males, the queen should be brought to the stud. The two should be placed together for short periods so that their behavior can be observed. The manager can then separate the animals before either is injured if fighting occurs. The manager can also determine whether the queen is in estrus and can be confident that matings have actually taken place. This supervised mating scheme may be the best way to optimize conception, but it is labor intensive. Some managers prefer to house the queen and

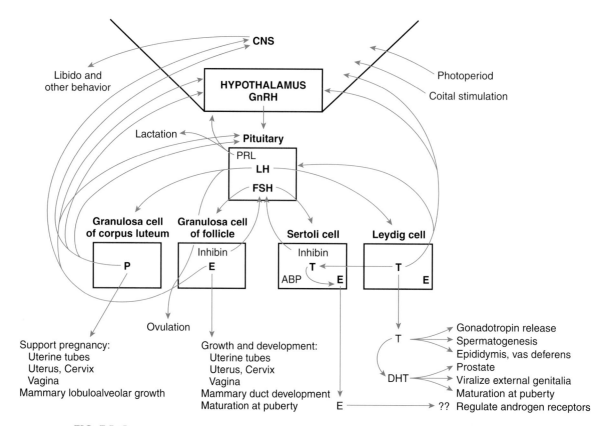

**FIG 56-4**
Hypothalamic-pituitary-gonadal axis. *ABP,* Androgen-binding protein; *DHT,* dihydrotestosterone; *E,* estrogen; *FSH,* follicle-stimulating hormone; *GnRH,* gonadotropin-releasing hormone; *LH,* luteinizing hormone; *P,* progesterone; *PRL,* prolactin; *T,* testosterone.

tom together and allow mating to occur ad libitum, without direct observation. In some large breeding colonies, harem, rather than individual, mating schemes are used. In the harem scheme, one or two toms are housed with many queens. This method is the least labor intensive but has the disadvantages of unknown breeding dates, unknown paternity if more than one tom is involved, and delayed recognition of subfertility in individual animals.

After ovulation the follicles luteinize and produce progesterone. This is the luteal phase of the cycle. Serum concentrations of progesterone rise 24 to 48 hours after ovulation and peak 25 to 30 days later. Luteal progesterone is necessary for the maintenance of pregnancy in both bitches and queens. Although it was generally thought that the primary source of progesterone during the latter part of pregnancy in cats was the feline placenta, Verstegen and colleagues (1993) have shown that the feline placenta either does not secrete progesterone or does so in amounts insufficient to maintain pregnancy. In cats, the life span of the corpus luteum is apparently influenced by the presence or absence of pregnancy. There apparently are pregnancy-specific luteotropic hormones from the feline placenta or pituitary. After the nonfertile induction of ovulation, the corpora lutea persist for about 30 to 40 days. The next cycle may begin any time thereafter, usually within 10 days. A re-

cent study found an average interestrous interval of 61 days in queens that were bred but did not conceive, whereas the average interestrous interval for nonbred queens was 22 days. Serum concentrations of progesterone were not determined in those cats. The corpora lutea continue to produce progesterone throughout the approximately 67-day gestation (Fig. 56-5), with the serum concentrations gradually declining during the second half of pregnancy. Although estrous behavior has been observed in pregnant queens, true superfetation has not been proved. Queens usually do not resume cycling while they are nursing a litter. Estrous behavior is usually evident 2 to 3 weeks after weaning, although this is quite variable. The postpartum estrus is shorter in duration and less fertile than others.

Litters typically consist of two to five kittens. Litter size and neonatal survival are best for queens age 1 to 5 years, provided that first parity occurs before 3 years of age. Litter size and neonatal survival usually improve after the first parity. However, if the first parity occurs after 3 years of age, litter size and neonatal survival usually remain poor. Reproductive performance declines after 6 years of age. Because of decreased fertility, decreased litter size, increased neonatal losses, and the increased prevalence of other illnesses in older queens, most should be retired from breeding after 8 years of age.

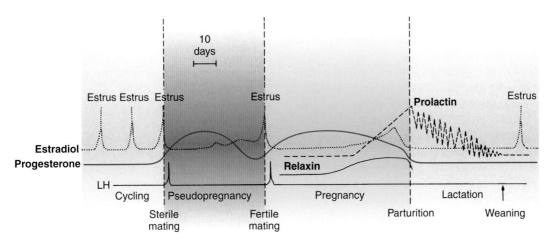

**FIG 56-5**
The feline estrous cycle.

## DIAGNOSTIC TESTS FOR THE FEMALE REPRODUCTIVE TRACT

### VAGINAL CYTOLOGY

The importance of exfoliative vaginal cytology in breeding management and in the evaluation of females with reproductive disorders cannot be overemphasized. Specimens may be obtained with a moistened, cotton-tipped swab or by flushing and aspirating a small volume of saline solution from the vagina. Specimens can be stained with any number of commercially available stains, including Wright's, Wright-Giemsa, modified Wright-Giemsa (Diff-Quik; Baxter Scientific, Chicago, Ill), trichrome, or new methylene blue. The number and morphologic characteristics of vaginal epithelial cells, WBCs, and RBCs are evaluated. The preparations are also examined for the presence of other material, such as bacteria, mucus, cellular debris, endometrial cells, neoplastic cells, or uteroverdin. Vaginal cytology is used to determine the present stage of the estrous cycle (see Fig. 56-2), to determine breeding (see p. 849) and whelping (see p. 891) dates, and to identify the nature of certain abnormal processes within the reproductive tract (see pp. 870-872).

### VAGINOSCOPY

Vaginoscopy is useful for determining the stage of the estrous cycle, evaluating anatomic abnormalities, determining the source of a vulvar discharge (vestibule, vagina, or uterus), and determining the nature and extent of lesions within the vestibule and vagina. Samples for cytologic, microbiologic, and histopathologic studies can easily be obtained through the endoscope. The endoscopic appearance varies with the stage of the estrous cycle. Endoscopic findings are assessed by comparing them to the normal anatomic features of the vagina, usually in conjunction with vaginal cytology.

The canine vagina is quite long. In Beagles, for example, it measures 10 to 14 cm in length and 1.5 cm in diameter, whereas in Newfoundlands the length may be up to 29 cm. The endoscopic equipment must be of the appropriate size for the particular female. Proctoscopes and cystoscopes designed for human pediatric or adult patients, or flexible fiberoptic endoscopic equipment of appropriate diameter can be used. Pediatric anoscopes or veterinary otoscopes may be narrow enough for use in queens and small bitches but are too short for examination of the cranial vagina and cervix.

In mature bitches, vaginoscopy is usually performed with the animal awake and standing, without sedation or anesthesia unless a biopsy is planned. Anesthesia is usually necessary for vaginoscopy in queens, very small bitches, and puppies. The perineum is inspected and cleansed. The endoscope is then lubricated with warm saline solution or with sterile, water-soluble lubricant. The clitoris and clitoral fossa must be avoided. Therefore the endoscope is passed in a dorsal direction through the dorsal commissure of the vulva. There may be slight resistance at the vestibulovaginal junction (see Fig. 57-2). The diameter of that area may be so narrow in prepubertal and neutered animals that the instrument cannot be safely passed. The angle of the speculum is adjusted to a more horizontal direction after it passes through the vestibulovaginal junction.

During proestrus the longitudinal folds of the vagina are edematous, round, and smooth. As new folds develop, the vaginal lumen becomes filled with folds. A clear, bright red fluid is seen in the vaginal lumen, sometimes in large amounts. As estrus approaches, the vaginal folds become lower and wrinkled. During estrus the folds appear sharp, angular, and crinkled. The mucosa is pale, and the vaginal lumen is wide. There is less luminal fluid than there is during proestrus. This fluid is clear and usually straw colored; however, it may continue to be bright red throughout estrus.

During diestrus (the luteal phase), the vaginal folds are low, round, and soft. The folds in the cranial vagina have a characteristic rosette appearance and may be mistaken for the cervix. Clear or opalescent mucus is present in the vaginal lumen during diestrus. The vaginal mucosa has streaks of hyperemia. During anestrus and in neutered bitches, the vaginal folds are low and round and do not fill the lumen. There is a thin mucus coating that gives the mucosa a translucent, pink-red appearance. In these animals the mucous membranes are thin and easily traumatized. Pinpoint submucosal hemorrhages may develop in response to seemingly gentle contact with the endoscope. During anestrus and in neutered animals there is usually some resistance to the passage of the endoscope unless the instrument is well lubricated.

In bitches, one of the vaginal folds, known as the *dorsal median postcervical fold,* is often mistaken for the cervix. This fold extends from the caudal-dorsal edge of the vaginal portion of the cervix along the dorsal midline and eventually blends into lesser folds of the vagina. It is composed of longitudinal and oblique smooth muscle bundles and irregularly arranged collagen. Unlike other folds of the vagina, the dorsal median fold has no elastic fibers. In Beagle-size bitches, this fold is 15 to 42 mm long and 2 to 10 mm wide, compared with the average vaginal length in the same bitches of 158 ± 30 mm. The lumen of the cranial vagina in this area is quite narrow. Because of its length, location, and inelastic nature, the dorsal median postcervical fold often prevents visualization and catheterization of the canine cervix.

The vaginal portion of the cervix is tubular, with small furrows radiating from the os, which give it the appearance of a star or rosette. The cervical os is not obviously patent, even if fluid is seen flowing through it, except during the puerperium. The vaginal lumen around the cervix and the cranial aspect of the dorsal median postcervical fold is quite narrow, and it is usually necessary to use small diameter (0.5 cm) instruments to visualize the cervix. The narrow pericervical vaginal lumen with the dorsal median postcervical fold, and the rosette appearance of the cranial vagina, can be confused with the cervix.

## VAGINAL BACTERIAL CULTURES

Bacterial infections of the reproductive tract are relatively common. Bacterial culture is indicated for the evaluation of many reproductive disorders, including infertility, purulent vulvar discharge, pyometra, metritis, and abortion and stillbirth. Because the uterus is normally sterile, the interpretation of uterine culture results is relatively straightforward. Unfortunately, because of the extreme difficulty in catheterizing the cervix in the bitch or queen, uterine samples are usually obtained only during laparotomy. Vaginal cultures are often performed in lieu of uterine cultures. To minimize contamination from the vestibule and caudal vagina, samples for bacterial culture should be obtained from the cranial vagina using a guarded culture swab (e.g., those manufactured by Kalayjian Industries, Long Beach, Calif., and Nasco, Fort Atkinson, Wis) or through a sterile speculum.

The canine vagina has normal bacterial flora, which are listed in Table 56-1. The normal flora of the feline vagina are very similar. *Staphylococcus* spp., *Streptococcus canis,* and *Escherichia coli* are the most common organisms recovered from queens. In normal bitches and queens, mixed populations of these organisms are usually recovered in small numbers.

Most of the organisms that comprise the normal vaginal flora are also potential pathogens. Several studies have shown

 **TABLE 56-1**

**Normal Bacterial Flora of the Canine Vagina**

**Aerobic Bacteria**

*Escherichia coli*
Coagulase-positive and coagulase-negative staphylococci
α- and β-hemolytic streptococci
Nonhemolytic streptococci
*Proteus*
*Bacillus*
*Corynebacterium*
*Pseudomonas*
*Klebsiella*
*Neisseria*
*Micrococcus*
*Haemophilus*
*Moraxella*
*Pasteurella*
*Acinetobacter*
*Flavobacterium*
*Lactobacillus*
*Enterobacter*

**Anaerobic Bacteria**

*Bacteroides melaninogenicus*
*Corynebacterium*
*Haemophilus aphrophilus*
*Bacteroides*
*Enterococcus*
*Peptostreptococcus* (hemolytic and nonhemolytic)
*Mycoplsma**
*Ureaplasma**

*See discussion of these infectious agents in Chapter 63.

that there are no differences among the bacterial isolates from normal fertile bitches, infertile bitches, and bitches with evidence of genital disease. Isolation of opportunistic pathogens from the vagina is therefore not proof of infection. Thus the results of vaginal cultures and the potential role of the isolated organisms in the pathogenesis of the clinical signs must be interpreted cautiously. *Brucella canis* is always considered a pathogen, even in the absence of clinical signs. A heavy growth of a single organism may also be significant. The role of *Mycoplasma* spp. and *Ureaplasma* spp. in reproductive disorders in cats and dogs is unclear at this time.

## VIROLOGY

Canine herpesvirus and feline herpesvirus I (feline viral rhinotracheitis) can cause respiratory disease in adult animals (see p. 228), as well as genital lesions (see p. 934), apparent failure to conceive, abortion, and neonatal death. Respiratory disease and neonatal death are the most common manifestations of herpes infection. Rarely, vesicular lesions may be found on the mucosa of the vestibule or prepuce of infected animals. The most important route of transmission is oronasal contact with infected secretions. Transplacental and venereal transmission is much less important. The virus can be isolated from nasal, conjunctival, tracheal, vaginal, or preputial scrapings from symptomatic animals. Because canine herpesvirus is poorly immunogenic, virus-neutralizing antibodies are present in small amounts for short periods. The finding of any detectable titer in the presence of compatible clinical signs is therefore considered significant. In queens, panleukopenia, feline infectious peritonitis, and feline leukemia virus infection are reported to be potential causes of infertility.

## ASSESSMENT OF REPRODUCTIVE HORMONES

Measurement of serum concentrations of reproductive hormones can be useful in evaluating animals with suspected or known reproductive disorders. Because all of the reproductive hormones are released in cyclic, episodic, or pulsatile manners, the results of hormone testing must always be interpreted in that light. Often the results of a single determination are not diagnostic because the phase of the cyclic release at the time of sample collection is unknown. For that reason, repetitive determinations performed over the course of hours, days, or weeks, or provocative testing, may be necessary. Most hormone assays, such as radioimmunoassays (RIAs), chemiluminescent, or enzyme-linked immunosorbent assays (ELISAs), depend on immunologic reactions. Errors can result if antibodies or antigens in homologous assay systems are not species specific or if species-specific interference with antibody binding occurs in heterologous systems. For these reasons, it is critical that each laboratory validate its procedures and determine reference ranges for each species and each hormone to be tested.

### Progesterone

Measurement of the serum progesterone concentration can be used to identify functional corpora lutea, to confirm that ovulation occurred, to monitor diestrus and, in bitches, to approximate the time of impending ovulation.

In bitches the serum progesterone concentration increases to more than 1 to 2 ng/ml (approximately 3 to 6 nmol/L) at or shortly before the preovulatory LH surge. Therefore serial determinations of the serum progesterone concentration during proestrus to identify an increase above 2 ng/ml could be used to estimate the time of ovulation, which follows the LH surge by about 2 days. Obviously the results of progesterone determination must be known promptly to be clinically applicable. Point-of-care ELISA kits for progesterone determination are available (Status Pro, Progest Assay; Synbiotics Corp., San Diego, Calif, Ovucheck; Cambridge Veterinarian Science, Littleport, Ely, U.K., and PreMate, Camelot Farms, College Station, Tex). When compared with the RIA determination of progesterone concentrations, one such kit was found on average to be 86% accurate. Comparisons of other kits with RIA have yielded similar results; nevertheless, some veterinarians have found the ELISA progesterone kits to be useful for serial progesterone determinations. The Canine Ovulation Timing Test (ICG-Status-Pro; Synbiotics Corp., San Diego, Calif), which is marketed for use in dogs,

has been found to be useful in assessing serum progesterone concentrations in cats. The kit was found to have an 11% error rate when compared with RIA determinations of the feline progesterone concentration. Additional critical studies of the ELISA progesterone assays for use in cats and dogs are needed, because an accurate, rapid method of progesterone determination would have many clinical applications. Many endocrinology laboratories perform RIA or chemiluminescence progesterone assays on a same-day basis.

As discussed earlier, serum progesterone concentrations remain at basal levels of less than 1 ng/ml (3.2 nmol/l) during proestrus in the bitch until the preovulatory LH surge. Coincident with the LH surge there is an increase in the serum progesterone concentration above basal levels. The magnitude of the concentration at the time of the LH surge, at the time of ovulation, and throughout diestrus varies within and among animals and between individual cycles. The progesterone concentration increases rapidly after ovulation in both the bitch and queen and plateaus 2 to 4 weeks later (see Figs. 56-1 and 56-5). It then gradually declines as the luteal phase (diestrus) continues, reaching basal levels of less than 1 ng/ml (approximately 3 nmol/L) in nonpregnant bitches 60 to 90 days after the LH surge. In the nonpregnant queen that did ovulate, the progesterone concentration declines to basal levels by 30 to 40 days after ovulation.

Because it is important to identify the fertile period when mature oocytes are available for fertilization in order to maximize conception rates in bitches and because determining serum concentrations of LH is less convenient than determining progesterone concentrations (see p. 856), interpretation of periovulatory progesterone concentrations is of interest. It is generally accepted that the concentration first exceeds 2 ng/ml (approximately 6 nmol/L) at the time of the LH surge in the bitch. After the initial rise in the progesterone concentration, variations within and among bitches and among laboratory procedures make comparison and interpretation of absolute values less than precise.

Some investigators have recommended insemination of the bitch 3 to 6 days after the initial rise in the progesterone concentration is detected, whereas others have recommended timing insemination to a specific progesterone concentration. The ELISA kits semiquantitatively determine progesterone concentrations, yielding results in low, middle, and high ranges. The low range is usually less than 2 ng/ml (approximately 6.4 nmol/L), the middle range is approximately 2 ng/ml to 5 to 7 ng/ml, and the high range is greater than approximately 7 ng/ml (approximately 22.3 nmol/L), depending on the manufacturer of the kit. Therefore a value in the middle range would correlate with the LH surge. If so, fertilization could occur 4 or more days later. If quantitative (RIA) progesterone determinations are available, the fertile period can be estimated. One study showed that the interval between the time when a serum progesterone concentration of more than 5 ng/ml (approximately 16 nmol/L) is first detected and the time of fertilization is 36 to 108 hours. Analysis of several independent breeding trials in which serum concentrations of progesterone were determined on the days of insemination revealed that pregnancy rates were best when insemination was performed when serum progesterone concentrations were greater than 8 ng/ml (approximately 25.4 nmol/l) and up to 19 to 26 ng/ml (approximately 60 to 80 nmol/L). Serum concentrations of progesterone greater than 8 ng/ml (25.4 nmol/L) are interpreted to indicate that ovulation has occurred.

Finding the increased serum concentrations of progesterone indicative of ovulation would be of interest in females suspected of having ovulatory failure. In the case of queens, this may be due to inadequate copulatory stimulation to induce the LH surge. The adequacy of luteal function during pregnancy can be monitored by determining serum progesterone concentrations once weekly for about 9 weeks after breeding or until parturition. This would be of interest in females in which inadequate luteal function was the suspected cause of unexplained abortion. In pregnant bitches (but not necessarily in pregnant queens), parturition occurs within 48 hours after serum concentrations of progesterone decrease below 1 to 2 ng/ml (approximately 3 to 6 nmol/L). Therefore impending parturition might be predicted by monitoring the serum progesterone concentration. This information would be of use in the management of dystocia and the planning of cesarean sections.

## Estradiol

Measurement of the estradiol concentration may be considered to help identify follicular ovarian cysts, estrogen-secreting ovarian or testicular tumors, and estrous cycles in females suspected of having silent or unobserved heats. Serum concentrations of estradiol are about a thousandfold less than those of progesterone. Typical mean serum estradiol concentrations in the bitch are 5 to 10 pg/ml during anestrus, 10 to 20 pg/ml during early proestrus, and 50 to 100 pg/ml during late proestrus. Estradiol concentrations are decreased during estrus and diestrus. Sporadic increases in the estradiol concentrations into the early proestrus range occur during anestrus (see Fig. 56-1).

Unfortunately, estradiol concentrations are often at or below the limits of detection of the assays used by many commercial endocrine laboratories. Estradiol concentrations also fluctuate widely and rapidly, and the high concentrations that occur during proestrus may only be detectable for a day or two. Pathologic increases in estradiol production, such as occur in animals with ovarian follicular cysts or Sertoli cell tumors, may still be less than the detectable limits of many assays. For these reasons, the measurement of estradiol concentrations often does not yield diagnostic results. A simple, accurate means of gauging estrogenic activity in the female is to evaluate vaginal epithelial cells for signs of cornification (see Fig. 56-2). All things considered, vaginal cytology is often preferable to determination of serum concentrations of estradiol in females. The preputial epithelium is also responsive to estrogen, exhibiting changes similar to those of the vaginal epithelium. This had led to speculation that exfoliative preputial cytologic tests may be helpful for demonstrating estrogen-secreting testicular tumors in male dogs.

## Gonadotropins: Luteinizing Hormone and Follicle-Stimulating Hormone

The pituitary gonadotropins are released in episodic pulses, the frequency and amplitude of which influence the mean concentrations. Mean concentrations are the values usually reported in the literature and those used for laboratory reference ranges. However, there is often considerable variation among laboratories in the absolute values of gonadotropin concentrations. Therefore whenever one is considering normal physiologic events, relative changes in gonadotropin concentrations are often as informative as absolute values. For the same reasons, the results of a gonadotropin determination (an absolute number) in an individual clinical animal must be interpreted in light of the standards for that particular laboratory, not the values reported by others. The gonadotropins are usually measured using RIAs. ELISA tests are also available for the measurement of canine LH concentrations (Reprokit, Sanofi, Overland Park, Kan, and Status LH, Synbiotics-ICG, Malvern, Pa). Although these appear to be useful for measuring canine LH concentrations, the results of comparisons of the ELISA assays with RIAs have yet to be reported.

Pulses of LH reportedly occur every 1 to 8 hours. During late anestrus in bitches, both the pulse frequency and amplitude of LH increase, which is thought to cause the onset of proestrous ovarian follicle development. Concentrations of FSH and LH are low during most of proestrus (see Fig. 56-1), and they both increase as a preovulatory surge about 1 or 2 days after the estradiol concentrations peak. This preovulatory surge may involve a tenfold to fortyfold increase in the LH concentration and a twofold to twentyfold increase in the FSH concentration. Both concentrations are low after the surge, although the LH concentration may occasionally increase during diestrus. The FSH concentration may increase slightly during late pregnancy. During anestrus the FSH concentration is elevated, whereas the LH concentration is not until late anestrus. FSH concentrations are highest during late anestrus and near the time of the LH surge. To identify animals with inadequate gonadotropin secretion, repetitive determinations of LH concentrations, such as three samples every 20 minutes, are more likely than a single determination to distinguish normal from abnormal animals. The secretory capacity of the pituitary gonadotropins can also be assessed by determining LH (and/or FSH) before and after administration of gonadotropin-releasing hormone (GnRH).

The interactions of hypothalamic GnRH, the pituitary gonadotropins LH and FSH, and the gonadal hormones estradiol, progesterone, and testosterone are referred to as the *hypothalamic-pituitary-gonadal axis* (see Fig. 56-4). Positive and negative feedback loops exist between each of these glands, all of which must function properly for normal reproduction to occur. In addition to the hypothalamic, pituitary, and ovarian interactions, sensory input from the vagina (copulatory stimulation that induces the LH surge) and the eyes (photoperiod) is necessary in queens (see p. 851). Measurement of the serum LH concentration can be used to evaluate the pituitary-gonadal axis and to predict ovulation. After oophorectomy in bitches, the LH and FSH concentrations are chronically increased to levels similar to those seen during the preovulatory surge. This is due to the lack of negative feedback from the ovarian gonadal hormones. The LH concentration reportedly exceeds 30 ng/ml within 1 month of oophorectomy. Elevated serum LH concentrations have been identified in intact bitches with ovarian dysplasia and would be expected in animals with primary ovarian failure resulting from any cause. Conversely, low serum concentrations of LH are expected at certain times of the normal ovarian cycle. Evaluation of LH concentrations is helpful in distinguishing between ovariectomized and sexually intact bitches. This is of importance to veterinarians, humane societies, and animal shelters that work with animals of unknown medical histories and that want to ensure that adopted animals are neutered without subjecting them to unnecessary laparotomy. The finding of a low serum concentration of LH in a single blood sample confirms the presence of negative feed back from ovarian tissue to the pituitary and hence the need for ovariectomy. The commercially available ELISA test (ICG Status-LH canine ovulation timing test, Synbiotics Corp., San Diego, Calif) is suitable for this purpose. A high concentration of LH in a single sample is not necessarily a reliable indicator of ovariectomy because it could also represent the normal pulsatile release of LH throughout the ovarian cycle.

Identification of the preovulatory LH surge would be a useful tool in canine breeding management, because ovulation occurs approximately 48 hours after the LH surge, and oocyte maturation is complete by about 48 hours after that. Therefore the period in which fertilization can occur begins approximately 4 days after the LH surge. Because the LH surge lasts only 24 to 72 hours, frequent sampling (i.e., at least once every 24 hours) is essential to ensure that it is not missed. Because such frequent blood sampling is inconvenient and expensive, progesterone concentrations are often assessed in lieu of LH to identify the preovulatory increase. Because LH appears in urine, urinary LH concentrations have been measured in bitches to identify the LH surge. When it is detected, the increase in urinary LH concentrations has been synchronous with the plasma LH peak, but urinary LH concentrations are not always detectable. When an increased urinary LH has been detected, it has been at least as transient as the serum LH peak. The FSH concentration is rarely measured in small animal practice, primarily because appropriate assays are usually not commercially available.

## Gonadotropin-Releasing Hormone

GnRH, which is secreted by the hypothalamus, controls pituitary secretion of FSH and LH in both male and female animals. However, the GnRH concentration is rarely measured in the clinical assessment of the male or female reproductive system. Exogenous GnRH administration can be used to evaluate the pituitary-gonadal axis and to determine whether functional gonads are present in the animal. After the administration of GnRH to normal dogs and cats, there is a prompt (by 30 minutes) increase in the serum concentrations of LH, with the magnitude of the response influenced by the stage of the reproductive cycle and the dose of the drug. For

example, a single intramuscular dose of 5 μg of GnRH causes a twentyfold increase in serum LH concentrations in anestrous queens, compared with a 100-fold increase in estrous queens (Table 56-2). A linear dose-response relationship between 5, 25, and 50 μg doses of GnRH and serum concentrations of LH was identified in anestrous Labrador bitches (mean body weight, 28.7 kg). The higher dose caused a greater increase, which peaked later (30 minutes versus 15 minutes) and lasted longer than that seen at the lower doses (Table 56-3).

Theoretically, in normal animals, once the serum concentration of gonadotropins increases in response to GnRH, serum concentrations of gonadal hormones should also increase. However, the degree of gonadal responsiveness varies with the stage of the reproductive cycle. For example, according to Chakraborty and colleagues (1979), a single intramuscular dose of 5, 10, or 25 μg of GnRH given to anestrous queens does not cause detectable follicular development, and ovulation does not occur. Because ovarian follicles are the source of estradiol, and corpora lutea, which form after ovulation, are the source of progesterone, the measurement of serum concentrations of estradiol or progesterone after GnRH administration in anestrous cats would be of little diagnostic value. On the other hand, a single intramuscular dose of 25 μg of GnRH is expected to cause ovulation in

## TABLE 56-2

**Serum Concentrations of LH (ng/ml) in Queens***

|  | TIME 0 | 30 MINUTES |
|---|---|---|
| Estrous | 5.2 ± 1.1 | 536.8 ± 104.8 |
| Anestrous | 5.7 ± 1.8 | 114.2 ± 26.5 |

From Chakraborty PK et al: Serum luteinizing hormone and ovulatory response to luteinizing hormone–releasing hormone in estrous and anestrous domestic cats, *Lab Anim Sci* 29:338, 1979.
*Before and after 5 μg of GnRH IM.
*LH*, Luteinizing hormone; *GnRH*, gonadotropin-releasing hormone.

## TABLE 56-3

**Mean Maximal Change in Serum Concentrations of LH After Various Doses of GnRH in Anestrous Labrador Bitches**

| DOSE | TIME OF PEAK LH | MEAN CHANGE IN LH (ng/ml) | MEAN PEAK LH (ng/ml) |
|---|---|---|---|
| 5 μg | 15 min | 6.5 ± 0.5 | 8.5 ± 0.5 |
| 25 μg | 15 min | 17.2 ± 3.7 | 18.7 ± 3.2 |
| 50 μg | 30 min | 44.6 ± 7.8 | 39.7 ± 7.8 |

Data from Chakraborty PK et al: Responsiveness of anestrous Labrador bitches to GnRH, *Proc Soc Exp Biol Med* 154:125, 1977.
*LH*, Luteinizing hormone; *GnRH*, gonadotropin-releasing hormone.

estrous queens, with a subsequent increase in the progesterone concentration 5 to 7 days later.

Likewise, GnRH causes ovulation and a subsequent increase in the progesterone concentration only if administered during estrus to bitches with mature ovarian follicles. Serum concentrations of progesterone should not change substantially in response to GnRH administration at other times of the cycle. Changes in estradiol concentrations in bitches after single and multiple administrations of FSH fluctuate so frequently and so widely, as they do during spontaneous cycles, that the mean concentrations tend to remain at pretreatment levels. Similarly, peak mean concentrations of estradiol were not detected for 10 to 23 days after multiple doses of GnRH were given to anestrous bitches. Even then, peak concentrations were much lower than those reported to occur during normal spontaneous cycles.

In oophorectomized females, serum concentrations of estradiol should be essentially undetectable before and after GnRH administration. Although the change in serum estradiol concentrations in response to GnRH in intact bitches is extremely variable, any incremental change is indicative of the presence of ovarian tissue. This finding could be of use to animal shelters wanting to determine the reproductive status of stray dogs before adoption. An increase in the serum estradiol concentration in response to GnRH indicates the presence of ovarian tissue; however, the converse is not true, in that lack of response to GnRH and undetectable resting estradiol concentrations are possible findings in normal, intact bitches at any phase of the ovarian cycle except during the follicular phase.

Failure of serum LH concentrations to increase after GnRH administration points to the possibility of a pituitary problem. GnRH administration can also be used to induce estrus in the bitch and queen (see p. 868). If a bitch or queen with persistent anestrus has an appropriate increase in the LH concentration but fails to begin cycling after pulsatile GnRH administration, prior ovariohysterectomy or gonadal dysfunction is suspected.

### Relaxin

Relaxin is produced primarily by the placenta, therefore a finding of elevated serum concentrations of relaxin is a very specific indicator of pregnancy. Using a rapid immunomigration (RIM) test (Witness Relaxin; Synbiotics Corp., San Diego, Calif), relaxin is detectable in pregnant bitches about 26 to 31 days after the LH surge. False-negative results occur if the test is performed too early during gestation. Although the manufacturer suggests that the test can be useful 21 days after breeding, it is a more sensitive indicator of pregnancy when performed 30 or more days after breeding. It is possible that a small litter size could yield a negative result. Relaxin disappears from the blood following abortion. Although pregnant cats also produce relaxin, this test has not yet been validated for accuracy in cats.

### RADIOLOGY AND ULTRASONOGRAPHY

Radiology and ultrasonography are useful for evaluating the ovaries, uterine wall thickness, and intrauterine contents; for confirming pregnancy; and for assessing fetal viability. The normal uterus and ovaries in a nonpregnant animal are not detected by routine abdominal radiography. During normal anestrus they may be difficult to identify by ultrasonography. Increased size and density and an abnormal shape of the uterus may be detected by either technique (Fig. 56-6). Ultrasonography can be used to evaluate the thickness of the uterine wall and the intrauterine contents. Ultrasonography may also help identify ovarian cysts in animals with persistent anestrus (nonfunctional or luteal cysts) or persistent estrus and hyperestrogenism (follicular cysts). It may be able to identify ovarian neoplasia as well.

Because of the difficulty involved in catheterizing the cervix, contrast studies of the uterus and uterine tubes (i.e., hysterosalpingography) are rarely done in bitches and queens. Positive-contrast vaginography, using a Foley catheter and a water-soluble contrast agent (e.g., Renografin [diatrizoate sodium and diatrizoate meglumine]), is easily performed, but general anesthesia is necessary. Vaginography can be considered if vaginoscopy fails to clearly identify strictures, anatomic defects, masses, or foreign material in the vagina.

### KARYOTYPING

Karyotyping is the determination of the chromosomal pattern of an animal. The chromosomes are obtained from cells, most commonly lymphocytes from peripheral blood, which have been induced to undergo mitosis. Cells from any tissue can theoretically be used for chromosomal analysis, but the limiting factor is the viability of the cells themselves and the ease with which they can be induced to divide. Lymphocytes can usually survive in heparinized blood at room temperature for overnight delivery to a cytogenetics laboratory. Tissue samples remain viable only if handled in special media such as tissue culture media kept at proper temperatures. The laboratory should be consulted before sample collection to ensure that the samples are properly handled and that the laboratory will be able to process them immediately upon arrival, as well as to find out the current cost. An example of such a laboratory is the University of Minnesota Veterinary Cytogenetics Laboratory, Department of Veterinary Pathobiology (St. Paul, MN 55108).

Some intersex conditions and developmental abnormalities of the reproductive tract may be associated with chromosomal anomalies (e.g., XXX, XO). These animals are usually seen because of abnormal external genitalia, infertility, or persistent anestrus. Karyotype analysis can be performed if a congenital rather than an acquired cause is suspected and if routine diagnostic tests have failed to identify the cause of the reproductive dysfunction.

### LAPAROSCOPY AND CELIOTOMY

Exploratory celiotomy is often the most cost-effective way to diagnose and treat intersex animals. In all other circumstances, however, diagnostic laparoscopy or exploratory celiotomy should not be done until a noninvasive diagnostic evaluation of the bitch or queen with a reproductive disorder has been completed. Laparoscopy and celiotomy allow

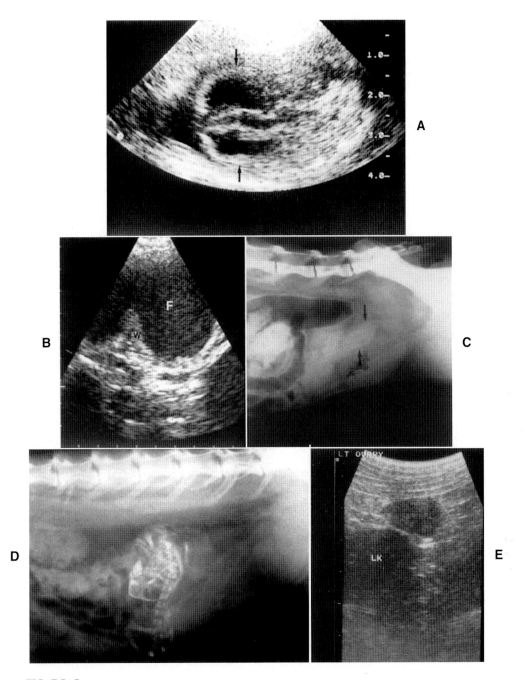

**FIG 56-6**
**A,** Sonogram of canine gestational sac *(arrows)* at 29 days. Scale is in centimeters.
**B,** Sonogram of canine pyometra showing thickened uterine wall *(W)* and lumen distended
with fluid *(F).* **C,** Radiograph of feline pyometra showing fluid-filled uterus *(arrows).* **D,** Radiograph of mummified fetus. **E,** Sonogram of 1.8 × 1.2 cm ovary with corpora lutea in a
normal 3-year-old Weimaraner 30 days after estrus. The serum progesterone concentration
was 64 nmol/L. *LK,* Left kidney. (**A** Courtesy Dr. Tom Bell, East Lansing, Mich.)

gross visualization of the reproductive tract, bacterial culture
of the uterine lumen, and full-thickness biopsy of the uterus.
The patency of the uterine horn and possibly uterine tube lumina might be determined by infusion of sterile saline solution. Laparoscopy and celiotomy are best performed during
anestrus to fully appreciate persistent pathologic changes in
the uterus.

## FEMALE INFERTILITY

An accurate history is critical to the evaluation of a female
animal suspected to be infertile. The history-taking should
investigate as many details of previous cycles as possible, including the dates of onset of each cycle, the female's behavior
during estrus, the dates and methods of previous insemina-

TABLE 56-4

**Historical Information for Female Infertility**

1. What is the present stage of the estrous cycle?
2. Description of previous cycles
   Age at puberty
   Dates of onset of previous cycles
   Lengths of previous cycles
   Behavior during proestrus and estrus
       Attractive to males?
       Allow mounting?
       Did intromission occur?
       Did insemination occur?
   Dates of insemination: How were these dates chosen?
       Predetermined day of season
       Behavioral changes
       Vaginal cytologic findings
       Ovulation timing
   Method of insemination
       Natural
       Artificial with fresh, chilled, or frozen semen
3. Assess male fertility
   Outcome of breeding to different males, if any
   Has this male ever sired a litter? When?
   Healthy litters from other females bred by him near the
       time of breeding the female in question?
   Results of recent semen evaluation
4. Events after breeding or after unbred cycles
   Early pregnancy diagnosis?
       When?
       What method?
           Physical/behavioral changes?
           Palpation?
           Ultrasound?
   Mammary development, overt false pregnancy?
   Vulvar discharge?
   Abortion?
   Parturition
       Length of gestation
       Dystocia?
       Litter size
       Health and survival of puppies or kittens
5. Previous diagnosis and treatment
   Tests performed and their results
       *Brucella canis*
       Thyroid profile
       Feline leukemia virus
   Medications administered
       Dose
       Route
       Frequency
   Correlate with stage of estrous cycle
6. Nonreproductive problems, diagnostic tests, and/or
   medication
       In this individual animal (e.g., glucocorticoids)
       In the kennel or cattery (e.g., feline viral
           rhinotracheitis infection)

tions, the fertility of the studs used, and the events following breeding (Table 56-4). A complete physical examination should be performed to identify (1) potential causes of infertility outside the reproductive tract; (2) other abnormalities that might adversely affect the health of the female or the pregnancy itself should conception occur; and (3) congenital and heritable defects that should exclude this female from a breeding program.

The reproductive tract is then examined. Mammary glands are carefully palpated to assess their size and consistency and the character of any secretions. The vulva is inspected to determine if there are structural abnormalities or any discharge. The labia are separated so that the vestibular mucosa and clitoris (in bitches) can be visualized. The uterus is palpated transabdominally. A vulvar discharge may be more apparent after abdominal palpation. The vestibule and posterior vagina should be palpated with a gloved finger in bitches of adequate size. Rectal palpation may help determine the extent of abnormal structures within the vagina.

The history and physical examination findings determine the nature of any additional diagnostic tests performed. Historic or physical abnormalities outside the reproductive tract should be investigated. A complete blood count (CBC), serum biochemistry panel, and urinalysis provide excellent information regarding the overall metabolic health of the animal and could reasonably be included as a routine part of the evaluation of infertility. All dogs should be tested for *B. canis* (see p. 936) before breeding and before infertility is evaluated further. Only normal, healthy animals in excellent condition should be bred.

The reproductive history often dictates the nature of the diagnostic approach. Perhaps most important are establishing the cycling behavior and interestrous interval of the female, identifying the criteria used to determine when the female is bred, and determining the female's behavior during mating. Typically one of the following four descriptions applies: failure to cycle, abnormal interestrous interval, abnormal proestrus-estrus, or normal cycles (Fig. 56-7).

## FAILURE TO CYCLE

There are two subcategories of animals with persistent anestrus. *Primary anestrus* refers to females 24 months of age or older that have never cycled. *Secondary anestrus* applies to females that have previously cycled but no longer are. An animal that has never cycled may be a normal prepubertal animal less than 24 months of age, may be experiencing "silent" heats, may have a congenital gonadal or chromosomal anomaly, or may have a concurrent disorder that is preventing estrous cycles. Exposure to light may be inadequate to initiate and maintain cyclicity in queens with persistent anestrus. Gonadal dysfunction, concurrent metabolic disorders or medications, and advancing age should be considered in females that were cycling in the past.

Diagnostic tests for persistent anestrus are usually delayed until a female is 2 years of age because of the probability that she is a normal prepubertal animal. Some veterinarians be-

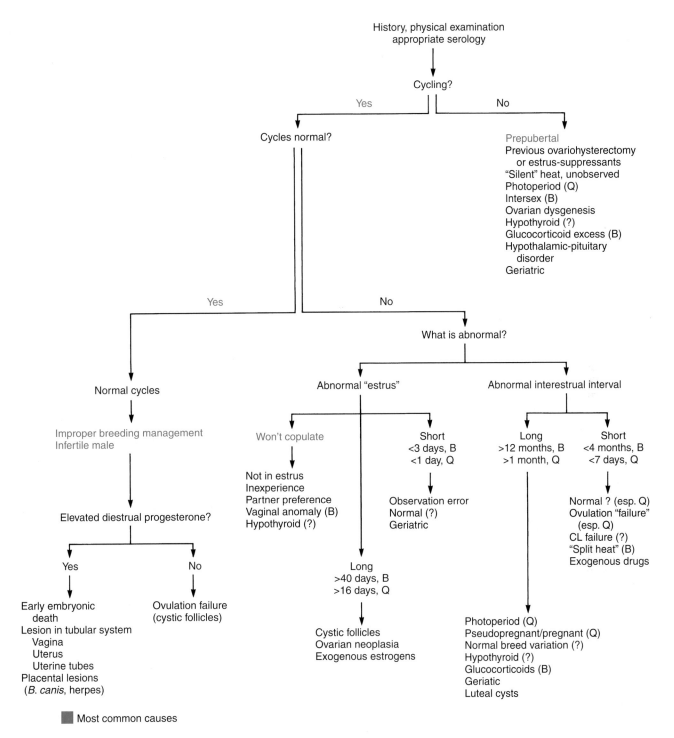

**FIG 56-7**
Diagnostic approach to female infertility. *B*, Bitch; *Q*, queen.

lieve that an initial undetected or "silent" first heat cycle is common in bitches. If so, this could explain why some young bitches appear to have persistent anestrus. Unobserved or silent heats may be detected retrospectively by measuring the serum progesterone concentration. If the concentration is greater than 2 ng/ml (approximately 6.4 nmol/L) in a bitch, a cycle has occurred within the last 60 to 90 days. The finding of high serum concentrations of progesterone in a supposedly anestrous queen indicates that unobserved estrus has occurred and also that either unobserved mating or spontaneous ovulation occurred within the past 30 to 40 days. Clinical signs of false pregnancy (see p. 886) would also indicate that an undetected cycle occurred approximately 45 days earlier in the queen or approximately 60 days earlier in the bitch.

A silent cycle could be detected prospectively by examining vaginal cytology every 1 to 2 weeks. Noncycling females should be housed with cycling females whenever possible, because the pheromones from cycling females may induce noncycling females to cycle. Queens should be exposed to the proper photoperiod for at least 2 months before further testing is done.

Persistent anestrus may result from suppression of function of the hypothalamic-pituitary-ovarian axis. Hypothyroidism, exogenous glucocorticoid therapy, and concurrent metabolic disease are commonly reported but rarely confirmed causes in bitches. Thyroid function is assessed by measuring serum concentrations of the thyroid hormones and canine thyroid-stimulating hormone (cTSH) (see Chapter 51). The role of hypothyroidism in infertility in the bitch has not been thoroughly evaluated. Exogenous glucocorticoids are commonly administered to animals, and they cause many alterations in reproductive function, including prolonged anestrus and abortion. The history should be reviewed to determine if the animal could have received glucocorticoid treatment. In mature bitches, increased serum alkaline phosphatase activity in conjunction with relatively normal alanine aminotransferase activity is suggestive of supraphysiologic amounts of glucocorticoids. If there is still doubt about excess endogenous or exogenous glucocorticoids, adrenocortical function can be assessed with an adrenocorticotropic hormone (ACTH) stimulation test (see p. 789). The presence of other concurrent metabolic disease is determined with a CBC, serum biochemistry panel, and urinalysis.

Persistent anestrus may also result from a primary abnormality anywhere within the hypothalamic-pituitary-gonadal axis, including intersex conditions, ovarian dysgenesis, and progesterone-secreting luteal cysts or ovarian tumor. It may also result from previous ovariohysterectomy. The functional status of the hypothalamic-pituitary-ovarian axis can be evaluated by measuring serum LH concentrations before and after GnRH administration (see p. 856). Females with ovarian dysgenesis or that have undergone oophorectomy reportedly have chronically increased serum concentrations of LH. Serum progesterone concentrations can be determined to assess functional luteal cysts. Ultrasonographic evaluation of the ovaries may identify ovarian abnormalities such as cysts or neoplasia. Many phenotypically female intersex animals have detectable anatomic abnormalities of the clitoris, vestibule, and/or vagina. If the findings from physical and endoscopic examinations of these areas are normal, a human chorionic gonadotropin (hCG) or GnRH stimulation test (see p. 912), done to assess the serum concentrations of testosterone could be used to demonstrate the presence of testicular tissue. Karyotyping can also be performed (see p. 858), although intersex animals may have normal karyotypes. Abnormal karyotypes have been found in bitches and queens with ovarian dysgenesis.

Induction of estrus (see p. 868) may be tried if other diagnostic tests have failed to identify the cause of persistent anestrus. Exploratory celiotomy or laparoscopy, done to assess the gross appearance of the reproductive tract and to obtain biopsy specimens of the internal genitalia, should be considered only after all noninvasive diagnostic methods have been tried.

## PROLONGED INTERESTROUS INTERVAL

Interestrous intervals of greater than 12 months in bitches and greater than 1 month in cycling queens are usually considered abnormal, although long interestrous intervals may be a normal breed variation, as seen in the Basenji, Tibetan Mastiff, and Dingo dogs, which often cycle only once a year. Pregnancy and pseudopregnancy lengthen the interestrous interval in queens. Prolonged interestrous intervals may also occur with increasing age or may signify an underlying disorder. Many of the causes of persistent anestrus, such as glucocorticoid administration in bitches and inadequate photoperiods in queens, may also cause a prolonged interestrous interval. Silent heats should also be considered. The diagnostic workup in such animals should include a thorough review of the estrus identification techniques used by the owner, identification of medications being administered to the animal, assessment of the overall metabolic health of the animal (i.e., CBC, biochemistry panel, urinalysis), and an evaluation of thyroid gland and adrenocortical function in bitches.

## SHORT INTERESTROUS INTERVAL

Abnormally short interestrous intervals of less than 4 months are occasionally seen in bitches. Many of them are infertile, perhaps because the endometrium does not have time to recover from the previous cycle, a process that takes 120 to 150 days. Infertility in these animals presumably results from failure of the embryo to implant. In some breeds, most notably the German Shepherd, and in some individual animals an interestrous interval of 4 to 4.5 months may be normal and may not interfere with fertility. However, interestrous intervals of less than 4 months are usually associated with infertility. The administration of gonadotropins, prostaglandin $F_{2\alpha}$, prolactin antagonists, or estrogen can artificially shorten the interestrous interval. In most bitches, however, the cause of short interestrous intervals is not discovered.

A short interestrous interval must be differentiated from a "split heat" cycle in bitches. Split heats are characterized by normal proestrus that stops abruptly before progressing to estrus. Two to 4 weeks later, proestrus begins again and progresses through normal, fertile estrus. Split heats are a normal phenomenon that can occur in any bitch during any estrus. Split heats are seen most often in pubertal bitches that have normal proestrus and estrus during subsequent cycles. Rarely do split heats occur repeatedly in an individual bitch. Split heats do not cause infertility, except in the sense that the initial proestrus frustrates breeding management.

Additional diagnostic tests are usually not performed in bitches with confirmed short interestrous intervals. Administration of an androgen such as methyltestosterone to prevent estrus for at least 6 months could be considered. Theoretically, androgens should have no effect on the endometrium, which would then have time to recover from the last cycle. Even though estrus can easily be delayed with treatment, affected bitches usually remain subfertile. The use of progestins such as megestrol acetate to delay the next cycle cannot be recommended because of their effects on the endometrium (see p. 866). Breeding on the first estrus occurring after the discontinuation of therapy is important, because short interestrous intervals frequently resume. The role of genetics in this problem is not known.

## ABNORMAL PROESTRUS AND ESTRUS

The most common abnormalities of proestrus and estrus are refusal to allow mating, prolonged estrus, and abnormally short estrus. Females that are not in estrus refuse mating. An occasional bitch or queen exhibits partner preference by refusing to mate with one male but readily mating with another. Inexperienced and timid females may also be reluctant to breed. Bitches with hypothyroidism reportedly may not exhibit normal behavior during estrus. In bitches, physical abnormalities of the vulva or vagina are common causes of refusal to mate. Physical abnormalities include vaginal strictures, congenital defects in the vulva and vagina (see p. 872), vaginal hyperplasia/prolapse (see p. 875), and rarely, vaginal neoplasia.

Vaginal cytologic studies should be performed to identify the present stage of the cycle (see Fig. 56-2). As just mentioned, females that are not in estrus will not accept mating. Digital palpation of the vulva, vestibule, and vagina can identify vaginal prolapse and most vaginal strictures and congenital defects. Vaginoscopy should be performed if digital palpation fails to identify a cause for the refusal to allow mating.

Vaginal strictures that are identified during anestrus should always be palpated again during estrus to determine their actual significance. Annular vaginal strictures are commonly located immediately cranial to the external urethral orifice, at the anatomic junction between the vestibule and the vagina. The vestibulovaginal junction is normally the narrowest part of the posterior tract. During anestrus this normal narrowing may be mistaken for an annular stricture. The diameter of the vestibulovaginal junction normally increases significantly during proestrus and estrus, making differentiation from a true stricture easy at this stage of the cycle. Similarly, normal vaginal examination findings during anestrus do not exclude the possibility of vaginal hyperplasia/prolapse, which occurs only at times of estrogenic stimulation, as a potential cause for reluctance to mate. Artificial insemination can be used to breed otherwise normal estrual females that refuse to mate, as well as those with vaginal hyperplasia/prolapse. Physical abnormalities other than vaginal hyperplasia/prolapse should be surgically corrected if the female is to remain in the breeding program. Surgery is best performed during anestrus. The genetics of congenital vaginal and vulvar anomalies are unknown.

## PROLONGED ESTRUS

Although proestrus and estrus each last an average of 9 days, proestrus lasting as long as 17 days and estrus lasting 21 days have been observed in normal, fertile bitches. Understandably many owners become concerned if a season (proestrus plus estrus) lasts longer than 3 weeks. Nevertheless, a season is not considered abnormally long in bitches until it reaches 35 to 40 days. In queens, estrus lasting longer than 16 days is considered abnormal. This must not be confused with the normal, multiple cycles that occur in queens.

Prolonged proestrus/estrus is usually caused by functional follicular cysts (Fig. 56-8), although ovarian neoplasia and

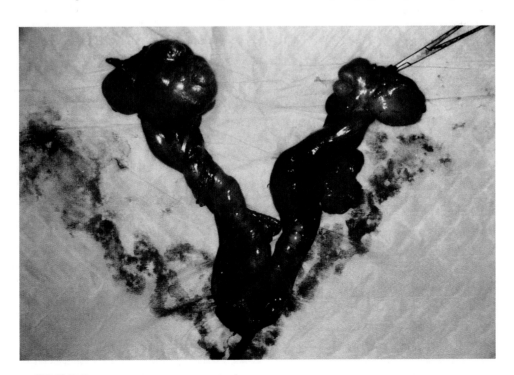

**FIG 56-8**
Cystic ovaries and uterus with cystic endometrial hyperplasia from 2-year-old Mastiff in heat for 12 weeks.

exogenous estrogen administration should also be considered. Vaginal cytology should be performed to confirm that estrogenic stimulation is present and thus that it could reasonably be considered the cause of the behavioral and physical signs. Abdominal ultrasonography, documentation of increased serum estrogen concentrations, or exploratory celiotomy can be performed to identify follicular ovarian cysts. Usually, however, the diagnosis is based on the historic, physical, vaginal cytologic, and ultrasound findings. Spontaneous regression of follicular cysts may occur; watchful waiting for 2 to 4 weeks should often be the initial therapeutic approach in the bitch with suspected follicular ovarian cysts. The cyst or cysts can be manually ruptured via celiotomy in those bitches with persistent or enlarging cysts. Induction of ovulation can be attempted using GnRH (Cystorelin; 2.2 μg/kg IM, once daily for 3 days); however, the results have been variable. If mature follicles are present and induced to ovulate, signs of estrus should resolve in 5 to 7 days. Ovariohysterectomy should be considered for those females that fail to respond promptly to medical management for cystic ovaries, because the prognosis for fertility is guarded and continued estrogenic stimulation may be harmful to the uterus and bone marrow. Ovarian neoplasia is uncommon in bitches and queens. Surgical excision is the treatment of choice. If treatment with exogenous estrogenic drugs is the cause of persistent estrus, it should be discontinued.

## SHORT ESTRUS

Abnormally short estrus of less than 3 days in bitches or less than 1 day in queens is most often the result of an error in observation or recognition of estrus. Females older than 6 to 8 years of age may experience erratic cycles, including short estrus. A split heat cycle should also be considered in bitches with an apparently short estrus. Short estrus may be normal in some animals. Methods of proestrus and estrus detection should be changed in females with a truly short estrus so that they can be bred at the appropriate time. This would usually entail beginning vaginal cytologic studies or teasing with a stud well before the expected onset of the next estrus and continuing this until the first day of estrus is identified. Combining this with ovulation timing, as determined by serum progesterone or LH concentrations, may be helpful in identifying the optimal time for insemination.

## NORMAL CYCLES

Infertility in a female otherwise normal in all aspects of the reproductive cycle may result from improper breeding management; infertility in the male; lesions in the vagina, uterus, or uterine tubes; infection of the reproductive tract; early embryonic death; or advancing age. Conception rates and litter size are greatest, and neonatal mortality is lowest, in bitches (Beagles) between 2 and 3.5 years of age. Reproductive performance in queens is best between 1 and 6 years of age. After 5 years of age in Beagles and 6 years of age in queens, conception rates and litter size decline and neonatal mortality begins to increase. Because of this age-related decrease in fertility, an extensive diagnostic evaluation of older females may not be warranted.

A common cause of apparent infertility in the normally cycling female is infertility in the male. Because male fertility can be so easily evaluated (see p. 913), the male should be evaluated before an extensive diagnostic evaluation of the female is undertaken. A solid history that the male sired litters that were born shortly before *and* shortly after mating with the bitch in question would provide good circumstantial evidence against male infertility. Semen evaluation would provide information about the male's current status.

The most common causes of infertility in females with normal estrous cycles are improper timing of insemination and poor semen quality. In well-managed colonies of normal dogs, conception rates of better than 90% can be expected. A thorough history concerning breeding management, particularly how the owner determines when to breed, is imperative. In bitches, most often the day for first insemination is a predetermined day after the onset of proestrus (commonly the tenth day) rather than a day chosen on the basis of the presence of behavioral or cytologic signs of the actual onset of estrus or the identification of hormonal indicators of impending ovulation. If a particular bitch has a short proestrus, for example, the tenth day may actually be at the end of estrus rather than at the beginning.

Determination of the first day of estrus is essential during an investigation of possible problems with breeding management as the cause of infertility. The first day of estrus can be identified on the basis of behavioral or vaginal cytologic changes, but it cannot be recognized unless the bitch is initially examined before that time (i.e., during proestrus). We recommend vaginal cytology beginning on the first or second day of proestrus, continuing every 2 to 3 days until about 50% to 60% cornification, at which time we assess serum concentrations of progesterone for ovulation timing. Vaginal cytology may be continued until diestrus occurs (see p. 850). Vaginal cytology performed in early proestrus may also identify pathologic processes within the reproductive tract that could contribute to infertility (see pp. 853 and 870). Bacterial culture of specimens from the anterior vaginal vault can also be performed at this time (see p. 854).

Allowing only one mating or allowing several matings only during a short time (i.e., 24 hours) are common causes of infertility in bitches. This is especially true if the mating is not performed near the fertile period. Unlike the situation in queens, breeding a bitch several times during the same day appears to offer no advantage over breeding a single time on a given day. Breeding management schemes were discussed earlier (p. 849). Conception rates are improved by performing at least two inseminations, usually 24 to 48 hours apart, during the fertile period. Litter size may also increase when multiple breedings are made possible. In queens the frequency of mating is a more important determinant of ovulation, and thus conception, than is the day of the cycle on which mating occurs.

Vaginal cytology identifies estrus but does not necessarily identify when ovulation occurs during estrus. Obtaining the specimen for cytologic evaluation may induce ovulation in some estrous queens, but this is apparently not a common occurrence. In bitches, the serum progesterone or LH concentrations (see p. 855) are very helpful for approximating the time of ovulation and determining when breeding should commence.

After the female has been appropriately bred, she should be examined 20 to 30 days later to determine whether she is pregnant. Pregnancy can be diagnosed on the basis of abdominal palpation or ultrasonographic findings. Ultrasonography is preferable to abdominal palpation in previously infertile animals because results can be documented on film and fetal viability can be assessed. If the female is not pregnant, the serum progesterone concentration should be determined to confirm that ovulation occurred (see p. 855). Low serum concentrations (less than 2 to 5 ng/ml or approximately 6.4 to 16 nmol/L) suggest ovulation failure or premature luteolysis. The cause of ovulation failure may be an ovarian abnormality or, in the case of queens, inadequate coital stimulation. Premature luteolysis, or failure of the corpora lutea to maintain progesterone production, should result in fetal resorption if it occurs before day 35 of gestation. Premature luteolysis is a theoretic consideration as the cause of low diestrual serum concentrations of progesterone. To differentiate ovulation failure from premature luteolysis, serum progesterone concentrations are serially determined using quantitative methods (e.g., RIA) from the time of proestrus through diestrus. Progesterone concentrations that never exceed 8 ng/ml (approximately 25 nmol/L) suggest ovulation failure, whereas premature luteolysis is reflected by a more rapid decline than normal from high postovulatory concentrations of progesterone.

To determine whether early embryonic death is occurring, the clinician should attempt earlier diagnosis of pregnancy using ultrasonography (see p. 888), beginning after gestation day 10 or 14 in cats or dogs, respectively. If pregnancy is found, this obviously indicates that ovulation and conception occurred. However, false negative results may occur because it is very difficult to detect sonographic evidence of pregnancy that early in gestation. Initial negative results should be reevaluated because pregnancy cannot be conclusively ruled out before gestation days 24 to 28. Serum concentrations of relaxin may also be determined. Detecting relaxin in an animal that was no longer pregnant would indicate very recent embryonic death.

Hypothalamic or pituitary dysfunction would be unlikely causes of ovulation failure in the female that is otherwise cycling normally. More likely, hypothalamic or pituitary malfunction would be manifest as abnormal cycles. When a female with normal cycles is known to have been bred appropriately during estrus to a male that is known to be fertile and when ovulation has been confirmed by the finding of elevated serum progesterone concentrations during diestrus, the hypothalamic-pituitary-gonadal axis is considered intact (see Fig. 56-4). Lesions within the müllerian duct derivatives (vagina, uterus, uterine tubes), the placenta, or the conceptus itself are then likely to be the source of the infertility.

Lesions in the müllerian duct derivatives include conditions that interfere with gamete or zygote transport or that create an inhospitable environment. Obstruction of the uterine tubes, for example, could prevent fertilization; or, if fertilization occurred, the obstruction could prevent the zygote from moving into the uterus. These are in fact some of the mechanisms by which estrogens ("mismating shots") exert their antifertility effects. Developmental defects in the vagina, such as agenesis or vertical vaginal septa (see p. 872), impede or prevent sperm transport. Theoretically, spermicidal agents such as infectious organisms, medications used for douching, or antisperm antibodies in cervical mucus can also be present in the vagina and can be the source of infertility. Although there is no doubt that these agents play a role in infertility in some species, their clinical importance in small animal reproduction is not known. The uterus may also be incapable of supporting pregnancy because of disorders such as cystic endometrial hyperplasia or bacterial endometritis.

Early embryonic death can occur because of abnormalities in the placenta, the embryo itself, or the dam (see p. 900). Infectious agents are an important cause of early embryonic death. Although many agents are capable of causing placentitis or fetal death, *B. canis* in bitches and herpesvirus in queens are the foremost such agents. Many commonly used medications such as glucocorticoids and certain antibiotics also cause embryonic death. In addition, some congenital fetal anomalies cause early embryonic death because they are incompatible with continued survival.

The diagnostic approach in a normally cycling female that has been appropriately bred to a fertile male and that is known to have ovulated should begin with a review of the history to identify potential causes of early embryonic death. Special attention should be paid to medications administered to the female and to signs of infectious disease in the colony. Serologic tests for herpesvirus and *B. canis* should be performed. Vaginal lesions can easily be excluded as the cause of infertility by vaginoscopy and vaginal cytology. The presence of antisperm antibodies in the female has not yet been documented as a cause of infertility in dogs or cats. However, were they to occur, the problem could be circumvented by breeding with a different male. In lieu of cultures of specimens from the uterine lumen, anterior vaginal cultures should be performed. Bacterial infections should be treated appropriately prior to breeding. The potential teratogenic or abortifacient effects of medications should always be considered. Finally, exploratory celiotomy can be performed during anestrus to visualize the reproductive tract, to assess the patency of the uterus and uterine tubes, to obtain uterine specimens for culture, and to obtain full-thickness uterine biopsy specimens for histologic assessment.

## ESTRUS SUPPRESSION AND POPULATION CONTROL

In the United States and Canada, ovariohysterectomy and castration are the most common methods of population control in dogs and cats. They are permanent and relatively expensive, invasive procedures. In an attempt to reduce the number of unwanted (i.e., relinquished by their owners) and stray animals euthanized at animal shelters, many shelters mandate surgical sterilization as part of the adoption agreement. Unfortunately, postadoption compliance with sterilization agreements has been universally poor. The concept of preadoption sterilization has received much attention. This concept has been especially attractive to shelters if sterilization could be done at a very young age (6 to 8 weeks), well before puberty and the time when there is any chance of accidental pregnancy occurring, and while the animal is still young enough to be highly adoptable. Safe and effective anesthetic and surgical techniques have since been described and the results evaluated. Several studies have shown that the physical and behavioral traits of animals neutered at 7 weeks of age are the same as those in animals neutered at the more conventional age of 7 months. However, neutered animals, whether gonadectomy is performed at 7 weeks or 7 months of age, have decreased metabolic rates, increased body weight, delayed physeal closure, and less developed secondary sex characteristics than do age-matched, sexually intact controls. The decreased metabolic rate is synonymous with decreased caloric requirements and a predisposition to obesity relative to that in intact animals. The decreased caloric requirements are evidently not a result of diminished physical activity, because no differences in activity between spayed and intact cats have been observed.

In studies of animals sterilized at 6 to 8 weeks of age, the animals have primarily been evaluated for only 12 to 24 months, therefore the longer-term effects, if any, of "early" neutering remain unknown. Although early neutering is safe and effective, the effect of preadoption sterilization on the overpopulation of unwanted pets is likely to be minimal, because only a small percentage of pets (5%, estimated by the Massachusetts Society for the Prevention of Cruelty to Animals; 8%, estimated from animal shelter data and data from a household survey in St. Joseph County, Ind) are originally acquired from animal shelters.

Less expensive, permanent methods of sterilization, especially to control the population of unwanted dogs and cats, have been investigated, including tubal ligation, vasectomy, the injection of occlusive-sclerosing agents into the testis or epididymis, and immunologic methods that induce anti-LH and anti–zona pellucida antibodies. Although tubal ligation and vasectomy are effective ways to prevent pregnancy, they both require anesthesia and a degree of technical expertise that make them somewhat expensive and impractical for the large scale application necessary for population control. The physical and behavioral changes associated with sexual maturity, such as urine marking by males and continued estrous cycles in females, are not affected by vasectomy or tubal ligation. Owners may or may not consider this desirable.

The injection of sclerosing agents into the epididymis causes ejaculates to be azoospermic in about 35 days in dogs. Some, but not all, of the agents cause severe tissue reactions and local posttreatment complications in some animal species but not in others. Intraepididymal injection of the

sclerosing agent chlorhexidine digluconate (4.5%) has apparently been helpful in controlling the free-roaming domestic dog populations in the Galapagos Islands. The same agent caused azoospermia after 140 days in half of the domestic cats treated. Intraepididymal injections are easy and inexpensive to perform, but their effectiveness in population control has yet to be investigated except as just described.

The induction of anti-LH antibodies delays puberty in bitches and suppresses spermatogenesis in male dogs, but the response is so variable that a single protocol for anti-LH vaccination has not been established. There is also the risk that anti-LH antibodies may have antithyrotropin (TSH) effects, because the two substances are structurally similar, including identical $\alpha$-subunits. The potential anti-TSH activity of anti-LH antibodies has not been investigated. Another immunologic method of sterilization is vaccination with zona pellucida. The zona pellucida is the acellular coating around ova, and vaccination with it has been found to consistently produce high anti–zona pellucida titers and prevent conception in bitches. Significant ovarian abnormalities also develop, including ovarian cysts of various types and prolonged proestrus/estrus. After the introduction of any foreign antigen, antigen-antibody complexes may form and damage the kidneys. This has not been investigated for any of the immunologically based methods of fertility control. The continuous administration of GnRH antagonists or agonists (by downregulation of GnRH receptors) suppresses the pituitary-gonadal axis, but problems with drug delivery and expense currently make them impractical.

Owners sometimes desire temporary suppression of estrus. Progestins and androgens can inhibit the release or synthesis of gonadotropins in dogs and cats and thereby prevent estrus. GnRH analogues reversibly inhibit reproductive function in male and females by down-regulating LH and FSH receptors, thereby suppressing the pituitary-gonadal axis.

## MEGESTROL ACETATE

Megestrol acetate (Ovaban; Schering-Plough Co., Kenilworth, NJ) is the only progestin approved for estrus control in bitches in the United States. It is not approved for use in cats. In some European countries, oral and injectable progestins such as medroxyprogesterone acetate (MPA) and proligestone are commonly used to prevent estrus. Progestins are most reliable in preventing estrus if treatment is initiated during anestrus and are less reliable if administered during early proestrus. The recommended dosage of megestrol acetate during anestrus is 0.5 mg/kg of body weight for 32 consecutive days for the bitch and 2.5 mg/wk for up to 18 months for the queen. If given during the first 3 days of proestrus in an attempt to discontinue that stage of the cycle, the recommended dosage is 2.2 mg/kg for 8 consecutive days in the bitch. However, the bitch should be confined until the bloody vulvar discharge has stopped. If the queen is entering estrus, a dosage of 5 mg daily for 3 days, followed by 2.5 to 5 mg/week for 10 weeks, has been suggested. No more than two consecutive estrous cycles should be suppressed, and the drug should be given only to postpubertal bitches and queens. The onset of the next estrus varies but usually occurs 2 to 9 months after megestrol acetate is discontinued. Preliminary studies have shown that the slow-release subdermal implant of levonorgestrel (Norplant; Wyeth-Ayerst, Philadelphia, Pa) is effective in suppressing estrus for 12 months in cats, with no adverse effects except the development of cystic endometrial hyperplasia. Three of four cats exhibited estrus and conceived within 54 days of implant removal.

Progestins, including megestrol acetate, have many undesirable effects that commonly occur at therapeutic doses. In the reproductive system, progestins cause cystic endometrial hyperplasia with an increased propensity for the formation of pyometra. Their use is also associated with mammary hyperplasia and an increased incidence of mammary tumors. When progestin therapy is discontinued, signs of false pregnancy may develop (see p. 886). Other adverse effects in bitches and queens include diabetes mellitus, acromegaly, and adrenocortical suppression. In the bitch, some progestins (MPA and proligestone) act as glucocorticoid agonists, and long-term treatment with high doses may result in iatrogenic hyperadrenocorticism, including steroid hepatopathy. In the bitch, diabetes mellitus and acromegaly are caused by progestin-induced growth hormone secretion. Alopecia, thinning of the skin, and discoloration of the hair at the site of progestin injection have also been observed. For all these reasons, we recommend against the use of progestins for estrus suppression.

## ANDROGENS

Mibolerone (Cheque; Pharmacia Co.) was the only androgen approved for estrus suppression in bitches in the United States. It is no longer available. Although not approved for this use, various forms of testosterone (intramuscularly administered testosterone propionate; orally administered methyltestosterone) are routinely administered to Greyhound bitches during training and racing. Prolonged anestrus occurs in some of these bitches after they are retired from the track and androgen therapy is discontinued. Adverse effects of androgens, including mibolerone, are clitoral hypertrophy (sometimes with permanent ossification), mucopurulent vulvar discharge, and vaginitis. Liver enzyme activity can also be increased. These effects are usually reversible after mibolerone is discontinued, but they may persist for months to years. Masculinization of female fetuses, which is irreversible, occurs if androgens are administered to pregnant females. Additional androgenic effects include an apparent increase in muscle mass and aggressiveness.

The use of abortifacients to abort unwanted puppies and kittens is discussed in Chapter 59.

## GnRH AGONISTS

The GnRH agonist deslorelin (Peptech Animal Health, Sydney, Australia) has been shown to effectively suppress reproductive function for periods of more than a year in male and female dogs and cats when administered as a slow-release subcutaneous implant. Although not currently available for such use, there is active research ongoing. Depending on the stage of the cycle at which the drug is implanted, it can initially induce an estrus cycle. This unwanted effect can be overcome by the simultaneous administration of a progestin such as megestrol acetate. Another GnRH agonist, nafarelin, is also effective in estrus suppression in bitches.

## OVARIAN REMNANT SYNDROME

Occasionally, queens and bitches resume or continue to exhibit behavioral and physical signs of estrus after oophorectomy. The most common cause is remnant ovarian tissue that has regained folliculogenesis and estrogen production. The presence of high concentrations of estrogen can be detected using vaginal cytology to identify cornification of epithelial cells (see Fig. 56-2). In the absence of exogenous estrogens, the finding of clinical signs typical of estrus, along with vaginal cytology consistent with estrus, confirms the presence of ovarian remnants and justifies a recommendation for exploratory celiotomy to find and remove the ovarian remnants. If additional confirmation of the ovarian remnant syndrome is desired before exploratory surgery, the remnant ovary's ability to ovulate and produce progesterone can be evaluated. Measuring serum concentrations of progesterone 5 to 7 days after expected ovulation does this. Progesterone concentrations of greater than 2 ng/ml (6.4 nmol/L) are indicative of spontaneous ovulation and the presence of corpora lutea. Conversely, ovulation can be induced while the female is in heat by administering hCG (10 IU/kg IM in bitches; 250 IU/queen IM) or GnRH (0.5 μg/kg IM in bitches; 25 μg/cat IM). Five to 7 days later the serum progesterone concentration should exceed 2 ng/ml if functional ovarian tissue is present.

Of 46 cases reported by Miller (1995), ovarian remnants were left more often in cats (n = 29) than in dogs (n = 17). Twenty of the animals had bilateral remnants. In all cases, the remnants were found in the usual anatomic location for ovaries, not in aberrant or ectopic places. The cause of ovarian remnant syndrome is evidently the surgical technique. The time from oophorectomy to the resumption of cycling was found to vary from weeks to more than 5 years. These findings are similar to those described in other reports. Treatment consists in the surgical removal of the ovarian remnants. Ovarian remnants are often small. They may be easier to identify if follicles (i.e., when the female is in heat) or corpora lutea (i.e., shortly after ovulation) are present rather than during the interestrous period (i.e., anestrus).

Granulosa cell tumors are also reported to occur in ovarian remnants, as well as in intact females. Dogs with estrogen-producing ovarian tumors may have clinical signs of estrus, bone marrow toxicity, or dermatologic changes, or a combination of these. Estrogen-producing ovarian tumors would not be expected to respond to exogenous hCG or GnRH administration. Dogs with progesterone-producing granulosa cell tumors may show mammary gland development and may have cystic endometrial hyperplasia. The finding of elevated serum concentrations of progesterone would confirm the presence of ovarian tissue.

## ESTRUS INDUCTION

Estrus induction has been attempted in bitches in clinical settings to shorten the normal interestrous interval, in bitches and queens to treat prolonged anestrus, and to time pregnancy and parturition for the owners' convenience. In research settings, estrus induction has been used to synchronize estrus for embryo transfer. Some estrus-induction protocols are associated with superovulation, as revealed by evaluation of ovarian follicles, but even so, litter size is apparently not increased.

### THE QUEEN

The photoperiod can be manipulated to induce estrus in queens. Continuous exposure to 12 to 14 hours of light of at least 50 foot candles and to 10 to 12 hours of dark per day causes normal, mature queens to begin cycling within 4 to 8 weeks. Housing anestrous queens with cycling queens also helps to induce estrus. If the hormonal induction of estrus is to be attempted, the queen should first be exposed for several months to a minimum of 12 hours of light per 24 hours.

In one protocol for the hormonal induction of estrus in mature queens, 2 mg of FSH is administered intramuscularly once daily until signs of estrous behavior are noted, or for a maximum of 5 days. Lower doses of FSH may be equally effective (2 mg on day 1; 1 mg on days 2 and 3; 0.5 mg on days 4 and 5). An alternative is to administer a GnRH analog (1 μg/kg SQ q8h [Decapeptyl; Organon, West Orange, N.J.]) until signs of estrous behavior are noted, or for a maximum of 10 days. hCG (250 IU IM) may be given on the first 2 days of estrus to induce ovulation. The administration of ultrapurified porcine FSH (2.5 IU divided into five daily SQ doses for 5 days, 1.25 IU of porcine FSH and 250 IU of hCG on day 6, and 250 IU of hCG on day 7) has been observed to result in superovulation and an ovulation rate of 73%. Mating with a tomcat should begin at the onset of estrus and can also be used to induce ovulation.

### THE BITCH

Results of studies of methods to induce estrus in bitches have been extremely variable. Although there are no recognized predictors of success, there are some predictors of failure. For example, it is less likely for fertile estrus to be induced and pregnancy to occur if bitches are in the luteal phase of the cycle (diestrus) or are under the influence of androgens. Of the many methods of estrus induction described to date, most have involved the administration of gonadotropins or GnRH, with or without estrogen priming. None has been found to be routinely effective in inducing fertile estrus. Exogenous gonadotropins can overstimulate the ovaries, interfere with ovulation, and cause the formation of cystic follicles. Recently, dopaminergic agonists have been investigated. The mechanisms by which they might induce estrus are not known, but

direct stimulation of the hypothalamic-pituitary axis is theorized. Dopaminergic agonists suppress prolactin secretion, but it is thought that change in the prolactin concentration or change in its effect on the ovaries is not the mechanism by which estrus is induced. Until a reliable, safe method of estrus induction is found and thoroughly investigated, estrus induction should probably be reserved for bitches with pathologic anestrus rather than being used for manipulating the cycle for owner convenience.

The pulsatile administration of GnRH is a fairly reliable method of estrus induction in bitches, but it is impractical in a clinical setting. Preliminary work performed by Cain and colleagues (1989) involving the use of an intermittently and subcutaneously administered GnRH analog (d-Trp[6]-GnRH; Decapeptyl [Organon]) has yielded promising results. In this method, 1 μg/kg of the GnRH analog is administered subcutaneously to the sexually mature bitch every 8 hours until the onset of estrus. Once estrus occurs, the dosage is reduced to 0.5 μg/kg, given subcutaneously every 8 hours for an additional 3 days. Breeding should begin on day 1 of estrus. Using this technique, proestrus usually begins on the fourth or fifth day of treatment, and estrous behavior usually begins 9 to 11 days after the onset of treatment. Seventy-five percent of postpubertal bitches bred using this protocol conceived. One bitch failed to maintain pregnancy to term. All mature bitches in this study were known to have had at least one spontaneous estrous cycle. This high rate of successful estrus induction does not hold for animals with pathologic anestrus caused by pituitary or ovarian lesions that are unresponsive to GnRH.

Estrogens alone can apparently induce estrus and ovulation in normally cycling, anestrous bitches. In this method, beginning on or after day 95 of anestrus, 5 mg of diethylstilbestrol (DES) is administered daily through 2 days after the onset of proestrus. All five bitches treated with this method came into estrus and conceived. DES treatment was maintained for 6 to 9 days (average, 7.4 days). Proestrus lasted for 0 to 2 days (average, 1.5 days). Although the treated bitches cycled promptly in response to DES therapy and earlier than expected based on the average duration of anestrus of the colony, a potential weakness of the study is that prostaglandin $F_{2\alpha}$ ($PGF_{2\alpha}$) was administered to some bitches during their preceding diestrus. $PGF_{2\alpha}$ is known to shorten the interestral interval.

Suppression of prolactin with dopamine agonists suppresses luteal function and increases LH pulsatility in bitches. Prolactin antagonists such as bromocriptine and cabergoline can thereby induce estrus, but the cycles are often nonfertile despite hormonal variations similar to those in normal cycles. This is apparently especially true when bitches are treated less than 30 days after the LH surge. In a study of six bitches that had not experienced an estrus cycle for 13 to 30 months, all were successfully induced to cycle and ovulate. The five that were bred became pregnant. They were treated with cabergoline (Galastop, Ceva Vetem, Milan, Italy; Dostinex, Pharmacia, Kalamazoo, Mich) at a dosage of 5 μg/kg given orally once daily through the first 2 days of proestrus. The duration of treatment ranged from 4 to 34 days, with a mean of 16 days. There were no adverse effects observed. Others have suggested that continuing treatment through the first 4 to 5 days of proestrus is important for success.

## INDUCTION OF OVULATION

The hormonal induction of ovulation may be indicated for females with ovulation failure as shown by low diestrous serum concentrations of progesterone or for those with persistent estrus caused by ovarian follicular cysts. Ovulation induction is part of some estrus induction protocols. However, the hormonal induction of ovulation succeeds only if mature ovarian follicles are present.

### THE QUEEN

In the queen, ovulation can be induced hormonally or mechanically, providing there is sufficient vaginal stimulation to induce the LH surge. The intramuscular administration of 250 IU of hCG or 25 μg of GnRH (Cystorelin; Ceva [Abbott Labs, North Chicago, Ill]) on the first 2 days of estrus is recommended, although a single 25 μg dose of GnRH is known to cause an LH surge in normal cats. Probing the vagina with a smooth rod such as a thermometer or with a cotton swab four to eight times, at 5- to 20-minute intervals, may also stimulate an LH surge. The probing need last only 2 to 5 seconds. As with natural breedings, repeated stimulation on several days is most likely to induce ovulation. The successful stimulation of ovulation does not shorten that estrus; rather, it delays the onset of the next cycle. Pseudopregnancy occurs if the queen ovulates but does not conceive. Estrus usually resumes 45 days (range, 35 to 70 days) after the nonfertile induction of ovulation.

### THE BITCH

Unlike the induction of ovulation in the queen, the induction of ovulation in the bitch must be done hormonally. Potential agents include hCG (22 IU/kg IM); GnRH (50 to 100 μg IM); or GnRH (Cystorelin, Ceva; 2.2 μg/kg IM). hCG and GnRH are given on the first day of estrus, as determined by the behavior of the bitch and vaginal cytology. Success can be confirmed by the finding of a serum progesterone concentration of greater than 5 ng/ml in early diestrus. For the treatment of follicular cystic ovarian disease in the bitch, 2.2 μg/kg of GnRH is administered intramuscularly for 3 days. However, the results of this treatment have been disappointing.

## Suggested Readings

Baldwin CJ et al: The contraceptive effects of levonorgestrel in the domestic cat, *Lab Anim Sci* 44:261, 1994.

Bjurström L et al: Long-term study of aerobic bacteria of the genital tract in breeding bitches, *Am J Vet Res* 53:665, 1992.

Bjurström L et al: Long-term study of aerobic bacteria of the genital tract in stud dogs, *Am J Vet Res* 53:670, 1992.

Cain JL et al: Induction of ovulation in bitches with pulsatile or continuous infusion of GnRH, *J Reprod Fertil Steril* Suppl 39:143, 1989.

Chakraborty PK et al: Serum luteinizing hormone and ovulatory response to luteinizing hormone–releasing hormone in estrous and anestrous cats, *Lab Anim Sci* 29:338, 1979.

Concannon PW et al, editors: Dog and cat reproduction, contraception and artificial insemination, *J Reprod Fertil Suppl* 39, 1989.

Concannon PW et al, editors: Fertility and infertility in dogs, cats and other carnivores, *J Reprod Fertil Suppl* 47, 1993.

Concannon PW et al, editors: Reproduction of dogs and cats and exotic carnivores, *J Reprod Fertil Suppl* 51, 1997.

Concannon PW et al, editors: Advances in reproduction of dogs and cats and exotic carnivores, *J Reprod Fertil Suppl* 57, 2001.

Davidson AP, editor: Clinical theriogenology, *Vet Clin North Am Small Anim Pract* 31:2 2001.

Gobello C et al: Use of cabergoline to treat primary and secondary anestrus in dogs, *J Am Vet Med Assoc* 220:1653, 2002.

Greene CE, editor: *Infectious diseases of the dog and cat,* ed 2, Philadelphia, 1990, WB Saunders.

Handelman C et al: Evaluation of a test for plasma relaxin in pregnant and nonpregnant bitches, *Proceedings of the 18th ACVIM Forum,* Seattle, 2000, p 722.

Johnston SD et al, editors: *Canine and feline theriogenology,* Philadelphia, 2001, WB Saunders.

Löfstedt RM et al: Evaluation of a commercially available luteinizing hormone test for its ability to distinguish between ovariectomized and sexually intact bitches, *J Am Vet Med Assoc* 220:1331, 2002.

Miller DM: Ovarian remnant syndrome in dogs and cats: 46 cases (1988-1992), *J Vet Diagn Invest* 7:572, 1995.

Patronek GJ et al: Dynamics of dog and cat populations in a community, *J Am Vet Med Assoc* 210:637, 1997.

Purswell BJ: Pharmaceuticals used in canine reproduction, *Semin Vet Med Surg* 9:54, 1994.

Rijnberk A, editor: *Clinical endocrinology of dogs and cats,* Boston, 1996, Kluwer Academic.

Root MV et al: Estrous length, pregnancy rate, gestation and parturition lengths, litter size and juvenile mortality in the domestic cat, *J Am Anim Hosp Assoc* 31:429, 1995.

Verstegen JP et al: Regulation of progesterone during pregnancy in the cat: studies on the roles of corpora lutea, placenta and prolactin secretion, *J Reprod Fertil Suppl* 47:165, 1993.

Verstegen JP et al: The ovarian cycle and oestrus induction in the bitch, prostate diseases in the male dog, *Proceedings of the Annual Conference of the Society for Theriogenology and American College of Theriogenology,* Colorado Springs, 2002, p 321.

# CHAPTER 57

# Disorders of the Vagina and Uterus

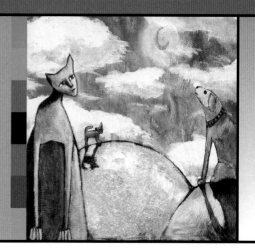

## CHAPTER OUTLINE

DIAGNOSTIC APPROACH TO VULVAR
DISCHARGE, 870
HEMORRHAGIC VULVAR DISCHARGE, 870
PURULENT VULVAR DISCHARGE, 872
MUCOID VULVAR DISCHARGE, 872
UTEROVERDIN AND CELLULAR DEBRIS, 872
CONGENITAL ANOMALIES OF THE VAGINA
AND VULVA, 872
VAGINITIS, 874
VAGINAL HYPERPLASIA AND PROLAPSE, 875
DISORDERS OF THE UTERUS, 877
CYSTIC ENDOMETRIAL HYPERPLASIA
AND PYOMETRA, 877

## DIAGNOSTIC APPROACH TO VULVAR DISCHARGE

The significance of a vulvar discharge is determined by its cellular composition, its source, and the stage of the reproductive cycle. A vulvar discharge is normally expected in bitches during proestrus and estrus, during parturition, and for as long as 6 weeks postpartum (lochia). Scant vulvar discharge is also normal in queens at these times; but, because of the fastidious nature of most queens, it is often not observed. The cellular composition of the vulvar discharge is used to classify it as hemorrhagic, purulent, mucoid, uteroverdin, or cellular debris (Table 57-1).

The diagnostic approach should be designed to determine the origin of the vulvar discharge (i.e., uterus, vagina, or vestibule) and the cause. Initially it includes a thorough history-taking, physical examination, vaginal cytology, and vaginoscopy. During the history-taking the stage of the reproductive cycle and the overall health of the bitch should be established. A complete physical examination including inspection of the discharge and vulva and palpation of the reproductive tract is then performed. Historical findings such as malaise, weight loss, vomiting, or polydipsia-polyuria are suggestive of systemic illness, as are physical findings such as fever and dehy-

dration. They deserve prompt attention. Disorders confined to the vulva, vestibule, or vagina rarely cause signs other than vulvar discharge, licking of the vulva, or pollakiuria. Physical abnormalities are usually confined to these areas. In contrast, disorders of the uterus frequently result in systemic signs of illness in addition to a vulvar discharge.

The character of the vulvar discharge is determined by vaginal cytology (see Table 57-1). The characteristic appearance of endometrial cells easily distinguishes them from other cells seen on vaginal cytologic preparations. They are columnar and have a basal nucleus and foamy cytoplasm (Fig. 57-1). The presence of endometrial cells indicates uterine involvement. They may be found in animals with cystic endometrial hyperplasia, even in the absence of an overt vulvar discharge, or, less commonly, in lochia and in animals with metritis. The source of the vulvar discharge is confirmed by physical examination of the vulva and endoscopic examination of the vestibule and vagina. If a uterine source of the discharge is suspected, abdominal radiography and/or ultrasonography of the uterus should also be performed. Further diagnostic tests may be indicated once the origin and probable cause of the discharge have been established.

## HEMORRHAGIC VULVAR DISCHARGE

Red blood cells (RBCs) are commonly found in normal and abnormal vulvar discharges. Their significance is determined by the other types of cells that are also present in the discharge. A serosanguineous discharge originating from the uterus is normal during proestrus and estrus. In addition to the plentiful RBCs, the cytologic findings during proestrus and estrus include numerous mature (cornified) superficial vaginal epithelial cells, indicating an estrogenic influence (see Figs. 56-2 and 57-1, B). White blood cells (WBCs) and extracellular bacteria may also be present. The administration of exogenous estrogen and the pathologic production of estrogens by ovarian follicular cysts or ovarian neoplasia can cause similar findings.

If RBCs are the predominant cytologic finding in the absence of cornified vaginal epithelial cells, a cause for hemor-

## TABLE 57-1

**Differential Diagnoses for Vulvar Discharge Based on Predominant Cytologic Characteristics**

### Cornified (Mature or Superficial) Epithelial Cells

Normal proestrus
Normal estrus
Contamination with squamous epithelium
　Skin or clitoris
Abnormal source of estrogen
　Exogenous
　Ovarian follicular cyst
　Ovarian neoplasia

### Peripheral Blood

Subinvoluted placental sites
Uterine or vaginal neoplasia
Trauma to reproductive tract
Uterine torsion
Coagulopathies

### Mucus

Normal late diestrus or late pregnancy
Normal lochia
Mucometra
Androgenic stimulation
(Idiopathic?)

### Cellular Debris

Normal lochia
Abortion

### Neutrophils

Nonseptic (no organisms seen)
　Normal first day of diestrus
　Vaginitis
　(Metritis or pyometra possible but unlikely)
Septic (organisms seen)
　Vaginitis
　Metritis
　Pyometra
　Abortion

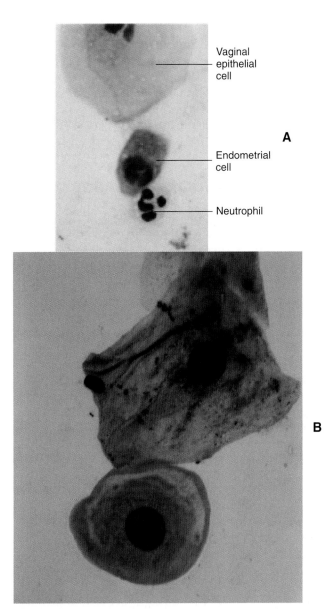

**FIG 57-1**
**A,** Canine endometrial cell with vaginal epithelial cell and neutrophil. **B,** Intermediate and superficial vaginal epithelial cells for comparison of size and morphology.

---

rhage, such as vaginal lacerations, uterine and vaginal neoplasia, subinvoluted placental sites, uterine torsion, and coagulopathies, should be sought. Vaginal lacerations or other trauma to the reproductive tract is uncommon but may occur during breeding or as a result of vaginoscopy or obstetric procedures. Foreign material in the vagina, such as foxtail awns, may cause a hemorrhagic discharge, but more typically the discharge associated with foreign material is predominantly purulent.

Leiomyoma is the most common neoplasm of the vagina and uterus in geriatric bitches and queens. It often causes hemorrhage. However, because leiomyomas do not exfoliate readily, neoplastic cells are usually not seen on cytologic preparations. Bitches with transmissible venereal tumors are more likely to be examined because of a mass protruding from the vulva than because of a vulvar discharge (see p. 937). Neoplastic cells exfoliate readily from transmissible venereal tumors, so the diagnosis is easily made on the basis of cytologic findings.

When placental sites do not involute properly, the lochia is more hemorrhagic and persists longer than usual. This condition is known as *subinvolution of placental sites (SIPS)* (see p. 897). The cytologic appearance of SIPS consists of RBCs with a mucoid background and some cellular debris. Uterine torsion is uncommon in bitches and queens. When it does occur, it almost always involves a near-term pregnancy. Although bleeding from the vulva is certainly not common in animals with coagulation defects, it has been observed as the sole site of bleeding in some bitches with coagulopathies. Finally, it is wise to remember that RBCs often accompany inflammatory processes in which WBCs are the predominant cytologic abnormality. If the number of WBCs exceeds that expected in peripheral blood, a cause of inflammation (WBCs) rather than of bleeding (RBCs) should be sought.

## PURULENT VULVAR DISCHARGE

Purulent and mucopurulent vulvar discharges are characterized by polymorphonuclear cells (PMNs), which are the predominant cell type found in bitches and queens with an inflammation of the reproductive tract. If bacteria are also present, the exudate is referred to as *septic*. Large numbers of PMNs without signs of degeneration or sepsis are often found during the first day or two of diestrus. This normal diestrual return of WBCs to the vaginal smear can be differentiated from inflammation of the reproductive tract by the absence of clinical signs, the temporal correlation with recent estrus, and the prompt disappearance of WBCs within 48 hours of the onset of diestrus.

A nonseptic exudate is often found in prepubertal bitches with vaginitis (see p. 874). Androgenic stimulation (exogenous testosterone or an intersex condition) can also cause a nonseptic inflammation. Because the vagina has a normal resident population of bacteria, nonseptic processes can become septic at any time. Other causes of nonseptic and septic vulvar discharges include vulvitis, vaginitis, pyometra (see p. 877), metritis (see p. 896), abortion (see p. 900), and a uterine stump granuloma or abscess. If vulvitis or vaginitis is the cause of the discharge, hyperemia, edema, or other mucosal lesions of the vulva or vagina are expected findings during physical and endoscopic examination. A finding of vulvitis or vaginitis does not exclude the possibility of a concurrent uterine abnormality.

## MUCOID VULVAR DISCHARGE

Mucus is the predominant component of the normal postpartum discharge, lochia. It may also be present during normal late pregnancy and possibly in small amounts during the nonpregnant luteal phase. Cervicitis and mucometra can cause a mucoid vulvar discharge. In rare instances, no apparent cause can be found in some bitches with small amounts of mucous discharge.

## UTEROVERDIN AND CELLULAR DEBRIS

Uteroverdin is the dark green heme pigment normally found in the placenta. It is identified macroscopically rather than microscopically. Its presence in a vulvar discharge indicates that placental separation has occurred. This is normal during stage

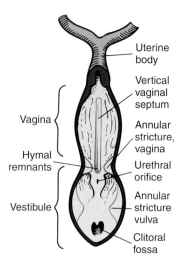

ANOMALOUS STRUCTURES

**FIG 57-2**
Anatomic location of normal structures and common congenital anomalies of the canine vagina and vulva. (Redrawn from Miller ME et al, editors: *Anatomy of the dog,* Philadelphia, 1964, WB Saunders.)

II of parturition and during the first few hours postpartum. Cellular debris and mucus are expected microscopic findings in lochia and accompany uteroverdin. When uteroverdin is present before the onset of stage II labor, it indicates that serious placental damage has occurred. If uteroverdin is still present after the first 12 postpartum hours, it may indicate that placental tissue has been retained. Cellular debris is often the predominant component of the discharge that accompanies abortion and also of the discharge that accompanies the metritis associated with retained fetal or placental tissue.

## CONGENITAL ANOMALIES OF THE VAGINA AND VULVA

The müllerian ducts are the embryologic origin of the vagina, uterus, and uterine tubes. The vestibule, urethra, and urinary bladder develop from the urogenital sinus. The genital folds also form part of the vestibule. The genital tubercle gives rise to the clitoris, and the genital swellings become the labia (vulva). The fusion of the müllerian ducts with the urogenital sinus forms the hymen, which is composed of two epithelial surfaces separated by a thin layer of mesoderm. In bitches the hymen normally disappears before birth.

The abnormal formation or disappearance of the hymen can result in a vertical band of tissue or in an annular fibrous stricture at the vestibulovaginal junction (Fig. 57-2). Abnormal or incomplete fusion of the paired müllerian ducts can result in the formation of an elongated vertical septum that bisects the vagina or in the formation of a vaginal diverticulum (pouch). Vaginal diverticula are uncommon. Complete duplication of parts of the urogenital tract, including a true double vagina, has been reported, but this is extremely rare. Abnormal fusion of the genital folds with the genital swellings can result in the formation of strictures within the vestibule and vagina. Hypoplasia or agenesis of parts of the reproductive tract also occurs. All these congenital anomalies of the vagina and vulva have been found in bitches, but they are apparently extremely rare in queens. With the exception of abnormalities of the vulva and vestibule, these congenital anomalies are located immediately anterior to the external urethral orifice.

## Clinical Features

Congenital anomalies of the vagina and vulva may cause no clinical signs, or they may be associated with chronic vaginitis. Occasionally they are associated with urinary incontinence, presumably because urine accumulates anterior to the lesion (urine pooling) and then flows out of the vagina. In breeding bitches, vulvar-vaginal anomalies may cause infertility or refusal to mate, or, if intromission is tolerated by the bitch, the male may dismount and refuse to breed once he encounters the lesion.

## Diagnosis

Congenital anomalies of the vagina and vulva are easily and most accurately identified by digital palpation. Because most anomalies are located just anterior to the urethral orifice, they are readily accessible to digital palpation and short endoscopic equipment such as an otoscope. Except for annular anomalies, they are almost always located on the midline. Vaginoscopy (see p. 853) is useful for evaluating congenital anomalies, but the endoscope can inadvertently be passed beside and beyond the lesion, especially in larger bitches. Vaginography (see p. 858) can also be performed. Abdominal radiography or ultrasonography can be performed to identify vaginal diverticula.

## Treatment

Treatment is unnecessary if a congenital anomaly is causing no clinical signs. Before the treatment of annular strictures is considered, the bitch should be evaluated during proestrus and estrus. This is because the junction of the vestibule and the vagina is normally so narrow during anestrus, especially in pubescent bitches, that it may be mistaken for a stricture. During proestrus and estrus the normal vestibulovaginal junction relaxes considerably and is easily differentiated from a true stricture. Some strictures in the vestibule-vulva also "relax" during estrus.

Anomalies of the vulva and vagina that are causing clinical signs should be corrected surgically during anestrus. Thin bands of persistent hymenal tissue can sometimes be broken using digital pressure alone. Some annular strictures are amenable to bougienage. Surgical repair is necessary for the treatment of other annular strictures and vaginal septa, and this can usually be achieved through an episiotomy. Celiotomy may be necessary to correct a vaginal diverticulum. The prognosis for the resolution of clinical signs after surgi-

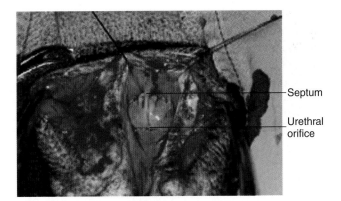

**FIG 57-3**
Vaginal septum.

cal correction of vaginal septa (Fig. 57-3) and hymenal remnants is excellent. Animals with annular strictures may be prone to fibrosis and restricture. Because hypoplasia or agenesis cannot be rectified, affected animals should be neutered to prevent additional complications, such as cystic endometrial hyperplasia. The role that heredity plays in the development of congenital vaginal and vulvar anomalies in bitches is unknown, but it is known that certain vaginal anomalies are inherited in mice.

**Clitoral hypertrophy.** In the female, the clitoris develops from the genital tubercle, as does the penis in the male. Under the influence of androgens the canine clitoris may enlarge and even ossify. This can be caused by exposure of female fetuses to androgens or progestins during gestation, by exogenous androgen administration to female animals of any age, or by endogenous androgen production from testicular tissue in intersex animals. Clitoral hypertrophy may go unnoticed. More commonly, however, the enlarged clitoris protrudes from the vulva. This is often first apparent when the female is near puberty or after the administration of exogenous androgens. A mucoid discharge is common, as is licking of the area. There may be a history of recurrent urinary tract infection. Physical examination will demonstrate the abnormal clitoris, which occasionally will have a distinctly phallic shape. When present, ossification is usually palpable. The vulva may have a normal appearance and position, or it may be ventrally displaced anywhere along the line of the prepuce in the male (Fig. 57-4). The vestibule-vagina may not be patent in females exposed in utero. Treatment is to remove the source of androgen if it still exists. If the clitoris is ossified, it is not likely to regress even in the absence of androgens. Unless it is clear that the female has been treated with androgens and was previously normal, such as might be the case with racing greyhound bitches, affected animals should be evaluated for the presence of an intersex condition. Exploratory laparotomy with the intent of removing the gonads and internal genitalia may be the most cost-effective approach. Clitorectomy may also be performed if needed to eliminate the clinical signs.

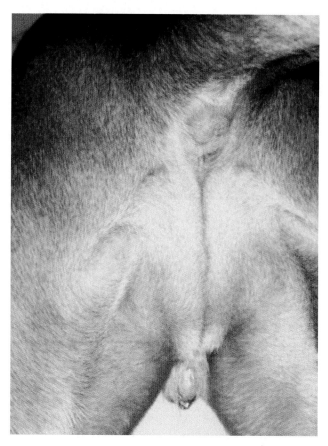

**FIG 57-4**
Clitoral hyperplasia in a 1-year-old Weimaraner examined because of recurrent urinary tract infection and vulvar discharge. Note the ventral displacement of the vulva. Testes and uterus were found at surgery. Gonadectomy, hysterectomy, and clitorectomy were curative.

## *VAGINITIS*

### Etiology

Vaginitis (i.e., inflammation of the vagina) occurs in sexually intact or neutered bitches of any age or breed during any stage of the reproductive cycle. It is rare in queens. Vaginitis may result from bacterial or viral infections; immaturity of the reproductive tract; androgenic stimulation; chemical irritation, such as that caused by urine; or mechanical irritation, such as that caused by foreign material, neoplasia, or anatomic abnormalities of the vagina or vestibule.

### Diagnosis

The diagnosis is based primarily on the historical and physical finding of a mucoid (white), mucopurulent (white-yellow), or purulent (yellow-green) vulvar discharge, which is present in 90% of bitches with vaginitis. Licking the vulva and pollakiuria are much less common additional clinical signs; both are present in about 10% of affected animals. The vulvar discharge of vaginitis rarely contains blood. The diagnosis can be substantiated by vaginal cytology and by vaginoscopy. The cytologic finding in an animal with vaginitis is nonseptic or septic inflammation without hemorrhage. The extent and gross appearance of the vaginal inflammation can be assessed by vaginoscopy. Vaginoscopy is especially useful for identifying anatomic abnormalities and other types of mechanical irritation that may predispose the animal to vaginitis.

The bacterial organisms isolated from bitches with vaginitis are usually quantitatively and qualitatively similar to the normal bacterial flora of the canine vagina. Therefore the recovery of these organisms, many of which are potential pathogens, does not constitute prima facie evidence of infection. The results of bacterial culture and sensitivity testing are used to guide the formulation of a rational therapeutic plan rather than to establish the diagnosis of vaginitis.

Additional diagnostic tests are useful for excluding or evaluating disorders other than, or in addition to, vaginitis. They are not useful for establishing the diagnosis of vaginitis per se. For example, hemograms from bitches with vaginitis are normal. If abnormalities on the hemogram are found, they can be attributed to lesions other than vaginitis. As expected, voided urine specimens from bitches with vaginitis contain many more inflammatory cells than do urine samples obtained by cystocentesis.

Urinary tract disorders should be excluded in animals with a history of pollakiuria. Although they are not associated with vaginitis in young bitches, urinary tract infection and urolithiasis, which are both common causes of pollakiuria, can occur in any young dog, irrespective of vaginitis.

### Treatment

**Prepubertal bitch.** The clinical findings, treatment, and prognosis of canine vaginitis vary according to the age of the bitch. In bitches less than 1 year of age, physical and historical abnormalities almost always consist only of the vulvar discharge and inflammation of the vulva and vagina. Vaginal cytologic findings are most often nonseptic in nature. Systemic or topical antibiotics, douches, and perineal cleansing have all been recommended as treatments, but 90% of young bitches recover from vaginitis with or without treatment. Therefore, if the historical and physical abnormalities in young bitches are limited to a vulvar discharge without blood, further diagnostic tests and treatment are usually not necessary. Most such animals recover spontaneously as they reach physical maturity. However, young bitches with any additional historical or physical abnormalities should be evaluated using the approach described for the mature bitch.

The role of estrus, if any, in the resolution of vaginitis in young bitches is unclear. In some bitches there is a temporal relationship between the onset of estrous activity and the resolution of vaginitis. However, vaginitis resolves spontaneously in most young bitches before their first estrous cycle. The effect of ovariohysterectomy on the resolution or persistence of vaginitis in the prepubertal bitch has not been reported. There is no evidence that ovariohysterectomy hastens the resolution of vaginitis. Because estrus may cause vaginitis to resolve (or conversely, the absence of estrus may cause vaginitis to persist), consideration should be given to delaying ovariohysterectomy until after a young bitch with chronic vaginitis has had her first estrus.

**Mature bitch.** Vaginitis is associated with identifiable predisposing abnormalities in approximately 70% of bitches older than 1 year. The key to the successful therapy of vaginitis in mature bitches is the identification and elimination of concurrent abnormalities. Of the identifiable abnormalities in mature bitches, physical abnormalities of the genital tract are the most common (35%). They are found during physical and endoscopic examinations and include vulvar anomalies, clitoral hypertrophy, vaginal strictures, vertical bands of tissue in the vagina, vaginal atresia, and vaginal neoplasia. Disorders of the urinary tract, including urinary tract infection and urinary incontinence, are the next most commonly (26%) identified abnormalities in mature bitches with vaginitis. Therefore vaginoscopy, vaginal cytology, and analysis and culture of urine obtained by cystocentesis should always be included in the evaluation of mature animals with vaginitis.

The resolution of vaginitis in mature bitches is directly related to the elimination of the underlying disorder. For example, the animal is usually cured of the vaginitis if anatomic abnormalities are corrected surgically. Treatment with systemic antibiotics is often beneficial, especially in animals with a known bacterial infection elsewhere, such as in the urinary tract. However, the clinical signs of vaginitis recur if antibiotic therapy is stopped unless the underlying abnormality is eliminated.

Approximately one third of mature bitches have no identifiable abnormalities other than vaginitis. Fortunately, most of these animals recover spontaneously, although it may take months or years to do so. The clinical signs in many are lessened by intermittent, systemic antibiotic therapy. Antibiotics should be chosen on the basis of the results yielded by culture and susceptibility testing of urine and anterior vaginal specimens. If a heavy growth (>100 colony-forming units) of a single organism is isolated from the vagina, it is usually considered to be a pathogen. However, as stated earlier, the organisms recovered from bitches with vaginitis are usually quantitatively and qualitatively the same as those that constitute normal vaginal flora. Ampicillin, trimethoprim-sulfonamides, clavulanate-amoxicillin, enrofloxacin, and cephalosporins are usually effective against gram-positive and gram-negative organisms isolated from the urogenital tract. Tetracycline and chloramphenicol can also be considered for the eradication of gram-negative infections. Several of these antibiotics, however, are contraindicated during pregnancy (see p. 897) and therefore should not be administered during diestrus in breeding animals. The efficacy of vaginal douches in the treatment of canine vaginitis is unknown. Douching should not be performed during proestrus or estrus in brood bitches because the douche solutions may be spermicidal.

The role of estrus, if any, in resolving vaginitis in mature bitches is unknown. The signs of vaginitis continue to improve in some mature bitches with each succeeding cycle. In others there is no apparent change in response to estrus. The effects of ovariohysterectomy on vaginitis in mature bitches are even less clear. In most bitches, ovariohysterectomy has no apparent therapeutic effect on the outcome. Signs of vaginitis occur after ovariohysterectomy in some previously healthy bitches.

**Chronic, nonresponsive vaginitis.** Animals with chronic vaginitis in which an underlying cause cannot be found and that do not recover in response to appropriate therapy remain a source of frustration. Findings from prior diagnostic tests should be reviewed to ensure that nothing was inadvertently overlooked or excluded by assumption. Bacterial culture of specimens from the anterior vagina and of urine should be repeated to identify the possible development of resistant organisms. Repeated vaginoscopy may identify lesions that were not present during prior evaluations. Vaginal biopsy, preferably performed at the site of visible lesions or inflammation, is indicated to establish the character of the lesions (e.g., plasmacytic-lymphocytic inflammation, neoplasia, vesicular lesions with inclusion bodies). The finding of vesicular lesions, especially those consisting of cells that have intranuclear inclusions, may indicate the presence of a herpesvirus infection. A finding of plasmacytic-lymphocytic inflammation may support a trial of therapy with systemic glucocorticoids. Uterine stump abscess or pyometra should be considered in the spayed bitch with chronic vaginitis. Ultrasonographic evaluation of the uterus and vagina can identify concurrent uterine lesions and assess the thickness of the vaginal wall. If a specific lesion cannot be found, long-term antibiotic therapy may be necessary to control rather than cure bacterial vaginitis.

Veterinarians often recommend the use of commercially available (over-the-counter) douches containing dilute vinegar or povidone-iodine for the treatment of canine vaginitis. There are no published results of studies demonstrating the efficacy, or the lack thereof, of vaginal douching in the treatment of canine vaginitis. Certainly douching is indicated only after causes of vaginitis such as anatomic defects or foreign material have been excluded. Beneficial effects of douching may be derived from the mechanical flushing or dilution of exudate and organisms, by altering the pH such that bacterial growth is inhibited, and/or from direct antimicrobial activity of the solution. However, none of the beneficial effects can be realized unless an adequate volume of douche solution is instilled into the vagina. Given the anatomy of the canine vagina, the discomfort of vaginitis, and the need for adequate animal restraint, many pet owners are unable to instill douches into the vagina. Often the solutions are instilled only into the vestibule. In addition, repeated, unsuccessful attempts at douching may only aggravate the inflammation, cause additional discomfort, and worsen the restraint problems. Until the efficacy of vaginal douching in bitches is clearly demonstrated, perhaps it should be reserved for animals in which it will at least do no harm.

## VAGINAL HYPERPLASIA AND PROLAPSE

During proestrus and estrus the vagina becomes edematous and hyperplastic. Sometimes the change is so severe that vaginal tissue protrudes out of the vulva (Fig. 57-5). This condition has

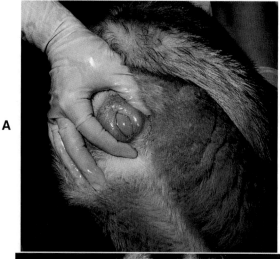

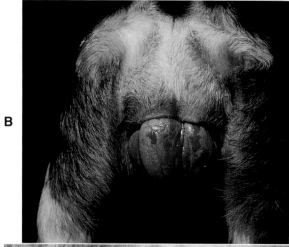

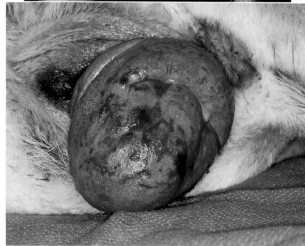

**FIG 57-5**
Vaginal hyperplasia and prolapse. **A,** Type I, edema.
**B,** Type II. **C,** Type III.

been referred to as *vaginal hyperplasia* or *vaginal prolapse,* because these are the most prominent physical and microscopic findings. The swelling initially results from the accumulation of edema fluid; therefore some theriogenologists have recommended that the condition be called *vaginal edema.* The pro-

lapse, or protrusion, of this edematous, hyperplastic tissue must not be confused with the prolapse of the vagina or uterus that occurs rarely during parturition.

Vaginal hyperplasia and prolapse occur in bitches exclusively during times of estrogenic stimulation. Therefore they are identified during proestrus and estrus. Prolapse recurs in a few bitches at the end of diestrus or at parturition, a time when additional estrogen may be secreted. The amount of edema and hyperplasia is extremely variable. It may be identified only during vaginal palpation (type I vaginal prolapse; see Fig. 57-5, *A*), or it may protrude from the vulva (type II vaginal prolapse; see Fig. 57-5, *B*). Although the tissue protruding from the vulva may be quite massive, it usually involves only 1 cm or so of the length of the vaginal floor, immediately cranial to the external urethral orifice. The width is variable, in that sometimes it consists of a stalklike attachment and sometimes it involves more of the width of the vaginal floor. Much less commonly the hyperplastic tissue involves the circumference of the vagina (type III; see Fig. 57-5, *C*). In this instance also the edematous hyperplastic tissue is located at the level of the urethral orifice; the rest of the vagina is normal.

## Diagnosis

The diagnosis of vaginal prolapse is made on the basis of the history and physical examination findings. Bitches may be seen because they refuse to allow intromission, or they may be seen because of the mass protruding from the vulva. The history indicates that they are in proestrus or estrus. If it does not, estrogenic stimulation can be confirmed by vaginal cytology. If there is doubt, the hyperplastic tissue can be differentiated from vaginal neoplasia on the basis of findings yielded by the cytologic examination of material obtained by fine-needle aspiration of the tissue.

Digital palpation of the vagina shows that the mass originates from the ventral vagina, immediately cranial to the urethral orifice. All other areas of the vagina are normal. If the edematous tissue is small enough to be contained within the vagina and vestibule, it is usually very smooth, glistening, and pale pink to opalescent (edematous). If the tissue protrudes from the vulva, it is dry, dull, and wrinkled. With continued exposure, fissures and ulcers may develop.

## Treatment

The treatment of vaginal edema is primarily supportive. The edema and hyperplasia will resolve spontaneously when the follicular phase of the cycle and the ovarian production of estrogen are over. This can be hastened by ovariohysterectomy. Ovariohysterectomy also prevents the recurrence of vaginal hyperplasia and prolapse. After oophorectomy, the edema and hyperplasia will resolve, usually within 5 to 7 days. The induction of ovulation using gonadotropin-releasing hormone (see p. 869) can be attempted, but no results of studies have been published showing that doing so hastens recovery. Artificial insemination (see p. 940) can be performed if vaginal hyperplasia and prolapse prevent copulation. Despite the fact that the edematous hyperplastic tissue lies over the external urethral orifice, urine flow is rarely impeded.

Exposed edematous tissue must be protected from trauma and infection if the mucosa is damaged. This is usually accomplished by applying topical antibiotic (e.g., bacitracin-neomycin-polymyxin) or antibiotic-steroid creams and cleaning the tissue (warm saline solution, or warm water and pHisoHex) as needed. An Elizabethan collar may be used to prevent self-mutilation, but this is rarely necessary. Attention should also be paid to the underlying perineal and vulvar skin, which may be subject to maceration. Potentially irritating bedding such as straw or wood chips should be removed. Severely damaged or necrotic tissue should be surgically excised.

Surgical resection of the edematous tissue has been considered in brood bitches, but this should probably be reserved for extremely valuable animals. The hemorrhage that results is usually significant, despite excellent surgical technique. The resection of hyperplastic tissue also does not prevent recurrence during subsequent estrous cycles, although the severity of the prolapse may be markedly reduced. We have seen one bitch with recurrent hyperplasia and prolapse in which the prolapse did not resolve despite ovariohysterectomy after the fourth recurrence. Resection was the only recourse.

It is common for vaginal hyperplasia and prolapse to recur during each estrus, although each episode is not always of the same severity. Because of its recurrent nature and the care required to manage severe cases, affected animals are not the best brood bitches. The role that heredity plays, if any, in the development of vaginal hyperplasia and prolapse is not known, but it appears to be at least familial in nature.

## DISORDERS OF THE UTERUS

The clinical signs of disorders of the uterus are variable and nonspecific. For example, there may be no clinical signs associated with congenital anomalies such as segmental aplasia. Rather, it may be an incidental finding at the time of elective ovariohysterectomy. Conversely, in cycling animals segmental aplasia may be the cause of fluid retention within the uterine lumen or the cause of infertility. Many uterine disorders are manifest by the presence of an abnormal vulvar discharge. Specimens collected from the vagina, or less commonly from the uterus itself via transcervical catheterization, are useful in evaluating uterine disease. The presence of endometrial cells on vaginal cytology specimens indicates uterine involvement. Specimens obtained from the uterus of normal bitches contained a few WBCs throughout the cycle, including neutrophils, lymphocytes, and macrophages. Bacteria were observed only during proestrus and estrus. Spermatozoa were found during estrus and early pregnancy in mated animals. Uterine enlargement may cause abdominal discomfort and abdominal distention. Uterine disorders often cause signs of systemic illness, especially when infection exists.

Uterine neoplasia is rare in dogs and cats. Leiomyoma is the most common neoplasm. Rarely, adenocarcinoma has been reported. Uterine neoplasia may be an incidental finding, or it may be associated with sangineous vulvar discharge, anorexia, weight loss, and abdominal discomfort and en-largement. The diagnosis is made by the finding of uterine enlargement on abdominal palpation, abdominal radiography, and ultrasonography. Treatment is ovariohysterectomy. The prognosis for leiomyoma is good, except when its physical location may preclude complete excision. The prognosis for uterine carcinoma is poor because metastasis is often present. Focal, benign uterine masses, such as adenomyosis, have also rarely been reported in geriatric bitches.

Uterine torsion is a life-threatening condition that occurs most commonly in the near-term gravid uterus in bitches and queens. As such, it is a life-threatening cause of dystocia. One or both horns may be involved. Torsion of the nongravid uterus has been reported in conjunction with other uterine pathologic findings, such as hematometra and pyometra. Clinical signs include sanguineous vulvar discharge, abdominal distention, abdominal pain, lethargy, and fever. The diagnosis is suspected on the basis of physical examination and ultrasonographic findings. It is confirmed at surgery. There may be severe metabolic complications depending on the duration and severity of the torsion. Treatment is ovariohysterectomy and intensive supportive therapy.

Metritis is discussed in Chapter 59.

## CYSTIC ENDOMETRIAL HYPERPLASIA AND PYOMETRA

### Etiology

Cystic endometrial hyperplasia (CEH)–pyometra complex is a potentially life-threatening disorder of the uterus. Progesterone normally stimulates the growth and secretory activity of endometrial glands. This can result in the development of CEH with fluid accumulation in the endometrial glands and the uterine lumen. Progesterone also diminishes myometrial activity, which may foster the retention of luminal fluid. As expected, CEH develops during or shortly after the luteal phase of the cycle (diestrus) when the ovarian production of progesterone is high, as well as after the administration of exogenous progestins. If the animal is examined at this stage in the pathogenesis of CEH-pyometra complex, before bacterial invasion occurs, CEH alone or in association with hydrometra or mucometra is found.

Bacteria, presumably of vaginal origin, are able to colonize the abnormal uterus, resulting in the development of pyometra. *Escherichia coli* is the organism most commonly isolated from bitches and queens with pyometra. Although bacterial infection does not initiate the pathogenesis of CEH-pyometra, it is the cause of most of the morbidity and mortality associated with pyometra. There is no apparent correlation between the severity of the clinical signs and the type of organisms isolated from bitches with pyometra; however, uteri infected with strains of *E. coli* that had cytotoxic necrotizing factor 1 (CNF 1) had the most severe histologic lesions. Bitches with pyometra are immunosuppressed. They have higher concentrations of circulating immune complexes, immunoglobulins, and lysozymes and depressed lymphocyte blastogenesis compared with normal animals. Sera from affected animals suppress the function of lymphocytes from normal dogs.

Why some animals have this pathologic response to progesterone and others do not is unknown. If there is a genetic component to the development of pyometra, it has not been reflected by substantially increased breed-specific risks in two large Scandinavian studies (Egenvall and colleagues [2001]; Niskanen and colleagues [1978]). However, mixed-breed dogs and Dachshunds apparently had lower risks. Pyometra was found in 12 of 3000 (0.4%) free-roaming queens of unknown age that were evaluated in a trap-neuter-return program. The risk of developing pyometra increases with age, presumably because of repeated hormonal stimulation of the uterus. Reported mean ages of bitches with pyometra range from 6.5 to 8.5 years. Analysis of survival rates in Swedish dogs indicates that, on average, 23% to 24% of bitches will develop pyometra by age 10 years. Parity has also been identified as a risk factor. There is a sixfold increased risk in nulliparous bitches compared with primiparous or multiparous animals.

Previous hormonal therapy is also a risk factor. CEH can be experimentally induced with exogenous progestins. Recent data from Europe, where surgical sterilization of bitches is uncommon relative to the United States, found no apparent increased risk in bitches treated with progestins for estrous suppression. This was attributed to substantially lower doses than were used experimentally and to the use of synthetic products, such as proligestone, that have a much lower binding specificity. Estrogens also increase the risk of pyometra, particularly when given during diestrus (when progesterone is high), such as would be done to prevent pregnancy following misalliance. It is known that estrogen increases the number of progesterone receptors in the uterus. Some have speculated that this might make it more susceptible to develop pathologic change. After the fact (i.e., after pyometra already exists), however, the luminal epithelium has been so disrupted that comparisons with normal have been difficult. Studies of uterine estrogen and progesterone receptors during the development of CEH-pyometra have apparently not been done. Younger bitches that develop pyometra are more likely than older bitches to have been treated with estrogens. In the study by Niskanen and colleague (1998), the average age of 953 bitches with pyometra was 8.5 years, except for those treated with estrogens, whose average age was 5.5 years.

## Clinical Features

Pyometra is classified as *open* or *closed* depending on whether there is a vulvar discharge. In normal bitches the cervix is patent during all stages of the cycle. The true status of the cervix and cervical "patency" are rarely investigated in animals with pyometra; nevertheless, use of the terms *open cervix* and *closed cervix* persists. The clinical signs stem from the infection in the uterus and tend to be more severe in a bitch or queen in which the uterus is not draining. A purulent vulvar discharge, which is usually also bloody, is present in animals with open pyometra. Partial to complete inappetence, lethargy, and vomiting occur in animals with pyometra. Polyuria-polydipsia is also a common finding in bitches but

not in queens. The most common physical finding is the septic vulvar discharge, which is present in the majority of animals with pyometra. Affected animals are often dehydrated. Fever is found in only 20% of bitches and queens with pyometra. The uterus is usually palpably abnormal, especially if the cervix is closed and the uterus is not draining. If pyometra goes untreated, septicemia, endotoxemia, or both can develop. Affected animals may be moribund, with hypothermia and shock.

## Diagnosis

Pyometra is diagnosed on the basis of the occurrence of clinical signs in a sexually mature female during or shortly after diestrus or after exogenous progestin administration, the presence of a septic vulvar discharge, and the identification of a fluid-filled uterus on abdominal radiographs or sonograms (see Figs. 56-6, *B* and *C*, and 57-6). A complete blood count, serum biochemistry profile, and urinalysis are necessary to detect the metabolic abnormalities associated with sepsis and to evaluate renal function.

Neutrophilia with a shift toward immaturity, monocytosis, and evidence of WBC toxicity are the most common findings on the complete blood count. The total WBC count may be as high as 100,000 to 200,000/μl. In severe sepsis

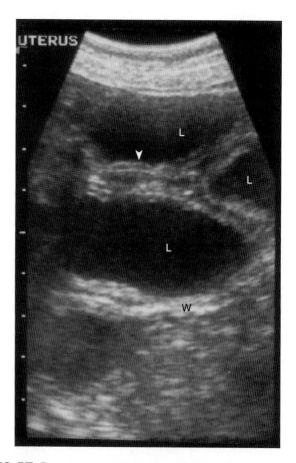

**FIG 57-6**
Sonogram of pyometra. *L*, Fluid-filled uterine lumen; *W*, uterine wall; *arrow*, endometrial cysts.

there may be a leukopenia with a degenerative left shift. A mild normocytic, normochromic, nonregenerative anemia is usually also evident.

Biochemical abnormalities include hyperproteinemia, hyperglobulinemia, and azotemia. Occasionally, alanine aminotransferase and alkaline phosphatase activities are mildly to moderately increased, presumably because of septicemia or hypoxia. Urinalysis findings include isosthenuria and/or proteinuria in one third of the bitches with pyometra. Bacteriuria is common. Many of the changes involving the kidney are thought to be secondary to immune complex glomerulonephritis, which results in proteinuria, and bacterial endotoxin interference with the renal tubular response to antidiuretic hormone, which results in isosthenuria. Other as yet unknown factors may be contributory. These renal abnormalities are potentially reversible once bacteria are eradicated.

Vaginal cytology reveals a septic exudate, sometimes containing endometrial cells (see Fig. 57-1). Cytologic findings are usually abnormal even if there is no visible discharge. Results of bacterial culture and sensitivity testing of the uterine exudate identify the offending organism and the appropriate antibiotic therapy.

Abdominal radiography or ultrasonography or both should always be performed to confirm the presence of pyometra and rule out pregnancy, because the goals of treatment of a pregnancy complicated by uterine infection may be quite different from those of treatment for pyometra. Both conditions occur during the diestrous stage of the cycle. Mature neutrophilia, anemia, and hyperglobulinemia may be found in normal, pregnant animals. Pregnant animals are not always healthy, and the presence of a septic vulvar discharge does not preclude the possibility of coexistent pregnancy. Uterine infection during pregnancy does not invariably result in the death of all fetuses. Even in the event of overt abortion, the entire litter is not always lost.

The radiographic appearance of pyometra and the gravid uterus are essentially identical until fetal calcification is detectable after 40 or more gestational days. After approximately days 42 to 45, abdominal radiographs can be used to differentiate pregnancy, in which calcified fetal skeleton can be identified, from pyometra, in which there are no identifiable fetuses. Ultrasonography can be used at any time to identify fetal structures, to assess the viability of the fetuses, to identify exudate in the lumen of the uterus, and to assess the thickness of the uterine wall.

## Treatment

Treatment of CEH-pyometra must be prompt and aggressive if the animal's life is to be saved. Septicemia, endotoxemia, or both can develop at any time, if they do not already exist. Intravenous fluid therapy is indicated to correct existing deficits, to maintain adequate tissue perfusion, and to improve renal function. Aggressive fluid therapy will be needed for animals in septic shock. Several studies have shown that the prognosis worsens if azotemia is not corrected in dogs before the surgical treatment of pyometra. Antibiotic therapy should begin immediately. A broad-spectrum, bactericidal antibiotic with efficacy against *E. coli,* such as trimethoprim-sulfonamides, ampicillin, or clavulanate-amoxicillin, should be administered until the results of bacterial culture and sensitivity testing are available. The appropriate antibiotic is then continued for 2 to 3 weeks.

It is thought that large doses of a glucocorticoid (prednisolone sodium succinate, 15 to 30 mg/kg, or dexamethasone, 4 to 6 mg/kg, given once intravenously or repeated at 4- to 6-hour intervals if shock persists) may be helpful for animals in septic or endotoxic shock. Glucocorticoids are most beneficial if administered early and in conjunction with other specific corrective measures (i.e., intravenous fluids, antibiotic therapy). Glucocorticoid therapy delayed for more than 4 hours after the experimental induction of bacterial or endotoxic shock has been observed to be associated with a marked reduction in the beneficial effects. Likewise, repeated doses become progressively less effective in improving the chances of survival. The role of glucocorticoids in the treatment of endotoxic shock associated with pyometra is not known.

As soon as the fluid deficits are corrected and antibiotic therapy has been initiated, definitive treatment for pyometra should begin. Ovariohysterectomy is the treatment of choice for pyometra in bitches and queens. Despite appropriate treatment, morbidity of 5% to 8% and mortality of 4% to 20% are reported. This is not unexpected, given the serious metabolic derangements caused by pyometra. Nevertheless, ovariohysterectomy is the only reasonable choice for animals that are critically ill, because surgical extirpation is immediate, whereas evacuation of infected uterine contents with medical therapy is not. Ovariohysterectomy is curative, barring complications resulting from anesthesia, surgery, or progression of the disease itself.

**Prostaglandin therapy.** Medical management of pyometra with prostaglandin $F_{2\alpha}$ ($PGF_{2\alpha}$) could be considered for valuable brood stock that are not critically ill. Prostaglandins are not approved for use in small animals in the United States. Prostaglandins of the F series cause myometrial contractions that can evacuate the uterine contents if the cervix is patent. The cervix normally dilates in response to pressure exerted against it. There is some risk, however, that the cervix will not dilate as rapidly as necessary to allow the uterine contents to escape in the bitch or queen with closed pyometra. Uterine rupture or the leakage of intraluminal contents into the abdomen through the uterine tubes is then possible. Prostaglandins also cause luteolysis or suppress ovarian steroidogenesis, which removes the source of the progesterone responsible for causing the disorder.

Prostaglandin therapy is more effective for the treatment of bitches and queens with existing uterine drainage, recognized by the presence of a vulvar discharge (i.e., open cervix), than for those without discharge (i.e., closed cervix). To treat pyometra in bitches or queens, natural $PGF_{2\alpha}$ (Lutalyse; Pharmacia, Kalamazoo, Mich) is administered subcutaneously, once or twice daily, at a dose of 0.1 to 0.25 mg/kg until the uterus is completely empty. It takes at least 3 to 5 days of treatment before this occurs. The volume of vulvar discharge should increase as the uterus empties. The discharge usually also becomes less purulent and more mucoid or sanguineous as treatment continues. Uterine size should return toward normal as the uterus empties, but CEH itself may persist. Uterine size can be assessed by abdominal palpation, radiography, or ultrasonography. Treatment should be continued for more than 5 days if necessary. There is some evidence that fertility is poorer in animals requiring treatment for longer than 5 or 6 days. Ovariohysterectomy should probably be reconsidered for animals needing prolonged treatment and for those that have a recurrence.

Adverse reactions are common in animals receiving $PGF_{2\alpha}$ therapy and include panting, salivation, emesis, defecation, urination, mydriasis, and nesting behavior (Table 57-2). Intensive grooming behavior and vocalization may also be seen in the queen. Adverse reactions usually develop within 5 minutes of $PGF_{2\alpha}$ administration and last for 30 to 60 minutes. The severity of reactions is directly related to the dose administered and inversely related to the number of days of therapy. Adverse reactions tend to become milder with subsequent injections.

The median lethal dose of $PGF_{2\alpha}$ is 5.13 mg/kg in dogs. Severe respiratory distress and ataxia were reported to develop in cats given 5 mg/kg, but none died. The suppression of progesterone would be advantageous in the treatment of pyometra. Unfortunately, the luteolytic doses of $PGF_{2\alpha}$ are associated with undesirable systemic effects. Because of the side effects, alternatives to $PGF_{2\alpha}$ are being sought. The synthetic prostaglandins, such as cloprostenol and fluprostenol, are more potent than the naturally occurring $PGF_{2\alpha}$, and they have fewer systemic effects in other species. However, appropriate dosages and their efficacy in the treatment of pyometra in dogs and cats have yet to be established. Because prolactin is luteotropic, the addition of a prolactin antagonist, such as bromocriptine or cabergoline, might allow the dose of prostaglandin, and thus its side effects, to be reduced. Investigations of combination prostaglandin-prolactin antagonist therapy have yielded mixed results. Investigations using the antiprogestin aglepristone, a competitive inhibitor of progesterone receptor binding, have yielded positive results from its use in the treatment of canine pyometra. However, the progesterone-receptor inhibitors are not yet available for veterinary use in the United States (see discussion of abortifacients, Chapter 59).

The justification for the medical, rather than surgical, treatment of pyometra is the owner's desire for offspring from the affected female. Bitches and queens should be bred during their next cycle using optimal breeding management techniques (see pp. 849 and 851). However, this may be somewhat more important for bitches than for queens, because bitches will have progesterone stimulation, the factor initiating CEH-pyometra, for at least 60 days after every cycle, whether or not conception occurs. Progesterone production would occur in queens only after copulation-induced ovulation or after spontaneous ovulation. Pregnancy rates of 80% to 90% are reported for bitches that have received $PGF_{2\alpha}$ therapy for open-cervix pyometra. The age of the bitch and the severity of the CEH and uterine pathologic condition affect pregnancy rates. Younger bitches are most likely to become pregnant on subsequent cycles. In one report, only one of four bitches with closed-cervix pyometra was successfully treated in this way. Pregnancy rates of 71% to 88% are reported for queens that receive $PGF_{2\alpha}$ therapy for open pyometra. The successful medical treatment of closed pyometra in queens has apparently yet to be reported in the English language literature. The interestrous interval after $PGF_{2\alpha}$ therapy in bitches may be shorter than usual.

Pyometra can be expected to recur after $PGF_{2\alpha}$ therapy. Although there are only a few reports of posttreatment uterine biopsy findings, CEH has been found in bitches and queens after $PGF_{2\alpha}$ therapy for pyometra. It is unknown, however, whether this represents a persistence or recurrence of CEH, because the animals had cycled after treatment. Recurrence rates of 77% during a 27-month period are reported for bitches. A recurrence rate of 15% is reported for queens. Therefore, because reproductive performance is limited by recurrence, the desired number of offspring should be obtained as soon as possible. Although there are a few reports of the successful medical treatment of recurrent pyometra in bitches and queens, ovariohysterectomy is usually recommended.

 TABLE 57-2

**Effects of Prostaglandin $F_{2\alpha}$ in Dogs and Cats**

**Doses of 0.1 to 0.25 mg/kg**

Myometrial contractions
± Luteolysis (see text)
Vomiting
Micturition
Defecation
Panting
Resting
Grooming (cats)
Vocalization (cats)
Change in pupil size

**Doses of 1 to >5 mg/kg**

Ataxia
Collapse
Hypovolemic shock (dogs)
Respiratory distress (cats)
Death (canine $LD_{50}$ 5.13 mg/kg)

### Suggested Readings

Concannon PW et al, editors: Fertility and infertility in dogs, cats and other carnivores, *J Reprod Fertil Suppl* 47, 1993.

Concannon PW et al, editors: Reproduction of dogs and cats and exotic carnivores, *J Reprod Fertil Suppl* 51, 1997.

Concannon PW et al, editors: Advances in reproduction of dogs and cats and exotic carnivores, *J Reprod Fertil Suppl* 57, 2001.

Davidson AP, editor: Clinical theriogenology, *Vet Clin North Am Small Anim Pract* 31:2, 2001.

Dhaliwal GK et al: Uterine bacterial flora and uterine lesions in bitches with cystic endometrial hyperplasia (pyometra), *Vet Rec* 143:659, 1998.

Dhaliwal GK et al: Oestrogen and progesterone receptors in the uterine wall of bitches with cystic endometrial hyperplasia/pyometra, *Vet Rec* 145:455, 1999.

Egenvall A et al: Breed risk of pyometra in insured dogs in Sweden, *J Vet Intern Med* 15:530, 2001.

Faldyna M et al: Immunosuppression in bitches with pyometra, *J Small Anim Pract* 42:5, 2001.

Fantoni DT et al: Intravenous administration of hypertonic sodium chloride solution with dextran or sodium chloride solution for treatment of septic shock secondary to pyometra in dogs, *J Am Vet Med Assoc* 215:1283, 1999.

Feldman EC: The cystic endometrial hyperplasia/complex and infertility in female dogs. In Ettinger SJ et al, editors: *Textbook of veterinary internal medicine,* ed 5, Philadelphia, 2000, WB Saunders, p 1549.

Johnston SD et al, editors: *Canine and feline theriogenology,* Philadelphia, 2001, WB Saunders.

Kyles AE et al: Vestibulovaginal stenosis in dogs: 18 cases (1987-1995), *J Am Vet Med Assoc* 209:1889, 1996.

Lightner BA et al: Episioplasty for the treatment of perivulvar dermatitis or recurrent urinary tract infection in dogs with excessive perivulvar skin folds: 31 cases (1983-2000), *J Am Vet Med Assoc* 219:1577, 2001.

Meyers-Wallen VN: CVT update: inherited disorders of the reproductive tract in dogs and cats. In Bonagura JD: *Kirk's current veterinary therapy XIII,* Philadelphia, 2000, WB Saunders, p 904.

Misumi K et al: Uterine torsion in two non-gravid bitches, *J Small Anim Pract* 41:468, 2000.

Murphy ST et al: Uterine adenocarcinoma in the dog: a case report and review, *J Am Anim Hosp Assoc* 30:440, 1994.

Niskanen M et al: Associations between age, parity, hormonal therapy and breed, and pyometra in Finnish dogs, *Vet Rec* 143:493, 1998.

Ridyard AE et al: Successful treatment of uterine torsion in a cat with severe metabolic and homeostatic complications, *J Feline Med Surg* 2:115, 2000.

Ritt MG et al: Successful treatment of uterine torsion and fetal retention in a postparturient Great Pyrenees bitch with septic peritonitis and prothrombotic complications, *J Am Anim Hosp Assoc* 3:537, 1997.

Scott KC et al: Characteristics of free-roaming cats evaluated in a trap-neuter-release program, *J Am Vet Med Assoc* 221:1136, 2002.

Stöcklin-Gautschi NM et al: Identification of focal adenomyosis as a uterine lesion in two dogs, *J Small Anim Pract* 42:413, 2001.

Watts JR et al: Endometrial cytology of the normal bitch throughout the reproductive cycle, *J Small Anim Pract* 39:2, 1998.

# CHAPTER 58

# Disorders of the Mammary Gland

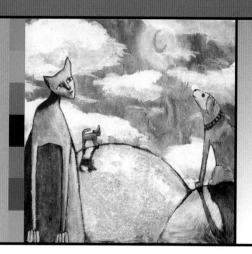

## CHAPTER OUTLINE

MASTITIS, 882
GALACTOSTASIS, 882
GALACTORRHEA, 883
FELINE MAMMARY HYPERPLASIA
AND HYPERTROPHY, 883
MAMMARY NEOPLASIA, 884

## MASTITIS

Bacterial infection of the mammary glands, mastitis, can occur in one or more lactating glands in postpartum bitches. Mastitis is uncommon in bitches that are lactating because of false pregnancy. It is rare in queens. The clinical signs are variable in severity and include warm, firm, swollen, painful glands. Fever, anorexia, and dehydration are often noted. Crying, unthrifty puppies may be what the owner notices first, because bitches that are ill with mastitis may neglect them. In severe cases, abscesses or gangrene of the glands can develop. The diagnosis is determined on the basis of these physical findings in a lactating female, and on the septic appearance of the mammary secretions. *Escherichia coli,* staphylococci, and β-hemolytic streptococci are the organisms most frequently isolated.

The treatment of mastitis includes antibiotics, fluid therapy, and supportive care. It should be aggressive to ensure that the bitch can resume her maternal duties as soon as possible. Adequate water and caloric intake is crucial to ensure continued milk production. During lactation, food and water needs are often double what they were during gestation. This should be taken into account when planning fluid therapy. Intravenous fluid therapy is indicated whenever even mild dehydration is present. Warm compresses applied to affected glands several times a day can reduce swelling and pain, and this should be included in the treatment of mastitis.

There are several factors to consider in the choice of antibiotics, including the susceptibility of the infecting organisms, the ability of the antibiotic to achieve high concentrations in milk, and the effects of the drug on the nursing neonate (see Table 59-3). Amoxicillin and cephalosporins can

be used if the results of bacterial culture are not known, because they are likely to achieve reasonable concentrations in the infected gland, they are likely to be effective against the most common organisms, and they are reasonably safe for neonates. Penicillin is also a reasonable choice, but it is not likely to be effective against *E. coli* infections. Antibiotic therapy should continue only as long as necessary to ensure that the mastitis resolves. This should occur within 7 days. In addition to fluid and antibiotic therapy, mammary abscesses and gangrene should be treated surgically.

Whether continued nursing is beneficial or desirable has not been critically evaluated, but it is recommended that pups continue nursing as long as the dam is willing and able to provide adequate nutrition. Monitoring the weight gain of the puppies, which should be about 10% of the birth weight per day, can assess this. The pups should also be watched closely for other signs of illness. If present, supplemental feeding or hand-rearing of the puppies should be considered.

Inflammatory carcinoma of a mammary gland may have a physical appearance similar to that of mastitis. However, inflammatory carcinoma is most likely to occur in geriatric animals, and there is no association with lactation. Whenever inflammation and/or abnormal secretions are present in nonlactating glands, mammary neoplasia should be strongly considered as the cause.

## GALACTOSTASIS

Galactostasis (i.e., the accumulation and stasis of milk within the mammary gland) is another cause of warm, firm, swollen, painful glands. Unlike mastitis, in galactostasis the mammary secretions are not infected and the dam is not ill. Milk is simply being produced faster than it can be comfortably stored. Galactostasis occurs most often at the time of weaning and occasionally at the time of peak lactation when production transiently exceeds the needs of the neonates. Galactostasis may also occur with false pregnancy (see Chapter 59).

Treatment is not indicated for the transient galactostasis that occasionally occurs early during lactation. If treatment is necessary for galactostasis that occurs at weaning, it is directed toward reducing milk production and relieving discomfort. Milk production diminishes as food and water intake is restricted. Therefore reducing the caloric and water intake to amounts appropriate to maintain ideal body weight and normal hydration during anestrus (i.e., neither pregnant nor lactating) is helpful in treating, as well as preventing, the galactostasis that occurs at weaning. Gradual rather than abrupt weaning is also helpful. Massaging or expressing the mammary glands may stimulate prolactin release and promote continued lactation. Therefore this should be avoided. Warm compresses may help relieve swelling and discomfort but may also stimulate further prolactin release.

## GALACTORRHEA

Galactorrhea refers to lactation that is not associated with pregnancy and parturition. It is the most common clinical manifestation of false pregnancy in the bitch (see Chapter 59). Galactorrhea of false pregnancy occurs in late diestrus, after the withdrawal of exogenous progestins, or after oophorectomy performed during diestrus. This galactorrhea is self-limiting and usually does not require treatment. Because any stimulation of the mammary glands, such as massage, the application of warm or cold compresses, or the bitch licking the glands, can promote lactation, these should be avoided. Withholding food for 24 hours, followed by a grad-

ual return to normal maintenance quantities, helps reduce lactation. Dopamine agonists such as bromocriptine or cabergoline inhibit prolactin secretion and thereby inhibit lactation. They are effective in reducing the lactation associated with false pregnancy in bitches but are not approved for this use in the United States (see Chapter 59).

## FELINE MAMMARY HYPERPLASIA AND HYPERTROPHY

Feline mammary hyperplasia (fibroepithelial hyperplasia, fibroadenoma, fibroadenomatosis) is characterized by the rapid, abnormal growth of mammary tissue. Hyperplasia of both epithelial and mesenchymal tissues is evident microscopically. It is most common in young, cycling queens that may or may not be pregnant (Fig. 58-1). It has also been observed in neutered male and neutered female cats that are receiving exogenous progestins. There is a strong temporal relationship between the onset of mammary hyperplasia and progesterone stimulation. Although progesterone exposure (endogenous or exogenous) precedes the development of this condition, serum progesterone concentrations may be normal at the time of diagnosis. Feline mammary hyperplasia is considered a benign condition, but its behavior and appearance may mimic those of mammary neoplasia. Therefore histologic evaluation of a biopsy specimen of an involved mammary

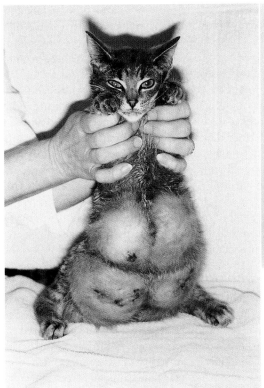
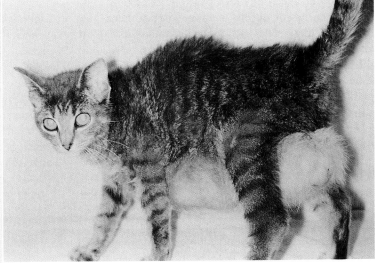

**FIG 58-1**
Mammary hyperplasia of 6 weeks' duration in a 5-month-old queen.

gland is often recommended if there is any doubt. Treatment consists of removing the source of the progesterone. Although successful pregnancy and nursing of kittens were reported in one queen with mammary hyperplasia, ovariohysterectomy is usually recommended, irrespective of the pregnancy status. It is often performed through a flank incision rather than through the usual midline approach, because of the massive size of the glands. The hyperplastic tissue resolves over several weeks following oophorectomy. Mastectomy may be indicated if the abnormal mammary tissue has outgrown its blood supply and become necrotic, or when remission does not occur after progesterone withdrawal.

## MAMMARY NEOPLASIA

### Etiology

Mammary neoplasms account for about half of all tumors in bitches. Although they are less prevalent in queens, mammary neoplasms are still the third most common tumor type in cats. They primarily affect older animals with a mean age of about 10 years. Most affected animals are intact females or females that have undergone oophorectomy late in life. Mammary tumors are rare in males and in young animals of either sex.

Early ovariohysterectomy is strongly protective against the development of mammary tumors. Bitches neutered before their first estrous cycle are at no greater risk for mammary tumors than are males. After 2.5 years of age or after the second estrous cycle, ovariohysterectomy is no longer protective in bitches. The age after which ovariohysterectomy is no longer beneficial for queens is unknown, but there is no doubt that intact queens are at much greater risk than are neutered ones. The progestins used to suppress estrus promote hyperplastic and neoplastic changes in the feline and canine mammary glands. Benign mammary tumors are found in more than 70% of bitches receiving long-term progestin treatment. About half of mammary tumors in bitches are benign, whereas feline mammary tumors are almost always malignant.

### Clinical Features

Mammary tumors are usually discrete, firm, and nodular. They may be found anywhere along the mammary chain. The size is extremely variable, ranging from a few millimeters to many centimeters in diameter. Multiple glands are involved more than half of the time. The tumors may adhere to the overlying skin but usually are not attached to the underlying body wall. Malignant tumors are more likely than benign tumors to be attached to the body wall and covered by ulcerated skin. About 25% of feline mammary tumors are covered by ulcerated skin. Abnormal secretions can often be expressed from the nipples of affected glands. The regional lymph nodes (axillary or inguinal) may be enlarged if metastasis has occurred. The remainder of the physical examination findings are often unremarkable. There may be evidence of tumor cachexia in animals with advanced neoplasia. Owners often discover mammary tumors in their pets months before they seek veterinary attention.

### Diagnosis

A diagnosis of mammary neoplasia is the most likely one in an older female with any kind of nodule in the mammary gland. Excisional biopsy is the method of choice to confirm the diagnosis. Cytologic examination of specimens obtained by fine-needle aspiration often yields equivocal results. Before any excisional biopsy is performed, radiographs of the thorax should be evaluated for evidence of pulmonary metastasis. If evidence of pulmonary metastasis is found, a justifiably grave prognosis can be given, even in the absence of histologic confirmation of mammary neoplasia.

Once a decision is made to pursue further diagnostic and therapeutic measures, the overall health of the animal and the tumor burden are assessed. Malignant mammary tumors frequently metastasize to the regional lymph nodes and to the lungs. Less commonly, hepatic metastasis occurs. Metastasis to distant sites can also occur, but this rarely happens in the absence of local lymph node or pulmonary involvement. Radiologic imaging and careful palpation are used to evaluate the tumor burden. The animal's overall health is assessed with a complete blood count, biochemistry profile, and urinalysis.

### Treatment

The treatment of mammary neoplasia is surgical excision of all abnormal tissue. Controversy persists as to the preferred surgical technique: nodule excision, simple mastectomy, or radical mastectomy. If nodulectomy is chosen, apparently normal surrounding tissue should always be included and submitted for histopathologic evaluation for evidence of tumor invasion. If there is evidence of extension beyond the nodule, mastectomy should be performed. There is no difference in the survival times after simple versus radical mastectomy in bitches and queens; however, the disease-free interval may be longer in cats that have undergone radical mastectomies. Excised mammary tumors should always be submitted for histopathologic examination because the prognosis is markedly affected by the tumor type. Ovariohysterectomy performed at the time of mastectomy has no effect on 2-year survival rates in bitches. There are also no differences in survival among bitches that undergo ovariohysterectomy before mastectomy, bitches that undergo ovariohysterectomy at the time of mastectomy, and bitches that undergo mastectomy alone.

### Histopathology

Approximately half of the mammary tumors in bitches are benign. Some of these benign tumors show evidence of cellular atypia within the parenchyma and are considered precancerous. Precancerous changes in bitches are associated with a ninefold increase in the risk of mammary adenocarcinoma developing at a later date, compared with the risk in animals with nodules with normal cellular characteristics, in which the risk of malignant mammary tumors subsequently developing is no greater than that in animals with no previous mammary nodules. In contrast, benign mammary tumors are rare in cats. More than 80% of feline mammary tumors are classified as adenocarcinomas.

Adenocarcinoma is the most common malignant mammary tumor in bitches and queens. If the neoplastic cells are confined to the duct epithelium (carcinoma in situ), the prognosis after surgery is good. The prognosis is somewhat worse if neoplastic cells are found beyond the boundary of the duct system but not in blood or lymphatic vessels. The prognosis is even worse if neoplastic cells are found in blood or lymphatic vessels. If neoplastic cells are found in the regional lymph nodes, the disease-free interval is shortened significantly.

The amount of invasion beyond the duct epithelium is not the only finding of prognostic importance. Nuclear differentiation affects the recurrence rates, even within the same stage of invasion. The recurrence rate 2 years after mastectomy in bitches with poorly differentiated (i.e., anaplastic) tumors is 90% versus rates of 68% and 24% in animals with moderately differentiated and well-differentiated tumors, respectively.

Tumor size is the single most important prognostic indicator in bitches and queens with mammary adenocarcinomas treated by surgery alone. In bitches, tumors less than 3 cm in diameter are associated with the best prognosis, with about a 35% recurrence rate after 2 years, compared with an 80% recurrence rate for larger tumors. In queens, tumors less than 2 cm in diameter are associated with the longest disease-free intervals after mastectomy (median survival time of 4.5 years).

In queens, mammary tumors are almost exclusively carcinomas. In bitches, other malignant tumors of the mammary gland, such as inflammatory carcinoma, sarcomas, and carcinosarcomas, are occasionally found, but they are much less common than are adenocarcinomas. Inflammatory carcinoma is a fulminant malignant disease associated with a grave prognosis in bitches and queens.

## Adjunct Therapy

Because the surgical excision of malignant mammary tumors is not curative, the effectiveness of adjunct therapies has been investigated. Although there are no data at present to support the beneficial effects of all such therapies in bitches or queens,

chemotherapy (see Chapter 79) is often used as an adjunct to the surgical treatment of mammary tumors. In some species, adjunct hormonal therapy has been helpful in slowing mammary tumor growth. The antitumor effects are presumably mediated by hormone receptors in tumor tissue. Despite some differences between normal and neoplastic mammary tissue in dogs, the general mechanism by which estrogen and progesterone receptor expression is modulated is similar among normal tissue, benign tissue, and well-differentiated adenocarcinoma. These tissues express estrogen receptors or progesterone receptors, or both. Undifferentiated malignant mammary tumors have significantly lower receptor concentrations and are more likely to express only one or the other receptor. This could explain why some benign mammary masses and well-differentiated adenocarcinomas appear to be hormone sensitive, whereas others do not. Tamoxifen competitively binds estrogen receptors and has been used for its antiestrogenic effects in the treatment of mammary neoplasia in women. Unlike the situation in humans, tamoxifen is known to have estrogenic effects in dogs. In a study of the use of tamoxifen as adjunct therapy for canine mammary neoplasia, no beneficial antitumor effects were proved but 56% of the treated dogs showed adverse estrogenic effects.

## Suggested Readings

Donnay I et al: Comparison of estrogen and progesterone receptor expression in normal and tumor mammary tissues from dogs, *Am J Vet Res* 56:1188, 1995.

Johnston SD et al, editors: *Canine and feline theriogenology,* Philadelphia, 2001, WB Saunders.

Kitchell BE: Mammary tumors. In Bonagura JD, editor: *Kirk's current veterinary therapy XII,* Philadelphia, 1995, WB Saunders.

Moe L: Population-based incidence of mammary tumours in some dog breeds, *J Reprod Fertil Suppl* 57:439, 2001.

Morris JS et al: Use of tamoxifen in the control of canine mammary neoplasia, *Vet Rec* 133:539, 1993.

Selman PJ et al: Comparison of the histologic changes in the dog after treatment with the progestins medroxyprogesterone acetate and proligestone, *Vet Q* 17:128, 1995.

Yamagami T et al: Influence of ovariohysterectomy at the time of mastectomy on the prognosis for canine malignant mammary tumours, *J Small Anim Pract* 37:462, 1996.

# False Pregnancy, Disorders of Pregnancy, Parturition, and the Postpartum Period

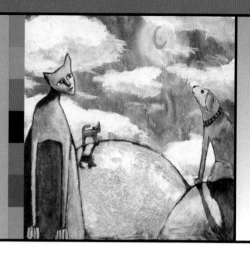

## CHAPTER OUTLINE

FALSE PREGNANCY, 886
NORMAL EVENTS IN PREGNANCY
AND PARTURITION, 887
  Fertilization and implantation, 887
  Corpora luteal function and serum progesterone
    concentrations, 888
  Litter size, 888
  Confirmation of pregnancy, 888
  Alterations in bitch and queen during pregnancy, 890
  Gestation length, 891
  Parturition, 891
  Predicting labor, 891
  Stages of labor, 891
DYSTOCIA, 892
POSTPARTUM DISORDERS, 895
  Agalactia, 895
  Puerperal hypocalcemia (puerperal tetany, eclampsia), 896
  Metritis, 896
  Subinvolution of placental sites, 897
ABORTIFACIENTS (MISMATING), 898
  Estrogens, 898
  Prostaglandins, 899
  Alternative treatments, 899
FETAL RESORPTION-ABORTION-STILLBIRTH
COMPLEX, 900
NEONATAL MORBIDITY AND MORTALITY, 901
  Environmental factors, 901
  The dam, 902
  The neonate, 902

## *FALSE PREGNANCY*

### Etiology

False pregnancy is a clinical phenomenon in which a female that was not pregnant exhibits maternal behavior and lactation at the end of diestrus (i.e., luteal phase). It occurs commonly in intact, cycling bitches and is considered to be normal. The terms *false pregnancy, pseudopregnancy,* and *psuedocyesis* are of-

ten used interchangeably, but none is really an accurate reflection of the situation in bitches in which the clinical signs occur during what would have been the postpartum period, not during what would have been the pregnant period (i.e., luteal phase) of the cycle. *Peudopregnancy* refers specifically to the nonpregnant luteal phase, usually in reference to an animal that is induced to ovulate by coitus, when serum concentrations of progesterone remain high despite the absence of pregnancy. Progesterone causes mammary gland development and weight gain, irrespective of pregnancy status, but not lactation nor the other behavioral and physical changes of false pregnancy.

Prolactin is the cause of the lactation and the maternal behavior of false pregnancy, but the mechanisms by which it does so are not completely understood. Prolactin concentrations increase during the second half of pregnancy. In bitches, it is the main luteotropic hormone during that time. Many hormones influence prolactin secretion. Serotonin, thyrotropin-releasing hormone (TRH), oxytocin, and others act as prolactin-releasing factors. Dopamine is considered to be the main prolactin inhibitory factor. Progesterone inhibits prolactin secretion via negative feedback. In bitches, false pregnancy is caused by the declining serum progesterone concentration associated with the end of the luteal phase, which in turn causes an increase in serum prolactin concentration, just as occurs at parturition. Because the bitch ovulates spontaneously and always enters a long luteal phase, false pregnancy is a common phenomenon in cycling bitches. It is uncommon in queens, because they must first have been induced to ovulate (presumably by copulation) but have not conceived (i.e., pseudopregnancy); they then have a decline in the progesterone concentration appropriate to stimulate prolactin release. In bitches, false pregnancy also occurs after the withdrawal of exogenous progestins and after oophorectomy performed during diestrus.

False pregnancy is considered a normal phenomenon in bitches. It is not associated with any reproductive abnormalities, including cycle irregularities, pyometra, or infertility. Quite the contrary, the occurrence of false pregnancy provides evidence that ovulation took place during the preceding cycle and that the hypothalamic-pituitary-gonadal axis is intact. Why some bitches are more prone to developing clinical signs and why the severity of the clinical signs vary from cycle to cycle are not known. Although serum concentrations of prolactin do increase when progesterone is withdrawn, they are not always elevated to the same degree, nor are they always found to remain elevated by the time bitches are evaluated for false pregnancy. Furthermore, at similar prolactin concentrations some bitches show clinical signs of false pregnancy and others do not. Some individual predisposition toward the development of false pregnancy apparently exists.

In addition, factors relating to nutrition influence the occurrence of false pregnancy. For example, Labrador bitches fed the calories required to maintain ideal body condition had significantly more episodes of false pregnancy during a 6-year study period than did those fed 75% of maintenance calories.

## Clinical Features

False pregnancy is characterized by the display of maternal behavior such as nesting, the adoption of inanimate objects or other animals, mammary gland development, and galactorrhea (i.e., milk production not associated with pregnancy and parturition). Additional, often more troublesome, clinical signs from the owner's perspective include restlessness, irritability, abdominal enlargement, anorexia, and vomiting.

## Diagnosis

False pregnancy is diagnosed based on the historical and physical findings in a nonpregnant bitch or, less commonly, in a queen at the end of diestrus. It may also occur after oophorectomy during diestrus and when exogenous progestins are discontinued. Abdominal radiography or ultrasonography could be considered to exclude pregnancy.

## Treatment

The clinical signs of false pregnancy are self-limiting and usually resolve after 2 or 3 weeks. Treatment is usually not necessary. Self-nursing (i.e., licking the mammary glands) and the application of warm or cold compresses or other stimuli to the mammary glands can promote lactation and should be avoided. Withholding food for 24 hours, followed by a gradual (i.e., 3 to 5 days) increase back to usual quantities, helps to reduce lactation. Mild tranquilization can be considered for bitches showing significant aggressive behavior; however, phenothiazines should not be used in this situation because they can increase prolactin secretion.

As mentioned earlier, false pregnancy is a normal, self-limiting phenomenon in bitches that usually does not require treatment. Before treatment of false pregnancy is undertaken, it is essential that the diagnostic evaluation be sufficient to rule out pregnancy because all treatments for false pregnancy will be deleterious to pregnancy, should it exist. When treatment is needed, drugs that inhibit prolactin release, such as dopamine agonists and serotonin antagonists, are effective in ameliorating the behavioral and physical signs of false pregnancy in bitches. They are not marketed for veterinary use in the United States. The dopamine agonists bromocriptine and cabergoline have been used. The suggested dose for bromocriptine (Parlodel; Sandoz, East Hanover, N.J.) is 10 to 100 µg/kg

orally twice a day for 10 to 14 days. Vomiting is a very common side effect. Reducing the dose and administering the drug after meals may help. Cabergoline rarely causes vomiting. An oral dose of cabergoline (Galastop; Boehringer Ingelheim, Richfield, Conn; Dostinex, Parmacia, Kalamazoo, Mich) of 5 µg/kg daily is reported to cause improvement in 3 to 4 days, with the signs resolving by 7 days. This appears to be the drug of choice at this time. The serotonin antagonist metergoline (Contralac; Virbac Laboratories, Carros, France) also inhibits prolactin secretion. The suggested dose is 0.1 to 0.2 mg/kg twice daily for 8 days. It does not cause vomiting but can cause hyperexcitability, aggression, and whining. Rarely, cabergoline may also cause increased aggression.

Progestins, such as megestrol acetate, and androgens suppress prolactin secretion and can thereby diminish the clinical manifestations of false pregnancy. As would be expected, however, clinical signs often recur after progestins are withdrawn. This is because declining concentrations of progesterone are an important stimulus for prolactin release. Therefore progestins are not recommended as a treatment for false pregnancy.

If severe signs of false pregnancy persist for longer than the expected 2 to 3 weeks, bitches should be evaluated for hypothyroidism (see Chapter 51). TRH stimulates prolactin release in some species, including dogs. Primary hypothyroidism is associated with increased hypothalamic TRH secretion. In some hypothyroid bitches an increased secretion of prolactin, presumably in response to increased TRH secretion, may result in excessive galactorrhea if false pregnancy occurs. Thyroid hormone replacement therapy causes the galactorrhea to resolve in these bitches.

False pregnancy may recur with subsequent estrous cycles. Ovariohysterectomy performed during late anestrus prevents recurrence. Ovariohysterectomy should not be performed during diestrus because false pregnancy can occur as a result of removing the ovarian source of progesterone. When false pregnancy does occur after ovariohysterectomy, it is likely to be more persistent than in intact bitches. Furthermore, in bitches spayed during an episode of false pregnancy, the condition may be prolonged, sometimes for years. Spaying during false pregnancy is therefore contraindicated. Cabergoline treatment has been beneficial in the majority of these cases of prolonged false pregnancy, even though prolactin concentrations were at basal levels in many animals. This suggests that the beneficial effects may be mediated at the tissue level, irrespective of serum concentrations. If signs of false pregnancy become recurrent in a spayed animal, the possibility of an ovarian remnant should be considered.

# NORMAL EVENTS IN PREGNANCY AND PARTURITION

## FERTILIZATION AND IMPLANTATION

In the bitch, fertilization occurs in the uterine tubes, where the fertilized ova then develop into 32- to 64-cell blastocysts before entering the uterus. Blastocysts enter the uterus about 10 days (range, 3 to 14 days) after a single, fertile mating.

During the ensuing week, the blastocysts move within the uterus, ultimately becoming equally spaced within both uterine horns. Implantation occurs 11 to 23 days after a single fertile mating (18 to 20 days after the luteinizing hormone [LH] peak).

A similar sequence of events occurs in the queen, although the timing is slightly different. This is to be expected, because the copulatory induction of ovulation ensures that insemination, ovulation, and fertilization occur over a less variable length of time than those in the bitch. It takes 4 to 5 days for the fertilized ova to be transported the length of the uterine tubes. The blastocysts migrate within the uterus for 6 to 8 days before implantation occurs, around 12 to 14 days after a fertile mating. Implantation may occur later if estrus was artificially induced.

## CORPORA LUTEAL FUNCTION AND SERUM PROGESTERONE CONCENTRATIONS

Functional corpora lutea (CLs) are essential throughout pregnancy in the bitch and queen. The serum progesterone concentration can be used to assess corpora luteal function. After ovulation, it should be greater than 5 to 8 ng/ml (approximately 16 to 25 nmol/L) and should continue to increase for the next 15 to 25 days (see Fig. 56-1). The serum progesterone concentration remains at peak levels for 7 to 14 days and then gradually declines throughout the remainder of pregnancy. In pregnant bitches a rapid, prepartum drop in the concentration to less than 2 ng/ml (approximately 6.4 nmol/L) is consistently found within 48 hours of whelping. Those nonpregnant bitches exhibiting clinical signs of false pregnancy may show a similar rapid decrease in the progesterone concentration. Otherwise, the decline in the serum progesterone concentration in nonpregnant bitches is more gradual and may not reach anestrual levels of 0.2 to 0.5 ng/ml (approximately 0.6 to 1.6 nmol/L) for 60 to 90 days. The luteal secretion of progesterone depends on both pituitary LH and prolactin. During the second half of the canine pregnancy, prolactin is the main luteotropic factor. No known luteotropic or luteolytic factors are found in the canine uterus or placenta.

A similar trend in the corpora luteal secretion of progesterone is observed in queens during early diestrus, but the life span of CLs is influenced by pregnancy, or its absence. After the nonfertile induction of ovulation, the CLs reportedly persist for only 30 to 50 days. If pregnancy results, the CLs continue to produce progesterone throughout gestation (see Fig. 56-5). As in the bitch, prolactin is luteotropic in the queen. Because prolactin secretion in pregnant queens begins around day 35 of pregnancy and because pseudopregnant queens do not secrete prolactin, it may be the pregnancy-specific luteotrope in cats. Serum concentrations of prolactin and relaxin increase during the second half of pregnancy in bitches and queens.

The pattern of progesterone secretion has several important clinical ramifications in bitches and queens. First, the progesterone concentration increases after ovulation, regardless of whether the queen or the bitch is pregnant. Therefore serum progesterone concentrations can be measured to as-

sess the function of the CLs but not to assess the pregnancy status of the bitch or queen. Second, the decline in the serum progesterone concentration at the end of diestrus is believed responsible in part for inducing the clinical signs of false pregnancy (see p. 886). Third, the stimulatory effects of progesterone on growth hormone secretion and uterine endometrial development may predispose older, intact bitches to diabetes mellitus and cystic endometrial hyperplasia (see p. 877), respectively.

## LITTER SIZE

Many factors influence litter size. In the bitch, litter size varies according to breed, with smaller breeds tending to have smaller litters than larger breeds. However, the typical litter size for a particular breed is not easy to verify. Using data from more than 700,00 litters registered by the American Kennel Club, one study defined "typical" litter size as the mean of the litter sizes recorded for the breed ±1 standard deviation of the mean, expressed in whole numbers. Using that method, a "typical" litter size for Labradors and Golden Retrievers ranged from 5 to 10 pups, with 70% of the litters containing 7 or more pups. "Typical" litter size for the Chihuahua and Yorkshire terrier was 2 to 5 pups, with 80% of litters having 4 pups or less.

Conception rates and litter size are greatest and neonatal mortality is lowest in Beagles between 2 and 3.5 years of age. After 5 years of age, conception and litter size decline and neonatal mortality begins to increase. Litter size also varies with parity, with the largest litters at third and fourth parity. Nutrition influences reproductive success. Bitches fed a commercially prepared diet containing 20% fat with an omega-6 to omega-3 fatty acid ratio of 5:1 had larger litters and fewer stillbirths than did those fed diets with less fat. In the queen, litters typically consist of two to five kittens. Litter size and neonatal survival are best in queens 1 to 5 years of age, provided that first parity occurs before 3 years of age. Litter size and neonatal survival usually improve after first parity. If first parity occurs after 3 years of age, however, litter size and neonatal survival usually remain poor. Reproductive performance declines after 6 years of age.

## CONFIRMATION OF PREGNANCY

Pregnancy can be confirmed by abdominal palpation, ultrasonography, and radiologic studies. Abdominal palpation is easily, quickly, and inexpensively performed. Although this is the most subjective method of pregnancy diagnosis, it is a reliable method for those skilled in palpation. The ease with which the abdomen can be accurately palpated is influenced by such factors as the amount of body fat, the body conformation, and the temperament of the animal, whereas these factors have little influence on the accuracy of other methods of pregnancy diagnosis. However, uterine enlargement caused by pregnancy cannot be accurately differentiated from uterine enlargement caused by some other process, such as pyometra, based on abdominal palpation findings alone.

In Beagle bitches, uterine swellings that represent uterine edema, embryonic membranes, and early placental development are about 1 cm in diameter at 20 days after breeding. By 30 days after breeding the uterine swellings are about 3 cm in diameter. By 35 days the gestational sacs are becoming elongated and the uterus is more diffusely enlarged, making it more difficult to detect pregnancy by palpation at that time. Allen and colleague (1981) have reported that abdominal palpation performed between 26 and 35 days of gestation is 87% accurate in identifying bitches that are pregnant and 73% accurate in identifying bitches that are not pregnant.

Real-time ultrasonography is an excellent method of pregnancy detection in bitches and queens. It is usually necessary to shave the abdominal hair to obtain good image quality. Scanning is easy to perform and requires minimal animal restraint. Pregnancy can be diagnosed if the gestational sac or fetal structures are identified (see Fig. 56-6, *A*; Fig. 59-1). The gestational sac appears as a spheric, anechoic structure, surrounded by a hyperechoic wall comprised of the uterus and placenta. Hyperechoic fetal structures are seen within the gestational sac. Although it has been reported that the gestational sac can be identified as early as 10 days after the last breeding in the bitch and 11 days after breeding in the queen, pregnancy is not reliably detected until 24 to 28 days after breeding in bitches and until 20 to 24 days after breeding in queens. At that time, fetal structures and cardiac activity are usually detected within the gestational sacs. Ultrasonography is reported to be 99.3% accurate in detecting pregnancy in bitches if performed 28 days after breeding. However, it is not particularly accurate in the estimation of litter size.

For several reasons, ultrasonography is the preferred method of pregnancy diagnosis in animals with reproductive disorders. First, if performed at the appropriate time, ultrasonography is more accurate than is abdominal palpation. Second, the results can be recorded on film. Third, fetal viability can be assessed. The first fetal cardiac activity is detectable 23 to 29 days after the LH peak in bitches and 18 to 25 days after copulation in cats. Canine fetal heart rates average 214 ± 13 beats

per minute (bpm) in early pregnancy, increasing to 238 ± 16 bpm by day 40, and declining to 218 ± 7 bpm from day 60 to parturition. Feline fetal heart rates are relatively stable throughout pregnancy, averaging 228 ± 36 bpm. Fetal movement characterized by dorsiflexion of the head and extension of the limbs is common in both species after day 33 to 39. After day 55, fetal anatomy is obvious (Fig. 59-2). Nonviable fetuses show no motion and within 1 day of death lose identifiable morphology. After death the fetal size decreases and it assumes the appearance of an ovoid mass of heterogeneous echogenicity (Fig. 59-3).

The fetal placental unit produces relaxin, beginning about 20 to 26 days of gestation. It is pregnancy specific, and the detection of increased serum relaxin concentrations can be used for pregnancy diagnosis in dogs. Using a rapid immunomigration (RIM) test (Witness Relaxin; Synbiotics, San Diego, Calif) relaxin is detectable in pregnant bitches about 26 to 31 days after the LH surge. False negative results occur if the test is performed too early during gestation. Although the manufacturer suggests that the test can be useful 22 to 27 days after breeding, it is a more sensitive indicator of pregnancy when performed 30 or more days after breeding. Relaxin disappears from the blood after abortion, but this decline can occur over several days after fetal death. During that time, the relaxin assay would yield a false positive result for viable pregnancy. Although pregnant cats also produce relaxin, this RIM test has not yet been validated for accuracy in cats. Serum fibrinogen concentrations increase in pregnant bitches at or just before the increase in the relaxin concentration. Although this is a consistent finding in pregnant bitches from 30 to 50 days of gestation, fibrinogen is an acute-phase reactant protein that can increase in concentration in response to inflammation of any cause. It is not specific to pregnancy.

Abdominal radiography can be used to confirm pregnancy after the fetal skeleton has calcified sufficiently to be detected on radiographs. This usually happens approximately 40 to 45

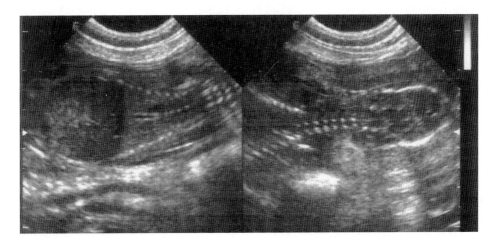

**FIG 59-1**
Sonograms of canine pregnancy, 40 days after first breeding (dorsal view). Fetal spine and ribs appear on left image. On right image, cervical spine and outline of fetal skull are shown.

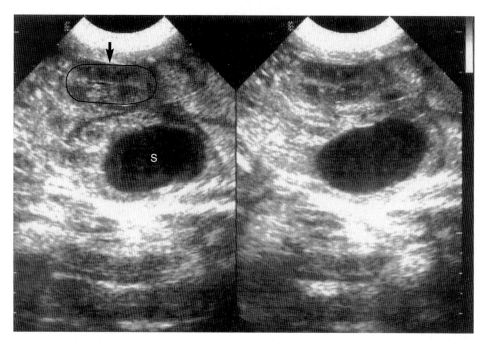

**FIG 59-2**
Sonogram of 59-day canine fetus. Fetal kidney *(arrow)* and stomach *(S)*.

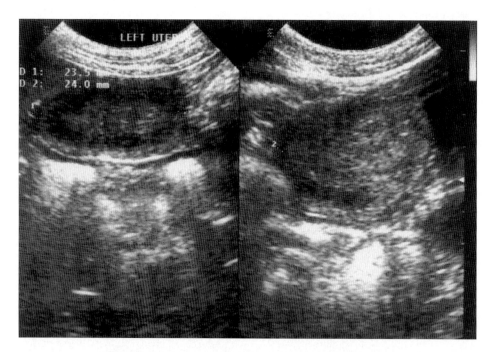

**FIG 59-3**
Sonogram of resorbing fetus, 30 days after first breeding.

days after breeding in the bitch and 35 to 40 days after breeding in the queen. Because abdominal radiographs are taken later, they are usually not used for pregnancy diagnosis *per se.* They are used to estimate fetal numbers, to assess the viability of the fetuses if ultrasonography is not available, to identify problems that might lead to dystocia, and to confirm the remaining presence of fetuses in the bitch or queen examined because of dystocia.

## ALTERATIONS IN BITCH AND QUEEN DURING PREGNANCY

Body weight and caloric needs steadily increase throughout pregnancy, especially during the last trimester, in both bitches and queens. Animals that are underweight may have difficulty maintaining body condition and milk production after parturition. Conversely, obesity is known to contribute to the development of dystocia and increased neonatal mortality. In bitches the packed cell volume (PCV) declines to 40% by day 35 and to less than 35% at term. Red blood cell (RBC) numbers, the hemoglobin concentration, and PCV decline throughout pregnancy in queens as well, but the absolute numbers are often still within the normal range.

## GESTATION LENGTH

Gestation length, defined as the interval from a fertile mating to parturition, averages 66 days (range, 64 to 71 days) in queens. Because the bitch ovulates spontaneously at any time during estrus, prediction of gestation length is more variable and depends on the criteria used to determine when a fertile mating occurred. The gestation length is 63 days $\pm$ 7 days if calculated from the date of first breeding to parturition, 65 $\pm$ 1 day if calculated from the LH peak, and 57 $\pm$ 3 days if calculated from the first day of cytologically confirmed diestrus (see p. 850). Gestation length appears to vary somewhat according to breed of dog as well.

## PARTURITION

In the bitch, maternal cortisol (and probably also fetal cortisol) concentration and maternal prostaglandin (PG) $F_{2\alpha}$ concentration increase before parturition. The increase in the $PGF_{2\alpha}$ concentration is thought to cause luteolysis and a subsequent decrease in the serum progesterone concentration to less than 1 ng/ml (approximately 3 nmol/L) 24 hours before parturition. Although a similar prepartum decline in the serum progesterone concentration is seen in queens, basal concentrations are apparently not necessary for parturition to be initiated. The decrease in the serum progesterone concentration probably causes placental dislocation, a further increase in $PGF_{2\alpha}$ secretion, and enhanced uterine sensitivity to oxytocin. Oxytocin is released in response to pressure against the cervix. In both bitches and queens a prepartum increase in the prolactin concentration is seen, which is probably also a result of the decreased serum progesterone concentration. Postpartum, prolactin secretion is stimulated by suckling. In queens the serum estradiol concentration increases before parturition.

## PREDICTING LABOR

In bitches, identifying the first day of diestrus on the basis of vaginal cytologic findings (see p. 850) can be used to predict when labor should occur, because most bitches whelp 57 days, $\pm 3$ days after day 1 of diestrus. Parturition is expected to occur 65 days, $\pm 1$ day after the LH surge. Because the serum concentrations of progesterone decrease from more than 3 ng/ml (approximately 9 nmol/L) to less than 1 ng/ml (approximately 3 nmol/L) during the 24 hours before labor in bitches, the progesterone concentration could be used to predict parturition.

Alternatively, because the decrease in the serum progesterone concentration just before whelping causes a transient drop in the rectal temperature in most bitches, measuring the rectal temperature is a useful way to predict impending labor. The usual recommendation is for owners to monitor rectal temperature two to three times daily during the last 2 weeks of gestation to establish a baseline. Temperature decreases below baseline by 2° to 3° F (1.1° to 1.7° C) 6 to 18 hours before parturition. In small breeds it may drop as low as 95° F (35° C), in medium-size breeds as low as 96.8° F (36° C), and in large breeds to 98.6° F (37° C). When the drop in temperature is identified, it is usually a reliable indication that parturition will soon occur. In some bitches, the temperature fluctuates. In a study of 100 canine pregnancies where rectal temperature was taken approximately every 12 hours, the prepartum drop in rectal temperature was not detected in 19 animals before the delivery of the first pup. A prepartum drop in the rectal temperature of queens is an inconsistent finding. Many, but not all, queens refuse to eat during the last 24 to 48 hours of gestation. This is a good indicator of impending parturition. If obvious signs of labor are not present within 24 hours of the rectal temperature drop in near-term bitches or of the loss of appetite in near-term queens, the gravid female should be examined.

## STAGES OF LABOR

Three stages of labor exist in bitches and queens. Stage I is characterized by nesting behavior, restlessness, shivering, and anorexia. Bitches usually pant. The cervix dilates during Stage I. No external signs of uterine or abdominal contractions exist. However, uterine contractions can be documented using external pressure transducers (tocodynamometers) that are strapped around the belly. During pregnancy, uterine contractions are slow and tonic in nature. During stage I of parturition, uterine contractions increase in frequency, duration and strength. These changes are coincident with the decline in progesterone concentrations, the decline in rectal temperature, and the change in behavior of the bitch. As determined by changes in rectal temperature and change in the dam's behavior, stage I normally lasts for 6 to 12 hours. As determined by the change in uterine contractions until the delivery of the first pup, the duration of stage I was reported to be 13 to 24 hours in one study (n=5) and to average 12 hours in another (n=100).

Stage II is characterized by obvious abdominal contractions, passage of amnionic fluid and delivery of the puppy or kitten. Rectal temperature rises to normal. Stage II is usually accomplished in 3 to 6 hours. It may last as long as 12 hours in some bitches. In queens, it may rarely last 24 hours. There may be intermittent, active abdominal straining for several hours before the birth of the first neonate. Constant, unrelenting straining is not normal. Usually less than 1 hour passes between the delivery of subsequent puppies or kittens. The dam may rest for as long as 1 hour or so between births, with no active straining during that time. Occasionally, 12 to 24 hours pass between the births of apparently healthy kittens, but this is not normal for puppies. Guidelines for differentiating normal parturition from dystocia are described on p. 893.

The placenta is normally passed within 5 to 15 minutes of the birth of each neonate. This is stage III. The dam removes the amniotic membranes and cleans the neonate, severing the umbilical cord and eating the placenta. If the dam fails to remove the fetal membranes from the neonate's face, the owner should. Cleaning the neonate is important maternal behavior necessary for bonding between the dam and her offspring; thus the dam should be encouraged to do it. All placentas should be passed within 4 to 6 hours. If the owner is attending, the umbilical cord should be clamped and cut about 1 cm from the body wall. If bleeding occurs, the cord can be ligated.

# DYSTOCIA

Dystocia, or difficult birth, has an overall prevalence of approximately 5% to 6% of pregnancies in bitches and queens. In certain breeds, however, the prevalence is much higher, approaching 18% in Devon rex cats in the United Kingdom and 100% in Bulldogs in the United States. With the exception of those breeds at high risk, dystocia might be considered a relatively uncommon cause of morbidity or mortality in bitches and queens, accounting for less than 1% of emergency admissions. However, it is the most common periparturient problem requiring emergency care and a major cause of neonatal mortality in puppies and kittens. Overall mortality rates from birth to weaning average 12% (range 10% to 30%) in puppies and 12.8% in kittens, but 65% of those losses occur at parturition and during the first week of life as a result of stillbirth, fetal stress, and hypoxia during birth.

There appears to be an increased risk of dystocia in aged bitches, but no relationship between age and dystocia has been found in queens. In both dogs and cats, purebred animals are more likely to have dystocia than are mixed breeds. Dolicocephalic (e.g., Siamese type) and brachycephalic (e.g., Persian type) are at greater risk for dystocia than mesocephalic (e.g., domestic short hair [DSH] type) cats. In dogs, chondrodysplastic breeds and those selected for large heads are at greater risk. Within breeds, certain individuals are at greater risk than others. For example, in both the Boston and Scottish Terriers, breeds with decidedly different head conformation, bitches with a dorsoventral flattening (i.e., vertical diameter ≤ horizontal diameter) of the pelvic canal are more likely to have obstructive dystocia than bitches with normal pelvic conformation (i.e., vertical diameter > horizontal diameter).

When normal parturition is used as a criterion in selection of breeding bitches or queens, the occurrence of dystocia within the colony can be decreased, demonstrating that breed alone is not the determinant. The majority (71%) of privately owned queens presented for dystocia have dystocia during more than one pregnancy, whereas in a large commercial colony of DSH cats, the incidence of dystocia was only 0.4%. Small litter size predisposes to dystocia in bitches for a variety of reasons. A negative correlation between litter size and puppy size exists: the smaller the litter, the larger the individual pup. Conversely, a very large litter may overstretch the uterus. Litter size has no bearing on the occurrence of dystocia in queens.

Dystocia may be fetal or maternal in origin. It may or may not be associated with obstruction. The two most common causes of dystocia in small animals are (1) uterine inertia and (2) fetal malpresentation. Of these, uterine inertia is by far the most common, accounting for about 60% and 72% of all

cases in queens and bitches, respectively. Uterine inertia is failure to develop and maintain uterine contractions sufficient for normal progression of labor. Uterine inertia has a variety of potential causes (e.g., genetic, age, nutrition, metabolic). With the exception of mechanical obstruction that results in myometrial exhaustion and secondary uterine inertia, the specific cause is not usually identified. Other causes of nonobstructed dystocia include fetal death and maternal anxiety. Fetal death accounts for 1% to 4.5% of dystocia without obstruction in bitches and queens, respectively. Extreme anxiety can inhibit normal progression of labor. How often this contributes to dystocia is not known.

Maternal causes of obstructive dystocia relate primarily to abnormalities in size or shape of the pelvic canal. These abnormalities may be congenital or acquired, involving the bony or soft tissue structures. Uterine torsion is also a differential. Fetal causes of obstructive dystocia are primarily caused by malpresentation. Malpresentation is the most common fetal cause of dystocia in bitches and queens, accounting for approximately 15% of cases. Fetal oversize (i.e., > 4% to 5% of dam's body weight) or monstrosity (i.e., congenital deformities causing large abnormal shape) may also cause obstruction, as can cephalopelvic disproportion (i.e., large fetal head/small maternal pelvic canal).

## History

Early recognition and correction of dystocia is critical to optimal neonatal survival. A common error made by owners and veterinarians is to delay intervention based on the fact that the dam does not appear to "be in trouble." The decision to delay is usually made without regard to the well-being of the fetuses, which are often severely stressed long before the dam shows clinical signs relating to the demise of her fetuses. It has been shown that neonatal mortality is directly correlated to duration of labor. For example, one study found that if delivery was complete within 1 to 4.5 hours of the onset of stage II labor, puppy mortality was 5.8%; whereas, neonatal mortality was 13.7% after 5 to 24 hours of stage II labor. In a different study, puppy mortality from birth to 7 days of age decreased from 33% to 6% as a result of fetal monitoring and early intervention during parturition. Among the multiparous bitches in that study, neonatal mortality decreased from 42% to 12%.

An accurate history is crucial to the successful management of dystocia. In particular the length of gestation, known predisposition to or previous occurrence of dystocia, the progression through the stages of labor, and any indication of illness in the dam must be investigated. This would include information on rectal temperature monitoring, behavior of the dam, presence of vulvar discharge, presence and characterization of contractions, presence of placental membranes or fetal parts at the vulva, any puppy or kitten born, and the duration of each of these events. Breeders should be asked if they have already administered any drugs or performed any obstetric procedures.

The dam should be examined if the expected due date has arrived and no signs of labor exist, irrespective of a lack of maternal discomfort or illness. This is to ensure that all is well with the fetuses and to determine if continued watchful waiting is a reasonable approach. The due date (i.e., normal length of gestation) in queens is 65 ± 2 days, with a reported range of 62 to 71 days from the first breeding. Normal gestation in bitches is 63 ± 7 days from the first breeding, 57 ± 3 days from the first day of cytologic diestrus, and 65 ± 1 day from the LH surge, as determined by serum concentrations of LH or by the initial rise above basal anestrual progesterone concentrations. The drop in rectal temperature to less than 99° F in a full-term bitch and anorexia in a full-term queen are indicators of stage I labor. If stage I has not progressed to stage II within 12 hours, the dam should be examined, irrespective of lack of other signs of labor or maternal illness.

Ultrasonography is ideal for assessment of fetal well-being. Normal canine fetal heart rates are 170 to 230 bpm. Fetal kittens' heart rates are 190 to 250 bpm. Fetal movement is observed from about day 40 of gestation onward. Normal fetuses are quite active near term. Subjectively, this activity seems to increase during ultrasonographic examination. Fetal movement and heart rates are decreased as a result of stress and hypoxemia. In fetal pups, heart rates below normal are associated with poor neonatal survival unless pups are delivered promptly. It has been shown that heart rates <150 to 160 bpm indicate fetal stress. When heart rates are less than 130 bpm, there is poor survival unless pups are delivered within 1 to 2 hours. There is high neonatal mortality among pups with fetal heart rates less than 100 bpm unless they are immediately delivered.

Presumably the situation is similar in cats, taking the normally faster feline heart rate into account. Using ultrasonography, previously recognizable fetal anatomy begins to be lost within 24 hours of fetal death. The overall size of the fetal mass decreases and condenses into a heterogeneous echotexture (see Fig. 59-3). The precise gestational age cannot be determined based on ultrasonographic findings, but fetal maturity can be assessed by the development, or lack thereof, of fetal organs (see Fig. 59-2).

The onset of stage II of labor is recognized by the return of rectal temperature to normal, the presence of strong abdominal contractions, and the passage of amnionic fluid. Any sign of illness in the pregnant female is reason to recommend that she be examined. Other findings of concern are the presence of a vulvar discharge, fetal membranes, or a partially delivered fetus (Table 59-1).

Partially delivered puppies or kittens need prompt attention if they are to survive. The passage of amnionic fluid is an indication of stage II labor, irrespective of obvious abdominal contractions. The first pup should be born within 2 to 3 hours of amnionic fluid. A dark green discharge in bitches or red-brown discharge in queens originates from the placenta. Its presence indicates that at least one placenta has begun to separate. If a pup or kitten has not been delivered within 2 to 4 hours, the dam should be examined. A bright yellow vulvar discharge is meconium. Passage of meconium is indicative of severe fetal stress. It is often associated with fetal aspiration of amnionic fluid and a grave prognosis for neona-

 TABLE 59-1

### Indicators of Dystocia

Any sign of illness in full-term female
History of previous dystocia
Known predisposition to dystocia
More than 24 hours since rectal temperature drop in full-term bitch
More than 24 hours of anorexia in full-term queen
Abnormal vulvar discharge
Failure to progress from stage I to stage II after 12 hours
Partially delivered fetus for more than 10-15 minutes
More than 3 hours of stage II labor before birth of first neonate
More than 1 hour of active labor between births
Constant, unrelenting, unproductive straining of 20-30 minutes
Labor appears to have stopped before entire litter delivered

tal survival. A purulent discharge may be found if uterine infection or fetal maceration exist. Viable fetuses may also be present.

Weak, intermittent straining lasting more than 2 to 4 hours before the first puppy or kitten is born, or lasting longer than 1 hour between births, is cause for concern. Strong, persistent straining lasting longer than 20 to 30 minutes without delivery of a pup or kitten is not normal. If more than 12 hours of stage II have elapsed, or conversely, if labor appears to have stopped before the entire litter is delivered, the dam should be examined. Cats have been observed to deliver live kittens over 24 to 40 hours, with no obvious straining or discomfort between kitten births. Even though live kittens are often born, such prolonged delivery is associated with increased neonatal morbidity and mortality and therefore should probably not be considered normal. The average duration of labor was reported to be 16 hours in one colony, but kitten mortality was 29%. In dogs, the outcome for the bitch and the puppies is favorable when the dam is healthy, the fetal heart rates are normal, when stage I is less than 6 hours in duration, and the duration of stage II is less than 12 hours. When stage II lasts longer than 12 hours but less than 24 hours, the prognosis for puppy survival is poor, although the prognosis for the bitch is still fine. If stage II lasts longer than 24 hours, the puppies are likely to die and morbidity for the bitch is increased. Fetal heart rates less than 150 to 160 bpm or illness in the bitch is also associated with worsening prognosis.

## Diagnosis

The historical and physical findings are diagnostic of dystocia. A complete physical examination should be performed to assess the overall health of the dam. The first step is to examine the perineum for evidence of a partially delivered fetus, which requires immediate attention. There may be a bulge in the perineum dorsal to the vulva, or there may be fetal limbs or tail protruding from the vulva. When it is determined that no partially delivered fetus is present, the physical examination of the dam proceeds as usual. All abnormalities should be addressed. For example, hyperthermia may be caused by the exertion of labor, but infection, especially of the mammae or uterus, should be considered. Regardless of cause, dehydration must be corrected.

The abdomen is palpated to evaluate uterine size, tone, and the presence of fetuses. Fetal movement and uterine contractions may be felt, but their adequacy cannot be assessed by palpation alone. The inability to detect movement or contractions via abdominal palpation is not necessarily cause for concern. The perineum is examined for the presence and character of any discharge. In bitches, a digital vaginal exam should be performed to assess for the presence of a fetus in the birth canal. If one is found, it should be delivered immediately. If none is found, the dorsal wall of the vagina should be stroked, because doing so often stimulates abdominal contractions. This procedure has been referred to as "feathering." The cervix is not palpable per vaginum. Puppies or kittens stuck in the vagina may be delivered by obstetric manipulation or with the aid of episiotomy. The mammary glands are palpated to assess the presence and character of secretions. Some primiparous bitches may not have obvious milk. Lactation begins within 24 hours of parturition. Multiparous bitches and queens may have colostrum during the last week of gestation.

Systemic illness in the dam should be pursued as usual for any ill animal. A complete blood count (CBC) and biochemical profile would be reasonable. Mild anemia (i.e., PCV around 35%) and a slight mature neutrophilia are normal in full-term bitches. Specimens should be submitted promptly so that results might be available when the other diagnostic evaluations (see following) are complete.

After assessing maternal health by physical examination, the fetuses are assessed by radiology and ultrasonography. The number, size, shape, location, posture, and presentation of any remaining fetuses are often best determined by radiographs. A cause for obstruction, such as large fetus or fetal monstrosity, an abnormal pelvic canal, or fetal malposition may be identified. Fetal viability is difficult to assess on radiographs (Table 59-2). Intrafetal gas may be detectable as early as 6 hours after death. The bones of the fetal skeleton and head may collapse as early as 48 hours after death. However, the absence of those radiographic signs is not diagnostic of life or death. The number of fetuses remaining cannot be accurately determined with ultrasonography; however, ultrasonography is ideal for assessment of fetal viability (see previous discussion).

## Treatment

When it has been determined that an "overdue" dam is healthy and the fetuses are healthy (as determined by the presence of fetal movement and normal heart rates), serum concentrations of progesterone could be determined. This would be especially helpful in situations where information by which the actual length of gestation might be calculated is

## TABLE 59-2

**Radiographic Signs of Fetal Death**

Absence of continued uterine enlargement before fetal skeletons are detected
Absence of continued fetal growth after initial detection of fetal skeletons
Demineralization or inadequate mineralization of fetal skeleton for gestational age
Overlap of skull bones, collapse of axial skeleton, or misalignment of fetal bones
Intrauterine or intrafetal gas

lacking. The finding of progesterone that is greater than 2 ng/ml (6 nmol/L) would indicate that the pregnancy has not yet reached full term. Intervention should be delayed and watchful waiting should continue for several hours. If 24 hours pass with no progression of labor, all parameters should be reassessed. This watchful waiting does *not* apply to dams already in stage II of labor. Animals in stage I of labor are expected to progress to stage II in less than 12 to 24 hours.

Sometimes all other parameters are found to be normal except one of the fetuses is not moving or has a heart rate of 150 to 160 bpm or less. The dam and the other fetuses are healthy. In that situation the benefits of prompt intervention in an attempt to save all the fetuses should be weighed against the cost and risk of intervention to the dam and the potential risk of not intervening to the rest of the litter. For example, the decisions made in a situation where all but one of 10 puppies are apparently normal might be different from the decisions made under identical circumstances but a litter size of only 2. The owner's attitude about the relative value of each puppy or kitten in the litter and about stillbirth or neonatal death must be considered.

Treatment is dictated by the presence or absence of obstruction and by the health of the fetuses. If obstruction or serious fetal compromise exists, Caesarean section is indicated without delay. If no obstruction exists, medical management may be attempted in healthy dams with no signs of fetal stress. Several studies have found that 65% to 80% of bitches and queens presented for dystocia were treated with Caesarean section. Medical management was successful in resolving the dystocia in only 20% to 30% of canine and feline cases. Maternal mortality was 1% of 808 bitches undergoing Caesarean section.

Exercise often stimulates abdominal contractions. For that reason, some have recommended that the owners walk the bitch up and down the stairs or around the house before loading her in the car for the drive to the veterinary hospital. A partially delivered fetus should be delivered within 10 minutes. Care must be taken to avoid disarticulating the extremities. Liberal amounts of lubrication should be used. Rotating the fetus 45 degrees to take advantage of the widest diagonal part of the pelvic canal may be helpful. Gently alternating (i.e., rocking) traction from left to right may help relieve shoulder or hip lock. Traction should be applied in a ventral direction that follows the natural conformation of the vestibule. It may be helpful to lift vulvar lips upward while pressing the pup downward.

A vaginal exam should be performed in all dams of adequate size to determine if a fetus is lodged in the vagina and to stimulate the vagina (i.e., "feathering") in hopes of initiating abdominal contractions. If the dam is extremely nervous, consider mild sedation.

### No obstruction and healthy dam and fetuses

Oxytocin increases the frequency of uterine contractions. Especially at higher doses it can cause sustained contraction. During uterine contraction the blood supply to the placenta is diminished. This contributes to placental separation, fetal hypoxia, and fetal acidosis. Therefore indiscriminant use of oxytocin contributes to stillbirth and neonatal mortality. The goal of oxytocin therapy is to increase the frequency of uterine contractions to normal. This is best accomplished while the uterine contractions are being monitored. Unfortunately this is often not done in veterinary medicine. Recent studies where uterine monitoring has been done have demonstrated that the large doses of oxytocin that have traditionally been recommended are not necessary. Current recommendations are to administer small doses, 0.25 to 4.0 U per dog, intramuscularly (IM). (In our colony of mixed breed dogs weighing 35 to 45 lb, we administer 0.25 U. We do not monitor uterine pressure.) Labor should progress (i.e., straining begins) within 30 minutes and a pup should soon be delivered. If so, the clinician may repeat administration of oxytocin as needed to perpetuate normal parturition (see previous guidelines). Repeated doses should not be administered if a normal labor pattern is not established. In one study monitoring uterine contractions of whelping bitches, the mean total cumulative dose of oxytocin used was 7.7 U. In another, the mean total cumulative dose of oxytocin was 4 U. If the animal does not respond to oxytocin administration within 30 to 45 minutes, it is unlikely that further treatment will be beneficial (see following discussion of calcium). High doses and/or frequent administration of oxytocin are contraindicated, because they cause sustained uterine contractions that delay the expulsion of fetuses and compromise placental blood flow. Placental separation may also occur. These actions contribute to fetal and neonatal mortality.

Myometrial contraction is dependent upon the influx of calcium ions. Generally speaking, calcium administration increases the strength of uterine contractions even in the absence of documented hypocalcemia. For this reason, some have recommended the routine administration of calcium gluconate in the management of nonobstructive dystocia in bitches with weak, ineffective uterine contractions. It has been recommended by some that 10% calcium gluconate be administered before the administration of oxytocin. If normal labor does not resume, oxytocin is added. Calcium gluconate, 0.2 ml/kg or less, or 1 to 5 ml/dog, is administered subcutaneously (SC) or intravenously (IV). The label directions must be followed precisely because some preparations are too irri-

tating to be administered by routes other than IV. If the IV route is chosen, calcium is administered slowly (1 ml/min), while auscultating the heart. Administration should be immediately discontinued if bradycardia or dysrhythmia occur. If labor progresses (i.e., straining begins) calcium may be repeated as needed or continued with oxytocin. When uterine monitoring is used as a guide, the mean total cumulative dose of 10% Ca gluconate administered to bitches was 3 ml.

Before uterine monitoring was available, doses of 1.5 to 20 ml were reported. Higher doses or bolus IV administration of Ca gluconate should be reserved for animals with documented clinical signs or laboratory evidence of hypocalcemia. When medical management fails to initiate a normal labor pattern, Caesarean section should be performed without delay.

Caesarean section is indicated, without delay, irrespective of fetal heart rate, in the following circumstances: obstruction (e.g., fetal oversize, fetal malposition, uterine torsion or rupture); fetal compromise exists; medical management (e.g., Ca/oxytocin administration) has failed; continued pregnancy or labor might be harmful to the dam; or maternal illness already exists. (See Suggested Readings for information on surgical and anesthetic techniques for Caesarean section.)

At the time of this writing, at least one company provides fetal and uterine monitoring services for veterinarians: Veterinary Perinatal Specialties, www.whelpwise.com.

## POSTPARTUM DISORDERS

Mastitis is an important postpartum disorder. It is discussed in Chapter 58.

### AGALACTIA

Agalactia is the absence of milk production or secretion. Normal milk production and secretion are dependent on many factors including genetics, nutrition, psychologic, and anatomic. Prolactin stimulates milk production. Oxytocin stimulates milk letdown. Primary agalactia refers to a situation where the gland is incapable of producing milk or the ducts are incapable of flow. More commonly, the gland and ducts are normal but other factors have diminished the capacity for production or inhibited milk letdown. Animals that are in poor body condition may have difficulty establishing and maintaining lactation. Caloric and water needs during lactation are as much as double that needed during gestation. To ensure that the needs of both gestation and lactation are met, a high-energy diet, appropriate for reproduction and lactation, should be fed from the time of breeding onward. Unlike multiparous animals that may have colostrum that is easily expressed during the last week of gestation, primiparous animals do not always have colostrum that is easy to express at the time of parturition; however, colostrum is almost always present within 24 hours of parturition. Anxiety will inhibit milk letdown. Sedation may be considered in those situations. Phenothiazines increase prolactin secretion, which would be beneficial. Oxytocin, 0.5 to 2.0 U SC every 2 hours has also been suggested for milk letdown. It is available for this purpose in people in the form of a nasal spray. Puppies or kittens are returned to nurse 30 minutes after oxytocin is administered. Metoclopramide stimulates prolactin secretion and has been successfully used to enhance lactation. Doses of 0.1 to 0.2 mg/kg (PO or SC) every 6 to 8 hours until lactation is adequate have been suggested. An oral dose of 0.5 mg/kg every 8 hours may be administered, but this dose may be more than is necessary. Treatment is usually needed for only a day or two. Meanwhile, other nutritional and psychologic factors should be corrected.

## PUERPERAL HYPOCALCEMIA (PUERPERAL TETANY, ECLAMPSIA)

Puerperal hypocalcemia is an acute, life-threatening hypocalcemia that occurs in the postpartum period. Although it is often called eclampsia, eclampsia in women is not the same condition as puerperal hypocalcemia in animals, although both are characterized by convulsions. Eclampsia refers to the convulsions that are associated with preeclampsia, a condition of pregnant women characterized by hypertension, proteinuria, edema, consumptive coagulopathy, sodium retention, and hyperreflexia. Convulsions (i.e., eclampsia) occur if the preeclampsia is uncontrolled. Preeclampsia usually occurs during the last trimester. Its pathogenesis is not fully understood, but the primary lesion is pregnancy-induced glomerular ischemia, which in turn causes the other physiologic derangements. Delivery of the fetus is the definitive treatment for eclampsia.

In contrast, puerperal hypocalcemia in bitches and queens occurs in the postpartum period, and the signs are a direct result of hypocalcemia. The cause of the hypocalcemia is usually undetermined, but it could result from such problems as maternal calcium loss to the fetal skeletons and to the milk, poor use of dietary calcium, and parathyroid gland atrophy caused by improper diet or dietary supplements. Clinical signs of puerperal hypocalcemia typically develop during peak lactation (i.e., 1 to 3 weeks postpartum) in small bitches nursing large litters. The dam is otherwise healthy, and the neonates are thriving. Puerperal hypocalcemia can, however, occur in cats, in any breed of dog, with any size litter, and at any time during lactation; rarely it occurs during late gestation in bitches. In queens, hypocalcemia may be seen as a preparturient event. The clinical signs of the prepartum hypocalcemia in cats are identical to those in the postpartum bitch, except that hypothermia was common in the cats.

### Clinical Features

The clinical signs are caused by the hypocalcemia and include panting, trembling, muscle fasciculations, weakness, and ataxia. These early clinical signs quickly progress (e.g., within hours) to tetany with tonic-clonic convulsions and opisthotonos. Heart rate, respiratory rate, and rectal temperature are increased, especially during convulsions. Clinical signs are rapidly progressive and may be fatal if the animal goes untreated.

### Diagnosis

Puerperal hypocalcemia is diagnosed based on the finding of appropriate clinical signs in a heavily lactating female. It can be confirmed by measuring the serum concentrations of calcium, which will be below the reference range. Because the clinical signs in postpartum bitches are so suggestive, treatment is usually initiated before, or without, laboratory confirmation. Laboratory confirmation would be necessary in a prepartum animal. Although severe hypoglycemia could cause similar clinical signs, it is a rare postpartum disorder in the bitch or queen.

### Treatment

Treatment consists of the slow, IV administration of a 10% solution of calcium gluconate, to effect. The total dose is usually 3 to 20 ml, depending on the size of the bitch or queen. Because calcium is cardiotoxic, the animal's heart must be closely monitored for the development of dysrhythmias and bradycardia during treatment. Calcium administration must be stopped immediately if any cardiac abnormalities are detected. If additional calcium is still needed, it can be administered after the cardiac rhythm has normalized, but the rate of administration should be much slower. The response to treatment is dramatic, and clinical signs resolve during IV calcium administration.

Some veterinarians have recommended that the same amount of calcium necessary to initially control clinical signs be mixed 50:50 with sterile saline solution and administered SC before the dam is sent home. If this is done, a salt other than calcium chloride must be used. Puppies or kittens should then not be allowed to nurse for 12 to 24 hours. Oral calcium (gluconate, carbonate, or lactate), 1 to 3 g daily, should be administered for the duration of lactation. The dam's diet should also be adjusted as necessary to ensure that it is nutritionally complete, balanced, and appropriate for lactation. Ad libitum feeding, or at least feeding three times a day, is recommended. Some veterinarians also recommend that dams be given vitamin D supplementation, but this must be done with caution because hypercalcemia can occur in response to overzealous vitamin D supplementation (see Chapter 55). Usually a balanced diet with additional oral calcium suffices to prevent hypocalcemia. If hypocalcemia recurs, the puppies should be weaned.

### Prevention

Several steps can be taken to prevent puerperal hypocalcemia in the bitch and queen: First, a high-quality, nutritionally balanced and complete diet should be fed to the bitch or queen during pregnancy and lactation. Oral calcium supplementation during gestation is contraindicated because it may worsen, rather than prevent, postpartum hypocalcemia. The bitch or queen should also have access to food and water ad libitum during lactation. If necessary, the dam can be physically separated from the neonates for 30 to 60 minutes several times a day to encourage her to eat. Supplemental feeding of the litter with milk replacer early in lactation and with solid food after 3 to 4 weeks of age may be helpful, especially for large litters.

## METRITIS

Metritis is an acute bacterial infection of the uterus that occurs postpartum. It may occur after abortion, dystocia, retention of placental or fetal tissues, obstetric procedures, or normal parturition. Bacteria that ascend from the vagina are the cause. Affected animals are febrile and have a fetid, septic uterine discharge. Dehydration, septicemia, endotoxemia, shock, or a combination of these can occur. Neglected, crying neonates are often one of the earliest signs of maternal illness, including metritis.

## Diagnosis

The diagnosis is based primarily on the historical and physical findings. The septic nature and the uterine source of the exudate can be confirmed by cytologic and endoscopic studies, if necessary. Bacterial culture and sensitivity testing of the uterine discharge should be performed. Abdominal radiography or ultrasonography (or both) should be done to evaluate the uterine contents (e.g., fetal remnants) and to assess the integrity of the uterus.

## Treatment

Because neonatal survival is more likely to be optimal with the dam in the home environment than in the hospital, metritis should be promptly and aggressively treated to minimize the hospital stay. Infected uterine contents can be removed surgically by ovariohysterectomy or by hysterotomy with lavage, or medically with the administration of ecbolic agents (e.g., oxytocin, $PGF_{2\alpha}$). The decision to manage metritis either medically or surgically is determined by the health of the bitch or queen, the integrity of the uterus, and the owner's desire for the animal to be able to reproduce in the future.

Regardless of the approach taken, appropriate IV fluids to correct existing deficits, maintain tissue perfusion, and provide for the additional demands of lactation, together with a broad-spectrum, bactericidal antibiotic, should be administered. The antibiotic should be chosen based on results of a culture of the uterine exudate obtained from the anterior vagina. When choosing an antibiotic, the clinician must also consider the potential deleterious effects of that antibiotic on the neonates, because it is assumed that the antibiotic will reach the neonates through the milk. Penicillins, amoxicillins, and cephalosporins generally are considered safe for the neonate. Chloramphenicol and tetracyclines should not be used (Table 59-3).

Ovariohysterectomy should be performed if the clinician sees evidence that the uterus has ruptured. Extreme abdominal discomfort, radiographic or ultrasonographic signs of fluid in the abdomen, and peritonitis are suggestive of uterine rupture. Ovariohysterectomy or hysterotomy is usually recommended if placental or fetal tissues remain in the uterus.

The medical management of metritis includes the administration of an ecbolic agent to promote the evacuation of infected uterine contents. Oxytocin and $PGF_{2\alpha}$ are two such agents that can be considered. Oxytocin (5 to 20 IU IM q24h or q12h) for several days is likely to be most effective if administered in the early postpartum period when the uterus is most sensitive to it. Natural $PGF_{2\alpha}$ (0.1 to 0.25 mg/kg SC q24h or q12h; Lutalyse; Pharmacia, Kalamazoo, Mich) is also

## TABLE 59-3

### Antimicrobial Therapy for Neonates

**Drugs with Known Safety**

Amoxicillin-clavulanate
Amoxicillin
Cephalosporins
Erythromycin
Penicillins
Tylosin

**Safety Not Established**

Clindamycin
Lincomycin

**Drugs Known to Cause Undesirable Effects**

Aminoglycosides
Chloramphenicol
Ciprofloxacin
Enrofloxacin
Nalidixic acid
Nitrofurantoin
Norfloxacin
Polymyxin
Sulfonamides
Tetracyclines
Trimethoprim

effective. Treatment should continue until the uterus is empty, which usually takes at least 2 days. Adverse reactions to $PGF_{2\alpha}$ therapy may be seen (see Table 57-2). Neither medication has been observed to have deleterious effects on lactation or on the neonates.

## SUBINVOLUTION OF PLACENTAL SITES

In the bitch, normal postpartum involution of the uterus occurs over 12 weeks. The placental sites and the entire endometrium slough. By the ninth week the uterine horns are uniformly contracted and the surface sloughing is complete. Replacement of the endometrial lining continues until the twelfth postpartum week, at which time involution is complete. The sloughed material makes up the normal, postpartum vulvar discharge known as *lochia*. Immediately after whelping, lochia contains large amounts of the placental blood heme pigment called uteroverdin. This makes the lochia dark green for the first few hours ($<12$ hours). Thereafter the lochia is reddish or red-brown and contains cellular debris and mucus. The volume of lochia diminishes quickly, and within a few weeks it is an intermittent (several times a day) spotting of reddish or red-brown mucoid material.

If subinvolution of placental sites (SIPS) occurs, this causes persistent postpartum hemorrhage lasting 7 to 12 or more weeks. Usually a fairly constant (as opposed to intermittent) bloody vulvar discharge is present, although the volume is usually very small. SIPS is most common in primiparous bitches less than 3 years of age, but it can occur in older multiparous animals as well. It has not been reported in cats. The cause is unknown.

### Diagnosis

Affected bitches are healthy and physically normal, except for a small amount of bloody vulvar discharge. The blood loss from SIPS is not severe. If the clinician is concerned, the CBC can be evaluated, keeping in mind the normal decline in the PCV that occurs during pregnancy. Vaginal cytology (see p. 870) can be used to differentiate the vulvar discharge associated with SIPS from lochia and from the discharge associated with metritis. Cytologically, evidence of hemorrhage is found. Decidua-like multinucleated giant cells may also be seen. SIPS is diagnosed based on the historical, physical, and cytologic findings. It can be confirmed by histopathologic examination of the placental sites, but this is rarely necessary. Normally involuted placental sites and SIPS can be found in the same uterus.

Bitches with SIPS rarely require treatment. Recovery is spontaneous, and subsequent fertility is not affected. Ovariohysterectomy is curative. The administration of ergonovine maleate or natural $PGF_{2\alpha}$ (e.g., Lutalyse) may diminish bleeding, but neither drug has been adequately investigated for the treatment of SIPS in dogs. They are not likely to affect the trophoblast-like cells. Progestin therapy has also been suggested, but its undesirable effects on the endometrium outweigh any potential benefit in this situation. If anemia is severe enough to require treatment, a diagnosis other than SIPS should be considered.

## ABORTIFACIENTS (MISMATING)

Queens and bitches may occasionally mate at an undesirable time or with an undesirable male. The dilemma is then how to prevent the birth of unwanted puppies or kittens without offending the moral sensibilities of the owner and veterinarian or threatening the health of the dam and her future reproductive capabilities. The safest approach to preserve the health of the female and her future reproductive capability may be to do nothing to interfere with the results of a misalliance. It is possible that conception will not occur as a result of the single, unwanted mating. It is noteworthy that Feldman and colleagues (1993) found that 30 (62%) of 48 bitches examined 30 to 35 days after a misalliance were not pregnant. Ovariohysterectomy performed during the first 3 to 4 weeks of pregnancy is no more dangerous than at other stages of the reproductive cycle. This is an effective, but permanent, method of preventing the birth of an unwanted litter. Ovariohysterectomy during pregnancy (i.e., diestrus) may cause galactorrhea (see False Pregnancy, p. 886). A third option is to use an abortifacient (Table 59-4).

### ESTROGENS

In some species, estrogens are known to interfere with conception and pregnancy by hastening the deterioration of ova,

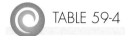

## TABLE 59-4

**Therapeutic Options for Canine Misalliance**

Do nothing
    Thirty of 48 (62%) dogs seen 30 to 35 days after misalliance not pregnant
Ovariohysterectomy (may cause galactorrhea)
Estrogen not recommended
    Estradiol cypionate (ECP) once (maximum dose, 1 mg)
        22 µg/kg (75% success)
        44 µg/kg (100% success)
        Pyometra (25% of cases)
Natural $PGF_{2\alpha}$ (Lutalyse)
    0.1-0.25 mg/kg SC q8-12h to effect (3-9 days) 30 to 35 days after breeding; monitor with ultrasound *or*
    0.15-0.25 mg/kg SC q12h for 4 days; begin day 8-15 of cytologic diestrus; monitor progesterone concentration (<3 nmol/L; <1 ng/dl)
    Cats: after day 45, 0.25 mg/kg SC q24h or q12h for 5 days (may produce side effects)
Bromocriptine: 30 µg/kg PO for 5-6 days, after day 35-40
Cabergoline: 5 µg/kg PO q24h for 5 days, week 7 or later
Cloprostenol: from day 25 after LH surge
    1 µg/kg SC every other day, plus cabergoline 5 µg/kg PO q24h, to effect *or*
    2.5 µg/kg SC once, plus cabergoline 5 µg/kg PO q24h for 10 days
Mifepristone (RU 486): beginning day 32, 2.5 mg/kg PO q12h, to effect
Aglepristone: 2 SC doses (10 mg/kg) 24 hours apart, day 0-45 after breeding; 97% success

delaying transport of the ova through the tubulouterine junction, and altering implantation. Oral diethylstilbestrol (DES) is ineffective in preventing pregnancy if given orally for 7 days at a dose of 75 mg/kg. It has been observed to prevent pregnancy in less than 25% of bitches treated during proestrus, estrus, or diestrus. Estradiol cypionate (ECP) (22 µg/kg up to 1 mg maximum dose, IM once) has been observed to prevent pregnancy in 50% of bitches treated in estrus and in 75% of bitches treated in early diestrus (see Table 59-4). At a dose of 44 µg/kg up to a maximum dose of 1 mg, pregnancy is prevented in bitches treated during estrus and early diestrus.

Although ECP is reasonably effective in preventing pregnancy, its use is strongly discouraged for the following reasons: First, pyometra develops in 25% of bitches given ECP during diestrus. Estrogens can also cause fatal aplastic anemia, prolong the duration of behavioral estrus, and predispose cystic ovarian follicles. These effects are dose dependent, but aplastic anemia develops in some bitches given the recommended dose. If ECP is used, it should not be administered during diestrus, as determined by vaginal cytologic findings; the total dose of ECP should not exceed 1 mg; and the dose should never be repeated. For these reasons, ECP is no longer approved for use in dogs in the United States.

## PROSTAGLANDINS

PGs have been used to terminate unwanted pregnancy in dogs and cats. They are not approved for use in small animals in the United States. In one protocol, treatment is begun 30 to 35 days after breeding, once pregnancy is confirmed. Beginning treatment after pregnancy is confirmed avoids the unnecessary treatment of nonpregnant females. Unfortunately, the later in gestation, the more likely the fetuses will be expelled by overt abortion rather than be reabsorbed. In bitches, natural $PGF_{2\alpha}$ (0.1 to 0.25 mg/kg; Lutalyse, Pharmacia, Kalamazoo, Mich) is administered SC two to three times daily beginning 30 to 35 days after breeding and continuing until abortion is complete, which is accomplished in 3 to 9 days (see Table 59-4). In queens, 0.2 to 0.5 mg/kg of natural $PGF_{2\alpha}$ SC twice daily for 5 days, beginning about day 45 of gestation, was effective in three of four queens. Treatment was discontinued after 5 days because of side effects.

Adverse reactions to $PGF_{2\alpha}$ (see Table 57-2) can be worrisome, even though they usually become less severe as therapy progresses. In both bitches and queens, the onset of abortion induced by this protocol is followed closely by the production of a vulvar discharge. The discharge is noticed more often than the actual abortion itself. Therefore abdominal ultrasonography should be performed whenever a vulvar discharge develops to confirm abortion and to identify fetuses remaining in the uterus. If treatment is stopped when only part of the litter is aborted, the remaining fetuses may be carried to term. Abdominal palpation has proved unreliable in determining whether fetuses are still present in the uterus. Because of the adverse reactions that can occur, the possibility that the entire litter may not be aborted, and the possibility of live puppies being born if abortion occurs near term, hospitalization of the bitch has been recommended.

Another protocol involves administration of $PGF_{2\alpha}$ to bitches early in diestrus. The advantage of early treatment is that fetuses are resorbed, rather than expelled. Postabortion sequelae such as vulvar discharge are also minimal compared with those in bitches treated after day 30 to 35 of gestation. The protocol is begun no sooner than day 8 of cytologic diestrus, up to day 15 of diestrus. Natural $PGF_{2\alpha}$ (Lutalyse, Pharmacia, Kalamazoo, Mich) is administered twice daily for 4 days (0.25 mg/kg SC q12h). The serum progesterone concentrations are determined at the end of the 4-day treatment and again 15 to 20 days later. Fetal death is likely if the serum progesterone concentration declines and remains below 2 ng/ml (approximately 6.4 nmol/L). If the progesterone concentration is greater than 2 ng/ml after treatment, luteolysis is not complete, in which case the pregnancy status should be assessed with ultrasonography, or a second course of treatment should be administered. Termination of early pregnancy with $PGF_{2\alpha}$ in bitches is about 85% effective. After $PGF_{2\alpha}$ treatment given anytime during diestrus, the interestrual interval may be shortened by 1 to 4 months.

## ALTERNATIVE TREATMENTS

Because prolactin is luteotropic, antiprolactin drugs such as bromocriptine and cabergoline can suppress serum progesterone concentrations and terminate pregnancy if used as single agents. When given after 7 weeks of gestation in bitches, a single daily dose of 5 μg/kg of cabergoline causes abortion in 3 to 5 days with no side effects. Unfortunately, at this late stage of gestation, recognizable fetal parts or live fetuses that die shortly thereafter may be passed. Parturition was prevented in 12 of 14 feral cats given cabergoline in their feed at a dose of either 25 μg/day for 5 days or 50 μg/day for 3 days.

In an attempt to minimize its side effects, $PGF_{2\alpha}$ has been used in combination with bromocriptine or cabergoline. Treatment began 25 days after breeding, once pregnancy had been confirmed, and continued until abortion occurred. When given at 0.1 to 0.2 mg/kg SC once daily with 15 to 30 μg/kg bromocriptine (Parlodel; Sandoz, East Hanover, N.J.) orally twice daily, abortion occurred in 5 days on average. When the same dose of bromocriptine was given with the PG analog cloprostenol (Estrumate; Schering-Plough, Atlanta, Ga) at 1 μg/kg SC every 48 hours, the mean time to abortion was about 4 days. Fewer side effects were noted with cloprostenol than with $PGF_{2\alpha}$, but both were effective in terminating pregnancy. Although doses of 2.5 μg/kg of cloprostenol cause similar side effects to natural $PGF_{2\alpha}$, they resolve in about 30 minutes without treatment. When started 22 to 28 days after breeding, a single SC dose of 2.5 μg/kg of cloprostenol on day 1 of treatment, combined with either 5 μg/kg cabergoline orally once daily for 10 days, or 30 μg/kg orally three times daily for 10 days, was effective in terminating canine pregnancy. Fetuses were resorbed. A brown serosanguineous discharge lasted for 4 to 21 days. Interestral interval was shortened by about 70 days. Subsequent fertility was not affected. After the initial injection of cloprostenol, side effects were so minimal that treatment on an outpatient basis could be considered.

Dexamethasone is an effective abortifacient in bitches, as it is in sheep and cattle. We do not recommend it for that purpose, rather it is mentioned here as a warning to clinicians to avoid the use of glucocorticoids during pregnancy. The mechanism of glucocorticoid-induced abortion has not been fully investigated in dogs, but the serum progesterone concentrations are known to decline to less than 2 ng/ml during treatment. When 0.2 mg/kg of dexamethasone is administered orally twice a day beginning on day 30 to 35, no fetal parts are observed to be expelled. However, if treatment is started after day 45, live fetuses that die within a few hours can be passed. Treatment is associated with development of a mucoid, red-brown vulvar discharge, polydipsia and polyuria, and anorexia. Additional study is needed to determine whether the postabortion uterus is normal and to evaluate subsequent fertility. In cattle a glucocorticoid-induced abortion is associated with an increased risk of retained placenta. Because glucocorticoids are teratogenic, if they fail to cause abortion, puppies with facial or other deformities could be born.

Mifepristone (RU 486) and its relative aglipristone are competitive inhibitors of the progesterone receptor. Mifepristone has been shown to be efficacious and safe for pregnancy termination in bitches (see Table 59-4). Aglipristone is available in Europe for pregnancy termination in bitches. It has an efficacy of 97% if given SC (two injections 24 hours apart) anytime from copulation to day 45. Unfortunately, neither is currently available for veterinary use in the United States.

## FETAL RESORPTION-ABORTION-STILLBIRTH COMPLEX

### Clinical Features

Embryonic death, abortion, and stillbirths can occur because of maternal, fetal, or placental abnormalities. If embryonic death occurs early in gestation, usually no outward signs are seen (e.g., vulvar discharge). Females may be presented for evaluation because of apparent failure to conceive (i.e., infertility) rather than because of suspected fetal death. Progesterone causes mammary development and weight gain regardless of whether pregnancy exists. Therefore bitches in which early embryonic death has occurred may continue to appear pregnant for 60 or more days. If early pregnancy is lost in queens, the CLs regress in 30 to 50 days; thus any appearance of pregnancy diminishes after that time. Queens are likely to resume cycling. If fetal death occurs in the latter half of pregnancy, often a vulvar discharge is present. The later in gestation fetal death occurs, the more obvious it becomes that fetal parts are being expelled.

### Etiology

Maternal factors thought to be associated with fetal death and abortion in bitches or queens include maternal infections, hypothyroidism, immune-mediated hemolytic anemia, immune-mediated thrombocytopenia and other bleeding disorders, herniation or torsion of the gravid uterus, and abdominal trauma. Apparent luteal insufficiency is also discussed as a cause of abortion, but it is rarely documented in bitches or queens. Determination of serial serum progesterone concentrations would be the first step in documenting this problem. Certain drugs that may be used to treat or prevent maternal illness are also known to be toxic to pregnant females, to be teratogenic, to cause fetal death, or to cause abortion (Table 59-5).

Infectious agents can cause fetal death and abortion through their effects on the dam, the fetus, or the placenta. Other than interrupting pregnancy, many of these pathogens cause minimal clinical signs of maternal illness. Bacteria reported to cause fetal death and abortion in bitches include *Brucella abortus, Escherichia coli,* and *Brucella canis,* β-hemolytic *Streptococcus, Leptospira, Campylobacter, Salmonella,* and *Mycoplasma* spp. (see p. 935). Experimental infection with *Toxoplasma gondii* has also been found to cause abortion in bitches and queens.

Viral agents are the most commonly reported infectious cause of abortion in queens. Viruses implicated in feline abortion include feline leukemia virus (FeLV), feline infectious peritonitis virus (i.e., coronavirus), and feline herpesvirus (i.e., rhinotracheitis) and calicivirus. Canine distemper virus and canine herpesvirus are reported to cause abortion in bitches.

 TABLE 59-5

**Examples of Drugs with Probable or Known Risk to Pregnancy in Dogs and Cats**

**Hormones**

| | |
|---|---|
| Androgens | Excessive thyroid |
| Bromocriptine | hormone replacement |
| Estrogens | Glucocorticoids |
| | Prostaglandins |

**Antimicrobials**

| | |
|---|---|
| Aminoglycosides | Enrofloxacin |
| Amphotericin-B | Griseofulvin |
| Chloramphenicol | Metronidazole |
| Ciprofloxacin | Oxytetracycline |
| Doxycycline | Tetracycline |

**Nonsteroidal Antiinflammatory Drugs**

**Anticonvulsants**

**Anticancer Drugs**

**Ansesthetics/Preanesthetics**

Barbiturates
Diazepam
Halothane
Methoxyflurane

**Antiparasitic Drugs**

Amitraz
Levamisole
Thiacetarsamide
Trichlorfon

**Miscellaneous**

| | |
|---|---|
| Captopril | Methocarbamol |
| Dantrolene | Methscopolamine |
| Dimethylsulfoxide (DMSO) | Mitotane (o,'p'-DDD) |
| Diphenoxylate | Nitroglycerin |
| Excessive vitamins | Nitroprusside |
| Isoproterenol | Propranolol |
| Loperamide | Thiazide diuretics |

Fetal anomalies and chromosomal aberrations are reported to be a major cause of spontaneous abortion in humans. Anatomic abnormalities are found in 20% of kittens that are stillborn or that die during the first 3 days of life. Most congenital fetal anomalies have no identifiable cause. Some are known to be heritable. Some are caused by environmental factors such as exposure to teratogens. Chromosomal anomalies have been poorly investigated as a cause of spontaneous abortion in domestic animals, but they have been identified in some stillborn kittens and puppies.

### Diagnosis

The diagnostic efforts are directed toward finding the cause so that (1) the dam and any remaining viable fetuses can be treated properly, (2) the problem can be avoided during the subsequent pregnancies of this particular female, and (3) the rest of the colony can be protected from similar occurrences. The diagnostic approach should begin with a thorough history-taking concerning such factors as changes in the bitch's or queen's environment, the recent addition of new animals to the house or kennel, the vaccination status of the animal, current drug therapy being given, and dietary supplements being administered. This should provide clues to possible exposure to infectious agents and teratogens. Many of the potential causes of fetal resorption-abortion-stillbirth can be excluded or identified during a careful history taking.

The dam should be thoroughly examined for signs of illness and for the presence of remaining fetuses. Bitches and queens may abort part of a litter and carry the rest to term. Abdominal palpation, radiologic studies, and ultrasonography can help in determining the status of the uterine contents. Of the three, ultrasonography is most helpful in assessing the viability of any remaining fetuses. The metabolic status of the dam or queen should be determined with appropriate laboratory tests, such as a CBC, a serum biochemistry profile, and urinalysis. A sample of the uterine discharge obtained from the anterior vagina should be submitted for bacterial culture and antibiotic sensitivity testing. Appropriate serologic tests (e.g., *Brucella* titer, FeLV, feline immunodeficiency virus [FIV]) should also be performed on the dam.

The abortus and placenta should be submitted for gross, microscopic, and microbiologic examinations. This complete postmortem examination of the abortus is the single most helpful procedure when one is attempting to identify the causes of fetal abortion-stillbirth. Chromosomal analysis of the fetus can also be considered, but this is rarely performed (see p. 858).

Hereditary causes of fetal anomalies may be difficult to prove. Knowledge of the hereditary defects common to the breed is an important aspect of such investigations. The breeding records of related animals should be scrutinized to determine whether there have been similar occurrences. If any are found, hereditary causes become more likely. If birth defects occur in subsequent litters from the same dam and sire, both should be eliminated from the breeding program. If hereditary causes and environmental causes (i.e., exposure to teratogens) can be ruled out, the dam and sire can reasonably be bred again because most birth defects have no identifiable cause, occur sporadically as isolated events, and do not recur in subsequent pregnancies.

### Treatment

Therapy for the aborting female is supportive and symptomatic, unless a cause can be found. If viable fetuses remain, the pregnancy can be allowed to continue. If not, any remaining contents of the uterus should be removed by ovariohysterectomy or through the administration of ecbolic agents. Oxytocin (1 to 10 U IM) and natural $PGF_{2\alpha}$ (0.1 to 0.25 mg/kg SC) promote uterine evacuation. Antibiotics should be administered as soon as appropriate specimens for microbiologic and serologic studies have been obtained. In many bitches and queens, fetal resorption-abortion-stillbirth is an isolated event with no identifiable cause or treatment. Subsequent breedings are often uneventful.

## NEONATAL MORBIDITY AND MORTALITY

The first 2 weeks of life are the most precarious for puppies and kittens. Almost all preweaning losses occur during this time and are highest during the first 3 days. Many of those early deaths are related to prolonged parturition and fetal stress. Depending on the management practices and the breeds involved, typically 10% to 15% of all full-term neonates are lost. Losses as high as 30% are also reported, but this is unacceptably high. Stillbirths account for about half of these losses. Ideally, postweaning losses should not exceed 1% to 1.5%. Early preweaning neonatal vulnerability is influenced most by the dam and by the environment into which the neonates are born.

A thorough history, including the events of parturition, is followed by examination of the affected neonate, its dam and littermates, and the environment. Examination of only the affected neonate is insufficient. The importance of a thorough postmortem examination to identify the cause of any unexplained death cannot be overemphasized. The findings determine how to treat or protect the remaining littermates or the dam, how to protect the rest of the colony, and, finally, how to prevent recurrence in future litters of this dam.

### ENVIRONMENTAL FACTORS

The environmental factors of greatest concern are sanitation, control of infectious diseases, appropriate environmental temperature and humidity, and adequate privacy. Environmental temperatures of 29.4° C (85° F) and humidity of 55% to 65% are often recommended for puppies and kittens. However, these must be adjusted for each colony. For example, maintenance of the recommended temperature and humidity does not prevent neonates from becoming chilled if the environment is also damp or drafty. Conversely, some heavy-coated breeds can be uncomfortably warm and may refuse to "cuddle" their young if the temperature is as high as that recommended. Many household pets, both bitches and queens, rear healthy litters in homes where room temperatures are 21.1° to 23.9° C (70° to 75° F) with an ambient humidity. Heat sources can also be used to obtain a temperature of 26.7° to 29.4° C (80° to 85° F) in part of the whelping box. The dam can then move herself and the litter to whatever temperature is appropriate. Whenever heat sources are used, however, extreme caution must be exercised. Because neonatal reflexes and mobility are both extremely limited, puppies and kittens can easily be burned.

Privacy is usually provided in the form of a whelping or kittening box that is placed in a suitably warm and quiet room. The box should be large enough to allow the dam to lie comfortably away from the litter but small enough to keep the young safely confined. The dam should be able to easily enter and leave the box. Bedding should be provided so that the dam can nest.

The whelping-kittening box provides an identifiable, private place for the dam and shelter for the litter.

A quiet, familiar, private environment is important for several reasons. Primarily, the dam must feel secure and safe. If she is nervous or frightened, labor may be prolonged and milk letdown may be inhibited, both of which contribute to the occurrence of neonatal losses. The dam may also spend excessive energy protecting her young and moving them from place to place, rather than caring for them. She may injure or cannibalize them. Visitors should not be allowed for the first 3 days. By 4 days, most dams are relaxed and willing to tolerate visitors, but they should not be excessive. Frequent, gentle handling of the young after 4 days is encouraged because it seems to improve their socialization with people.

The second reason for providing a private environment is to restrict exposure to infectious diseases. Other animals in the colony should never be allowed to mingle with the newborns. The nursery should be attended by a limited number of people who pay strict attention to washing their hands and equipment before coming in contact with the young.

## THE DAM

The dam provides all the necessities of early life: warmth, nutrition, and sanitation. The outcome of pregnancy depends largely on the overall health of the dam. Only healthy animals in excellent physical condition should be bred. The breeding of aged dams should be discouraged. Neonatal mortality is greatest in litters born to older, heavier dams and to queens that are older than 3 years at the time of first parity. Vaccinations, deworming, and other health maintenance measures should be completed before breeding or after weaning. Anything affecting the dam is also likely to affect the neonate. Ill or neglected puppies and kittens are often the first sign of maternal illness. Two fairly common postpartum disorders that are often evidenced by neonatal neglect are mastitis (see p. 882) and metritis (see p. 896). If one neonate is ill, the entire litter and the dam should be examined.

## THE NEONATE

Newborn puppies and kittens should be round and sleek, with good muscle tone and pink mucous membranes. Respiratory rates are 15 to 35 breaths/min. Heart rates are greater than 200 bpm for the first 2 weeks. Neonatal puppies and kittens are incapable of thermoregulation until they are 2 weeks old. The normal rectal temperature at birth is 35.6° to 36.1° C (96° to 97° F). It gradually increases to 37.8° C (100° F) by 7 days of age.

The normal birth weight of kittens is 100 g ±10 g. The minimum expected weight gain is 7 to 10 g/day. By 6 weeks of age, kittens should weigh at least 500 g. The normal birth weight of puppies varies with the breed, ranging from 100 to 750 g. Puppies should gain 5% to 10% of their birth weight per day, such that by 10 to 12 days of age they weigh twice their birth weight. Neonates with less-than-normal birth weights are often ineffective at nursing, and the death rate is highest in these animals. Some normal neonates may not nurse well during the first 24 hours; however, they should learn quickly and begin gaining weight by the second day of life. Weight loss is not normal.

## Clinical Features of Neonatal Illness

The most common clinical signs of neonatal illness are persistent crying; decreased activity, including decreased nursing; failure to gain weight; a dry, rough haircoat; and decreased muscle tone. Crying for more than 20 minutes is abnormal. It may indicate that the neonate is cold, hungry, neglected, or ill. Eventually the ill neonate will quit crying and become increasingly less active. Like crying, decreased activity is an early, but nonspecific, sign of neonatal illness.

If littermates pile on top of one another, they are probably cold. If they are widely separated, not touching each other or the dam, they may be too warm, or conversely, they may be so cold that the dam has culled them. If, in the absence of infection, the skin and mucous membranes of neonates are hyperemic or if animals older than 2 weeks of age are panting, they are probably too hot.

Failure to gain weight at the expected rate is another sign of neonatal illness. Supplemental bottle or tube feeding of milk replacer should be initiated in such animals. A foster mother, if another lactating female is available, should be considered, especially if the failure to gain weight is a result of inadequate lactation or maternal neglect. If the neonate loses more than 10% of its birth weight, the chances for survival are very poor.

A dry, rough haircoat can be a sign of neonatal illness or maternal neglect. Decreased muscle tone, resulting in a limp or flat appearance, is a grave sign. Other signs of illness (e.g., dehydration, cyanosis, pale mucous membranes) are interpreted in the same way in neonates as they are in older animals. However, the signs of illness in the neonate should always be viewed with greater concern than they are in the adult, because signs in neonates usually progress in a matter of hours, as opposed to days in older animals.

## Common Causes of Neonatal Mortality

Causes of death in neonates can be divided into infectious and noninfectious causes. Noninfectious causes account for most deaths in neonates from 0 to 3 days of age. They include hypothermia, hypoglycemia, stillbirth and anatomic abnormalities, and trauma.

**Hypothermia.** Hypothermia is a common cause of neonatal death. Immediately after birth puppies' temperatures plummet unless they are vigorously attended. They also have significant mixed metabolic and respiratory acidosis, which is likely to worsen if hypothermia persists. The importance of a proper environmental temperature and of adequate maternal care to maintain body temperature cannot be overemphasized. As noted earlier, puppies and kittens can become chilled in a damp, drafty environment, even though the temperature is appropriate. Clipping the hair on the ventrum of dams with very heavy coats, such as Siberian Huskies, may enable them to better recognize cool temperatures and be more willing to snuggle with their young. A sign of hypothermia is crying followed by decreasing activity. Dams may cull cold puppies and kittens as if they were already dead.

Hypothermic neonates should be warmed slowly until their rectal temperature is 36.1° to 36.7° C (97° to 98° F). As the neonate is warmed, it becomes more active. Once it is warmed, the dam will usually accept it again. Neonates that do not begin to respond during the first few hours are unlikely to do so and usually die. The cause of hypothermia must be found and eliminated.

**Hypoglycemia.** Hypoglycemia is another common cause of neonatal mortality. Neonates have fewer gluconeogenic precursors and less ability to generate or use other energy sources than adults do. They also have a much greater glucose requirement. Therefore increases in demand or reductions in intake may precipitate hypoglycemia more easily. Clinical signs include weakness and decreased activity, crying, bradycardia, respiratory distress, convulsions, and coma.

Anything that interferes with the quality or quantity of the dam's milk can cause hypoglycemia. Hypothermia lower than 34.4° C (94° F) can also cause hypoglycemia in the neonate because digestive functions then cease. Septicemia is another cause of hypoglycemia. Glucose solutions should be used to treat hypoglycemia while the cause is being sought. They are usually administered orally, so they need not be isotonic. Caloric needs are not met by glucose solutions; thus feedings with milk replacer or milk should be reinstituted as soon as possible. Hypothermia must be corrected, however, before oral milk or milk replacer can be digested and absorbed.

**Stillbirths and anatomic abnormalities.** Stillbirths, anatomic abnormalities, and low birth weights can account for more than 50% of kitten deaths in some colonies. The causes should be determined whenever possible to prevent this from happening in subsequent litters. Females that consistently produce offspring with low birth weights should be retired from breeding.

**Trauma.** Trauma and infection can occur in neonates of any age, but they are the more common causes of death in those older than 4 days. Trauma may account for as much as 37% of neonatal deaths in puppies and kittens. The dam can cause accidental puncture wounds, umbilical herniation, or crushing. Most commonly it is nervous or frightened dams that bite or cannibalize their puppies or kittens. Every effort should therefore be made to provide a stress-free environment so that the entire litter is not killed. Tranquilization may be considered to calm very anxious dams. Dams that exhibit this behavior toward one or more litters should be culled from the breeding program.

**Infection.** Although the dam and other adults in the colony may show no clinical signs of disease, they are usually the source of the infectious agents. The neonates can become infected in utero, during passage through the birth canal, through the umbilicus, or through the oronasal route. Poor environmental conditions, inadequate sanitation practices, and the intermingling of animals of all ages increase the neonates' exposure to infectious agents. Infectious agents known to cause neonatal death are listed in Table 59-6.

A thorough postmortem examination is the best means of establishing the diagnosis of infectious causes of neonatal illness and death. Some infectious agents produce a character-

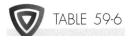

### TABLE 59-6

**Infectious Causes of Neonatal Morbidity and Mortality**

**Viral Causes**

Parvovirus
Feline leukemia virus
Herpesvirus
Canine adenovirus I
Canine distemper virus
(Role of coronavirus and rotavirus not established)

**Bacterial Causes**

*Escherichia coli*
Hemolytic and nonhemolytic *Streptococcus* spp.
*Staphylococcus*
*Bordetella* spp.
*Pasteurella* spp.
*Salmonella* spp.
*Brucella* spp.
*Campylobacter* spp.

**Parasitic Causes**

*Toxocara* spp.
*Ancyclostoma* spp.
*Giardia* spp.
*Coccidium* spp.
*Cryptosporidium* spp.

istic pathology that can be identified by gross examination. For example, hemorrhagic and necrotizing renal lesions are found in puppies with canine herpesvirus infection and adult parasites are found in the intestinal tract of animals dying of parasitism. More commonly, however, additional testing is usually necessary to establish the definitive diagnosis. Samples of liver, spleen, lung, and gastrointestinal tract should routinely be submitted for histopathologic examination, bacterial culture, and virus isolation. If obvious lesions are found during the gross examination, specimens of them should be submitted as well. For some infectious diseases, such as brucellosis, it may be helpful to perform serologic tests or cultures on the dam or other colony members to establish the source or extent of infection.

### Suggested Readings

Allen WE et al: Detection of pregnancy in the bitch: a study of abdominal palpation, A-mode ultrasound, and Doppler ultrasound techniques, *J Small Anim Pract* 22:609, 1981.

Aroch et al: Paresis and unusual electrocardiographic signs in a severely hypomagnesaemic, hypocalcemic lactating bitch, *J Small Anim Pract* 39:299, 1998.

Baldwin CJ: Pregnancy termination in the domestic cat using natural prostaglandins, *Proceedings of the Annual Conference of the Society for Theriogenology and American College of Theriogenology,* San Antonio, Tex, 1995, p 169.

Bouchard G, Sinclair Research Center, Columbia, Mo. Personal communication, 2002.

Caldow GL et al: Abortion in foxhounds and a ewe flock associated with *Salmonella montevideo* infection, *Vet Rec* 142:138, 1998.

Concannon PW et al, editors: Fertility and infertility in dogs, cats and other carnivores, *J Reprod Fertil Suppl* 47, 1993.

Copley K: Comparison of traditional methods for evaluating parturition in the bitch versus using external uterine and fetal monitors, *Proceedings of the Annual Conference of the Society for Theriogenology and American College of Theriogenology,* Colorado Springs, Colo, 2002, p 375.

Cortese L et al: Hyperprolactinemia and galactorrhea associated with primary hypothyroidism in a bitch, *J Small Anim Pract* 38:572, 1997.

Davidson AP, editor: Clinical theriogenology, *Vet Clin North Am* 31:209, 2001.

Drobatz KJ et al: Eclampsia in dogs: 31 cases (1995-1998), *J Am Vet Med Assoc* 217:216, 2000.

England GCW: Complications of treating presumed psuedopregnancy in pregnant bitches, *Vet Rec* 142:369, 1998.

England GCW et al: *Manual of small animal reproduction and neonatology,* Cheltenham, UK, 1998, British Small Animal Veterinary Association.

Fascetti AJ et al: Preparturient hypocalcemia in four cats, *J Am Vet Med Assoc* 215:1127, 1999.

Feldman EC et al: Prostaglandin induction of abortion in pregnant bitches after misalliance, *J Am Vet Med Assoc* 202:1855, 1993.

Gardil CM et al: Pregnancy diagnosis in the bitch. In Bonagura JD, editor: *Kirk's current veterinary therapy XIII,* Philadelphia, 2000, WB Saunders, p 918.

Gobello C et al: Dioestrous ovariectomy: a model to study the role of progesterone in the onset of canine pseudopregnancy, *J Reprod Fertil Suppl* 57:55, 2001.

Gobello C et al: Use of prostaglandins and bromocriptine mesylate for pregnancy termination in bitches, *J Am Vet Med Assoc* 220:1017, 2002.

Harvey MJA et al: A study of the aetiology of pseudopregnancy in the bitch and the effect of cabergoline therapy, *Vet Rec* 144:433, 1999.

Johnson CA: Dystocia, *Compendium's Standards of Care: Emergency and Critical Care* 3:8, 2001.

Johnston SD et al, editors: *Canine and feline theriogenology,* Philadelphia, 2001, WB Saunders.

Kelley R: Canine reproductive management: factors affecting litter size, *Proceedings of the Annual Conference of the Society for Theriogenology and American College of Theriogenology,* Colorado Springs, Colo, 2002, p 291.

Lawler DF et al, editors: Pediatrics, *Vet Clin North Am Small Anim Pract* 17:505, 1987.

Lawler DF et al: Influence of restricted food intake on estrous cycles and pseudopregnancies in dogs, *Am J Vet Res* 60:820, 1999.

Linde-Forsberg C et al: Abnormalities in pregnancy, parturition and the periparturient period. In Ettinger SJ et al, editors: *Textbook of veterinary internal medicine,* ed 5, Philadelphia, 2000, WB Saunders, p 1527.

Moon PF et al: Perioperative management and mortality rates of dogs undergoing Caesarean section in the United States and Canada, *J Am Vet Med Assoc,* 213:365, 1998.

Onclin K et al: Comparisons of different combinations of analogues of $PGF_{2\alpha}$ and dopamine agonists for the termination of pregnancy in dogs, *Vet Rec* 144:416, 1999.

Schweizer CM et al: Medical management of dystocia and indications for cesarean section in the bitch. In Bonagura JD, editor: *Kirk's current veterinary therapy XIII,* Philadelphia, 2000, WB Saunders, p 933.

Slatter DH, editor: *Textbook of small animal surgery,* Philadelphia, 1985, WB Saunders.

van der Weyden et al: Physiological aspects of pregnancy and parturition in dogs, *J Reprod Fert Suppl* 39:211, 1989.

van Vuuren M et al: Characterization of a potentially abortigenic strain of feline calicivirus isolated from a domestic cat, *Vet Rec* 144:636, 1999.

Yeager AE et al: Ultrasonography of the reproductive tract of the female dog and cat. In Bonagura JD, editor: *Kirk's current veterinary therapy XII,* Philadelphia, 1995, WB Saunders, p 1040.

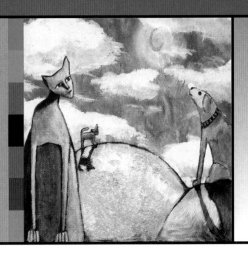

# CHAPTER 60

# Disorders of Male Fertility

## CHAPTER OUTLINE

NORMAL SEXUAL DEVELOPMENT
AND BEHAVIOR, 905
    Testicular descent, 905
    Puberty, 905
    Reproductive physiology, 905
    Age-related effects, 906
    Breeding behavior, 907
DIAGNOSTIC TECHNIQUES TO ASSESS
REPRODUCTIVE FUNCTION, 907
    Semen collection and evaluation, 907
    Bacterial culture of semen, 911
    Radiography and ultrasonography, 912
    Testicular aspiration and biopsy, 912
    Hormonal evaluation, 912
DIAGNOSTIC APPROACH TO INFERTILITY, 913
    Physical examination, 914
    Semen evaluation, 914
OLIGOZOOSPERMIA AND AZOOSPERMIA, 915
CONGENITAL INFERTILITY, 916
ACQUIRED INFERTILITY, 916

## NORMAL SEXUAL DEVELOPMENT AND BEHAVIOR

### TESTICULAR DESCENT

The age at which testicular descent normally occurs in dogs or cats has not been firmly established. In cats, testicular descent appears to be a prenatal event. In dogs, it is a postnatal event that should occur by 10 days of age. Cryptorchidism (see p. 922) should be suspected if the testes are not palpable within the scrotum by 8 weeks of age.

### PUBERTY

Sexual and physical maturity usually coincide in males. Puberty occurs around 9 to 10 months of age in tomcats. The same is generally true for dogs, but the large and giant breeds mature more slowly. The onset of puberty is signaled by the development of masculine physical characteristics and sexual behavior, such as the mounting of less-dominant members of the colony and territorial urine marking. Semen quality and serum concentrations of testosterone gradually approach those of mature males, although prepubescent males may be fertile.

### REPRODUCTIVE PHYSIOLOGY

The testis has three functional compartments (interstitial, basal, adluminal) that are controlled by, and in turn provide feedback to, the hypothalamus, the pituitary, and each other (see Fig. 56-4). The Leydig cells, which produce testosterone, estradiol, and other hormones, are located in the interstitial compartment. Luteinizing hormone (LH) stimulates the Leydig cells to produce pregnenolone from cholesterol. Within the Leydig cells, pregnenolone is then metabolized into the other steroid hormones, the most important of which are testosterone and estradiol.

Testosterone promotes the development of the vas deferens and epididymis, initiates and maintains all aspects of spermatogenesis, supports libido, and regulates the secretion of gonadotropin-releasing hormone (GnRH) by the hypothalamus and gonadotropins (LH, follicle-stimulating hormone [FSH]) by the pituitary. The testicular concentrations of testosterone are much greater (50 times or more) than those of serum. The administration of testosterone or other androgenic steroids for pharmacologic purposes results in suppression of the hypothalamic-pituitary-testicular axis and thus a diminishment of all the functions of testosterone just listed. The end result may be sterility.

Testosterone also serves as a prohormone for dihydrotestosterone and estradiol, which are formed in the testes, as well as in peripheral tissues. These metabolites of testosterone act directly at the tissue of origin, such as the prostate, or enter the circulation and act elsewhere. Dihydrotestosterone causes the prostate to mature, the external genitalia to develop and grow, and the male secondary sex characteristics to develop at puberty. Most of the estradiol in adult males is formed by the extragonadal aromatization of circulating testosterone, and the remainder is secreted directly by the testes.

The second functional compartment of the testis is the basal compartment. It is composed of spermatogonia and Sertoli cells. Cytoplasmic processes from Sertoli cells extend from the lamina propria of the seminiferous tubules (basal compartment) to the tubular lumen. These cytoplasmic processes surround the developing germ cells in the basal and adluminal compartments. Sertoli cell function is regulated by FSH and testosterone. Sertoli cells produce several substances that are necessary for spermatogenesis and for normal spermatid maturation. In fact, spermatogenesis is regulated by the effects of FSH on Sertoli cells, not by any direct effect of FSH on germ cells. Specific functions of Sertoli cells vary according to the developmental stage of the germ cells they surround. These may also vary depending on the species of animal.

Sertoli cells convert testosterone, produced by the Leydig cells, to estradiol. This is especially apparent in prepubertal animals. Most of the testicular estradiol in adults appears to originate from Leydig cells. The role of estradiol in male reproduction is unclear. Along with testosterone, it is involved in the regulation of gonadotropin secretion. In some instances, estrogens augment the effects of androgens, such as in the canine prostate, where estradiol regulates the number of dihydrotestosterone receptors. In the mammary gland estrogens seem to have antiandrogenic effects.

Sertoli cells also produce a substance known as *androgen-binding protein,* which is thought to moderate the effects of testosterone. It may also be involved in the transport of testosterone within the testis and epididymis. Sertoli cells also produce the hormones inhibin and activin. Inhibin causes a decrease in FSH secretion by the pituitary. Activin has the opposite effect on FSH secretion. The fetal and neonatal Sertoli cells produce müllerian inhibiting substance, which causes müllerian ducts to regress during sexual differentiation.

## Spermatogenesis

*Spermatogenesis* refers to the maintenance of spermatogonial numbers and the differentiation of spermatogonia (germ cells) into spermatozoa. It takes place within the seminiferous tubules (Fig. 60-1). Both proliferating and noncommitted spermatogonia are located nearest the tubular basement membrane. As the germ cells mature into spermatocytes and eventually spermatids, they move toward the tubular lumen, such that the most differentiated cells are nearest the lumen. The adluminal compartment, which is the third functional compartment of the testis, contains the primary spermatocytes and spermatids.

Eight to 10 different stages of sperm development, or cellular associations, have been identified in dogs. They comprise several stages of maturation of spermatogonia, then several stages of maturing spermatocytes, and finally several stages of maturing spermatids. A cross section of any given normal seminiferous tubule contains all of these different stages of developing spermatozoa.

In addition to the proliferating spermatogonia, there is a population of noncommitted spermatogonia that are called

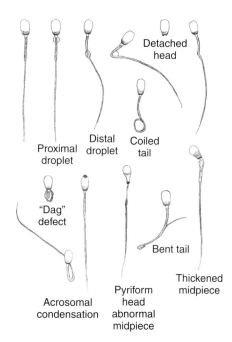

**FIG 60-1**
Morphologic appearance of canine spermatozoa.

$A_0$-*spermatogonia.* These spermatogonia remain in "reserve" and, unlike proliferating spermatogonia, are quite resistant to damage by toxins and radiation. The recovery of spermatogenesis that occurs after testicular injury results from the repopulation of the germinal epithelium by the progeny of the $A_0$-spermatogonia. Approximately 62 days elapse from the time $A_0$-spermatogonia begin to differentiate into mature spermatogonia until the time mature spermatozoa are released into the tubular lumen. This is the duration of spermatogenesis in dogs. It then takes approximately 14 days for spermatozoa to become fully mature and motile in the epididymis. The duration of spermatogenesis in cats is unknown. Frequent ejaculation does not influence daily sperm production, but it does influence the number of sperm ejaculated by depleting the extragonadal reserves in the epididymis and vas deferens.

## AGE-RELATED EFFECTS

Reportedly, semen quality and libido tend to decline with advancing age, especially in geriatric males. No age-related changes in concentrations of steroid hormones and gonadotropin concentrations were found in dogs. Although males are fertile long past 6 years of age, they often are less active in breeding programs. This is primarily because they are replaced by younger males with similar or preferred phenotypic and genotypic qualities. Because other health problems often develop in older animals, their physical ability to mate may decline. Undesirable behavior is cited as a common reason for retiring older tomcats from breeding colonies.

# BREEDING BEHAVIOR

Much of normal breeding behavior is learned by dogs and cats. Consequently, early breeding experiences help to determine a male's future success as a stud. There is usually one dominant male in any specific territory. Even if all males are given equal opportunity, most of the breedings will be done by the dominant male of the colony. Establishing dominance and territory is usually a prerequisite to mating; therefore the standard practice is to bring the female to the male. Because successful studs must be physically, sexually, and socially mature, it is usually recommended that males not enter a breeding program until they are at least 12 months old, even though puberty may have occurred months earlier. Dogs that are used in an artificial insemination program may become so accustomed to semen collection that they are no longer interested in natural service.

Ideally a sexually inexperienced male should first be exposed to a docile, experienced female in his own territory. Virgin males should be expected to have unproductive nervous energy. They usually make many unsuccessful attempts to mount before achieving intromission. This first encounter should be short and well supervised so that the male does not become frustrated or exhausted by his unsuccessful attempts to copulate, or worse, become intimidated or actually injured by an aggressive female. There may be an advantage to introducing the breeding pair early in or before estrus so that it is not urgent that insemination occur immediately. However, the physical and psychologic well-being of the male must be protected during such an introduction, because any attempts to actually copulate will be actively rebuffed by females that are not in estrus.

Both male dogs and cats initially approach the female's face. If the male is not rebuffed, he then investigates the perineum. The amount of foreplay varies among individual animals and breeding pairs. The tomcat typically grasps the queen's neck near her shoulders and straddles her with his front feet. The neck grasp is thought to be necessary to restrain the female and to properly position both animals' rear quarters to allow intromission to occur. The rear quarters are then straddled, and intromission occurs.

Because the canine os penis maintains rigidity, intromission can and does occur before the penis is actually erect. During erection the bulbus glandis of the canine penis swells twofold to threefold, filling the vestibule and preventing separation of the breeding pair. The first two seminal fractions begin to be ejaculated shortly after intromission, during the rapid pelvic thrusting. Soon after the dog's pelvic thrusting subsides, he dismounts and faces away from the bitch, but the erect penis, having turned 180 degrees in a horizontal plane, remains in the bitch. This is known as the *postcoital lock* or *tie*. Ejaculation, primarily of the third fraction, which consists of prostatic fluid, continues during the tie. The tie persists until the dog's erection subsides 15 to 30 minutes or more later. If the dog's penis is erect before intromission, complete intromission is not possible and a tie will not occur. Some dog owners refer to this as an "outside tie." In this situation, the entire ejaculate may not be deposited in the bitch.

# DIAGNOSTIC TECHNIQUES TO ASSESS REPRODUCTIVE FUNCTION

## SEMEN COLLECTION AND EVALUATION
### Indications

Semen is collected and evaluated if artificial insemination is to be performed, if semen is to be preserved by freezing, as a routine part of a breeding soundness examination, and for evaluation of male infertility. Cytologic evaluation of the ejaculate is also used to evaluate diseases of the prostate, testes, and epididymides.

### Technique

The quality of the ejaculate varies with the collection technique, the degree of sexual arousal, the frequency of ejaculation, age, testicular size, and the amount of seminal fluid collected. General anesthesia and electroejaculation are usually required to obtain semen from cats. Although the procedure is not difficult, it does require an electroejaculation unit and therefore is not commonly performed in clinical practice. Some cats can also be trained to ejaculate into an artificial vagina, but again this is not usually performed in clinical practice.

Semen is easily collected from dogs, especially those with previous breeding experience. The dog is encouraged to ejaculate by manually stimulating the penis through the prepuce or artificial vagina. The presence of an estrual bitch may improve the quality of the ejaculate, especially in inexperienced or timid dogs. The collection area should be quiet and free from distractions, with secure footing for the animals.

Canine semen is ejaculated in three fractions. The first fraction is composed of a few drops of a clear fluid that originates from the prostate. Certain dogs may ejaculate several milliliters of this presperm fraction. The second fraction is the sperm-rich fraction. The volume varies from 0.5 to 5 ml, depending on testicular size and individual variation. The sperm-rich fraction appears cloudy and opalescent. Usually no attempt is made to separate the first two fractions.

The third and largest fraction is prostatic fluid, of which there may be as much as 30 ml. Normal prostatic fluid is clear and easily differentiated from the milky, sperm-rich fraction. For routine semen evaluation and artificial insemination, it is only necessary to collect enough prostatic fluid to ensure that the entire sperm-rich fraction has been ejaculated.

Semen must be handled carefully. All equipment should be clean and free of contaminants, including water and excessive lubricant. The sample must be protected against sudden changes in temperature. Normal dog semen can usually be handled at room temperature for 15 to 30 minutes without adverse effects. Nevertheless, the sample should be processed promptly. Slides and coverslips should be maintained at 37° C.

The semen sample is evaluated from the standpoint of its volume, color, and the concentration, motility, and morphology of the spermatozoa. Complete cytologic examination, pH determination, alkaline phosphatase determination, and bacterial culture of the ejaculate may also be indicated. Because feline semen is rarely evaluated in clinical practice, the interested reader is referred to Howard (1992) and Johnston and colleagues (2001) for additional information (see Suggested Readings). The discussion that follows pertains only to dogs, except as otherwise indicated. However, the principles discussed are applicable to animals in general.

## Volume

The seminal volume is determined directly from the calibrated tube into which the sample is collected. Volumes tend to be smaller in young dogs than in mature dogs. Volume does not usually correlate with fertility unless the animal fails to ejaculate an adequate amount of the sperm-rich fraction. For intravaginal artificial insemination a minimal volume of 2 to 10 ml may be necessary, because the spermatozoa may be deposited some distance from the cervix; however, this has not yet been thoroughly investigated. Conversely, for intrauterine insemination, a volume of 4 ml or less is used. This is accomplished by centrifugation of the sample to concentrate the number of sperm/unit volume.

## Color

The color is assessed by direct visualization. Dog semen is normally white to opalescent and opaque. If it is yellow, this may indicate the presence of urine. To avoid urine contamination, dogs should not be allowed to micturate immediately before semen collection. Some males urinate during ejaculation, which is not normal. They are usually subfertile. Red or brownish semen usually contains blood. Blood in an ejaculate usually originates from the prostate, or it results from damage to small surface vessels of the erect penis that has occurred during collection. The latter source of hemorrhage can easily be excluded by prompt inspection of the penile surface. If there are many inflammatory cells in the semen, this may cause it to be flocculated or yellow-green. Inflammatory cells can originate from anywhere in the urinary or genital tract, including smegma from the prepucial cavity. If an ejaculate with many inflammatory cells is obtained, a quantitative culture for bacteria and *Mycoplasma* organisms should be performed. Dogs should also be tested for *Brucella canis* infection (see p. 936). Any abnormally colored samples should be closely examined to determine the cause. Cytologic evaluation of the semen is important.

## Spermatozoa Concentration

The volume and thus the concentration are influenced most by the (essentially) sperm-free prostatic fluid. For this reason, the number of sperm in the total ejaculate, rather than the number of sperm per milliliter of semen, is assessed. The number of sperm may be determined with spectrophotometric methods. However, in many veterinary practices the number of sperm is determined using a hemocytometer and white blood cell (WBC)/platelet dilution pipettes (Unopette; Becton-Dickinson and Co., Rutherford, N.J.) that dilute the sample 1:100. Highly concentrated samples can be diluted with red blood cell (RBC) pipettes, which dilute the sample 1:200. The concentration of spermatozoa is determined by counting the cells of the diluted sample in a hemocytometer. It may be unnecessary to dilute oligozoospermic samples before counting.

The actual counting method used to determine the concentration varies among laboratories. Most methods are equally acceptable, provided the principles of the hemocytometer are kept in mind: the hemocytometer has nine 1 mm squares ($1 \times 1$ mm) etched on it; the center 1 mm square has 25 subdivisions; and the coverslip is 0.1 mm above the etched surface. When using the WBC technique, the spermatozoa in the outer four squares are usually counted. When using the RBC technique, the spermatozoa in five of the 25 subdivisions of the center square ($5/25 = 1/5$ mm$^2$) are counted. Whatever the method, the following factors are used to calculate the number of spermatozoa per milliliter:

**Number of sperm counted:**
Chamber is 0.1 mm deep—multiply by 10.
X mm squares were counted—divide by X.
Sample was diluted—multiply by dilution factor.
1 ml = 1000 mm$^3$—multiply by 1000.

The number of sperm per milliliter of ejaculate is then multiplied by the volume (milliliters) of the ejaculate to obtain the number of sperm per ejaculate. The number of sperm per ejaculate in normal dogs is $250 \times 10^6$ to $2000 \times 10^6$.

The breed of dog, size of the testes, and frequency of ejaculation affect the number of sperm ejaculated. Because the spermatogenic potential is directly related to testicular size, smaller breeds of dogs are expected to have fewer sperm per ejaculate than large breeds of dogs. Although it has been stated that testicular sperm production is also directly related to body weight, this holds only for animals with a normal conformation and body weight. The relationship between sperm production and body weight is lost in obese dogs. Frequent ejaculation depletes extragonadal reserves, causing a reduction in the number of sperm ejaculated. As a general rule, a total number of less than $200 \times 10^6$ sperm in any sample from a mature dog should be considered abnormally low (oligozoospermic), regardless of the breed of dog or frequency of ejaculation.

## Motility

To assess spermatozoal motility, a drop of undiluted semen is placed on a warm slide, covered with a warm coverslip, and examined by phase-contrast or light microscopy using the $40\times$ and $100\times$ objectives. Very concentrated samples should be diluted with warm 2.9% sodium citrate or phosphate-buffered saline solution to permit careful evaluation of individual spermatozoa. The percentage of motile sperm is then estimated. In the normal dog, more than 70% of the sperm should show rapid, steady, progressively forward motility. Although not a precise measure, assessment of motility is considered a critical part of semen evaluation because it gauges spermatozoa function and viability. Very poor samples can be distinguished from very good ones.

*Asthenozoospermia* is the term used to denote low motility. A decrease in the percentage of motile sperm is one of the first detectable changes after testicular injury. It may also be found in the setting of incomplete ejaculation. The percentage of motile sperm and the vigor of the movement can be spuriously diminished if the sample is exposed to excessive heat or cold, contaminated equipment, inflammatory cells, or bacteria. The motility of sperm ejaculated after a long sexual rest may also be poor because of aging of the cells. In addition, sperm in semen that has been chilled or frozen usually does not regain its original motility when warmed. In the case of chilled semen, the percentage of motility may be similar to that seen in fresh semen, but the individual sperm usually move with less vigor. Both the percentage and the speed of motility are usually diminished in thawed, frozen semen. Side-to-side oscillation may be a reflection of chilling, or it may be an artifact, representing the jostling of nonmotile sperm by motile ones. Spermatozoa that move in circles usually do so because of morphologic defects in the tail or midpiece.

## Morphology

The sperm head is composed of the nucleus, which is covered proximally by the acrosome. The equatorial segment of the head represents thinning of the acrosome. The postacrosomal sheath and cell membrane cover the sperm head distally. The sperm tail is composed of the neck, midpiece, principal piece, and end piece. Often the principal piece and end piece together are referred to as the *tail.* The neck is composed of laminated fibers and implantation plates that connect the midpiece to the head at the implantation fossa. A mitochondrial helix surrounds the axoneme of the midpiece. The axoneme is composed of nine microtubule doublets surrounding a central pair of singlet microtubules. A fibrous sheath of nine outer dense fibers surrounds the axoneme of the principal piece. The outer dense fibers gradually dissipate and the end piece begins where the fibrous sheath ends. During spermatogenesis, residual midpiece cytoplasm is extruded at the level of the midpiece.

*Teratozoospermia* refers to abnormal spermatozoal morphology. Primary abnormalities are usually attributed to abnormal spermatogenesis in the testicle, whereas secondary abnormalities are attributed to errors in epididymal maturation or to improper sample handling. Because the morphologic abnormality does not always reflect the site of the lesion, the abnormality should be described specifically, as well as classified as primary or secondary. This may make the interpretation and comparison of samples more accurate. Abnormalities are also classified according to their effect on fertility as being either major or minor in importance.

Although many stains can be used to evaluate sperm morphology, the most common are eosin-nigrosin stains. One drop of semen and one drop of stain are mixed together on a slide and then smeared across several slides. These are allowed to dry and then examined microscopically under oil immersion. A minimum of 100, but preferably 200, spermatozoa is classified as being normal or abnormal (Fig. 60-2). Abnormalities in the size and shape of the head, acrosome, midpiece, or proximal tail, and proximal droplets are usually considered the most severe. Loose or detached heads or acrosomes that are otherwise normal, distal droplets, as well as bent tails, are considered less severe, although they may be the first abnormalities noted after a testicular insult. Less than 20% of the spermatozoa should have morphologic abnormalities. Electron microscopy may provide additional useful information in selected cases.

Bent tails may be caused by cold shock and by the use of a stain or diluent of improper pH or osmolality. The finding of normal motility in a sample with excessive numbers of bent tails should suggest the possibility that the bent tails were caused by the stain, because sperm with bent tails usually cannot move with a straight, forward progression. Abnormalities resulting from improper sample handling should not be found in subsequent, properly handled samples. Persistence of morphologic abnormalities is an indication for further diagnostic evaluation, including semen culture and possibly testicular biopsy (see pp. 911 and 912).

## Cytology

Cells other than spermatozoa found in semen samples should be examined cytologically. Additional slides can be prepared and stained appropriately (e.g., Wright's stain) to evaluate these cells. Cytologic examination of the third fraction of the ejaculate is very helpful in the evaluation of prostatic disorders. A finding of RBCs indicates hemorrhage, whereas a finding of WBCs and macrophages indicates inflammation somewhere in the urogenital tract. The number of WBCs in normal dog semen is apparently less than 2000 per milliliter. Dogs with leukospermia should be tested for *B. canis.* Some epithelial cells are normally present in dog semen, and their numbers increase with sexual rest. If excessive numbers of cells other than spermatozoa are found, further diagnostic assessment of the urogenital tract may be warranted. Crystals may be found in samples contaminated with urine or with talc from the collection equipment.

## Seminal pH

The pH of canine seminal plasma and of prostatic fluid normally ranges from 6.3 to 7.0 and from 6.0 to 7.4, respectively, even in the presence of genital tract disease. Therefore determination of the seminal or prostatic fluid pH is rarely of diagnostic importance in dogs. However, the prostatic fluid pH can be used to determine the optimal antibiotics for treating prostatitis, because penetration of the blood-prostate barrier depends on the degree of ionization and the lipid solubility of the drug. Feline seminal plasma has a pH of about 6.6.

## Seminal Alkaline Phosphatase

The seminal alkaline phosphatase activity in whole semen from normal dogs is reportedly 4000 to 5000 IU/L or greater. The canine epididymis is the source of seminal alkaline phosphatase. Therefore the enzyme can be used as an indicator that epididymal fluid is present in the ejaculate. Azoospermic dogs with low seminal alkaline phosphatase activity may have a bilateral obstruction distal to the epididymides, or ejaculation may have been incomplete. Alkaline phosphatase activity in seminal fluid is determined by the same methods used to

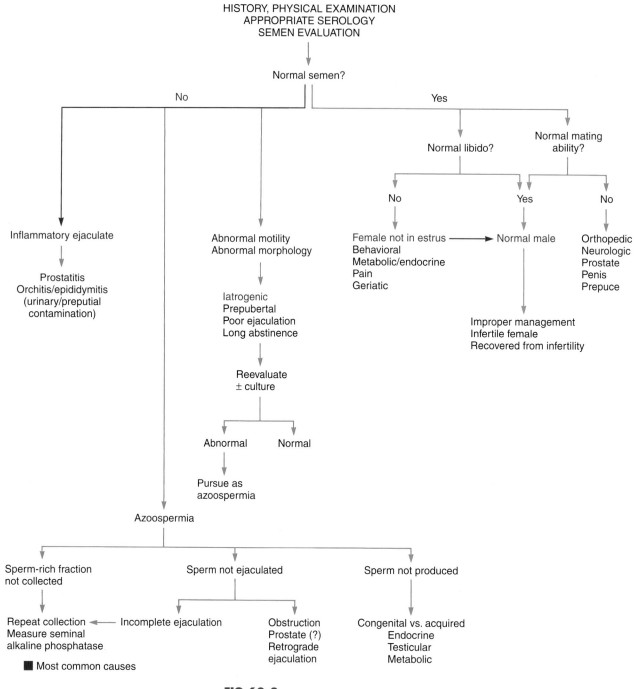

**FIG 60-2**
Diagnostic approach to male infertility.

determine alkaline phosphatase activity in serum. The fraction of feline semen originating from the testis/epididymis also has high concentrations of alkaline phosphatase.

### Interpretation of Semen Evaluation

The seminal characteristics thought to correlate best with fertility are the total number of sperm per ejaculate, motility, and the morphology of spermatozoa. Semen quality is ultimately determined primarily on the basis of these findings. However, the dog's age, testicular size, and frequency of ejac-

ulation must also be considered. The finding of normal semen is not proof of normal fertility, however, because the male must also have a normal libido and normal mating ability. Nevertheless, a dog with normal semen is expected to successfully impregnate a bitch if other factors are favorable. On the other hand, the finding of abnormal semen does not necessarily indicate sterility unless there is azoospermia or complete, true necrozoospermia.

Interestingly, the seminal characteristics of 28 fertile Labrador Retrievers, Golden Retrievers, and German Shepherd Dogs, 2 to 9.5 years of age, that had sired litters before and within 6 months after semen evaluation were not always found to be within the expected normal ranges. In these dogs, motility ranged from 65% to 95% (mean, 89.5%). Total sperm counts ranged from $36 \times 10^6$ to $630 \times 10^6$ (mean, $332.75 \times 10^6$). Normal morphology was found in 62% to 90% (mean, 78.2%) of the spermatozoa. Semen quality in some of these dogs, especially the total spermatozoal output, was less than the usually accepted minimal standard, yet in breeding trials these dogs were found to be fertile. Oettlé (1995) found that if the percentage of morphologically normal sperm was less than 60%, conception rates were very poor, with only 2 of 15 (13%) bitches conceiving.

The quality of a semen sample is a reflection of (1) spermatozoal production during the past 62 days, (2) epididymal maturation during the past 14 days, (3) the extragonadal sperm reserves, which take up to 7 days to be replenished in normal dogs, and (4) the spermatozoal output of that particular ejaculation. Although it has been stated that prolonged abstinence contributes to poor semen quality because of spermatozoa senescence, it is unlikely that abstinence alone causes previously normal semen quality to diminish to the point of oligozoospermia and less than 60% normal morphology and motility. To help establish a prognosis or to resolve doubt about the cause of an unsatisfactory sample, the dog should be reevaluated several times over a period of at least 2 months. Recovery from a testicular insult may not be reflected by improved seminal quality for more than 3 to 5 months.

## BACTERIAL CULTURE OF SEMEN

Quantitative and qualitative culture of the semen is indicated (1) if inflammatory cells are identified in the semen; (2) as part of the diagnostic evaluation of infertility in the male; and (3) in dogs with suspected bacterial prostatitis, epididymitis, or orchitis. Bacterial prostatitis is thought to be a common cause of infertility in dogs. For culture results to be meaningful, an aseptic technique and sterile collection devices should be used. Several techniques are used for culturing semen. Ideally the second and third fractions of the ejaculate are collected into separate sterile tubes, and the fractions are cultured individually. In most dogs the first fraction consists of only a few drops of fluid and is difficult to separate from the second fraction.

Culturing each fraction separately may help show whether the infection is in the testes and epididymis (second fraction) or in the prostate gland (third fraction). The sperm-rich fraction and the prostatic fraction should yield fewer than 100 colony-forming units (CFUs) of bacteria per milliliter in the normal dog. Normal feline seminal plasma apparently can contain more than 10,000 CFUs of bacteria. Results of semen cultures must be interpreted in conjunction with the clinical signs, the results of the cytologic evaluation of the ejaculate, and the total number and variety of species of bacteria grown.

The normal bacterial flora of the prepuce and urethra must also be taken into consideration. The number of CFUs per milliliter of semen attributable to urethral contamination

## TABLE 60-1

### Normal Preputial and/or Distal Urethral Flora

| CANINE | FELINE |
|---|---|
| *Acinetobacter* sp. | *Bacillus* sp. |
| *Bacillus* sp. | *Enterococcus* sp. |
| *Corynebacterium* sp. | *Escherichia coli* |
| *Escherichia coli* | *Klebsiella oxytoca* |
| *Flavobacterium* sp. | *Proteus mirabilis* |
| *Haemophilus* sp. | *Pseudomonas aeruginosa* |
| *Klebsiella pneumoniae* | *Serratia odorifera* |
| *Moraxella* sp. | *Staphylococcus* sp. |
| *Mycoplasma* sp.* | *Streptococcus* sp. |
| *Proteus mirabilis* | *Yersinia intermedia* |
| *Pseudomonas aeruginosa* | |
| *Staphylococcus aureus* | |
| *Staphylococcus epidermidis* | |
| *Streptococcus canis* | |
| *Streptococcus equisimilis* | |
| *Viridans streptococci* | |

From Johnston SD: Disorders of the external genitalia of the male. In Ettinger SJ, editor: *Textbook of veterinary internal medicine,* ed 3, Philadelphia, 1989, WB Saunders, p 1882.
*See discussion in text.

reportedly varies from 100 to 10,000. The normal flora of the urethra and prepuce of the dog consists predominantly of aerobic organisms and, to a lesser extent, *Mycoplasma* (see p. 935), *Ureaplasma,* and anaerobic organisms (Table 60-1). These are the same organisms most frequently isolated from dogs with bacterial prostatitis, orchitis, or epididymitis. To limit contamination from the preputial cavity, the preputial orifice should be cleansed and smegma flushed off the surface of the penis before semen is collected. A separate culture of the material from a urethral swab, obtained before ejaculation, can be used to identify urethral organisms. Alternatively, the first fraction and the initial portion of the second fraction of the ejaculate can be discarded (i.e., not submitted for culture). The number of urethral organisms contained in the later seminal fractions tends to be reduced. Most of the bacterial organisms isolated from normal feline semen collected by electroejaculation are normal preputial flora. Culture for *B. canis* should specifically be requested in dogs with epididymitis or orchitis.

Anaerobic organisms are not commonly isolated from abnormal canine semen and as such are not routinely included in the culture request. Infection with anaerobic organisms should be considered if bacteria or inflammatory cells are seen on cytologic preparations of the ejaculate but cultures for aerobic bacteria are negative. Samples for anaerobic culture must be handled promptly and carefully using such media as Anaerobic Culturette (Becton-Dickinson, Rutherford, N.J.). The veterinarian should contact the microbiology laboratory to obtain specific instructions concerning the submission of anaerobic cultures. *Mycoplasma* and *Ureaplasma* organisms can constitute the normal flora of the canine pre-puce and distal urethra. Their role in causing reproductive disease in the male remains to be fully clarified.

# RADIOGRAPHY AND ULTRASONOGRAPHY

In the evaluation of male reproductive disorders, radiography is used primarily to assess the size of the prostate gland and to identify metastatic lesions in the dog with suspected prostatic adenocarcinoma. Ultrasonography provides valuable information concerning changes in the reproductive tract. It can be used to identify and characterize lesions within the prostate, testis, and epididymis; to help determine the cause of testicular or scrotal swelling; to assess the size of the vas deferens; and to help establish the location of undescended testes. Finally, ultrasonography can assist in directing the insertion of biopsy needles for obtaining specimens of the prostate gland or focal lesions within the testis or epididymis.

# TESTICULAR ASPIRATION AND BIOPSY

Testicular biopsy or aspiration and epididymal aspiration are usually reserved for animals that have been thoroughly investigated by other noninvasive means but in which no cause of infertility has been identified. Aspiration, biopsy, or both are indicated early in the evaluation of animals with discrete, focal lesions or in those with marked changes in the consistency of the testis or epididymis.

The cytologic evaluation of testicular aspirates can identify inflammatory cells, sperm, neoplastic cells, and infectious agents. Testicular aspiration is usually reserved for the evaluation of palpable abnormalities. A disadvantage of this technique is that tissue architecture is not preserved, and the progression of spermatogenesis cannot be assessed. Fine-needle (i.e., 25 g of tissue) aspiration of the testes is performed in a manner similar to the aspiration of other masses. Sedation may be required in some dogs and is usually recommended for animals undergoing epididymal aspiration. In the absence of equipment to collect semen from cats, cytologic evaluation of a testicular aspirate could be used to confirm the presence of sperm.

If a testicular biopsy specimen is obtained, seminiferous tubule architecture, the progression of spermatogenesis, and interstitial and Sertoli cell numbers can be evaluated. It can also be used to determine whether there is inflammation or neoplasia within the testicular parenchyma. It has been shown that biopsy of a normal testis has no deleterious effect on semen quality. General anesthesia is required for animals undergoing testicular biopsy. The initial surgical approach is similar to that used for open castration except that the testis is not lifted out through the skin incision. When the proper vaginal tunic and the adherent tunica albuginea are incised, normal testicular tissue promptly bulges through the incision site. This bulging testicular tissue is excised for histopathologic and microbiologic evaluation. The proper vaginal tunic–tunica albuginea is closed. Then the common vaginal tunic is closed, the testis is replaced in the scrotum, and the closure is as in a routine castration. Alternatively, the skin is incised with a scalpel, the testis is immobilized, and a Tru-Cut biopsy needle

(Travenol Laboratories, Inc., Deerfield, Ill) is pushed through the tunic into testicular tissue. After testicular biopsy, we routinely rinse residual scrub material off the scrotum and periscrotal area as soon as the skin is closed. An ice pack is immediately applied to the area and left in place until the dog recovers from anesthesia.

A portion of the biopsy specimen should be submitted for histopathologic evaluation, and because the technique is aseptic, a portion of the specimen can also be submitted for bacterial culture. Testicular tissue for histopathologic evaluation must not be fixed in formalin because artifacts are produced. Zenker's, Bouin's, glutaraldehyde, and Karnovsky's fixative are recommended, depending on whether tissues are to be embedded in paraffin or plastic. Some have suggested that glutaraldehyde is preferred over Bouin's for the epididymis. It is recommended that the pathologist be consulted regarding the preferred fixative before obtaining the specimen.

Complications from testicular aspiration or biopsy are not common if a careful, gentle, and aseptic technique is used. Swelling and local skin irritation can be minimized by rinsing away residual scrub solutions and applying cold compresses to the biopsy site. Some of the potential complications could seriously affect the future fertility of the dog. These include infection, hemorrhage, the formation of sperm granulomas, swelling, and local hyperthermia. Incisional biopsy provides larger tissue specimens than does Tru-Cut biopsy, but there also is greater histologic evidence of damage to testicular parenchyma in animals in which this method is used. All pertinent noninvasive tests should be performed before biopsy is considered.

# HORMONAL EVALUATION

## Testosterone

The serum testosterone concentration is most frequently measured to determine the presence and functional status of the testes. Concentrations in anestrous bitches and castrated males are usually less than 0.2 ng/ml, whereas those in intact males range from 0.5 to 9 ng/ml. Because testosterone is released in an episodic manner, a single determination is often not helpful. For example, testosterone concentrations were undetectable in 8 of 63 samples collected from seven normal fertile male cats. Provocative testing is necessary to adequately assess testosterone production. This is done by measuring the serum testosterone concentration before and after the administration of human chorionic gonadotropin (hCG) or GnRH. The protocols and reference ranges vary among laboratories, therefore consultation with the laboratory is important. In one hCG stimulation protocol, the serum testosterone concentration is measured before and 4 hours after the administration of hCG (44 IU/kg IM in dogs; 250 IU IM per cat). Resting serum testosterone values in intact male dogs are 0.5 to 5 ng/ml and less than 0.05 to 3 ng/ml in intact male cats. Four hours after hCG administration, the serum testosterone concentration is 4.6 to 7.5 ng/ml in intact male dogs and 3.1 to 9 ng/ml in intact male cats. Assuming that the pituitary is normal and capable of responding, GnRH can be used instead of hCG. In this test the serum testosterone is 3.7 to 6.2 ng/ml 1 hour after 2.2 mg/kg of GnRH has been administered intramuscularly to intact male dogs. It is 5 to 12 ng/ml in intact male cats 1 hour after an intramuscular dose of 25 mg. An increase in the serum testosterone concentration in a supposedly castrated male or intersex animal indicates the presence of testicular tissue. Animals with only one testis, such as a unilateral cryptorchid in which the scrotal testis has been removed, and intersex animals may have values between baseline and those typically found in normal males after GnRH administration.

Penile spines begin to appear in intact male cats at about 12 weeks of age; they regress by 6 weeks after castration. Because the development and maturation of penile spines are androgen dependent, they serve as a bioassay for the presence of testosterone. The finding of penile spines indicates the presence of testicular tissue and justifies a presumptive diagnosis of cryptorchidism in tomcats that do not have palpable testes in the scrotum.

## Luteinizing Hormone

The serum LH concentration can be measured to assess pituitary-gonadal interactions. The serum LH concentration in normal male dogs reportedly ranges from 0.2 ng/ml to less than 20 ng/ml. LH pulses occur about every 100 minutes during daylight hours and approximately every 80 minutes during darkness. Repetitive determinations of LH concentrations, such as three samples every 20 minutes, are more likely than a single determination to distinguish normal from abnormal animals, but this technique is also more expensive. Castrated males frequently have serum LH concentrations of more than 30 ng/ml. After the administration of GnRH, serum concentrations of LH should increase, as discussed on p. 857. Failure to do so would be consistent with a pituitary lesion.

## Follicle-Stimulating Hormone

Measurement of serum FSH concentrations has also been used to assess pituitary-gonadal function. Normal FSH concentrations in healthy dogs reportedly range from 20 to 293 ng/ml, whereas castrated dogs and some dogs with severe oligozoospermia or azoospermia have values in excess of 250 ng/ml. In the latter dogs the increased FSH concentrations are thought to result from the fact that the failing testes are no longer able to secrete adequate amounts of inhibin. Inadequate pituitary FSH (and LH) can cause oligozoospermia-azoospermia, a condition known as *hypogonadotropic hypogonadism*. Although measurement of FSH concentrations may be helpful in localizing the lesion in dogs with oligozoospermia-azoospermia, canine-specific FSH assays are not readily available.

## DIAGNOSTIC APPROACH TO INFERTILITY

Normal seminal quality, normal desire to breed (libido), and normal ability to mate are all necessary for normal fertility in males. Therefore the diagnostic approach to infertility must investigate all three of these factors (see Fig. 60-2). The diag-

nostic approach begins with a complete history-taking and physical examination. The history-taking should assess the male's past breeding performance, breeding management, fertility of the females to which he has been bred, and current or previous health problems (Table 60-2). Some common drugs and metabolic disorders that are known to affect male fertility are listed in Table 60-3. Dogs achieving pregnancy rates of less than 75% when bred to apparently normal females using proper breeding management should probably be evaluated for subfertility. Pregnancy rates of 85.4% ± 12.4% have been reported for privately owned, fertile stud dogs in which two matings/estrus were done. Better than 90% pregnancy rates are achieved in well-managed commercial breeding colonies, but these rates stem from the fact that individual dogs with lower rates are likely to be promptly culled from such colonies.

Assessment of the male's libido and mating ability can help narrow the differential diagnoses. A normal male may appear to lack libido if he is not in his established territory; if he is less dominant than the female or another male in the immediate vicinity; if he is inexperienced or frightened; or if he prefers a different partner. Some normal males show no interest until the female is actually in estrus, as opposed to proestrus. Dogs that are accustomed to semen collection may no longer be interested in natural service despite normal arousal and a willingness to ejaculate. Daily ejaculation, especially over a week or two, and ejaculation more often than twice a day are other factors that can diminish the libido of normal male dogs. Such frequent ejaculation does not diminish libido in tomcats. Excessive endogenous or exogenous glucocorticoids, stress, and pain can also cause decreased libido in dogs. Libido also appears to decrease with advancing age.

Some animals may exhibit normal arousal and mount, only to dismount before attempting intromission. It is often difficult to determine whether this behavior is caused by

## TABLE 60-2

**Historical Information for Male Infertility**

1. Previous breeding performance
   Libido
   Mating ability
   Dates of breeding, the outcome, and litter size
   Results of previous semen evaluation
2. Previous breeding management
   Methods of insemination
   Date of insemination chosen by
       Predetermined day of season?
       Behavioral changes?
       Vaginal cytology findings?
       Ovulation timing?
3. Fertility of the female
   Previously produced pups?
   Subsequently produced pups?
4. Other health problems, test results, and medications

TABLE 60-3

**Common Drugs and Metabolic Disorders Affecting Male Reproduction**

| DISORDER | CAUSE |
|---|---|
| Decreased luteinizing hormone (LH), testosterone, sperm output, seminal volume and libido; increased sperm abnormalities | Glucocorticoids Hyperadrenocorticism |
| Decreased LH, testosterone, and spermatogenesis | Estrogens Androgens Anabolic steroids Cimetidine |
| Decreased testosterone, libido, and sperm count | |
| Decreased testosterone and libido | Spironolactone Anticholinergics Propranolol Digoxin Verapamil Thiazide diuretics Chlorpromazine Barbiturates Diazepam Phenytoin Primidone |
| Decreased testosterone | Progestagens Ketoconazole |
| Decreased spermatogenesis | Amphotericin B Many anticancer drugs |
| Decreased libido and sperm count; abnormal semen | Diabetes mellitus |
| Decreased libido and sperm count | Renal failure Stress |

inadequate libido or by inadequate mating ability. This behavior is often exhibited when a vaginal abnormality is encountered and also in some males accustomed to semen collection. Painful conditions often diminish libido, as well as interfere with mating ability. Generally, mating ability is determined by physical, mechanical, and neurologic factors governing mounting, erection, intromission, and ejaculation. Orthopedic disorders of the rear legs, spine and, less commonly, the front legs may prevent mounting or intromission but do not usually affect libido and ejaculatory ability. Semen collection and artificial insemination could be used in such animals.

## PHYSICAL EXAMINATION

A complete physical examination should be performed to assess the animal's overall health and identify congenital or heritable abnormalities that should be grounds for excluding the male from the breeding program. Many metabolic and physical abnormalities can adversely affect spermatogenesis, libido, and mating ability. The testes and epididymides are palpated to determine their size, shape, consistency, and location. In situations of unilateral disease, there is urgency to establish and correct the cause before the condition affects the contralateral testis. This can occur by direct extension of the disease process itself or as a result of local swelling, pressure, and hyperthermia, all of which are deleterious. The canine prostate is palpated per rectum and transabdominally. The penis and prepuce are palpated and inspected. Because the penis must be extruded from the prepuce for a thorough examination to be performed, as well as for semen to be collected in dogs, the two are often performed together. This is contraindicated if the history indicates the animal may have a penile lesion that could be aggravated by sexual arousal.

Anatomic abnormalities reported to cause difficulty in mating include phimosis, a persistent penile frenulum, an abnormally short os penis in dogs, and entanglement of the penis in preputial hair in cats. Male cats that fail to grasp the female's neck in the proper location may not be in the correct position for intromission. This is seen in some inexperienced males and in mating pairs with disparate body lengths. Male dogs are often reluctant to breed bitches with anatomic abnormalities of the vulva or vagina. Usually neither shows outward signs of discomfort other than failure to mate; thus it may be difficult to discern whether intromission does not occur because of a female or a male problem.

A thorough neurologic and orthopedic examination, especially of the rear limbs, should be performed. Neurologic disorders can interfere with mounting, erection, intromission, and ejaculation. For example, motor nerve dysfunction can cause difficulty with mounting and intromission. Semen collection for artificial insemination may be possible in such animals. Sensory or autonomic disturbances can cause difficulty with erection (and therefore with intromission in cats) and ejaculation. Semen collection by electrical stimulation may or may not be possible in such animals, depending on the location of the lesion.

## SEMEN EVALUATION

The semen of infertile males should be submitted for culture, and *B. canis* testing should be performed in dogs (p. 936). Males with a history of infertility but that currently have normal semen, normal libido, and normal mating ability are normal. Such males may have recovered from their previous infertility, the breeding management (e.g., timing of insemination) could have been inappropriate, or the females may have been infertile. Normal males should be bred again to fertile females using optimal breeding management. If the semen is abnormal, further evaluation of the reproductive tract is indicated. Semen is judged to be abnormal if inadequate numbers of sperm are found; if the motility of sperm is inadequate; if sperm morphology is abnormal; or if the semen contains other cells (WBCs, macrophages, RBCs). Semen evaluation is discussed in detail on p. 907.

Abnormal motility (asthenozoospermia) and morphology (teratozoospermia) are often the first indicators of gonadal damage, irrespective of the cause. Morphologically abnormal sperm often do not have normal motility. Causes include primary testicular disease, metabolic disorders, transient insults (e.g., fever), incomplete ejaculation, and iatrogenic causes. Sperm in semen from young dogs and from dogs that have not mated for a long time may show poor motility, and the semen may contain more than the usual number of morphologically abnormal sperm. Iatrogenic causes include temperature shock, exposure of the semen sample to a stain of improper pH and osmolality, and exposure of the sample to latex rubber, plastics, and other spermicidal agents.

The semen should be reevaluated in the next 4 to 7 days (or sooner if an iatrogenic cause is suspected); care should be taken at that time to ensure that the entire sperm-rich fraction is ejaculated and collected and that the sample is not damaged by improper handling. If abnormalities persist, semen culture and a metabolic evaluation (e.g., complete blood count [CBC], serum biochemistry profile, urinalysis) are indicated. If a cause is not identified, semen should be reevaluated in 2 to 3 months before additional testing is done. If the problem persists, additional testing is indicated as is done for the evaluation of acquired infertility (see p. 916).

## OLIGOZOOSPERMIA AND AZOOSPERMIA

A decrease in the total number of sperm per ejaculate may occur with or without abnormalities in sperm morphology or motility. Sperm numbers may be less than normal (oligozoospermia), or sperm may be completely absent (azoospermia). The degree of arousal influences the number of sperm ejaculated. Therefore using an estrual female for teasing should be considered when one is evaluating a male with a low sperm count. The frequency of ejaculation can also affect the number of sperm ejaculated in that it depletes extragonadal reserves, causing the concentration of sperm in each ejaculate to be reduced. In dogs ejaculated once daily for 2 to 3 days, the number of sperm per ejaculate is reduced by as much as 50% relative to dogs that have not ejaculated for 7 or more days. The total number of sperm per ejaculate, however, may still be within the normal range (i.e., more than $250 \times 10^6$ per ejaculate). After 7 to 10 days of daily ejaculation, the number will be less than normal. This may be important when evaluating a popular stud. If semen is collected from dogs more than once daily, especially if the time between collections is brief, the sperm numbers and libido decline drastically by the second or third collection. Normal dogs can ejaculate two to three times weekly for 2 weeks or once weekly for 6 weeks and show no significant decrease in the number of sperm per ejaculate.

The collection of semen by either electroejaculation or artificial vagina once weekly for 4 weeks does not adversely affect the total number of sperm ejaculated by cats. However, the retrograde ejaculation of significant numbers of sperm occurs during electrical stimulation. Healthy male cats can copulate three times daily for 4 to 5 days with no change in the resultant conception rates or litter sizes. Frequent copulation, as often as five times per hour for the first 2 hours of exposure to an estrual queen, is normal in cats. Unlike dogs, such frequent copulation is not associated with diminishing libido in tomcats. In the absence of equipment to collect semen from cats, the presence of spermatozoa in the ejaculate can be confirmed by examining a vaginal cytology specimen obtained from the queen after copulation.

The concentration of sperm per ejaculate may also decline because of abnormalities in spermatogenesis or ejaculation. The clinician must always exclude the possibility that the entire sperm-rich fraction was not collected before proceeding further. This is ensured by repeat semen collection (see following section). Spermatogenesis is a complex process that can be affected by environmental factors such as scrotal temperature; metabolic disorders, especially endocrinopathies; toxins and drugs; and infection. A thorough history-taking and physical examination, standard laboratory tests, and semen culture help to identify these possibilities. In addition, oligozoospermia and azoospermia may result from primary testicular failure, bilateral obstruction of the vas deferens or epididymides, or retrograde ejaculation. Because a bilateral obstruction could occur at the level of the prostate gland, the prostate should be carefully evaluated. Measuring the seminal alkaline phosphatase activity (see p. 909) should help determine whether epididymal fluid is present in the ejaculate. If the seminal alkaline phosphatase activity is high, this shows that epididymal contents have been ejaculated and obstruction to flow from the epididymides is apparently not the cause of the low sperm count.

Retrograde ejaculation of semen into the urinary bladder rather than out the urethra is thought to be neurogenic in origin, perhaps resulting from inadequate pressure in the proximal urethra or neck of the bladder. Some spermatozoa normally pass retrograde during ejaculation but substantially more do so during electroejaculation than during natural copulation. In the event of pathologic retrograde ejaculation, the volume of semen or the number of spermatozoa discharged is lower than normal. Retrograde ejaculation is diagnosed on the basis of the finding of excessive numbers of sperm in the urinary bladder after ejaculation. This is likely to be easiest to assess when an animal has an empty bladder before ejaculation. Some sperm are normally found in urine, but large numbers, especially approaching those in discharged semen, are considered abnormal. Treatment with α-adrenergic drugs (e.g., pseudoephedrine, 4 to 5 mg/kg PO q8h or twice, 3 hours and 1 hour, before breeding) to increase urethral tone in dogs with retrograde ejaculation has been recommended, but experience with this treatment is limited.

The treatment of oligozoospermia and azoospermia depends on finding and eliminating the cause. Unfortunately this is not always possible. As a general rule, azoospermic males tend to remain azoospermic, especially if testicular size is also less than normal. The finding of small testes in an infertile male suggests the presence of congenital hypoplasia or of acquired testicular atrophy or fibrosis, none of which is likely to be reversible. Oligozoospermia may or may not progress to azoospermia, depending on the cause. Because recovery from a testicular insult is slow and because canine spermatogenesis takes 62 days, the animal could reasonably be evaluated every 2 months for a year to determine the trend in the numbers of sperm per ejaculate before pronouncing him irreversibly sterile.

Oligozoospermic males may be subfertile rather than infertile. It is assumed that sperm reserves and spermatogenesis are poor in oligozoospermic males, therefore they should be bred judiciously. This means adequate time between breedings to allow sperm reserves to be replenished, infrequent ejaculation during estrus, insemination at the optimal time on the basis of vaginal cytology and ovulation timing (serum progesterone concentration) in the female, and breeding only to healthy, fertile females. Dogs with as few as $20 \times 10^6$ to $100 \times 10^6$ sperm per ejaculate have been reported to successfully impregnate normal, fertile bitches when ejaculation has been limited to twice, done at a 2-day interval late in estrus. Intrauterine, rather than intravaginal, insemination may also be considered (see Chapter 64).

## CONGENITAL INFERTILITY

Congenital infertility should be considered in azoospermic animals that have no history of siring a litter or other reproductive activity. Abnormalities of the hypothalamic-pituitary-gonadal axis, such as hypogonadotropic hypogonadism; anatomic abnormalities of the wolffian duct system, such as atresia; and disorders of sexual differentiation, such as intersex, are possible causes. The phenotypic, gonadal, and chromosomal sex of the animal can be determined by endocrinologic evaluation (serum testosterone and LH concentrations), karyotyping, gonadal biopsy, and evaluation for internal genitalia (e.g., uterus). Gonadal biopsy specimens can show whether the gonad is truly a testis and whether spermatogenesis is present. The external genitalia can be examined by physical methods. The internal genitalia (müllerian and wolffian duct derivatives) can be examined by ultrasonography, laparoscopy, or laparotomy. If an animal with congenital infertility is found to be a genotypic and phenotypic male, the diagnostic plan is the same as that for males with acquired infertility.

## ACQUIRED INFERTILITY

Animals with acquired infertility are known, or at least thought, to have previously been fertile (they have sired litters) or capable of producing normal semen (previous semen evaluation). In some instances the onset of infertility or subfertility may be identified by a review of the breeding record, looking for a diminution in litter sizes and conception rates. In other cases the time of onset of infertility is never determined. A thorough history-taking and physical examination, measurement of the *B. canis* titer in dogs, and semen evaluation should be done, paying special attention to the possibility of toxin- or drug-induced infertility, excessive stress, or excessive frequency of ejaculation.

If excessive numbers of WBCs (leukozoospermia) are found in the semen, the site of contamination (urine, pre-putial cavity) or of the inflammatory process must be determined (e.g., testes, epididymides, prostate). The third fraction of the canine ejaculate should be submitted separately for cytologic and microbiologic examination (see p. 911). *B. canis* should be excluded by appropriate cultures and serologic tests (p. 936). Ultrasonography with or without fine-needle aspiration of the testis or prostate may be helpful in localizing the lesion.

The semen should be cultured for aerobic and anaerobic bacteria and *Mycoplasma*. Bacterial infection of the testes, epididymides, or scrotum causes alterations in spermatogenesis as a result of the destructive properties of the organisms themselves and as a result of local swelling and hyperthermia. The role of bacterial prostatitis in canine infertility is unclear, but most theriogenologists consider bacterial prostatitis to be a common, potentially reversible, cause of infertility. Appropriate antibiotic therapy should be initiated if the semen culture is positive for pathologic numbers of bacteria. Appropriate antimicrobial therapy should continue for a minimum of 2 to 4 weeks, or longer in the case of chronic bacterial prostatitis.

If the history, physical examination, semen evaluation, and semen culture findings fail to establish the diagnosis, a thorough metabolic and endocrine evaluation should be done before more invasive procedures are performed. Such diagnostic tests include a CBC, serum biochemistry profile, urinalysis, and adrenal function tests (i.e., adrenocorticotropic hormone stimulation test). Assessment of the hypothalamic-pituitary-testicular axis, done by assessing LH and testosterone concentrations, may also be warranted (see p. 912). According to Dekrester and colleague (1997), no cause for infertility can be found in 30% to 40% of infertile men with abnormal semen analysis findings.

Testicular aspiration or biopsy (see p. 912) can be considered if other, noninvasive diagnostic tests have failed to identify the cause and the abnormalities in sperm morphology or concentrations have not diminished after several months. Seminiferous tubule architecture, spermatogenesis, interstitial cell numbers, and the presence or absence of inflammation and etiologic agents within the testicular parenchyma can be assessed in testicular biopsy specimens. A portion of the biopsy specimen should also be submitted for bacterial culture. The following histologic lesions have been identified in dog testes: neoplasia (see p. 924), suppurative and nonsuppurative inflammation, mycotic orchitis, lymphocytic orchitis, granulomatous orchitis, spermatogenic arrest, and testicular degeneration. There is limited information available on cats other than information on the testicular changes associated with aging.

Noninflammatory, degenerative conditions of the testes vary in severity from diminished spermatogenesis to a complete absence of germ cells and collapse of the seminiferous tubules. Sometimes only Sertoli cells remain. The less severe lesions are potentially reversible if the underlying cause can be eliminated. Unfortunately, the histologic appearance of testicular specimens obtained from animals with degenerative conditions of the testes rarely indicates the initiating cause. Chemical toxins and thermal and radiation injury can all cause testicular degeneration that may progress to testicular atrophy. The Leydig and Sertoli cells may be spared. Libido is maintained if the Leydig cells are not affected. Chronic testicular infection can also result in testicular degeneration. In this event, evidence of the etiologic agents and inflammation may no longer be present.

Testicular biopsy specimens from cats older than 7 years show diminished spermatogenesis and degeneration of seminiferous tubules compared with the findings in younger cats. These are considered typical age-related changes. Testicular atrophy is common in dogs older than 10 years. Diabetes mellitus, glucocorticoid excess, excessive androgen and estrogen levels, and deficient gonadotropin levels can all cause diminished spermatogenesis and testicular atrophy in dogs. Because the underlying cause of testicular degeneration is usually not elucidated by histopathologic studies and because testicular atrophy (the end stage of degeneration) is considered irreversible, testicular biopsy may be unwarranted in animals with testes that are already substantially smaller than normal.

Suppurative inflammation of the testes is characterized by an infiltration of neutrophils. Macrophages and giant cells are also found. Bacterial or mycotic infections are the usual cause (see p. 921). Viral orchitis, which occurs in some species, has not been reported in dogs. Some bacterial infections, such as *B. canis* infection, cause nonsuppurative orchitis involving lymphocytes and plasma cells rather than neutrophils. Immune-mediated reactions to sperm, mycotic infection, and *B. canis* infection are the most common causes of granulomas in the canine testicle.

If lymphocytes and plasma cells are found, the orchitis is usually thought to be immune mediated, but this does not exclude the possibility that infection was the initiating cause. For example, the antisperm antibodies produced as a result of *B. canis* infection are thought to play a major role in the pathogenesis of the orchitis. Because the antigens that are unique to spermatozoa are usually not accessible to immune surveillance, anything that disrupts the integrity of the seminiferous tubules or the blood-testis barrier has the potential to expose sperm antigens and incite an immune response. By this mechanism, testicular trauma, infection, or neoplasia may cause lymphocytic orchitis. Often the cause of canine lymphocytic orchitis is not found, and sterility ultimately occurs. Foci of lymphocytes can be found in testicular biopsy specimens from apparently normal cats of all ages. The significance of these is unknown, but they are most prevalent in cats older than 8 to 9 years of age.

## Suggested Readings

Axnér E et al: Sperm morphology is better in the second ejaculate than in the first in domestic cats electroejaculated twice during the same period of anesthesia, *Theriogenology* 47:929, 1997.

Davidson AP: Clinical theriogenology, *Vet Clin North Am* 31:2, 2001.

Dekrester DM et al: The Y chromosome and spermatogenesis, *N Engl J Med* 336:576, 1997.

England GGCW et al: *Manual of small animal reproduction and neonatology,* Cheltenham, UK, 1998, British Small Animal Veterinary Association.

Greene CE, editor: *Infectious diseases of the dog and cat,* ed 2, Philadelphia, 1990, WB Saunders.

Griffin JE: Androgen resistance: the clinical and molecular spectrum, *N Engl J Med* 326:611, 1992.

Howard J: Feline semen analysis and artificial insemination. In Kirk RW et al, editors; *Current veterinary therapy XI,* Philadelphia, 1992, WB Saunders, p 929.

Johnson CA et al: Morphology stain-induced spermatozoal abnormalities, *Proceedings of the Annual Conference of the Society of Theriogenology and the American College of Theriogenology,* San Diego, 1991, p 238.

Johnson CA et al: Effect of $^{131}$I-induced hypothyroidism on indices of reproductive function in adult male dogs, *J Vet Intern Med* 13:104, 1999.

Johnston SD et al: Canine reproduction, *Vet Clin North Am* 21:3 1991.

Johnston SD et al: *Canine and feline theriogenology,* Philadelphia, 2001, WB Saunders.

Linde-Forsberg C: Hints on semen freezing, cryoextenders and frozen semen artificial insemination. *Proceedings of the Annual Conference of the Society of Theriogenology and the American College of Theriogenology,* Colorado Springs, Colo, 2002, p 303.

Meyers-Wallen VN: CVT update: inherited disorders of the reproductive tract in dogs and cats. In Bonagura JD, editor: *Kirk's current veterinary therapy XIII,* Philadelphia, 2000, WB Saunders, p 904.

Oettlé EE: Sperm abnormalities and fertility in the dog. In Bonagura JD, editor: *Kirk's current veterinary therapy XII,* Philadelphia, 1995, WB Saunders, p 1060.

Peters MAJ et al: Aging, testicular tumours and the pituitary-testis axis in dogs, *J Endocrinol* 166:153, 2000.

Root Kerstritz MV et al: The effects of stains and investigators on assessment of morphology of canine spermatozoa, *J Am Anim Hosp Assoc* 34:348, 1998.

# CHAPTER 61

# Disorders of the Penis, Prepuce, and Testes

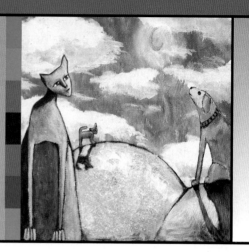

## CHAPTER OUTLINE

ACQUIRED PENILE DISORDERS, 918
    Penile trauma, 918
    Priapism, 918
    Miscellaneous acquired disorders, 919
CONGENITAL PENILE DISORDERS, 919
    Persistent penile frenulum, 919
    Miscellaneous congenital disorders, 919
PREPUTIAL DISORDERS, 920
    Balanoposthitis, 920
    Phimosis, 920
    Paraphimosis, 920
TESTICULAR DISORDERS, 921
    Orchitis and epididymitis, 921
    Cryptorchidism, 922
    Testicular torsion, 923
    Testicular neoplasia, 924

## ACQUIRED PENILE DISORDERS

### PENILE TRAUMA

Traumatic injury of the penis occurs in dogs and cats as a result of fighting, being hit by cars, jumping onto rather than over barriers, and mating trauma. Hematomas, lacerations, and fracture of the os penis are injuries that may occur. Penile injuries are usually very painful. Other clinical signs include swelling, bruising, and hemorrhage. The prepuce may or may not be similarly affected, depending on whether the penis was extruded (as it would be if erect) when the injury occurred. The diagnosis is made on the basis of the findings yielded by visual examination of the penis and radiographic examination of the penile urethra and os penis. The integrity of the urethra should be evaluated by retrograde urethrography whenever significant penile trauma is identified. Ultrasonography and color-flow Doppler may help differentiate penile hematoma from priapism.

Treatment includes cleansing of the wounds and débridement if necessary. Lacerations may have to be closed surgically using absorbable sutures. An antibiotic cream should be applied to the surface of the penis, and the penis should be protruded from the prepuce twice daily until the lesions are healed. This is done to prevent adhesions from forming between the penis and the prepuce. Sexual arousal and other types of excitement must be avoided until the penile lesion is completely healed, because erection before then is likely to result in hemorrhage and possibly dehiscence.

Fractures of the canine os penis are often associated with a urinary outflow tract obstruction or a urethral tear. In addition to the local signs associated with the trauma, these animals may have signs referable to a distended urinary bladder or postrenal uremia. The treatment adopted depends on the severity of the urethral damage and fracture displacement. As an emergency treatment, the urinary bladder may be decompressed by cystocentesis. An indwelling urethral catheter may be placed while the urethra heals. Urethral tears should be sutured if necessary. Urethrotomy or urethrostomy could be considered in some circumstances to temporarily or permanently divert urine flow. Systemic antibiotics should be administered to prevent urinary tract infection. Displaced fractures of the os penis can be immobilized with orthopedic wires. Immobilization is not required in animals with fractures that are not displaced, because the penis itself provides adequate support. Occasionally calluses that form during the healing of the os penis obstruct the urethra. It may be necessary to amputate the penis in the event of severe penile trauma.

### PRIAPISM

Priapism is abnormal, persistent erection that is not associated with sexual arousal. The cause is not always identified, but the result is occlusion of venous outflow and filling of the corpora cavernosa with blood. During the normal process of erection, relaxation of sinusoidal smooth muscle and increased flow through the arteries and arterioles facilitate rapid filling of the sinusoidal system, which in turn compresses the venous channels and occludes outflow. During the process of detumescence, the trabecular smooth muscle contracts, enabling the venous channels to reopen, and the trapped blood is expelled. Fortunately, priapism occurs rarely in dogs and cats. Although it is uncommon, it must be corrected promptly because stagnated blood in the cavernous sinuses will eventually clot, which will not promptly resolve even when venous draining is reestablished. In addition, ischemic necrosis is common.

Some high-strung dogs transiently develop erections when they are excited for any reason. This is not priapism. These transient erections in highly excitable dogs usually diminish as the dog matures. If not, castration is usually curative, with or without behavioral modification. Priapism is also different from the erection that occasionally persists for longer than expected in some dogs after copulation or semen collection. In these cases, if the estrual bitch is still present, she should be removed from the premises. The male dog should be taken out of the room in which copulation or semen collection took place. These are often sufficient distractions, and the erection subsides. If not, sedation or application of cold water compresses could be considered. Priapism should also be differentiated from other causes of penile swelling, such as hematoma or edema. Penile hematomas usually form as a result of trauma or bleeding disorders. Edema usually occurs as a result of paraphimosis. Simple visual inspection and palpation of the penis are usually sufficient means to differentiate the conditions. An ultrasound and/or color-flow Doppler examination may help differentiate hematoma from priapism.

The neurophysiology of erection includes sympathetic innervation provided by the hypogastric nerve, parasympathetic innervation provided by the pelvic nerve, and somatic and sensory input provided by the pudendal nerve. Parasympathetic innervation is considered responsible for stimulating erection, and sympathetic innervation is considered responsible for stimulating ejaculation. Spinal cord lesions, general anesthesia, and phenothiazine administration are reported causes of priapism in animals and men. Thromboembolism is also reported as a cause of priapism in dogs and cats. If it occurs at the base of the penis, venous occlusion from any cause could result in priapism. In many cases, the cause of priapism is undetermined.

Nonischemic priapism may respond to pharmacologic treatment with anticholinergic or antihistaminic agents, such as diphenhydramine and benztropine. Benztropine contains the active ingredients of atropine and diphenhydramine; a dose of 0.015 mg/kg intravenously has been suggested for dogs. The β-adrenergic agonist terbutaline has also been used successfully in the treatment of priapism in men. Clotting of the blood trapped in the canvernous sinuses, ischemia, and necrosis develop quickly. Therefore pharmacologic intervention, if it is to be successful, must be done early, within hours. Unfortunately, many of the reported cases in dogs and cats were not presented to veterinarians until the condition had been present for days to weeks, by which time necrosis necessitated penile amputation or perineal urethrostomy. Surgical drainage and intracorporeal lavage have also been reported successful treatments.

During priapism the penis should be protected against additional damage or irritation that may perpetuate the problem or invite the development of sequelae, such as edema, thrombosis, fibrosis, penile paralysis, or necrosis. Physical treatments include cleansing the penis, the application of an-

tibiotic cream, and attempts to maintain the penis within the prepuce until the condition subsides.

## MISCELLANEOUS ACQUIRED DISORDERS

Vesicles, ulcers, pyogranulomatous lesions, warts, and neoplasia of the penis have been identified in dogs. The clinical signs are similar and include a preputial discharge, excessive licking of the prepuce or penis, or a mass protruding from the prepuce. These lesions are differentiated on the basis of the findings revealed by visual examination, exfoliative cytologic studies, bacterial and fungal cultures, and biopsy. In our experience, penile warts often resolve spontaneously after biopsy of the lesion. The cause of vesicular lesions is uncertain. Canine herpesvirus has been implicated but is usually not documented. Lymphoid follicle hyperplasia may be confused with vesicles unless the tissues are examined microscopically. Ulcers and pyogranulomatous lesions are uncommon. They seem to be associated with infection (see Balanoposthitis section, p. 920).

## *CONGENITAL PENILE DISORDERS*

## PERSISTENT PENILE FRENULUM

Under the influence of testosterone the surfaces of the glans penis and the preputial mucosa normally separate before or within months of birth, depending on the species of animal. If this separation does not occur, connective tissue persists between the penis and the prepuce. In dogs the persistent penile frenulum is usually located on the ventral midline of the penis. A persistent penile frenulum may cause no clinical signs, or it may be associated with preputial discharge or excessive licking of the prepuce. Persistent frenulum may cause the penis to deviate ventrally or laterally so the dog is unable or unwilling to mate. The diagnosis is made by visual examination. Treatment is surgical excision, which can often be done using sedation with local anesthesia because the frenulum tends to be a sheer, avascular membrane.

Persistence of the adhesions of the prepuce and penis is seen in male cats that are castrated between 7 weeks and 5 months of age. The prevalence of this condition in the general cat population, irrespective of neuter status or age at castration, is unknown. Failure of the glans penis and preputial mucosa to separate prevents the penis from being fully extruded or causes deviation of the erect penis (Fig. 61-1). The clinical significance, if any, of the failed penile-preputial separation seen in some cats neutered at very young ages remains to be determined.

## MISCELLANEOUS CONGENITAL DISORDERS

Congenital penile disorders other than a persistent penile frenulum are rare. Penile hypoplasia has been noted in dogs and cats. Some affected animals have had an abnormal complement of sex chromosomes. In most, the penile hypoplasia has been an incidental finding. In one dog it was associated with urine pooling in the preputial cavity.

Hypospadia is a developmental defect in closure of the urethra, resulting in one or more abnormal openings into the

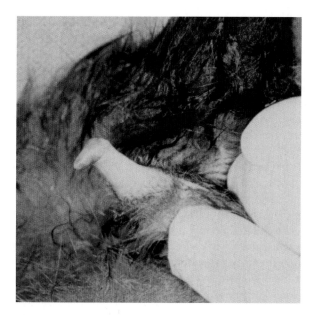

**FIG 61-1**
Failure of complete separation of penile and preputial mucosa in a cat.

urethra. The urethra closes under the influence of dihydrotestosterone. Hypospadia results from an androgen receptor defect. The urethra can fail to close anywhere along its length. The prepuce and sometimes the scrotum are simultaneously and similarly affected. Hypospadia has been noted in dogs. Besides the abnormal appearance of the external genitalia, clinical signs include urinary incontinence and urinary tract infection. Affected animals may have additional congenital anomalies. Surgical correction may be considered.

Diphallia, or duplication of the penis, has been reported in dogs and cats.

## PREPUTIAL DISORDERS

### BALANOPOSTHITIS

Inflammation or infection of the preputial cavity, balanoposthitis, is very common in dogs and rare in cats. The offending organisms are usually members of the normal preputial flora (see Table 60-1), although infection with canine herpesvirus and *Blastomyces* has also been reported. Balanoposthitis usually causes no clinical signs other than a purulent preputial discharge. The volume of the discharge and the degree of purulence are extremely variable, from a scant white smegma to a copious green pus. The discharge associated with uncomplicated balanoposthitis is not sanguineous. The diagnosis of balanoposthitis is made on the basis of the findings revealed by physical examination of the preputial cavity and penis. The penis should be thoroughly examined in a search for foreign material, neoplasia, ulceration, or inflammatory nodules. Cultures and cytologic studies are rarely performed, unless herpesvirus or fungal infection is suspected because of the vesicular appearance of the lesions or the presence

of similar lesions elsewhere on the body. The treatment of balanoposthitis is conservative. Cleansing the preputial cavity with antiseptic solutions (e.g., chlorhexidine, povidone-iodine [Betadine]) seems to be helpful. Topical antibacterial medications may be instilled into the preputial cavity. Castration usually results in diminished preputial secretions.

### PHIMOSIS

Phimosis is a condition in which the penis is trapped within the preputial cavity. It usually occurs as a congenital defect where the preputial opening is abnormally small and the penis cannot protrude. Phimosis is uncommon in cats and dogs. It may be recognized in young animals as a cause of a urinary outflow tract obstruction or of the dribbling of urine that has accumulated in the preputial cavity. Phimosis may be recognized in an affected male when it is unable to copulate. It is treated by surgically enlarging the preputial orifice. The preputial hairs of long-haired cats may entangle the preputial orifice, causing clinical signs similar to phimosis. It is treated by clipping the preputial hairs.

### PARAPHIMOSIS

Paraphimosis is a condition in which the penis is prevented from retracting back into the preputial cavity. It occurs most frequently after an erection in dogs. Therefore it is seen quite often after semen collection and occasionally after copulation. Paraphimosis may occur in long-haired cats when the penis becomes entangled in the preputial hairs. Otherwise it is uncommon in cats. The protruded penis usually becomes trapped because the prepuce has turned in on itself (Fig. 61-2, *A* and *B*). Presumably this occurs because the skin or hair at the preputial orifice adheres to the surface of the penis and is pulled into the preputial cavity as an erection subsides. The preputial skin then compromises the circulation to the protruded penis.

The signs of paraphimosis depend primarily on its duration. Initially the exposed penis is normal in appearance and nonpainful (see Fig. 61-2, *A* and *B*). However, after several minutes the exposed penis becomes edematous (Fig. 61-2, *C*) and increasingly painful. In addition to the damage caused by continued poor circulation, the exposed penis is subject to trauma. The surface becomes dry, and fissures may develop. The urethra is usually not damaged. The unexposed penis and the uninvolved prepuce are normal and nonpainful. Long-standing paraphimosis may result in gangrene or necrosis.

Paraphimosis is diagnosed on the basis of the findings during visual inspection. The exposed penis may have become so painful that sedation or anesthesia is required so that examination and treatment can be performed, although this is not usually necessary. Treatment involves returning the prepuce to its normal configuration, restoring circulation to the penis, and replacing the penis in the preputial cavity. This is accomplished by gently sliding the prepuce in a posterior direction, such that more of the glans penis is protruded. The prepuce is thus retracted until the cranial aspect of the prepuce "unfolds" and the preputial orifice is exposed (see Fig.

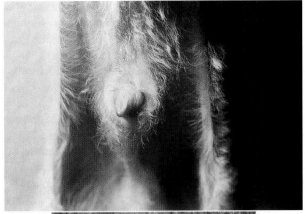

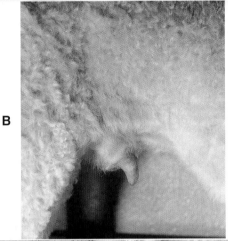

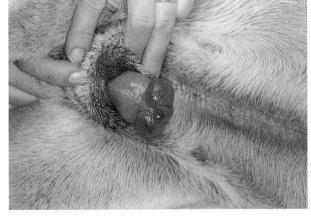

**FIG 61-2**
**A** and **B,** Ventral and lateral views of paraphimosis in a dog before edema develops. Note the inverted preputial opening. **C,** Edema of the tip of the penis as a result of paraphimosis. Note that retraction of the prepuce enabled it to evert into its normal configuration.

61-2, *C*). Circulation to the penis usually improves immediately after the prepuce is restored to its normal configuration. Penile edema then begins to subside. The surface of the penis is cleansed or débrided as necessary. Topical antibiotic or an antibiotic-steroid cream may be applied if the penile mucosa has been damaged. Even though some penile edema may still be present, the prepuce usually slides easily over it and the pe-

nis is thus replaced in the preputial cavity. Water-soluble lubricant should be applied as necessary to accomplish this. If, even after circulation is restored, the edematous tissue is of sufficient magnitude that the prepuce cannot slide over it, application of pressure with a cool water compress is usually effective in resolving the edema.

Rarely is it necessary to enlarge the preputial orifice. If it is, an incision is made on the ventral midline of the prepuce, and after the penis is in place, the incision is closed in separate layers. The penis will usually stay within the preputial cavity, and penile swelling quickly subsides. The degree of swelling can be assessed by palpating the penis through the prepuce if there is concern that protruding the penis from the preputial cavity will be unduly painful. Rarely does the still-swollen penis protrude from the prepuce. The preputial orifice may be temporarily (1 to 24 hours) sutured closed, but there is then the risk that urine will accumulate in the preputial cavity during this time. If the penis has become necrotic or gangrenous, penile amputation is indicated.

Conditions other than paraphimosis may also cause the penis to protrude from the prepuce. These include priapism, phimosis, an abnormally short prepuce in dogs, and a ring of preputial tissue in cats. Penile trauma may cause penile hematomas to form. The swelling associated with the extravasation of blood may be sufficiently severe to cause the penis to protrude. Treatment is conservative and consists in protecting the exposed penis from trauma. The preputial orifice may also be temporarily closed, as described in the preceding paragraph. If possible, the hematoma is allowed to resolve spontaneously; otherwise it can be drained surgically. Foreign material within the preputial cavity or around the glans penis may also cause the penis to protrude. Therefore the preputial cavity to its fornix and the entire glans penis should always be examined in an animal with penile or preputial disease.

## TESTICULAR DISORDERS

### ORCHITIS AND EPIDIDYMITIS
#### Etiology

The testis or epididymis can become infected via the hematogenous route, through the ascension of pathogens from elsewhere in the urogenital tract, or as a result of penetrating wounds. Although infection of one does occur without involvement of the other, the causative organisms typically are the same. Extension or progression of infection from the epididymis to the testis, or vice versa, is common. For this reason, they are discussed together. Orchitis-epididymitis is more common in dogs than in cats. Aerobic bacteria are most often implicated. *Mycoplasma, Brucella canis* (see p. 936), *Blastomyces, Ehrlichia,* Rocky Mountain spotted fever, and feline infectious peritonitis are also reported to infect the testes, epididymides, or scrotum. Bacterial infection of the testes, epididymides, or scrotum causes alterations in spermatogenesis as a result of the destructive properties of the organisms themselves and as a result of local swelling, inflammation, and hyperthermia.

## Clinical Features

The clinical signs of orchitis-epididymitis vary with the chronicity of the infection. Acute infections are usually associated with swelling of the scrotum and the scrotal contents and are painful. The affected epididymis or testis is enlarged, firm, and warm. The scrotal skin may be inflamed, and dogs may lick the scrotum excessively. Fever and lethargy may be present in animals with systemic infections. Conversely, some affected animals may show minimal discomfort and the acute phase may be unnoticed by the owner. The scrotum is usually normal in animals with chronic orchitis-epididymitis. The testis becomes soft and atrophic. The epididymis may seem more firm and prominent than normal, especially if the testis is primarily affected. Infertility is common in animals with either acute or chronic orchitis-epididymitis, and it may be the presenting complaint.

## Diagnosis

Orchitis-epididymitis is diagnosed on the basis of physical examination, ultrasonography (Fig. 61-3), cytology, and culture findings. Specimens for culture and cytology may be obtained by collection of semen or by fine-needle aspiration of the testis (see p. 912). Semen from dogs with active orchitis-epididymitis contains many inflammatory cells (leukospermia) and abnormal spermatozoa. Bacteria or other infectious agents, however, are usually not seen during cytologic evaluation of semen. They are more commonly observed in specimens obtained by fine-needle aspiration. In animals with chronic infection and atrophy of the testes, the number of inflammatory cells and spermatozoa decreases, eventually resulting in azoospermia. Serologic tests for *B. canis* should always be performed in dogs with these clinical and cytologic findings. A thorough evaluation of the prostate gland is also warranted.

Semen cultures in dogs with active bacterial orchitis-epididymitis usually yield more than $10^5$ colony-forming units per milliliter of semen. However, culture results must be interpreted in light of the normal urethral flora and other clinical and cytologic findings. Microbiologic cultures may be negative in animals with chronic orchitis-epididymitis. This is frequently the case in animals with chronic *B. canis* infection. Therefore negative culture results do not necessarily exclude infection as the inciting cause. The results of cytologic and microbiologic evaluation of semen from dogs with orchitis-epididymitis are indistinguishable from those of prostatitis. Further, prostatitis and orchitis-epididymitis may be concurrent. Therefore the prostate should always be thoroughly evaluated (see p. 927) by palpation, ultrasonography, and cytologic evaluation of the third fraction of the ejaculate or specimens obtained by fine-needle aspiration of the prostate.

## Treatment

Appropriate antimicrobial therapy should be initiated on the basis of culture results. Antibiotics to consider pending results of sensitivity testing are those that are usually effective against the common urogenital organisms. These antibiotics include enroflaxacin, amoxicillin, clavulanate-amoxicillin, chloramphenicol, and trimethoprim-sulfonamide, which are effective against either gram-negative or gram-positive organisms. Cephalosporins and tetracycline can also be considered. Antimicrobial therapy, determined on the basis of the results of culture and sensitivity testing, should continue for a minimum of 2 weeks. Soaking the scrotum in cool water may help to minimize the damage caused by hyperthermia and swelling. The prognosis for the recovery of fertility is poor in dogs or cats with orchitis and epididymitis, regardless of the causative organism. Orchiectomy effectively decreases the burden of infection and should be considered if fertility appears to be irreversibly lost. In cases of unilateral involvement, unilateral orchiectomy may be the best way to protect the apparently unaffected gonad. Antibiotics should be administered regardless of whether surgery is performed.

## CRYPTORCHIDISM

The normal time of testicular descent has not been firmly established in dogs or cats. In cats, testicular descent appears to be a prenatal event. In dogs, testicular descent occurs by 10 days of age, although there may be some breed-related variations. If the testis is not palpable within the scrotum by 8 weeks of age, cryptorchidism is diagnosed. Unilateral cryptorchidism is more common than bilateral cryptorchidism in both dogs and cats. The undescended testis is found in the abdomen or in the subcutaneous tissues in the inguinal area with about equal frequency. There is no apparent difference in the prevalence of right- or left-sided unilateral cryptorchidism in dogs or cats. Bilaterally undescended testes are most often found in the abdomen. True monorchidism (congenital absence of one testis) is extremely rare. The true incidence of cryptorchidism in the population is unknown, but its prevalence in both dogs and cats in various hospital populations is reportedly between 1% and 2%. Cryptorchidism was found in 44 (2.6%) of 1679 dogs from a pet store. Of 466 dogs brought in for elective castration, 46 (9.9%) were crypt-

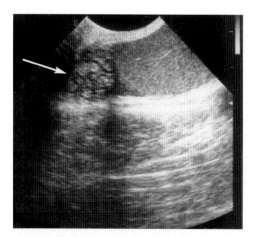

**FIG 61-3**
Sonogram of abnormal canine epididymis *(arrow)* typical of suppurative epididymitis. Normal-appearing testis is to the right.

orchid, whereas 6 of 613 (1%) cats brought in for elective castration were cryptorchid. However, it is possible that castration was requested because the animals were cryptorchid. Therefore the prevalence of cryptorchidism among animals brought in for castration may actually be greater than it is in the rest of the hospital population. However, of 2289 free-roaming male cats evaluated in a trap-neuter-return program, none was monorchid, whereas 43 (1.9%) were cryptorchid.

There is no doubt that cryptorchidism is hereditary in dogs and cats, because (1) it occurs most commonly in certain breeds (Toy and Miniature Poodles, Yorkshire Terriers, Chihuahuas, Boxers, Pomeranians, Miniature Schnauzers, Pekingese, Maltese, Shetland Sheepdogs, Cairn Terriers, Persian cats); (2) it occurs more often in certain families than in others; and (3) the prevalence of the trait can be increased or decreased by selecting for or against affected animals, respectively. The exact mode of inheritance is not known, however. The simplest model consistent with the evidence available is a sex-limited, autosomal recessive mode of inheritance. The expression of the trait is limited to males, but the genetic defect is not linked to the sex chromosomes. Therefore both males and females carry the gene and can pass it on to their offspring. Obviously, only the homozygous males are phenotypically abnormal (cryptorchid) and therefore readily identifiable, because homozygous females cannot express the trait.

According to this model, all male offspring born to a homozygous (cryptorchid) male × homozygous female cross would be affected (cryptorchid), and all the females would carry the gene as homozygotes. A heterozygous × heterozygous cross would result in one quarter of the male offspring being cryptorchid, one half of the males being phenotypically normal heterozygous carriers, and one quarter of the males being phenotypically and genotypically normal. All the female offspring would obviously be phenotypically normal, but three quarters of them would carry the gene (one half as heterozygotes and one fourth as homozygotes). The greater the number of offspring born to any genotypic cross, the greater the likelihood that the proportions of affected and unaffected animals would actually be realized. This is especially true for a trait such as cryptorchidism, in which the only marker for the gene is the abnormal phenotype, which is expressed only in homozygous males. Therefore, with the exception of a homozygous × homozygous cross, some litters are likely to contain all phenotypically normal males, whereas other litters from the same dam and sire will have affected males. However, the inheritance of cryptorchidism may well be more complicated than that explained by the simple autosomal recessive, sex-limited model, providing yet another possible explanation for why each litter from the same breeding pair does not always have the same phenotypic result.

The undescended testis is not normal. Spermatogenesis is usually completely absent, especially in intraabdominal testes, because of the high intraabdominal temperature. Spermatogenesis does not fully recover, even if the testis descends into the scrotum at a later time. Because interstitial cells continue to produce testosterone, libido is usually normal. Bilaterally cryptorchid animals are sterile; therefore they are effectively removed from the gene pool. The scrotal testis of an animal with unilateral cryptorchidism should be normal. Although the number of spermatozoa in the ejaculate of animals with unilateral cryptorchidism is less than that of normal animals, they usually are fertile. Therefore unilaterally cryptorchid males will perpetuate the trait if allowed to breed. For this reason, cryptorchid animals should be castrated.

There is no known medical treatment that can reliably cause cryptorchid testes to descend. Occasionally favorable results have been noted in male dogs and in boys treated with human chorionic gonadotropin. Such reports generally stimulate renewed controversy and discussion in both the human medical and veterinary communities. However, it is generally believed that the apparent success is actually the result of the coincidental spontaneous descent of mobile testes that were located very near the scrotum. There appear to be no reports of the successful medical management of intraabdominal cryptorchidism in any species. Castration of cryptorchid dogs is recommended. Ultrasonography may be helpful in locating the retained testis (Fig. 61-4).

In dogs, testicular neoplasia is reported to be as much as 13 times more likely to develop in undescended than in descended testes (Fig. 61-5), and because testicular neoplasia, even in scrotal testes, is so common in older dogs, this represents a significant risk. Castration of cryptorchid dogs while they are young is therefore recommended. Peters and colleague (2002) estimated the expected life span of a young cryptorchid dog undergoing "prophylactic" castration compared with its estimated expected life span if it were not castrated. The life expectancy was calculated based on the estimated risks associated with castration of a young cryptorchid dog and the estimated risks associated with the eventual development of testicular neoplasia. Using this model, the authors predicted no significant difference in life span if the cryptorchid dog was castrated while he was young and healthy or at the time testicular neoplasia occurred. Whether this mathematic model accurately reflects actual survival of dogs with and without testicular neoplasia is not known. The quality of life for affected versus unaffected dogs was not considered in this study. Testicular neoplasia is rare in cats, regardless of the location of the testes. See p. 924.

## TESTICULAR TORSION

Testicular torsion more commonly affects intraabdominal testes than scrotal testes. The clinical signs are related to the acute abdominal pain that results. It is treated by castration. If torsion of a scrotal testis occurs, pain is also the major clinical sign. There is also scrotal and testicular swelling, which can be quite pronounced. Often the spermatic cord is thickened. Ultrasonographic examination of the affected testes and spermatic cord usually reveals the abnormal course of the spermatic vessels. Treatment is unilateral orchiectomy. Spermatogenesis is irreparably damaged as a result of ischemia within 1 to 2 hours of testicular torsion. Although some recovery is possible, fibrosis usually occurs.

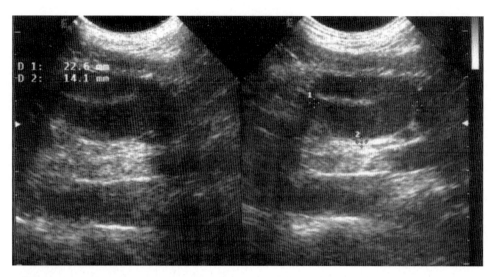

**FIG 61-4**
Sonogram showing an intraabdominal cryptorchid testis in a dog. (Courtesy Dr. Gustavo Sepulveda, East Lansing, Mich.)

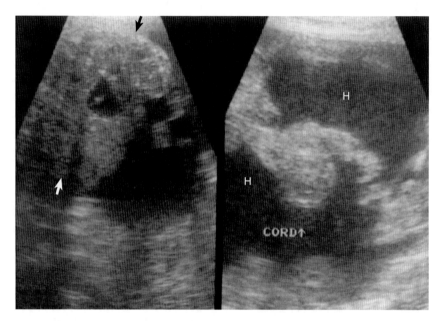

**FIG 61-5**
Abdominal ultrasound image of a neoplastic, undescended testis *(left image, arrows)* with invasion of the spermatic cord *(right image)* and peritoneal hemorrhage *(H)*.

## TESTICULAR NEOPLASIA

### Classification

Testicular tumors are very common in old dogs, second only to skin tumors. In most dogs, testicular tumors are found incidentally. Testicular tumors are extremely rare in cats. In dogs, Sertoli cell tumors, Leydig cell (interstitial cell) tumors, and seminomas occur with about equal frequency. Most testicular tumors in dogs are benign. The mean age of animals at the time of diagnosis is about 10 years. Nearly 100% of interstitial cell tumors and 75% of seminomas occur in descended testes, whereas 60% of Sertoli cell tumors occur in unde-

scended testes. Likewise, 60% of tumors occurring in undescended testes are Sertoli cell tumors.

Sertoli cell tumors are usually 1 mm to 5 cm in diameter, although they may become much larger. Ten to twenty percent of Sertoli cell tumors metastasize, usually to the lumbar or iliac lymph nodes. Dogs with Sertoli cell tumors are usually seen because of inguinal or scrotal enlargement. Intraabdominal tumors may cause abdominal enlargement or signs of testicular torsion. Some dogs are seen because of the paraneoplastic syndromes (Table 61-1) associated with estrogen production by the Sertoli cell tumor. Ten to fifteen percent of

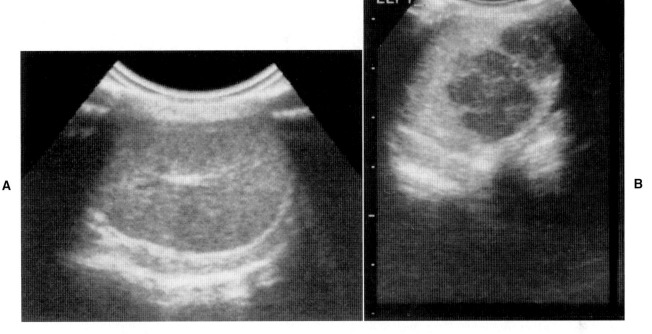

**FIG 61-6**
**A,** Sonogram of normal right testis and, **B,** left testis with a seminoma in an infertile, 9-year-old English Bulldog. After hemicastration the dog sired a litter of nine pups. Hatch marks are 1 cm.

TABLE 61-1

**Paraneoplastic Syndromes Associated with Hyperestrogenism**

Alopecia
Pigmentation
Feminization of males: gynecomastia, pendulous scrotum and prepuce
Squamous metaplasia of the prostate
Bone marrow suppression: anemia, thrombocytopenia, leukopenia
Depressed spermatogenesis
Testicular atrophy

dogs with Sertoli cell tumors have bone marrow hypoplasia leading to anemia, thrombocytopenia, leukopenia, or a combination of these.

Interstitial cell tumors are usually 1 to 2 cm in diameter; they rarely metastasize and rarely cause clinical signs. They are most often found incidentally during physical examination, castration, or necropsy. They may secrete hormones and cause paraneoplastic syndromes. Seminomas are usually confined to one testis, although metastasis has been reported to occur in 6% to 11% of cases. They may be incidental findings or grow to a size at which scrotal or inguinal enlargement is obvious.

## Diagnosis

The diagnosis of testicular neoplasia is usually straightforward. The index of suspicion is highest in old, cryptorchid males. The diagnosis is most challenging in animals (erroneously) assumed by their owners to have been previously castrated because they do not have scrotal testes. Neoplasia is suspected if a mass is palpated in a testis or in the mid or caudal abdomen of a cryptorchid dog or if signs of feminization are present. Less commonly the dog may be seen because of poor fertility, testicular atrophy of the contralateral testis, prostatic disease, or hematologic or dermatologic abnormalities.

Ultrasonography is helpful in evaluating the testes of animals in which testicular neoplasia is suspected but not palpable, as well as in differentiating intratesticular from extratesticular causes of scrotal enlargement. Testicular tumors have a variable echo texture (Fig. 61-6). Tumors less than 3 cm in diameter usually appear hypoechoic. The larger tumors tend to disrupt normal testicular architecture and may contain focal areas of ischemic necrosis; thus large testicular tumors usually have mixed echogenicity. Ultrasonography and radiology can be used to evaluate intraabdominal testes (see Figs. 61-4 and 61-5), but testes similar in size to the diameter of the small bowel are difficult to identify.

Fine-needle aspiration of palpable testicular masses is easily performed, but it is rarely done when the index of suspicion of neoplasia is high, because tissue specimens can be obtained at the time of castration. Nevertheless, cytologic examination of aspirated material can be very helpful in differentiating a testicular neoplasm from other masses such as abscess or granuloma. Fine-needle aspiration should be considered if dogs have less-than-classic clinical signs of testicular neoplasia or if owners are reluctant to consider castration.

Exfoliative cytologic studies of the preputial mucosa can be done to identify estrogenic stimulation, such as may occur in animals with Sertoli cell tumors. Like the vaginal epithelium, the preputial mucosa becomes cornified as a result of the estrogenic influence. Specimens are obtained by inserting a cotton-tipped swab into the preputial cavity and gently scraping the preputial mucosa. The penis itself should be avoided. Specimens are then processed as they are for vaginal cytologic studies (see p. 853). If the preputial mucosal epithelial cells are found to be cornified, this indicates estrogenic stimulation, which, in the absence of a history of administration of exogenous estrogens, indicates the presence of an estrogen-secreting tumor. This would most likely be of testicular origin, but pathologic production of sex hormones by the adrenal gland has also been reported in dogs with hyperadrenocorticism.

## Treatment

The treatment for all testicular tumors is castration. If there is unilateral involvement in a stud dog, hemicastration may be considered. However, semen quality may not improve after removal of the neoplastic testis. After castration, a definitive diagnosis is made on the basis of the results from the histopathologic evaluation of the affected testis. Dogs with bone marrow suppression may need supportive care, such as a blood transfusion to treat anemia or thrombocytopenia. Systemic antibiotics may be necessary to help prevent infection in granulocytopenic animals. The prognosis for bone marrow recovery is guarded to poor. Improvement often takes months. Treatment of metastatic lesions with surgery or chemotherapy or both may be considered, but the prognosis is grave (see Chapters 78 and 79).

## Suggested Readings

Axnér E et al: Reproductive disorders in 10 domestic male cats, *J Small Anim Pract* 37:394, 1996.

Griffin JE: Androgen resistance—the clinical and molecular spectrum, *N Engl J Med* 326:611, 1992.

Johnston SD et al: *Canine and feline theriogenology,* Philadelphia, 2001, WB Saunders.

Lue TF: Erectile dysfunction, *N Engl J Med* 342:1802, 2000.

Meyers-Wallen VN: CVT update: inherited disorders of the reproductive tract in dogs and cats. In Bonagura JD, editor: *Kirk's current veterinary therapy XII,* Philadelphia, 2000, WB Saunders, p 904.

Nielen AL et al: Heritability estimations for diseases, coat color, body weight, and height in a birth cohort of Boxers, *Am J Vet Res* 62:1198, 2001.

Peters MA et al: Aging, testicular tumours and the pituitary-testis axis in dogs, *J Endocrinol* 166:153, 2000.

Peters MA et al: Decision analysis tree for deciding whether to remove an undescended testis from a young dog, *Vet Rec* 150:408, 2002.

Root-Kustritz MV: Theriogenology question of the month (priapism), *J Am Vet Med Assoc* 214:1483, 1999.

Ruble RP et al: Congenital abnormalities in immature dogs from a pet store: 253 cases (1987-1988), *J Am Vet Med Assoc* 202:633, 1993.

Scott KC et al: Characteristics of free-roaming cats evaluated in a trap-neuter-return program, *J Am Vet Med Assoc* 221:1136, 2002.

Syme HM et al: Hyperadrenocorticism associated with excessive sex hormone production by an adrenocortical tumor in two dogs, *J Am Vet Med Assoc* 219:1725, 2001.

# CHAPTER 62

## Disorders of the Prostate Gland

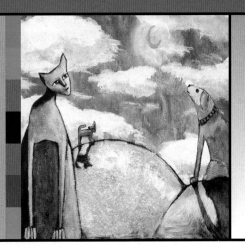

## CHAPTER OUTLINE

OVERVIEW, 927
BENIGN PROSTATIC HYPERPLASIA, 928
SQUAMOUS METAPLASIA OF THE PROSTATE, 930
BACTERIAL PROSTATITIS AND PROSTATIC ABSCESS, 930
    Chronic bacterial prostatitis, 931
PARAPROSTATIC CYSTS, 932
PROSTATIC NEOPLASIA, 932

## OVERVIEW

Disorders of the prostate gland are common in dogs but very rare in cats. They include benign prostatic hyperplasia, squamous metaplasia, bacterial prostatitis, prostatic abscess, prostatic and paraprostatic cysts, and prostatic neoplasia.

### Clinical Features

The clinical signs of the prostatic diseases are similar because each causes some degree of prostatic enlargement or inflammation (Table 62-1). The most common clinical signs include tenesmus, blood dripping from the urethra independent of urination, hematuria, and recurrent urinary tract infections. In a study by Read and colleagues (1995), 28 of 88 dogs with prostatic disease were presented because of urethral bleeding. In 20 of the 28, urethral bleeding was the only clinical sign. Additional, nonspecific signs, such as fever, malaise, and caudal abdominal pain, are often present in animals with bacterial infections and neoplasia of the prostate gland. Prostatic adenocarcinoma may cause an animal's gait to be abnormal as a result of pelvic and lumbar vertebral metastatic lesions. Other nonspecific signs of prostatic enlargement may stem from its mechanical interference with other abdominal organs. Less commonly, prostatic diseases may cause urethral obstruction, infertility, or urinary incontinence.

### Diagnosis

Physical examination of the prostate gland is accomplished by abdominal and rectal palpation. The enlarged prostate is rarely located completely within the pelvic canal. Palpation is done to assess the size, shape, symmetry, consistency, and movability of the prostate, as well as to detect any discomfort. The clinical signs and physical findings will usually localize the disease process to the prostate gland, but they are not able to differentiate among the various prostatic conditions.

Abdominal radiography, ultrasonography, prostatic cytologic studies, bacterial culture, biopsy, or a combination of these studies is usually required to differentiate the specific prostatic disorders. Abdominal radiographs help define the size, shape, and position of the prostate. Atalan and colleagues (1999) suggested that prostatic length of greater then 70% of the distance from the sacral promontory to the pelvic brim on the lateral abdominal radiograph is indicative of prostatomegaly. Prostatic depth is an unreliable indicator of prostatic size. In 34 dogs with prostatic disease, prostatic length ranged from 3.5 to 8.3 cm (mean, 5.4 cm) and depth was 2.4 to 7.0 cm (mean, 4.3 cm). The radiographic appearance of the sublumbar lymph nodes, lumbar vertebrae, and bony pelvis should be examined for evidence of metastasis. A positive-contrast cystourethrogram can be performed if it is difficult to differentiate an abnormal prostate from the urinary bladder and to assess the prostatic urethra. Ultrasonography provides additional information about the homogeneity of the prostatic parenchyma, the urethral diameter, and the diffuse or focal nature of the disease (Fig. 62-1). Atalan and colleagues (1999) studied prostatic size by ultrasonography in 154 normal dogs of various ages and breeds. Length ranged from 1.8 to 5.0 cm (mean, 2.9 cm), depth ranged from 1.4 to 3.6 cm (mean, 2.3 cm), and width ranged from 1.4 to 4.3 cm (mean, 2.5 cm). Not surprisingly, the authors found a positive correlation between prostatic size and age, and also body weight. The finding of urethral invasion or destruction on contrast radiologic studies or ultrasonograms is highly suggestive of prostatic neoplasia. Other radiographic and ultrasonographic findings do not differentiate cysts from abscesses, or hyperplasia from metaplasia, prostatitis, or diffuse neoplasia.

Prostatic material for cytologic and microbiologic examination can be obtained by several methods. Prostatic massage is performed by placing a urethral catheter into the urinary bladder and removing the urine. An aliquot of urine is saved

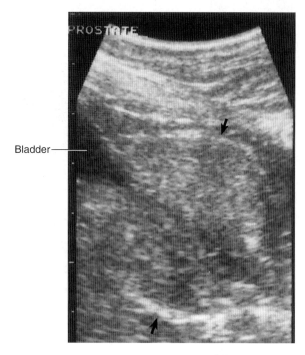

**FIG 62-1**
Sonogram of normal canine prostate *(arrows)* of an English Setter. Hatch marks represent 1 cm.

 TABLE 62-1

**Clinical Signs of Prostatic Disease**

**Common Signs**

Blood dripping from urethra without micturition
Tenesmus
Recurrent urinary tract infections
Hematuria

**Less Common Signs**

Pain
Fever
Urethral obstruction
Infertility
Gait abnormalities

for future comparison. The catheter is then withdrawn to the level of the prostate, the prostate is thoroughly massaged per rectum, and additional material is aspirated through the catheter. The prostatic urethra can be lavaged with sterile saline solution if an inadequate volume is recovered. The premassage and postmassage specimens are analyzed and compared. A urethral brush may also be used to obtain material for cytologic and microbiologic evaluation. In this method the brush is passed through a urinary catheter to the level of the prostate, as determined by rectal palpation. The prostatic urethra is then "brushed."

Prostatic massage is easily performed; however, samples are always contaminated by material from the urinary blad-

der. There is also a risk of rupturing prostatic abscesses or liberating septic emboli during massage. Because prostatic fluid normally refluxes into the urinary bladder, urinary tract infection is usually present whenever there is bacterial prostatitis. Conversely, urinary tract infection can exist in the absence of prostatitis. If a urinary tract infection is present, microbiologic examination of the prostatic portion (third fraction) of the ejaculate to confirm the presence of bacterial prostatitis is more accurate than examination of specimens obtained by massage. The prostatic fraction of the ejaculate (see p. 909) can also be evaluated cytologically.

Neoplastic cells are often not recovered in specimens obtained by ejaculation or prostatic massage, except for the latter in cases of urethral invasion. Fine-needle aspiration or biopsy of the prostate gland, or both, may be required to establish the diagnosis. Fine-needle aspiration is performed to obtain specimens for cytology and culture for any of the other prostatic disorders, as well as neoplasia. Fine-needle aspiration is usually performed percutaneously, with or without ultrasound guidance. A transrectal approach for fine-needle aspiration has also been described. The percutaneous approach is generally safe and simple, although some veterinarians have been reluctant to perform fine-needle aspiration of the prostate for fear that the abdomen might be contaminated with infected or neoplastic material. Although there is a potential for peritoneal contamination or inadvertent penetration of surrounding structures to occur, these risks are minimal if a careful technique, especially with ultrasound guidance, is used. There were no complications from percutaneous fine-needle aspiration of the prostate in 30 dogs evaluated for prostatic disease by Kay and colleagues (1989) or in 77 dogs evaluated by Teske and colleague (1996). In the same studies, the only complication of ultrasound-guided biopsy of the prostate was mild, transient hematuria that required no treatment. Biopsy is the most definitive, but also the most invasive, diagnostic procedure for differentiating prostatic diseases. Prostatic biopsy is performed through a celiotomy or percutaneously using ultrasound guidance.

## BENIGN PROSTATIC HYPERPLASIA

Benign prostatic hyperplasia (BPH) is the most common prostatic disorder in the dog. It represented 58% of all the prostatic disorders diagnosed at Murdoch University Veterinary Hospital (Read and colleague, 1995). BPH is found in most intact male dogs older than 6 years of age. It occurs as a result of androgenic stimulation; specifically, it is mediated by dihydrotestosterone. Why some males are affected and others are not is unknown. BPH may be subclinical, or tenesmus and prostatic bleeding reflected by blood dripping from the urethra in the absence of urination or by hematuria may occur (see Table 62-1).

### Diagnosis

The diagnosis of BPH is suggested when tenesmus, a sanguineous urethral discharge, hematuria, or a combination of

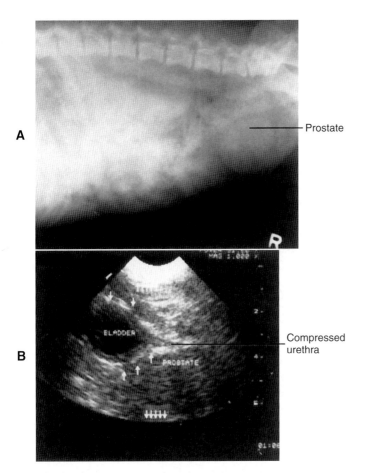

**FIG 62-2**
Benign prostatic hyperplasia. **A,** Radiograph and **B,** sonogram from the same dog showing urethral compression. *Single arrows,* bladder; *multiple arrows,* prostate.

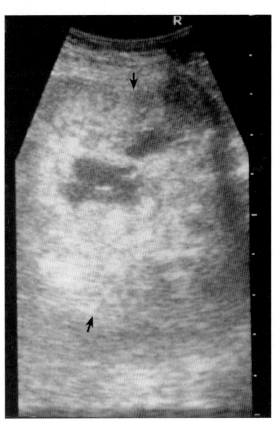

**FIG 62-3**
Sonogram of the cystic, hyperechoic prostate of a German Shepherd Dog with prostatomegaly (5.7 × 4.6 cm) resulting from benign prostatic hyperplasia. Hatch marks represent 1 cm.

these is found in an otherwise healthy, middle-aged or older, intact dog with symmetric prostatomegaly. Less commonly, dogs with BPH may be evaluated because of blood in the semen. The prostate gland is not painful when palpated. Radiologic studies confirm the presence of prostatomegaly (Fig. 62-2, *A*). Ultrasound studies should show diffuse, relatively symmetric involvement throughout the prostate (Figs. 62-2, *B,* and 62-3). Small, multiple, diffuse, cystic structures are commonly seen on ultrasound images obtained in dogs with BPH. Initially, prostatic enlargement is due primarily to glandular hyperplasia. This progresses to cystic hyperplasia. In a study of asymptomatic dogs with BPH, cysts were found during prostatic ultrasonography in 14%. The size of the cysts ranged from 0.7 to 1.2 cm by 1.5 to 2.4 cm. The cystic fluid was aspirated, and 42% had positive cultures. Cytologic examination of massage, ejaculate, or aspirate specimens reveals evidence of hemorrhage and perhaps mild inflammation but no evidence of sepsis or neoplasia. The diagnosis of BPH could be confirmed by histopathologic studies of biopsy specimens, in which hyperplastic changes, often including microscopic cysts, are found, but biopsy is rarely necessary.

## Treatment

Treatment is not necessary for asymptomatic BPH, but castration is the treatment of choice for dogs showing clinical signs of BPH. Prostatic involution is usually evident within a few weeks of castration and is complete by 12 weeks after the source of androgens is removed. Prostatic bleeding usually resolves in about 4 weeks.

Castration may not be a feasible treatment option for breeding males. Such animals can be treated with antiandrogens, but this is not as effective as castration in resolution of the clinical signs, and the results are only temporary. Relapse occurs after such drugs are discontinued. Cysts can be treated by fine-needle aspiration under ultrasound guidance. The fluid should be submitted for bacterial culture because many cultures are found to be positive for bacteria (see later discussion of chronic bacterial prostatitis).

Estrogen therapy to reduce prostatic hyperplasia, although initially effective, is not recommended, because repeated low doses, as well as overdosage, of estrogen can induce squamous metaplasia of the prostate, which in turn can cause the prostate to enlarge and only worsen the clinical signs. In addition, estrogens may enhance the cystic changes within the prostate and depress spermatogenesis by inhibiting hypothalamic gonadotropin-releasing hormone (GnRH) and pituitary gonadotropin secretion. The dose-dependent and idiosyncratic toxic effect of estrogens on canine bone marrow is well known.

Progestins have antiandrogenic effects. At high doses they depress spermatogenesis and spermatozoal motility, increase morphologic defects in spermatozoa, and depress serum testosterone concentrations, despite having no apparent effect on serum luteinizing hormone (LH) concentrations. Progestins reportedly also have no apparent effect on libido in dogs, despite the fact that they suppress serum testosterone concentrations. Megestrol acetate at a dosage of 0.5 mg/kg orally, given once daily for 10 days to 4 weeks, has been reported to cause the clinical signs of BPH to resolve without adverse effects on fertility in dogs. Long-term use has not been evaluated. Delmadinone acetate is another progestin that is used to treat BPH. It is administered at a dose of 1.5 mg/kg subcutaneously at weeks 0, 1, and 4. This causes adrenal suppression for up to 21 days after the last dose, but no change in glucose tolerance or growth hormone. It is not as effective as castration in resolving prostatic bleeding.

A single subcutaneous injection of 3 mg/kg of medroxyprogesterone acetate (MPA) was found to relieve the clinical signs of BPH in most dogs treated (84%). Treated dogs were evaluated for 27 weeks, during which time semen quality was not affected. Serum testosterone concentrations were decreased after week 5, but this apparently caused no problems with semen quality or libido. Clinical signs of BPH reappeared 10 to 24 months after MPA treatment. The effects on fertility of repeated or long-term use of MPA for the treatment of BPH have apparently not been reported. In addition to the likelihood of adverse effects of long-term progestin therapy on reproductive function, the effects of progestins on adrenal function, growth hormone secretion, and insulin and glucose homeostasis (see Chapter 52) should be considered.

Finasteride (Proscar; Propecia; Merck, West Point, Pa) inhibits 5-α-reductase, thereby inhibiting the conversion of testosterone to dihydrotestosterone. The most appropriate dose of finasteride for the treatment of BPH in dogs has not been determined. The dose for men with BPH is 5 mg/day. Doses of 0.1 to 0.2 mg/kg daily or 5 mg/dog/day orally have been studied. Clinical signs began to improve after 1 week of treatment. Prostatic size was demonstrably and significantly decreased by 8 weeks of treatment. Prostatic fluid volume decreased; otherwise, there was no effect on semen quality. Libido and ejaculation were unaffected. Serum testosterone concentration was unchanged, but serum dihydrotestosterone concentrations were significantly decreased. After 4 to 6 months of treatment, all dogs that were subsequently bred sired litters. Histopathologic preparations of the prostate specimens from treated dogs showed evidence of atrophy of the prostatic epithelium and fibromuscular stroma. Although the changes induced by finasteride were found to have reversed by 6 months after the termination of treatment, the prostate glands had not returned to pretreatment sizes. At the 0.1 to 0.2 mg/kg doses, adverse effects were not reported. The 5 mg oral daily dose is a substan-

tially higher dose for dogs than for men. Once the appropriate dose is determined, finasteride may prove useful for the treatment of BPH in stud dogs, in which castration is not a treatment option. Finasteride is teratogenic. Therefore pregnant women must not handle the drug.

An extract of the berry of the saw palmetto plant (*Serenoa repens*) has been used to treat some of the urine retention symptoms of BPH in men. It is available over the counter. After 91 days of treatment of dogs with BPH, there was no effect on weight, volume, or histologic findings in the prostate. The radiographic and ultrasonographic appearance of the prostate did not change. There was no change in semen quality, libido, or serum testosterone concentrations. No adverse effects were noted. Contrary to the situation in men, urine retention is a rare manifestation of BPH in dogs.

## SQUAMOUS METAPLASIA OF THE PROSTATE

Estrogen-secreting Sertoli cell tumors (see p. 924) or, rarely, adrenal tumors and exogenous estrogen therapy, may cause squamous metaplasia of the prostatic epithelium and diminish the movement of prostatic fluid within prostatic ducts. The net effect is enlargement of the prostate gland and a propensity for fluid to accumulate within the gland. The clinical signs and physical examination findings may be identical to those seen in the setting of BPH. Additional signs of hyperestrogenism (see Table 61-1) may also be present. A testicular mass may be palpable or cryptorchidism may be identified during physical examination.

### Diagnosis

Squamous metaplasia is tentatively diagnosed on the basis of the history and physical examination findings. Increased numbers of squamous epithelial cells are often found in ejaculated or aspirated prostatic specimens. If necessary, the diagnosis can be confirmed by the findings from studies of fine-needle aspiration or prostatic biopsy specimens.

### Treatment

Squamous metaplasia is treated by removing the source of estrogen. This is accomplished by the castration of animals with testicular tumors or the discontinuation of estrogenic drugs. The effects of the estrogen other than those on the bone marrow are potentially reversible. Unilateral castration might be considered for a dog that still has potential value as a stud, although it may take some time for the hypothalamic-pituitary-gonadal axis to recover.

## BACTERIAL PROSTATITIS AND PROSTATIC ABSCESS

Bacterial infection of the prostate gland may be acute or chronic, and overt prostatic abscesses may develop in animals with such infections. Normally the prostate is protected against bacterial colonization by the local production of secretory immunoglobulin A (IgA), the production of prostatic antibacterial factor, and the removal of organisms through frequent micturition. Presumably, the diseased prostate (cystic hyperplasia, squamous metaplasia) is more prone to infection than the normal gland. The most common route of infection is the ascension of urethral flora. A hematogenous route of infection is also possible. The organisms most commonly isolated from the infected prostate are *Escherichia coli*, *Staphylococcus*, *Streptococcus*, and *Mycoplasma*. Occasionally *Proteus* spp., *Pseudomonas*, or anaerobic organisms are found.

## Clinical Features

Animals with acute bacterial prostatitis or prostatic abscess usually have a history of an acute onset of severe illness, with abdominal pain and perhaps a hemorrhagic preputial discharge. Fever, dehydration, and pain on palpation of the prostate are usually present. Septicemia and endotoxemia can develop.

## Diagnosis

Bacterial prostatitis and prostatic abscess are diagnosed on the basis of the findings from physical examination and ultrasonography, culture of prostatic fluid or urine, and cytologic studies of material obtained by prostatic aspiration. Prostatic size may not be markedly changed in dogs with prostatitis. Asymmetry, prostatomegaly, and fluctuant areas are usually palpable in animals with prostatic abscesses. A neutrophilic leukocytosis with a variable shift toward immaturity, signs of toxicity in the neutrophils, and monocytosis are typically shown by a complete blood count in animals with acute infections or abscesses. Ultrasonographic examination of the prostate identifies intraparenchymal, fluid-filled spaces consistent with abscesses.

Prostatic fluid obtained by ejaculation is a good specimen for bacterial culture and sensitivity testing. Cultures of prostatic specimens from dogs with bacterial prostatitis usually yield greater than $10^{3-5}$ colony-forming units per milliliter, in which case prostatic infection is easily differentiated from urethral contamination. However, dogs with acute prostatitis or abscess usually have too much pain and are too ill to ejaculate. Prostatic specimens obtained by fine-needle aspiration, preferably with ultrasound guidance, are also fine. Alternatives include culture of urine, because normally some prostatic fluid refluxes into the bladder. Urinalysis usually shows hematuria, pyuria, and/or bacteriuria. When urinalysis findings are abnormal, urine should always be submitted for culture and sensitivity testing. Usually, cultures of urine and prostatic material grow the same organisms. Although specimens for culture can also be obtained by prostatic massage, extreme caution should be exercised when massaging the prostate of animals with acute bacterial prostatitis or prostatic abscess because of the risk of rupturing an abscess or the risk of a septic embolism developing. Cytologic evaluation of the prostatic material should be performed. This usually reveals inflammation with evidence of sepsis and hemorrhage, with macrophages found in animals with chronic infection.

Unlike the situation in men, prostatic fluid pH, specific gravity, and cholesterol and zinc concentrations typically are not abnormal in dogs with prostatitis.

## Treatment

Antibiotics are the principal mode of therapy for bacterial prostatitis. The blood-prostate barrier is quite effective in preventing many drugs from penetrating into the prostatic parenchyma. The reason for this is that the pH of the fluid compartment containing the antibiotic affects the pKa of the drug and thus its degree of ionization. The degree of ionization in turn determines the lipid solubility of the drug, which is the major factor determining the extent to which a drug penetrates the blood-prostate barrier. Prostatic fluid is often weakly acidic; therefore antibiotics that are weak bases are the ones most likely to penetrate into the parenchyma of the gland. The pH does not affect the lipid solubility of some drugs. Erythromycin, clindamycin, oleandomycin, trimethoprim-sulfonamide (or sulfa), chloramphenicol, carbenicillin, enrofloxacin, and ciprofloxacin are the agents most capable of achieving therapeutic concentrations in the prostate.

Acute bacterial prostatitis and prostatic abscesses are serious, life-threatening disorders. Treatment must be prompt and aggressive. In addition to antibiotics, fluid therapy is necessary to correct dehydration and shock. Despite aggressive therapy, the morbidity and mortality associated with prostatic abscesses are high. Large prostatic abscesses are treated most effectively by surgical drainage. The abscess may also be drained by fine-needle aspiration under ultrasound guidance. Antibiotic treatment for acute prostatitis and prostatic abscesses should be continued for 2 to 3 weeks. Urine or prostatic fluid should be recultured within a few days of discontinuing antibiotic therapy and again 2 to 4 weeks later to be certain the infection has resolved. Castration should be considered. It can be performed whenever the dog's hemodynamic and metabolic status are stable enough for general anesthesia. Prostatic abscessation has been reported to recur in about 10% of treated dogs.

## CHRONIC BACTERIAL PROSTATITIS

Chronic bacterial prostatitis may be asymptomatic, except for recurrent urinary tract infection. Physical abnormalities may be limited to the urinary tract. Prostatic size and shape may be normal, or the prostate may be asymmetric and more firm than normal. It may or may not be painful to palpation. Dogs with chronic bacterial prostatitis are usually willing to ejaculate. Prostatic fluid and urine should be submitted for cytologic and microbiologic examination.

Chronic bacterial prostatitis may be difficult to eradicate. Antibiotic therapy should be continued for at least 4 weeks. Cultures should be repeated during and for several months after discontinuing antibiotic therapy to ascertain whether resistance to antibiotics or persistent infection has developed. Castration is beneficial in the treatment of chronic bacterial prostatitis.

Cystic structures within the prostate are found in some dogs with BPH (see earlier discussion). Many of these cysts are found to have asymptomatic infection. The organisms most commonly isolated are *E. coli, Streptococcus viridans,* and *Mycoplasma,* sometimes in mixed populations. In a study by Marquez Black and colleagues (1998), urine cultures were positive when the cyst fluid cultures were positive, except in one case in which mixed infection *Mycoplasma* was not isolated from the urine when it was from the prostatic cyst. Furthermore, asymptomatic bacterial urinary tract infection was identified in several of the dogs that had negative prostatic cyst cultures. These findings emphasize the importance of urine cultures in the overall management of prostatic disease.

## PARAPROSTATIC CYSTS

Paraprostatic cysts apparently develop from remnants of the müllerian duct or as a result of the tremendous enlargement of an existing cyst (prostatic retention cyst). In the former situation the rest of the prostate gland is essentially normal, whereas in the latter situation, cystic benign hyperplasia usually exists. Often the origin of the cyst is obscure. Paraprostatic cysts are located outside the prostatic parenchyma but are attached to the gland by a stalk or adhesions. These cysts can become extremely large and cause signs, including tenesmus, stemming from mechanical interference with abdominal viscera.

### Diagnosis

A paraprostatic cyst should be considered in the dog with a large caudal-abdominal mass. The mass may be difficult to differentiate from the urinary bladder unless cystography is performed (Fig. 62-4). Fine-needle aspiration of the paraprostatic cyst usually yields a sterile, yellow-to-serosanguineous fluid showing minimal evidence of inflammation.

### Treatment

The treatment of choice is surgical excision of the cyst and castration. In situations where the cyst cannot be completely excised, omentalization is recommended. If this fails to resolve the problem, marsupialization could be performed. Marsupialization is considered a poor alternative to extirpation and to omentalization because it is not curative in and of itself, and the permanent fistula may become infected.

## PROSTATIC NEOPLASIA

Prostatic adenocarcinoma is the most common neoplasm of the canine prostate. It occurs in older dogs, with a mean age of 10 years at the time of diagnosis. Transitional cell carcinoma arising in the urinary tract may also invade the prostate. The clinical signs and biologic behavior of both tumors in the prostate gland are similar. Prostatic adenocarcinoma is locally invasive and metastasizes to the sublumbar lymph nodes, bony pelvis, and lumbar vertebrae. The link between previous castration and the development of prostatic adenocarcinoma is unclear, but 45% of affected dogs have been previously castrated, which is higher than the percentage of castrated dogs in the general hospital population of dogs. Prostatic neoplasia

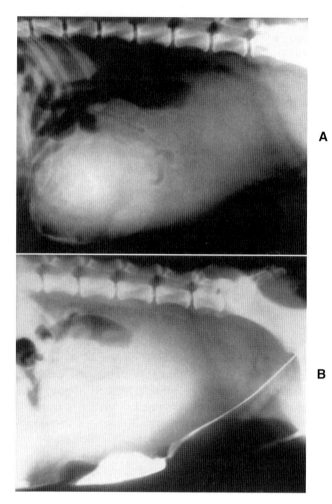

**FIG 62-4**
Very large, partially calcified, paraprostatic cyst. **A,** Survey radiograph and **B,** cystourethrogram showing bladder displacement.

was the only prostatic disease found in the neutered males of a population of 177 dogs with prostatic disease. A benign prostatic adenoma has been reported in one intact male dog. Prostatic adenocarcinoma is rarely reported in cats.

### Clinical Features

Clinical signs include tenesmus and dyschezia, stranguria, pain, gait abnormalities, and weight loss. Palpation of the prostate usually elicits pain. The gland is usually not dramatically enlarged, but the shape may be irregular and the consistency somewhat firmer than normal. Because prostatic involution, resulting in a small gland, occurs within 12 weeks of castration, prostatic neoplasia should be the primary consideration in a previously castrated male found to have a "normal" or large size prostate. Urinary obstruction rarely occurs in dogs as a result of prostatic diseases other than prostatic neoplasia, but it is fairly common in those with cancer.

### Diagnosis

The diagnosis of prostatic neoplasia is suggested by the history, physical, and radiographic findings. Prostatic adenocarcinoma is usually hyperechoic relative to the normal prostate, but this is not pathognomonic. The finding of urethral invasion demonstrated by contrast radiologic studies or ultrasonography is highly suggestive of neoplasia. The diagnosis is confirmed by fine-needle aspiration or biopsy findings. Neoplastic cells may be found in specimens aspirated through a urethral catheter, especially if the tumor is transitional cell carcinoma or prostatic adenocarcinoma that has invaded the urethra. Usually, however, neoplastic cells are not found in massage or ejaculate specimens. The serum and seminal plasma concentrations of acid phosphatase and prostate-specific antigen are not different between normal dogs and dogs with prostatic disease. Although prostate-specific esterase concentrations are higher in dogs with prostatic disease than in normal dogs, this finding is not specific to the cause of prostatic disease.

## Treatment

The prognosis for animals with prostatic adenocarcinoma is grave. To date, surgical (prostatectomy), chemotherapeutic, hormonal, and radiation therapy have been largely unsuccessful in improving the quality or length of life.

## Suggested Readings

Atalan G et al: Comparison of ultrasonographic and radiographic measurements of canine prostate measurements, *Vet Radiol Ultrasound* 40:408, 1999.

Atalan G et al: Ultrasonographic estimation of prostate size in normal dogs and relationship to bodyweight and age, *J Small Anim Pract* 40:119, 1999.

Barsanti JE et al: Effects of an extract of *Serenoa repens* on dogs with hyperplasia of the prostate gland, *Am J Vet Res* 61:880, 2000.

Court EA et al: Effects of delmadinone acetate on pituitary-adrenal function, glucose tolerance and growth hormone in male dogs, *Aust Vet J* 76:555, 1998.

Dorfman M et al: CVT update: treatment of canine bacterial prostatitis. In Bonagura JD, editor: *Kirk's current veterinary therapy XII*, Philadelphia, 1995, WB Saunders, p 1029.

Johnston SD et al, editors: *Canine and feline theriogenology*, Philadelphia, 2001, WB Saunders.

Kay ND et al: Cytological diagnosis of canine prostatic disease using urethral brush technique, *J Am Anim Hosp Assoc* 25:517, 1989.

Marquez Black G et al: Prevalence of prostatic cysts in adult, large-breed dogs, *J Am Anim Hosp Assoc* 34:177, 1998.

Rawlings CA et al: Use of partial prostatectomy for treatment of prostatic abscesses and cysts in dogs, *J Am Vet Med Assoc* 211:868, 1997.

Read RA et al: Urethral bleeding as a presenting sign of benign prostatic hyperplasia in the dog: a retrospective study (1979-1993), *J Am Anim Hosp Assoc* 31:261, 1995.

Sirinarumitr K: Effects of finasteride on size of the prostate gland and semen quality in dogs with benign prostatic hypertrophy, *J Am Vet Med Assoc* 218:1275, 2001.

Teske E et al: Zur Aussagekraft der Zytologie bei der Diagnostik des Prostatakarzinoms beim Heyrd, *Kleintierpraxis* 41:239, 1996.

# CHAPTER 63

# Genital Infections and Transmissible Venereal Tumor

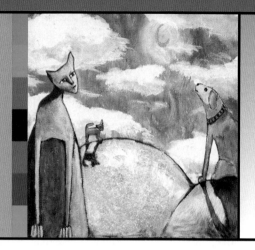

## CHAPTER OUTLINE

GENITAL INFECTION, 934
    Herpesvirus infection, 934
    *Mycoplasma* and *Ureaplasma*, 935
    *Brucella canis*, 936
CANINE TRANSMISSIBLE VENEREAL TUMOR, 938

## *GENITAL INFECTION*

### HERPESVIRUS INFECTION
#### Clinical Features

Although herpesviruses are generally species specific, they cause similar clinical syndromes in most species of animals. Mild respiratory tract disease is the most common clinical sign of herpesvirus infection in dogs and cats older than 12 weeks of age. The lesions are usually limited to the mucosal surfaces of the oropharynx. Occasionally, the manifestations of feline herpesvirus (FHV) type I (i.e., rhinotracheitis) may be severe and include conjunctivitis, corneal ulceration, and fatal pneumonia. The severity of the clinical signs is directly related to the immunocompetence of the host. Pregnant females, animals with compromised immune systems, and neonates are at greatest risk of infection and illness. Because herpesviruses are spread primarily by aerosolization and direct contact with oronasal secretions, the population density, segregation of life stages, and sanitation of the facility influence the severity of disease within the colony. The prevalence of canine herpesvirus (CHV) is estimated to be 10% to 15% in single-pet households and as high as 85% in kennels. Once infected, animals are considered infected for life. The infection may remain latent or be expressed at any time. Nasal secretions, even from asymptomatic carriers, are considered epizootiologically the most important routes of transmission. Venereal transmission of CHVs and FHVs is rare.

In neonates, herpesvirus infection causes fulminant multiple-organ failure and death. Neonates become infected either in utero or through exposure to infected secretions of the dam or through postnatal exposure to infected older members of the colony. Neonatal herpesvirus infection is one of the most common manifestations of CHV infection in a breeding colony. Neonates nursing seropositive bitches are resistant to infection.

Abortion, stillbirths, and infertility have been observed in dogs and cats with herpesvirus infection. CHV has been suggested as the causative organism of vesicular lesions of the vagina and prepuce, but isolation of the virus from spontaneously occurring genital cases is rarely reported. The experimental intravaginal inoculation of CHV and FHV has been observed to produce vesicular lesions in their host species. CHV has been recovered from semen and can be transmitted venereally.

Different types of herpesvirus have been identified in some species. The primary route of transmission and the clinical signs vary according to the type. For example, equine herpesvirus type 3 is transmitted venereally and causes genital lesions, whereas equine herpesvirus type 4 is transmitted by the aerosol route and causes rhinopneumonitis. Similar differences in the routes of transmission and pathogenicity are found among the various types of human herpesviruses. Although only one CHV has been described, the possibility that the more common respiratory and neonatal manifestations are caused by a different type of CHV than the less common genital form should be considered. FHV type 2 has been implicated in feline lower urinary tract disease and has many similarities to bovine herpesvirus type 4. The relationship between the two is being investigated.

#### Diagnosis

As stated earlier, the most common clinical signs of herpesvirus infection in dogs and cats are respiratory. From the standpoint of reproductive disease, herpesvirus infection should be considered in cases of acute neonatal death, as a potential cause of abortion, and as a potential cause of vesicular lesions of the mucosal surfaces of the genitalia in adult animals. Genital herpes is very uncommon relative to respiratory infection in dogs and cats. The diagnosis can be confirmed by the finding of the characteristic intranuclear inclusion bodies in tissue sections, by serologic studies, and by virus isolation.

The diagnosis of CHV infection is most easily established in cases of neonatal death. The clinical signs and postmortem lesions are very characteristic in this setting. Grossly, the lesions consist of multifocal, diffuse hemorrhages and gray discoloration of parenchymal organs, especially the kidney, liver, and lungs. Microscopically, multifocal, necrotizing lesions are found. The virus can be isolated from many organs, especially the adrenals, lung, liver, kidneys, and spleen. In cases of neonatal death, chilled (not frozen) samples from the liver, kidney, and spleen should be submitted for virus isolation and formalin fixed for histopathologic examination. The whole abortus or placenta can be submitted chilled for virus isolation. Although FHV infection causes abortion in pregnant cats, the virus is usually not recoverable from aborted material. Intranuclear inclusions are found in histologic specimens from the uterus, placenta, and aborted fetus of infected queens. CHV has been isolated from various organs of dead canine fetuses.

In cases of suspected herpes-induced genital lesions, swabs from the affected area should be submitted on ice for virus isolation. Some laboratories have found that herpesviruses are more easily recovered from rayon-Dacron swabs (Dacron-tipped applicators; Baxter, Deerfield, Ill) than from wooden cotton-tipped swabs. This is especially important if the virus concentration is low.

Herpesvirus has usually not been isolated beyond 2 to 3 weeks after the primary infection. Therefore virus isolation is not a very useful diagnostic test for chronic infection, unless viral recrudescence has occurred. The genital lesions can be biopsied. Histopathologic findings typical of herpesvirus infection include the vesicles produced by profound degeneration of epithelial cells. Acantholysis is marked. Inclusions may be found but are less common in the material from genital lesions than in nasal epithelium or kidney tissue.

Because genital lesions have not been reported for cats with naturally occurring FHV infection, virus isolation can be attempted from nasal and conjunctival swabs. Samples should be collected during the first week of illness, because the virus is usually not recoverable in animals with chronic infection. Conjunctival smears may show intranuclear inclusions if fluorescent antibody techniques are used. However, the inclusions are transient and difficult to detect. The histopathologic appearance of FHV is characteristic and similar to that of CHV; however, intranuclear inclusions are reliably found only early in infection.

Herpesviruses induce a weak systemic humoral response in the host, with antibody titers rising and falling quickly (4 to 8 weeks) after infection. Titers are relatively low in the setting of both FHV (1:8 to 1:64) and CHV (1:2 to 1:32) infection. The detection of antibody titers indicates exposure to herpesvirus (or the presence of maternal antibodies in animals less than 6 weeks old). Titers are not indicative of viral shedding. If seropositive animals also show typical clinical signs, this is considered diagnostic for herpesvirus infection.

### Prevention and Control

From the standpoint of healthy reproduction, herpesvirus infection is prevented and controlled by changing management practices. Crowded conditions should be eliminated. Her-

pesviruses are very labile, and commonly available disinfectants are effective in destroying them. Sanitation and hygiene should be improved. Animals should be segregated according to life stages. Pregnant females and neonates should be isolated from all other colony members. Although a bitch infected late in pregnancy is likely to suffer neonatal losses, she is also likely to acquire some immunity, which will protect her subsequent litters. For that reason, neonatal CHV usually is not a recurrent problem in an individual bitch. Neonatal CHV may remain a colony problem, however, unless management practices are changed. Modified-live and killed vaccines against FHV (e.g., against feline rhinotracheitis) are available. No vaccine against CHV exists.

## MYCOPLASMA AND UREAPLASMA

*Mycoplasma* and *Ureaplasma* are members of the normal genital flora of dogs, being found in the vagina, prepuce, and distal urethra. *Mycoplasma* has been isolated from 59% of vaginal cultures, 80% of preputial samples, and 27% of semen samples from normal dogs in kennels with pregnancy rates of 88% to 90%. Of the numerous aerobic organisms isolated from these dogs, *Mycoplasma* constituted about 9% of the vaginal isolates, 11% of the preputial isolates, and 3% of the seminal isolates. In comparison, bacterial cultures yielded no growth of aerobic organisms in about 14% of preputial samples, 70% of semen samples, and 5% of vaginal samples. Although many species of *Mycoplasma* and *Ureaplasma* have been isolated from diseased animals, few have been shown conclusively to be pathogenic. Perhaps a preexisting pathologic condition is necessary for an opportunistic infection to develop. *Mycoplasma* infection has been reported to cause conjunctivitis, polyarthritis, abscesses, and urinary tract infection in cats. In dogs, pneumonia, urinary tract infection, colitis, and reproductive disorders have been associated with *Mycoplasma* and *Ureaplasma* infection.

Experimental inoculation of the reproductive tract with *Mycoplasma canis* causes endometritis in bitches and orchitis and epididymitis in dogs. Although *M. canis* has been recovered from bitches with spontaneously occurring endometritis and from infertile dogs with leukospermia, the causative role of the *Mycoplasma* is not clear. In a survey of 136 bitches and dogs, there was no difference between the prevalence of *Mycoplasma* isolated from normal animals and the prevalence of *Mycoplasma* isolated from animals with reproductive disorders.

In that same study, *Ureaplasma* organisms were isolated only in association with *Mycoplasma*. Although *Ureaplasma* were found more often in bitches with purulent vulvar discharges than in normal bitches, the difference was not statistically significant. *Ureaplasma* were significantly more prevalent in the prepuce of infertile dogs than in the prepuce of normal dogs, but results of semen cultures in both groups were the same. Additional studies of the role of *Mycoplasma* and *Ureaplasma* in reproductive disorders of dogs and cats are needed.

Because *Mycoplasma* and *Ureaplasma* are members of the normal canine genital flora, and because they are isolated with equal frequency from normal dogs and dogs with reproductive disorders, *Mycoplasma* or *Ureaplasma* infection should not be diagnosed based on culture results alone. The clinical signs and cytologic findings should also be consistent with an infectious process. *Mycoplasma* and *Ureaplasma* are fragile organisms. A special medium such as Amies must be used for culture studies, and samples should be placed on ice and arrive at the laboratory within 24 hours. Susceptibility testing is rarely available. Usually the organisms are susceptible to tetracycline, chloramphenicol, and fluoroquinolones. Erythromycin, lincomycin, and the aminoglycosides are less effective. Unfortunately, many of these antibiotics are contraindicated during pregnancy and lactation. Antibiotic therapy should continue for 2 to 3 weeks, or longer if a bacteriostatic antibiotic is chosen. Isolation, and even culling, of infected animals has been recommended for the control of *Mycoplasma* infection in a kennel, but such extreme measures are not usually necessary.

## BRUCELLA CANIS

*Brucella canis* is a small, gram-negative coccobacillus. Natural infection is limited to *Canidae* and rarely humans. *B. canis* is capable of penetrating any mucous membrane, but the oral, conjunctival, and vaginal membranes are the most important in the natural transmission of the disease. The oronasal transmission of aerosolized organisms from aborted material is one of the most important modes of transmission because of the large numbers of organisms contained therein. Females transmit the disease during estrus, at breeding, transplacentally, and after abortion. The organism is also shed in the milk and urine of infected females, but in lower numbers. Nevertheless, urine is a potential route of transmission, especially if animals are housed in groups.

*B. canis* can be transmitted in semen, especially during the first 6 to 8 weeks of infection when the number of organisms in seminal fluid is very high. Later in infection the number of organisms recovered from semen is lower, but shedding persists for 60 weeks to 2 years. The urinary excretion of *B. canis* coincides with the onset of bacteremia and persists for at least 3 months. The urine of infected male dogs can contain enough organisms to be a source of infection. *B. canis* can also be transmitted on contaminated fomites.

Once the mucous membrane is penetrated, *B. canis* is phagocytosed by macrophages and transported to the lymphoid and genital tissues. Bacteremia is present 1 to 4 weeks after infection and persists for 6 months to 5.5 years. With infection, the animal experiences transient lymphoid tissue hyperplasia and hyperglobulinemia. Because *B. canis* is an intracellular organism, cell-mediated immunity is the most important defense against infection. Nonprotective antibody titers develop 4 to 12 weeks after infection and persist for as long as the bacteremia is present. Titers decline after the bacteremia subsides, even though the organism is still present in tissues.

### Clinical Features

*B. canis* infection primarily affects reproduction. Abortion, especially late in gestation, in an otherwise healthy afebrile bitch, is the most common clinical sign of *B. canis* infection in females. Abortion in infected animals can occur at any time during gestation. Early embryonic death and conception failure are also reported. Occasionally a litter in an infected bitch is carried to term, but the pups usually die within a few days of birth.

The most common clinical sign of *B. canis* infection in males is infertility. Scrotal and epididymal enlargement are usually transient early in infection. Testicular enlargement is uncommon; testicular atrophy occurs in animals with chronic infection. Abnormalities in seminal quality occur within 5 weeks of infection and become pronounced by 8 weeks. White blood cells, macrophages, sperm agglutination, and abnormal sperm morphology are found. By 20 weeks of infection, more than 90% of the sperm may be abnormal. Eventually testicular atrophy develops. Azoospermia with evidence of resolution of the inflammation is found in the semen.

Occasionally, *B. canis* infects other tissues. Uveitis, diskospondylitis, osteomyelitis, and dermatitis have been noted in animals with *B. canis* infection. Infection of these other tissues is associated with clinical signs related to disease of these organ systems.

### Diagnosis

The diagnosis of *B. canis* infection is suggested by the history, seminal abnormalities in the male, and the relative absence of physical abnormalities. The organism must be isolated and identified for the diagnosis to be confirmed. *B. canis* grows slowly on the conventional media used for other brucellae. Specimens must not be contaminated, because faster-growing organisms will overgrow *B. canis*. The concentration of organisms is very high in aborted material and the postabortion vulvar discharge, making them the preferred specimens to culture. If these specimens are not available, blood, urine, or semen can be cultured. Polymerase chain reaction (PCR) techniques have also been used to confirm the diagnosis.

Hemoculture is the best method for identifying early (2 to 8 weeks) infection. The number of bacteria in blood usually remains very high for at least 6 months after infection. As mentioned earlier, the bacteremia subsides as the infection becomes chronic; thus blood cultures are not always positive. Semen cultures are most helpful during the first 3 months of infection, when the number of organisms in semen is high. Urine cultures may be positive, especially in males. The organism can also be recovered from lymph nodes, spleen, liver, bone marrow, prostate, epididymis, placenta, and the lumen of the gravid or postabortion uterus.

Although isolation of the organism is the definitive diagnosis, it is a time-consuming procedure. It is also impractical for the routine screening of asymptomatic animals. For this reason, serologic testing is the most frequently used screening diagnostic procedure for *B. canis* infection. Serologic tests use either cell wall (i.e., somatic) or cytoplasmic (i.e., internal) antigens. Antibodies to the cell wall antigens are first detectable 3 to 10 weeks after infection. Although many serologic tests for *B. canis* exist, standardized antigen and standardized diagnostic protocols are not available. Therefore the magnitude of the titers and the accuracy of results vary greatly among laboratories.

The rapid slide agglutination test (RSAT), the tube agglutination test (TAT), and some of the agar gel immunodiffusion (AGID) tests use cell wall antigen. The cell wall antigens are common to many of the *Brucella* spp. and to several other bacteria, including *Pseudomonas aeruginosa* and *Staphylococcus* spp. Therefore the test results are not specific to *B. canis* and false-positive results are possible. A positive result from any of these tests must therefore be confirmed by other methods as truly reflecting *B. canis* infection. An enzyme-linked immunosorbent assay (ELISA) has been reported to be very specific and sensitive for evaluating infected dogs, but it is not yet commercially available.

Despite its lack of specificity, the RSAT (D-Tec CB; Synbiotics, Kansas City, Mo) has the tremendous advantage of being easy, quick to perform, and highly sensitive. False-negative RSAT results are rare (1%) in animals that have been infected long enough to develop antibodies to cell wall antigens. Treatment with antibiotics also may cause negative culture and serology results, despite persistence of the organism in tissues. Titers decline in chronic infection.

AGID tests that use cytoplasmic antigen are highly specific for *Brucella* infection. Only other brucellae share these internal antigens. Antibodies to cytoplasmic antigens are not detected for 8 to 12 weeks after *B. canis* infection, but they may persist for up to 12 months after the bacteremia has ceased. During this time other test results are often negative. Disadvantages of the AGID test are the complexity of the procedure and the fact that it is less sensitive than the RSAT or TAT. A positive result from an AGID test using *B. canis* cytoplasmic antigen would also occur in animals with *Brucella suis* or *Brucella abortus* infection, but this is probably not of great clinical concern because they are both rare in dogs compared with *B. canis* infection.

## Treatment

Because of the intracellular location of *B. canis*, antibiotic therapy rarely results in a cure. Bacteremia often recurs days to months after treatment. Minocycline or a combination of tetracycline and dihydrostreptomycin for 2 to 4 weeks has been the most commonly recommended treatment. However, because dihydrostreptomycin is no longer available, some clinicians have recommended using gentamicin and doxycycline, though therapeutic trials of these agents have not been conducted. The fluoroquinolones have been shown to be effective against *B. canis* in vitro, but in vivo experience is limited. Evidence shows that, despite therapy, the organism is not cleared from the prostate.

The results of cultures and serologic testing become negative in animals with chronic infection and in those receiving antibiotic therapy, despite the persistence of *B. canis* in tissues in both instances; thus it is difficult to ascribe the declining titers and negative culture findings to treatment rather than to the natural progression of the disease. Finally, testicular damage is usually irreversible. Because the chance of successful treatment is so uncertain and because infected animals remain a source of infection for other dogs and people, treatment is ill advised. Treated dogs are readily susceptible to reinfection. If treatment is attempted, infected animals should be neutered to minimize the shed of organisms. No vaccine exists.

## Prevention and Control

*B. canis* is insidious. No readily recognizable signs appear until animals have been infected for weeks or months, during which they have exposed other members of the colony to the infection. Eventually *B. canis* infection will devastate the reproductive performance of the individual animal and the kennel. In kennels with infected animals, conception rates can decline to as low as 30%; the proportion of pregnancies ending in abortion can reach 80%; litter size (Beagles) can decline from a previous average of six pups to one pup per litter; and the number of pups surviving to weaning age can reach zero. Obviously, the risk of inadvertent exposure to asymptomatic, infected animals that are brought into the colony, even briefly, is too great to leave to chance.

The RSAT is recommended for the routine screening of asymptomatic animals, because it is so sensitive. If enough time for antibody production has elapsed, if the animal is not so chronically infected that the titers have declined, and if no antibiotics have been administered, animals that do not have the infection should be correctly identified by this test. As noted earlier, the RSAT lacks specificity, and positive test results must always be confirmed by other diagnostic methods. All animals should be tested before breeding. New members to be added to the colony should be quarantined for 8 to 12 weeks until the results of at least two tests performed at 4-week intervals are negative. Animals with any of the symptoms of *B. canis* infection should never be admitted to the colony for any reason until *B. canis* infection is positively excluded as the cause. As with asymptomatic animals, it may take as long as 3 months to be certain that the animal is not infected.

When an animal is found to be positive based on the RSAT or other screening test, especially if clinical signs compatible with *B. canis* infection are seen, the animal should be isolated from the rest of the colony and the entire kennel should be quarantined until the results can be verified. The definitive diagnosis is made only based on the isolation and identification of the organism. An AGID test that uses cytoplasmic antigens may also be helpful, as discussed earlier.

If the infection is confirmed, the positive animal should be eliminated from the colony and all other colony members tested monthly. Positive animals are eliminated. Monthly colony-wide testing of all remaining animals, including those with negative results to the previous month's test, continues until results are negative in all the remaining animals for 3 consecutive months. Because of the biologic behavior of the infection, it is expected that additional positive animals will be found for several months. The prevalence of infected animals in the colony is usually not significantly lowered until testing and culling have continued for 4 to 5 months.

Testing and culling are time-consuming and expensive, even in small colonies. Many are tempted to try treating the disease rather than to accept the immediate losses incurred by culling. Treatment is made all the more attractive by reports of success. As mentioned earlier, bacteremia and serologic titers diminish in response to antibiotic therapy, and many treated bitches successfully conceive and carry a healthy litter to term during that time. However, it must be emphasized that no study to date has shown that 100% of the animals respond to treatment. In addition, in studies in which animals were evaluated by culturing internal organs or blood 6 or more months after treatment, many were found to still harbor the organism despite negative serologic test results. These animals were therefore not cured. Even when the best possible results have been obtained, some treated animals have remained infected and continue to contaminate the kennel. Treated dogs are also readily reinfected. Several studies of spontaneously occurring infection have shown that *B. canis* cannot be eliminated from the colony, even if infected animals are strictly isolated, until infected animals are actually culled.

Because of the cost of treatment, the cost of maintaining subfertile or infertile animals, the overall decrease in the reproductive efficiency of the colony, the decrease in the number of puppies surviving to weaning, and the persistence of infection in the colony, it is ultimately more economical to test and cull than to attempt treatment. The same has been shown to be true for *Brucella ovis* infection in flocks of sheep.

A different approach might be considered for a household pet than for a breeding animal. Antibiotic therapy plus neutering should essentially eliminate the genital secretions and the shedding of organisms by this route, but this does not absolutely exclude the possibility that the animal might remain a source of infection for other dogs or human members of the household. *B. canis* does not readily infect people, but more than 40 cases have been reported since the 1960s. Most often the source of infection is the person's own pet. Laboratory personnel have also acquired the disease from infected specimens. In some instances the source of human infection has not been found. It is recommended that immunocompromised people avoid contact with infected dogs.

The prevalence of *B. canis* infection in people in the United States is unknown, because, as in dogs, it may not be isolated from blood cultures, especially after antibiotic therapy. The antibodies to *B. canis* also are not detected by some of the common serologic tests for *B. suis*, *B. abortus*, or *Brucella melitensis*. Conversely, cross-reactivity among serologic tests for some other *Brucella* spp. is seen. In this situation, *B. canis* infection would not be differentiated from infection with other *Brucella* spp. Finally, although human brucellosis is a notifiable disease, the Centers for Disease Control (CDC) does not require speciation. After peaking at more than 300 cases in 1975, the number of cases of human brucellosis in the United States has declined and remained relatively stable at approximately 100 cases per year through 2001. How many of these cases represent human infection with *B. canis* is unknown, but literature from the CDC describes it as "rare." In a study of human brucellosis in Texas from 1977 to 1986, *B. canis* infection was found in 4 of the 331 patients with brucellosis. *B. melitensis* accounted for 66% of the cases and was associated with the consumption of unpasteurized goat milk products.

# CANINE TRANSMISSIBLE VENEREAL TUMOR

## Etiology

Transmissible venereal tumor (TVT) is a contagious round-cell tumor of mesenchymal origin. Venereal transmission is most common. It occurs primarily on the mucosal surfaces of the external genitalia of male and female dogs, but it can be transplanted to other sites and transmitted to other dogs by licking and by direct contact with the tumor. Primary TVTs have been found on the skin and in the oral and anal mucous membranes. These neoplastic cells contain 57 to 62 chromosomes, instead of the normal canine complement of 78. The prevalence of TVT seems to vary greatly with the geographic area. It has been reported from many countries throughout the world. Some TVTs regress spontaneously, but most do not. Some TVTs metastasize to the regional lymph nodes, the perineum, or the scrotum. Metastasis seems to be more likely in animals with tumors that have been present for longer than 1 month. Rarely, metastasis to distant sites such as the lungs, abdominal viscera, or central nervous system (CNS) occurs.

## Clinical Features

TVTs have a fleshy, hyperemic appearance. Initially they appear as a raised area. As they grow they acquire a cauliflower-like shape and may reach a diameter of 5 cm or larger. They are often quite friable and bleed easily. TVTs in males are most often found on the bulbus glandis area of the penis, but they may appear anywhere on the penile or preputial mucosa. Affected animals are usually examined because of a mass on the external genitalia, but they may also be seen because of a preputial or vulvar discharge.

## Diagnosis

The diagnosis of TVT is strongly suspected based on the physical appearance of the tumor on the external genitalia. Differential diagnoses, especially in animals with nongenital lesions, include other round-cell tumors such as mast cell tumor, histiocytoma, and lymphoma. Pyogranulomatous lesions of the genitalia may also have a similar gross appearance. The diagnosis of genital TVT is easily confirmed by exfoliative cytologic studies, fine-needle aspiration, or histopathologic findings. The cytologic appearance is very characteristic and consists of a homogeneous population of large round or oval cells with a small nuclear-to-cytoplasmic ratio, prominent nucleoli, and vacuolated cytoplasm; mitotic figures are common. The differentiation of TVT from other round-cell tumors is less confident when the lesion is not on the genitalia.

## Treatment

TVTs respond to several chemotherapeutic agents. However, vincristine, administered once weekly as a single agent (see

Chapter 79), is extremely effective, has a low toxicity, and is financially acceptable to most owners. It is administered for two treatments beyond the time when the tumor disappears. The total duration of treatment is usually 4 to 6 weeks. Complete remission is achieved in more than 90% of dogs treated with vincristine, and they usually remain disease free. TVTs are also extremely sensitive to radiation therapy. Although surgical excision results in long-term control, relapses occur in as many as 50% of animals.

## Suggested Readings

Carmichael LE et al: Canine brucellosis: a diagnostician's dilemma, *Semin Vet Med Surg (Small Anim)* 11:161, 1996.

Carpenter TE et al: Economics of *Brucella ovis* control in sheep: epidemiologic simulation model, *J Am Vet Med Assoc* 190:977, 1987.

Greene CE, editor: *Infectious diseases of the dog and cat,* ed 2, Philadelphia, 1990, WB Saunders.

Johnson CA: Management of *Brucella canis* outbreaks in breeding kennels. In Bonagura JD, editor: *Kirk's current veterinary therapy XII,* Philadelphia, 1995, WB Saunders, p 1094.

Johnston SD et al: *Canine and feline theriogenology,* Philadelphia, 2001, WB Saunders.

Shin S et al: Canine brucellosis caused by *Brucella canis.* In Carmichael LE, editor: *Recent advances in canine infectious disease,* International Veterinary Information Service, 1999, http://www.ivis.org.

Taylor JP et al: The changing epidemiology of human brucellosis in Texas, 1977-1986, *Am J Epidemiol* 130:160, 1989.

## CHAPTER 64

# Artificial Insemination and Frozen Semen

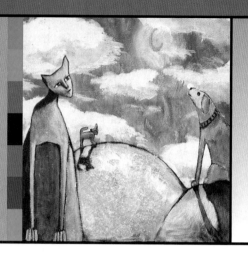

## CHAPTER OUTLINE

PRINCIPLES, 940
TECHNIQUE, 941
FRESH SEMEN, 942
FROZEN SEMEN, 942
CHILLED EXTENDED SEMEN, 943
CAT SEMEN, 943

## PRINCIPLES

Artificial insemination (AI) is used in dogs primarily when natural breeding cannot be accomplished. Transporting semen, rather than live animals, to distant geographic locations is a great advantage of AI over natural service. AI is also used when behavioral problems, such as partner preference, or physical problems, such as vaginal prolapse, prevent copulation of the desired pair. Some dog breeders prefer AI because they believe that the risk of breeding trauma is minimized and that the stud is less likely to be exposed to infectious diseases carried by the bitch. In addition, a single ejaculate with sufficient numbers of spermatozoa can be divided and used to inseminate several bitches. Although the number of viable spermatozoa necessary to maintain conception rates and litter size has not been determined for dogs, 150 to 200 $\times$ 10⁶ viable spermatozoa is considered the minimum desirable number for intravaginal insemination. However, pregnancies produced by intrauterine insemination have been achieved under ideal conditions with as few as 20 $\times$ 10⁶ fresh spermatozoa and 30 to 35 $\times$ 10⁶ normal frozen-thawed spermatozoa.

Several factors determine the success of AI, including the reproductive health of the animals, the quality of the semen, the timing and the number of inseminations, and the technical skills of the person performing the insemination. First and foremost is the reproductive health of the male and female. Normal animals are expected to be willing and able to breed. However, various causes of reluctance to breed, which are discussed in the sections on infertility (see pp. 859 and 913), may make AI necessary. On the other hand, the problem that necessitated AI may also adversely affect fertility.

Second, the timing of insemination is critical. Animals may be brought in for AI because the usual behavioral signs of estrus are not manifested or recognized. In such cases, estrus can be identified by exfoliative vaginal cytology (see p. 853) and ovulation can be estimated by serum luteinizing hormone (LH) or progesterone concentrations. Ideally, several inseminations are planned for a particular estrous cycle, because it has been shown that conception rates and litter size are better if bitches are bred two or three times than if they are bred only once. If only two inseminations are included in the stud fee, which is a common practice, the second insemination would ideally occur 48 or more hours after the first insemination during the fertile period unless frozen-thawed semen is being used (see p. 942).

Insemination at the time fertilizable ova are present greatly improves the chances of conception. Ovulation cannot be determined on the basis of vaginal cytology, but it can be predicted on the basis of the changes in the serum concentrations of LH or progesterone (see p. 855). Progesterone or LH concentrations are determined serially during proestrus and early estrus. The preovulatory luteinization that occurs in bitches is reflected by an increase in serum concentrations of progesterone above 2 ng/ml (approximately 6 nmol/L). This coincides with the LH surge. Because this initial rise in the progesterone concentration is a preovulatory event, and because oocytes must mature for about 2 days after ovulation before fertilization can occur, at least one of the inseminations should take place approximately 4 days after the initial increase in the progesterone concentration is detected. Alternatively, insemination is best performed when serum progesterone concentrations are 30 to 60 nmol/L (approximately 10 to 20 ng/ml). Ovulation timing is especially worthwhile in situations in which pregnancy is urgently desired by the owner and poor fertility is expected (e.g., because frozen semen is being used or because animals are subfertile or aging).

The reproductive health of the breeding animals, the quality of the semen, and the timing and number of inseminations affect fertility, regardless of whether AI or natural insemination is used. The technical aspects (collection, handling, and deposition of semen) of AI add a new set of variables to the already variable determinants of fertility. Prostatic fluid and other seminal components are known to have deleterious effects on spermatozoa during long-term storage. If immediate AI with fresh semen is to be performed, this is probably of little importance. Prostatic fluid, the third fraction of the ejaculate, is not collected with the sperm-rich fraction when semen is being collected for AI, except to ensure that the entire sperm-rich fraction was collected.

Whenever semen is handled, it must be protected from spermicidal agents. These include water, lubricants, some plastics, and some types of rubber. The latex rubber of which artificial vaginas are made (see p. 907) may also be spermicidal. It is necessary to lubricate the artificial vagina to prevent the penis from being damaged by the device, and the lubricant can be spermicidal. In addition, some, but not all, plastics from which some urine cups or centrifuge tubes are made have been shown to diminish sperm motility. Certain plastics liberate aldehydes or contain mold retardants or other chemicals that are potentially spermicidal. Because the use of at least some potentially spermicidal agents cannot be avoided, contact of the semen with them must be minimized. Centrifugation has also been shown to decrease motility and alter the acrosomes and viability.

While the semen is being handled, it must be protected from sudden changes in temperature. Freshly ejaculated canine semen is most effectively protected against temperature shock by working at room temperature and inseminating promptly after collection. Spermatozoa in normal, nonextended dog semen usually maintain normal motility for at least 15 minutes at room temperature. Chilled and frozen semen must be protected against damage during chilling, freezing, and thawing. This is accomplished by adding a protective "semen extender" to the sample and by careful attention to cooling, freezing, and thawing rates. Semen extenders have been formulated to provide nutritional support for the sperm cells, to buffer pH changes that occur because of continued metabolic activity, to maintain physiologic osmotic pressure, to prevent bacterial growth, to protect cells from cold shock during chilling, and to limit cell damage during freezing and thawing.

## TECHNIQUE

Regardless of whether freshly ejaculated, chilled, or frozen-thawed semen is used for AI, the principles are the same. First, the (thawed) sample is examined microscopically to determine its quality. A complete semen evaluation can be performed (see p. 907), but more typically the number of normal motile sperm is estimated by microscopic examination of a drop of semen. The semen should be gently mixed before the drop is removed to ensure that a representative sample is obtained. The slide and coverslip should be warm (37° C) so that motility is not artifactually diminished by cooling. It has been assumed that motile sperm are viable and that nonmotile sperm are not. However, although the former is certainly true, the latter may not be. It is also recognized that all live sperm are not necessarily capable of fertilization. Certainly, insemination with dead sperm serves no useful purpose.

The effects of various morphologic defects on fertility have not been thoroughly evaluated in dogs, but the use of samples containing more than 30% to 40% abnormal spermatozoa is known to result in very poor pregnancy rates. There is a correlation between motility and morphology, with abnormal spermatozoa more likely to be nonmotile than normal spermatozoa. Spermatozoa with proximal droplets appear to lack the capacity to fertilize, but fertility is apparently not affected if spermatozoa have distal droplets. The total number of normal, motile spermatozoa inseminated is the critical seminal determinant of conception rates and litter size in dogs.

It is important to document semen quality before insemination, because the success of the insemination will be no better than the quality of the semen. Knowing that semen quality is poor, the owner may then wish to use different semen. Although pregnancies are occasionally achieved using fresh semen of inferior quality, the litter size is usually smaller. Usually no litters result if frozen-thawed semen of poor quality is used. In addition, once inseminated, the bitch should not be bred to a different male during that cycle, because paternity will then be uncertain unless DNA testing is done.

Once the decision to use this semen is made, the sample is gently mixed and aspirated into a syringe of suitable size for the volume to be inseminated. Vaginal insemination is acceptable for fresh and chilled semen but not for frozen-thawed semen because conception rates are very poor in that case. A volume of 2 to 10 ml, depending on the breed, is customarily used for vaginal insemination. The insemination pipette is passed into the cranial vagina, as close as possible to the cervix. Because the canine cervix is difficult to catheterize (see p. 853), the pipette is not typically passed into the uterus unless special equipment is used. Given the length of the canine vagina, the AI pipette should be at least 10 to 25 cm long (depending on the breed) to ensure that semen is deposited in the cranial vagina. Standard bovine AI pipettes work well for bitches. They are 18 or 22 inches (45 or 55 cm) long but can easily be cut to the desired length if needed. Raw edges can be smoothed by heating them with a flame. It takes gentle maneuvering to pass the pipette to the level of the cervix. A gloved finger can serve as a guide as the pipette passes through the vestibule and posterior vagina. Some veterinarians also believe that vaginal massage promotes uterine contractions. Some have recommended that the bitch's rear quarters be elevated (so that her spine is nearly vertical) throughout the insemination procedure.

Once the pipette is in position, the semen is gently injected through it, followed by the gentle injection of air to ensure that none of the sample remains in the pipette. The pipette is then removed, and the bitch's rear quarters are elevated for 10 to 15 minutes to promote the flow of semen toward the cervix and hasten the arrival of sperm in the uterine horns. The bitch should not be restrained or lifted in a manner that applies pressure on the abdomen, because some of the semen sample may then be forced out the vagina.

Intrauterine, rather than intravaginal, insemination is important if frozen-thawed semen, which has a very short life span, is being used, because fewer spermatozoa may then be needed for conception and because the spermatozoa do not then need to traverse the cervix. It has been estimated that to achieve the same results, at least 10 times the number of viable sperm are needed for vaginal AI than for intrauterine AI. A special canine AI catheter, the Norwegian catheter (Norske Pelsdyrforlag A/L, Oslo, Norway), has been designed for transcervical intrauterine insemination. Others have described using an endoscope to guide a catheter to the cervical os. Transcervical insemination is performed in the awake, standing bitch. Finally, intrauterine insemination can be accomplished surgically, through a minilaparotomy, or laparoscopically. Intrauterine insemination can also be used for fresh and chilled semen, where it would offer the same advantages as for the more fragile frozen-thawed semen.

## FRESH SEMEN

Freshly ejaculated semen is used far more often than chilled or frozen semen. The AI of semen of normal quality should yield conception rates and litter sizes similar to those associated with natural service, provided that the semen is not damaged during the process and that the timing and the placement (i.e., cranial vagina) of the inseminate are appropriate. Pregnancy rates associated with natural service in privately owned dogs (as opposed to those observed in commercial or laboratory settings) are reported to be 85% to 90%. Pregnancy rates of 84% have been achieved through the vaginal AI of fresh semen. Results are poorer if semen of inferior quality is used. In addition, although conception may still occur, litter sizes are usually smaller. The American Kennel Club (AKC) will register litters conceived by AI with freshly ejaculated semen. It is not necessary that a veterinarian perform the collection and insemination; however, the breeder is required to complete an additional registration form.

## FROZEN SEMEN

The cryopreservation of semen is the only way in which semen, and therefore the genetic potential of valuable male animals, can be saved indefinitely. Using frozen semen, litters can be sired by a dog long after his death. In addition, semen can be collected and stored whenever it is convenient to do so, in contrast to natural service, in which the timing is determined by the availability of cycling females. The frozen semen, rather than the animals, can also be shipped to distant geographic locations when convenient. In contrast, the timing of shipping of animals and of chilled semen is dictated by the female's estrous cycle. A further drawback of natural breeding that can be circumvented by using frozen semen is that there may be great demand for stud service at some times of the year and none at other times.

The progressive motility of spermatozoa after thawing and the total sperm dose are the most important seminal factors in determining fertility using frozen-thawed semen. Unfortunately, the variables routinely assessed in fresh semen, with

the possible exception of proximal cytoplasmic droplets, are of little value in predicting the post-thaw motility of semen of normal quality. The post-thaw quality of inferior samples is usually substantially worse than the pre-freeze quality.

Conception rates achieved using frozen semen vary according to the extender used, the sperm-processing techniques used (pellets versus straws, freezing rates, thawing rates), the number of viable sperm, the timing and frequency of insemination, and the site of insemination (intravaginal, intrauterine). Pregnancy rates achieved with vaginal insemination using frozen-thawed semen of good quality under field conditions have been about 30%, whereas pregnancy rates of 70% to 84% have been achieved when intrauterine insemination has been performed during the optimal time (i.e., 2 to 5 days after ovulation). Conception rates reportedly vary according to the extender used. At present, it is not clear which extender is most ideal for canine semen. Data from studies of proprietary frozen semen should be interpreted and compared cautiously, however, until further objective evaluations in which variables such as the AI technique, timing of insemination, and post-thaw semen quality are controlled.

Practicing veterinarians are more likely to be involved with the insemination, rather than the freezing, of semen. (See Concannon and colleague [1989] for an overview of the technical aspects of the cryopreservation of semen.) A list of semen collection and storage facilities in the United States can be obtained from the AKC. The collection and storage facility releases frozen semen on the authorization of the owner of the semen. It is shipped in a small tank primed with liquid nitrogen, known as a "dry shipper." If the semen is to be stored for longer than a few days before use, it will probably be safer if it is transferred to a tank in which it can be submerged in liquid nitrogen.

The semen should be accompanied by information from the collection and storage facility regarding the number of sperm in each straw or vial and the recommendations for thawing the semen. The latter is important because the thawing rates and temperatures have a significant effect on the post-thaw motility. The ideal rates and temperatures are influenced by the ingredients in the extender. Although the number of studies from different laboratories is limited, the data indicate that faster thaw rates at higher temperatures (such as 75° C for 12 seconds or 70° C for 6 seconds) are generally better than slow rates at lower temperatures (1° C for 120 seconds or 23° C for several minutes). Because variations of even a few degrees or a few seconds affect the post-thaw motility, the instructions from the supplier must be followed exactly.

As is clear from the preceding discussion, thawing begins as soon as the semen is no longer submerged in the liquid nitrogen. Therefore the semen must not be removed from the liquid nitrogen until all the other equipment is prepared for the proper thawing process. The samples must never remain in contact with the high temperatures used for thawing for longer than is recommended. Even normal, freshly ejaculated dog sperm are quickly killed by high temperatures. Poor post-thaw thermoresistance has been a problem with canine semen. It has been shown that if dog semen with an immediate post-thaw motility of 50% is incubated at 23° or 37° C for 2 hours, sperm motility decreases to 20%. By 6 hours, the post-thaw motility is zero. In contrast, bull semen incubated at 37° C has an immediate post-thaw motility of about 50%, a motility of 40% to 50% at 3 hours, and a motility of 20% by 8 hours of incubation.

After thawing and before insemination, a drop of semen should be examined to assess motility (see p. 908). The post-thaw motility is affected by the pre-freeze quality of the semen and by the extender, freezing technique, and thawing process used. Most laboratories strive to attain post-thaw motilities of 50% to 60%. This is usually possible only for semen of excellent quality. Semen with a pre-freeze motility of less than 70% is unlikely to yield satisfactory results after it has been frozen. Poor post-thaw motility may be partially compensated for by inseminating the animal with greater numbers of sperm than originally planned for that breeding. The post-thaw motility and the total sperm dose are the best predictors of the fertilizing capability of canine frozen semen identified thus far. Unlike in some species, the post-thaw acrosomal integrity and sperm morphology are apparently not predictors of fertility in dogs.

Because frozen-thawed semen has a short life span of less than 24 hours and apparently has difficulty migrating through the cervix, the timing of insemination and the placement of the semen are especially critical. Every available tool (vaginal cytology, measurement of serum LH or progesterone concentrations) should be used to determine the optimal time for insemination. Intrauterine insemination is clearly superior to intravaginal insemination. Intrauterine insemination may be accomplished by transcervical catheterization or by a surgical approach to the uterine horns.

Each dog registry club has its own rules and regulations regarding the registration of puppies conceived from frozen semen. These regulations may be subject to change, and they may differ depending on whether domestic or imported frozen semen is used. Likewise, there are regulations governing the importation and exportation of semen from one country to another. The AKC will register litters conceived by AI with frozen semen. However, insemination must be performed by a veterinarian, and certification from the owner of the semen, the owner of the bitch, and the veterinarian must be provided for registration. Since 1999 the AKC also requires DNA identification of the male. The Canadian Kennel Club will register litters of recognized breeds conceived by AI with fresh, chilled, or frozen semen. It requires certification from the veterinarian who collected the semen, the veterinarian who inseminated the semen, the owner of the sire, and the owner of the dam. Semen cannot be imported into Canada until approval is obtained from the Veterinary Director General of Agriculture Canada. The Field Dog Stud Book and the United Kennel Club also register litters born from frozen semen.

## CHILLED EXTENDED SEMEN

Properly extended canine semen may remain fertile for several days at refrigeration temperatures. The advantage of chilled semen over natural breeding is that the semen, rather than the animals, can be transported. The advantage of chilled semen over frozen semen is that the conception rates are better. Concannon and colleague (1989) described several extenders that have been used for the cold storage of dog semen. They are similar to those used for freezing semen, except that glycerol is omitted. Glycerol is the most commonly used cryoprotectant, but although it protects sperm from freezing damage, it depresses sperm fertility. Extender, equipment, and instructions for their use and for collecting, chilling, and inseminating semen are available from several commercial sources (Fresh Express ICG, Synbiotics, San Diego Calif; Cryogenetics Laboratory of New England, Chester Springs, Pa; International Canine Semen Bank, Portland, Ore; Canine Cryobank, Encinitas, Calif).

The sperm-rich portion of the ejaculate is collected with as little prostatic fluid as possible. The quality of the semen should be evaluated before proceeding further. Instructions from commercially available systems should be followed exactly. Typically, one part of semen is diluted with one to five parts of extender at 23° to 35° C. The ratio of semen to extender depends on the type of extender and the volume of the ejaculate. The extended semen is then cooled in a standard refrigerator to 5° C over 30 minutes to several hours. The rate of cooling is very important to sperm survival and protection against cold shock. Rapid cooling should be avoided. This is accomplished by placing the extended semen in a warm or room temperature water bath in the refrigerator, according to instructions. The rate of cooling is influenced by the size of the sample, the size and shape of the container, and the volume and temperature of the water bath. These variables are adjusted for each sample, as necessary, to achieve the proper rate of cooling. The sample should not be chilled below 4° C.

Properly extended and cooled semen of good quality can be stored at 5° C for 12 to 24 hours, and usually longer. Chilled semen is slowly warmed to room temperature before insemination. Pregnancy rates of 50% to 70% are reported for the use of various extenders with chilled semen and vaginal insemination. Motility should always be evaluated before insemination. If possible, the dose should be adjusted to ensure adequate numbers of motile sperm. The AKC will register litters from chilled, extended semen.

## CAT SEMEN

AI with fresh or frozen feline semen is rarely performed in clinical practice. The same principles apply to cats as to dogs, but the collection of semen is more difficult. Domestic cats have served as the reproductive model for the big cats, especially endangered species. Therefore information is available on semen collection, semen freezing, AI, estrous induction, embryo transfer, and in vitro fertilization in domestic cats used in research facilities. The interested reader is referred to the review by Howard (1992).

## Suggested Readings

Axnér E: Mating and artificial insemination in domestic cats. In England GCW et al, editors: *Manual of small animal reproduction and neonatology,* Cheltenham, UK, 1998, British Small Animal Veterinary Association, p 105.

Concannon PW et al: Canine semen freezing and artificial insemination. In Kirk RW, editor: *Current veterinary therapy X,* Philadelphia, 1989, WB Saunders, p 1247.

Concannon PW et al, editors: Reproduction of dogs and cats and exotic carnivores, *J Reprod Fertil Suppl* 51:99, 1997.

Concannon PW et al, editors: Advances in reproduction of dogs and cats and exotic carnivores, *J Reprod Fertil Suppl* 57:151, 341, 2001.

Farstad W: Mating and artificial insemination in the dog. In England GCW et al, editors: *Manual of small animal reproduction and neonatology,* Cheltenham, UK, 1998, British Small Animal Veterinary Association, p 95.

Goodman M: Ovulation timing: concepts and controversies, *Vet Clin North Am* 31:219, 2001.

Howard J: Feline semen analysis and artificial insemination. In Kirk RW et al, editors: *Current veterinary therapy XI,* Philadelphia, 1992, WB Saunders, p 929.

Johnston SD et al, editors: *Canine and feline theriogenology,* Philadelphia, 2001, WB Saunders. Semen collection, evaluation and preservation in the dog, p 287; semen collection and evaluation in the cat, p 508.

Linde-Forsberg C: Hints on dog semen freezing, cryoextenders, and frozen semen artificial insemination, *Proceedings of the Annual Conference of the Society for Theriogenology and American College of Theriogenology,* Colorado Springs, CO, 2002, p 303.

Root-Kustritz MV et al: Artificial insemination in the bitch. In Bonagura JD, editor: *Kirk's current veterinary therapy XIII,* Philadelphia, 2000, WB Saunders, p 916.

Wilson MS: Transcervical insemination techniques in the bitch, *Vet Clin North Am* 31:291, 2001.

## Drugs Used in Reproductive Disorders

| DRUG | TRADE NAME | USE | CANINE DOSE | FELINE DOSE |
|---|---|---|---|---|
| Bromocriptine | Parlodel, Sandoz | False pregnancy | 10 µg/kg, PO, q12h, 10-14 days | |
| | Lactafal, Eurovet BV | Abortifacient | Combined with cloprostenol, see below | |
| Carbergoline | Galastop, Beringer-Ingeheim | False pregnancy | 5 µg/kg, PO, q24h, 4-7 days | |
| | Dostinex, Pharmacia | Abortifacient | Combine with cloprostenol, see below | |
| | | Abortifacient, late gestation | 5 µg/kg, PO, q24h, 3-5 days begin after gestation day 49 | |
| | | Estrus induction during anestrus | 5 µg/kg, PO, q24h, until 2 days after onset of proestrus | |
| Calcium gluconate, 10% solution | Various | Puerperal hypocalcemia | 10%, slow IV, to effect, (3-20 ml) | Same |
| Calcium gluconate, lactate, or carbonate | Example: Tums | Maintain eucalcemia during lactation | 1-3 g, PO, q24h | 500-600 mg, PO, q24h |
| Cloprostenol | Estrumate, Mallinckrodt | Abortifacient 25 days after LH surge | 1 µg/kg, SC, q48h, **plus** bromocriptine, 30 µg/kg, PO, q8h **OR** **plus** cabergoline, 5 µg/kg, PO, q24h | |
| Finasteride | Proscar, Merck Propecia, Merck | Benign prostatic hyperplasia | Preliminary recommendations: 0.1 mg/kg **OR** 5 mg/dog, PO, q24h | |
| GnRH | Cystorelin, Abbott | Ovulation induction during estrus | 50-100 µg/dog, IM, once | 25 µg/cat, IM, once or twice, q24h |
| | | Follicular ovarian cysts | 2.2 µg/kg, IM, q24h, 3 days | |

### Drugs Used in Reproductive Disorders—cont'd

| DRUG | TRADE NAME | USE | CANINE DOSE | FELINE DOSE |
|---|---|---|---|---|
| hCG | Various | Ovulation induction during estrus | 10-20 IU/kg, IM, once | 250 IU/cat, IM, once or twice, q24h |
| Medroxyprogesterone | Depo-Provera, Pharmacia | Benign prostatic hyperplasia | 3 mg/kg, SC, once | |
| Megestrol acetate | Ovaban, Shering | Benign prostatic hyperplasia | 0.5 mg/kg, PO, q24h, 10 or more days | |
| Metergoline | Contralac, Vibrac | False pregnancy | 0.1 mg/kg, PO, q12h, 8 days | |
| PGF$_{2\alpha}$ | Lutalyse, Pharmacia | Treat pyometra | 0.1-0.25 mg/kg, SC, q12-24h until uterus is empty | Same |
| | | Abortifacient, late gestation | 0.1-0.25 mg/kg, SC, q8-12h, begin $\geq$ gestation day 35, continue until abortion complete | 0.25-0.5 mg/kg, SC, q12h, begin $\geq$ gestation day 45, continue until abortion complete |
| | | Abortifacient, early gestation | 0.25 mg/kg, SC, q12h, 4 days, begin during cytologic diestrus days 8-15, monitor progesterone | |

CHAPTER **65**

# The Neurologic Examination

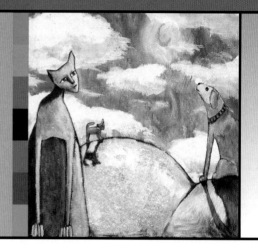

**CHAPTER OUTLINE**

FUNCTIONAL ANATOMY OF THE NERVOUS
SYSTEM, 946
SCREENING NEUROLOGIC EXAMINATION, 948
   Diagnostic approach, 957
   Animal history, 957
   Disease onset and progression, 958

## FUNCTIONAL ANATOMY OF THE NERVOUS SYSTEM

A systematic examination of the nervous system is perhaps the most important diagnostic step in the evaluation of dogs or cats with neurologic signs. In many cases the diagnosis depends on accurate localization of the lesion that is based on results of the neurologic examination (Table 65-1). To assess neurologic examination findings, one must have some basic knowledge of the structure and function of the nervous system, including an understanding of lower motor neuron (LMN), upper motor neuron (UMN), and sensory pathways.

### Lower Motor Neuron

The LMN is the efferent neuron that directly connects the central nervous system (CNS) to a muscle to generate movement (Fig. 65-1). The LMN is composed of nerve cell bodies in the spinal cord gray matter and brainstem nuclei as well as peripheral nerves and cranial nerves formed from their axons. The spinal cord is arranged in a segmental fashion, with each spinal cord segment generating one pair of spinal nerves (left and right), each of which has a dorsal (sensory) and ventral (motor) root (Fig. 65-2).

Damage to any component of the LMN results in the appearance of neurologic signs in the muscles normally innervated by that particular LMN. These "LMN signs" include decreased muscle tone, rapid muscle atrophy, decreased or absent spinal reflexes, and flaccid paresis (weakness) or paral-

ysis (loss of motor function). Most muscles are innervated by peripheral nerves that originate in more than one spinal cord segment, such that damage to one spinal cord segment is likely to cause paresis (weakness), rather than paralysis, and decreased, rather than absent, reflexes. Lesions of peripheral nerves may cause more profound dysfunction.

### Upper Motor Neuron

Those motor systems originating in the brain to control the LMN are called the *upper motor neurons* (see Fig. 65-1). UMNs are responsible for initiating and maintaining normal movement and for regulating the muscle tone used to support the body. Components of the UMN include nerve cell bodies in the cerebral cortex, basal nuclei, and brainstem, as well as the motor tracts, or pathways, in the brainstem and spinal cord white matter, which relay information from the higher centers to the LMN. These pathways cross the midline in the rostral brainstem, so that lesions of the spinal cord or brainstem result in ipsilateral (same-side) deficits in the limbs, whereas cerebral cortical lesions result in contralateral (opposite-side) deficits.

Damage to the UMN nuclei or tracts will cause loss of the normal UMN regulation of LMNs, resulting in the development of "UMN signs" in all muscles caudal to the site of the lesion. These UMN signs include increased extensor muscle tone, increased spinal reflexes, and spastic paresis or paralysis. Associated sensory signs can reflect the interruption of sensory tracts responsible for mediating proprioception (position sense) and pain perception.

### Sensory Pathways

Sensory nerves that detect touch, temperature, and pain are distributed to the surface of the body and limbs. There are also sensory nerves responsible for proprioception that originate in the skin, muscles, tendons, and joints. The nerve cell bodies of most of these sensory nerves are located in the ganglia of dorsal nerve roots entering the spinal cord (see Fig. 65-2). Sensory pathways (long tracts) responsible for medi-

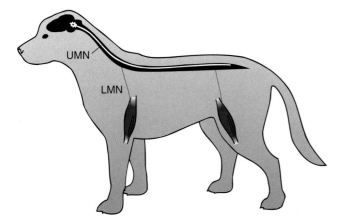

**FIG 65-1**
The upper motor neuron *(UMN)* and lower motor neuron *(LMN)* systems are responsible for mediating normal motor function.

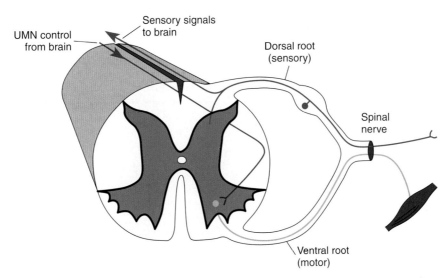

**FIG 65-2**
A single spinal cord segment.

 TABLE 65-1

**Steps in Neurologic Diagnosis**

1. Describe the neurologic abnormalities.
2. Localize the lesion.
3. Describe any concurrent nonneurologic disease.
4. Characterize the onset and progression of the neurologic disease.
5. Generate a list of differential diagnoses.
6. Use ancillary tests, if needed, to make a diagnosis and gauge the prognosis.

ating sensation and conscious and unconscious proprioception ascend the spinal cord and brainstem to the brain. Most of the tracts responsible for conveying information regarding conscious proprioception ascend the ipsilateral spinal cord and cross over in the brainstem to reach the contralateral cerebrum. Damage to the sensory pathways in the spinal cord disrupts the transmission of sensory and proprioceptive in-

formation to the brain (UMN), resulting in signs of ataxia, or incoordination, and the loss of conscious proprioception caudal to the site of the lesion. If spinal cord lesions are serious enough to cause paralysis, there may also be some loss of superficial sensation.

In addition to the sensory pathways responsible for relaying information to UMN centers regarding sensory input and proprioception, there are multisynaptic, small-diameter, bilateral crossing tracts deep in the white matter of the spinal cord that project to the cerebral cortex and are involved in the conscious perception of noxious stimuli (deep pain). These tracts are very resistant to compressive injury, so loss of the ability to perceive deep pain is a reliable indicator of very severe spinal cord injury.

Damage to a segmental sensory neuron, a dorsal nerve root, or the sensory portion of a peripheral nerve results in anesthesia or decreased sensation in the innervated region of the skin, allowing the lesion to be precisely localized on the basis of skin sensation mapping. In some cases there is pain at the site if there is a compressive or irritative lesion of the nerve root or peripheral nerve.

# SCREENING NEUROLOGIC EXAMINATION

A screening neurologic examination takes only a few minutes (Table 65-2). Abnormalities of mentation, posture, and gait are initially evaluated. Postural reactions are then evaluated. If abnormalities are detected, evaluation of muscle tone, spinal reflexes, urinary tract function, and sensory perception aids in lesion localization. Finally, cranial nerves are evaluated, and if necessary, localization of a lesion within the brain is attempted.

## Mental State

A decreased level of consciousness, such as depression, stupor, or even coma, may occur as a result of a metabolic disturbance, cerebral cortical disease, compression or inflammation of the brainstem, or disruption of the pathways between the brainstem and the cerebral cortex (Table 65-3). Behavioral changes such as delirium or agitation can indicate the presence of cerebral cortical disease or a metabolic encephalopathy. Seizures always indicate a problem in the brain, although this problem may be secondary to a metabolic or toxic condition.

## Posture

A normal upright posture is maintained through the integration of multiple CNS pathways and spinal reflexes (see Postural Reactions). Abnormal postures reflect a disruption of this normal integration. A continuous head tilt with resistance to straightening is usually associated with an abnormality of the vestibular system (Fig. 65-3). A wide-based stance is common in all forms of ataxia and may be seen in generalized weakness (Fig. 65-4). In animals that are acutely recumbent after trauma, extensor posturing can indicate severe neurologic disease (Fig. 65-5).

## Gait

A clinical evaluation of gait involves observation of the animal's movements during walking and running on a flat, nonslippery surface. Abnormalities of gait include proprioceptive deficits, paresis, circling, ataxia, and dysmetria. To assess gait, the animal should be walked slowly back and forth, with frequent turns and circling. Abnormalities of proprioception may cause an animal to stand or walk with a foot knuckled over on its dorsal surface or may cause scuffing of the nails during walking or running. Paresis or paralysis can be seen in diseases of the cerebral cortex, brainstem, spinal cord, peripheral spinal nerves, or muscles. Tight circling associated with a head tilt usually indicates vestibular disease (Fig. 65-6). Compulsive pacing or circling without a head tilt and accompanied by delirium is most indicative of a lesion involving the ipsilateral forebrain (cerebral cortex, thalamus, hypothalamus).

Animals with LMN disease typically exhibit weakness with a short-strided gait, making them appear lame, whereas animals with UMN lesions have delayed protraction, a prolonged stiff-spastic stride, and remarkable ataxia. Ataxia, or incoordination, may be caused by lesions of the cerebellum, vestibular system, or spinal cord proprioceptive pathways (see

## TABLE 65-2

### Neurologic Examination

Mental state
Posture
Gait
   Proprioceptive deficits
   Paresis or paralysis
   Circling
   Ataxia
   Dysmetria
Postural reactions
   Proprioceptive positioning
   Hopping
   Wheelbarrowing
   Hemiwalking
Spinal reflexes
Muscle tone
Sensation and pain
Urinary tract function
Cranial nerves

## TABLE 65-3

### Disorders of Consciousness

| STATE | CHARACTERISTIC |
|---|---|
| Normal | Alert; responds appropriately to environmental stimuli |
| Depression | Awake but relatively unresponsive to environmental stimuli |
| Delirium | Alert, overactive; responds inappropriately to stimuli |
| Stupor | Asleep except when aroused by strong (often painful) stimuli |
| Coma | A state of deep unconsciousness from which the animal cannot be aroused even with noxious stimuli |

Chapter 67). Limb or head movements that are too long (hypermetria) or too short (hypometria) usually indicate the presence of cerebellar or spinocerebellar pathway lesions.

## Postural Reactions

The complex series of responses that maintain an animal in an upright position are called *postural reactions*. These reactions involve multiple CNS pathways and spinal reflexes that are integrated to maintain normal posture and body position. Sensory pathways responsible for conveying information regarding conscious and unconscious proprioception originate in the skin, muscles, tendons, and joints and ascend the spinal cord, relaying this information to the brain. Most of these pathways ascend the ipsilateral spinal cord and cross the midline in the

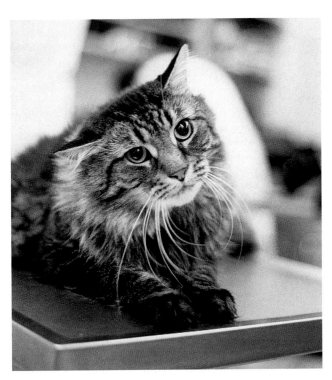

**FIG 65-3**
Right-sided head tilt in an adult cat with right-sided peripheral vestibular disease caused by otitis media/interna.

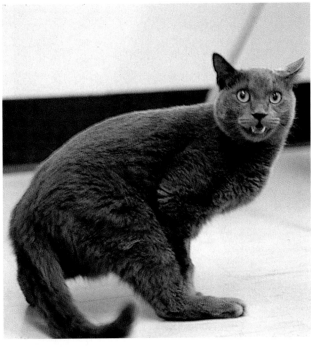

**FIG 65-4**
Ataxia with wide-based stance and excessive limb abduction in a young adult domestic short-haired cat after spinal trauma that caused traumatic disk herniation at the T13-L1 intervertebral space.

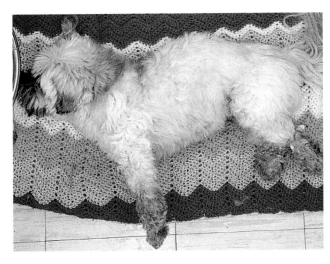

**FIG 65-5**
Schiff-Sherrington posture in a 9-year-old Lhaso Apso caused by traumatic fracture and luxation of the spine at T11-T12, with damage to the spinal cord at that site. There was a loss of proprioception, loss of voluntary motion, and loss of deep pain in the rear limbs, with increased reflexes. The forelimbs were neurologically normal except for increased extensor tone.

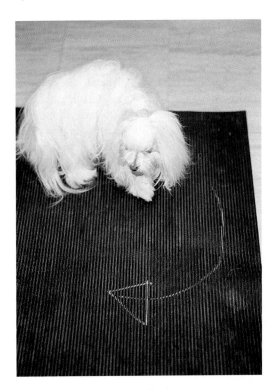

**FIG 65-6**
Tight circling and head tilt to the right in a 3-year-old Maltese with inflammatory disease affecting the right forebrain and brainstem.

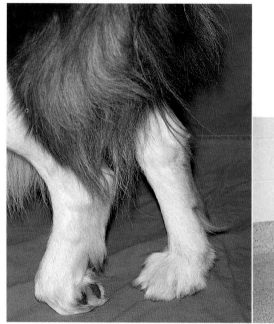
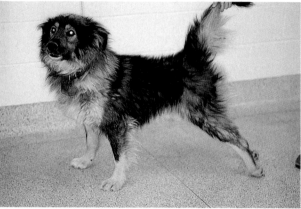

**FIG 65-7**
Postural reaction testing. **A,** Conscious proprioception (knuckling) is evaluated by placing the dorsal surface of the animal's paw on the floor while the animal's weight is supported. The normal response is an immediate return to a normal position. **B,** This 9-year-old Norwegian Elkhound–cross has lost conscious proprioception in both pelvic limbs as a result of a degenerative myelopathy affecting the thoracolumbar spinal cord. Although this dog is still able to move his limbs, there is no response to knuckling of the pelvic limbs.

brainstem. Abnormalities detected during the manipulations performed to test postural reactions do not provide precise localizing information but are sensitive indicators of neurologic dysfunction somewhere along the neurologic pathway. A careful and systematic evaluation of postural reactions may detect subtle deficits not observed during routine gait examination and should allow the examiner to determine whether each limb is neurologically normal or abnormal. Postural reaction testing should include conscious proprioceptive positioning (knuckling), hopping, wheelbarrowing, and hemiwalking (Fig. 65-7). For the purpose of localization, abnormalities of conscious proprioception are usually interpreted as UMN signs, which must then be confirmed with testing of the spinal reflexes.

## Muscle Tone

Muscle atrophy and muscle tone should be assessed as part of the neurologic examination. Muscle atrophy can occur slowly as a result of disuse or rapidly as a result of a lesion of the LMN supplying a muscle. If focal muscle atrophy is detected, it can be useful in localizing lesions of the peripheral nerve, nerve roots, or spinal cord, because the spinal cord segment origin of each of the peripheral nerves responsible for innervating individual muscles is well known. Muscle tone is tested by gently flexing and extending the joints. Muscle tone is decreased in animals with lesions of the LMN, whereas extensor muscle tone is increased with UMN lesions.

Schiff-Sherrington posture, or syndrome, is characterized by markedly increased muscle tone and hyperextension of the thoracic limbs occurring in conjunction with normal forelimb proprioception. This posture is most commonly seen in dogs with severe acute mid to caudal thoracic spinal cord lesions causing UMN paralysis of the rear limbs (see Fig. 65-5). The forelimb hyperextension results from interruption of ascending inhibitory impulses originating in the border cells of the lumbar gray matter. These border cells are present in the dorsolateral part of the ventral gray matter from L1 to L7 (most from L2 to L4), and axons from these cells ascend in the spinal cord to affect the forelimbs. These cells are normally responsible for tonic inhibition to the extensor muscle alpha motor neurons in the cervical intumescence. Loss of this ascending inhibition as a result of spinal cord injury results in hyperextension of the forelimbs. Although there is hyperextension of the forelimbs, these dogs can use their forelimbs normally when hopped or wheelbarrowed. Although the Schiff-Sherrington posture is usually seen with severe spinal cord injury causing UMN paralysis of the rear legs, the posture does not suggest that there has been irreversible damage. Deep pain perception in the rear limbs is a much better prognostic indicator for return to function.

## Spinal Reflexes

The integrity of the sensory and motor components of the reflex arc and the influence of descending UMN pathways are

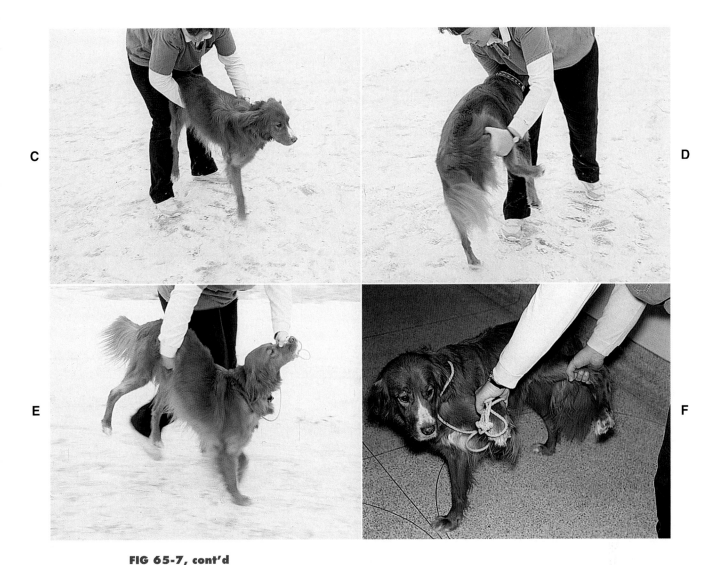

**FIG 65-7, cont'd**
**C,** Forelimb hopping. The animal is supported under the abdomen, and one thoracic limb is lifted from the ground. The animal is moved laterally toward the limb being evaluated. The normal animal responds by quickly lifting and replacing the limb under its body as it moves laterally. **D,** Pelvic limb hopping. The animal is supported under the chest, and one pelvic limb is lifted. The animal is leaned and moved laterally toward the limb being evaluated. The normal animal responds by quickly lifting and replacing its limb under the body as it moves laterally. **E,** Wheelbarrowing. The animal is supported under the abdomen and moved forward. The head may be elevated to remove visual input and accentuate proprioceptive abnormalities, as shown here. **F,** Hemiwalking. The front and rear limbs on one side are lifted, and forward and lateral walking movements are evaluated.

evaluated during examination of the spinal reflexes. Each reflex is recorded as absent, depressed, normal, or exaggerated. If an injury within the reflex arc damages the neuromuscular junction, the peripheral nerve, or the spinal cord segments responsible for mediating the reflex, the reflex is lost and other LMN signs such as decreased muscle tone and rapid muscle atrophy are seen (Table 65-4). The unilateral loss of a reflex strongly indicates that the lesion is in the peripheral nerve or nerve roots rather than in the spinal cord.

Loss of a reflex allows very precise localization of the site of injury. On the other hand, if a lesion occurs in the brain or spinal cord cranial to a reflex arc, it disconnects the reflex from its normal UMN inhibition, resulting in UMN signs such as hyperreflexia and increased muscle tone in all limbs caudal to the lesion (see Table 65-4). The finding of UMN signs confirms the presence of a neurologic lesion but only localizes the lesion to any region cranial to the spinal cord segments responsible for mediating the reflex being tested.

The spinal reflexes that are most useful in dogs and cats include the patellar reflex, the sciatic reflex, the pelvic limb withdrawal (flexor) reflex, and the thoracic limb withdrawal (flexor) reflex (Table 65-5; Fig. 65-8). The panniculus reflex

TABLE 65-4

Summary of Upper Motor Neuron and Lower Motor Neuron Signs

| CHARACTERISTIC | UPPER MOTOR NEURON | LOWER MOTOR NEURON |
|---|---|---|
| Muscle tone | Normal or increased | Decreased |
| Spinal reflexes | Normal or increased | Decreased |
| Motor function | Spastic paresis to paralysis caudal to lesion | Flaccid paresis to paralysis at site of lesion |
| Muscle atrophy | Mild—disuse | Severe—neurogenic |
| Gait | Delayed protraction | Weak, unable to support weight |
| | Long stride | |
| | Stiff, spastic | Short strided |
| | Ataxic | Appears lame |
| | Excessive abduction of limbs during turning | May bunny-hop |

TABLE 65-5

Spinal Reflexes

| REFLEX | STIMULUS | NORMAL RESPONSE | SPINAL CORD SEGMENTS |
|---|---|---|---|
| Thoracic limb withdrawal | Pinch foot of forelimb | Withdraw limb | C6, C7, C8, T1, (T2) |
| Patellar | Strike patellar ligament | Extension of stifle | L4, L5, L6 |
| Pelvic limb withdrawal | Pinch foot of rear limb | Withdraw limb | L6, L7, S1, (S2) |
| Sciatic | Strike sciatic nerve between greater trochanter and ischium | Flexion of stifle and hock | L6, L7, S1, (S2) |
| Cranial tibial | Strike belly of cranial tibial muscle just below proximal end of tibia | Flexion of hock | L6, L7 |
| Perineal | Stimulate perineum with pinch | Anal sphincter contraction, ventroflex tail | S1, S2, S3, pudendal nerve |
| Bulbourethral | Compress vulva or bulb of penis | Anal sphincter contraction | S1, S2, S3, pudendal nerve |
| Panniculus | Stimulate skin over dorsum just lateral to vertebral column | Twitch of cutaneous trunci muscle | Response will be absent caudal to a spinal cord lesion that disrupts the superficial pain pathway; used to localize lesions between T3 and L3 |

*( ),* Variable contribution.

(Fig. 65-9) can be used to more precisely localize severe spinal cord lesions between T3 and L3. The perineal reflex and the bulbourethral reflex are used to evaluate the sacral segments and the pudendal nerve. Other reflexes are found inconsistently in normal animals, so they are not routinely evaluated.

The spinal reflexes and the spinal cord segments responsible for mediating each reflex are listed in Table 65-5. Limb reflexes are judged to be absent (0), decreased (1), normal (2), or increased (3). The results of reflex tests and muscle tone can then be used to characterize the neurologic abnormalities in each limb as either UMN or LMN in origin and to localize spinal cord lesions to a particular region of the spinal cord (Table 65-6). In many cases it is only possible to determine that a reflex is normal to increased (i.e., it is not de-

creased). However, in the face of obvious abnormalities of postural reactions, such a finding should enable the examiner to characterize the lesion as UMN in origin and to localize the lesion as described.

The panniculus reflex is a contraction (twitch) of the cutaneous trunci muscle that occurs in response to a cutaneous stimulus or pinch along the dorsum. Sensory nerves from the skin enter the spinal cord through the dorsal root, and the signal ascends the spinal cord through a superficial pain pathway. If the spinal cord is intact between the site of stimulation and the C8-T1 segments, a synapse occurs at C8-T1, stimulating motor neurons of the lateral thoracic nerve and causing the cutaneous trunci muscle to contract. In spinal cord lesions causing paralysis, the ascending pathway may be

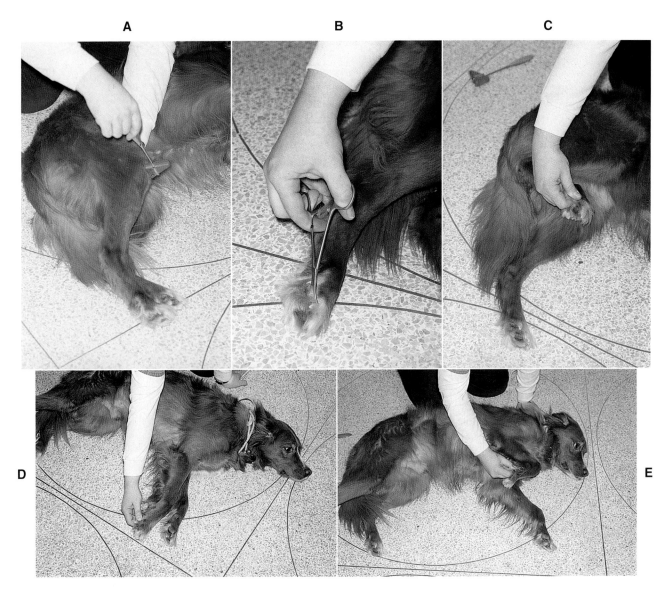

**FIG 65-8**
Assessment of limb reflexes. **A,** Patellar reflex. Strike the straight patellar ligament, resulting in a reflex "kick" extension of the stifle. Pelvic limb withdrawal reflex. Pinch the toe **(B),** resulting in limb flexion **(C).** Assess flexion in all of the joints of the limb. It may be necessary to apply a forceps to the nail base to provide adequate stimulation. Thoracic limb withdrawal reflex. Pinch the toe **(D),** resulting in limb flexion **(E).** Assess flexion in all the joints of the limb.

disrupted such that no panniculus reflex is elicited if the skin is pinched caudal to the level of the lesion, but stimulation of the skin cranial to the lesion does elicit a response. Because the sensory nerves that supply the skin enter the cord one or two vertebrae cranial to the dermatome stimulated (see Fig. 65-9), the cord lesion is predictably slightly cranial to the site where the panniculus reflex is lost. This reflex does not always accurately reflect the location of the lesion, however, so the response should be interpreted in light of other clinical findings when one is attempting to localize a spinal cord lesion. The sensory pathways of the panniculus reflex are bilateral

and crossing, so that the panniculus response is elicited bilaterally when skin on only one side of the cord is pinched. The panniculus reflex can also be used to evaluate the gray matter of the C8-T1 spinal cord segments, the corresponding ventral nerve roots, and the spinal nerves in animals with thoracic limb injuries (see Chapter 73).

## Sensation

When there is severe loss of motor function caused by a spinal cord lesion, the ability of the animal to feel a painful stimulus (skin pinch) should be assessed to map out areas of

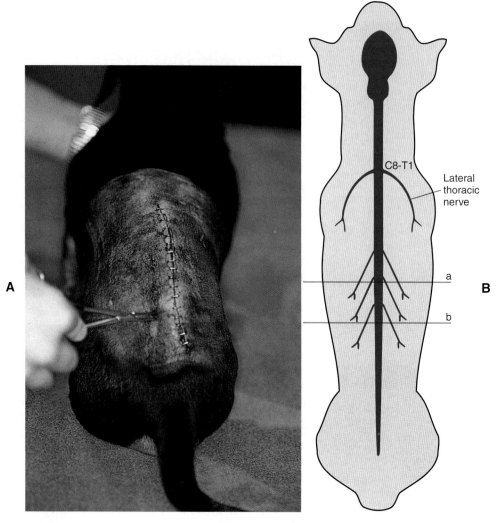

**FIG 65-9**
Panniculus reflex. **A,** Pinch the dorsal skin with a hemostat just lateral to the spine. If the spinal cord is not injured between the site of stimulation and the C8-T1 spinal cord segments, this will lead to a bilateral twitch of the cutaneous trunci muscle. The reflex may be absent caudal to a severe spinal cord lesion. **B,** The spinal sensory nerves course caudally so that the dermatomes for skin sensation lateral to the vertebral column are caudal to their own vertebral bodies. A spinal cord lesion at site *a* will therefore result in loss of the panniculus response caudal to site *b*.

 TABLE 65-6

Localization of Spinal Cord Disease

| Cranial cervical spinal lesion (C1-C5) | Thoracolumbar spinal cord lesion (T3-L3) | Sacral spinal cord lesion (S1-S3) |
|---|---|---|
|   UMN signs in rear limbs |   UMN signs in rear limbs |   Normal forelimbs |
|   UMN signs in forelimbs |   Normal forelimbs |   Normal patellar reflexes |
| Caudal cervical spinal lesion (C6-T2) | Lumbosacral spinal cord lesion (L4-S3) |   Loss of sciatic function |
|   UMN signs in rear limbs |   LMN signs in rear limbs |   Loss of perineal sensation and reflexes |
|   LMN signs in forelimbs |   Loss of perineal sensation and reflexes | |
| |   Normal forelimbs | |

*UMN,* Upper motor neuron; *LMN,* lower motor neuron.

sensory loss. Decreased sensation in the limbs caudal to a spinal cord lesion is common in animals with severe spinal cord compression and damage causing complete paralysis (loss of voluntary motion). If superficial pain (toe or skin pinch with fingers) does not elicit a behavioral response, the animal's ability to perceive deep pain is tested by applying an intense noxious stimulus sufficient to elicit a behavioral response (e.g., hemostat applied to nail base). A response such as turning the head, vocalizing, or trying to bite indicates that there is some functional neurologic connection between the toe and the brain (Fig. 65-10). It is important to remember that withdrawal of the limb indicates only an intact reflex arc (peripheral nerve and spinal cord segments), whereas a behavioral response requires intact peripheral nerve and spinal cord segments, as well as intact pathways for deep pain perception in the spinal cord, brainstem, and forebrain. Deep pain fibers in the spinal cord are small, bilateral, and multisynaptic and are located deep within the spinal cord, such that loss of deep pain sensation due to a compressive lesion indicates very severe spinal cord damage.

If LMN paralysis of a limb is present, superficial sensation should be assessed by pinching the skin of the limb with a hemostat. Damage to a peripheral nerve or the sensory nerve roots that innervate a region can result in local anesthesia or decreased sensation. If abnormalities are located, the boundaries of normal and abnormal sensation should be "mapped." By identifying anesthetic regions and comparing these results with established maps of cutaneous regions deriving sensory innervation from individual nerves (dermatomes), an LMN neurologic defect can be precisely localized (see Chapter 73).

## Pain/Hyperpathia

A region of painfulness or hyperpathia can be detected in an animal by palpating and manipulating its limbs, neck, spine, muscles, bones, and joints. If pain is present, this could indicate inflammation or the rapid distortion of tissues (e.g., meninges, nerve roots) at that site and can help to precisely localize a lesion.

Neck pain is a sign commonly associated with compressive or inflammatory diseases of the cervical spinal cord. Animals with neck pain will typically have a guarded horizontal neck carriage and will be unwilling to turn their neck to look to the side; they will instead pivot their entire body. As part of every routine neurologic examination, the presence or absence of cervical hyperesthesia (painful response to a normally nonpainful stimulus) should be assessed by deep palpation of the vertebrae and cervical spinal epaxial muscles and by resistance to flexion, hyperextension, and lateral flexion of the neck (Fig. 65-11). Anatomic structures that can cause neck pain include the meninges, nerve roots, intervertebral disks, joints, bones, and muscles (Table 65-7). Neck pain has also been recognized as a clinical symptom of intracranial disease, particularly of forebrain mass lesions.

Pain in other regions of the vertebral column may help to localize lesions caused by intervertebral disk disease, diskospondylitis, or neoplasia. Dogs and cats with disease of the

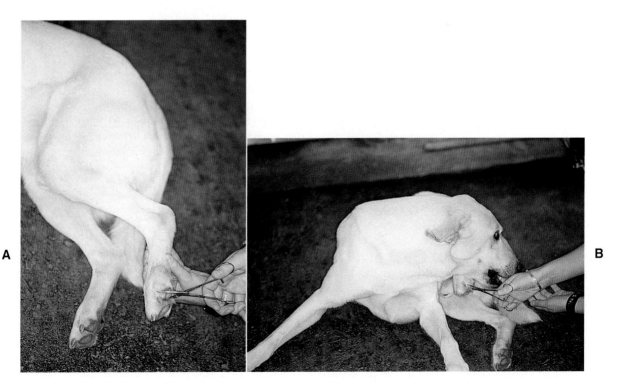

**FIG 65-10**
Evaluation of deep pain. Pinch the toe **(A)** to assess whether this elicits a behavioral response **(B).** Absent deep pain sensation indicates the presence of severe spinal cord damage.

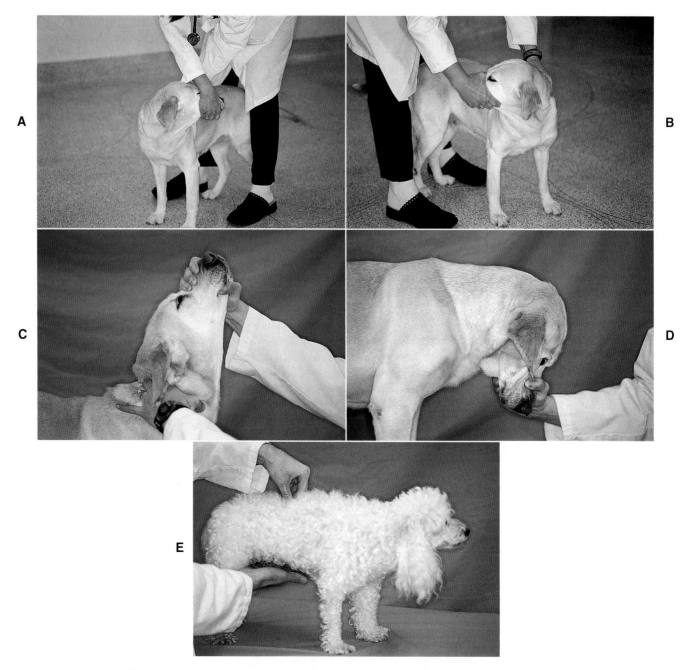

**FIG 65-11**
Testing for cervical and thoracolumbar spinal pain by (**A** to **D**) manipulating the neck through a full range of motion and (**E**) applying pressure through deep palpation of the vertebral bodies and spinal epaxial muscles.

thoracolumbar spine may experience pain when pressure is applied over the affected vertebrae. These animals may also resist abdominal palpation, with the apparent abdominal pain reflecting their vertebral or spinal hyperpathia. Cauda equina compression that is caused by a tumor, disk, or ligamentous proliferation causes pain in the lumbosacral region (see p. 1038). This can be demonstrated in affected dogs by applying direct pressure over the lumbosacral junction or by applying dorsal traction to the tail (see Fig. 72-18).

Muscular pain should be assessed by manipulating the limbs and by palpating individual muscle groups. During palpation it is important to attempt to differentiate pain that originates within the muscle from that caused by bone or joint abnormalities. Muscle disorders that are associated with pain are primarily the inflammatory diseases, such as immune-mediated polymyositis, masticatory myositis, and infectious myositis caused by the protozoal organisms *Toxoplasma* and *Neospora*. Ischemic myopathy, as occurs in animals with

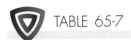

## TABLE 65-7

**Causes of Neck Pain**

**Muscle**

Myositis (immune, infectious)
Muscle injury

**Bone**

Fracture/luxation
Diskospondylitis
Vertebral osteomyelitis
Neoplasia

**Joint (Facetal Joints)**

Polyarthritis (immune, infectious)
Degenerative joint disease (osteoarthritis)

**Intervertebral Disk**

Disk degeneration/prolapse

**Nerve Root**

Neoplasia
Compression (by disk, tumor, fibrous tissue)

**Meninges**

Neoplasia
Inflammation (immune, infectious)

**Brain**

Mass lesion (neoplasia, inflammatory)

thrombosis affecting the arterial blood supply to a muscle group, can also result in severe muscular cramping and pain on palpation.

### Urinary Tract Function

Severe lesions of the spinal cord are often associated with urinary tract dysfunction. Some idea of urinary tract function can be gained from the animal's history. The bladder should be palpated, and the ease with which urine can be expressed assessed. A flaccid, easily expressed bladder with absent or diminished perineal and bulbourethral reflexes is found with lesions of the LMN (S1-S3 spinal cord segments, pudendal nerve, pelvic nerve) (see Table 65-5). UMN lesions cranial to the sacral segments typically result in a tense bladder that is difficult to express owing to increased urethral sphincter tone. Detrusor-urethral dysynergia may be observed with lumbosacral lesions in some dogs.

### Cranial Nerves

Cranial nerve dysfunction may result from a disorder affecting a single nerve, a diffuse polyneuropathy affecting multiple nerves, or a cluster of abnormalities, as may be seen in animals with a disease affecting the ear or the brainstem.

Cranial nerve examination is not difficult. The cranial nerves that are most often affected can be evaluated quickly (Table 65-8). If findings yielded by the preliminary examination indicate the presence of an abnormality, a more thorough examination of all the cranial nerves can be undertaken (Table 65-9; see also Suggested Readings).

### Localization Within the Brain

If a dog or cat has a neurologic abnormality above the foramen magnum, the examiner should attempt to further localize the disease to one of five clinically important regions of the brain. These include (1) the cerebral cortex; (2) the diencephalon, composed of the thalamus and hypothalamus; (3) the brainstem; (4) the vestibular system; and (5) the cerebellum. The abnormality is localized on the basis of the neurologic signs of disease in each region (Table 65-10).

### Lesion Localization

After the neurologic examination is completed, an animal's mentation, cranial nerves, forelimbs, rear limbs, perineum, anus, and bladder should be characterized as normal or abnormal. By determining whether the neurologic abnormality in each limb is UMN or LMN in origin, neurologic lesions can be localized to a particular region of the spinal cord. If LMN signs are present in a single limb, the lesion can be even more precisely localized by determining the muscles affected and, if sensory nerves are also affected, by testing sensation in dermatomes. If focal hyperpathia is detected, that may help to more precisely localize a lesion. If disease above the foramen magnum is present, particular clinical findings allow it to be localized to a specific region of the brain. It is very important to always try to account for all detected neurologic abnormalities on the basis of a single lesion. Occasionally, however, this is impossible because the animal has multiple foci of disease or a diffuse disorder.

## DIAGNOSTIC APPROACH

Once a neurologic lesion has been localized, it is necessary to generate a list of likely differential diagnoses. This can be done after considering the signalment of the animal, its history, the nature of the onset of neurologic signs, and the speed at which these signs progress. When generating this list of differential diagnoses, it is important to consider all of the possible mechanisms or causes of disease affecting the nervous system (Table 65-11).

## ANIMAL HISTORY

The age, gender, breed, and lifestyle of the animal may provide clues regarding the underlying disease. Young animals are most likely to be seen because of congenital or hereditary disorders; they are also at high risk for intoxications and infectious diseases. Older animals are more susceptible to neoplastic diseases and many of the known degenerative disorders. Certain breeds are predisposed to particular disorders. For example, the small brachycephalic breeds, as well as some of the toy breeds, are most commonly found to have hydrocephalus.

TABLE 65-8

Quick Assessment of Cranial Nerve Function

| PHYSICAL EXAMINATION FINDING | CRANIAL NERVE(S) INVOLVED |
|---|---|
| Blind | II (brain, retina) |
| Loss of menace | II (VII, cerebellum) |
| Asymmetric pupils | II, III (sympathetic innervation, parasympathetic innervation) |
| Asymmetric eyes in palpebral fissure | III, IV, VI |
| Atrophy of temporal/masseter muscles | V (motor) |
| Dropped jaw, loss of jaw tone | V (motor) |
| Decreased facial sensation (inside ear, lip pinch, nasal mucosa, cornea) | V |
| Lip droop, ear droop | VII |
| Inability to blink | VII |
| Head tilt | VIII |
| Spontaneous resting nystagmus | VIII |
| Deafness | VIII |
| Difficulty swallowing | IX, X |
| Loss of gag reflex | IX, X |
| Laryngeal paralysis | IX, X |
| Weakness, asymmetry of tongue | XII |

 TABLE 65-9

Cranial Nerve Function

| CRANIAL NERVE | SIGNS OF LOSS OF FUNCTION |
|---|---|
| I (olfactory) | Loss of ability to smell |
| II (optic) | Loss of vision, dilated pupil, loss of pupillary light reflex (direct and consensual when light shone in affected eye) |
| III (oculomotor) | Loss of pupillary light reflex on affected side (even if light shone in opposite eye), dilated pupil, ventrolateral strabismus |
| IV (trochlear) | Slight dorsomedial eye rotation |
| V (trigeminal) | Atrophy of temporalis and masseter muscles, loss of jaw tone and strength, dropped jaw (if bilateral), analgesia of innervated areas (face, eyelids, cornea, nasal mucosa) |
| VI (abducent) | Medial strabismus, impaired lateral gaze, poor retraction of globe |
| VII (facial) | Lip, eyelid, and ear droop; loss of ability to blink; loss of ability to retract lip; possibly decreased tear production |
| VIII (vestibulocochlear) | Ataxia, head tilt, nystagmus, deafness |
| IX (glossopharyngeal) | Loss of gag reflex, dysphagia |
| X (vagus) | Loss of gag reflex, laryngeal paralysis, dysphagia |
| XI (accessory) | Atrophy of trapezius, sternocephalicus, and brachiocephalicus muscles |
| XII (hypoglossal) | Loss of tongue strength |

In addition, some of the congenital and inherited disorders have only been seen in a certain breed. Dogs engaging in particular competitive or working activities (hunting, herding, racing, jumping) may be at increased risk for numerous specific activity-related injuries. Exposure to trauma, toxins, and infectious disorders can be ascertained through careful history taking.

## DISEASE ONSET AND PROGRESSION

Evaluation of the onset and progression of neurologic signs is of primary importance in prioritizing the differential diag-

noses (Table 65-12). The onset of signs may be peracute, subacute, or chronic. In peracute disorders the time of onset of the neurologic signs can be pinpointed exactly, and the signs reach maximal intensity within minutes or hours of onset. The signs then remain static or may abate with time. Examples of such disorders include trauma, vascular disorders such as infarcts or hemorrhage, and intoxications. Acute exacerbations of a more chronically progressive disease, such as a brain tumor that hemorrhages, may also result in an acute clinical presentation. A thorough history should identify animals that were not entirely normal before the acute deterioration.

## TABLE 65-10

### Characteristics That Aid in Localizing Brain Lesions

**Cerebral Cortex**

Altered behavior, mental status
May pace or circle to side of lesion
May head-press
Gait usually relatively normal
May have postural reaction, and proprioceptive deficits on side opposite lesion
Cortical blindness (blind with normal pupils and pupillary light reflexes) on side opposite lesion
Seizures

**Diencephalon (Thalamus and Hypothalamus)**

Altered mental status: aggression, disorientation, hyperexcitability, depression, coma
Postural reaction and proprioceptive deficits on side opposite lesion
Abnormalities of eating, drinking, sleeping, or temperature (hypothalamus)
Diabetes insipidus

**Brainstem (Mesencephalon, Pons, Medulla Oblongata)**

Altered mental status: severe depression or coma
Ipsilateral hemiparesis or quadriparesis and ataxia
Multiple ipsilateral cranial nerve deficits
Cerebellopontine angle lesion: V, VII, VIII

**Vestibular System**

Head tilt, asymmetric ataxia (incoordination), falling, rolling toward side of lesion
Possibly spontaneous or positional abnormal nystagmus, with fast phase away from side of lesion
Ipsilateral ventrolateral strabismus
Important to differentiate central from peripheral vestibular disease (see Chapter 70)

**Cerebellum**

Normal mental status
Ataxia, head tremor, intention tremor, dysmetria
Normal strength
Normal proprioceptive positioning
Menace response may be lost on side of lesion
Exaggerated limb responses (hypermetria), goose-stepping gait

## TABLE 65-11

### DAMNIT–VP Scheme: Mechanisms of Disease

| | |
|---|---|
| **D** | Degenerative |
| **A** | Anomalous |
| **M** | Metabolic, malformation |
| **N** | Neoplastic, nutritional |
| **I** | Infectious, inflammatory, immune, iatrogenic, idiopathic |
| **T** | Traumatic, toxic |
| **V** | Vascular |
| **P** | Parasitic |

## TABLE 65-12

### Characterization of Disease Processes Based on Onset and Progression

**Peracute, Nonprogressive**

External trauma
Hemorrhage
Infarct
Internal trauma (disk, fracture)

**Subacute, Progressive**

Infectious inflammatory disease
Noninfectious inflammatory disease
Rapidly growing tumors (e.g., lymphoma, metastatic neoplasia)

**Chronic Progressive**

Most tumors
Degenerative disorders
Metabolic disorders

Subacute illnesses may progress over days to weeks. Inflammatory diseases of the CNS and some of the more rapidly progressive neoplasms (e.g., lymphomas, metastatic malignancies) fall into this category. Most tumors, degenerative disorders, and metabolic disorders are more chronic and insidious in onset and only slowly progress over many weeks to months.

## Systemic Signs

Identification of a concurrent disease or systemic abnormalities may aid in the diagnosis of neoplastic, metabolic, or inflammatory disorders. A complete physical examination and ophthalmologic evaluation, including a fundus-scopic examination, should be performed in every animal with suspected neurologic disease. This is important in order to find clues to the cause of the nervous system disease, to exclude disorders that may mimic nervous system disease, and to identify concurrent disorders that affect the prognosis. Ancillary diagnostic tests are performed to further evaluate animals with neurologic disease in order to arrive at a specific diagnosis.

## Suggested Readings

Chrisman CL: *Problems in small animal neurology,* Philadelphia, 1991, Lea & Febiger, p 11.

DeLahunta A: *Veterinary anatomy and clinical neurology,* Philadelphia, 1983, WB Saunders, p 175.

Lane IF: Diagnosis and management of urinary retention, *Vet Clin North Am Small Anim Pract* 30:24, 2000.

Moore MP: Approach to the patient with spinal disease, *Vet Clin North Am Small Anim Pract* 22:751, 1992.

Oliver JE et al: *Handbook of veterinary neurology,* Philadelphia, 1993, WB Saunders, p 1.

Shores A et al: Neurologic examination and localization. In Slatter DH, editor: *Textbook of small animal surgery,* Philadelphia, 1993, WB Saunders, p 984.

Thomas WB: Initial assessment of patients with neurologic dysfunction, *Vet Clin North Am Small Anim Pract* 30:1, 2000.

Wheeler SJ et al: *Small animal spinal disorders: diagnosis and surgery,* London, 1994, Times Mirror International, p 8.

## CHAPTER 66

# Diagnostic Tests
# for the Neuromuscular
# System

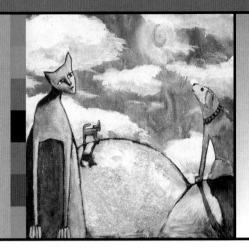

## CHAPTER OUTLINE

HEMATOLOGY, 961
SERUM BIOCHEMISTRY PROFILE, 961
URINALYSIS, 961
RADIOGRAPHY, 961
CEREBROSPINAL FLUID ANALYSIS, 962
CONTRAST-ENHANCED RADIOGRAPHY, 965
ELECTRODIAGNOSTIC TESTING, 970
BIOPSY OF MUSCLE AND NERVE, 972
IMMUNOLOGIC AND SEROLOGIC TESTS, 973

## HEMATOLOGY

Routine screening hematologic tests may be of some benefit in dogs and cats with neurologic disease. For example, a leukocytosis suggests inflammatory disease. Severe inflammation and a left shift might be expected in the setting of bacterial meningitis or encephalitis. Lymphopenia and inclusion bodies within red blood cells (RBCs), and lymphocytes may be seen in dogs with acute canine distemper virus infection. Microcytosis with or without thrombocytopenia is a common finding in dogs with portosystemic shunts. Occasionally, concurrent leukemia is detected in an animal with brain or spinal cord lymphoma based on a complete blood count (CBC). In most cases, however, hematologic findings are unremarkable in dogs and cats with disease confined to the central nervous system (CNS).

## SERUM BIOCHEMISTRY PROFILE

A serum biochemistry profile is most useful in determining the likelihood of metabolic abnormalities as the cause of neuropathies, encephalopathies, and seizures. Diabetes mellitus, hypoglycemia, hypocalcemia, hypokalemia, and uremia can be eliminated from the list of differential diagnoses if the biochemistry panel is found to be normal. On the other hand, the finding of a greatly increased serum cholesterol concentration may prompt the performance of further diagnostic

tests for hypothyroidism (see Chapter 51) as the cause of the neurologic signs observed. The finding of high liver enzyme activities (i.e., alanine aminotransaminase, serum alkaline phosphatase) or hypoalbuminemia may prompt consideration of liver disease and hepatic encephalopathy. In this event, liver function tests should be considered (see p. 487). Evidence of hepatocellular disease may also suggest a multisystemic disease such as toxoplasmosis. If high serum muscle enzyme activities (i.e., creatinine kinase, aspartate aminotransaminase) are found, muscle damage or inflammation is suspected, and this should prompt an evaluation for myositis.

## URINALYSIS

If azotemia is present, it is critically important to determine the urine specific gravity to differentiate primary renal from prerenal causes. Volume depletion with hypernatremia and prerenal azotemia is commonly found in animals that stop drinking because of intracranial disease. In addition, ammonium biurate crystals are found in the urine of some dogs and cats with portosystemic shunts.

## RADIOGRAPHY

Radiographs of the thorax and abdomen can be useful as screening tests for infectious and neoplastic diseases and as a means of evaluating liver size. They are noninvasive tests that should be performed routinely in animals in which these types of diseases are suspected.

Spinal radiographs are necessary and useful in the diagnosis of disk disease, diskospondylitis, and some neoplastic diseases affecting the vertebrae or spinal cord. Rarely a growing peripheral nerve tumor causes its vertebral foramen to enlarge, thereby aiding in the diagnosis. In most cases, general anesthesia is required to obtain lateral and ventrodorsal radiographs of sufficient quality to permit subtle abnormalities to be detected. Radiographs should be centered on the region of clinical interest based on the findings from the neurologic examination.

Although skull radiographs are a low-yield procedure, they should be performed in animals with disease above the foramen magnum, because occasionally the finding of an area of lysis, a region of tumor calcification, or an intranasal mass aids in the diagnosis of primary or secondary neoplasia of the CNS.

# CEREBROSPINAL FLUID ANALYSIS

## Indications

Analysis of the cerebrospinal fluid (CSF) is one of the best ways to evaluate the brain and spinal cord and arrive at a diagnosis. A CSF examination is indicated in any animal with certain or suspected neurologic disease in which a diagnosis is not readily apparent, including dogs and cats with a suspected intracranial disorder as the cause of a seizure disorder, with fever and axial pain, or with progressive signs of deteriorating mentation. It should always be done before myelography to rule out inflammatory disease. CSF analysis is not usually indicated in animals with metabolic abnormalities, obvious disc disease, CNS anomalies, or trauma causing neurologic signs.

## Contraindications

If the proper technique is followed, the procedure for obtaining CSF is safe and simple. The animal is first placed under general anesthesia and the puncture site is prepared in a sterile fashion, thereby minimizing the risk of damage resulting from animal movement and the risk of iatrogenic infections. Spinal puncture is contraindicated in an animal that is an obvious anesthetic risk or that has a severe coagulopathy, in which hemorrhagic complications are likely. Greatly increased intracranial pressure, manifested by deterioration of mentation, may place an animal at increased risk for brain herniation. Unfortunately, noninvasive means of achieving a diagnosis are often not readily available; thus even those animals suspected to have a high intracranial pressure routinely undergo spinal puncture. Endotracheal intubation, hyperventilation, and the intravenous (IV) administration of mannitol (1 to 3 g/kg over 30 minutes as a 20% solution) and dexamethasone (0.25 to 1 mg/kg) may reduce the risk of herniation in these animals. These precautions should be routinely taken whenever anesthetizing animals with abnormal mentation suggestive of increased intracranial pressure.

## Technique

In dogs and cats the most reliable source of CSF for analysis is the cerebellomedullary cistern. The L5-L6 site used for lumbar myelography may also be used, but it is more difficult to obtain a large volume of uncontaminated fluid from this site. Although it has been stated that CSF obtained from the cerebellomedullary cistern best reflects the nature of intracranial disease, whereas fluid from a lumbar tap is most useful in characterizing disease of the spinal cord, diagnostically the two are not very different. Lumbar CSF from normal dogs may have a slightly higher protein content and lower nucleated cell count than CSF obtained from the cerebellomedullary cistern.

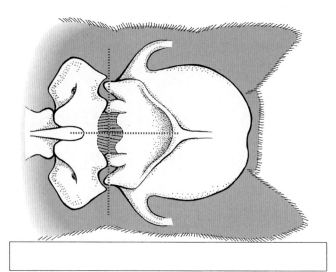

**FIG 66-1**
Landmarks for cerebrospinal fluid (CSF) collection at the cerebellomedullary cistern. The site of needle entry is at the intersection of the dorsal midline and the most cranial aspect of the wings of the atlas.

With the animal under general anesthesia, the back of its neck between the ears from the occipital protuberance to C2 should be prepared as for surgery. If the clinician is right-handed, the animal should be placed in right lateral recumbency with its neck flexed so that the median axis of the head is perpendicular to the spine. The nose should be elevated slightly so that its midline is parallel to the surface of the table. With the thumb and third finger of the left hand, the clinician should palpate the cranial edges of the wings of the atlas and draw an imaginary line at their most cranial aspect.

The examiner can then use the left index finger to palpate the external occipital protuberance and draw a second imaginary line caudally from that site along the dorsal midline. The needle should be inserted where the two imaginary lines intersect (Fig. 66-1).

A 1½ or 3 inch (3.75 to 7.5 cm) long, styletted spinal needle is then directed straight in through the skin, perpendicular to the spine, and into the underlying tissues. Lateral motion of the needle must be avoided to prevent damage to the spinal cord. The needle is advanced 1 to 2 mm at a time and the stylette removed to look for CSF fluid. While the right hand is used to remove the stylette, the thumb and first finger of the left hand, which is rested against the spine for support, should grasp and stabilize the hub of the needle. A sudden loss of resistance may be felt as the dorsal atlantooccipital membrane and the dura mater and arachnoid mater are penetrated simultaneously (Fig. 66-2). This is not a reliable sign, however, because the level at which the subarachnoid space is reached varies greatly with the breed and individual animal. It is often very close to the skin surface in toy breeds and some cats.

If the needle strikes bone, it should be withdrawn, the landmarks reassessed, and the procedure repeated. If whole blood appears in the spinal needle, the needle should be withdrawn and the procedure repeated with another sterile nee-

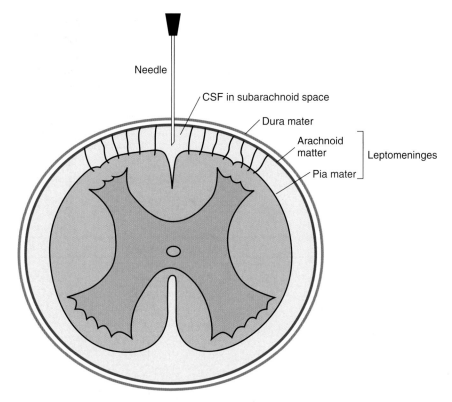

**FIG 66-2**
Transverse section showing the relationship among the meninges, the cerebrospinal fluid (CSF), and the spinal cord. The tip of the needle is in the subarachnoid space, as it would be for CSF collection or myelography.

dle. When CSF is observed, pressure can be measured, if desired, using a manometer. Alternatively the fluid can just be allowed to drip directly from the needle into a test tube. The clinician should check with the laboratory to determine the tube preferred for collection of the CSF. The amount of CSF collected ranges from 0.5 to 3 ml, depending on the size of the animal. Simultaneous jugular vein compression may hasten flow. Blood in the CSF may be the result of the disease or of the tap. If it is caused by the procedure, the amount of blood should decrease as the CSF drips from the needle. If this occurs, some of the less contaminated fluid should be collected in a second tube for cytologic evaluation. Mild CSF contamination with hemorrhage (<10 RBCs/μl) does not alter the CSF protein and leukocyte determinations. Grossly hemorrhagic CSF should always be collected into a tube containing ethylenediaminetetraacetic acid (EDTA) to prevent clotting.

## Analysis

Normal CSF is clear and colorless. A cell count should be performed and a cytologic preparation made for examination as soon as possible, because white blood cells (WBCs) in the CSF deteriorate rapidly. Refrigerating the sample can slow cellular degeneration. If the sample must be stored for longer than 1 hour before analysis, the specimen should be refrigerated to slow cellular degeneration. The addition of autologous serum (10% by volume of the sample) will preserve CSF

so that cytologic analysis 24 to 48 hours after collection will yield reliable results, but a separate sample must be saved for protein analysis.

Once the fluid is collected, a total cell count is performed and the concentration of RBCs and WBCs is determined. The normal range of values varies with each laboratory, but in general there should be less than two WBCs per microliter. Cytologic analysis of CSF is necessary even if the WBC count is normal, because there may be abnormal cell types or organisms present.

A concentration procedure is usually required to obtain sufficient cells for cytologic assessment if the CSF WBC count is less than 500 cells per microliter. Cytocentrifuge concentration of CSF is available in most institutions and commercial laboratories, and results are best if samples are processed within 30 minutes of collection or if samples are preserved as described earlier. Alternatively, an in-clinic sedimentation technique can be used, in which 0.5 ml of CSF is allowed to sediment over a region of a slide within a sedimentation chamber that is attached to the slide with paraffin or Vaseline (Fig. 66-3). The CSF supernate is then gently aspirated with a needle and syringe and can be used for protein or antibody titer determination. Any remaining fluid is then removed by applying blotting paper to the fluid edge, and the slide is quickly dried by vigorously waving it in the air. Once the slide is dry, the remaining paraffin or Vaseline should be scraped off. Slides should be evaluated by a veterinary cytopathologist.

**FIG 66-3**

A sedimentation chamber can be made from a cut section of a glass vacutainer or plastic specimen tube that is attached to a glass microscope slide with paraffin or Vaseline. Cerebrospinal fluid (CSF) (0.5 ml) is placed in the chamber. After 30 minutes the supernate is gently aspirated with a needle and syringe and the slide is dried rapidly. The slide is then fixed, and the paraffin or Vaseline is removed with a scalpel.

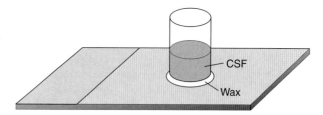

TABLE 66-1

Cerebrospinal Fluid in Various Neurologic Diseases

| CONDITION | WBC | WBC DIFFERENTIAL | TOTAL PROTEIN |
|---|---|---|---|
| Normal | <2 cells/μl (dog) | Mononuclear cells | <25 mg/dl |
| Steroid-responsive suppurative meningitis | +++ | Neutrophils (mature, nontoxic) | +++ |
| Breed-associated meningeal vasculitis | +++ | Neutrophils (mature, nontoxic) | +++ |
| Granulomatous meningoencephalitis | ++ | Lymphocytes, monocytes, occasional plasma cells. Occasional anaplastic mononuclear cell with lacy cytoplasm. Neutrophils in 60% (< 20% of cells) | ++ |
| Pug Dog meningoencephalitis | +++ | Small lymphocytes | ++ |
| Bacterial meningitis | +++ | Neutrophils (toxic), bacteria | +++ |
| Canine distemper | + | Small lymphocytes | + |
| Rabies | + | Small lymphocytes | + |
| Toxoplasmosis | ++ | Lymphocytes, macrophages, occasional PMNs; may see organism—occasionally see eosinophils >50% | ++ |
| Neosporosis | ++ | Lymphocytes, monocytes, occasional PMNs; may see organism—occasionally see eosinophils >50% | ++ |
| Cryptococcosis | ++ | Neutrophils, mononuclears, occasionally eosinophils; organisms in 60% | ++ |
| Rocky Mountain spotted fever (RMSF) | + | Neutrophils | + |
| Ehrlichiosis infection | ++ | Lymphocytes | + |
| Feline infectious peritonitis | +++ | Mixed mononuclear neutrophils | +++ |
| CNS parasite migration | + | Mononuclears, neutrophils, occasionally eosinophils | + |
| Brain or spinal cord infarct | N or + | Mononuclear cells, neutrophils | + |
| CNS neoplasia (except lymphoma, meningioma) | N or + | Mononuclear cells | + |
| Meningioma | N or ++ | Mononuclear cells, neutrophils | ++ |
| CNS lymphoma | ++ | Lymphocytes, neoplastic cells | + |
| Hydrocephalus | N | Normal | N |
| Lissencephaly | N | Normal | N |
| Degenerative myelopathy | N | Normal | N or + |
| Intervertebral disk prolapse | N | Normal | N or + |
| Polyradiculoneuritis | N | Normal | N or + |

*PMN*, Polymorphonuclear neutrophil.

| | WBC count (WBC/μl) | Protein (mg/dl) |
|---|---|---|
| N = normal | <6 (dog); <2 (cat) | <25 |
| + = mild increase | <50 | 25-50 |
| ++ = moderate increase | 50-100 | 50-100 |
| +++ = marked increase | 100 | >100 |

If the slide cannot reach a commercial laboratory within a few hours, it should be fixed and stained with Diff-Quik Differential Stain Set (American Scientific Products) or with Wright's or Giemsa stain.

Most of the cells in the CSF of normal dogs and cats are monocytoid cells and lymphocytes. Small numbers of macrophages can be seen, but the numbers are dramatically increased in some diseases. Occasional neutrophils and eosinophils are present, but these cells should not normally make up more than 10% of the cell population. The typical CSF findings in some specific disorders in dogs and cats are summarized in Table 66-1. It is important to realize, however, that the CSF cytologic findings must always be interpreted in relation to the signalment, history, and clinical findings.

If blood contamination is severe, it can influence the cytologic findings, but even grossly apparent iatrogenic contamination with peripheral blood will have only a minor impact on WBC count and protein analysis. To approximate the maximum effect blood contamination will have on the WBC count in CSF, 1 WBC per microliter can be expected for every 100 RBCs per microliter.

The protein content of the collected CSF should be determined and, whenever possible, protein electrophoresis performed. An increase in the CSF protein content can occur in diseases that disrupt the blood-brain barrier, cause local necrosis, interrupt normal CSF flow and absorption, or result in intrathecal globulin production. Information from CSF protein electrophoresis can be used to determine whether the high protein content in CSF is a result of blood-brain barrier disruption, the intrathecal production of immunoglobulin, or both. CSF protein electrophoresis patterns typical of inflammation, degeneration, and neoplasia of the CNS have been established and can be used with some degree of accuracy to predict the mechanism of disease involved. The amount of immunoglobulins in CSF can also be quantified using radial immunodiffusion, which helps differentiate inflammatory from noninflammatory disorders. Guidelines for interpreting results of CSF protein analyses are found in the Suggested Readings.

Whenever the CSF is cellular, it should be submitted for Gram's staining and culture. In cases in which canine distemper, Rocky Mountain spotted fever (RMSF), borreliosis, ehrlichiosis, neosporosis, or toxoplasmosis is likely, CSF titers of these agents can be compared with the serum titers. Such paired titers are recommended, because CSF immunoglobulin concentrations may vary with those in serum, especially if the CSF specimen has been contaminated with blood or the blood-brain barrier has been disrupted.

# CONTRAST-ENHANCED RADIOGRAPHY

## Myelography

In animals with clinical evidence of spinal cord disease or compression, myelography may be required to confirm, localize, and characterize the lesion. This procedure is particularly valuable for identifying herniated disks, compression of the spinal cord, and tumors of the cord. Myelography should be reserved for animals in which surgery or radiotherapy is being contemplated; thus precise localization of the lesion is necessary.

To perform myelography, an iodinated contrast material is injected into the subarachnoid space. However, this should only be done after it has been confirmed that the CSF is not inflammatory, because myelography can worsen the inflammation and clinical symptoms in an animal with meningitis.

The contrast materials commonly used for this purpose are iohexol (Omnipaque; Winthrop-Breon Laboratories, New York), and iopamidol (Isovue; E.R. Squibb and Sons, Princeton, N.J.). Iohexol and iopamidol (0.25 to 0.45 ml/kg of 180 to 240 mgI/ml contrast media) are associated with a low (<10%) prevalence of postmyelographic adverse effects, such as seizure, hyperesthesia, and vomiting.

The choice between cisternal and lumbar puncture for myelography depends on the suspected lesion location, the technical ease with which either can be done, and the personal preference of the clinician. Cisternal myelography is technically easier to perform, but the contrast agent must be injected slowly to prevent apnea. In addition, contrast material may not be able to flow past obstructive lesions caudal to the cervical region. If lumbar myelography is being performed, the contrast material can be injected under increased pressure to delineate obstructive lesions of the lumbar or thoracic cord.

When performing cisternal myelography, the contrast material can be injected slowly at the cerebellomedullary cistern and allowed to flow caudally the length of the spinal subarachnoid space. Needle removal and elevation of the animal's head, neck, and thorax promote caudal flow, resulting in opacification of the caudal limit of the subarachnoid space within 10 minutes. The needle is inserted using the same technique and landmarks as for cisternal puncture for CSF collection. The bevel is directed caudally. During myelography the flow of the contrast agent is visualized fluoroscopically (when available) and radiographs are taken directly over each region of interest.

Lumbar myelography is performed with the needle at the L4-L5 or L5-L6 site. To insert the needle for lumbar myelography, the animal is placed in lateral recumbency with its trunk flexed. Foam cushions are placed between its limbs and beneath the lumbar region to achieve true lateral positioning, and survey radiographs are taken to ensure that the exposure and positioning are correct. A 3½ inch (8.75 cm) spinal needle is inserted at the cranial edge of the dorsal spinal process of the L5 or L6 vertebra (Fig. 66-4). The needle is then passed in a smooth motion through the spinal cord into the subarachnoid space ventral to it. The animal's tail and pelvic limbs may twitch when the cord is penetrated. The contrast agent is injected only if spinal fluid is obtained, because intramedullary injection could result in severe myelomalacia and inadvertent leakage of some contrast material epidurally can make it difficult to interpret a lumbar myelogram. A small test volume (0.2 ml) of contrast medium can be injected and lateral radiography or fluoroscopy performed to make sure the needle is positioned correctly.

Seizures occasionally occur in an animal after it recovers from anesthesia for myelography. Seizures are most common

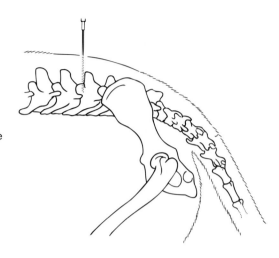

**FIG 66-4**
Landmarks for cerebrospinal fluid (CSF) collection from a lumbar site. The needle is inserted at the cranial edge of the dorsal spinal process of the L6 vertebra.

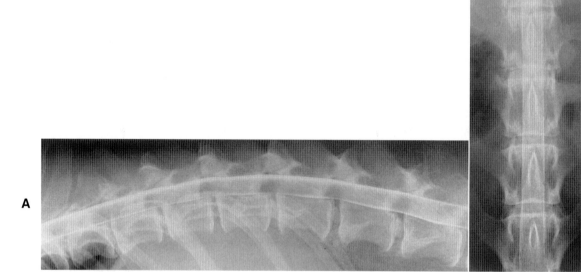

A    B

**FIG 66-5**
Lateral **(A)** and ventrodorsal **(B)** views of a normal myelogram of the thoracolumbar region in a dog. Multiple calcified intervertebral discs can be seen, but no spinal cord compression is evident. (Courtesy Dr. John Pharr, University of Saskatchewan.)

in dogs larger than 29 kg and when greater than two injections of contrast are administered. These seizures can usually be controlled with diazepam (5 to 20 mg IV).

Neurologic deterioration occasionally occurs after myelography. Large-breed dogs with cervical vertebral instability/

malformation spondylomyelopathy, dogs and cats with inflammatory CNS disease or extradural tumors, and dogs with degenerative myelopathy are most often affected. Fortunately this deterioration is usually transient. Myelography will cause some inflammation in the subarachnoid space, even in normal ani-

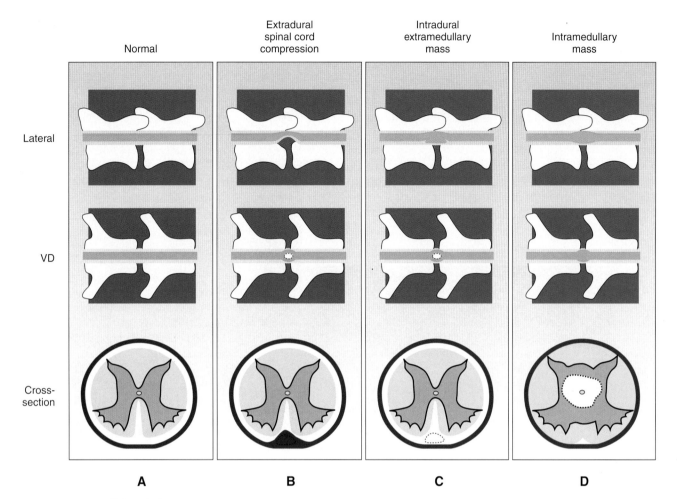

| | Normal | Extradural spinal cord compression | Intradural extramedullary mass | Intramedullary mass |
|---|---|---|---|---|
| Lateral | | | | |
| VD | | | | |
| Cross-section | | | | |
| | **A** | **B** | **C** | **D** |

**FIG 66-6**

The myelographic appearance of extradural, intradural-extramedullary, and intramedullary spinal cord masses. **A,** Normal myelogram. **B,** Ventral extradural spinal cord compression. The leading edge of the contrast material tapers toward the spinal cord, away from the bone on the lateral view. The dorsal column is thinned in this region. On the ventrodorsal view the spinal cord appears widened or flattened, resulting in narrow columns of contrast material. **C,** Ventral intradural, extramedullary spinal cord compression. The leading edge of the contrast material expands and outlines the lesion, tapering toward the spinal cord and toward the bony margin of the osseous canal, resulting in a filling defect at the site of the lesion and the appearance of a "golf tee sign." On the ventrodorsal view the spinal cord appears widened or flattened, resulting in narrow columns of contrast material. **D,** Intramedullary mass or swelling. The leading edges of the contrast material taper toward the bony margin of the osseous canal on both views, with diverging columns of contrast material indicating spinal cord enlargement.

mals, with mild to severe increases in the total WBC count and increases in the neutrophil count and the CSF protein content within 24 hours. Therefore it is important that CSF analysis be performed before myelography to avoid interference with the cytologic studies of CSF.

A normal myelogram will show contrast material filling the subarachnoid space. It appears as a column of contrast agent on each side of the cord on ventrodorsal views and in the ventral and dorsal columns on lateral views (Fig. 66-5). In normal myelograms often a slight elevation and thinning of the ventral column of the contrast agent can be seen as it passes over the intervertebral disc space; however, a wide dorsal column remains, indicating that spinal cord compression is not present. Based on the features of the myelogram, a lesion can be characterized as an extradural spinal cord compression, an intradural but extramedullary compression, or an intramedullary swelling (Figs. 66-6 and 66-7).

## Epidurography

Epidurography is one of the diagnostic-imaging modalities used for evaluating lumbosacral disease in the dog. This is

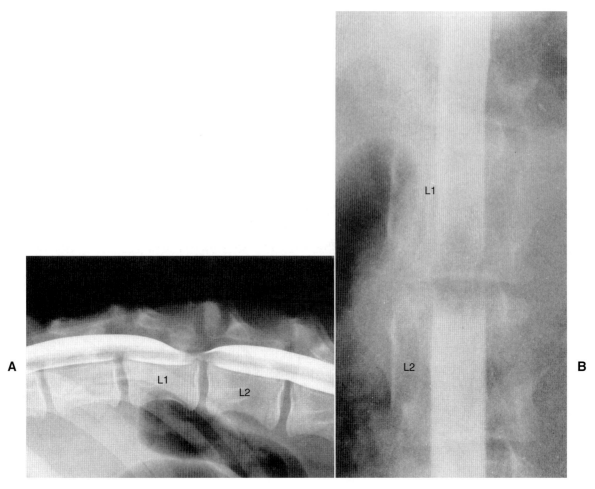

**FIG 66-7**
Lateral **(A)** and ventrodorsal **(B)** views of a myelogram in a 5-month-old German Shepherd with a 3-week history of progressive ataxia. A dorsally located extradural compression of the spinal cord within the caudal portion of the L1 vertebra can be seen. At necropsy the dog was found to have a single focal cartilaginous exostosis of the roof of the L1 vertebra.

because, in most dogs, the dural sac ends cranial to the lumbosacral junction, making myelography of limited value in an evaluation of this region (Fig. 66-8).

To perform epidurography, with the animal under general anesthesia, the skin over the sacrum and first two caudal vertebrae is aseptically prepared. An epidural puncture is made at S3-Cd1 or between the first and second caudal vertebrae (Cd1-Cd2). The needle is advanced to the ventral aspect of the spinal canal with the bevel directed cranially. Contrast material (0.1 to 0.2 ml/kg) of the same type as that used for myelography is injected into the epidural space. Lateral radiographs are obtained just before the end of injection with the pelvis in flexed, neutral, and hyperextended positions. Additional contrast material (0.1 ml/kg) may have to be injected for each additional view. A radiograph in the dorsoventral position should also be obtained. Epidurography appears to be safe, and adverse effects have not been noted. However, it may be difficult to interpret the findings

without experience, because the well-defined lines and columns of contrast seen in myelograms are not normally seen in epidurograms (Fig. 66-9).

## Pneumoventriculography

Pneumoventriculography has been historically useful for confirming the presence of hydrocephalus in small animals. In this technique a needle is inserted into the lateral ventricle through the skull or through an open fontanelle (Fig. 66-10). The needle should not be inserted more than half the distance from the calvarium to the floor of the cranial cavity, as determined by radiographs. In an animal with marked hydrocephalus, the widely dilated ventricle is entered almost immediately after skin puncture. A small amount (0.5 to 2 ml) of fluid is removed and replaced by air to outline the ventricles. The air bubble rises to the top of the ventricular system and allows the thickness of the remaining rim of cerebral cortex to be evaluated.

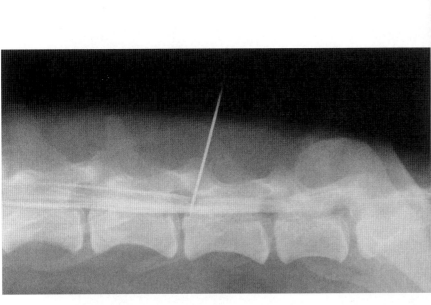

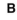

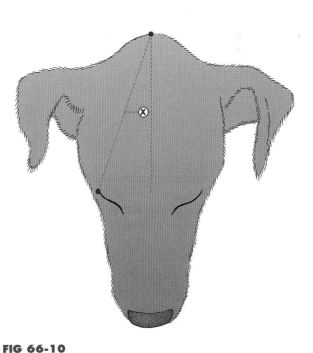

A

B

**FIG 66-8**
Lateral **(A)** and ventrodorsal **(B)** views of a normal myelogram in the lumbar region of a dog. Note that the dural sac ends within the body of the L7 vertebra, making it impossible to evaluate the spinal canal at the lumbosacral junction in this study.

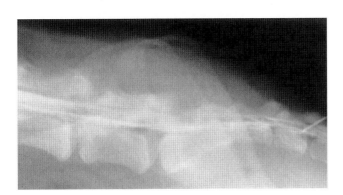

**FIG 66-9**
Normal canine epidurogram. (Courtesy Dr. John Pharr, University of Saskatchewan.)

**FIG 66-10**
Landmarks for inserting a needle into the lateral ventricle for the injection of air for pneumoventriculography. The midpoint of a line connecting the external occipital protuberance and the lateral angle of the eye is determined. A line is then traced from that site medially toward the midline. The skull is entered on that line 3 to 5 mm from the midline.

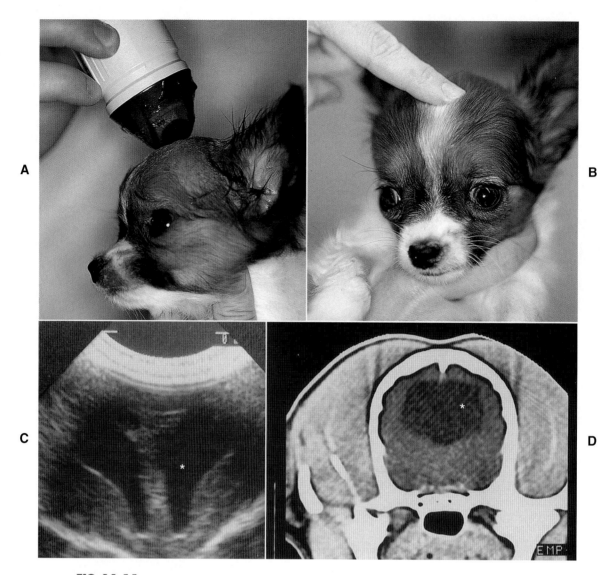

**FIG 66-11**
Ultrasound image **(A** and **C)** of a young Papillon with hydrocephalus and open fontanelles **(B).** Computerized tomography (CT) scan **(D)** of the head of a dog with hydrocephalus. *, Dilated lateral ventricles. **(D** Courtesy Dr. Greg Daniel, University of Tennessee.)

Pneumoventriculography has been largely replaced by ultrasonography performed through open or incomplete fontanelles or ultrasonography performed through the temporal bones in neonates. Computed tomography (CT), and magnetic resonance imaging (MRI) (Fig. 66-11) are also used to evaluate the ventricular system in dogs and cats.

## Computerized Tomography and Magnetic Resonance Imaging

CT and MRI are available for the diagnosis of neurologic disease at most major veterinary referral centers and in some larger communities. These techniques are noninvasive and are valuable in the localization, identification, and characterization of many brain and spinal cord lesions (Figs. 66-12 and 66-13). CT is most useful for identification and characterization of bony abnormalities of the vertebral bodies and skull. MRI can be used to determine very small density differences in brain and spinal cord tissues. These techniques allow precise topographic mapping of lesions, making them very valuable tools in the evaluation of compressive lesions of the brain, spinal cord, or cauda equina when surgery is being considered.

## *ELECTRODIAGNOSTIC TESTING*

### Electromyography

Electromyography (EMG) can be used to identify diseases affecting the spinal or cranial lower motor neuron cell body, its nerve root or peripheral nerves, the neuromuscular junc-

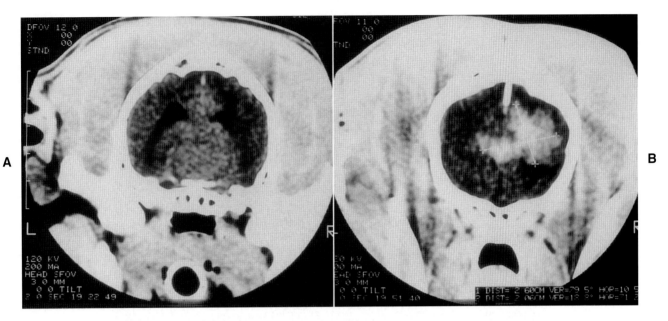

**FIG 66-12**
Computerized tomography (CT) scan of the head of a 9-year-old Golden Retriever with behavioral changes and seizures, showing distortion of the right lateral ventricle **(A)**. CT scan after injection of organic iodide **(B)** shows an extensive irregular mass. Four months later at necropsy, granulomatous meningoencephalitis was found at this site.

tion, and muscle fibers. Normal muscle is electrically silent. As a needle is inserted into normal muscle, a short burst of electrical activity is elicited, which stops when the needle insertion is stopped. Severance, destruction, or demyelination of the peripheral nerve results in the development of spontaneous fibrillations and positive sharp waves (i.e., denervation potentials) and prolonged insertional activity in affected muscles 5 to 7 days after denervation. These changes may also be seen in primary muscle disorders, but other characteristic EMG changes are observed in many muscle diseases (e.g., myositis, myotonia). EMG should be considered to confirm a suspected diagnosis of a muscle disorder, to localize peripheral nerve disease or damage, or to identify abnormal muscles for subsequent biopsy. If multifocal or diffuse neuromuscular disease is suspected based on the findings from the needle EMG examination, nerve stimulation studies may be performed to further characterize the underlying disease.

## Nerve Conduction Velocities

The conduction velocity of motor nerves can be determined by stimulating a nerve at two separate sites and recording the time it takes for an evoked muscle potential to occur. By measuring the distance between the two sites and the difference in the time it takes for the evoked potentials to appear, the motor nerve conduction velocity in that segment of nerve can be determined. The conduction velocity of sensory nerves can be measured using a similar technique. Slow conduction times are seen in demyelinating disorders, allowing the diagnosis of peripheral neuropathies and

polyneuropathies. Nerves that have been injured or avulsed and that have degenerated (onset typically 4 to 5 days after injury) do not conduct an impulse; thus nerve conduction velocity testing can be used to diagnose and localize peripheral nerve injuries.

## Electroretinography

An electroretinogram (ERG) is a recording of the electrical response of the retina to a flashing light stimulus. It is an objective way to evaluate retinal function. The ERG is abnormal with degenerative disorders of the retina, but is normal if the lesion causing visual dysfunction is located caudal to the retina (in the optic nerves, optic chiasm, optic tract, or cerebral cortex). Electroretinography is most widely used as a test to evaluate the retina in dogs before cataract removal.

## Brainstem Auditory Evoked Response

The brainstem auditory evoked response (BAER) depicts the response of nervous tissues to an auditory stimulus. The response is a series of waveforms representing activity beginning in the cochlea and being relayed up the auditory pathway in the brainstem. Lesions of the sense organ itself, the peripheral vestibulocochlear nerve, and the brainstem caudal to the midbrain cause characteristic changes in the response, aiding in lesion localization. The BAER has been used widely for detecting unilateral and bilateral deafness and brainstem masses in dogs.

## Electroencephalography

Electroencephalography provides a graphic record of the electrical activity of the cerebral cortex, but it rarely reveals the

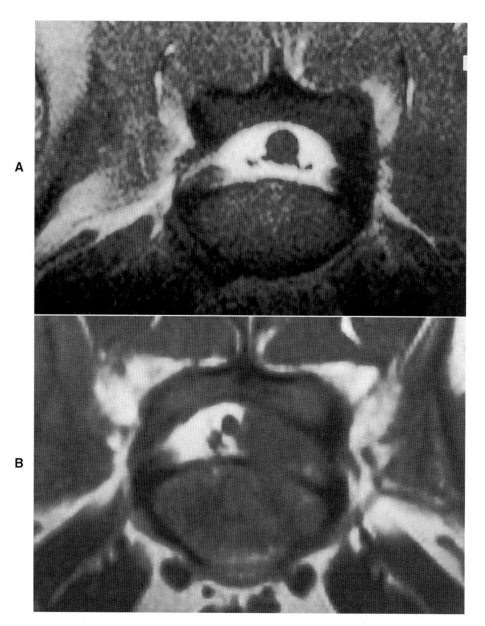

**FIG 66-13**
Magnetic resonance imaging (MRI) scans (transverse T1 images) of the caudal lumbar region of **(A)** a normal dog and **(B)** a Golden Retriever with prolapsed disc material within the vertebral canal. (Courtesy Dr. John Pharr, University of Saskatchewan.)

cause of the lesion. Electroencephalography may help determine whether a cerebral disorder is focal or diffuse.

## BIOPSY OF MUSCLE AND NERVE

### Muscle Biopsy

Muscle biopsy specimens are obtained in an effort to confirm clinical and electrophysiologic evidence of neuromuscular disease and may reveal the cause. For best results, muscle that is affected should be biopsied. The excised muscle fibers should be maintained in a slightly stretched state if electron microscopy is to be performed, but this is not absolutely essential for routine histopathologic and histochemical studies.

Histologic studies may reveal inflammatory or neoplastic changes and the etiologic agent if the disease is infectious.

Many muscle disorders cannot be diagnosed unless the muscle specimens undergo histochemical staining and alterations in fiber types are analyzed. When stained for myofibrillar adenosine triphosphatase, normal muscle has a checkerboard appearance, with light fibers (type I) alternating with the darker type II myofibers. Some myopathies result in a selective loss of one fiber type. Denervation with reinnervation, as occurs in many neuropathies, results in "type grouping," in which the normal checkerboard pattern disappears and large clusters of fibers of the same type appear. To perform myofiber analysis, biopsy specimens must be specially processed and immediately frozen.

Samples should be sent to a laboratory with a special interest in muscle disorders, to ensure that optimal results are obtained and accurately interpreted. Clinicians should contact the laboratory that will process and analyze the biopsy to learn the proper technique of obtaining and preparing specimens and the other procedures to be followed.

## Nerve Biopsy

It may be useful to obtain nerve biopsy specimens in an effort to evaluate peripheral nerve disorders. Fascicular nerve biopsy specimens are used whenever possible, leaving most of the nerve trunk intact. It is important to biopsy nerves that are affected. The common peroneal nerve and the ulnar nerve are the mixed (i.e., motor and sensory) nerves most commonly biopsied. As with muscle biopsy specimens, nerve biopsy specimens require special handling to ensure that maximal information is obtained. Samples should be laid out on a piece of wooden tongue depressor and pinned at each end to keep them gently stretched. They should then be fixed in 2.5% glutaraldehyde for electron microscopy or buffered 10% formalin for light microscopy. Fresh nerve samples can be frozen in liquid nitrogen and stored for biochemical analysis.

## IMMUNOLOGIC AND SEROLOGIC TESTS

### Canine Distemper

The finding of an increased titer of anticanine distemper virus antibody in CSF relative to that in serum is definitive proof of distemper encephalitis or myelitis, because the antibody is locally produced within the CNS.

Immunofluorescent techniques may be applied to cytologic smears prepared from conjunctival, tonsillar, and respiratory epithelium or CSF. These slides are fixed in acetone and stained directly or indirectly with fluorescein-conjugated anti–canine distemper virus antibody and examined by fluorescence microscopy. Antigen in extraneural tissues is most readily detectable early in infection when systemic disease is clinically evident. As the antibody titers rise, the antibody may bind and mask antigen in infected cells, resulting in false-negative results, although distemper antigen can still be detected in CSF cells in most cases. These techniques and a similar immunoperoxidase technique may also be used for diagnosing distemper based on histologic findings in biopsied tissues.

### Toxoplasmosis

Approximately 30% of healthy dogs and cats have antibody against *Toxoplasma gondii*. Increased IgG antibody titers to *T. gondii* merely indicate prior infection. A serial fourfold rise in the serum IgG titer over a 3-week period is suggestive of an active infection with the organism. With the availability of enzyme-linked immunosorbent assays to detect IgM antibody and circulating *T. gondii* antigens, the ability to detect recent or ongoing infections serologically has improved. In spite of this, many dogs and cats with CNS toxoplasmosis have negative antibody titers at the time of diagnosis. Measurement of *T. gondii* IgM antibody in the CSF as compared with the serum may be the best means of diagnosis in some cases.

### Neospora Caninum

The finding of a serial fourfold rise in serum IgG titer against *N. caninum* is diagnostic proof of infection. Antibody levels in the CSF may also be increased in neurologic disease resulting from this organism.

### Ehrlichiosis and Rocky Mountain Spotted Fever

Serologic testing has been the traditional method used to confirm a diagnosis of *Ehrlichia canis* infection, and it involves the use of an immunofluorescent assay test that measures the serum IgG concentration. A positive titer indicates infection. Test results may be negative early in infection. Infection with *Rickettsia rickettsii*, the pathogen that causes RMSF, can be diagnosed by the finding of an increased serum concentration of IgM against this organism or a rising IgG antibody titer. Occasionally, RMSF can be diagnosed based on the finding of the organism in tissue biopsy specimens detected using direct immunofluorescent testing. Use of the polymerase chain reaction to detect deoxyribonucleic acid (DNA) from the infecting organisms may be more sensitive and specific in identifying active infection than the serologic tests routinely performed (see p. 1236).

### Antinuclear Antibody Test and Lupus Erythematosus (LE) Cell Test

Readers are referred to pp. 1214 and 1220 for a description of the antinuclear antibody test and the LE cell test.

### Antiacetylcholine Receptor Antibody

Autoantibodies to canine or feline muscle acetylcholine receptors can be demonstrated by immunoprecipitation radioimmunoassay in most dogs and cats with acquired myasthenia gravis (see p. 1059).

### Antibody Directed Against Type IIM Myofibers

Autoantibody directed against Type IIM myofibers can be demonstrated in the serum of most dogs with masticatory muscle myositis (see p. 1062).

### Cryptococcus Latex Agglutination Test

Readers are referred to p. 1288 for a description of the *Cryptococcus* latex agglutination test.

### Suggested Readings

Braund KG: Nerve and muscle biopsy techniques, *Prog Vet Neurol* 2:35, 1994.

Chrisman CL: Cerebrospinal fluid analysis, *Vet Clin North Am Small Anim Pract* 22:781, 1992.

Kirkberger RM: Recent developments in canine lumbar myelography, *Compend Cont Educ Pract Vet* 16:847, 1994.

Rand JA: The analysis of cerebrospinal fluid in cats. In Bonagura JD et al, editors: *Kirk's current veterinary therapy XII*, Philadelphia, 1995, WB Saunders.

Sande RD: Radiography, myelography, computed tomography and magnetic resonance imaging of the spine, *Vet Clin North Am Small Anim Pract* 22:811, 1994.

# CHAPTER 67

# Disorders of Locomotion

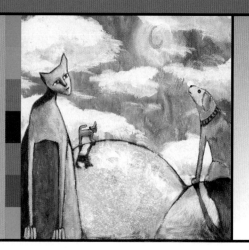

## CHAPTER OUTLINE

ATAXIA, 974
PARESIS AND PARALYSIS, 974
    Localizing spinal cord lesions, 975
    Generalized lower motor neuron paresis and paralysis, 976
    Episodic weakness, 976
DYSMETRIA AND HYPERMETRIA, 977
INVOLUNTARY ALTERATIONS IN MUSCLE TONE, 980
    Dyskinesias, 980
    Tremors, 980
    Opisthotonos and tetanus, 980
    Myoclonus, 981

## ATAXIA

Ataxia, or incoordination, is seen whenever the sensory pathways responsible for transmitting the signals that control proprioception are disrupted. This most commonly occurs as a result of spinal cord disease but may also result from cerebellar or vestibular dysfunction.

Ataxia is a loss of coordination of muscular function that results in staggering and irregular muscular movements. Most often, affected animals tend to cross their limbs so that they interfere with each other during walking. Limbs may be abducted excessively during turning, and movements may be exaggerated or hypermetric (Fig. 67-1). In addition, the weight-bearing phase of walking may be prolonged because of the delayed protraction of affected limbs. The degree of paresis and ataxia is often graded on a five-point scale (Table 67-1).

The initial diagnostic approach in an ataxic animal must focus on localizing the disease to the cerebellum, the vestibular system, or a region of the spinal cord (Fig. 67-2). Incoordination and a loss of balance in association with head tilt and nystagmus are seen in animals with disease of the vestibular system (Chapter 70).

Ataxia, or incoordination, of the head, neck, and all four limbs with preservation of strength is usually caused by a lesion in the cerebellum. The cerebellum processes sensory information concerning position and movement and coordi-

nates that movement. Without cerebellar function, voluntary movement can still occur, but the animal is unable to regulate the rate, range, and force of these movements. Head, neck, and limb movements are jerky and uncontrolled. There is an overreaching and high-stepping gait (hypermetria). The diagnostic approach taken in animals with signs of cerebellar disease is outlined later in this chapter (see Dysmetria and Hypermetria).

Ataxia of the limbs in an animal with spinal cord disease is usually accompanied by some degree of weakness or paresis caused by interruption of descending upper motor neuron (UMN) tracts (see Paresis and Paralysis). Evaluation of spinal reflexes, muscle tone, and conscious proprioception, together with the motor deficits identified, facilitates lesion localization within the spinal cord.

## PARESIS AND PARALYSIS

Any disturbance of the normal mechanism for initiating voluntary movement will cause paresis (weakness) or paralysis, depending on the severity and location of the lesion. Unilateral lesions of the cerebral cortex generally cause very mild, almost undetectable, hemiparesis of the limbs on the contralateral (opposite) side of the body accompanied by slightly abnormal postural reactions in these limbs. Ipsilateral (same-side) hemiparesis and postural reaction deficits are more severe when lesions occur in the brainstem. The finding of other signs such as cranial nerve deficits and altered mentation helps to differentiate a brainstem lesion from a spinal cord lesion.

Ataxia and paresis or paralysis of all four limbs without neurologic evidence of brain or brainstem disease are seen in animals with focal cervical spinal cord lesions or in those with multifocal or diffuse spinal cord disease affecting primarily UMN tracts. There will also be mild to markedly increased muscle tone and increased spinal reflexes in the affected limbs.

Diffuse disease of the lower motor neuron (LMN), including the spinal cord nerve cell bodies, the ventral nerve roots, and the spinal nerves or peripheral nerves, as well as disease of the neuromuscular junction, will result in LMN

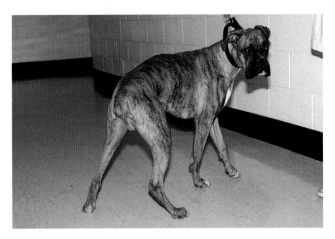

**FIG 67-1**
Wide-based stance and excessive limb abduction indicative of ataxia in a 2-year-old Boxer with *Neospora caninum* meningoencephalomyelitis affecting the cervical spinal cord and cerebellum.

  TABLE 67-1

Clinical Grading in Animals with Rear Limb Paresis and Ataxia

| GRADE | CLINICAL FINDINGS |
|---|---|
| 0 | No purposeful movement—paraplegia |
| 1 | Unable to stand to support weight; when supported by tail, there is slight voluntary movement of rear limbs; severe paraparesis |
| 2 | Unable to stand to support weight; when assisted, moves limbs readily but stumbles and falls; moderate paraparesis and ataxia |
| 3 | Can stand to support weight but frequently stumbles and falls; "drunken sailor gait"; mild paraparesis and ataxia |
| 4 | Can stand to support weight and walk with minimal paraparesis and ataxia |
| 5 | Normal strength and coordination |

paresis or paralysis without remarkable ataxia. Most animals with strictly LMN disease are aware of their limb position, and if their weight is supported by the examiner, postural reactions, including conscious proprioception, are normal as long as voluntary movement is still present. Muscle tone is decreased and spinal reflexes are depressed in dogs and cats with LMN diseases. Generalized weakness with normal postural reactions, normal reflexes, and no ataxia are seen in animals with metabolic, cardiorespiratory, or muscular system disorders.

## LOCALIZING SPINAL CORD LESIONS

Once a complete neurologic examination has been performed and postural reactions, proprioception, strength, muscle tone,

and spinal reflexes have all been assessed, it is possible to identify the location of a spinal cord lesion. Functionally the spinal cord can be divided into four regions: the cranial cervical spinal cord (C1-C5), the *cervical intumescence* (C6-T2), the thoracolumbar region (T3-L3), and the lumbar intumescence (L4-S3) (Table 67-2).

A focal cranial cervical (C1-C5) spinal cord lesion may be mild or severe. Irritation or inflammation of the meninges in this region without compression or damage to the spinal cord parenchyma results in cervical pain without neurologic deficits. A mild compressive lesion of the cranial cervical spinal cord results in ataxia and paresis of all four limbs; however, because the nerve fibers to the rear limbs are more superficial in the cord than those to the forelimbs, rear limb signs are usually worse than forelimb signs. Lesions that primarily affect the central C1-C5 spinal cord (intramedullary neoplasia, infarcts, hydromyelia) will sometimes cause UMN weakness that is present in all four limbs but is most dramatic in the forelimbs (central cord syndrome). Compressive lesions of the C1-C5 cord cause postural reaction deficits, including decreased conscious proprioception. The animal will be incoordinated and may stand so that all four paws are knuckled over on the dorsum. Muscle tone is normal to increased in all four limbs, and all spinal reflexes are normal to hyperactive. A unilateral lesion of the cervical cord results in signs only in the ipsilateral rear limbs and forelimbs.

A lesion of the spinal cord between C6 and T2 results in paresis of all four limbs and ataxia that is most pronounced in the rear limbs. This region is known as the cervical intumescence (swelling) because the spinal cord is larger in this region, since this is where all of the important spinal nerves originate to form the peripheral nerves of the brachial plexus. The spinal cord segments directly supplying the nerves of the brachial plexus are affected in this region, along with the spinal cord UMN tracts to the rear limbs. With a lesion between C6 and T2, the forelimbs may appear to be more severely paretic (weak) than the rear limbs. The forelimbs lose muscle tone and strength, and the muscles rapidly atrophy. The spinal reflexes in the forelimbs may be depressed or absent (LMN signs), whereas those in the rear limbs are normal to hyperactive (UMN signs). Proprioception in the rear limbs decreases as the UMN tracts are disrupted. Unilateral lesions produce signs confined to the ipsilateral side. Horner's syndrome may be seen if the T1-T2 region is involved (see p. 987), and the ipsilateral panniculus reflex may be lost if the C8-T1 spinal cord segments, nerve roots, or peripheral nerve is damaged. Because the phrenic nerve originates at C5 to C7, a severe lesion in this region could cause diaphragmatic paralysis. Occasionally, forelimb signs are very subtle in an animal with a compressive lesion of the cervicothoracic cord, even though the UMN signs to the rear limbs are remarkable, making it difficult to differentiate disease at this site from a T3-L3 lesion. Atrophy of the muscles over the scapula may be the most prominent LMN signs in animals with a mild C6-T2 lesion.

A lesion of the spinal cord between T3 and L3 results in paresis and UMN signs (increased tone, hyperactive reflexes) in the rear limbs (see Table 67-2). Postural reactions, including

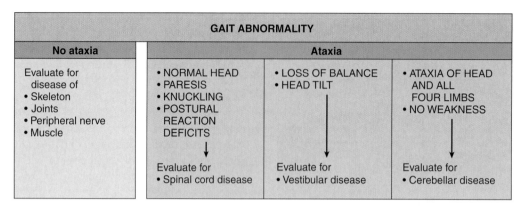

**FIG 67-2**
Diagnostic approach to a dog or cat with a gait abnormality.

TABLE 67-2

Neurologic Findings in Dogs and Cats with Spinal
Cord Lesions

| SITE OF LESION | THORACIC LIMBS | PELVIC LIMBS |
|---|---|---|
| C1-C5 | UMN | UMN |
| C6-T2 | LMN | UMN |
| T3-L3 | Normal | UMN |
| L4-S3 | Normal | LMN |

*UMN,* Upper motor neuron signs; *LMN,* lower motor neuron signs.

conscious proprioception, are abnormal in the rear limbs, whereas the forelimbs are completely neurologically normal. As compressive lesions of the spinal cord in this region become more severe, there is a predictable worsening of the neurologic deficits (Fig. 67-3; see also Table 67-1). A lesion affecting the lumbar intumescence (cord segments L4 to S3) causes LMN paralysis (decreased tone, loss of reflexes) in the rear limbs, but the forelimbs remain normal.

Spinal cord disorders may be caused by anomalies, degenerative conditions, neoplasia, inflammatory diseases, external trauma, internal trauma resulting from disk extrusion, and infarction. (See Chapter 72 for a discussion of specific spinal cord disorders and the diagnostic approach taken in dogs and cats with spinal cord disease.)

## GENERALIZED LOWER MOTOR NEURON PARESIS AND PARALYSIS

Generalized weakness or paralysis with loss of reflexes is seen in diffuse diseases that affect the LMN (i.e., diseases that affect the peripheral nerves, the spinal nerves or nerve roots, or the nerve cell bodies in the ventral gray matter of the spinal cord bilaterally at both cervical and lumbosacral intumescences) or in diseases that prevent neuromuscular transmission. In many conditions the rear limbs are affected more severely at first, with the paralysis ascending until all four limbs are af-

fected. Muscle tone is decreased, and spinal reflexes are decreased or absent. The gait is stiff, stilted, and choppy as the animal tries to maintain its limbs under its center of gravity for support. Sensation may be normal or abnormal, depending on whether sensory nerves are affected. In dogs and cats with peripheral neuropathies affecting primarily sensory axons, ataxia or self-mutilation without loss of reflexes may be seen. Diseases causing signs of diffuse LMN paralysis include congenital and familial disorders of demyelination and axonal degeneration; inflammatory immune-mediated disorders of nerves; polyneuropathies associated with metabolic, toxic, or neoplastic disease; and neuromuscular junction toxicity, as seen in botulism and tick-induced paralysis (see Chapter 73).

## EPISODIC WEAKNESS

Episodic weakness that worsens with exercise and abates with rest may be secondary to disorders of skeletal muscle or the neuromuscular junction, cardiopulmonary disease, rupture of vascular neoplasms, and several metabolic imbalances that affect the central nervous system (CNS) (Table 67-3). Apparent weakness can also be a manifestation of orthopedic and articular diseases if pain makes the animal reluctant to exercise.

Many inflammatory, degenerative, and metabolic conditions of muscle cause weakness that worsens with exercise and abates with rest, appearing episodic (see Chapter 74). Myasthenia gravis, a disorder causing impaired neuromuscular transmission, is characterized by weakness exacerbated by exercise and alleviated by rest (see p. 1059).

Cardiopulmonary disease may cause decreased exercise tolerance and weakness. Severe respiratory tract disease occasionally results in the development of peripheral hypoxemia with subsequent weakness and exercise intolerance. Congestive heart failure, cardiac tamponade, and severe bradyarrhythmias and tachyarrhythmias may cause cardiac output to be decreased, such that peripheral hypoxemia, weakness, and collapse occur when the animal is exercised or stressed. Auscultation of the heart and lungs, palpation of the peripheral arterial pulses, and examination of mucous membrane color may be useful in detecting cardiopulmonary dis-

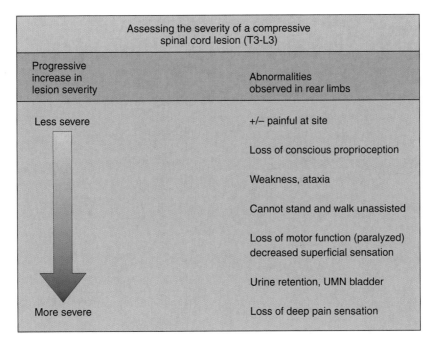

**FIG 67-3**
Assessing the severity of a compressive lesion of the T3-L3 spinal cord.

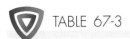 TABLE 67-3

**Common Causes of Episodic Weakness or Collapse**

Cardiac disease
Respiratory disease
Episodic hemorrhage (e.g., ruptured hemangiosarcoma)
Hypoglycemia
Hypoadrenocorticism
Polymyositis
Other myopathies
Myasthenia gravis
Orthopedic or articular disease

ease, particularly if these examinations are performed during an episode of collapse or weakness. Thoracic radiographs, an electrocardiogram (ECG), and cardiac ultrasound may also reveal abnormalities. Some spontaneous episodic disturbances in heart rhythm can result in episodes of weakness and collapse but can be difficult to diagnose unless an ECG is performed immediately before the collapse or continuous ambulatory ECG monitoring can be done. Rupture of vascular tumors, such as a hemangiosarcoma, into the peritoneal cavity is a common cause of episodic weakness and collapse in large-breed dogs. Palpation of the tumor, recognition of the associated hemoperitoneum, or identification of a regenerative anemia a few days after recovery supports this diagnosis (see p. 1142).

Hypoglycemia is the most common metabolic cause of generalized episodic weakness. In addition, hypoadrenocor-

ticoid animals may have episodes of collapse and weakness associated with hypotension and shock, which resolve after fluid and/or glucocorticoid therapy, or both. In the initial stages of the disease, clinical signs may become apparent only when the dog is stressed or exercised, because of the blunted adrenal gland response to corticotropin. These disorders are discussed in Chapters 52 and 53.

## DYSMETRIA AND HYPERMETRIA

The cerebellum coordinates the muscle groups of the body so that movements are smooth and accurate. Information concerning the position of the limbs is transmitted up the spinal cord to the cerebellum through the spinocerebellar tracts. Damage to the cerebellum results in a broad-based stance, loss of balance, ataxia, tremor, hypermetria, and dysmetria without paresis. The animal is unable to judge distances or control the range of head movements. When it attempts to perform a certain movement, it makes a series of jerking and bobbing movements (intention tremor). The gait is choppy and uncoordinated (dysmetria), and exaggerated flexion and extension of the limbs (hypermetria) are common. A fine tremor of the head and body may be present at rest. The animal is strong but uncoordinated. All postural reactions, spinal reflexes, and sensations are normal if the animal is supported. In most cases the cranial nerve examination findings are normal. The menace reflex may be lost. Damage to the very superficial spinocerebellar tracts in the cervical spinal cord will produce limb signs very similar to those seen in animals with cerebellar disease, since the UMN influence of the cerebellum to the limbs is lost. Affected dogs

TABLE 67-4

### Disorders Resulting in Signs of Cerebellar Disease

Acute, nonprogressive disorders
    Trauma
    Infarction
Subacute, progressive disorders
    Infectious inflammatory diseases
    Granulomatous meningoencephalitis (dogs)
Chronic, slowly progressive disorders
    Neoplasia
    Degeneration (see Table 72-5)
Young animal—present at birth, static
    Panleukopenia (kittens)
    Herpesvirus (puppies)
    Cerebellar hypoplasia (see Table 67-5)
    Malformations
Young animal—progressive
    Neonatal abiotrophy (see Table 67-5)
    Postnatal abiotrophy (see Table 67-5)
    Metabolic storage diseases (see Table 67-6)
    Degeneration (see Table 72-5)

 TABLE 67-5

### Inherited and Congenital Cerebellar Syndromes

**Cerebellar Hypoplasia (Present at Birth, Not Progressive)**

Chow Chow
Irish Setter
Wire-Haired Fox Terrier
Boston Terrier
Labrador Retriever
Bull Terrier
Weimaraner
Dachshund
Miniature Poodle
Beagle
Silky Terrier
Siberian Husky
Poodle

**Neonatal Abiotrophy (Very Early Onset, Progressive)**

Samoyed
Beagle
Irish Setter
Miniature Poodle
Bernese Mountain Dog
Rhodesian Ridgeback
Jack Russell Terrier

**Postnatal Abiotrophy (Later Onset, Progressive)**

Airedale Terrier, 12 weeks old at onset
Australian Kelpie, 6 to 12 weeks old at onset
Beagle, 3 to 14 weeks old at onset
Bernese Mountain Dog, 6 months old at onset
Border Collie, 6 to 8 weeks old at onset
Brittany Spaniel, 2.5 to 13 years old at onset
Bull Mastiff, 4 to 28 weeks old at onset
Bull Terrier, 3 months old at onset
Cairn Terrier, 8 to 24 weeks old at onset
Cocker Spaniel, 8 to 12 weeks old at onset
Cocker Spaniel, 6 to 14 months old at onset
English Springer Spaniel, 6 to 16 weeks old at onset
German Shepherd Dog, 6 to 16 weeks old at onset
Golden Retriever, 8 to 12 weeks old at onset
Gordon Setter, 6 to 24 months old at onset
Great Dane, 8 to 12 weeks old at onset
Kerry Blue Terrier, 9 to 16 weeks old at onset
Labrador Retriever, 8 to 17 weeks old at onset
Rottweiler, 7 to 8 weeks old at onset
Rough Collie, 4 to 12 weeks old at onset
Samoyed, 6 months at onset
Isolated cases in many breeds

and cats will show ataxia, dysmetria, and hypermetria of all four limbs but no head tremor or other brain signs. Animals with a lesion in the flocculonodular lobe of the cerebellum may exhibit paradoxical central vestibular signs (head tilt to the side opposite the lesion, nystagmus with the fast phase directed to the side opposite the lesion, and abnormal postural reactions on the side of the lesion).

### Etiology

Most of the intracranial disorders that cause seizures (see p. 992) can also cause cerebellar diseases. Cerebellar dysfunction may occur in any animal of any age as a result of trauma, hemorrhage, infarction, infectious or inflammatory disease, granulomatous meningoencephalitis (dogs), or primary or metastatic neoplasia (Table 67-4). These are most common in adult animals, however. Vascular and traumatic disorders occur acutely and either remain static or abate with time. Inflammatory and neoplastic disorders invariably progress over time.

Congenital cerebellar hypoplasia has been documented in several breeds (Table 67-5). Clinical signs are present as soon as affected animals begin to ambulate, and one or more animals in a litter may be affected. The cause of these malformations is unknown, and a genetic basis has not been documented. Virus-induced cerebellar malformations in kittens (panleukopenia virus induced) and puppies (herpesvirus induced) also occur, causing cerebellar dysfunction that becomes apparent very early in life. Clinical signs in these syndromes do not progress, which helps to differentiate them from cerebellar neuronal abiotrophy (see Table 67-5).

Cerebellar neuronal abiotrophy is a syndrome of premature degeneration of cells within the cerebellum that has been observed in several breeds of dogs and cats and is suspected to have a hereditary basis (see Table 67-5). Clinical signs may be

present at birth or appear at a young age and then worsen with time. Progressive signs of cerebellar dysfunction may also be seen in animals affected by more generalized neurodegenerative conditions (see Table 72-3) or metabolic storage diseases (Table 67-6). The presence of neurologic signs unrelated to the cerebellar deficit enables these conditions to be differentiated from syndromes of cerebellar abiotrophy.

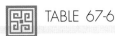 TABLE 67-6

Metabolic Storage Diseases

| DISORDER | SIGNALMENT | CLINICAL SIGNS |
|---|---|---|
| **Metabolic Storage Diseases Causing Seizures in Dogs and Cats** | | |
| GM$_2$ gangliosidosis | German Shorthair Pointers, other dogs, cats, 6-12 mo | Dementia, blindness, seizures |
| Ceroid lipofuscinosis | English Setters, Border Collies, Salukis, 1-2 yr; Chihuahuas, 6-12 mo; Cocker Spaniels, Dachshunds, 6-18 mo; Siamese cats | Dementia, blindness, seizures, ataxia, head tremor, hypermetria |
| Neuronal glycoproteinosis | Poodles, Basset Hounds, Beagles, mixed breed, other, 5-12 mo | Dementia, seizures |
| **Metabolic Storage Diseases Causing Cerebellar Signs in Dogs and Cats** | | |
| GM$_1$ gangliosidosis | Siamese and Korat cats, Beagles, English Springer Spaniels, Portuguese Water Dogs, others, 3-6 mo | Ataxia, head tremors, spastic quadriparesis |
| Sphingomyelinosis (Niemann-Pick disease) | Siamese and domestic short-haired cats, Poodles, others, 4-6 mo | Ataxia, head tremors, hypermetria ± dementia and ± LMN paralysis |
| Type C Niemann-Pick Disease | Kittens | Ataxia, hypermetria, head tremors |
| Glucocerebrosidosis (Gaucher's disease) | Australian and Silky Terriers, Abyssinian cats, 6-8 mo | Ataxia, tremors, hyperactivity |
| α-Mannosidosis | Persian, domestic short-haired cats, birth-10 mo | Ataxia, dysmetria, head tremor ± hepatomegaly and ± gingival hyperplasia |
| Globoid cell leukodystrophy (Krabbe's disease) | West Highland White Terriers, Cairn Terriers, Coonhounds, Beagles, Poodles, cats, 4-12 mo | Ataxia, tremor, proprioception loss, LMN, paralysis |
| **Metabolic Storage Diseases Causing Other Signs in Dogs and Cats** | | |
| Fucosidosis | English Springer Spaniel, 12 mo | Dementia, ataxia, proprioception loss, blindness, hoarseness, dysphagia |
| Glycogen storage disease, type 3 | German Shepherd Dog, 2 mo | Weak, exercise intolerance, slow growth, hepatomegaly |
| Glycogenosis IV | Norwegian Forest cats 5-12 mo | Perinatal death, hyperthermia, muscle twitches, muscle atrophy, tetraplegia |
| Glycogen storage disease, type 7 | English Springer Spaniel, 8-12 mo | Weak, hemolysis, hemoglobinuria |
| Mucopolysaccharidosis I | Domestic short-haired cat, 10 mo; rare dog, 3-6 mo | Facial dysmorphism, corneal opacity, lameness |
| Mucopolysaccharidosis VI | Siamese cat, Domestic short-haired cat, Miniature Pinscher, 4-7 mo | Facial dysmorphism, xyphosis, corneal opacity, lameness, paraparesis |

## Diagnostic Approach

Cerebellar dysfunction can usually be identified during a neurologic examination. Congenital hypoplasia, malformations, or abiotrophy should be suspected in puppies or kittens that are otherwise alert and active but have signs of cerebellar dysfunction. There is no therapy for these disorders. Progressive disorders such as the abiotrophies, metabolic storage diseases, and degenerative disorders will become more extensive with time, usually resulting in an inability to ambulate, leading to euthanasia.

If other neurologic abnormalities are present, especially in an adult dog or cat with cerebellar dysfunction, inflammatory or neoplastic diseases should be considered. A complete physical and ophthalmologic examination, clinicopathologic tests (complete blood count, biochemistry profile, urinalysis), and thoracic and abdominal radiographs may identify an underlying disease. If abnormalities are not detected, cerebrospinal fluid (CSF) analysis should be performed in an attempt to establish a diagnosis (see Table 66-1). Skull radiographs are not very useful for evaluating dogs with cerebellar disease unless a bony tumor or skull fracture is suspected. If available, computed tomography (CT) or magnetic resonance imaging (MRI) may be used to visualize the cerebellum and identify malformations, neoplasms, or granulomas. A degenerative disease is suspected if all test results are normal in an adult dog or cat. Neuraxonal dystrophy and other degenerative disorders affecting the cerebellum have been observed in Rottweilers, Chihuahuas, Jack Russell Terrier puppies, and

Scottish Terriers, as well as sporadically in other breeds and in cats (see Table 72-3). Such disorders can be definitively diagnosed only on the basis of the findings from cerebellar biopsy or postmortem examination.

## INVOLUNTARY ALTERATIONS IN MUSCLE TONE

Tremors, tetany, tetanus, opisthotonos, dyskinesias, and myoclonus are all involuntary alterations of muscle tone. Tremors are a mild form of tetany characterized by involuntary muscle trembling or quivering, whereas tetany is characterized by severe generalized muscle twitching that may progress to seizures. Tetanus is a sustained tonic contraction of the muscles without twitching. Opisthotonos is a very severe form of tetanus in which spasm of the limb and neck muscles results in lateral recumbency with dorsiflexion of the neck and extensor rigidity of the limbs. Myoclonus is the rhythmic repetitive contraction of a particular group of muscles. Forelimb extensor rigidity occurring in association with UMN paralysis of the rear limbs is occasionally seen in dogs with acute, severe thoracic or thoracolumbar spinal cord injury and is termed *Schiff-Sherrington syndrome* (see Fig. 65-5).

### DYSKINESIAS

Dyskinesias are disorders of the CNS that result in involuntary movements in a fully conscious individual. These movement disorders have only occasionally been described in dogs and cats. Episodes typically involve unpredictable episodic involuntary limb hyperextension or hyperflexion. There is no altered consciousness, no preceding aura, and no apparent postictal phase. Anticonvulsant therapy is ineffective for preventing or terminating an episode. In humans, dyskinesias are usually the result of structural disease affecting the basal ganglia.

### TREMORS

A tremor is a rhythmic, oscillatory movement of a body part. Intention tremors of the head, usually associated with cerebellar disease, substantially worsen when the head nears a target during goal-oriented movement such as attempts to eat, drink, or sniff an object.

A toxic cause should be suspected in an animal with severe generalized tremors or tetany of acute onset (see Table 69-2). Strychnine, metaldehyde, chlorinated hydrocarbons, mycotoxins, and organophosphates are the most common toxic causes of tremors and tetany. Metabolic disturbances such as hypoglycemia and hypocalcemia can also cause tremors and tetany.

Head and body tremors unassociated with a metabolic or toxic disorder may arise acutely in young adult (5 months to 3 years of age), predominantly white dogs of small breeds (Maltese, West Highland White Terrier, Beagle). The tremors in these "shaker dogs" develop rapidly over 1 to 3 days and then occur continually, worsening with excitement and disappearing during sleep. There is no weakness, and neurologic

findings are usually normal, although nystagmus, dysconjugate eye movements, head tilt, or seizures have been observed in a few dogs. All clinicopathologic test results are normal. Occasionally, CSF analysis reveals a mild lymphocytosis. Hydrocephalus of questionable significance has been documented in a few dogs. In the few cases where necropsy was performed, histology has revealed a mild, nonsuppurative encephalomyelitis with some perivascular cuffing. In some dogs the tremors decrease and may subside 1 to 3 months after onset, even without treatment, but they persist for life in other dogs. Diazepam (0.5 mg/kg PO q8h) and corticosteroids (prednisone, 2 to 4 mg/kg/day PO) administered early in the disease may result in rapid clinical improvement, with most dogs showing dramatic improvement within 4 or 5 days. Treatment should be tapered gradually over 4 or 5 months, with the drug doses titrated to control the clinical signs. A few dogs suffer relapse months to years later, requiring retreatment. Some dogs require lifelong low-dose therapy with corticosteroids and diazepam. The cause of this syndrome is unknown.

Congenital tremor syndromes can occur as a result of metabolic storage diseases or congenital spongy degeneration of the CNS, or in association with abnormal or deficient myelination (dysmyelinogenesis). A congenital diffuse tremor syndrome associated with dysmyelinogenesis has been observed in puppies. Affected puppies stand with a wide-based stance and show whole-body tremors that worsen with exercise or excitement. The syndrome that has been most extensively studied occurs in male Springer Spaniels. These puppies have a severe generalized tremor that is progressive, usually resulting in death within 2 to 4 months. Similar syndromes have been recognized in the Weimaraner, Bernese Mountain Dog, Samoyed, Dalmatian, and Chow Chow, as well as sporadically in other breeds. Clinical signs usually begin within the first 4 weeks of life. Diagnosis is based on the signalment and clinical findings in the absence of other neurologic deficits and of clinicopathologic abnormalities. In the Springer Spaniel and the Samoyed this has been shown to be a sex-linked, recessively inherited trait. In the Chow Chow and in mildly affected dogs of other breeds, gradual clinical recovery may occur within 1 to 3 months without treatment.

Trembling of the pelvic limbs may develop in old dogs (senile tremors) that are weak but otherwise neurologically normal. The trembling disappears at rest but is apparent when the animals stand, and it worsens with exercise. Results of all tests are normal, and there is no effective treatment. Diagnostically it is important to rule out electrolyte disturbances, hypothyroidism, hypoadrenocorticism, hip dysplasia, and lumbosacral disease.

### OPISTHOTONOS AND TETANUS

Loss of consciousness occurring in association with tetanus and opisthotonos (decerebrate rigidity) is seen in dogs and cats with severe brainstem disease caused by infection, trauma, or neoplasia. Brainstem disease in these animals is suspected on the basis of the history, neurologic findings, and results of clinicopathologic tests. CSF analysis and CT or MRI can be used to make a diagnosis. Opisthotonos and tetanus with no altered state of consciousness may be seen in animals with mild strychnine poisoning (see p. 995), after trauma to the rostral cerebellum, and in *Clostridium tetani* infection.

*C. tetani* produces spores that persist for long periods in the environment. If a deep wound or an area of tissue damage becomes contaminated with these spores, the spores may be anaerobically converted to a vegetative form and a toxin produced. Within a few hours the toxin ascends peripheral nerves to the spinal cord, where it blocks the release of neurotransmitter from the inhibitory interneurons (Renshaw cells). The extensor muscles are thereby released from inhibition, resulting in tetany. Cats are more resistant to the toxin than dogs are.

Clinical signs of tetanus appear 5 to 20 days after wound infection. Animals with mild or early tetanus show a stiff gait, erect ears, an elevated tail, and contraction of the facial muscles (risus sardonicus) (Fig. 67-4). The signs may be most severe in the area of the body adjacent to where the toxin is being produced. In severe disease the animal is recumbent and shows extensor rigidity of all four limbs, opisthotonos, and occasionally seizures. The animal may die as a result of an inability to ventilate adequately. Tetanus is diagnosed on the basis of clinical signs and the history of a recent wound. It is difficult to isolate *C. tetani* from wounds, and this is not critical for the diagnosis.

Treatment should consist of rest, immediate wound debridement, antibiotics, neutralization of the toxin, and intensive supportive care. Initially, aqueous penicillin G is administered intravenously (40,000 U/kg), after which the procaine salt is given by intramuscular injection (40,000 U/kg q12h). Alternatively, metronidazole (10 to 15 mg/kg q8h) may be administered; it is bactericidal against most anaerobes and achieves a therapeutic concentration even in necrotic tissues. Antibiotics are administered for 2 weeks or until clinical recovery occurs.

A test dose of tetanus antitoxin (equine origin) is injected intradermally 15 to 30 minutes before the administration of a treatment dose. If no wheal develops, the antitoxin is administered intravenously (1000 U/kg; maximum, 20,000 U). This dose is not repeated, because a therapeutic blood concentration persists for 7 to 10 days after a single injection, and repeated administration of antitoxin increases the chance of an anaphylactic reaction. The injection of a small dose of antitoxin (1000 U) just proximal to the wound site may be beneficial in dogs and cats with localized tetanus.

The animal is maintained in a quiet, dark environment. Muscle spasms are controlled with diazepam (0.5 to 1 mg/kg IV or PO, as needed) and chlorpromazine (0.5 mg/kg IV q8h) or acepromazine (0.1 to 0.2 mg/kg IM q6h). Phenobarbital (2 mg/kg q8h IV or IM) or pentobarbital (5 to 15 mg/kg IV to effect) may be administered as needed. IV fluids are administered, and nutritional support is achieved using nasogastric or gastrotomy tube feeding. The animal is hand-fed as soon as it is able to prehend food and swallow. In some animals, urinary and fecal retention must be managed by repeated catheterization and enemas. Improvement is usually notice-

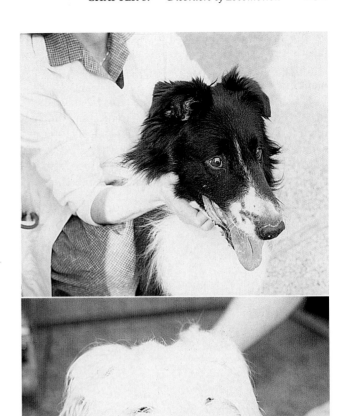

**FIG 67-4**
Tetanus in two dogs, with the erect ears and risus sardonicus resulting from contraction of the head and facial muscles. Both dogs had wounds on a forelimb, which were presumed to be the site of entry of the toxin.

able within 1 week, but signs may persist for 3 to 4 weeks. The prognosis is poor if the signs progress rapidly; many severely affected animals die of respiratory failure within 5 days of the appearance of signs.

## MYOCLONUS

Myoclonus is a rhythmic, shocklike, repetitive contraction of a portion of a muscle, an individual muscle, or a group of muscles occurring as often as 60 times per minute. These rhythmic contractions do not abate during sleep or general anesthesia (unlike tremors). Limb and facial muscles are most often involved. Myoclonus is most commonly associated with canine distemper meningoencephalomyelitis. Distemper-related myoclonus may be the sole sign, or it may occur in association with other neurologic signs. Other focal inflammatory or neoplastic lesions of the spinal cord can also rarely produce myoclonus. Evaluation in such animals is approached in the same way as that for any CNS disorder. The prognosis for resolution of the myoclonus is grave.

Familial reflex myoclonus has been recognized in 4- to 6-week-old Labrador Retriever puppies. Clinical signs include intermittent spasms of the axial and appendicular muscles with occasional episodes of opisthotonos. These signs worsen when the animal is stressed or excited. Treatment with diazepam and clonazepam has not been successful. The prognosis for recovery is grave.

## Suggested Readings

Berry WL: Episodic weakness in dogs, *Compend Contin Educ Pract Vet* 12:141, 1990.

Coates JR et al: Congenital and inherited neurologic disorders in dogs and cats. In Bonagura JD et al, editors: *Kirk's current veterinary therapy XII,* Philadelphia, 1995, WB Saunders.

deLahunta A: Abiotrophies in domestic animals: a review, *Can J Vet Res* 54:65, 1990.

Parker AJ: "Little white shakers" syndrome: generalized sporadic acquired tremors of adult dogs. In Bonagura JD et al, editors: *Kirk's current veterinary therapy XII,* Philadelphia, 1995, WB Saunders.

Wheeler SJ et al: *Small animal spinal disorders: diagnosis and surgery,* St Louis, 1994, Mosby.

# CHAPTER 68

## Abnormalities of Mentation, Loss of Vision, & Pupillary Abnormalities

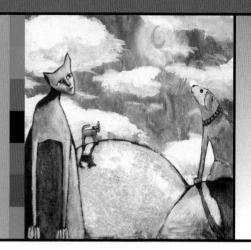

### CHAPTER OUTLINE

MENTATION, 983
HEAD TRAUMA, 983
LOSS OF VISION AND PUPILLARY
ABNORMALITIES, 984
    Optic neuritis, 985
    Optic chiasm and occipital cortex, 986
    Anisocoria, 986
    Horner's syndrome, 987
    Protrusion of the third eyelid, 987

## MENTATION

Abnormal behavior, delirium, and compulsive behavior are seen in dogs and cats with lesions of the cerebral cortex, metabolic encephalopathies, or intoxications. Disorders affecting the brainstem, thalamus, or cerebral cortex can also cause severe depression, stupor, and coma in conjunction with cranial nerve and postural reaction abnormalities (see Table 65-3).

When presented with a dog or cat with abnormal mentation, the clinician must first ascertain whether the problem is purely behavioral or is an indication of an actual neurologic abnormality. The history obtained from the owner regarding the animal's normal behavior and the circumstances preceding the onset of signs may help differentiate a behavioral from a neurologic problem. The finding of neurologic deficits in addition to the mentation problem confirms the existence of an abnormality within the nervous system.

Intoxication with household toxins, insecticides, rodenticides, and prescription or illicit drugs must be considered in any dog or cat with neurologic signs that were acute at onset. The index of suspicion should be particularly high when a previously healthy dog or cat experiences sudden onset of neurologic signs. Anxiety and delirium may be observed early in such animals, with other neurologic and systemic signs seen concurrently or subsequently. A history of exposure is helpful in establishing the diagnosis but is rarely obtained. As such, therapy in these animals is usually supportive and de-signed to buy time until the effects of the offending substance have dissipated (see Table 69-3).

Any animal showing episodic or chronic abnormalities of mentation should be evaluated for a metabolic encephalopathy such as hepatic disease, hypoglycemia, severe uremia, or hyperosmolality caused by diabetes mellitus or hypernatremia. Cerebral cortical disorders that cause abnormalities of mentation include anomalies (e.g., hydrocephalus, lissencephaly), inflammatory diseases (e.g., meningitis, encephalitis), degenerative disorders (see Table 72-5), primary or metastatic brain tumors, external trauma, and vascular disorders (e.g., feline ischemic encephalopathy, canine vascular accident). The diagnostic evaluation of dogs and cats with suspected cerebral cortical disease is discussed in more detail on p. 991.

## HEAD TRAUMA

The outcome in animals with head trauma depends largely on the location and severity of the initial injury, although secondary events can include progressive edema, ischemia, and death. Severe bilateral miosis (i.e., pupil constriction but normal responses to light) and diminished consciousness may indicate the existence of acute severe brain damage and increased intracranial pressure. Dilated pupils, an absent pupillary light reflex (PLR), stupor, coma, or an abnormal respiratory pattern usually indicates significant brainstem involvement, and the prognosis in such animals is grave, regardless of therapy. Development of brainstem signs minutes to hours after the initial trauma usually indicates forebrain herniation stemming from progressive edema or continuing hemorrhage. The primary goal of treatment in animals with severe head trauma is to prevent rising intracranial pressure, worsening neuronal edema and ischemia, and herniation. These complications usually develop slowly over several hours, so animals with severe head trauma should be treated and monitored closely for at least 48 hours before their condition is considered stable.

Treatment usually includes observation and supportive care (Table 68-1). A patent airway should be established and

## TABLE 68-1

### Management of Intracranial Injury

Establish patent airway, administer oxygen
Examine, assess, and treat concurrent injuries
Treat shock
    IV fluids, colloids
    Glucocorticoids
Administer glucocorticoids
    Methylprednisolone sodium succinate: 30 mg/kg IV
    once, then q6h or administer constant infusion
    (5 mg/kg/hr) for 6 hours
                or
    Dexamethasone sodium phosphate: 1 mg/kg once
Antibiotics if open wound or craniotomy

**If Severe Initial Injury or Deterioration:**

Administer diuretics
    20% Mannitol: 1 g/kg IV over 30 minutes (can repeat
    in 3 hours)
    Furosemide (Lasix): 1.0-2.0 mg/kg IV 15 minutes later
Elevate head 30 degrees
Treat seizures with diazepam, barbiturates
± Dimethyl sulfoxide: 1 g/kg IV over 30 minutes
Consider craniotomy

---

oxygen administered. Physical and neurologic examinations should be performed to assess the extent of the injury and identify concurrent life-threatening problems that should be addressed. Shock should be treated. Although it is important to avoid overhydration-induced exacerbation of cerebral edema, blood pressure must be restored to normal levels as soon as possible. Volume replacement fluids such as hetastarch (6%) may be a better choice for volume replacement than large volumes of crystalloid fluids.

Little evidence supports the routine use of corticosteroids (e.g., prednisone, dexamethasone) using standard dosing protocols in patients with head trauma. Administration of high doses of methylprednisolone sodium succinate (SoluMedrol) during the first 6 hours after presentation may be beneficial (see Table 68-1). In cases where SoluMedrol is not available, a single dose of intravenous (IV) dexamethasone may be administered. If the animal has open wounds or if craniotomy is considered, then antibiotics should be administered.

In animals with very severe initial injury or in those in which neurologic signs worsen despite initial therapy, more intensive treatment is recommended (see Table 68-1). Diuretics should be administered to decrease cerebral edema and lower intracranial pressure. The administration of mannitol followed by furosemide produces a very marked decrease in intracranial pressure within 10 minutes that generally lasts for 3 to 5 hours. The continued administration of oxygen by mask or intranasally is indicated. Although some references recommend mechanical hyperventilation to lower intracranial pressure, this may be deleterious to patients whose increased intracranial pressure is not caused by hypercarbia-induced intracranial vasodilation. Hyperventilation in the first 24 hours after injury may decrease cerebral blood flow and worsen ischemic injury to the brain. Diazepam and barbiturates are the best drugs for seizure control or for sedation and anesthesia. Narcotic analgesics should not be administered because they cause hypoventilation and increase intracranial pressure. In recumbent patients, the head should be elevated approximately 15 to 30 degrees to improve cerebral venous outflow. Although clinicians have conflicting opinions regarding its efficacy, the IV administration of dimethyl sulfoxide has been recommended as a way to decrease the cerebral metabolic rate, stabilize lysosomal membranes, and scavenge damaging free radicals. Finally, craniotomy can be performed if the clinician sees evidence of increasing intracranial pressure (e.g., progressive worsening of mentation) despite medical therapy and support. Ideally the decision to operate is based on results of computerized tomography (CT) or magnetic resonance imaging (MRI). Surgery can be beneficial to decompress, to evacuate hematomas, to remove bone fragments, or to lavage a penetrating wound such as a bite.

## LOSS OF VISION AND PUPILLARY ABNORMALITIES

Loss of vision or pupillary abnormalities may be detected during the physical examination of an animal seen because of some other neurologic dysfunction or may be the primary reason for presentation. Owners rarely recognize a visual deficit until it is bilateral and complete, at which time the animal may be brought in because of an apparent sudden onset of blindness. When an animal is evaluated because of loss of vision, it is important to first determine whether the animal is actually blind. One way of doing this is to determine its response to a menacing gesture. However, the absence of a response could be a result of poor vision, an altered mental state, or cerebellar disease; it could also be normal in a puppy or kitten. It is therefore often more useful to observe the animal's response to the environment, including its ability to negotiate doorways and stairs, and the attention it pays to rolling or falling objects. If unilateral vision loss is suspected, the normal eye should be covered during testing.

Evaluation of PLR may help localize the lesion within the visual pathway. The direct response (i.e., constriction of the stimulated pupil) and consensual response (i.e., constriction of the unstimulated pupil) should be evaluated in a darkened room with a bright, focal light source. The localization of lesions based on vision and PLRs is summarized in Table 68-2. Lesions of the eye or optic nerve result in a loss of vision in the affected eye and no direct or consensual PLR. If the opposite eye is normal, then illumination of that visual (i.e., normal) eye will result in normal pupillary responses in both eyes. It is important to realize that ocular or optic nerve disease must be very severe for the PLR to be abolished completely. Even animals that are functionally blind as a result of progressive retinal atrophy or optic neuritis will sometimes have an intact direct and consensual PLR in response to a bright light. Pupils may, however, be more dilated than normal in room light in these animals.

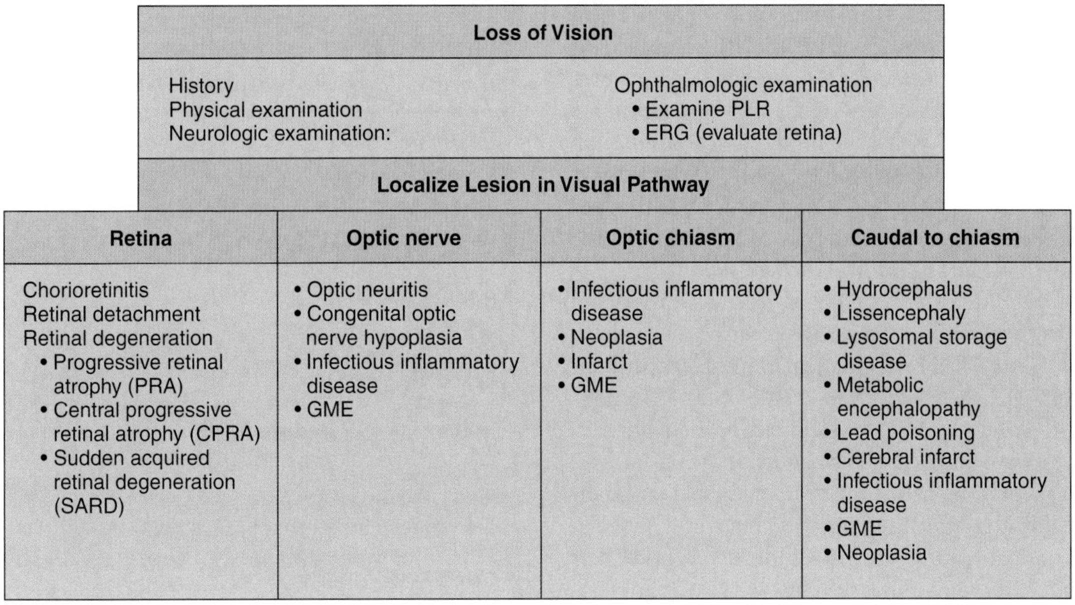

| Loss of Vision | | |
|---|---|---|
| History<br>Physical examination<br>Neurologic examination: | | Ophthalmologic examination<br>• Examine PLR<br>• ERG (evaluate retina) |
| Localize Lesion in Visual Pathway | | |

| Retina | Optic nerve | Optic chiasm | Caudal to chiasm |
|---|---|---|---|
| Chorioretinitis<br>Retinal detachment<br>Retinal degeneration<br>  • Progressive retinal<br>    atrophy (PRA)<br>  • Central progressive<br>    retinal atrophy (CPRA)<br>  • Sudden acquired<br>    retinal degeneration<br>    (SARD) | • Optic neuritis<br>• Congenital optic<br>  nerve hypoplasia<br>• Infectious inflammatory<br>  disease<br>• GME | • Infectious inflammatory<br>  disease<br>• Neoplasia<br>• Infarct<br>• GME | • Hydrocephalus<br>• Lissencephaly<br>• Lysosomal storage<br>  disease<br>• Metabolic<br>  encephalopathy<br>• Lead poisoning<br>• Cerebral infarct<br>• Infectious inflammatory<br>  disease<br>• GME<br>• Neoplasia |

**FIG 68-1**
Diagnostic approach to a dog or cat with loss of vision.

TABLE 68-2

Localization of Visual Pathway Lesions Based on Vision and Pupillary Light Reflexes

| LOCATION OF COMPLETE LESION | VISION IN RIGHT EYE | VISION IN LEFT EYE | LIGHT RESPONSE EITHER EYE | LIGHT IN LEFT EYE |
|---|---|---|---|---|
| Right retina/eye* | Absent | Normal | No response in either eye | Both pupils constrict |
| Bilateral retina/eye* | Absent | Absent | No response in either eye | No response in either eye |
| Right optic nerve | Absent | Normal | No response in either eye | Both pupils constrict |
| Bilateral optic nerves | Absent | Absent | No response in either eye | No response in either eye |
| Optic chiasm (bilateral) | Absent | Absent | No response in either eye | No response in either eye |
| Lesion caudal to optic chiasm (right lateral geniculate nucleus, right optic radiation, or right occipital cortex) | Normal | Absent | Both pupils constrict | Both pupils constrict |
| Bilateral lesion caudal to optic chiasm | Absent | Absent | Both pupils constrict | Both pupils constrict |
| Right oculomotor nerve | Normal | Normal | Left pupil constricts; right is dilated, no response | Left pupil constricts; right is dilated, no response |

*Retinal or eye lesions must be very severe to cause loss of pupillary light reflexes (PLRs).

Most of the optic nerve axons cross in the optic chiasm so that impulses generated by the retina of an eye primarily project to the opposite optic tract, lateral geniculate nucleus, optic radiations, and visual cortex. If the animal has a lesion caudal to the optic chiasm, pupils will be normal in size and normal direct and consensual PLRs will be seen; however, there will be a consistent loss of vision in the eye on the side opposite the brain lesion.

Blindness can occur with or without other systemic or neurologic signs of illness. Glaucoma, retinal detachment, and sudden acquired retinal degeneration (SARD) are all frequent causes of acute blindness in dogs. If the loss of vision has been localized anterior to the optic chiasm, it is therefore critically important to evaluate the eye to determine the source of the blindness. A thorough ophthalmologic examination should be performed to evaluate the anterior and posterior segments of the eye, the retina, and the optic disc. An electroretinogram (ERG) can be performed to further evaluate the retina. If the retina appears normal and the ERG is normal in an animal with blindness localized anterior to the chiasm, a lesion of the optic nerve must be suspected.

## OPTIC NEURITIS

Inflammation is the most common condition affecting the optic nerve (Fig. 68-1). Optic neuritis can be the result of infectious agents, inflammatory diseases, neoplasia, and idiopathic causes. Typically swollen, out-of-focus optic disks with or without associated hemorrhage will be seen. When optic neuritis occurs posterior to the globes (i.e., retrobulbar), the visible portion of the optic nerves (i.e., optic disks, papilla) is not remarkably affected so that the fundiscopic examination is normal. A normal ERG will be needed to differentiate blindness caused by bilateral retrobulbar optic neuritis from that caused by SARD, where there may only be very subtle retinal changes but the ERG will be extinguished.

Although optic neuritis is frequently seen as an isolated idiopathic immune-mediated disorder affecting one or both optic nerves, it may also be a manifestation of systemic illness (Table 68-3). When seen in association with infectious disorders of the central nervous system (CNS), it is common to see progressive neurologic deficits outside the visual system. Most cases of optic neuritis have no definable cause; diagnosis is made after infectious, inflammatory, and neoplastic disorders are ruled out during a thorough workup for systemic and intracranial disease. This workup should include a complete blood count (CBC), serum chemistry profile, urinalysis, heartworm antigen test, serologic screening for infectious diseases, thoracic radiography, and cerebrospinal fluid (CSF) collection and analysis. If all test results are normal, primary immune-mediated optic neuritis is tentatively diagnosed.

Treatment with orally administered corticosteroids should be initiated whenever a diagnosis of primary optic neuritis is established. If a favorable response is seen after 1 week (i.e., improved vision and PLRs), then the dose of steroids should be gradually decreased over 2 to 3 weeks until alternate-day therapy is achieved. If no initial response to steroid therapy is seen, then the prognosis for the return of vision is poor. Untreated optic neuritis leads to irreversible optic nerve atrophy and permanent blindness. Even if appropriate therapy is instituted, many cases will progress or relapse. The owner should always be warned that there might be an undetected underlying CNS disorder that could cause other neurologic signs to develop.

## OPTIC CHIASM AND OCCIPITAL CORTEX

Lesions of the optic chiasm result in a failure of transmission of the visual image, causing blindness with abnormal PLRs. Bilateral lesions of the optic chiasm may be seen in animals with spontaneous infarcts, infectious inflammatory disease, pituitary tumors, or meningiomas (see Fig. 68-1; Fig. 68-2). Lesions caudal to the chiasm in the lateral geniculate nucleus, optic radiations, or visual cortex create an inability to interpret the image, resulting in a normal fundic examination, normal ERG, normal PLRs (direct and consensual), and blindness in the eye opposite the side of the lesion. Causes of intracranial (i.e., central or cortical) blindness include trauma-induced hemorrhage and edema, vascular infarcts, granulomatous meningoencephalitis (GME), infectious encephalitis (especially canine distemper, systemic mycoses, *T. gondii,* and feline infectious peritonitis [FIP]), and CNS neoplasia. Congenital disorders (e.g., hydrocephalus, lissencephaly, polymicrogyria, lysosomal storage disease), lead

### TABLE 68-3

**Disorders Associated with Optic Neuritis**

**Infectious Disease**

Canine distemper
Toxoplasmosis
Feline infectious peritonitis
Cryptococcosis
Blastomycosis
Systemic aspergillosis
Bacterial disease
Feline leukemia virus

**Inflammatory Disease**

Systemic lupus erythematosus
Granulomatous meningoencephalitis
Steroid-responsive suppurative meningitis

**Neoplastic Disease**

Systemic
Intracranial

**Idiopathic Optic Neuritis**

intoxication, and metabolic encephalopathies may cause diffuse or bilateral visual disturbances that are localized to the occipital cortex. Diagnostic evaluation for intracranial blindness should include thorough physical, ophthalmologic, and neurologic examinations; a laboratory database; CSF analysis; and CT or MRI evaluation (see Fig. 68-2).

## ANISOCORIA

When pupils are asymmetrical, it is necessary to decide whether it is the constricted or the dilated pupil that is abnormal. A unilateral miotic (i.e., constricted) pupil is most often seen in primary ocular diseases such as uveitis, in painful ocular diseases such as severe keratitis, and as a manifestation of the loss of sympathetic innervation to the eye (i.e., Horner's syndrome). The anisocoria seen in animals with Horner's syndrome is more pronounced when the animal is examined in a darkened room, as the normal pupil dilates. In animals with one abnormal mydriatic pupil, the pupil on the normal side may be slightly miotic because of the excessive amount of light entering through the abnormally dilated pupil, causing consensual constriction of the normal pupil.

Unilateral mydriasis (i.e., pupil dilatation) that does not resolve when light is directed into either eye can be seen in animals with glaucoma, in geriatric animals with iris atrophy, and in animals with lesions of the oculomotor nerve. The anisocoria in these animals is most pronounced when the animal is examined in ambient light. The motor component of the PLR is the parasympathetic lower motor neuron (LMN) located in the oculomotor nerve. The finding of a mydriatic, unresponsive pupil in an animal with no other neurologic or

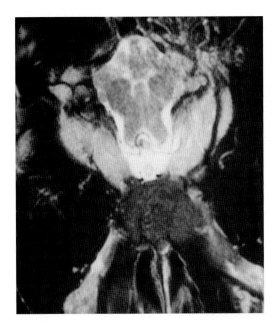

**FIG 68-2**
Neoplasm of the optic chiasm identified with magnetic resonance imaging (MRI) in a 7-year-old Doberman with an acute onset of bilateral blindness, loss of pupillary light reflexes (PLRs), and no other neurologic deficits.

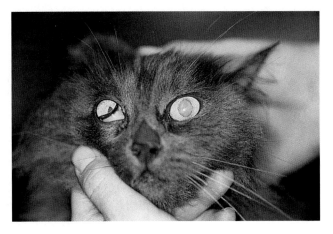

**FIG 68-3**
Horner's syndrome in a domestic short-haired cat with otitis media/interna.

ophthalmologic signs warrants evaluation and observation, because some tumors that initially impinge only on the oculomotor nerve grow and eventually compress the midbrain, resulting in hemiparesis and other abnormalities. It is recommended that cats be tested for feline leukemia virus (FeLV) antigen, because unilateral involvement of the short ciliary nerve to the iris has been documented in this disease.

The finding of unilateral or bilateral pupil dilatation in cats and dogs has also been associated with dysautonomia (i.e., Key-Gaskell syndrome), an autonomic polyganglionopathy. In these animals the iris constrictor muscle is hypersensitive as a result of denervation, so instilling one drop of very dilute (0.05% to 0.1%) pilocarpine in the affected eye causes the pupil to constrict within 45 minutes (see Chapter 73).

## HORNER'S SYNDROME

Horner's syndrome results from an interruption of the sympathetic innervation to the eye. The affected pupil is miotic, whereas the pupil in the other eye is normal. In addition to the small pupil, other components of Horner's syndrome are drooping of the upper eyelid (i.e., ptosis) and an inward sinking of the eyeball (i.e., enophthalmos). The third eyelid is often partially protruded (i.e., prolapsed nictitans) (Table 68-4; Fig. 68-3).

Horner's syndrome can result from injury to the sympathetic innervation to the eye anywhere along its pathway (Table 68-5; Fig. 68-4). The upper motor neuron (UMN) system involves a pathway originating in the hypothalamus and midbrain that courses through the brainstem and cervical cord to terminate on the preganglionic cell bodies in the

 TABLE 68-4

**Components of Horner's Syndrome**

| | |
|---|---|
| Miosis | Enophthalmos |
| Ptosis | Prolapsed nictitans |

 TABLE 68-5

**Common Causes of Horner's Syndrome**

**Upper Motor Neuron (UMN) Causes (Rare)**

Intracranial neoplasia, trauma, infarct
Cervical spinal cord lesion
Intervertebral disc protrusion
Neoplasm
Fibrocartilaginous embolism
Trauma

**Preganglionic Causes (First Neuron)**

Spinal cord lesion T1-T4 (trauma, neoplasia,
    fibrocartilaginous embolism)
Brachial plexus avulsion
Thoracic spinal nerve root tumor
Cranial mediastinal mass
Cervical soft-tissue neoplasia, trauma
Skull base trauma

**Postganglionic Causes (Second Neuron)**

Otitis media/interna
Neoplasia in middle ear
Retrobulbar injury, neoplasia

**Unknown Causes**

Idiopathic

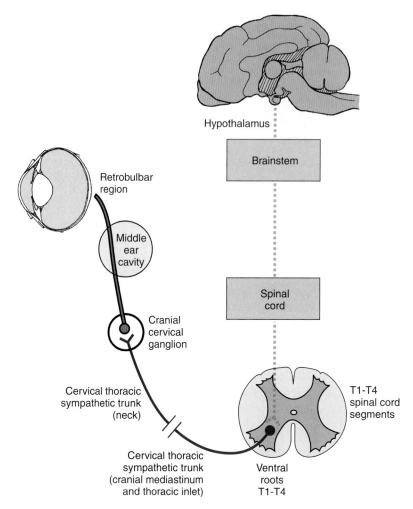

**FIG 68-4**
Sympathetic innervation to the eye. An injury anywhere along this pathway will result in Horner's syndrome.

thoracic spinal cord. UMN lesions in the brainstem or cervical spinal cord are a relatively rare cause of Horner's syndrome but may occur secondary to trauma, infarction, neoplasia, or inflammatory disease. Ipsilateral hemiplegia and other concurrent neurologic abnormalities would be expected in these animals.

The preganglionic cell bodies are located in the intermediate gray column of the first three or four segments of the thoracic spinal cord. Injury to the spinal cord between T1 and T4 (especially T1) can therefore result in a partial or mild LMN paresis of the forelimb, UMN signs in the rear limb on that side, and an ipsilateral Horner's syndrome. These signs can be seen in dogs and cats with spinal trauma, disc protrusion, neoplasia, or infarct of the cranial thoracic spinal cord.

The axons from the preganglionic cell bodies in these spinal cord segments leave the T1-T4 spinal cord in the ventral nerve roots and join the spinal nerves arising from those cord segments. Avulsion of the roots or spinal nerves of T1-T4, as commonly occurs in dogs and cats with brachial **plexus** avulsion secondary to automobile-induced trauma, results in a Horner's syndrome on the same side as a LMN-

paralyzed thoracic limb (Fig. 68-5). Horner's syndrome is also commonly seen in dogs with nerve sheath tumors originating in the cranial thoracic spinal nerves (especially T1).

Before the spinal nerves branch, the preganglionic axons of the sympathetic nervous system leave the spinal nerves and join the thoracic sympathetic trunk, which courses ventrolateral to the vertebral column inside the thorax. Thoracic inlet or cranial mediastinal lesions such as lymphoma or thymoma may cause Horner's syndrome and no other neurologic deficits.

The axons continue to course cranially within the vagosympathetic trunk in the cervical region. Bite wounds to the neck, neoplasia (e.g., thyroid adenocarcinoma), or errors made during thyroidectomy or surgery for intervertebral disc disease may injure the preganglionic axons. Horner's syndrome (but no other neurologic deficits) may develop in such animals.

Just ventral and medial to the tympanic bulla at the base of the skull, the preganglionic axons terminate in the cranial cervical ganglion and synapse with the postganglionic cell bodies. The postganglionic axons for ocular innervation course ros-

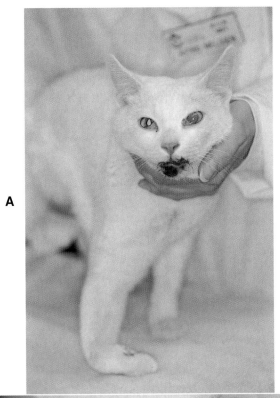

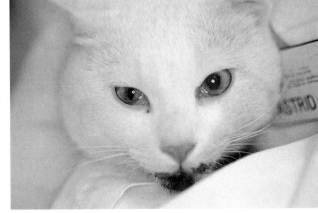

**FIG 68-5**
Horner's syndrome **(A)** in a domestic short-haired cat with traumatic right brachial plexus avulsion **(B).**

Pharmacologic testing has been recommended to help localize the cause of Horner's syndrome in dogs and cats (Table 68-6). This testing can be used to help determine whether a lesion is of the first (i.e., preganglionic) or second (i.e., postganglionic) neuron of the LMN portion of the pathway. Testing involves the topical application of indirect- or direct-acting sympathomimetics and observation of pupillary responses. The response to indirect-acting agents (e.g., hydroxyamphetamine) can be inconsistent, however, so usually only a direct-acting agent (e.g., phenylephrine) is used for pharmacologic localization.

A very dilute concentration of a direct-acting sympathomimetic (0.1% phenylephrine: stock 10% solution diluted 1:100 with saline solution) is applied to both eyes. This dilute solution does not normally induce pupillary dilation. Dilation of the affected pupil will occur within 20 minutes in an animal with a postganglionic lesion, because of the denervation hypersensitivity that occurs when the postganglionic neuron is damaged. If no dilation occurs in either pupil after application of the very dilute phenylephrine solution, one drop of full strength (10%) phenylephrine should be applied in both eyes to confirm that dilation is possible. Dilation of the abnormal pupil with the 0.1% solution and both pupils with the 10% solution suggests a postganglionic lesion (middle ear, retrobulbar) causing the Horner's syndrome. Although, theoretically, pharmacologic testing should be helpful in localizing the site of neuron injury in animals with Horner's syndrome, results of pharmacologic testing can be equivocal and may not always contribute practical information regarding the cause or the prognosis.

The diagnostic approach in an animal with Horner's syndrome should include a complete physical examination and ophthalmologic, neurologic, and otoscopic examinations. Thoracic and cervical radiography should be performed. Clinicopathologic testing, including CSF analysis and advanced diagnostic imaging (e.g., CT, MRI), should be considered if spinal or intracranial disease is suspected. When a postganglionic lesion is suspected, radiographs of the skull should be performed to evaluate the middle ear for signs of otitis media, neoplasia, or trauma. The cause of Horner's syndrome cannot be determined in approximately half of all dogs and cats who develop a Horner's syndrome and no other neurologic deficits. The syndrome resolves spontaneously in some animals.

## PROTRUSION OF THE THIRD EYELID

In dogs and cats the third eyelid may protrude over the corneal surface in the presence of corneal or conjunctival irritation or space-occupying orbital disease. This may also occur if the animal experiences a decrease in periorbital mass as a result of dehydration or a loss of retrobulbar fat or the clinician detects a loss of volume within the eye (i.e., microphthalmos, phthisis bulbi).

Protrusion of the third eyelid is a conspicuous feature of Horner's syndrome (with miosis) and also of dysautonomia (with mydriasis). Systemic illness or tranquilization can also result in third eyelid protrusion in some dogs and cats. A

trally through the tympanooccipital fissure into the middle ear, where they are closely associated with the ventral surface of the petrosal bone. Otitis media or neoplasia (e.g., squamous cell carcinoma in cats) within the middle ear commonly results in Horner's syndrome, together with signs of a peripheral vestibular disturbance and sometimes facial paralysis.

The postganglionic sympathetic axons are further distributed via the ophthalmic nerve to the smooth muscle of the periorbita, the eyelids, the third eyelid, and the iris muscles. Rarely, retrobulbar injury, neoplasia, or an abscess can result in some loss of sympathetic innervation to the eye and Horner's syndrome.

## TABLE 68-6

Pharmacologic Localization of Horner's Syndrome

| | | RESPONSE OF AFFLICTED PUPIL | |
| AGENT | RESPONSE OF NORMAL PUPIL | PREGANGLIONIC LESION | POSTGANGLIONIC LESION |
| --- | --- | --- | --- |
| 0.1% Phenylephrine (10% stock solution Neo-Synephrine, Winthrop; 1:100 saline) Apply 2 drops topically; evaluate at 20 minutes | No dilation | No dilation | No dilation |

peculiar syndrome (e.g., Haw syndrome) has been observed in cats, in which a dramatic bilateral third eyelid protrusion of no obvious cause is observed. This syndrome occurs most often in cats less than 2 years of age. Affected cats are usually in good health otherwise, although digestive disturbances or heavy intestinal parasite loads have occasionally been documented. The instillation of sympathomimetic drops causes the membrane to rapidly retract. The condition resolves spontaneously within several weeks or months.

### Suggested Readings

Chrisman CL: *Problems in small animal neurology,* Philadelphia, 1991, Lea & Febiger, p 237.

Collins BK et al: Autonomic dysfunction of the eye, *Semin Vet Med Surg (Small Anim)* 5:24, 1990.

deLahunta A: Neuro-ophthalmology. In Ettinger SJ et al, editors: *Textbook of veterinary internal medicine,* Philadelphia, 1995, WB Saunders.

Hamilton HL et al: *Diagnosis of blindness. Current veterinary therapy XIII,* Philadelphia, 2000, WB Saunders, p 1038.

Mattson A et al: Clinical features suggesting hyperadrenocorticism associated with sudden acquired retinal degeneration syndrome in a dog, *J Am Anim Hosp Assoc* 28:199, 1992.

Morgan RV et al: Horner's syndrome in dogs and cats: 49 cases (1980-1986), *J Am Vet Med Assoc* 194:1096, 1989.

Roberts SM: Assessment and management of the ophthalmic emergency, *Compend Cont Educ Pract Vet* 7:739, 1985.

Szymanski C: The eye. In Holzworth J, editor: *Diseases of the cat,* Philadelphia, 1987, WB Saunders.

# CHAPTER 69

# Seizures

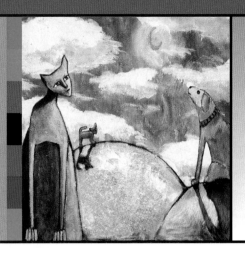

## CHAPTER OUTLINE

OVERVIEW AND DIAGNOSTIC APPROACH, 991
DISORDERS RESULTING IN SEIZURES, 994
    Metabolic disorders, 994
    Toxins, 994
    Congenital malformations, 994
    Degenerative diseases, 995
    Neoplasia, 996
    Inflammatory diseases, 999
    Vascular diseases, 999
    Feline ischemic encephalopathy, 999
    Trauma/scar–related epilepsy, 1000
    Thiamine deficiency, 1000
    Epilepsy, 1000
ANTICONVULSANT THERAPY, 1001
    Anticonvulsant drugs, 1001
    Alternative therapies, 1004
EMERGENCY THERAPY FOR DOGS AND CATS
IN STATUS EPILEPTICUS, 1004

## OVERVIEW AND DIAGNOSTIC APPROACH

A seizure or convulsion is the clinical manifestation of excessive or hypersynchronous electrical activity in the cerebral cortex. This electrical event results in a loss or derangement of consciousness, altered muscle tone, jaw chomping or trismus, salivation, and often involuntary urination and defecation. Most dogs and cats have tonic-clonic, generalized (symmetric) motor seizures in which the animal experiences a period of extremely increased extensor muscle tone (tonus), falls into lateral recumbency, and then has periods of tonus alternating with periods of relaxation (clonus), resulting in rhythmic contractions of muscles manifested as paddling or jerking of the limbs and chewing movements (Table 69-1). In some cases the actual seizure may be preceded by minutes to hours of unusual behavior (preictal phase), including hiding, attention seeking, or agitation. In other animals, seizures start during sleep or may be triggered by a specific stimulus or event (repetitive noise, flickering light). Estrus, certain drugs (especially phenothiazines), stress, and excitement can all precipitate seizures in a predisposed animal. In most animals, each seizure is followed by a short period of disorientation (postictal phase), during which ataxia, blindness, pacing, and delirium are common.

Less common than generalized, symmetric tonic-clonic seizures in dogs and cats are focal partial motor seizures (see Table 69-1). These seizures arise in part of one cerebral hemisphere, resulting in asymmetric signs that may include turning of the head away from the side of the lesion and focal twitching or tonic-clonic contractions of the contralateral facial or limb muscles. These seizures may ultimately become generalized. Although it is often stated that partial motor seizures are usually associated with structural brain disease, close observation of dogs with idiopathic epilepsy reveals that many experience focal seizures with secondary generalization.

Psychomotor seizures are focal seizures manifested as stereotypic paroxysms of abnormal behavior, such as rage, hysteria, hyperesthesia, self-mutilation, tail chasing, and fly biting. Without event-triggered electrodiagnostic testing, however, it is very difficult to distinguish these seizures from compulsive stereotypic behavior. In some cases, consciousness is impaired (complex focal seizures) or the seizure progresses to a generalized symmetric tonic-clonic seizure, aiding diagnosis.

Seizure disorders are classified according to their cause as being intracranial or extracranial in origin or idiopathic (Table 69-2). Idiopathic, or primary, epilepsy is diagnosed in approximately 25% to 30% of dogs having seizures. These animals have no identifiable extracranial or intracranial cause and are said to have primary epileptic seizures. Approximately 35% of dogs with seizures have an identifiable abnormality within their brain (anomaly, inflammation, neoplasia, etc.), that is causing seizures, and these dogs are said to have secondary epileptic seizures. Extracranial causes such as the ingestion of toxins or metabolic or endocrine derangements result in reactive epileptic seizures. Seizure activity always indicates a functional or structural abnormality of the cerebrum, particularly of the frontal or temporal lobes.

It is important to evaluate the animal's signalment and history, as well as the onset and progression of a seizure disorder,

TABLE 69-1

**Classification of Seizures**

**Generalized**

*Tonic-clonic:* tonic phase followed by rhythmic muscle contraction/paddling
*Tonic:* generalized muscular rigidity
*Clonic:* rhythmic muscular contractions, no tonic phase
*Atonic:* total loss of muscle tone
*Myoclonic:* brief rhythmic contractions of individual muscle groups

**Focal (May Progress to Generalized)**

*Simple focal seizures (no loss of consciousness)*
Rhythmic muscle contractions
Chewing/licking at body
Fly biting
Autonomic signs (vomiting, diarrhea, abdominal pain)
Behavioral abnormalities, rage
*Complex focal seizures (consciousness impaired)*

TABLE 69-2

**Common Disorders Resulting in Seizures**

**Extracranial Causes (Reactive Epileptic Seizures)**

Toxins
Metabolic diseases
Hypoglycemia
Liver disease
Hypocalcemia
Hyperlipoproteinemia
Hyperviscosity
Electrolyte disturbances
Hyperosmolality
Severe uremia

**Intracranial Causes (Secondary Epileptic Seizures)**

Congenital malformations
Hydrocephalus
Lissencephaly
Neoplasia
　Primary brain tumors
　Metastatic tumors
Inflammatory disease
Infectious inflammatory disease
Granulomatous meningoencephalitis
Necrotizing encephalitis
Vascular disease
Hemorrhage
Infarct
Scar tissue
Metabolic storage diseases (see Table 67-6)
Degenerative conditions (see Table 72-5)

**Idiopathic Epilepsy (Primary Epileptic Seizures)**

to determine the most likely differential diagnoses. Congenital structural disorders such as hydrocephalus and lissencephaly, as well as infectious inflammatory diseases of the brain, are most likely to be the cause of a seizure disorder in a very young animal. In aging animals, cerebral neoplasia, vascular accidents, and acquired metabolic disturbances are more likely causes. Idiopathic epilepsy initially causes seizures in affected dogs and cats between 6 months and 3 years of age; thus it is not a likely diagnosis in a dog or cat with seizures that begin late in life.

The onset, course, duration, and frequency of the seizure disorder may help to narrow the differential diagnosis list (Fig. 69-1). An acute onset of frequent severe seizures, with or without concurrent neurologic abnormalities, most likely indicates a toxic, vascular, infectious, metabolic, or neoplastic process. A chronic, intermittent seizure disorder with no other clinical signs or neurologic deficits is most consistent with idiopathic epilepsy or a nonprogressive intracranial structural lesion (scar, anomaly).

Complete physical, ophthalmologic, and neurologic examinations should be obtained in all dogs and cats evaluated because of seizures. The neurologic examination should be interpreted with caution if it is performed during the postictal phase, when transient neurologic abnormalities are common. Results of these examinations may be useful in determining whether the cause of the seizures is extracranial or intracranial and, if intracranial, may help to localize the lesion within the brain (see Table 65-9). The results may also be completely normal, as is typical for dogs and cats with idiopathic epilepsy, and as may be the case in a variety of other disorders.

The diagnostic evaluation of an animal experiencing seizures may include screening tests (i.e., complete blood count [CBC], biochemistry panel, and urinalysis) for metabolic and toxic disorders and a more thorough workup to identify infectious or neoplastic diseases and intracranial causes of seizures (see Fig. 69-1). The diagnostic tests selected ultimately depend on the historical and physical examination findings, especially the age of the animal, the nature of any other neurologic abnormalities or clinical signs, and the frequency of the seizures. Dogs older than 5 years of age at the time of their first seizure, those with an initial interictal period of less than 4 weeks, and those with partial seizures are most likely to have an underlying intracranial or extracranial cause for their seizures.

A diagnostic workup may not be warranted in an animal with a clinically or historically obvious toxic cause for seizures; therapy is simply initiated. Routine clinicopathologic screening tests (CBC, fasting serum biochemistry panel, and urinalysis) are recommended in a young animal (6 months to 3 years) with a history of one seizure in which physical, neurologic, and ophthalmologic examination findings are normal. In some cases a liver function test such as a fasting and postprandial bile acid determination is performed to rule out a portosystemic shunt and to obtain baseline information regarding liver function (see Chapter 36). A more extensive diagnostic evaluation is rarely warranted at the time of first presentation in a young animal if results of these tests are normal. The

Seizures

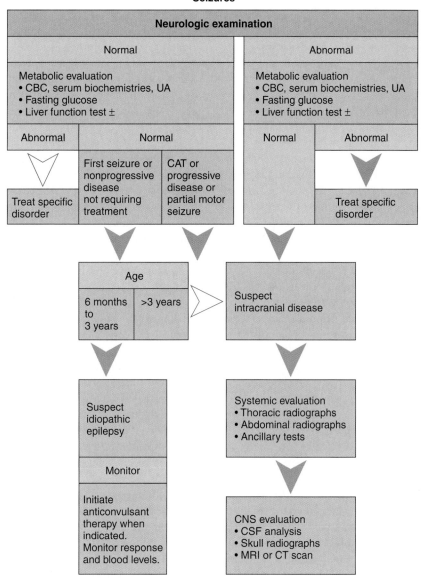

**FIG 69-1**
Diagnostic approach used in dogs or cats with seizures.

owner is instructed to monitor the animal for further seizures and to keep a record of seizure frequency, duration, characteristics, and associated activities or environmental factors.

Routine clinicopathologic screening tests, as well as thoracic and abdominal radiography and abdominal ultrasonography, are recommended in older animals seen after a single seizure, in any animal with severe or progressively worsening seizures, and in all animals with neurologic or systemic abnormalities detected interictally. This extensive testing is performed in an effort to identify a metabolic, neoplastic, or infectious cause for seizures. Additional diagnostic tests for infectious diseases (feline leukemia virus antigen, feline immunodeficiency virus, *Neospora* and *Toxoplasma* serology) may be warranted in some cases.

Once most metabolic and systemic diseases have been ruled out, intracranial disorders must be considered. In a young adult (<4 to 5 years old), neurologically normal dog with a nonprogressive, intermittent seizure disorder of 1 or more years' duration, idiopathic epilepsy is most likely, and an extensive intracranial workup may not be warranted unless the seizure disorder worsens or changes. In all other cases an evaluation for intracranial disease should be performed. This consists of cerebrospinal fluid (CSF) collection and analysis, and referral for special neuroradiographic studies (computed tomography [CT], magnetic resonance imaging [MRI]). Because idiopathic epilepsy is uncommon in the cat, evaluation for intracranial disease is warranted in every cat with an undiagnosed seizure disorder.

## *DISORDERS RESULTING IN SEIZURES*

### METABOLIC DISORDERS

Hypoglycemia, hepatic encephalopathy, hypocalcemia, and primary hyperlipoproteinemia may cause seizures in dogs and cats. Other metabolic alterations, including hyperviscosity syndromes (e.g., multiple myeloma, polycythemia), severe electrolyte disturbances (e.g., hypernatremia), hyperosmolality (e.g., untreated diabetes mellitus), heat stroke, and prolonged severe uremia, also occasionally cause seizures (see Table 69-2). In many of these disorders, intermittent nonneurologic clinical signs and physical examination findings point toward an extracranial cause of the seizures. Most metabolic encephalopathies also intermittently or permanently alter consciousness, manifesting as confusion, delirium, or depression at least intermittently. Results of a CBC, serum biochemistry panel, and urinalysis often help establish the diagnosis. Hepatic encephalopathy resulting from portosystemic shunting can occasionally cause seizures in the absence of other clinical or clinicopathologic abnormalities, especially in cats, so evaluation of liver function is an important component of the initial evaluation for metabolic causes of seizures. More detailed information on the diagnosis and management of these metabolic disorders is contained elsewhere in this text.

### TOXINS

Common toxic agents that cause seizures in dogs and cats include strychnine, metaldehyde, chlorinated hydrocarbons, organophosphates, lead, and occasionally ethylene glycol (Table 69-3). The clinical signs of intoxication in dogs and cats are usually severe, are rapid in onset, and steadily worsen. An intoxication causing seizures is diagnosed on the basis of a history of ingestion of or exposure to a toxin or the finding of characteristic clinical signs. In most cases, immediate emergency treatment for seizures is required and is the same as that described for status epilepticus (Table 69-4). In addition, treatment to remove the toxin, prevent its absorption, and speed its elimination is recommended (Table 69-5).

### CONGENITAL MALFORMATIONS

#### Hydrocephalus

Hydrocephalus is the condition in which the cerebral ventricular system is enlarged secondary to an increased amount of CSF, with secondary compression or atrophy of the surrounding neurologic tissue. Most cases are congenital. Dog breeds at risk include the Maltese, Yorkshire Terrier, English Bulldog, Chihuahua, Lhasa Apso, Pomeranian, Toy Poodle, Cairn Terrier, Boston Terrier, Pug, Chow Chow, and Pekingese. Cats are occasionally affected.

Many affected animals have an obviously enlarged head and palpably open fontanelles (Fig. 69-2). Care must be taken not to overinterpret these findings, however, because open fontanelles and mild, asymptomatic hydrocephalus may be "normal" in some of these breeds.

Animals with symptomatic hydrocephalus are slow learners and may seem dull or depressed. They may have episodes of abnormal behavior or delirium and cortical blindness. Seizures occur in animals with severe symptomatic hydrocephalus or in previously asymptomatic animals that are decompensated by mild trauma or infection. Possible neurologic findings include tetraparesis, slow postural reactions, decreased proprioception, and hyperactive reflexes; there may also be bilateral divergent strabismus.

Hydrocephalus is suspected on the basis of characteristic signs and physical examination findings in a young animal of a typical breed. If fontanelles are open, ultrasound examination of the brain can be performed through the openings, and this can determine the size of the lateral ventricles and confirm the diagnosis (see Fig. 66-11). If the fontanelles are small or closed, ultrasound scanning is more difficult but may still be attempted through the temporal bone in young animals. Alternatively, CT, MRI, or pneumoventriculography can be performed to detect ventricular enlargement. If severe hydrocephalus is present, all of these tests are useful for making a diagnosis. In animals with mild or moderate hydrocephalus, there is very little correlation between ventricular size and clinical signs.

Long-term management of neurologic signs using corticosteroids (prednisone, 0.5 mg/kg PO q48h) can be attempted. Seizures may be controlled with anticonvulsant therapy as described for epilepsy (see p. 1001). The prognosis for a normal life is poor if neurologic signs are present. Surgical drainage and placement of a permanent ventriculoperitoneal shunt has been successful in a few cases.

Acute, severe, and progressive neurologic signs occasionally occur in dogs and cats with hydrocephalus. This is probably the result of a sudden increase in intracranial pressure. Hence, it is important to rapidly lower intracranial pressure in these animals. If fontanelles are open, a ventricular tap can be performed 3 to 5 mm off midline as described for pneumoventriculography (see p. 968) and a small volume of CSF (0.1 to 0.2 ml/kg) can be removed. Mannitol (20% solution, 1 g/kg IV over 30 minutes), furosemide (2 mg/kg SC), and corticosteroids (dexamethasone, 2 to 4 mg/kg, or methylprednisolone sodium succinate, 30 mg/kg IV) are administered immediately after the tap, and long-term medical management is initiated.

#### Lissencephaly

Lissencephaly is a rare condition in which the sulci and gyri fail to develop normally, resulting in a smooth cerebral cortex. Cerebellar hypoplasia may be seen in association with this malformation. Lissencephaly has been recognized primarily in the Lhasa Apso, although Wire-Haired Fox Terriers and Irish Setters are occasionally affected. Behavioral abnormalities and visual deficits are common. These animals are also very difficult to train and may not be housebroken. If seizures occur, they usually are not prominent until the end of the first year of life. Diagnosis may be suspected on the basis of the electroencephalogram, which reveals slow-wave, high-voltage

TABLE 69-3

Intoxications Resulting in Acute Neurologic Dysfunction

**Strychnine**

*Common use:* rat, mole, gopher, and coyote poison
*Clinical findings:* stiff extension of legs and body, erect ears, tetanic spasms induced by auditory stimuli
*Diagnosis:* history of access or ingestion, characteristic signs, chemical analysis of stomach contents
*Treatment:* vomiting (if no neurologic signs), gastric lavage, diazepam as needed, pentobarbital to effect; establish diuresis

**Metaldehyde**

*Common use:* snail, slug, and rat poison
*Clinical findings:* anxiety, hyperesthesia, tachycardia, hypersalivation, muscle fasciculations, and tremors; not worsened by auditory stimuli; nystagmus in cats; may convulse; depression, respiratory failure
*Diagnosis:* history of access or ingestion, characteristic signs, acetaldehyde odor on breath, analysis of stomach contents
*Treatment:* gastric lavage, pentobarbital to effect, endotracheal tube and ventilation if necessary; establish diuresis

**Chlorinated Hydrocarbons**

*Common use:* agricultural products and insecticides; lipid-soluble products are usually absorbed through skin
*Clinical findings:* apprehension, hypersensitivity, hypersalivation, exaggerated response to stimuli, muscle twitching of face and neck progressing to severe fasciculations and tremors; tonic-clonic seizures may occur
*Diagnosis:* history of access, characteristic signs, insecticide smell to haircoat, analysis of stomach contents
*Treatment:* wash with warm soapy water to prevent further exposure; if ingested (rare), gastric lavage and instill activated charcoal; pentobarbital to effect

**Organophosphates and Carbamates**

*Common use:* insecticides
*Clinical findings:* excessive salivation, lacrimation, diarrhea, vomiting, and miosis; twitching of facial and tongue muscles, progressing to extreme depression and tonic-clonic seizures
*Diagnosis:* history of exposure, characteristic signs, analysis of stomach contents, low serum acetylcholinesterase activity

**Organophosphates and Carbamates—cont'd**

*Treatment:* prevent further exposure; wash if topical exposure; gastric lavage and activated charcoal if ingested; atropine (0.2 mg/kg IV initially and 0.2 mg/kg SC as needed q6-8h); pralidoxime (20 mg/kg IM q12h) if within 48 hours of exposure or if was dermal exposure

**Lead**

*Common use:* ubiquitous in environment in linoleum, rug padding, old lead-based paints (before 1950s), putty and caulking material, roofing materials, batteries, grease, used motor oil, golf balls, fishing sinkers, pellets, and lead shot
*Clinical findings:* gastrointestinal signs of anorexia, abdominal pain, vomiting and diarrhea, and megaesophagus; neurologic signs of hysteria, aggression, nervousness, barking, tremors, seizures, blindness, hypermetria and nystagmus (cats), and dementia
*Diagnosis:* history of exposure, characteristic signs, CBC changes (basophilic stippling of RBCs, increase in nucleated RBCs); blood lead level (heparinized tube: >0.5 ppm [50 mg/dl], diagnostic; >0.25 ppm, suggestive); radiographs may reveal radiopaque material in gastrointestinal system
*Treatment:* emetics, gastric lavage, activated charcoal, enemas; surgery or endoscopy if lead in stomach; specific: calcium ethylenediaminetetraacetic acid (Ca EDTA) to chelate lead and hasten excretion (25 mg/kg IV q6h as 10 mg Ca EDTA/ml in dextrose for 2-5 days); establish diuresis; alternative treatment: succimer (10 mg/kg PO for 10-14 days; Chemet; Sandofi Pharm, N.Y.)

**Ethylene Glycol**

*Common use:* automobile antifreeze, color film processing solutions
*Clinical findings:* ataxia, severe depression, polyuria-polydipsia, vomiting; seizures are rare
*Diagnosis:* history of exposure, characteristic signs, severe metabolic acidosis, calcium oxalate crystalluria; eventually, decreased urine production and acute renal failure; diagnosis and treatment of this disorder are discussed in detail in Chapter 44

patterns over all areas of the cerebral cortex and paroxysmal wave patterns. For a definitive diagnosis to be rendered, MRI, brain biopsy, or necropsy must be performed.

## DEGENERATIVE DISEASES

Metabolic storage diseases are fatal neurodegenerative disorders resulting from an inherited deficiency of enzymes within the lysosomes of the cells of the nervous system (see Table 67-6). Undigestible material builds up within the affected lysosomes and results in cell death. Dogs and cats with some of the rare lysosomal storage diseases such as $GM_2$ gangliosidosis, ceroid lipofuscinosis, and neuronal glycoproteinosis have seizures as a predominant feature of their neurologic dysfunction. Delirium and irritability are common. Signs

TABLE 69-4

**Status Epilepticus Treatment in Dogs and Cats**

1. If possible, insert an IV CATHETER.
2. Administer DIAZEPAM (2.0 mg/kg RECTALLY if no IV access).
   If IV access is possible, administer 0.5 to 1.0 mg/kg; maximum: 20 mg.
   Repeat this dose every 5 minutes if ineffective or if seizures recur.
   Administer maximum of four doses if necessary and proceed to steps 3 and 4.
3. SODIUM PENTOBARBITAL (3-15 mg/kg IV slowly to effect)
   or
   PROPOFOL (4-8 mg/kg IV slowly to effect)
   Administer if needed to stop the seizure activity.
4. Administer PHENOBARBITAL (2-4 mg/kg IV or IM) even if did not need step 3.
5. Maintain a patent AIRWAY and monitor respirations.
6. Assess body TEMPERATURE. If >41.4° C (>105° F), cool with cold water.
   **If hyperthermic, if suspect cerebral edema, or if seizure activity was prolonged (>15 minutes),** administer:
   MANNITOL (1.0 g/kg IV over 15 minutes)
   and
   GLUCOCORTICOIDS
   Methylprednisolone sodium succinate (30 mg/kg IV)
   or
   Dexamethasone sodium phosphate (1 mg/kg IV)
   and
   THIAMINE (2 mg/kg IM)
7. COLLECT BLOOD for analysis.
   Determine blood glucose concentration. If low, administer 2 ml/kg of 50% dextrose IV.
   If suspect hypocalcemia, administer 0.5 to 1.0 ml/kg of 10% calcium gluconate IV slowly to effect.
   Determine electrolyte and calcium concentrations and acid-base status; correct any abnormalities.
   Initiate IV FLUIDS (0.9% saline at 10 ml/kg/hr).
8. QUESTION THE OWNER regarding:
   Possible trauma
   Toxin exposure
   Previous seizures
   Medications
   Systemic or neurologic signs in past few weeks
9. If TOXIN is suspected, treat to decrease absorption and speed elimination (see Tables 69-3 and 69-5).
10. If the cause of the seizures has not been determined and resolved, or if the animal has idiopathic epilepsy, maintain seizure control until the animal has recovered sufficiently to accept oral phenobarbital using:
    DIAZEPAM as an IV drip (0.5 mg/kg/hr) in saline
    or
    PHENOBARBITAL (2-4 mg/kg IM q8h)
    or
    PENTOBARBITAL as an IV drip (2.0-5.0 mg/kg/hr to effect) in saline

develop in young animals and are progressive and severe. Histopathologic examination of biopsy specimens from affected organs can show characteristic changes, but enzyme assays are required to establish the diagnosis. The prognosis is poor because of the progressive nature of these disorders. No treatment is currently available. An autosomal recessive mode of inheritance is common. Leukodystrophies, hypomyelinating disorders, and spongy degeneration of the white matter occur as familial disorders in young dogs. Some of these degenerative disorders are associated with seizures. Diagnosis requires biopsy.

## NEOPLASIA

Neoplasms of the brain are common in dogs and cats. They usually result in the gradual onset of slowly progressive neurologic signs, but clinical signs may arise acutely if hemorrhage or edema occurs in association with the tumor. With the exception of lymphoma, which can occur in animals of any age, most primary and metastatic brain tumors occur in middle-aged and older animals. All breeds are affected, with a greatly increased incidence of glial tumors in Boxers and Boston Terriers. Meningiomas are common in old cats.

Brain tumors may cause signs by destroying adjacent tissue, by increasing intracranial pressure, or by causing hemorrhage or obstructive hydrocephalus. Seizures are a prominent clinical feature. Circling, ataxia, and head tilt are less common. Increasing intracranial pressure will cause progressive loss of consciousness and a change in mentation, so that the owner may report that the dog or cat has become dull, depressed, and "old." Progressive subtle neurologic signs are sometimes present for weeks or months before the onset of seizures. In rare instances a small, slow-growing cerebral cortical tumor will cause seizures without detectable interictal neurologic deficits. Acutely progressive behavioral changes, seizures, or motor deficits are seen in some dogs and cats with primary or metastatic brain neoplasms; presumably these signs are related to tumor-related intracranial hemorrhage.

Neurologic examination most commonly reveals evidence of a focal neurologic abnormality. Compulsive circling toward the side of the lesion and abnormal postural reactions, vision, and proprioception on the side opposite the lesion are common.

Intracranial neoplasia should be suspected in any older animal showing a slow, insidious progression of clinical signs

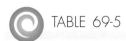

## TABLE 69-5

Emergency Treatment of Intoxications

| **Prevent Further Absorption of Intoxicant** | **Prevent Further Absorption of Intoxicant—cont'd** |
|---|---|
| ***Remove intoxicant from skin and haircoat*** | ***Gastric lavage—cont'd*** |

**Prevent Further Absorption of Intoxicant**

***Remove intoxicant from skin and haircoat***

If:    1. Toxin was cutaneously absorbed.
How:   1. Remove flea collar if that is source of toxin.
       2. Wash animal in warm, soapy water; rinse and repeat.
       3. Flush with warm water for 10 minutes.

***Induce emesis***

If:    1. Ingestion of intoxicant occurred less than 3 hours before presentation.
       2. Product ingested was not a petroleum distillate, strong acid, or strong base.
       3. Animal has a normal gag reflex and is not convulsing or very depressed (danger of aspiration).
How:   1. At home can recommend syrup of ipecac, 6.6 ml/kg. Use this in cats.
       2. Administer apomorphine subcutaneously (0.08 mg/kg) or in conjunctival sac (1 crushed tablet or 1 disk [6 mg]: rinse eye with saline solution after emesis).
       3. Administer xylazine (cats; 0.44 mg/kg IM).
Save vomitus for analysis.

***Gastric lavage***

If:    1. Ingestion of intoxicant occurred less than 3 hours before presentation.
       2. Attempts to produce emesis were unsuccessful or emesis was not recommended.
How:   1. Induce anesthesia and place cuffed endotracheal tube.
       2. Lower head relative to body.
       3. Pass a large-bore stomach tube to level of stomach.

**Prevent Further Absorption of Intoxicant—cont'd**

***Gastric lavage—cont'd***

       4. Use water (5-10 ml/kg body weight) for each washing; aspirate with syringe.
       5. Repeat 10 times.
Save stomach contents for analysis.

***Gastrointestinal adsorbents***

How:   1. If gastric lavage has been performed, administer activated charcoal slurry (10 ml/kg of 1 g of activated charcoal/5 ml of water) as last lavage. Let this sit for 20 minutes, then administer a cathartic.
       2. If gastric lavage was not performed, administer slurry (dose as above) via stomach tube or administer tablets of activated charcoal.

***Cathartics***

How:   1. Sodium sulfate 40% solution should be administered (1 g/kg PO) 30 minutes after activated charcoal is administered.

***Diuresis***

How:   1. Administer saline solution to effect diuresis.
       2. Mannitol (20% solution, 1-2 g/kg IV) or furosemide (2-4 mg/kg IV) may be added to enhance diuresis if needed.

**Administer Specific Antidotes**

See Table 69-3.

**Supportive and Symptomatic Care**

---

or demonstrable neurologic deficits. A careful physical examination should be performed, looking for potential sites of primary neoplasia. Particular attention should be paid to the lymph nodes, spleen, skin, mammary chain, and prostate gland. A CBC, serum biochemistry panel, urinalysis, radiography of the thorax and abdomen, and abdominal ultrasonography should be performed to look for metabolic disorders and evidence of a primary or metastatic tumor. Most dogs with metastatic tumors in the brain that are causing seizures have detectable pulmonary metastatic lesions.

Skull radiography should be performed with the animal under general anesthesia. Although this is a low-yield procedure in dogs and cats with seizures, it may occasionally reveal calcified superficial tumors (usually meningiomas) or nasal tumors invading the cribriform plate and encroaching on the brain. If the means are available, CT and MRI are much more valuable imaging techniques for detecting and characterizing intracranial tumors. These techniques are noninvasive and can provide valuable information regarding the size, location, and density of tumors. Currently the tumor type cannot be reliably ascertained using these imaging techniques, and in some cases granulomatous disease (granulomatous meningoencephalitis [GME]) can be indistinguishable from neoplasia, making it necessary to rely on other test results for making a definitive diagnosis (see Fig. 66-12). Stereotactic CT-guided biopsy of brain tumors has been described and, when available, can result in a definitive diagnosis without invasive intracranial surgery.

CSF collection and analysis should be performed to differentiate neoplastic from inflammatory disease of the central nervous system (CNS). Animals with evidence suggesting increased intracranial pressure (i.e., progressively deteriorating

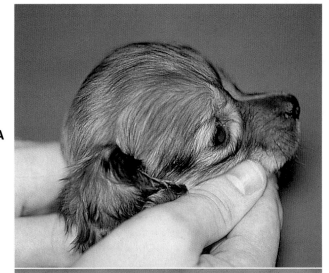

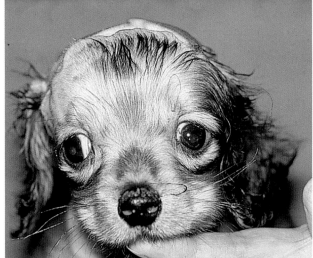

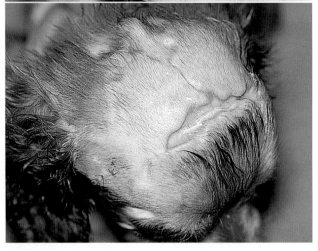

**FIG 69-2**
**A** and **B,** Hydrocephalus in a Chihuahua puppy. Note the greatly enlarged, domed skull and the divergent strabismus. **C,** The open skull sutures (fontanelles) are visible in this puppy after surgical drainage of the lateral ventricles with a ventriculoperitoneal shunt.

mentation) should first be treated aggressively to lower their intracranial pressure (see Chapter 66) to decrease the risk of brain herniation. CSF analysis is necessary, but results are rarely diagnostic for neoplasia, because intracranial masses seldom exfoliate cells into the CSF. The classic CSF findings in an animal with CNS neoplasia include an increase in the CSF protein concentration and a normal nucleated cell count (i.e., albuminocytologic dissociation) (see Table 66-1). These changes are found in approximately half of all dogs with brain neoplasms. The CSF cell count, when it is increased, is usually less than 50 white blood cells (WBCs)/μl, but counts as high as 150 WBCs/μl may be seen, especially in animals with meningiomas. The predominant cell type in most cases is the mononuclear cell, although a larger percentage of neutrophils may be seen in a few dogs and cats with meningiomas. As just noted, neoplastic cells are rarely observed in the CSF of dogs and cats with intracranial tumors, with lymphoma being an exception. CSF cell counts of more than 500/μl, consisting entirely of neoplastic cells, are common in dogs and cats with intracranial lymphoma. Quantitative evaluation of the CSF protein content can help differentiate between inflammatory and neoplastic brain conditions. In both conditions there is an increased concentration of albumin in the CSF because of a break in the blood-CSF barrier. However, the CSF from dogs with brain tumors tends to also have high alpha and beta globulin concentrations, whereas the CSF from dogs with inflammatory conditions, such as GME, has high gamma globulin concentrations. When the CSF is inflammatory, CSF bacterial culture and serology or polymerase chain reaction (PCR) for likely organisms may be worthwhile.

Treatment for brain tumors depends on the tumor type, tumor location, growth history, neurologic signs, and associated morbidity and mortality. Once identified with CT or MRI, some small, superficially located, well-encapsulated, benign cerebral tumors, dorsal cerebellar tumors, and bony tumors of the skull are amenable to surgical removal. In particular, there has been some success in the removal of feline cerebral meningiomas. In dogs, although meningiomas are superficially located and histologically benign, they are not well encapsulated, so surgical removal is more difficult and is associated with a high rate of recurrence. Specific chemotherapy and radiotherapy for lymphoma is possible, but most of the available chemotherapeutic agents do not cross the blood-brain barrier. The intrathecal administration of cytosine arabinoside and methotrexate may be considered, but the prognosis for recovery is poor and complications are frequent (see Chapter 80). Some nonlymphoid brain tumors respond to systemic chemotherapy with nitrosoureas (carmustine [BCNU] or lomustine [CCNU]).

Traditional radiotherapy using orthovoltage, cobalt 60, or megavoltage is often used as an adjunct to surgery of resectable tumors and as the sole therapy for nonresectable primary (nonmetastatic) brain tumors in dogs. Many dogs that are stable neurologically before therapy show some clinical improvement. Remissions in excess of 1 year are common in dogs with certain brain tumors (e.g., meningioma) treated with radiotherapy or combined surgery and radiotherapy. Boron neutron capture therapy (BNCT) has been used to increase the radiation dose that can be administered to tumor cells while sparing normal brain cells. An important drawback of radiotherapy is that multiple anesthesias and access to a referral center involved in this form of therapy are required.

Most intracranial neoplasms are not resectable, so the treatment of brain tumors is primarily directed at improving the quality and length of life. Symptomatic or supportive therapy includes corticosteroids and anticonvulsants. Corticosteroids decrease the edema surrounding the tumor and may improve CSF absorption, thereby decreasing intracranial pressure. In the event of an acute exacerbation of tumor-related clinical signs, a single high intravenous (IV) dose of dexamethasone (1 mg/kg) or methylprednisolone sodium succinate (20 to 40 mg/kg) should be administered. Maintenance doses of prednisone (0.5 mg/kg PO q48h) can be given later, as needed, to control clinical signs. Phenobarbital is the anticonvulsant of choice for animals with seizures. The initial dose is 2 mg/kg given orally twice a day. Subsequent changes in the dose should be based on the animal's response to therapy and the blood phenobarbital concentrations (see p. 1001).

## INFLAMMATORY DISEASES

All of the infectious inflammatory disorders discussed in Chapter 71 can cause encephalitis and result in seizures. Infectious inflammatory disorders are progressive and are nearly always associated with interictal neurologic abnormalities. GME, a noninfectious inflammatory disease in dogs, can also cause seizures, with or without concurrent interictal neurologic deficits. Pug encephalomyelitis commonly causes seizures and other signs of cerebral cortical dysfunction. Feline polioencephalomyelitis may cause seizures in some affected cats. (See Chapter 71 for more information concerning the clinical manifestations, diagnosis, and therapy for these inflammatory disorders.)

## VASCULAR DISEASES

Spontaneous infarction and hemorrhage occasionally occur in the CNS of dogs and cats. Older dogs; dogs with renal failure or hypothyroidism; and cats with renal failure, hyperthyroidism, or primary hypertension may be predisposed. Intracranial hemorrhage and infarction may also occur secondary to septic emboli, neoplasia, coagulopathies, heartworm disease, or vasculitis. The onset of seizures or other neurologic abnormalities is peracute, and these problems are nonprogressive. Results of physical examination, clinicopathologic evaluation, thoracic radiography, skull radiography, and CSF analysis may be unremarkable, aside from the neurologic abnormalities, or may reflect the underlying disease process. Occasionally the CSF is xanthochromic, with erythrophagia apparent cytologically. MRI may be an effective means of making an antemortem diagnosis. Short-term corticosteroid therapy as for head trauma (see Table 68-1) may be indicated for the first 24 hours once an infectious cause has been excluded through appropriate diagnostic test-

ing. Mannitol may be used acutely to decrease edema and lower intracranial pressure. Ideally, surgical drainage of large, localized hematomas should be considered. Most mildly or moderately affected animals show dramatic improvement during the first 3 to 10 days after the onset of signs, although some never return to a normal functional status.

## FELINE ISCHEMIC ENCEPHALOPATHY

Feline ischemic encephalopathy (FIE) is a syndrome of acute cerebral cortical dysfunction caused by cerebral infarction in cats. The portion of the cortex supplied by the middle cerebral artery is most commonly affected. Adult cats of any breed and either gender are affected. Most cases of FIE are diagnosed during the summer months, and the prevalence of this disorder seems to be highest in cats living in the northeastern United States with access to the outdoors. Cats are presented because of a peracute onset of asymmetric neurologic abnormalities, including delirium, aggression, circling to the side of the lesion, ataxia, and seizures. There may be a loss of proprioception and hyperactive reflexes (UMN signs) in the limbs opposite the side of the lesion, and the cat may be blind but have normal pupillary light reflexes (cortical blindness) on the side opposite the lesion. FIE should be suspected in any cat with an acute onset of nonprogressive unilateral cerebral cortical dysfunction and no history of trauma or systemic illness. Physical examination typically reveals no abnormalities other than the neurologic signs. Ophthalmologic examination, clinicopathologic evaluation, and skull radiography findings are also normal. CSF is normal cytologically, with a normal or only slightly increased protein content, making inflammatory disease unlikely. MRI may be the best method of documenting the infarcted region.

Histopathology reveals extensive acute necrosis and edema of the cerebral cortex, apparently resulting from acute infarction of the middle cerebral artery. As well, in many cats, there are histopathologic features compatible with aberrant migration of *Cuterebra* fly larvae. The larvae apparently enter the brain through the nasal cavity and, once within the CNS, elaborate a toxic factor that causes neurologic damage and vasospasm, leading to brain infarction. Acutely, corticosteroids and mannitol can be administered intravenously to decrease the edema associated with the vascular lesion (see Table 68-1). If seizures occur, anticonvulsants should be administered (see p. 1001). Specific treatment of the migrating parasite is possible and may be warranted in young and middle-aged cats from endemic areas with acute lateralizing cerebral cortical signs in the summer. Treatment is with diphenhydramine (4 mg/kg IM), followed 2 hours later with dexamethasone (0.1 mg/kg IV) and ivermectin (400 µg/kg SC). This treatment is repeated 48 hours later. Most cats show marked improvement in 2 to 7 days, whether or not the ivermectin treatment is initiated. Complete recovery occurs in approximately 50% of cats. Permanent neurologic sequelae may include aggressive behavior or recurrent seizures, often resulting in euthanasia.

## TRAUMA/SCAR-RELATED EPILEPSY

Trauma may cause seizures at the time of severe damage to the cerebral cortex (see Chapter 68), or seizures may begin weeks or months after the initial head injury when a cerebral scar serves as an epileptogenic focus.

Scar tissue–related acquired epilepsy can occur following an inflammatory, traumatic, toxic, metabolic, or vascular insult. If a history of significant trauma or infection can be ascertained, the event usually precedes the onset of the seizure disorder by 6 months to 3 years. Findings from physical and neurologic examinations, clinicopathologic tests, and CSF analysis are normal. MRI is not usually able to detect a structural abnormality, and even necropsy will not reliably demonstrate a lesion. The treatment is the same as for idiopathic epilepsy (i.e., anticonvulsant therapy), but the prognosis for seizure control in some large-breed dogs may be better for those with scar-related acquired epilepsy than for those with idiopathic epilepsy.

## THIAMINE DEFICIENCY

Thiamine (vitamin $B_1$) deficiency may occur in cats fed uncooked all-fish diets that contain thiaminase. It may also occur in cats after a period of illness and anorexia. Experimentally it is very difficult to cause thiamine deficiency in dogs, and it is almost never seen clinically except in racing sled dogs fed a diet high in raw fish. Thiamine deficiency results in abnormal glucose metabolism in the brain, encephalopathy, and hemorrhage of brainstem nuclei. Clinical signs initially include ataxia, weakness, and depression. Ventroflexion of the head and neck, dementia, head tilt, nystagmus, and seizures are also seen in affected animals. The tentative diagnosis is based on the history, signalment, and clinical signs and is further supported by the remission of signs within 24 hours of the administration of thiamine (2 mg/kg/day). Treatment is continued for 5 days or until the deficiency can be corrected.

## EPILEPSY

Epilepsy is a syndrome of recurrent seizures not associated with progressive intracranial disease. It can be caused by an inherited functional problem in the brain (i.e., primary, or idiopathic, epilepsy) or result from a static cerebral anomaly or scar.

### Idiopathic Epilepsy

Idiopathic (primary, inherited) epilepsy is the most common cause of seizures in the dog. It is characterized by repeated episodes of seizures with no demonstrable cause. Affected dogs are normal between seizures; an inherent neurotransmitter imbalance is the suspected underlying cause. Idiopathic epilepsy is uncommon in cats; most seizure disorders in cats have an identifiable underlying structural cause, such as neoplasia or encephalitis.

Idiopathic epilepsy is inherited in German Shepherd Dogs, Belgian Tervurens, Keeshonds, Beagles, and Dachshunds. On the basis of pedigree analysis, a genetic basis is also strongly suspected in Labrador Retrievers, Golden Retrievers, and Collies. Epilepsy is also commonly seen in Saint Bernards, Cocker Spaniels, Irish Setters, Boxers, Siberian Huskies, Springer Spaniels, Alaskan Malamutes, Border Collies, Shelties, Miniature Poodles, and Wire-Haired Fox Terriers. It is seen sporadically in almost all breeds, in mixed-breed dogs, and in cats.

The initial onset of seizures usually occurs between 6 months and 3 years of age, although seizures are not observed until 5 years of age in some dogs. In most breeds it seems that the younger the age at the onset of a seizure disorder, the more difficult the disorder will be to control. A difficult-to-control seizure disorder develops at a very young age in some purebred dogs (e.g., 8- to 12-week-old Cocker Spaniels), but such animals may then "outgrow" the problem by 4 to 6 months of age. This form of epilepsy is termed *juvenile epilepsy*.

The seizures in dogs and cats with idiopathic epilepsy are usually generalized tonic-clonic and last from 1 to 2 minutes. Simple or complex focal seizures with or without secondary generalization may also occur, with certain individuals exhibiting more than one type of seizure (see Table 69-1). Some Miniature Poodles and Labrador Retrievers initially exhibit a mild, generalized type of seizure in which they do not lose consciousness but appear anxious and are unable to walk, experiencing either uncontrollable trembling or muscular rigidity as they attempt to crawl; many of these dogs will develop more classical generalized tonic-clonic seizures later in life. Seizures caused by idiopathic epilepsy typically recur at regular intervals, with weeks or months intervening between the seizures. With aging, the frequency and severity of seizures may increase, especially in large-breed dogs. In some dogs, particularly those of large breeds, seizures can eventually occur in clusters, in which multiple seizures occur during a 24-hour period. Clusters of seizures are not usually seen in association with the first seizure in dogs with idiopathic epilepsy, except in Border Collies, Dalmatians, and German Shepherd Dogs. If more than two seizures occur in the first week of a seizure disorder, a progressive intracranial or extracranial cause should be sought.

Findings from a complete physical, neurologic, and ophthalmologic evaluation and results of routine clinicopathologic tests are normal in animals with idiopathic epilepsy. Idiopathic epilepsy is the most likely diagnosis in a young adult, neurologically normal animal with a nonprogressive intermittent seizure disorder of 1 or more years' duration. More extensive diagnostic testing may not be necessary in these animals unless the disorder progresses or changes. Metabolic and systemic evaluation, CSF analysis, and advanced diagnostic imaging (CT or MRI) should be considered in animals with neurologic abnormalities between seizures, in animals that are not of the typical age or breed to have idiopathic epilepsy, and in animals that do not show a seizure pattern typical of idiopathic epilepsy.

Anticonvulsant medication is the only treatment for idiopathic epilepsy. However, not every animal with idiopathic epilepsy requires anticonvulsant therapy. Animals that have had only one seizure and animals that have very short, nonviolent, infrequent seizures probably do not require treatment unless their condition worsens. Dogs treated early in the course of their epilepsy may have better long-term control of their seizures compared with dogs that are allowed to have many seizures before treatment is initiated. It is speculated that each time an animal has a seizure, it increases the likelihood that more severe seizures will develop that may become nonresponsive to medication or that may lead to status epilepticus, a life-threatening condition in which seizure activity is sustained (see p. 1004).

## ANTICONVULSANT THERAPY

Anticonvulsant therapy is indicated for dogs and cats with severe seizures, cluster seizures, individual seizures that occur more often than once every 12 to 16 weeks, increasingly frequent seizures, or status epilepticus. Owners of affected animals must participate in the decision whether to start anticonvulsant medication. They must be willing to commit themselves to fairly rigid medication schedules, frequent reevaluations, and the expense of medication and office visits. Many owners are willing to take on this commitment if there is a chance that some seizure control can be obtained.

The first step in the initiation of therapy is client education regarding idiopathic epilepsy and the objectives of therapy. Complete control or cure of idiopathic epilepsy is rarely possible. However, partial control with a decrease in the frequency and severity of seizures is a realistic goal that can be accomplished in 70% to 80% of animals. Owners should keep a log detailing the frequency and severity of seizures so that the effects of the medication can be monitored. Adverse effects of the medication and plans for monitoring blood concentrations and dose adjustments should be discussed with owners. Emergency situations that can arise, such as status epilepticus, should also be described, and the owners given specific recommendations regarding the actions they should take should these situations arise. A minimum database, including a CBC, serum biochemistry profile, and urinalysis, should always be obtained before the start of anticonvulsant therapy. In many cases a liver function test is also recommended. Phenobarbital and potassium bromide are the initial drugs of choice for treating dogs and cats with epilepsy. Whenever possible, animals should be treated with a single anticonvulsant drug to decrease the prevalence of adverse effects, to optimize owner compliance, and to decrease overall costs of drugs and monitoring. The clinical response and therapeutic drug concentrations should be monitored to determine the proper dose of anticonvulsant drug for the individual animal. If the initial drug is ineffective in spite of optimal serum drug concentrations, then another antiepileptic drug should be added or substituted (Table 69-6).

## ANTICONVULSANT DRUGS

### Phenobarbital

Phenobarbital (PB) has been considered the drug of choice for the initial and ongoing treatment of seizures in dogs and cats for decades. PB is a relatively safe, effective, and inexpensive anticonvulsant drug. The initial dosage is 2.0 mg/kg given orally twice a day. After 2 to 4 weeks of therapy, the animal

should be examined and its trough blood PB concentration determined. Steady-state serum and tissue concentrations of drug are achieved after 7 to 10 days of therapy. Plasma concentrations peak approximately 4 hours after administration, although in most dogs there is not much difference between peak and trough PB concentrations.

The trough serum concentration of PB is evaluated; ideally, this should be measured just before the morning dose is administered in a fasting animal. The trough serum PB concentration should be in the therapeutic range of 25 to 35 μg/ml (107 to 150 μmol/L ) in dogs and 10 to 30 μg/ml (45 to 129 μmol/L) in cats. If the serum concentration is too low, the dose of PB should be increased by approximately 25% (Fig. 69-3; see also Table 69-6) and the trough serum concentration

 TABLE 69-6

**Guidelines for Anticonvulsant Therapy in Dogs**

1. Initiate treatment with phenobarbital (PB; 2.0 mg/kg PO q12h).
2. If seizures continue to occur after 48 hours of treatment, double the dose.
3. At least 10 days after initiating therapy, measure the trough (pre-pill) serum PB concentration. If the concentration is less than 20 μg/ml (86 μmol/L), increase the PB dose by 25% and reevaluate the serum concentration 2 weeks later. Repeat until the trough serum PB concentration is between 20 and 30 μg/ml (86 to 130 μmol/L).
4. If seizures are adequately controlled, maintain the dose and monitor the serum PB concentration twice a year and the liver enzymes/function once a year.
5. If seizures continue to occur in spite of an adequate trough serum PB concentration, measure the serum PB peak (4 hours post-pill) and trough (pre-pill) concentrations. If there is more than a 25% variation, increase PB administration to three times a day.
6. If seizures continue to occur, increase the PB dose further to achieve a therapeutic concentration in the high range (30 to 35 μg/ml; 130 to 150 μmol/L).
7. If seizures continue to occur, add potassium bromide (KBr) therapy (15 mg/kg PO q12h with food).
8. If seizures are controlled but the dog is severely sedated, decrease the PB dose by 20%.
9. If seizures continue to occur, increase the dose of KBr to 20 mg/kg PO q12h.
10. Measure the trough KBr concentration in 3 to 4 months. It should be between 1.0 and 2.0 mg/ml (10 to 20 mmol/L).

$$\text{New dose to be administered} = \frac{\text{(old dose)} \times \text{(target SDC)}}{\text{patient SDC}}$$

**FIG 69-3**
Formula for calculating the adjusted dose of phenobarbital to be administered to a dog. *SDC,* Serum drug concentration.

determined again 2 to 4 weeks later. If the serum concentration is still inadequate, the dose of PB should be gradually increased while the blood concentration is monitored to achieve therapeutic concentrations. The dose necessary to achieve this serum concentration may vary dramatically among animals and even within a given animal. Blood PB concentrations should be reevaluated 2 to 4 weeks after any change in dosage. Serum separator tubes should not be used to collect serum for therapeutic drug monitoring, however, because their use could cause the serum concentration of PB to be underestimated. If the measured blood concentration of PB is adequate, the dog or cat should then be observed through two or three cycles of seizures, and if control is determined to be acceptable, therapy is maintained at that dosage.

Long-term dosing of PB can be complicated by the drug's induction of hepatic microsomal enzyme activity. PB increases its own elimination, so that dosage increases are usually required, especially during the first few months of therapy. Blood PB concentrations should be reevaluated routinely every 6 months, 2 to 4 weeks after any change in dosage, and whenever two or more seizures occur between scheduled PB evaluations.

If an animal has several seizures while it is receiving a stable dose of PB, the serum concentration of PB should be measured. Most "drug failures" are actually the result of inadequate serum anticonvulsant concentrations stemming from poor owner compliance or altered drug metabolism. Although twice-daily administration of PB is sufficient in most dogs and cats, the half-life of the drug may be shortened in some animals, resulting in fluctuations in the plasma drug concentration during the day. This problem can be identified by measuring peak (4 hours post-pill) and trough (pre-pill) drug concentrations. If the serum concentration varies greatly (>25%) during the day, then every-8-hour dosing is recommended, if this is practical. If seizures are uncontrolled despite therapeutic serum drug concentrations, then the dosage of PB should be gradually increased until the blood concentrations reach the high end of the therapeutic range. In these animals, peak and trough PB concentrations should be determined to avoid problems with toxicity. Severe hepatotoxicity has been documented in dogs treated with PB, especially in those with serum concentrations maintained at the high end of the therapeutic range (>35 µg/ml; >150 µmol/L). Increasing the serum PB concentration beyond this upper level will rarely benefit seizure control. Additional or alternative drug therapy may be warranted.

The most common adverse effects of PB include polyuria, polydipsia, and polyphagia. Owners should be advised to avoid overfeeding animals receiving this anticonvulsant, even though their pet seems ravenous. During the first 7 to 10 days of therapy, sedation, depression, and ataxia may also be pronounced; these adverse effects should resolve with time (10 to 21 days) as the animal acquires a tolerance for the sedative effects of the drug. Hyperexcitability can occur as an idiosyncratic effect in up to 40% of dogs and cats treated. Many animals acquire a dependence on the drug, and sudden withdrawal of the drug will precipitate seizures, so it is important for owners to consistently administer the drug once treatment is started.

Veterinary reevaluation is recommended every 6 to 12 months to assess the effectiveness of the drug regimen, the serum concentration of PB, liver enzyme activities, and liver function. PB is a potent inducer of hepatic enzymes, and mild to moderate elevations in serum alkaline phosphatase (ALP) and alanine transaminase (ALT) activities are seen in most dogs receiving the anticonvulsant. Significant hepatotoxicity is uncommon but is most likely to occur when peak serum PB concentrations are high. Clinical features of significant hepatotoxicity include anorexia, sedation, ascites, and occasionally icterus. Laboratory testing typically reveals a large increase in ALT, decreased serum albumin, and abnormal bile acids. If the serum PB concentration in the blood increases while the animal is being maintained on a stable dose of drug, diminished liver function must be suspected and liver function tests performed. Liver function testing is recommended every 6 months in all animals receiving PB. If liver function deteriorates, then an alternate anticonvulsant must be administered.

Rarely, PB administration can cause leukopenia, with or without thrombocytopenia and anemia. These abnormalities may represent an idiosyncratic reaction rather than a dose-related effect, and they usually resolve after the drug is discontinued.

PB increases the biotransformation of drugs metabolized by the liver, decreasing the systemic effects of many drugs administered concurrently. PB also increases the rate of thyroid hormone elimination, decreasing total and free $T_4$ concentrations. Thyroid hormone supplementation is recommended only if clinical signs of hypothyroidism develop (see Chapter 51). Drugs that inhibit microsomal enzymes (e.g., chloramphenicol, tetracycline, cimetidine, ranitidine, enilconazole) may dramatically inhibit the hepatic metabolism of PB, resulting in increased serum concentrations of PB, potentially causing toxicity.

Seizures are controlled in 70% to 80% of dogs and most cats treated with PB monotherapy if serum PB concentrations are maintained within the target range. If seizures continue to occur at an unacceptable frequency or severity despite adequate serum concentrations, therapy with additional drugs must be considered. The addition of a second drug (usually potassium bromide) to the therapy of an animal refractory to PB treatment decreases seizure numbers by 50% or more in approximately 70% to 80% of dogs (see Table 69-6).

### Potassium Bromide

Control of refractory seizures can be improved through the addition of potassium bromide (KBr) to already-established PB therapy in animals with poorly controlled seizures despite adequate serum concentrations of PB. KBr is also effective as a single agent in some animals that do not tolerate PB and is considered by many to be the initial drug of choice (as monotherapy) for some dogs with idiopathic epilepsy. The drug also seems to be effective in many cats with refractory seizures. Bromide is excreted unchanged by the kidney. It is not metabolized by the liver and does not cause hepatotoxicity.

The half-life of bromide is long (dog, 25 days; cat, 11 days), so there is a long lag period between the initiation of treatment and a therapeutic response. If KBr is the only anti-convulsant therapy to be administered to a dog with a severe or progressive seizure disorder, or if toxicity to PB has necessitated an immediate switch in drugs and the rapid achievement of therapeutic serum concentrations of KBr, a loading dose of KBr should be administered. A recommended protocol is as follows: (1) administer 60 to 80 mg/kg of KBr orally twice a day for 5 days with food, followed by (2) the administration of maintenance doses of KBr (15 mg/kg q12h with food) and therapeutic serum monitoring. When used as monotherapy, a trough therapeutic blood KBr concentration of 2.0 to 3.0 mg/ml (20 to 30 mmol/L) is desired. It is important to recognize that chloride competes with bromide for renal excretion, so increases in dietary chloride intake can dramatically increase bromide elimination and decrease seizure control.

When KBr is being administered as monotherapy to an animal with a less severe or less progressive seizure disorder, or when KBr is administered to an animal refractory to PB despite a steady-state concentration of PB within the therapeutic range, there is no need to rapidly achieve therapeutic serum concentrations of KBr (see Table 69-6), and KBr is administered at a maintenance rate (15 mg/kg q12h with food). Whenever possible, PB is continued at the already-established dose. Blood concentrations of PB and KBr should be monitored 1 month and 4 months after the initiation of therapy and every 6 to 9 months thereafter. A trough therapeutic blood KBr concentration of 1.0 to 2.0 mg/ml (10 to 20 mmol/L) is desired. Serum PB concentrations should also be maintained in the mid–therapeutic range in animals receiving KBr and PB.

Adverse effects of KBr include polyuria, polydipsia, and polyphagia. Sedation, incoordination, anorexia, and constipation also occur. Limb stiffness, lameness, and muscle weakness can occur at high serum levels of the drug and will generally resolve if the dose is decreased. Vomiting is a very common problem caused by gastric irritation from the hyperosmolality of the drug; this toxicity can be diminished by further splitting the daily dose (into four equal doses) and by feeding a small amount of food with each dose. Pancreatitis occasionally occurs. Chronic severe bronchitis has been documented in some cats receiving KBr monotherapy. Dramatic sedation can occur in dogs being concurrently treated with PB; this can be decreased, if necessary, by lowering the PB dose by 25%. If more serious neurotoxicity occurs, saline solution can be administered intravenously to increase the renal excretion of bromide. Biochemical abnormalities are not common in animals treated with KBr monotherapy, but because some laboratory assays cannot distinguish bromide from chloride, there may be an artifactual increase in measured chloride in dogs or cats being treated with KBr.

KBr is not manufactured for use in animals and is not approved for use in animals in the United States. It may be obtained as a reagent-grade chemical and dissolved in water to achieve a concentration of 250 mg/ml or reformulated into a gelatin capsule. Those doing so must exercise caution, however, because there have been some reports of tingling sensations in the extremities and peripheral neuropathies developing in people who handle the drug.

## Diazepam

Diazepam (Valium; Roche, Nutley, N.J.) is of limited use as a primary anticonvulsant in dogs because of its expense, its very short half-life, and the rapid development of tolerance to its anticonvulsant. This drug has, however, been shown to be of some benefit for the long-term management of seizures in cats, since tolerance to its anticonvulsant effect does not seem to occur in that species. The only common adverse effect is sedation, although idiosyncratic severe, life-threatening hepatotoxicity has been documented in cats receiving daily diazepam for 5 to 11 days. This potentially fatal reaction warrants close owner observation of appetite and attitude, and periodic monitoring of liver enzymes in all cats treated with diazepam. PB and KBr may be better choices for chronic anticonvulsant therapy. Diazepam can be administered orally (0.3 to 0.8 mg/kg q8h) to achieve trough blood concentrations of 200 to 500 ng/ml.

Diazepam also has a place in the at-home treatment of dogs with idiopathic epilepsy and cluster seizures. In dogs with a recognizable preictal phase or an aura preceding the seizure, diazepam (10 to 30 mg) may be administered orally to decrease the severity of the impending seizure cluster. Alternatively, the injectable preparation of diazepam (5 mg/ml) can be administered rectally (1 mg/kg) by the owner just after each seizure, to a maximum dose of 3 mg/kg in 24 hours. Each dose administered can be doubled in dogs being chronically treated with PB, since this will increase diazepam clearance. At-home rectal administration of diazepam can decrease the occurrence of cluster seizures and the development of status epilepticus, as well as dramatically decrease the need for owners to seek expensive emergency treatment for their epileptic dogs. Diazepam dispensed for at-home rectal administration should be stored in a glass vial, since plastic will adsorb the drug, decreasing its effectiveness. For administration the drug can be drawn into a syringe and injected through a 1-inch plastic teat cannula or rubber catheter directly into the rectum. Nasal administration of aerosolized diazepam for rapid effect is also being evaluated—the ideal product preparation and protocol have not yet been established.

## Clonazepam and Clorazepate

Clonazepam and clorazepate have characteristics very similar to those of diazepam, the more commonly administered benzodiazepine. Although these drugs are highly effective anticonvulsants, they have a very short duration of action, they are very expensive, and the development of tolerance to their antiseizure effects is common. Cross-tolerance between benzodiazepines is common, so chronic use of one of these drugs for seizure control may limit the effectiveness of diazepam for emergency treatment. Clonazepam (Klonopin; Roche, Nutley, N.J.; 0.5 to 1.5 mg/kg PO q8-12h) has been administered with some success to dogs in which seizure control with PB alone has not been adequate. Blood concentrations should be monitored, and a serum concentration of 0.01 to 0.08 mg/ml achieved. Clorazepate dipotassium (Traxene; Abbott Laboratories; 1 to 2 mg/kg PO q12h) has been shown to have anticonvulsant effects in dogs and is less likely to induce tolerance than clonazepam, but it is very expensive. Clinical results in dogs that are refractory to PB have not been promising. Neither of these drugs has gained wide acceptance as a primary anticonvulsant for dogs or cats.

## Valproic Acid

The combination of sodium valproate and PB results in improved seizure control in some large-breed dogs with idiopathic epilepsy that are refractory to PB monotherapy. The combination has not been evaluated in cats. Clinical results have been obtained in dogs at dosages much lower than those required to obtain serum concentrations known to be therapeutic in humans. Valproic acid (Depakene; Abbott Laboratories, North Chicago, Ill) may be administered at a dosage of 20 to 60 mg/kg orally twice a day to three times a day. Long-term adverse effects are uncommon, although alopecia and rapidly fulminating fatal hepatic necrosis have been documented.

## Felbamate

Felbamate (Felbatol) administration can be beneficial in dogs refractory to anticonvulsant therapy with PB or KBr. The recommended starting dose is 15 mg/kg every 8 hours. The dose can be increased in 15 mg/kg increments until the seizures are adequately controlled. Therapeutic blood monitoring is not very useful, since an ideal target range has not been established. Side effects have not been reported in dogs, but aplastic anemia and hepatotoxicity have been reported in humans.

## ALTERNATIVE THERAPIES

Approximately 20% to 25% of dogs treated for epilepsy using standard anticonvulsant therapy are never well controlled despite attempts at therapeutic drug monitoring and appropriate dose adjustments. It is important to evaluate poorly controlled animals for underlying metabolic or intracranial disease that could be specifically treated. Alternative treatments could also be considered in these animals, including the feeding of hypoallergenic diets, acupuncture, surgical division of the corpus callosum, and vagus nerve stimulation.

## EMERGENCY THERAPY FOR DOGS AND CATS IN STATUS EPILEPTICUS

As noted earlier, status epilepticus is a series of seizures without periods of intervening consciousness. It constitutes a medical emergency, and immediate seizure control is re-
quired, because continuous seizure activity of 20 minutes or longer has been shown to result in permanent neuronal damage. The goals of treatment are to stabilize the animal, stop the seizure activity, protect the brain from further damage, and allow recovery from the systemic effects of prolonged seizure activity. Oxygen is administered, as well as fluid therapy and supportive care, to minimize systemic effects, including hyperthermia, lactic acidosis, hypoxemia, cardiac arrhythmias, and pulmonary edema. Diazepam is administered (intravenously or rectally) to stop the seizures and is followed by barbiturates to prevent seizure recurrence. Thiamine, an important cofactor for anaerobic metabolism, may be administered. Corticosteroids and mannitol are also recommended to decrease the brain edema secondary to prolonged seizure activity. Details regarding the treatment of status epilepticus are outlined in Table 69-4.

## *Suggested Readings*

Dewey CW et al: Primary brain tumors in dogs and cats, *Compend Contin Educ Pract Vet* 22(8):756, 2000.

Evans SM et al: Radiation therapy of canine brain masses, *J Vet Intern Med* 7:216, 1993.

Forrester SD et al: Current concepts in the management of canine epilepsy, *Compend Contin Educ Pract Vet* 11:811, 1989.

Gallagher JG et al: Prognosis after surgical excision of cerebral meningiomas in cats: 17 cases (1986-1992), *J Am Vet Med Assoc* 203:1437, 1993.

Glass EN et al: Clinical and clinicopathologic features in 11 cats with *Cuterebra* larval myiasis of the central nervous system, *J Vet Intern Med* 12:365, 1998.

Joseph RJ et al: Canine cerebrovascular disease: clinical and pathological findings in 17 cases, *J Am Anim Hosp Assoc* 24:569, 1988.

Lane B et al: Medical management of recurrent seizures in dogs and cats, *J Vet Intern Med* 4:26, 1990.

Patterson JS et al: Neurologic manifestations of cerebrovascular atherosclerosis associated with primary hypothyroidism in a dog, *J Am Vet Med Assoc* 186:499, 1985.

Podell M: The use of diazepam per rectum at home for the acute management of cluster seizures in dogs, *J Vet Intern Med* 9:68, 1995.

Rivers WJ et al: Hydrocephalus in the dog: utility of ultrasonography as an alternate diagnostic imaging technique, *J Am Anim Hosp Assoc* 28:333, 1992.

Thomas WB: Idiopathic epilepsy in dogs, *Vet Clin North Am Small Anim Pract* 30(1):183, 2000.

# CHAPTER 70

## Head Tilt

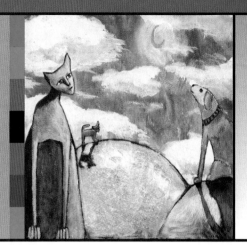

### CHAPTER OUTLINE

GENERAL CONSIDERATIONS, 1005
LOCALIZATION OF THE LESION, 1005
PERIPHERAL VESTIBULAR DISEASE, 1006
BILATERAL PERIPHERAL VESTIBULAR DISEASE, 1009
CENTRAL VESTIBULAR DISEASE, 1009
CONGENITAL NYSTAGMUS, 1009

## GENERAL CONSIDERATIONS

Head tilt is a common neurologic abnormality in dogs and cats. It indicates a lesion of the vestibular system, which consists of central and peripheral parts.

The peripheral vestibular system includes receptors in the inner ear within the petrous temporal bone of the skull and the vestibular portion of cranial nerve VIII, which carries information from these receptors to the brainstem. The central vestibular structures include the brainstem vestibular nuclei in the medulla oblongata and neurons in the flocculonodular lobe of the cerebellum. Abnormalities involving the central or peripheral vestibular system cause head tilt, circling, ataxia, rolling, and an involuntary rhythmic movement of the eyes (i.e., nystagmus).

## LOCALIZATION OF THE LESION

Because different disorders affect the central and peripheral vestibular systems, one should always attempt to localize disease to one of these systems (Table 70-1). Problems of balance resulting in incoordination are prominent in animals with vestibular disease. The head tilt (ear pointed toward the ground) is on the same side as the lesion. Tight circling, falling, and rolling toward the side of the lesion are common in such animals. A ventral deviation of the eye (i.e., strabismus) may be seen on the same side as the lesion when the nose is elevated. Vomiting, salivation, and other signs of motion sickness are common in dogs and cats with disease of either the central or peripheral vestibular systems.

When the head of a normal animal is turned to the side, the eyes drift slowly away from the direction the head is turning and then quickly jerk back toward the direction of movement. The fast phase of this *physiologic nystagmus* is in the direction of the head movement. In cats and dogs with central or peripheral vestibular disease, a pathologic *spontaneous nystagmus* develops with its fast phase toward the side opposite the vestibular lesion. Spontaneous nystagmus in a horizontal or rotatory direction may be seen in peripheral or central vestibular disease.

Spontaneous vertical nystagmus or nystagmus that changes in character or direction with changes in body position indicates central vestibular disease. As compensation occurs, spontaneous pathologic nystagmus often resolves within several days in animals with acute vestibular dysfunction. Nystagmus that is only elicited when the animal is placed on its side or back is termed *positional nystagmus* and may be seen in dogs and cats with either peripheral or central vestibular disease.

Animals with peripheral or central vestibular disease often have decreased extensor muscle tone in the forelimbs and rear limbs on the side of the lesion and increased extensor tone in the limbs on the side opposite the lesion. These abnormalities result in a tendency for the animal to fall or roll toward the side of the lesion. However, animals with peripheral vestibular disease have no loss of proprioception or strength and postural reactions (e.g., knuckling, hopping) are normal, although difficult to perform because of the impaired balance. Central vestibular disease should be suspected if the animal has actual proprioceptive abnormalities. Deficits in this animal would be expected on the same side as the brainstem lesion.

The finding of concurrent nervous system abnormalities aids in the localization of lesions. The nerve fibers of the facial nerve and the sympathetic innervation to the eye pass through the middle ear. Many diseases that affect the peripheral vestibular system within the inner ear therefore also affect these nerves within the middle ear and result in ipsilateral (i.e., same sided) facial nerve paralysis (i.e., inability to blink or move lip or ear on affected side) or Horner's syndrome (i.e., miosis, enophthalmos, ptosis) (see p. 987; Fig. 70-1).

The presence of cranial nerve abnormalities other than facial nerve paralysis and Horner's syndrome in an animal with

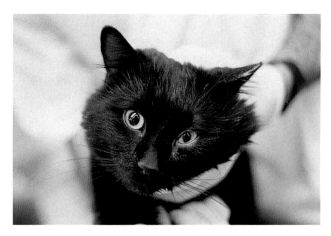

**FIG 70-1**
Adult cat with peripheral vestibular disease and Horner's syndrome on the left side caused by otitis media/interna.

## TABLE 70-1

Vestibular Disease

### Central and Peripheral Vestibular Disease

Incoordination
Head tilt toward side of lesion
Falling/rolling toward side of lesion
± Ventral strabismus on side of lesion
Vomiting, salivation
Spontaneous nystagmus (fast phase away from lesion)
Nystagmus may intensify with changes in body position

### Peripheral Vestibular Disease

Nystagmus is horizontal or rotatory
No change in nystagmus direction with changes in head position
Postural reactions and proprioception normal
Concurrent Horner's syndrome, cranial nerve VII paralysis with involvement of the middle/inner ear; other cranial nerves normal

### Central Vestibular Disease

Nystagmus horizontal, rotatory, or vertical
Nystagmus direction may change direction with changes in head position
Abnormal postural reactions and proprioception may be seen on side of lesion
Multiple cranial nerve deficits may be seen

## TABLE 70-2

Disorders Causing Head Tilt

### Central Vestibular Disease

Trauma or hemorrhage
Infectious inflammatory disorders
Granulomatous meningoencephalitis (dogs)
Neoplasia
Vascular infarct
Thiamine deficiency

### Peripheral Vestibular Disease

Otitis media/interna
Middle ear tumors/feline nasopharyngeal polyps
Trauma
Congenital vestibular syndromes
Geriatric canine vestibular disease
Feline idiopathic vestibular syndrome
Aminoglycoside ototoxicity
Hypothyroidism(?)

vestibular disease usually indicates central (i.e., brainstem) disease. Neoplasms or granulomas located at the cerebellomedullary angle may result in simultaneous dysfunction of the vestibular, facial, and trigeminal nerves. The trigeminal nerve (i.e., facial sensation) should always be assessed during the neurologic examination of any animal with vestibular signs. Other cranial nerve deficits, proprioceptive abnormalities, head tremor, or hypermetria all suggest central vestibular disease.

Central vestibular lesions involving primarily the caudal cerebellar peduncle or the flocculonodular lobe of the cerebellum can cause paradoxical vestibular signs, in which the head tilt and the fast phase of nystagmus are both directed toward the side opposite the lesion. Dysmetria, hypermetria, or proprioceptive abnormalities occur in the limbs on the side of the lesion, helping to localize the disease to the correct side. Head bobbing and intention tremors are occasionally seen.

## PERIPHERAL VESTIBULAR DISEASE

Peripheral vestibular disease is much more common in dogs and cats than central disease and generally carries a better prognosis. Peripheral vestibular disease occurs as a congenital problem in many breeds of dogs and cats; it can also result from infection, neoplasia, polyps, or trauma affecting the vestibular nerve in the middle and inner ear; from aminoglycoside-induced receptor degeneration (rare); or from a transient idiopathic syndrome in the adult cat or geriatric dog (Table 70-2). Peripheral vestibular disease with or without facial nerve paralysis may also occur in association with a hypothyroid-associated polyneuropathy in dogs.

### Etiology

**Otitis media-interna.** Extension of otitis external to otitis media-interna is a very common cause of peripheral vestibular disease in dogs and cats. Bacteria can directly infect the middle and inner ear, or the bacteria can produce toxins that inflame the labyrinth. The vestibular signs are consistent with a unilateral peripheral vestibular lesion. In addition to vestibu-

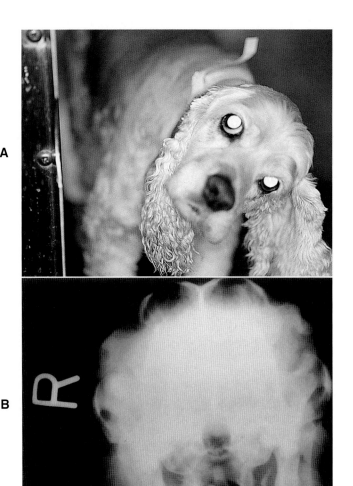

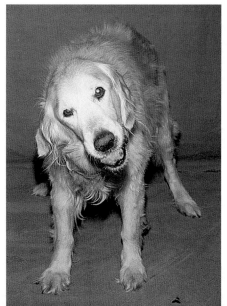

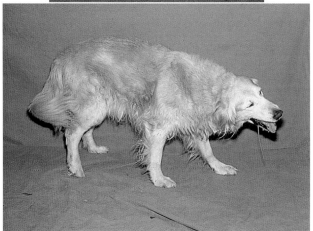

**FIG 70-2**
**A,** Adult Cocker Spaniel with left peripheral vestibular disease caused by otitis media/interna. **B,** Radiograph reveals thickening of the left bulla wall with an increase in density within the bulla. Osteotomy of the ventral bulla revealed bilateral otitis media/interna.

**FIG 70-3**
**A** and **B,** A 12-year-old Golden Retriever with head and body tilt caused by geriatric canine vestibular disease.

lar signs, facial nerve paralysis or Horner's syndrome affecting the same side may be identified during a neurologic examination (see Fig. 70-1; Fig. 70-2). There may be obvious otitis externa, an abnormal or ruptured tympanic membrane, and pain when the bulla is palpated, but occasionally otoscopic examination is normal. The diagnosis and treatment of otitis media/interna are discussed on p. 1051.

**Geriatric canine vestibular disease.** Geriatric canine vestibular disease (i.e., old dog vestibular disease), an idiopathic syndrome, is the most common cause of unilateral peripheral vestibular disease in old dogs. The mean age of onset is 12.5 years, and the disorder is characterized by the very sudden onset of unilateral peripheral vestibular signs. Head tilt, ataxia, and falling may be mild or severe (Fig. 70-3); nystagmus is horizontal or rotatory. Proprioception and postural

reactions are normal, although they may be difficult to assess. No other neurologic abnormalities are observed, and all of the other cranial nerves are normal. Approximately 30% of affected dogs also have transient nausea, vomiting, and anorexia.

Any older dog with a peracute onset of unilateral peripheral vestibular disease with no other neurologic abnormalities should be suspected to have geriatric canine vestibular disease. A careful physical examination, neurologic examination, and otoscopic examination should be performed. Further extensive diagnostic testing is often delayed for a few days while the dog is supported and monitored for improvement.

The diagnosis of geriatric canine vestibular disease is based on the exclusion of other causes of peripheral vestibular dysfunction and on the alleviation of clinical signs with time.

The spontaneous nystagmus usually resolves within a few days and is replaced by a transient positional nystagmus in the same direction. The ataxia gradually abates during 1 to 2 weeks, as does the head tilt. The head tilt is rarely permanent.

The prognosis for recovery is excellent; no therapy is recommended. Occasionally vomiting is severe, and H1 histaminergic receptor antagonists (diphenhydramine, 2 to 4 mg/kg SC q8h), M$_1$ cholinergic receptor antagonists (chlorpromazine, 1 to 2 mg/kg os q8h), or vestibulosedative drugs (meclizine, 1 to 2 mg/kg os q24h) are administered for 2 to 3 days to alleviate the emesis associated with motion sickness. Recurrent attacks are unusual but may occur on the same side or on the opposite side.

**Feline idiopathic vestibular syndrome.** Feline idiopathic vestibular syndrome is an acute, nonprogressive disorder similar to the idiopathic geriatric vestibular syndrome that occurs in dogs. It is a common disorder affecting cats of any age. The disease may be more prevalent in the summer and early fall and in certain geographic locations, particularly the northeastern United States, suggesting a possible role for an infectious or parasitic cause. This syndrome is characterized by the peracute onset of peripheral vestibular signs, such as severe loss of balance, disorientation, falling and rolling, a head tilt, and spontaneous nystagmus, with no abnormalities of proprioception or in other cranial nerves. The diagnosis is based on the clinical signs and the absence of ear problems or other disease. If radiographs of the tympanic bullae and petrous temporal bone are obtained, the findings are normal, as are the results of cerebrospinal fluid (CSF) analysis. Spontaneous improvement is usually seen within 2 to 3 days, with a complete return to normal within 2 to 3 weeks.

**Neoplasia.** Tumors of the bullae or bony labyrinth may damage or involve the peripheral vestibular structures and result in peripheral vestibular signs. Likewise, tumors within the ear canal (e.g., squamous cell carcinoma, ceruminous gland adenocarcinoma) may spread locally and result in vestibular disease. Less commonly, neurofibroma or neurofibrosarcoma of the peripheral nerve (cranial nerve VIII) may result in slowly progressive peripheral vestibular signs.

In addition to the signs of peripheral vestibular disease, facial nerve paralysis or Horner's syndrome is common when tumors are located in the middle and inner ear. These tumors are usually evident on skull radiographs as a soft tissue density within the bulla or a region of associated bone lysis. Diagnosis can be confirmed by biopsy findings. Because of the invasive nature of most of these tumors, total resection is difficult but radiotherapy or chemotherapy may be beneficial in some animals (see Chapters 78 and 79).

**Congenital vestibular syndromes.** Purebred dogs and cats that show peripheral vestibular signs before 3 months of age are likely to have a congenital vestibular disorder. Congenital unilateral peripheral vestibular syndromes have been recognized in the German Shepherd, Doberman Pinscher, Akita, English Cocker Spaniel, Beagle, Smooth Fox Terrier, and Tibetan Terrier, as well as in Siamese, Burmese, and Tonkinese cats. Clinical signs may be present at birth or develop during the first few months of life. Head tilt, circling,

and ataxia may initially be severe; however, with time, compensation is common and many affected animals make acceptable pets. The diagnosis is based on the early onset of signs. If ancillary tests such as radiography and CSF analysis are performed, findings are normal. Deafness may accompany the vestibular signs, particularly in the Doberman Pinscher, the Akita, and the Siamese cat.

**Aminoglycoside ototoxicity.** Aminoglycoside antibiotics rarely cause degeneration within the vestibular and auditory systems of dogs and cats. This ototoxicity is usually associated with the administration of high doses or the prolonged use of these antibiotics, particularly in animals with impaired renal function. Degeneration within the vestibular system may result in unilateral or bilateral peripheral vestibular signs and loss of hearing. In most cases the vestibular signs resolve if therapy is discontinued immediately, but deafness may persist.

**Chemical ototoxicity.** Many drugs and chemicals are potentially toxic to the inner ear, but the actual prevalence of ototoxicity in dogs and cats is low. Whenever vestibular dysfunction becomes evident immediately after instilling a substance in an ear canal, the product should be removed and the ear canal flushed with copious quantities of saline. Vestibular signs will usually resolve within a few days or weeks.

**Hypothyroidism.** Hypothyroidism has been implicated as a possible cause of peripheral vestibular disease in adult dogs. Other signs of hypothyroidism may or may not be present. Clinicopathologic testing may show abnormalities suggestive of hypothyroidism (e.g., mild anemia, hypercholesterolemia). The diagnosis is established through thyroid function testing (see Chapter 51). The response to replacement thyroid hormone is variable.

**Inflammatory polyps.** Inflammatory polyps are discussed on p. 232.

## Diagnosis

In an animal in which peripheral vestibular disease is suspected, the external ear canal and tympanic membrane on the affected side should be examined carefully. The finding of a ruptured, bulging, or cloudy tympanic membrane is suggestive of disease of the middle and possibly inner ear. The region of the osseous bullae and the temporomandibular joints (TMJs) should be palpated carefully to determine existence of asymmetry or pain. If possible, the pharynx should be examined visually and by palpation. In animals in which idiopathic vestibular syndromes are suspected, it may be appropriate to let time pass to assess the reversibility of the signs rather than to perform further diagnostic tests. Further diagnostic evaluation is warranted in animals that do not improve with cage rest and time (3 to 5 days) or in animals with other evidence of middle or inner ear disease.

Clinicopathologic tests (i.e., complete blood count [CBC], serum biochemistry panel, urinalysis) rarely contribute information that can be used as the basis for diagnosing a peripheral vestibular disorder, although test results occasionally suggest hypothyroidism. Radiography of the tympanic bullae and bony labyrinth should be performed with the animal under anesthesia to search for evidence of chronic infection, trauma, inflammatory polyps, or neoplasia (see Fig. 70-2).

Ventrodorsal, left and right lateral oblique, and open-mouth views are all used. Alternatively, computerized tomography (CT) or magnetic resonance imaging (MRI) can be used to evaluate the middle and inner ear. If these examinations do not reveal abnormalities and the signalment, onset, or progression of clinical signs does not support a diagnosis of an idiopathic vestibular syndrome, CSF analysis should be performed to evaluate for central vestibular disease. Brainstem auditory evoked response testing may provide information that can help in localizing the lesion within the vestibular system (see discussion of brainstem auditory evoked response testing on p. 971).

## BILATERAL PERIPHERAL VESTIBULAR DISEASE

There may be no discernible head tilt in animals with bilateral peripheral vestibular disease. Affected animals typically have a wide-based stance and are ataxic, although their conscious proprioception is normal. The animals may fall or circle to either side, and they usually ambulate in a crouched position with a wide side-to-side swinging of the head. No spontaneous or positional nystagmus is observed; in most cases, normal vestibular eye movements are also lost. Some affected animals are deaf because the cochlear portion of cranial nerve VIII is involved as well. If the animal is held suspended by the pelvis and lowered toward the ground, there may be no normal extension of the thoracic limbs toward the floor. Instead, an affected animal may curl its head and neck toward the sternum. Differential diagnoses that must be considered in animals with bilateral vestibular disease include an idiopathic or congenital syndrome, trauma, ototoxicity, inner ear infections, and hypothyroidism. The diagnostic workup is the same as that used in dogs and cats with unilateral peripheral vestibular disease.

## CENTRAL VESTIBULAR DISEASE

Central vestibular disease is much less common in dogs and cats than peripheral vestibular disease and generally carries a poor prognosis. Central vestibular disease can be caused by any inflammatory, neoplastic, vascular, or traumatic disorders of the central nervous system (CNS) (see Table 70-2). In particular, granulomatous meningoencephalitis (dogs), Rocky Mountain spotted fever (RMSF) (dogs), and feline infectious peritonitis (cats) seem to have a predilection for this part of the brain.

A standard workup for intracranial disease is performed in animals that clearly have central vestibular disease. A complete physical, neurologic, and ophthalmologic examination is essential to look for evidence of disease elsewhere in the body. Clinicopathologic testing and thoracic and abdominal radiography are warranted to search for neoplastic or infectious inflammatory systemic disease. Finally, diagnostic imaging and CSF analysis should be considered. Advanced diagnostic imaging, particularly using MRI, is effective for the identification of abnormalities in dogs and cats with central vestibular disease. (See Chapter 66 for a more thorough discussion of the diagnostic approach taken in animals with intracranial disease.)

### Metronidazole Toxicity

Signs of metronidazole toxicity can occur in dogs after the administration of this drug at high doses (>60 mg/kg/day) for 3 to 14 days. The signs occur acutely and include vertical nystagmus, ataxia, anorexia, and vomiting. The ataxia may be very severe, making walking impossible. Seizures and head tilt occasionally occur. Treatment consists of stopping the medication and providing supportive care. The prognosis is good for recovery.

## CONGENITAL NYSTAGMUS

A fine oscillating or pendular nystagmus not associated with other features of vestibular disease such as head tilt or ataxia is occasionally seen as a congenital syndrome. The speed and force of the nystagmus are equal in both directions of movement. This has been recognized in entire litters of puppies. It may also accompany other congenital abnormalities of the visual system, particularly in Siamese and Himalayan cats and Belgian Sheepdogs.

### Suggested Readings

Chrisman CL, editor: Head tilt, circling, nystagmus and other vestibular deficits. In *Problems in small animal neurology,* Philadelphia, 1991, Lea & Febiger.

deLahunta A, editor: Vestibular system—special proprioception. In *Veterinary neuroanatomy and clinical neurology,* Philadelphia, 1983, WB Saunders.

Schunk KL et al: Peripheral vestibular syndrome in the dog: a review of 83 cases, *J Am Vet Med Assoc* 182:1354, 1983.

Thomas WB: Vestibular dysfunction, *Vet Clin North Am Small Anim Pract* 30(1):227, 2000.

# CHAPTER 71

# Encephalitis, Myelitis, and Meningitis

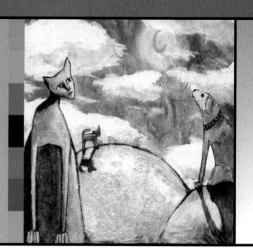

## CHAPTER OUTLINE

SYNOPSIS OF CLINICAL FEATURES, 1010
STEROID-RESPONSIVE SUPPURATIVE
MENINGITIS, 1010
MENINGEAL VASCULITIS, 1012
GRANULOMATOUS MENINGOENCEPHALITIS, 1012
PUG MENINGOENCEPHALITIS, 1013
FELINE POLIOENCEPHALOMYELITIS, 1013
FELINE IMMUNODEFICIENCY VIRUS
ENCEPHALOPATHY, 1014
BACTERIAL MENINGITIS AND MYELITIS, 1014
CANINE DISTEMPER VIRUS, 1015
RABIES, 1016
FELINE INFECTIOUS PERITONITIS, 1016
TOXOPLASMOSIS, 1017
NEOSPOROSIS, 1017
LYME DISEASE, 1018
MYCOTIC INFECTIONS, 1018
RICKETTSIAL DISEASES, 1018
PARASITIC MENINGITIS, MYELITIS,
AND ENCEPHALITIS, 1018

## SYNOPSIS OF CLINICAL FEATURES

Bacterial, viral, protozoal, mycotic, rickettsial, and parasitic pathogens are all recognized as etiologic agents of inflammatory central nervous system (CNS) disease in dogs and cats. In addition, a variety of meningitis syndromes that have no identifiable etiology exist in dogs. These include a steroid-responsive suppurative meningitis of young dogs, meningeal vasculitis, granulomatous meningoencephalomyelitis, and pug meningoencephalitis. Many veterinary professionals consider these syndromes to have an immunologic basis.

The clinical signs of CNS inflammation vary and depend on both the anatomic location and the severity of inflammation. Individual syndromes often have characteristic constellations of clinical signs. Cervical pain and rigidity are common in dogs with meningitis of any etiology and may be manifested by reluctance to walk, a boardlike stance, an arched spine, and resistance to passive manipulation of the head, neck, and limbs (Fig. 71-1). Fever is common. Inflammation of the spinal cord (myelitis) or brain (encephalitis) will result in neurologic deficits, localizing the disease to a particular region of the CNS.

Cerebrospinal fluid (CSF) analysis is necessary to confirm a suspected diagnosis of inflammatory disease of the CNS. Analysis of the cells found in the CSF, together with the clinical and neurologic findings, may aid in determining the etiology of the inflammation in an individual case. A reliable correlation exists between changes seen in the CSF and pathologic changes in the CNS and meninges (see Table 66-1). In addition to the determination of cell types, analysis of CSF protein, CSF culture, and antibody titers for likely infectious agents may occasionally be of diagnostic value. These results, together with the use of other appropriate ancillary diagnostic tests, allow diagnosis of a specific disorder and the initiation of prompt appropriate treatment (Table 71-1).

## STEROID-RESPONSIVE SUPPURATIVE MENINGITIS

Suppurative meningitis responsive to corticosteroid treatment is the most common form of meningitis diagnosed in most veterinary hospitals. Large dogs younger than 2 years old are most often affected, but middle-aged and older dogs are occasionally affected. Clinical signs include fever, cervical rigidity, and vertebral pain. Affected dogs are alert and systemically normal. Neurologic deficits are uncommon, but they may occur in untreated or in inadequately treated dogs. Peripheral neutrophilia is usually present, although neutropenia is occasionally documented. CSF analysis shows increased protein concentration and a severe neutrophilic pleocytosis (usually >500 cells/µl; 75% to 100% neutrophils). High IgA concentrations are found in the CSF and serum, aiding diagnosis. Early in the course of the disease, CSF may be normal and CSF collected from dogs after initial treatment with corticosteroids may show nearly normal cell counts

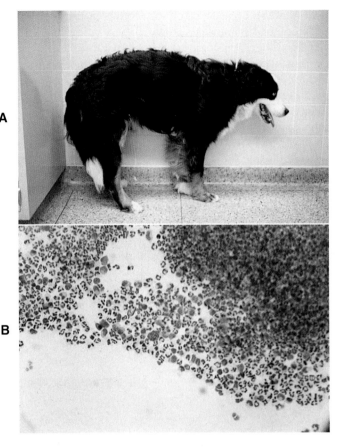

**FIG 71-1**

**A,** A young Bernese Mountain Dog with meningeal vasculitis stands with an arched spine and is reluctant to walk because of pain. **B,** CSF from this dog is inflammatory, with a dramatic neutrophilic pleocytosis. (From Meric S et al: Necrotizing vasculitis of the spinal pachyleptomeningeal arteries in three Bernese Mountain Dog littermates, *J Am Anim Hosp Assoc* 22:463, 1986.)

TABLE 71-1

**Ancillary Tests in the Diagnosis of Infectious Inflammatory CNS Disease**

| DISORDER SUSPECTED | ANCILLARY DIAGNOSTICS |
|---|---|
| Acute distemper (D) | Conjunctival scrapings |
| | Funduscopic examination |
| | Thoracic radiographs |
| | CSF antibody titer |
| | Skin biopsy immunohistochemistry |
| Bacterial (D, C) | Ear/throat/eye examination |
| | Thoracic radiographs |
| | Cardiac ultrasound |
| | Skull/spinal radiographs |
| | Blood/urine cultures |
| | CSF culture |
| Toxoplasmosis (D, C) | Funduscopic examination |
| | ALT, AST, CK activities |
| | CSF, serum titers |
| Neosporosis (D) | Funduscopic examination |
| | AST, CK activities |
| | CSF, serum titers |
| Feline infectious peritonitis (C) | Funduscopic examination |
| | Ophthalmologic examination |
| | Serum globulin |
| | Abdominal palpation/ultrasound |
| | Coronavirus antibody CSF and serum |
| | Coronavirus PCR or CSF |
| Cryptococcosis (D, C) | Funduscopic examination |
| | Thoracic radiographs |
| | Skull radiographs |
| | Nasal swab cytology |
| | Test for capsular antigen in serum |
| | CSF culture |
| Rocky Mountain spotted fever (D) | Thoracic radiographs |
| | CBC, platelet count |
| | Skin biopsy: IFA |
| | Serum titer (demonstrate rise) |
| Ehrlichiosis (D) | CBC, platelet count |
| | Serum titer |
| | Funduscopic examination |

*D,* Dog; *C,* cat.

and a predominance of mononuclear cells within 24 to 48 hours of initiating therapy. Some affected dogs also have immune-mediated polyarthritis. Bacterial cultures of the CSF and blood are negative. To date, no etiologic agent has been identified.

The clinical signs are not responsive to antibiotic therapy, although an initial waxing and waning course may give the impression of antibiotic response. Treatment with corticosteroids consistently and rapidly alleviates the signs of fever and pain. Dogs not treated early in the course of the disease may develop neurologic deficits associated with spinal cord infarction and meningeal fibrosis; treatment may not resolve all of the signs in these dogs. Corticosteroids should be administered initially at immunosuppressive dosages (e.g., prednisone, 2 to 4 mg/kg/day). The corticosteroid treatment should be tapered to alternate-day therapy and decreasing dosages over a period of 1 to 2 months. Long-term corticosteroid therapy is not necessary in most cases. Slower tapering of the corticosteroid dosage is appropriate in dogs that re-

lapse. Therapy for 4 to 6 months may be necessary, but the prognosis for survival and complete resolution is excellent. Dogs with aseptic meningitis that do not respond well to treatment with prednisone alone may benefit from the addition of azathioprine (Imuran; Burroughs Wellcome, Research Triangle Park, N.C.; 2.2 mg/kg/day) to their treatment for 4 to 8 weeks.

The rapid and reliable response to therapy has made neurologic tissues from affected dogs generally unavailable for examination. The signs are thought to be due to idiopathic, immune-mediated meningeal vasculitis, similar to that described in the following section as a breed-associated syndrome.

## MENINGEAL VASCULITIS

Severe necrotizing vasculitis of the CNS occurs in Beagles, Boxers, Bernese Mountain Dogs, and German Short-Haired Pointers as a breed-associated syndrome. The classical meningeal signs are fever, cervical rigidity, and spinal pain. Progression to neurologic signs, including paralysis, blindness, and seizures, may rarely occur. CSF analysis reveals increased protein concentration and an extreme neutrophilic pleocytosis (see Fig. 71-1). Some affected dogs have concurrent immune-mediated polyarthritis.

Long-term treatment with corticosteroids (prednisone, 2 to 4 mg/kg/day PO initially, then 1 mg/kg q48h) is effective in most dogs. More aggressive immunosuppressive therapy with azathioprine (2 mg/kg PO q24-48h) has been effective in some refractory cases. The prognosis must be considered guarded for dogs that are severely affected and those that do not respond rapidly and completely to immunosuppressive therapy. Resolution of the disorder after 4 to 6 months of treatment without the need for continuing medication has been recognized in some Bernese Mountain Dogs and most German Short-Haired Pointers. Multiple littermates are commonly affected, and many affected dogs have been closely related, suggesting a hereditary basis for the disorder.

Postmortem examination reveals extensive suppurative leptomeningitis in association with severe arteritis and fibrinoid necrosis of the small and medium-sized arteries of the meninges. Tissue ischemia and hemorrhage may be extensive in dogs with neurologic signs. Affected Beagles consistently manifest similar pathologic changes in the coronary vessels, and if they experience repeated acute painful episodes, they may develop splenic, hepatic, and renal amyloidosis.

## GRANULOMATOUS MENINGOENCEPHALITIS

Granulomatous meningoencephalitis (GME) is an idiopathic inflammatory disorder of the CNS of dogs with proposed infectious, immune, and neoplastic etiologies. GME occurs primarily in young adult dogs of small breeds, with Poodles and Terriers most commonly affected. Large-breed dogs are occasionally affected. Most dogs with GME are 2 to 6 years of age, although the disease may affect older or younger dogs. Cats are not affected.

Focal and disseminated forms of the disease occur. The focal form induces clinical signs suggestive of a single enlarging space-occupying mass in the brain or spinal cord. Signs have an insidious onset and are slowly progressive. Focal GME has a predilection for the brainstem, cerebral cortex, cerebellum, or cervical spinal cord. The disseminated form of GME most commonly affects the lower brainstem, the cervical spinal cord, and the meninges. Signs of disseminated GME usually occur acutely and are rapidly progressive. Neurologic dysfunction and severe pain from meningeal involvement are common with both forms. There is also an ocular form of

GME that can occur alone or, more often, in combination with focal or disseminated disease.

Clinical signs reflect the location and nature of the lesion. Prominent features may include cervical pain, suggesting meningeal involvement, or brainstem signs such as nystagmus, head tilt, blindness, or facial and trigeminal paralysis. Ataxia, seizures, circling, and behavior change are also common. Many dogs with the disseminated form of GME have a fever and peripheral neutrophilia but no other evidence of systemic disease. The disseminated form of the disease has an acute to subacute onset and can be very rapidly progressive over a 1- to 8-week period, with 25% of the cases progressing to death within 1 week. The focal form is more insidious, with progression over 3 to 6 months.

CSF analysis reveals an increase in protein concentration and a mild to marked pleocytosis, consisting primarily of lymphocytes, monocytes, and occasional plasma cells (Fig. 71-2). Reticulum cells, anaplastic mononuclear cells with abundant lacy cytoplasm, are sometimes present. Neutrophils are seen in two thirds of the samples, usually making up less than 20%

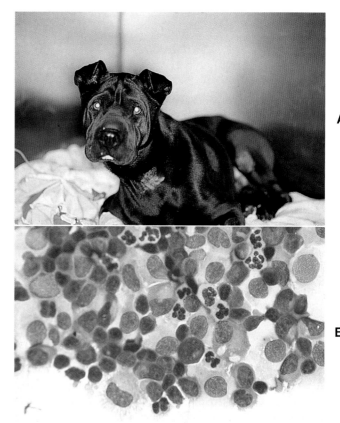

**FIG 71-2**

**A,** A young Sharpei with incoordination, depression, vertical nystagmus, and a slight head tilt resulting from disseminated GME. **B,** CSF from this dog has increased cellularity—primarily lymphocytes, monocytes, plasma cells, and neutrophils.

of the cells but occasionally predominating. A single sample of CSF is sometimes normal. CSF electrophoresis typically shows evidence of blood-brain barrier disruption, and chronically affected dogs have dramatically increased intrathecal production of gamma globulins. Evaluation for infectious causes of meningoencephalomyelitis through culture and appropriate serology should precede a presumptive diagnosis of GME. Computed tomography (CT) or magnetic resonance imaging (MRI) may show one or more contrast enhancing masses in the brain or spinal cord. Definitive diagnosis requires biopsy or necropsy for histologic examination.

Corticosteroids can occasionally halt or reverse the progression of clinical signs. The administration of prednisone (1 to 2 mg/kg/day) has a dramatic response in some animals, particularly those with a slower progression of clinical signs. After the clinical signs stabilize, the dose of prednisone may be lowered gradually. More aggressive chemotherapy using cyclophosphamide (2.2 mg/kg PO q48h) or cytosine arabinoside (50 mg/m$^2$ body surface area twice daily for 2 days SC or IV, then 100 mg/m$^2$ SC once per week) is rarely effective. Recently leflunomide (Arava; Aventis Pharma, Bridgewater, N.J.), a pyrimidine synthesis inhibitor, has been used with some success to treat dogs with GME. This drug is administered at an initial dose of 4 mg/kg/day, and the dose is adjusted to maintain a trough plasma level of 20 μg/ml (usual maintenance dose is 0.5 mg/kg/day). Radiation therapy may greatly benefit some dogs with focal intracranial masses resulting from GME. Most cases improve with treatment but relapse quickly, and the prognosis for permanent recovery is poor.

The characteristic microscopic lesion of GME is inflammatory cell accumulation and/or proliferation around blood vessels in the CNS. Dense aggregations of cells may form a whorling perivascular pattern, with perivascular cuffs composed of histiocytes, lymphocytes, plasma cells, and occasional neutrophils and multinucleate giant cells. Sometimes a marked epithelioid differentiation of histiocytes within the lesion exists, resulting in the formation of discrete nests of these cells within the perivascular cuff. In the disseminated form, lesions are widely distributed throughout the CNS. In the focal form, granulomatous nodules coalesce to form a space-occupying mass that compresses and invades adjacent CNS parenchyma, resulting in necrosis, glial cell reaction, and edema.

## PUG MENINGOENCEPHALITIS

A breed-specific necrotizing meningoencephalitis of the cerebral cortex is common in the Pug, in which a genetic predisposition is likely. Affected dogs first show clinical signs between 9 months and 7 years of age. Recently a disorder with an identical clinical course and pathologic features has been described in the Maltese. A pathologically similar disorder has also been described in the Yorkshire terrier, but in this breed brainstem lesions predominate.

Dogs with acute pug meningoencephalitis are presented with a sudden onset of seizures and neurologic signs referable to the cerebrum and meninges. Dogs may have difficulty walking, or may be weak or lack coordination. They may also circle, have a head tilt or head press, exhibit blindness with normal pupillary light reflexes, or show signs of cervical rigidity and pain. These neurologic signs progress rapidly, and within 5 to 7 days the dogs develop uncontrollable seizures or become recumbent, unable to walk, and comatose.

Dogs with the more slowly progressive form of this disease are also commonly presented with a generalized or partial motor seizure, but these dogs are usually neurologically normal following the seizure. Seizures then recur at varying intervals from a few days to a few weeks, followed by the development of other neurologic signs referable to the cerebral cortex. Survival has generally been only a few weeks, with a maximum survival of less than 6 months from the time of initial presentation.

A diagnosis of pug meningoencephalitis should be suspected on the basis of signalment and characteristic clinical and clinicopathologic features. Hematologic and serum biochemistry findings are unremarkable. CSF analysis reveals a high protein concentration and an increased nucleated cell count, with the predominant cell type being the small lymphocyte. Definitive diagnosis requires autopsy or brain biopsy. Histopathologically, a nonsuppurative necrotizing meningoencephalitis affects primarily the cerebral hemispheres with widespread leptomeningitis, characterized by perivascular accumulations of lymphocytes, plasma cells, and macrophages. These pathologic findings are most suggestive of a viral etiology, but no viral agents have been isolated. An autoantibody directed against brain tissue has been identified in the CSF of a few affected dogs.

No specific treatment exists for this disease. Treatment with antiepileptic doses of phenobarbital may decrease the severity and frequency of the seizures for a short period of time. Corticosteroids are commonly administered but do not appear to alter the course of this disease in most animals. As the disease progresses, treatment becomes ineffective, or the interictal signs become too severe, and affected dogs are euthanized.

## FELINE POLIOENCEPHALOMYELITIS

A nonsuppurative encephalomyelitis most compatible with a viral etiology has been identified as a cause of progressive seizures or spinal cord signs in young adult cats. Affected cats range from 3 months to 6 years of age, with most cats being younger than 2 years old. Affected animals have a subacute to chronic progressive course of neurologic signs. Pelvic limb hyperreflexia may accompany ataxia and paresis of the pelvic limbs, and intention tremors of the head and seizures may occur. Seizures and behavior change may be the only signs observed in some cats.

Clinicopathologic findings are normal in most cats. CSF analysis reveals a mild increase in CSF mononuclear cells and a normal or slightly increased CSF protein concentration.

Definitive diagnosis can be confirmed only at necropsy. Lesions are confined to the CNS and are found in the spinal cord, cerebral cortex, brainstem, and cerebellum. These lesions include perivascular cuffing with mononuclear cells, lymphocytic meningitis, neuronophagia, and the formation of glial nodules. White matter degeneration and demyelination are also present. The prognosis is poor, although reports exist of spontaneous recovery from a clinically similar disorder in a few cats.

## FELINE IMMUNODEFICIENCY VIRUS ENCEPHALOPATHY

Neurologic abnormalities associated with feline immunodeficiency virus (FIV) encephalopathy in cats include behavioral and mood changes, seizures, and twitching of the face and tongue. Depression, persistent staring, and inappropriate elimination are common. A presumptive diagnosis of FIV encephalopathy is made on the basis of suggestive clinical signs, positive FIV serology, and exclusion of other neurologic diseases. CSF analysis reveals an increase in lymphocytes and normal or only slightly increased CSF protein concentration. FIV antibodies can be demonstrated in the CSF of most affected cats. Care must be taken to avoid blood contamination of the CSF during collection, because serum antibody titers are higher than those in the CSF. Culture of freshly collected CSF may yield the virus. Zidovudine (20 mg/kg PO q12h) administration may reduce the severity of neurologic impairment in some cats.

## BACTERIAL MENINGITIS AND MYELITIS

Bacterial infection of the CNS is rare in dogs and cats. It may result from local extension of infection from adjacent structures such as ears, eyes, sinuses, nasal passages, or areas of osteomyelitis. Hematogenous dissemination from extracranial foci may also occur in animals with bacterial endocarditis, omphalophlebitis, prostatitis, metritis, diskospondylitis, pyoderma, or pneumonia. Local extension and hematogenous dissemination of bacterial infection to the CNS may be most common in dogs and cats with underlying immunodeficiency. Bacteria most often implicated include *Staphylococcus aureus*, *Staphylococcus epidermidis*, *Staphylococcus albus*, *Pasteurella multocida*, *Actinomyces*, and *Nocardia*.

Clinical signs of bacterial infection of the CNS may include cervical rigidity, hyperesthesia, pyrexia, vomiting, and bradycardia; seizures may also occur. Additional neurologic deficits, such as paresis, paralysis, hyperreflexia, blindness, nystagmus, and head tilt, are common; these suggest parenchymal involvement. The clinical course is variable. However, once the meningitis occurs, it can progress rapidly.

Physical examination of an animal with bacterial meningitis may reveal a focus of underlying infection. These animals are almost always systemically ill. Shock, hypotension, and disseminated intravascular coagulation may be present. The

complete blood count (CBC) may be normal or have an elevated leukocyte count or may be indicative of sepsis. Definitive diagnosis requires CSF analysis and bacterial culture.

CSF analysis reveals increased protein concentration and a predominantly neutrophilic pleocytosis that may be severe (see Table 66-1). Bacterial infection should be suspected whenever degenerate neutrophils are present in the CSF, although in many cases the neutrophils are mature and nontoxic. Treatment with antibiotics before CSF is collected may result in lowering of the CSF cell count and a predominance of mononuclear cells. Intracellular bacteria are rarely identified in cytologic preparations of CSF (Fig. 71-3). In humans, 70% to 90% of all cases of bacterial meningitis have positive CSF cultures, and 40% to 60% also have positive blood cultures. The rate of organism recovery from dogs and cats is difficult to determine because of the paucity of reported cases, but it seems that recovery rates are much lower than in humans. Every case with suspected bacterial meningitis, even if bacteria are not visualized on cytology, requires CSF analysis; CSF anaerobic and aerobic bacterial culture; blood and urine bacterial cultures; ophthalmologic and otic examination; screening radiographs of the spine, skull, and

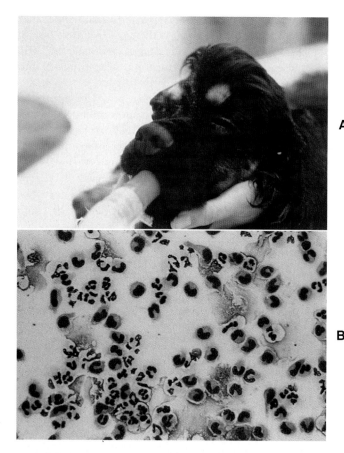

**A**

**B**

**FIG 71-3**
**A,** A 4-year-old Cocker Spaniel with a chronic retrobulbar abscess developed fever and severe depression. **B,** CSF from this dog reveals septic inflammation. Postmortem examination confirmed communication between the retrobulbar abscess and the CNS.

thorax; and abdominal ultrasound examination. The presence of systemic illness or the identification of a focus of infection in a dog or cat with inflammatory CSF should prompt immediate treatment for suspected bacterial infection of the CNS. Therapy usually is initiated before the culture results are available.

Bacterial meningitis is a life-threatening infection and requires rapid and aggressive treatment. Appropriate therapy of CNS infections is based on identification of the causative organism and choosing an appropriate antimicrobial agent. Chloramphenicol, trimethoprim-sulfadiazine, and the quinolones can penetrate into the CNS in therapeutic concentrations. Metronidazole is also effective and is the drug of choice whenever anaerobic infection is likely. In the presence of inflammation, ampicillin, penicillin, and amoxicillin with clavulonic acid also reach adequate concentrations. Although some of the third-generation cephalosporins (cefotaxime) are expensive, most penetrate the CNS well and are effective against many infectious agents, including gram-negative bacteria. Whenever possible, use of a bactericidal antibiotic to which the organism is sensitive and that will reach adequate concentrations in the CSF is recommended. Although chloramphenicol reaches high concentrations in the CNS, its bacteriostatic nature may lead to a high incidence of treatment failures and relapses. Cats treated with this drug often lose their appetite and develop gastrointestinal signs. If concurrent anticonvulsant therapy is required, combined therapy with chloramphenicol may be toxic because of the inhibition of hepatic metabolism of phenobarbital.

When the organism involved is not known, treatment is initiated with trimethoprim-sulfadiazine (15 mg/kg PO q12h) and either ampicillin (22 mg/kg IV q6h or PO) or metronidazole (10 mg/kg PO q8h). Alternatively an appropriate third-generation cephalosporin or quinolone can be administered. Treatment response is monitored by the resolution of clinical signs or the reevaluation of CSF. Antibiotic therapy should continue for at least 2 to 4 weeks past the resolution of clinical signs.

The response to antibiotic therapy is variable, and relapses are common. The prognosis should be considered guarded, because even with appropriate therapy many animals die. However, treatment should be attempted, because some cases respond dramatically to therapy and have complete resolution of their neurologic defects.

## CANINE DISTEMPER VIRUS

Widespread vaccination has substantially decreased the incidence of canine distemper virus (CDV) infections in many regions, but outbreaks still occur among unvaccinated dogs and sporadically in vaccinated dogs. Canine distemper (CD) is usually seen as a multisystemic disease that may include multifocal progressive involvement of the CNS. Clinical signs vary, depending on virulence of the virus strain, environmental conditions, and host age and immune status. Most CDV infections are probably subclinical or are associated with mild signs of upper respiratory tract infection that resolves without therapy.

Young, unvaccinated dogs are most commonly affected by severe generalized distemper. In these dogs there may initially be overt nonneurologic signs, including ocular and nasal discharge, coughing, dyspnea, vomiting, and diarrhea. Neurologic signs begin 1 to 3 weeks after dogs start to recover from systemic illness and may include hyperesthesia, cervical rigidity, seizures, cerebellar or vestibular signs, tetraparesis, and ataxia. Seizures can be of any type, depending on the region of the brain affected, but "chewing gum" seizures caused by polioencephalomalacia of the temporal lobes are commonly described. Myoclonus, a repetitive rhythmic contraction of a group of muscles resulting in repetitive flexion of a limb or contractions of the muscles of mastication, is often referred to as *distemper chorea* and is most commonly associated with distemper encephalomyelitis. In young dogs infected while their permanent teeth are developing, enamel hypoplasia (brown discoloration) of the teeth will be noted. Older animals may develop a more subacute to chronic encephalomyelitis with neurologic signs, including progressive tetraparesis or vestibular dysfunction, in the absence of systemic signs.

CDV is diagnosed on the basis of history, physical examination, and laboratory findings. In many animals a history of mild to severe gastrointestinal and respiratory illness precedes the onset of neurologic signs. Results of a CBC may be normal or may reveal a persistent lymphopenia; distemper inclusions can sometimes be found in the circulating lymphocytes and erythrocytes. Optic neuritis, chorioretinitis, and retinal detachment may be detected during an ophthalmologic examination. Irregular, ill-defined, gray-to-pink densities in the tapetal or nontapetal region suggest acute or active chorioretinitis, whereas well-defined hyperreflective regions are more indicative of chronic infection with scarring.

Immunofluorescent techniques, using anti-CDV antibodies, may reveal CDV in cytologic smears prepared from conjunctival or respiratory epithelium (see pp. 973 and 1273). Positive fluorescence in conjunctival epithelium is usually detected only early in an infection, before the development of neurologic signs. Virus may be detected past these initial stages in epithelial cells and macrophages obtained from the lower respiratory tract by tracheal wash. The virus persists for up to 60 days in the skin, footpads, and CNS; thus fluorescent antibody or immunoperoxidase techniques can detect it when they are applied to biopsy or necropsy specimens for diagnosis. Biopsy of the haired skin of the dorsal neck can be used for antemortem immunohistochemical testing to confirm acute and subacute infection with CDV. Reverse-transcriptase polymerase chain reaction (RT-PCR) can also be used to detect CDV in the serum, whole blood, or CSF of affected dogs.

Distemper meningoencephalitis characteristically causes an increase in protein concentration and a mild lymphocytic pleocytosis in the CSF; occasionally the CSF is normal or more indicative of an inflammatory process (increased neutrophils). Increased protein concentration in the CSF has been identified primarily as anti-CDV antibody. Measured CDV antibody titer in the CSF may be increased relative to the serum titer. Monoclonal antibody techniques can be used to detect the CD antigen in cells from the CSF in many cases.

Treatment of acute CDV meningoencephalomyelitis is supportive, nonspecific, and frequently unrewarding. Progressive neurologic dysfunction usually necessitates euthanasia. Anticonvulsant therapy has been recommended to control seizures. Antiinflammatory doses of glucocorticosteroids (0.5 mg/kg q12h for 10 days, then taper) may be used to control other neurologic signs in the absence of systemic disease; however, their beneficial effects are not well documented.

Prevention of CDV infection through routine vaccination is usually very effective (see Chapter 102). CDV can, however, develop with exposure following stress, illness, or immunosuppression, even in a currently vaccinated dog. Meningoencephalitis has been reported in a few dogs 7 to 14 days after vaccination with modified live virus-canine distemper vaccines (MLV-CDV) vaccines. Particular batches of vaccines may be implicated, but vaccination of immunosuppressed neonates, particularly those with a known or suspected parvoviral infection, should be avoided.

## RABIES

Rabies virus infection usually produces fatal encephalomyelitis in dogs and cats. The source of rabies infection is generally considered to be the bite of an infected animal that has rabies virus in the saliva. Bats, raccoons, skunks, and foxes most commonly serve as the source of rabies exposure.

Rabies can have a wide range of clinical signs, making it difficult to differentiate from other acute, progressive encephalomyelitis syndromes. Because of its public health significance, rabies should be on the list of differential diagnoses considered in every animal with rapidly progressing neurologic dysfunction.

In naturally occurring rabies the initial signs may include behavior changes of depression, dementia, or aggression. Excessive salivation, difficulty swallowing, and multiple cranial nerve deficits are usually seen, suggesting brainstem disease. Ataxia and rear limb paresis progressing to flaccid quadriparesis are common. There may be a history of contact with a known rabid animal. Animals may shed rabies virus in the saliva for up to 14 days before the onset of clinical signs. The incubation period from the time of the bite to the onset of clinical signs is extremely variable (1 week to 8 months). However, once neurologic signs are seen, the disease is rapidly progressive, with death occurring within 7 days in most animals.

Any unvaccinated animal with an acute, rapidly progressive course of neurologic disease should be considered a rabies suspect and handled with caution. Clinicopathologically there is no feature specific to rabies. The CBC and serum biochemistry analysis are normal. CSF analysis reveals increased mononuclear cells and protein concentration, as might be expected with any viral encephalomyelitis. CSF antibody titers compared with serum titers may aid in diagnosis. Finding a

positive immunoglobulin G (IgG) titer for rabies in the CSF is good evidence for rabies infection, because CSF titers will not increase with vaccination alone. Rabies fluorescent antibody tests may be performed on cytology smears from the nasal mucosa and cornea or on skin biopsy tissue of the sensory vibrissae in the maxillary region. A negative result on these tests does not eliminate the possibility of rabies, particularly in the early stages of disease. If rabies is truly a major differential diagnosis, all ancillary testing requires great caution, if it is performed at all. Wearing gloves, masks, and protective clothing is important while performing the neurologic examination and collecting and testing samples from any animal suspected of having rabies. The variable but occasionally very short incubation period makes rapid diagnosis critical, particularly in cases of human exposure. Diagnosis is usually made by examination of brain tissue obtained after death. Direct immunofluorescent antibody testing for the virus is performed. If that test is negative but there has been human exposure, mouse inoculation studies are done to verify the negative fluorescent antibody test.

In addition to naturally occurring rabies encephalomyelitis, syndromes of vaccine-induced rabies rarely have been recognized in the dog and cat. Occasionally a flaccid quadriparesis without cranial nerve deficits develops 10 to 21 days after rabies virus vaccination in dogs. This syndrome is typical of immunologically mediated acute polyradiculoneuritis, and the prognosis for recovery is excellent. Less commonly, a rapidly progressive encephalomyelitis is recognized in dogs after rabies vaccination. The prognosis for recovery from this disorder is poor. Cats with vaccine-induced rabies typically develop rear limb paresis in the leg in which the vaccine was administered. This progresses to flaccid paralysis of both rear limbs and finally to rigidity in all four limbs, cranial nerve deficits, and dementia. Euthanasia is recommended, because the prognosis for recovery is grave. Fortunately, vaccinations have been extremely effective in reducing the prevalence of rabies in pet dogs and cats and in decreasing the incidence of rabies infection in humans. MLV and inactivated products are available and are relatively safe and effective when used as directed.

Dogs and cats should receive their first rabies vaccine after 12 weeks of age and then again 1 year later. Subsequent boosters are administered every 1 to 3 years, depending on the vaccine used and local public health regulations (see Chapter 99). Rarely, soft-tissue sarcomas have developed in cats at the site of rabies virus prophylactic inoculation.

## FELINE INFECTIOUS PERITONITIS

Progressive neurologic involvement is common in cats affected with the dry form of feline infectious peritonitis (FIP) (see p. 1275). Cerebellar signs may predominate, but other common abnormalities include rear limb paralysis and ataxia, central vestibular signs, seizures, and tetraparesis. Neurologic FIP is most common in cats younger than 2 years of age and in cats older than 9 years of age. Most affected cats have a fever and systemic signs such as anorexia and depression. Concurrent anterior uveitis and chorioretinitis are common and should raise the suspicion of this disease. Careful abdominal palpation may reveal organ distortion caused by granulomas in the abdominal viscera.

Typically the CBC reveals an inflammatory leukogram. Serum globulin concentrations may be very high. Tests for coronavirus antibody are often nondiagnostic; although an extremely high serum titer in the presence of typical clinical findings suggests a diagnosis of FIP, a negative titer does not rule out FIP. Typical findings on CSF analysis include nonseptic inflammation with many neutrophils, macrophages, and lymphocytes (>100 cells/μl; >70% PMN) and an increase in CSF protein concentration (>200 mg/dl). In a few cases, however, CSF will be normal or only slightly inflammatory. Coronavirus antibody will usually be positive in the CSF, and coronavirus can often be detected in the CSF and affected tissue using RT-PCR. MRI and CT may reveal multifocal granulomatous lesions and secondary hydrocephalus in many cats. The prognosis for cats with CNS FIP is very poor. Some palliation may be achieved with immunosuppressive and antiinflammatory medications (see p. 1277).

## TOXOPLASMOSIS

*Toxoplasma gondii* is a common protozoan parasite that infects many animals but rarely causes clinical symptoms of disease. Clinical manifestations of *Toxoplasma* infection may be associated with young age or immunosuppression (e.g., FIV infection). Toxoplasmosis in dogs and cats can affect the lung, liver, muscle, CNS, and eyes. Ocular lesions such as uveitis and chorioretinitis are especially common in cats.

Neurologic signs are uncommon in dogs and cats with toxoplasmosis. Clinical signs depend on the location of the lesion(s) in the cerebrum, cerebellum, brainstem, spinal cord, or muscles. Cases have been described with a wide variety of neurologic signs, including hyperexcitability, depression, tremor, paresis, paralysis, and seizures. Weakness, muscle pain, fever, and increased creatine kinase (CK) have been seen in cats with *Toxoplasma* myositis. A syndrome of protozoal polyradiculoneuritis and myositis restricted to the rear limbs, causing neurogenic atrophy and progressive hind limb hyperextension, has been recognized in young dogs. Also, a rapidly progressive lower motor neuron paralysis similar to acute idiopathic polyradiculoneuritis has been seen in dogs infected with *T. gondii*. Many dogs originally thought to have *Toxoplasma* myositis, neuritis, or meningoencephalitis have later been shown to have been affected by *Neospora caninum*.

CSF analysis often reveals increases in protein concentration and a nucleated cell count. Lymphocytes and monocytes usually predominate, although neutrophils may be seen. Eosinophils may be the predominant cell in a few infected dogs and cats. An increase in macrophages or monocytoid cells with abundant foamy cytoplasm is a characteristic finding. *T. gondii*–specific antibody can be detected in the CSF of some infected cats but does not always indicate active CNS

toxoplasmosis. Rarely, cytologic examination of the CSF reveals *T. gondii* organisms within host cells, allowing a definitive diagnosis of toxoplasmosis.

Antemortem diagnosis of CNS toxoplasmosis may be difficult. If other organ systems are involved, biopsy of affected extraneural tissue may allow identification of the organism. A fourfold rise in IgG titer in two serum samples taken 3 weeks apart or a single elevated IgM titer supports a diagnosis of toxoplasmosis. Unfortunately, subclinically infected dogs and cats occasionally have high antibody titers, and antibodies may be absent in animals with severe clinical disease (see Chapter 104).

Recommended treatment for meningoencephalomyelitis caused by toxoplasmosis in dogs and cats consists of clindamycin hydrochloride (10 mg/kg/day q8h for at least 4 weeks). This drug has been shown to cross the blood-brain barrier and has been used with success in a limited number of animals. Trimethoprim-sulfadiazine (15 mg/kg PO q12h) can be used as an alternate anti-*Toxoplasma* drug, especially in combination with pyrimethamine (1 mg/kg/day). The prognosis for recovery should be considered grave in animals with profound neurologic dysfunction. Affected cats should be routinely tested for concurrent FeLV and FIV infections. Neurologic, ocular, and muscular manifestations of toxoplasmosis are not usually associated with patent infection and oocyte shedding in cats, so isolation of affected animals is not necessary.

## NEOSPOROSIS

*Neospora caninum* is a protozoan that can cause neuromuscular disease similar to that caused by *T. gondii*. Naturally occurring infections have been reported in the dog. Although domestic cats are susceptible experimentally, naturally occurring disease in this species has not been recognized. Adult dogs may have multifocal CNS involvement, polymyositis, and polyneuritis, usually in association with disseminated systemic disease affecting the liver and lung. Paraparesis, multifocal CNS disease, cerebellar signs, and seizures are reported. A rapidly progressive lower motor neuron paralysis similar to acute idiopathic polyradiculoneuritis has also been seen in adult dogs infected with *N. caninum*. Most affected puppies are evaluated for protozoal polyradiculoneuritis and myositis restricted to the rear limbs causing neurogenic atrophy and progressive hind limb hyperextension and rigid contracture. Multiple puppies in a litter are often affected.

Hematologic and biochemical findings vary and depend on the organ systems involved. CSF findings have included mild increases in protein concentration and leukocyte count, with monocytes and lymphocytes predominating; some neutrophils and eosinophils may be present. The organism may rarely be found in the CSF or in biopsy specimens. Specific antibodies may be detected in the CSF, or a rising titer may be measured in the serum to support the diagnosis. Immunocytochemical staining can be used to differentiate *Neospora* from *Toxoplasma* in tissue biopsies. Treatment with clindamycin hydrochloride (10 mg/kg/day q8h for at least 4 weeks) is most effective in dogs without severe neurologic signs. Multifocal signs, rapid progression of signs, pelvic limb rigid hyperextension, and delayed treatment are all associated with a poor prognosis for recovery.

## LYME DISEASE

Lyme neuroborreliosis, resulting from infection of the CNS by the spirochete *Borrelia burgdorferi,* has been reported occasionally in dogs. Most affected dogs have had concurrent polyarthritis, lymphadenopathy, and fever. Signs of neurologic system involvement have included aggression, other behavior changes, and seizures. CSF analysis has been normal or only slightly inflammatory in the limited cases reported. There may be an increase in anti–*B. burgdorferi* immunoglobulin in the CSF compared with a paired serum titer, indicating intrathecal antibody production in affected dogs. Lyme neuroborreliosis, a well-documented manifestation of Lyme disease in humans, should be considered in the differential diagnosis of disease involving the CNS in dogs from endemic regions. Early antibiotic treatment may be effective, but it is important to select an antibiotic that is thought to act against the spirochete and that is capable of reaching high concentrations in the CSF (see p. 1084 and Chapter 98).

## MYCOTIC INFECTIONS

Disseminated systemic mycotic infections may occasionally involve the CNS and eyes. Clinical signs depend on the fungus involved and include gastrointestinal, respiratory, or skeletal problems in conjunction with neurologic signs. The most common neurologic signs are depressed mentation and seizures; a fundic examination may reveal chorioretinitis. Typical abnormalities on CSF analysis include a neutrophilic pleocytosis and increased protein content. Therapy may be attempted (see Chapter 103); however, the prognosis is poor when the nervous system is involved.

It is uncommon for systemic mycoses to present with only neurologic signs. The exception is *Cryptococcus neoformans,* which has a predilection for the CNS in the dog and cat (see p. 1287). Infection occurs via extension from the nose through the cribriform plate in the cat and via hematogenous dissemination of severe disease in the dog or cat.

In cases of *C. neoformans* meningoencephalitis, CSF analysis reveals increased protein concentration and cell counts. A neutrophilic pleocytosis is most common, but eosinophils have been reported. Organisms can be visualized in the CSF in approximately 60% of cases. Fungal culture of the CSF should be considered in dogs with inflammatory CSF in which no organisms are visible. Detection of capsular antigen in the CSF or serum of affected animals using a latex agglutination test may also be a useful aid to diagnosis (see p. 1287). Cytologic examination of nasal exudate, draining tracts, enlarged lymph nodes, and granulomas located extraneurally may yield the diagnosis. The organism is readily visible using

Gram's stain, India ink, or Wright's stain. Drugs commonly used to treat systemic cryptococcal infection include itraconazole, fluconazole, and amphotericin B. The prognosis is considered poor for treatment of the neurologic form of this disease, although some success has been reported in cats using either itraconazole or fluconazole (see Chapter 103).

## RICKETTSIAL DISEASES

Rocky Mountain spotted fever (RMSF), caused by *Rickettsia rickettsii,* and ehrlichiosis, caused by *Ehrlichia canis,* commonly involve the CNS of dogs, causing meningoencephalomyelitis. Neurologic signs are seen in approximately 30% of dogs with both diseases, but the signs are most severe in dogs with RMSF. Neurologic abnormalities in dogs with RMSF tend to be more acute and progressive than those seen with ehrlichiosis. Neurologic signs include hyperesthesia, cervical rigidity, mental changes, ataxia, vestibular signs, stupor, and seizures. Neurologic abnormalities have not been recognized in dogs without concurrent systemic disease (see p. 1265). Signs of systemic disease depend on the degree of involvement of other organ systems but may include fever, anorexia, depression, vomiting, oculonasal discharge, cough, and lymphadenopathy.

Although the number of cases reported is small, neutrophils seem to predominate in the CSF of dogs with RMSF, whereas lymphocytes predominate in ehrlichiosis; the CSF is normal in some dogs with each disease. Serologic testing is essential to confirm the diagnosis of rickettsial infection and to differentiate between these two diseases. CSF titers can be determined and compared with serum titers to document CNS infection and intrathecal antibody production, but the titer may be negative in acutely infected dogs. Treatment with tetracycline (22 mg/kg PO q8h) is effective in most cases of acute ehrlichiosis and RMSF. Doxycycline (5 to 10 mg/kg PO or IV q12h), a lipid-soluble tetracycline, achieves high concentrations in the CSF and may be useful in cases with CNS involvement. Chloramphenicol (25 to 50 mg/kg PO or IV q8h) may also be effective. Enrofloxacin is very effective in dogs with RMSF. Dramatic clinical improvement should be expected within 24 to 48 hours of initiating treatment. The presence of neurologic signs may slow recovery, and in some cases the neurologic damage is irreversible.

## PARASITIC MENINGITIS, MYELITIS, AND ENCEPHALITIS

Meningitis and meningoencephalitis caused by aberrant parasite migration have been reported in the dog and cat. In these diseases, migration and growth of parasites can result in extensive damage to the neural parenchyma. An eosinophilic CSF pleocytosis should prompt consideration of parasitic migration through the CNS, although several more common neurologic disorders should also be considered, including intracranial neoplasia, toxoplasmosis, neosporosis, and GME. An apparently immune-mediated eosinophilic meningitis has also been described in young dogs, particularly Golden Retrievers. Diagnostic evaluation of animals with eosinophilic CSF should include a fundic examination, CBC, serum biochemistry profile, urinalysis, serum and CSF titers for *Toxoplasma* and *Neospora*, thoracic and abdominal radiographs, abdominal ultrasound, fecal flotation, and heartworm antigen testing. CT and MRI may document necrosis along the path of parasite migration within the CNS. Definitive diagnosis of parasitic CNS disease requires pathologic demonstration of the parasite in the CNS. Empirical treatment with ivermectin should be considered if parasite migration is likely (ivermectin, 200 to 300 μg/kg PO or SC every 2 weeks for 3 treatments). Antiinflammatory treatment with prednisone may also be indicated.

## Suggested Readings

Dubey JP: Neospora caninum: a look at a new *Toxoplasma*-like parasite of dogs and other animals, *Compend Contin Educ Pract Vet* 12(5):653, 1990.

Dubey JP et al: Neonatal *Neospora caninum* infection in dogs: isolation of the causative agent and experimental transmission, *J Am Vet Med Assoc* 193(10):1259, 1988.

Irving G et al: Long-term outcome of 5 cases of corticosteroid responsive meningomyelitis, *J Am Anim Hosp Assoc* 26:324, 1990.

Lappin MR et al: Clinical feline toxoplasmosis, *J Vet Intern Med* 3:139, 1989.

Meric SM: Canine meningitis, *J Vet Intern Med* 2(1):26, 1988.

Meric SM: Breed-specific meningitis in dogs. In Kirk RW, editor: *Current veterinary therapy XI*, Philadelphia, 1992, WB Saunders.

Munana KR et al: Prognostic factors for dogs with granulomatous meningoencephalomyelitis: 42 cases (1982-1996), *J Am Vet Med Assoc* 212(12):1902, 1998.

Ryan K et al: Granulomatous meningoencephalitis, *Compend Contin Educ Small Anim Pract* 23(7):644, 2001.

Shell LG: Canine distemper, *Compend Contin Educ Pract Vet* 12(2):173, 1990.

Tipold A et al: Steroid responsive meningitis-arteritis in dog: long term study of 72 cases, *J Small Anim Pract* 35:311, 1994.

Thomas WB et al: Retrospective evaluation of 38 cases of canine distemper encephalomyelitis, *J Am Anim Hosp Assoc* 29:129, 1993.

Vandevelde M et al: The neurologic form of canine distemper. In Kirk RW, editor: *Current veterinary therapy XI*, Philadelphia, 1992, WB Saunders.

# CHAPTER 72

## Disorders of the Spinal Cord

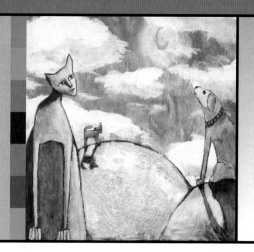

### CHAPTER OUTLINE

GENERAL CONSIDERATIONS, 1020
ACUTE SPINAL CORD DYSFUNCTION, 1021
    Trauma, 1021
    Hemorrhage/infarction, 1024
    Acute intervertebral disk disease, 1024
    Fibrocartilaginous embolism, 1030
SUBACUTE PROGRESSIVE SPINAL CORD
DYSFUNCTION, 1031
    Infectious inflammatory disease, 1031
    Noninfectious inflammatory disease, 1031
    Diskospondylitis, 1031
CHRONIC PROGRESSIVE SPINAL CORD
DYSFUNCTION, 1034
    Neoplasia, 1034
    Intraspinal articular cysts, 1036
    Type II intervertebral disk disease, 1036
    Degenerative myelopathy, 1037
    Cauda equina syndrome, 1038
    Cervical vertebral instability/malformation (wobbler
      syndrome), 1040
PROGRESSIVE SPINAL CORD DYSFUNCTION
IN YOUNG ANIMALS, 1043
    Neuronal abiotrophies and degenerations, 1043
    Metabolic storage diseases, 1043
    Atlantoaxial instability and luxation, 1046
CONGENITAL SPINAL CORD DYSFUNCTION:
NONPROGRESSIVE SIGNS, 1047
    Spina bifida, 1047
    Caudal agenesis of Manx cats, 1047
    Spinal dysraphism, 1047
    Syringomyelia/hydromyelia, 1048

## GENERAL CONSIDERATIONS

Spinal cord disorders can be caused by anomalies, degeneration, neoplasia, inflammatory conditions, external trauma, internal trauma from disk extrusion, hemorrhage, or in-
farction (Table 72-1). Clinical signs frequently include focal or generalized pain, paresis, or paralysis and, occasionally, an inability to urinate. Examination of the signalment, history, onset, and progression of the disease can provide valuable information necessary for establishing a likely cause. Congenital malformations are present at birth, do not progress, and are often breed-associated. Traumatic and vascular disorders are acute and nonprogressive. Acute spinal cord compression may result from trauma, atlantoaxial subluxation, or intervertebral disk disease. More progressive disease is expected in infectious or noninfectious inflammatory disease. Tumors and degenerative processes are usually slowly progressive.

Lesions in the spinal cord may be localized based on a neurologic examination (see Chapter 65). Once localized, further diagnostic testing may be necessary to establish an etiology. Vertebral radiographs may identify vertebral malformations, subluxation caused by trauma, diskospondylitis, vertebral fractures, intervertebral disk disease, and vertebral neoplasia. It is important to recognize that spinal cord segments do not correlate directly with vertebral location in the dog and cat (Table 72-2; Fig. 72-1). The spinal cord ends within the L6 vertebral body in most dogs and within L7 in most cats. The nerve roots of the thoracic and lumbar spinal cord segments always exit the vertebral canal just caudal to the vertebra of the same number.

The spinal cord segments involved in a lesion are identified through a careful neurologic examination; then radiographs are taken of the vertebral bodies that house those spinal cord segments. Normal radiographs may warrant cerebrospinal fluid (CSF) analysis to look for evidence of neoplasia or inflammation. A myelogram, epidurogram, or other diagnostic imaging technique (e.g., computerized tomography [CT], magnetic resonance imaging [MRI]) may be performed to identify a compressive or expansive lesion in the spinal canal. Some cases may require surgical exploration of the site to achieve a diagnosis, gauge prognosis, and recommend treatment. If results of CSF analysis and diagnostic imaging are normal, vascular and degenerative diseases should be suspected.

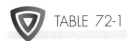

## TABLE 72-1

### Common Causes of Spinal Cord Dysfunction

**Acute**

Trauma
Hemorrhage/infarction
Type I intervertebral disk herniation
Fibrocartilaginous embolism

**Subacute/Progressive**

Infectious inflammatory diseases
Noninfectious inflammatory diseases
Diskospondylitis

**Chronic Progressive**

Neoplasia
Type II intervertebral disk protrusion
Degenerative myelopathy
Cauda equina syndrome
Cervical vertebral malformation/malarticulation

**Progressive in Young Animals**

Neuronal abiotrophies and degenerations
Metabolic storage diseases
Atlantoaxial luxation

**Congenital (Constant)**

Spina bifida
Caudal agenesis of Manx cats
Spinal dysraphism

## TABLE 72-2

### Localization of Spinal Cord Segments Within Vertebral Bodies in the Dog

| SPINAL CORD SEGMENT | VERTEBRAL BODY |
| --- | --- |
| C1-C5 | C1-C4 |
| C6-T2 | C4-T-2 |
| T3-L3 | T2-L3 |
| L4 | L3-L4 |
| L5, L6, L7 | L4-L5 |
| S1-S3 | L5 |
| Caudal | L6-L7 |
| Cauda equina spinal nerves | L5-sacrum |

## ACUTE SPINAL CORD DYSFUNCTION

### TRAUMA

Traumatic injuries to the spinal canal are common, with fractures and luxations of the spine and traumatic disk protrusion being most frequent. Severe spinal cord bruising and edema can occur secondary to trauma, even without disruption of the bony spinal canal.

### Clinical Features

The clinical signs associated with spinal trauma are acute and generally nonprogressive. Animals are usually in pain, and other evidence of trauma (e.g., lacerations, abrasions, fractures) may be present. Neurologic findings depend on lesion location and severity. Neurologic examination should determine the location and extent of the spinal injury. Excessive manipulation or rotation of the animal should be avoided until the vertebral column is determined to be stable.

### Diagnosis

The diagnosis of trauma is readily made based on history and physical examination findings. A thorough and rapid physical examination is important to determine whether the animal has life-threatening, nonneurologic injuries that should be addressed immediately. Concurrent problems may include shock, pneumothorax, pulmonary contusions, diaphragmatic rupture, ruptured biliary system, ruptured bladder, orthopedic injuries, and head trauma. Concern that the animal may have vertebral column instability warrants the use of a stretcher or board to restrain, examine, and transport the dog or cat in lateral recumbency.

The neurologic examination can be performed with the animal in lateral recumbency but will be limited to evaluation of mental status, cranial nerves, posture, muscle tone, voluntary movement, spinal reflexes, the panniculus reflex, and pain perception. Dogs with severe thoracic spinal cord lesions may exhibit the Schiff-Sherrington posture (see Fig. 65-5). The most important prognostic indicator after spinal trauma is the presence or absence of deep pain sensation. If deep pain is absent caudal to a traumatic spinal cord lesion, the prognosis for return of neurologic function is poor.

The neurologic examination allows determination of the neuroanatomic site of the lesion in most cases. Survey radiographs can then be used to more specifically localize the lesion, assess the degree of vertebral damage and displacement, and to aid in prognosis. Manipulation or twisting of unstable areas of the spine must be avoided during radiography. If the animal is recumbent or restrained on a board, then lateral and cross-table ventrodorsal views allow assessment for the presence or absence of fractures or an unstable vertebral column.

The *entire* spine should be assessed radiographically. Lower motor neuron (LMN) signs in a limb can mask an upper motor neuron (UMN) lesion located more cranially in the spinal cord; therefore radiographic and clinical evaluation are important. Most spinal fractures and luxations occur at the junction of mobile and immobile regions of the spine, such as the lumbosacral junction or the thoracolumbar, cervicothoracic, atlantoaxial, or atlantooccipital regions. When necessary, myelography or other advanced diagnostic imaging can be used to determine the site and degree of spinal cord compression in potential surgical candidates.

A three-compartment model is useful for assessing radiographs of spinal fractures to determine the degree of stability and the need for surgery (Fig. 72-2). The vertebral body is divided into three compartments, and radiographs are evaluated to assess which of the three compartments are damaged.

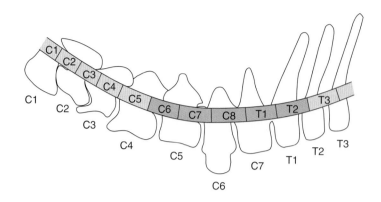

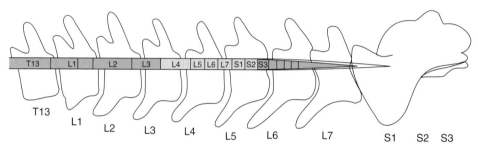

**FIG 72-1**
Position of the spinal cord segments within the cervical, cranial thoracic, and lumbar vertebrae. The cervical intumescence (C6-T2) and the lumbar intumescence (L4-S3) are highlighted.

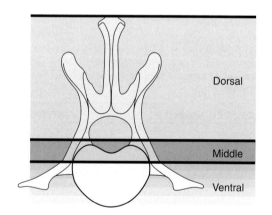

**FIG 72-2**
Illustration of the three-compartment model for radiographic evaluation of spinal fractures. The dorsal compartment includes the articular facets, laminae, pedicles, spinous processes, and supporting ligaments. The middle compartment contains the dorsal longitudinal ligament, the dorsal annulus, and the floor of the spinal canal. The ventral compartment consists of the remainder of the vertebral body and the annulus, the nucleus pulposus, and the ventral longitudinal ligament. When two or three of the compartments are damaged or displaced, surgical stabilization is indicated.

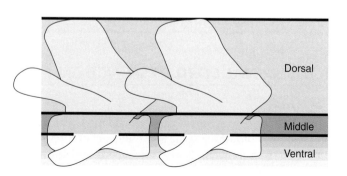

When two of the three compartments are damaged or displaced, the fracture is considered unstable. Unstable fractures generally require surgical intervention. If a fracture is radiographically stable and no compression is documented using myelography or advanced imaging techniques (i.e., MRI, CT), then conservative management is optimal.

Pelvic and sacral fractures present unique considerations. Indications for pelvic fracture repair include the presence of articular fractures, disruption of major weight-bearing structures, and fragment displacement causing collapse of the pelvic canal. Decompressive and exploratory spinal surgery must be considered whenever evidence of spinal nerve compression (i.e., severe pain with or without neurologic deficits) is seen. Dogs and cats with sacral fractures and denervation of the tail nearly always have some denervation of the pelvic viscera. An intact perineal reflex, anal tone, and perineal sensation but a LMN bladder (i.e., large, easily expressed) indicates that the pudendal nerve is intact but the more fragile pelvic nerve has been damaged. These animals have a much better chance of recovery than those with loss of anal tone and perineal sensation.

## Treatment

Primary treatment of acute spinal injury involves the immediate intravenous (IV) administration of highly soluble corticosteroids (Fig. 72-3) and evaluation for and treatment of other life-threatening injuries. Gastrointestinal adverse effects of corticosteroids (including bleeding) are common, and these adverse effects should be monitored and may be decreased by concurrent administration of an $H_2$-receptor blocker (ranitidine 2 mg/kg PO or IV q8h or famotidine 0.5 mg/kg PO or IV q24h; see p. 397), a proton pump inhibitor (omeprazole 0.7 to 1.5 mg/kg/day), or a synthetic prostaglandin E1 analog (misoprostol 2 to 5 µg/kg PO q8h) and a mucosal protectant (sucralfate 0.25 to 1 g PO q8h) (see Tables 30-7 and 30-8). Controlled studies have not demonstrated efficacy of mannitol, dimethyl sulfoxide, naloxone, or other substances when administered after spinal cord trauma.

Surgery may be necessary to stabilize an unstable vertebral column or to decompress a compressed spinal cord. Animals with spinal cord contusion (no apparent compression) unassociated with bone damage rarely benefit from surgical decompression. Progression of clinical signs in spite of medical therapy may warrant further diagnostic imaging or surgical intervention. Because of the extremely poor prognosis for recovery, euthanasia is generally recommended when the animal experiences complete functional loss (characterized by paralysis) and loss of deep pain sensation. Indications for surgical treatment and detailed discussion of surgical procedures and nonsurgical management are outlined in the Suggested Readings at the end of this chapter.

Intensive nursing care is critically important in dogs and cats managed conservatively (and important postoperatively in animals requiring surgery). Splinting for stabilization and forced cage rest may be required. Narcotic analgesics (oxymorphone 0.05 mg/kg IM or butorphanol 0.2 mg/kg SC prn)

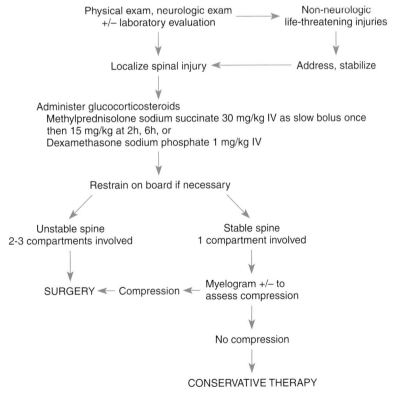

**FIG 72-3**
Algorithm for the management of acute spinal trauma.

may be administered. Thickly padded, clean, dry cages and frequent turning of the patient will help to prevent pressure sores. All impaired limbs should be moved repeatedly through a full range of motion many times each day. Maintenance of an indwelling urinary catheter ensures a dry animal but may increase the risk of urinary tract infection, particularly when kept in place for longer than 3 days. When long-term care is necessary, the bladder should be gently expressed or catheterized and emptied four to six times daily and urinary tract infections treated as they occur. In animals with UMN bladders (see p. 957) or those with urethral spasm, medical therapy (phenoxybenzamine 1 mg/kg q8h and diazepam 1.25 to 2.5 mg/kg q8h) may help to relax the urethral sphincter, making bladder expression easier and less traumatic. When an animal starts to regain voluntary motion in the limbs, physical therapy is increased; hydrotherapy or swimming stimulates voluntary movement, improves circulation to the limbs, and cleans the skin.

## Prognosis

Prognosis for recovery depends on the site and severity of injury. Animals that have intact voluntary motion after traumatic spinal cord injury have a good prognosis for return of full function. Animals that are paralyzed but retain deep pain and normal bladder function have a fair prognosis for recovery, although they may have residual neurologic deficits. Lesions of the white matter producing strictly UMN signs seem to have a better prognosis than lesions affecting clinically important LMNs. Unstable cervical vertebral fractures are associated with very high mortality at the time of trauma and also in the perioperative period. Animals that have lost deep pain sensation after suffering spinal trauma have a very poor prognosis for recovery. If deep pain sensation is gone for at least 48 hours before treatment or if a patient has lost deep pain sensation while experiencing greater than 100% displacement of the vertebral canal, that animal has virtually no chance of functional recovery (i.e., walking). In any animal with paralysis caused by a spinal cord injury, if no signs of improvement are evident by 21 days after injury, the prognosis for recovery is poor.

## HEMORRHAGE/INFARCTION

Nontraumatic hemorrhage into the spinal canal causing acute neurologic deficits and sometimes pain (i.e., hyperesthesia) has been recognized in young dogs with Hemophilia A, dogs of any age with von Willebrand's disease, dogs and cats with acquired bleeding disorders (i.e., warfarin intoxication, thrombocytopenia), dogs with vascular anomalies (i.e., aneurysms, arteriovenous fistulas), and dogs and cats with primary or metastatic spinal neoplasia (i.e., lymphoma, hemangiosarcoma). Hemorrhage can be subdural or epidural. Signs occur acutely and are minimally progressive, with neurologic signs reflecting the site and severity of spinal cord damage. Antemortem diagnosis usually requires advanced diagnostic imaging (i.e., MRI), although identification of a systemic bleeding disorder or neoplasia can suggest the diagnosis. In addition to treatment to resolve the cause of bleeding, significant acute

spinal cord compression caused by hemorrhage should be treated with surgical decompression whenever possible.

Spinal cord infarction is a rare cause of neurologic dysfunction in dogs and cats. Signs occur acutely and are referable to the site and severity of the vascular compromise. Blood stasis, endothelial irregularity, hypercoagulability, and impaired fibrinolysis are all known predisposing factors for thromboembolism (see pp. 134, 310, and 1199). Cardiomyopathy, hyperadrenocorticism, protein-losing nephropathy, immune-mediated hemolytic anemia, heartworm disease, and disseminated intravascular coagulation have all been associated with an increased risk of systemic thrombosis and can occasionally result in regional spinal cord infarction. Treatment consists of general supportive care and medications to decrease the risk of further infarction; however, antemortem definitive diagnosis is difficult.

## ACUTE INTERVERTEBRAL DISK DISEASE

Acute rupture of an intervertebral disk, whereby a large mass of disk material (i.e., nucleus pulposus) herniates through the annular fibers and enters the spinal canal, bruising or compressing the spinal cord, is classified as a Hansen's type I disk (Fig. 72-4; for type II disk, see p. 1836). This type of disk injury is most common in small breeds of dogs such as the Dachshund, Toy Poodle, Pekingese, Beagle, Welsh Corgi, Lhasa Apso, Shih Tzu, and Cocker Spaniel. In these breeds, chondroid degeneration of the intervertebral disks, including mineralization of the nucleus, commonly occurs at a young age, predisposing to acute disk rupture in dogs between 3 and 6 years of age. Acute type I disk injuries are also occasionally diagnosed in large-breed dogs, particularly in Basset Hounds, Doberman Pinschers with caudal cervical vertebral instability, and in German Shepherds. Intervertebral disk disease is a rare cause of clinically evident spinal cord compression in the cat, with predominantly acute type I disk prolapse occurring in older cats (mean age, 9.8 years) in the lower thoracic and lumbar regions (most common, L4/L5).

## Clinical Features

Some dogs with acute intervertebral disk disease have spinal pain and no accompanying neurologic deficits. Others suffer severe concussive and compressive injury to the spinal cord from the disk extrusion and have varying degrees of spinal cord injury. The clinical signs observed depend on the location of the spinal injury, the severity of cord damage, and the degree of spinal cord compression (see Fig. 67-3, Table 67-1).

Most disk extrusions occur in the caudal thoracic or lumbar spine, with 65% of all acute thoracolumbar disk lesions in the dog occurring between T11 and L2. Intervertebral disk extrusions causing spinal cord compression in this region result in UMN signs to the rear limbs (see p. 950) with normal forelimbs. Intervertebral disk extrusions at an intumescence (C6 to T2 or L4 to S3) result in LMN signs in the corresponding limbs and are associated with a more guarded prognosis for return to function. Disk extrusion caudal to the L6 vertebra, causing compression of the cauda equina, is generally associated with a positive response to decompressive therapy.

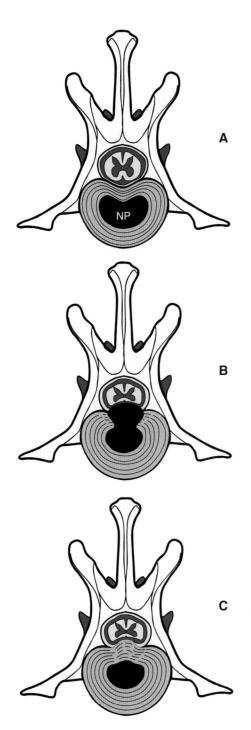

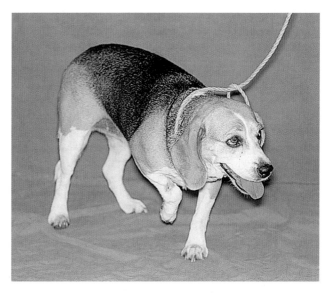

**FIG 72-5**
Adult Beagle with neck and shoulder pain secondary to cervical intervertebral disk prolapse. Lifting of the limb has been referred to as *root signature*.

**FIG 72-4**
**A,** The normal relationship between the intervertebral disk and the spinal cord. *NP,* Nucleus pulposus; *AF,* annulus fibrosus. **B,** Hansen type I disk extrusion, where the *NP* herniated into the vertebral canal through a damaged *AF.* **C,** Hansen type II disk protrusion, with bulging of the annulus into the vertebral canal.

Cervical disk disease (C1 to C5) most commonly causes neck pain without associated neurologic deficits, even when large masses of disk material extrude into the spinal canal. The larger diameter of the vertebral canal in this region makes severe spinal cord compression secondary to cervical disk extrusion uncommon. When significant spinal cord compression is present, UMN signs occur in all four legs. The C2/3 disk is most frequently involved, with the prevalence progressively decreasing from C3/4 to C7/T1. The C6/7 disk is more commonly affected in large-breed dogs as a component of cervical vertebral malformation malarticulation syndrome (also known as *wobbler syndrome*).

Pain is a prominent feature in most dogs with intervertebral disk disease. The extruded material irritates or compresses the nerve roots and meninges, causing pain. Dogs with cervical disk extrusions commonly resist movement or manipulation of their neck and stand at rest with the head and neck lowered. One forelimb may be lifted if caudal cervical (C5/6 to C7/T1) disk prolapse results in irritation of the nerve roots to that limb or spasm of the cervical muscles; this lifting is called *root signature* (Fig. 72-5). Disk extrusions in the region of the cervical or lumbar intumescence commonly compress the nerve roots supplying clinically important peripheral nerves, resulting in lameness and occasional muscle atrophy, even in the absence of significant spinal cord compression.

Pain from thoracolumbar disk disease characteristically results in arching of the back and tensing of the abdominal muscles, mimicking abdominal pain such as may be seen with pancreatitis or an acute surgical abdomen. In addition to pain, weakness and paralysis are commonly observed in dogs with acute thoracolumbar intervertebral disk extrusion. The severity of the initial signs and the speed with which they progress are related not only to the volume of disk material extruded and the degree of resultant spinal cord compression, but also to the force of the extrusion (see Fig. 67-3). In some dogs, evidence of pain and subtle weakness resulting from partial disk rupture and mild spinal cord compression may be present for a few days or weeks before mild trauma or movement results in the extrusion of more disk material causing paralysis. The neurologic signs observed in dogs and cats with intervertebral disk disease are usually bilaterally symmetric.

## Diagnosis

Disk disease causing neurologic dysfunction should be suspected based upon the signalment, history, physical examination, and neurologic findings. Trauma and fibrocartilaginous embolism (FCE) are the major differential diagnoses to be considered, but clinical and historical features can generally differentiate these conditions. Neurologic examination and detection of a specific area of spinal pain are used to localize the lesion to a particular region of the spinal cord. Spinal radiographs can then be taken in an awake animal to look for evidence of disk disease and to rule out other diseases (e.g., diskospondylitis, lytic vertebral tumor, fracture) if the diagnosis is in doubt. It is important to realize that careful positioning of the suspected disk space in the center of the beam, with the dog anesthetized, is usually necessary for radiographic diagnosis of subtle lesions. Radiographs under general anesthesia are usually only recommended in a potential surgical candidate, when preparations have been made for further diagnostic imaging and perhaps decompressive surgery during the same anesthetic episode.

Not all herniated intervertebral disks are apparent on survey radiographs, even when optimal positioning and technique are achieved. Observation of calcified disk spaces confirms the presence of generalized intervertebral disk disease but does not necessarily pinpoint the site of the extrusion causing neurologic dysfunction. Radiographic changes consistent with herniation of an intervertebral disk in the thoracolumbar region include a narrowed or wedged disk space, a small or cloudy intervertebral foramen (i.e., "horse's head"), narrowing of the facetal joints, and a calcified density within the spinal canal above the involved disk space (Figs. 72-6 and 72-7).

Radiographs in dogs with cervical disk herniation usually demonstrate narrowing of the intervertebral space and dorsal displacement of mineralized disk material (Fig. 72-8).

Myelography or advanced diagnostic imaging (i.e., CT, MRI) will usually be required to definitively localize an extruded vertebral disk in animals in which surgery is being considered.

Analysis of CSF should always precede a myelogram, even in dogs with classic signs of cervical or thoracolumbar disk disease. Inflammatory and neoplastic lesions of the CNS can result in very similar clinical findings to those seen with disk extrusion, but they have very different recommended therapies and outcomes. CSF analysis in a dog with disk herniation may reveal very slight increases in protein concentration and cell count, or it may be normal. Subarachnoid injection of myelographic contrast material will exacerbate CNS inflammation caused by infections or immune-mediated disorders and will even induce inflammation in normal animals, making it difficult to interpret CSF collected days to weeks after myelography.

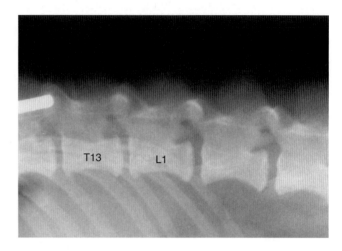

**FIG 72-6**
Lateral plain radiograph of vertebral column of a 4-year-old Pekingese with acute intervertebral disk prolapse. The intervertebral space between T13 and L1 is narrowed, the intervertebral foramen ("horse's head") is small, and a calcified density can be seen in the spinal canal above the T13-L1 disk space.

CT or MRI may be used to further delineate a compressive disk lesion identified myelographically, or may be used as the sole technique for detecting and characterizing a disk lesion, particularly in regions where myelographic interpretation can be difficult and precise anatomic localization is important (e.g., caudal cervical, lumbosacral regions) (Fig. 72-9).

## Treatment

Treatment of acute intervertebral disk extrusion may be nonsurgical or surgical. Nonsurgical treatment is usually prescribed in an animal that has a single acute episode of back or neck pain without neurologic deficits, and occasionally in dogs with mild neurologic deficits resulting from thoracolumbar disk disease. Strict cage confinement is the most important part of nonsurgical treatment. If pain is very severe, nonsteroidal antiinflammatory drugs (NSAIDs) (see Table 76-1) or narcotic analgesics (oxymorphone 0.05 mg/kg IM or butorphanol 0.2 mg/kg SC prn) may be administered for the first 3 days of treatment. It is important to realize, however, that these drugs will decrease pain, resulting in increased activity by the patient and increased risk of further prolapse of disk material. Whenever analgesics are administered, the animal should remain hospitalized to enforce cage rest and allow close observation for neurologic deterioration. It is important that animals being treated nonsurgically be evaluated at least twice a day for deterioration in neurologic status. If the symptoms do not improve within 5 to 7 days or if even minor deterioration in neurologic status is seen, then surgical therapy is indicated.

Strict cage confinement should be continued at home for 3 to 4 weeks, followed by 3 weeks of house confinement and leash exercise. Dogs with cervical disk disease should wear a harness

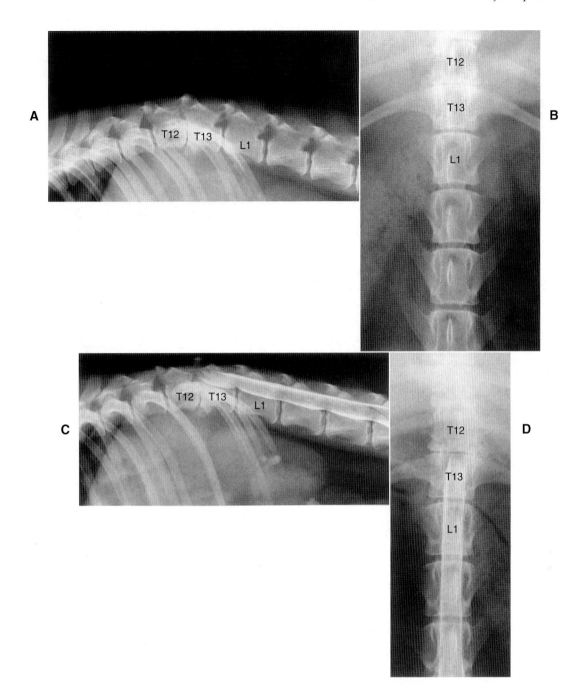

**FIG 72-7**
Lateral, **A,** and ventrodorsal, **B,** plain radiographs of the vertebral column of an 8-year-old Miniature Schnauzer with acute paralysis after a chronic history of intermittent back pain. Marked collapse of the intervertebral space at T12-T13, a small intervertebral foramen, and clouding of the foramen is evident. The T13-L1 space is also slightly narrowed. **C** and **D,** Myelography confirms the presence of a significant extradural mass at T12-T13, located ventrally and on the right, causing considerable cord compression and displacement. A minimal extradural mass effect exists as well at T13-L1 without significant compression. Surgery confirmed spinal cord compression by the disk material at T12-T13.

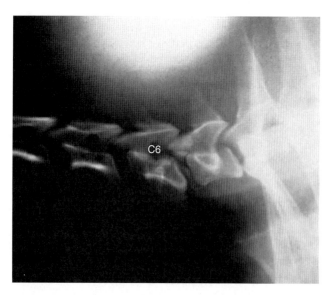

**FIG 72-8**
Lateral radiograph of the cervical vertebral column of an adult dog showing acute intervertebral disk prolapse at C6-C7 site. The intervertebral space is narrowed, and a calcified density can be seen in the spinal canal above the disk space. (Courtesy Dr. C. Fries, University of Saskatchewan.)

instead of a collar when walking. After the prescribed confinement period, there should be a gradual increase in monitored exercise and (if necessary) a weight reduction program.

Advantages of nonsurgical treatment are that it is inexpensive and can be carried out at home.

Most walking dogs (80% to 100%) with thoracolumbar disk disease (i.e., grade 1 or 2) (Table 72-3) respond well. Recovery rates in nonambulatory (i.e., grades 3 and 4) dogs treated medically range from 43% to 50%, although their recovery time may be quite prolonged. Dogs treated medically always face some risk that they may deteriorate markedly in the hours and days after presentation, worsening their long-term prognosis for recovery. Even if dogs recover from an acute episode, nearly 30% of dogs treated nonsurgically have a recurrence in the future.

## Thoracolumbar Disk Disease

Most dogs recover from their first episode of disk-related thoracolumbar back pain with routine nonsurgical management as described previously. Many of these dogs, however, have repeated episodes of pain in the subsequent weeks and months if surgery is not performed. Persistent or recurrent pain is an indication for surgical intervention. Even in the absence of neurologic deficits, most of these dogs have myelographically visible extruded disk material in the spinal canal. If warranted, a decompressive hemilaminectomy should be performed. Although controversial, fenestration of the affected site and surrounding high-risk disk spaces (T11/12 to L2/3) may also be recommended concurrently to decrease the chances of future disk extrusions.

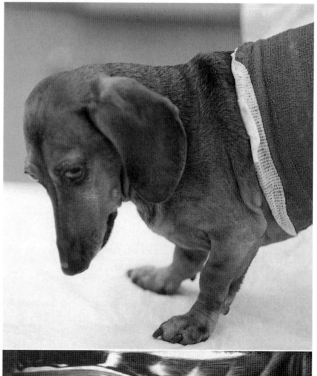

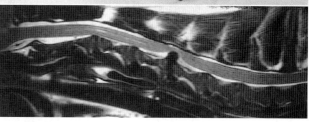

**FIG 72-9**
A 7-year-old Dachshund **(A)** with a 3-week history of severe neck pain and mild proprioceptive deficits in the left rear limb. Magnetic resonance imaging (MRI) revealed prolapse of the C3-C4 intervertebral disk, with significant spinal cord compression at that site **(B).**

Dogs that have acute thoracolumbar pain, proprioceptive abnormalities, and rear limb weakness but that can still support weight and walk (i.e., grade 2 disk disease) are treated initially with strict in-hospital cage rest for 3 days. Dogs are monitored carefully, and decompressive surgery is recommended if the neurologic signs deteriorate. In most cases these dogs deteriorate within 6 to 12 hours, and surgery is clearly indicated. Although many veterinarians routinely treat these dogs with corticosteroids (prednisone 0.1 to 0.2 mg/kg PO q12h) for the first few days, little evidence suggests that this influences the long-term outcome. Prednisone treatment is associated with high risk of serious gastrointestinal adverse effects, and it alters CSF cellularity, making it difficult to subsequently diagnose the cause of the dog's signs (i.e., granulomatous meningoencephalitis [GME], neoplasia) if the initial presumptive diagnosis of disk disease is incorrect. Dogs with suspected thoracolumbar disk disease that improve markedly with 3 days of conservative therapy (without corticosteroids)

TABLE 72-3

Classification of Dysfunction: Canine Thoracolumbar
Disk Disease

| GRADE | CLINICAL FINDINGS |
|---|---|
| 1 | Painful<br>No neurologic deficits |
| 2 | Ataxia<br>Conscious proprioceptive deficits<br>Paraparesis |
| 3 | Severe paraparesis (cannot stand or walk) |
| 4 | Paraplegia<br>Loss of urinary/fecal continence<br>Loss of superficial sensation, panniculus |
| 5 | Paraplegia<br>Incontinence<br>Loss of deep pain sensation |

 TABLE 72-4

Classification of Dysfunction and Treatment
Recommendations: Canine Cervical Disk Disease

| GRADE | CLINICAL FINDINGS | TREATMENT |
|---|---|---|
| 1 | Single episode<br>of pain | Cage rest<br>± Analgesics |
| 2 | Recurrent episodes<br>of pain | Surgery<br>Decompression<br>Fenstration |
| 3 | Neck pain and neuro-<br>logic deficits | Surgery<br>Decompression<br>Fenstration |

can then be treated at home with strict rest as described. Any dog that does not significantly improve within 5 to 7 days should be considered a surgical candidate.

Dogs with severe proprioceptive and motor deficits and an inability to support weight or walk at the time of initial examination (i.e., grades 3, 4, and 5 disk disease) and those that deteriorate during medical management should receive intensive IV corticosteroid therapy immediately (e.g., methylprednisolone sodium succinate 30 mg/kg or dexamethasone 0.25 mg/kg) and undergo rapid surgical decompression. Any delay in decompression will worsen the prognosis for recovery. Decompression is accomplished through a laminectomy, and disk material is removed from the spinal canal. In addition to surgical decompression, disk fenestration at adjacent high-risk sites (T11 to L3) may be recommended to help decrease the likelihood of subsequent herniations in dogs with apparent generalized disk disease.

Dogs that are unable to move their limbs voluntarily (grades 4 and 5 disk disease) should be assessed carefully for the presence of conscious perception of deep pain. In some dogs it is difficult to determine whether there really is complete loss of sensation. Whenever an animal has been truly analgesic for longer than 48 hours, the prognosis for recovery, regardless of therapy, is poor and euthanasia is often recommended. Dogs that have lost deep pain perception for a shorter time (<48 hours) have a guarded prognosis for recovery, but up to 50% may recover and become ambulatory. Surgical exploration is recommended for decompression.

Euthanasia is recommended if significant myelomalacia is detected at the time of surgery.

Acute, forceful, intervertebral disk extrusions can cause considerable intramedullary hemorrhage and edema. In some dogs initially presented for a rapid onset of complete paralysis resulting from thoracolumbar disk disease, hemorrhage, edema, and ischemia cause progressive spinal cord damage; re-

sulting in progressive myelomalacia of the cord cranial and caudal to the original lesion (i.e., ascending descending myelomalacia). This disorder should be suspected when the line demarcating the loss of panniculus reflex moves cranially or the patellar and withdrawal reflexes are lost in the rear limbs of a dog that previously had UMN signs in the rear limbs. Most affected dogs are also very anxious and experience a great deal of pain. This condition affects approximately 3% to 6% of dogs with severe thoracolumbar disk extrusions; it becomes evident 24 to 36 hours after the initial paralysis. When ascending descending myelomalacia is recognized, euthanasia should be recommended, because no chance for recovery exists, and affected dogs will die within a few days of respiratory paralysis.

## Cervical Disk Disease

Treatment decisions in dogs with cervical disk disease are based on the severity of disease noted at the time of presentation (Table 72-4). Dogs with a single episode of acute pain are usually managed conservatively as described on p. 1026. Although many dogs respond initially, approximately 40% of these dogs will have a recurrence in the future. Even if cervical pain is the only clinical finding, most dogs with cervical intervertebral disk prolapse have a large amount of disk material within the spinal canal and will benefit from surgery to remove it. Dogs with repeated episodes of cervical pain, cervical pain that does not resolve with cage rest, and neurologic deficits caused by cervical disk disease should always be treated surgically. Myelography or MRI to locate the lesion, followed by one dose of glucocorticoids (methylprednisolone sodium succinate 30 mg/kg or dexamethasone 0.25 mg/kg) and prompt surgical decompression using a ventral slot procedure is recommended. Ventral slot decompression of caudal cervical disks is occasionally associated with postoperative vertebral luxation causing neck pain and worsening of neurologic deficits, so surgical distraction and stabilization is often recommended when ventral slot decompression is performed in this region. At the time of surgical decompression, cervical disk fenestration may be performed at other sites in an attempt to prevent future cervical disk extrusions.

## Postoperative Care

Postsurgical management of dogs with neurologic deficits secondary to cervical or thoracolumbar disk herniation involves good general nursing care. The animals must be kept clean and confined, with supervised exercise as desired. Pressure sores should be prevented through the use of padded bedding and frequent turning. Narcotic analgesics (oxymorphone 0.05 mg/kg IM, butorphanol 0.2 mg/kg IV or SC) may be administered for 24 to 48 hours and the skeletal muscle relaxant, methocarbamol (20 mg/kg PO q8-12h), can be used to relieve muscle spasm if necessary.

Care of the urinary bladder is important to prevent cystitis and detrusor atony. Complete bladder emptying at least four times daily by manual expression or catheterization is necessary in dogs that have lost bladder function. In dogs with UMN bladders, medical treatment with phenoxybenzamine and diazepam can lower sphincter pressure, facilitating manual expression and attempts by the animal to void.

Massage of the limbs and passive physiotherapy, including limb abduction, may help prevent neurogenic atrophy and muscle fibrosis in the paraplegic animal. Towel walking of paraparetic dogs and sling or harness walking of dogs with cervical disease can improve attitude and promote early use of the affected limbs. Once the skin incision has healed, swimming may be instituted to encourage movement. In dogs with a prolonged anticipated recovery period, use of a paraplegic cart can provide a stimulus for recovery (Fig. 72-10). Improvement in neurologic function usually occurs within 1 week of surgery. No improvement after 21 days signals that the prognosis for recovery is poor.

## FIBROCARTILAGINOUS EMBOLISM

Acute infarction and ischemic necrosis of the spinal cord parenchyma can occur as a result of fibrocartilage lodging in the very small arteries and veins supplying the spinal cord parenchyma and leptomeninges. This very acute, nonprogressive phenomenon can affect any region of the spinal cord and result in paresis or paralysis.

The cause of FCE is unknown. The fibrocartilaginous material that makes up the embolus appears to originate in the nucleus pulposus of the intervertebral disk. How this fibrocartilaginous material gains access to the spinal cord blood vessels is still a matter of debate. Concurrent clinically significant intervertebral disk degeneration is not common.

This disorder is most common in medium-sized and large-breed dogs. It has also been described in small-breed dogs (especially the Miniature Schnauzer) and a few cats. Most affected dogs are middle aged, with the majority of cases from 3 to 7 years of age. A few dogs younger than 1 year of age have been recognized with FCE. No gender predilection exists.

## Clinical Features

The onset of neurologic signs is very sudden. Occasionally, signs may progressively worsen for 2 to 6 hours. In approximately half of all cases, FCE occurs immediately after minor trauma or during exertion.

Neurologic examination reflects a focal spinal cord lesion. The deficits observed depend on the region of spinal cord affected and the severity of cord involvement. The thoracolumbar cord and lumbosacral intumescence are affected with equal frequency. The cervical cord is affected less frequently, but it is the site most often affected in small breeds of dogs. Neurologic dysfunction may be mild or severe. Asymmetry is common, with the right and left sides affected to different degrees. Dogs commonly cry out as though in pain at the onset of signs, and dogs evaluated within 2 to 6 hours of onset will sometimes exhibit focal spinal hyperpathia (i.e., painfulness), but this resolves quickly so that most affected dogs are not painful by the time they are brought to a veterinarian, even on manipulation of their spine. The lack of pain and the asymmetry are very helpful in differentiating FCE from other disorders that cause acute nonprogressive neurologic dysfunction, such as acute intervertebral disk protrusion, trauma, and diskospondylitis.

## Diagnosis

FCE is suspected based on the signalment, history, and recognition of acute, nonprogressive, nonpainful spinal cord dysfunction. Radiographs of the affected spinal region assist in ruling out diskospondylitis, fractures, lytic vertebral neoplasia, and intervertebral disk disease. Radiographs are normal in dogs and cats with FCE. CSF is usually normal, although an increase in protein (especially albumin) concentration may be observed in some (50%) cases. In the first 24 hours after the onset of clinical signs, a few dogs have a mild increase in neutrophil numbers within the CSF. Myelography is usually normal, although some animals may exhibit subtle focal cord swelling. Myelography is most useful to rule out compressive lesions of the spinal cord for which surgery might be indicated, such as fractures, disk protrusion, and neoplasia.

CT has not been useful in the diagnosis of FCE but is also helpful in excluding a compressive myelopathy. MRI may re-

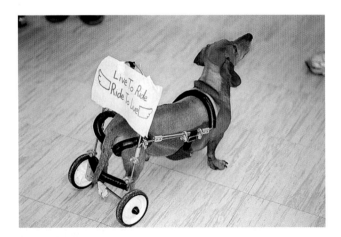

**FIG 72-10**
The use of a paraplegic cart can provide a stimulus for recovery and improve mobility and attitude in paralyzed dogs recovering from thoracolumbar disk surgery.

veal focal cord density changes in severely affected dogs, but mild lesions will not be evident. The diagnosis of FCE can only be made by exclusion of compressive and inflammatory acute spinal cord disorders (Fig. 72-11).

### Treatment

Treatment for FCE consists of nonspecific supportive measures and nursing care as described for paralyzed dogs. Most affected dogs are large breeds, making this management difficult. Although corticosteroids have been recommended and used, their effect on outcome has not been documented. In animals brought to the clinician during first 6 hours of paralysis, it may be reasonable to treat aggressively with one dose of corticosteroids as recommended for the initial treatment of acute spinal cord trauma. Most clinical improvement takes place within the first 7 to 10 days after the onset of neurologic signs, although it may take 6 to 8 weeks for a complete return to function. If no improvement is seen within 21 days, it is unlikely that the dog or cat will improve.

### Prognosis

Approximately 50% of dogs and cats with FCE recover sufficiently to be returned to their owners as acceptable pets. The prognosis is best for recovery in dogs and cats with intact deep pain sensation and strictly UMN signs, including increased muscle tone and hyperactive reflexes. Dogs and cats that have involvement of the spinal cord at the brachial or lumbosacral intumescence (C6 to T2 or L4 to S3) exhibit LMN signs, such as rapid muscle atrophy, loss of muscle tone, and diminished reflexes in the affected limbs. Urinary and fe-cal incontinence may be present if the lumbosacral cord is involved. Animals with severe LMN signs or absent deep pain sensation have a very poor prognosis for satisfactory recovery from FCE.

## SUBACUTE PROGRESSIVE SPINAL CORD DYSFUNCTION

### INFECTIOUS INFLAMMATORY DISEASE

All of the infectious inflammatory diseases discussed in Chapter 71 can result in myelitis (i.e., spinal cord inflammation), leading to progressive neurologic signs suggesting multifocal or focal spinal cord damage. CSF analysis is necessary to confirm that inflammatory disease is present. Additional diagnostic tests may be necessary to identify an etiology (see Chapter 71).

### NONINFECTIOUS INFLAMMATORY DISEASE

Noninfectious inflammatory diseases, specifically GME, breed-associated meningeal vasculitis, steroid-responsive suppurative meningitis, and feline polioencephalomyelitis, can affect the spinal cord. Cervical pain is a constant feature of steroid-responsive meningitis and breed-associated meningeal vasculitis. Neurologic deficits are variable, being most common with GME and uncommon with steroid-responsive meningitis. CSF analysis is necessary to confirm inflammatory myelitis, and additional tests are required to rule out infectious etiologies. See Chapter 71 for more information on these syndromes.

### DISKOSPONDYLITIS

Diskospondylitis is an infection of the intervertebral disks with concurrent osteomyelitis in the adjacent end plates and vertebral bodies. In most dogs and cats with diskospondylitis, no underlying cause for the disorder can be determined. The mode of introduction of organisms is thought to be hematogenous in nearly all cases, with extension from a local site or migration of an inhaled foreign body responsible for a small number of cases. Urinary tract infections, dermatitis, bacterial endocarditis, prostatitis, dental disease, and orchitis may serve as primary sites of infection, resulting in bacteremia and dissemination of bacteria through the blood to the vertebrae. Subchondral vascular loops may slow circulation in the vertebral epiphysis, promoting blood sludging and colonization by blood-borne organisms. The infection then spreads by local extension to the disk.

Numerous causative organisms have been isolated from dogs and cats with diskospondylitis. Among the most common are the coagulase-positive *Staphylococcus* spp., *Streptococcus* spp., *E. coli*, and *Brucella canis* (in dogs). The fungal organisms *Aspergillus terreus* and *Paecilomyces varioti* have been isolated from a few cases. *Actinomyces* spp. have been implicated in diskospondylitis caused by grass awn migration.

Diskospondylitis occurs most often in medium- to large-breed dogs of any age. German Shepherds and Labrador

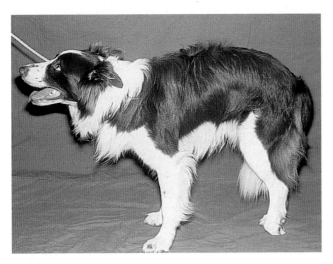

**FIG 72-11**
This adult Border Collie had an acute onset of lameness, decreased conscious proprioception, and hyporeflexia in the left rear limb while retrieving a Frisbee. The limb was not painful, and radiographs, cerebrospinal fluid (CSF), and myelogram were all normal. A presumptive diagnosis of fibrocartilaginous embolism (FCE) involving the lumbar and sacral spinal cord segments on the left side was made. This dog recovered uneventfully within a 3-week period.

Retrievers may have an increased prevalence of this disorder. Diskospondylitis is very rarely diagnosed in cats; no known age or breed predilection exists. Males are affected more often than females in both species.

## Clinical Features

The most common presenting complaint is spinal pain. Palpation of the affected region of the spine often allows localization of the lesion. Systemic signs such as fever, anorexia, depression, and weight loss occur in 30% of affected dogs, but hematologic inflammatory changes are rarely observed. Secondary (i.e., reactive) polyarthritis may occur, resulting in a generally stiff, stilted gait in some dogs.

Neurologic deficits in dogs and cats with diskospondylitis are uncommon and do not correlate with the degree of spinal cord compression. Neurologic dysfunction can result from spinal cord compression by proliferating bone, granulation tissue, and fibrous connective tissue at the site of infection from vertebral subluxation or from inflammation extending from the underlying bone to the meninges and spinal cord. Extension of actual infection to the neurologic tissues is extremely rare, except in animals with diskospondylitis secondary to foreign body (usually grass awn) migration. Dogs with grass awn–associated diskospondylitis often have other evidence of infection, which may include pyothorax, draining paralumbar tracts, or palpable sublumbar lymph nodes or abscesses.

## Diagnosis

The diagnosis of diskospondylitis is suspected after physical examination and confirmed by radiographic examination of the affected vertebrae. Radiographic changes of diskospondylitis characteristically involve the ventral structures of affected vertebrae. Changes include end plate erosion and focal lysis of one or both vertebral end plates, collapse of the disk space, proliferative bony changes adjacent to the disk space, and sclerosis at the margins of bone loss (Fig. 72-12). The most commonly affected sites are the midthoracic, caudal cervical, thoracolumbar, and lumbosacral spine. It is common for diskospondylitis to affect more than one disk space (Fig. 72-13), so survey radiographs of the entire spine are recommended. Radiographic signs of diskospondylitis may not be apparent for several weeks after the onset of clinical signs. MRI evidence of diskospondylitis will precede radiographically apparent lesions.

Blood culture is the most rewarding noninvasive method of isolating the organism responsible for the vertebral infection, yielding the organism in approximately half of the cases. Cardiac, urogenital, and hepatic systems should be evaluated as potential sources of infection. Although culture of the urine is often positive (25%), it does not reliably yield the organism responsible for the diskospondylitis. Percutaneous needle aspiration of the infected disk during general anesthesia using fluoroscopy has been effective in yielding positive cultures in some cases with negative blood and urine cultures. A spinal needle is guided into the disk space using fluoroscopy or CT and a small amount of sterile saline (0.3 to 0.5 ml) is injected

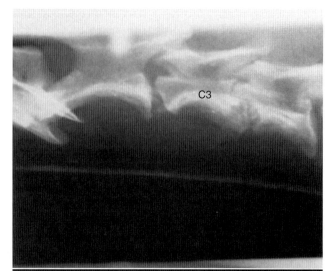

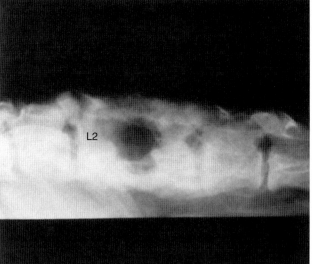

**FIG 72-12**
**A,** Lateral radiograph of cervical vertebral column of adult dog showing diskospondylitis between the third and fourth cervical vertebrae (C3 and C4). **B,** Lateral radiograph of lumbar vertebral column of an adult Pointer showing severe chronic diskospondylitis between the second and third lumbar vertebrae (L2 and L3). (**A,** Courtesy Dr. C. Fries, University of Saskatchewan.)

and then aspirated for culture. *Brucella* serology or PCR should be considered in all affected dogs because of the public health significance (see p. 1317), despite its very low prevalence (<10%) in the United States and Canada.

## Treatment

Initial treatment of diskospondylitis usually consists of antibiotics, cage rest, and antibiotics. If an organism is isolated, susceptibility testing should guide antibiotic therapy. If an organism is not found, initial treatment attempts should be directed against *Staphylococcus* spp. Bactericidal antibiotics with a spectrum against gram-positive organisms and the ability to con-

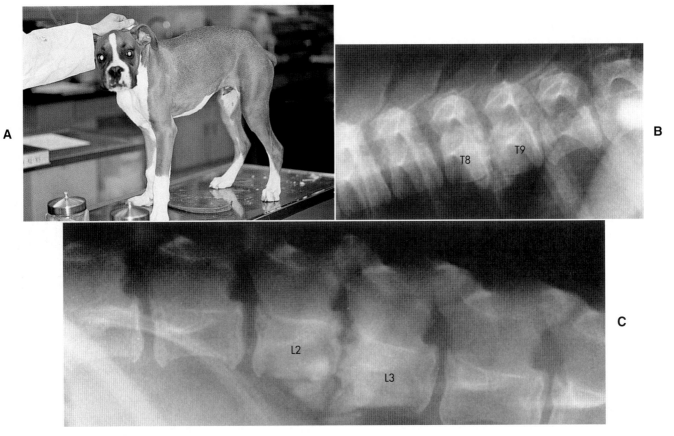

**FIG 72-13**
**A,** A 5-month-old Boxer puppy with back pain resulting from diskospondylitis. **B** and
**C,** Lateral spinal radiographs reveal lesions at T8-T9 and L2-L3, with destruction of adjacent
vertebral body end plates, collapse of the intervertebral disk spaces, shortening of the
vertebral bodies, and new bone production around the ends of the affected vertebral bodies.

centrate in bone are recommended. First-generation cephalosporins (cefazolin 25 mg/kg IV q8h, cephalexin 22 mg/kg PO q8h) and amoxicillin with clavulanate (Clavamox 12.5 to 25 mg/kg PO q8h) have been effective. Quinolones can be added if gram-negative organisms are suspected. Penicillin is the antibiotic of choice for *Actinomyces* infections associated with grass awn migration. Antibiotics are administered parenterally for the first 3 days whenever fever, neurologic deficits, or rapidly progressing signs are present. Antibiotic therapy is continued orally for at least 8 weeks, up to 6 months, if necessary. Most dogs show very rapid clinical improvement within the first week of treatment.

Animals that worsen or do not improve after 5 days of antibiotic therapy must be reevaluated. Failure to respond could be the result of infection with *B. canis* (dog), with another organism not sensitive to the antibiotic selected, or with a mycotic organism. If multiple sites of vertebral infection exist, changing to another broad-spectrum bactericidal antibiotic is a potential treatment. If only one site is involved, vertebral body fine needle aspiration or surgery to obtain a culture should be considered.

Dogs and cats with severe paresis or paralysis may not improve neurologically after conservative medical therapy. CSF analysis and myelography or MRI should be considered to rule out meningitis and determine the degree of spinal cord compression. Decompressive surgery and curettage for culture followed by stabilization may be necessary if severe neurologic deficits are still present 5 to 10 days after initiating antibiotic therapy and myelography reveals severe spinal cord compression. The prognosis is guarded in dogs and cats with severe neurologic dysfunction, regardless of treatment. When grass awn migration and diskospondylitis resulting from *Actinomyces* spp. occur, surgical removal of the grass awn followed by antibiotic treatment of the cultured organism is ideal, but it is rarely feasible. Most cases are instead treated with ampicillin (22 mg/kg PO q8h), amoxicillin (20 mg/kg PO q8h) or Clavamox (12.5 to 25 mg/kg PO q8h) for a minimum of 6 months, and sometimes for life.

In addition to antibiotic therapy, the patient's activity should be restricted to minimize discomfort and decrease the chance of pathologic fracture and luxation. Analgesics may be administered for 3 to 5 days if absolutely necessary, but their use will make it difficult to assess the efficacy of antibiotic therapy and may make it more difficult to enforce strict cage rest.

Dogs and cats treated medically should be reevaluated clinically and radiographically every 3 weeks. With time, the lytic process should resolve and the affected vertebrae should fuse. Antibiotics should be administered for a minimum of 8 weeks. Ideally, blood cultures should be repeated 2 weeks after antibiotic therapy is discontinued, and radiographs should be reevaluated 2 months after treatment is completed. Most treated animals do not relapse, unless the diskospondylitis is caused by grass awn migration.

# CHRONIC PROGRESSIVE SPINAL CORD DYSFUNCTION

## NEOPLASIA

Tumors that grow and compress or damage spinal cord parenchyma frequently cause chronic, progressively worsening signs of spinal cord dysfunction. Spinal tumors can be primary or metastatic. The most common tumors affecting the spinal cord in the dog are extradural tumors arising from the vertebral body (e.g., osteosarcoma, chondrosarcoma, fibrosarcoma, myeloma) and extradural soft tissue tumors, including metastatic hemangiosarcoma or carcinoma, liposarcoma, and lymphoma. Intradural extramedullary tumors such as meningiomas and peripheral nerve sheath tumors (see p. 1049) are also common, comprising 35% of all spinal tumors. Intramedullary tumors (i.e., astrocytomas, ependymomas, metastatic tumors) are relatively rare in the dog, with the exception of metastatic hemangiosarcoma. Extradural lymphoma is the only common spinal tumor in the cat.

Spinal tumors occur with equal frequency in males and females and can occur in any breed of dog or cat, although large-breed dogs are most often affected. Most spinal cord tumors are found in middle-aged and older dogs, with the mean age at the time of diagnosis being 5 to 6 years. Two noteworthy exceptions are lymphoma, which can affect dogs of any age, and neuroepithelioma, a primary intradural extramedullary tumor that has a predilection for T10 to L1 in young dogs, particularly German Shepherds and Golden Retrievers. In addition, vertebral osteomas may occur in young dogs and result in spinal cord compression, as can cartilaginous exostoses, benign proliferative lesions of the bone indistinguishable from neoplasia except by biopsy (see Fig. 66-7; Fig. 72-14). Spinal lymphoma is most common in young (mean age, 4 years) adult feline leukemia (FeLV)-positive cats. Certainly spinal neoplasia cannot be eliminated as a differential diagnosis strictly based on signalment.

### Clinical Features

Clinical signs are usually insidious and related to the location of the tumor. Early diagnosis is difficult because neurologic abnormalities are not clinically apparent until there has been significant compression of the spinal cord. Many animals have months of slowly progressive clinical signs before a diagnosis is made. Pain may be a prominent feature in dogs and cats with nerve root tumors encroaching on the spinal cord, tumors involving the meninges, and aggressive tumors involving bone. Progressively worsening lameness and pain on

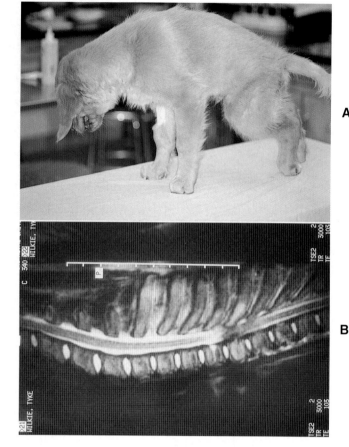

**FIG 72-14**
**A,** A 3-month old Golden Retriever puppy with spinal pain and progressive upper motor neuron (UMN) signs in both rear limbs resulting from a vertebral osteoma. **B,** Magnetic resonance imaging (MRI) showing severe compressive spinal cord damage from the caudal aspect of the T4 vertebral body extending caudally through the T6 vertebral body.

limb manipulation (i.e., radicular pain, root signature) without initial neurologic deficits are common in dogs with peripheral nerve sheath tumors involving nerve roots in the cervical or lumbar intumescence. An ipsilateral Horner's syndrome and/or loss of the panniculus reflex may be seen if the thoracic nerve roots are involved. Pain is not a common feature of intramedullary spinal cord primary tumors or metastases.

Differential diagnoses must include other disorders that can cause slowly progressive neurologic dysfunction, including type II disk protrusion, degenerative myelopathy (DM), and diskospondylitis. Highly malignant extradural tumors such as lymphoma and primary or metastatic intramedullary tumors may cause rapidly progressive neurologic signs similar to inflammatory spinal cord diseases. On rare occasions, rapidly growing intradural tumors cause hemorrhage into the cord and an acute onset of paralysis; this is most common in dogs with metastatic spinal cord malignancies (e.g., hemangiosarcoma, adenocarcinoma). Spontaneous fractures of ver-

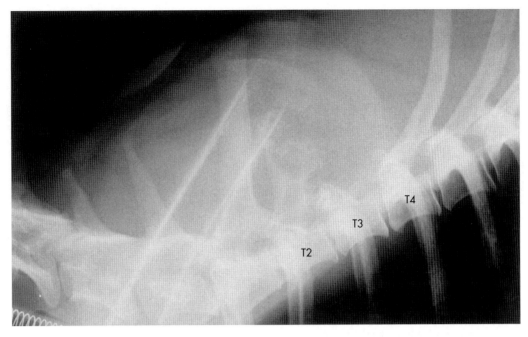

**FIG 72-15**
Lateral spinal radiograph from a 2-year-old Irish Setter with a 1-week history of progressive ataxia and a 12-hour history of upper motor neuron (UMN) paralysis of the rear limbs and Schiff-Sherrington syndrome. The entire spinous process of T3, the roof of T3, and most of the spinous process of T2 are destroyed, most consistent with a neoplastic process. An undifferentiated sarcoma at this site was identified on postmortem examination.

tebrae damaged by tumor may also result in an acute onset of pain and neurologic dysfunction.

## Diagnosis

Neoplasia may be suspected after evaluation of the signalment, history, physical examination, screening blood tests, and plain radiographs. Definitive diagnosis frequently requires CSF analysis, further diagnostic imaging (i.e., myelography, CT, MRI), and histopathologic evaluation of the lesion. Whenever a neoplasm is considered as a differential diagnosis, a complete physical examination is necessary to look for sites of primary tumor. Fundic examination, palpation of lymph nodes, and rectal examination should be performed, and thoracic and abdominal radiographs should be taken to identify a primary tumor site or metastasic lesions. Ultrasonographic examination of the spleen, liver, and heart should be performed in dogs whenever metastatic hemangiosarcoma is suspected. Most dogs with spinal cord lymphoma have multicentric disease, so aspiration of the lymph nodes and examination of peripheral blood or bone marrow smears is warranted. A high percentage of cats with spinal lymphoma are FeLV-positive (> 80%), and many have obvious systemic disease and hematologic evidence of bone marrow involvement.

Survey radiographs of the affected region of the spine are recommended. Spinal tumors are usually not visible unless osteolysis (e.g., myeloma) is obvious or bone proliferation in association with the tumor (e.g., osteosarcoma) is seen (Fig. 72-15). Tumors within the vertebral canal may occasionally cause a loss of bone density, resulting in an apparent widening of the vertebral canal. Occasionally, a pressure-induced enlargement of the intervertebral foramen is seen at the site where a nerve root tumor enters the spinal canal.

Performance of CSF analysis should precede myelography. In spinal tumors, the CSF may reveal slight increases in protein concentration with or without increases in mononuclear cell numbers, but this finding is inconsistent and nonspecific. CSF from the lumbar region is more likely to be abnormal (>85%) than CSF from the cerebellomedullary cistern (>25%). Neoplastic cells are rarely identified, although cats with intradural lymphoma will often have diagnostic CSF with a pleocytosis consisting almost entirely of neoplastic lymphocytes (Fig. 72-16). Cats with the more common extradural lymphoma typically have normal CSF, whereas dogs with extradural lymphoma commonly have extensive meningeal infiltration and diagnostic CSF. Other tumor types rarely exfoliate into the fluid sufficiently to make a diagnosis. Fine needle aspiration of extradural lesions under fluoroscopy has been used to successfully diagnose lymphoma. Myelography is a fairly reliable method to identify and localize spinal tumors (see Fig. 66-7). Standard lateral and dorsoventral or ventrodorsal views should be examined. Occasionally additional oblique views can help to further define the lesion. Based on the myelogram, lesions can be characterized as intramedullary, extramedullary-intradural, or extradural (see Fig. 66-6). This classification is important when making

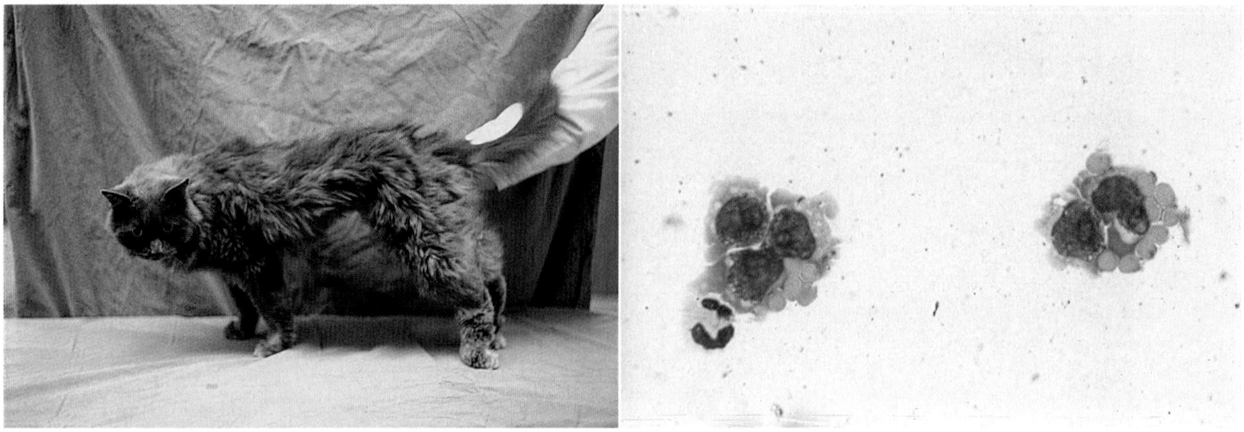

**FIG 72-16**
**A,** A 2-year-old cat with a 5-day course of progressive rear limb ataxia and upper motor neuron (UMN) paresis. **B,** Cerebrospinal fluid (CSF) revealed an increased cell count consisting predominantly of neoplastic lymphoid cells.

therapeutic recommendations. Where available, advanced imaging techniques (i.e., CT, MRI) can add valuable information regarding precise tumor location and degree of spinal cord involvement, which may be important when considering surgical treatment and/or radiation therapy.

### Treatment

Surgical decompression and attempts at complete tumor excision are usually limited to well-encapsulated intradural extramedullary tumors. Feline noninvasive intradural extramedullary meningiomas may have a good prognosis after surgical excision. Extradural tumors of bone origin usually cannot be removed without creating overwhelming compromise of the structural integrity of the vertebral canal. Even with aggressive surgical treatment of vertebral tumors, local recurrence and metastases are common. Intramedullary tumors cannot usually be treated successfully because of their intimate involvement with neural tissue. Chemotherapy and radiation therapy as primary or postoperative adjuvant therapies have met with limited success in the treatment of spinal tumors in dogs and cats. Radiation therapy may be of some benefit in dogs and cats with spinal lymphoma. Corticosteroids, although they have little effect on most tumors, can decrease tumor-associated edema and result in remarkable temporary improvement. Lymphoreticular tumors such as lymphoma and myeloma can be treated with traditional chemotherapy protocols, although only a few of the drugs used cross the blood-brain barrier (e.g., corticosteroids, cytosine arabinoside) and the long-term prognosis is poor (see Chapter 82).

### INTRASPINAL ARTICULAR CYSTS

Cysts arising from the joint capsule of spinal facetal joints can, through enlargement, cause chronic progressive focal compression of the spinal cord or nerve roots. These cysts can result from an out pouching of the synovium (i.e., synovial cysts) or they may arise from mucinous degeneration of periarticular connective tissue (i.e., ganglion cysts). Synovial cysts and ganglion cysts are clinically indistinguishable and both arise sec-

ondary to degenerative changes in the facetal joints. Degenerative changes occur because of congenital malformations, vertebral instability, or after trauma. Signs are referable to the site and degree of resulting spinal cord or nerve root compression. Young giant breeds of dogs such as Mastiffs and Great Danes most commonly develop single or multiple cysts in the cervical region, which cause an UMN myelopathy and occasionally cervical pain. Older dogs, particularly German Shepherds, have been identified with thoracolumbar or lumbosacral articular cysts that cause spinal cord or cauda equina compression. Radiographs reveal degenerative changes of the articular facets. CSF analysis reveals normal cytology and slightly increased protein (i.e., albuminocytologic dissociation) consistent with a noninflammatory chronic compressive myelopathy. Myelography reveals focal extradural compression. MRI is necessary to identify the facetal joints as the origin of the cysts and to precisely localize the cysts before surgical therapy. Treatment consists of spinal cord decompression, cyst drainage, and arthrodesis of the facetal joint, with excellent results.

### TYPE II INTERVERTEBRAL DISK DISEASE

Fibroid degeneration of the intervertebral disk occurs in some dogs as part of the aging process. Partial rupture of the disk annulus allows prolapse of a small amount of disk nucleus into the annulus fibrosus. This, in conjunction with an accompanying fibrotic reaction, results in a round, domelike bulging of the dorsal surface of the disk into the spinal canal (see Fig. 72-4). Repetitive partial prolapse and the accompanying response cause slowly progressive signs of spinal cord compression. This type of disk protrusion (i.e., Hansen's type II) is seen most commonly in aging large-breed dogs, particularly German Shepherds, Labrador Retrievers, and Doberman Pinschers but has also been recognized occasionally in small-breed dogs.

### Clinical Features

Clinical signs result primarily from spinal cord compression, although spinal discomfort is apparent in a few dogs. Thoracolumbar type II disk disease is most common, resulting in UMN signs to the rear limbs with normal forelimbs. Cervical type II disk disease (and type I extrusion) may be seen in Doberman Pinschers, particularly in association with the cervical vertebral malformation-malarticulation syndrome (i.e., wobbler syndrome; see p. 1040). In these dogs, thoracic and pelvic limbs are affected, with neurologic signs most prominent in the pelvic limbs. Cervical pain is present if nerve roots are compressed or when concurrent type I disk herniation is present.

## Diagnosis

Slowly progressive signs of spinal cord dysfunction should prompt consideration of type II disk disease, DM, neoplasia, and diskospondylitis as differential diagnoses. Neurologic examination should allow localization of the lesion.

Radiographs of the spine may help to identify type II disk disease but may be normal in some affected dogs. Disk space narrowing, osteophyte production, and end-plate sclerosis are commonly seen at multiple sites; thus they are not very helpful in localizing the lesion. A myelogram or advanced imaging technique (i.e., CT, MRI) is necessary to determine the extent and location of the lesion and to distinguish disk protrusion from spinal neoplasia and DM.

## Treatment

Treatment with corticosteroids (prednisone 0.2 mg/kg PO q24-48h) may result in neurologic improvement for a short time in dogs with type II disk protrusion. This treatment is not curative, however, and surgery is recommended as the definitive treatment. Ventral decompression is performed if the cervical vertebrae are affected, whereas hemilaminectomy for decompression at the site is usually attempted for type II disks in the thoracolumbar spine. Effective surgical decompression is often difficult to achieve because of the chronic nature of the lesion and the difficulty encountered in removal of the dorsal annulus. The goal of therapy is to stabilize the animal's neurologic status. The spinal cord has usually undergone considerable chronic compression before clinical signs appear; thus full recovery is rare. A few dogs experience temporary or permanent worsening of clinical signs postoperatively.

## DEGENERATIVE MYELOPATHY

A degenerative disorder of the spinal cord white matter characterized by widespread myelin and axon loss occurs most often in aging German Shepherds. DM has been recognized in dogs from 5 to 14 years of age and has rarely been seen in old dogs of other large breeds and in cats. A DM-like disorder has also been identified in the Pembroke Welsh Corgi. The thoracic and thoracolumbar spinal cord segments are most severely affected in all affected breeds; thus the neurologic findings suggest a lesion between T3 and L3.

## Etiology

The cause of DM is uncertain. Some have speculated that deficiencies of nutrients or vitamins are responsible for the widespread demyelination and degeneration of axons ob-

served histologically. An inherited cause has also been proposed in the German Shepherd. Whatever the initiating event, DM is generally considered to be an immune-mediated neurodegenerative disease similar to multiple sclerosis in humans. Depressed cell-mediated immunity and an increase in circulating immune complexes are consistent findings in dogs with DM, and spinal cord deposition of immunoglobulin and complement has been documented in association with histologic lesions of the disease.

## Clinical Features

Clinically, DM results in a slowly progressive (e.g., 6 months to 2 years) UMN paraparesis and ataxia of the rear limbs. A loss of conscious proprioception results in knuckling of the toes, wearing of the dorsal nail surfaces of the digits of the rear limbs, and severe posterior ataxia.

Increased muscle tone and hyperactivity of the rear limb tendon reflexes result in localization of the problem to the spinal cord between T3 and L3 spinal cord segments. Thoracic limbs are normal and urinary and fecal continence are maintained until very late in the course of the disease. Neurologic deficits in the rear limbs may be asymmetric. In a very small number of cases (<10%), a decrease or loss of pelvic limb reflexes is observed late in the course of the disease as a result of involvement of the dorsal spinal nerve roots important for the afferent arm of the reflex.

## Diagnosis

A diagnosis of DM is suspected in any large-breed dog with slowly progressive spinal ataxia and UMN weakness in the rear limbs. Affected dogs are systemically normal, and no site of localizable spinal pain exists. Differential diagnoses include neoplasia, type II disk disease, and musculoskeletal disease (e.g., severe hip dysplasia, bilateral anterior cruciate ligament rupture).

The antemortem diagnosis of DM is one of exclusion. Radiographs of the spine are normal, as is CSF analysis, although a slight increase in CSF protein concentration may be found. If electrodiagnostic tests are performed, spinal cord–evoked potentials may reveal abnormal spinal cord conduction, whereas EMG is normal. Myelography or other diagnostic imaging is necessary to rule out the presence of spinal cord compression or focal spinal cord neoplasia. Normal spinal radiographs, a cytologically normal CSF, and a normal myelogram in an older dog with slowly progressive UMN signs to the pelvic limbs warrant a diagnosis of DM.

## Treatment

No effective treatment exists for dogs with DM. Corticosteroids and other immunosuppressive agents have been used without long-term benefit. In fact, the administration of corticosteroids can cause muscle wasting and exacerbation of the muscle weakness in this disease. Some investigators have advocated vitamin (i.e., vitamin E, vitamin B complex, vitamin C) and omega-3 fatty acid supplementation. Exercise may be helpful in slowing the progression of the disease. Walking, running, and swimming for 30 minutes every other day is recommended. Some studies report success after the administration of aminocaproic acid (EACA) (Amicar; Lederle Laboratories,

American Cyanamide, Wayne, N.J.), 500 mg by mouth every 8 hours. This drug blocks the final common pathway of tissue inflammation and may slow or halt the progression of DM in a few cases. Drawbacks of EACA therapy include gastrointestinal irritation, high cost, and a need to treat for 2 to 3 months before response to treatment is detectable. Administration of EACA in combination with the potent antioxidant acetylcysteine (25 mg/kg administered as a 5% solution PO q8h for 14 days, then every other day) has also been recommended. In the absence of other effective treatments for DM, these unproven treatments should be considered.

## CAUDA EQUINA SYNDROME

In dogs the last three lumbar spinal cord segments (L5, L6, L7) are within the fourth lumbar vertebra, the sacral segments (S1, S2, S3) are within the body of the fifth lumbar vertebra, and the coccygeal segments are within the sixth lumbar vertebra. Nerve roots from these lumbar, sacral, and coccygeal segments of the spinal cord exit the spinal canal through the intervertebral foramina caudal to the vertebrae with the same number; thus they must course a considerable distance within the vertebral canal caudal to the point of termination of the spinal cord (Fig. 72-17). This collection of nerve roots descending in the vertebral canal is termed the *cauda equina.* The spinal nerves from the sacral and caudal segments overlie the lumbosacral junction, so compressive diseases of this region are likely to involve the L7, sacral, and caudal nerves.

Compression of the nerves of the cauda equina can occur secondary to intervertebral disk protrusion, tumor, diskospondylitis, vertebral or sacral osteochondrosis, congenital bony malformation, or progressive proliferation of tissues in the lumbosacral region (i.e., degenerative lumbosacral stenosis). Acquired type II disk prolapse with progressive lumbosacral stenosis occurring secondary to spinal instability, bone remodeling, and soft tissue proliferation in older, large-breed dogs is the most common cause of cauda equina compression. German Shepherds, Labrador Retrievers, and Belgian Malinois, particularly those used as working dogs, are most often affected with the disorder. It primarily affects male dogs over the age of 5 years.

Genetic predisposition, conformation, physical activity, and vertebral malformations are all factors proposed to cause increased mechanical stress on the intervertebral disk at the lumbosacral junction, promoting type II disk prolapse. Loss of the structural strength of the disk worsens instability at the site, resulting in proliferative changes in the articular facets, joint capsules, and the interarcuate ligament (i.e., ligamentum flavum). These proliferative changes result in further narrowing of the vertebral canal, compression of the cauda equina, and compression of the nerve roots as they exit the foramina.

### Clinical Features

Compression of the cauda equina results in a very characteristic constellation of clinical signs. Affected dogs are slow to rise from a prone position and reluctant to run, sit up, jump,

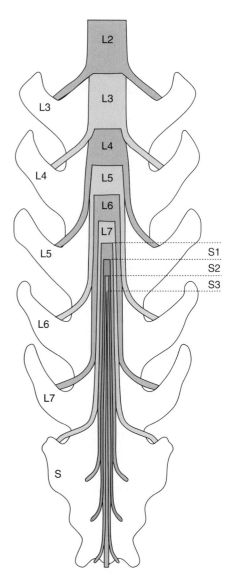

**FIG 72-17**
The anatomy of the cauda equina region in the dog. L5-L7 spinal cord segments sit within the L4 vertebra. S1-S3 spinal cord segments are within the L5 vertebra, and the coccygeal segments are within L6. Nerve roots from all of the lumbar, sacral, and coccygeal spinal cord segments leave the canal through the intervertebral foramen just caudal to the vertebra with the same number so that these nerve roots course a considerable distance within the vertebral canal.

or climb stairs. Rear limb lameness and weakness worsen with exercise as the blood vessels accompanying the spinal nerve roots within the already crowded intervertebral foramen dilate and further compress the nerve roots (i.e., neurogenic intermittent claudication). Affected dogs may be reluctant to raise or wag their tails. Hyperesthesia or paresthesia of the perineum may develop, with self-inflicted moist dermatitis of the perineum and tail base. Urinary and fecal incontinence rarely occur.

The most consistent physical examination finding is pain elicited by deep palpation of the dorsal sacrum or by dorsiflexion of the tail or hyperextension of the lumbosacral region (Fig. 72-18). If no neurologic deficits exist, it can be difficult to distinguish affected dogs from those with pain and lameness caused by diskospondylitis, prostatic disease, gracilis muscle contracture, or degenerative joint disease resulting from dysplasia or cranial cruciate ligament rupture. Rear limb weakness, atrophy of the muscles of the caudal thigh and distal limb (i.e., sciatic innervation), and a decrease in limb flexion (especially hock flexion) during the withdrawal reflex are seen when lumbosacral spinal canal narrowing progresses to cause compression of the L7, sacral, and caudal spinal nerves. The patellar reflex may appear increased in some dogs because of a loss of tone in the opposing caudal thigh muscles. Urinary dysfunction can occur because of interference with pelvic and pudendal nerve (S1 to S3) function, resulting in urine dribbling and a large, flaccid bladder that is easily expressed. A few dogs develop reflex dysynergia, where although they recognize that they have a full bladder and posture and strain to urinate, only a small volume or an interrupted stream of urine is produced with a large residual volume.

## Diagnosis

Clinical findings are often the primary basis for reaching a diagnosis in affected dogs, because many of the routinely available diagnostic tests may be difficult to interpret. Spinal radiographs are useful to rule out causes of cauda equina compression (e.g., diskospondylitis, lytic vertebral neoplasia, fracture/luxation) and to identify predisposing factors for degenerative stenosis (e.g., sacral osteochondrosis, vertebral malformations). Radiographs most commonly reveal end plate sclerosis and spondylosis of the ventral and lateral margins of the L7 and S1 vertebral end plates (Fig. 72-19). Narrowing or collapse of the L7-S1 intervertebral disk space may occur. Ventral displacement of the body of S1 relative to L7 has also been reported. Caution is critical when interpreting radiographs of this region, because these same abnormalities are common in clinically normal dogs.

CSF collection and analysis to rule out inflammatory CNS disease should be performed before administration of radiographic contrast material for further diagnostic imaging. Myelography is sometimes useful for documenting cauda equina compression, but it will not be diagnostic in those dogs (20%) where the dural sac ends cranial to the lumbosacral junction or in dogs where the primary lesion is lateral compression of the spinal nerves at the intervertebral foramen. Lesions overlying the sacrum or tail may be better delineated by epidurography (see Fig. 72-19) or diskography. Electromyography (EMG) of the pelvic limb, paraspinal, and tail muscles, when available, can suggest denervation of the muscles innervated by the cauda equina, confirming a clinical suspicion of cauda equina compression. EMG can also be used to detect polymyositis and polyneuropathy in dogs where the diagnosis is in question. When available, MRI provides the most sensitive, accurate, and noninvasive means of evaluating the lumbosacral region, allowing visualization of all components potentially involved in cauda equina com-

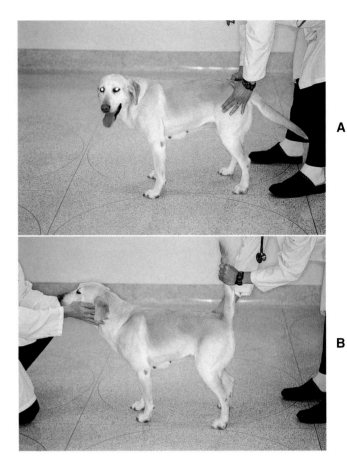

**FIG 72-18**
Dogs affected by cauda equina syndrome will often experience pain upon **(A)** deep palpation of the dorsal sacrum and **(B)** dorsiflexion of the tail.

pression (see Fig. 72-19). The use of MRI to characterize the anatomic components of compression is especially important when surgical treatment is being considered.

## Treatment

Restriction of exercise and the administration of analgesics or antiinflammatory drugs may result in temporary improvement in dogs with clinical signs limited to pain and lameness. More definitive treatment involves lumbosacral dorsal laminectomy, excision of compressing tissues, and L7 to S1 foraminotomy when necessary. Decompression together with a distraction-fusion technique has been advocated for patients with significant collapse of the lumbosacral space and foramen causing entrapment and compression of the L7 nerve root. Descriptions of the surgical procedures are provided in the Suggested Readings listed at the end of this chapter. Rapid relief from pain occurs in most dogs. Strict confinement is important for 4 to 8 weeks postoperatively followed by a gradual return to exercise and work. The prognosis is excellent for resolution of lameness and mild neurologic deficits. Most dogs with mild-to-moderate deficits will return to working function. Dogs with severe LMN deficits or incontinence are likely to have permanent deficits.

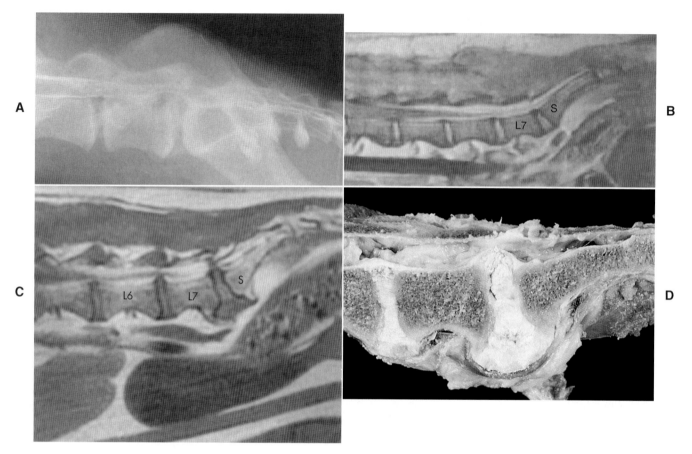

**FIG 72-19**
**A,** Epidurogram revealing a large ventral epidural mass at L7-S1 in a 5-year-old Dalmatian. The height of the vertebral canal is reduced by well over 50%. **B,** Normal midline sagittal T1 on a magnetic resonance image (MRI) scan of the lumbar spine of a dog. (The image reveals the high signal intensity *[white]* of the nucleus pulposus and the epidural fat, in contrast to the lesser signal density of the spinal cord and the nerve roots of the cauda equina *[darker]*.) **C,** MRI from a dog with lumbosacral pain showing T1-weighted midline sagittal, displacement of epidural fat and ventral and dorsal compression of the nerve roots at the L7-S1 disk space. Spondylosis deformans ventral to the L7-S1 intervertebral disk space and disk protrusion at the L6-L7 space can also be seen. **D,** Postmortem dissection of the lumbosacral region of a German Shepherd with acquired degenerative lumbosacral stenosis and type II disk protrusion. The vertebral canal is compromised at the lumbosacral junction, resulting in compression of the nerves of the cauda equina. (**A,** Courtesy Dr. John Pharr, University of Saskatchewan. **B** and **C,** Courtesy Dr. Greg Daniel, University of Tennessee.)

# CERVICAL VERTEBRAL INSTABILITY/MALFORMATION (WOBBLER SYNDROME)

*Canine wobbler syndrome* is a term used to describe caudal cervical spinal cord and nerve root compression in large-breed dogs that occurs secondary to developmental malformations, instability, or instability-associated changes in the spinal canal. Vertebral canal narrowing can be the result of malformed vertebral laminae, hypertrophy of the ligamentum flavum, articular facet enlargement, periarticular soft tissue hypertrophy, or a combination of these. In addition, changes in the vertebral body and end plates can result in instability that leads to intervertebral disk failure and the de-

velopment of type II disk protrusions or occasionally type I disk herniation.

Typically, Great Danes and Doberman Pinschers are affected, but the condition has been reported in many large breeds of dogs. Males may be affected more often than females. Age at presentation varies from 7 weeks to 10 years. Stenosis of the cranial aspect of the cervical vertebrae (usually C4, C5, or C6) and articular facet deformities are the most common abnormalities in young Great Danes. Vertebral column instability with spinal cord compression by secondary soft tissue hypertrophy or disk, with or without cervical vertebral malformation (usually C5, C6, or C7), is more commonly recognized in middle-aged and older Dobermans and

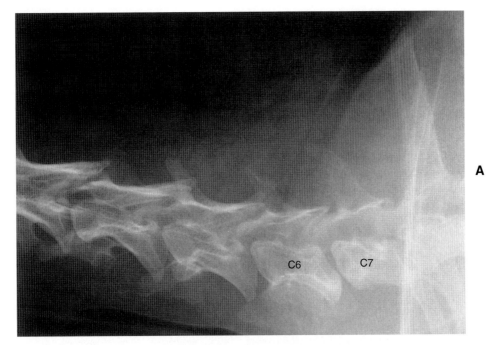

**FIG 72-20**
**A,** Radiographs of the cervical region in a 6-year-old Doberman Pinscher "wobbler" with a sudden onset of ataxia, paraparesis, proprioceptive deficits and hyperreflexia in the rear limbs, and mild cervical pain. A slight narrowing of the C6-C7 disk space can be seen; the vertebral canal is stenotic within the cranial aspect of C6 and C7.

*Continued*

in older dogs of other breeds. Genetic predisposition, overnutrition, and conformation have all been implicated in the development of this disorder.

## Clinical Features

A slowly progressive course of paresis and an incoordinated or wobbling gait, particularly in the pelvic limbs, is characteristic of this disorder. Scuffing of the toenails or a stiff gait in the forelimbs may also be present. Slowly progressive deterioration is common, but occasionally a traumatic episode results in an acute exacerbation of clinical signs. At the time of examination, neurologic deficits can be localized to the cervical spinal cord. A broad-based stance is often noted in the rear limbs. Dogs may be mildly ataxic with subtle loss of conscious proprioception, or they may be tetraplegic. Rear limbs are invariably more severely affected than forelimbs, perhaps because of the superficial position of the UMN pathways to the pelvic limbs. Resistance to dorsal extension of the cervical spine is common, but overt cervical pain is rare unless secondary disk prolapse has occurred. Lameness and muscle atrophy in one thoracic limb or pain when traction is applied to a limb (i.e., root signature; see Fig. 72-5) suggests that nerve root compression is present. Although increased tone commonly exists in the forelimbs, neurologic deficits can be subtle or undetectable. In some cases involving the caudal cervical spine, the only evidence of LMN disease in the forelimbs is pronounced muscle atrophy of the supraspinatus and infraspinatus muscles over the scapula.

## Diagnosis

The diagnosis is suspected based on signalment, history, and clinical findings. Radiographs, CSF analysis (i.e., normal CSF), and myelography allow definitive diagnosis and facilitate exclusion of other potential differential diagnoses, including neoplasia, disk disease, DM, GME, and infectious inflammatory disease. All affected animals should be evaluated for systemic disease, particularly Dobermans who may have concurrent hypothyroidism, von Willebrand's disease, or cardiomyopathy.

Radiologic diagnosis of wobbler syndrome usually requires proper positioning under general anesthesia. Although radiographs may be normal in some dogs with wobbler syndrome, most dogs have some radiographic changes, including tipping of the craniodorsal aspect of the vertebral body into the spinal canal on the lateral radiographic view, stenosis of the vertebral canal at the cranial aspect of the vertebra, collapsed disk spaces, and degenerative changes of the articular facets (Fig. 72-20, *A*). In the middle-aged Doberman, the disorder is often associated with the presence of chronic degenerative disk disease (i.e., type II disk) involving C5/6 or C6/7.

Cervical myelography is used to establish the diagnosis, determine the site of spinal cord attenuation, and judge the severity of the condition (see Fig. 72-20, *B* and *C*). Myelography or MRI should be performed whenever surgery is a treatment consideration. These tests allow visualization of cord compression dorsally by a hypertrophied ligamentum flavum, ventrally by the hypertrophied dorsal annulus fibrosus, laterally by the

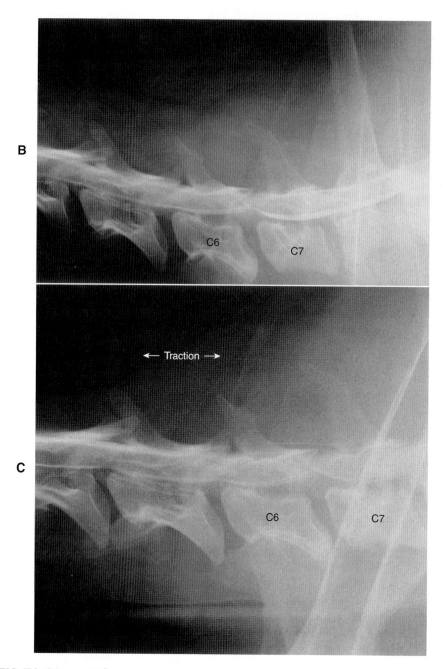

**FIG 72-20, cont'd**
**B,** Myelography shows spinal cord compression by a ventral extradural mass at C6-C7 that is not altered significantly with traction, **(C).** Surgery revealed a large amount of disk material within the vertebral canal at this site.

malformed articular facets, and circumferentially by stenosis of the vertebral canal. Standard lateral and ventrodorsal myelographic views should be evaluated, in addition to views taken while traction is applied to the neck. Compressive lesions noted on the routine views that are markedly reduced with traction are "dynamic" lesions, usually caused by redundant annulus fibrosus or ligamentous tissue (Fig. 72-21). "Static" lesions that do not improve are most often due to herniation of nucleus pulposus (type I disk) or bony malformations (see Fig. 72-20). Rational decisions regarding therapy and prognosis can be

made after determining whether compression is at one site or many, is primarily dorsal or ventral, and is static or dynamic.

## Treatment

The clinical course of untreated wobbler syndrome is chronically progressive. Medical or surgical therapy can be used to attempt to relieve clinical signs. Severe exercise restriction in conjunction with corticosteroids may result in temporary improvement in neurologic function. Sometimes long-term management of dogs with minimal or mild signs of neuro-

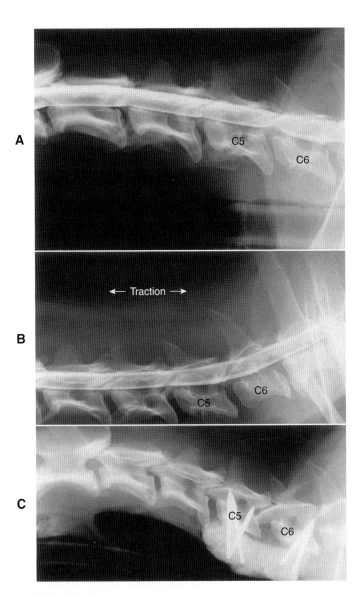

**FIG 72-21**
**A,** Cervical myelogram of an 11-year-old Doberman/ Weimaraner cross with a chronic history of nonpainful ataxia and hypermetria of all four limbs. Narrowing of the C5-C6 disk space and thinning of the dorsal contrast column over this site (in association with dorsal deviation and thinning of the ventral contrast column) can be seen. **B,** The dramatic resolution of this spinal cord compression in the traction view suggests a dynamic compression by a bulging annulus fibrosus or ligamentum flavum. **C,** Surgery was performed to maintain traction on the spine at this site.

logic dysfunction is satisfactory with corticosteroid therapy alone (prednisone 0.5 mg/kg PO q12h for 2 days; then 0.5 mg/kg once every day for 2 days; then 0.5 mg/kg once every other day for 14 days; then 0.25 mg/kg once every other day for 2 months). Restricted exercise is important, and the dog should wear a chest harness instead of a collar.

Although initial improvement is common after medical therapy, the underlying compression and instability persist and generally progress without more definitive treatment.

Surgical treatment is recommended in mildly affected cases if the condition does not improve or continues to deteriorate during medical management. Surgical treatment is recommended in all severely affected dogs. The main factor determining the specific surgical procedure to be recommended is the appearance of the cord myelographically, especially on the traction view. If the only lesion identified is a static ventral spinal cord compression resulting from disk herniation, then ventral decompression is performed. If a single dynamic lesion is causing compression, such as a bulging annulus (ventrally) or a hypertrophied ligamentum flavum (dorsally), then a distraction/fusion technique is used to pull the vertebral bodies apart and maintain the separation, decreasing spinal cord compression and relieving pressure on the nerve roots (see Fig. 72-21). The method used will depend on the number of sites involved and surgeon preference. If the imaging studies indicate static dorsal compression of the spinal cord resulting from vertebral malformation or articular process osteophytes, then a dorsal decompressive technique must be attempted.

### Prognosis

Dogs with wobbler syndrome have extremely variable prognoses, depending on their neurologic status, the temporal course of their disease, and the specific abnormalities that are present. Surgical results in ambulatory animals with a short history and only one lesion can be good, with up to 80% success reported. Multiple lesions, chronic disease, and an inability to walk are all associated with a poor prognosis.

## PROGRESSIVE SPINAL CORD DYSFUNCTION IN YOUNG ANIMALS

### NEURONAL ABIOTROPHIES AND DEGENERATIONS

Neuronal abiotrophies and degenerative disorders of the nervous system have been recognized in a few breeds of dogs (Table 72-5). Progressive neurologic dysfunction usually begins early in life. In disorders affecting the spinal cord, clinical signs involving the rear limbs are often noted early in the course of disease but progression to tetraparesis may occur. Some disorders primarily affect white matter and result in UMN signs. Other disorders result in LMN paralysis. The disorders are diagnosed based on the typical clinical course, the signalment, and the lack of any definable etiology on screening blood tests, spinal radiographs, CSF analysis, myelography, and other diagnostic testing. Diagnosis is confirmed by necropsy examination in most cases. No treatment is available.

### METABOLIC STORAGE DISEASES

A large group of rare disorders, characterized pathologically by the accumulation of metabolic products in cells caused by a genetically based enzyme deficiency, may result in signs of spinal cord dysfunction (see Table 67-5). The enzyme deficiency itself or the accumulation of the metabolic intermediates within cells causes a gradual progression of neurologic signs, ending in death.

## TABLE 72-5

Congenital, Familial, and Idiopathic Degenerative Disorders of the Nervous System

**Predominantly Brain or Spinal Cord UMN Signs**
**Hereditary Afghan myelopathy**

ONSET: 3 to 13 months of age
CLINICAL SIGNS: Rapidly progressive rear limb paresis, ataxia, increased tone, hyperreflexia (initially); progresses to tetraplegia
PATHOLOGY: Extensive demyelination of spinal cord axons (especially thoracic)

**Boxer central-peripheral neuropathy**

ONSET: 6 months of age
CLINICAL SIGNS: Progressive severe ataxia and hypermetria; signs begin in rear limbs, progress to include forelimbs; loss of proprioception, weakness, patellar areflexia, normal flexor reflexes
EMG: Normal
NCV: Normal or slightly reduced
Evoked muscle action potential: Low amplitude

**Spongiform degeneration of the gray matter of Bull Mastiffs**

ONSET: 4 to 7 weeks of age
CLINICAL SIGNS: Ataxia, proprioceptive deficits, hypermetria, head tremors, visual deficits, dementia

**Multisystem neuronal degeneration in Cocker Spaniels**

ONSET: 10 to 14 months of age
CLINICAL SIGNS: Progressive abnormal behavior, anxiety, cerebellar ataxia, intention tremor
PATHOLOGY: Neuronal degeneration in the brain and brainstem

**Leukodystrophy of Dalmatians**

ONSET: 3 to 5 months of age
CLINICAL SIGNS: Visual deficits, progressive ataxia
PATHOLOGY: Brain atrophy, cavitation of white matter of cerebral hemispheres

**Hereditary ataxia in Jack Russell and smooth-coated Fox Terriers**

ONSET: 2 to 6 months of age
CLINICAL SIGNS: Weakness, rear limb incoordination, progressing to ataxia of all four limbs and hypermetria; signs may stabilize
PATHOLOGY: Bilaterally symmetric spinal cord degeneration predominantly involving the spinocerebellar tracts

**Spongy degeneration of the white matter in Labrador Retrievers**

ONSET: 4 to 6 months of age
CLINICAL SIGNS: Progressive forelimb rigidity, opisthotonic posturing, cerebellar ataxia
PATHOLOGY: Spongiform degeneration in CNS cerebellar peduncles, cerebral white matter, and peripheral nerves

**Predominantly Brain or Spinal Cord UMN Signs—cont'd**
**Labrador Retriever axonopathy**

ONSET: 3 to 4 weeks of age
CLINICAL SIGNS: Pelvic limb gait short strided, adducted, and crouched; forelimbs wide-based and stiff; hypermetria; progressive for 4 to 5 months, then static, ± head tremor
PATHOLOGY: Spinal cord white matter degeneration

**Leukoencephalomyelopathy in Rottweilers**

ONSET: 1.5 to 4 years of age
CLINICAL SIGNS: Very slow progression (years) of ataxia, tetraparesis, hypermetria, weakness, loss of proprioception; hyperactive reflexes
PATHOLOGY: Demyelination of spinal cord, caudal cerebellar peduncle, and lower brainstem

**Neuroaxonal dystrophy in Rottweilers**

ONSET: 3 months to 6 years of age
CLINICAL SIGNS: Very slowly progressive disorder; initially clumsy gait, forelimb hypermetria progressing to obvious cerebellar ataxia, head intention tremor, and nystagmus; normal conscious proprioception, not weak
PATHOLOGY: Spheroids in granular level of cerebellum, vestibular nuclei, and spinal cord; similar syndromes in young Chihuahuas, Jack Russell terriers, Collies, and tricolor cats

**Central axonopathy of Scottish Terriers**

ONSET: 10 to 12 weeks of age
CLINICAL SIGNS: Generalized body tremors, ataxia, progress to paraparesis
PATHOLOGY: Neuroaxonal dystrophy, axonopathy

**Degenerative myelopathy**

AFFECTED: Older (>5 years of age) German Shepherds, Siberian Huskies, Chesapeake Bay Retrievers, other large-breed dogs; rarely seen in cats
CLINICAL SIGNS: Slowly progressive loss of proprioception; UMN paralysis of the pelvic limbs
PATHOLOGY: Diffuse demyelination of all white matter tracts of spinal cord, particularly in thoracic region (focal areas of cerebellum, cerebrum, brainstem also involved)

**Metabolic storage diseases:**

See Table 67-6

**Cerebellar atrophy and abiotrophy:**

See Table 67-4

**Congenital vestibular disorders:**

See Chapter 70

*UMN,* Upper motor neuron; *EMG,* electromyography; *NCV,* nervous condition velocity; *CNS,* central nervous system; *LMN,* lower motor neuron.

TABLE 72-5

Congenital, Familial, and Idiopathic Degenerative Disorders of the Nervous System—cont'd

**Predominantly LMN Signs**

**Hereditary polyneuropathy of Alaskan Malamutes**

ONSET: 7 to 18 months of age
CLINICAL SIGNS: Slowly progressive weakness, exercise intolerance, muscle atrophy, hyporeflexia, megaesophagus, laryngeal paralysis

**Progressive axonopathy of Boxers**

ONSET: 2 to 3 months of age
CLINICAL SIGNS: Pelvic limb ataxia, hypotonia, hyporeflexia progressing to tetraparesis ± cerebellar signs
PATHOLOGY: Axonal swellings in dorsal and ventral nerve roots, peripheral nerves, spinal cord

**Laryngeal paralysis of Bouvier des Flandres**

ONSET: 4 to 8 months of age
CLINICAL SIGNS: Exercise intolerance, inspiratory stridor, dyspnea, laryngeal paralysis
PATHOLOGY: Axonal degeneration in recurrent laryngeal nerves, neuronal loss in nucleus ambiguous; autosomal dominant inheritance

**Spinal muscular atrophy of Brittany Spaniels**

ONSET: 1 to 6 months of age
CLINICAL SIGNS: Weakness and atrophy of proximal limb muscles; rapid or slow progression to tetraplegia, loss of reflexes, tendon contracture
PATHOLOGY: Neuronal degeneration of selected brainstem nuclei and ventral gray matter of spinal cord

**Neuronal chromatolysis of Cairn Terriers**

ONSET: 3 to 7 months of age
CLINICAL SIGNS: Initially episodic pelvic limb collapse with spontaneous resolution; rear limb weakness, loss of patellar reflexes, progress to tetraparesis; ataxia, hypermetria, head tremors
PATHOLOGY: Central and peripheral widespread chromatolytic degeneration and focal myelomalacia

**Motor neuron disease in cats**

ONSET: Adult cats >6 years
CLINICAL SIGNS: Progressive weakness, cervical ventroflexion, dysphagia, muscle atrophy, loss of reflexes (late)
PATHOLOGY: Degeneration of ventral horn of spinal cord and ventral nerve roots

**Dalmatian laryngeal paralysis and polyneuropathy**

ONSET: 2 to 6 months of age
CLINICAL SIGNS: Acute respiratory distress, syncope, gagging, coughing, laryngeal paralysis, megaesophagus, muscle weakness, muscle atrophy, hyporeflexia
PATHOLOGY: Focal loss of myelinated fibers, distal polyneuropathy

**Predominantly LMN Signs—cont'd**

**Distal polyneuropathy of Doberman Pinschers**

ONSET: Adult (3 to 5 years of age), slow progression
CLINICAL SIGNS: Initial tendency to flex one or the other pelvic limb while standing ("dancing Doberman"); atrophy of gastrocnemius, semitendinosus, semimembranosus; rear limb weakness, one-half decrease in conscious proprioception, one-half normal hyperreflexia
EMG: Positive sharp waves and fibrillation potentials in gastrocnemius with advanced disease
NCV: Normal
PATHOLOGY: Type II muscle fiber atrophy in advanced disease; may be a primary muscle disorder

**Progressive neurogenic muscular atrophy in English Pointers**

ONSET: 18 to 23 weeks of age
CLINICAL SIGNS: Trembling, pelvic limb weakness, hoarse, progressing over 2 to 3 months to stumbling, tetraplegia, extreme muscle atrophy (especially shoulder), hyporeflexia
EMG: Denervation

**Giant axonal neuropathy in German Shepherds**

ONSET: 14 to 16 months of age
CLINICAL SIGNS: Progressive rear limb paresis, proprioceptive deficits, depressed patellar reflexes, atrophy of distal pelvic limb muscles, megaesophagus, hoarse, fecal incontinence
PATHOLOGY: Axonal swellings containing neurofilaments

**Spinal muscle atrophy of German Shepherds**

ONSET: 12 to 14 weeks of age
CLINICAL SIGNS: Forelimb weakness, severe muscle atrophy
PATHOLOGY: Symmetric ventral horn degeneration confined to the cervical intumescence

**Hypomyelinating polyneuropathy of Golden Retrievers**

ONSET: 7 weeks of age
CLINICAL SIGNS: Hind limb weakness, crouched stance, muscle atrophy, depressed postural reactions

**Spinal muscular atrophy in Maine Coon Cats**

ONSET: 15 to 17 weeks of age
CLINICAL SIGNS: Progressive muscle weakness and atrophy, fasciculations
PATHOLOGY: Neurogenic muscle atrophy, loss of large motor neurons in ventral horns of spinal cord

**Distal sensorimotor polyneuropathy in Rottweilers**

ONSET: Adult (1 to 4 years of age)
CLINICAL SIGNS: Paraparesis slowly progressing to tetraparesis, hyporeflexia, hypotonia, muscle atrophy in distal limb muscles
PATHOLOGY: Degeneration of myelinated and unmyelinated peripheral axons

*Continued*

TABLE 72-5

Congenital, Familial, and Idiopathic Degenerative Disorders of the Nervous System—cont'd

**Predominantly LMN Signs—cont'd**
*Spinal muscular atrophy in Rottweilers*

ONSET: 4 weeks of age
CLINICAL SIGNS: Rapid progression of weakness, loss of proprioception, hyporeflexia, severe denervation atrophy, megaesophagus
PATHOLOGY: Degeneration of motor neurons in gray matter of spinal cord

*Laryngeal paralysis in Siberian Husky dogs, crosses, and Alaskan Husky dogs*

ONSET: 6 weeks
CLINICAL SIGNS: Inspiratory dyspnea, stridor, exercise intolerance, laryngeal paralysis
PATHOLOGY: Not documented

*Spinal muscular atrophy of Swedish Lapland Dogs*

ONSET: 5 to 7 weeks of age
CLINICAL SIGNS: Weakness, then rapid progression to flaccid tetraplegia with severe muscle atrophy; spinal reflexes are decreased
EMG: Denervation potentials
PATHOLOGY: Neuronal degeneration of spinal cord ventral gray matter and ventral nerve roots

*Inherited hypertrophic neuropathy in Tibetan Mastiffs*

ONSET: 7 to 10 weeks of age
CLINICAL SIGNS: Rapidly progressing weakness, loss of muscle tone, hyporeflexia, tetraplegia; cranial nerves normal

**Predominantly LMN Signs—cont'd**
*Inherited hypertrophic neuropathy in Tibetan Mastiffs—cont'd*

NCV: Slow because of extensive demyelination of peripheral nerves
PATHOLOGY: Extensive, chronic demyelination

*Metabolic storage diseases:*

See Table 67-6

**Disorders of the Sensory Nerves**
*Long-haired Dachshund sensory neuropathy*

ONSET: 6 weeks of age
CLINICAL SIGNS: Hind limb ataxia, decreased superficial and deep sensation, loss of proprioception, urinary incontinence; no paresis, no muscle atrophy, normal tendon reflexes
EMG: Motor
NCV: Normal
Sensory NCV: Absent
PATHOLOGY: Loss of myelinated fibers, degeneration of unmyelinated sensory nerve fibers

*Sensory neuropathy of English Pointers*

ONSET: 2 to 12 months of age
CLINICAL SIGNS: Loss of sensation, particularly distal limbs; self-mutilation; normal gait and reflexes

Spinal signs are usually UMN in nature, although peripheral nerve involvement may occur. Cortical signs (e.g., seizures) and cerebellar signs (e.g., hypermetria) are common. Signs are gradually progressive and usually obvious within the first year or two of life. Metabolic storage diseases are diagnosed based on the typical clinical course and signalment, the lack of any other identifiable etiology, and (in some cases) organomegaly, abnormal appearance, blindness, and other readily identifiable clinical abnormalities resulting from the accumulation of metabolic product in extraneural sites.

## ATLANTOAXIAL INSTABILITY AND LUXATION

Normally the dens (i.e., odontoid process) of the axis (C2) is held firmly against the floor of the atlas (C1) by ligaments. Malformation or absence of the dens or a loss of the intervertebral ligamentous support can be seen as a congenital defect in many small breeds of dogs, including the Yorkshire Terrier, Miniature or Toy Poodle, Chihuahua, Pomeranian, Pekingese, and rarely in large-breed dogs and in cats. The malformation and resultant atlantoaxial instability can lead to acute at-

lantoaxial luxation as a consequence of minor trauma. Alternatively, congenital deformity of the dens may produce slowly progressive clinical signs of spinal cord compression in a young adult dog as the supporting ligaments gradually stretch, causing instability and spinal cord compression before complete luxation occurs. In young dogs with congenital atlantoaxial instability, mild trauma may precipitate a sudden onset of cervical pain, tetraparesis, or paralysis. In any normal dog, severe trauma could result in traumatic luxation or fracture in this region and similar clinical findings.

### Clinical Features

Clinical signs include neck pain, low head carriage, ataxia, and tetraparesis. Paralysis is rare. Some dogs have a persistent head tilt or turn. Atlantoaxial luxation secondary to malformation should be suspected in any young (i.e., 6 to 18 month old) toy-breed dog with a history of cervical pain, tetraparesis, or tetraplegia. Atlantoaxial luxation should be considered as a possible differential diagnosis in any dog with evidence for high cervical spinal cord disease, particularly in those with a history of trauma.

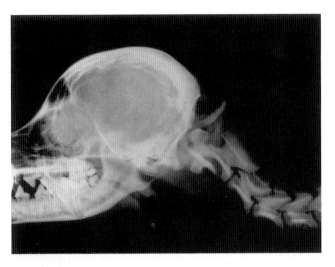

**FIG 72-22**
Atlantoaxial subluxation in a 7-month-old Bichon Frise. The dens rises well above its normal position, consistent with rupture of its ligament and compression of the cervical spinal cord. The space between the arch of the atlas and the spinous process of the axis is increased. This dog had a chronic history of intermittent cervical pain and severe upper motor neuron (UMN) tetraparesis.

Physical examination reveals UMN signs to all four limbs and cervical pain. Dogs with atlantoaxial luxation typically keep their necks in extension and resist flexion of the high cervical region. Manipulation of the spine should be avoided, because it can exacerbate motor dysfunction.

## Diagnosis

Radiographic examination should be performed initially without anesthesia when atlantoaxial luxation is suspected to prevent inadvertent overflexion or twisting of an unstable cervical spine. Lateral and oblique lateral views may aid in demonstrating absence or deformity of the dens. Instability with significant luxation can be recognized on a lateral view as widening of the space between the dorsal arch of the atlas and the dorsal spinous process of the axis on the lateral view and dorsal displacement of the body of the axis (Fig. 72-22). In cases of congenital luxation the dens may be recognized as abnormal, and fracture of the dens may be apparent in traumatic luxations. If preliminary radiographs are not diagnostic, the animal should be anesthetized and the radiographs repeated with the head gently flexed. This may allow demonstration of the instability. Extreme care is critical when manipulating an animal suspected of having atlantoaxial instability under anesthesia, because rotation or excessive flexion of the neck may result in further spinal cord compression, respiratory paralysis, and death. Splinting the animal's head and neck in extension before anesthesia is recommended to prevent excessive flexion during induction of anesthesia and intubation. Incidental radiographic findings in affected toy and miniature breeds may include malformations of the atlas with fusion to the occipital bones (i.e., occipitoatlantoaxial

malformation) or a larger-than-normal foramen magnum (i.e., occipital dysplasia), neither of which should alter the diagnostic or therapeutic plan nor the prognosis.

### Treatment

Treatment as for acute spinal cord trauma (see p. 1023) is recommended followed by internal surgical stabilization using a dorsal or ventral technique. Surgical procedures are described in detail in the Suggested Readings listed at the end of this chapter.

### Prognosis

The prognosis for recovery is good in dogs less than 2 years of age with voluntary motor function and conscious perception of pain.

## CONGENITAL SPINAL CORD DYSFUNCTION: NONPROGRESSIVE SIGNS

### SPINA BIFIDA

Spina bifida results from embryonic failure of fusion of the two halves of the dorsal spinous processes of the vertebrae. Although spina bifida may occur anywhere along the spinal canal, the lumbosacral segment and the sacrococcygeal junction are most often affected. This malformation is most common in English Bulldogs and Manx cats. In the Manx cat the condition is an autosomal recessive trait and may be associated with caudal agenesis. The development of neurologic signs is variable. When clinical signs are present, they include rear limb paresis, fecal and urinary incontinence, loss of perineal sensation, and decreased tone of the anal sphincter. No therapy is available.

### CAUDAL AGENESIS OF MANX CATS

Congenital malformations of the sacrococcygeal spinal cord and vertebrae are common in tailless Manx cats. Clinical signs result from agenesis or dysgenesis of the caudal vertebrae and sacral spinal cord. These signs include hopping or crouched pelvic limb gait, fecal and urinary incontinence, and chronic constipation.

### SPINAL DYSRAPHISM

Spinal dysraphism is an inherited congenital malformation of the spine. It results from an abnormality of development of the structures of the spinal cord along the central plane. The malformation includes a dilated or absent central canal, cavitation in the white matter, and the abnormal presence of ventral gray column cells across the median plane between the central canal and the ventral median fissure. Spinal dysraphism is recognized most commonly in Weimaraners, although other breeds are occasionally affected.

Clinical signs are present at birth. Affected dogs have a symmetric, bunny-hopping pelvic limb gait, a wide-based stance, and depressed proprioception. The patellar reflex is normal. The pelvic limb flexor reflex stimulated in one limb usually elicits simultaneous flexion of both pelvic limbs. Clinical signs caused by spinal dysraphism do not progress, and mildly affected dogs can live a normal life.

## SYRINGOMYELIA/HYDROMYELIA

Cystic accumulations of fluid within the spinal cord causing compression of adjacent parenchyma are being recognized with increasing frequency as advanced diagnostic imaging techniques (i.e., CT, MRI) are used for neurologic diagnosis. Syringomyelia is the development of a CSF-filled cavity anywhere within the cord, and hydromyelia is the accumulation of excessive CSF within a dilated central canal. These disorders can develop as a result of altered CSF pressures within the spinal canal, a loss of spinal cord parenchyma, or secondarily to obstructed CSF flow caused by congenital malformations or inflammatory or neoplastic obstruction of CSF flow.

Clinical signs reflect the site and degree of spinal cord parenchymal destruction. Ataxia and paresis are common. With cervical lesions, UMN signs are more pronounced in the rear limbs if the dorsal and lateral portions of the cord are affected. When the spinal cord damage is more centrally located, ataxia and paresis will often be more significant in the forelimbs than in the rear limbs (i.e., central cord syndrome). Spinal pain may be seen because of stretching of nerve roots or meninges. Scoliosis occasionally develops as LMN cell body damage within the cord causes asymmetric denervation of the paraspinal muscles, resulting in vertebral deviation. Cervical paresthesia and scratching has been noted in Cavalier King Charles Spaniels with bony malformations causing overcrowding of the foramen magnum, resulting in syringohydromyelia.

Diagnosis requires advanced diagnostic imaging. MRI is superior to CT for demonstration of the intraparenchymal spinal cord abnormalities. Treatment is controversial. Early surgical intervention to decompress the fluid accumulation and reestablish normal CSF flow or shunting is ideal but is rarely effective. Medical therapy consists of the administration of prednisone and acetazolamide to decrease CSF production.

## Suggested Readings

Adams WH et al: Magnetic resonance imaging of the caudal lumbar and lumbosacral spine in 13 dogs (1990-1993), *Vet Radiol Ultrasound* 36(1):3, 1995.

Applewhite AA et al: Potential central nervous system complications of von Willebrand's disease, *J Am Anim Hosp Assoc* 35:423, 1999.

Bagley RS: Spinal fracture or luxation, *Vet Clin North Am Sm Anim Pract* 30(1):133, 2000.

Bagley RS et al: Exogenous spinal trauma: Surgical therapy and aftercare, *Comp Cont Ed Sm An Pract Vet* 22(3):218, 2000.

Bagley RS et al: Syringomyelia and hydromyelia in dogs and cats, *Comp Cont Educ Sm An Pract Vet* 22(5):471, 2000.

Barclay KB et al: Immunohistochemical evidence for immunoglobulin and complement deposition in spinal cord lesions in degenerative myelopathy in German Shepherd Dogs, *Can J Vet Res* 58: 20, 1994.

Braund KG: Neoplasia of the nervous system, *Compend Cont Ed Pract Vet* 6:717, 1984.

Chambers JN: Lumbosacral degenerative stenosis. In Kirk RW, editor: *Current veterinary therapy XI*, Philadelphia, 1992, WB Saunders.

Clemmons RM: Degenerative myelopathy. In Kirk RW, editor: *Current veterinary therapy X*, Philadelphia, 1989, WB Saunders.

Clemmons RM: Degenerative myelopathy, *Vet Clin North Am* 22(4):965, 1992.

Cook JR et al: Atlantoaxial luxation in the dog, *Compend Cont Ed Pract Vet* 3(3):242, 1981.

Fingeroth JM: Treatment of canine intervertebral disk disease: recommendations and controversies. In Bonagura JD et al, editors: *Current veterinary therapy XII*, Philadelphia, 1995, WB Saunders.

Griffiths IR: Central nervous system trauma. In Oliver JE et al, editors: *Veterinary neurology*, Philadelphia, 1987, WB Saunders.

Hawthorne JC et al: Fibrocartilaginous embolic myelopathy in Miniature Schnauzers, *J Am Anim Hosp Assoc* 37: 374, 2001

Kornegay JN: Intervertebral disk disease: treatment guidelines. In Bonagura JD et al, editors: *Current veterinary therapy XII*, Philadelphia, 1995, WB Saunders, p 1146.

Lincoln JD: Cervical vertebral malformation/malarticulation syndrome in large dogs, *Vet Clin North Am* 22(4):923, 1992.

Luttgen P: Neoplasms of the spine, *Vet Clin North Am* 22(4):973, 1992.

McCarthy RJ et al: Atlantoaxial subluxation in dogs, *Compend Cont Educ Pract Vet* 17(2):215, 1995.

Moore MP: Discospondylitis, *Vet Clin North Am* 22(4):1027, 1992.

Munana KR et al: Intervertebral disk disease in cats, *J Am Anim Hosp Assoc* 37:384, 2001.

Neer TM: Fibrocartilaginous emboli, *Vet Clin North Am* 22(4):1017, 1992.

Penwick RC: Fibrocartilaginous embolism and ischemic myelopathy, *Compend Cont Ed Pract Vet* 11(3):287, 1989.

Schulman AJ et al: Canine cauda equina syndrome, *Compend Cont Ed Pract Vet* 10(7):835, 1988.

Seim H: Diagnosis and treatment of cervical vertebral instability-malformation syndromes. In Bonagura JD: *Kirk's current veterinary therapy XIII*, Philadelphia 2000, WB Saunders, p 992.

Shores A: Spinal trauma: pathophysiology and management of traumatic spinal cord injuries, *Vet Clin North Am* 22(4):859, 1992.

Simpson ST: Intervertebral disk disease, *Vet Clin North Am* 22(4): 889, 1992.

Sisson AF et al: Diagnosis of cauda equina abnormalities by using electromyography, discography and epidurography in dogs, *J Vet Int Med* 6:253, 1992.

Thomas WB: Diskospondylitis and other vertebral infections, *Vet Clin North Am Small Anim Pract* 30(1):169, 2000.

Toombs JP: Cervical intervertebral disk disease in dogs, *Compend Cont Educ Pract Vet* 14(11):1477, 1992.

Vangundy T: Canine wobbler syndrome, part 1, pathophysiology and diagnosis, *Compend Cont Ed Pract Vet* 11(2):144, 1989.

Wheeler SJ: Lumbosacral disease, *Vet Clin North Am* 22(4):937, 1992.

Wheeler SJ, Sharp NJH: *Small animal spinal disorders*, London, 1994, Times Mirror International.

# CHAPTER 73

# Disorders of Peripheral Nerves and the Neuromuscular Junction

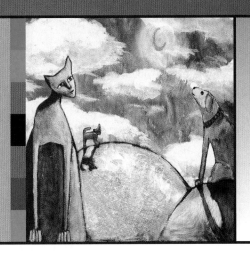

## CHAPTER OUTLINE

FOCAL NEUROPATHIES, 1049
    Traumatic neuropathies, 1049
    Peripheral nerve tumors, 1049
    Facial nerve paralysis, 1051
    Trigeminal nerve paralysis, 1053
HYPERCHYLOMICRONEMIA, 1054
ISCHEMIC NEUROMYOPATHY, 1054
POLYNEUROPATHY, 1055
ACUTE POLYRADICULONEURITIS, 1056
TICK PARALYSIS, 1057
BOTULISM, 1058
PROTOZOAL POLYRADICULONEURITIS, 1058
DYSAUTONOMIA, 1059
MYASTHENIA GRAVIS, 1059

## FOCAL NEUROPATHIES

### TRAUMATIC NEUROPATHIES

Traumatic neuropathies are common. They result from mechanical blows, fractures, pressure, stretching, laceration, and the injection of agents into or adjacent to the nerve. Diagnosis is usually straightforward and is based on the history and clinical findings. Individual nerves or a group of adjacent nerves may be damaged. Traumatic radial nerve paralysis, complete avulsion of the entire brachial plexus, and sciatic nerve injury are most common in the dog and cat (Table 73-1; Fig. 73-1).

Electrodiagnostic testing, when available, can be used to evaluate the extent of nerve damage. In 5 to 7 days after denervation of a muscle, electromyography detects denervation action potentials (i.e., increased insertional activity and spontaneous action potentials) in the muscles normally supplied by the damaged nerve (see Table 73-1). Nerve conduction studies proximal and distal to the site of injury are useful in assessing nerve integrity.

When an animal is presented with a peripheral nerve injury, careful mapping and assessment of cutaneous sensation and motor function help to determine the precise location of the injury, and sequential mapping can be used to monitor progress (see Fig. 73-1). The regenerative ability of a nerve is proportional to the continuity of connective tissue structures remaining around the damaged portion of the nerve. If adequate connective tissue scaffolding is left, axonal regeneration can occur at a rate of 1 to 4 mm/day. The closer a nerve injury is to the innervated muscle, the better the chances are of recovery. If a nerve is entirely disrupted, the prognosis for regeneration is poor.

Physical therapy such as swimming, limb manipulation, and massage helps delay muscle atrophy and tendon contracture and speed return of function in animals with incomplete lesions. Self-mutilation may become a problem 2 to 3 weeks after injury, because regeneration of sensory nerves can result in abnormal sensation lasting 7 to 10 days. Lack of improvement in motor function after 1 month warrants consideration of amputation of the affected limb or, when feasible, arthrodesis for limb salvage.

## PERIPHERAL NERVE TUMORS

Peripheral nerve sheath tumors (i.e., schwannomas, neurofibromas, neurofibrosarcomas) involve the peripheral nerves and nerve roots of dogs and (rarely) cats. These tumors are a relatively common cause of lameness and neuropathy when they involve the nerves of the brachial plexus. Lymphoma may also involve the nerve roots or peripheral nerves of dogs and cats.

### Clinical Features

Clinical signs depend on the tumor location and the nerves involved. Trigeminal nerve sheath tumors are occasionally seen and result in ipsilateral atrophy of the temporalis and masseter muscles. More commonly, tumors involve the spinal nerve roots in the lower cervical and upper thoracic region and the peripheral nerves of the brachial plexus, resulting in lameness, muscle atrophy, and pain. Intermittent or persistent lameness and lifting of the affected leg may occur. The insidious onset of these tumors may make it difficult to differentiate them from lameness caused by a vague musculoskeletal injury or nerve root compression caused by intervertebral disk disease. With progression of the tumor, atrophy, weakness, and

TABLE 73-1

**Traumatic Neuropathies**

| PERIPHERAL NERVES DAMAGED | MOTOR DYSFUNCTION | SKIN REGION OF SENSATION LOSS | MUSCLES AFFECTED |
|---|---|---|---|
| **Lesions of Nerves of the Thoracic Limb** | | | |
| Peripheral radial nerve damage (at level of digital elbow) | Loss of carpus and digit extension; may walk on dorsal paw or carry limb | Cranial and lateral forearm and dorsal forepaw | Extensor carpi radialis, ulnaris lateralis, digital extensors |
| Brachial plexus avulsion (proximal damage): | | | |
| Suprascapular nerve ([C5], C6, C7) | Loss of shoulder extension; muscle atrophy over scapular spine | None | Supraspinatus, infraspinatus |
| Axillary nerve ([C6], C7, C8) | Reduced shoulder flexion; deltoid muscle atrophy | Small area dorsolateral brachium | Deltoideus, teres major, teres minor, subscapularis |
| Musculocutaneous nerve (C6, C7, C8) | Reduced elbow flexion | Medial forearm | Biceps brachii, brachialis, coracobrachialis |
| Radial nerve (C7, C8, T1, [T2]) | Reduced extension of elbow, carpus, and digits; cannot support weight | Cranial and lateral forearm, from toes to elbow | Triceps brachii, extensor carpi radialis, ulnaris lateralis, digital extensors |
| Median nerve (C8, T1, [T2]) | Reduced flexion of carpus and digits | None | Flexor carpi radialis, digital flexors |
| Ulnar nerve (C8, T1, [T2]) | Reduced flexion of carpus and digits | Caudal forearm (toes to elbow); lateral digits | Flexor carpi ulnaris, deep and digital flexor |
| **Lesions of Nerves of the Pelvic Limb** | | | |
| Femoral nerve damage (L4, L5, L6) | Inability to extend stifle; cannot support weight; atrophy of quadriceps; loss of patellar reflex | Medial limb (toes to thigh) | Iliopsoas, quadriceps, sartorius |
| Sciatic nerve paralysis (L6, L7, S1, [S2]) | Reduced flexion and extension of hip; loss of stifle flexion; loss of hock flexion and extension hock dropped; paw is knuckled, but weight bearing does occur; absent withdrawal reflex; atrophy of cranial, tibial, semimembranosus, and semitendinosus muscles | All regions below stifle except medial surface | Biceps femoris, semimembranosus, semitendinosus |
| Tibial branch (L7, S1, [S2]) | Dropped hock | Caudal plantar (stifle to paw) | Gastrocnemius, popliteus, digital flexors |
| Peroneal branch (L6, L7, S1, S2) | Stands knuckled; no cranial tibial reflex | Cranial and dorsal limb (stifle to paw) | Peroneus longus, digital extensors, cranial tibial |

[ ], Variable contribution.

loss of reflexes may occur as the affected peripheral nerve is destroyed. Tumors involving the T1-T3 nerve roots may interrupt the sympathetic pathway and result in ipsilateral Horner's syndrome.

Tumors of a peripheral nerve in the brachial plexus are not readily palpable, although pain may be evident on palpation of the axillary region. Tumors originating from a nerve root in an intradural location may extend peripherally through the intervertebral foramen and affect adjacent peripheral nerves of the extremity. The tumor may eventually expand within the vertebral canal, causing spinal cord compression and upper motor neuron (UMN) signs caudal to the site of the lesion.

## Diagnosis

Radiographs of the spine are indicated if a neoplasm involving a spinal nerve root is suspected. Nerve sheath tumors rarely cause bony changes, although expanding tumors that pass through an intervertebral foramen may cause widening of the foramen as a result of pressure necrosis. Myelography is useful to identify spinal cord compression. Electromyography and nerve conduction velocity determinations may confirm the presence of a peripheral nerve lesion and aid localization. Advanced diagnostic imaging (computed tomography [CT], magnetic resonance imaging [MRI]) may be the best diagnostic tests to characterize the lesion once it has been localized and to determine options for treatment (Fig. 73-2).

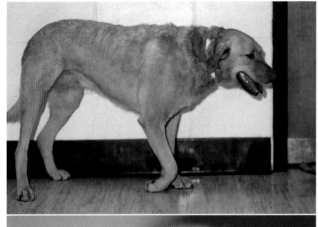

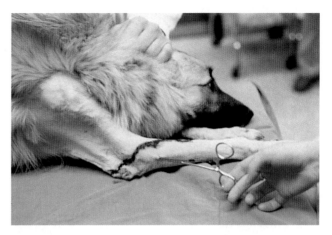

**FIG 73-2**
Mapping the region of sensory loss is important in localizing lesions and monitoring improvement. This dog has a brachial plexus avulsion, so he has lost superficial sensation on the limb distal to the elbow.

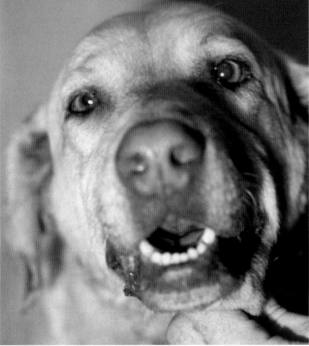

**FIG 73-1**
**A,** Traumatic brachial plexus avulsion in a Chesapeake Bay Retriever. **B,** Horner's syndrome in the same dog.

## Treatment

The treatment of choice for a nerve sheath tumor is surgical removal. Removal can result in a cure in a few cases. Extensive neurologic damage by the tumor, damage affecting several spinal nerves or nerve roots, or severely atrophied muscles may require amputation of the limb. Nerve root tumors that have progressed to cause spinal cord compression usually involve multiple nerve roots, are rarely completely resectable, and are associated with a poor prognosis. Postoperative irradiation may be indicated in an attempt to slow tumor recurrence.

## FACIAL NERVE PARALYSIS

Facial nerve paralysis is recognized frequently in dogs and cats. In 75% of dogs and 25% of cats with acute facial nerve paraly-

sis, there are no associated neurologic or physical abnormalities and no underlying cause can be found, prompting a diagnosis of idiopathic facial nerve paralysis. Canine hypothyroidism can occasionally be associated with a mononeuropathy involving the facial nerve. Traumatic injury to the facial nerve can also occur at the level of the brainstem or peripherally as the nerve courses through the petrous temporal bone.

The most common identifiable cause of facial nerve paralysis, however, is damage to branches of the facial nerve within the middle ear secondary to inflammation, infection, or neoplasia. Otitis media and otitis interna usually occur from extension of bacterial otitis externa, particularly in breeds predisposed to chronic bacterial otitis externa (e.g., Cocker Spaniels, German Shepherd Dogs, and Setters). Foreign bodies (e.g., grass awns), malignant tumors (in both dogs and cats), and benign nasopharyngeal polyps (in cats) involving the middle ear can also cause facial nerve paralysis.

### Clinical Features

Clinical manifestations of facial nerve paralysis include an inability to close the eyelid, move the lip, or move the ear. Affected animals are unable to blink spontaneously or in response to visual or palpebral sensory stimulation. Keratoconjunctivitis sicca may develop following loss of facial nerve–stimulated lacrimal gland secretion. Drooping of the ear and lip as a result of loss of muscle tone on the affected side is common (Fig. 73-3). Many dogs and cats with facial nerve paralysis caused by middle ear disease also develop peripheral vestibular signs and/or Horner's syndrome because of the close proximity of the nerves in the area of the middle and inner ear. Rarely, a syndrome of hemifacial spasm with facial muscle contracture and lip retraction may occur, either acutely as a result of facial nerve irritation or chronically because of muscle atrophy and contracture in animals with long-standing facial nerve paralysis (Fig. 73-4).

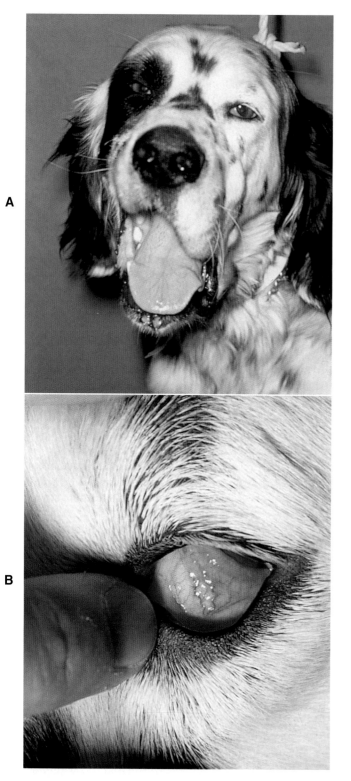

**FIG 73-3**
Idiopathic facial nerve paralysis in a 4-year-old English Setter. Note the drooping lip and ear, **A,** and the inability to blink, **B.** The paralysis resolved in 14 days without therapy.

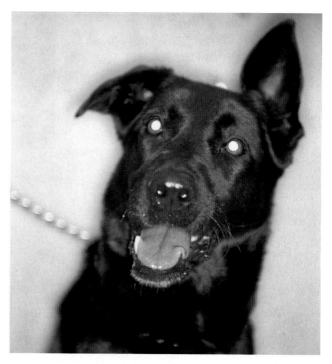

**FIG 73-4**
Contraction of the muscles on the left side of the face developed in an adult dog with a 2-month history of idiopathic left-sided facial nerve paralysis. Note the erect left ear and nasal deviation to the left.

## Diagnosis

Idiopathic facial nerve paralysis can be diagnosed only after excluding all other causes. A complete neurologic examination should be performed to ensure that there are no other cranial nerve deficits, ataxia, or proprioceptive deficits suggesting a brainstem lesion. Clinicopathologic testing (complete blood count [CBC], serum biochemistry profile, urinalysis) is required to evaluate for systemic or metabolic disease. A suspicion of hypothyroidism warrants evaluation of thyroid function (see Chapter 51).

All dogs and cats with facial nerve paralysis should be evaluated carefully for disease of the middle and inner ear. Careful otoscopic examination is important, even if general anesthesia is required. Most animals with otitis media or otitis interna have obvious otitis externa and a tympanic membrane that appears abnormal or ruptured, but occasionally the otoscopic examination is normal.

Skull radiographs should be evaluated for changes in the tympanic bullae suggesting chronic inflammatory disease, trauma, or tumor. Ventrolateral, oblique, lateral, and open-mouth radiographs of the skull are necessary. Radiographic evidence of otitis media and otitis interna includes increased thickness of the bones of the tympanic bullae and petrous temporal bone and increased soft-tissue density within the tympanic bullae (Fig. 73-5; see also Fig. 70-2). Radiographs very commonly appear normal in animals with acute infections. CT and MRI may be more sensitive techniques for de-

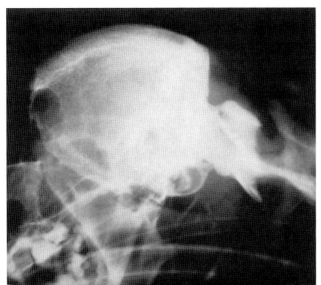

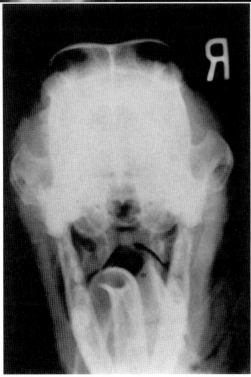

**FIG 73-5**
Skull radiographs of a 4-year-old Cocker Spaniel with bilateral otitis media resulting in bilateral facial nerve paralysis. Both bullae chambers are opacified, and the left bulla is thickened by irregular and slightly indistinct new bone. (Courtesy Dr. A. Remedios, University of Saskatchewan.)

tecting small amounts of fluid in the middle ear. Radiographic evidence of soft-tissue density within the bullae and associated bone lysis suggests tumor. Nasopharyngeal polyps in cats result in radiographic evidence of soft tissue within the bullae, but no bone lysis.

Following radiographs, while the animal is still under general anesthesia, the external ear canal and the tympanic membrane should be carefully examined using an otoscope or a small endoscope. The ear canal should be flushed with a warm 0.9% saline solution until the fluid obtained is clear and the tympanic membrane can be visualized. A sample should be obtained from inside the middle ear for culture and cytology. If the tympanic membrane is intact, the external ear should be thoroughly cleaned and then myringotomy performed just caudal to the malleus with a 22-gauge, 3.5-inch spinal needle attached to a 6 ml syringe inserted through the tympanic membrane at the 6 o'clock position. Myringotomy relieves pressure and pain and allows collection of material for cytology and culture. If exudate is not obtained, 0.5 to 1.0 ml of sterile saline can be instilled and then aspirated. If the tympanic membrane is already ruptured, a similar procedure can be performed to obtain a sample.

### Treatment

No treatment exists for idiopathic facial nerve paralysis. If keratoconjunctivitis sicca is present, the eye should be medicated as needed. The paralysis may be permanent, or spontaneous recovery may occur in 2 to 6 weeks.

If evaluation of the middle and inner ear reveals bony lysis or extensive soft-tissue proliferation, this suggests that neoplasia could be the cause of facial nerve paralysis. A biopsy should be performed, and surgery to debulk or remove the tumor should be considered. The prognosis for cure with feline benign inflammatory nasopharyngeal polyps in this location is excellent. Tumors of the bulla, bony labyrinth, ear canal, or peripheral nerve are less likely to be treated effectively using surgery alone. Radiotherapy or chemotherapy may be beneficial in some cases.

Medical treatment of dogs and cats with bacterial otitis media and otitis interna can be attempted but is rarely effective. Systemic antibiotics are administered for 4 to 6 weeks, with the choice of antibiotic based on culture and sensitivity results. Pending culture results, antibiotic treatment can be initiated using a broad-spectrum antibiotic such as a first-generation cephalosporin (cephalexin, 22 mg/kg PO q8h), a combination of amoxicillin and clavulanic acid (Clavamox, 12.5 to 25 mg/kg PO q8h), or enrofloxacin (5 mg/kg PO q12h).

If conservative treatment does not resolve the infection, or if there is radiographic evidence of fluid or tissue in the tympanic bulla or chronic bone changes in the bulla, ventral bulla osteotomy should be performed, followed by a course of antibiotic therapy. Early recognition of inflammation together with prompt initiation of appropriate therapy results in a good prognosis for recovery. The facial nerve paralysis may be permanent in spite of treatment. Failure to treat otitis media and otitis interna can result in ascent of the infection up the nerves into the brainstem, leading to progression of neurologic signs and death.

## TRIGEMINAL NERVE PARALYSIS

Paralysis of the motor component of cranial nerve V results in the sudden onset of an inability to close the jaw. The mouth hangs open, and the animal cannot prehend food.

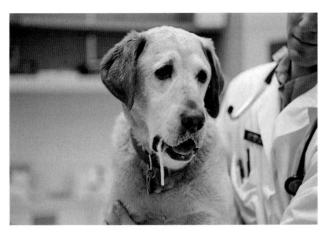

**FIG 73-6**
Idiopathic trigeminal nerve motor paralysis resulting in a dropped jaw and excessive drooling in a 9-year-old Labrador Retriever. The paralysis resolved in 14 days without therapy.

Swallowing is usually normal. In the idiopathic form, no obvious sensory deficit is present. Severe rapid atrophy of the muscles of mastication may occur (Fig. 73-6).

Idiopathic trigeminal paralysis is seen in middle-aged and older dogs and rarely in cats. The diagnosis relies on clinical signs and on ruling out other possible causes. Rabies and other inflammatory CNS diseases are unlikely in the absence of other clinical signs. Neoplastic and traumatic disorders are not usually bilateral, although bilateral motor trigeminal nerve infiltration has been reported in a dog with multicentric lymphoma.

The etiology of this idiopathic disorder is unknown. If biopsy of the nerve is performed, it reveals bilateral nonsuppurative neuritis of all motor branches of cranial nerve V associated with demyelination. Treatment consists of supportive care. Most dogs can drink and maintain their hydration if they are given water in a deep container such as a bucket. Hand-feeding may be necessary. The prognosis is excellent, with most animals recovering completely within 2 to 4 weeks.

## HYPERCHYLOMICRONEMIA

Peripheral neuropathies have been observed in cats of all ages with defective lipoprotein lipase function and delayed clearance of chylomicrons from the circulation. Most clinical signs of the resulting hyperchylomicronemia are related to the formation of lipid deposits (xanthomas) in the skin and other tissues. These xanthomas may compress a nerve against bone, resulting in neuropathology. Horner's syndrome and tibial and radial nerve paralysis are most often seen. Clinicopathologic testing reveals fasting hyperchylomicronemia and blood that looks like "cream-of-tomato soup." Diagnosis is by biopsy of the xanthomas or measurement of lipoprotein lipase concentration. The neurologic signs are reversible if hyperchylomicronemia can be controlled by feeding affected cats a low-fat, high-fiber diet.

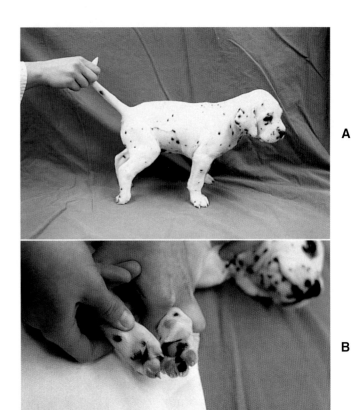

**FIG 73-7**
**A,** Acute, severe LMN paralysis of the rear limbs occurred in this 6-week-old Dalmatian puppy. The limbs were cool, and no femoral pulses were palpable. **B,** The footpads on the front feet were warm and pink, whereas those on the rear feet were cool and pale. Ultrasound examination revealed a caudal aortic thrombus.

## ISCHEMIC NEUROMYOPATHY

Caudal aortic thromboembolism causes paralysis from ischemic damage to affected muscles and peripheral nerves. Ischemia is caused by vasoconstriction of the collateral circulation to the limbs as a result of release of thromboxane $A_2$ and serotonin from platelets in the clot. Caudal aortic thromboembolism is common in cats and rare in dogs. An acute onset of lower motor neuron (LMN) pelvic limb paralysis or paresis is seen. Femoral pulses are weak or absent. The legs and feet are cool, and the pads are no longer pink (Fig. 73-7). Hemorrhage does not occur when a toenail is cut short on an affected foot. The affected muscles are swollen and painful. Flaccidity and complete areflexia of the rear limbs are common, although occasionally the patellar reflex is maintained. Within hours, rigid extension of the legs may occur as a result of contracture of ischemic muscle. A disorder associated with hypercoagulability can usually be identified in dogs (see p. 1199). Endocarditis, neoplasia, nephrotic syndrome, hyperadrenocorticism, and heartworm disease should be considered. In cats, cardiomyopathy is most common.

## POLYNEUROPATHY

Polyneuropathies affect more than one group of peripheral nerves, resulting in generalized LMN signs that include flaccid muscle weakness or paralysis, marked muscle atrophy, decreased muscle tone, and reduced or absent reflexes. Proprioceptive deficits may be evident if the sensory portions of the nerves are severely affected. Polyneuropathies may be seen in association with hypothyroidism, diabetes mellitus (especially in cats), and insulinomas; as a manifestation of systemic lupus erythematosus (SLE); and as a paraneoplastic condition in association with a variety of neoplasms in dogs. Chronic inflammatory demyelinating polyneuropathies with no identifiable underlying cause and a presumed immune-mediated pathogenesis have been identified in dogs and cats. Chronic organophosphate intoxication may result in a polyneuropathy. In addition, a number of breed-associated degenerative peripheral neuropathies are usually congenital and presumed to have a hereditary basis (see Table 72-5). Some of these disorders are undoubtedly the result of disorders of intermediary metabolism or impaired energy utilization.

Diagnosis of a polyneuropathy should be suspected in any dog or cat with chronic progressive development of the LMN signs of weakness, muscles atrophy, and diminished spinal reflexes. When available, electrodiagnostic testing aids in the diagnosis. Electromyography reveals evidence of denervation, and nerve conduction velocity is decreased in affected nerves. Biopsy of a peripheral nerve may be necessary to confirm the diagnosis. When the diagnosis of polyneuropathy is made, it is important to investigate known etiologies to attempt to reach a specific diagnosis (Table 73-2).

All dogs and cats with a confirmed peripheral neuropathy require evaluation for diabetes mellitus. Clinical signs of diabetic polyneuropathy are usually subtle or inapparent in the dog but may be dramatic in the cat. Weakness of the rear limbs, reluctance to jump, a plantigrade pelvic limb stance, and weakness of the tail are characteristic (Fig. 73-8). Physical examination findings may include rear limb hyporeflexia and marked muscle atrophy. The onset of signs is generally rapid, developing within less than a week in most cases. The diagnosis of diabetic polyneuropathy is probable when these neurologic signs are observed in a cat with diabetes mellitus. Diagnosis can be confirmed with biopsies of muscle and distal nerves. If diabetic polyneuropathy is recognized early, neurologic signs may improve if the diabetes can be regulated.

Dogs with polyneuropathy should be evaluated for hypothyroidism, because hypothyroid polyneuropathy has been implicated as a cause of diffuse LMN paralysis, unilateral peripheral vestibular disease, facial nerve paralysis, laryngeal paralysis, and megaesophagus in dogs. Nerve and muscle biopsies in affected dogs may show neuronal degeneration and regeneration, as well as muscle fiber type grouping that is most indicative of neurogenic atrophy. In some hypothyroid dogs with mononeuropathies or polyneuropathies, neurologic signs resolve once supplementation with thyroid hormone is initiated (Fig. 73-9).

### TABLE 73-2

**Disorders of Peripheral Nerves and the Neuromuscular Junction Causing Paresis**

| | |
|---|---|
| **Focal** | Traumatic disorders |
| | Peripheral nerve tumors |
| | Idiopathic facial nerve paralysis |
| | Idiopathic trigeminal neuritis |
| | Hyperchylomicronemia |
| | Ischemic neuromyopathy |
| | Ehrlichiosis |
| **Generalized (Chronic)** | Inherited degenerative disorders (see Table 72-5) |
| | Idiopathic polyneuropathy |
| | Metabolic disorders |
| |     Diabetes mellitus |
| |     Hypothyroidism |
| | Paraneoplastic syndromes |
| |     Insulinoma |
| |     Other tumors |
| | Manifestation of SLE or other immune-mediated disease |
| | Chronic organophosphate intoxication |
| | Ehrlichiosis (?) |
| **Generalized (Acute)** | Acute polyradiculoneuritis (Coonhound paralysis) |
| | Tick paralysis* |
| | Botulism* |
| | Protozoal polyradiculoneuritis |
| | Dysautonomia |
| **Episodic** | Myasthenia gravis* |

*Disorder of the neuromuscular junction.

Hypoglycemia in an older animal with polyneuropathy should raise an index of suspicion for an insulin-secreting tumor, which has been associated with a paraneoplastic polyneuropathy in dogs. Other neoplastic processes should also be considered in dogs and cats with polyneuropathies with no identifiable cause. This situation may warrant careful physical examination, thoracic and abdominal radiographs, abdominal ultrasonography, lymph node aspirates, and bone marrow examination. Polyneuropathy has been recognized in several dogs with multicentric lymphoma or disseminated carcinoma. In some cases, removal of the offending neoplasm is associated with resolution of the clinical signs of polyneuropathy.

Rarely, dogs are identified with a mononeuropathy or polyneuropathy and concurrent positive serologic or polymerase chain reaction (PCR) testing for *Ehrlichia canis*, but with no other clinical signs indicating ehrlichiosis. In some dogs the neuropathy resolves after appropriate treatment with doxycycline (5 mg/kg PO q12h) or imidocarb dipropionate (5 mg/kg IM twice, 14 days apart), making active ehrlichiosis likely.

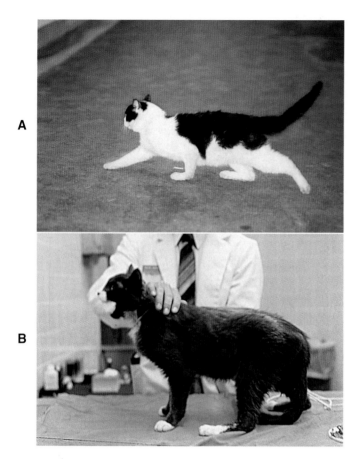

**FIG 73-8**
Plantigrade stance in **A,** an 11-year-old cat and **B,** a 6-year-old cat with polyneuropathy caused by diabetes mellitus.

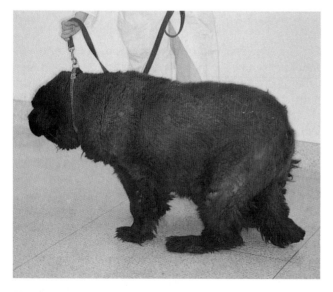

**FIG 73-9**
Plantigrade stance and weak gait in a 6-year-old Newfoundland Dog with severe hypothyroid neuropathy. All neurologic signs and weakness resolved, and the dog lost 60 pounds within 12 months of thyroid hormone supplementation.

Some toxins, including organophosphates, heavy metals, and industrial chemicals, can cause polyneuropathies. Organophosphates, in particular, can have a delayed neurotoxic effect. A dying back neuropathy and demyelination may develop 1 to 6 weeks after excretion of most of the chemical. Exposure to the toxin may have been a single severe exposure, often with the development of severe clinical signs, or chronic mild to moderate exposure repeated over weeks or months without acute signs. Affected animals are weak but do not have classic autonomic signs of organophosphate intoxication, such as salivation, vomiting, diarrhea, or miosis. With chronic exposure, hair, blood, fat, or liver samples may contain the toxin. Plasma acetylcholinesterase activity is low. Toxic neuropathies may be suspected on the basis of results of nerve biopsy. Spontaneous improvement should occur in 3 to 12 weeks, provided that the toxic substance is removed and reexposure is prevented.

Finally, systemic immune-mediated disease such as SLE may cause a polyneuropathy. Screening tests should include evaluation of a CBC, measurement of protein in the urine (i.e., protein/creatinine ratio), and analysis of synovial fluid. Skin lesions should be biopsied, and blood should be submitted for an antinuclear antibody (ANA) titer. Immunosuppressive therapy should be initiated if there is evidence of immune-mediated disease (see p. 1216). A number of chronic, inflammatory, demyelinating polyneuropathies have been observed in dogs and cats; these disorders may resolve spontaneously or with corticosteroid therapy. Unfortunately, many polyneuropathies have been identified in dogs and cats, with no identifiable underlying cause and poor response to immunosuppressive therapy.

## ACUTE POLYRADICULONEURITIS

Acute polyradiculoneuritis (Coonhound paralysis) is the acute polyneuropathy most commonly diagnosed in dogs. The disease affects dogs of any breed and gender, and most affected dogs are adults. A similar disease occurs rarely in cats.

The popular name *Coonhound paralysis* results from the fact that in most of the early cases the syndrome was thought to result from exposure to raccoon saliva. Coonhounds used for hunting were bitten by a raccoon and subsequently (7 to 10 days later) developed the syndrome. Raccoon saliva injection does not reliably produce the disorder but has been shown to induce the disease in a few susceptible dogs. It is hypothesized that the disorder results from an immune response against some component of raccoon saliva (Fig. 73-10).

Acute polyradiculoneuritis also occurs in many dogs and cats with no possible exposure to raccoons. Previous systemic illness or vaccination (particularly rabies vaccination) has been implicated as an initiating factor in some of these cases, but in many cases no initiating factor can be identified. The pathologic manifestation includes extensive demyelination, inflammatory cell infiltration, and disruption of axons (especially the ventral roots) and peripheral spinal nerves. The disease is very similar to allergic neuritis and Guillain-Barré syndrome in humans, making an immunologic pathogenesis suspect.

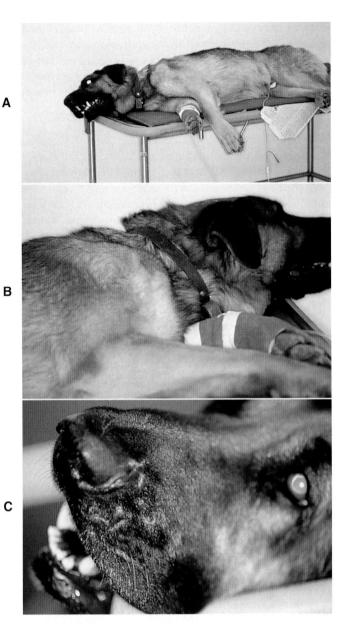

**FIG 73-10**
A 4-year-old German Shepherd Dog with **A,** rapidly progressive ascending LMN paralysis, **B,** severe appendicular muscle atrophy, and **C,** healing facial wounds presumed to be from an encounter with a raccoon. The tentative diagnosis in this dog was acute polyradiculoneuritis. Supportive care was initiated, and the dog returned to normal after a prolonged recovery lasting 3 months.

## Clinical Features

Clinical signs of weakness and hyporeflexia are sometimes preceded by a change in character of the bark; dogs sound hoarse. Rear limb weakness occurs and ascends rapidly, with a flaccid symmetric tetraplegia developing in most cases. The time from initial signs to complete paralysis may be as short as 12 hours or as long as 1 week. Neurologic examination reveals remarkably decreased muscle tone and rapid

muscle atrophy. Motor impairment is more remarkable than sensory loss. Some dogs seem to be hyperesthetic, reacting vigorously to mild stimulation such as palpation of the muscles or pinching of the toes. This hyperesthesia is a feature of polyradiculoneuritis that does not occur in association with tick paralysis or botulism, the two major differential diagnoses. Spinal reflexes are diminished or absent; the perineal reflex is normal, and bladder and rectum functions remain normal. As a rule, cranial nerves are not involved; no problems with chewing or swallowing exist; neither do any pupillary abnormalities. A small percentage of very severely affected dogs have concurrent bilateral facial nerve paralysis. Paralyzed dogs maintain their appetites and are afebrile. In a few dogs, respiratory paralysis may result in death.

## Diagnosis

The diagnosis is suspected on the basis of clinical and neurologic findings. When available, electromyography reveals diffuse denervation after 6 or more days of paralysis, and motor nerve conduction velocities are slow in affected nerves. CSF is usually normal, although a mild increase in protein concentration may occur. Pathologic changes are most marked in the ventral nerve roots and spinal nerves, with leukocyte infiltration, demyelination, and axonal degeneration predominating.

## Treatment

No specific treatment exists for this disorder. Corticosteroid treatment has not proved beneficial. Supportive therapy is very important; the animal may require assistance in sitting up to eat and drink. If possible, the dog should be kept on an air mattress, waterbed, lounge chair, or bed of straw and turned periodically to prevent lung atelectasis and pressure sores.

## Prognosis

Most dogs begin to improve after the first week, but recovery occasionally takes months. The prognosis for recovery is good. Some dogs never recover completely, and the prognosis for complete recovery in the cat appears to be poor. Affected animals that have recovered may be prone to recurrences, particularly if exposed again to the initiating antigen.

## TICK PARALYSIS

A flaccid, rapidly ascending motor paralysis has been recognized in dogs infested with certain species of ticks. The common wood ticks *Dermacentor variabilis* and *Dermacentor andersoni* are most often incriminated in the United States (*Ixodes* spp. in Australia). The feeding of a female tick results in the elaboration and circulation of a salivary neurotoxin that interferes with acetylcholine release at the neuromuscular junction. Not all strains of each species of tick generate the toxin, and not all infested animals become paralyzed. Signs occur within 5 to 9 days after tick attachment.

## Clinical Features

Dogs with tick paralysis exhibit a rapid progression from pelvic limb weakness to recumbency over 24 to 72 hours, resulting in complete LMN paralysis. Loss of muscle tone and spinal reflexes occurs without significant muscle atrophy. Pain is perceived normally, and no evidence of hyperesthesia exists. In most cases the cranial nerves are not significantly affected. An altered voice, cough, and dysphagia may occur, and mild jaw and facial weakness may be recognized. Without treatment, death from respiratory paralysis occurs in 1 to 5 days.

## Diagnosis

Tick paralysis is diagnosed on the basis of the history, clinical signs, and knowledge of the geographic region. Sometimes a tick can be found on the animal, and diagnosis is confirmed by documenting rapid improvement following tick removal. When electromyography is available, it reveals the absence of spontaneous activity (no denervation potentials). Diminished amplitude of the muscle action potential occurs in response to a single supramaximal stimulus, as would be expected with a defect in neuromuscular transmission.

## Treatment

Removal of a tick or dipping the animal in an insecticidal solution results in dramatic recovery within 24 to 72 hours. The prognosis for complete recovery is good when the proper diagnosis is made.

# BOTULISM

Botulism is rarely recognized in dogs and has not been clinically seen in cats. It results from the ingestion of spoiled food or carrion containing a preformed type C neurotoxin produced by the bacterium *Clostridium botulinum*. This toxin blocks the release of acetylcholine from the neuromuscular junction, resulting in complete LMN paralysis. Clinical signs occur hours to days following ingestion of the toxin.

## Clinical Features

A progressive, ascending LMN paralysis affecting spinal and cranial nerves is seen with botulism. Dogs are profoundly weak and have loss of muscle tone and absent spinal reflexes, but no muscle atrophy. Proprioception and pain perception are normal, without hyperesthesia. Extensive cranial nerve involvement is common. Affected dogs may drool, cough, and have difficulty prehending food. Regurgitation resulting from megaesophagus is common. Mydriasis and loss of the palpebral response may be seen in severely affected dogs.

## Diagnosis

The diagnosis is based on clinical findings and/or a history of ingestion of spoiled food. The incubation period is less than 6 days. Botulism is especially likely if an outbreak of LMN paralysis is seen in a group of dogs. Rabies must be considered as a differential diagnosis in severely affected dogs, but it is usually rapidly progressive and associated with abnormal mentation. Weakness of the muscles of the face, jaw,

and pharynx is much more pronounced with botulism than would be expected with acute polyradiculoneuritis or tick paralysis. Electrodiagnostic studies are as described for tick paralysis (see Diagnosis under Tick Paralysis). Botulinum toxin (types C and D) may be demonstrated in the blood, vomitus, or feces from affected dogs.

## Treatment

No specific treatment for botulism exists. The administration of laxatives and enemas may help remove unabsorbed toxin from the gastrointestinal tract if ingestion was recent. Oral broad-spectrum antibiotics may help reduce the intestinal population of clostridial organisms. Administration of commercially available trivalent antitoxin (types A, B, and E) is not likely to be effective. Type C antitoxin is recommended for dogs but is not readily available. Most dogs recover in 1 to 3 weeks with supportive care.

# PROTOZOAL POLYRADICULONEURITIS

Progressive LMN paralysis has been documented secondary to polyradiculoneuritis caused by *Toxoplasma gondii* or *Neospora caninum*. Rapidly progressive flaccid paralysis with hyporeflexia and dysphagia similar to tick paralysis or botulism has been recognized in a few adult dogs and litters of puppies with protozoal polyradiculoneuritis. Electromyography in these dogs reveals denervation secondary to extensive involvement of the ventral nerve roots.

*N. caninum* has also been associated with a syndrome of polyradiculoneuritis and myositis affecting only the rear limbs of young dogs. There is progressive rear limb LMN paresis with loss of patellar and (eventually) withdrawal reflexes and some pain on muscle palpation. Over time, quadriceps muscle contraction occurs, fixing the rear limbs in rigid extension.

Increases in serum creatine kinase (CK) and aspartate transaminase (AST) activities are common with either of these clinical presentations of protozoal polyradiculoneuritis, because concurrent myositis is usually present. CSF analysis may reveal inflammatory changes and occasionally the presence of organisms. In cats with toxoplasmosis, uveitis and chorioretinitis may be seen. Dogs and cats with toxoplasmosis or neosporosis may exhibit evidence of systemic disease, including liver enzyme (alanine aminotransferase) increases or pulmonary involvement. Serology may be positive, but it can be difficult to interpret. Definitive diagnosis requires biopsy of the affected muscles and nerves. A mononuclear inflammatory reaction and many organisms are typically seen. Immunocytochemical stains can be performed to distinguish between *Toxoplasma* and *Neospora*. Some success has been reported in dogs treated with clindamycin (5.5 to 11 mg/kg PO, SC, or IM q12h), but severely affected animals are unlikely to respond.

# DYSAUTONOMIA

Dysautonomia is a disorder of the autonomic nervous system that has historically caused widespread morbidity and mortality in cats in the United Kingdom and has more recently been recognized in dogs and a few cats in the United States, particularly in the Midwest. Pathologic lesions in the autonomic ganglia are consistent with a toxic etiology, but the cause remains unknown. Clinical signs reflect a loss of neurons in the sympathetic and parasympathetic nervous systems, particularly involving the urinary, alimentary, and ocular systems.

## Clinical Features

Young cats and dogs are most often affected. Affected animals have a rapid onset of clinical signs, which progress over 48 hours. Clinical signs include depression, anorexia, dilated pupils that do not respond to light, prolapse of the nictitating membrane, constipation, and regurgitation caused by megaesophagus. Mucous membranes of the eyes, mouth, and nose are dry. Other potential signs include bradycardia, weakness, proprioceptive deficits, and loss of the anal reflex. Dysuria and urine retention due to bladder atony are reported in most dogs (80% to 100%) and some cats (17% to 40%) with dysautonomia.

## Diagnosis

Diagnosis is suspected on the basis of the observed clinical signs. Thoracic and abdominal radiographs may reveal megaesophagus, aspiration pneumonia, and a largely distended urinary bladder. The bladder is easily expressed, suggesting diminished urethral sphincter tone. Anal tone may be decreased as well. Pharmacologic testing of the pupillary light reflex and the bladder should support the diagnosis. Ocular administration of very dilute (0.05% to 0.1%) pilocarpine (Isoptocarpine 1%, Alcon Laboratories, diluted with saline) produces dramatic miosis within 30 to 45 minutes in affected dogs because of the phenomenon of denervation hypersensitivity. Administration of bethanechol (0.04 mg/kg) enables many affected animals to void normally and completely. Definitive diagnosis requires the demonstration of lesions within the autonomic nervous system at postmortem examination. A loss of nerve cell bodies results in decreased neuron density in all autonomic ganglia, especially the pelvic, mesenteric, and ciliary ganglia.

## Treatment

Treatment is supportive and includes the administration of fluids, force-feeding, lubricating eye ointments, enemas, and bladder emptying. Bethanecol administration may improve urinary function, and pilocarpine may be administered to stimulate tear production and relieve photophobia. Some animals recover spontaneously, but the prognosis is generally poor, with a mortality rate of greater than 70%.

# MYASTHENIA GRAVIS

Myasthenia gravis (MG) is a neuromuscular disorder characterized by weakness that is exacerbated by exercise and alleviated by rest. Two forms have been described: congenital and acquired. The congenital form of MG results from an inherited deficiency of acetylcholine receptors (ACHRs) at the postsynaptic membranes in skeletal muscle. Signs of impaired

neuromuscular transmission first become evident in puppies or kittens 3 to 8 weeks old. The disorder has been recognized in English Springer Spaniels, Smooth-Haired Fox Terriers, Jack Russell Terriers, and a few cats. An unusual, poorly classified transient congenital myasthenic syndrome has also been identified in Miniature Dachshunds the signs in these dogs resolve with maturation.

The acquired form of MG is a common immune-mediated disorder in which antibodies are directed against the nicotinic ACHRs of skeletal muscle, resulting in impaired neuromuscular transmission. Antibodies bind to the receptors, reducing the sensitivity of the postsynaptic membrane to the transmitter acetylcholine.

The acquired form of MG affects dogs of all breeds and both genders. German Shepherd Dogs, Golden Retrievers, Labrador Retrievers, and Dachshunds are most commonly affected, but this may merely reflect the popularity of these breeds. Breeds that seem to be at increased risk for acquired MG relative to their popularity include Akitas, some terrier breeds, German Shorthaired Pointers, and Chihuahuas. Cats are rarely affected, but breed predispositions include the Abyssinian and Somali. A bimodal age distribution occurs with young dogs (mean age: 2 to 3 years) and old dogs (mean age: 9 to 10 years), making up most of the affected population.

## Clinical Features

The characteristic clinical abnormality in most animals with MG is appendicular muscle weakness that worsens with exercise and improves with rest. Mentation, postural reactions, and reflexes are normal, although reflexes may be fatiguable with repeated stimulation. Additional signs seen in affected dogs and cats may include excessive salivation and regurgitation caused by megaesophagus (seen in 90% of dogs with acquired MG). Megaesophagus is not found as consistently in cats with MG as in dogs, and it is less common in congenitally affected animals than in those with acquired MG. Dysphagia, hoarse character of the bark or meow, persistently dilated pupils, or facial muscle weakness may also be seen.

A focal form of MG, with clinical signs attributable to megaesophagus but no appendicular weakness, has been reported in dogs. Dogs with focal MG exhibit weakness of the pharyngeal, laryngeal, and/or facial muscles. They may have a fatiguable palpebral reflex. Approximately 25% to 40% of all dogs with adult-onset megaesophagus actually suffer from acquired focal MG. This disorder should always be considered as a differential diagnosis early in the course of evaluation of dogs with megaesophagus.

An acute, fulminating form of acquired MG has also been recognized, causing a rapid onset of severe appendicular muscle weakness. Affected animals are often unable to stand and cannot even raise their head. This form of MG is usually associated with severe megaesophagus and aspiration pneumonia. Profound muscle weakness and severe pneumonia may lead to respiratory failure and death.

## Diagnosis

MG should be considered as a differential diagnosis in any dog with generalized muscular weakness and in all dogs with acquired megaesophagus. Definitive diagnosis is made by demonstrating circulating antibodies against acetylcholine receptors. This test is readily available (Comparative Neuromuscular Laboratory, University of California, San Diego) and is positive in 90% of all dogs and cats with acquired disease and in 98% of those with generalized acquired disease. False-positive results have not been documented. Although the serum anti-ACHR antibody titer does not correlate directly with the severity of clinical signs, dogs with focal MG tend to have lower titers and dogs with acute fulminating MG have the highest titers. Rarely, dogs with acquired MG are negative for circulating ACHR antibodies, but immune complexes can be demonstrated at the neuromuscular junction using immunocytochemical methods. These dogs may have very-high-affinity antibody that remains bound to ACHRs and does not circulate, or antibodies directed against junctional antigens other than ACHRs.

When results of the serum test for antibodies are not yet available, or in animals with suspected congenital disease, support for the diagnosis of MG can be gained by demonstrating a positive response to administration of the ultra-short-acting anticholinesterase edrophonium chloride (Tensilon) (Table 73-3). This drug inhibits enzymatic hydrolysis of acetylcholine at the neuromuscular junction, increasing the effective concentration of acetylcholine and the duration of its effect in the synaptic cleft, optimizing the opportunities for successful interactions between acetylcholine and the ACHRs. Most animals with MG exhibit obvious improvement in clinical signs (e.g., resolution of weakness) within 30 to 60 seconds after administration of edrophonium chloride, with the effect lasting approximately 5 minutes. Some dogs with other myopathic and neuropathic disorders may also show some minor improvement, but a dramatic unequivocal response is very suggestive of MG. A failure to respond does not rule out MG. The response can be difficult to assess in dogs and cats with focal MG; many cats with generalized MG have an unpredictable response, and approximately 50% of dogs with acute fulminating MG do not respond to Tensilon, because they have experienced marked antibody-mediated destruction of ACHRs.

Electromyography (showing a decremental response of muscle action potentials to repetitive nerve stimulation) can be performed as an aid to reaching a definitive diagnosis of MG. However, whenever possible, anesthesia should be avoided in animals with megaesophagus because of the risk of aspiration during recovery.

Thoracic radiographs should be assessed for megaesophagus, aspiration pneumonia, or thymoma, and the animal should be evaluated for underlying or associated immune-mediated and neoplastic disorders. If a cranial mediastinal mass is identified, fine-needle aspiration cytology should be used to confirm the suspicion that it is a thymoma—a tumor that has been identified in less than 5% of dogs with acquired MG and in more than 25% of cats. Concurrent immune-mediated disorders are common in dogs with MG, including hypothyroidism, immune-mediated thrombocytopenia, immune-mediated hemolytic anemia, hypoadrenocorticism, polymyosi-

 TABLE 73-3

**Tensilon Test Protocol**

1. Place an intravenous catheter.
2. Premedicate with atropine (0.04 mg/kg IM) to minimize muscarinic side effects.
3. Have equipment available for intubation and ventilation.
4. Exercise to the point of detectable weakness.
5. Administer Tensilon (edrophonium chloride) IV:
   0.1-0.2 mg/kg (dogs)
   0.2 mg/kg (cats)

tis, and SLE. MG may also develop as a paraneoplastic disorder in association with a wide variety of tumors, including hepatic carcinoma, anal sac adenocarcinoma, osteosarcoma, cutaneous lymphoma, and primary lung tumors. Acquired drug-induced MG has also been documented in hyperthyroid cats being treated with methimazole.

## Treatment

Treatment of acquired MG includes supportive care and the administration of anticholinesterase drugs and occasionally immunosuppressive agents. Surgical removal should be considered in animals with a thymoma, since many animals will have a decrease in ACHR antibody titer and dramatic resolution of their signs following thymectomy. Animals with megaesophagus and regurgitation should be maintained in an upright position during feeding and for 10 to 15 minutes after feeding to facilitate the movement of esophageal contents into the stomach, decreasing the chance of aspiration (Fig. 73-11). If severe regurgitation remains a problem, a gastrostomy tube can be placed to assist in the delivery of nutrients, fluids, and medications. Whenever aspiration pneumonia is present, a transtracheal wash (see p. 264) should be performed for culture and then aggressive treatment for the pneumonia should be initiated using antibiotics, fluids, nebulization, and coupage. One should avoid the use of antibiotics that can impair neuromuscular transmission (ampicillin, aminoglycosides).

Anticholinesterase drugs are commonly administered in an attempt to improve muscular strength. Pyridostigmine bromide (Mestinon, 1 to 2 mg/kg PO q8h) has been used in dogs. In cats, pyridostigmine bromide syrup (5 mg/kg PO q12h, diluted 1:1 with water to decrease gastric irritation) has been recommended. For both dogs and cats, the dose must be individualized on the basis of clinical response. Ideally, feeding should be timed to coincide with peak drug effect. In dogs initially unable to tolerate oral medication because of severe megaesophagus, neostigmine methylsulfate (Prostigmin, 0.01 to 0.04 mg/kg IM q6-8h) can be used.

If an animal appears to be responding to anticholinesterase treatment and then deteriorates, anticholinesterase under-

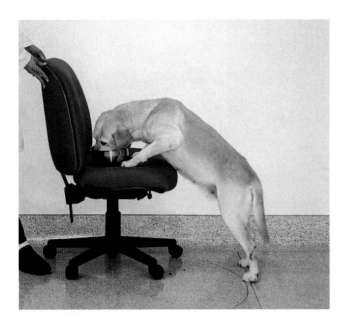

**FIG 73-11**
Upright feeding in animals with megaesophagus facilitates emptying of esophageal contents into the stomach. Animals should be maintained in this position for 10 to 15 minutes after eating.

dosage (myasthenic crisis) and anticholinesterase overdosage (cholinergic crisis) should be suspected. Clinically these two therapeutic problems are indistinguishable. An edrophonium (Tensilon) test allows the clinician to distinguish between them. The animal in a myasthenic crisis improves following edrophonium administration, whereas the condition of an animal in a cholinergic crisis becomes transiently worse or does not change following edrophonium administration.

Corticosteroids are sometimes administered to animals with MG in an attempt to decrease the production of antibodies against ACHRs. The administration of corticosteroids and other immunosuppressive drugs has been associated with an improved outcome in some dogs with acquired MG, but whenever possible their administration should be delayed until the animal is stable and aspiration pneumonia has resolved. Corticosteroids, if administered at high doses, commonly cause transient worsening of muscular weakness in dogs with MG. Therapy should always be initiated with a low dose (prednisone, 0.5 mg/kg/day) and the dosage gradually increased over 2 to 4 weeks to the level required for immunosuppression (2 to 4 mg/kg/day). The administration of azathioprine (Imuran, 2 mg/kg/day) as the sole immunosuppressive agent or in combination with prednisone has been associated with a positive clinical response and a decrease in ACHR antibody in a number of dogs.

## Prognosis

Response to medical management of MG can be good if aspiration pneumonia is not severe and the complications of aspiration and anticholinesterase overdosage are avoided. Severe aspiration pneumonia, persistent megaesophagus, acute fulminating MG, and the presence of a thymoma or an underlying neoplasm are all associated with a poor prognosis for recovery. Most affected dogs die of either acute fatal aspiration or euthanasia within 12 months of diagnosis. Anticholinesterase drugs can effectively control appendicular muscle weakness in most animals, but their effect on esophageal function is variable. Dogs and cats without significant aspiration pneumonia may respond to immunosuppressive drugs such as prednisone and azathioprine. When evaluating medical treatments for MG, it is important to recognize that many dogs with acquired MG will go into a spontaneous permanent clinical remission at an average of 6.4 months after diagnosis (range 1 to 18 months), regardless of the treatment used. Remission is unlikely to occur in animals with MG occurring secondary to a thymoma or other neoplasm. Although there is no consistent relationship between disease severity and serum ACHR antibody concentration among animals, sequential antibody determinations in an individual animal can be correlated with disease progression or remission; thus it is recommended that ACHR antibody concentrations be measured and monitored every 4 to 8 weeks in animals being treated for MG.

## Suggested Readings

Braund KG et al: Toxoplasma polymyositis/polyneuropathy—a new clinical variant in two mature dogs, *J Am Anim Hosp Assoc* 24:93, 1988.

Coates JR et al: Congenital and inherited neurologic disorders of dogs and cats. In Bonagura JD, editor: *Current veterinary therapy XIII*, Philadelphia, 2001, WB Saunders, p 1111.

Cornelissen JMM et al: Type C botulism in five dogs, *J Am Anim Hosp Assoc* 21:401, 1985.

Jones BR: Hyperchylomicronemia in the cat. In Bonagura JD et al, editors: *Kirk's current veterinary therapy XII*, Philadelphia, 1995, WB Saunders.

Kern TJ et al: Facial neuropathy in dogs and cats: 95 cases, *J Am Vet Med Assoc* 191(12):1604, 1987.

Kocan AA: Tick paralysis, *J Am Vet Med Assoc* 192(11):1498, 1988.

Longshore RC et al: Dysautonomia in dogs: a retrospective study, *J Vet Intern Med* 10(3):103, 1996.

Shell L: Otitis media and interna. In Bonagura JD et al, editors: *Kirk's current veterinary therapy XII*, Philadelphia, 1995, WB Saunders.

Shelton GD: Myasthenia gravis and other disorders of neuromuscular transmission, *Vet Clin North Am Small Anim Pract* 32(1):188, 2002.

Shelton GD et al: Acquired myasthenia gravis: selective involvement of esophageal, pharyngeal and facial muscles, *J Vet Intern Med* 4(6):181, 1990.

Towell TL et al: Endocrinopathies that affect peripheral nerves of dogs and cats, *Compend Contin Educ Pract Vet* 16(2):157, 1994.

# CHAPTER 74

# Disorders of Muscle

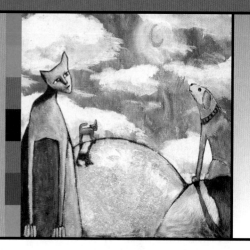

## CHAPTER OUTLINE

INFLAMMATORY MYOPATHIES, 1062
    Masticatory myositis, 1062
    Canine idiopathic polymyositis, 1063
    Feline idiopathic polymyositis, 1064
    Dermatomyositis, 1064
    Protozoal myositis, 1065
METABOLIC MYOPATHIES, 1065
    Glucocorticoid excess, 1065
    Hypothyroidism, 1065
    Hypokalemic polymyopathy, 1065
INHERITED MYOPATHIES, 1066
    Muscular dystrophy, 1066
    Hereditary Labrador Retriever myopathy, 1067
    Myotonia, 1067
    Miscellaneous, 1068

## INFLAMMATORY MYOPATHIES

### MASTICATORY MYOSITIS

Masticatory muscle myositis (MMM) is a widely reported inflammatory disorder involving primarily or exclusively the muscles of mastication in the dog. The masticatory muscles are composed primarily of a unique myofiber (Type 2M) that is not present in limb muscles. In dogs with MMM, necrosis and phagocytosis are limited to these fibers and circulating IgG is directed against the unique myosin component of these fibers. The etiology of masticatory myositis is unknown but the nature of the inflammatory infiltrate in diseased muscle, the response to immunosuppressive doses of corticosteroids, and the identification of autoantibodies (i.e., antitype 2M myofibers) in some affected dogs suggest an immune-mediated mechanism. Masticatory myositis can occur in any breed of dog, but the German Shepherd, the retrieving breeds, the Doberman Pinscher, and other large breeds of dogs are most commonly affected. Primarily, young or middle-aged dogs are affected, and no apparent gender predilection exists. The disorder has not been documented in cats.

### Clinical Features

The acute form of the disease involves recurrent painful swelling of the muscles of mastication, particularly the temporalis and masseter muscles. Exophthalmus may occur, caused by pressure on retrobulbar tissues from the swollen musculature. Pyrexia, submandibular and prescapular lymphadenopathy, and tonsillitis are variably present. Dogs are reluctant to eat and may salivate profusely. Most dogs are presented for anorexia and depression. Palpation of the muscles of the head and attempts to open the mouth are met with resistance because of pain.

The chronic form of masticatory myositis is more commonly recognized than the acute form. Affected dogs have progressive, severe atrophy of the temporal and masseter muscles, resulting in a skull-like appearance of their heads. They may have difficulty opening their mouths to eat, but they are otherwise bright, alert, and systemically normal (Fig. 74-1). The globes may sink deep into the orbits because of the dramatic loss of muscle mass (Fig. 74-2). The chronic form may occur after repeated acute episodes of masseteric myositis or without any history of signs related to acute episodes.

### Diagnosis

Diagnosis is suspected based on the clinical findings. In the acute form, various disorders affecting the teeth, eyes, mouth, and temporomandibular joints must be considered. Severe, nonpainful atrophy of the masticatory muscles in the chronic disease must be differentiated from atrophy caused by trigeminal neuropathy or widespread polymyositis.

A hemogram may reveal mild anemia and neutrophilic leukocytosis; occasionally a peripheral eosinophilia is found. Serum creatine kinase (CK), aspartate aminotransferase (AST), and globulin concentrations may be increased, particularly in the acute phase of the disease. Proteinuria sometimes occurs. Circulating antibodies against Type 2M fibers can be detected in the serum of over 80% of dogs with MMM. Electromyography (EMG) can help confirm the presence of muscle disease restricted to the masticatory muscles, although it is normal in a few chronically affected dogs when

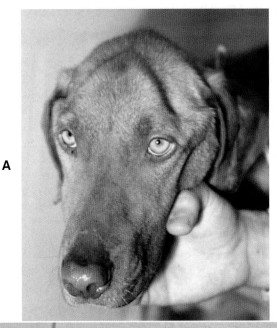

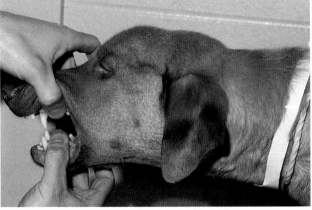

**FIG 74-1**
Masticatory muscle myositis (MMM) causing **(A)** severe temporalis and masseter muscle atrophy and **(B)** inability to open the mouth more than a few centimeters in an adult Vizsla.

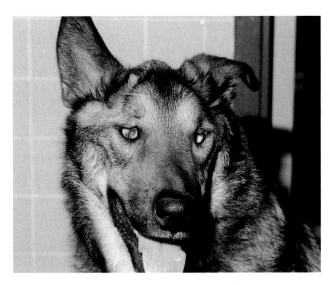

**FIG 74-2**
Dramatic muscle atrophy in a dog with masticatory muscle myositis (MMM) has resulted in retraction of the globes into the orbits.

most of the muscle has been replaced by fibrous connective tissue. Histopathologic evaluation of a muscle biopsy establishes the diagnosis of masticatory myositis. In addition to the submission of formalin-fixed biopsies, muscle tissue should be frozen or chemically fixed (e.g., using acetone) to permit the subsequent use of histochemical and immunohistochemical stains to identify antibody bound to Type 2M muscle fibers.

### Treatment

The administration of corticosteroids (prednisone, 1 to 2 mg/kg PO q12h) should result in rapid clinical remission. After approximately 3 weeks, the dose of corticosteroids can be decreased (to 1 mg/kg q24h) and then gradually tapered over 4 to 6 months to the lowest possible alternate-day dose. Inadequate dosing or treatment for an insufficient period of time is associated with a high rate of relapse. Dogs that do not respond adequately to corticosteroid therapy or relapse each time the dose is decreased may benefit from the use of other immunosuppressive drugs such as Azathioprine (Imuran; Burroughs Wellcome, Research Triangle Park, N.C.) given 2 mg/kg orally once a day, then every 48 hours. Dogs treated aggressively have a good prognosis for recovery. They should be carefully monitored for relapse (using jaw mobility and discomfort and serum CK), particularly as the corticosteroid dose is tapered. Lifelong treatment may be required.

Historically it was recommended that dogs with chronic atrophic myositis have their jaws opened by force under anesthesia to stretch the fibrous tissue and muscle. This practice is no longer recommended, because it does not improve clinical outcome, it increases the inflammation in torn muscle fibers, and it carries an inherent risk of iatrogenic mandibular luxation or fracture.

## CANINE IDIOPATHIC POLYMYOSITIS

Idiopathic polymyositis (PM) is a diffuse inflammation of skeletal muscle presumed to be an autoimmune process. Large-breed adult dogs are most commonly affected, with many reported cases in German Shepherds.

### Clinical Features

Mild-to-severe weakness that may be exacerbated by exercise is the most common feature. The animal may exhibit lameness or a stiff, stilted gait. Muscles are painful in some dogs, whereas nonpainful, severe atrophy occurs in others. Affected dogs may regurgitate as a result of megaesophagus. Occasionally, dysphagia, excessive salivation, and a weak bark occur. Signs may be intermittent in mild cases or early in the course of the disease. Some dogs with acute severe disease are pyrexic and experience generalized pain. Neurologic examination reveals normal proprioception, spinal reflexes, mental status, and cranial nerves. Muscle atrophy is usually prominent, especially involving the temporalis and masseter muscles. A unique form of polymyositis confined to the extraocular muscles resulting in acute bilateral exophthalmus has recently been described in young dogs.

## Diagnosis

The diagnosis of idiopathic polymyositis is based on clinical signs, CK determination, EMG, and muscle biopsy. High serum CK (twofold to 100-fold increase) and AST activities are seen in most affected dogs at rest and even more dramatic increases are common after exercise. Gamma globulins may also be increased. EMG can be performed to document that multiple muscle groups are involved and to select a severely affected muscle for biopsy. EMG changes include prolonged insertional activity, positive sharp waves, fibrillation potentials, and bizarre high-frequency discharges.

A definitive diagnosis of idiopathic polymyositis requires muscle biopsy. Typical histopathologic findings include multifocal necrosis and phagocytosis of Type 1 and Type 2 myofibers, perivascular lymphocytic and plasmacytic infiltration, and evidence of muscle regeneration and fibrosis. An occasional muscle biopsy is normal because of the multifocal patchy nature of the disease. This should not preclude a diagnosis of myositis if the clinical findings, EMG, and serum CK and AST activities suggest the diagnosis.

Generalized systemic immune-mediated disease (e.g., systemic lupus erythematosus), neoplasia, and infectious myositis (e.g., *Toxoplasma, Neospora* organisms) must be eliminated as initiating causes whenever polymyositis is diagnosed. A CBC, synovial fluid analysis, urinalysis, serum ANA titer, serology, and/or immunohistochemical staining of muscle biopsies for protozoal antigens should be performed. Assessment of thoracic radiographs and abdominal ultrasound should focus on a search for neoplasia and identification of megaesophagus and aspiration pneumonia. Lymph node aspirates and bone marrow biopsy may be indicated. If all of these tests are normal, a diagnosis of idiopathic polymyositis is made.

## Treatment

Prednisone administration (1 to 2 mg/kg q12h for 14 days, then q24h for 14 days, then q48h) results in dramatic clinical improvement and recovery of most dogs. If megaesophagus is present, upright feeding of small meals (Fig. 73-11) may be beneficial to prevent aspiration, and aspiration pneumonia, if it occurs, should be treated with antibiotics. Prednisone treatment should continue for at least 4 to 6 weeks at decreasing doses, with long-term treatment for 12 months or longer occasionally required. Azathioprine should be administered if an inadequate response to prednisone is seen.

## Prognosis

The prognosis is good for recovery in dogs without severe megaesophagus or aspiration pneumonia if no underlying neoplastic cause for the polymyositis is identified.

## FELINE IDIOPATHIC POLYMYOSITIS

An acquired inflammatory disorder of skeletal muscle similar to canine polymyositis has been described in a few cats. Affected cats between 6 months and 14 years of age experience a sudden onset of weakness with pronounced ventral neck flexion, an inability to jump, and a tendency to sit or lie down after walking short distances. Muscle pain may be evident. Neurologic examination reveals normal mentation, cranial nerves, proprioception, and reflexes.

Diagnosis is suspected based on clinical features, increases of serum CK and AST activities, and multifocal EMG abnormalities. Many affected cats (70%) are slightly hypokalemic, suggesting a possible relationship between this disorder and hypokalemic polymyopathy (see p. 1065). Some clinical features of PM also mimic mild thiamine deficiency; thus evaluation of the response to treatment of affected cats with thiamine (10 to 20 mg/day IM) and correction of hypokalemia are recommended before proceeding with extensive diagnostic testing for polymyositis.

Serum titers against *Toxoplasma gondii* should be evaluated, as should tests for feline leukemia virus antigen and feline immunodeficiency virus antibody. A complete drug history should be obtained to eliminate the possibility of drug-induced PM. Thoracic and abdominal radiographs and abdominal ultrasound should be considered to look for an underlying neoplastic cause of the PM. Muscle biopsy reveals myofiber necrosis and phagocytosis, muscle regeneration, variation in muscle fiber size, lymphocytic inflammation, and fibrosis. Empiric treatment for *Toxoplasma* myositis is sometimes recommended (Clindamycin 12.5 to 25 mg/kg PO q12h)—if the animal has a dramatic response to Clindamycin, the treatment should be continued for at least 6 weeks. It is important to realize, however, that spontaneous recovery or remission is observed in at least one-third of all cats with PM. Corticosteroid therapy (prednisone, 4 to 6 mg/kg/day initially, tapered over 2 months) may aid recovery in some cats. Recurrences are common.

The cause of this myopathy in cats is not known. Inclusion bodies have been identified in muscle fibers of some affected animals, causing speculation of viral infection. The literature includes reports of several adult cats with polymyositis in association with thymoma. The relationship of this disorder to hypokalemic polymyopathy is unknown. In some cases the changes found on muscle biopsy and the animal's response to corticosteroids suggest an immune basis for this disorder.

## DERMATOMYOSITIS

Dermatomyositis is an uncommon disease characterized by dermatitis and polymyositis. Familial canine dermatomyositis has been reported in juvenile rough-coated and smooth-coated Collies and in Shetland Sheepdogs (i.e., Shelties). Sporadic cases have been observed in a few other breeds, including Welsh Corgis, Australian Cattle Dogs, and Border Collies. The disease has not been recognized in cats. Skin lesions include erythema, ulcers, crusts, scales, and alopecia on the inner surfaces of pinnae and on the head and skin surfaces subjected to trauma (e.g., tail, elbows, hocks, sternum) (Fig. 74-3). Mild pruritus may occur. Histopathologic findings include hydropic degeneration of basal cells and separation of the dermoepidermal junction. A perivascular mononuclear infiltrate may be seen. Dermatologic lesions appear during the first 3 months of life and may improve or resolve with time. The course often fluctuates.

Dogs severely affected by dermatomyositis may develop signs of muscle disease, including generalized muscle atrophy, facial palsy, decreased jaw tone, weakness, and a stiff gait. Mentation, proprioception, and reflexes are normal. Dysphagia is common, and regurgitation as a result of megaesophagus may occur. EMG reveals spontaneous myofiber discharges, including fibrillation potentials, positive sharp waves, and bizarre high-frequency discharges in affected muscles. Nerve conduction velocities are normal. Muscle biopsies reveal myofiber necrosis with mononuclear cell infiltrates, atrophy, regeneration, and fibrosis. Some dogs with relatively severe dermatologic lesions exhibit no evidence of muscle disease.

Biopsies of skin and muscle, as well as EMG, may confirm a diagnosis of dermatomyositis. Breeding should not occur in dogs with confirmed dermatomyositis. Response of affected dogs to treatment with immunosuppressive doses of corticosteroids varies.

## PROTOZOAL MYOSITIS

Myositis caused by *T. gondii* can occur alone or in conjunction with myelitis, meningitis, or polyradiculoneuritis in dogs and cats, and similar syndromes caused by *Neospora caninum* can occur in the dog (see Chapters 71 and 73). Lesions can be found in the lung, liver, eye, central nervous system (CNS), and muscle.

Clinical signs referable to protozoal myositis typically include muscle pain, swelling or atrophy, and weakness. Increases in CK and AST activities are common, and serum titers

for the offending organism may be positive. EMG may reveal spontaneous activity in affected muscles (definitive diagnosis requires muscle biopsy). A mononuclear inflammatory reaction is present, and organisms are often seen. Immunohistochemical stains can be used to identify the organisms and to differentiate between *T. gondii* and *N. caninum* in affected dogs. Success has been reported in the treatment of protozoal myositis with clindamycin (12.5 to 25 mg/kg PO q12h) for 14 days, but more prolonged treatment (4 to 6 weeks) may be advisable.

## METABOLIC MYOPATHIES

In addition to the myopathies associated with infectious and inflammatory disease, myopathies may accompany hyperadrenocorticism (i.e., Cushing's disease), the administration of exogenous corticosteroids, and perhaps hypothyroidism. In cats a myopathy associated with hypokalemia has been recognized.

### GLUCOCORTICOID EXCESS

Glucocorticoid excess has been associated with an acquired degenerative myopathy. Spontaneous hyperadrenocorticism or exogenous administration of glucocorticoids, especially in high doses, can result in the syndrome. Muscle weakness and atrophy are common. Rarely, affected dogs develop limb rigidity, stiff gait, and hyperextension of all four limbs.

Diagnosis is suspected based on a history of exogenous steroid administration or clinical findings consistent with steroid excess (e.g., polyuria, polydipsia, hair loss, pendulous abdomen, thin skin). Diagnostic tests for hyperadrenocorticism (i.e., adrenocorticotropic hormone stimulation test; see Chapter 53) may confirm the diagnosis. Control of excess glucocorticoids may result in some clinical improvement; however, in most dogs the prognosis is poor for complete resolution of the myopathy.

### HYPOTHYROIDISM

Hypothyroidism may be associated with a subclinical myopathy in dogs. Some have speculated that the weakness and reduced exercise tolerance seen in hypothyroid dogs is related to this myopathy. Electrodiagnostic findings are normal.

### HYPOKALEMIC POLYMYOPATHY

A polymyopathy linked to total body potassium depletion has been recognized in cats of all breeds, ages, and genders. Cats with chronic renal failure and those consuming acidifying diets are most commonly affected, but cats with polyuria or polydipsia secondary to hyperthyroidism and cats with anorexia from any etiology may also be at risk. Severe total body depletion of potassium occurs secondary to decreased dietary intake or increased urinary excretion of potassium. A similar syndrome has been reported in Burmese kittens, with a probable hereditary basis.

The predominant clinical feature in all of these cats is weakness characterized by persistent ventroflexion of the neck (Fig. 74-4); a stiff, stilted gait; and reluctance to move.

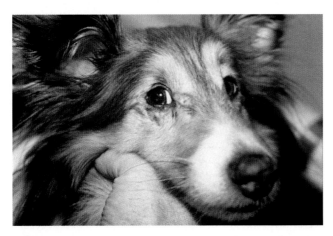

**FIG 74-3**
A Shetland Sheepdog with typical skin lesions of dermatomyositis. This dog also had megaesophagus and generalized muscular weakness.

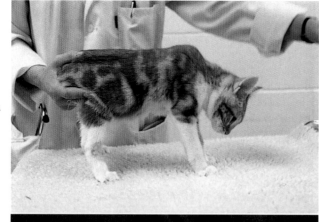

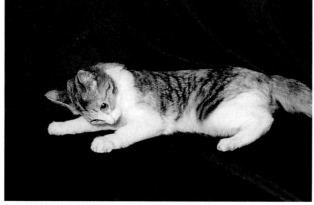

**FIG 74-4**
Feline hypokalemic myopathy resulting in weakness and cervical ventroflexion in **(A)** a kitten with congenital renal disease and **(B)** a hyperthyroid cat. The weakness resolved in both cats after potassium supplementation.

Some cats exhibit excessive scapular movement during walking. Muscle pain may be apparent, but the neurologic examination is otherwise unremarkable, with normal postural reactions and spinal reflexes. Clinical signs may have an acute onset and be episodic. Serum CK activity is usually high (10 to 30 times normal), serum potassium concentration is decreased (<3.5 mEq/L), and increased fractional urinary excretion of potassium may occur. Many affected cats have renal disease, so serum urea and creatinine concentrations may be increased. Interpretation of these parameters and the urine specific gravity can be difficult, because the hypokalemia can itself decrease renal blood flow and GFR, interfering with urine-concentrating mechanisms.

Mild diffuse EMG changes, including increased insertional activity, positive sharp waves, fibrillation potentials, and high frequency discharges have been recorded in affected cats. Muscle biopsies show mild myonecrosis or are normal, helping to distinguish this condition from the more obviously inflammatory polymyositis.

Signs of hypokalemic polymyopathy usually resolve after parenteral or oral supplementation of potassium. Oral treatment with potassium gluconate is recommended for mildly affected cats (Kaon Elixir; Adria Laboratories, Columbus, Ohio) at a dose of 2.5 to 5.0 mEq/cat twice a day for 2 days, then once a day. The dose administered is adjusted based on serum potassium levels. Cats with more dramatic hypokalemia (<2.5 mEq/L) or those with severe muscular weakness causing respiratory compromise require parenteral administration of lactated Ringer's solution, intravenously [IV] or subcutaneously [SC] supplemented with at least 80 mEq/L of potassium chloride per liter of fluid. IV supplementation of potassium should not exceed 0.5 mEq/kg/hour. Oral supplementation with potassium gluconate may be beneficial long-term. Monitoring serum potassium concentration periodically is recommended.

## *INHERITED MYOPATHIES*

### **MUSCULAR DYSTROPHY**

The muscular dystrophies (MDs) are a group of inherited myopathies characterized by progressive degeneration of skeletal muscle. Originally described in the Golden Retriever, dystrophic conditions have now been characterized in many breeds of dogs including the Irish Terrier, Samoyed, Rottweiler, Belgian Shepherd, Miniature Schnauzer, Pembroke Welsh Corgi, Alaskan Malamute, Wire-Haired Fox Terrier, German Shorthaired Pointer, Brittany Spaniel, and the Rat Terrier. Dystrophin, a crucial cytoskeletal protein, is lacking in the skeletal and cardiac muscle of affected dogs.

The clinical syndrome is similar in all affected breeds, although the clinical severity and precise genetic mutation leading to MD may be different in each breed. In many breeds, including the Golden Retriever and the Irish Terrier, an X-linked inheritance has been documented, causing the disease to be clinically apparent in male dogs and carried by female dogs.

Golden Retriever muscular dystrophy (GRMD) has been well described. Despite the fact that all affected male dogs have the same genetic lesion, the severity of clinical expression is variable. Puppies with GRMD are often stunted even before weaning. Abduction of the elbows, a bunny-hopping gait, and difficulty opening the mouth may be noted. With time, affected puppies develop a progressively more stilted gait, exercise intolerance, a plantigrade stance, atrophy of the truncal, limb and temporalis muscles, and muscle contractures. Muscle strength deteriorates until approximately 6 months of age, when the signs tend to stabilize. Proprioceptive positioning and spinal reflexes are normal, but spinal reflexes may be difficult to elicit if muscle fibrosis and joint contractures occur. Severely affected dogs may develop pharyngeal or esophageal dysfunction. Cardiac failure occurs occasionally.

MD should be suspected when typical clinical signs are seen in a young male puppy of a predisposed breed. Serum CK levels are markedly increased as early as 1 week of age and peak at 6 to 8 weeks of age. Very dramatic increases in CK occur after exercise. EMG reveals pseudomyotonic discharges in most muscles by 10 weeks of age. Biopsies reveal marked myofiber size variation, necrosis, and regeneration with multifocal myofiber mineralization. Immunocytochemical studies document the absence of the sarcolemmal protein dystrophin. No effective treatment exists.

An X-linked MD has also been reported in the cat. Clinical signs first appear at 5 to 6 months of age. Affected cats exhibit marked generalized muscular hypertrophy, protrusion of the tongue, excessive salivation, stiff gait, and bunny hopping. Megaesophagus is common. Serum CK is greatly elevated (often >30,000 U/L). Diagnosis requires muscle biopsy and dystrophin immunostaining.

## HEREDITARY LABRADOR RETRIEVER MYOPATHY

Hereditary Labrador Retriever myopathy (HLRM) is a degenerative myopathy inherited as an autosomal recessive trait in males and females of the breed (also called *autosomal recessive muscular dystrophy* [ARMD]). Although the age of onset of signs is variable (6 weeks to 6 months), signs usually become evident at 3 to 4 months of age. A low head carriage (i.e., ventroflexion); muscular weakness; and a stiff, stilted gait are common (Fig. 74-5). The back may be arched, and a bunny-hopping gait may develop with exercise. Activity, excitement, exercise, and cold temperatures exacerbate the clinical signs and may precipitate collapse. Affected dogs often have carpal overextension, carpal valgus deformity, and splaying of their toes. Muscle atrophy may be marked, especially in the proximal limbs and the muscles of mastication.

Affected dogs are bright and alert. Their muscles are not painful, and although they are weak, conscious proprioception is normal. Spinal reflexes are generally reduced or absent, even in mildly affected dogs. Megaesophagus causing regurgitation has been seen in a few affected dogs. Serum CK activity is usually normal. Electrodiagnostic testing reveals spontaneous myofiber discharges and normal nerve conduction velocity. Muscle biopsy is required to confirm the diagnosis. The predominant histologic change is myofiber atrophy with a paucity of Type 2 myofibers (sometimes called *Type 2 myofiber deficiency*). In most cases the clinical signs stabilize between 6 and 12 months of age, so many of these dogs remain functional as pets.

## MYOTONIA

Myotonia is a rare disorder of muscle that has been recognized in Chow Chows, Staffordshire Bull Terriers, Labrador Retrievers, Rhodesian Ridgebacks, Great Danes, and individual dogs of a number of breeds. Affected kittens have also been identified. Myotonia, by definition, is the continued active contraction and delayed relaxation of muscle. It results from hyperexcitable muscle membranes and is characterized clinically by generalized muscle stiffness and hypertrophy that begins at a young age (i.e., 2 to 6 months).

Dogs with myotonia are neurologically normal. No abnormalities of proprioception or mentation exist. Cold weather, excitement, and exercise exacerbate the clinical signs. Affected dogs may remain in rigid recumbency for up to 30 seconds if they are suddenly placed in lateral recumbency.

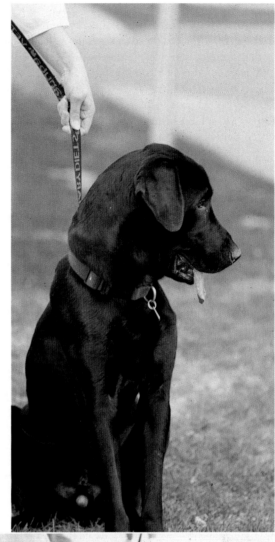

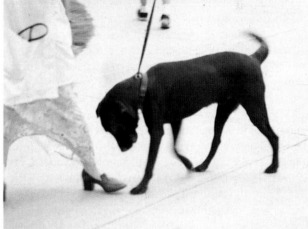

**FIG 74-5**
A 1-year-old Labrador Retriever with Hereditary Labrador Retriever myopathy (HLRM) exhibiting proximal muscle atrophy; a stiff, stilted gait; and ventroflexion of the neck that worsens with exercise.

Serum CK and AST activities may be increased, indicating muscle fiber necrosis. Bizarre high-frequency discharges that wax and wane ("dive bomber sound") are revealed by EMG and, when present, confirm the diagnosis. Muscle biopsy alone is rarely diagnostic. Membrane-stabilizing agents such as procainamide (10 to 30 mg/kg PO q6h) and phenytoin (20 to 35 mg/kg by PO q12h) and the sodium channel blocker, mexiletine (Mexitil; Boehringer Ingelheim: 8 mg/kg PO q8h), have been beneficial in the treatment of some cases. The avoidance of cold temperatures is also advised. Most dogs are euthanized because of the severity of their signs.

## MISCELLANEOUS

A number of genetically based noninflammatory myopathies have been described in dogs and cats. Some of the most common clinical signs include exercise intolerance; muscular weakness; a stiff, stilted gait; muscle tremors; and muscle atrophy. These disorders can result from deficiencies of the enzymes necessary for normal muscle metabolism, abnormalities of muscle membranes, or dysfunctional ion channels. Establishing the precise cause of a metabolic myopathy can be difficult because of the wide range of biochemical abnormalities that can arise and the codependence of all of the structural proteins making up a muscle fiber. Sometimes metabolic testing can be beneficial; for example, inappropriate lactic acidosis in association with exercise intolerance suggests mitochondrial dysfunction. Evaluation of plasma lactate and pyruvate before and after exercise and quantitative analysis of urinary organic acids and plasma, urine and muscle carnitine may help to determine the affected biochemical pathway. This testing, although expensive, is recommended for the investigation of all dogs with unexplained weakness and exercise-induced collapse. Histologic and ultrastuctual examination of skeletal muscle can also aid diagnosis.

Various glycolytic pathway enzyme deficiencies have been described in dogs. These include a glycogen storage disease in Lapland dogs, a debranching enzyme deficiency in German Shepherds and an inherited decrease in phosphofructokinase in English Springer Spaniels.

Defects in oxidative metabolism in muscle can result in a lipid storage myopathy, producing an abnormal accumulation of lipid in skeletal muscle. Adult dogs are affected, with signs ranging from poorly localizable pain and exercise intolerance to severe muscle weakness and atrophy. Serum CK and AST activities are often normal. Muscle biopsy reveals a vacuolar myopathy with increased intramyofiber lipid. These lipid storage myopathies may accompany deranged carnitine metabolism, mitochondrial defects, or disorders of fatty acid oxidation. Dogs in which low muscle carnitine levels are doc-

umented, whether this is primary or secondary, may benefit from oral L-carnitine supplementation (50 mg/kg q12h).

Mitochondrial myopathies resulting in collapse and severe lactic acidosis have been identified in Clumber and Sussex Spaniels because of an inability to oxidize pyruvate. Similar disorders have been recognized in the Old English Sheepdog and the Cavalier King Charles Spaniel. Affected young dogs (i.e., 3 to 4 months old) develop marked lactic acidemia and hyperthermia ($>42°$ C, $>107°$ F) after only mild-to-moderate exercise. Young Great Danes may exhibit a syndrome of muscle atrophy, weakness, and exercise-induced collapse (i.e., central core myopathy), also thought to result from a defect in oxidative metabolism.

A group of metabolic myopathies in which nemaline rods accumulate in myofibers have been reported in a group of related cats and in dogs with an apparently inherited myopathy. Affected animals usually begin to show signs during the first year of life, including weakness, reluctance to move, a hypermetric gait, muscle atrophy, and hyporeflexia. Muscle biopsy reveals the characteristic histologic changes, but the actual metabolic abnormality has not been identified.

Malignant hyperthermia is a rare hypermetabolic disorder of skeletal muscle, resulting from a genetic defect of intracellular calcium homeostasis. In genetically susceptible dogs, exertional, thermal, anoxic, or mechanical stresses or the administration of halothane anesthesia or succinylcholine will result in dramatic muscular contraction, lactic acidemia, and hyperthermia. Definitive diagnosis relies on physiologic testing on specially prepared muscle biopsies or identification of the defective gene in affected dogs.

### Suggested Readings

Braund KG: Skeletal muscle biopsy, *Semin Vet Med Surg (Small Anim)* 4(2):108, 1989.

Braund KG et al: Toxoplasma polymyositis/polyneuropathy—a new clinical variant in two mature dogs, *J Am Anim Hosp Assoc* 24:93, 1988.

Dow SW et al: Hypokalemia in cats: 186 cases (1984-1987), *J Am Vet Med Assoc* 194(11):1604, 1989.

Gilmour MA et al: Masticatory myopathy in the dog: a retrospective study of 18 cases, *J Am Anim Hosp Assoc* 28:300, 1992.

Klopp LS et al: Autosomal recessive muscular dystrophy in Labrador Retrievers, *Comp Cont Educ Sm Anim Pract* 22(2):121, 2000.

LeCouteur R et al: Metabolic and endocrine myopathies of dogs and cats, *Semin Vet Med Surg (Small Anim)* 4(2):146, 1989.

Shelton DG: Disorders of neuromuscular transmission, *Semin Vet Med Surg (Small Anim)* 4(2):126, 1989.

Smith MO: Idiopathic myositides in dogs, *Semin Vet Med Surg (Small Anim)* 4(2):156, 1989.

Taylor SM: Selected disorders of muscle and the neuromuscular junction, *Vet Clin North Am Sm Anim Pract* 30(1):59, 2000.

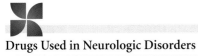

## Drugs Used in Neurologic Disorders

| DRUG NAME (TRADE NAME) | PURPOSE | RECOMMENDED DOSE DOG | CAT |
|---|---|---|---|
| Acetylpromazine (Acepromazine) | Restraint, sedation, relaxation | 0.1-0.2 mg/kg IM q6h | 0.1-0.2 mg/kg IM q6h |
| Activated Charcoal (1 g/5 ml water) | Gastrointestinal adsorbent | 10 ml/kg | 10 ml/kg |
| Acetylsalicylic acid (Aspirin) | Analgesia, antiinflammatory Antithrombotic | 25 mg/kg PO q8h 10 mg/kg PO q6h | 10 mg/kg PO q48h 10 mg/kg PO q48h |
| Aminocaproic Acid (Amicar) | Antiinflammatory for degenerative myelopathy | 500 mg PO q8h | Not evaluated |
| Ampicillin | Antibiotic | 22 mg/kg PO q8h or 22 mg/kg IV, SC, IM q6h | 22 mg/kg PO q8h or 22 mg/kg IV, SC, IM q6h |
| Apomorphine | Emetic | 0.08 mg/kg SC or 6 mg (1 crushed tablet) in conjunctival sac | Use alternative (xylazine) |
| Atropine | Antidote for cholinergic toxins | 0.5 mg/kg IV, then 1.5 mg/kg SC q6-8h | 0.5 mg/kg IV, then 1.5 mg/kg SC q6-8h |
| Azathioprine (Imuran) | Immune-mediated diseases | 50 mg/m² (approx. 2.2 mg/kg) PO q6h | 0.2 mg/kg PO q48h |
| Bethanechol (Urecholine) | Treat bladder atony | 0.04 mg/kg PO, SC q8h | 0.04 mg/kg PO, SC q8h |
| Calcium EDTA (Versenate) (1 g/100 ml D₅W) | Lead poisoning antidote | 25 mg/kg SC q6h | 25 mg/kg SC q6h |
| Calcium gluconate (10%) | Treating hypocalcemia | 0.5-1.0 ml/kg IV | 0.5-1.0 ml/kg IV |
| Cefadroxil | Antibiotic | 22 mg/kg PO q12h | 22 mg/kg PO |
| Cephalexin (Keflex) | Antibiotic | 20-40 mg/kg PO q8h | 20-40 mg/kg PO q8h |
| Cephalothin (Keflin) | Antibiotic | 25 mg/kg IV, IM, SC q6h | 25 mg/kg IV, IM, SC q6h |
| Chloramphenicol | Antibiotic | 25-50 mg/kg PO, IV q6-8h | 12.5-25 mg/kg PO, IV q12h |
| Chlorazepate dipotassium (Traxene) | Anticonvulsant | 1 mg/kg q12h | Unknown |
| Chlorpromazine (Thorazine) | Muscle relaxation | 0.5 mg/kg IV q8h | 0.5 mg/kg IV q8h |
| Cimetidine (Tagamet) | H₂ blocker antacid | 5 mg/kg PO, IM, IV q8h | 5 mg/kg PO, IM, IV q8h |
| Clonazepam (Clonapin) | Anticonvulsant | 0.5 mg/kg PO q8-12h | Not evaluated |
| Clindamycin (Cleocin) | Antibiotic | 10-15 mg/kg PO q12h | 10-15 mg/kg PO q12h |
| Cloxacillin (Tegopen) | Antibiotic | 10-15 mg/kg PO, IV q6h | 10-15 mg/kg PO, IV q6h |
| Dexamethasone | Acute spinal cord or brain edema | 2-4 mg/kg IV | 2-4 mg/kg IV |
| | Antiinflammatory/ antiedema | 0.1-1.0 mg/kg PO, IV, SC (see specific disorder) | 0.1-1.0 mg/kg PO, IV, SC (see specific disorder) |
| Dextrose (50%) | Treating hypoglycemia | 2 ml/kg | 2 ml/kg |
| Diazepam (valium) | Anticonvulsant | | |
| | Status epilepticus | 5-20 mg IV (repeat if needed) | 5 mg IV (repeat if needed) |
| | Chronic seizure management | 0.5-1 mg/kg PO q8h | 0.3-0.8 mg/kg PO q8h |
| | Muscle relaxant | 0.5-1 mg/kg PO q8h | 0.3-0.8 mg/kg PO q8h |
| Dimethyl sulfoxide (DMSO) | Cerebral edema treatment | 1 g/kg IV/30 min | 1 g/kg IV/30 min |
| Diphenhydramine HCl (Benadryl) | Antiemetic (vestibular disease) | 2-4 mg/kg SC | 1-2 mg/kg SC |
| Doxycycline (Vibramycin) | Antibiotic | 5-10 mg/kg PO, IV q12h | 5-10 mg/kg PO, IV q12h |
| Edrophonium chloride (Tensilon) | Tensilon test—myasthenia gravis | 0.1-0.2 mg/kg IV | 0.2 mg/cat IV |
| Enrofloxacin (Baytril) | Antibiotic | 5 mg/kg PO, SC, IV q12h | 2-5 mg/kg PO, SC, IV q12h |
| Folinic acid | Pyrimethamine toxicity | 0.5-5 mg/day | 0.5-5 mg/day |
| Furosemide (Lasix) | Diuretic, antiedema | 2-4 mg/kg IV, IM, SC q6h | 2-4 mg/kg IV, IM, SC q6h |
| Ipecac Syrup | Emetic | 6.6 ml/kg PO | 6.6 ml/kg PO |

*Continued*

Drugs Used in Neurologic Disorders—cont'd

| DRUG NAME (TRADE NAME) | PURPOSE | RECOMMENDED DOSE | |
|---|---|---|---|
| | | **DOG** | **CAT** |
| Mannitol (20% solution over 30 minutes) | Cerebral edema treatment | 1-3 g/kg | 1-3 g/kg |
| Methocarbamol (Robaxin) | Muscle relaxant | 20 mg/kg PO q8-12h | None |
| Methylprednisolone sodium succinate (SoluMedrol) | Spinal, brain trauma | 20-40 mg/kg IV | 20-40 mg/kg IV |
| Metronidazole (Flagyl) | Antibiotic | 10-15 mg/kg PO q8h | 10-15 mg/kg PO q8h |
| Neostigmine bromide (Prostigmin) | Myasthenia gravis | 0.5 mg/kg q12h | None |
| Neostigmine methylsulfate (Stiglyn) | Myasthenia gravis | 0.01-0.04 mg/kg IM q6-8h | None |
| Penicillin G | Antibiotic | | |
| Aqueous (K or Na) | | 40,000 U/kg IV q6h | 40,000 U/kg IV q6h |
| Procaine | | 40,000 U/kg IM, SC q12h | 40,000 U/kg IM, SC q12h |
| Pentobarbital (Nembutal) | Anticonvulsant/anesthetic | 5-15 mg/kg IV to effect | 5-15 mg/kg IV to effect |
| Phenobarbital | Anticonvulsant | 0.5-2 mg/kg IV, IM, PO q8h | 0.5-2 mg/kg IV, IM, PO q8h |
| Phenoxybenzamine (Dibenzyline) | Adrenogenic α blocker | 0.25-0.5 mg/kg PO q8-12h | 2.5-7.5 mg/cat PO q8-12h |
| Phenylbutazone (Butazolidin) | Analgesia | 5-10 mg/kg PO q8h (max. 800 mg/day) | None |
| Potassium bromide | Anticonvulsant | 30-40 mg/kg PO q6h | 30 mg/kg PO q6h |
| Potassium gluconate (Kaon Elixir) | Hypokalemia | None | 2.5-5.0 mEq/cat PO q12h |
| Pralidoxime chloride (2 PAM, Protopam) | Organophosphate intoxication | 20 mg/kg IM q12h | 20 mg/kg IM q12h |
| Prednisone | Immunosuppression | 2-4 mg/kg/day PO | 2-6 mg/kg/day PO |
| | Antiinflammatory/ antiedema | 0.5-0.75 mg/kg PO | 0.5-0.75 mg/kg PO |
| Primidone | Anticonvulsant | 10 mg/kg PO q8h—not recommended as first choice | None |
| Pyrimethamine | Toxoplasmosis | 0.25-0.5 mg/kg PO q12h | 0.25-0.5 mg/kg PO q12h |
| Pyridostigmine bromide (Mestinon) | Myasthenia gravis | 2 mg/kg PO q8-12h | 0.5 mg/kg PO q12h |
| Sodium sulfate (40%) | Cathartic | 1 g/kg PO | 1 g/kg PO |
| Tetracycline hydrochloride | Antibiotic | 22 mg/kg PO q8h | 22 mg/kg PO q8h |
| Thiamine (vitamin B1) | Thiamine deficiency | 10-100 mg IM, PO q6h | 10-50 mg IM, PO q6h |
| Trimethoprim-sulfadiazine (Tribrissen) | Antibiotic | 15 mg/kg PO or SC q12h | 15 mg/kg PO or SC q12h |
| Valproic Acid (Depakene) | Anticonvulsant | 20-60 mg/kg PO q8-12h | Not evaluated |
| Xylazine (Rompun) | Emetic (cats) | Not recommended | 0.44 mg/kg IM |

C H A P T E R 75

# Clinical Manifestations of and Diagnostic Tests for Joint Disorders

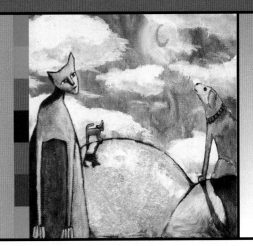

## CHAPTER OUTLINE

GENERAL CONSIDERATIONS, 1071
CLINICAL MANIFESTATIONS, 1071
DIAGNOSTIC TESTS, 1073
    Clinical pathology, 1073
    Radiography, 1073
    Synovial fluid collection and analysis, 1073
    Synovial fluid culture, 1076
    Synovial membrane biopsy, 1077
    Immunologic and serologic tests, 1077

## GENERAL CONSIDERATIONS

Disorders affecting the joints can be divided into two major categories: noninflammatory and inflammatory (Table 75-1). Noninflammatory joint diseases include developmental, degenerative, neoplastic, and traumatic processes. These disorders are discussed in greater detail in surgery textbooks and the Suggested Readings at the end of this chapter. Inflammatory joint diseases include infectious and immune-mediated processes.

## CLINICAL MANIFESTATIONS

Animals with joint disease are usually presented with a history of lameness or gait abnormality. Traumatic or developmental disorders of the joint typically involve only one joint, so the lameness is consistently described in the same limb. A shifting-leg lameness is commonly reported with disorders affecting multiple joints. When pain is severe in multiple joints (e.g., polyarthritis), the animal may refuse to walk, or it may cry in pain when moved or touched, making it difficult to differentiate joint disease from other serious musculo-skeletal and neurologic disorders causing pain (Fig. 75-1). In addition to lameness, clinical signs of immune-mediated

inflammatory joint disease may include cyclic fevers, stiffness, neck pain, and reluctance to exercise. Many affected animals are presented with a vague history of decreased appetite, weakness, or fever and no apparent lameness. Inflammatory joint disease is one of the most common causes of fever and nonspecific inflammation in dogs, and because many affected dogs do not have obvious joint pain or detectable joint swelling, it is important to maintain a high index of suspicion for polyarthritis when evaluating dogs and cats with nonspecific illness.

Animals with nonspecific pain, a stiff gait, reluctance to exercise, or fever of unknown origin require a complete physical examination. When pain is noted, it is important to make an attempt to localize the origin of the pain. Thorough palpation of the muscles, bones, and joints of each limb is important. Palpation of the bones themselves often elicits pain in animals following trauma and in those dogs affected by panosteitis, hypertrophic osteodystrophy, osteomyelitis, or bone neoplasia. Palpation of affected muscles elicits pain in most animals with myositis or strain/sprain injuries. Pain on palpation or manipulation of the neck could indicate a variety of spinal cord or vertebral abnormalities, intracranial disease, meningitis, or polyarthritis—inflammation of the intervertebral facetal joints can manifest as neck or back pain.

Many animals with joint disease will experience obvious joint pain. Flexing and extending the affected joint may reveal a restricted range of motion, discomfort, and crepitation, suggesting articular wear, the presence of osteophytes, or other periarticular changes most common in degenerative or erosive joint disease. The stability of the painful joint should be evaluated to assess the integrity of the supporting ligaments. Although dramatic joint swelling due to effusion will be apparent in some dogs with joint disease (Fig. 75-2), many dogs with immune-mediated inflammatory polyarthritis will not have appreciable joint swelling. A joint that feels normal on palpation can still be severely affected by joint disease.

The initial diagnostic tests for dogs and cats with suspected joint disease typically include radiographs and synovial fluid

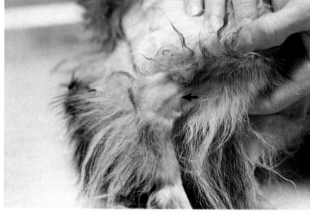

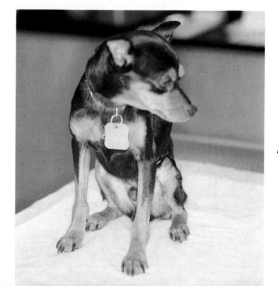

**FIG 75-1**
**A,** A 7-year-old Shetland Sheepdog was referred for suspected paralysis. The dog was neurologically normal but refused to rise because of joint pain resulting from idiopathic immune-mediated polyarthritis. **B,** The hock joint is visibly swollen.

 TABLE 75-1

**Classification of Common Joint Disorders in Dogs and Cats**

| |
|---|
| **Noninflammatory Joint Disease** |
| Developmental |
| Degenerative |
| Traumatic |
| Neoplastic |
| **Inflammatory Joint Disease** |
| Infectious |
| Noninfectious (immune) |
|  Nonerosive |
|  Erosive |

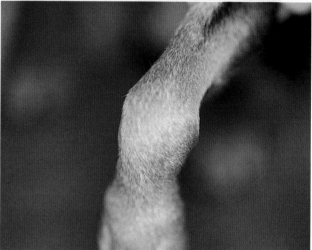

**FIG 75-2**
**A,** A 4-year-old Miniature Pinscher was referred for intermittent fever and depression during the previous year. All joints are palpably and visibly swollen, particularly the carpus **(B).**

analysis. Radiographs are taken to evaluate for degenerative, lytic, or erosive changes. Synovial fluid must be collected and analyzed in order to differentiate inflammatory joint disease from noninflammatory conditions (see Table 75-1 and p. 1073).

When inflammatory joint disease is identified, it is important to first eliminate infectious diseases as differential di-

agnoses. Infectious agents causing arthritis include bacteria, *Mycoplasma* spp., bacterial L-forms, spirochetes, rickettsial agents, and fungi. Diagnostic tests to assist in diagnosis may include a complete blood count (CBC); urinalysis; culture of urine, blood, and synovial fluid; and rickettsial (i.e., *Ehrlichia* spp. Rocky Mountain spotted fever [RMSF] and Lyme disease titers). Thoracic radiographs and fungal serology may also be warranted. Once infectious causes of polyarthritis have been ruled out, the immune-mediated conditions should be considered.

Noninfectious, immunologically mediated arthritis is common in dogs and uncommon in cats. Immune-mediated polyarthritis syndromes can be characterized as being erosive or nonerosive on the basis of physical examination findings and results of radiographs of affected joints.

Immune-mediated, nonerosive polyarthritis is the most common form of inflammatory joint disease recognized in dogs. It occurs as a result of immune-complex deposition within the synovium, leading to a sterile synovitis. Most often it is an idiopathic syndrome, but it may also occur as a feature of systemic lupus erythematosus (SLE) or secondary to prolonged antigenic stimulation (reactive polyarthritis) caused by chronic infection, neoplasia, or administration of drugs. In addition, a few breed-associated syndromes of polyarthritis or polyarthritis/meningitis/myositis are thought to have a genetic basis in dogs (see p. 1088).

Whenever noninfectious, nonerosive inflammatory joint disease is identified, it is important to obtain a thorough history regarding recent drug administration. In addition, a battery of tests is required to look for evidence of chronic infection or neoplasia (e.g., CBC, thoracic and abdominal radiographs, ophthalmologic examination, bacterial culture of urine and blood, cardiac ultrasonography, abdominal ultrasound) or SLE (e.g., CBC, platelet count, urine protein/creatinine ratio, antinuclear antibody [ANA] titer). Normal results on these tests warrant a diagnosis of idiopathic immune-mediated polyarthritis.

Rheumatoid arthritis is an uncommon erosive immune-mediated polyarthritis characterized by progressive joint destruction. Aseptic inflammatory joint disease in a dog with radiographic evidence of joint destruction warrants consideration of this disease. Serologic testing for rheumatoid factor and synovial membrane biopsy are required to establish this rare diagnosis.

Feline polyarthritis is uncommon. Infectious arthritis has been reported as resulting from bacteria, including bacterial L-forms and *Mycoplasma* spp., and calicivirus. Two forms of chronic progressive polyarthritis (erosive and nonerosive) have also been identified in male cats in association with feline leukemia virus and feline syncytium-forming virus infections. Noninfectious immunologically mediated polyarthritis resulting from SLE does occur occasionally in cats.

## DIAGNOSTIC TESTS

### CLINICAL PATHOLOGY

Evaluation of routine clinical pathology is indicated when polyarthritis is suspected. Depending on the underlying etiology, abnormal findings may include anemia, leukocytosis, thrombocytopenia, hypoproteinemia, proteinuria, and changes in the urinalysis consistent with urinary tract infection. Normal clinical pathology does not rule out polyarthritis.

### RADIOGRAPHY

Radiographic abnormalities of the joints and periarticular region are expected in animals with degenerative joint disease (DJD), chronic septic arthritis, and rheumatoid arthritis. Radiographs from patients with infectious polyarthritis caused by rickettsial agents, Lyme disease, or viruses are similar to radiographs from patients with immune-mediated nonerosive polyarthritis—typically the only abnormalities seen are mild joint capsule distention and associated soft-tissue swelling.

Results of the physical examination usually help to identify which joints should be radiographically evaluated. Suspected immune-mediated erosive polyarthritis warrants evaluation of the hocks and carpi. Each joint evaluated requires two views (i.e., lateral and anterior/posterior). Radiographs of the thorax and abdomen are recommended in dogs and cats with inflammatory joint disease to evaluate for underlying infectious or neoplastic disease. In addition, radiographs of the spine are used to screen for diskospondylitis as a cause for immune-mediated or infectious polyarthritis.

Radiography is an important tool, but it is limited. Many of the bony changes seen with DJDs and erosive immune disease are not apparent for weeks to months after the onset of signs. Although positive findings contribute a great deal to the diagnosis, negative findings should be interpreted with caution. Sequential radiographic studies may be warranted in animals in which a diagnosis of nonerosive polyarthritis is uncertain or in cases that do not respond to appropriate therapy.

## SYNOVIAL FLUID COLLECTION AND ANALYSIS

Synovial fluid collection and analysis is a valuable aid in establishing a diagnosis of canine and feline joint disease. It is of greatest value in confirming the presence of disease within a joint and differentiating inflammatory from noninflammatory disorders. Synovial fluid collection and analysis may also provide information regarding a specific diagnosis.

### Collection Method

Arthrocentesis requires little in the way of expertise or equipment, involves minimal risk to the animal, is inexpensive to perform, and has a high diagnostic yield. In dogs and cats, although synovial fluid can sometimes be collected without sedation or anesthesia, light tranquilization or sedation is usually used to prevent the animal from moving during sample collection and contaminating the sample. Whenever polyarthritis is suspected, synovial fluid should be analyzed from at least six joints. Immunologically mediated disease tends to be most prominent in the distal small joints, such as the hock and carpus, whereas septic joint disease is more often detected in the larger proximal joints. Even if only one joint is clinically affected, synovial fluid should be collected from multiple joints.

The hair should be clipped from the area, and the skin washed as for surgery. Wearing sterile gloves is necessary if the area where the needle will be inserted is to be palpated. Arthrocentesis in dogs and cats typically requires a 25-gauge needle attached to a 3 ml syringe (Fig. 75-3). A 22-gauge, 1½-inch needle is used for the shoulder, elbow, and stifle joints of larger dogs. Large dogs may require a 3-inch spinal needle to enter the hip joint.

Landmarks for arthrocentesis vary according to personal preference, but recommended approaches are outlined in Fig. 75-4. Following aseptic preparation, the needle attached to the syringe is inserted into the joint. Once the tip of the needle is in the joint, gentle negative pressure is applied to the syringe. Only a very small amount of joint fluid (one to three drops) is needed for the critical determination of viscosity, estimated cell count, differential white blood cell (WBC) count, and culture. The negative pressure on the syringe is released before withdrawal of the needle through the skin. The appearance of blood should prompt immediate release of

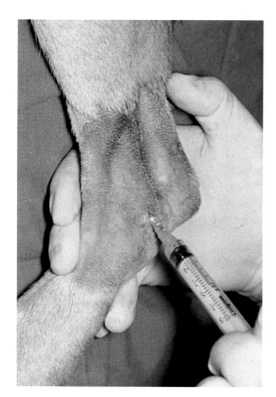

**FIG 75-3**
Arthrocentesis is performed using a small-gauge needle attached to a 3-ml syringe.

**FIG 75-4**
Schematic representation of recommended sites for arthrocentesis in the dog and cat. **A,** Carpus: partially flex the joint. Palpate and enter the anteromedial aspect of the carpometacarpal or radiocarpal space. **B,** Hock: anterior approach. Palpate the space between the tibia and tibiotarsal bone on the anterolateral surface of the hock; insert the needle in the shallow, palpable space. **C,** Hock: lateral approach. Partially flex the joint and insert the needle under the lateral malleolus of the fibula. **D,** Elbow: insert the needle just medial to the lateral epicondylar ridge proximal to the olecranon process. Advance parallel to the olecranon process into the olecranon fossa. **E,** Shoulder: lateral approach. Insert the needle just distal to the acromion process, direct the needle distally, medially, and posteriorly. **F,** Shoulder: cranial approach. Insert the needle just medial to the greater tubercle, ventral to the supraglenoid tubercle of the scapula. **G,** Stifle: insert the needle just lateral to the straight patellar ligament distal to the patella. Direct the needle medially and proximally toward the center of the joint. **H,** Coxofemoral: abduct and medially rotate the limb. Insert the needle dorsal to the greater trochanter; angle ventrally and caudally.

suction and withdrawal of the needle. Slides are made immediately (Fig. 75-5), using one drop of synovial fluid for each slide.

When possible, a sample should also be collected and saved for culture and sensitivity in a sterile tube or else should be directly inoculated into an enrichment media. When larger samples of synovial fluid are obtained, the remaining fluid can be placed in a test tube containing ethylenediaminetetraacetic acid (EDTA) for precise cell counts and further analysis.

## Analysis of Gross Appearance

Normal synovial fluid is clear and colorless. Cloudiness or turbidity is seen in any condition that causes red blood cells (RBCs) or WBCs to enter the joint in high numbers. Color change may be an indication of blood contamination or a pathologic condition. Hemorrhage from an earlier puncture attempt or an ongoing disease process results in a diffuse red discoloration of the synovial fluid, whereas blood from a traumatic tap does not appear to be homogeneously mixed with the joint fluid. A yellowish fluid (xanthochromia) usually indicates previous hemorrhage into the joint and is occasionally seen in degenerative, traumatic, and inflammatory joint diseases.

Normal synovial fluid is very viscous. It forms a long string when allowed to drop from the tip of a needle onto a slide (Fig. 75-6). A thin or watery consistency indicates that the synovial fluid is deficient in polymerized hyaluronic acid. This

may occur following dilution by serum or through degradation by an intense intraarticular inflammatory reaction.

## Analysis of Microscopic Appearance

Cytologic evaluation is the most important aspect of synovial fluid analysis. Usually only a few drops of synovial fluid are collected, and estimates of cell numbers are made from a stained direct smear of the fluid. Occasionally a large volume of fluid is obtained. In this case a hemocytometer is used for absolute cell counts, using physiologic saline as the diluting fluid, because the diluting fluid normally used with a hemocytometer for counting nucleated cells (2% acetic acid) precipitates the hyaluronate in the fluid, resulting in a mucin clot. Smears of synovial fluid should still be submitted in addition to the fluid preserved in EDTA, because the cells in synovial fluid may degenerate with time.

Normal synovial fluid contains between 100 and 3000 WBCs/μl; mononuclear cells predominate. One to three mononuclear cells per high-power (100×) field may be seen on a smear of normal synovial fluid. Estimates of WBC numbers in synovial fluid require comparing the average number of WBCs per microscope field on a slide of the synovial fluid with the average number of WBCs per microscope field on a blood smear with a known WBC count (Fig. 75-7). Experienced clinicians find simple microscopic scanning of a stained slide of synovial fluid sufficient to estimate cell numbers as normal, mildly increased, or greatly increased.

Normal synovial fluid has a mixture of large and small mononuclear cells that frequently contain many vacuoles and granules. An occasional neutrophil may be observed, but these cells should represent less than 10% of the total. If blood

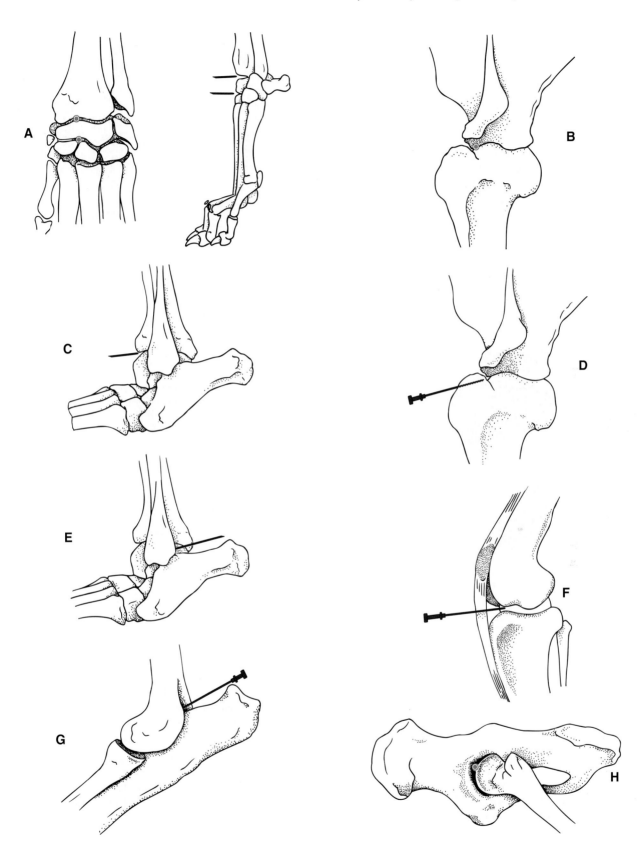

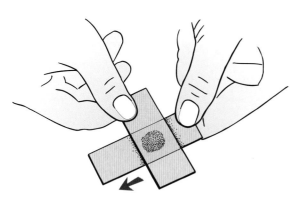

**FIG 75-5**
Preparing a smear of synovial fluid. A drop of fluid is placed onto a slide. A second slide is used to gently spread the fluid using a pull smear technique.

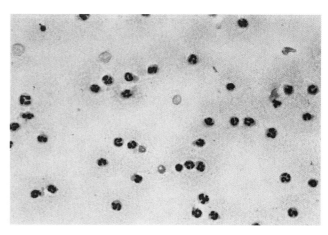

**FIG 75-8**
Synovial fluid with an increased nucleated cell count consisting primarily of neutrophils from an adult dog with idiopathic immune-mediated polyarthritis.

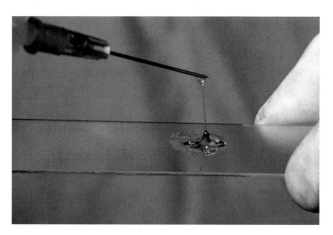

**FIG 75-6**
Normal synovial fluid is clear and viscous.

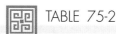 TABLE 75-2

**Synovial Fluid Cytology in Common Joint Disorders**

|  | WBC/μl | % PMN |
|---|---|---|
| Normal | 200-3000 | <10 |
| Degenerative | 1000-5000 | 0-12 |
| Traumatic | Variable | <25 |
| Septic | 40,000-280,000 | 90-99 |
| Rheumatoid arthritis (erosive) | 6000-80,000 | 20-80 |
| Immune mediated (nonerosive) | 4000-370,000 | 15-95 |

PMN, Polymorphonuclear neutrophil leukocytes.

$$\text{Estimated nucleated cell count} = \frac{\text{WBC count in peripheral blood}}{\text{WBC per average microscopic field of blood smear}} \times \text{WBC per average microscopic field in smear of synovial fluid}$$

**FIG 75-7**
Formula for calculating the approximate nucleated cell count in a synovial fluid sample.

contamination of normal synovial fluid has occurred, less than 1 neutrophil should be present for every 500 RBCs contaminating the fluid. The presence of platelets indicates recent hemorrhage or blood contamination. Hemosiderin-laden macrophages and erythrophagia confirm prior hemorrhage.

An increased nucleated cell count consisting primarily of mononuclear cells is seen in many chronically diseased joints and in joints that have been traumatized or have undergone degenerative change (Table 75-2). An increase in the number of neutrophils within a joint indicates inflammation of the synovial lining. The more inflamed the synovium is, the greater is the concentration of WBCs in the synovial fluid, and the greater the percentage of neutrophils (Fig. 75-8).

In addition to the actual or estimated WBC count and WBC differential, cytologic evaluation of the cells in the joint fluid is important. Neutrophils in the synovial fluid of dogs and cats with immune-mediated disease have a normal appearance. In acute or severe cases of septic arthritis, it is common to see bacteria within the cells, and neutrophils in the joint may be toxic, ruptured, and degranulated. Organisms may be observed within the cells in the synovial fluid from animals with rickettsial polyarthritis. Occasionally in dogs with SLE-induced polyarthritis, lupus erythematosus (LE) cells can be seen within the synovial fluid (Fig. 75-9).

## SYNOVIAL FLUID CULTURE

Bacteria are the most common cause of joint infection. Septic arthritis sometimes is diagnosed on the basis of the appearance of toxic changes within neutrophils and the identification of

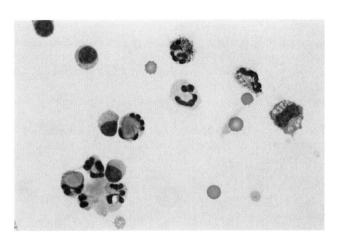

**FIG 75-9**
Synovial fluid from an adult German Shepherd Dog with polyarthritis. Some of the cells are LE cells containing phagocytized, opsonized, amorphous nuclear material. Finding these LE cells supports a diagnosis of SLE.

bacteria on stained smears of synovial fluid. Some organisms such as *Mycoplasma* spp. do not, however, induce characteristic cytologic abnormalities. Any joint fluid with an increased nucleated cell count and a high percentage of neutrophils warrants a culture. Synovial fluid should be submitted for aerobic and anaerobic culture and for specific *Mycoplasma* spp. culture. Direct bacterial culture of synovial fluid is positive in only approximately half of all cases of septic arthritis, so failure to grow bacteria in synovial fluid does not rule out septic arthritis. The diagnostic yield can be greatly improved (85% to 100% positive) if synovial fluid is collected and inoculated into broth-enrichment media (such as thioglycolate blood culture bottles), incubated for 24 hours, and then recultured. Microbiologic culture of blood, urine, and synovial membrane biopsy specimens should also be considered to improve chances of recovering the offending organism.

## SYNOVIAL MEMBRANE BIOPSY

Performing synovial membrane biopsy can support a diagnosis already suspected on the basis of the history, physical examination, radiographic studies, and synovial fluid analysis. It may also be used to collect a sample for microbiologic culture in cases of suspected septic arthritis. Examination of the synovial membrane is especially valuable in the diagnosis of neoplasia and in the differentiation of infectious arthritis from the immune-mediated disorders. An undetermined cause of joint disease or ineffective routine therapy warrants synovial membrane analysis.

Synovial membrane biopsies may be obtained by needle biopsy or surgical arthrotomy. Surgical excision of a wedge of synovial membrane allows visualization of the entire joint and selection of a specific site from which to obtain the biopsy. Needle biopsy of the synovial membrane is quick and minimally traumatic, but samples are small and easily obtained only from the stifle joint. Techniques for both procedures are described in the Suggested Readings listed at the end of this chapter.

## IMMUNOLOGIC AND SEROLOGIC TESTS

### Lyme Disease Titers

Infection with the spirochete *Borrelia burgdorferi,* the etiologic agent for Lyme disease polyarthritis, causes an antibody response that can be detected using an indirect fluorescent antibody (IFA) test or an enzyme-linked immunosorbent assay (ELISA). Dogs with clinical signs of Lyme disease generally have high titers, but asymptomatic dogs in endemic areas may also have titers greater than 1:8000. A positive antibody titer therefore merely indicates exposure to the organism and cannot be used to diagnose active disease. The varied, nonspecific clinical signs of Lyme arthritis warrant questioning of the significance of a positive titer. A diagnosis of Lyme disease polyarthritis must rely on a combination of the history (i.e., recent exposure to an area in which the disease is enzootic), clinical signs, elimination of other known causes of polyarthritis, serologic testing, and response to therapy (see p. 1084).

### Rickettsial Titers

Serologic testing plays an important role in the diagnosis of RMSF (see p. 1265) and canine ehrlichiosis (see p. 1267). The microscopic immunofluorescence method is the most commonly used serologic test to diagnose RMSF. Markedly increased IgG titers support the diagnosis. Titers may not increase for 2 to 3 weeks after exposure; thus a negative or low titer does not rule out RMSF. A second sample obtained 3 weeks later should be evaluated if the initial titer is nondiagnostic. A fourfold increase between acute and convalescent titers is expected in active infections.

The IFA test is a reliable, highly sensitive, and specific serologic test for detecting *Ehrlichia canis* infection; any positive titer usually indicates active infection. Rarely, a dog with polyarthritis is seronegative for *E. canis* but positive using polymerase chain reaction (PCR).

### Systemic Lupus Erythematosus

Tests used to help identify SLE include the LE cell test and the ANA test. The LE cell test requires identification of the LE cell, which is a neutrophil or other WBC that has phagocytized opsonized nuclear material. The cytoplasm of these cells is filled with amorphous purple material. The LE cell test reliability is laboratory dependent, requiring an experienced technician. The test has been reported to be positive in the blood of 30% to 90% of dogs with SLE. The LE cell test may also be positive in other immune or neoplastic disorders. In rare instances, in a dog with SLE-induced polyarthritis, LE cells are detected in the synovial fluid and are considered convincing evidence of this disorder (see Fig. 75-9).

The ANA test detects circulating antibodies to nuclear material. These antibodies are the most prominent of the autoantibodies associated with canine and feline SLE. The ANA test is a sensitive indicator for the diagnosis of SLE and is positive (>1:10) in 90% of SLE cases. The ANA is constant from day to day and is less steroid labile than the LE cell test. Unfortunately, a positive ANA test is not specific for SLE, and false-positive results may be seen in dogs and cats with many other systemic inflammatory or neoplastic diseases.

## Rheumatoid Factor

The laboratory test for rheumatoid factor (RF) detects serum agglutinating antibody against IgG that is chemically or immunologically bound to a particulate carrier such as latex beads or sheep RBCs. A simple slide agglutination test is performed, and the result is positive if visible agglutination occurs. Results vary greatly among the different test systems currently in use. A titer of 1:16 or higher is generally considered positive, regardless of the test system used. A titer of 1:8 is considered suspect and should be repeated. Some normal dogs have positive tests of low titer (1:2, 1:4). The reliability of the test increases with the severity and chronicity of the disease. The test is reported to be positive in 20% to 70% of dogs with rheumatoid arthritis. Any disease associated with systemic inflammation and immune-complex generation and deposition can result in weak, false-positive results.

## Suggested Readings

Ellison RS: The cytologic examination of synovial fluid, *Semin Vet Med Surg* 3(2):133, 1988.

Hardy RM et al: Arthrocentesis and synovial membrane biopsy, *Vet Clin North Am* 4(2):449, 1974.

Lewis RM et al: *Veterinary clinical immunology,* Philadelphia, 1989, Lea & Febiger.

Pedersen NC et al: Joint diseases of dogs and cats. In Ettinger SJ, editor: *Textbook of veterinary internal medicine,* Philadelphia, 1989, WB Saunders.

Schrader SC: The use of the laboratory in the diagnosis of joint disorders in dogs and cats. In Bonagura JD et al, editors: *Kirk's current veterinary therapy XII,* Philadelphia, 1995, WB Saunders.

Schrader SC et al: Disorders of the skeletal system. In Sherding RG, editor: *The cat: diseases and clinical management,* New York, 1989, Churchill Livingstone.

Werner LL: Arthrocentesis and joint fluid analysis: diagnostic applications in joint diseases of small animals, *Compend Contin Ed Pract Vet* 1(11):855, 1979.

# CHAPTER 76

# Disorders of the Joints

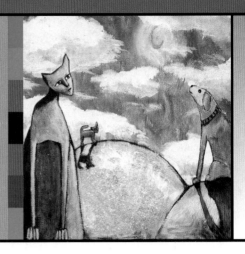

## CHAPTER OUTLINE

NONINFLAMMATORY JOINT DISEASE, 1079
  Degenerative joint disease, 1079
INFECTIOUS INFLAMMATORY JOINT DISEASES, 1081
  Septic (bacterial) arthritis, 1081
  *Mycoplasma* polyarthritis, 1083
  Bacterial L form–associated arthritis, 1083
  Rickettsial polyarthritis, 1084
  Lyme disease, 1084
  Fungal arthritis, 1084
  Viral arthritis, 1085
NONINFECTIOUS INFLAMMATORY JOINT
DISEASES—NONEROSIVE, 1085
  Systemic lupus erythematosus–induced polyarthritis, 1085
  Reactive polyarthritis, 1086
  Idiopathic, immune-mediated, nonerosive
    polyarthritis, 1086
  Breed-specific polyarthritis syndromes, 1088
  Lymphoplasmacytic synovitis, 1088
NONINFECTIOUS INFLAMMATORY JOINT
DISEASES—EROSIVE, 1089
  Rheumatoid arthritis, 1089
  Erosive polyarthritis of Greyhounds, 1091
  Feline chronic progressive polyarthritis, 1091

## NONINFLAMMATORY JOINT DISEASE

### DEGENERATIVE JOINT DISEASE
#### Etiology

Degenerative joint disease (DJD) is a chronic, progressive, minimally inflammatory disorder of joints that results in articular cartilage damage and degenerative and proliferative changes. Normal articular cartilage is made up of a collagen and protein matrix that is produced, assembled, and maintained by a relatively small number of chondrocytes. The initiating damage to the articular cartilage may be an idiopathic phenomenon or result from identified abnormal mechanical stresses acting on the joint. These abnormal stresses may stem from congenital deformities, abnormal conformation, or trauma. Disruption of the normal articular surface, or joint instability, can change the normal wear pattern of the articular cartilage and accelerate the turnover of the articular matrix. Although this process is predominantly noninflammatory, it is accelerated by cytokines and prostaglandins released by synovial cells into the joint. The joint capsule thickens, and periarticular osteophytes form in the body's attempt to improve joint stability.

DJD is the most common joint disorder diagnosed in dogs. In contrast, lameness resulting from DJD is rarely diagnosed in cats, probably because mild-to-moderate DJD is usually subclinical in this species.

### Clinical Features

The clinical signs of DJD are usually insidious in onset and confined to the musculoskeletal system, with no associated systemic signs. Lameness and stiffness may initially be prominent only after periods of overexertion and may worsen in cold and damp weather. Mildly affected dogs may "warm out" of their lameness with exercise. As DJD progresses, function is lost as a result of fibrosis and pain, which leads to decreased exercise tolerance, constant lameness, and, in severe cases, muscular atrophy. Either a single joint or multiple joints may be affected.

### Diagnosis

DJD is usually diagnosed based on history, physical examination findings, and characteristic radiographic features. Clinical examination may reveal pain in the affected joint or joints, decreased range of motion, crepitation on flexion and extension of the joint, and (perhaps) appreciable joint swelling. Radiographic changes characteristic of DJD include joint effusion, subchondral bone sclerosis, subchondral cyst formation, joint space narrowing, periarticular osteophyte formation, and bone remodeling (Fig. 76-1). It is often difficult to appreciate collapse of the cartilage (or so-called joint space narrowing) radiographically, because radiographs are usually taken while traction is being applied to the limb. Often a predisposing condition is identified, such as trauma, rupture of supporting ligaments, poor conformation, or a congenital deformity. DJD is not associated with the fever, leukocytosis, and

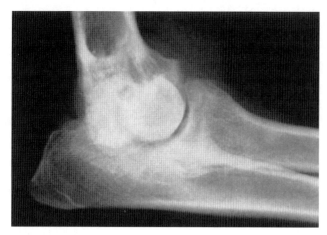

**FIG 76-1**
Close-up mediolateral radiograph of left elbow joint of a 14-month-old female German Shepherd with severe degenerative changes secondary to a fragmented coronoid process.

 TABLE 76-1

Nonsteroidal Antiinflammatory Drugs Used to Treat Degenerative Joint Disease in Dogs

| DRUG NAME | TRADE NAME | DOSE |
|---|---|---|
| Acetylsalicylic acid | Aspirin | 10-20 mg/kg PO q8-12h |
| Carprofen | Rimadyl | 2.2 mg/kg PO q12h |
| Etodolac | Etogesic | 10-15 mg/kg PO q24h |
| Meloxicam | Metacam | 0.2 mg/kg once, then 0.1 mg/kg/day PO |
| Piroxicam | Feldene | 0.3 mg/kg PO q48h |

depression commonly seen in animals with inflammatory joint disease.

If synovial fluid analysis is performed in a dog with DJD, it typically reveals minimal or no inflammation in the affected joints. Analysis of synovial fluid from acute and chronically affected joints may reveal an increase in the volume and a slight decrease in the viscosity of the fluid. The total white blood cell (WBC) count may be normal or slightly increased, but it rarely exceeds 5000 cells/μl. Characteristically, lymphocytes constitute 70% to 80% and neutrophils less than 12% of the cells. Partial cranial cruciate ligament ruptures in the dog are sometimes associated with increases in the cell count and the numbers of neutrophils, indicating an inflammatory reaction (see Lymphoplasmacytic Synovitis, p. 1088).

### Treatment

The goals of treatment in dogs with DJD are to alleviate discomfort and to prevent further degeneration. If possible, factors that are augmenting articular cartilage stresses or joint laxity are eliminated. Surgical intervention may be necessary to stabilize the joint or correct a deformity and to relieve discomfort. Medical treatment is symptomatic and nonspecific. Weight reduction may decrease the stresses acting on the joint. Rest often helps to decrease the discomfort associated with acute exacerbations of disease. High-impact exercise, such as running and jumping, should be discouraged, whereas low-impact exercise done in moderation, such as swimming and leash walking, is recommended to maintain the animal's strength and mobility. Other forms of physical therapy may include passive range of motion exercises, cold (acute) or heat (chronic) therapy, muscle and joint massage, ultrasound, and electrical stimulation.

Pharmacologic therapies may be used to decrease further degradation of the articular cartilage, inhibit the release of inflammatory mediators, and control pain. Corticosteroids are potent antiinflammatory agents, and they will decrease

the release of degradative enzymes from chondrocytes and synovial cells. However, they are not widely recommended for the treatment of DJD, because they markedly inhibit the chondrocyte synthesis of proteoglycans and collagen, resulting in matrix depletion and progression of DJD.

The nonsteroidal antiinflammatory drugs (NSAIDs) are often recommended for the treatment of DJD because of their antiinflammatory and analgesic effects. The primary action of most NSAIDs is reversible inhibition of cyclooxygenase, preventing synthesis of the prostaglandins responsible for pain and inflammation. The discovery of two forms of cyclooxygenase (COX-1 and COX-2) may explain some of the differences in efficacy and toxicity among some of the available NSAID agents. Greater inhibition of COX-2 by an NSAID is associated with improved control of inflammation and decreased potential for gastric irritation and ulceration. Buffered aspirin (10 to 20 mg/kg PO q8-12h) is the NSAID most often administered to dogs. Aspirin is an effective analgesic and antiinflammatory; however, chronically it may impair cartilage repair, and reports of adverse gastrointestinal effects (e.g., vomiting, nausea) are common. Misoprostol (2.5 mg/kg PO q8h), a synthetic PGE1 analog can be administered concurrently to decrease gastrointestinal tract irritation. Carprofen (Rimadyl), a NSAID with a more favorable COX-2:COX-1 ratio, is very effective and is associated with fewer gastrointestinal side effects; although duodenal ulceration has been documented in a few treated dogs and idiosyncratic hepatic necrosis rarely occurs. Etodolac, Piroxicam, and Meloxicam have also been used to successfully treat dogs with DJD (Table 76-1). Other NSAIDs can be used in dogs, but many are associated with a higher prevalence of gastrointestinal adverse effects.

Chondroprotective agents are similar in chemical composition to the mucopolysaccharides that make up the articular cartilage. They may protect articular cartilage by increasing matrix production or by decreasing matrix degradation in dogs with DJD. Adequan (polysulfated glycosaminoglycans; Luitpold Pharm, Shirley, N.Y.) has been administered with some success (2 to 5 mg/kg IM every 4 days for four to eight treatments, then every 30 days). An orally administered combination of glucosamine HCl, chondroitin sulfate and manganese ascorbate has also been recommended (Cosequin RS, 1 to 2 tablets/day in cats or small dogs; Cosequin DS, 2 to 4 tablets/day in large dogs; Nutramax Labs, Baltimore, Md). Alternatively oral glucosamine (15 to 20 mg/kg q12h) and chondroitin sulfate (15 to 20 mg/kg q12h) can be purchased separately and administered. To achieve the maximum theoretic benefit from these products, they should be administered before DJD has occurred. Therefore they may be indicated for the treatment of dogs that have sustained trauma or undergone surgery that is known to have damaged articular cartilage. Clinical trials are necessary to evaluate their efficacy.

# INFECTIOUS INFLAMMATORY JOINT DISEASES

## SEPTIC (BACTERIAL) ARTHRITIS
### Etiology

Septic arthritis can result from a blood-borne infection or from direct inoculation of a joint as a result of surgery, foreign-body penetration, or trauma. Infection of multiple joints generally indicates that the septic polyarthritis is secondary to bacteremia originating from a local site of infection in the body. This hematogenous spread of bacterial infection is uncommon, except in immunosuppressed animals or neonates. Polyarticular septic arthritis is most commonly seen in neonatal kittens secondary to omphalophlebitis that has occurred because the queen has severed the umbilical cord too close to the abdominal wall. Direct inoculation of bacteria into a joint, causing monoarticular septic arthritis, is much more common in dogs and cats. *Staphylococcus* spp., *Streptococcus* spp., and coliform organisms are most commonly incriminated in the dog, and *Pasteurella* spp. are most commonly identified in cats. Septic arthritis, regardless of the cause, is more common in dogs than cats, is most common in large-breed dogs, and more frequently affects males than females.

### Clinical Features

Animals with septic polyarthritis are often systemically ill, febrile, and depressed. The affected joints are usually very painful, especially when manipulated, and may be palpably distended with synovial fluid. The periarticular soft tissues may be inflamed and edematous as well. Septic arthritis stemming from bacteremia usually involves one or a few of the large proximal joints. In contrast, the smaller distal joints are more commonly involved in immune-mediated arthritis, which is the primary differential diagnosis (Table 76-2).

### Diagnosis

For septic arthritis to be diagnosed, bacteria must be identified in cytologic preparations of synovial fluid or cultured in synovial fluid, blood, or urine from an animal with appropriate clinical signs and inflammatory joint disease. Synovial fluid obtained by arthrocentesis is often yellow, cloudy, or bloody. The joint fluid is less viscous than normal as a result

## TABLE 76-2

### Classification of Polyarthritis in Dogs

**Infectious**

Bacterial
*Mycoplasma*
Rickettsial
Lyme borreliosis
Fungal

**Noninfectious, Inflammatory**
***Nonerosive***

Idiopathic, immune-mediated polyarthritis
Systemic lupus erythematosus
Reactive polyarthritis (bacterial, fungal, parasitic, neoplastic, enterohepatic, drug reaction, vaccine induced)
Breed-associated syndromes
　Polyarthritis (Akita, Boxer, Weimaraner)
　Polyarthritis/meningitis (Akita, Bernese Mountain Dog, German Shorthair Pointer, Beagle)
　Polyarthritis/polymyositis (Spaniels)
Lymphoplasmacytic synovitis

***Erosive***

Rheumatoid arthritis
Erosive polyarthritis of Greyhounds

of the dilution and degradation of synovial mucin by bacterial hyaluronidase and the enzymes released from the inflammatory cells within the joint. Because it is common for synovial fluid from infected joints to clot rapidly, a portion of the fluid should be immediately placed in an anticoagulant (i.e., ethylenediaminetetraacetic acid [EDTA]) tube for future cytologic evaluation if an adequate sample is obtained. Smears of the fluid should also be made for the purpose of Gram's and differential staining.

Cytologically, animals with septic arthritis show a marked increase in the number (40,000 to 280,000/ml) of nucleated cells in the synovial fluid, with neutrophils predominating (<90%). In very acute or severe cases, it is common to see bacteria within the cells and the neutrophils may be toxic, ruptured, and degranulated. Organisms that do not cause rapid destruction of articular cartilage (i.e., streptococci, *Mycoplasma*) may not cause remarkable toxic or degenerative changes in synovial fluid neutrophils. In chronic infections, bacteria may no longer be evident and the neutrophils may appear healthy.

Synovial fluid should be cultured for aerobic and anaerobic bacteria. A few drops of fluid should be removed from the joint and the smears stained for cytologic analysis. A larger sample should then be obtained from an affected joint for culture. Direct bacterial culture of the synovial fluid is positive in approximately half of all animals with septic arthritis—improved diagnostic yield may be obtained by inoculating

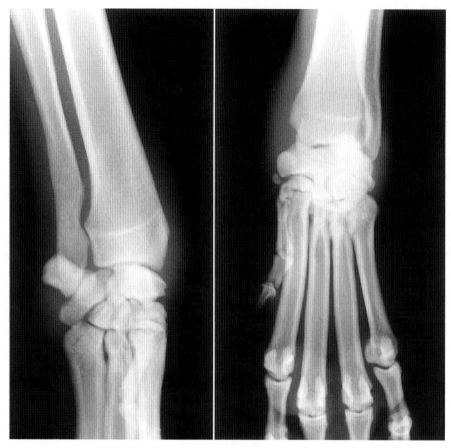

**FIG 76-2**
Radiographs of the swollen left carpus of a 2-year-old Bull Mastiff with a 1-week history of lameness caused by septic arthritis. Surgical exploration revealed two porcupine quills within the infected joint.

synovial fluid into blood culture medium (9:1 ratio) and incubating it for 24 hours at 37° C before inoculation. Bacteria can also be recovered from cultures of synovial membrane biopsy, blood, or urine specimens.

Radiographic changes of the involved joints in septic arthritis may be minimal or nonspecific initially and limited to thickening of the joint capsule, widening of the joint space, and irregular thickening of periarticular soft tissues (Fig. 76-2). In chronic infections, cartilage degeneration, periarticular new bone formation, a marked periosteal reaction, and subchondral bone lysis may be seen (Fig. 76-3).

If septic arthritis is suspected and the animal has no history of direct inoculation of the joint with bacteria, a septic site in the body should be sought. Radiography of the thorax, abdomen, and spine and cardiac and abdominal ultrasonography are especially helpful in identifying a focal site of infection. If possible, cultures of material from any suspected site of infection should be performed.

## Treatment

The goals of therapy are to rapidly resolve the bacterial infection and to remove intraarticular accumulations of enzymes and fibrin debris. Identifiable systemic sources of infection should also be eliminated. Antibiotics should be administered as soon as possible after all samples are collected in an animal suspected of having septic arthritis. Until culture results are available, a broad-spectrum, β-lactamase–resistant antibiotic such as a first-generation cephalosporin (e.g., cephalexin, 20 to 40 mg/kg q8h) or clavamox (Smith Kline-Beecham Animal Health; Exton, Pa) (12 to 25 mg/kg q8h) is indicated. Initially the antibiotic can be administered parenterally, followed by long-term oral administration. Quinolones should be used if gram-negative organisms are suspected. Animals with acute septic arthritis can be treated conservatively initially with joint drainage and systemic antibiotics; however, if dramatic improvement is not seen within 3 days, surgery should be performed. Chronic infections, suspected intraarticular foreign bodies and postoperative joint infections are all indications for immediate surgical débridement and lavage. A minimum of 6 weeks of antibiotic therapy is administered, and cage rest is recommended to facilitate healing of articular cartilage.

## Prognosis

The prognosis for a return to normal function depends on the severity of the damage to the articular cartilage at the time

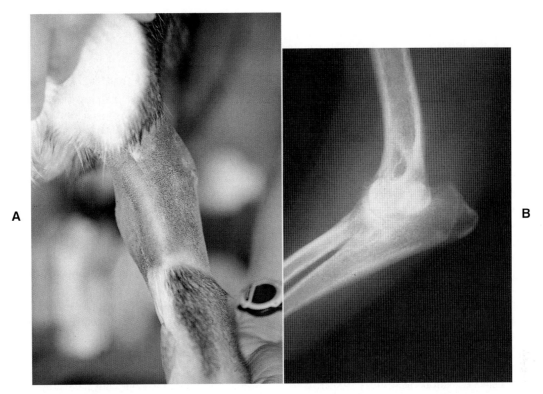

**FIG 76-3**

**A,** A Very swollen elbow in a Husky-cross dog with a 3-month history of a nonweight-bearing lameness not responding to antibiotics. **B,** Radiographs reveal marked swelling within the joint and diffuse periosteal proliferation. Synovial fluid showed septic inflammation, and surgical exploration revealed a single porcupine quill within the joint. The dog recovered completely.

the infection is brought under control. Secondary DJD commonly occurs.

## MYCOPLASMA POLYARTHRITIS

*Mycoplasma* spp. are normal inhabitants of the upper respiratory and urogenital tracts of most species and are generally considered nonpathogenic. Systemic *Mycoplasma* infection may occasionally occur in debilitated or immunosuppressed animals, but the prevalence of *Mycoplasma* arthritis is low. *Mycoplasma gatea* and *Mycoplasma felis* are the two organisms that have been rarely associated with clinical disease in cats.

*Mycoplasma* polyarthritis results in a chronic polyarthritis indistinguishable from idiopathic immune-mediated, nonerosive polyarthritis. Clinical signs include lameness, joint pain, depression, and fever. Synovial fluid analysis reveals an increased nucleated cell count consisting predominantly of nondegenerate neutrophils. Routine aerobic and anaerobic cultures of joint fluid are negative, because *Mycoplasma* organisms are deficient in cell walls and cannot revert to a parental state. Diagnosis is made based on the isolation of organisms from synovial fluid cultured in special *Mycoplasma* medium. Treatment with tetracycline (22 mg/kg PO q8h), doxycycline (5 mg/kg PO or IV q12h), tylosin (20 mg/kg PO q8h), or chloramphenicol (dogs, 25 to 50 mg/kg PO q8h; cats, 10 to 15 mg/kg q12h) should be effective.

## BACTERIAL L FORM–ASSOCIATED ARTHRITIS

A rare syndrome of pyogenic subcutaneous (SC) abscesses with associated polyarthritis has been observed in cats. This syndrome appears to be infectious in nature and transmitted from one cat to another by bite wounds. No age or gender predilection exists. A bacterial L–form mutant bacteria that has lost its cell wall but can revert to its original form has been implicated. Affected cats have swollen, painful joints and fever. Fistulating SC wounds develop over the affected joints. Exudate from the joints or the SC abscesses contains degenerate and nondegenerate neutrophils and macrophages. Cultures for aerobic and anaerobic bacteria, *Mycoplasma,* and fungal organisms are all negative. Specific L-form media must be used to grow the organism. Radiographically, severely affected joints show extensive soft tissue swelling, periosteal proliferation, and destruction of articular cartilage and subchondral bone, resulting in subluxation and joint space collapse. Electron microscopic studies and antibiotic sensitivity testing can yield findings that help support a diagnosis of L-form bacterial infection. Rarely, cats are concurrently infected with feline leukemia virus (FeLV) or feline immunodeficiency virus (FIV). Treatment with doxycycline (5 mg/kg q12h) or chloramphenicol (10 to 15 mg/kg q12h) is effective, with improvement noted within 48 hours. Therapy should continue for 10 to 14 days.

## RICKETTSIAL POLYARTHRITIS

Two rickettsial diseases of dogs, ehrlichiosis and Rocky Mountain spotted fever (RMSF), are occasionally associated with nonerosive polyarthritis, but in most cases concurrent systemic signs are obvious (see Chapter 101). Joint pain and effusion are noted, and increased numbers of nondegenerate neutrophils are identified in the joint fluid; occasionally, *Ehrlichia* morulae can be identified in cytologic preparations of joint fluid. Fever and polyarthritis may be the only clinical abnormalities in dogs with ehrlichiosis, although hematologic abnormalities such as mild thrombocytopenia and anemia are common. Serologic testing has not reliably identified affected dogs; studies using the polymerase chain reaction (PCR) technique may be more sensitive.

Dogs with polyarthritis caused by RMSF are more likely to show a variety of clinical signs, including fever, petechiae, lymphadenopathy, neurologic signs, edema of the face or extremities, and pneumonitis. Hematologic abnormalities, including thrombocytopenia, are common. Diagnosis is made based on the results of serologic testing.

### Treatment

Both disorders are treated with either doxycycline (5 mg/kg PO q12h) or chloramphenicol (25 to 50 mg/kg PO or IV q8h). Empirical antibiotic treatment is warranted in dogs from endemic areas with confirmed polyarthritis and typical signs of rickettsial disease. Concurrent glucocorticoid therapy (prednisone, 0.5 to 2.0 mg/kg/day) may be necessary in some dogs with confirmed rickettsial polyarthritis if antimicrobial therapy alone does not eliminate the fever, lameness, and joint swelling.

## LYME DISEASE

### Etiology

The tick-borne spirochete *Borrelia burgdorferi* can cause a multisystemic illness in dogs (i.e., Lyme disease) that may include fever, lymphadenopathy, myocarditis, inflammatory joint disease, and glomerulonephritis. The disease is poorly documented in cats, despite evidence of seropositivity in the species. Ticks of the genus *Ixodes* transmit the spirochete. Although the disease has been seen in dogs throughout North America, most confirmed cases have occurred in dogs from the northeastern and mid-Atlantic states, with Minnesota, Wisconsin, California, and Oregon accounting for most of the remaining cases. The rate of veterinary diagnosis of Lyme disease polyarthritis far exceeds its actual prevalence.

### Clinical Features

Most dogs bitten by ticks infected with *B. burgdorferi* never show clinical signs of illness. Host immunodeficiency may play a role in the development of clinically apparent disease. Acute polyarthritis is the most common form of Lyme *borreliosis* diagnosed in dogs. The major clinical features are lameness, fever, lymphadenopathy, and anorexia. These signs occasionally resolve after a few days but may then recur periodically. Acute signs of illness are reported to be most common during the summer months. Complete heart block, re-

nal failure, and neurologic signs (e.g., seizure, behavior change) are rarely reported.

### Diagnosis

Complete blood counts (CBCs) and radiographic images of the thorax, abdomen, and joints are usually normal during the acute phase of the illness. Synovial fluid analysis reveals an increase in the nucleated cell count (mean, 46,300/μl), with nondegenerate neutrophils predominating (43% to 85%). Although clinical signs such as fever, joint distention, and lameness may wax and wane, synovial fluid analysis findings remain consistently abnormal. Attempts to culture *B. burgdorferi* from the blood, urine, and synovial fluid of affected dogs are usually unsuccessful. The identification of *Borrelia* organisms in biopsy specimens of diseased tissues (e.g., synovium, kidney) using direct immunofluorescent techniques supports the diagnosis, but the means of doing this are often not available.

Serologic tests for antibodies directed against the spirochete are available and consist of an indirect fluorescent antibody test and an enzyme-linked immunosorbent assay. A positive antibody titer only constitutes evidence of exposure to the agent and is not indicative of disease. Clinical illness does not develop in many dogs exposed to the infectious agent. Although most dogs with acute polyarthritis caused by Lyme disease have high antibody titers, some dogs are seronegative early in the disease. Vaccination against *B. burgdorferi* can cause an increase in antibody titer, making it difficult to differentiate immunized dogs from those that are naturally exposed; Western blot testing can, however, distinguish between naturally exposed and vaccinated dogs.

Lyme disease polyarthritis should only be diagnosed if the animal has a history of recent potential exposure, the synovial fluid is confirmed to be inflammatory and sterile, serologic testing is positive, and a prompt and permanent response to appropriate antibiotic therapy is seen. The diagnosis can be supported by the identification of *Borrelia* organisms in biopsy specimens of tissues prepared using special stains and monoclonal antibodies.

### Treatment

Antibiotics are the treatment of choice. Doxycycline (5 mg/kg PO q12h), Amoxicillin (22 mg/kg PO q12h), ampicillin (22 mg/kg PO q8h), Clavamox (12.5 to 25 mg/kg PO q8-12h) and Cephalexin, 20 to 40 mg/kg PO q8h) are all effective. Treatment during the acute stage of the disease should result in very rapid clinical improvement (i.e., within 2 to 3 days). Treatment for at least 3 to 4 weeks is advised. Failure to recognize acute disease or the institution of inappropriate treatment can allow chronic disease to develop, including relapsing polyarthritis, glomerulonephritis, and cardiac abnormalities.

### Prevention

The prevention of Lyme disease is discussed in Chapter 99.

## FUNGAL ARTHRITIS

Fungal arthritis is very rare. When it does occur, it is usually as an extension of fungal osteomyelitis caused by *Coccidioides*

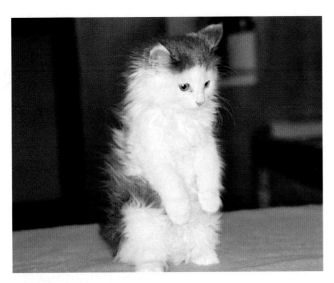

**FIG 76-4**
Presumed calicivirus polyarthritis in a 10-week-old kitten exhibiting swollen joints, lameness, and fever 6 days after modified-live virus vaccination.

*immitis, Blastomyces dermatitidis,* or *Cryptococcus neoformans.* More commonly a reactive, immunologically mediated, culture-negative polyarthritis occurs in dogs and cats with systemic fungal infections.

## VIRAL ARTHRITIS

### Calicivirus

Natural calicivirus infection and attenuated live calicivirus vaccination have been associated with the development of transient polyarthritis in 6- to 12-week-old kittens. Clinical signs include lameness, stiffness, and fever, which usually resolve spontaneously after 2 to 4 days (Fig. 76-4). Some kittens go on to develop overt calicivirus infection, with glossal and palatine vesicles or ulcers and signs of upper respiratory tract disease. Synovial fluid analysis reveals a mildly to greatly increased nucleated cell count, with small mononuclear cells and macrophages predominating, some of which contain phagocytosed neutrophils. Two specific strains of calicivirus have been implicated. Isolation of the virus from affected joints has been unrewarding, although the virus can be found in the oropharynx of some infected cats.

## NONINFECTIOUS INFLAMMATORY JOINT DISEASES—NONEROSIVE

Noninfectious inflammatory joint diseases are very common in the dog and rare in the cat. These immune-mediated polyarthritis syndromes are routinely classified as being erosive or nonerosive based upon radiographic evidence of joint destruction, although the erosive (rheumatoid arthritis [RA]-like) conditions are very rare. The nonerosive immune-mediated polyarthritis syndromes are all thought to be me-

diated through immune complex formation and deposition. Immune-mediated nonerosive polyarthritis can occur as a feature of systemic lupus erythematosus (SLE), secondary to chronic antigenic stimulation from chronic infection, neoplasia, or drugs (i.e., reactive polyarthritis), or it can occur as an idiopathic syndrome. Breed-associated syndromes of polyarthritis or polyarthritis/meningitis or polyarthritis/myositis also exist and are thought to have a genetic basis.

## SYSTEMIC LUPUS ERYTHEMATOSUS–INDUCED POLYARTHRITIS

SLE is an immune complex disease of unknown etiology. In SLE, autoantibodies against tissue proteins and deoxyribonucleic acid (DNA) form, and complexes of host antigens and autoantibodies result in the formation of circulating immune complexes. These circulating immune complexes pass through endothelial cell junctions and are trapped in the underlying basement membrane, where they induce inflammation that causes organ system dysfunction and the resultant clinical signs (see Chapter 94).

SLE has been well documented in dogs and to a lesser extent in cats. Any breed of dog may be affected, but the incidence may be increased in Spitzes, Shetland Sheepdogs, Collies, German Shepherds, Beagles, and sporting breeds. Most affected dogs are 2 to 4 years old. The familial clustering of cases that is seen may indicate a hereditary factor. Although SLE is an uncommon cause of polyarthritis in dogs compared with idiopathic immune-mediated polyarthritis, its effects on other organ systems can be devastating; therefore accurate diagnosis is important.

### Clinical Features

The clinical manifestations of SLE vary with the organ involved and include intermittent fevers, polyarthritis, glomerulonephritis, skin lesions, hemolytic anemia, immune-mediated thrombocytopenia, myositis, and polyneuritis. Polyarthritis is the most common manifestation, occurring in 70% to 90% of dogs with SLE. Some dogs show no signs of their joint disease, and their polyarthritis is detected during screening tests performed as a workup for fever or after other evidence of immune disease (e.g., anemia, proteinuria) is identified. More often, animals show generalized stiffness or a shifting leg lameness that suggests polyarthritis. A sterile, nonerosive arthritis occurs in SLE, with distal joints (i.e., hocks, carpi) usually more severely affected than proximal joints. Synovial fluid analysis reveals an increased WBC count (5000 to 350,000/ml) consisting primarily of nondegenerate neutrophils (>80%). In rare instances, LE cells are detected in the synovial fluid (Fig. 75-9).

### Diagnosis

SLE should be suspected in any dog or cat with noninfectious polyarthritis. A CBC, platelet count, biochemistry profile, urinalysis, urine protein/creatinine ratio determination, and careful physical examination should be performed in every animal with polyarthritis to search for other manifestations of this disease. Laboratory tests that may aid in the diagnosis of SLE polyarthritis include the LE cell test (positive in 30% to 90% of cases) and the antinuclear antibody (ANA) test (positive in 55% to 90% of cases). An animal may be said to have SLE if one or more of these "specific" diagnostic tests (e.g., ANA, LE) are positive and the animal has two or more of the clinical abnormalities known to be associated with SLE (e.g., polyarthritis, glomerulonephritis, anemia, thrombocytopenia, dermatitis) (see Chapter 94). When two or more of the common clinical syndromes are recognized but none of the serologic tests are positive, the dog is determined to have a SLE-like multisystemic immune-mediated disease.

### Treatment

Treatment for SLE-associated polyarthritis is the same as that used for idiopathic, immune-mediated polyarthritis (see p. 1088). If the animal is clinically normal and synovial fluid is noninflammatory after 6 months of therapy, it may be worthwhile to discontinue medications, because long periods of drug-free remission can occur.

### Prognosis

The prognosis is good from the standpoint of controlling the polyarthritis, but multisystemic involvement (particularly glomerulonephritis) may progress despite therapy, occasionally resulting in the death of the animal.

## REACTIVE POLYARTHRITIS

Reactive polyarthritis is a relatively common manifestation of immune complex diseases seen in association with chronic bacterial, fungal, or parasitic infection; neoplasia; drug administration; or disease of the gastrointestinal tract. Reactive polyarthritis may occur secondary to any chronic inflammatory disorder or persistent antigenic stimulus. Arthritis is a common manifestation of the immune complex disease seen in association with bacterial endocarditis, pleuritis, diskospondylitis, and dirofilariasis. Drug-induced polyarthritis has been documented in dogs and cats receiving a variety of drugs, including sulfadiazine-trimethoprim, phenobarbital, erythropoietin, penicillin, cephalexin, and routine vaccinations. Careful questioning of the owners regarding recently administered medications is important. Polyarthritis can also be seen as a consequence of neoplasia—squamous cell carcinoma, mammary adenocarcinoma, and other tumors have been implicated.

Although the underlying condition is often obvious, a veterinarian does not see some animals until the polyarthritis makes them reluctant to walk. It is important therefore to perform a thorough physical examination of every animal with polyarthritis and to obtain a complete history regarding the administration of medications and the presence or absence of systemic signs. Screening tests (i.e., CBC, thoracic and abdominal radiography, abdominal ultrasonography, culture of urine and blood, cardiac ultrasonography, determination of rickettsial and Lyme disease titers, heartworm test [dogs], FeLV and FIV tests [cats]) will then need to be performed to evaluate for infectious causes of polyarthritis and for underlying chronic infections, neoplasia, or SLE (Fig. 76-5).

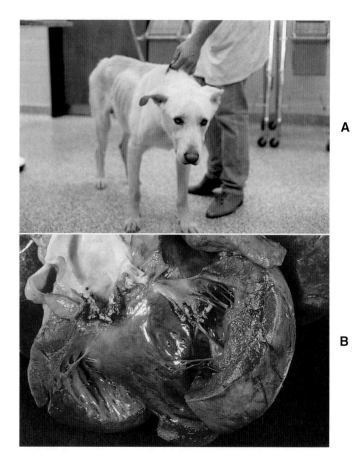

**FIG 76-5**
A 2-year-old German Shepherd/Labrador Retriever cross with reactive polyarthritis **(A).** The dog was seen because of a 3-month history of shifting leg lameness and weight loss. There was joint swelling and pain and a grade IV/VI diastolic cardiac murmur. Synovial fluid was inflamed but sterile. A cardiac ultrasound study revealed bacterial endocarditis of the aortic valve **(B).**

Clinical signs in dogs with reactive polyarthritis may include cyclic fevers, stiffness, and lameness. There may also be some clinical features attributable to their underlying primary disorder. Synovial fluid analysis typically reveals an increase in the WBC count and the percentage of neutrophils in affected joints. Even if the primary inflammatory disease is infectious, culture of the synovial fluid is negative, indicating an immunologically mediated cause. Radiographically the only finding is joint swelling.

Treatment must be directed at eliminating the underlying disease or antigenic stimulus. If this can be done, the polyarthritis usually resolves. In addition, short-term, low-dose corticosteroid therapy (prednisone, 0.25 to 1.0 mg/kg/day) may be warranted to control the synovitis in severe cases.

## IDIOPATHIC, IMMUNE-MEDIATED, NONEROSIVE POLYARTHRITIS

Nonerosive, noninfectious polyarthritis in which a primary or underlying disease cannot be identified is referred to as idiopathic, immune-mediated polyarthritis. This disorder can

**Joint Pain**

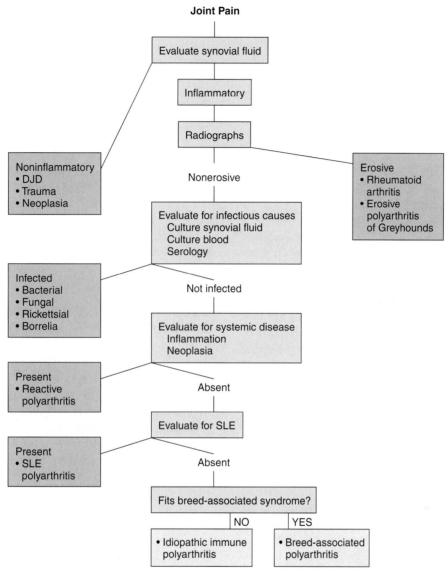

**FIG 76-6**
Algorithm for diagnostic evaluation of dogs with joint pain.

only be diagnosed by ruling out the other causes of polyarthritis, and it is the most common form of polyarthritis diagnosed in dogs (see Table 76-2). It is especially common in sporting and large breeds. Dogs of any age can be affected, but the incidence peaks at 2.5 to 4.5 years. In contrast, idiopathic, immune-mediated, nonerosive polyarthritis is uncommon in cats.

## Clinical Features

The clinical signs of idiopathic, immune-mediated, nonerosive polyarthritis may include cyclic fevers, stiffness, and lameness with no response to antibiotics. Cervical pain and vertebral hypersensitivity may reflect intervertebral facetal joint involvement or the presence of concurrent meningitis. Signs may be subtle, and the diagnosis may be missed if the index of suspicion for polyarthritis is not high. Many animals are seen because of a history of decreased appetite or because

of fever of unknown origin (see Chapter 95). Multiple joints are usually involved, with the small distal joints (i.e., carpus, hock) affected most severely. Disease affecting only the elbow joint has also been recognized. It is common for no palpable joint effusion or localizable pain to be experienced.

## Diagnosis

Idiopathic, immune-mediated, nonerosive polyarthritis is diagnosed based on the results of synovial fluid analysis, the lack of significant radiographic changes in affected joints, failure to identify an infectious cause, and the absence of evidence to support a diagnosis of SLE or reason to suspect reactive polyarthritis (Fig. 76-6). A CBC commonly reveals neutrophilia, although neutropenia is occasionally noted and some dogs have a normal CBC. Radiographic findings are normal or limited to joint and periarticular swelling with no bone or cartilage abnormalities. Synovial fluid is thin and may be turbid. Nucleated cell counts are increased (4000 to 370,000 cells/μl), and nondegenerate neutrophils predominate (usually >80%). In animals with less severe or fluctuating disease and animals that have received corticosteroids, there may be a lower WBC count and a lower percentage of neutrophils (15% to 80%). Blood, urine, and synovial fluid cultures are typically negative for bacteria and *Mycoplasma.*

If nonseptic, nonerosive polyarthritis is diagnosed, a thorough evaluation for an underlying immune-mediated disease should be performed. Dogs and cats with idiopathic polyarthritis are usually ANA negative and do not have evidence of immune disease affecting other systems (e.g., anemia, thrombocytopenia, proteinuria, skin disease) as would be present in SLE. If synovial biopsies are performed, specimens show a neutrophilic synovitis initially, but as the disease becomes chronic, lymphocytes, plasma cells, and macrophages predominate and villous hyperplasia may occur.

## Treatment

Glucocorticoids are the initial treatment of choice for dogs and cats with idiopathic, immune-mediated polyarthritis. Prednisone treatment alone results in remission in 50% of the cases. The initial dose is 2 to 4 mg/kg/day administered orally for 2 weeks. The dose is then decreased to 1 to 2 mg/kg daily and administered for another 2 weeks. If at the end of this time the animal is clinically normal and the inflammation in the synovial fluid has subsided, the animal is given 1 to 2 mg/kg every 48 hours. This dose is maintained for 4 weeks and then further tapered if the synovial fluid is found to be cytologically normal.

It is recommended that synovial fluid be evaluated monthly during initial therapy. Synovial fluid should be determined to be noninflammatory before each decrease in drug dose. If the joints are not inflamed, the drug doses may be tapered monthly and (rarely) discontinued. In dogs receiving a stable dose of medication, synovial fluid should be evaluated every 4 to 6 months. Most animals need at least alternate-day prednisone therapy for the remainder of their lives. If a dog can be maintained on a low, alternate-day dose of prednisone (<0.5 mg/kg every other day) for 2 months and the synovial fluid is not inflammatory, it may be possible to discontinue all therapy.

Azathioprine (Imuran; Burroughs Wellcome, Research Triangle Park, N.C.) should be administered to dogs with clinical signs or inflammation of synovial fluid that persists despite prednisone therapy. Azathioprine may also be used in dogs that relapse when the prednisone dose is decreased. Azathioprine (2.2 mg/kg) is administered once daily for 4 to 6 weeks and then only on alternate days if the animal is doing well clinically and the synovial fluid is no longer inflammatory. Corticosteroids can be administered concurrently (as described earlier). The major toxicity of azathioprine is myelosuppression; thus a CBC and platelet count should be performed initially every 2 weeks and then every 6 to 8 weeks. Hepatic enzyme activities should also be monitored to facilitate the early detection of hepatotoxicity. Dogs treated with Azathioprine and prednisone may also be at increased risk for developing pancreatitis. In addition to medical treatment, management should initially include restricted exercise, followed by regular gentle exercise and weight control. Chondroprotective agents may also prove beneficial.

## Prognosis

The prognosis for animals with idiopathic, immune-mediated, nonerosive polyarthritis is good. One animal in 50 is very difficult to treat and keep in remission. Additional therapies such as cyclophosphamide, leflonamide, or chrysotherapy should be considered in these animals. For a further discussion of immunosuppressive treatment, see p. 1216. Dogs that require long-term (4 to 5 years) high-dose immunosuppressive drug therapy for this disorder may develop symptomatic DJD secondary to chronic low-grade synovial inflammation or the detrimental effects of corticosteroids on cartilage synthesis and repair.

## BREED-SPECIFIC POLYARTHRITIS SYNDROMES

Immune-mediated polyarthritis, with or without disease involving other organ systems, has been shown to be a problem in a number of breeds. A heritable polyarthritis has been documented in Akitas less than 1 year of age and sporadically in Boxers and Weimaraners. Many of these dogs have a concurrent meningitis resembling the meningeal vasculitis syndromes seen in a few other breeds (see Chapter 71). ANA tests are negative in these animals, and generally they respond poorly to immunosuppressive therapy. In contrast, polyarthritis that accompanies meningeal vasculitis in some Bernese Mountain dogs, German Shorthair Pointers, and Beagles often responds completely to immunosuppressive therapy. Familial polyarthritis with a concurrent myositis has been rarely reported in a few Spaniel breeds. These animals respond poorly to therapy.

Progressive renal amyloidosis and polyarthritis has been documented in the Sharpei and is known as "Sharpei fever" or "Sharpei hock" syndrome. The disease affects growing pups or adult dogs and is characterized initially by episodic fever and swelling of the hock or carpal joints. Over time, renal or hepatic failure develops in affected dogs as a result of amyloidosis. To assess the severity of the renal disease, it is recommended that the urinary protein loss be monitored using urine protein/creatinine ratios. Steroid treatment has been of little value in these dogs and may actually hasten the development of amyloidosis.

## LYMPHOPLASMACYTIC SYNOVITIS

Lymphoplasmacytic synovitis is a rare syndrome affecting the stifle joints of dogs. Clinical signs are limited to acute or chronic lameness involving one or both rear limbs. Immune-mediated synovitis is associated with cruciate ligament degeneration and rupture, and it must be differentiated from more conventional causes of cruciate rupture such as trauma or instability. Affected animals are in good body condition and are not systemically ill; CBC is normal. Synovial fluid is thin and turbid, with an increased nucleated cell count (5000 to 20,000 cells/ml, but occasionally >200,000/ml). Lymphocytes and plasma cells predominate in the synovial fluid in most affected dogs. Characteristic histopathologic changes seen in the synovial lining and cruciate ligaments include lymphocytic and plasmacytic infiltration and villous hyperplasia. Some investigators have estimated that perhaps as many as 10% of cruciate ruptures in dogs are caused by this immunologic disorder, but this is a controversial claim. It is difficult to assess, because partial tears or ruptures of the cruciate ligament can themselves initiate an inflammatory reaction directed against the collagen of the ligament, resulting in mildly inflammatory synovial fluid. Anticollagen antibodies have also been identified in serum and synovial fluid from some dogs with cruciate ligament rupture. Biopsy of ligament and synovium should be performed at the time of surgical exploration and repair in all dogs with nontraumatic cruciate ligament ruptures. Treatment is the same as that for idiopathic polyarthritis and also includes surgical stabilization of the affected stifles and synovectomy of diseased intraarticular tissue. Antiinflammatory therapy with colchicine (0.03 mg/kg PO q24h) is also occasionally administered.

## NONINFECTIOUS INFLAMMATORY JOINT DISEASES—EROSIVE

### RHEUMATOID ARTHRITIS (RA)

A disorder resembling human RA rarely results in erosive polyarthritis and progressive joint destruction in dogs. Small and toy breeds are most commonly affected. The age of onset is variable (i.e., 9 months to 13 years), but most affected dogs are young or middle-aged. Initially the disease is indistinguishable from idiopathic nonerosive polyarthritis, but the joints are destroyed over time (weeks to months), with distal joints most severely affected.

### Etiology

The precise etiology of canine RA is unknown. Most current theories have been extrapolated from what is known about RA in people, where rheumatoid factors (i.e., IgM and IgG autoantibodies) are directed against altered host IgG, binding to the Fc portion of the altered Ig molecule to form immune complexes. Canine RA may result when a triggering event or inciting antigen initiates an immune reaction against endogenous antigens, causing immune complexes to form. Immune complexes are deposited in the synovium, resulting in complement activation, the chemotactic attraction of inflammatory cells, the intraarticular release of cytokines, synovial cell proliferation, and progressive, severe, erosive inflammatory joint disease. Granulation tissue arises from the inflamed synovium and extends across the joint underneath the articular cartilage. This vascular granulation tissue (i.e., pannus) begins to erode cartilage, and joint swelling and periarticular inflammation cause the joint capsule to stretch and collateral ligaments to rupture.

### Clinical Features

Affected dogs initially have signs indistinguishable from those of other forms of polyarthritis. Fever, depression, anorexia, and reluctance to exercise are common. Joint-related clinical signs such as joint pain and stiff gait are prominent. In the early stages, signs may be sporadic, and stiffness is generally worse after rest and improves with mild exercise. The joints may appear normal or may be swollen and painful. The joints most commonly affected are the carpi, hocks, and phalanges, although elbows, shoulders, and stifles can also be affected. Early radiographic evaluation of affected joints reveals periarticular swelling with minimal evidence of bony change. As the disease progresses, clinical examination reveals crepitus, laxity, luxation and deformity of affected joints (Fig. 76-7).

Radiographic features include periarticular osteoporosis, narrowing of the joint space stemming from a loss of articular cartilage, and focal irregular radiolucent cystlike areas of subchondral bone destruction (Fig. 76-8). Joint space collapse, marginal erosions, and subluxations and luxations are common in the late stages.

### Diagnosis

RA should be suspected in any dog with noninfectious, erosive polyarthritis. In RA the synovial fluid in affected joints is thin, cloudy, and hypercellular (6000 to 80,000 WBC/$\mu$l; mean, 30,000/$\mu$l). Neutrophils are usually the predominant cell (20% to 95%; average, 74%) although in some animals mononuclear cells predominate. Culture of the synovial fluid is negative. Whenever possible the synovial fluid should be collected during a period when the dog is most symptomatic, as the cyclical nature of the disease could make diagnosis difficult.

Serologic tests for RA detect circulating antibody (i.e., rheumatoid factor [RF]) against denatured or immune complexed IgG. A titer of 1:16 or higher is considered positive,

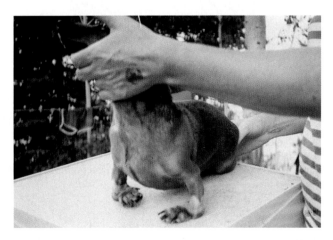

**FIG 76-7**
Complete collapse of both carpi resulting in luxation and severe distortion of the forelimbs in a Dachshund with rheumatoid arthritis (RA). (Courtesy Dr. D. Haines, University of Saskatchewan.)

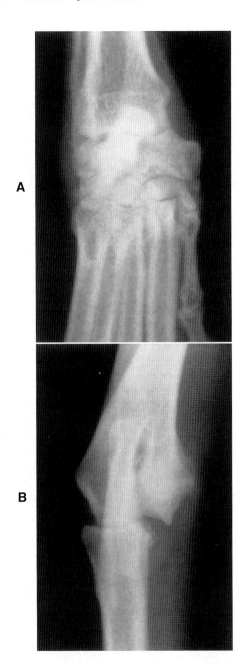

**FIG 76-8**
**A,** Close-up dorsopalmar radiograph of the left carpal joint of a mature female Shetland Sheepdog with rheumatoid arthritis (RA). The intercarpal cartilage spaces have thinned laterally, an osteophyte is present on the lateral aspect of the fourth carpal bone, and mild soft tissue swelling is evident. **B,** Close-up craniocaudal radiograph of the right elbow from the same dog shows medial subluxation of the humerus, new bone deposition on the medial epicondyle and adjacent humeral metaphysis, a small osteophyte on the medial coronoid process, and a narrowed cartilage space.

with tests positive in 20% to 70% of affected dogs. Weak false-positive results may be seen in the setting of other systemic inflammatory diseases and even in dogs with DJD. Synovial biopsy may help to establish the diagnosis. Histologically, synovial thickening, hyperplasia, and proliferation synovitis with pannus formation characterizes RA. The pannus is composed

primarily of proliferating activated synoviocytes, lymphocytes, plasma cells, macrophages, and neutrophils. Culture of the synovial biopsy is negative. RA is diagnosed based on the typical clinical findings and radiographic features, characteristic synovial fluid features, a positive RF test result, and the typical histopathologic changes seen in a synovial biopsy specimen.

**Treatment**

Early treatment of RA is important to prevent irreversible changes and progressive disease. Medical treatment usually includes immunosuppressive drugs, gold salts, and chondroprotective agents. Despite their antiinflammatory and immunosuppressive effects, systemic corticosteroids do not seem to have any effect on the long-term progression of RA in people, and the response in dogs is variable. Initially most dogs are treated with prednisone (2 to 4 mg/kg/day PO for 14 days, then 1 to 2 mg/kg/day for 14 days) and azathioprine (2.2 mg/kg/day), administered as described for the treatment of refractory idiopathic, nonerosive polyarthritis (see p. 1086). Oral chondroprotective agents (Cosequin or glucosamine and chondroitin sulfate) are routinely administered. Subjective improvement has also been observed in dogs receiving injectable chondroprotective agents (e.g., Adequan).

After 1 month of therapy, the dog is reexamined and synovial fluid is evaluated. If the fluid is noninflammatory, the corticosteroid dose is decreased to 1 to 2 mg/kg orally every 48 hours and treatment with azathioprine is continued. If the fluid is still inflammatory, then daily administration of prednisone (1 to 2 mg/kg) and azathioprine (2.2 mg/kg) continues and methotrexate (2.5 mg/m² PO q48h) may be added to treatment. Monthly evaluation of synovial fluid is recommended. If inflammation of the synovial fluid persists after 2 months, additional therapy such as gold salts should be attempted. Aurothioglucose (Solganal; Schering Corp., Kenilworth, N.J.) is given at a dose of 1 mg/kg IM once weekly for 10 weeks or until remission occurs, followed by 1 mg/kg IM every 30 days. Toxicity is uncommon but may include fever, thrombocytopenia, leukopenia, dermatitis, glomerulonephritis, and stomatitis. The oral preparation Auranofin (Ridaura; Smith Kline & French, Philadelphia, Pa) is less effective and is very expensive. Leflunomide (Arava; Aventis Pharma, Bridgewater, N.J.), a pyrimidine synthesis inhibitor, has recently been used with some success to treat dogs with RA when administered at an initial dose of 4 mg/kg/day and the dose is adjusted to maintain a trough plasma level of 20 µg/ml (usual maintenance dose is 0.5 mg/kg/day).

Some therapeutic success may be expected if treatment is initiated before joint damage is severe. In most cases, however, damage to the articular cartilage is severe before the diagnosis is made. Many dogs require additional therapy to control joint discomfort. Palliative treatment with aspirin or other NSAIDs has been recommended (see Table 76-1), but the additive gastrointestinal toxicities of corticosteroids and NSAIDs must be considered. The concurrent administration of misoprostol can help to decrease gastrointestinal adverse effects. RA is a relentlessly progressive disorder, and even with appropriate therapy most dogs show deterioration with time. Surgical proce- dures can occasionally be used to improve joint stability and pain. Synovectomy, arthroplasty, joint replacement, and arthrodesis may decrease painfulness and improve function.

## EROSIVE POLYARTHRITIS OF GREYHOUNDS

An erosive, immune-mediated polyarthritis occurs in Grey- hounds from 3 to 30 months of age. This disorder is primar- ily seen in Australia. The proximal interphalangeal joints and other distal joints are most commonly affected. The articular cartilage erodes in the absence of pannus formation and lysis of subchondral bone. The same therapy as that used for the treatment of idiopathic, immune-mediated, nonerosive poly- arthritis is sometimes effective (see p. 1088). Some evidence shows that this disorder is associated with infection with *My- coplasma spumans,* leading to a recommendation that anti- *Mycoplasma* agents such as tylosin (15 mg/kg PO q8h) should be administered in affected animals.

## FELINE CHRONIC PROGRESSIVE POLYARTHRITIS

Polyarthritis is rarely recognized in cats. Clinical signs may in- clude fever, lethargy, reluctance to walk, and swollen, painful joints. The finding of nonerosive polyarthritis in a cat should prompt evaluation for an infectious cause (e.g., *Mycoplasma gatea, Borrelia burgdorferi, Calicivirus*) or for other evidence of SLE, which is a rare condition in cats. Investigation for an underlying neoplastic or inflammatory condition should be complete before a diagnosis of idiopathic immune-mediated nonerosive polyarthritis can be made in the cat. This rare con- dition seems to respond well to corticosteroids alone in most cats. Cyclophosphamide, chlorambucil, and gold salts have been used in some refractory cases with success.

In contrast to dogs, most cats with polyarthritis have ero- sive joint disease. This can result from septic arthritis, bacte- rial L–form infection (see p. 1314), or a syndrome known as *chronic progressive polyarthritis.* Feline chronic progressive polyarthritis occurs exclusively in male cats. The pathogene- sis of the disorder is not well understood but may involve in- fection with feline syncytia–forming virus (FeSFV) and FeLV (or occasionally FIV). The disorder cannot be experimentally induced by infection with these viruses, but it may result from immune complexes forming as a result of interactions be- tween the viruses and the cat's immune system. Two clinical variants of this disorder affect cats: (1) a proliferative peri- osteal arthritis that predominantly affects young adult cats and (2) a more severe, deforming erosive arthritis that pri- marily affects older cats.

The periosteal proliferative form occurs in 1- to 5-year- old male cats and is characterized by the acute onset of fever, joint pain, lymphadenopathy, and edema of the skin and soft tissues overlying the joint. Initially the radiographic changes are mild and include soft tissue swelling and mild periosteal proliferation. With time the periosteal proliferation worsens and periarticular osteophytes, subchondral cysts, and collapse of the joint space with fibrosis and ankylosis may be noted.

Synovial fluid analysis initially reveals inflammation with an increased WBC count, particularly neutrophils. As the disease becomes chronic, the numbers of lymphocytes and plasma cells increase.

The deforming type of chronic progressive polyarthritis is rare and occurs in old male cats. In this variant the polyar- thritis is insidious in onset, with the slow development of lame- ness and stiffness. Deformation of the carpal and distal joints is common. Severe subchondral central and marginal ero- sions, luxations, and subluxations can be seen radiographi- cally, which can lead to joint instability and deformities. Cy- tologic findings in synovial fluid are less remarkable than those in the periosteal proliferative form and consist of a mild-to-moderate increase in inflammatory cells (i.e., neu- trophils, lymphocytes, macrophages).

### Diagnosis

The diagnosis is based on the typical signalment, clinical signs, radiographic features, and results of synovial fluid analysis. Tests for FeSFV (when available) and FeLV may be positive. In addition, cultures of synovial fluid are negative, and no evidence of an underlying disorder causing a reactive polyarthritis is seen.

### Treatment

Treatment with prednisone (4 to 6 mg/kg/day) may slow the progression of these diseases. If the cat shows clinical im- provement after 2 weeks, the dose of the prednisone is de- creased to 2 mg/kg daily. Alternate-day prednisone therapy (1 to 2 mg/kg) is adequate in some cats. Combination therapy with cyclophosphamide (50 mg/m² PO, 4 days on, 3 days off) or chlorambucil (Leukeran; Burroughs Wellcome; 20 mg/m² PO every 2 weeks) may aid in the long-term control of the disorder. The prognosis is good for a favorable response to therapy and temporary improvement but not for complete control. Lifetime therapy is required. Other FeLV-related dis- orders commonly develop in FeLV-positive cats.

### *Suggested Readings*

Appel MJG: Lyme disease in dogs and cats, *Compend Cont Educ Pract Vet* 12:617, 1990.

Appel MJG et al: CVT update: canine Lyme disease. In Bonagura JD et al, editors: *Kirk's current veterinary therapy XII,* Philadelphia, 1995, WB Saunders.

Arnoczky SP et al: Degenerative joint disease. In Slatter DH, editor: *Textbook of small animal surgery,* Philadelphia, 1985, WB Saunders.

Bennett D: Immune-based erosive inflammatory joint disease of the dog: canine RA, *Small Anim Pract* 28:779, 1987.

Bennett D: Treatment of the immune based inflammatory arthropathies of the dog and cat. In Bonagura JD et al, editors: *Kirk's current veterinary therapy XII,* Philadelphia, 1995, WB Saunders.

Bennett D et al: Bacterial infective arthritis in the dog, *Small Anim Pract* 29:207, 1988.

Carro T: Polyarthritis in cats, *Compend Cont Educ Pract Vet* 16(1):57, 1994.

Cowell RL et al: Ehrlichiosis and polyarthritis in three dogs, *J Am Vet Med Assoc* 192:1093, 1988.

Greene RT: An update on the serodiagnosis of canine Lyme *borreliosis, J Vet Intern Med* 4:167, 1990.

Greene RT: Lyme *borreliosis*. In Greene CE, editor: *Infectious diseases of the dog and cat,* Philadelphia, 1990, WB Saunders.

Griffin DW et al: Synovial fluid analysis in dogs with cruciate ligament rupture, *J Am Anim Hosp Assoc* 28:277, 1992.

Hopper PE: Immune-mediated nonerosive arthritis in the dog. In Kirk RW, editor: *Current veterinary therapy X,* Philadelphia, 1989, WB Saunders.

Levy SA et al: Canine Lyme *borreliosis, Compend Cont Educ Pract Vet* 15:833, 1993.

Lewis RM: RA, *Vet Clin North Am Small Anim Pract* 24:697, 1994.

Lipowitz AJ: Immune-mediated articular disease. In Slatter DH, editor: *Textbook of small animal surgery,* Philadelphia, 1985, WB Saunders.

Manley PA: Treatment of degenerative joint disease. In Bonagura JD et al, editors: *Kirk's current veterinary therapy XII,* Philadelphia, 1995, WB Saunders.

Romatowski J: Comparative therapeutics of canine and human RA, *J Am Vet Med Assoc* 185:558, 1984.

Rosendal S: Mycoplasmal infections. In Greene CE, editor: *Infectious diseases of the dog and cat,* Philadelphia, 1990, WB Saunders.

## Drugs Used in Joint Disease

| DRUG NAME (TRADE NAME) | PURPOSE | RECOMMENDED DOSE | |
|---|---|---|---|
| | | DOG | CAT |
| Acetylsalicylic acid (Aspirin) | Analgesia, antiinflammatory | 25 mg/kg PO q8h | 10 mg/kg PO q48h |
| | Antithrombotic | 10 mg/kg PO q12h | 10 mg/kg PO q12h |
| Amoxicillin | Antibiotic | 20 mg/kg PO, SC, IV q12h | 20 mg/kg PO, SC, IV q12h |
| Ampicillin | Antibiotic | 22 mg/kg PO q8h or 22 mg/kg IV, SC, IM q6h | 22 mg/kg PO q8h or 22 mg/kg IV, SC, IM q6h |
| Auranofin (Ridaura) | Immune-mediated diseases | 0.5-0.2 mg/kg PO q12h (max. 9 mg/day) | None |
| Aurothioglucose (Solganal) | Immune-mediated diseases | 1 mg/kg IM weekly × 10 weeks then q30d | 1 mg/kg IM weekly × 10 weeks then q30d |
| Azathioprine (Imuran) | Immune-mediated diseases | 50 mg/m² (approx. 2.2 mg/kg) q24h | 0.2 mg/kg PO q48h |
| Carprofen (Rimadyl) | Analgesia Antiinflammatory | 2.2 mg/kg PO q12h | Not evaluated |
| Ceftriaxone sodium | Antibiotic | 20 mg/kg IV q12h | 20 mg/kg IV q12h |
| Cephalexin (Keflex) | Antibiotic | 20-40 mg/kg PO q8h | 20-40 mg/kg PO q8h |
| Chloramphenicol | Antibiotic | 25-50 mg/kg PO, IV q6-8h | 25 mg/kg PO q12h |
| Cyclophosphamide (Cytoxan) | Immune-mediated diseases | 50 mg/m² (approx. 2.2 mg/kg), 4 days on 3 off or q48h | 50 mg/m², 4 days on 3 off or q48h |
| Doxycycline (Vibramycin) | Antibiotic | 5-10 mg/kg PO or IV q12h | 5-10 mg/kg PO or IV q12h |
| Erythromycin | Antibiotic | 10 mg/kg PO q8h | 10 mg/kg PO q8h |
| Ketoprofen (Anafen) | Analgesia Antiinflammatory | 1-2 mg/kg PO q24h | 1-2 mg/kg PO q24h |
| Minocycline (Minocin) | Antibiotic | 25 mg/kg PO q12h | None |
| Oxytetracycline | Antibiotic | 20 mg/kg PO q8h | 20 mg/kg PO q8h |
| Penicillin G | Antibiotic | | |
| Aqueous (K or Na) | | 40,000 U/kg IV q6h | 40,000 U/kg IV q6h |
| Procaine | | 40,000 U/kg IM, SC q12h | 40,000 U/kg IM, SC q12h |
| Phenylbutazone (Butazolidin) | Analgesia | 1.0-5.0 mg/kg PO q8h | None |
| Polysulfated glycosaminoglycan (Adequan) | Chondroprotective | 2-5 mg/kg IM q4d × 4 treatments, then q30d | None |
| Prednisone | Immunosuppression | 2-4 mg/kg/day PO | 2-6 mg/kg/day PO |
| | Antiinflammatory/ antiedema | 0.5-0.75 mg/kg PO | 0.5-0.75 mg/kg PO |
| Sodium aurothiomalate (Myochrysine) | Immune-mediated diseases | 1 mg/kg IM weekly | None |
| Tetracycline HCl | Antibiotic | 22 mg/kg q8h | 22 mg/kg PO q8h |
| Tylosin (Tylan) | Antibiotic | 20 mg/kg PO q8h | 22 mg/kg PO q8h |

CHAPTER 77

# Cytology

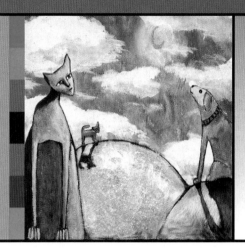

## CHAPTER OUTLINE

GENERAL CONSIDERATIONS, 1093
FINE-NEEDLE ASPIRATION, 1093
IMPRESSION SMEARS, 1094
STAINING OF CYTOLOGIC SPECIMENS, 1094
INTERPRETATION OF CYTOLOGIC SPECIMENS, 1094
    Normal tissues, 1094
    Hyperplastic processes, 1094
    Inflammatory processes, 1094
    Malignant cells, 1095
    Lymph nodes, 1098

## GENERAL CONSIDERATIONS

Evaluation of a cytologic specimen obtained by fine-needle aspiration (FNA) in small animals with suspected neoplastic lesions often yields information that can be used to make a definitive diagnosis, thereby circumventing the need to perform a surgical biopsy. At our hospital, almost every mass or enlarged organ is evaluated cytologically before a surgical biopsy is performed, because the risks and costs associated with FNA are considerably lower than those associated with surgical biopsy.

Clinically applicable diagnostic cytologic techniques are summarized in this chapter, with emphasis on sample collection and the cursory interpretation of the specimens. Although some clinicians are able to obtain sufficient diagnostic information, a board-certified veterinary clinical pathologist should always evaluate a cytologic specimen before one makes prognostic or therapeutic decisions.

## FINE-NEEDLE ASPIRATION

In FNA, a single cell suspension is obtained using a small-gauge needle (i.e., 23 to 25 gauge) of the appropriate length

for the desired target organ or mass; this needle can be coupled to a 12 or 20 ml sterile, dry, plastic syringe. Tissues easily accessible using this technique include the skin and subcutis, deep and superficial lymph nodes, spleen, liver, kidneys, lungs, thyroid, prostate, and intracavitary masses of unknown origin (e.g., mediastinal mass).

If one is aspirating superficial masses, sterile preparation of the site is not necessary. However, clipping and sterile surgical preparation should always be done if one is aspirating organs or masses within body cavities. Once the mass or organ has been identified by palpation or radiography, it should be manually isolated; manual isolation is not necessary when performing ultrasound- or fluoroscopy-guided FNAs. A needle coupled to a syringe is then introduced into the mass or organ, and suction is applied to the syringe three or four times. If the size of the mass or lesion allows it, the needle is then redirected two or three times and the procedure is repeated. Before withdrawing the needle and syringe, one should release the suction so as not to aspirate blood that would contaminate the sample or air that would make the sample irretrievable from the barrel of the syringe. The needle is then detached, air is aspirated into the syringe, the needle is recoupled, and the sample is expelled onto a glass slide. In most cases no material is seen in the syringe, and the amount of cells present within the hub of the needle is usually adequate to obtain four to eight good-quality smears. When one is using the "needle alone" technique, the mass or lesion is isolated as described and the needle is inserted into the lesion four to six times. This allows one to core out small samples, which will be completely contained within the hub of the needle. Once a sample has been obtained, a clean, disposable syringe is loaded with air and coupled to the needle, and the specimen is then gently expelled onto slides.

An aspiration gun (or handle) facilitates the acquisition of specimens by FNA, particularly in hard-to-reach areas such as a solitary small mass in the abdominal cavity. I use a 12 or 20 ml AspirGun (The Everest Co., Linden, N.J.), which easily fits onto a Monoject syringe.

Superficial ulcerated masses can easily be sampled by scraping their surface with a sterile scalpel, wooden tongue depressor, or gauze. Smears are then made either by touching a glass slide onto the ulcerated lesion (see Impression Smears, below) or by further scraping the surface with a tongue depressor and transferring the material thus obtained onto the slide. "Pull" smears made using two glass slides are preferable over "push" smears. Once the smears have been made, they are air-dried and stained using any of the techniques described below.

## IMPRESSION SMEARS

Impression smears of surgical specimens or open lesions are commonly used in practice. At our clinic, we evaluate numerous intraoperative impression smears to determine the therapeutic course to follow in a given patient.

When making impression smears from surgical specimens, the clinician first gently blots the tissue onto a gauze pad or paper towel to remove any blood or debris, then gently grasps it with forceps from one end. Touch imprints are made on a glass slide by gently touching the slide with the tissue specimen. I usually make two or three rows of impressions along the slide and then stain it. It is advisable to submit a different tissue specimen for histopathologic evaluation.

## STAINING OF CYTOLOGIC SPECIMENS

Several staining techniques are practical for in-office use, including rapid Romanowsky's (e.g., Diff-Quik; various manufacturers) and new methylene blue (NMB) stains. Most commercial laboratories use Romanowsky's stains, such as Wright's or Giemsa.

There are remarkable differences between these staining techniques. Romanowsky's stains are slightly more time-consuming, but they produce better cellular detail and offer worse contrast between nucleus and cytoplasm; moreover, the smears can be permanently archived. NMB, on the other hand, is a quick stain (it takes literally seconds to stain a smear), but it is not permanent, which means that slides cannot be saved for consultation; moreover, cellular details are not as sharp as they are on Romanowsky-stained smears. In addition, because nuclear DNA and RNA stain extremely well with this technique, most cells appear "malignant." I frequently use Diff-Quik to get both a quick appreciation of the quality of the sample and, possibly, to arrive at a tentative diagnosis. This frequently allows a tentative diagnosis to be made while the client is still in the office. The main difference between rapid hematologic stains (e.g., Diff-Quik) and Giemsa or Wright-Giemsa stains is that, in a variable proportion of canine and feline mast cell tumors, the former do not stain the granules. In addition, rapid hematologic stains may not stain granules in some large granular lymphocytes (LGLs).

## INTERPRETATION OF CYTOLOGIC SPECIMENS

Although the clinician should strive to be able to evaluate cytologic specimens proficiently, the ultimate cytologic diagnosis should be made by a board-certified veterinary clinical pathologist. The following are guidelines for cytologic interpretation.

### NORMAL TISSUES

#### Epithelial Tissues

Most epithelial cells, particularly those of the glandular or secretory epithelium, tend to cling together (i.e., they have desmosomes), forming clusters. Individual cells are easily identifiable and are round or polygonal; nuclei and cytoplasms are well differentiated. Most cells in Romanowsky's-stained smears have blue cytoplasm and round nuclei.

#### Mesenchymal Tissues

Cells from mesenchymal tissues (e.g., fibroblasts, fibrocytes, chondroblasts) are difficult to obtain in routine FNA material or tissue scrapings because they are usually surrounded by intercellular matrix. Mesenchymal cells are typically spindle shaped, polygonal, or oval and have irregular nuclei; cytoplasmic boundaries are usually indistinct; and cell clumps are seen rarely.

#### Hematopoietic Tissues

A detailed morphologic description of circulating blood cells is beyond the scope of this chapter. Briefly, however, most cells from hemolymphatic organs are round, individual cells (with no tendency to clump); they have a blue cytoplasm on Romanowsky's-stained smears, and a variable nuclear size; most nuclei are round or kidney shaped. Tissue such as bone marrow has cells in different stages of development (i.e., from blasts to well-differentiated circulating cells).

### HYPERPLASTIC PROCESSES

Hyperplasia of different tissues commonly results in enlargement of glandular organs and lymphoid structures. The cytologic features of epithelial and lymphoid hyperplasia differ; lymphoid hyperplasia is discussed on p. 1098. Cytologically, hyperplastic changes may be difficult to recognize, because they may mimic either normal or neoplastic tissues. Care should be taken when evaluating specimens from organs such as enlarged prostates or thickened urinary bladders, because the high degree of hyperplasia and dysplasia may appear to indicate malignancy.

### INFLAMMATORY PROCESSES

Most inflammatory reactions are characterized cytologically by the presence of inflammatory cells and debris in the smear. The type of cell present depends on the etiologic agent (e.g., neutrophils in pyogenic infections, eosinophils in parasitic or allergic reactions) and the duration of the inflammatory

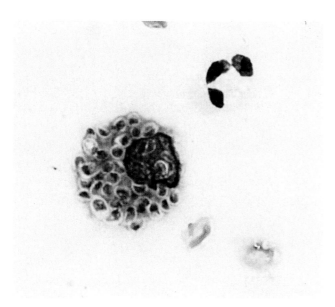

## FIG 77-1
Photomicrograph of a *Histoplasma capsulatum*–laden macrophage obtained from an ulcerated mucocutaneous lesion in a 6-year-old female, spayed, black Labrador Retriever. (×1000.)

**TABLE 77-1**

**Cytologic Characteristics of Malignant Neoplasms**

Large nuclei
Fine chromatin pattern
One or more nucleoli
Anisokaryosis
Monomorphism
Pleomorphism
Anisocytosis
Cytoplasmic vacuolization
Cytoplasmic basophilia
Multinucleated giant cells
Phagocytosis
Heterotopia

process (i.e., acute processes are usually characterized by a predominance of granulocytes, whereas macrophages and lymphocytes predominate in chronic processes). The following pathogens are frequently identified in cytologic specimens: *Histoplasma, Blastomyces, Cryptococcus, Coccidioides, Aspergillus/Penicillium, Toxoplasma, Leishmania,* other rickettsial agents (e.g., salmon poisoning), bacteria, and *Demodex* (Fig. 77-1).

## MALIGNANT CELLS

The cells that make up most normal organs and tissues (with the exception of bone marrow precursors) are well differentiated, in that most of them are similar in size and shape; they have a normal nuclear:cytoplasmic (N:C) ratio; the nuclei usually have condensed chromatin and no nucleoli; and the cytoplasm may exhibit features of differentiation (e.g., keratin formation in squamous epithelium).

Malignant cells have one or more of the following features (Table 77-1): a decreased N:C ratio (i.e., larger nucleus and smaller cytoplasm); a delicate chromatin pattern; nucleoli (usually multiple); anisokaryosis (i.e., cells have nuclei of different sizes); nuclear molding (i.e., a nucleus in a multinucleated cell is compressed by a neighboring one); morphologic homogeneity (i.e., all cells look alike); pleomorphism (i.e., cells in different stages of development); vacuolization (primarily in malignant epithelial tumors); anisocytosis (i.e., cells are of different sizes); multinucleated giant cells; and, occasionally, phagocytic activity. Another feature of malignancy is heterotopia (i.e., the presence of a given cell type where it is not found anatomically); for example, epithelial cells can appear in a lymph node only as a consequence of metastasis

from a carcinoma. In addition, malignant cells tend to be morphologically different from the progenitor cell population (Table 77-1). On the basis of the predominant cytologic features, malignancies can be classified as carcinomas (epithelial), sarcomas (mesenchymal), or round (or discrete) cell tumors (Fig. 77-2).

### Carcinomas

Most carcinomas are composed of round or polygonal cells that tend to cling together, forming clusters. Their cytoplasms are usually deep blue, and vacuolization is evident in most adenocarcinomas. Cytoplasmic boundaries are difficult to recognize, and the cells look like a mass of protoplasm rather than a sheet of individual cells. In squamous cell carcinomas, cells are usually individualized, have a deep blue cytoplasm (with an occasional eosinophilic fringe), and have no vacuoles. Nuclei in both adenocarcinomas and squamous cell carcinomas are large, with a fine chromatin pattern and evident nucleoli (Fig. 77-3).

### Sarcomas

The cytologic features of sarcomas vary according to the histologic type. However, most mesenchymal tumors have spindle shaped, polygonal, polyhedral, or oval cells, with a reddish blue to dark blue cytoplasm and irregularly shaped nuclei. Most cells are individualized, although clumping may occur. The cells in most sarcomas have a tendency to form "tails," and the nuclei protrude from the cytoplasm (Fig. 77-4). The presence of spindle-shaped or polygonal cells with a vacuolated blue-gray cytoplasm is highly suggestive of hemangiosarcoma. Intercellular matrix (e.g., osteoid, chrondroid) is found occasionally; in these two tumor types, the cells are usually round or ovoid. Multinucleated giant cells are common in some sarcomas in cats (Fig. 77-5).

As a general rule, because sarcoma cells do not exfoliate easily, aspirates of these masses may yield false-negative results. Therefore, if a mass is clinically suspected to be a sarcoma and

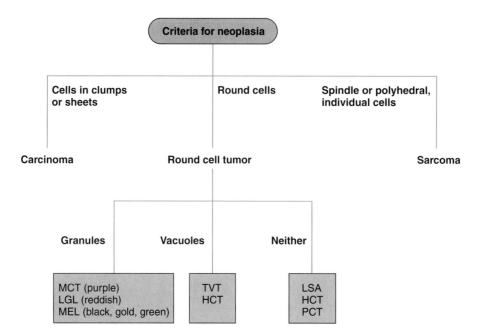

**FIG 77-2**
Flow chart for the cytologic diagnosis of tumors in dogs and cats. *MCT,* Mast cell tumor; *LGL,* large granular lymphoma; *MEL,* melanoma; *TVT,* transmissible venereal tumor; *HCT,* histiocytoma; *LSA,* lymphoma; *PCT,* plasma cell tumor.

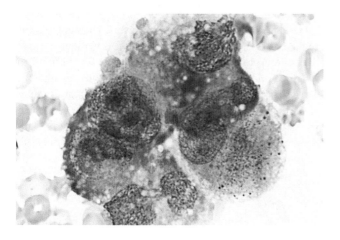

**FIG 77-3**
Photomicrograph of pleural fluid from an older female Irish Setter showing a cluster of deeply basophilic cells, with vacuolated cytoplasm, anisocytosis, anisokaryosis, and prominent nucleoli. The cytologic diagnosis was carcinomatosis (i.e., metastatic adenocarcinoma of unknown origin). (×1000.)

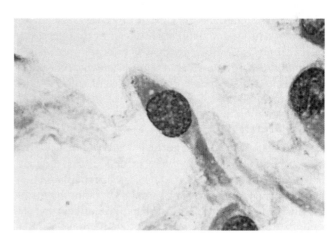

**FIG 77-4**
Photomicrograph of a fine-needle aspirate of a firm, lobulated, subcutaneous mass in an older dog. The cells are spindle shaped, have "tails," and do not associate with other cells. The nuclei appear to be protruding from the cytoplasm. (×1000.) The cytologic diagnosis is spindle cell sarcoma. Histopathologic findings were diagnostic for fibrosarcoma.

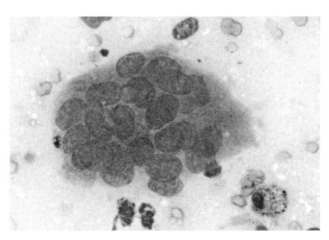

**FIG 77-5**
Photomicrograph of a multinucleated giant cell from a soft tissue sarcoma in a 13-year-old cat with tumor-associated hypercalcemia that resolved after surgical excision of the primary mass. (×400.)

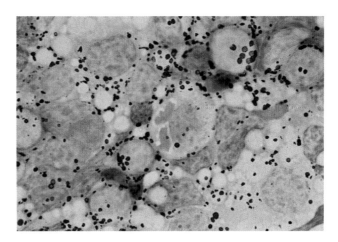

**FIG 77-7**
Photomicrograph of an impression smear from a mesenteric lymph node in an old cat evaluated because of vomiting and diarrhea. Note the large round cells with red, large cytoplasmic granules. The diagnosis was lymphoma of large granular lymphocytes. (×1000.)

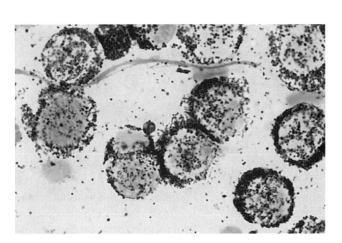

**FIG 77-6**
Photomicrograph of a fine-needle aspirate from a subcutaneous mass in an older Boxer with multiple dermoepidermal and subcutaneous masses and marked multifocal lymphadenopathy. Note the monomorphic population of round cells containing purple granules. The cytologic diagnosis was mast cell tumor. (×1000.)

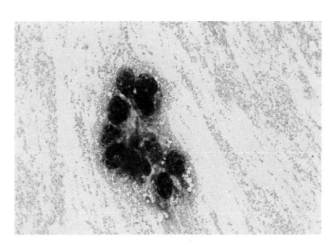

**FIG 77-8**
Photomicrograph of a fine-needle aspirate from a mass in the oral cavity of a 10-year-old Schnauzer. Note the dark, fine granules in the cytoplasm. The diagnosis was melanoma. (×1000.)

FNA findings are negative, a core biopsy specimen of the mass should be obtained.

## Round (Discrete) Cell Tumors

Tumors composed of a homogeneous population of round (or discrete) cells are referred to as *round* (or *discrete*) *cell tumors*. These tumors are common in dogs and cats and include lymphomas, histiocytomas, mast cell tumors, transmissible venereal tumors, plasma cell tumors, and malignant melanomas; as discussed above, osteosarcomas and chondrosarcomas can be composed of round cells. Round cell tumors are easily diagnosed on the basis of cytology; the presence or absence of cytoplasmic granules or vacuoles aids in the classification of round cell tumors (see Fig. 77-2).

The cells that make up mast cell tumors (Fig. 77-6), LGL lymphomas (Fig. 77-7), and melanomas (Fig. 77-8) usually have cytoplasmic granules; cells in neuroendocrine tumors can also have granules. When hematologic stains are used, the granules are purple in mast cell tumors; red in LGL lymphomas; and black, green, brown, or yellow in melanomas. Lymphomas (Fig. 77-9), histiocytomas (Fig. 77-10), plasma cell tumors, and transmissible venereal tumors do not have cytoplasmic granules. Cytoplasmic vacuoles are common in transmissible venereal tumors and in histiocytomas.

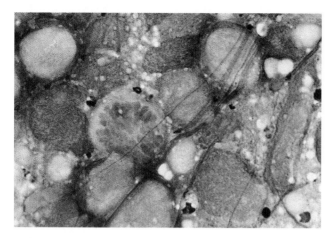

**FIG 77-9**
Photomicrograph of a fine-needle aspirate from the kidney of a middle-aged Boxer with bilateral renomegaly. Note the monomorphic population of round cells, with large nuclei, prominent nucleoli, and no cytoplasmic granules or vacuoles. The cytologic diagnosis was lymphoma. (×1000.)

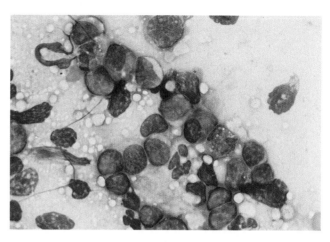

**FIG 77-11**
Photomicrograph of a fine-needle aspirate from a reactive lymph node in a dog. Note the heterogeneous population of lymphoid cells (small, medium, and large), plasma cells, and macrophages. (×1000.)

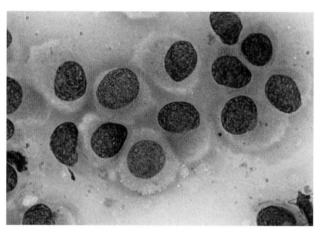

**FIG 77-10**
Photomicrograph of a fine-needle aspirate from a small, round, dermoepidermal mass in the head of a 1-year-old dog. Note the large round cells with abundant clear cytoplasm and fine chromatin pattern. The diagnosis was histiocytoma. (×1000.)

Briefly, lymphomas are characterized by a monomorphic population of individual, undifferentiated round cells with large nuclei, a coarse chromatin pattern, and one or two nucleoli; occasional cells can be vacuolated (see Fig. 77-9). Cells in histiocytomas are similar to those in lymphomas except that the chromatin pattern is fine rather than coarse, they have more abundant cytoplasm, and they are frequently vacuolated (see Fig. 77-10). Because inflammation is an important component of histiocytomas, inflammatory cells (i.e., neutrophils, lymphocytes) are commonly found in these tumors. Mast cell tumors are distinctive in that the cytoplasm of the cells contains purple (metachromatic)

granules, which can be so numerous as to obscure the nuclear features; eosinophils are also a common feature in these tumors. Mast cell granules may be absent in poorly differentiated tumors.

## LYMPH NODES

Cytologic evaluation of lymph node aspirates is commonly done in practice. At our clinic, a cytologically based diagnosis is obtained in approximately 90% of dogs and 60% to 75% of cats with lymphadenopathy. If the cytologic findings of an enlarged lymph node are inconclusive, the node should be surgically excised and submitted for histopathologic evaluation.

When evaluating cytologic specimens prepared from lymph node aspirates or impression smears, the clinician should keep in mind that these organs react to a variety of stimuli following a distinct pattern. In general, four cytologic patterns are recognized: normal lymph node, reactive or hyperplastic lymphadenopathy, lymphadenitis, and neoplasia.

### Normal Lymph Node

Cytologic specimens from normal nodes are composed predominantly (75% to 90%) of small lymphocytes. These cells are approximately 7 to 10 μm in diameter (1 to 1.5 times the diameter of a red blood cell) and have a dense chromatin pattern and no nucleoli. The remaining cells are macrophages, lymphoblasts, plasma cells, and other immune cells.

### Reactive or Hyperplastic Lymphadenopathy

Lymphoid tissues reacting to different antigenic stimuli (e.g., bacterial, immunologic, neoplastic, fungal) are cytologically similar in that the cell population is composed of a mixture of small, intermediate, and large lymphocytes; lymphoblasts; plasma cells; and macrophages (Fig. 77-11). In addition, other cell types may be present, depending on the specific agent (e.g., eosinophils in parasitic or allergic reactions). The first impression when evaluating a reactive or hyperplastic node cytologically is that of a heterogeneous population of cells. The presence of cells in different stages of development indicates that the lymphoid tissue is undergoing polyclonal expansion (i.e., response to multiple antigens).

## Lymphadenitis

Inflammatory processes affecting the lymph nodes produce cytologic changes similar to the ones seen in reactive lymphadenopathy, although there is a profusion of inflammatory cells (e.g., neutrophils in suppurative infections) and degenerative changes (e.g., pyknosis, karyorrhexis) in most cell lines. The etiologic agents may be visualized.

## Neoplasia

Neoplastic cells can appear in a lymph node either as a result of lymphatic or vascular dissemination (i.e., metastasis from a primary tumor distal to the node) or as a primary process affecting these structures (i.e., lymphomas). Cytologic features of metastatic lymph node lesions consist of a reactive pattern and the presence of neoplastic cells; in advanced metastatic lesions, it is frequently difficult to identify normal lymphoid cells. The morphology of the metastatic cells depends on the primary tumor type. As discussed above, lymphomas are characterized by a monomorphous population of large, immature lymphoid cells; these cells are usually large and have an abnormally low N:C ratio, coarse chromatin, and evident nucleoli (see Fig. 77-9).

## Suggested Readings

Baker R et al: *Color atlas of cytology of the dog and cat,* St Louis, 2000, Mosby.

Barton CL: Cytologic diagnosis of cutaneous neoplasia: an algorithmic approach, *Compend Contin Educ* 9:20, 1987.

Cowell RL et al: *Diagnostic cytology and hematology of the dog and cat,* ed 2, St Louis, 1999, Mosby.

Mills JN: Lymph node cytology, *Vet Clin North Am* 19:697, 1989.

Morrison WB et al: Advantages and disadvantages of cytology and histopathology for the diagnosis of cancer, *Semin Vet Med Surg* 8:222, 1993.

Radin MJ et al: *Interpretation of canine and feline cytology,* Wilmington, Del, 2001, the Gloyd Group.

Raskin RE et al: *Atlas of canine and feline cytology,* Philadelphia, 2001, WB Saunders.

Wellman ML: The cytologic diagnosis of neoplasia, *Vet Clin North Am* 20:919, 1990.

## CHAPTER 78

# Principles of Cancer Treatment

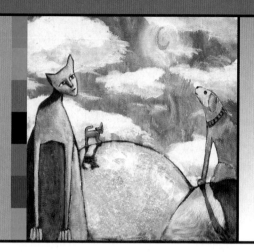

## CHAPTER OUTLINE

GENERAL CONSIDERATIONS, 1100
PATIENT-RELATED FACTORS, 1100
OWNER-RELATED FACTORS, 1100
TREATMENT-RELATED FACTORS, 1101

## GENERAL CONSIDERATIONS

Over the past several decades, a variety of therapeutic modalities have been used in dogs and cats with cancer (Table 78-1). However, until two or three decades ago, surgery remained the mainstay of cancer treatment for pets. Today, nonresectable or metastatic malignancies can be treated with varied degrees of success, using some of the modalities listed in Table 78-1.

When evaluating a cat or a dog with malignancy, the clinician should bear in mind that in most cases owners elect to treat their pets, if given the option. Although euthanasia still remains a reasonable choice in some small animals with cancer, every effort should be made to investigate other (treatment) options.

Depending on the tumor type, biologic behavior, and clinical stage, a clinician may recommend one or more of the treatments listed in Table 78-1. However, in addition to tumor-related factors, many other factors influence the selection of the optimal treatment for an animal with cancer. These include patient-related, owner-related, and treatment-related factors.

## PATIENT-RELATED FACTORS

It is important to remember that the best treatment for a particular tumor does not necessarily constitute the best treatment for a particular patient or the best treatment from the owner's perspective. The most important patient-related factor to be considered is the animal's general health and activity or performance status (Table 78-2). For example, a cat or dog with markedly diminished activity and severe constitu-

tional signs (i.e., poor performance status) may not be a good candidate for aggressive chemotherapy or for the repeated anesthetic episodes required for external beam radiotherapy. Age by itself is not a factor that should be considered when discussing cancer therapy with the owner (i.e., "age is not a disease"). For example, a 14-year-old dog in excellent health is a better candidate for chemotherapy or radiotherapy than a 9-year-old dog with chronic renal failure or decompensated congestive heart failure. Patient-related factors should be addressed before one institutes specific cancer treatment (e.g., correct the azotemia, improve the nutritional status with enteral feeding).

## OWNER-RELATED FACTORS

Owner-related factors play an important role in determining the treatment to be implemented in small animals with cancer. Every clinician is aware of the significance of the owner-pet bond. This bond is so important that it often dictates the treatment approach used in a given patient. For example, owners may be so apprehensive about having their dog with lymphoma receive chemotherapy that they refuse such treatment; thus the optimal treatment cannot be used in this patient.

In my experience owners should be made a part of the medical team that treats their pet. If they are assigned tasks to perform at home, such as measuring the tumors to monitor the response to treatment, taking their pet's temperature daily, and monitoring their pet's performance status, they assume responsibility for the fate of their pet and are therefore quite cooperative. The clinician should also be constantly available to answer concerned pet owners' questions and guide them through difficult times. The clinician should discuss all potential treatment options with the owner, emphasizing the pros and cons of each (e.g., beneficial effects and potential for adverse effects of treatment A versus B versus C versus no treatment). The clinician should also clearly explain what will (or should) happen during the pet's treatment (including a thorough description of the potential adverse effects). By observing these easy steps, the clinician usually cul-

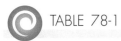

## TABLE 78-1

### Treatment Options for Animals with Cancer

Surgery
Radiotherapy
Chemotherapy
Immunotherapy (biologic response modifiers)
Hyperthermia
Cryotherapy
Phototherapy
Photochemotherapy
Thermochemotherapy
Nonconventional (alternative)

## TABLE 78-2

### Modified Karnovsky's Performance Scheme for Dogs and Cats

| GRADE | ACTIVITY/PERFORMANCE |
|---|---|
| 0—Normal | Fully active, able to perform at pre-disease level |
| 1—Restricted | Restricted activity from predisease level but able to function as an acceptable pet |
| 2—Compromised | Severely restricted activity level; ambulatory only to the point of eating but consistently defecating and urinating in acceptable areas |
| 3—Disabled | Completely disabled; must be force-fed; unable to confine urinations and defecations to acceptable areas |
| 4—Dead | |

Modified from International Histological Classification of Tumors of Domestic Animals, *Bull World Health Organ* 53:145, 1976.

tivates realistic expectations on the part of the owner and ensures that the interaction with the owner is smooth and uneventful. As discussed in later paragraphs, the option of euthanasia should also be addressed at this time, either as an immediate option or as an option if treatments fail.

Another very important owner-related factor is finances. In general the treatment of a cat or dog with disseminated or metastatic malignancy is "expensive," as judged by the average clinician. However, it is the owner who should determine whether this treatment is indeed "expensive." It is relatively common for an owner to spend $2000 to $7000 to treat a dog or cat with surgery, radiotherapy, or chemotherapy. In other words, all treatment options should be described to the client, regardless of their cost. Occasionally owners spend what most people consider to be exorbitant amounts of money to treat their pet with cancer or other diseases.

## TREATMENT-RELATED FACTORS

There are several important treatment-related factors to be considered when planning cancer therapy. First, the specific indication should be considered. Surgery, radiotherapy, and hyperthermia are treatments aimed at eradicating a locally invasive tumor with a low metastatic potential (and potentially curing the animal), although they can be used palliatively in dogs or cats with extensive (bulky) disease or in those with metastatic disease. On the other hand, chemotherapy usually does not constitute a curative treatment, although palliation of advanced disease can easily be accomplished for several tumor types. Immunotherapy (the use of biologic response modifiers) also constitutes an adjuvant or palliative approach (i.e., tumors are not cured by immunotherapy alone). In general it is best to use an aggressive treatment when the tumor is first detected (because this is when the chances of eradicating every single tumor cell are the highest) rather than to wait until the tumor is in an advanced stage—that is, to "treat big when the disease is small."

In most cases, the highest success rates are obtained by combining two or more treatment modalities. For example, the combination of surgery and chemotherapy (with or without immunotherapy) has resulted in a significant prolongation of disease-free survival in dogs with osteosarcoma of the appendicular skeleton and in dogs with splenic hemangiosarcoma. Similarly, the combination of radiotherapy and hyperthermia has resulted in a prolongation of disease-free survival in dogs with fibrosarcoma of the oropharynx.

The complications and adverse effects of different treatments also constitute treatment-related factors to be considered when planning therapy. Complications of chemotherapy are addressed in Chapter 80. As discussed later, the animal's quality of life should be maintained (or improved) during cancer treatment. At our clinic, this is the first priority in a cat or a dog with cancer receiving treatment. Our motto is: "The patient should feel better with the treatment than with the disease."

Cancer treatment can be either palliative or curative. Given the current paucity of information regarding specific tumor types and treatments, it is also possible that these two approaches will sometimes overlap (i.e., a treatment initially thought to be palliative may result in cure or vice versa). As discussed earlier, every effort should be made to eradicate every single cancer cell in the body (i.e., obtain a cure) shortly after diagnosis. This means taking immediate action rather than a wait-and-see attitude. With very few exceptions, malignancies do not regress spontaneously. Therefore, by delaying treatment in an animal with confirmed malignancy, one is only increasing the probability that the tumor will disseminate locally or systemically, thereby decreasing the likelihood of a cure. As discussed earlier, surgery, radiotherapy, and hyperthermia are potentially curative treatments, whereas chemotherapy and immunotherapy are usually palliative.

If a cure cannot be obtained, the two main goals of treatment are to induce remission while achieving a good quality of life. The term *remission* refers to shrinkage of the tumor. If one is objectively evaluating the effects of therapy, one should measure the tumor or tumors and assess the response using the criteria given in Table 78-3. The quality-of-life issue is quite important in small animal oncology (see preceding paragraphs). In a quality-of-life survey of owners whose pets had undergone chemotherapy for nonresectable or metastatic malignancy conducted in our clinic, more than 80% responded that the quality of life of their pets was maintained or improved during treatment. If a good quality of life cannot be maintained (i.e., the animal's performance status deteriorates), the treatment being used should be modified or discontinued.

Palliative treatments are quite acceptable for small animals with cancer and to their owners. For example, even though chemotherapy rarely achieves a cure for most tumors, we can provide a cat or dog (and its owner) with a prolonged, good-quality survival. Although these patients ultimately die of tumor-related causes, the owners are usually pleased to have a pet that is asymptomatic for a long time. Another common example that is frequently forgotten is palliative surgery; for example, in dogs or cats with ulcerated mammary carcinomas and small pulmonary metastases, we formerly recommended euthanasia. However, we now know that performing a mastectomy or lumpectomy (even if the owners decline chemotherapy) will likely result in several months of good-quality survival, until the metastatic lesions finally cause respiratory compromise. In another example, dogs with apocrine gland adenocarcinoma of the anal sacs and metastatic sublumbar lymphadenopathy benefit from surgical resection of the primary tumor even if adjuvant chemotherapy or lymphadenectomy will not be considered. Removal of the primary mass improves clinical signs of straining in these patients; since the colon and rectum are compressed ventrally by the enlarged lymph nodes and laterally or dorsally by the primary mass, removal of one of the lesions easily alleviates clinical signs. Moreover, we have successfully performed sublumbar (or iliac) lymphadenectomies in dogs with metastatic apocrine gland adenocarcinoma of the anal sacs, resulting in survival times of 1 to 3 years.

Needless to say, the clinician should also address the presence of paraneoplastic syndromes even if specific antineoplastic therapy is not contemplated. For example, treatment of humoral hypercalcemia of malignancy with diphosphonates (bisphosphonates) causes remarkable improvement in the quality of life of affected dogs. We have used either etidronate (Didronel, Procter and Gamble Pharmaceuticals, Cincinnati, Ohio, at a dosage of 10 to 20 mg/kg PO q12h) or pamidronate (Aredia, Novartis Pharmaceuticals, East Hannover, N.J., at a dosage of 1.3 to 1.5 mg/kg IV q6-8wk) in dogs with tumor-associated hypercalcemia in which the neoplastic disease could not be surgically removed or that had failed chemotherapy. In most dogs, serum calcium concentrations could be maintained within normal limits, and we did not detect any appreciable toxicity.

Finally, most cats and dogs with cancer are treated using a team approach. This team includes the pet, the owner, the medical oncologist, the oncologic nurse, the surgical oncologist, the radiotherapist, the clinical pathologist, and the pathologist. A smooth interaction among the members of the team results in marked benefits for the pet and its owner.

 TABLE 78-3

**Criteria Used to Assess Tumor Response to Treatment**

Complete remission (CR): complete disappearance of all tumors
Partial remission (PR): decrease in the bidimensional tumor diameter by more than 50%
Stable disease (SD): less than 25% variation in bidimensional tumor diameter
Progressive disease (PD): increase in the bidimensional tumor diameter by more than 25%

## Suggested Readings

Couto CG: Principles of cancer treatment. In Nelson RW et al: *Essentials of small animal internal medicine,* St Louis, 1992, Mosby–Year Book.

Lagoni L et al: *The human-animal bond and grief,* Philadelphia, 1994, WB Saunders.

LaRue SM et al: Recent advances in radiation oncology, *Compend Contin Educ Pract Vet* 15:795, 1993.

Page RL et al: Clinical indications and applications of radiotherapy and hyperthermia in veterinary oncology, *Vet Clin North Am* 20:1075, 1990.

Withrow SJ: The three rules of good oncology: biopsy! biopsy! biopsy! *J Am Anim Hosp Assoc* 27:311, 1991.

# CHAPTER 79

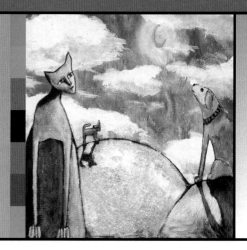

# Practical Chemotherapy

## CHAPTER OUTLINE

CELL AND TUMOR KINETICS, 1103
BASIC PRINCIPLES OF CHEMOTHERAPY, 1103
INDICATIONS AND CONTRAINDICATIONS
OF CHEMOTHERAPY, 1105
MECHANISM OF ACTION OF ANTICANCER
DRUGS, 1106
TYPES OF ANTICANCER DRUGS, 1106

## CELL AND TUMOR KINETICS

To better understand the effects of chemotherapy on both neoplastic and normal tissues, it is necessary to have a basic understanding of cell biology and tumor kinetics. As a general rule, the biologic characteristics of neoplastic cells are similar to those of their normal counterparts, with the main difference being that neoplastic cells usually do not undergo terminal differentiation. Hence, the cell cycles of normal and neoplastic cells are similar.

The mammalian cell cycle has two apparent phases: mitosis and the resting phase. The resting phase is actually composed of four phases (Fig. 79-1):

1. Synthesis phase *(S):* DNA is synthesized.
2. Gap 1 phase *(G1):* RNA and the enzymes needed for DNA production are synthesized.
3. Gap 2 phase *(G2):* the mitotic spindle apparatus forms.
4. Gap 0 phase *(G0):* this is the true resting phase.

The mitosis phase is termed the *M phase.*

Oncogenes serve as checkpoints between different phases of the cell cycle.

Several terms must be defined before chemotherapy is discussed. The *mitotic index (MI)* refers to the proportion of cells in the process of mitosis within a tumor; the pathologist quite often provides information about the mitotic activity in a given tumor sample, reported as the MI or as the number of mitoses per high-power field (or per X number of high-power fields). The *growth fraction (GF)* refers to the proportion of proliferating cells within a tumor and cannot be quantified in a patient. The *doubling time (DT)* refers to the time it takes for a tumor to double in size; it can be calculated by using sequential measurements of the tumor volume [$V = \pi/6 \times$ (mean diameter)$^3$] seen on radiographs or ultrasonograms or determined by direct palpation. In dogs the DT ranges from 2 days (for metastatic osteosarcoma) to 24 days (for metastatic melanoma), whereas in humans it ranges from 29 days (for malignant lymphomas) to 83 days (for metastases from breast cancer). The DT depends on the time spent in mitosis, the cell cycle duration, the GF, and the cell loss resulting from death or metastasis. Given our knowledge of tumor kinetics, by the time a pulmonary metastatic nodule is visualized on radiographs, it consists of 200,000,000 cells, weighs less than 150 mg, and has already divided 25 to 35 times. A 1 cm palpable nodule has $10^9$ tumor cells (1,000,000,000) and weighs 1 g (Fig. 79-2). As a general rule, most nonneoplastic tissues (with the exception of bone marrow stem cells and intestinal crypt epithelium) have a low GF, low MI, and prolonged DT, whereas most neoplastic tissues have a high MI, high GF, and short DT (at least initially) (see Fig. 79-2).

Surgical cytoreduction (debulking) of a tumor that has reached a plateau of growth decreases the total number of cells, thus increasing the MI and GF and shortening the DT through yet unknown mechanisms (Fig. 79-3). In theory, this renders the neoplasm more susceptible to chemotherapy or radiotherapy.

## BASIC PRINCIPLES OF CHEMOTHERAPY

Chemotherapeutic agents predominantly kill cells in rapidly dividing tissues. To exploit the tumoricidal effect of different chemotherapeutic drugs, it is common practice to combine three or more drugs to treat a given malignancy. These drugs are selected on the basis of the following principles: each should be active against the given tumor type; each should act by a different mechanism of action; and they should not have superimposed toxicities. It is customary to name the protocol after the first letters of each drug in the combination (e.g., *VAC* for *v*incristine, doxorubicin [or *A*driamycin], and *c*yclophosphamide). As a general rule, combination chemotherapy

### FIG 79-1

Mammalian cell cycle. Cells in mitosis *(M)* can differentiate and subsequently die (the rule in normal tissues); they can also progress to $G_0$ (true resting phase), from which they can be recruited by a variety of stimuli (see text). $G_1$, Gap 1; *S*, DNA synthesis; $G_2$, gap 2; $G_0$, resting phase.

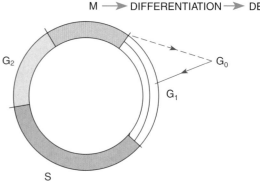

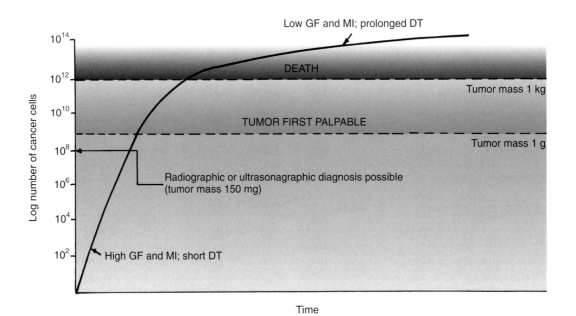

### FIG 79-2

Tumor (cell) kinetics. Additional information on tumor kinetics can be found in the text. *GF,* Growth fraction; *MI,* mitotic index; *DT,* doubling time. (From Couto CG: Principles of chemotherapy. In *Proceedings of the Tenth Annual Kal Kan Symposium for the Treatment of Small Animal Diseases: Oncology,* Kalkan Foods, Inc, Vernon, Calif, 1986, p 37.)

### FIG 79-3

The effect of surgical or radiotherapeutic intervention on tumor kinetics. After cytoreduction, cells are recruited from the $G_0$ phase and the tumor returns to the exponential phase. *XRT,* radiation therapy; *GF,* growth factor; *MI,* mitotic index; *DT,* doubling time. (From Couto CG: Principles of chemotherapy. In *Proceedings of the Tenth Annual Kal Kan Symposium for the Treatment of Small Animal Diseases: Oncology,* Kalkan Foods, Inc, Vernon, Calif, 1986, p 37.)

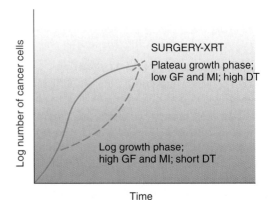

results in more sustained remissions and prolonged survival times, as compared with those achieved using single-agent chemotherapy; this is thought to result from the fact that multichemotherapy delays (or even prevents) the development of drug-resistant clones. However, some exceptions to this rule include the treatment of dogs with osteosarcoma using cisplatin, carboplatin, or doxorubicin as single agents; the treatment of dogs with chronic lymphocytic leukemia using chlorambucil alone; and the treatment of dogs with transmissible venereal tumors with vincristine alone.

Another general concept of chemotherapy from the standpoint of cell kinetics is that it is more effective in a relatively small tumor than in a large one, even though the inherent sensitivity to the drug, or drugs, may be the same. As can be seen in Fig. 79-3, a small tumor (e.g., $10^6$ cells) is more likely than a larger one (e.g., $10^{11}$ cells) to be completely eradicated by the drugs, because the smaller mass has a higher MI, a higher GF, and consequently a shorter DT than the larger mass (i.e., more cells are actively dividing at a given time).

Despite continued controversy, the doses of most chemotherapeutic agents are still determined on a body surface area (BSA) basis; exceptions will be listed in same chapter. This appears to provide a more constant metabolic parameter for comparing doses across species. It can be calculated using the following formula:

$$\frac{\text{Weight (g)}^{2/3} \times \text{K (constant)}}{10^4} = \text{m}^2 \text{ BSA}$$

The constant is 10.1 for the dog and 10 for the cat. Table 79-1 is a conversion table of weight (in kilograms) to BSA (in squared meters) for dogs. Table 79-2 is a conversion table of pounds (and kilograms) to BSA for cats. When drugs such as doxorubicin are being used, doses determined on the basis of BSA usually lead to adverse effects in very small dogs (i.e., those under 10 kg) and cats. A dose determined on the basis of weight (e.g., 1 mg/kg) is more appropriate in such small animals.

## INDICATIONS AND CONTRAINDICATIONS OF CHEMOTHERAPY

Chemotherapy is primarily indicated for animals with systemic (e.g., lymphoma, leukemias) or metastatic neoplasms, although it can also be used for the management of nonresectable, chemoresponsive neoplasms that have historically proved refractory to radiotherapy or hyperthermia (primary chemotherapy). It can also be used as an adjuvant treatment after partial surgical debulking of a neoplasm (e.g., partial excision of an undifferentiated sarcoma) and is indicated for the control of micrometastatic disease after the surgical excision of a primary neoplasm (e.g., cisplatin, carboplatin, or doxorubicin therapy after limb amputation in dogs with osteosarcoma; VAC after splenectomy for dogs with hemangiosarcoma). Chemotherapy can also be administered intracavitarily in dogs and cats with

## TABLE 79-1

### Conversion of Body Weight to Body Surface Area in Dogs

| BODY WEIGHT (kg) | BODY SURFACE AREA (m²) |
|---|---|
| 0.5 | 0.06 |
| 1 | 0.10 |
| 2 | 0.15 |
| 3 | 0.20 |
| 4 | 0.25 |
| 5 | 0.29 |
| 6 | 0.33 |
| 7 | 0.36 |
| 8 | 0.40 |
| 9 | 0.43 |
| 10 | 0.46 |
| 11 | 0.49 |
| 12 | 0.52 |
| 13 | 0.55 |
| 14 | 0.58 |
| 15 | 0.60 |
| 16 | 0.63 |
| 17 | 0.66 |
| 18 | 0.69 |
| 19 | 0.71 |
| 20 | 0.74 |
| 21 | 0.76 |
| 22 | 0.78 |
| 23 | 0.81 |
| 24 | 0.83 |
| 25 | 0.85 |
| 26 | 0.88 |
| 27 | 0.90 |
| 28 | 0.92 |
| 29 | 0.94 |
| 30 | 0.96 |
| 31 | 0.99 |
| 32 | 1.01 |
| 33 | 1.03 |
| 34 | 1.05 |
| 35 | 1.07 |
| 36 | 1.09 |
| 37 | 1.11 |
| 38 | 1.13 |
| 39 | 1.15 |
| 40 | 1.17 |
| 41 | 1.19 |
| 42 | 1.21 |
| 43 | 1.23 |
| 44 | 1.25 |
| 45 | 1.26 |
| 46 | 1.28 |
| 47 | 1.30 |
| 48 | 1.32 |
| 49 | 1.34 |
| 50 | 1.36 |

TABLE 79-2

**Conversion of Body Weight to Body Surface Area in Cats**

| BODY WEIGHT (lb) | BODY WEIGHT (kg) | BODY SURFACE AREA (m²) |
|---|---|---|
| 5 | 2.3 | 0.165 |
| 6 | 2.8 | 0.187 |
| 7 | 3.2 | 0.207 |
| 8 | 3.6 | 0.222 |
| 9 | 4.1 | 0.244 |
| 10 | 4.6 | 0.261 |
| 11 | 5.1 | 0.278 |
| 12 | 5.5 | 0.294 |
| 13 | 6.0 | 0.311 |
| 14 | 6.4 | 0.326 |
| 15 | 6.9 | 0.342 |
| 16 | 7.4 | 0.356 |
| 17 | 7.8 | 0.371 |
| 18 | 8.2 | 0.385 |
| 19 | 8.7 | 0.399 |
| 20 | 9.2 | 0.413 |

malignant effusions or neoplastic involvement of the cavity/ area in question (e.g., intrathecally administered cytosine arabinoside in dogs and cats with lymphoma of the central nervous system; intrapleurally administered cisplatin or 5-fluoruracil in dogs with pleural carcinomatosis). Finally, neoadjuvant, or primary, chemotherapy is the approach used in animals with bulky tumors not amenable to surgical excision. After the drugs cause the tumor to shrink, the tumor can be surgically excised; chemotherapy is then continued to eliminate any residual neoplastic cells (e.g., fluoruracil, doxorubicin, cyclophosphamide [FAC] chemotherapy for dogs with thyroid adenocarcinoma; VAC chemotherapy for dogs with subcutaneous hemangiosarcomas).

As a general rule, chemotherapy should not be used as a substitute for surgery, radiotherapy, or hyperthermia; nor should it be used in animals with severe underlying multiple-organ dysfunction (or it should be used cautiously, with a dose modification), because this increases the risk of systemic toxicity.

## MECHANISM OF ACTION OF ANTICANCER DRUGS

The effects of anticancer drugs on a neoplastic cell population follow first-order kinetic principles (i.e., the number of cells killed by a drug or drug combination is directly proportional to one variable—the dose used). These drugs kill a constant proportion of cells, rather than a constant number of cells. Therefore the efficacy of a drug or drug combination

depends on the number of cells in a given tumor (e.g., a drug combination that kills 99% of the cells in a tumor containing 100,000,000 [$10^9$] cells leaves 1,000,000 [$10^6$] viable cells).

As discussed in the following paragraphs, different types of anticancer drugs kill tumor cells by different mechanisms. Drugs that kill only dividing tumor cells (i.e., that do not kill cells in the $G_0$ phase) by acting on several phases of the cycle are termed *cell cycle phase–nonspecific drugs*. Alkylating agents belong to this group. Drugs that selectively kill tumor cells during a given phase of the cell cycle are termed *cell cycle phase–specific drugs*. Most antimetabolites and plant alkaloids are phase-specific drugs. Finally, drugs that kill neoplastic cells regardless of their cycle status (i.e., they kill both dividing and resting cells) are termed *cell cycle–nonspecific drugs*. These latter drugs are extremely myelosuppressive (e.g., nitrosoureas) and are infrequently used in veterinary medicine.

## TYPES OF ANTICANCER DRUGS

Anticancer drugs are commonly classified into the following categories. Most of these drugs are also currently available as generic products:

- Alkylating agents
- Antimetabolites
- Antitumor antibiotics
- Plant alkaloids (or mitotic inhibitors)
- Hormones
- Miscellaneous agents

*Alkylating agents* cross-link DNA, thus preventing its duplication. Because they mimic the effects of radiotherapy, they are also referred to as *radiomimetics*. These drugs are active during several phases of the cell cycle (i.e., they are cell cycle phase-nonspecific) and are more active if given intermittently at high doses. The major toxicities of these drugs are myelosuppressive and gastrointestinal in nature. Alkylating agents commonly used in pets with cancer include the following:

- Cyclophosphamide (Cytoxan; Mead-Johnson, Evansville, Ind)
- Chlorambucil (Leukeran; Burroughs Wellcome, Research Triangle Park, N.C.)
- Melphalan (Alkeran; Burroughs Wellcome)
- Cisplatin (Platinol; Bristol-Myers Oncology, Evansville, Ind); *SHOULD NOT BE USED IN CATS!*
- Carboplatin (Paraplatin; Bristol-Myers Oncology)

*Antimetabolites* exert their activity during the S phase of the cell cycle (cell cycle phase-specific) and are more active if given repeatedly at low doses or as continuous intravenous infusions. These drugs are structural analogs of naturally occurring metabolites (fake metabolites) that substitute for normal purines or pyrimidines. The major toxicities of these drugs are myelosuppressive and gastrointestinal. The following antimetabolites are commonly used in small animals with cancer:

- Cytosine arabinoside (Cytosar-U; Upjohn, Kalamazoo, Mich)
- Methotrexate (Methotrexate; Lederle, Wayne, N.J.)
- 5-Fluorouracil (5-FU; Roche, Nutley, N.J.); *SHOULD NOT BE USED IN CATS!*
- Azathioprine (Imuran; Burroughs Wellcome)

*Antitumor antibiotics* act by several mechanisms (i.e., cell cycle phase nonspecific), the most important of which appears to be DNA damage produced by free radicals or by a topoisomerase-II–dependent mechanism. There are now several synthetic or semisynthetic antibiotics. The major toxicities of these drugs are myelosuppressive and gastrointestinal in nature; doxorubicin and actinomycin D are extremely caustic if given perivascularly, and the former has cumulative cardiotoxic effects. Antitumor antibiotics include the following:

- Doxorubicin (Bedford Labs, Bedford, Ohio)
- Bleomycin (Blenoxane; Bristol-Myers)
- Actinomycin D (Cosmegen; Merck Sharp & Dohme, West Point, Pa)
- Mitoxantrone (Novantrone; Lederle)

*Plant alkaloids* are derived from the periwinkle plant (*Vinca rosea*) and the May apple plant (*Podophyllum peltatum*). Vinca derivatives disrupt the mitotic spindle and are therefore cell cycle phase-specific (active during M phase), whereas *Podophyllum* derivatives cross-link DNA. The major toxicity is perivascular sloughing if the agent extravasates. Etoposide should not be administered intravenously, because the vehicle (Tween 80) causes anaphylaxis.

Commonly used plant alkaloids include the following:

- Vincristine (Oncovin; Eli Lilly, Indianapolis, Ind)
- Vinblastine (Velban; Eli Lilly)
- Etoposide, or VP-16 (VePesid; Bristol-Myers)

*Hormones* are commonly used for the treatment of hemolymphatic malignancies or endocrine-related tumors. Commonly used hormones include the following:

- Prednisone

With the exception of corticosteroids, hormones are not recommended as antineoplastics, because they are associated with relevant adverse effects in animals.

*Miscellaneous agents* consist of drugs with a mechanism of action that is either unknown or differs from those of agents already described. Miscellaneous agents commonly used in small animals with cancer include the following:

- DTIC (DTIC; Dome, Westhaven, Conn)
- L-Asparaginase (Elspar; Merck Sharp & Dohme)

## Suggested Readings

Chabner BA et al: *Cancer chemotherapy and biotherapy: principles and practice*, ed 2, Philadelphia, 1996, Lippincott-Raven.

Couto CG: Principles of chemotherapy. In *Proceedings of the Tenth Annual Kal Kan Symposium for the Treatment of Small Animal Diseases: Oncology*, Kalkan Foods, Inc, Vernon, Calif, 1986, p 29.

Helfand SC: Principles and applications of chemotherapy, *Vet Clin North Am* 20:987, 1990.

Moore AS: Recent advances in chemotherapy for non-lymphoid malignant neoplasms, *Compend Contin Educ Pract Vet* 15:1039, 1993.

Vail DM: Recent advances in chemotherapy for lymphoma in dogs and cats, *Compend Contin Educ Pract Vet* 15:1031, 1993.

# CHAPTER 80

# Complications of Cancer Chemotherapy

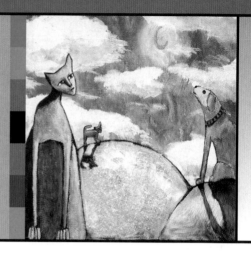

## CHAPTER OUTLINE

GENERAL CONSIDERATIONS, 1108
HEMATOLOGIC TOXICITY, 1108
GASTROINTESTINAL TOXICITY, 1111
HYPERSENSITIVITY REACTIONS, 1112
DERMATOLOGIC TOXICITY, 1112
PANCREATITIS, 1113
CARDIOTOXICITY, 1114
UROTOXICITY, 1114
HEPATOTOXICITY, 1115
NEUROTOXICITY, 1115
PULMONARY TOXICITY, 1115
ACUTE TUMOR LYSIS SYNDROME, 1115

## GENERAL CONSIDERATIONS

Most anticancer agents are relatively nonselective in that they kill not only rapidly dividing neoplastic tissues but also some of the rapidly dividing normal tissues in the host (e.g., villus epithelium, bone marrow cells). In addition, similar to other commonly used agents (e.g., digitalis glycosides), most anticancer agents have low therapeutic indices (i.e., narrow therapeutic/toxic ratios).

Because anticancer agents follow first-order kinetic principles (i.e., the fraction of cells killed is directly proportional to the dose used), increasing the dose of a particular drug increases the proportion of the neoplastic cells killed, but it also enhances its toxicity. This is commonly seen when a tumor relapses and higher doses of a previously prescribed chemotherapeutic agent are administered.

Because toxicity generally tends to affect rapidly dividing tissues, given the short doubling times of bone marrow and villus epithelial cells, myelosuppression and gastrointestinal signs are the most common toxicities encountered in practice. Other rare complications of chemotherapy include anaphylactoid (or anaphylactic) reactions, dermatologic toxicity, pancreatitis, cardiotoxicity, pulmonary toxicity, neurotoxicity, hepatopathies, and urotoxicity. Table 80-1 lists anticancer drugs commonly used in small animals and their toxicities.

Several factors can potentiate the effects of anticancer agents and thereby enhance their toxicity. For example, drugs that are excreted primarily through the kidneys (e.g., cisplatin, carboplatin, methotrexate) are more toxic to animals with renal disease; thus a dose reduction or the use of an alternative drug is usually recommended in such cases.

In addition to the direct effects of some drugs on different organ systems, rapid killing of certain neoplastic cells (i.e., lymphoma cells) can lead to sudden metabolic derangements that result in acute clinical signs mimicking those of drug toxicity (i.e., depression, vomiting, diarrhea). This syndrome is referred to as acute tumor lysis syndrome (ATLS) (see p. 1115).

In general, cats appear to be more susceptible than dogs to some of the adverse effects of chemotherapy (e.g., anorexia, vomiting) but not to others (e.g., myelosuppression). Certain breeds of dogs, including Collies and Collie crosses, Old English Sheepdogs, Cocker Spaniels, and West Highland White Terriers, also appear to be more prone to some of the acute adverse reactions to chemotherapy (i.e., gastrointestinal signs, myelosuppression) than the general dog population.

The overall prevalence of toxicity of different chemotherapy protocols is considerably lower in dogs and cats (approximately 5% to 40%) than in humans (75% to 100%) treated with similar drugs or combinations. A recent survey of owners whose pets had been treated with a variety of chemotherapy protocols at The Ohio State University Veterinary Teaching Hospital revealed that more than 80% considered their pets' quality of life to be equal to or better than that before the start of chemotherapy.

## HEMATOLOGIC TOXICITY

The high mitotic rate and growth fraction (i.e., 40% to 60%) of the bone marrow cells predispose this organ to relevant toxicity from anticancer drugs. Hematologic toxicity constitutes the most common complication of chemotherapy, and often the severe and potentially life-threatening cytopenias that occur necessitate the temporary or permanent discontinuation of the offending agent or agents. Table 80-1 lists agents commonly implicated in this type of toxicity.

TABLE 80-1

Toxicity of Anticancer Agents in Cats and Dogs

| TOXICITY | DOX | BLEO | ACT | CTX | LEUK | CISP | MTX | araC | 5-FU | L-asp | VCR | VBL | DTIC |
|---|---|---|---|---|---|---|---|---|---|---|---|---|---|
| Myelosuppression | S | N | M | M/S | N/M | M | M/S | M/S | M | N/M | N/M | M/S | M/S |
| Vomiting/diarrhea | M/S | N | M | M | N/M | M/S | M/S | N/M | N/M | N | N/M | N/M | M/S |
| Cardiotoxicity | M/S | N | N | N/? | N | N | N | N | N | N | N | N | N |
| Neurotoxicity | N | N | N | N | N | N | N | N | M | N/M? | N/M | N | N |
| Hypersensitivity | M/S | N | N | N | N | N | N | N | N | M/S | N | N | N |
| Pancreatitis | M | N | N | N/M | N | N | N | N/M | N | M/S | N | N | N/M |
| Perivascular sloughing | S | N | M/S | N | NA | N/M | N | N | N/M | N | M/S | M/S | M/S |
| Urotoxicity | ? | N | N | M/S | N | M/S | M | N | N | N | N | N | N |

*DOX*, Doxorubicin; *BLEO*, bleomycin; *ACT*, actinomycin D; *CTX*, cyclophosphamide; *LEUK*, chlorambucil; *CISP*, cisplatin; *MTX*, methotrexate; *araC*, cytosine arabinoside; *5-FU*, 5-fluorouracil; *L-asp*, L-asparaginase; *VCR*, vincristine; *VBL*, vinblastine; *DTIC*, dacarbazine; *S*, severe; *N*, none; *M*, mild to moderate, *NA*, not applicable; *?*, questionable.

It is easy to anticipate the cell line that will be affected, based on the bone marrow transit times and circulating half-lives of blood-formed elements. For example, the bone marrow transit time and circulating half-life of red blood cells in the dog are approximately 7 and 120 days, those of the platelets are 3 days and 4 to 6 days, and those of granulocytes are 6 days and 4 to 8 hours, respectively. On the basis of this, neutropenia would occur first, followed by thrombocytopenia. Chemotherapy-induced anemia is rare in dogs and cats and, if it occurs, is of late onset (3 to 4 months after initiation of therapy). Other patient-related factors (e.g., malnutrition, old age, concurrent organ dysfunction, prior extensive chemotherapy) and tumor-related factors (e.g., bone marrow infiltration, widespread parenchymal organ metastases) can also affect the degree of myelosuppression.

Although thrombocytopenia is probably as common as neutropenia, it is rarely severe enough to cause spontaneous bleeding, and therefore it is not discussed at length here. In general, in most dogs with chemotherapy-induced thrombocytopenia, the platelet counts remain above 50,000 cells/μl. Spontaneous bleeding usually does not occur until platelet counts are less than 30,000/μl. The protocols currently used at our clinic that are associated with predictable thrombocytopenia are doxorubicin and dacarbazine (ADIC) and D-MAC (see Cancer Chemotherapy Protocols table at the end of Part 11) in dogs; platelet counts associated with these protocols are usually less than 50,000/μl. Platelet counts between 50,000 and 75,000/μl are common in dogs receiving melphalan (Alkeran) or lomustine chronically. Chemotherapy-induced thrombocytopenia is extremely rare in cats. Thrombocytosis is common in cats and dogs receiving vincristine (Oncovin).

Neutropenia usually constitutes the dose-limiting cytopenia and occasionally leads to life-threatening sepsis in dogs; although neutropenia does occur in cats receiving chemotherapy, it rarely leads to the development of clinically recognizable sepsis. The nadir of neutropenia for most drugs (i.e., lowest point in the curve) usually occurs 5 to 7 days after treatment, and the neutrophil counts return to normal within 36 to 72 hours of the nadir. With certain drugs, the nadir of neutropenia is delayed (i.e., approximately 3 weeks for carboplatin). Dogs with neutrophil counts less than 2000 cells/μl should be closely monitored for the development of sepsis, although overwhelming sepsis rarely occurs in animals with neutrophil counts of more than 1000 cells/μl. The development of sepsis in neutropenic cats is extremely rare.

The pathogenesis of sepsis in neutropenic animals is as follows: first, the chemotherapy-induced death and desquamation of gastrointestinal crypt epithelial cells occur simultaneously with myelosuppression; next, enteric bacteria are absorbed through the damaged mucosal barrier into the systemic circulation; and finally, because the number of neutrophils in the circulation is not sufficient to phagocytose and kill the invading organisms, multiple organs become colonized with the bacteria and death ensues unless the animal is treated appropriately.

It is important to identify the septic neutropenic animal using laboratory means, since the cardinal signs of inflammation (i.e., redness, swelling, increased temperature, pain, abnormal function) may be absent because there are not enough neutrophils to participate in the inflammatory process. The same holds true for radiographic changes compatible with inflammation; for example, dogs with neutropenia and bacterial pneumonia diagnosed on the basis of cytologic and microbiologic findings in transtracheal wash material often have normal thoracic radiograph findings (Fig. 80-1). As a general rule, if a severely neutropenic animal (neutrophil count <500/μl) is evaluated because of pyrexia (>104° F [>40° C]), the fever should be attributed to bacterial pyrogens until proved otherwise and the patient should be treated aggressively with antimicrobial therapy (see following paragraphs).

All dogs and cats undergoing chemotherapy should be up-to-date in their vaccines; it is controversial whether the use

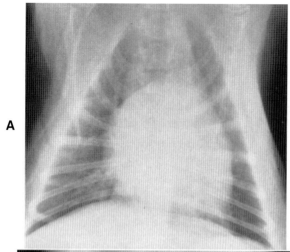

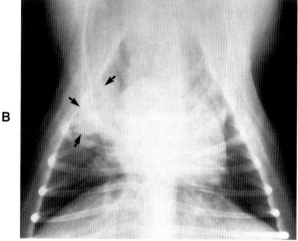

**FIG 80-1**
Thoracic radiographs from a 5-year-old, male, castrated Boston Terrier with multicentric lymphoma treated with doxo-rubicin and dacarbazine (ADIC) chemotherapy. This dog presented as an emergency because of depression, fever, and mild bilateral nasal discharge. The neutrophil count on admission was 1500/μl. **A,** Thoracic radiograph findings were considered normal at the time, but a transtracheal wash specimen contained bacteria. **B,** Two days later, when the neutrophil count increased to 16,300/μl, focal areas of pneumonia became evident. (From Couto CG: Management of complications of cancer chemotherapy, *Vet Clin North Am* 20:1037, 1990, with permission.)

of modified-live vaccines should be avoided because of the potential for inducing illness in immunosuppressed animals. Recent evidence suggests that dogs with cancer undergoing chemotherapy have protective serum antibody titers for commonly used vaccines.

Hematologic monitoring of the patient receiving chemotherapy constitutes the most effective way to prevent (or anticipate) severe, life-threatening sepsis or bleeding secondary to myelosuppression. Complete blood counts (CBCs) should be obtained weekly or every other week (depending on the treatment protocol), and the myelosuppressive agent or

agents should be temporarily discontinued (or the dose decreased) if the neutrophil count decreases to less than 2000 cells/μl or if the platelet count decreases to less than 50,000 cells/μl. Discontinuing the offending agent or agents for two or three administrations usually allows sufficient time for the cell counts to return to normal. When therapy is reinstituted, it is recommended that only 75% of the initial dose be given and the doses increased during the next 2 to 3 weeks until the initially recommended dose (or a dose that does not produce marked cytopenias) is reached. Obviously, the drawback of discontinuing chemotherapy is the potential for tumor relapse, so the clinician and owner must weigh the pros and cons of temporarily discontinuing treatment.

Clinically, neutropenic animals can be classified as febrile or afebrile. Neutropenic, febrile animals should be managed aggressively, because they are usually septic. Thus fever in a neutropenic patient constitutes a medical emergency. The following protocol is the one currently used in such patients at our clinic. First, a thorough physical examination is performed to search for a septic focus, an indwelling intravenous (IV) catheter is placed aseptically, and IV fluids are administered as required. All anticancer agents are discontinued immediately, with the exception of corticosteroids, which should be discontinued gradually because acute hypoadrenocorticism can develop in animals receiving steroid therapy if the drug is abruptly discontinued. Blood samples for a CBC and determination of the serum electrolyte, blood glucose, and blood urea nitrogen concentrations are obtained immediately. A urine sample for urinalysis and bacterial culture is also obtained. Two or three sets of aseptically collected blood samples can be obtained at 30-minute intervals for aerobic and anaerobic bacterial cultures and antibiotic susceptibility tests, although this is usually not necessary because the bacterial isolates are quite predictable (see following paragraph) and because the results of these tests will not be available for several days. After the second set of samples for blood cultures is collected, therapy with an empirical bactericidal antibiotic combination is instituted. We use a combination of amikacin (15 to 20 mg/kg IV q24h) and cephalothin (22 mg/kg IV q8h), or enrofloxacin (5 to 10 mg/kg IV q24h) and ampicillin (22 mg/kg IV q8h) because most bacterial isolates in such animals are Enterobacteriaceae and staphylococci, organisms commonly susceptible to these agents. Once the neutrophil count returns to normal and the animal's condition is clinically normal (usually within 72 to 96 hours), the antibiotic combination is discontinued and the animal is allowed to go home, with instructions to the owner to administer sulfadiazine-trimethoprim (ST) at a dosage of 13 to 15 mg/kg by mouth (PO) every 12 hours or enrofloxacin (5 to 10 mg/kg PO q24h) for 5 to 7 days. When the patient returns for additional chemotherapy, the dose of the offending agent or agents should be decreased by 15% to 20%.

At our clinic the yield for three sets of blood cultures in dogs with cancer, fever, and normal-to-high neutrophil counts is approximately 40%, whereas it is approximately 30% in dogs with cancer, fever, and neutropenia. Isolates in the former group usually include *Streptococcus* spp., *Staphy-*

*lococcus* spp., *Enterobacter* spp., *Klebsiella* spp., and *Escherichia coli,* in decreasing order of frequency. In neutropenic, febrile dogs the isolates include mainly *Klebsiella* spp. *and E. coli; Staphylococcus* spp. is isolated in less than 20% of the dogs.

Neutropenic, afebrile, asymptomatic patients can be treated as outpatients by discontinuing the drug or drugs as described earlier and administering ST (13 to 15 mg/kg PO q12h). The patient that is afebrile but has constitutional signs should be considered to be septic and treated as described in previous paragraphs. If the neutropenia is not severe (i.e., >2000 cells/μl), no therapy is required and the animal should only be observed by the owner. Owners should be instructed to take their pet's rectal temperature twice daily and to call the veterinarian if pyrexia develops, in which case the animal is treated as neutropenic and febrile. ST eliminates the aerobic intestinal flora but preserves the anaerobic bacteria, which are an important component of the local defense system because of their ability to produce local antibiotic factors. In addition, ST is active against many pathogens isolated from animals with cancer, and it achieves therapeutic blood and tissue concentrations and also high intragranulocytic concentrations.

Myelosuppression may be alleviated through the use of lithium carbonate (10 mg/kg PO q12h) in dogs, or recombinant human granulocyte colony–stimulating factor (G-CSF; Neupogen; AmGen, Thousand Oaks, Calif; 5 μg/kg subcutaneously [SQ] q24h) in dogs and cats. Although several studies have reported on the beneficial role of G-CSF or granulocyte-macrophage colony–stimulating factor (GM-CSF) in dogs and cats, it is unlikely that these agents will find their way into the clinic owing to their high cost (approximately $50 to $150/day) and the fact that dogs and cats can mount an antibody response to this protein of human origin and inactivate it; moreover, in dogs with chemotherapy-induced neutropenia the activity of endogenous G-CSF is extremely high, and neutrophil counts return to normal within 36 to 72 hours, the same interval reported for "response" to G-CSF. In our clinic G-CSF is typically reserved for patients that received accidental chemotherapy overdoses and in which the predicted duration of neutropenia is unknown.

## GASTROINTESTINAL TOXICITY

Although less common than myelosuppression, gastrointestinal toxicity is a relatively common complication of cancer chemotherapy in pets. From a clinical standpoint, two major types of gastrointestinal complications can occur: gastroenterocolitis and the combination of anorexia, nausea, and vomiting.

Although results of controlled studies are not available, nausea and vomiting are not apparently as common in pets as they are in humans receiving similar drugs and dosages. Drugs associated with nausea and vomiting in dogs or cats include dacarbazine (DTIC), cisplatin, doxorubicin (primarily in cats), methotrexate, actinomycin D, cyclophosphamide, and 5-fluorouracil (5-FU) (see Table 80-1).

Acute anorexia, nausea, and vomiting caused by injectable drugs are usually prevented by administering the offending agents by slow IV infusion. If these problems persist despite this, antiemetics such as metoclopramide (Reglan; A.H. Robins, Richmond, Va) can be given at a dosage of 0.1 to 0.3 mg/kg IV, SQ, or PO every 8 hours, or prochlorperazine (Compazine; Smith Kline & French Laboratories, Philadelphia, Pa) can be administered at a dosage of 0.5 mg/kg intramuscularly (IM) every 8 to 12 hours. Other antiemetics that may be effective in dogs with chemotherapy-induced emesis are butorphanol (Torbugesic; Fort Dodge Labs, Fort Dodge, Iowa) at a dosage of 0.3 to 0.4 mg/kg IM or IV every 6 to 8 hours and ondansetron (Zofran; Glaxo, Research Triangle Park, N.C.) at a dosage of 0.1 mg/kg IV immediately before chemotherapy and every 6 hours thereafter; the latter is extremely expensive for use in dogs. (For additional information on this subject, see Chapter 30.) Two drugs, methotrexate and cyclophosphamide, that are commonly administered PO can also cause anorexia, nausea, and vomiting. Methotrexate commonly causes anorexia and vomiting 2 or 3 weeks after the start of therapy in dogs; these adverse effects are usually controlled with metoclopramide given at the dosage just described. If these problems persist, methotrexate treatment may need to be discontinued. Cyclophosphamide tends to induce anorexia or vomiting in cats. Cyproheptadine (Periactin; Merck Sharp & Dohme, West Point, Pa) at a dosage of 1 to 2 mg (total dose) PO every 8 to 12 hours is quite effective as an appetite stimulant and antinausea agent in cats.

It is rare for gastroenterocolitis to develop in animals receiving anticancer agents. Drugs that occasionally cause mucositis include methotrexate, 5-FU, actinomycin D, and doxorubicin. It occurs rarely in association with other alkylating agents, such as cyclophosphamide. Of the drugs mentioned in the previous paragraphs, only doxorubicin and methotrexate appear to be of clinical importance. On the basis of our experience, Collies and Collie crosses, Old English Sheepdogs, Cocker Spaniels, and West Highland White Terriers appear to be extremely susceptible to doxorubicin-induced enterocolitis.

Doxorubicin-induced enterocolitis is characterized by the development of hemorrhagic diarrhea (with or without vomiting), primarily of the large bowel type, 3 to 7 days after the administration of the drug. Supportive fluid therapy (if necessary) and treatment with therapeutic doses of bismuth subsalicylate–containing products (Pepto-Bismol, 3 to 15 ml or 1-2 tabs PO q8-12h) are generally effective in controlling the clinical signs in dogs, which usually resolve in 3 to 5 days. The administration of Pepto-Bismol from days 1 to 7 of the treatment may alleviate or prevent these signs in dogs at risk for gastroenterocolitis (i.e., one of the breeds mentioned, an animal with a history of this toxicity). The use of bismuth subsalicylate should be avoided in cats. Gastroenteritis associated with the PO administration of methotrexate usually occurs a minimum of 2 weeks after the animal has been receiving this drug; the treatment is the same as that used for doxorubicin-induced enterocolitis.

## HYPERSENSITIVITY REACTIONS

Acute type I hypersensitivity reactions occasionally occur in dogs receiving parenteral L-asparaginase or doxorubicin and are common in dogs treated with IV etoposide; in the latter, there is a reaction to the solubilizing agent (Tween 80). The reaction to doxorubicin does not appear to be a true hypersensitivity reaction, however, because this agent can induce direct mast cell degranulation independently of immunoglobulin E (IgE) mediation. Etoposide can be safely administered to dogs PO. Hypersensitivity reactions to anticancer agents are extremely rare in cats and thus are not discussed.

Clinical signs in dogs with hypersensitivity reactions to anticancer agents are similar to those in dogs with other types of hypersensitivity reactions (i.e., they are primarily cutaneous and gastrointestinal in nature). Typical signs appear during or shortly after administration of the agent and include head shaking (caused by ear pruritus), generalized urticaria and erythema, restlessness, occasionally vomiting or diarrhea, and rarely collapse caused by hypotension.

Most systemic anaphylactic reactions can be prevented by pretreating the patient with $H_1$ antihistamines (i.e., diphenhydramine, 1 to 2 mg/kg IM 20 to 30 minutes before administration of the drug) and by administering certain drugs (e.g., L-asparaginase) SQ or IM rather than IV. If the agent cannot be given by any other routes (i.e., doxorubicin), it should be diluted and administered by slow IV infusion.

The treatment of acute hypersensitivity reactions includes immediate discontinuation of the agent and the administration of $H_1$ antihistamines (i.e., diphenhydramine, 0.2 to 0.5 mg/kg by slow IV infusion), dexamethasone sodium phosphate (1 to 2 mg/kg IV), and fluids if necessary. If the systemic reaction is severe, epinephrine (0.1 to 0.3 ml of a 1:1000 solution IM or IV) should be used. Once the reaction subsides (and if it was mild), the administration of certain drugs, such as doxorubicin, may be continued. Injectable $H_1$ antihistamines should be used with caution in cats (if at all), because they can cause acute central nervous system depression leading to apnea.

## DERMATOLOGIC TOXICITY

It is rare for anticancer agents to cause dermatologic toxicity in small animals. However, three types of dermatologic toxicities can occur: local tissue necrosis (caused by extravasation), delayed hair growth and alopecia, and hyperpigmentation.

Local tissue necrosis resulting from the extravasation of vincristine, vinblastine, actinomycin D, or doxorubicin is occasionally seen in dogs receiving these drugs but is extremely rare in cats. The pathogenesis of this toxicity is poorly understood, but it is thought to be mediated by release of free radicals; however, these drugs are extremely caustic if given perivascularly, causing moderate to severe tissue necrosis. As a consequence, every effort should be made to ensure that these drugs are administered intravascularly. In addition to this complication, some retrievers (e.g., Labrador and Golden

 TABLE 80-2

**Recommendations for the Management of Perivascular Injections of Caustic Anticancer Drugs in Cats and Dogs**

1. Do not remove the IV catheter.
2. Administer 10 to 50 ml of sterile saline solution through the catheter (in an attempt to dilute the agent).
3. With a 25-gauge needle, administer 10 to 20 ml of sterile saline solution SQ in the affected area.
4. Inject 1 to 4 mg of dexamethasone sodium phosphate SQ in the affected area (in an attempt to stabilize lysosomal and plasma membranes).
5. Apply cold compresses or ice packs to the area for 48 to 72 hours (to cause vasoconstriction and prevent local dissemination of the drug and to decrease local tissue metabolism).

*IV,* Intravenous; *SQ,* subcutaneously.

Retrievers) appear to experience pruritus or discomfort around the site of the IV injection even when the drug is known to have been administered intravascularly. This pain and discomfort frequently lead to licking and to the development of a pyotraumatic dermatitis ("hot spot") within hours of the injection. In these dogs, applying a bandage over the injection site or placing an Elizabethan collar prevents this type of reaction.

To prevent or minimize the probability of extravascular injection of caustic drugs, they should be administered through small-gauge (22- to 23-gauge), indwelling, IV, over-the-needle catheters or through 23- to 25-gauge butterfly catheters. We use the former to administer doxorubicin and the latter to administer the vinca alkaloids and actinomycin D. Caustic drugs should be properly diluted before administration (i.e., vincristine to a final concentration of 0.1 mg/ml and doxorubicin to a concentration of 0.5 mg/ml) and the patency of the intravascular injection site ensured by intermittently aspirating until blood appears in the catheter. If the site is not patent, the catheter should be placed in another vein. Recommendations for the management of extravascular injections are listed in Table 80-2.

If, despite these precautions, a local tissue reaction occurs, it develops approximately 1 to 7 days after the perivascular injection of vinca alkaloids or actinomycin D and 7 to 15 days after doxorubicin extravasation. Tissue necrosis resulting from doxorubicin extravasation is far more severe than that associated with the extravasation of other agents, because the drug is extremely caustic and persists in tissues for up to 16 weeks. Clinical signs include pain, pruritus, erythema, moist dermatitis, and necrosis of the affected area; severe tissue sloughing may occur (Fig. 80-2). If local tissue reactions develop, they can be treated as follows:

1. Apply an antibiotic ointment (with or without corticosteroids) to the affected area.
2. Bandage the area (and replace bandages daily).

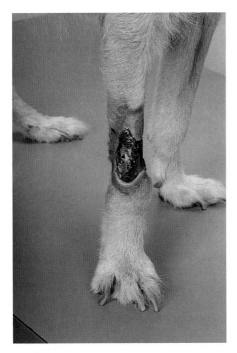

**FIG 80-2**
Tissue necrosis after extravascular injection of doxorubicin in a dog. Note the full-thickness sloughing of the area.

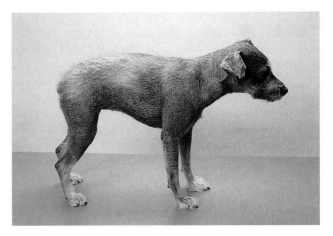

**FIG 80-3**
Alopecia in a 7-year-old Schnauzer undergoing doxorubicin and dacarbazine (ADIC) chemotherapy. Note the short and light-colored hair coat.

3. Prevent self-mutilation by placing an Elizabethan collar or a muzzle.
4. If there is no bacterial contamination (ruled out on the basis of negative bacterial cultures), 10 to 20 mg of methylprednisolone acetate (Depo-Medrol; Upjohn-Pharmacia, Kalamazoo, Mich) can be injected SQ in the affected area to alleviate pruritus and inflammation.
5. If severe necrosis or gangrene caused by anaerobic contamination occurs, the area should be surgically debrided.
6. In the event of severe doxorubicin-induced soft tissue necrosis, the affected limb may have to be amputated.

In dogs and cats undergoing chemotherapy, delayed hair growth is more common than alopecia. This is in contrast to the situation in human patients, in whom severe scalp alopecia is a predictable complication of therapy. Because most chemotherapeutic agents affect rapidly dividing tissues, cells in the anagen (growth) phase of the hair cycle are usually affected. Therefore hair is slow to regrow in areas that were clipped or shaved before or during chemotherapy. Excessive shedding is also common.

Alopecia occurs predominantly in woolly-haired (coarse-haired) dogs, such as Poodles, Schnauzers, and Kerry Blue Terriers (Fig. 80-3). It affects primarily the tactile hairs in short-haired dogs and cats. Although the exact reason why chemotherapy-induced alopecia occurs in woolly-haired dogs is unknown, a prolonged anagen phase and synchronous hair growth, comparable to those occurring in human scalp hair, may make these dogs prone to this toxic effect. Drugs commonly associated with delayed hair growth and alopecia in-clude cyclophosphamide, doxorubicin, 5-FU, 6-thioguanine, and hydroxyurea (Hydrea; E.R. Squibb & Sons, Princeton, N.J.). Alopecia and delayed hair growth usually resolve shortly after discontinuation of the offending agent.

It is rare for anticancer agents to induce hyperpigmentation in dogs, and this is extremely rare in cats. Cutaneous hyperpigmentation affecting the face, ventral abdomen, and flanks is common in dogs receiving doxorubicin- and bleomycin-containing protocols.

## PANCREATITIS

Pancreatitis is a well-recognized entity in human patients undergoing chemotherapy. Offending drugs in humans include corticosteroids, azathioprine, 6-mercaptopurine, L-asparaginase, cytosine arabinoside, and combination chemotherapy. Sporadic reports of pancreatitis in dogs (but not in cats) receiving chemotherapeutic and immunosuppressive agents have also appeared in the literature.

We have documented acute pancreatitis in several dogs receiving L-asparaginase or combination chemotherapy. Dogs in the latter group were receiving COAP (cyclophosphamide, vincristine, cytosine arabinoside, prednisone), ADIC (doxorubicin, DTIC); or VAC (vincristine, doxorubicin, cyclophosphamide) chemotherapy. Clinical signs developed 1 to 5 days after the start of chemotherapy and consisted of anorexia, vomiting, and depression. Physical examination findings in these dogs were unremarkable, and abdominal pain was rare. Serum lipase and amylase activities were high in all the animals, and ultrasonographic evidence of pancreatitis was detected in approximately one half of the dogs. The animals were treated with IV fluids, and the clinical signs resolved within 3 to 10 days in most dogs.

It is difficult to prevent chemotherapy-induced pancreatitis, because it is not a predictable complication. As a general precaution, we refrain from using L-asparaginase in dogs at high risk for pancreatitis (i.e., overweight, middle-age to older female dogs). As a further precaution, dogs receiving drugs with the potential to cause pancreatitis should be fed a low-fat diet.

## CARDIOTOXICITY

Cardiotoxicity is a relatively uncommon complication of doxorubicin therapy in dogs; it is extremely rare in cats. Two types of doxorubicin-induced cardiac toxicity are observed in dogs: an acute reaction occurring during or shortly after administration and a chronic cumulative toxicity. Acute doxorubicin toxicity is characterized by cardiac arrhythmias (mainly sinus tachycardia) that develop during or shortly after administration. This phenomenon is thought to stem from doxorubicin-induced, histamine-mediated catecholamine release, because the sinus tachycardia and hypotension can be prevented by pretreatment with $H_1$ and $H_2$ antihistamines. Several weeks or months after repeated doxorubicin injections, persistent arrhythmias, including ventricular premature contractions, atrial premature contractions, paroxysmal ventricular tachycardia, second-degree atrioventricular blocks, and intraventricular conduction defects, develop. These rhythm disturbances are usually associated with the development of a dilated cardiomyopathy, similar to that which occurs spontaneously in Dobermans and Cocker Spaniels.

The hallmark of chronic doxorubicin toxicity is a dilated cardiomyopathy that develops after a total cumulative dose of approximately 240 mg/m$^2$ is exceeded in the dog. The histologic lesions seen in dogs with doxorubicin-induced cardiomyopathy consist of vacuolation of myocytes, with or without myofibril loss. Clinical signs of toxicity in dogs are those of congestive heart failure (usually left-sided). Therapy consists of discontinuation of the offending drug and the administration of cardiac drugs such as digitalis glycosides or nonglycoside inotropic agents. Once cardiomyopathy develops, the prognosis is poor, because the myocardial lesions are irreversible.

It is critical to monitor patients receiving doxorubicin to prevent fatal cardiomyopathy. In this respect, dogs (and possibly) cats with underlying rhythm disturbances or impaired myocardial contractility, as shown by decreased fractional shortening on M-mode or Doppler echocardiograms, should not receive doxorubicin. It is also recommended that animals receiving doxorubicin undergo echocardiographic evaluation every three doxorubicin cycles (9 weeks) to assess myocardial contractility and that the drug be discontinued if decreased fractional shortening occurs. Endomyocardial biopsy specimens are commonly obtained in people receiving doxorubicin in an effort to detect submicroscopic lesions, but this is impractical in dogs. Monitoring serum troponin concentrations to detect early myocardial damage from doxorubicin is currently being evaluated.

Several protocols have been devised in an attempt to minimize doxorubicin-induced cardiomyopathy in dogs. Unfortunately only two have shown promise in minimizing or preventing cardiomyopathy. Of these, weekly low-dose doxorubicin therapy in humans has been found to be associated with a significantly lower frequency of histologic changes than the conventional 3-week schedule has been. I have been able to administer total cumulative doses of 500 mg/m$^2$ to two dogs using a 10 mg/m$^2$ weekly protocol. However, recent reports describe a loss of antitumor activity when using weekly low-dose doxorubicin in dogs with lymphoma. A new compound, dexrazoxane (Zinacard, Upjohn-Pharmacia, Kalamazoo, Mich), offers a promising means of reducing the chronic cardiotoxicity induced by doxorubicin; doses in excess of 500 mg/m$^2$ have been administered to dogs receiving the agent without causing significant cardiotoxicity.

## UROTOXICITY

The urinary tract in small animals is rarely affected by adverse reactions to anticancer agents. Only two specific complications are of clinical importance in pets with cancer: nephrotoxicity and sterile hemorrhagic cystitis. Transitional cell carcinomas of the urinary bladder associated with chronic cyclophosphamide therapy have also been reported in dogs.

Nephrotoxicity is rarely observed in dogs and cats undergoing chemotherapy. Although several potentially nephrotoxic drugs are commonly used in these species, only doxorubicin (primarily in cats), cisplatin (in dogs), and intermediate to high doses of methotrexate (in dogs) are of concern to clinicians. Doxorubicin may be a nephrotoxin in cats, and the limiting cumulative toxicity in this species may be renal rather than cardiac. Doxorubicin may cause nephrotoxicosis in dogs with preexisting renal disease and in those concomitantly receiving other nephrotoxins, such as aminoglycoside antibiotics or cisplatin. The administration of cisplatin using forced diuresis protocols minimizes the prevalence of nephrotoxicity in dogs.

Sterile hemorrhagic cystitis is a relatively common complication of long-term cyclophosphamide therapy in dogs; rarely, it may also occur acutely after a single dose of cyclophosphamide. This toxicity is not clinically relevant in cats. Acute clinical signs and urinalysis changes compatible with sterile hemorrhagic cystitis developed after the first injection in three dogs treated at our clinic with IV cyclophosphamide, 100 mg/m$^2$, and four dogs receiving PO cyclophosphamide, 300 mg/m$^2$. Sterile cystitis apparently results from the irritating effects of one of the cyclophosphamide metabolites (acrolein). It develops in approximately 5% to 25% of dogs and 1% to 3% of cats treated with cyclophosphamide, usually after an average of 18 weeks of therapy. Furosemide or prednisone administered concomitantly with cyclophosphamide appears to decrease the prevalence of cystitis.

Forced diuresis appears to minimize the severity of this complication or prevent it. I usually recommend administering the cyclophosphamide in the morning, allowing the pet to urinate frequently (if it is an indoor dog), salting the food, and administering prednisone on the same day that the animal receives the cyclophosphamide (if the protocol calls for prednisone administration).

Clinical signs of sterile hemorrhagic cystitis are similar to those of other lower urinary tract disorders and include pollakiuria, hematuria, and dysuria. Urinalysis typically reveals blood and mildly to moderately increased numbers of white blood cells, but no bacteria. Treatment of this complication consists of discontinuing the cyclophosphamide, forcing diuresis, diminishing the inflammation of the bladder wall, and preventing secondary bacterial infections. The cystitis resolves in most dogs within 1 to 4 months after the cyclophosphamide is discontinued. I administer furosemide (Lasix) at a dosage of 2 mg/kg PO every 12 hours for its diuretic effects, prednisone at a dosage of 0.5 to 1 mg/kg PO every 24 hours for its antiinflammatory (and diuretic) effect, and an ST combination at a dose of 13 to 15 mg/kg PO every 12 hours to prevent secondary bacterial contamination. If the clinical signs worsen despite this approach, the instillation of 1% formalin solution in water into the bladder can be attempted. Gross hematuria resolved within 24 hours and did not recur in two dogs thus treated. The intravesical infusion of a 25% to 50% dimethylsulfoxide solution may also alleviate the signs of cystitis in dogs.

## HEPATOTOXICITY

Chemotherapy-induced hepatotoxicity is extremely rare in dogs and cats. With the exception of the hepatic changes induced by corticosteroids in dogs, to my knowledge only methotrexate, cyclophosphamide, lomustine, and azathioprine (Imuran; Burroughs Wellcome, Research Triangle Park, N.C.) have been implicated as or confirmed to be hepatotoxins in dogs. In my experience, the hepatotoxicity caused by anticancer drugs in small animals is of little or no clinical relevance, with the exception of lomustine.

A recent report describes a low prevalence of hepatotoxicity (<10%) in dogs receiving lomustine (CCNU) for lymphoma or mast cell tumors. We have documented marked increases in alanine transaminase (ALT) activities (>1000 IU/L) and mild increases in alkaline phosphatase (ALP) activities (<500 IU/L) within 3 weeks of starting lomustine therapy in five dogs with mast cell tumors ($N = 3$) or granulomatous meningoencephalitis ($N = 2$). In two dogs, ALT activity decreased within 2 to 3 weeks of discontinuing the offending agent; in one dog with a grade 2 metastatic mast cell tumor, we elected to continue treatment, and the patient developed end-stage liver disease after 18 months on the drug.

Dogs with immune-mediated disorders receiving chronic azathioprine therapy rarely develop increases in liver enzyme activities that respond to discontinuation of the drug.

## NEUROTOXICITY

Anticancer agent–induced neurotoxicity is also extremely rare in dogs and cats. Neurotoxicosis occurs infrequently in dogs

receiving 5-FU, although it is common in cats (for this reason, this drug should not be used in cats). Neurotoxicity can also occur in dogs and cats that ingest 5-FU intended for human use (i.e., prescribed for the owners). Clinical signs occur shortly (3 to 12 hours) after ingestion of the drug and consist primarily of excitation and cerebellar ataxia, resulting in death in approximately one third of the dogs and in most cats. Neurotoxicity was also documented in 25% of dogs receiving a combination of actinomycin D, 5-FU, and cyclophosphamide (the CDF protocol) for the management of metastatic or nonresectable carcinomas at our clinic. This prevalence is considerably higher than that seen in association with the use of 5-FU in combination with other drugs and may be a result of drug interactions.

## PULMONARY TOXICITY

Pulmonary toxicity is extremely rare in dogs and cats receiving chemotherapy. To my knowledge, only cisplatin has been documented as a cause of pulmonary toxicity in cats. Acute signs of dyspnea leading to death occur within 48 to 96 hours of the administration of cisplatin in this species. Necropsy findings consist of pulmonary and mediastinal edema and microangiopathic changes in the pulmonary vasculature. Because of the risk of this serious toxicity, cisplatin should not be used in cats; carboplatin, a cisplatin derivative, does not cause pulmonary toxicity in this species.

## ACUTE TUMOR LYSIS SYNDROME

In human patients the rapid lysis of certain tumor cells (e.g., lymphoma cells) shortly after chemotherapy may lead to a syndrome of hyperuricemia, hyperphosphatemia, and hyperkalemia, either singly or in combination. This clinical entity is referred to as *acute tumor lysis syndrome* and is thought to be secondary to the release of high quantities of intracellular phosphate, uric acid, and nucleic acid metabolites. The intracellular concentration of phosphorus in human lymphoma and leukemic cells is four to six times higher than that in normal lymphocytes, and the same appears to be true for dogs.

In dogs, ATLS has been reported to occur only in association with lymphomas treated with chemotherapy, radiation therapy, or both and is characterized by hyperphosphatemia, with or without azotemia, hyperkalemia, hypocalcemia, metabolic acidosis, and hyperuricemia. It is rare in cats. Clinical signs include depression, vomiting, and diarrhea and occur within hours of the start of chemotherapy.

We have documented clinically evident ATLS after chemotherapy in eight dogs with lymphoma, during a period in which approximately 1200 to 1500 dogs with lymphoma were treated with chemotherapy. In most dogs the pretreatment serum creatinine concentrations or the tumor burden was high; one of the dogs had high liver enzyme activities. Within 1 to 7 days of the start of chemotherapy, lethargy, vomiting,

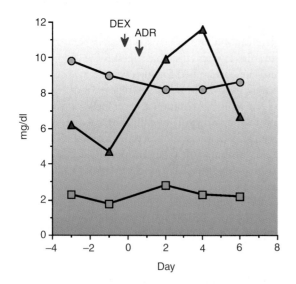

**FIG 80-4**
Serum phosphorus (△), calcium (○), and creatinine (□) concentrations in a dog with acute tumor lysis syndrome after chemotherapy for a primary pulmonary lymphoma. Note the increase in the serum phosphorus concentrations, with a mild decrease in the calcium concentrations and minor increases in the serum creatinine concentrations. *DEX,* Dexamethasone; *ADR,* doxorubicin. (From Couto CG: Management of complications of cancer chemotherapy, *Vet Clin North Am* 20:1037, 1990, with permission.)

and bloody diarrhea developed in affected dogs and the serum phosphorus concentrations increased markedly (Fig. 80-4). Aggressive fluid therapy and the correction of acid-base and electrolyte disturbances resulted in resolution of the clinical signs within 3 days in six dogs; the remaining two dogs died of ATLS.

## Suggested Readings

Couto CG: Management of complications of cancer chemotherapy, *Vet Clin North Am* 20:1037, 1990.

Crow SE et al: Cyclophosphamide-induced cystitis in the dog and cat, *J Am Vet Med Assoc* 171:259, 1977.

Harvey HJ et al: Neurotoxicosis associated with use of 5-fluorouracil in five dogs and one cat, *J Am Vet Med Assoc* 171:277, 1977.

Knapp DW et al: Cisplatin toxicity in cats, *J Vet Intern Med* 1:29, 1988.

Laing EJ et al: Acute tumor lysis syndrome following treatment of canine lymphoma, *J Am Anim Hosp Assoc* 24:691, 1988.

Laing EJ et al: Treatment of cyclophosphamide-induced hemorrhagic cystitis in five dogs, *J Am Vet Med Assoc* 193:233, 1988.

Weller RE: Intravesical instillation of dilute formalin for treatment of cyclophosphamide-induced cystitis in two dogs, *J Am Vet Med Assoc* 172:1206, 1978.

# CHAPTER 81

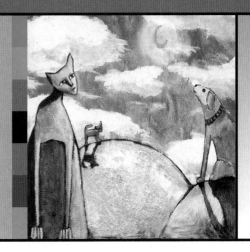

# Approach to the Patient with a Mass

## CHAPTER OUTLINE

APPROACH TO THE CAT OR DOG WITH A SOLITARY MASS, 1117

APPROACH TO THE CAT OR DOG WITH A METASTATIC LESION, 1118

APPROACH TO THE CAT OR DOG WITH A MEDIASTINAL MASS, 1119

## APPROACH TO THE CAT OR DOG WITH A SOLITARY MASS

It is common for the practicing veterinarian to evaluate a clinically healthy cat or dog in which a single mass is found during a routine physical examination or in which the owner has detected a mass and is concerned about it. The mass can be superficial (e.g., enlarged prescapular lymph node, subcutaneous mass) or deep (e.g., splenic mass, enlarged mesenteric lymph node), and often the clinician wonders how to proceed and what to recommend to the owner.

In this situation there are several possible approaches that one can take:

1. Do nothing and see if the mass "goes away."
2. Evaluate the mass cytologically.
3. Evaluate the mass histopathologically.
4. Do a complete workup, including complete blood count (CBC), serum biochemistry tests, radiography, abdominal ultrasonography, and urinalysis.

The first option (i.e., do nothing and see if the mass goes away) is not really an option because the presence of any mass is abnormal, and it should therefore be evaluated. As a general rule, most masses, with the notable exception of inflammatory lesions, do not regress spontaneously.

At our clinic, the typical first step in evaluating a solitary mass is to perform fine-needle aspiration (FNA) to obtain material for cytologic evaluation (see Chapter 77). Using this simple, relatively atraumatic, quick, and inexpensive procedure, we can arrive at a highly presumptive or definitive diagnosis in the vast majority of animals. Once we have identified the nature of the mass (i.e., benign neoplastic, malignant neoplastic, inflammatory, or hyperplastic), we can recommend additional tests to the owner.

Performing a biopsy for histopathology constitutes another valid alternative. However, the cost, the trauma to the patient, and the time it takes for the pathologists' report to become available make this a less attractive option than FNA. An intensive workup of a cat or dog with a solitary mass (i.e., option 4) may not be warranted, because additional diagnostic information regarding the mass is rarely gained from these procedures. However, the presence of metastatic lesions on thoracic radiographs may suggest that the mass in question is a malignant tumor.

If a cytologic diagnosis of a benign neoplasm is made (e.g., lipoma), the clinician faces two options: to do nothing and observe the mass or to surgically excise it. Because benign neoplasms in cats and dogs are rarely premalignant (with the notable exception of solar dermatitis /carcinoma in situ preceding the development of squamous cell carcinomas in cats), if a benign neoplasm is definitively diagnosed, a sound approach is to recommend a wait-and-see attitude. If the mass enlarges, becomes inflamed, or ulcerates, then surgical excision is recommended. However, the clinician should keep in mind that most benign neoplasms are easier to excise when they are small (i.e., it is not advisable to wait until the mass becomes quite large). To some owners, the option of surgically excising the mass shortly after diagnosis is more appealing.

If a cytologic diagnosis of malignancy is obtained (or if the findings are "suggestive of" or "compatible with" malignancy), additional workup is warranted. Different approaches are indicated, depending on the cytologic diagnosis (i.e., carcinoma versus sarcoma versus round cell tumor). However, with the exception of mast cell tumors (i.e., pulmonary metastases are extremely rare in dogs and cats with this tumor type), thoracic radiographs should be obtained to search for metastatic disease in dogs and cats with most types of malignant neoplasms. Two lateral views and a ventrodorsal (or dorsoventral) view are recommended to increase the likelihood of detecting metastatic lesions. If available, a computed tomography (CT) scan may be obtained, because it can detect masses smaller than those detectable on plain radiography.

Plain radiographs of the affected area may also be indicated to look for soft tissue and bone involvement. Abdominal ultrasonography (or radiography) may be indicated for further staging in animals with certain neoplasms (e.g., hemangiosarcoma, intestinal neoplasms, mast cell tumors). A CBC, serum biochemistry profile, and urinalysis may provide additional clinical information (e.g., paraneoplastic syndromes, concurrent organ failure).

If the mass is malignant and there is no evidence of metastatic disease, surgical excision is usually recommended. If there are metastatic lesions and the pathologist feels comfortable with the cytologic diagnosis, chemotherapy constitutes the best viable option (see Chapter 78). However, as discussed in Chapter 78, surgical resection of the primary mass (e.g., mammary carcinoma) in a patient with metastatic lesions may provide considerable palliation and prolong good-quality survival. If an assertive diagnosis cannot be made on the basis of the cytologic findings, an incisional or excisional biopsy of the mass is advisable. In our clinic, we typically do not recommend euthanasia in dogs and cats with metastatic lesions and good quality of life, because survival times in excess of 6 months (without chemotherapy) are common in animals with certain metastatic neoplasms.

## APPROACH TO THE CAT OR DOG WITH A METASTATIC LESION

Often radiographic or ultrasonographic evidence of metastatic cancer is found during the routine evaluation of an animal with a suspected or confirmed malignancy or during the evaluation of a cat or dog with obscure clinical signs. In such instances the clinician should be familiar with both the biologic behavior of the common neoplasms and with their characteristic radiographic and ultrasonographic patterns (Table 81-1). Suter and colleagues (1974) have described the typical radiographic appearances of various metastatic malignancies. In addition, the owner should be questioned regarding any prior surgeries in the pet (e.g., excision of a "benign-looking" mass that was disposed of but may have been the primary malignancy).

If a cytologic or histopathologic diagnosis of malignancy has already been made and the metastatic lesions are detected while staging the animal, treatments can be recommended to the owner at this point (assuming that the metastatic lesions have arisen from the previously diagnosed primary tumor). If the metastatic lesions are detected during the evaluation of a cat or dog with vague clinical signs and no history of neoplasia, cytologic or histopathologic evaluation of one or more of these lesions should be performed so that one can best advise the owner as to the appropriate course of action.

A cytologic diagnosis of metastatic lung lesions can usually be obtained through blind percutaneous FNA of the lungs. To do this, the area to be aspirated (i.e., the one with the highest density of lesions radiographically) is clipped and aseptically prepared. With the animal in sternal recumbency or standing, a 25 gauge, 2 to 3 inch (5 to 7.5 cm) nee-

 TABLE 81-1

**Metastatic Behavior of Some Common Neoplasms in Dogs and Cats**

| NEOPLASM | SPECIES | COMMON METASTATIC SITES |
|---|---|---|
| HSA | D | Liver, lungs, omentum, kidney, eye, CNS |
| OSA | D | Lungs, bone |
| SCC—oral | C, D | Lymph nodes, lungs |
| aCA—mammary | C, D | Lymph nodes, lungs |
| aCA—anal sac | D | Lymph nodes |
| aCA—prostate | D | Lymph nodes, bone, lungs |
| TCC—bladder | D | Lymph nodes, lungs, bone |
| MEL—oral | D | Lymph nodes, lungs |
| MCT | D | Lymph nodes, liver, spleen |
| MCT | C | Spleen, liver, bone marrow |

*aCa,* Adenocarcinoma; *C,* cat; *CNS,* central nervous system; *D,* dog; *HSA,* hemangiosarcoma; *MEL,* malignant melanoma; *MCT,* mast cell tumor; *OSA,* osteosarcoma; *SCC,* squamous cell carcinoma; *TCC,* transitional cell carcinoma.

dle (depending on the size of the animal) coupled to a 12 to 20 ml syringe is rapidly advanced through an intercostal space along the cranial border of the rib to the depth required (previously determined on the basis of the radiographs). Suction is applied two or three times and then released; the needle is then withdrawn. Smears are made as described in Chapter 77. When aspirating lungs, it is common to obtain a fair amount of air or blood, or both, in the syringe. Complications associated with this technique include pneumothorax (animals should be closely observed for 2 to 6 hours after the procedure and dealt with accordingly if pneumothorax develops) and bleeding. As a general rule, FNA of the lungs should not be performed in cats or dogs with coagulopathies.

If an FNA of the lungs fails to yield a diagnostic sample, a lung biopsy performed with a biopsy needle (under ultrasonographic or CT guidance) or through a thoracotomy should be contemplated. This procedure is associated with an extremely low morbidity and should be recommended if owners are considering treatment.

Metastatic lesions in other organs or tissues (e.g., liver, bone) can also be diagnosed on the basis of FNA findings. The clinician should remember that nodular lesions of the liver or spleen in dogs with a primary malignancy should not necessarily be considered metastatic. FNA or biopsies of such lesions frequently reveal normal hepatocytes (i.e.; reactive hepatic nodule), or extramedullary hematopoiesis/lymphoreticular hyperplasia, respectively. In the case of bone metastases, an aspirate can be obtained using an 16 or 18 gauge bone marrow aspiration needle; if a cytologic diagnosis cannot be made, a core (needle) biopsy can be performed.

As discussed in Chapter 78, we can now fairly successfully treat cats and dogs with metastatic neoplasms using chemotherapy. To do this, however, we need to know the histologic (or cytologic) tumor type. It should always be kept in mind that euthanasia is a viable option for some owners.

## APPROACH TO THE CAT OR DOG WITH A MEDIASTINAL MASS

Several lesions are found as anterior mediastinal masses (AMMs) during physical examination or plain thoracic radiography (Table 81-2). Some of these lesions are malignant neoplasms, therefore diagnosis and treatment should be approached aggressively in such animals.

### Clinicopathologic Features and Diagnosis

When one is evaluating a cat or dog with an AMM, there are several issues to be considered before one recommends a specific treatment. As discussed previously (see Chapter 78), the treatment prescribed depends on the specific tumor type (i.e., surgical excision may be curative for dogs and cats with thymomas, whereas chemotherapy is indicated for those with lymphoma). Because lymphomas and thymomas are the most common AMMs in small animals, the ensuing discussion is limited to these two neoplasms. Other neoplasms that originate in anterior mediastinal structures include chemodectomas (heart base tumors), ectopic thyroid carcinomas, and lipomas, among others. Nonneoplastic lesions of the mediastinum include mainly thymic or mediastinal hematomas and ultimobranchial cysts.

Paraneoplastic syndromes, such as generalized or focal myasthenia gravis, polymyositis, exfoliative dermatitis, and second neoplasms, have been well characterized in cats and dogs with thymoma. Aplastic anemia, a paraneoplastic syndrome common in humans with thymoma, has not been recognized in small animals with this tumor type. Hypercalcemia is a common finding in dogs with mediastinal lymphoma, but it can also occur in those with thymoma.

In cats the age at the time of presentation points to a specific diagnosis. That is, anterior mediastinal lymphomas are more common in young cats (1 to 3 years old), whereas thymomas are more common in older cats (8 to 10 years old). It is also important to know the feline leukemia virus (FeLV) status in this species, because most cats with mediastinal lymphomas are viremic (i.e., FeLV-positive), whereas most cats with thymoma are not.

Most AMMs in dogs are diagnosed in older animals (over 5 to 6 years of age), therefore age cannot be used as a means of distinguishing between lymphomas and thymomas. However, a large proportion of dogs with mediastinal lymphomas are hypercalcemic, whereas most dogs with thymoma are not (although hypercalcemia also occurs in dogs with this neoplasm). Peripheral lymphocytosis can be present in dogs and cats with either lymphoma or thymoma. The presence of neuromuscular signs in a dog or cat with an AMM suggests the existence of a thymoma.

Thoracic radiographs are of little help in differentiating thymomas from lymphomas. The two neoplasms are similar

## TABLE 81-2

**Anterior Mediastinal Masses in Cats and Dogs**

| LESION | CAT | DOG | COMMENTS |
|---|---|---|---|
| Thymoma | Common | Common | See text |
| Lymphoma | Common | Common | See text |
| Thyroid adenocarcinoma | Rare | Rare | |
| Lipoma | ? | Rare | Low radiographic density |
| Branchial cysts | Rare | Rare | Cystic on ultrasound |
| Thymic hematomas | ? | Rare | Traumatic, rodenticides? |
| Heart base tumors | ? | Rare | Brachiocephalic breeds |

?, Questionable.

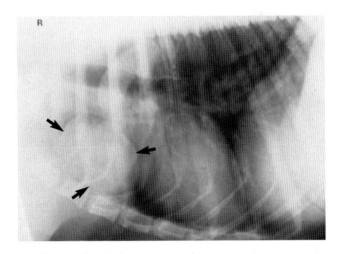

**FIG 81-1**
Typical radiographic features of thymoma *(arrows)* in a dog. The mass originates in the ventral mediastinum, unlike most lymphomas, which originate in the dorsal mediastinal region. Percutaneous fine-needle aspiration of this mass yielded findings diagnostic for thymoma, and the dog underwent a thoracotomy with complete resection of the mass.

in appearance, although lymphomas appear to originate more frequently in the dorsal anterior mediastinum, whereas thymomas originate more often in the ventral mediastinum (Fig. 81-1). The prevalence of pleural effusions in dogs and cats with either thymomas or lymphomas appears to be similar; thus the finding cannot be used as means to distinguish between these two tumor types.

Ultrasonographic evaluation of the AMM should be attempted before more invasive diagnostic techniques are used. Ultrasonographically, most thymomas have a mixed echogenicity, with discrete hypoechoic to anechoic areas that correspond to true cysts on cross section. The lack of a supporting stroma in lymphomas usually confers a hypoechoic to an-echoic density to the mass, which therefore looks diffusely "cystic." In addition to aiding in the presumptive diagnosis of a given tumor type, ultrasonography provides information regarding the resectability of the mass and assists in obtaining a specimen for cytologic evaluation (see next paragraph).

Transthoracic FNA of AMMs constitutes a relatively safe and reliable evaluation technique. After sterile preparation of the thoracic wall overlying the mass (see Chapter 77), a 2- to 3-inch (5- to 7.5-cm), 25-gauge needle coupled to a syringe is used to aspirate the mass. This can be done blindly (if the mass is so large that it is pressing against the interior thoracic wall) or guided by radiography (using three views to establish a three-dimensional location), fluoroscopy, or ultrasonography. Despite the fact that there are large vessels within the anterior mediastinum, postaspiration bleeding is extremely rare if the animal remains motionless during the procedure. Alternatively, if the mass is large enough to be in close contact with the internal thoracic wall, a transthoracic needle biopsy can be performed to allow histopathologic evaluation.

Cytologically, lymphomas are composed of a monomorphic population of lymphoid cells that are mostly immature (i.e., low nuclear-to-cytoplasmic ratio, dark blue cytoplasm, clumped chromatin pattern, and nucleoli); in cats, most cells in anterior mediastinal lymphomas are heavily vacuolated and resemble human Burkitt's lymphoma cells (Fig. 81-2). Occasionally, mediastinal lymphomas are composed primarily of large granular lymphocytes. Thymomas are cytologically heterogeneous and are composed primarily of a population of small lymphocytes (although large blasts are sometimes present) and, occasionally, a distinct population of epithelial-like cells that are usually polygonal or spindle shaped and can be identified either as individual cells or in sheets. Hassall's corpuscles are rarely seen in Wright's-stained cytologic preparations. Plasma cells, eosinophils, neutrophils, mast cells, macrophages, and melanocytes are all occasionally seen.

### Treatment

As discussed in preceding paragraphs, anterior mediastinal lymphomas are best treated with chemotherapy (see Chapter 82). Radiotherapy can also be used in conjunction with chemotherapy to induce a more rapid remission. However, in my experience, the combination of radiotherapy and chemotherapy does not offer any advantages over chemotherapy alone, and it may indeed be detrimental to the animal, given that many cats and dogs with anterior mediastinal lymphoma have severe respiratory compromise at the time of presentation. Chemical restraint of these animals for radiotherapy may further compound this problem.

Because most thymomas are benign, surgical excision is usually curative. Although in some reports the perioperative morbidity and mortality of this procedure are high (Atwater and colleagues, 1994), in our experience, most patients that undergo thoracotomies for removal of a thymoma do well and are released from the hospital in 3 to 4 days. Radiotherapy can successfully shrink thymomas, although complete,

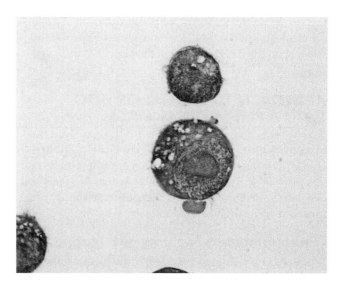

**FIG 81-2**
Cytologic characteristics of feline mediastinal lymphoma. Note the dark cytoplasm with abundant vacuoles typical of this neoplasm in cats. (×1000.)

long-lasting remission is rarely achieved. It is possible that this is because the radiotherapy eliminates only the lymphoid component of the neoplasm but the epithelial component remains unchanged. Chemotherapy may be beneficial in selected cats and dogs with nonresectable thymomas or in those in which repeated anesthetic episodes or a major surgical procedure poses a severe risk. We have used combination chemotherapy protocols commonly used for dogs and cats with lymphoma (i.e., cyclophosphamide, vincristine, cytosine arabinoside, and prednisone [COAP]; cyclophosphamide, vincristine, and prednisone [COP]; and cyclophosphamide, doxorubicin, vincristine, and prednisone [CHOP]; see Chapter 82) in a limited number of cats and dogs with cytologically diagnosed thymomas. As with radiotherapy, however, chemotherapy may only eliminate the lymphoid cell population, thus rarely resulting in complete or long-lasting remissions.

If a definitive diagnosis of thymoma or lymphoma cannot be obtained, the clinician has two therapeutic options: (1) to perform a thoracotomy and excise the mass; or (2) to initiate chemotherapy for lymphoma (COP, COAP, or CHOP). In the latter case, if no remission (or only a partial remission) is observed 10 to 14 days after the start of chemotherapy, the mass is most likely a thymoma, and surgical resection should be considered.

### Suggested Readings

Aronsohn MG et al: Clinical and pathologic features of thymoma in 15 dogs, *J Am Vet Med Assoc* 184:1355, 1984.
Atwater SW et al: Thymoma in dogs: 23 cases (1980-1991), *J Am Vet Med Assoc* 205:1007, 1994.
Bellah JR et al: Thymoma in the dog: two case reports and review of 20 additional cases, *J Am Vet Med Assoc* 183:1095, 1983.

Carpenter JL et al: Thymoma in 11 cats, *J Am Vet Med Assoc* 181:248, 1982.

Liu S et al: Thymic branchial cysts in the dog and cat, *J Am Vet Med Assoc* 182:1095, 1983.

Rae CA et al: A comparison between the cytological and histological characteristics in thirteen canine and feline thymomas, *Can Vet J* 30:497, 1989.

Scott DW et al: Exfoliative dermatitis in association with thymoma in 3 cats, *Fel Pract* 23:8, 1995.

Suter PJ et al: Radiographic recognition of primary and metastatic pulmonary neoplasms of dogs and cats, *J Am Vet Radiol Soc* 15:3, 1974.

# CHAPTER 82

# Lymphoma in the Cat and Dog

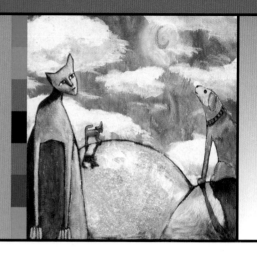

## CHAPTER OUTLINE

ETIOLOGY AND EPIDEMIOLOGY, 1122
CLINICAL FEATURES, 1122
DIAGNOSIS, 1125
TREATMENT, 1126

Lymphoma (malignant lymphoma, lymphosarcoma) is a lymphoid malignancy that originates from solid organs (e.g., lymph nodes, liver, spleen); this distinguishes lymphomas from lymphoid leukemias, which originate in the bone marrow (see Chapter 83).

## Etiology and Epidemiology

It has been reported that approximately 70% of cats with lymphoma have feline leukemia virus (FeLV) infection (Table 82-1). Although the prevalence of viremia in cats with lymphoma varies with the anatomic form of presentation (see later discussion), in general, young cats with lymphoma are FeLV-positive, whereas older cats are FeLV-negative. However, over the past few years, the prevalence of FeLV infection in cats with lymphoma seen at our clinic has been decreasing. Feline immunodeficiency virus (FIV) infection increases the risk of developing lymphoma in cats; cats infected with FIV are almost six times more likely to develop lymphoma than noninfected cats, whereas cats coinfected with FeLV and FIV are more than 75 times more likely to develop lymphoma than noninfected cats (Shelton and colleagues, 1990).

In dogs, the etiology of lymphomas is considered multifactorial, because no single etiologic agent has been identified. However, a genetic component is evident, in that the neoplasm is highly prevalent in certain bloodlines. There is also a distinct breed-related predisposition to lymphoma in dogs, with some breeds, such as Boxer, Basset Hound, Rottweiler, Cocker Spaniel, St. Bernard, Scottish Terrier, Airedale Terrier, English Bulldog, and Golden Retriever, being at high risk. At our clinic the breeds most commonly affected are Golden Retrievers, Cocker Spaniels, and Rottweilers.

The age of cats with lymphoma at the time of presentation is bimodal, with the first peak occurring in cats that are ap-

proximately 2 years of age and the second one occurring in cats that are approximately 10 to 12 years of age. The cats that make up the first peak are mainly FeLV-positive, whereas those that make up the second peak are predominantly FeLV-negative. As mentioned before, the prevalence of FeLV-positive cats with lymphoma continues to decrease a our clinic. The mean age of FeLV-positive cats with lymphoma when first seen is 3 years, whereas the mean age of FeLV-negative cats with lymphoma is 7 to 8 years. Most dogs with lymphoma are middle-age or older (6 to 12 years of age).

## Clinical Features

There are four anatomic forms of presentation in cats and dogs with lymphoma:

1. *Multicentric,* characterized by generalized lymphadenopathy; hepatic, splenic, or bone marrow involvement; or a combination of these
2. *Mediastinal,* characterized by mediastinal lymphadenopathy, with or without bone marrow infiltration
3. *Alimentary,* characterized by solitary, diffuse, or multifocal gastrointestinal tract infiltration, with or without intraabdominal lymphadenopathy
4. *Extranodal,* affecting any organ or tissue (e.g., renal, neural, ocular, cutaneous)

The distribution of the different anatomic forms differs between cats and dogs. The multicentric form is the most common in dogs, accounting for more than 80% of all the lymphomas in this species. In cats the mediastinal and alimentary forms are more common than the multicentric and extranodal forms. At our clinic, alimentary lymphoma is found in more than 70% of the cats with this neoplasm.

The clinical findings in cats and dogs with lymphoma are related to the anatomic form of the presentation. Animals with the *generalized* or *multicentric form* are evaluated because of vague, nonspecific clinical signs; frequently, the owners detect one or more subcutaneous masses (i.e., enlarged lymph nodes) during grooming in an otherwise healthy pet, and this prompts them to seek veterinary care. Occasionally, dogs and cats with lymphoma are evaluated because of nonspecific clinical signs, such as weight loss, anorexia, and lethargy. If the enlarged lymph nodes mechanically obstruct lymph drainage, edema occurs; if they compress the airway, coughing is the main presenting complaint.

Physical examination of cats and dogs with multicentric lymphoma usually reveals massive generalized lymphadenopathy, with or without hepatomegaly, splenomegaly, or extranodal lesions (e.g., ocular, cutaneous, renal, neural). The affected lymph nodes are markedly enlarged (5 to 15 times their normal size), painless, and freely movable. A syndrome of reactive (hyperplastic) lymphadenopathy that occurs in cats can mimic the clinicopathologic features of multicentric lymphoma (see p. 1200).

Cats and dogs with *mediastinal lymphoma* are usually evaluated because of dyspnea, coughing, or regurgitation (the latter is more common in cats) of recent onset. Polyuria and polydipsia are common presenting complaints in dogs with mediastinal lymphoma and hypercalcemia; tumor-associated hypercalcemia is extremely rare in cats with lymphoma. The respiratory and upper digestive tract signs are caused by compression from enlarged anterior mediastinal lymph nodes, although malignant pleural effusion can contribute to the severity of the respiratory tract signs. On physical examination, the abnormalities are usually confined to the thoracic cavity and consist of decreased bronchovesicular sounds, normal pulmonary sounds displaced to the dorsocaudal thoracic cavity, a dull sound heard on percussion of the ventral thoracic cavity, and a noncompressible anterior mediastinum (in cats). Unilateral or bilateral Horner's syndrome may occur in

cats (and occasionally dogs) with mediastinal lymphoma. Some dogs with mediastinal lymphoma have marked head and neck edema due to compression from enlarged lymph nodes (anterior vena cava syndrome).

Cats and dogs with an *alimentary lymphoma* usually display gastrointestinal tract signs, such as vomiting, anorexia, diarrhea, and weight loss. Occasionally, signs compatible with an intestinal obstruction or peritonitis (caused by rupture of a lymphomatous mass) occur. Physical examination typically reveals intraabdominal masses (e.g., enlarged mesenteric or ileocecocolic lymph nodes, or intestinal masses) and thickened bowel loops (in patients with diffuse small intestinal lymphoma). Rarely, polypoid lymphomatoid masses can protrude through the anus in cats and dogs with colorectal lymphoma.

The clinical signs and physical examination findings in cats and dogs with *extranodal lymphomas* are extremely variable and depend on the location of the mass or masses. In general, the clinical signs stem from the compression or displacement of normal parenchymal cells in the affected organ (e.g., azotemia in renal lymphoma, variable neurologic signs in central nervous system [CNS] lymphoma). The typical clinical signs and physical examination findings in cats and dogs with extranodal lymphomas are summarized in Table 82-2. Common extranodal forms in dogs include cutaneous and ocular lymphomas; in cats they include nasopharyngeal, ocular, renal, and neural lymphomas.

*Cutaneous lymphoma* is one of the most common extranodal forms of lymphoma in dogs; it is the most common extranodal lymphoma in dogs at our clinic, but it is rare in cats. The clinical signs and characteristics of the lesions are extremely variable, and they can mimic any primary or secondary skin lesion. Dogs with mycosis fungoides (an epidermotropic T-cell lymphoma) are usually first evaluated because of chronic alopecia, desquamation, pruritus, and erythema, eventually leading to plaque and tumor formation. Mucocutaneous and mucosal lesions are relatively common, but generalized lymph node involvement may not be seen initially. A characteristic lesion in dogs with this form of lymphoma is a circular, raised, erythematous, donut-shaped, dermoepidermal mass that contains normal skin in the center. Most of the cats with cutaneous lymphoma reported in the literature have been negative for FeLV viremia.

## TABLE 82-1

Prevalence of Feline Leukemia Virus Infection in Cats with Lymphoma

| ANATOMIC FORM | FeLV POSITIVE (%) |
|---------------|-------------------|
| Alimentary | 30 |
| Mediastinal | 90 |
| Multicentric | 80 |
| Cutaneous | 0 |

## TABLE 82-2

Clinical Signs and Physical Examination Findings in Dogs and Cats with Extranodal Lymphomas

| ORGAN INVOLVED | CLINICAL PRESENTATION | PHYSICAL FINDING(S) |
|----------------|----------------------|---------------------|
| CNS | Solitary or multifocal CNS signs | Any neurologic finding |
| Eye | Blindness, infiltrates, photophobia | Infiltrates, uveitis, RD, glaucoma |
| Kidney | PU/PD, azotemia, erythrocytosis* | Renomegaly, renal masses |
| Lung | Coughing, dyspnea | None, radiographic changes |
| Skin | Any primary or secondary lesion | Any primary or secondary lesion |

*CNS,* Central nervous system; *RD,* retinal detachment; *PU/PD,* polyuria/polydipsia.
*Only in dogs.

*Ocular lymphoma* occurs in both dogs and cats. Ocular involvement in dogs is commonly associated with the multicentric form, whereas both primary ocular involvement and ocular involvement associated with the multicentric form are common in cats. A variety of signs and lesions may be present in these animals, including photophobia, blepharospasm, epiphora, hyphema, hypopyon, ocular masses, third eyelid infiltration, anterior uveitis, chorioretinal involvement, and retinal detachment.

*Nasopharyngeal lymphoma* is relatively common in cats but is extremely rare in dogs. Clinical signs are similar to those seen in cats with any upper respiratory tract disorder and include sneezing, unilateral or bilateral nasal discharge (ranging from mucopurulent to frankly hemorrhagic), stertorous breathing, exophthalmos, and facial deformity; this is one of the most common forms of presentation of extranodal lymphoma seen in cats at our clinic.

*Renal lymphoma* is relatively common in cats but rare in dogs. Cats with this anatomic form are first evaluated because of vague clinical signs, usually secondary to chronic renal failure. On physical examination the cat is emaciated and usually anemic and has large, irregular, and firm kidneys; both kidneys are commonly affected. There is a purported association between renal and CNS lymphoma in cats, to the point that some clinicians recommend using antineoplastic drugs that achieve high CNS concentrations (i.e., cytosine arabinoside, lomustine) in the treatment of cats with renal involvement in an attempt to prevent secondary CNS dissemination. This association has not been recognized at our clinic.

Cats and dogs with *neural lymphoma* are evaluated because of a variety of neurologic signs that reflect the location and extent of the neoplasms. Although CNS signs are most common, peripheral nerve involvement may occur occasionally in cats. Three forms of presentation are clinically recognized: solitary *epidural* lymphoma, *neuropil* (intracranial or intraspinal) lymphoma (also called *true CNS lymphoma*), and *peripheral nerve* lymphoma. The solitary epidural lymphoma is common in young, FeLV-positive cats. Neural lymphomas can be primary (e.g., epidural lymphoma), or they may be secondary to the multicentric form; as discussed earlier, secondary CNS lymphoma may be common in cats with the renal form. A relatively common presentation is that of a CNS relapse in dogs that have been receiving chemotherapy for multicentric lymphoma for months to years; these patients develop acute onset of neurologic signs, typically while the multicentric neoplasm is still in remission. This late CNS relapse is likely related to the fact that most drugs used to treat lymphoma do not cross the blood-brain barrier when used at standard doses; thus the CNS becomes a sanctuary for tumor cells.

A variety of differential diagnoses should be considered in a cat or dog with suspected lymphoma. The clinician should always bear in mind that lymphomas are great imitators; they can mimic numerous different neoplastic and nonneoplastic disorders. The differential diagnoses in cats and dogs with lymphoma are similar to those in patients with leukemia (see p. 1135).

Occasionally, dogs with lymphoma are evaluated because of clinical signs secondary to a paraneoplastic syndrome (i.e., molecularly mediated distant effects of the neoplasm). Paraneoplastic syndromes that have been encountered in dogs with lymphoma include hypercalcemia, monoclonal and polyclonal gammopathies, immune cytopenias, polyneuropathy, and hypoglycemia. Only hypercalcemia and gammopathies have been documented in cats with this neoplasm, although they are considerably less frequent than in dogs. Of all these syndromes, only humoral hypercalcemia of malignancy in dogs is of clinical relevance.

**Hematologic and serum biochemical features.** A variety of nonspecific hematologic and serum biochemical abnormalities can be detected in cats and dogs with lymphoma. The hematologic abnormalities result from the infiltration of bone marrow with neoplastic cells, splenic hypofunction or hyperfunction (caused by neoplastic infiltrates), chronic disease, or paraneoplastic immune-mediated abnormalities (i.e., immune hemolytic anemia or thrombocytopenia, both of which are rare). Certain hematologic abnormalities (i.e., monocytosis, leukemoid reactions) may result from the local or systemic production of bioactive substances by the tumor cells (e.g., hematopoietic growth factors, interleukins). The serum biochemical abnormalities result either from the production of bioactive substances by the tumor cells (i.e., paraneoplasia) or from organ failure secondary to neoplastic infiltration. In general the complete blood count (CBC) and biochemical profile are not diagnostic in cats and dogs with lymphoma.

Common hematologic abnormalities include anemia, leukocytosis, neutrophilia (with or without a left shift), monocytosis, abnormal lymphoid cells in peripheral blood (i.e., lymphosarcoma cell leukemia), thrombocytopenia, isolated or combined cytopenias, and leukoerythroblastic reactions, among others. Lymphocytosis is rare in dogs and cats with lymphoma; when present, it is usually of low magnitude (i.e., <10,000 to 12,000/$\mu$l).

Serum biochemical abnormalities are more common in dogs than in cats with lymphoma and consist mainly of hypercalcemia and gammopathies. Hypercalcemia is one of the most common paraneoplastic abnormalities in dogs with lymphoma, occurring in approximately 20% to 40% of the patients; it is extremely rare in cats; it is more prevalent in dogs with mediastinal lymphoma than in those with the multicentric, alimentary, or extranodal forms. In most dogs with lymphoma and hypercalcemia, the tumor is of T-cell origin.

The molecular mechanism underlying hypercalcemia in dogs with lymphoma is still not agreed on, but in most cases hypercalcemia is thought to occur as a result of the production of a parathormone-like protein, called *PTHrp (PTH-related protein)*, by the neoplastic cells. Markedly increased serum concentrations of 1,25-vitamin D have been documented in human patients with lymphoma and hypercalcemia. We have recently recognized a similar condition in five dogs with lymphoma and hypercalcemia (most of the dogs were Boxers with mediastinal lymphoma).

Hyperproteinemia is another paraneoplastic abnormality that rarely occurs in cats and dogs with lymphoma. It may be secondary to the production of a monoclonal protein by the lymphoma cells and can result in the development of hyperviscosity syndromes. Polyclonal gammopathies may also be present in cats and dogs with lymphoma.

**Imaging.** Radiographic abnormalities in cats and dogs with lymphoma vary with the different anatomic forms but in general are secondary to lymphadenopathy or organomegaly (i.e., hepatomegaly, splenomegaly, renomegaly); occasionally the infiltration of other organs (e.g., lungs) may lead to the appearance of additional radiographic abnormalities.

Radiographic changes in cats and dogs with multicentric lymphoma include sternal or tracheobronchial lymphadenopathy or both; interstitial, bronchoalveolar, or mixed pulmonary infiltrates; pleural effusion (rare); intraabdominal lymphadenopathy (e.g., mesenteric or iliac); hepatomegaly; splenomegaly; renomegaly; or intraabdominal masses. Rarely, lytic or proliferative bone lesions are identified on plain abdominal or thoracic radiographs.

In cats and dogs with mediastinal lymphoma, radiographic changes are usually limited to the finding of an anterior (or, more rarely, posterior) mediastinal mass, with or without pleural effusion. In cats and dogs with alimentary lymphoma, abnormalities are rarely detected on plain abdominal radiographs (<50%). When present, they vary in nature but include mainly hepatomegaly, splenomegaly, and midabdominal masses. Positive contrast–enhanced radiography of the upper gastrointestinal tract usually reveals abnormalities in most animals. In a series of dogs with alimentary lymphoma evaluated at our clinic, abnormalities were found in all dogs that underwent positive contrast–enhanced radiography of the upper gastrointestinal tract and included mucosal irregularities, luminal filling defects, and irregular thickening of the wall, suggestive of infiltrative mural disease.

Gray scale ultrasonography constitutes an invaluable tool for evaluating cats or dogs with suspected or confirmed intraabdominal lymphoma. The technique is also helpful in the evaluation of mediastinal masses in both species (see p. 1119). Changes in the echogenicity of parenchymal organs (i.e., liver, spleen, kidneys) detected by this technique usually reflect changes in organ texture secondary to neoplastic infiltration. In addition, enlarged lymphoid structures or organs can easily be identified using this technique. Several abnormalities are commonly detected ultrasonographically in cats and dogs with intraabdominal lymphoma; these include hepatomegaly, splenomegaly, changes in the echogenicity of liver or spleen (mixed echogenicity or multiple hypoechoic areas), intestinal thickening, lymphadenopathy, splenic masses, and effusion. In a study of 11 cats with alimentary lymphoma evaluated ultrasonographically at our clinic, we found hypoechoic masses of the gastric or intestinal wall, focal or diffuse gastric wall thickening, a symmetrical thickening of the intestinal wall, loss of the normal layered appearance of the gastrointestinal wall, and abdominal lymphadenopathy. Fine-needle aspiration and needle biopsy can also be easily performed using this technique to guide the placement of the needle.

 TABLE 82-3

**TNM Staging System for Dogs and Cats with Lymphoma**

| STAGE | CLINICAL FEATURES |
|---|---|
| I | Solitary lymph node involvement |
| II | More than one lymph node enlarged but on one side of the diaphragm (i.e., cranial or caudal) |
| III | Generalized lymph node involvement |
| IV | Stage III findings, plus hepatomegaly and/or splenomegaly |
| V | Any of the above, plus bone marrow or extranodal involvement |
| substage a: | asymptomatic |
| substage b: | sick |

*TNM,* Tumor node metastasis.

## Diagnosis

The clinical signs and physical examination findings described in preceding paragraphs are usually suggestive of lymphoma. However, before instituting therapy, the diagnosis should be confirmed cytologically or histopathologically. In addition, a minimum database consisting of a CBC, serum biochemistry profile, and urinalysis should be obtained if the owners are contemplating treatment.

In most cats and dogs with multicentric, superficial extranodal, mediastinal, or alimentary lymphoma, a diagnosis can easily be obtained by fine-needle aspiration cytologic studies of the affected organs or lymph nodes. The techniques for fine-needle aspiration and the cytologic features of lymphoma are described in detail in Chapter 77.

In our practice, lymphomas can be diagnosed cytologically in approximately 90% of dogs and 70% to 75% of cats so evaluated (i.e., usually in only 10% of the dogs and 25% to 30% of the cats is it necessary to perform a histopathologic evaluation of a surgically excised lymph node or mass to establish a diagnosis). Until there is conclusive evidence that the histopathologic classification of canine and feline lymphomas offers prognostic information, the surgical removal of a lymph node or extranodal mass for histopathologic evaluation in an animal with a cytologic diagnosis of lymphoma is not necessarily indicated. A diagnosis based on cytologic findings rather than on histopathologic findings yielded by an excisional lymph node biopsy also offers two major benefits: (1) it is associated with minimal or no morbidity, and (2) it is financially acceptable to most owners (i.e., approximate cost of a lymph node aspirate is $40 to $50; the cost for biopsy and histopathologic evaluation is $200 to $300).

After a diagnosis of lymphoma is confirmed, it is customary to stage the disease to obtain a prognosis. A staging system devised by the World Health Organization has been used for the past two decades for the staging of cats and dogs with lymphoma (Table 82-3). In this system, derived from the TNM (tumor, node, metastasis) staging system for neoplasms in humans, clinical and clinicopathologic information from the patient is used in an attempt to determine the extent of disease and correlate it with the prognosis. Unfortunately, it cannot be used prognostically (i.e., animals with stage I disease have survival times similar to those of animals with stage IV disease). The only prognostic information of clinical relevance in this system is the fact that asymptomatic (i.e., substage a) dogs with lymphoma have better prognosis than "sick" (i.e., substage b) dogs. A staging system that takes into account tumor bulk and FeLV status in cats with lymphoma provides some prognostic information when cats are treated with a specific chemotherapy protocol (Mooney and colleagues, 1989). Until a new system is devised, we recommend determining the prognosis on the basis of the patient's overall clinical condition, the FeLV status (in cats), and any constitutional signs or severe hematologic and biochemical abnormalities the patient may have. Another important issue is that even though a specific staging protocol may be of some prognostic value in patients treated with a given chemotherapy protocol, it may not be so when a different drug combination is used. Moreover, at this time there is a paucity of information as to whether more aggressive protocols would be effective in dogs and cats with "advanced stage" lymphoma.

I recommend performing at least a CBC, a serum biochemistry profile, and a urinalysis in all cats and dogs with lymphoma whose owners are contemplating therapy. In addition, an FeLV and an FIV test should be performed in cats. The resulting minimum database can provide a wealth of information that can help the owner (and the clinician) decide whether to treat the patient. In addition, once a decision to treat the pet has been made, the nature of any clinicopathologic abnormalities usually dictates the treatment or treatments used. For example, in a dog with pronounced cytopenias caused by lymphomatous infiltration of the bone marrow, a highly myelosuppressive chemotherapy combination almost certainly will result in severe neutropenia and sepsis; thus it should be avoided.

In cats and dogs with suspected lymphoma of the neuropil, it is advisable to perform cerebrospinal fluid (CSF) analysis and advanced imaging (i.e., computed tomography [CT] scan or magnetic resonance imaging [MRI]). The finding of high numbers of neoplastic lymphoid cells and an increased protein concentration in a CSF sample is diagnostic for lymphoma. Because of their poor accessibility, the diagnosis of extradural masses usually requires the collection of a surgical specimen for cytologic or histopathologic evaluation.

Immunophenotyping of canine and feline lymphoma has become routine for most oncologists. Most dogs with T-cell lymphoma treated with standard combination chemotherapy have a worse prognosis for remission and survival than dogs with B-cell tumors; however, at this time, protocols specifically designed for T-cell lymphomas are not available.

## Treatment

Once a cytologic or histopathologic diagnosis of lymphoma is established, the prognosis and potential therapeutic options should be discussed with the pet's owner. Remission rates in

cats and dogs with lymphoma treated with various chemotherapy protocols are approximately 65% to 75% and 80% to 90%, respectively. Most cats with lymphoma treated with multiple-agent chemotherapy protocols are expected to live 6 to 9 months; approximately 20% of the cats live more than 1 year. Most dogs with lymphoma treated in a similar fashion are expected to live 12 to 16 months; approximately 20% to 30% of the dogs are alive 2 years after diagnosis. The approximate survival times in untreated cats and dogs with lymphoma are 4 to 8 weeks. Probably the most important reason for the shorter survival times in cats than in dogs with lymphoma is that remissions appear to be difficult to reinduce once the tumor has relapsed. In addition, the retrovirus-associated nonlymphomatous disorders that affect cats with lymphoma lead to shortened survival times (i.e., FeLV infection is a negative prognostic factor in cats with lymphoma).

In my experience, even if an animal has stage I nodal or extranodal lymphoma at the time of presentation, systemic dissemination of the disease usually occurs weeks to months after diagnosis. Therefore the mainstay of treatment for animals with lymphoma is chemotherapy, given the fact that lymphomas are (or will be) systemic neoplasms. Surgery or radiotherapy or both can be used to treat localized lymphomas before or during chemotherapy. General guidelines for the management of patients with lymphoma are presented here. The protocols recommended in this chapter have been used at our clinic with a success rate comparable to those of other treatments published in the literature.

The treatment of cats and dogs with lymphoma is divided into several phases, or strategies: induction of remission, intensification, maintenance, and reinduction of remission or "rescue" (Table 82-4). Immediately after diagnosis, a relatively aggressive multiple-agent chemotherapy protocol (cyclophosphamide, vincristine [Oncovin], cytosine arabinoside, prednisone [COAP]) is used to *induce remission*. During this phase, which lasts 6 to 8 weeks, the animals are evaluated weekly by a veterinarian, at which time they receive an intravenous (IV) injection of an antimitotic agent (vincristine) in addition to undergoing a routine physical examination (with or without a CBC). If at the end of this phase the patient is considered to be in complete remission (CR) (i.e., all neoplastic masses have completely disappeared), the *maintenance* phase is initiated. During this phase, a multiple-agent chemotherapy protocol consisting of three drugs (chlorambucil [Leukeran], methotrexate, prednisone [LMP]) administered orally is used, so that the animal requires less intensive monitoring (once every 6 to 8 weeks). In my experience, maintenance chemotherapy is necessary when using COP-based protocols.

The reinduction continues until the tumor relapses (i.e., is out of remission), at which time the *reinduction* phase begins. This phase is similar to the induction phase, in that intensive treatments are used. Once remission is obtained, the patient is started again on a modified maintenance protocol (at The Ohio State University we typically use the LMP protocol for routine maintenance, but we substitute cytarabine [Cytosar] for the methotrexate at a dosage of 200 to 300 mg/m$^2$ subcutaneously

TABLE 82-4

**Chemotherapy Protocols Used to Treat Dogs and Cats\* with Lymphoma at The Ohio State University Veterinary Teaching Hospital**

**1. Induction of Remission**

*COAP protocol†*

Cyclophosphamide (Cytoxan): 50 mg/m² PO q48h in dogs or 200-300 mg/m² PO q3wk in cats

Vincristine (Oncovin): 0.5 mg/m² IV weekly

Cytosine arabinoside (Cytosar-U): 100 mg/m² daily as an IV drip or SQ for only 2 days in cats and 4 days in dogs

Prednisone: 50 mg/m² PO q24h for 1 week, then 20 mg/m² PO q48h

**2. Intensification**

**Dogs**

L-Asparaginase (Elspar): 10,000-20,000 IU/m² IM (one or two doses)

or

Vincristine (Oncovin): 0.5-0.75 mg/m² IV q1-2wk

**Cats**

Doxorubicin (Adriamycin): 1 mg/kg IV q3wk

or

Mitoxantrone (Novantrone): 4-6 mg/m² IV q3wk

**3. Maintenance‡**

*LMP protocol*

Chlorambucil (Leukeran): 20 mg/m² PO q2wk

Methotrexate (Methotrexate): 2.5 mg/m² PO 2 or 3 times per week

Prednisone: 20 mg/m² PO q48h

*COAP protocol*

Use as above every other week for six treatments, then every third week for six additional treatments, then try to maintain the animal on one treatment every fourth week. Maintenance therapy is continued until the tumor relapses.

**4. Rescue**

**Dogs**

*D-MAC protocol (14-day cycle)*

Dexamethasone: 0.5 mg/lb (0.23 mg/kg) PO or SQ on days 1 and 8

Actinomycin D (Cosmegen): 0.75 mg/m² as IV push on day 1

Cytosine arabinoside (Cytosar): 200-300 mg/m² as IV drip over 4 hours *or* SQ on day 1

Melphalan (Alkeran): 20 mg/m² PO on day 8§

*AC protocol (21-day cycle)*

Doxorubicin (Adriamycin): 30 mg/m² (or 1 mg/kg for dogs under 10 kg) IV on day 1

Cyclophosphamide (Cytoxan): 100-150 mg/m² PO on days 15 and 16

**4. Rescue—cont'd**

**Dogs—cont'd**

*ADIC protocol (cycle is repeated every 21 days)*

Doxorubicin (Adriamycin): 30 mg/m² (or 1 mg/kg for dogs under 10 kg) IV on day 1

Dacarbazine (DTIC): 700-1000 mg/m² in IV infusion (over 6-8 hours) on day 1

*CHOP protocol (21-day cycle)*

Cyclophosphamide (Cytoxan): 200-300 mg/m² PO on day 10

Doxorubicin (Adriamycin): 30 mg/m² (or 1 mg/kg for dogs under 10 kg) IV on day 1

Vincristine (Oncovin): 0.75 mg/m² IV on days 8 and 15

Prednisone: 20-25 mg/m² PO q48h

**Cats**

*MiC protocol (21-day cycle)*

Mitoxantrone (Novantrone): 4-6 mg/m² as IV drip over 4-6 hours on day 1

Cyclophosphamide (Cytoxan): 200-300 mg/m² PO on day 10 or 11

*AC protocol (21-day cycle)*

Doxorubicin (Adriamycin): 1 mg/kg IV on day 1

Cyclophosphamide (Cytoxan): 200-300 mg/m² PO on day 10 or 11

*MiCA protocol (21-day cycle)*

Mitoxantrone (Novantrone): 4-6 mg/m² in IV drip over 4-6 hours on day 1

Cyclophosphamide (Cytoxan): 200-300 mg/m² PO on day 10 or 11

Cytosine arabinoside (Cytosar-U): 200 mg/m² in IV drip over 4-6 hours (mixed in the same bag with mitoxantrone) on day 1

*CHOP protocol (21-day cycle)*

Cyclophosphamide (Cytoxan): 200-300 mg/m² PO on day 10

Doxorubicin (Adriamycin): 1 mg/kg IV on day 1

Vincristine (Oncovin): 0.5 mg/m² IV on days 8 and 15

Prednisone: 20-25 mg/m² PO q48h

**5. "Low-Budget" Protocols**

Prednisone: 50 mg/m² PO q24h for 1 week; then 25 mg/m² PO q48h

Chlorambucil (Leukeran): 20 mg/m² PO q2wk

Lomustine (CCNU; Ceenu): 60-90 mg/m² PO q3wk in dogs; 10 mg (total dose) q3wk in cats

Prednisone and chlorambucil: doses as above

Prednisone and lomustine: doses as above

\*Unless otherwise specified, protocols can be used in both dogs and cats.

†Use for 6-10 weeks, then use LMP.

‡Use until relapse occurs, then go to "rescue."

§After four doses, substitute Leukeran (20 mg/m² PO q2wk) for Alkeran.

[SQ] every other week when maintenance is induced for a second time). If at the end of the induction phase the patient is not in CR, it is recommended that *intensification* with L-asparaginase be done before the maintenance phase is initiated. In addition to the chemotherapeutic approach discussed in this section, a variety of protocols have been used successfully in the treatment of cats and dogs with lymphoma. (See Suggested Readings for additional information.) It costs approximately $800 to $1000 to treat a cat with uncomplicated lymphoma, whereas it costs $1500 to $2500 to treat a 65- to 70-lb (30- to 32-kg) dog.

**Induction of remission.** Our protocol of choice for the induction of remission is COAP. The agents in this protocol consist of cyclophosphamide vincristine (Oncovin; Eli Lilly, Indianapolis), cytosine arabinoside (Cytosar-U; Upjohn-Pharmacia, Kalamazoo, Mich), and prednisone; these four drugs are also currently available as generic products. The dosages are specified in Table 82-4. These drugs belong to four different categories, have different mechanisms of action, and do not have superimposed toxicities (with the exception of cyclophosphamide and cytosine arabinoside, which are myelosuppressive; but the latter is used only for a short period); thus they fulfill the basic criteria of multiple-agent chemotherapy described in Chapter 79. The cytosine arabinoside is usually administered by the SQ route, because, given its short half-life and S-phase–specific mechanism of action, an IV bolus injection results in minimal cell kill; SQ administration of this drug is painful in cats (and in some dogs). IV infusion of the agent is also associated with myelosuppression. The induction phase lasts 6 to 8 weeks, and weekly visits to the veterinarian are necessary during this time.

During the induction phase, toxicity is minimal (<15% to <20%) and client compliance is high, because most of the toxic signs are hematologic (i.e., cytopenias) and usually do not result in clinical signs that can be detected by the owners. The dose-limiting toxicity of this induction protocol is hematologic (i.e., myelosuppression leading to neutropenia); the neutrophil nadir usually occurs around day 7 or 8, which is explained by the fact that two myelosuppressive agents (i.e., cyclophosphamide and cytosine arabinoside) are given during the initial 2 to 4 days of treatment. In most cases the neutropenia is mild (2000 to 3500 cells/μl). The neutropenia is severe if the animals have neoplastic bone marrow infiltration before the initiation of treatment, have FeLV- or FIV-associated myelodysplasia or other retrovirus-associated bone marrow disorders, or receive the cytosine arabinoside by constant-rate IV infusion rather than by the SQ route. Treatment changes to be made in cats and dogs in which neutropenia develops are described on p. 1110. Gastrointestinal toxicity is minimal to nonexistent; however, cats receiving cyclophosphamide occasionally become anorectic. Consequently, we administer this drug once every 3 weeks in cats (as opposed to every other day in dogs) (Table 82-4). If anorexia develops, treatment with cyproheptadine (Periactin; Merck Sharp & Dohme, West Point, Pa), an antiserotonin compound, at a dosage of 1 to 2 mg per cat PO every 8 to 12 hours is indicated. Hair loss is also minimal, and it occurs primarily in

woolly-haired dogs (e.g., Poodle, Bichon Frise); cats (and some dogs) may shed their tactile hairs during treatment.

During this phase, owners are instructed to monitor their pet's appetite and activity level, to measure their lymph nodes (if superficial lymphadenopathy was present initially), and to take their pet's rectal temperature daily (pyrexia is usually secondary to neutropenia and sepsis). If pyrexia develops, owners are instructed to contact their veterinarian so that their pet can undergo a complete physical examination and CBC (for additional information see Chapter 80). Treatment with COAP results in CR within 1 to 14 days of the start of therapy in most animals (>85% in dogs, >70% to >75% in cats). This remission is usually maintained throughout the induction phase.

In dogs with diffuse alimentary lymphoma and those with mycosis fungoides or mucocutaneous lymphoma, we use a more aggressive doxorubicin-containing protocol (CHOP; see Table 82-4), because, in my experience, the response rate to COAP is low. This protocol is more expensive and is more likely to cause adverse effects than the COAP protocol. We have recently seen encouraging responses to lomustine (CCNU) in a limited number of dogs with epidermotropic lymphoma (see Table 82-4).

In dogs and cats with multicentric (or any other anatomic form of) lymphoma coexisting with neurologic signs, we usually use the COAP protocol but administer the cytosine arabinoside as a continuous IV infusion (200 mg/m² as an IV infusion over 24 hours for 1 to 4 days) in an attempt to increase the concentration of this drug in the CNS. This protocol tends to cause marked myelosuppression in cats, so we typically administer cytosine arabinoside as a 12- to 24-hour infusion (200 mg/m²) in this species. More information on the treatment of dogs and cats with suspected or confirmed CNS lymphoma is given later in this chapter.

**Maintenance.** The protocol recommended for the maintenance phase of treatment is LMP ("lump"), which consists of chlorambucil (Leukeran; Burroughs Wellcome, Research Triangle Park, N.C.), methotrexate (Methotrexate; Lederle, Wayne, N.J.), and prednisone (see Table 82-4). These three drugs also act by three different mechanisms of action, have different toxicities, and have proved effective as single agents in cats and dogs with lymphoma. The advantages of this protocol include its reduced cost compared with the cost of the induction phase; its ease of administration (all the drugs are administered orally by the owners); its minimal toxicity; and the fact that intensive monitoring by a veterinarian is not necessary.

The toxicities associated with LMP maintenance chemotherapy are minimal. Of the three drugs in this protocol, methotrexate is the only one that is associated with moderate to severe toxicity. In approximately 25% of dogs and cats receiving methotrexate, gastrointestinal tract signs consisting of anorexia, vomiting, or diarrhea develop. Anorexia and vomiting are more common than diarrhea and usually occur after the patient has been receiving the drug for more than 2 weeks. In these cases, treatment with an antiemetic, such as metoclopramide (Reglan; A.H. Robins, Richmond, Va), on the days the animal receives the methotrexate, at a dosage of 0.1 to 0.3 mg/kg PO every 8 hours, alleviates or eliminates the upper gastrointestinal tract signs. In cases of methotrexate-associated diarrhea, treatment with a bismuth subsalicylate–containing product (Pepto-Bismol) may also alleviate or eliminate the signs; however, it may be necessary to discontinue the drug. Hematologic toxicity associated with LMP therapy is minimal to nonexistent. In a very small proportion of cats (i.e., <5%) receiving chlorambucil for weeks to months, serum biochemical abnormalities consistent with cholestasis that resolve on discontinuation of the drug may develop.

During this phase the patient is examined every 6 to 8 weeks, at which time a complete physical examination and a CBC are performed. As with the induction protocols, owners are instructed to monitor their pet's activity, appetite, behavior, rectal temperature, and lymph node size.

Most animals treated with this protocol remain in remission for approximately 3 to 6 months. If a relapse occurs, reinduction of remission (as discussed next) is instituted. After reinducing remission, animals can be treated with a modified maintenance protocol, as described in previous paragraphs.

**Reinduction of remission or rescue.** Virtually every dog and cat with lymphoma treated with maintenance chemotherapy eventually relapses; this generally occurs 6 to 8 months after the start of induction therapy, but it can occur within weeks of starting the maintenance phase or years after the original diagnosis was made. At this time, reinduction of remission is indicated. In our experience, remission can be reinduced one to four additional times in most dogs with relapsing lymphoma. Reinduction of remission is usually not as successful in cats as in dogs (i.e., remission cannot be reinduced in most cats with relapsing lymphoma). Therefore the following discussion on "rescue" pertains mostly to dogs with lymphoma.

There are numerous "rescue" protocols described in the literature, and as a general rule, the practitioner may have difficulty deciding what protocol to choose. For example, if a dog is being treated with the LMP maintenance protocol and the tumor starts to relapse (i.e., either the owner or the clinician notes that the lymph nodes are just enlarging), we typically add vincristine (0.5 mg/m² IV q2wk) on the weeks the patient is not receiving chlorambucil; if tumor growth is arrested but remission is not obtained, we increase the dose of vincristine to 0.75 mg/m² every 2 weeks. This intervention alone frequently results in a long-lasting remission. If the patient is examined when the tumor has progressed to an advanced stage, we usually recommend administering L-asparaginase, as described in Table 82-4.

We currently used the D-MAC protocol (see Table 82-4), consisting of dexamethasone, melphalan (Alkeran; Burroughs Wellcome, Research Triangle Park, N.C.), cytosine arabinoside (Cytosar-U), and actinomycin D (Cosmegen; Merck Sharp & Dohme, West Point, Pa) as our "trump card" for rescue. This protocol results in an approximately 80% remission rate in dogs with relapsing lymphoma treated at our clinic; it has a relatively low toxicity compared with that of

doxorubicin-containing protocols; and it is necessary for the owner to go the veterinarian only once every 2 weeks (instead of every week). Because the long-term use of melphalan is associated with moderate to severe chronic thrombocytopenia, chlorambucil (Leukeran), 20 mg/m², is substituted for melphalan after four cycles. If complete or partial remissions are achieved after the administration of four to six cycles of D-MAC, the patient can be started on a maintenance protocol again.

If the response to D-MAC is poor (i.e., disease progresses), we recommend using the ADIC or CHOP protocol (see Table 82-4). Our protocol calls for two or three cycles of ADIC or CHOP once the tumor has relapsed; if CR is obtained, the patient is started on maintenance chemotherapy at the end of the second or third ADIC or CHOP cycle. The maintenance protocol in these animals also includes LMP, with the possible addition of vincristine (0.5 to 0.75 mg/m² IV once weekly to every other week, alternating weeks with the Leukeran) or cytosine arabinoside (200 to 400 mg/m² SQ every other week, alternating weeks with the Leukeran).

After a second relapse occurs, D-MAC, ADIC, or CHOP is administered for two additional cycles, as described in the preceding paragraph. In our experience, after the second and third relapses, the percentage of animals in which remission can be easily reinduced decreases with each subsequent cycle. This likely stems from the development of multiple-drug resistance by the tumor cells. Other protocols that have been successful in reinducing remission in dogs with lymphoma are listed in Table 82-4. Although the probability of reinducing remission is considerably lower in cats than in dogs, one of the protocols listed in Table 82-4 can be used for this purpose.

In cats, doxorubicin- or mitoxantrone-containing protocols are commonly used in our clinic with some degree of success (see Table 82-4); asparaginase-containing protocols may also be used, but in my experience they are not as effective as in dogs.

**Intensification.** If a dog is undergoing induction therapy but only partial remission (PR) is obtained, intensification with one or two doses of L-asparaginase (Elspar) (10,000 to 20,000 IU/m² IM repeated once at a 2- to 3-week interval) may be indicated. This drug can rapidly induce CR in most dogs with lymphoma that have shown only PR while receiving COAP. Asparaginase should not be used in dogs with a history of pancreatitis or in those that are at high risk for acute pancreatitis (i.e., obese, middle-age, female dogs). L-Asparaginase appears to be less effective in cats than in dogs; doxorubicin (1 mg/kg IV q3wk) or mitoxantrone (4 to 6 mg/m² IV q3wk; Novantrone; Lederle, Wayne, N.J.) can be used as intensifying agents in cats.

**Management of solitary and extranodal lymphomas.** The clinician faces a problem when confronted with a dog or cat with a solitary lymphoma, regardless of whether it is nodal (i.e., stage Ia disease) or extranodal (i.e., a solitary cutaneous mass). Should the mass (or lymph node) be treated as other solitary malignancies are treated (i.e., by wide surgical excision)? Should the patient be treated primarily with chemotherapy? Should the patient be treated with a combination of surgery, irradiation, and chemotherapy? Unfortunately, there are no correct answers to these questions.

In my experience, "solitary" lymphomas become (or already are) systemic in most animals. Although cures have been achieved through the surgical excision or irradiation of solitary lymphomas, they are extremely rare. Therefore we do not underestimate the malignant behavior of this neoplasm by treating the patient only with a local treatment modality, such as surgery or radiotherapy. The following guidelines can be used in this subset of patients:

1. If the tumor is easily resectable (e.g., cutaneous mass, superficial lymph node, intraocular mass) and the surgical procedure does not pose a considerable risk to the patient, the mass should be resected and the animal treated with chemotherapy.
2. If the mass is difficult or impossible to resect, or if a major surgical procedure would pose an undue risk for the animal, a fine-needle aspirate or needle biopsy specimen of the mass should be obtained and the animal treated with chemotherapy (with or without radiotherapy of the primary lesion).

Radiotherapy constitutes an excellent treatment for dogs and cats with solitary lymphomas, because lymphoma cells are extremely radiosensitive. Marked responses (CR or PR) are seen within hours or days of the start of such treatment. Different sources and protocols have been used in cats and dogs with lymphoma, but in general, 3 to 5 Gy (300 to 500 rad) per fraction is delivered, for a total of six to ten fractions (total dose, 30 to 50 Gy [3000 to 5000 rad]). As discussed previously, this treatment can be used in conjunction with chemotherapy. Special settings in which radiotherapy is beneficial include CNS lymphomas (see following paragraphs) and upper airway lymphomas that cause respiratory compromise.

Another decision the clinician must make if chemotherapy is to be used is which protocol to use and for how long. There are also no certain guidelines for this. We use a standard induction chemotherapy protocol (COAP) in most cats and dogs with solitary lymphoma after they have undergone surgical excision or irradiation. After completion of the induction phase, the animals are treated with a maintenance protocol (LMP) and remission is reinduced as necessary (as in other forms of lymphoma). In our experience, early relapses occur in most animals treated with only maintenance chemotherapy protocols after the surgical excision of solitary lymphomas.

***Central nervous system lymphoma.*** The treatment of choice for cats and dogs with primary or secondary epidural lymphoma is radiotherapy plus multiple-agent chemotherapy. If radiotherapy facilities are not available, multiple-agent chemotherapy is an effective alternative approach. It is my clinical impression that the surgical excision of such masses does not provide a significant advantage over chemotherapy alone or radiotherapy plus chemotherapy, given the fact that the latter two forms of treatment consistently induce rapid remis-

sions (i.e., within 12 to 36 hours of the initiation of therapy). However, because surgery may be necessary to confirm the diagnosis, surgical excision of the mass is usually attempted at that time. If radiotherapy is available, three doses per week of 3.6 to 4 Gy, to a total of 25 to 30 Gy, are indicated. The COAP protocol alone has been effective in inducing remission in cats with epidural lymphoma.

In cats and dogs with lymphoma of the neuropil (i.e., true CNS lymphoma), chemotherapy with or without radiotherapy is the preferred protocol. In animals in which it is possible to localize the lesion (i.e., by neurologic examination, computed tomography, or magnetic resonance imaging), radiotherapy should be used in conjunction with chemotherapy. If this is not possible, diffuse craniospinal irradiation can be performed (3.6 to 4 Gy three times per week, for a total of 25 to 30 Gy).

Intrathecal chemotherapy can be used in cats and dogs with confirmed or highly likely neuropil lymphoma. The drug of choice is cytosine arabinoside (Cytosar-U) because it is almost nontoxic, it is inexpensive, and it is easy to administer. This drug is administered intrathecally at dosages of 20 to 40 mg/m$^2$ once or twice weekly, after the removal of an equivalent amount of CSF, for a total of six to eight doses. Lactated Ringer's solution or CSF should be used to dilute the drug. Once diluted, the remaining drug should be discarded or used within 24 hours for systemic administration only (the vial should never be reused for intrathecal injection). A strict aseptic technique should be used during administration. Responses to intrathecal cytosine arabinoside treatment are usually quite spectacular. Dogs and cats that are tetraparetic, demented, or comatose usually regain normal neurologic status within 6 to 48 hours of receiving the first dose of this agent. In addition, disappearance of the neoplastic cells from the CSF can be documented within hours of the injection.

If radiotherapy or intrathecal chemotherapy cannot be used because the anesthesia necessary poses a high risk to the animal, systemic chemotherapy can be used with some degree of success. Protocols used in such animals should include cytosine arabinoside, because, besides the corticosteroids, it is one of the few drugs that appears to attain high CSF concentration with minimal systemic toxicity. The cost of treatment is also relatively low. The cytosine arabinoside should be administered as a slow IV drip, because it has a relatively short half-life and it is a cell cycle phase-specific agent (i.e., it kills only cells that are synthesizing; therefore prolonged administration results in more cells being exposed to the drug). The CSF concentrations reached when it is administered by this route are similar to those in blood. The doses used range from 200 to 400 mg/m$^2$ during 1 to 4 days of continuous infusion. Because the administration of cytosine arabinoside by this route is commonly associated with marked myelosuppression that may lead to neutropenia and sepsis, prophylactic antibiotics may be indicated (see Chapter 80). We have been able to induce clinical and cytologic remission (i.e., normal neurologic status and disappearance of neoplastic cells from CSF) in several cats and dogs with primary or secondary CNS lymphoma treated with COAP (using cytosine arabinoside as an IV infusion). An alternative drug that crosses the blood-brain barrier and is effective in eliminating lymphoma cells is lomustine (CCNU; see Table 82-4) administered at a dosage of 60 to 90 mg/m² PO every 3 weeks in dogs and at a dosage of 10 mg every 3 weeks in cats; we have seen marked improvement or disappearance of neurologic signs in dogs with lymphoma treated with this drug.

Despite the fact that remissions are easily attained in dogs and cats with CNS lymphoma, they are relatively short in duration compared with the duration of remissions in dogs and cats with disease in other anatomic locations. Most dogs and cats with CNS lymphoma relapse within 2 to 4 months of diagnosis; however, prolonged remissions (i.e., 6 to 12 months) can occur.

***Ocular lymphoma.*** Ocular lymphoma can be treated using a variety of modalities. However, the eye behaves similarly to the blood-brain barrier in that adequate intraocular concentrations of chemotherapeutic agents are usually difficult to attain. If the clinician and the owner want to try to preserve the animal's eye, there are several alternatives to enucleation. One of these is subconjunctival chemotherapy using cytosine arabinoside. The dosages and precautions are similar to those that pertain to the intrathecal administration of this drug (see previous section), including the use of lactated Ringer's solution to dilute the drug. These injections can be administered once or twice per week for a total of 2 to 4 weeks. In the limited number of animals we have treated using this approach, responses were rapid and sustained and ocular complications minimal to nonexistent. As in animals with CNS lymphoma, the administration of cytosine arabinoside as a slow IV drip usually results in remission of the tumor. Lomustine should also be effective in dogs and cats with intraocular lymphoma.

***Cutaneous lymphoma.*** Cutaneous lymphoma is the most common extranodal form of lymphoma in dogs seen at the Veterinary Teaching Hospital of The Ohio State University. In dogs with cutaneous involvement secondary to multicentric lymphoma, we use a standard chemotherapy protocol (i.e., COAP). In dogs with mycosis fungoides, "histiocytic" cutaneous lymphoma, or mucocutaneous epidermotropic lymphoma we use doxorubicin-containing protocols (i.e., CHOP; see Table 82-4) because these dogs usually fail treatment with standard drug combinations. Although we have used retinoids to treat dogs with this form of disease, they are rarely beneficial. As mentioned above, lomustine has been effective in dogs with mycosis fungoides or other epidermotropic lymphomas.

***Alimentary lymphoma.*** We use standard chemotherapy protocols (i.e., COAP) in dogs and cats with solitary mural or nodal (e.g., mesenteric or ileocecocolic lymph node) involvement. Even though surgery is not necessarily indicated for these dogs and cats, a fair number are referred after exploratory surgery and an incisional or excisional biopsy has been performed. In general the response in these animals is good. Dogs and cats with diffuse intestinal lymphoma usually respond poorly to chemotherapy. Responses to doxorubicin-containing protocols (i.e., CHOP) appear to be better than

those to COAP, although survival times are short (4 to 6 months). Dogs with colorectal lymphoma and cats with gastric lymphoma tend to respond extremely well to COAP chemotherapy; we have documented remission times in excess of 3 years in these subsets of patients.

**"Low-budget" lymphoma protocols.** Quite frequently the clinician is evaluating a dog or cat with lymphoma that should benefit from chemotherapy, but because of finances or other issues (e.g., time commitment) the owners are not interested in the standard multiagent chemotherapy approach. Because most of these patients are asymptomatic, they would benefit from some form of therapy. In our clinic we have use either prednisone alone, prednisone and chlorambucil, chlorambucil alone, lomustine alone, or prednisone and lomustine quite successfully in these patients. Although the duration of remission is shorter than when using COP-based protocols, most of these patients (and their owners) enjoy prolonged (i.e., months), good-quality survivals. These protocols are listed in Table 82-4.

## Suggested Readings

Baskin CR et al: Factors influencing first remission and survival in 145 dogs with lymphoma: A retrospective study, *J Am Anim Hosp Assoc* 36:404, 2000.

Carter RF et al: Chemotherapy of canine lymphoma with histopathologic correlation: doxorubicin alone compared to COP as first treatment regimen, *J Am Anim Hosp Assoc* 23:587, 1987.

Chun R et al: Evaluation of a high-dose chemotherapy protocol with no maintenance therapy for dogs with lymphoma, *J Vet Intern Med* 14:120, 2000.

Cotter SM: Treatment of lymphoma and leukemia with cyclophosphamide, vincristine, and prednisone. I. Treatment of dogs, *J Am Anim Hosp Assoc* 19:159, 1983.

Cotter SM: Treatment of lymphoma and leukemia with cyclophosphamide, vincristine, and prednisone. II. Treatment of cats, *J Am Anim Hosp Assoc* 19:166, 1983.

Couto CG: Canine lymphomas: something old, something new, *Compend Cont Educ Pract Vet* 7:291, 1985.

Couto CG: Extranodal lymphomas. In Kirk RW, editor: *Current veterinary therapy IX: small animal practice,* Philadelphia, 1986, WB Saunders.

Couto CG et al: Gastrointestinal lymphoma in 20 dogs, *J Vet Intern Med* 3:73, 1989.

Grooters AM et al: Ultrasonographic appearance of feline alimentary lymphoma, *Vet Radiol Ultrasound* 35:468, 1994.

Jeglum KA et al: Chemotherapy for lymphoma in cats, *J Am Vet Med Assoc* 190:174, 1987.

Keller E et al: Evaluation of prognostic factors and sequential combination chemotherapy for canine lymphoma, *J Vet Intern Med* 7:289, 1993.

Loar AS: The management of feline lymphosarcoma, *Vet Clin North Am* 14:1299, 1984.

MacEwen EG et al: Some prognostic factors for advanced multicentric canine lymphosarcoma, *J Am Vet Med Assoc* 190:564, 1987.

Madewell BR: Diagnosis, assessment of prognosis, and treatment of dogs with lymphoma: sentinel changes (1973-1999), *J Vet Intern Med* 13:393, 1999.

Mooney SC et al: Renal lymphoma in cats: 28 cases (1997-1984), *J Am Vet Med Assoc* 191:1473, 1987.

Mooney SC et al: Treatment and prognostic factors in lymphoma in cats: 103 cases (1977-1981), *J Am Vet Med Assoc* 194:696, 1989.

Moore AS et al: Lomustine (CCNU) for the treatment of resistant lymphoma in dogs, *J Vet Intern Med* 13:395, 1999.

Postorino N et al: Single-agent therapy with adriamycin for canine lymphoma, *J Am Anim Hosp Assoc* 25:221, 1989.

Shelton GH et al: Feline immunodeficiency virus and feline leukemia virus infection and their relationships to lymphoid malignancies in cats: a retrospective study, *J AIDS* 3:623, 1990.

Teske E et al: Prognostic factors for treatment of malignant lymphoma in dogs, *J Am Vet Med Assoc* 205:1722, 1994.

Vail DM: Recent advances in chemotherapy for lymphoma in dogs and cats, *Compend Cont Educ Pract Vet* 15:1031, 1993.

Wellman ML et al: Lymphoma involving large granular lymphocytes in cats: 11 cases (1982-1991), *J Am Vet Med Assoc* 201:1265, 1992.

# CHAPTER 83

# Leukemias

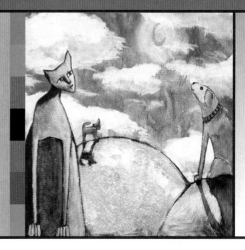

## CHAPTER OUTLINE

DEFINITIONS AND CLASSIFICATION, 1133
LEUKEMIAS IN DOGS, 1133
    Acute leukemias, 1134
    Chronic leukemias, 1136
LEUKEMIAS IN CATS, 1138
    Acute leukemias, 1138
    Chronic leukemias, 1139
MYELODYSPLASTIC SYNDROMES, 1140

## DEFINITIONS AND CLASSIFICATION

Leukemias are malignant neoplasms that originate from hematopoietic precursor cells in the bone marrow. These cells are unable to undergo terminal differentiation, therefore they self-replicate as a clone of usually immature (and nonfunctional) cells. The neoplastic cells may or may not appear in peripheral circulation, thus the confusing terms *aleukemic* and *subleukemic* are used to refer to leukemias in which neoplastic cells proliferate within the bone marrow but are absent or scarce in the circulation.

Leukemias can be classified philogenetically into two broad categories according to the cell line they originate from: *lymphoid* and *myeloid* (or nonlymphoid) (Table 83-1). The term *myeloproliferative disease* or *disorder* has also been used to refer to myeloid leukemias (mainly to the acute forms). On the basis of their clinical course and the cytologic features of the leukemic cell population, leukemias can also be classified as *acute* or *chronic*. Acute leukemias are characterized by an aggressive biologic behavior (i.e., death ensues shortly after diagnosis if the patient is not treated) and by the presence of immature (blast) cells in bone marrow or blood, or both. Chronic leukemias have a protracted, often indolent course, and the predominant cell is a well-differentiated, late precursor (i.e., lymphocyte in chronic lymphocytic leukemia and neutrophil in chronic myeloid leukemia). In dogs (and possibly in cats), chronic myeloid leukemia (CML) can undergo *blast transformation* (blast crisis), during which the disease behaves like an acute leukemia and is usually refractory to therapy. Blast crises do not appear to occur in dogs or cats with chronic lymphocytic leukemia (CLL).

Acute leukemias may be difficult to classify morphologically as myeloid or lymphoid based on evaluation of Giemsa- or Wright's-stained blood or bone marrow smears, because poorly differentiated blasts look similar under the light microscope. In veterinary medicine, cytochemical stains are used routinely in several diagnostic laboratories to establish whether the blasts are lymphoid or myeloid and also to subclassify myeloid leukemias, as described later (i.e., myeloid versus monocytic versus myelomonocytic). These cytochemical stains reveal the presence of different enzymes in the cytoplasm of the blasts, which aids in establishing their origin (Table 83-2).

Immunophenotyping of canine and feline leukemic cells using monoclonal antibodies is now available in teaching institutions and some commercial diagnostic laboratories; however, clinical correlations between immunophenotype and prognosis have not yet been established.

A classification scheme for acute leukemia in people was devised by a group of French, American, and British investigators (the FAB scheme) and was based on the morphologic features of the cells in Giemsa-stained smears of blood and bone marrow and the clinical presentation and biologic behavior of the disease. Because this scheme has not yet proved to be prognostically or therapeutically applicable to cats or dogs, it is not discussed here (see the Suggested Readings for additional information on the FAB scheme).

The term *preleukemic syndrome or myelodysplastic syndrome* (MDS or myelodysplasia) refers to a syndrome of hematopoietic dysfunction that precedes the development of acute myelogenous leukemia by months to years. The syndrome is characterized by cytopenias and a hypercellular bone marrow and appears to be more common in cats than in dogs. The clinical and hematologic features of cats and dogs with MDS are discussed at the end of this chapter.

## LEUKEMIAS IN DOGS

In dogs, leukemias constitute fewer than 10% of all hemolymphatic neoplasms and are therefore considered rare.

TABLE 83-1

Classification of Leukemias in Dogs and Cats

| CLASSIFICATION | SPECIES |
|---|---|
| **Acute Leukemias** | |
| ***Acute myeloid (myelogenous) leukemia (AML)*** | |
| Undifferentiated myeloid leukemia (AML-M$_0$) | D, C |
| Acute myelocytic leukemia (AML-M$_{1-2}$) | D, C |
| Acute progranulocytic leukemia (AML-M$_3$) | – – |
| Acute myelomonocytic leukemia (AMML; AML-M$_4$) | D, C |
| Acute monoblastic/monocytic leukemia (AMoL; AML-M$_5$) | D, C |
| Acute erythroleukemia (AML-M$_6$) | C, D? |
| Acute megakaryoblastic leukemia (AML-M$_7$) | D, C |
| ***Acute lymphoblastic leukemia (ALL)*** | |
| ALL-L$_1$ | D, C |
| ALL-L$_2$ | D, C |
| ALL-L$_3$ | C, D? |
| Acute leukemia of large granular lymphocytes (LGL) | D, C? |
| **Subacute and Chronic Leukemias** | |
| Chronic myeloid (myelocytic) leukemia (CML) | D>C |
| Chronic myelomonocytic leukemia (CMML) | D |
| Chronic lymphoid (lymphocytic) leukemia (CLL) | D>C |
|    Large granular lymphocyte (LGL) variant | D |
| Subacute (chronic) myelomonocytic leukemia | D |

*D*, Dog; *C*, cat.

 TABLE 83-2

Cytochemical Stains in Acute Leukemic Cells from Dogs and Cats

| CYTOCHEMICAL STAIN | AML | AMoL | AMML | ALL |
|---|---|---|---|---|
| MPO | + | – | ± | – |
| CAE | + | – | ± | – |
| ANBE | – | + | ± | –(+) |
| LIP | – | + | ± | – |
| LAP | + | – | ± | –(+) |

*AML,* Acute myelogenous leukemia (AML-M$_{0-2}$); *AMoL,* acute monoblastic/monocytic leukemia (AML-M$_5$); *AMML,* acute myelomonocytic leukemia (AML-M$_4$); *ALL,* acute lymphoblastic leukemia; *MPO,* myeloperoxidase; *CAE,* chloroacetate esterase; *ANBE,* α-naphthyl butyrate esterase; *LIP,* lipase; *LAP,* leukocyte alkaline phosphatase; *+,* positive; *–,* negative; *±,* positive or negative.

At our hospital, however, the leukemia-to-lymphoma ratio is approximately 1:7 to 1:10. This ratio is artificially high, because most dogs with lymphoma are treated by their local veterinarians, whereas most dogs with leukemia are referred for treatment. Although most leukemias in dogs are consid-

 TABLE 83-3

Clinical Signs and Physical Examination Findings in Dogs and Cats with Acute Leukemias*

| FINDING | DOG | CAT |
|---|---|---|
| **Clinical Sign** | | |
| Lethargy | >70 | >90 |
| Anorexia | >50 | >80 |
| Weight loss | 30-40 | 40-50 |
| Lameness | 20-30 | ? |
| Persistent fever | 30-50 | ? |
| Vomiting/diarrhea | 20-40 | ? |
| **Physical Examination Finding** | | |
| Splenomegaly | >70 | >70 |
| Hepatomegaly | >50 | >50 |
| Lymphadenopathy | 40-50 | 20-30? |
| Pallor | 30-60 | 50-70? |
| Fever | 40-50 | 40-60? |

*?,* Unknown.

*Results are expressed as the approximate percentage of animals showing the abnormality.

ered to be spontaneous in origin, radiation and viral particles have been identified as possible etiologic factors in dogs with this disease.

## ACUTE LEUKEMIAS

### Prevalence

Acute myeloid leukemias are more common than acute lymphoid leukemias in dogs, constituting approximately three fourths of the cases of acute leukemia. It should be remembered, however, that morphologically (i.e., as determined by evaluation of a Wright's- or Giemsa-stained blood or bone marrow smear), most acute leukemias are initially classified as lymphoid. After cytochemical staining of the smears or immunophenotyping is performed, approximately one third to one half of them are then reclassified as myeloid. Approximately half of the dogs with myeloid leukemia are found to have myelomonocytic differentiation when cytochemical staining or immunophenotyping is performed (see Table 83-2).

### Clinical Features

The clinical signs and physical examination findings in dogs with acute leukemia are usually vague and nonspecific (Table 83-3). Most owners seek veterinary care when their dogs become lethargic or anorectic or when persistent or recurrent fever, weight loss, shifting limb lameness, or other nonspecific signs develop; neurologic signs occur occasionally. Splenomegaly, hepatomegaly, pallor, fever, and mild generalized lymphadenopathy are commonly detected during routine physical examination. The spleen in these dogs is usually markedly enlarged, and it has a smooth surface on palpation. Careful inspection of the mucous membranes in dogs with

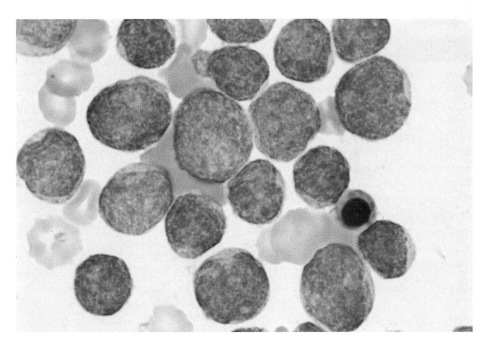

**FIG 83-1**
Blood smear from a dog with acute lymphoblastic leukemia and a white blood cell count of approximately 1,000,000/µl. Note the predominance of large, immature lymphoid cells with large nuclei, clumped chromatin, and nucleoli. (×1000.)

acute leukemia often reveals petechiae or ecchymoses, or both, in addition to pallor. Icterus may also be detected if marked leukemic infiltration of the liver has occurred. The generalized lymphadenopathy seen in dogs with acute leukemia is usually mild, in contrast to that seen in dogs with lymphoma, in which the lymph nodes are massively enlarged. In other words, the hepatosplenomegaly is of higher magnitude than the lymphadenopathy. Most dogs with leukemia also have constitutional signs (i.e., they are clinically ill), whereas most dogs with lymphoma are asymptomatic. Although it is usually impossible to distinguish between acute myeloid and acute lymphoid leukemia on the basis of physical examination findings alone, some subtle differences do exist: mainly, shifting limb lameness, fever, and ocular lesions are more common in dogs with acute myeloid leukemia, whereas neurologic signs are more common in dogs with acute lymphoid leukemia.

### Hematologic Features

Marked hematologic changes are usually present in dogs with acute leukemia. Couto (1985) and Grindem and colleagues (1985b) have published detailed reviews of the hematologic features of dogs with acute leukemia. Briefly, abnormal (leukemic) cells are observed in the peripheral blood of most dogs with acute myeloid leukemia (AML) and acute lymphoblastic leukemia (ALL), although this is slightly more common in the latter (i.e., circulating blasts are absent in some dogs with AML) (Fig. 83-1). Isolated cytopenias, bicytopenias, or pancytopenia is present in almost all dogs with AML and ALL. Leukoerythroblastic reactions are detected in approximately half of dogs with AML but are rare in dogs

with ALL. The total white blood cell (WBC) and blast counts are highest in dogs with ALL (median, 298,200/µl; range, 4000 to 628,000/µl), and as a general rule, only dogs with ALL have WBC counts greater than 150,000/µl. Most dogs with AML and ALL are anemic, but dogs with acute monoblastic/monocytic leukemia (AMoL or AML-M$_5$) have the least severe anemia (packed cell volume of 30% versus 23% in all other groups). Most dogs with acute leukemias are also thrombocytopenic, although the thrombocytopenia also appears to be less severe in dogs with AML-M$_5$ (median, 102,000/µl; range, 39,000 to 133,000/µl).

### Diagnosis

A presumptive diagnosis in dogs with acute leukemia is usually made on the basis of the history and physical examination findings; a complete blood count (CBC) is usually confirmatory, although the hematologic changes in dogs with "aleukemic leukemia" may resemble those of ehrlichiosis or other bone marrow disorders. To evaluate the extent of the disease, a bone marrow aspirate or biopsy is indicated. Splenic, hepatic, or lymph node aspirates for cytologic evaluation can also be obtained easily, although the information yielded may not help in establishing the diagnosis or prognosis. For example, if a dog has mild generalized lymphadenopathy and the only laboratory sample submitted is a lymph node, spleen, or liver aspirate, the finding of undifferentiated blasts in the smear points toward a cytologic diagnosis of either acute leukemia or lymphoma (i.e., the neoplastic lymphoid cells in lymphoma and leukemia are indistinguishable morphologically); indeed, it is quite common for the clinical pathologist to issue a diagnosis of lymphoma, because it is the most common of the two diseases. In these cases, further clinical and clinicopathologic information (i.e., the degree and extent of lymphadenopathy, presence and degree of hepatosplenomegaly, hematologic and bone marrow biopsy or aspiration findings) is required to establish a definitive diagnosis.

It may be difficult to diagnose the tumor type in a dog with generalized lymphadenopathy, hepatosplenomegaly, and a low number of circulating lymphoblasts. The main differential diagnoses are ALL and lymphoma with circulating blasts (lymphosarcoma cell leukemia). It is important to differentiate between these two disorders, because the prognosis for dogs with lymphoma is considerably better than that for dogs with leukemia. These two entities may be difficult to distinguish on the basis of the clinical, hematologic, and cytologic information obtained, but the following guidelines can be used to try to arrive at a definitive diagnosis:

1. If the lymphadenopathy is massive, the dog more likely has lymphoma.
2. If the dog is systemically ill, it more likely has ALL.
3. If bicytopenia or pancytopenia is present, ALL is the more likely diagnosis.
4. If the percentage of lymphoblasts in the bone marrow is more than 40% to 50%, the dog more likely has ALL.
5. If hypercalcemia is present, the more likely diagnosis is lymphoma.

When the neoplastic cells are poorly differentiated, cytochemical staining or immunophenotyping is required to establish a definitive diagnosis (see Table 83-2). This is important if the owner is contemplating treatment, because the therapy and prognosis for dogs with AML are different from those for dogs with ALL (i.e., the survival time in dogs with AML is shorter than that in dogs with ALL).

Besides lymphoma, differential diagnoses in dogs with acute or chronic leukemias include other disorders of the mononuclear-phagocytic or hematopoietic systems, such as malignant or systemic histiocytosis, systemic mast cell disease (mast cell leukemia), rickettsial diseases (i.e., canine ehrlichiosis), bartonellosis, hemobartonellosis, storage diseases, and tuberculosis.

The following basic principles of diagnosis apply to all dogs with suspected leukemia:

1. If cytopenias or abnormal cells are present in peripheral blood, a bone marrow aspirate or biopsy specimen should be obtained.
2. If the spleen or liver is enlarged, a fine-needle aspirate of the affected organs should be obtained for cytologic evaluation.
3. If blasts are present, blood and bone marrow specimens should be submitted to a veterinary referral laboratory for cytochemical staining or immunophenotyping.
4. Other diagnostic tests (e.g., serologic tests or polymerase chain reaction [PCR] testing for *Ehrlichia canis*) should be performed if appropriate.

The diagnosis of acute leukemia can be extremely straightforward (i.e., a dog that is evaluated because of weight loss, lethargy, hepatosplenomegaly, pallor, and central nervous system [CNS] signs and that has a WBC of more than 500,000/μl, most of which are blasts, is most likely to have ALL), or it may represent a challenge (i.e., a dog with unexplained cytopenias of prolonged duration in which aleukemic AML-M₁ subsequently develops).

### Treatment

The treatment of dogs with acute leukemias is usually unrewarding. Most dogs with these diseases respond poorly to therapy, and prolonged remissions are rare. Treatment failure usually stems from one or more of the following factors:

1. Failure to induce remission (more common in AML than in ALL)
2. Failure to maintain remission
3. The presence or development of organ failure resulting from leukemic cell infiltration; this precludes the use of aggressive combination chemotherapy (i.e., because of enhanced toxicity)
4. The development of fatal sepsis or bleeding, or both, caused by already existing or treatment-induced cytopenias

Prolonged remissions in dogs with AML treated with chemotherapy are extremely rare. In most dogs with AML, remissions in response to any of the protocols listed in Table 83-4 are rarely observed. If animals do respond, the remission is usually extremely short-lived, and survival rarely exceeds 3 months. In addition, more than half of the dogs die during induction as a result of sepsis or bleeding. Further, the supportive treatment required in these patients (e.g., blood component therapy, intensive care monitoring) is financially unacceptable to most owners, and the emotional strain placed on the owner is also quite high. Therefore owners should be aware of all these factors before deciding to treat their dogs.

The prognosis may be slightly better in dogs with ALL; however, responses to treatment and survival times in such dogs are considerably lower than those in dogs with lymphoma. The remission rates in dogs with ALL are approximately 20% to 40%, in contrast with those in dogs with lymphomas, which approach 90%. Survival times with chemotherapy in dogs with ALL are also shorter (average, 1 to 3 months) than those in dogs with lymphoma (average, 12 to 18 months). Untreated dogs usually live less than 2 weeks. Chemotherapy protocols used in dogs with acute leukemia are listed in Table 83-4.

## CHRONIC LEUKEMIAS

### Prevalence

In dogs, CLL is far more common than CML; in addition, the latter is poorly characterized. At our hospital, we evaluate approximately six to eight dogs with CLL a year, whereas we evaluate approximately one dog with CML every 3 to 5 years. CLL is one of the leukemias most commonly diagnosed at diagnostic referral laboratories.

TABLE 83-4

**Chemotherapy Protocols for Dogs and Cats with Acute Leukemias**

### Acute Lymphoblastic Leukemia

1. Vincristine, 0.5 mg/m² IV once a week
   Prednisone, 40-50 mg/m² PO q24h for a week; then 20 mg/m² PO q48h
2. Vincristine, 0.5 mg/m² IV once a week
   Prednisone, 40-50 mg/m² PO q24h for a week; then 20 mg/m² PO q48h
   Cyclophosphamide, 50 mg/m² PO q48h
3. Vincristine, 0.5 mg/m² IV once a week
   Prednisone, 40-50 mg/m² PO q24h for a week; then 20 mg/m² PO q48h
   L-Asparaginase, 10,000-20,000 IU/m² IM or SQ once every 2-3 weeks
4. Vincristine, 0.5 mg/m² IV once a week
   Prednisone, 40-50 mg/m² PO q24h for a week; then 20 mg/m² PO q48h
   Cyclophosphamide, 50 mg/m² PO q48h
   Cytosine arabinoside, 100 mg/m² SQ daily for 2-4 days*

### Acute Myelogenous Leukemias

1. Cytosine arabinoside, 5-10 mg/m² SQ q12h for 2-3 weeks; then on alternate weeks
2. Cytosine arabinoside, 100 mg/m² SQ daily for 2-6 days
   6-Thioguanine, 50 mg/m² PO q24-48h
3. Cytosine arabinoside, 100 mg/m² SQ daily for 2-6 days
   6-Thioguanine, 50 mg/m² PO q24-48h
   Doxorubicin, 10 mg/m² IV once a week
4. Cytosine arabinoside, 100-200 mg/m² in IV drip over 4 hours
   Mitoxantrone, 4-6 mg/m² in IV drip over 4 hours; repeat every 3 weeks

*The daily dose should be divided into two to four daily administrations.

## Clinical Features

Like their acute counterparts, the clinical signs in dogs with CLL or CML are vague and nonspecific; however, there is a history of chronic (i.e., months), vague clinical signs in approximately half of the dogs with chronic leukemia. Many cases of chronic leukemia are diagnosed incidentally during routine physical examination and clinicopathologic evaluation (i.e., dogs are asymptomatic). Clinical signs in dogs with CLL include lethargy; anorexia; vomiting; polyuria-polydipsia; enlarged lymph nodes; intermittent diarrhea or vomiting; and weight loss. As mentioned above, over half of the dogs with CLL are asymptomatic. Physical examination findings in dogs with CLL include mild generalized lymphadenopathy, splenomegaly, hepatomegaly, pallor, and pyrexia. The clinical signs and physical examination findings in dogs with CML appear to be similar to those in dogs with CLL.

A terminal event in dogs with CLL is the development of a diffuse large cell lymphoma, termed *Richter's syndrome*. This is characterized by a massive, generalized lymphadenopathy and hepatosplenomegaly. Once this multicentric lymphoma develops, chemotherapy-induced, long-lasting remissions are difficult to obtain and survival times are short.

*Blast crisis,* which involves the appearance of immature blast cells in blood and bone marrow, occurs in humans and dogs with CML months to years after the initial diagnosis is made. In humans these blasts are of either myeloid or lymphoid phenotype; the origin of the blast cell in dogs with blast crises has not been determined. Blast crises occurred in five of 11 dogs with CML described in the literature (Leifer and colleagues, 1983). Blast crises do not appear to occur in dogs with CLL.

## Hematologic Features

The most common hematologic abnormality in dogs with CLL is a marked lymphocytosis resulting in leukocytosis. The lymphocytes are usually morphologically normal, although large granular lymphocytes (LGL) are occasionally present. The lymphocyte counts range from 8000/µl to more than 100,000/µl, but lymphocyte counts of more than 500,000/µl are rare. In addition to the lymphocytosis, which may be diagnostic in itself (i.e., a dog with a lymphocyte count of 100,000/µl most certainly has CLL), anemia is detected in more than 80% of the dogs and thrombocytopenia in approximately half of the dogs. Although cytologic evaluation of bone marrow aspirates in dogs with CLL usually reveals the presence of many morphologically normal lymphocytes, normal numbers of lymphocytes are occasionally detected. This is probably because the lymphocytosis in some animals with CLL stems from disorders of recirculation rather than from the increased clonal proliferation of lymphocytes in the bone marrow.

Monoclonal gammopathies are found in approximately two thirds of dogs with CLL in which serum is evaluated using protein electrophoresis (Leifer and colleagues, 1986). The monoclonal component is usually IgM, but IgA and IgG components have also been reported. This monoclonal gammopathy can lead to hyperviscosity. Rarely, dogs with CLL have paraneoplastic, immune-mediated blood disorders (e.g., hemolytic anemia, thrombocytopenia, neutropenia).

The hematologic features of CML in dogs are poorly characterized but include leukocytosis with a left-shift down to myelocytes (or occasionally myeloblasts), anemia, and possibly thrombocytopenia, although thrombocytosis can also occur. The hematologic findings seen during a blast crisis are indistinguishable from those seen in dogs with AML or ALL.

## Diagnosis

Absolute lymphocytosis is the major diagnostic criterion for CLL in dogs. Although other diseases (e.g., ehrlichiosis, babesiosis, leishmaniasis, Chagas' disease, Addison's disease) should be considered in the differential diagnosis of dogs with mild lymphocytosis (i.e., 7000 to 20,000/µl), marked lymphocytosis (i.e., more than 20,000/µl) is almost pathognomonic for CLL. If the physical examination and hematologic abnormalities discussed in previous paragraphs (i.e., mild lymphadenopathy, splenomegaly, monoclonal gammopathy, anemia) are found, this may help establish a diagnosis of CLL in dogs with lymphocytosis, although all these changes can also be present in dogs with chronic ehrlichiosis (see Chapter 101).

The diagnosis of CML may be challenging, particularly because this syndrome is poorly characterized in dogs. Some of the markers used to diagnose CML in humans are of no use in dogs. For example, the Philadelphia 1 chromosome and the alkaline phosphatase score are used in humans to differentiate CML from leukemoid reactions (i.e., CML cells have the Philadelphia 1 chromosome, and the alkaline phosphatase content of the neutrophils increases in the setting of leukemoid reactions and decreases in the setting of CML). Unfortunately the Philadelphia 1 chromosome has not been identified in dogs, and mature canine (and feline) neutrophils lack alkaline phosphatase. Therefore a final diagnosis of CML should be made only after the clinical and hematologic findings have been carefully evaluated and the inflammatory and immune causes of neutrophilia have been ruled out.

## Treatment

The clinician usually faces the dilemma of whether to treat a dog with CLL. If the dog is symptomatic, has organomegaly, or has concurrent hematologic abnormalities, treatment with an alkylator (with or without corticosteroids) is indicated. If there are no paraneoplastic syndromes (i.e., immune hemolysis or thrombocytopenia, monoclonal gammopathies), I recommend using single-agent chlorambucil (Leukeran) at a dosage of 20 mg/m² given orally once every 2 weeks (Table 83-5). If there are paraneoplastic syndromes, the addition of corticosteroids (prednisone, 50 to 75 mg/m² PO q24h for 1 week, then 25 mg/m² PO q48h) may be beneficial.

Because the growth fraction of neoplastic lymphocytes in CLL appears to be low, a delayed response to therapy is common. In a high proportion of dogs with CLL treated with chlorambucil or chlorambucil and prednisone, it may take more than 1 month (and as long as 6 months) for the hematologic and physical examination abnormalities to resolve. This is in contrast to dogs with lymphoma and acute leukemias, in which remission is usually induced in 2 to 7 days.

The survival times in dogs with CLL are quite long. Indeed, even without treatment, survival times of more than 2 years are common. More than two-thirds of the dogs with CLL treated with chlorambucil (with or without prednisone) at our clinic have survived in excess of 2 years. In fact, most dogs with CLL do not die of leukemia-related causes but rather from other geriatric disorders.

The treatment of dogs with CML using hydroxyurea (see Table 83-5) may result in prolonged remission, provided a blast crisis does not occur. However, the prognosis does not appear to be as good as that for dogs with CLL (i.e., survivals of 4 to 15 months with treatment). The treatment of blast crises is usually unrewarding. A novel therapeutic approach targeting tyrosine kinase in the neoplastic cells of humans with CML using gleevec (STI571) has shown to be beneficial in inducing remission; however, the drug appears to be hepatotoxic in dogs and will probably be of little use in this species until new analogues are developed.

# LEUKEMIAS IN CATS

## ACUTE LEUKEMIAS
### Prevalence

True leukemias are rare in the cat, constituting only 15% to 35% of all hematopoietic neoplasms. Although exact figures regarding the incidences of leukemias and lymphomas are not available for cats, the practitioner is likely to see considerably more leukemias in cats than in dogs.

If cytochemical staining (or immunophenotyping) is used to classify acute leukemias in cats, approximately two-thirds are myeloid and one-third are lymphoid. However, in contrast to dogs, myelomonocytic leukemias ($M_4$) appear to be rare in cats.

Feline leukemia virus (FeLV) is commonly implicated as a cause of leukemias in cats; however, the role of feline immunodeficiency virus (FIV) in the pathogenesis of these neoplasms is still unclear. Overall, it is reported that approximately 90% of cats with lymphoid and myeloid leukemias test positive for FeLV p27 with enzyme-linked immunosorbent assay or immunofluorescence. As discussed in Chapter 82, because the prevalence of FeLV infection is decreasing, most cats with leukemia diagnosed in our clinic over the past few years have not been viremic for FeLV (i.e., they are FeLV-negative).

## Clinical Features

The clinical features and physical examination findings in cats with acute leukemias are similar to those in dogs and are summarized in Table 83-3. Shifting limb lameness and neurologic signs do not appear to be as common in cats as in dogs with myeloid leukemias.

## TABLE 83-5

### Chemotherapy Protocols for Dogs and Cats with Chronic Leukemias

**Chronic Lymphocytic Leukemia**

1. Chlorambucil, 20 mg/m² PO once every 2 weeks
2. Chlorambucil as above, plus prednisone, 50 mg/m² PO q24h for a week; then 20 mg/m² PO q48h
3. Cyclophosphamide, 200-300 mg/m² IV once every 2 weeks; vincristine, 0.5-0.75 mg/m² IV once every 2 weeks (alternating weeks with the cyclophosphamide); prednisone as in protocol 2, above this treatment is continued for 6-8 weeks, at which time protocol 1 or 2 can be used for maintenance

**Chronic Myelogenous Leukemia**

1. Hydroxyurea, 50 mg/kg PO q24h for 1-2 weeks; then q48h

## Hematologic Features

More than three-fourths of cats with AML and ALL have cytopenias; leukoerythroblastic reactions are common in cats with AML but extremely rare in those with ALL. In contrast to dogs, circulating blasts appear to be more common in cats with AML than in those with ALL.

Sequential studies of cats with myeloid leukemias have revealed that the cytomorphologic features can change from one cell type to another over time (e.g., sequential diagnoses of erythremic myelosis, erythroleukemia, and acute myeloblastic leukemia are common in a given cat). This is one of the reasons why most clinical pathologists prefer the term *myeloproliferative disorder* (MPD) to refer to this leukemia in cats.

## Diagnosis and Treatment

The diagnostic evaluation of cats with suspected acute leukemia follows the same general sequence as that for dogs. If the changes in the CBC are not diagnostic, a bone marrow aspirate can provide information that can confirm the diagnosis (Fig. 83-2). In addition, cats with suspected or confirmed acute leukemias should be evaluated for circulating FeLV p27 and for serum antibodies against FIV.

With treatment, cats with ALL apparently have better survival times than cats with AML. Survival times in cats with ALL treated with multichemotherapy range from 1 to 7 months.

There have been several published reports of cats with myeloid leukemias treated with single-agent or combination chemotherapy. The treatment protocols have included single-agent cyclophosphamide or cytosine arabinoside, as well as combinations of cyclophosphamide, cytosine arabinoside, and prednisone; cytosine arabinoside and prednisone; cyclophosphamide, vinblastine, cytosine arabinoside, and prednisone; and doxorubicin, cyclophosphamide, and prednisone. Survival times in these cats have usually ranged from 2 to 10 weeks, with a median of approximately 3 weeks. Therefore, as in dogs, intensive chemotherapy does not appear to be beneficial in cats with acute leukemias.

New alternatives for the therapy of feline MPD are currently being explored. Low-dose cytosine arabinoside (LDA) (10 mg/m² SQ q12h; Cytosar-U; Upjohn, Kalamazoo, Mich) has been used as an inductor of differentiation of the neoplastic clone. In several studies this treatment was observed to induce complete or partial remission in 35% to 70% of humans with MDS and MPD. Moreover, although myelosuppression was observed in some patients, the treatment was exceedingly well tolerated and associated with minimal toxicity.

We have treated several cats with MPD using LDA and in most have observed complete or partial remissions, with transient hematologic improvement. Although no major toxicities were seen, the remissions were short-lived (3 to 8 weeks).

## CHRONIC LEUKEMIAS

As discussed in previous paragraphs, chronic leukemias are extremely rare in cats. CLL is occasionally found incidentally during routine physical examination. More often cats with CLL are seen by a veterinarian because of a protracted history of vague signs of illness, including anorexia, lethargy, and gastrointestinal tract signs. In cats with CLL, mature, well-differentiated lymphocytes predominate in peripheral blood and bone marrow,

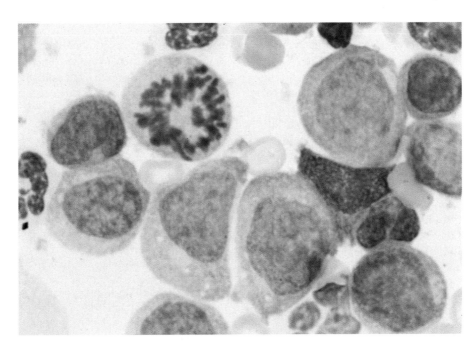

**FIG 83-2**
Bone marrow aspirate from a cat with peripheral blood cytopenias and absence of circulating blasts. Note the predominance of large immature myeloid cells, characterized by round to kidney-shaped nuclei. A mitotic figure is evident. (×1000.)

and the response to therapy appears to be good. Most cats with CLL evaluated at our clinic showed a complete remission in response to chlorambucil and prednisone treatment. As in dogs, CML is poorly characterized in cats.

# MYELODYSPLASTIC SYNDROMES

In humans, a variety of hematologic abnormalities and vague clinical signs characterized by cytopenias in the presence of a normocellular or hypercellular bone marrow may precede the development of AML by months to years. AML develops in approximately 10% to 45% of humans with MDS 1 month to 25 years after the initial diagnosis.

In addition to the morphologic abnormalities in blood and bone marrow, functional abnormalities of granulocytes and platelets have been well documented in humans with MDS. Therefore recurrent infections or spontaneous bleeding tendencies, or both, are common in such patients, even when the neutrophil and platelet counts are within normal limits. These abnormalities have also been observed in cats with MDS (see following paragraphs).

MDS has been recognized in both dogs and cats but appears to be more common in retrovirus-infected cats. All dogs have been lethargic, depressed, and anorectic. Physical examination findings have included hepatosplenomegaly, pallor, and pyrexia; hematologic changes have included pancytopenia or bicytopenia, macrocytosis, metarubricytosis, and reticulocytopenia. AML subsequently developed 3 months after the initial diagnosis of MDS in one of our patients (Couto and colleague, 1984). The cytologic bone marrow abnormalities were similar to those described in cats and are discussed in the following paragraphs. Some authors have proposed classifying dogs with primary myelodysplastic syndromes into those with refractory anemia and those with true myelodysplasia, following similar classification schemes used in humans (Weiss and colleague, 2000); however, because almost no clinical information was provided for the dogs evaluated, that classification scheme is of questionable clinical relevance.

Several reports of MDS in cats have appeared in the literature. More than 80% of cats in which the FeLV status has been investigated were found to be viremic. Most cats were evaluated because of nonspecific clinical signs such as lethargy, weight loss, and anorexia. Other signs, such as dyspnea, recurrent infections, and spontaneous bleeding, were observed in a few cats. Physical examination revealed hepatosplenomegaly in more than half of the cats; generalized lymphadenopathy and pyrexia were detected in approximately one third.

Hematologic abnormalities in cats with MDS are similar to those seen in dogs; they include isolated or combined cytopenias, macrocytosis, reticulocytopenia, metarubricytosis, and macrothrombocytosis. Morphologic changes in the bone marrow include a normal-to-increased cellularity, less than 30% blasts, an increased myeloid/erythroid ratio, dyserythropoiesis, dysmyelopoiesis, and dysthrombopoiesis. Megaloblastic red blood cell precursors are common, with occasional binucleated, trinucleated, or tetranucleated rubricytes or metarubricytes. The morphologic abnormalities in the myeloid cell line include giant metamyelocytes and asynchronous nuclear-cytoplasmic maturation.

Acute leukemia subsequently developed within weeks to months of the diagnosis in approximately one third of cats with MDS described in the literature. It is common for MDS to progress to AML in humans, with only isolated reports of progression to ALL. However, according to Maggio and colleagues (1978), in one series of 12 cats with MDS, ALL subsequently developed in nine. This may reflect the fact that cytochemical staining was not done to classify the leukemic cells, and cells were thus morphologically classified as lymphoid when they were indeed myeloid. However, because all the cats that showed progression to ALL were also viremic (with FeLV), the hematologic changes preceding the development of leukemia did not reflect a "spontaneous" hematologic disorder (as seen in humans and dogs) but were rather a manifestation of the morphologic and functional changes induced by FeLV.

The management of dogs and cats with MDS is still controversial. A variety of treatments have been used in humans with MDS; however, none has proved effective. Chemotherapy, supportive therapy, anabolic steroids, inductors of differentiation, hematopoietic growth factors, and androgenic steroids, among others, have been reported to be of benefit in some humans with MDS. Currently the preferred approach in humans is to treat them with supportive therapy and inductors of differentiation or hematopoietic growth factors. Because most patients are older, chemotherapy does not constitute the first treatment option, given its toxicity. We recommend using supportive therapy (e.g., fluids, blood components, antibiotics) and low-dose cytosine arabinoside as an inductor of differentiation (see Table 83-4). Recently, aclarubicin (5 mg/m$^2$ IV q24h for 5 days), a drug not currently available in the United States, was reported to be of benefit in a Shih Tzu with myelodysplasia (Miyamoto and colleagues, 1999).

## Suggested Readings

Bennett JM et al: Proposal for the classification of acute leukemias, *Br J Haematol* 33:451, 1976.

Blue JT et al: Non-lymphoid hematopoietic neoplasia in cats: a retrospective study of 60 cases, *Cornell Vet* 78:21, 1988.

Cotter SM: Treatment of lymphoma and leukemia with cyclophosphamide, vincristine, and prednisone. II. Treatment of cats, *J Am Anim Hosp Assoc* 19:166, 1983.

Couto CG: Clinicopathologic aspects of acute leukemias in the dog, *J Am Vet Med Assoc* 186:681, 1985.

Couto CG et al: Preleukemic syndrome in a dog, *J Am Vet Med Assoc* 184:1389, 1984.

Facklam NR et al: Cytochemical characterization of feline leukemic cells, *Vet Pathol* 23:155, 1986.

Grindem CB et al: Morphological classification and clinical and pathological characteristics of spontaneous leukemia in 10 cats, *J Am Anim Hosp Assoc* 21:227, 1985a.

Grindem CB et al: Morphological classification and clinical and pathological characteristics of spontaneous leukemia in 17 dogs, *J Am Anim Hosp Assoc* 21:219, 1985b.

Jain NC et al: Proposed criteria for classification of acute myeloid leukemia in dogs and cats, *Vet Clin Pathol* 20:63, 1991.

Leifer CE et al: Chronic myelogenous leukemia in the dog, *J Am Vet Med Assoc* 183:686, 1983.

Leifer CE et al: Chronic lymphocytic leukemia in the dog: 22 cases, *J Am Vet Med Assoc* 189:214, 1986.

Maggio L et al: Feline preleukemia: an animal model of human disease, *Yale J Biol Med* 51:469, 1978.

Matus RE et al: Acute lymphoblastic leukemia in the dog: a review of 30 cases, *J Am Vet Med Assoc* 183:859, 1983.

Miyamoto T et al: Long-term case study of a myelodysplastic syndrome in a dog, *J Am Anim Hosp Assoc* 35:475, 1999.

Weiss DJ: Flow cytometric and immunophenotypic evaluation of acute lymphocytic leukemia in dog bone marrow, *J Vet Intern Med* 15:589, 2001.

Weiss DJ et al: Primary myelodysplastic syndromes of dogs: a report of 12 cases, *J Vet Intern Med* 14:491, 2000.

Wellman ML et al: Lymphocytosis of large granular lymphocytes in three dogs, *Vet Pathol* 26:158, 1989.

# CHAPTER 84

## Selected Neoplasms in Dogs and Cats

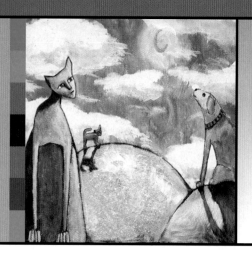

### CHAPTER OUTLINE

HEMANGIOSARCOMA IN DOGS, 1142
OSTEOSARCOMA IN DOGS AND CATS, 1144
MAST CELL TUMORS IN DOGS AND CATS, 1146
    Mast cell tumors in dogs, 1146
    Mast cell tumors in cats, 1149
OROPHARYNGEAL NEOPLASMS IN DOGS
AND CATS, 1149
    Oropharyngeal neoplasms in dogs, 1150
    Oropharyngeal neoplasms in cats, 1150
    Approach to dogs and cats with an oropharyngeal
      mass, 1150
INJECTION SITE SARCOMAS IN CATS, 1151

This chapter discusses the clinical approach to common tumors in dogs and cats; uncommon tumors will not be discussed in this textbook.

## HEMANGIOSARCOMA IN DOGS

Hemangiosarcomas (HSAs, hemangioendotheliomas, angiosarcomas) are malignant neoplasms that originate from the vascular endothelium. They occur predominantly in older dogs (8 to 10 years of age) and in males; German Shepherd Dogs and Golden Retrievers are at high risk for this neoplasm.

The spleen, right atrium, and subcutis are common sites of involvement at the time of presentation. In a review of 220 cases of HSA reported in the literature and diagnosed at our institution, approximately 50% of the tumors originated in the spleen, 25% in the right atrium, 13% in subcutaneous tissue, 5% in the liver, 5% in the liver-spleen–right atrium, and 1% to 2% simultaneously in other organs (i.e., kidney, urinary bladder, bone, tongue, prostate). The latter are referred to as *multiple tumor, undeterminable primary.*

In general, the biologic behavior of this neoplasm is highly aggressive, with most anatomic forms of the tumor infiltrating and metastasizing early in the disease. The only exception is that of primary dermal HSAs, which have a lower metasta-

tic potential than the tumors that originate in subcutaneous tissues.

### Clinical and Clinicopathologic Features

The nature of owners' complaints and the clinical signs at presentation are usually related to the site of origin of the primary tumor; to the presence or absence of metastatic lesions; and to the development of spontaneous tumor rupture, coagulopathies, or cardiac arrhythmias. More than one-half of the dogs with HSA are evaluated because of acute collapse after spontaneous rupture of the primary tumor or a metastatic lesion. Some episodes of collapse may stem from ventricular arrhythmias, which are relatively common in dogs with splenic or cardiac HSA. In addition, dogs with splenic HSA often are seen because of abdominal distention secondary to tumor growth or to hemoabdomen.

Dogs with cardiac HSA usually are presented for evaluation of right-sided congestive heart failure (caused by cardiac tamponade or obstruction of the posterior vena cava by a neoplasm) or cardiac arrhythmias (see Cardiovascular System Disorders section for additional information). Dogs with cutaneous or subcutaneous neoplasms are usually evaluated because of a lump.

Two common problems in dogs with HSA, regardless of the primary location or stage, are anemia and spontaneous bleeding. The anemia is usually the result of intracavitary bleeding or microangiopathic hemolysis (MAHA), whereas the spontaneous bleeding is usually caused by disseminated intravascular coagulation (DIC) or thrombocytopenia secondary to MAHA (see later discussion). HSA is so highly associated with clinical DIC that, at our hospital, dogs with DIC of acute onset but without an obvious primary cause are evaluated for HSA first.

Hemangiosarcomas are "hematologists' dreams" in that they are usually associated with a wide variety of hematologic and hemostatic abnormalities. Hematologic abnormalities in dogs with HSA have been well-characterized and include anemia; thrombocytopenia; the presence of nucleated red blood cells (RBCs), RBC fragments (schistocytes), and acanthocytes in the blood smear; and leukocytosis with neutrophilia, a left shift, and monocytosis. In addition, hemostatic abnormalities are also common in dogs with HSAs.

Twenty of twenty-four dogs with HSA (83%) evaluated at our clinic were anemic; more than one half had RBC fragmentation and acanthocytosis (Hammer and colleagues, 1991b). The pretreatment coagulograms of these 24 dogs were normal in only four dogs (17%). Most dogs (75%) had thrombocytopenia, with a mean platelet count of 137,000/μl. Approximately one-half of the coagulograms met three or more criteria for diagnosis of DIC, whereas less than 12% of them were compatible with microangiopathic thrombocytopenia. Approximately 25% of these dogs died as a result of their hemostatic abnormalities.

## Diagnosis

Hemangiosarcomas can be diagnosed cytologically on the basis of the appearance of fine-needle aspirates or impression smears. The neoplastic cells are similar to those in other sarcomas in that they are spindle-shaped or polyhedral, have large nuclei with a lacy chromatin pattern and one or more nucleoli, and a bluish gray, usually vacuolated cytoplasm (Fig. 84-1). Although HSA cells are relatively easy to identify in tissue aspirates or impression smears, they are extremely difficult to identify in HSA-associated effusions. The probability of establishing a cytologic diagnosis of HSA after evaluating effusions is less than 25%. A further problem with effusions is that a specimen may contain reactive mesothelial cells that may resemble neoplastic cells, leading to a false-positive diagnosis of HSA.

In general a presumptive clinical or cytologic diagnosis of HSA should be confirmed histopathologically. Because of the large size of some splenic HSAs, however, multiple samples (from different morphologic areas) should be submitted in appropriate fixative. Histochemically, HSA cells are positive for von Willebrand factor antigen in approximately 90% of the cases.

Metastatic sites can be detected radiographically, ultrasonographically, or on computerized tomography (CT). Our routine staging system for dogs with HSA includes a complete blood count (CBC), serum biochemistry profile, hemostasis screen, urinalysis, thoracic radiographs, abdominal ultrasonography, and echocardiography. The latter is used to identify cardiac masses and to determine the baseline fractional shortening before instituting doxorubicin-containing chemotherapy (see the section on Treatment and Prognosis).

Thoracic radiographs in dogs with metastatic HSA are typically characterized by the presence of interstitial or alveolar infiltrates, as opposed to the common "cannonball" metastatic lesions seen with other tumors. The radiographic pattern may be due to true metastases or to DIC and intrapulmonary bleeding, or adult respiratory distress syndrome (ARDS).

Ultrasonography constitutes a reliable way to evaluate dogs with suspected or confirmed HSA for intraabdominal disease. Neoplastic lesions appear as nodules with variable echogenicity, ranging from anechoic to hyperechoic (Fig. 84-2). Hepatic metastatic lesions can often be identified using this imaging technique. However, one should bear in mind that the "metastatic nodules" in the liver of a dog with a splenic mass may represent regenerative hyperplasia rather than true metastatic lesions.

## Treatment and Prognosis

Historically the mainstay of treatment for dogs with HSA has been surgery, although the results have been poor. Survival times vary with the location and stage of the tumor, but in general (with the exception of dermal HSAs), they are quite short (approximately 20 to 60 days, with a 1-year survival of <10%). Results of treatment combining surgery and postoperative adjuvant chemotherapy with doxorubicin; doxorubicin and cyclophosphamide (AC protocol); and vincristine, doxorubicin, and cyclophosphamide (VAC protocol) are better than with surgery alone. Median survival times range from 140 to 202 days.

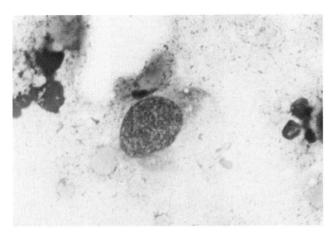

**FIG 84-1**
Cytologic features of canine hemangiosarcoma. Note the spindle-shaped cells, with a dark, vacuolated cytoplasm, and the fine nuclear chromatin pattern with prominent nucleolus. (×1000.)

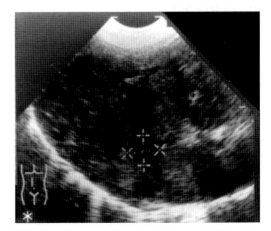

**FIG 84-2**
Ultrasonogram of an intraabdominal hemangiosarcoma.

The median survival times of dogs with HSA treated with the VAC protocol (see table on Cancer Chemotherapy Protocols on p. 1153) are approximately 190 days, with a 30% 1-year survival rate. Adverse effects associated with this protocol included myelosuppression, gastroenteritis, alopecia and hyperpigmentation, and cardiotoxicity. There was no apparent difference in the survival times between dogs with bulky disease (i.e., no surgical cytoreduction) and those that had undergone surgery. Recently, similar results were reported for dogs treated either with doxorubicin and cyclophosphamide or with doxorubicin alone. The coagulopathies in these dogs should be managed simultaneously, as discussed in Chapter 89.

Biologic response modifiers and antiangiogenic factors have recently been used in dogs with HSA in combination with doxorubicin-containing chemotherapy. Dogs receiving liposome-encapsulated MTP (muramyl tripeptide—the active immunomodulatory molecule in bacille Calmette-Guérin [BCG]) and AC chemotherapy after splenectomy for HSA had significantly longer survival times (277 days) than those receiving chemotherapy and placebo (144 days; Vail and colleagues, 1995). However, liposomal MTP is not readily available to the practicing veterinarian. Recently, minocycline, an antiangiogenic antibiotic, used at a dosage of 5 mg/kg by mouth every 24 hours, was added to the AC protocol in dogs with HSA (Sorenmo and colleagues, 2000); the median survival time was 170 days, similar to the median survival times obtained when using chemotherapy alone.

In summary, HSAs are usually diagnosed on the basis of historical, physical examination, and clinicopathologic findings, in conjunction with ultrasonographic and radiographic changes. A morphologic diagnosis can usually be made on the basis of cytologic or histopathologic findings. Although surgery is the preferred treatment, survival times in such animals are extremely short. Postoperative adjuvant chemotherapy using doxorubicin-containing protocols prolongs survival in dogs with this malignancy.

# OSTEOSARCOMA IN DOGS AND CATS

## Etiology and Epidemiology

Primary bone neoplasms are relatively common in dogs and rare in cats. Most primary bone tumors in dogs are malignant in that they usually cause death as a result of local infiltration (e.g., pathologic fractures or extreme pain leading to euthanasia) or metastasis (e.g., pulmonary metastases in osteosarcoma). In cats, most primary bone neoplasms, although histologically malignant, are cured by wide surgical excision (i.e., amputation). Neoplasms that metastasize to the bone are rare in dogs; some that occasionally metastasize to bones in dogs are transitional cell carcinoma of the urinary tract, osteosarcoma of the appendicular skeleton, hemangiosarcoma, mammary adenocarcinoma, and prostatic adenocarcinoma. Bone metastases are exceedingly rare in cats.

Osteosarcomas (OSAs) are the most common primary bone neoplasm in dogs. They can affect either the appendicular or axial skeletons, and they occur primarily in large-breed (and giant-breed), middle age to older dogs. Their biologic behavior is characterized by aggressive local infiltration of the surrounding tissues and rapid hematogenous dissemination (usually to the lungs). Although historically it was believed that OSAs of the axial skeleton had a low metastatic potential, it now appears that their metastatic rate is similar to that of the appendicular OSAs.

## Clinical Features

Appendicular OSAs occur predominantly in the metaphyses of the distal radius, distal femur, and proximal humerus, although other metaphyses can also be affected. As just mentioned, they typically affect male dogs of large (and giant) breeds, and owners seek veterinary care because of lameness or swelling of the affected limb. Physical examination usually reveals a painful swelling in the affected area, with or without soft tissue involvement. The pain and swelling can be acute in onset, leading to the presumptive diagnosis of a nonneoplastic orthopedic problem and thus considerably delaying diagnosis and definitive therapy for the neoplasm.

## Diagnosis

Radiographically, OSAs exhibit a mixed lytic-proliferative pattern in the metaphyseal region of the affected bone (Fig. 84-3). Adjacent periosteal bone formation leads to the devel-

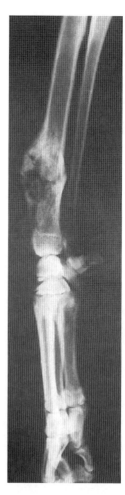

**FIG 84-3**
Radiographic appearance of a typical osteosarcoma of the radius in a dog. Note the lytic and proliferative changes characteristic of this neoplasm. (Courtesy RM Gamblin.)

opment of the so-called Codman's triangle, which is composed of the cortex in the affected area and the periosteal proliferation. OSAs typically do not cross the articular space, but occasionally they can infiltrate adjacent bone (e.g., ulnar lysis resulting from an adjacent radial OSA). Because other primary bone neoplasms and some osteomyelitis lesions can mimic the radiographic features of OSAs, biopsy specimens of every lytic or lytic-proliferative bone lesion should be obtained before the owners decide on a specific treatment. An exception to this rule is an owner who has already decided that amputation is the initial treatment of choice for that lesion (i.e., the limb is amputated and the lesion is submitted for histopathologic evaluation).

Once a presumptive radiographic diagnosis has been established and if the owners are contemplating treatment, thoracic and/or bone (i.e., skeletal survey) radiographs should be obtained to determine the extent of the disease. We usually obtain three radiographic views of the thorax and do not do a skeletal radiographic survey (or radionuclide bone scan). Only approximately 10% of dogs with OSA initially have radiographically detectable lung lesions; the presence of metastases is a strong negative prognostic factor.

The radiographic diagnosis can be confirmed before surgery (i.e., limb amputation or limb salvage) on the basis of the findings yielded either by fine-needle aspiration (FNA) (if there is considerable cortical lysis) or by aspiration of the affected area using a bone marrow aspiration needle. OSA cells are usually round or oval; have distinct cytoplasmic borders; have a bright blue, granular cytoplasm; and have eccentric nuclei with or without nucleoli (Fig. 84-4). A preamputation diagnosis can also be made after histopathologic evaluation of core biopsy specimens from the affected areas. To obtain a bone biopsy, a 13- or 11-gauge Jamshidi bone marrow biopsy needle (Monoject) is used with the animal under general anesthesia, and a minimum of two (and preferably three) cores of tissue are obtained from both the center of the lesion and the area between affected and unaffected

bone. The diagnostic yield of this procedure is quite high (approximately 70% to 75%).

As long as the owners understand the biologic behavior of the neoplasm (i.e., the high likelihood of their dog dying of metastatic lung disease within 4 to 6 months of amputation if no chemotherapy is used) and as long as the clinical and radiographic features of the lesion are highly suggestive of OSA, the limb can be amputated in the absence of a histopathologic diagnosis. However, the amputated leg (or representative samples) should always be submitted for histopathologic evaluation.

## Treatment and Prognosis

The treatment of choice for dogs with OSA is amputation with adjuvant single-agent or combination chemotherapy. The median survival time in dogs with appendicular OSA treated with amputation alone is approximately 4 months, whereas in dogs treated with amputation and cisplatin, amputation and carboplatin, or amputation and doxorubicin it is approximately 1 year. The dosages and the recommended ways of administering chemotherapy for dogs with OSA are given in the table on Cancer Chemotherapy Protocols (see p. 1153) and Table 84-1. At our hospital, we use either of the drugs mentioned above immediately after amputation for a total of four or five treatments. The cost of carboplatin chemotherapy is quite high (approximately $3 per milligram of drug, or roughly $30/kg of body weight).

A novel therapeutic approach for dogs with distal radial or ulnar OSAs consists of sparing the limb in affected dogs. Instead of amputation, the affected bone is resected and an allograft from a cadaver is used to replace the neoplastic bone; novel biomaterials are also currently being investigated for this purpose. The dogs are also treated with intravenous (IV) cisplatin, carboplatin, or doxorubicin and, in general, have almost normal limb function. The main complication is the development of osteomyelitis in the allograft; if that occurs, the limb frequently needs to be amputated. Survival times in dogs

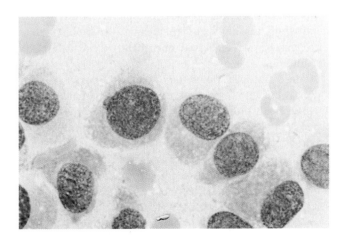

**FIG 84-4**
Characteristic cytologic features of osteosarcoma in a fine-needle aspirate of a lytic/proliferative lesion in the proximal scapula of a 12-year-old Wirehaired Terrier. Note the round to oval shape, eccentric nuclei with a fine chromatin pattern, and prominent nucleoli. (×1000.)

 TABLE 84-1

**Cisplatin Treatment Protocol for Dogs with Osteosarcoma**

1. Obtain a CBC, serum biochemistry profile, and urinalysis.
2. Place indwelling IV catheter, and perform 0.9% saline diuresis (120 to 150 ml/kg/day) for 8 hours.
3. Initiate cisplatin (Platinol) treatment (70 mg/m²); the dose of cisplatin is diluted in the volume of 0.9% saline solution to be administered over 8 hours, calculated on the basis of 120 to 150 ml/kg/24 hr (i.e., 40 to 50 ml/kg).
4. On completion of the cisplatin drip, 0.9% saline solution is administered for 8 additional hours as an IV drip.
5. The dog is discharged and readmitted every 3 weeks for further treatments.

*CBC,* Complete blood count; *IV,* intravenous.

treated with limb-sparing procedures are comparable to those in dogs that undergo amputation plus chemotherapy, with the added benefit to the owners of having a four-legged pet.

If owners are reluctant to allow the veterinarian to amputate the limb, local radiotherapy plus cisplatin, carboplatin, or doxorubicin may be of some benefit. However, in our limited experience, most dogs are eventually euthanized within 3 to 4 months of the initial diagnosis because of the development of pathologic fractures (i.e., after radiotherapy the tumor is not as painful; therefore the dog regains normal use of the limb and fractures the area), osteomyelitis, or metastatic lesions.

Chemotherapy apparently modifies the biologic behavior of the tumor, resulting in a higher prevalence of bone metastases and a lower prevalence of pulmonary metastases. Moreover, the doubling time (i.e., growth rate) of metastatic lesions appears to be longer than that in dogs that have not received chemotherapy, and there appear to be fewer metastatic nodules in treated than in untreated dogs. Therefore surgical removal of the metastatic nodules (i.e., metastasectomy) followed by additional cisplatin or carboplatin therapy may be recommended for a dog that has been treated with chemotherapy after amputation of the limb and in which one to three pulmonary metastatic lesions are detected (O'Brien and colleagues, 1993).

As discussed in previous paragraphs, the treatment of choice for OSAs in cats is limb amputation alone. Extremely long survival times (in excess of 2 years) are common in such cats. As discussed on p. 1115, cisplatin is extremely toxic in cats and should therefore not be used in this species. If necessary, carboplatin or doxorubicin can be used instead.

## MAST CELL TUMORS IN DOGS AND CATS

> Not one of them is like the other, don't ask me why, please ask your mother.
> From *One Fish, Two Fish, Red Fish, Blue Fish* by Dr. Seuss

Mast cell tumors (MCTs) are one of the most common skin tumors in dogs and are relatively common in cats. They originate from mast cells, which are intimately involved in the local control of vascular tone and which contain a large array of intracytoplasmic bioactive molecules, including heparin, histamine, leukotrienes, and several cytokines. Given their unpredictable biologic behavior, the term *mast cell tumor* is preferred to *mastocytoma* or *mast cell sarcoma*. Because of differences in the clinical and pathologic features of canine and feline MCTs, they are discussed separately.

### MAST CELL TUMORS IN DOGS

#### Etiology and Epidemiology

MCTs constitute approximately 20% to 25% of the skin and subcutaneous tumors seen by practicing veterinarians. Brachiocephalic breeds (Boxer, Boston Terrier, Bull Mastiff, En-

glish Bulldog) are at high risk for MCTs. These tumors are also more common in middle-aged to older dogs (mean age, approximately 8.5 years) than in younger dogs, but there is no gender-related predilection. MCTs have been found in sites of chronic inflammation or injury, such as burn scars.

### Clinical and Pathologic Features

MCTs occur either as dermoepidermal masses (i.e., a superficial mass that moves with the skin) or subcutaneous masses (i.e., the overlying skin moves freely over the tumor). Grossly, MCTs can mimic any primary or secondary skin lesion, including a macula, papula, nodule, tumor, and crust. Approximately 10% to 15% of all MCTs in dogs are clinically indistinguishable from the common subcutaneous lipomas. As a rule, an MCT cannot be definitively diagnosed until the lesion has been evaluated cytologically or histopathologically.

Most MCTs are solitary, although multifocal MCTs can occur in dogs. Regional lymphadenopathy caused by metastatic disease is also common in dogs with invasive MCTs. Occasionally splenomegaly or hepatomegaly is present in dogs with systemic dissemination.

Given the fact that mast cells produce a variety of bioactive (mainly vasoactive) substances, dogs with MCTs may be evaluated because of diffuse swelling (i.e., edema and inflammation around a primary tumor or its metastatic lesion), erythema, or bruising of the affected area. These episodes may be acute, and they may occur during or shortly after exercise or exposure to cold weather. Percutaneous FNA of an unexplained subcutaneous swelling in dogs should always be performed as part of the work-up.

A "typical" MCT is a dermoepidermal, dome-shaped, alopecic, and erythematous lesion. However, as discussed in previous paragraphs, MCTs rarely have a typical appearance. A clinical feature that may aid in the diagnosis of an MCT is Darier's sign, which is the erythema and wheal that form after the tumor is slightly traumatized (i.e., scraped or compressed).

Most dogs with MCTs have a normal CBC, although eosinophilia (sometimes marked), basophilia, mastocythemia, neutrophilia, thrombocytosis, or anemia, or a combination of these, may be present. Serum biochemistry abnormalities are uncommon.

From a histopathologic standpoint, MCTs are traditionally classified into three categories: well differentiated (grade 1), moderately differentiated (grade 2), and poorly differentiated (grade 3). Several studies have shown that dogs with grade 1 tumors treated with surgery or radiotherapy have longer survival times than identically treated dogs with grade 3 tumors, mainly because well-differentiated neoplasms have a lower metastatic potential (i.e., most tumors in dogs with systemic mast cell disease are grade 3). Special stains may be required to identify the typical intracytoplasmic granules in poorly differentiated neoplasms.

In addition to the grading of the tumor, the pathologist should provide the clinician with information regarding the completeness of the excision. A dog with an incompletely excised MCT is rarely cured by the initial surgical procedure and requires either a second surgery or irradiation of the affected area.

## Biologic Behavior

The biologic behavior of canine MCTs can be summed up in one word: unpredictable. Even though several criteria may help in establishing the biologic behavior of these neoplasms, they rarely apply to an individual dog (i.e., they may be meaningful from the statistical viewpoint).

In general, well-differentiated (grade 1), solitary cutaneous MCTs have a low metastatic potential and low potential for systemic dissemination. However, one may encounter a dog with several dozen cutaneous MCTs, which on histopathologic evaluation are well differentiated.

Grade 2 and 3 tumors have a higher metastatic potential and a higher potential for systemic dissemination than grade 1 MCTs. Metastases to the regional lymph nodes commonly occur (particularly in dogs with grade 3 tumors), although occasionally a tumor "skips" the draining lymph node and metastasizes to the second or third regional node (e.g., a digital MCT in the rear limb metastasizing to the iliac or sublumbar node). Pulmonary metastases are extremely rare. Although not evident from previously published clinical data, it appears that MCTs in certain anatomic locations are more aggressive than tumors in other areas. For example, distal limb (e.g., toe), perineal, inguinal, and extracutaneous (e.g., oropharyngeal, intranasal) MCTs appear to have a higher metastatic potential than similarly graded tumors in other regions (e.g., trunk, neck).

Another biologic characteristic of canine MCTs is that they may become systemic, behaving like a hematopoietic malignancy (i.e., a lymphoma or leukemia). These dogs usually have a history of a cutaneous MCT that was excised. Most dogs with systemic mast cell disease (SMCD) are evaluated because of lethargy, anorexia, vomiting, and weight loss in association with splenomegaly, hepatomegaly, pallor, and, occasionally, detectable cutaneous masses. The CBC in affected dogs commonly reveals cytopenias, with or without circulating mast cells.

MCTs can release bioactive substances that may cause edema, erythema, or bruising of the affected area. Gastrointestinal tract ulceration may also occur as a result of hyperhistaminemia (approximately 80% of dogs euthanized because of advanced MCTs have gastroduodenal ulceration). Therefore any dog with an MCT should undergo occult fecal blood testing. Profuse intraoperative and postoperative bleeding and delayed wound healing occur in some dogs as a consequence of the bioactive substances released from mast cells.

## Diagnosis

The evaluation of a dog with a suspected MCT should include FNA of the affected area. MCTs are extremely easy to diagnose cytologically. They consist of a monomorphic population of round cells with prominent intracytoplasmic purple granules; eosinophils are frequently present in the smear (see Fig. 77-6). In approximately one-third of MCTs, the granules do not stain with Diff-Quik; hence, if agranular round cells are found in a dermal or subcutaneous mass resembling an MCT, the clinician should stain the slide with Giemsa or Wright's stain to reveal the characteristic purple granules. A cytologic diagnosis of MCT allows the clinician to discuss treatment options with the owner and to plan therapeutic strategies (see the section on Treatment and Prognosis).

Although clinical pathologists will frequently state the degree of differentiation of the cells in a cytologic specimen of an MCT, that scheme does not necessarily correlate with the histopathologic grading system. In other words, a cytologic diagnosis of a well-differentiated MCT does not necessarily imply that it will be a grade 1 tumor when evaluated histopathologically (i.e., cytologic grading may not have the same prognostic implications as histopathologic grading).

The clinical evaluation of a dog with a cytologically confirmed MCT should include careful palpation of the affected area and its draining lymph nodes; abdominal palpation, radiography, or ultrasonography to search for hepatosplenomegaly; a CBC, serum biochemistry profile, and urinalysis; and thoracic radiography if the neoplasm is in the anterior one-half of the body (i.e., to detect intrathoracic lymphadenopathy). If lymphadenopathy, hepatomegaly, or splenomegaly is present, FNA of the enlarged lymph node or organ should be performed to detect mast cells (i.e., local neoplasm versus metastatic tumor versus SMCD).

The use of a buffy coat smear to search for circulating mast cells is controversial. It was thought that the presence of mast cells in a buffy coat smear indicated systemic dissemination and therefore a poor prognosis. However, dogs with a solitary, potentially curable MCT occasionally have low numbers of circulating mast cells that disappear from circulation shortly after the primary tumor is excised or irradiated. Moreover, a recent study revealed that circulating mast cells are more common in dogs with diseases other than MCTs; over 95% of the CBCs with circulating mast cells were from dogs with inflammatory disorders, regenerative anemia, tumors other than MCTs, and trauma (McManus, 1999). Also, dogs with MCT had significantly lower circulating mast cell counts (71 per buffy coat smear) than those with other diseases (276 per buffy coat smear). Cytologic evaluation of a bone marrow aspirate may therefore be more beneficial for staging purposes. Dogs with more than five mast cells per 500 nucleated cells are believed to have SMCD; however, bone marrow mast cells have also been documented to disappear after excision or irradiation of the primary tumor. Therefore there is disagreement as to the appropriate staging procedures in dogs with MCTs. At our clinic we do not use buffy coat smears or bone marrow aspirates routinely in dogs with MCT and a normal CBC; if cytopenias or leukoerythroblastic reactions are present, we perform a bone marrow aspirate.

As discussed previously, all dogs with MCTs should be tested for occult blood in the stool even if melena is not evident. There are several kits for this purpose (see p. 367). The presence of blood in the stool is suggestive of upper gastrointestinal tract bleeding. If this is found on repeat testing, the dog should be treated with $H_2$ antihistamines (i.e., famotidine, ranitidine) with or without a coating agent (i.e., sucralfate) (see Chapter 30). Once this clinical information is obtained, the tumor should be staged to determine the extent of disease (Table 84-2).

## Treatment and Prognosis

As discussed previously, it is imperative to know whether the mass the clinician is preparing to excise is an MCT, because this information is useful when discussing treatment options with the client and when planning the treatment strategy. Dogs with MCT can be treated with surgery, radiotherapy, or chemotherapy or a combination of these. However, the first two treatment options are potentially curative, whereas chemotherapy is usually only palliative. Treatment guidelines are provided in Table 84-3.

A solitary MCT in an area in which complete surgical excision is feasible should be removed by aggressive en bloc resection (i.e., 3 to 5 cm margins around and underneath the tumor). If a complete excision is obtained (according to the pathologist evaluating the specimen), the tumor is grade 1 or 2, and no metastatic lesions are present, there is usually no need for further treatment (i.e., the dog is most likely cured). If the excision appears incomplete, the clinician can take one of two courses of action: (1) perform a second surgery in an attempt to excise the remaining tumor (the excised area should be submitted for histopathologic evaluation to assess the completeness of excision); or (2) irradiate the surgical site (35 to 40 Gy delivered in 10 to 12 fractions). Both options appear to be equally effective, resulting in approximately 80% probability of long-term survival.

A solitary MCT in an area in which surgical excision is difficult or impossible, or at a site where the cosmetic or functional results are unacceptable (e.g., prepuce, eyelid), can be successfully treated with radiotherapy. Approximately two-thirds of dogs with a grade 1 or 2 localized MCT treated with radiotherapy alone are cured. Irradiation is also recommended for the management of tumors in "high-risk" areas. Intralesional injections of corticosteroids (triamcinolone [Vetalog], 1 mg intralesionally per centimeter of tumor diameter every 2 to 3 weeks) can also successfully shrink the tumor (although it is usually only palliative). Intralesional injections of deionized water have also been reported to be beneficial in managing local MCTs.

Once metastatic or disseminated MCTs (or SMCD) develop, a cure is rarely obtained. Treatment in these dogs consists of chemotherapy and supportive therapy and is aimed at palliating the neoplasm and its complications. Results of prospective studies of chemotherapy in dogs with MCTs have not been very encouraging; two chemotherapy protocols have been widely used (see table on Cancer Chemotherapy Protocols, p. 1154): (1) prednisone and (2) the CVP protocol (cyclophosphamide, prednisone, vinblastine). Over the past 2 years, lomustine (CCNU) has been used with a high degree of success in dogs with nonresectable, metastatic, or systemic MCTs. The probability of response is high (>50%), and we have documented remissions in excess of 18 months in dogs with metastatic grade 2 and 3 MCTs.

Traditionally, I used prednisone (see Table 84-3), with or without famotidine and/or sucralfate, in dogs with metastatic or nonresectable MCTs. Over the past 2 years I have added lomustine (CCNU) to the treatment protocol (see Table

## TABLE 84-2

**Clinical Staging Scheme for Dogs with Mast Cell Tumors**

| STAGE | DESCRIPTION |
|---|---|
| I | One tumor confined to the dermis without regional lymph node involvement<br>a. Without systemic signs<br>b. With systemic signs |
| II | One tumor confined to the dermis with regional lymph node involvement<br>a. Without systemic signs<br>b. With systemic signs |
| III | Multiple dermal tumors or a large infiltrating tumor with or without regional lymph node involvement<br>a. Without systemic signs<br>b. With systemic signs |
| IV | Any tumor with distant metastases or recurrence with metastases<br>a. Without systemic signs<br>b. With systemic signs |

## TABLE 84-3

**Treatment Guidelines for Dogs with Mast Cell Tumors**

| STAGE | GRADE | RECOMMENDED TREATMENT | FOLLOW-UP |
|---|---|---|---|
| I | 1, 2 | Surgical excision | Complete → observe<br>Incomplete → second surgery or radiotherapy |
| I | 3 | Chemotherapy* | Continue chemotherapy |
| II | 1, 2, 3 | Surgical excision or radiotherapy | CCNU and prednisone (see below)* |
| III, IV | 1, 2, 3 | Chemotherapy* | Continue chemotherapy |

*Prednisone, 50 mg/m² by mouth (PO) q24h for 1 week; then 20-25 mg/m² PO q48h indefinitely plus lomustine (CCNU, Ceenu), 60-90 mg/m² PO q3wk.

84-3), with extremely good results. Although lomustine is potentially myelosuppressive, clinically relevant cytopenias are extremely rare; however, a potential complication of lomustine therapy is hepatotoxicity (see Chapter 80), so chemistry profiles should be evaluated periodically.

I reserve CVP chemotherapy for patients that do not respond to the prednisone/lomustine combination. During CVP treatment, dogs should be monitored for the development of myelosuppression, as discussed on p. 1108. Chemotherapy should be continued indefinitely (i.e., until death or tumor relapse). Given the risk of sterile hemorrhagic cystitis developing in dogs receiving CVP, chlorambucil (Leukeran) should be substituted for cyclophosphamide after 8 to 12 weeks of treatment (see Chapter 80).

## MAST CELL TUMORS IN CATS

### Etiology and Epidemiology

Although MCTs are relatively common in cats, they rarely result in the considerable clinical problems seen in dogs with this neoplasm. Most cats with MCTs are middle-aged or older (median, 10 years old), there is apparently no gender-related predilection, and Siamese cats may be at high risk. Feline leukemia virus and feline immunodeficiency virus do not play a role in the development of this tumor.

As opposed to the dog, in which most of the MCTs are cutaneous or subcutaneous, there are two main forms of feline MCTs: visceral and cutaneous. There is controversy as to whether cutaneous forms are more common than visceral forms and whether both forms can coexist in the same cat. At our clinic the cutaneous form is considerably more common than the visceral form, and it is extremely rare for the cutaneous and visceral forms to coexist.

### Clinical and Pathologic Features

Visceral MCTs are characterized by either hemolymphatic or intestinal involvement. Cats with hemolymphatic disease are classified as having SMCD (or mast cell leukemia), because the bone marrow, spleen, liver, and blood are commonly involved. Most cats initially have nonspecific signs, such as anorexia and vomiting; abdominal distention caused by massive splenomegaly is a consistent feature. As in dogs, the hematologic abnormalities in cats with SMCD are extremely variable and include cytopenias, mastocythemia, basophilia, or eosinophilia, or a combination of these; however, a high percentage of cats may have normal CBCs. Cats with the intestinal form of SMCD usually are evaluated because of gastrointestinal signs such as anorexia, vomiting, or diarrhea. Abdominal masses are palpated in approximately one-half of these cats. Most tumors involve the small intestine, where they can be solitary or multiple. Metastatic disease affecting the mesenteric lymph nodes, liver, spleen, and lungs is commonly found at the time of presentation. Multiple intestinal masses in cats are most commonly associated with lymphoma and with MCT, although both neoplasms can coexist. Gastrointestinal tract ulceration has also been documented in affected cats.

Cats with cutaneous MCTs usually initially have solitary or multiple, small (2 to 15 mm), white to pink, dermoepidermal masses primarily in the head and neck regions, although solitary dermoepidermal or subcutaneous masses also occur in other locations. It has been reported that, on the basis of the clinical, epidemiologic, and histologic features, MCTs in cats can be classified as either mast cell–type MCTs (common) or histiocytic-type MCTs (rare). Cats with mast cell–type MCTs are usually more than 4 years of age and have solitary dermal masses; there is no apparent breed predilection. Cats with histiocytic-type MCTs are primarily Siamese cats under 4 years of age. Typically such cats have multiple (miliary) subcutaneous masses that exhibit a benign biologic behavior. Some of these neoplasms appear to regress spontaneously. We have never seen the histiocytic type of disease in cats treated at our clinic, even in Siamese cats with multiple dermoepidermal nodules. The subcutaneous MCTs commonly seen in dogs are extremely rare in cats. Unlike the situation in dogs, the histopathologic grade does not appear to correlate well with the biologic behavior of MCTs in cats (Molander-McCrary and colleagues, 1998).

### Diagnosis and Treatment

The diagnostic approach to cats with MCT is similar to that in dogs. As in dogs, some mast cells in cats are poorly granulated and the granules may not be easily identified during a routine cytologic or histopathologic evaluation.

The treatment for cats with MCTs is controversial. As a general rule, surgery is indicated for cats with a solitary cutaneous mass, for cats with two to five skin masses, and for cats with intestinal or splenic involvement. As discussed above, cutaneous MCTs in cats are less aggressive than in dogs, and in a large proportion of cats, removal of a solitary dermoepidermal MCT using a biopsy punch is curative; the same applies to cats with fewer than five dermoepidermal MCTs. The combination of splenectomy, prednisone, and chloramibucid (leukeran) treatment is recommended for cats with SMCD, in which survival times in excess of approximately 1 year are common; splenectomy alone does not result in prolonged survival. Surgical excision and prednisone treatment are recommended for cats with intestinal MCT. Prednisone alone (4 to 8 mg/kg PO q24-48h) may also be beneficial for cats with systemic or metastatic MCTs. Cats with multiple skin MCTs are best treated with prednisone, in the dosage just given. Although radiotherapy is as effective in cats as in dogs, it is rarely necessary in cats with this neoplasm. When an additional chemotherapeutic agent is needed in cats with MCTs, I usually use chlorambucil (Leukeran, 20 mg/m² PO q2wk); this drug seems to be quite effective and well-tolerated. In my limited experience, lomustine (CCNU) is not very effective in cats with MCTs.

## OROPHARYNGEAL NEOPLASMS IN DOGS AND CATS

Oropharyngeal neoplasms are common in dogs and cats, constituting approximately 5% of all malignancies. Most oropharyngeal neoplasms in dogs and cats are malignant, and most animals are evaluated because of halitosis, dysphagia, drooling, or pain; facial swelling is occasionally present. Given the differences in the clinical presentation, biologic behavior, and treatment of these tumors in dogs and cats, they are discussed separately. Treatment recommendations are also given in Chapter 78 and on p. 1154.

## OROPHARYNGEAL NEOPLASMS IN DOGS

There are four tumor types commonly found in the oropharyngeal cavity of dogs: malignant melanoma (MM), fibrosarcoma (FSA), squamous cell carcinoma (SCC), and epulides. MMs, FSAs, SCCs, and the acanthomatous epulides are malignant; the fibromatous and ossifying epulides are benign. MM, FSA, and SCC each constitute approximately 30% of all the oropharyngeal tumors; male dogs appear to be at high risk. Most oropharyngeal tumors in this species are predominantly treated with surgery, although radiotherapy is beneficial in some cases (see later discussion).

### Malignant Melanoma

MM is the most common oropharyngeal neoplasm noted in some studies and is most prevalent in middle-aged to older dogs with pigmented oral mucous membranes; males may be at increased risk. Typically these lesions are pigmented, glistening, solitary masses. They can occur anywhere in the oropharynx, but the gingiva and buccal or labial mucosae are the most common sites. Frequently MMs are nonpigmented or only partially pigmented. Given their aggressive biologic behavior, bone invasion and metastatic lesions are commonly found at the time of presentation. Bone invasion occurs in approximately two-thirds of dogs, and metastatic lesions in the regional lymph nodes or lungs or both are present in approximately one-half of the dogs. Most dogs with melanoma die as a result of recurrence or metastatic disease.

### Fibrosarcoma

FSAs are the second or third most common oropharyngeal neoplasm in most studies and occur predominantly in younger dogs (i.e., 2 to 6 years old); Golden Retrievers and Doberman Pinschers are at high risk for this neoplasm, and males are more frequently affected. The lesions are usually pink, sessile, fleshy, firm solitary masses in the gingiva or palate that deeply infiltrate the soft tissues and bone. In contrast to MMs, most FSAs are only locally invasive and have a low metastatic potential (<10% of dogs have metastatic lesions at presentation). Therefore complete surgical excision is usually curative (see the section on Treatment and Prognosis).

### Squamous Cell Carcinoma

SCCs represent the second or third most common oropharyngeal neoplasm in most series, and they occur predominantly in middle-aged to older dogs. They are either sessile, fleshy, friable masses or, more commonly, progressively ulcerative and infiltrative lesions (usually invading bone). Regional lymphadenopathy is common in affected dogs, although it is frequently caused by hyperplasia rather than by

metastatic disease. The biologic behavior of these tumors depends on the location. Most tumors in the rostral oropharynx are locally invasive and have a low metastatic potential, whereas most tumors in the caudal oropharyngeal cavity (e.g., tonsils, base of the tongue, soft palate, pharynx) display extremely rapid infiltrative and metastatic behaviors.

### Epulides

Epulides are usually benign fleshy tumors of the gingiva. Of the three histologic types, fibromatous and ossifying epulides are benign and thus can be cured by conservative surgery; acanthomatous epulides are locally invasive tumors that, if left untreated, can cause severe facial distortion and mechanically interfere with mastication. Acanthomatous epulides are common in the rostral mandibular or premaxillary gingiva of middle-aged to older female dogs; they are pink, sessile, fleshy masses that are deeply invasive (bone lysis by the tumor is common).

## OROPHARYNGEAL NEOPLASMS IN CATS

Most oropharyngeal tumors in cats are malignant; they consist primarily of SCCs (three-fourths) and FSAs (less than one-fourth). The gross morphologic features and biologic behavior of these neoplasms are similar to those in dogs (i.e., most SCCs are ulcerative, whereas most FSAs are proliferative). Bone invasion mimicking a primary bone tumor is common in cats with mandibular SCCs. Given cats' finicky eating behavior when ill, most patients with large oral tumors are malnourished at the time of presentation. Thus, in addition to tumor treatment, it is vital to provide nutritional support, with feeding done through a nasogastric tube or a percutaneous gastrostomy tube.

## APPROACH TO DOGS AND CATS WITH AN OROPHARYNGEAL MASS

As discussed previously, most cats and dogs with oropharyngeal tumors are evaluated because of halitosis, dysphagia, pain, or a facial deformity. The halitosis is usually caused by secondary anaerobic bacterial infection of the neoplasm and can be successfully eliminated by treatment with antibacterial agents such as clindamycin (5 mg/kg PO q12h) or metronidazole (20 to 25 mg/kg PO q12h) before a definitive treatment for the neoplasm is instituted.

Once an oropharyngeal mass or ulcer has been identified (frequently during dental care), a biopsy specimen should be obtained before a definitive treatment is instituted. It is extremely valuable to know the tumor type before one discusses the treatment options with the owner. For example, aggressive surgery (e.g., mandibulectomy or maxillectomy) is as effective as radiotherapy in dogs with an infiltrative acanthomatous epulis, although radiotherapy may be more acceptable to some owners who cannot cope with the potentially unacceptable cosmetic results of aggressive surgery.

FNAs for cytologic studies are not a very reliable diagnostic tool in dogs and cats with oral neoplasms, since they are frequently contaminated (i.e., there is an abundance of inflammatory cells) and some of these tumors do not yield cells easily. However, FNA of an enlarged regional lymph node should always be performed to rule out metastatic disease. Thoracic radiographs should also be obtained to search for pulmonary metastases. With the animal under general anesthesia, radiographs or a CT scan of the affected area should be obtained to determine the extent of bone involvement and thus plan a specific treatment. The radiographs or CT scan of the lesion is usually obtained at the time the biopsy is performed.

## Treatment and Prognosis

**Surgery.** The treatment of choice for patients with localized oropharyngeal tumors without metastases is aggressive surgical excision. Surgical excision is also indicated as a palliative measure in dogs with metastatic lesions. With the advent of maxillectomies and mandibulectomies almost two decades ago, a large proportion of dogs with tumors that would previously have been nonresectable can now be cured. These procedures are indicated for dogs and cats with oropharyngeal malignancies, because, given the high prevalence of bone invasion, these tumors can rarely be eliminated by a conservative procedure (i.e., "shaving off the tumor with a cautery knife"). The cosmetic and functional outcomes are usually well received by the clients; however, in my experience, these aggressive oral surgeries are better tolerated by dogs than by cats. In general, aggressive surgery is curative if a complete excision can be obtained during the first procedure (provided there are no metastatic lesions). One-year survival rates in dogs that undergo surgery alone are approximately 25% to 40% in those with FSAs and 20% to 25% in those with MMs. (See Suggested Readings for a description of the techniques and the results.)

**Radiotherapy.** Radiotherapy can be used successfully in some dogs and cats with oropharyngeal SCCs (e.g., those with a small gingival mass) and is usually curative in dogs with acanthomatous epulides. A second tumor may develop at the irradiated site (usually an SCC) in as many as 20% of such dogs cured with orthovoltage irradiation. Survival times in dogs with SCCs in the rostral oral cavity treated with radiotherapy are considerably better than those in dogs with SCCs involving the tonsils or tongue. More than one-half of the dogs in the former group may be cured with radiotherapy. Median survival times in dogs with tonsillar or lingual SCCs treated with surgery or radiotherapy are approximately 3 to 4 months.

Local control of SCCs in cats is rarely achieved using either surgery or radiotherapy; most cats die within 4 months of diagnosis, with less than 10% alive at 1 year. FSAs and MMs are typically considered radioresistant. However, radiotherapy in combination with hyperthermia provides long-term local control in more than one-half of the dogs with FSA so treated; it also provides long-term local control when combined with surgery. Response rates of more than 50% have been observed in dogs with MM of the oropharynx treated using recently introduced protocols of coarse fractionation.

**Chemotherapy.** As discussed in previous paragraphs, most oropharyngeal neoplasms are local diseases that may be cured with either surgery or radiotherapy. However, chemotherapy may be beneficial in some dogs and cats. Dogs with incompletely excised, nonresectable, or metastatic FSAs of a high to intermediate histologic grade may benefit from a combination of doxorubicin (Adriamycin, 30 mg/m² or 1 mg/kg for dogs <10 kg given IV q3wk) and dacarbazine (DTIC, 1 g/m² given as an IV drip over 8 hours immediately after the doxorubicin). Chemotherapy is rarely beneficial in dogs with SCCs or MMs. Various single-agent and combination protocols have been used in dogs with SCCs, but the results have been disappointing. In cats, a combination of mitoxantrone (Novantrone, 4 to 6 mg/m² IV q3wk) and cyclophosphamide (Cytoxan, 200 to 300 mg/m² PO 10 days after the mitoxantrone) or single-agent carboplatin (Paraplatin, 240 to 280 mg/m² IV q3wk) may be of benefit.

Single-agent dacarbazine (DTIC, 1 g/m² as an IV drip delivered over 8 hours and repeated q3wk), cisplatin (Platinol, 70 mg/m² as an IV drip q3wk), or carboplatin (Paraplatin, 300 mg/m² IV q3wk) may be beneficial in up to 10% of dogs with nonresectable or metastatic MM. A combination of radiotherapy, doxorubicin (30 mg/m² or 1 mg/kg for dogs <10 kg IV on day 1), and cisplatin (60 mg/m² IV on day 8), repeated every 3 weeks, has yielded promising preliminary results in dogs with tonsillar SCCs. For additional chemotherapy protocols see p. 1153.

## INJECTION SITE SARCOMAS IN CATS

An association between injections/vaccination and the development of sarcomas has been recently recognized in cats, and epidemiologic studies have confirmed the association. In this syndrome, FSA (or occasionally other types of sarcomas) develops in the subcutis or muscle or both of the interscapular region or the thigh, common sites of injection/vaccination. It is estimated that a sarcoma develops in one to two of 10,000 vaccinated cats. Although the exact pathogenesis is still unclear, both the adjuvants and the local immune response against the antigens have been implicated as causative agents.

A rapidly growing soft tissue mass develops in the region weeks to months after vaccination or injection in cats with injection site sarcomas (ISSs). A vaccine- or injection-associated inflammatory reaction may precede the development of this neoplasm. Therefore an ISS should be suspected in any cat with a superficial or deep mass in the interscapular or thigh regions, and every effort should be made to establish a diagnosis immediately. Although FNA findings may provide a definitive answer, more often a surgical biopsy is necessary, because sarcomas do not consistently exfoliate cells (see Chapter 77).

Although most FSAs in dogs and cats have a low metastatic potential, ISSs are quite aggressive and should be treated accordingly. Although studies are currently in progress, based on the results of studies reported in the literature and on the findings in cats seen at our clinic, the rate of metastasis of ISSs is high (probably as high as 50% to 70%). Pulmonary metastatic lesions can be detected at presentation in a high proportion of cats; we have also seen ocular metastases as the main presenting feature in a few cats with ISSs.

The treatment of choice for cats with ISS is aggressive surgical excision (see Chapter 78). Based on the maxim "cut it once, but cut it all," an en bloc resection (to include any biopsy tracts) should be performed immediately after the diagnosis is established, provided there is no metastatic disease. In a recent study, cats treated with aggressive surgery had significantly longer disease-free survival than cats treated with conservative surgery (274 versus 66 days); also, cats with tumors in the limbs had significantly longer disease-free survival than cats with tumors in the trunk (325 versus 66 days; Hershey and colleagues, 2000). Complete surgical excision of a relatively small ISS (i.e., <2 cm in diameter) is usually associated with long-term remissions. Although the role of postoperative adjuvant chemotherapy has not been thoroughly evaluated, cats with large or incompletely excised tumors may benefit from treatment with mitoxantrone and cyclophosphamide, doxorubicin and cyclophosphamide, or carboplatin (see the section on Approach to Dogs and Cats with an Oropharyngeal Mass). We have seen objective complete or partial responses in cats with nonresectable or metastatic ISS treated with doxorubicin/cyclophosphamide combinations or with carboplatin alone; some of these cats have been in remission for more than 1 year. If metastatic disease is already present, chemotherapy is not usually effective.

To obtain more information about this emerging disorder, a task force has been created and specific guidelines for vaccination sites have been developed (visit the website at http://www.vin.com/mainpub/feline/vaccines/fpvacmain.htm).

## Suggested Readings

Barber L et al: Combined doxorubicin and cyclophosphamide chemotherapy for nonresectable feline fibrosarcoma, *J Am Anim Hosp Assoc* 36:416, 2000.

Bateman KE et al: 0-7-21 Radiation therapy for the treatment of canine oral melanoma, *J Vet Intern Med* 8:267, 1994.

Birchard S et al: Aggressive surgery for the management of oral neoplasia, *Vet Clin North Am* 20:1117, 1989.

Blackwood L et al: Radiotherapy of oral malignant melanomas in dogs, *J Am Vet Med Assoc* 209:98, 1996.

Brown NO et al: Canine hemangiosarcoma: retrospective analysis of 104 cases, *J Am Vet Med Assoc* 186:56, 1985.

Clifford CA et al: Treatment of canine hemangiosarcoma: 2000 and beyond, *J Vet Intern Med* 14:479, 2000.

Couto CG: Oncology. In Sherding RG, editor: *The cat—diseases and management*, New York, 1988, Churchill Livingstone, p 589.

Couto CG et al: Review of treatment options for vaccine-associated feline sarcoma. In Vaccine-Associated Feline Sarcoma Symposium, *J Am Vet Med Assoc* 213:1426, 1998.

Esplin DG et al: Postvaccination sarcomas in cats, *J Am Vet Med Assoc* 202:1245, 1992.

Hammer AS et al: Efficacy and toxicity of VAC chemotherapy (vincristine, doxorubicin, and cyclophosphamide) in dogs with hemangiosarcoma, *J Vet Intern Med* 5:16, 1991a.

Hammer AS et al: Hemostatic abnormalities in dogs with hemangiosarcoma, *J Vet Intern Med* 5:11, 1991b.

Hershey AE et al: Prognosis for presumed feline vaccine-associated sarcoma after excision: 61 cases (1986-1996), *J Am Vet Med Assoc* 216:58, 2000.

Kass PH et al: Epidemiologic evidence for a causal relation between vaccination and fibrosarcoma tumorigenesis in cats, *J Am Vet Med Assoc* 203:396, 1993.

LaRue SM et al: Limb-sparing treatment for osteosarcoma in dogs, *J Am Vet Med Assoc* 195:1734, 1989.

Lester S et al: Vaccine-site associated sarcomas in cats: clinical experience and a laboratory review (1982-1993), *J Am Anim Hosp Assoc* 32:91, 1996.

Macy DW et al: Vaccine-associated sarcomas in cats, *Feline Pract* 23:24, 1995.

Macy DW et al: Mast cell tumor. In Withrow SJ et al, editors: *Clinical veterinary oncology*, Philadelphia, 1989, JB Lippincott.

McManus PM: Frequency and severity of mastocythemia in dogs with and without mast cell tumors: 120 cases (1995-1997), *J Am Vet Med Assoc* 215:355, 1999.

Molander-McCrary H et al: Cutaneous mast cell tumors in cats: 32 cases (1991-1994), *J Am Anim Hosp Assoc* 34:281, 1998.

O'Brien MG et al: Resection of pulmonary metastases in canine osteosarcoma: 36 cases, *Vet Surg* 22:105, 1993.

Ogilvie GK et al: Surgery and doxorubicin in dogs with hemangiosarcoma, *J Vet Intern Med* 10:379, 1996.

O'Keefe DA: Canine mast cell tumors, *Vet Clin North Am* 20:1105, 1990.

Prymak C et al: Epidemiologic, clinical, pathologic, and prognostic characteristics of splenic hemangiosarcoma and splenic hematomas in dogs: 217 cases (1985), *J Am Vet Med Assoc* 193:706, 1988.

Rassnik KM et al: Treatment of canine mast cell tumors with CCNU (lomustine), *J Vet Intern Med* 13:601, 1999.

Russell WO et al: A clinical and pathologic system for soft tissue sarcomas, *Cancer* 40:1562, 1977.

Salisbury SK et al: Long-term results of partial mandibulectomy for the treatment of oral tumors in 30 dogs, *J Am Anim Hosp Assoc* 24:285, 1988.

Sorenmo KU et al: Chemotherapy of canine hemangiosarcoma with doxorubicin and cyclophosphamide, *J Vet Intern Med* 7:370, 1993.

Sorenmo KU et al: Canine hemangiosarcoma treated with standard chemotherapy and minocycline, *J Vet Intern Med* 14:395, 2000.

Turrel JM et al: Prognostic factors for radiation treatment of mast cell tumors in 85 dogs, *J Am Vet Med Assoc* 193:936, 1988.

Vail DM et al: Liposome-encapsulated muramyl tripeptide phosphatidylethanolamine adjuvant immunotherapy for splenic hemangiosarcoma in the dog: a randomized multiinstitutional clinical trial, *Clin Cancer Res* 1:1165, 1995.

Withrow SJ et al: Mandibulectomy in the treatment of oral cancer, *J Am Anim Hosp Assoc* 19:273, 1983.

Cancer Chemotherapy Protocols Commonly Used at The Ohio State University Veterinary Teaching Hospital

I. Lymphoma
   A. Induction of remission
      1. COAP protocol
         Cyclophosphamide (Cytoxan): 50 mg/m$^2$ PO 4 days per week or q48h for 8 weeks in dogs; 200-300 mg/m$^2$ PO q3wk in cats
         Vincristine (Oncovin): 0.5 mg/m$^2$ IV once per week for 8 weeks
         Cytosine arabinoside (Cytosar-U): 100 mg/m$^2$ IV or SQ divided q12h for 4 days
         Prednisone: 40-50 mg/m$^2$ PO q24h for 1 week; then 20-25 mg/m$^2$ PO q48h for 7 weeks
         **In cats, cystosine arabinoside is administered for only 2 days and the remaining three drugs (cyclophosphamide, vincristine, prednisone) are administered for 6 weeks rather than 8 weeks.**
      2. COP protocol
         Cyclophosphamide (Cytoxan): 50 mg/m$^2$ PO 4 days per week or q48h; or 300 mg/m$^2$ PO q3wk*
         Vincristine (Oncovin): 0.5 mg/m$^2$ IV once per week
         Prednisone: 40-50 mg/m$^2$ PO q24h for 1 week; then 20-25 mg/m$^2$ PO q48h
      3. CLOP protocol
         As in COP protocol, but with the addition of L-asparaginase (Elspar) at a dosage of 10,000-20,000 IU/m$^2$ IM q4-6wk
      4. CHOP protocol (21-day cycle)
         Cyclophosphamide (Cytoxan): 200-300 mg/m$^2$ PO on day 10
         Doxorubicin (Adriamycin): 30 mg/m$^2$ IV or 1 mg/kg if <10 kg on day 1
         Vincristine (Oncovin): 0.75 mg/m$^2$ IV on days 8 and 15
         Prednisone: 40-50 mg/m$^2$ PO q24h on days 1-7; then 20-25 mg/m$^2$ PO q48h on days 8-21
         Sulfa-trimethoprim: 15 mg/kg PO q12h
   B. Maintenance
      1. Chlorambucil (Leukeran): 20 mg/m$^2$ PO every other week
         Prednisone: 20-25 mg/m$^2$ PO q48h
      2. LMP protocol: chlorambucil (Leukeran) and prednisone, as above, plus methotrexate; 2.5-5 mg/m$^2$ PO 2 or 3 times per week
      3. Chlorambucil (Leukeran): 20 mg/m$^2$ PO every other week
         Prednisone: 20-25 mg/m$^2$ PO q48h
         Cytosine arabinoside (Cytosar): 200-400 mg/m$^2$ SQ q2wk; alternating with Leukeran
      4. COP protocol used every other week for 6 cycles; then every third week for 6 cycles; then monthly thereafter
   C. "Rescue"
   DOGS
      1. D-MAC protocol (repeat continuously for 10-16 weeks)
         Dexamethasone: 0.5 mg/lb (0.23 mg/kg) PO or SQ on days 1 and 8
         Actinomycin D (Cosmegen): 0.75 mg/m$^2$ IV push on day 1
         Cytosine arabinoside (Cytosar): 200-300 mg/m$^2$ IV drip over 4 hours or SQ on day 1
         Melphalan (Alkeran): 20 mg/m$^2$ PO on day 8 (after 4 doses of melphalan, substitute Leukeran at the same dose)
      2. ADIC protocol
         Doxorubicin (Adriamycin): 30 mg/m$^2$ (or 1 mg/kg if <10 kg) IV q3wk
      3. L-Asparaginase (Elspar): 10,000-30,000 IU/m$^2$ IM q2-3wk
      4. CHOP protocol if second relapse in response to COAP protocol or if good response to Adriamycin was previously observed
   CATS
      1. Cytosine arabinoside (Cytosar-U): 100-200 mg/m$^2$/day IV drip for 1-2 days
         Mitoxantrone (Novantrone): 4 mg/m$^2$ in IV drip, mixed in the bag with the Cytosar
         Dexamethasone: 0.5-1 mg/lb (0.23-0.45 mg/kg) PO weekly; repeat q3wk
II. Acute lymphoid leukemia (ALL)
   COAP, CLOP, or COP protocols

---

*The duration of chemotherapy using this protocol varies.
*PO,* Orally; *IV,* intravenously; *SQ,* subcutaneously.

*Continued*

**Cancer Chemotherapy Protocols Commonly Used at The Ohio State University Veterinary Teaching Hospital—cont'd**

III. Chronic lymphocytic leukemia (CLL)
   1. Chlorambucil (Leukeran): 20 mg/m² PO every other week (with or without prednisone, 20 mg/m² PO q48h)
   2. Cyclophosphamide (Cytoxan): 50 mg/m² PO 4 days per week
      Prednisone: 20 mg/m² PO q48h
IV. Acute myelogenous leukemia
   1. Cytosine arabinoside (Cytosar-U): 100 mg/m²/day IV drip or SQ (divided q12h) for 4 days
      6-Thioguanine (6-TG): 40-50 mg/m² PO q24h or q48h
   2. Cytosar and 6-TG plus Adriamycin (10 mg/m² IV on days 2 and 4 of the cycle)
   3. Cytosine arabinoside (Cytosar-U): 100-200 mg/m²/day IV drip for 1-2 days
      Mitoxantrone (Novantrone): 4 mg/m² IV drip, mixed in the bag with the Cytosar
      Repeat q3wk
V. Chronic myelogenous leukemia
   1. Hydroxyurea (Hydrea): 50 mg/kg PO q24-48h until normal white blood count
VI. Multiple myeloma
   1. Melphalan (Alkeran): 2-4 mg/m² PO q24h for 1 week; then q48h
      Prednisone: 40-50 mg/m² PO q24h for 1 week, then 20 mg/m² PO q48h. Can also be given at 6-8 mg/m² PO
         for 5 days, repeating every 21 days
   2. As in III.2
VII. Mast cell tumors (systemic)
   1. Prednisone: 40-50 mg/m² PO q24h for 1 week; then 20-25 mg/m² PO q48h
   2. Lomustine (CCNU): 60-90 mg/m² PO q3wks (with or without prednisone as in 1)
   3. CVP protocol
      Vinblastine (Velban): 2 mg/m² IV once per week
      Cyclophosphamide (Cytoxan): 50 mg/m² PO q48h or 4 days per week
      Prednisone: 20-25 mg/m² PO q48h
VIII. Soft-tissue sarcomas—dogs
   1. ADIC protocol
      Doxorubicin (Adriamycin): 30 mg/m² IV (or 1 mg/kg if <10 kg) q3wk
      DTIC (dacarbazine): 700-1000 mg/m² IV drip for 6-8 hours; repeat q21 days
      Sulfa-trimethoprim: 15 mg/kg PO q48h q3wk
   2. VAC protocol (21-day cycle)
      Vincristine (Oncovin): 0.75 mg/m² IV on days 8 and 15
      Doxorubicin (Adriamycin): 30 mg/m² IV (or 1 mg/kg if <10 kg) on day 1
      Cyclophosphamide (Cytoxan): 200-300 mg/m² PO on day 10
      Sulfa-trimethoprim: 15 mg/kg PO q12h
IX. Soft-tissue sarcomas—cats
   1. AC protocol (21 day cycle)
      Doxorubicin (Adriamycin): 1 mg/kg IV on day 1
      Cyclophosphamide (Cytoxan): 200-300 mg/m² on day 10.
   2. VAC protocol (28-day cycle)
      Vincristine (Oncovin): 0.5 mg/m² IV on days 8, 15, and 22
      Doxorubicin (Adriamycin): 1 mg/kg IV on day 1
      Cyclophosphamide (Cytoxan): 200-300 mg/m² on day 10
   3. MiC protocol (21-day cycle)
      Mitoxantrone (Novantrone): 4-6 mg/m² in IV drip over 4 hours on day 1
      Cyclophosphamide (Cytoxan): 200-300 mg/m² PO on day 10

**Cancer Chemotherapy Protocols Commonly Used at The Ohio State University Veterinary Teaching Hospital—cont'd**

    4. MiCO protocol (21-day cycle)
       Mitoxantrone (Novantrone): 4-6 mg/m$^2$ in IV drip over 4 hours on day 1
       Cyclophosphamide (Cytoxan): 200-300 mg/m$^2$ PO on day 10
       Vincristine (Oncovin): 0.5-0.6 mg/m$^2$ IV on days 8 and 15
    5. Carboplatin (Paraplatin): 200-280 mg/m$^2$ IV q3wk

X. Osteosarcoma—dogs
    1. Cisplatin (Platinol): 50-70 mg/m$^2$ in IV drip q3wk. Prior intensive diuresis is required (see Table 84-1).
    2. Carboplatin (Paraplatin): 300 mg/m$^2$ IV q3wk
    3. Doxorubicin (Adriamycin): 30 mg/m$^2$ IV q2wk for 6 doses
    4. Doxorubicin and carboplatin as above, alternating drugs q3wks for 2-3 doses each

XI. Carcinomas—dogs
    1. CMF protocol
       5-Fluorouracil (5-FU): 150 mg/m$^2$ IV once per week
       Cyclophosphamide (Cytoxan): 50 mg/m$^2$ PO 4 days per week or q48h
       Methotrexate 2.5 mg/m$^2$ PO 2.3/week
    2. FAC protocol
       5-Fluorouracil (5-FU): 150 mg/m$^2$ IV on days 8 and 15
       Doxorubicin (Adriamycin): 30 mg/m$^2$ (or 1 mg/kg if <10 kg) IV on day 1
       Cyclophosphamide (Cytoxan): 200-300 mg/m$^2$ PO on day 10
       Sulfa-trimethoprim: 15 mg/kg PO q12h
    3. VAF protocol
       Vincristine (Oncovin): 0.75 mg/m$^2$ IV on days 8 and 15
       Doxorubicin (Adriamycin): 30 mg/m$^2$ (or 1 mg/kg if <10 kg) IV on day 1
       5-Fluorouracil (5-FU): 150 mg/m$^2$ IV on days 1, 8, and 15
    4. VAC protocol
    5. Cisplatin (Platinol): 70 mg/m$^2$ in IV drip q3wk. Prior intensive diuresis is required (see Table 84-1).

XII. Carcinomas—cats
    **5-Fluorouracil is toxic for the cat, producing severe, and often fatal, CNS signs. Cisplatin is also extremely toxic, causing acute pulmonary toxicity in this species.**
    1. Carboplatin (Paraplatin): 200-280 mg/m$^2$ IV q3wk
    2. AC protocol (21-day cycle)
       Doxorubicin (Adriamycin): 1 mg/kg IV on day 1
       Cyclophosphamide (Cytoxan): 200-300 mg/m$^2$ PO on day 10
    3. VAC protocol (28-day cycle)
       Vincristine (Oncovin): 0.5 mg/m$^2$ on days 8, 15, and 22
       Doxorubicin (Adriamycin): 1 mg/kg IV on day 1
       Cyclophosphamide (Cytoxan): 200-300 mg/m$^2$ on day 10
    4. MiC protocol (21-day cycle)
       Mitoxantrone (Novantrone): 4-6 mg/m$^2$ IV drip over 4 hours on day 1
       Cyclophosphamide (Cytoxan): 200-300 mg/m$^2$ PO on day 10
    5. MiCO protocol (21-day cycle)
       Mitoxantrone (Novantrone): 4-6 mg/m$^2$ IV drip over 4 hours on day 1
       Cyclophosphamide (Cytoxan): 200-300 mg/m$^2$ PO on day 10
       Vincristine (Oncovin): 0.5-0.6 mg/m$^2$ IV on days 8 and 15

# CHAPTER 85

# Anemia

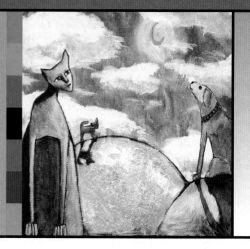

## CHAPTER OUTLINE

DEFINITION, 1156
CLINICAL AND CLINICOPATHOLOGIC
EVALUATION, 1156
PRINCIPLES OF MANAGEMENT OF THE ANEMIC
PATIENT, 1160
REGENERATIVE ANEMIAS, 1160
   Blood loss anemia, 1160
   Hemolytic anemia, 1160
NONREGENERATIVE ANEMIAS, 1164
   Anemia of chronic disease, 1165
   Bone marrow disorders, 1165
   Anemia of renal disease, 1166
   Acute and peracute blood loss or hemolysis (first 48
     to 96 hours), 1167
SEMIREGENERATIVE ANEMIAS, 1167
   Iron deficiency anemia, 1167
PRINCIPLES OF TRANSFUSION THERAPY, 1168
   Blood groups, 1168
   Crossmatching and blood typing, 1168
   Blood administration, 1168
   Complications of transfusion therapy, 1169

## DEFINITION

Anemia is defined as a decrease in the red blood cell (RBC) mass and in practical terms can be defined as a decrease in the packed cell volume (PCV), the hemoglobin (Hb) concentration, or the RBC count below reference values for the species. In special circumstances, anemia is diagnosed in a given animal with a PCV that has decreased over time, even though it may remain within reference values. Because the reference values reflect the actual status in 95% of the feline and canine population, occasionally an "abnormal" value is indeed normal for a particular animal, prompting a needless evaluation in search of other abnormalities. It should be em-phasized that anemia does not constitute a primary diagnosis; therefore every effort should be made to identify its cause.

## CLINICAL AND CLINICOPATHOLOGIC EVALUATION

When interpreting the PCV, Hb concentration, or RBC count, the clinician should keep in mind that in some situations these values are above (e.g., sight hounds) or below (e.g., puppyhood, pregnancy) the reference value for the species. From a practical standpoint, when evaluating the erythroid series, the clinician does not need to assess all the values in the complete blood count (CBC), because several provide identical information. For example, the PCV, Hb concentration, and RBC count provide the same type of information (i.e., an increase in the number of RBCs usually results in an increased PCV and Hb concentration, and vice versa). Thus, when evaluating the erythron in a CBC, the PCV is usually used as an indirect index of the RBC mass (or number).

The main clinical manifestations of anemia in cats and dogs include pale or icteric mucous membranes, lethargy, exercise intolerance, pica (mainly in cats), and decreased over-all activity (Table 85-1). These clinical signs can be acute or chronic and can vary in severity. Owners may also detect some of the adaptive changes to anemia, such as tachycardia or an increased precordial beat. Following are several impor-tant questions to ask the owner of an anemic cat or dog:

- Is the pet currently receiving any medication?—Certain drugs can cause hemolysis, gastrointestinal blood loss, or bone marrow hypoplasia.
- Have the owners detected any blood loss or dark (tarry) stool?—Gastrointestinal tract bleeding from a gastric ulcer or a tumor can lead to iron deficiency anemia (IDA).
- Have the owners noticed any fleas? Severe flea infestation can cause IDA.

## TABLE 85-1

### Clinical Manifestations of Anemia in Cats and Dogs

**History**

1. Family history
2. Exercise intolerance, syncopal episodes
3. Pallor, jaundice
4. Localized or generalized bleeding
5. Feline leukemia virus or immunodeficiency virus infection
6. Malnutrition, malabsorption
7. Chronic inflammation, cancer
8. Travel history

**Physical Examination**

1. Pallor, jaundice, petechiae, ecchymoses
2. Lymphadenopathy
3. Hepatomegaly, splenomegaly
4. Tachycardia, heart murmur, cardiomegaly, left-sided hypertrophy
5. Occult blood in the stool
6. Hematuria

## TABLE 85-2

### Drugs and Toxins that Have Been Associated with Anemia in Cats and Dogs

Acetaminophen
Antiarrhythmics
Anticonvulsants
Antiinflammatories (nonsteroidal)
Barbiturates
Benzocaine
Chemotherapeutic agents
Chloramphenicol
Cimetidine
Gold salts
Griseofulvin
Levamisole
Methimazole
Methionine
Methylene blue
Metronidazole
Penicillins and cephalosporins
Phenothiazines
Propylthiouracil
Propylene glycol
Sulfa derivatives
Vitamin K
Zinc

- Has the cat recently been tested for feline leukemia (FeLV) or immunodeficiency virus (FIV) infections?—Retroviruses can cause bone marrow hypoplasia, myelodysplasia, or leukemias, leading to blood cytopenias.
- Has the owner noticed any ticks on the dog?—Ehrlichiosis can cause bone marrow hypoplasia; babesiosis can cause hemolysis.
- Has the pet been vaccinated recently?—Modified-live vaccines can cause bleeding as a result of platelet dysfunction or thrombocytopenia, or they can be associated with immune-mediated hemolysis.
- Has the bitch received any "shots" for mismating recently?—Estrogen derivatives can cause bone marrow aplasia or hypoplasia.

In addition to these questions, a detailed travel and pharmacologic history should be obtained. Certain infectious diseases associated with anemia have a definitive geographic distribution (e.g., babesiosis in the southeastern part of the United States). Some drugs and toxins that have been associated with anemia in cats and dogs are listed in Table 85-2.

When evaluating a patient with pallor, it should be determined whether the condition is caused by hypoperfusion or by anemia (i.e., not every patient with pale mucous membranes is anemic). The simplest approach to determining this is to evaluate the PCV and the capillary refill time (CRT). Dogs and cats with cardiovascular disease and hypoperfusion usually have normal PCVs and additional clinical signs, whereas symptomatic anemic dogs typically have low PCVs. Occasionally, dogs and cats with congestive heart failure have dilutional anemia caused by intravascular fluid retention. The CRT may be difficult to evaluate in anemic cats and dogs because of the absence of contrast (resulting from pallor).

The clinician should also look for petechiae, ecchymoses, and evidence of deep bleeding in animals with pallor. These findings are suggestive of a platelet or clotting factor deficiency (as seen in animals with Evans's syndrome, disseminated intravascular coagulation [DIC], or acute leukemias; see Chapter 89), resulting in bleeding and secondary anemia. Particular attention should be paid to the lymphoreticular organs, such as the lymph nodes and spleen, because several disorders associated with anemia may also result in lymphadenopathy, hepatosplenomegaly, or both (Table 85-3). Abdominal radiographs in a dog with intravascular hemolysis may show metallic foreign bodies in the stomach, a potential source of zinc that frequently results in RBC lysis.

The degree of anemia may be helpful in establishing its cause. To this end, anemias are graded as follows:

| | **PCV** | |
| | **Dogs** | **Cats** |
|---|---|---|
| Mild | 30%-36% | 20%-24% |
| Moderate | 18%-29% | 15%-19% |
| Severe | <18% | <14% |

For example, if an anemic dog or cat has severe anemia, certain causes (i.e., bleeding, anemia of chronic disease, anemia of renal disease, iron deficiency anemia) can immediately be ruled out because none of those mechanisms are likely to result in such a severe decrease in the PCV; therefore the patient most likely has hemolysis or a bone marrow disorder.

## TABLE 85-3

**Disorders Commonly Associated with Anemia and Hepatomegaly, Splenomegaly, and/or Lymphadenopathy**

| DISORDER | FREQUENCY | SPECIES |
|----------|-----------|---------|
| Lymphoma | F | D, C |
| Hemobartonellosis | F | C > D |
| Acute leukemias | F | C, D |
| Ehrlichiosis | F* | D > C |
| Systemic mast cell disease | R | C > D |
| Bone marrow hypoplasia | R | C, D |
| Immune hemolytic anemia | F | D > C |
| Hypersplenism | R | D, C |

*Geographic variation.
*F,* Frequent; *R,* rare; *D,* dog; *C,* cat.

The severity of the clinical signs usually also correlates with the pathogenesis of the anemia. For example, a dog or cat with severe anemia and mild to moderate clinical signs more likely has a chronic cause of anemia (e.g., bone marrow disease); acute causes of severe anemia (e.g., hemolysis) result in clinical signs of marked severity, because the adaptive compensatory changes have not yet occurred.

As part of the evaluation of a patient's PCV, the plasma should be examined for evidence of icterus or hemolysis and the protein content should be determined with a refractometer. The microhematocrit tube should be carefully inspected for evidence of autoagglutination (see p. 1162), and a slide agglutination test should be performed (see below). It is also helpful to evaluate a blood smear to detect morphologic changes that may point the clinician toward the cause of the anemia.

Once it has been established that the patient is anemic, it should be determined whether the anemia is *regenerative* or *nonregenerative.* This is accomplished either by obtaining a reticulocyte count during a routine CBC or by evaluating a blood smear for the presence of polychromasia. This reflects the pathogenesis of the anemia, thereby dictating the most logical diagnostic and therapeutic approach (Table 85-4). In brief, *regenerative* anemias always stem from extra-marrow causes, because the presence of reticulocytes or polychromatophilic RBCs (i.e., immature RBCs) in the circulation is a clear indication of a functional bone marrow. Regenerative anemias can result only from hemolysis or blood loss. *Nonregenerative* anemias can be caused by bone marrow and extra-marrow disorders, such as erythroid hypoproliferation, chronic inflammatory disease, chronic renal disease, and acute hemorrhage or hemolysis (first 48 to 96 hours). Although traditionally iron deficiency anemias (IDAs) are classified as nonregenerative, most dogs with chronic blood loss leading to iron deficiency display a mild (to moderate) degree of regen-

eration, and the RBC indices are different than in other nonregenerative anemias (see below); therefore I prefer to classify IDA in a separate category. Regenerative anemias are usually acute, whereas nonregenerative anemias are either peracute (i.e., blood loss or hemolysis of less than 48 hours' duration) or chronic.

During the initial clinical evaluation of an anemic patient, examination of the blood smear usually suffices in determining whether the bone marrow is responding appropriately to the anemia (i.e., whether the anemia is regenerative). Several pieces of information can be acquired during the examination of a good-quality, properly stained blood smear, including the RBC size and morphology, the presence of autoagglutination, the approximate numbers and the morphology of white blood cells and platelets, the presence of nucleated RBCs, the presence of polychromasia (indicative of regeneration), and the presence of RBC parasites. The clinician can (and should) do this cursory evaluation of the blood smear, and the blood sample should be submitted to a diagnostic laboratory for further analysis and evaluation by a clinical pathologist. Some of the abnormalities detected during a careful examination of the blood smear and their clinical implications are summarized in Table 85-5. It is important to conduct this evaluation in a monolayer field (in which the erythrocytes are in a single layer and 50% of the cells are touching) under oil immersion lens.

A CBC and a reticulocyte count in an anemic patient provide more absolute data by which to assess the degree of regeneration. However, the information presented below must be used cautiously, because the number of reticulocytes should increase proportionally to the decrease in the PCV. For example, a reticulocyte count of 120,000/μl or of 4% represents an appropriate response for a dog with a PCV of 30% but not for one with a PCV of 10%. The following points generally hold true:

1. If the RBC indices are *macrocytic* and *hypochromic,* the anemia most likely is associated with the presence of high numbers of reticulocytes (which are larger and contain less Hb than mature RBCs); therefore the anemia is likely regenerative.
2. If the reticulocyte count is more than 100,000/μl and the anemia is mild to moderate, the anemia is likely regenerative.
3. If the reticulocyte index (RI) percentage is more than 3% and the anemia is mild to moderate, the anemia is likely regenerative.
4. RI calculations are presented in Table 85-6. In dogs, a RI greater than 3% usually supports regeneration.

As part of the evaluation of a patient with regenerative anemia, it is beneficial to determine the serum or plasma protein concentration, because blood loss usually results in hypoproteinemia, but hemolysis does not. Other physical examination and clinicopathologic findings that help distinguish blood loss from hemolytic anemias are listed in Table 85-7.

TABLE 85-4

Pathogenetic Classification of Anemias

| REGENERATIVE | SEMIREGENERATIVE | NONREGENERATIVE |
|---|---|---|
| Blood loss (after 48-96 hours)<br>Hemolysis | Iron deficiency anemia | Anemia of chronic disease<br>Anemia of renal disease<br>Bone marrow disorder<br>Blood loss/hemolysis (first 48-96 hours)<br>Endocrine anemia |

 TABLE 85-5

Interpretation of Morphologic Red Blood Cell Abnormalities in Cats and Dogs

| MORPHOLOGIC ABNORMALITY | COMMONLY ASSOCIATED DISORDERS |
|---|---|
| Macrocytosis | Regeneration, breed-related characteristic (Poodles); feline leukemia virus or immunodeficiency virus infection; dyserythropoiesis (bone marrow disease) |
| Microcytosis | Iron deficiency; breed-related characteristic (Akitas, Sharpeis, Shiba Inus); portosystemic shunt; polycythemia (erythrocytosis) |
| Hypochromia | Iron deficiency |
| Polychromasia | Regeneration |
| Poikilocytosis | Regeneration; iron deficiency; hyposplenism |
| Schistocytosis (fragments) | Microangiopathy; hemangiosarcoma; disseminated intravascular coagulation; hyposplenism |
| Spherocytosis | Immune hemolytic anemia; mononuclear phagocytic neoplasm; zinc toxicity |
| Acanthocytosis (spur cells) | Hemangiosarcoma; liver disease; hyposplenism |
| Ecchinocytosis (burr cells) | Artifact; renal disease; pyruvate kinase deficiency anemia |
| Elliptocytosis | Congenital elliptocytosis (dogs) |
| Heinz bodies | Oxidative insult to red blood cells |
| Howell-Jolly bodies | Regeneration; hyposplenism |
| Autoagglutination | Immune hemolytic anemia |
| Metarubricytosis | Breed-related characteristic (Schnauzers, Dachshunds); extramedullary hematopoiesis; regeneration; lead toxicity; hemangiosarcoma |
| Leukopenia | See text |
| Thrombocytopenia | See text |
| Pancytopenia | Bone marrow disorder; hypersplenism |

Modified from Couto CG et al: Hematologic and oncologic emergencies. In Murtaugh R et al, editors: *Veterinary emergency and critical care medicine,* St Louis, 1992, Mosby.

 TABLE 85-6

Calculation of the Reticulocyte Index in Dogs

1. $\dfrac{\text{Patient's PCV}}{45} \times \text{Reticulocyte percentage} = A$

   where 45 is the average PCV in the dog; this corrects for the artifact caused by the anemia (i.e., with a low PCV, the percentage of reticulocytes exaggerates the absolute number of cells).
2. If there is polychromasia in the blood smear, *divide A by 2* to correct for the maturation time in circulation.
3. If the results are >2.5, the anemia is regenerative.

From Couto CG et al: Hematologic and oncologic emergencies. In Murtaugh R et al, editors: *Veterinary emergency and critical care medicine,* St Louis, 1992, Mosby.
*PCV,* Packed cell volume.

TABLE 85-7

Criteria for Differentiating Blood Loss from Hemolytic Anemias

| VARIABLE | BLOOD LOSS | HEMOLYSIS |
|---|---|---|
| Serum (plasma) protein concentration | Normal-low | Normal-high |
| Evidence of bleeding | Common | Rare |
| Icterus | No | Common |
| Hemoglobinemia | No | Common |
| Spherocytosis | No | Common |
| Hemosiderinuria | No | Yes |
| Autoagglutination | No | Occasional |
| Direct Coombs' test | Negative | Usually positive (in IHA) |
| Splenomegaly | No | Common |
| RBC changes | No | Common (see Table 85-5) |

From Couto CG et al: Hematologic and oncologic emergencies. In Murtaugh R et al, editors: *Veterinary emergency and critical care medicine,* St Louis, 1992, Mosby.
*IHA,* Immune hemolytic anemia; *RBC,* red blood cell.

## PRINCIPLES OF MANAGEMENT OF THE ANEMIC PATIENT

The first basic principle of the management of anemic (or bleeding) patients is to collect *all* blood samples before instituting any therapy. Because the condition in most of these patients may constitute a true emergency at the time of presentation, often samples are not collected until the animal's condition has been completely stabilized, resulting in treatment-induced changes in hematologic or serum biochemical values.

As a general rule, because of the acute onset of these disorders, patients with regenerative anemias (i.e., blood loss or hemolysis) require more aggressive therapy than those with nonregenerative forms. Specific therapy should be instituted once the clinician has determined that the patient's condition is stable and whether the anemia is regenerative or not. The diagnosis and management of different forms of anemia in cats and dogs are discussed throughout the remainder of this chapter.

## REGENERATIVE ANEMIAS

### BLOOD LOSS ANEMIA

Acute blood loss results in reticulocytosis (i.e., regeneration) within 48 to 96 hours in normal dogs and cats. Therefore animals seen shortly after a traumatic injury and severe blood loss usually have nonregenerative anemias with low-to-normal serum (plasma) protein concentrations. The source of bleeding should be identified and the bleeding arrested; if the patient is bleeding as a result of a systemic hemostatic defect, it

should be identified and specific treatment should be initiated (see p. 1189). Aggressive intravenous (IV) fluid therapy with crystalloids or colloids, or the transfusion of blood or blood products is often required in patients with anemia caused by acute blood loss.

## HEMOLYTIC ANEMIA

In people, the bone marrow is capable of undergoing hyperplasia until its production rate is increased approximately sixfold to eightfold; the same is probably true for dogs and cats. As a consequence, a considerable number of RBCs have to be destroyed before anemia develops. As is the case in cats and dogs with blood loss anemia, patients with peracute hemolysis can be in a nonregenerative state at the time of presentation because the bone marrow has not yet been able to mount a regenerative response. In addition, in some dogs with immune-mediated hemolysis, the destruction of erythroid precursors in the bone marrow results in a lack of regeneration.

On the basis of their pathogenesis, hemolytic anemias can be classified as extravascular (i.e., the RBCs are destroyed by the mononuclear phagocytic cells) or intravascular (i.e., the RBCs are lysed by antibody-complement, drugs, toxins, or fibrin strands). On the basis of the age of the animal at onset, anemias can be classified as congenital or acquired (Table 85-8). Most dogs and cats with hemolytic anemia seen at our clinic have acquired extravascular hemolysis.

In *extravascular* hemolysis, RBCs are phagocytosed by the mononuclear-phagocytic system (MPS) in the spleen, liver, and bone marrow. Stimuli that trigger RBC phagocytosis consist mainly of intracellular inclusions, such as RBC parasites or Heinz bodies (the latter are commonly seen in cats) and membrane coating with immunoglobulin (Ig) G or M (common in dogs). Congenital RBC enzymopathies can also precipitate extravascular hemolysis. Once abnormal RBCs are recognized, the MPS rapidly phagocytoses them, resulting in a decrease in the number of circulating RBCs and the generation of cells with specific morphologic changes (e.g., spherocytes). Anemia develops if the destruction of RBCs continues. Spherocytes are RBC "leftovers," in that after a mononuclear-phagocytic cell takes a "bite" of cytoplasm and membrane, the membrane is resealed. Spherocytes are characteristic of immune hemolytic anemia (IHA), although they can occasionally be seen in other disorders. Immune hemolysis is the most common cause of extravascular hemolytic anemia in dogs at our hospital. Drug-associated hemolysis (e.g., β-lactam antibiotics) and hemobartonellosis are the two most common causes in cats, although IHA is becoming more common in this species. Other causes of extravascular hemolytic anemia in dogs and cats are listed in Table 85-8.

*Intravascular* hemolysis can occur as a consequence of direct RBC lysis caused by antibodies-complement (e.g., immune-mediated hemolysis), infectious agents (e.g., babesiosis), drugs or toxins (e.g., zinc in pennies minted after 1983, in pet carrier bolts, in other hardware, and in zinc oxide–containing ointments), metabolic imbalances (e.g., hypophosphatemia in dogs and cats with diabetes mellitus treated with insulin), or increased shearing of RBCs (i.e., microangiopathy, DIC). In-

## TABLE 85-8

**Causes of Hemolytic Anemia in Dogs and Cats**

| DISORDER | SPECIES | BREED |
|---|---|---|
| **Congenital (Inherited?)** | | |
| Pyruvate kinase deficiency | D, C | Basenji, Beagle, West Highland White Terrier, Cairn Terrier, Poodle, Dachshund, Chihuahua, Pug, American Eskimo, Abyssinian, Somali, domestic short-haired cat |
| Phosphofructokinase deficiency | D | English Springer Spaniel, Cocker Spaniel |
| Stomatocytosis | D | Alaskan Malamute, Miniature Schnauzer |
| Nonspherocytic hemolytic anemia | D | Poodle, Beagle |
| **Acquired** | | |
| Immune hemolytic anemia | D > C | All |
| Neonatal isoerythrolysis | C | British breeds, Abyssinian, Somali (other type B cats) |
| Microangiopathic hemolytic anemia | D > C | All |
| Infectious | | |
|    Hemobartonellosis | C > D | All |
|    Babesiosis | D > C | All |
|    Cytauxoonosis | C | All |
|    Ehrlichiosis | D > C | All |
| Hypophosphatemia | D, C | All |
| Oxidants | | |
|    Acetaminophen | C | All |
|    Phenothiazines | D, C | All |
|    Benzocaine | C | All |
|    Vitamin K | D, C | All |
|    Methylene blue | C > D | All |
|    Methionine | C | All |
|    Propylene glycol | C | All |
| **Drugs that Can Cause Immune Hemolysis** | | |
|    Sulfas | D > C | Doberman, Labrador Retriever |
|    Anticonvulsants | D | All |
|    Penicillins and cephalosporins | D > C | All |
|    Proplythiouracil | C | All |
|    Methimazole | C | All |
|    Antiarrhythmics? | D | All |
|    Zinc | D | All |

Modified from Couto CG et al: Hematologic and oncologic emergencies. In Murtaugh R et al, editors: *Veterinary emergency and critical care medicine*, St Louis, 1992, Mosby.

travascular hemolysis is considerably less common in dogs and cats than extravascular hemolysis, with the notable exception of DIC in dogs with hemangiosarcoma, zinc toxicity, and hypophosphatemia. Certain congenital enzymopathies in dogs also result in intravascular hemolysis.

Dogs with *congenital* (frequently familial) hemolytic anemias may have relatively prolonged clinical courses at the time of presentation, with the notable exception of English Springer Spaniels with phosphofructokinase deficiency–induced hemolysis, in which acute hemolytic episodes occur after they hyperventilate during exercise (i.e., alkaline hemolysis). Dogs and cats with *acquired* hemolytic anemias usually are evaluated because of acute clinical signs consisting of pallor with or without icterus (in my experience only ap-

proximately half of dogs and a lower percentage of cats with hemolytic anemia are icteric); splenomegaly may be a prominent finding. If there is associated thrombocytopenia (e.g., Evans's syndrome, DIC), petechiae and ecchymoses may be present. Clinical signs and physical examination findings associated with the primary disease can also be present in cases of secondary hemolytic anemias.

In the evaluation of dogs or cats with hemolytic anemia, a careful examination of the blood smear is mandatory. Morphologic abnormalities pathognomonic for or highly suggestive of a particular etiology are often detected in this way (see Table 85-5). The sample should also be tested for autoagglutination; this is done by placing a large drop of blood on a glass slide at room temperature and at 4° C. Agglutination can be distinguished from rouleaux formation by diluting the blood 5:1 in saline solution (this disaggregates rouleaux); rouleaux formation is common in cats but is extremely rare in dogs. A direct Coombs' test to detect RBC-bound immunoglobulins should always be performed in dogs and cats with suspected hemolysis (see below). As a general rule, the presence of Ig coating on the RBCs indicates that there is immune-mediated hemolysis. A positive Coombs' test result should be interpreted with caution, however, because certain drugs and hemoparasites can induce formation of antibodies that bind to the RBCs, thus causing secondary immune hemolysis (e.g., cats with hemobartonellosis). The pretreatment of an animal with corticosteroids may also result in decreased binding of Ig molecules to the surface of the RBC, thus resulting in false-negative results. Direct Coombs' tests are usually not necessary in animals with autoagglutination, because this phenomenon connotes the presence of immunoglobulins on the surface of the RBCs (i.e., "biologic" Coombs' test). Cryoagglutination (i.e., the agglutination of RBCs if the blood sample is refrigerated for 6 to 8 hours) occurs in a large proportion of cats with hemobartonellosis and is usually associated with IgM coating of the RBCs.

If an etiologic agent cannot be identified (i.e., RBC parasite, drug, pennies in the stomach), the patient should be treated for primary or idiopathic IHA while further test results (e.g., serologic tests or polymerase chain reaction [PCR] for hemoparasites) are pending. As mentioned previously, primary IHA is considerably more common in dogs than in cats; thus every effort should be made to identify a cause of hemolysis in cats, such as drugs or hemoparasites. The next section contains a detailed discussion of IHA.

Hemolytic anemias not associated with immune destruction of the RBCs are treated by removal of the cause (i.e., drug, infectious agent, gastric foreign body) and supportive therapy. Corticosteroids (see later discussion) can be administered to suppress MPS activity while the etiologic agent is being eliminated, although this is not always beneficial. Doxycycline (5 to 10 mg/kg PO q12-24h for 14 to 21 days) usually results in resolution of the signs in dogs and cats with hemobartonellosis and in dogs with ehrlichiosis.

## Immune Hemolytic Anemia

IHA constitutes the most common form of hemolysis in dogs. Although two pathogenetic categories of hemolytic anemia are recognized (primary or idiopathic, and secondary), most cases of IHA in dogs are primary (i.e., a cause cannot be found after exhaustive clinical and clinicopathologic evaluation). The immune-mediated destruction of RBCs can occur in association with drug administration (e.g., β-lactam antibiotics) or vaccination. With the exception of the immune hemolysis secondary to hemoparasitism, IHA is rare in cats (although its prevalence appears to be increasing). The clinical course in dogs is typically acute, but peracute presentations are also common.

In immune hemolytic anemia, the RBCs become coated primarily with IgG, which leads to the early removal of the coated cells by the MPS, mainly in the spleen and liver. As a

consequence, spherocytes are generated; therefore the presence of spherocytes in the blood smear of a dog with anemia is highly suggestive of IHA. Spherocytes are difficult to identify in cats.

Clinical signs in dogs with IHA include depression of acute (or peracute) onset, exercise intolerance, and pallor or jaundice, occasionally accompanied by vomiting or abdominal pain. Physical examination findings usually consist of pallor or jaundice, petechiae and ecchymoses (if immune thrombocytopenia is also present), splenomegaly, and a heart murmur. As noted in previous paragraphs, jaundice can be absent in dogs with IHA. A subset of dogs with acute (or peracute) IHA with icterus (and usually autoagglutination) shows clinical deterioration within hours or days of admission, resulting from multifocal thromboembolic disease or a lack of response to conventional therapy. We treat these dogs more aggressively than the typical dog with IHA (see p. 1163).

Hematologic findings in dogs with IHA typically include a strongly regenerative anemia, leukocytosis caused by neutrophilia with a left-shift and monocytosis, increased numbers of nucleated RBCs, polychromasia, and spherocytosis. The serum (plasma) protein concentration is usually normal to increased, and hemoglobinemia or bilirubinemia may be present (i.e., pink or yellow plasma). As noted previously, autoagglutination is prominent in some dogs. Thrombocytopenia is also present in dogs with Evans's syndrome or DIC.

The presence of polychromasia with autoagglutination and spherocytosis in a dog with illness and anemia of acute onset is virtually pathognomonic of IHA. In these cases a direct Coombs' test is usually not necessary to confirm the diagnosis. In dogs that do not have some of these physical examination and hematologic findings, a direct Coombs' test should be performed to detect Ig adsorbed to the RBC membrane.

The direct Coombs' test is negative in approximately 10% to 30% of dogs with IHA, yet they respond to immunosuppressive therapy (see following paragraph). In these cases, there may be enough Ig or complement molecules bound to the RBC membrane to induce the MPS to stimulate phagocytosis but not enough to result in a positive Coombs' test. It is generally accepted that hemolysis can occur in people with approximately 20 to 30 molecules of Ig bound to the RBC, whereas the direct Coombs' test can only detect more than 200 to 300 molecules of Ig per cell. Another explanation for the findings in this subset of patients is that the previous administration of exogenous corticosteroids has resulted in decreased antibody binding to the surface of the RBCs.

Immunosuppressive doses of corticosteroids (equivalent to 2 to 4 mg/kg of prednisone q12-24h in the dog and up to 8 mg/kg q12-24h in the cat) constitute the treatment of choice for primary IHA. Although dexamethasone can be used initially, it should not be used as maintenance therapy for prolonged periods because of its higher potential to cause gastrointestinal tract ulceration or pancreatitis, and because, if given on an alternate-day basis, it causes interference with the hypothalamic-pituitary-adrenal axis. In equivalent doses, dexamethasone does not appear to be more beneficial than prednisone in these animals.

A high percentage of dogs treated with corticosteroids show a marked improvement within 24 to 96 hours (Fig. 85-1). Corticosteroids act mainly by three different mechanisms: they suppress MPS activity, decrease complement and antibody binding to the cells, and suppress Ig production. The first two effects are rapid in onset (hours), whereas the third effect is delayed (1 to 3 weeks). Other effects of corticosteroids on the immune system are discussed on p. 1216.

We have observed a high number of dogs with acute or paracute IHA generally associated with icterus and autoagglutination that show a rapid deterioration and that usually die of thromboembolism of the liver, lungs, or kidneys despite aggressive corticosteroid therapy. I treat such animals with cyclophosphamide (Cytoxan; Mead Johnson, Evansville, Ind) at a dosage of 200 to 300 mg/m$^2$ given orally or intravenously in a single dose over 5 to 10 minutes, in conjunction with a single IV dose of dexamethasone sodium phosphate (1 to 2 mg/kg). I also advocate the use of prophylactic heparin therapy because dogs with hemolysis are at high risk for DIC and thrombosis. In our practice, we routinely use heparin therapy of 50 to 75 IU/kg given subcutaneously every 8 hours. These dosages of heparin usually do not result in therapy-related prolongation of the activated clotting time (ACT) or the activated partial thromboplastin time (Aptt), tests used routinely to monitor heparinization. If there is clinical evidence of thromboembolism (see p. 1199), I recommend using high-dose heparin (700 to 1000 IU/kg SQ q8h) or a dose that will cause the ACT to be prolonged up to 2.5 times the normal or the baseline value. Because dogs with IHA are at high risk for thromboembolic events, we refrain from placing central venous lines; thrombosis of the anterior vena cava commonly leads to severe pleural effusion in these dogs. If excessive bleeding occurs as a result of overheparinization, protamine sulfate can be administered by slow IV infusion (1 mg for each 100 IU of the last dose of heparin; 50% of the calculated dose is given 1 hour after the heparin and 25% 2 hours after the heparin). The remainder of the dose can be administered if clinically indicated. Protamine sulfate should be administered with caution in dogs, however, because it can cause acute anaphylaxis. Aggressive fluid therapy should be administered in conjunction with these treatments in an attempt to flush the microaggregates of agglutinated RBCs from the microcirculation. One must also bear in mind, however, that, depending on the degree of anemia, the resultant hemodilution may be detrimental to the patient. If deemed necessary, oxygen therapy should also be used.

We have recently used human intravenous Ig (0.5 to 1.5 g/kg IV infusion, single dose) with a high degree of success in dogs with refractory IHA. This treatment is aimed at blocking the Fc receptors in the MPS with a foreign immunoglobulin, thus minimizing the phagocytosis of antibody-coated RBCs. This treatment appears to have other immunomodulatory effects as well. However, the product is extremely expensive (approximately $600 to $700 per dose for a 10-kg dog), and it may not be readily available.

Drugs used for the maintenance treatment of dogs with IHA include prednisone (1 mg/kg PO q48h) and azathioprine (50 mg/m$^2$ PO q24-48h; Imuran; Burroughs Welcome, Research Triangle Park, N.C.), used either singly or in combination. Azathioprine is associated with few adverse effects, although close hematologic and serum biochemical monitoring is necessary because of its potential to suppress bone marrow function and cause a mild hepatopathy. A dose reduction is necessary if myelosuppression or hepatotoxicity occurs; occasionally azathioprine has to be discontinued in dogs with hepatotoxicity (see p. 1115).

In general, dogs (and possibly cats) with IHA require prolonged (often lifelong) immunosuppressive treatment. Whether an animal requires continuous treatment is determined on the basis of trial and error; decremental doses of the immunosuppressive drug or drugs are administered for a given period (usually 2 to 3 weeks), at which time the patient is reevaluated clinically and hematologically. If the PCV has not decreased (or it has increased) and the animal is clinically stable (or has shown improvement), the dose is reduced by 25% to 50%. This procedure is repeated until the drug or drugs are discontinued or the patient relapses; in the latter case, the previously used dosage that had beneficial effects is used again. In my experience, more than two thirds of dogs with IHA require lifelong treatment.

Alternative treatments for dogs with refractory IHA include therapeutic plasmapheresis, danazol (5 to 10 mg/kg PO q12h; Danocrine; Winthrop, New York, N.Y.), cyclosporine (10 mg/kg PO q12-24h; Sandimune, Sandoz, East Hanover, N.J.), and possibly splenectomy. However, splenectomy has rarely been of benefit in dogs with IHA treated at our clinic.

Chlorambucil (20 mg/m$^2$ PO q2wk; Leukeran, Burroughs Welcome, Research Triangle Park, N.C.) appears to be the best induction and maintenance agent in cats with IHA refractory

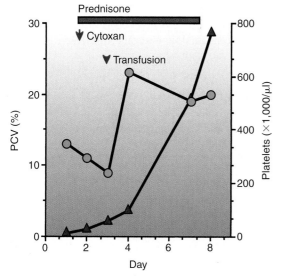

**FIG 85-1**

Response to treatment in a dog with immune hemolytic anemia and immune-mediated thrombocytopenia (Evans's syndrome). *PCV*, Packed cell volume; –●–, PCV; –△–, platelets; ↑, treatment administered.

to corticosteroids or in those in which corticosteroid-induced diabetes mellitus occurs. In my experience, azathioprine causes pronounced myelosuppression in this species.

One of the biggest dilemmas the clinician faces in the treatment of a dog with IHA is whether to administer a transfusion of blood or blood products. As a general rule, a transfusion should not be withheld if it represents a lifesaving procedure. However, because patients with IHA are already destroying their own antibody-coated RBCs, they may also be prone to destroying transfused RBCs (although this has not been scientifically proven). My recommendation is to administer a transfusion to any animal with IHA that is "in dire need of RBCs" (i.e., withholding a transfusion would result in the animal's death). We usually pretreat these patients with dexamethasone sodium phosphate (0.5 to 1 mg/kg IV), administer fluids through an additional IV catheter, and continue the heparin therapy. Although crossmatching is indicated, time is usually of the essence, therefore noncrossmatched blood is frequently administered; moreover, if the patient is autoagglutinating, the results of a crossmatch are difficult to interpret.

Another issue pertaining to transfusion in dogs with autoagglutinating IHA has to do with blood typing; if blood typing cards are used, the results will be false positive for DEA 1.1 (see Principles of Transfusion Therapy section, p. 1168). Finally, there is no rule of thumb (i.e., PCV value, lack of response to oxygen therapy) as to when to administer a transfusion. The clinician should use his or her best clinical judgment to determine when a transfusion of blood or blood products is necessary (i.e., does the patient exhibit tachypnea, dyspnea, orthopnea?). If available, packed RBCs should be used instead of whole blood, because they deliver a high oxygen-carrying capacity in a smaller volume, and their administration usually does not result in hypervolemia.

Recently, a polymer of bovine hemoglobin has become available for use in dogs with acute anemia that are in dire need of oxygen-carrying capacity (Oxyglobin; Biopure Corp., Cambridge, Mass). This compound has a long shelf-life; it does not require refrigeration, blood typing, or crossmatching. Administration of Oxyglobin typically results in clinical improvement of the signs associated with anemia, but the duration of response is limited (i.e., 2 or 3 days); because of the nature of this compound, the PCV does not increase after infusion (the hemoglobin concentration does increase). Some laboratory test results may be difficult to obtain after infusion of Oxyglobin due to interference with colorimetric analysis.

## NONREGENERATIVE ANEMIAS

With the exception of anemia of chronic disease (ACD), nonregenerative anemias do not appear to be clinically as common as regenerative forms in dogs, whereas the opposite is true in cats.

Five forms of nonregenerative anemia are typically recognized in cats and dogs (see Table 85-4). Because IDA can be mildly to moderately regenerative and the RBC indices are typically different from those in other forms of nonregenerative anemia (i.e., microcytic, hypochromic versus normocytic, normochromic) (see Tables 85-4 to 85-9), I prefer to classify it in a separate category. Anemia of endocrine disease is typically mild and usually is an incidental finding in dogs with hypothyroidism or hypoadrenocorticism; it is discussed in Chapters 51 and 53. In general, most nonregenerative anemias and IDA in cats and dogs are chronic, thus allowing for physiologic adaptation to the decrease in the RBC mass. As a consequence, these types of anemia may be detected incidentally during the routine evaluation of a cat or dog, which to the owner is asymptomatic. In many cases (e.g., ACD), the anemia is mild and clinical signs are absent. Although most nonregenerative anemias are chronic, two situations are commonly encountered in which this form of anemia is acute: acute blood loss (first 48 to 96 hours) and peracute hemolysis. In these two instances the bone marrow has not yet had time to mount a regenerative reticulocyte response.

When evaluating dogs and cats with symptomatic nonregenerative anemias of acute onset, the clinician should try to answer the following questions:

- Has this patient had an acute blood loss or does it have hemolytic anemia and has not yet been able to mount a regenerative response (i.e., less than 48 to 96 hours have elapsed since the event)?
- Does this patient have chronic anemia but is now symptomatic because of intercurrent disease (e.g., heart failure, sepsis)?

Most clinical and clinicopathologic abnormalities in cats and dogs with nonregenerative anemia have been discussed (see p. 1156). In general, the RBCs in dogs and cats with nonregenerative anemias are normocytic and normochromic; however, the RBCs are usually macrocytic and normochromic in cats with FeLV- or FIV-related hypoproliferative anemias. As discussed above, the RBC indices are microcytic and hypochromic in dogs and cats with IDA.

 TABLE 85-9

**Classification and Causes of Nonregenerative Anemia in Cats and Dogs**

Anemia of chronic disease
Bone marrow disorders
    Bone marrow (or erythroid) aplasia/hypoplasia
    Myelophthisis
    Myelodysplastic syndromes
    Myelofibrosis
    Osteosclerosis/osteopetrosis
Anemia of renal disease
Acute blood loss or hemolysis (first 48-96 hours)
Anemia of endocrine disorders
    Hypoadrenocorticism
    Hypothyroidism

The clinical evaluation of a cat or dog with nonregenerative anemia differs from that of a patient with regenerative forms because the absence of regeneration usually reflects primary or secondary bone marrow abnormalities (i.e., bone marrow disorder, ACD). Therefore, after extra-marrow causes have been ruled out, a bone marrow aspiration or biopsy is usually indicated in these animals.

## ANEMIA OF CHRONIC DISEASE

ACD constitutes the most common form of nonregenerative anemia in cats and dogs; however, because it is mild, it almost never results in clinical signs of anemia, and the patients are usually evaluated as a consequence of their primary disorder. ACD develops secondary to a variety of chronic inflammatory, degenerative, or neoplastic conditions. In most cats with ACD, the PCV values range from the high teens to the mid-twenties, whereas in dogs they range from the mid-twenties to the low thirties. Therefore ACD can usually be excluded in dogs with PCVs of less than 20% and in cats with PCVs of less than 17% to 18%. The RBC indices are normocytic and normochromic, and the CBC may also reflect the nature of the primary problem (e.g., leukocytosis, neutrophilia, monocytosis, hyperproteinemia resulting from a polyclonal gammopathy); some cats with ACD have microcytic hypochromic RBC indices, a condition that mimics IDA.

Sustained inflammatory or neoplastic processes cause iron to be sequestered within the bone marrow MPS, and it is therefore not available to the erythroid precursors for normal erythropoiesis. This unavailability of iron is mainly mediated by lactoferrin and other acute-phase reactants released from neutrophils during inflammation. In cats and dogs with ACD, the serum iron concentration and total iron-binding capacity (TIBC or transferrin concentration) are usually decreased, and the Hb saturation is low, but iron stores in the bone marrow are increased (Table 85-10). Although serum ferritin concentrations are the main feature that distinguishes ACD from IDA (i.e., high in ACD and low in IDA) in people, the results of ferritin assays in dogs with

IDA and ACD are not as clear-cut. Therefore, to conclusively differentiate ACD from IDA, it is important to evaluate bone marrow iron stores by performing Prussian blue staining. After a diagnosis of ACD has been confirmed, every effort should be made to identify the cause of the problem if it is not already evident.

Dogs and cats with ACD usually do not require specific or supportive therapy; treatment of the primary disorder causes the anemia to resolve. Although some have advocated the use of anabolic steroids in dogs and cats with ACD, these agents appear to be of little or no benefit.

## BONE MARROW DISORDERS

Neoplastic, hypoplastic, or dysplastic bone marrow disorders can result in anemia and other cytopenias. In these conditions, there is a "crowding out" of the normal erythroid precursors by neoplastic or inflammatory cells (i.e., myelophthisis), a paucity or absence of erythroid precursors (i.e., hypoplasia or aplasia, respectively), or a maturation arrest of the erythroid precursors (i.e., dysplasia). All these disorders, with the exception of pure red cell aplasia (PRCA) (see below in this chapter), typically affect more than one cell line, and the patients are bicytopenic or pancytopenic (see Chapter 88). In general, these disorders are chronic, and the clinical signs are those of anemia (see p. 1156), with or without signs of the underlying disorder. Although some information regarding the pathogenesis of this type of anemia is obtained by evaluating the clinical and hematologic data, a definitive diagnosis is usually made on the basis of the cytologic or histopathologic appearance of a bone marrow specimen and, possibly, the results of serologic tests or PCR for infectious agents (e.g., FeLV, FIV, *Ehrlichia canis*).

### Bone Marrow (or Erythroid) Aplasia-Hypoplasia

Bone marrow aplasia-hypoplasia is characterized by aplasia or hypoplasia of all the bone marrow cell lines (bone marrow aplasia-hypoplasia or aplastic pancytopenia) or of the erythroid precursor (RBC aplasia-hypoplasia or PRCA). This form of anemia (or combined cytopenias) can be caused by a variety of agents or disorders (Table 85-11). For additional discussion, please see Chapter 88. The following discussion pertains mainly to PRCA.

Clinically dogs and cats with PRCA are evaluated because of the clinical signs already discussed. In contrast to ACD, in which the degree of anemia, and thus the severity of the clinical signs, is mild, cats and dogs with PRCA usually have PCVs of less than 15% and are therefore symptomatic. Hematologically, severe (normocytic normochromic) nonregenerative anemia is usually the only abnormality; macrocytosis in the absence of reticulocytes is a consistent finding in cats with FeLV- or FIV-related PRCA, and mild microcytosis can occasionally be present in dogs with PRCA. The large RBC volume in cats with retroviral infections is attributed to the erythroid dysplasia or dyserythropoiesis induced by the virus. Occasionally dogs with PRCA have circulating spherocytes, pointing toward an immune basis for the anemia. The

---

▦ TABLE 85-10

**Distinguishing Features of Anemia of Chronic Disease and Iron Deficiency Anemia in Dogs**

| PARAMETER | ACD | IDA |
|---|---|---|
| Serum iron concentration | ↓ | ↓↓ |
| Total iron binding capacity | N | N↑ |
| Percentage saturation | ↓ | ↓↓ |
| Bone marrow iron stores | ↑ | ↓ |
| Platelet count | N, ↓, ↑ | ↑, ↑↑ |
| Fecal occult blood | N | +(−) |
| Ferritin | N | ↓ |

*ACD,* Anemia of chronic disease; *IDA,* iron deficiency anemia; ↓, low; ↓↓, markedly low; ↑, high; ↑↑, markedly high; *N,* normal; +(−), positive or negative.

TABLE 85-11

**Bone Marrow Disorders in Cats and Dogs**

Marrow (or erythroid) aplasia-hypoplasia
  FeLV (C)
  Immune mediated (D, C)
  Estrogen (D)
  Phenylbutazone (D)
  Other drugs (D, C)
  Idiopathic (D, C)
Myelophthisis
  Acute leukemias (D, C)
  Chronic leukemias (D > C)
  Multiple myeloma (D, C)
  Lymphoma (D, C)
  Systemic mast cell disease (C > D)
  Malignant histiocytosis (D > C)
  Metastatic carcinoma (rare D, C)
  Histoplasmosis (rare D, C)
Myelodysplastic syndromes
  FeLV (C)
  FIV (C)
  Preleukemic syndrome (D, C)
  Idiopathic (D, C)
Myelofibrosis
  FeLV (C)
  Pyruvate kinase–deficiency anemia (D)
  Idiopathic (D, C)
Osteosclerosis/osteopetrosis
  FeLV (C)

*FeLV,* Feline leukemia virus; *FIV,* feline immunodeficiency virus;
*D,* dog; *C,* cat.

direct Coombs' test is also positive in over half of these dogs, and their anemia responds to immunosuppressive therapy. Cats and dogs with bone marrow aplasia-hypoplasia are pancytopenic (see p. 1173).

In addition to the above, FeLV and FIV testing should be done in cats with PRCA. A bone marrow aspiration or biopsy specimen should also be obtained to rule out other bone marrow disorders.

The FeLV envelope protein p15E suppresses erythropoiesis in vitro and is postulated to cause PRCA in FeLV-infected cats. The anemia in these cats is usually chronic and severe (PCVs of 5% to 6% are relatively common), and despite supportive therapy, the condition of the patient deteriorates, leading the owners to request euthanasia. The supportive treatment of these cats includes whole blood or packed RBC transfusions as needed; usually the interval between transfusions shortens with each transfusion, until the cat needs transfusions weekly. Anabolic steroids may be beneficial in some cats, although there is no clinical evidence to support this. Interferon administered orally may improve clinical signs (without resolution of the anemia) in some of these cats (see Chapter 102).

FeLV-negative cats with PRCA often have a positive direct Coombs' test and frequently benefit from immunosuppres-

sive doses of corticosteroids, equivalent to 4 to 8 mg/kg of prednisone given orally every 24 hours. The use of human recombinant erythropoietin (Epo) (see later discussion) does not appear to be indicated in these cats, because their endogenous erythropoietin activity is higher than that of normal cats. In addition, the long-term use of human recombinant Epo usually leads to the development of anti-Epo antibodies and resultant refractory anemia.

PRCA of presumptive immune origin is relatively common in dogs and cats. The postulated mechanism is similar to that of IHA, except that in PRCA the antibodies (or cell-mediated immunity) are directed against the erythroid precursors. Humoral factors (antibodies) that block erythropoiesis in vitro have been well characterized in dogs with PRCA. As discussed previously, the direct Coombs' test result is positive in some of these dogs (60%) and cats (50%), and they respond well to immunosuppressive and supportive therapy. Bone marrow aspirates in dogs and cats with PRCA reveal either erythroid hypoplasia or hyperplasia of the early erythroid precursors and a "maturation arrest" at the rubricyte or metarubricyte stage. The same treatment as that used during the maintenance phase of IHA is recommended for these dogs (prednisone, 2 to 4 mg/kg PO q24-48h and/or azathioprine [Imuran], 50 mg/m² PO q24-48h). In cats, I have successfully used prednisone alone (as discussed in previous paragraphs) or in combination with chlorambucil (Leukeran) at a dosage of 20 mg/m² given orally every 2 weeks. Responses occur in approximately 70% to 80% of the patients, but clinical and hematologic recovery may take 2 to 3 months; long-term (lifelong) treatment is usually required. Supportive treatment and transfusions of blood or blood products are sometimes necessary. Because these patients are normovolemic, packed RBC transfusions are preferable. Also, as transfusions may need to be administered on an ongoing basis, crossmatching is recommended before the administration of each transfusion. It should be remembered in such animals receiving transfusions that one of the mechanisms of adaptation to chronic hypoxia (e.g., anemia) is an increase in the intraerythrocytic 2,3-diphosphoglycerate (2,3-DPG) concentration, resulting in a lower oxygen affinity (i.e., the delivery of oxygen to the tissues is facilitated). Therefore, because stored RBCs have lower concentrations of 2,3-DPG, the transfused cells have a higher affinity for oxygen. As a result, the transfusion of stored blood to a patient with chronic anemia may result in transient decompensation, because it usually takes approximately 24 hours for the transfused stored RBCs to regain 50% of the normal 2,3-DPG concentrations.

## Myelophthisis, Myelodysplastic Syndromes, Myelofibrosis, Osteosclerosis-Osteopetrosis

These disorders are discussed in Chapter 88.

## ANEMIA OF RENAL DISEASE

The kidney is the main site of the production of Epo, the principal stimulus of erythropoiesis. In addition, in dogs and cats with chronic renal failure, the life span of RBCs is considerably shorter and there is subclinical to clinical gastrointestinal tract bleeding; high levels of PTH also suppress erythropoiesis. Because of these factors, anemia is common in such patients. The anemia is usually normocytic, normochromic, with few or no reticulocytes. PCVs in dogs and cats with anemia of renal disease (ARD) are usually in the 20% to low 30% range, although PCVs in the teens are common. It should be remembered that the PCV in these patients is usually that low only after they have undergone intensive fluid therapy (i.e., upon presentation the anemia is not that severe, because the patients are markedly dehydrated).

Improvement in renal function may result in marginal increases in the RBC mass. The use of anabolic steroids has been advocated in cats and dogs with ARD, although the results of controlled clinical studies evaluating their use are not available. Human recombinant Epo (Epogen; Amgen, Thousand Oaks, Calif) has been used successfully to treat anemia in cats (and some dogs) with chronic renal failure. A dose of 100 to 150 IU/kg given subcutaneously twice weekly is administered until the PCV returns to a target value (usually 20% to 25%), then the interval between injections is lengthened for maintenance therapy. The PCV usually returns to normal within 3 to 4 weeks of the start of treatment. Given the fact that this Epo is foreign to dogs and cats, an appropriate antibody response usually nullifies the beneficial effects of long-term therapy (i.e., 6 to 8 weeks) in over 50% of the patients.

## ACUTE AND PERACUTE BLOOD LOSS OR HEMOLYSIS (FIRST 48 TO 96 HOURS)

After an acute episode of blood loss or hemolysis, it takes the bone marrow approximately 48 to 96 hours to release enough reticulocytes to result in regeneration. Therefore blood loss and hemolytic anemias are nonregenerative during the initial phases of recovery.

In most dogs and cats with acute blood loss, there is either historical or clinical evidence of profound bleeding. If no obvious cause of bleeding is found or if the patient is bleeding from multiple sites, the hemostatic system should be evaluated in search of a coagulopathy (see Chapter 89). Sites of internal bleeding should be evident after a complete physical examination is performed.

Once the bleeding has been arrested, the anemia typically resolves within days to weeks. The initial management of a bleeding episode should include supportive therapy and IV crystalloids or plasma expanders. If necessary, blood or packed RBCs, or hemoglobin solutions should be administered.

The management of dogs with peracute hemolysis was discussed earlier in the chapter.

## *SEMIREGENERATIVE ANEMIAS*

### IRON DEFICIENCY ANEMIA

IDA is traditionally classified as nonregenerative, even though mild-to-moderate regeneration usually occurs; moreover, as discussed above, the RBC indices in dogs and cats with IDA are microcytic and hypochromic, distinguishing it from other forms of nonregenerative anemia, which are normocytic and normochronic. When evaluating the CBC of a dog with microcytic hypochromic anemia, the clinician must remember that microcytosis occurs in some breeds (i.e., Akita, Shiba Inu, Sharpei) and in dogs with other disorders, such as portosystemic shunts (see Table 85-5).

This form of anemia is well characterized in dogs with chronic blood loss. In cats, IDA has been well documented only in weanling kittens, in which iron supplementation results in rapid resolution of the clinical and hematologic abnormalities; IDA is extremely rare in adult cats, and I have seen it only in association with chronic gastrointestinal (GI) blood loss. Given its rarity in cats, the following discussion of IDA pertains primarily to dogs.

Chronic blood loss leading to iron depletion is common in dogs with GI tract bleeding caused by neoplasia, gastric ulcers, or endoparasites (e.g., hookworms) and in those with heavy flea infestation. Other causes of chronic blood loss, such as urogenital bleeding and iatrogenic blood letting, are extremely rare. In my experience, the most common cause of symptomatic IDA in dogs (i.e., dogs that present for evaluation of signs associated with anemia) is GI neoplasia.

Typically dogs with IDA are evaluated because of the signs of the anemia or because of GI tract signs such as diarrhea, melena, or hematochezia. Occasionally, mild IDA is recognized during the routine evaluation of heavily parasitized dogs (mostly pups). Hematologically, most dogs with IDA have microcytic, hypochromic indices, mild reticulocytosis (1% to 5%), a high red blood cell distribution width (RDW) with an occasional bimodal population of RBCs, thrombocytosis, low serum iron and TIBC (transferrin) concentrations, an extremely low percentage of saturation (usually less than 10%), a low serum ferritin concentration, and low iron stores in the bone marrow (see Table 85-10). The RDW generated by a particle counter represents a histogram of RBC sizes; a high RDW is indicative of anisocytosis. The typical tetrad of hematologic abnormalities in dogs with IDA is microcytosis, hypochromia, mild regeneration, and thrombocytosis.

Because the most common cause of IDA in adult dogs is chronic gastrointestinal tract bleeding, the stools should always be evaluated for occult blood using commercially available kits (see Chapter 29); if the results are negative, they should be evaluated again two or three times during a period when the animal is not eating canned dog food (myoglobin in canned dog food can occasionally result in false-positive reactions). If occult blood is present in the stool, a GI tract neoplasm should be ruled out. Tumors commonly associated with IDA in dogs include leiomyomas, leiomyosarcomas, and lymphomas, although chronic blood loss can also occur in dogs with gastrointestinal tract carcinomas. Dogs with GI neoplasms may not exhibit clinical signs referable to the GI tract (e.g., vomiting, hematemesis); in fact, jejunal neoplasms are usually "silent" (i.e., lack of GI tract signs).

Another condition that can lead to IDA is chronic upper gastrointestinal tract bleeding secondary to gastroduodenal ulceration, although most of these dogs have overt clinical signs associated with the GI tract (e.g., vomiting, hematemesis, weight loss) (see p. 427). In pups or kittens with IDA, fecal flotation or a direct smear for hookworms and a thorough physical examination (i.e., search for fleas) are mandatory, because these are the two most common causes of IDA in young dogs and cats.

IDA usually resolves within 6 to 8 weeks after the primary cause has been eliminated. Oral or intramuscular iron supplementation is usually not necessary to hasten the resolution of the hematologic abnormalities; a sound diet usually achieves the same effect. As a general rule, if the cause can be eliminated, I do not use iron supplementation. While recovering from IDA, dogs and cats should be eating a sound, iron-containing diet. The dietary iron requirement for adult dogs and cats is approximately 1.3 mg/kg/day.

## PRINCIPLES OF TRANSFUSION THERAPY

The transfusion of whole blood or blood components (e.g., packed RBCs, platelet-rich plasma, fresh frozen plasma, cryoprecipitate, or plasma) is indicated in several clinical situations. Whole blood or packed RBC transfusion is most commonly required to restore the oxygen-carrying capacity in patients with anemia. Whole blood should be used if the anemic patient is hypovolemic or if it needs clotting factors, whereas packed RBCs are recommended for normovolemic dogs and cats with anemia (i.e., PRCA, ARD, hemolysis). Transfusion therapy should be used with caution in animals with IHA (see p. 1162), because a massive transfusion reaction may occur; in those patients, hemoglobin derivatives may be a better alternative.

Clotting factor deficiencies (see p. 1189) resulting in hemorrhage can be corrected through the administration of whole fresh blood (if a considerable blood loss has occurred) or, more ideally, of fresh or fresh frozen plasma. Cryoprecipitate contains high concentration of factor VIII (FVIII) and von Willebrand's factor (vWF), so it is typically used in dogs with hemophilia A or von Willebrand's disease. Cryo-poor plasma is a good source of clotting factors (except for FVIII and vWF) and albumin. Platelet-rich plasma or platelet transfusions, if available, can be used in dogs and cats with severe thrombocytopenia resulting in spontaneous bleeding. However, the platelet count of the recipient is rarely raised enough to halt bleeding. Platelet-rich plasma and platelet transfusions are of no benefit in patients with peripheral platelet destruction (e.g., immune-mediated thrombocytopenia), because the platelets are removed from the circulation immediately after the transfusion. Transfusion with whole fresh blood, platelet-rich plasma, or fresh frozen plasma is also indicated for the management of patients with DIC (see p. 1195).

Less frequently, plasma is prescribed to correct hypoalbuminemia. However, only rarely can relevant increases in the recipient's serum albumin concentration be achieved. Colloids or human albumin solutions are more effective in restoring plasma oncotic pressure.

## BLOOD GROUPS

Several blood groups have been recognized in dogs; these include dog erythrocyte antigen (DEA) 1.1 and 1.2 (formerly Blood Group A) and DEA 3 through 8. Dogs do not have naturally acquired antibodies against blood group antigens; they can only acquire them after receiving a transfusion or after pregnancy. Transfusion reactions can occur if blood positive for DEA 1.1, 1.2, or 7 is transfused (i.e., donors should be negative for those antigens); however, clinically relevant acute hemolytic transfusion reactions are quite rare in dogs.

Blood groups in cats include A, B, and AB. Cats tested in the United States have almost exclusively been A-type; the prevalence of B-type cats varies greatly from region to region and among breeds. Breeds in which 15% to 30% of the cats are B-type include Abyssinian, Birman, Himalayan, Persian, Scottish Fold, and Somali; breeds in which more than 30% of cats are B-type include the British Shorthair and the Devon Rex. Because fatal transfusion reactions commonly occur in B-type cats receiving A-type blood, cats should always be crossmatched or typed before receiving a transfusion. In those cases, a B-type cat should be used as a donor. All the B-type cats seen in our clinic in the past 5 years have been domestic short-haired cats. Blood typing is also vital in cattery situations to prevent neonatal isoerythrolysis in A- or AB-type kittens born to B-type queens.

## CROSSMATCHING AND BLOOD TYPING

Crossmatching is an alternative to blood typing in in-house donors or in animals that have had prior transfusions, in cats, or in animals that will require multiple transfusions. Crossmatching detects many incompatibilities but does not guarantee complete compatibility. The procedure for major and minor crossmatching is described in Table 85-12. Recently, rapid, cage-side blood typing cards for DEA 1.1 in dogs and for groups A and B in cats have become available (Rapid Vet-H, dms/laboratories, Flemington, N.J.).

## BLOOD ADMINISTRATION

Refrigerated blood may be warmed before or during administration, particularly in small dogs or cats; excessive heat should be avoided, however, because fibrinogen precipitation or autoagglutination may then occur. The administration set should have a filter in place (Travenol Laboratories, Deerfield, Ill) to remove clots and other particulate matter, such as platelet aggregates. The blood is usually administered via the cephalic, saphenous, or jugular veins. However, intraosseous infusion may be performed in small animals, neonates, or animals with poor peripheral circulation. To administer fluids or blood intraosseously, the skin over the femur is surgically prepared and the skin and periosteum of the femoral trochanteric fossa are anesthetized with 1% lidocaine. A bone marrow needle (18 gauge) is placed into the marrow cavity parallel to the shaft of the femur. Suction with a 10 ml syringe should yield marrow elements (fat, spicules, and blood), confirming correct placement of the needle. The blood is administered through a standard blood administration set.

TABLE 85-12

## Crossmatching Procedure for Dogs and Cats

1. Collect 2 ml of blood from donor and recipient in EDTA tubes.
2. Centrifuge samples at 3000 *g* for 1 minute; remove and retain plasma.
3. Resuspend RBCs in saline, centrifuge, and discard supernate; repeat three times.
4. Prepare a 2% RBC suspension with 0.02 ml of washed RBCs and 0.98 ml of saline.
5. Major crossmatch:
   Two drops of donor RBC suspension
   Two drops of recipient plasma
6. Minor crossmatch:
   Two drops of recipient RBC suspension
   Two drops of donor plasma
7. Control:
   Two drops of donor RBC suspension
   Two drops of donor plasma
8. Incubate major, minor, and control specimens at 25° C for 30 minutes.
9. Centrifuge all tubes at 3000 *g* for 1 minute.
10. Agglutination is a positive result.

*EDTA*, Ethylenediaminetetraacetic acid; *RBC*, red blood cell.

The recommended rate of administration is variable, but should not exceed 22 ml/kg/day (up to 20 ml/kg/hr can be used in hypovolemic animals). Dogs and cats in heart failure may not tolerate a rate of more than 5 ml/kg/day. To prevent bacterial contamination, blood should not be exposed to room temperature during administration for longer than 4 to 6 hours (i.e., blood is considered to be contaminated if it is at room temperature for more than 6 hours). If necessary, two smaller volumes of blood can be administered in succession. Blood should never be administered with lactated Ringer's solution because of the calcium chelation with citrate and consequent clot formation that may occur. Normal saline solution (0.9% NaCl) should be used instead. A simple rule of thumb to predict the increase in the recipient's PCV is to remember that 2.2 ml/kg (or 1 ml/lb) of transfused whole blood will raise the PCV by 1% if the donor has a PCV of approximately 40%.

## COMPLICATIONS OF TRANSFUSION THERAPY

Transfusion-related complications can be divided into those that are immunologically mediated and those that are of non-immunologic origin. Immune-mediated reactions include urticaria, hemolysis, and fever. Non-immune-mediated complications include fever resulting from the transfusion of improperly stored blood, circulatory overload, citrate intoxication, disease transmission, and the metabolic burden associated with the transfusion of aged blood. Signs of imme-

diate immune-mediated hemolysis appear within minutes of the start of transfusion and include tremors, emesis, and fever; these are rare in dogs but common in cats receiving incompatible blood products. Delayed hemolytic reactions are more common and are manifested primarily by an unexpected decline in the PCV after transfusion over days, in association with hemoglobinemia, hemoglobinuria, and hyperbilirubinemia. Circulatory overload may be manifested by vomiting, dyspnea, or coughing. Citrate intoxication occurs when the infusion rate is too great or the liver is not able to metabolize the citrate. Signs of citrate intoxication are related to hypocalcemia and include tremors and cardiac arrhythmias. If signs of a transfusion reaction are recognized, the transfusion must be slowed or halted.

## Suggested Readings

Andrews GA: Red blood cell antigens and blood groups in the dog and cat. In Feldman BF et al, editors: *Schalm's veterinary hematology,* ed 5, Philadelphia, 2000, Lippincott Williams & Wilkins, p 767.

Authement JM et al: Canine blood component therapy: product preparation, storage, and administration, *J Am Anim Hosp Assoc* 23:483, 1987.

Boyce JT et al: Feline leukemia virus–induced erythroid aplasia: in vitro hemopoietic culture studies, *Exp Hematol* 9:990, 1981.

Callan MB et al: Canine red blood cell transfusion practice, *J Am Anim Hosp Assoc* 32:303, 1996.

Duvall D et al: Vaccine-associated immune-mediated hemolytic anemia in the dog, *J Vet Intern Med* 10:290, 1996.

Feldman BF et al: Anemia of inflammatory disease in the dog: clinical characterization, *J Am Vet Med Assoc* 42:1109, 1981.

Giger U: Erythrocyte phosphofructokinase and pyruvate kinase deficiencies. In Feldman BF et al, editors: *Schalm's veterinary hematology,* ed 5, Philadelphia, 2000, Lippincott Williams & Wilkins, p 1020.

Giger U et al: Transfusion of type-A and type-B blood to cats, *J Am Vet Med Assoc* 198:411, 1991.

Harvey JW et al: Chronic iron deficiency anemia in dogs, *J Am Anim Hosp Assoc* 18:946, 1982.

Jacobs RM et al: Use of a microtiter Coombs' test for study of age, gender, and breed distributions in immunohemolytic anemia in the dog, *J Am Vet Med Assoc* 185:66, 1984.

Jonas LD et al: Nonregenerative form of immune-mediated hemolytic anemia in dogs, *J Am Anim Hosp Assoc* 23:201, 1987.

Klag AR et al: Idiopathic immune-mediated hemolytic anemia in dogs: 42 cases (1986-1990), *J Am Vet Med Assoc* 202:783, 1993.

Klein MK et al: Pulmonary thromboembolism associated with immune-mediated hemolytic anemia in dogs: ten cases (1982-1987), *J Am Vet Med Assoc* 195:246, 1989.

Stokol T et al: Pure red cell aplasia in cats: 9 cases (1989-1997), *J Am Vet Med Assoc* 214:75, 1999.

Stokol T et al: Idiopathic pure red cell aplasia and nonregenerative immune-mediated anemia in dogs:43 cases (1988-1999), *J Am Vet Med Assoc* 216:1429, 2000.

Weiser MG: Correlative approach to anemia in dogs and cats, *J Am Anim Hosp Assoc* 17:286, 1981.

Weiss DJ: Antibody-mediated suppression of erythropoiesis in dogs with red blood cell aplasia, *Am J Vet Res* 12:2646, 1986.

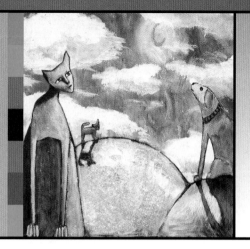

# CHAPTER 86

# Erythrocytosis

## CHAPTER OUTLINE

DEFINITION AND CLASSIFICATION, 1170
    Clinical and clinicopathologic findings, 1170
    Diagnosis and treatment, 1171

## DEFINITION AND CLASSIFICATION

*Erythrocytosis* is defined as an increase in the circulating red blood cells (RBCs) mass and is manifested hematologically as an increase in the packed cell volume (PCV) above reference values. Certain dog breeds, such as sight hounds, have PCVs above the reference range for the species; this also occurs in dogs that live at high altitudes. An increase in the RBC numbers may lead to severe hemorrheologic alterations, resulting in turn in clinical signs secondary to hyperviscosity. Although the term *polycythemia* is commonly used to refer to this hematologic abnormality, it is incorrect, because it actually means an increase in the numbers of all circulating cells (i.e., poly: multiple).

On the basis of its pathogenesis, erythrocytosis can be classified as either relative or absolute (Table 86-1). The term *relative erythrocytosis* refers to hemoconcentration (i.e., dehydration), and it is characterized by an increased PCV, usually in association with an increased serum or plasma protein concentration; in dogs and cats with relative erythrocytosis the RBC mass is normal. In *absolute,* or true, *erythrocytosis* there is an increase in the RBC mass; it can be classified as primary or secondary, depending on the cause and the serum erythropoietin (Epo) concentration or activity.

*Primary erythrocytosis* (polycythemia rubra vera [PRV]) results from an autonomous, Epo-independent proliferation of RBC precursors in the bone marrow. As a consequence, most dogs and cats with PRV have low to nondetectable serum Epo concentrations. *Secondary erythrocytosis* results from increased orthotopic (i.e., produced by the kidneys) or heterotopic (i.e., produced in sites other than the kidneys) Epo production. Orthotopic (i.e., physiologically appropriate) Epo production occurs in response to tissue hypoxia, such as that which occurs at a high altitude and in the settings of chronic cardiopulmonary disease, cardiovascular right-to-left shunts, and carboxyhemoglobinemia. Tumor-associated erythrocytosis (i.e., heterotopic

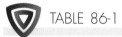

## TABLE 86-1

**Classification and Causes of Erythrocytosis in Cats and Dogs**

Relative erythrocytosis (pseudoerythrocytosis)
    Hemoconcentration
Absolute erythrocytosis
    Primary
        Polycythemia rubra vera
    Secondary
        Appropriate (i.e., secondary to decreased tissue
            oxygenation)
            Pulmonary disease
            Right-to-left cardiovascular shunts
            High altitude
            Hemoglobinopathies?
        Inappropriate (normal tissue oxygenation)
            Hyperadrenocorticism
            Hyperthyroidism
            Renal masses
            Neoplasms in other areas

?, Not well documented in cats or dogs.

or orthotopic Epo production) has been observed in people with a wide variety of neoplasms, in dogs with renal masses, and in a dog with a nasal fibrosarcoma. Hormonal stimuli may also trigger erythrocytosis in animals with normal tissue oxygenation, such as in dogs with hyperadrenocorticism and cats with hyperthyroidism. At our clinic, secondary erythrocytosis is more common in dogs, and PRV is more common in cats. However, erythrocytosis is rare in both species. Interestingly, although infiltrative renal diseases (e.g., lymphoma, feline infectious peritonitis) are common in cats, they rarely, if ever, result in secondary erythrocytosis.

### Clinical and Clinicopathologic Findings

The clinical signs may occur acutely and consist primarily of functional abnormalities of the central nervous system (i.e., behavioral, motor, or sensory changes); in cats, signs of a transverse myelopathy are common. A common manifestation of erythrocytosis in dogs is paroxysmal sneezing, attributed to in-

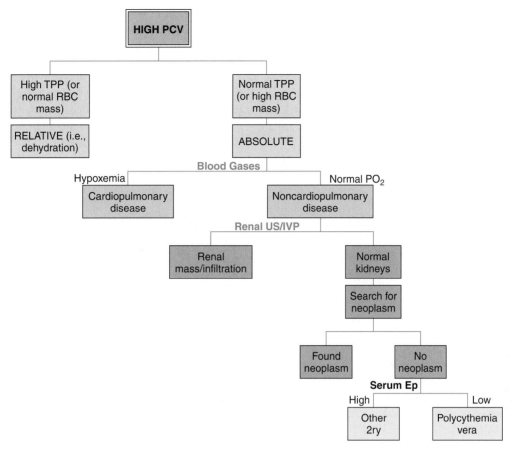

**FIG 86-1**
Diagnostic approach to the dog or cat with erythrocytosis. *PCV,* Packed cell volume; *TPP,* total plasma protein; *RBC,* red blood cell; *US/IVP,* ultrasonography/intravenous pyelography; *Ep,* erythropoietin; *2ry,* secondary.

creased blood viscosity in the nasal mucosa. Cardiopulmonary signs may occasionally be present. Although the erythrocytosis usually develops gradually, most affected animals do not exhibit clinical signs until the RBCs have reached a critical mass (or the PCV has reached a certain percentage). It is relatively common to find PCVs of 70% to 80% in cats and dogs with absolute erythrocytosis. Physical examination and historical findings in dogs and cats with erythrocytosis may also include bright red mucous membranes (plethora), erythema, polyuria, polydipsia, splenomegaly, renal masses, or a neoplasm elsewhere.

Hematologic abnormalities are usually limited to the erythrocytosis, although thrombocytosis may be present in cats and dogs with PRV. Microcytosis caused by relative iron deficiency (i.e., the erythron is extremely active and is relatively iron-deficient) is common in dogs with erythrocytosis.

## Diagnosis and Treatment

Relative erythrocytosis (i.e., dehydration) should be ruled out first. This is done primarily on the basis of the serum (or plasma) protein concentration, which is typically high in dogs and cats with this form of erythrocytosis. However, in certain circumstances, such as hemorrhagic gastroenteritis, dogs may have a high PCV but a relatively normal serum protein concentration. Radioisotopic RBC mass determinations are com-

monly performed in humans with erythrocytosis, but this test is usually not done in small animals.

The initial approach used in small animals with absolute erythrocytosis is to decrease the blood viscosity by reducing the number of circulating RBCs. This can be accomplished by performing therapeutic phlebotomies, in which a certain volume of blood (20 ml/kg) is collected from a central vein through a blood collection set. In cats a 19-gauge butterfly catheter coupled to a 60 ml syringe containing 500 to 600 U of heparin diluted in 3 to 5 ml of saline solution is usually used to collect blood from the jugular vein under chemical restraint. Gradual phlebotomy (5 ml/kg, repeated as needed) is recommended for animals with right-to-left shunts and erythrocytosis, because an increased RBC mass appears to be the body's way of enhancing oxygen delivery to the tissues and thereby compensating for the chronic hypoxemia in these animals. Because sudden decreases in blood volume can result in marked hypotension, a peripheral vein catheter can be used to administer an equivalent volume of saline solution at the same time that blood is being collected. As a result of its high viscosity, it may be extremely difficult to obtain blood through a relatively small (e.g., 19-gauge) catheter.

Once the patient's condition has been stabilized, the cause of the erythrocytosis should be sought (Fig. 86-1). The following approach is recommended for this. First, the patient's cardiopulmonary status should be evaluated (i.e., by auscultation, precordial palpation, thoracic radiography, echocardiography; see Chapters 1 and 2); an arterial blood sample should be obtained for blood gas analysis (i.e., to rule out hypoxemia). In some animals with erythrocytosis the blood viscosity is so high that the blood gas analyzer (which is usually flow-dependent) cannot generate results; in this event a therapeutic phlebotomy should be performed before a sample is resubmitted for testing (i.e., the blood oxygen content [$PO_2$] does not change after therapeutic phlebotomy). If the $PO_2$ is normal, excretory urography (intravenous pyelography), ultrasonography, or computerized tomography should be performed to determine whether there are masses or infiltrative lesions in the kidneys. If no such lesions are found, the patient most likely does not have renal secondary erythrocytosis, so a search for an extrarenal neoplasm should be conducted. A serum sample for determination of Epo activity (or concentrations) should be sent for analysis to a reliable laboratory (e.g., Dr. Urs Giger, Department of Genetics, School of Veterinary Medicine, University of Pennsylvania). In my experience, bone marrow evaluations of cats and dogs with erythrocytosis are unrewarding, because in most cases the only abnormality is a decreased myeloid/erythroid ratio resulting from erythroid hyperplasia.

If it is established that the animal has PRV, hydroxyurea (30 mg/kg PO q24h; Hydrea; E.R. Squibb & Sons, Princeton, N.J.) is administered for 7 to 10 days, after which the dose and dosing interval can be gradually decreased to fulfill the patient's needs. Phlebotomies should be repeated as dictated by the patient's clinical signs. If the final diagnosis is secondary erythrocytosis, the primary disorders should be treated (e.g., surgery for a renal mass).

Most dogs and cats with PRV have extremely long survival times (>2 years) if treated with hydroxyurea (with or without phlebotomies). Because this drug is potentially myelosuppressive, complete blood counts should be performed every 4 to 8 weeks and the dose decreased commensurate with the neutrophil count (see Chapter 80). The prognosis in dogs and cats with secondary erythrocytosis depends on the nature of the primary disease.

## Suggested Readings

Campbell KL: Diagnosis and management of polycythemia in dogs, *Compend Cont Educ* 12:443, 1990.

Cook SM et al: Serum erythropoietin concentrations measured by radioimmunoassay in normal, polycythemic, and anemic dogs and cats, *J Vet Intern Med* 8:18, 1994.

Giger U: Erythropoietin and its clinical use, *Compend Cont Educ* 14:25, 1992.

Hasler AH et al: Serum erythropoietin values in polycythemic cats, *J Am Anim Hosp Assoc* 32:294, 1996.

Peterson ME et al: Diagnosis and treatment of polycythemia. In Kirk RW, editor: *Current veterinary therapy VIII,* Philadelphia, 1983, WB Saunders.

Watson ADJ: Erythrocytosis and polycythemia. In Feldman BF et al: *Schalm's veterinary hematology,* ed 5, Philadelphia, 2000, Lippincott Williams & Wilkins, p 216.

# CHAPTER 87

# Leukopenia and Leukocytosis

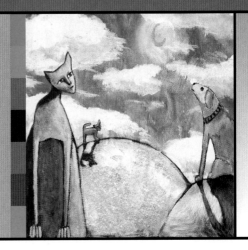

## CHAPTER OUTLINE

GENERAL CONSIDERATIONS, 1173
NORMAL LEUKOCYTE MORPHOLOGY
AND PHYSIOLOGY, 1173
LEUKOCYTE CHANGES IN DISEASE, 1174

Neutropenia, 1174
Neutrophilia, 1176
Eosinopenia, 1177
Eosinophilia, 1177
Basopenia, 1178
Basophilia, 1178
Monocytopenia, 1178
Monocytosis, 1178
Lymphopenia, 1179
Lymphocytosis, 1179

## GENERAL CONSIDERATIONS

The leukogram, evaluated as part of the complete blood count (CBC), includes a quantification of the total number of white blood cells (WBCs) and the differential WBC count. Although a specific disorder is rarely diagnosed on the basis of a leukogram, the information obtained may be useful in limiting the number of differential diagnoses or in predicting the severity of the disease and its prognosis. Sequential leukograms may also be helpful in monitoring a patient's response to therapy.

Using standard laboratory techniques, all nucleated cells are counted during a WBC count (including nucleated red blood cells [nRBCs]). Differential leukograms yielded by particle counters used at human referral laboratories are not valid for cats and dogs. *Leukocytosis* occurs if the WBC count exceeds the upper limit of normal for the species; *leukopenia* occurs if the WBC count is below the reference range.

A differential WBC count may be reported in either relative (percentages) or absolute numbers (number of cells per microliter). However, it is the *absolute* leukocyte numbers, rather than the percentages, that should always be evaluated, because the latter may be misleading, particularly if the WBC count is very high or very low. For example, a total WBC of 3000/$\mu$l and a differential WBC count of 90% lymphocytes and 10% neutrophils can lead to one of two conclusions:

1. On the basis of the percentages alone, the dog has lymphocytosis and neutropenia; in this situation, the clinician may erroneously "zoom in" on the "lymphocytosis" rather than the neutropenia.
2. On the basis of the absolute numbers, the dog has severe neutropenia (300 cells/$\mu$l) with a normal lymphocyte count (i.e., 2700 cells/$\mu$l).

Obviously the second conclusion reflects the actual clinical situation. The clinician should then concentrate on determining the cause of the neutropenia and ignore the normal lymphocyte count.

## NORMAL LEUKOCYTE MORPHOLOGY AND PHYSIOLOGY

From the morphologic standpoint, leukocytes can be classified as either polymorphonuclear or mononuclear. Polymorphonuclear cells include the neutrophils, eosinophils, and basophils, whereas the mononuclear cells include the monocytes and lymphocytes. Their basic morphologic and physiologic characteristics are reviewed elsewhere (Feldman and colleagues, 2000).

The following morphologic changes have important clinical implications and should thus be recognized:

1. Neutrophils may become toxic in response to injury; toxic neutrophils display characteristic cytoplasmic changes, including basophilia or granulation, vacuolation, and Döhle bodies (small, bluish cytoplasmic inclusions that consist of aggregates of endoplasmic reticulum).
2. Giant neutrophils, bands, and metamyelocytes are large, polyploidal cells that may result from skipped cell division; they represent yet another manifestation of toxic changes and are more common in cats than in dogs.

Other neutrophil morphologic abnormalities recognized during a careful examination of blood smears include the

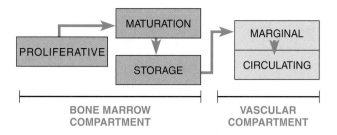

**FIG 87-1**
Theoretical neutrophil compartments in bone marrow and blood.

Pelger-Huët anomaly (cats and dogs) and Chédiak-Higashi syndrome (cats). The Pelger-Huët anomaly occurs when the nucleus of polymorphonuclear leukocytes fails to divide but the nuclear chromatin and cytoplasm maturation is complete (i.e., the nucleus has a band-like appearance with mature, clumped chromatin). Typically cats and dogs with this anomaly have profound "left-shifts" in the absence of clinical signs. On careful examination of the smear, however, the "left-shifted" cells are mature cells with nuclear hyposegmentation and not immature neutrophils. This anomaly may be acquired or inherited (autosomal dominant), but it is usually considered of minimal clinical relevance.

The Chédiak-Higashi syndrome, a lethal autosomal recessive condition of Persian cats with smoke-colored haircoats and yellow eyes, is characterized by enlarged neutrophilic and eosinophilic granules in association with partial albinism, photophobia, an increased susceptibility to infections, bleeding tendencies, and abnormal melanocytes.

Nuclear hypersegmentation (i.e., four or more distinct nuclear lobes) may result from a prolonged neutrophil transit time. It occurs in dogs with hyperadrenocorticism, cats and dogs receiving corticosteroid therapy, and cats and dogs with chronic inflammatory disorders. It may also be noted in Poodles with macrocytosis.

A basic review of neutrophil physiology follows. Three theoretical physiologic neutrophil compartments exist in the bone marrow (Fig. 87-1). The *proliferative* compartment is composed of dividing cells (i.e., myeloblasts, progranulocytes, myelocytes); it takes myeloblasts approximately 48 to 60 hours to mature into metamyelocytes. The *maturation* compartment consists of metamyelocytes and band neutrophils; the transit time through this compartment is 46 to 70 hours. The *storage* compartment is made up of mature neutrophils; the transit time in this compartment is approximately 50 hours, and it contains an estimated 5-day supply of neutrophils. Mature neutrophils leave the bone marrow by a random process that involves changes in cell deformability and adhesiveness.

Two neutrophil pools are present in the *vascular* compartment (see Fig. 87-1). The *marginal neutrophil pool* (MNP) consists of neutrophils that are adhered to the vascular endothelium (and are thus not counted during a CBC). The *circulating neutrophil pool* (CNP) consists of the neutrophils circulating in the blood (i.e., the cells counted during a differential WBC count). The *total blood neutrophil pool* is composed of the MNP and the CNP. In dogs the CNP is approx-

imately equal in size to that of the MNP. However, in cats the MNP is approximately two to three times the size of the CNP. The neutrophil has an average blood transit time of approximately 6 to 8 hours in dogs and 10 to 12 hours in cats, with all blood neutrophils replaced every 2 to 2.5 days. Once the neutrophils leave the blood vessel (by diapedesis), they normally do not return to the circulation and may be lost in the lungs, gut, other tissues, urine, or saliva.

## LEUKOCYTE CHANGES IN DISEASE

### NEUTROPENIA

*Neutropenia* is defined as an absolute decrease in the number of circulating neutrophils. It can result from decreased (or impaired) cell production within the bone marrow or from the increased margination or destruction of circulating neutrophils (Table 87-1). Neutropenia is relatively common in cats and dogs. The clinician should keep in mind, however, that normal cats may have neutrophil counts of 1800 to 2300/$\mu$l.

Clinical signs in neutropenic cats and dogs are usually vague and nonspecific; they include anorexia, lethargy, pyrexia, and mild gastrointestinal tract signs. Oral ulceration, a common feature of neutropenia in humans, does not seem to occur in small animals. Frequently neutropenia is an incidental finding in an otherwise healthy animal (i.e., the patient is asymptomatic). If the neutropenia is caused by peripheral neutrophil consumption (i.e., a septic process), most animals exhibit clinical signs. Dogs and cats with parvoviral enteritis have neutropenia in association with severe vomiting or diarrhea, or both. Occasionally cats and dogs with neutropenia can present in septic shock (i.e., pale, hypoperfused, hypothermic) and should be treated aggressively.

The evaluation of neutropenic cats and dogs should include a detailed drug history (e.g., estrogen or phenylbutazone in dogs, griseofulvin in cats; see Table 87-1), vaccination history (e.g., was the cat vaccinated against panleukopenia or the dog against parvoviral enteritis), a complete physical examination and imaging in search of a septic focus, serologic or virologic tests for infectious diseases (e.g., feline leukemia virus, feline immunodeficiency virus, canine ehrlichiosis, parvoviral enteritis), and, if necessary, bone marrow cytologic or histopathologic studies. Evaluating changes in a blood smear is important in establishing the pathogenesis of the neutropenia. For example, if a dog or cat has anemia and/or thrombocytopenia in association with the neutropenia, and particularly if the anemia is nonregenerative, a primary bone marrow disorder should be strongly suspected. If a dog or cat has regenerative anemia and spherocytosis in association with neutropenia, an immune-mediated disease should be considered a likely diagnosis. The presence of toxic changes in the neutrophils tends to suggest infection (i.e., toxic changes are usually absent in dogs and cats with steroid-responsive neutropenia or primary bone marrow disorders). Evaluation of sequential leukograms in neutropenic dogs and cats is helpful in excluding transient or cyclic neutropenia (or cyclic hematopoiesis).

## TABLE 87-1

Causes of Neutropenia in Cats and Dogs

| Decreased or Ineffective Production of Cells in the Proliferating Pool | Decreased or Ineffective Production of Cells in the Proliferating Pool—cont'd |
|---|---|
| Myelophthisis (neoplastic infiltration of the bone marrow)<br>  *Myeloproliferative disorders (D, C)*<br>  **Lymphoproliferative disorders (D, C)**<br>  Systemic mast cell disease (D, C)<br>  Malignant histiocytosis (D, C?)<br>  Myelofibrosis (D, C)<br>  *Metastatic carcinoma (D?, C?)*<br>Drug-induced neutropenia<br>  Anticancer and immunosuppressive agents (C, D)<br>  Chloramphenicol (C)<br>  **Griseofulvin (C)**<br>  Sulfa-trimethoprim (D, C)<br>  **Estrogen (D)**<br>  **Phenylbutazone (D)**<br>  *Phenobarbital (D)*<br>  Other<br>Toxins<br>  Industrial chemical compounds (inorganic solvents, benzene) (D, C)<br>  *Fusarium sporotrichiella toxin (C)*<br>Infectious diseases<br>  **Parvovirus infection (D, C)**<br>  *Retrovirus infection (feline leukemia virus, feline immunodeficiency virus) (C)*<br>  Myelodysplastic or preleukemic syndromes (C)<br>  Cyclic neutropenia (C)<br>  *Histoplasmosis (D, C)*<br>  **Ehrlichiosis (D, C)** | Infectious diseases—cont'd<br>  Toxoplasmosis (D, C)<br>  Early canine distemper virus infection (D)<br>  Early canine hepatitis virus infection (D)<br>Other<br>  Idiopathic bone marrow hypoplasia-aplasia (D, C)<br>  Cyclic neutropenia of gray Collies (D)<br>  Acquired cyclic neutropenia (D, C)<br>  **Steroid-responsive neutropenia (D, C)**<br><br>**Sequestration of Neutrophils in the Marginating Pool**<br><br>**Endotoxic shock (D, C)**<br>Anaphylactic shock (D, C)<br>Anesthesia (D?, C?)<br><br>**Sudden, Excessive Tissue Demand, Destruction, or Consumption**<br><br>Infectious diseases<br>  **Peracute, overwhelming bacterial infection (e.g., peritonitis, aspiration pneumonia, salmonellosis, metritis, pyothorax) (D, C)**<br>  Viral infection (e.g., canine distemper or hepatitis, preclinical stage) (D)<br>Drug-induced (D, C) (see above)<br>**Immune-mediated (D, C)**<br>Paraneoplastic (D)<br>"Hypersplenism" (D?) |

**Common;** *relatively common;* uncommon; *D,* dog; *C;* cat; *?,* poorly documented.

If the pathogenesis of neutropenia cannot be ascertained in an animal, sophisticated diagnostic techniques such as leukocyte nuclear scanning or kinetic studies can be performed. As noted earlier, normal cats can have low neutrophil counts. Therefore, if a cat with a neutrophil count of 1800 to 2300/µl is brought in for evaluation (or, more likely, if the "neutropenia" is detected during a routine hematologic evaluation), a conservative approach (i.e., repeat the CBC in 2 to 3 weeks) is indicated as long as no other clinical or hematologic abnormalities are found.

Because corticosteroid-responsive neutropenia has been well characterized in cats and dogs, if most infectious and neoplastic causes of neutropenia have been ruled out in an asymptomatic neutropenic animal, an in-hospital therapeutic trial of immunosuppressive doses of corticosteroids (prednisone, 2 to 4 mg/kg/day PO for dogs; 4 to 8 mg/kg/day PO for cats) can be instituted. Responses are usually observed within 24 to 96 hours of the start of treatment in such patients. Treatment is continued as it is for dogs with immune hemolytic anemia and other immune-mediated disorders (see Chapter 93) (Fig. 87-2).

Asymptomatic, afebrile neutropenic animals should be treated with broad-spectrum bactericidal antibiotics, because

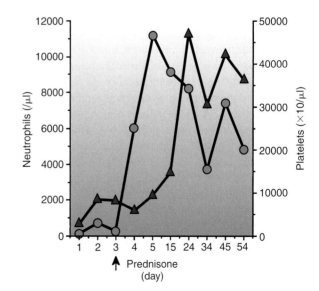

**FIG 87-2**

Response to therapy in a 6-year-old, female, spayed Airedale Terrier with steroid-responsive neutropenia and thrombocytopenia. Note the rapid response to immunosuppressive doses of prednisone. —●—, Polymorphonuclear neutrophils (µl); —△—, platelets (× 10³/µl).

they are at high risk for sepsis (see p. 1108). My drug of choice in dogs is a combination of a sulfa drug and trimethoprim at a dosage of 15 mg/kg given orally every 12 hours; another drug that can be used in both dogs and cats is enrofloxacin (Baytril; Bayer, Shawnee Mission, Kan) at a dosage of 5 mg/kg given orally every 12 to 24 hours. Antibiotics with an anaerobic spectrum should not be used because they deplete intestinal anaerobes, a protective bacterial population.

Neutropenic febrile (or symptomatic) cats and dogs should be treated with aggressive intravenous antibiotic therapy, as described on p. 1110. Our treatment of choice consists of cephalothin (20 mg/kg IV q8h) in combination with amikacin (15 mg/kg IV q24h); a combination of ampicillin (20 mg/kg IV q8h) and enrofloxacin (5 mg/kg IV q12-24h) is also effective in these patients.

Neutrophil production can be stimulated by the administration of human recombinant granulocyte colony-stimulating factor (G-CSF) (5 μg/kg SQ q24h). Although results are quite spectacular, the responses are usually short-lived because of the counteractive effects of anti-CSF antibodies produced by the affected dog or cat. Lithium carbonate (10 mg/kg PO q12h) can increase the neutrophil counts in dogs; the therapeutic trough serum concentration of lithium is 0.8 to 1.5 mmol/L. This drug should be used with caution in dogs with a decreased glomerular filtration rate, because it is primarily excreted by the kidneys. Lithium carbonate does not appear to be effective (and may be toxic) in cats.

## NEUTROPHILIA

*Neutrophilia* is defined as an absolute increase in the number of neutrophils, and it constitutes the most common cause of leukocytosis in dogs and cats. Several terms used to characterize neutrophilia are defined in the following paragraph.

The term *mature neutrophilia* refers to an increase in the number of segmented (mature) neutrophils without an increase in the number of immature forms (e.g., bands). *Neutrophilia with a left-shift* refers to an increase in the number of both mature and immature neutrophils (bands, more than 300/μl). A *regenerative left-shift* is a neutrophilia with increased numbers of immature neutrophils in which the number of immature forms does not exceed the number of mature neutrophils. A *degenerative left-shift* occurs when the number of immature forms exceeds that of mature neutrophils; the number of the latter may be normal, low, or high. Degenerative left-shifts are usually suggestive of an aggressive disease. Disorders commonly associated with degenerative left-shifts include pyothorax, septic peritonitis, bacterial pneumonia, pyometra, prostatitis, and acute pyelonephritis. A *leukemoid reaction* refers to a marked neutrophilia with a severe left-shift, which includes metamyelocytes and myelocytes. It indicates severe inflammatory disease and may be difficult to distinguish from chronic granulocytic (myelogenous) leukemia (see p. 1139).

Although a high percentage of cats and dogs with neutrophilia have underlying infectious disorders, neutrophilia is not synonymous with infection. Rather, neutrophilia in cats and dogs is commonly the result of inflammatory or neo-

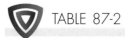

## TABLE 87-2

**Causes of Neutrophilia in Cats and Dogs**

Physiologic or epinephrine-induced neutrophilia
  **Fear (C)**
  Excitement (?)
  Exercise (?)
  *Seizures (D, C)*
  Parturition (?)
Stress- or corticosteroid-induced neutrophilia
  Pain (?)
  Anesthesia (?)
  **Trauma (D, C)**
  *Neoplasia (D, C)*
  **Hyperadrenocorticism (D)**
  Metabolic disorders (?)
  Chronic disorders (D, C)
Inflammation or increased tissue demand
  **Infection (bacterial, viral, fungal, parasitic) (D, C)**
  **Tissue trauma and/or necrosis (D, C)**
  **Immune-mediated disorders (D)**
  *Neoplasia (D, C)*
  *Metabolic (uremia, diabetic ketoacidosis) (D, C)*
  Burns (D, C)
  Neutrophil function abnormalities (D)
  Other (acute hemorrhage, hemolysis) (D, C)

**Common;** *relatively common;* uncommon; *D,* dog; *C,* cat; ?, poorly documented.

plastic processes. Several disorders resulting in neutrophilia are listed in Table 87-2.

It should be kept in mind that neutrophilia commonly results from endogenous epinephrine release (physiologic neutrophilia). This neutrophilia, which is associated with the release of neutrophils from the MNP, is transient (lasting 20 to 30 minutes after endogenous release of catecholamines) and is commonly associated with erythrocytosis and lymphocytosis (the latter primarily in cats).

The endogenous release or exogenous administration of corticosteroids results in a stress- or corticosteroid-induced neutrophilia, which is associated with decreased neutrophil egress from the vasculature and increased bone marrow release of neutrophils from the storage pool. Other hematologic changes typical of a stress leukogram include lymphopenia, eosinopenia, and monocytosis (the latter only occurs in dogs). These abnormalities are commonly seen in sick dogs and cats at our clinic.

Clinical signs in cats and dogs with neutrophilia are usually secondary to the underlying disorder. Pyrexia may or may not be present. If the patient has persistent neutrophilia, if the neutrophils display toxic changes (see p. 1173), or if a degenerative left-shift is present, every effort should be made to identify a septic focus or an infectious agent immediately. The workup in such animals should include a thorough physical examination (e.g., abscess); thoracic and abdominal radiography (e.g., pneumonia, pleural or abdominal effusion); abdominal ultrasonography (e.g., peritonitis, pancreatic or hepatic abscess); and the collection of blood, urine, fluid, or tissue samples for bacterial and fungal cultures. As discussed in previous paragraphs, autologous or allogeneic neutrophils labeled with radionuclides (i.e., technetium 99m or indium 111) can be injected intravenously and the septic focus, or foci, identified by gamma camera imaging.

The treatment of dogs and cats with neutrophilia is aimed at the primary cause. Empiric antibiotic therapy with a broad-spectrum bactericidal antibiotic (e.g., sulfa-trimethoprim, enrofloxacin, cephalosporin, amoxicillin) is an acceptable approach if a cause for the neutrophilia cannot be identified after exhaustive clinical and clinicopathologic evaluation.

## EOSINOPENIA

*Eosinopenia* is defined as an absolute decrease in the number of circulating eosinophils. It is commonly seen as part of the stress leukogram and is usually of little clinical relevance. Causes of eosinopenia are listed in Table 87-3.

## EOSINOPHILIA

*Eosinophilia* is defined as an absolute increase in the circulating eosinophil numbers. It is relatively common in small animals, and it can have a variety of causes, which are listed in Table 87-4. Because eosinophilia is quite common in parasitic disorders, no animal should undergo a thorough evaluation for eosinophilia before parasitic causes have been ruled out. In cats, flea infestation usually results in marked increases in the eosinophil count. In dogs, eosinophilia is frequently seen in those with roundworm and hookworm infestations or with dirofilariasis or dipetalonemiasis. Three additional relatively common causes of eosinophilia in cats include eosinophilic granuloma complex, bronchial asthma, and eosinophilic gastroenteritis. Eosinophilia can also occur in dogs and cats with mast cell tumors, but it is rare.

Clinical signs in dogs and cats with eosinophilia are related to the primary disorders rather than to the hematologic abnormality. Because eosinophilia is so commonly found in animals with parasitic diseases, clinical evaluation of these animals should be aimed mainly at excluding these disorders. Once this has been done, other causes of eosinophilia should be pursued (see Table 87-4) using the appropriate diagnostic procedures (e.g., tracheal wash for pulmonary infiltrates with eosinophils, endoscopic biopsy for eosinophilic gastroenteritis). Treatment is usually aimed at the primary disorder.

A syndrome in which there are high eosinophil counts in peripheral blood and tissue infiltration with eosinophils has been well documented in cats and in Rottweilers. This syndrome is termed *hypereosinophilic syndrome* and is usually indistinguishable from eosinophilic leukemia. These patients have primary gastrointestinal tract signs, although multisystemic signs are also common. In cats, treatment with immunosuppressive doses of corticosteroids, 6-thioguanine,

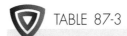

### TABLE 87-3

**Causes of Eosinopenia in Cats and Dogs**

Stress or corticosteroid induced (see Table 87-2)
Acute inflammation or infection
    Secondary to endogenous corticosteroid release

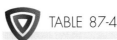

### TABLE 87-4

**Causes of Eosinophilia in Cats and Dogs**

Parasitic disorders
    *Ancylostomiasis (D)*
    **Dirofilariasis (D, C)**
    **Dipetalonemiasis (D)**
    **Ctenocephalidiasis (D, C)**
    Filaroidiasis (C)
    Aelurostrongylosis (C)
    *Ascariasis (D, C)*
    Paragonimiasis (D, C)
Hypersensitivity disorders
    **Atopy (D, C)**
    **Flea allergy dermatitis (D, C)**
    **Food allergy (D, C)**
Eosinophilic infiltrative disorders
    **Eosinophilic granuloma complex (C)**
    **Feline bronchial asthma (C)**
    Pulmonary infiltrates with eosinophils (D)
    **Eosinophilic gastroenteritis/colitis (D, C)**
    *Hypereosinophilic syndrome (D, C)*
Infectious diseases
    Upper respiratory tract viral disorders (C?)
    Feline panleukopenia (C?)
    Feline infectious peritonitis (C?)
    Toxoplasmosis (C)
    Suppurative processes (D, C)
Neoplasia
    *Mast cell tumors (D, C)*
    Lymphomas (D, C)
    Myeloproliferative disorders (C)
    Solid tumors (D, C)
Miscellaneous
    Soft tissue trauma (D?, C?)
    Feline urologic syndrome (C?)
    Cardiomyopathy (D?, C?)
    Renal failure (D?, C?)
    Hyperthyroidism (C?)
    Estrus (D?)

**Common;** *relatively common;* uncommon; D, dog; C, cat; ?, poorly documented.

TABLE 87-5

Causes of Basophilia in Cats and Dogs

**Disorders Associated with IgE Production/Binding**

Heartworm disease (**D,** C)
*Inhalant dermatitis (D, C)*

**Inflammatory Diseases**

**Gastrointestinal tract disease (D, C)**
**Respiratory tract disease (D, C)**

**Neoplasms**

*Mast cell tumors (D, C)*
Lymphomatoid granulomatosis (D, C)
Basophilic leukemia (D)

**Associated with Hyperlipoproteinemia**

Hypothyroidism (D?)

---

**Common;** *relatively common;* uncommon; *D,* dog; *C,* cat;
?, poorly documented.

---

 TABLE 87-6

Causes of Monocytosis in Cats and Dogs

**Inflammation**
Infectious disorders
  Bacteria
    **Pyometra (D, C)**
    **Abscesses (D, C)**
    **Peritonitis (D, C)**
    **Pyothorax (D, C)**
    **Osteomyelitis (D, C)**
    **Prostatitis (D)**
  Higher bacteria
    *Nocardia (D, C)*
    *Actinomyces (D, C)*
    Mycobacteria (D, C)
  Intracellular parasites
    Ehrlichia (D, C?)
    Hemobartonella (D, C)
  Fungi
    **Blastomyces (D, C)**
    **Histoplasma (D, C)**
    Cryptococcus (D, C)
    Coccidioides (D)
  Parasites
    Heartworms (D, C?)
Immune-mediated disorders
  **Hemolytic anemia (D, C)**
  Dermatitis (D, C)
  *Polyarthritis (D, C)*
Trauma with severe crushing injuries (D, C)
Hemorrhage into tissues or body cavities (D, C)
**Stress- or corticosteroid-induced (D)**
Neoplasia
  Associated with tumor necrosis (D, C)
  Lymphoma (D, C)
  Myelodysplastic disorders (D, C)
  Leukemias
    Myelomonocytic leukemia (D, C)
    Monocytic leukemia (D, C)
    Myelogenous leukemia (D, C)

---

**Common;** *relatively common;* uncommon; *D,* dog; *C,* cat;
?; poorly documented.

---

cytosine arabinoside, cyclophosphamide, and other anticancer agents (see Chapter 79) has been unrewarding, and most affected patients die within weeks of diagnosis. Clinical response to some of these drugs has been documented in Rottweilers.

## BASOPENIA

*Basopenia* is defined as an absolute decrease in the basophil number. Because basophils are rare in circulation, basopenia is not clinically relevant.

## BASOPHILIA

*Basophilia* is defined as an absolute increase in the basophil numbers and is commonly associated with eosinophilia. Because basophils are similar to tissue mast cells, their numbers increase in disorders characterized by excessive IgE production and binding and in a variety of nonspecific inflammatory disorders. Causes of basophilia are listed in Table 87-5.

## MONOCYTOPENIA

The term *monocytopenia* refers to an absolute decrease in circulating monocyte numbers. Monocytopenia is not clinically relevant.

## MONOCYTOSIS

*Monocytosis* refers to an absolute increase in monocyte numbers. It can occur in response to inflammatory, neoplastic, or degenerative stimuli. Although traditionally monocytosis has been observed primarily in chronic inflammatory processes, it is also common in acute disorders. Causes of monocytosis in cats and dogs are listed in Table 87-6. The monocytosis in dogs is typically more pronounced than that in cats.

Monocytosis is part of a stress leukogram in dogs, and it can result from a variety of bacterial, fungal, and protozoal diseases. In the Midwest, systemic fungal disorders (i.e., histo-

plasmosis and blastomycosis) are relatively common causes. Because monocytes are precursors of tissue macrophages, granulomatous and pyogranulomatous reactions commonly result in monocytosis (see Table 87-6). In addition, immune-mediated injury resulting in cell destruction (e.g., immune hemolysis, polyarthritis) and certain neoplasms (e.g., lymphomas) commonly cause monocytosis. Some neoplasms secrete colony-stimulating factors for monocytes and can result in marked monocytosis ($>5000/\mu l$).

The nature of the clinical evaluation in patients with monocytosis is similar to that in those with neutrophilia, in that it should concentrate on identifying infectious foci. If an

## TABLE 87-7

### Causes of Lymphopenia in Cats and Dogs

**Corticosteroid or stress induced (D, C)** (see also
 Table 87-2)
Loss of lymph
 **Lymphangiectasia (D, C)**
 **Chylothorax (D, C)**
Impaired lymphopoiesis
 **Chemotherapy (D, C)**
 **Long-term corticosteroid use (D, C)**
Viral diseases
 *Parvoviruses (D, C)*
 *Feline infectious peritonitis (C)*
 *Feline leukemia virus (C)*
 *Feline immunodeficiency virus (C)*
 Canine distemper (D)
 Canine infectious hepatitis (D)

**Common;** *relatively common;* uncommon; *D,* dog; *C,* cat;
?, poorly documented.

## TABLE 87-8

### Causes of Lymphocytosis in Cats and Dogs

**Physiologic or epinephrine induced (C)** (see Table
 87-2)
Prolonged antigenic stimulation
 Chronic infection
  **Ehrlichiosis (D, C?)**
  Chagas' disease (D)
  Babesiosis (D)
  Leishmaniasis (D)
 Hypersensitivity reactions (?)
 Immune-mediated disease (?)
 **Postvaccinal reaction (D, C)**
Leukemia
 **Lymphocytic (D, C)**
 **Lymphoblastic (C, D)**
 *Hypoadrenocorticism (D)*

**Common;** *relatively common;* uncommon; *D,* dog; *C,* cat;
?, poorly documented.

immune-mediated disorder is suspected, arthrocentesis to obtain fluid for analysis or other immune tests (see Chapter 92) should be performed. Treatment should be aimed at the primary disorder.

## LYMPHOPENIA

*Lymphopenia* is defined as an absolute decrease in the lymphocyte count. It constitutes one of the most common hematologic abnormalities in hospitalized or sick dogs and cats, in which it is attributed to the effects of endogenous corticosteroids (stress leukogram). Lymphopenia is also commonly identified in dogs and cats that have chronic loss of lymph, such as those with chylothorax or intestinal lymphangiectasia. It also constitutes a common feature of certain acute viral diseases (Table 87-7).

In general, cats and dogs with lymphopenia have obvious clinical abnormalities. As a general rule, it should be "ignored" (i.e., a diagnosis should not be pursued) in sick cats and dogs and in those receiving corticosteroids. The lymphocyte count should be reevaluated after the clinical abnormalities have resolved or steroid therapy has been discontinued. Contrary to popular belief, lymphopenia does not appear to predispose to infections.

## LYMPHOCYTOSIS

*Lymphocytosis* is defined as an absolute increase in lymphocyte numbers. It is common in several clinical situations, including fear (cats) (see Neutrophilia, above), vaccination (dogs and possibly cats), chronic ehrlichiosis (dogs), Addison's disease (hypoadrenocorticism) (dogs), and chronic lymphocytic leukemia. The lymphocytes are morphologically normal in all these disorders with the exception of vaccination reactions, in which reactive lymphocytes (larger cells with dark blue cytoplasm) are commonly seen. High numbers of morphologically abnormal (i.e., blast) lymphoid cells

are found in dogs and cats with acute lymphoblastic leukemia (see pp. 1134 and 1138).

In cats with marked lymphocytosis and neutrophilia, endogenous release of catecholamines should be ruled out as the cause of these hematologic abnormalities. If the cat is fractious and blood cannot be collected without a considerable struggle, a blood sample should be collected under chemical restraint

Recent vaccination should be ruled out in dogs with lymphocytosis and reactive lymphocytes in the blood smear. Most dogs with lymphocyte counts of more than 10,000 cells/μl have either chronic ehrlichiosis or chronic lymphocytic leukemia (CLL); lymphocyte counts of more than 20,000 cells/μl are extremely rare in dogs with ehrlichiosis (i.e., dogs with >20,000 lymphocytes/μl more like have CLL). A high proportion of these dogs also have hyperproteinemia caused by a monoclonal or polyclonal gammopathy (see p. 1139). The clinical and hematologic features of the two disorders are quite similar (i.e., cytopenias, hyperproteinemia, hepatosplenomegaly, lymphadenopathy). Serologic tests or polymerase chain reaction testing for *Ehrlichia canis* and findings yielded by a bone marrow aspiration may be helpful in differentiating between these two disorders. Bone marrow cytologic findings in dogs with chronic ehrlichiosis usually consist of generalized hematopoietic hypoplasia and plasmacytosis, whereas hypoplasia with increased numbers of lymphocytes is more common in dogs with chronic lymphocytic leukemia. Causes of lymphocytosis in cats and dogs are listed in Table 87-8.

### Suggested Readings

Carothers M et al: Disorders of leukocytes. In Fenner WR, editor: *Quick reference to veterinary medicine,* ed 3, New York, JB Lippincott, 2000, p 149.

Center SA et al: Eosinophilia in the cat: a retrospective study of 312 cases (1975 to 1986), *J Am Anim Hosp Assoc* 26:349, 1990.

Couto CG: Immune-mediated neutropenia. In Feldman BF et al, editors: *Schalm's veterinary hematology,* ed 5, Philadelphia, 2000, Lippincott Williams & Wilkins, p 815.

Couto GC et al: Disorders of leukocytes and leukopoiesis. In Sherding RG, editor: *The cat: diseases and clinical management,* ed 2, New York, 1994, Churchill Livingstone.

Feldman BF et al, editors: *Schalm's veterinary hematology,* ed 5, Philadelphia, 2000, Lippincott Williams & Wilkins.

Huibregtse BA et al: Hypereosinophilic syndrome and eosinophilic leukemia: a comparison of 22 hypereosinophilic cats, *J Am Anim Hosp Assoc* 30:591, 1994.

# CHAPTER 88

## Combined Cytopenias and Leukoerythroblastosis

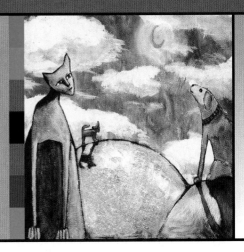

**CHAPTER OUTLINE**

DEFINITIONS AND CLASSIFICATION, 1181

## DEFINITIONS AND CLASSIFICATION

Combined cytopenias commonly result from decreased bone marrow production or, less frequently, from increased destruction or sequestration of circulating cells. Following are the definitions of several terms used throughout this chapter: *Bicytopenia* is a decrease in the numbers of two circulating blood cell lines (i.e., anemia and neutropenia, anemia and thrombocytopenia, neutropenia and thrombocytopenia). If all three cell lines are affected (i.e., anemia, neutropenia, thrombocytopenia), this is called *pancytopenia* (from the Greek *pan,* meaning "all"). In most cases, if anemia is present, it is nonregenerative. If regenerative anemia occurs in association with other cytopenias, usually the cause is peripheral destruction of cells. *Leukoerythroblastic reaction* (LER) (or leukoerythroblastosis) refers to the presence of immature white blood cells (WBCs) and nucleated red blood cells (nRBCs) in the circulation (i.e., nRBCs and a left shift). The WBC count is usually high, but it can be normal or low.

Cytopenias can develop as a result of the decreased production or increased peripheral destruction of the affected cell line or lines. In general, bicytopenias and pancytopenias result from primary bone marrow disorders (i.e., there is a problem in the "cell factory"; Table 88-1), although they may also result from peripheral blood cell destruction, such as occurs in sepsis, disseminated intravascular coagulation (DIC), and some immune-mediated blood disorders.

Leukoerythroblastic reactions result from a variety of mechanisms (Table 88-2), but in general the presence of immature blood cells in the circulation is secondary to their premature release from the bone marrow or from other hematopoietic organs (i.e., spleen, liver). This premature release can result from (1) an increased demand for blood cells (e.g., hemolytic anemia, blood loss, peritonitis), resulting in a shorter transit time through the bone marrow compartments, or (2) the crowding out of normal bone marrow precursors (e.g., leukemia, bone marrow lymphoma). They may also be prematurely released from a site of extramedullary hematopoiesis (EMH) (i.e., spleen, liver) as a result of the absence of normal feedback mechanisms.

### Clinicopathologic Features

The clinical signs and physical examination findings in dogs and cats with combined cytopenias or LERs are usually related to the underlying disorder rather than to the hematologic abnormalities per se, with the exception of pallor and spontaneous bleeding (i.e., petechiae, ecchymoses) secondary to anemia and thrombocytopenia, respectively. Pyrexia may be present if the patient is markedly neutropenic and is septic.

An important aspect of the clinical evaluation of these patients is the history. A detailed history should be obtained, with particular inquiries about the therapeutic use of drugs (e.g., estrogen or phenylbutazone in dogs, griseofulvin or chloramphenicol in cats), exposure to benzene derivatives, travel history, vaccination status, and exposure to other animals, among others. Most drugs that cause anemia or neutropenia can also cause combined cytopenias (see Tables 85-2 and 87-1).

The physical examination of dogs and cats with combined cytopenias may reveal the presence of spontaneous hemorrhages compatible with a primary hemostatic disorder (i.e., thrombocytopenia) or of pallor secondary to the attendant anemia. Several physical examination findings may help the clinician establish a more presumptive or definitive diagnosis in patients with cytopenias or LER. Of particular interest is the finding of male-feminizing signs in a male dog (usually a cryptorchid) with pancytopenia, which may indicate the presence of a Sertoli cell tumor or, less frequently, an interstitial cell tumor or a seminoma with secondary hyperestrogenism. The finding of generalized lymphadenopathy, hepatomegaly or splenomegaly, or intraabdominal or intrathoracic masses may direct the clinician toward a specific group of presumptive diagnoses. For example, the finding of a cranial or midabdominal mass in a dog with anemia, thrombocytopenia, and LER is highly suggestive of splenic hemangiosarcoma.

The presence of diffuse splenomegaly indicates that the spleen may be sequestering or destroying circulating blood

TABLE 88-1

### Causes of Bicytopenia and Pancytopenia in Dogs and Cats

**Decreased Cell Production**

Bone marrow hypoplasia-aplasia
  *Idiopathic*
  *Chemicals (e.g., benzene derivatives)*
  *Hormones (endogenous or exogenous estrogen)*
  **Drugs (chemotherapeutic agents, antibiotics, nonsteroidal antiinflammatories)**
  Radiation therapy
  **Immune-mediated**
  **Infectious** (parvovirus, feline leukemia virus, feline immunodeficiency virus, *Ehrlichia canis*)
Bone marrow necrosis
  **Infectious disorders** (sepsis, parvovirus)
  Toxins (mycotoxins)
  Neoplasms (acute and chronic leukemias, metastatic neoplasia)
  Other (hypoxia, DIC)
Bone marrow fibrosis-sclerosis
  Myelofibrosis
  Osteosclerosis
  Osteopetrosis
Myelophthisis
  Neoplasms
    **Acute leukemias**
    Chronic leukemias
    *Lymphoma*
    **Multiple myeloma**
    Systemic mast cell disease
    Malignant histiocytosis
    Metastatic neoplasms
  Granulomatous disorders
    *Histoplasma capsulatum*
    *Mycobacterium* spp.
    Storage diseases
Myelodysplasia

**Increased Cell Destruction and Sequestration**

Immune-mediated disorders
  **Evans's syndrome**
**Sepsis**
**Microangiopathy**
  **DIC**
  **Hemangiosarcoma**
*Splenomegaly*
  Congestive splenomegaly
  Hypersplenism
  *Hemolymphatic neoplasia*
  Other neoplasms

**Common;** *relatively common; uncommon. DIC,* Disseminated intravascular coagulation.

TABLE 88-2

### Causes of Leukoerythroblastosis in Dogs and Cats

**Extramedullary hematopoiesis***
**Immune hemolytic anemia**
*Blood loss anemia*
**Sepsis**
*Disseminated intravascular coagulation*
Chronic hypoxia (i.e., congestive heart failure)
Neoplasia
  **Hemangiosarcoma**
  Lymphoma
  *Leukemias*
  Multiple myeloma
Other
  Diabetes mellitus
  Hyperthyroidism
  Hyperadrenocorticism

**Common;** *relatively common;* uncommon.
*Extramedullary hematopoiesis may play a role in the pathogenesis of the leukoerythroblastic reaction in several of the disorders mentioned in the text.

cells or that EMH is occurring in response to a primary bone marrow disorder. Cytologic evaluation of spleen specimens obtained by percutaneous fine-needle aspiration is always indicated in dogs and cats with cytopenias and diffuse splenomegaly to determine whether the enlarged spleen is the cause or consequence of the cytopenias (see Chapter 90).

Serologic studies for PCR (polymerase chain reaction) are usually indicated in dogs and cats with bicytopenias or pancytopenias. Infectious diseases associated with bicytopenias and pancytopenias commonly diagnosed on the basis of or serologic PCR findings include ehrlichiosis in dogs and feline leukemia and feline immunodeficiency virus infections in cats. If the clinical and hematologic features of the case point toward an immune-mediated disease (i.e., presence of polyarthritis or proteinuria, spherocytosis) a direct Coombs' test and an antinuclear antibody test should be done (see Chapter 92). It is also helpful to submit fluid obtained from one or more joints for cytologic evaluation, because the presence of suppurative nonseptic arthritis indicates an immune pathogenesis or a rickettsial disease.

Because it is important to establish whether the cytopenia is the result of peripheral cell destruction or a bone marrow disorder, it is only logical to evaluate the "cell factory" if there is no evidence of RBC regeneration in the blood smear (see Chapter 85). Therefore bone marrow aspiration and ideally bone marrow core biopsy to obtain specimens for histopathologic studies should be performed in all dogs and cats with combined cytopenias, except for dogs with highly likely or confirmed Evans's syndrome and dogs and cats with DIC (i.e., the anemia is regenerative; thus it is assumed that the "factory" is working properly). Algorithms for the evaluation of bone marrow findings in dogs and cats with bicytopenia and pancytopenia are shown in Figs. 88-1 and 88-2. In pri-

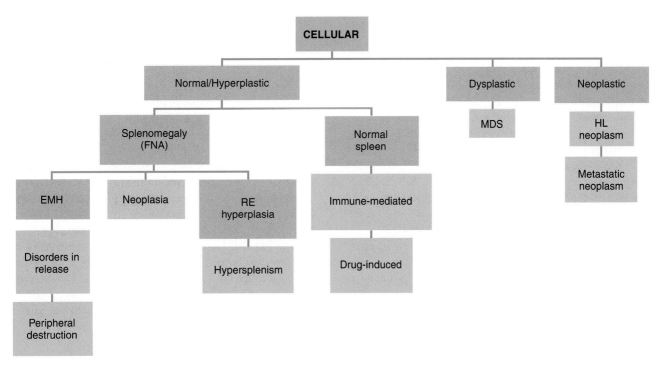

**FIG 88-1**
Algorithm for the diagnosis of a pancytopenic animal with hypercellular bone marrow. *FNA,* Fine-needle aspiration; *MDS,* myelodysplastic syndrome; *HL,* hemilymphatic; *EMH,* extramedullary hematopoiesis; *RE,* reticuloendothelium. Orange boxes indicate final diagnoses.

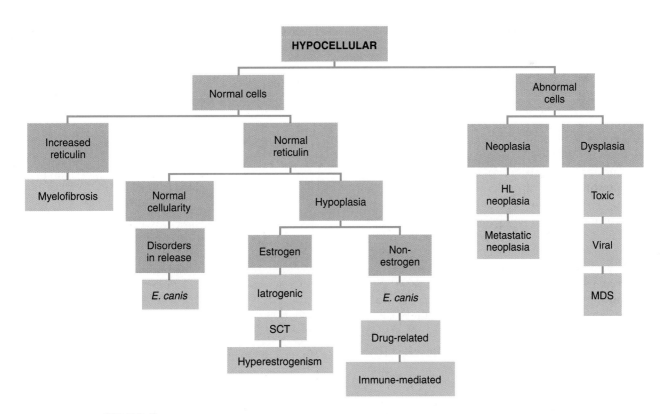

**FIG 88-2**
Algorithm for the diagnosis of a pancytopenic animal with hypocellular bone marrow. *HL,* Hemilymphatic; *MDS,* myelodysplastic syndrome; *SCT,* Sertoli cell tumor. Orange boxes indicate final diagnoses.

vate practice it is usually easier to obtain a bone marrow aspirate; bone marrow core biopsies are usually performed at referral institutions.

A bone marrow evaluation should also be part of the clinical work-up in animals with LERs, because it is important to determine whether the immature WBCs and RBCs in the circulation are secondary to a primary bone marrow disorder or to a disorder such as EMH. Because abdominal neoplasms, particularly hemangiosarcoma, are commonly associated with LERs in dogs, abdominal radiography or ultrasonography should be done. If diffuse splenomegaly is detected, percutaneous fine-needle aspiration of the spleen should be performed. If splenic or hepatic masses or both are present, the patient should be evaluated as described in Chapter 90.

**Bone marrow aplasia-hypoplasia.** Bone marrow aplasia-hypoplasia is a disorder characterized by peripheral blood cytopenias and by a paucity or absence of hematopoietic precursors in the bone marrow. As discussed earlier, bone marrow aplasia-hypoplasia is commonly associated with the administration of certain drugs, such as griseofulvin or chloramphenicol in cats and phenylbutazone or estrogen in dogs. It is also commonly associated with infectious diseases, such as canine ehrlichiosis and feline leukemia virus (FeLV) infection. A corticosteroid-responsive syndrome of combined cytopenias or pancytopenia has been recognized in dogs and cats in our clinic. Some patients with pancytopenia have a hypercellular bone marrow (see later discussion), suggesting that the cells are destroyed peripherally.

Bone marrow aspirates from dogs and cats with bone marrow aplasia or hypoplasia typically show hypocellularity or acellularity, and it is frequently necessary to perform a bone marrow biopsy to obtain specimens for histopathologic analysis so that a definitive diagnosis can be made. Once infectious diseases (e.g., *Ehrlichia canis* titer or PCR, FeLV p27 determination) and drug exposure have been ruled out, a therapeutic trial of immunosuppressive doses of corticosteroids (with or without other immunosuppressive drugs; see Chapter 93) is warranted. Anabolic steroids and erythropoietin do not appear to be beneficial in these patients.

**Myelophthisis.** Infiltration of the bone marrow with neoplastic or inflammatory cells can lead to the crowding out of normal hematopoietic precursors and hence to the development of peripheral blood cytopenias. Disorders resulting in myelophthisis are listed in Table 88-1. Often these animals are evaluated because of anemia, although fever and bleeding caused by neutropenia and thrombocytopenia, respectively, can also be presenting complaints. The presence of hepatomegaly, splenomegaly, or lymphadenopathy in a dog or cat with anemia or combined cytopenias is highly suggestive of some of the neoplastic or infectious disorders listed in Table 88-1.

A definitive diagnosis in dogs and cats with myelophthisis is obtained by evaluating the cytologic or histopathologic characteristics of a bone marrow specimen. Given the fact that certain neoplastic or granulomatous disorders can show a patchy or multifocal distribution, the findings yielded by a bone marrow core biopsy specimen are usually more reliable than those yielded by an aspirate. Once a cytologic or histopathologic diagnosis is obtained, treatment is aimed at the primary neoplasm (i.e., with chemotherapy) or infectious agent (see specific sections for detailed discussion).

**Myelodysplastic syndromes.** Myelodysplastic syndromes are discussed on p. 1140.

**Myelofibrosis, osteosclerosis, and osteopetrosis.** Fibroblasts or osteoblasts within the bone marrow can proliferate in response to retroviral infections, chronic noxious stimuli, or unknown causes, leading to fibrous (or osseous) replacement of the bone marrow cavity and thereby displacing the hematopoietic precursors. These syndromes are termed *myelofibrosis* and *osteosclerosis-osteopetrosis*, respectively. Although both syndromes are rare, they have been observed in FeLV-infected cats and in dogs with chronic hemolytic disorders, such as the pyruvate kinase deficiency anemia that occurs in Basenjis and Beagles. There are reports in the literature on a limited number of dogs and cats with myelofibrosis for which an obvious underlying cause was not found; these cases are considered idiopathic. A presumptive diagnosis of osteosclerosis/osteopetrosis is made on the basis of the presence of combined cytopenias together with increased osseous radiographic density and can be confirmed by means of a core biopsy of the bone marrow. Unfortunately, no effective treatment is available.

## Suggested Readings

Feldman BF et al: *Schalm's veterinary hematology,* ed 5, Philadelphia, 2000, Lippincott Williams & Wilkins.

Gilmour M et al: Investigating primary acquired pure red cell aplasia in dogs, *Vet Med* 86:1199, 1991.

Harvey JW: Canine bone marrow: normal hematopoiesis, biopsy techniques, and cell identification and evaluation, *Compend Cont Educ* 6:909, 1984.

Kunkle GA et al: Toxicity of high doses of griseofulvin in cats, *J Am Vet Med Assoc* 191:322, 1987.

Miura N et al: Bone marrow hypoplasia induced by administration of estradiol benzoate in male Beagle dogs, *Jpn J Vet Sci* 47:731, 1985.

Peterson ME et al: Propylthiouracil-associated hemolytic anemia, thrombocytopenia, and antinuclear antibodies in cats with hyperthyroidism, *J Am Vet Med Assoc* 184:806, 1984.

Scott-Moncrieff JCR et al: Treatment of nonregenerative anemia with human gamma-globulin in dogs, *J Am Vet Med Assoc* 206:1895, 1995.

Smith M et al: Radiophosphorus ($^{32}$P) treatment of bone marrow disorders in dogs: 11 cases (1970-1987), *J Am Vet Med Assoc* 194:98, 1989.

Watson ADJ et al: Phenylbutazone-induced blood dyscrasias suspected in three dogs, *Vet Rec* 107:239, 1980.

Weiss DJ: Antibody-mediated suppression of erythropoiesis in dogs with red blood cell aplasia, *Am J Vet Res* 47:2646, 1986.

# CHAPTER 89

# Disorders of Hemostasis

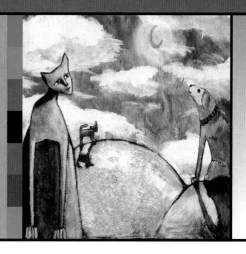

## CHAPTER OUTLINE

GENERAL CONSIDERATIONS, 1185
NORMAL HEMOSTASIS, 1185
CLINICAL MANIFESTATIONS OF SPONTANEOUS
BLEEDING DISORDERS, 1186
CLINICOPATHOLOGIC EVALUATION
OF THE BLEEDING PATIENT, 1187
MANAGEMENT OF THE BLEEDING PATIENT, 1189
PRIMARY HEMOSTATIC DEFECTS, 1190
    Thrombocytopenia, 1190
    Platelet dysfunction, 1192
SECONDARY HEMOSTATIC DEFECTS, 1194
    Congenital clotting factor deficiencies, 1194
    Vitamin K deficiency, 1194
MIXED (COMBINED) HEMOSTATIC DEFECTS, 1195
    Disseminated intravascular coagulation, 1195
THROMBOSIS, 1199

## GENERAL CONSIDERATIONS

Spontaneous or excessive bleeding is relatively common in small animals, but particularly in dogs. In general, a hemostatic abnormality is found to be the underlying cause of excessive bleeding in dogs and cats that have sustained trauma or are undergoing a surgical procedure and in dogs evaluated because of spontaneous bleeding tendencies (spontaneous bleeding is rare in cats with hemostatic abnormalities). Approaching these patients' condition in a logical and systematic fashion allows the clinician to confirm the presumptive diagnosis in most cases.

In addition to bleeding, abnormal hemostatic mechanisms can also cause thrombosis and thromboembolism, potentially leading to organ failure. Spontaneous bleeding disorders are extremely common in dogs evaluated at our clinic but are rare in cats. Thromboembolic disorders are rare in both cats and dogs. The most common disorder responsible for causing spontaneous bleeding in dogs seen at our clinic is thrombocytopenia, mainly of immune-mediated pathogenesis. Other common hemostatic disorders leading to spontaneous bleeding in dogs evaluated at our hospital include disseminated in-travascular coagulation (DIC) and rodenticide poisoning. Congenital clotting factor deficiencies resulting in spontaneous bleeding are rare. Although von Willebrand's disease (vWD) is commonly documented in certain breeds (see p. 1192), it rarely leads to spontaneous bleeding. Abnormalities in hemostasis screens are frequently noted in cats with liver disease, feline infectious peritonitis (FIP), or neoplasia; however, spontaneous bleeding tendencies are extremely rare in these patients. Decreased production of platelets (thrombocytopenia) or virus-induced thrombocytopathia resulting in spontaneous bleeding is occasionally seen in cats with retrovirus-induced bone marrow disorders.

## NORMAL HEMOSTASIS

Normally, injury to a blood vessel leads to immediate vascular changes (e.g., vasoconstriction) and to rapid activation of the hemostatic system. Exposure of circulating blood to subendothelial collagen results in rapid adhesion of platelets to the affected area. The adhesion of platelets to the subendothelium is mediated by adhesive proteins, such as von Willebrand factor (vWF) and fibrinogen. The platelets then aggregate and form the *primary hemostatic plug,* which is short-lived (seconds) and unstable. The primary hemostatic plug serves as a framework in which secondary hemostasis occurs.

Activation of the contact phase of the coagulation cascade occurs almost simultaneously with platelet adhesion and aggregation (Fig. 89-1) and leads to the formation of fibrin through the intrinsic coagulation cascade. A good mnemonic is to refer to the intrinsic system as the "dime store" coagulation cascade: "it is not $12, but $11.98" (for factors XII, XI, IX, and VIII). Factor XII is activated by contact with the subendothelial collagen and by the platelet plug; once it has been activated, fibrin, or the *secondary hemostatic plug,* forms. Prekallikrein (Fletcher factor) and high-molecular-weight kininogen are important cofactors for factor XII activation. The role of the contact phase of coagulation in vivo is questionable. The secondary hemostatic plug is stable and long-lasting. In addition, whenever tissue trauma occurs, the release of tissue procoagulants (collectively referred to as *tissue factor)* results in activation of the extrinsic coagulation cascade,

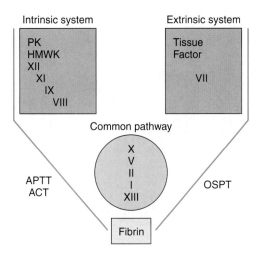

## FIG 89-1

The traditional intrinsic, extrinsic, and common coagulation pathways. *PK,* Prekallikrein; *HMWK,* high-molecular-weight kininogen; *APTT,* activated partial thromboplastin time; *ACT,* activated coagulation time; *OSPT,* one-stage prothrombin time.

also leading to the formation of fibrin (Fig. 89-1). Although the intrinsic, extrinsic, and common coagulation pathways have been well characterized, coagulation in vivo does not necessarily follow these pathways, in that factors XII and XI do not appear to be needed for the initiation of coagulation (e.g., dogs and cats with factor XII deficiency do not have spontaneous bleeding tendencies).

The stimuli that activate the contact phase of coagulation also activate the fibrinolytic and kinin pathways. Fibrinolysis is extremely important as a safeguard mechanism because it prevents excessive clot or thrombus formation. The activation of plasminogen into plasmin results not only in the destruction (lysis) of an existing clot (or thrombus) but also in interference with the normal clotting mechanisms (i.e., inhibition of platelet aggregation and of clotting factor activation in the affected area). Therefore excessive fibrinolysis usually leads to spontaneous bleeding.

Other systems that oppose blood coagulation also become operational once intravascular clotting has occurred. The best-characterized ones include antithrombin III (AT III), a protein synthesized by hepatocytes that acts as a cofactor for heparin and inhibits the activation of factors IX, X, and thrombin; and proteins C and S, two vitamin K–dependent anticoagulants also produced by hepatocytes. These three factors are some of the natural anticoagulants that prevent excessive clot formation.

## CLINICAL MANIFESTATIONS OF SPONTANEOUS BLEEDING DISORDERS

In the evaluation of a cat or dog with spontaneous or excessive bleeding, it is important that the clinician ask the owners several questions that may provide additional clues to the

## TABLE 89-1

Clinical Manifestations of Primary and Secondary Hemostatic Defects

| PRIMARY HEMOSTATIC DEFECT | SECONDARY HEMOSTATIC DEFECT |
| --- | --- |
| Petechiae common | Petechiae rare |
| Hematomas rare | Hematomas common |
| Bleeding in skin and mucous membranes | Bleeding into muscles, joints, and body cavities |
| Bleeding immediately after venipuncture | Delayed bleeding after venipuncture |

pathogenesis of the coagulopathy. These questions include the following:

- Is this the first bleeding episode?—If it is occurring in a mature animal, an acquired coagulopathy is suspected.
- Has the pet had any surgeries before this, and if so, did it bleed excessively?—If the pet has had previous bleeding episodes during elective surgeries, a congenital coagulopathy is suspected.
- Do any littermates have similar clinical signs? Was there increased perinatal mortality in the litter?—These findings also support a congenital coagulopathy.
- Has the pet recently been vaccinated with modified-live vaccines? (see Table 89-8)—Modified-live vaccines can cause thrombocytopenia or platelet dysfunction, or both.
- Is the pet currently receiving any medication (including aspirin or sulfas or other antibiotics that may cause thrombocytopenia or platelet dysfunction)?
- Does the pet have access to rodenticides or does it roam freely?—This may indicate rodenticide toxicity.

The clinical manifestations of primary hemostatic abnormalities are quite different from those of secondary hemostatic abnormalities (Table 89-1); indeed, the clinician would most likely have classified the type of coagulopathy on the basis of the physical examination findings and before submitting any samples for laboratory evaluation. This is rather easy to conceptualize by thinking about the normal coagulation mechanisms. For example, a primary hemostatic plug cannot form in a cat or dog with severe thrombocytopenia or platelet dysfunction. Because this plug is short-lived and eventually "covered" with fibrin (generated through the secondary hemostatic mechanisms), multiple, short-lived bleeds occur that are arrested as soon as fibrin is formed, resulting in multiple small and superficial hemorrhages. This is analogous to the result of turning on and off a faucet connected to a garden hose with multiple perforations (i.e., an irrigator): multiple "spurts" of water (i.e., blood) form adjacent to the hose (i.e., the vessel). On the other hand, a short-lived primary hemostatic plug can form in a cat or dog with severe clotting factor deficiencies (e.g., hemophilia, rodenticide poisoning), the main reason being that there are enough functional platelets, but fibrin cannot be generated. The result of this is a delayed continuous, long-

TABLE 89-2

Simple Cage-Side Tests for the Rapid Classification of Hemostatic Disorders

| TEST | RESULTS | MOST LIKELY DISORDER(S) IF PROLONGED (OR POSITIVE) |
|---|---|---|
| Platelet estimation in blood smear | Low | Thrombocytopenia |
| Activated coagulation time | Prolonged | Intrinsic/common system defect |
| Fibrin degradation products | Positive | Enhanced fibrinolysis; disseminated intravascular coagulation |
| Buccal mucosa bleeding time | Prolonged | Thrombocytopenia, thrombocytopathia |

lasting bleed, leading to hematoma formation or to bleeding into a body cavity. This is analogous to turning on a faucet connected to a regular garden hose with a single large opening; in this situation, water (i.e., blood) continues to flow and collect in large amounts next to the opening in the hose (i.e., vessel).

Spontaneous bleeding infrequently occurs in cats and dogs with excessive fibrinolysis. We have evaluated four dogs with protein-losing nephropathy and nephrotic syndrome in which spontaneous bleeding (i.e., petechiae and ecchymoses) appeared to result from enhanced fibrinolysis.

In cats and dogs with primary hemostatic defects (i.e., platelet or vascular disorders), therefore, the typical manifestations are those of superficial bleeding, consisting of petechiae, ecchymoses, bleeding from mucosal surfaces (e.g., melena, hematochezia, epistaxis, hematuria), and prolonged bleeding immediately after venipuncture. In clinical practice, the vast majority of primary hemostatic disorders are caused by decreased numbers of circulating platelets (thrombocytopenia). Occasionally, primary hemostatic defects result from platelet dysfunction (e.g., uremia, von Willebrand's disease [vWD], monoclonal gammopathies). Primary hemostatic defects caused by vascular disorders are extremely rare in cats and dogs.

Clinical signs in cats and dogs with secondary hemostatic defects (i.e., clotting factor deficiencies) consist of deep bleeding, including bleeding into body cavities and joints, and deep hematomas (most of which are discovered as a "lump"). Certain congenital "coagulopathies," including factor XII, prekallikrein, and high-molecular-weight kininogen deficiencies, result in a markedly prolonged activated coagulation time (ACT) or activated partial thromboplastin time (APTT) *without* spontaneous or prolonged bleeding.

Most secondary bleeding disorders seen in clinical practice are caused by rodenticide poisoning or liver disease; occasionally, selective congenital clotting factor deficiencies can also lead to spontaneous secondary bleeding disorders. A combination of primary and secondary bleeding disorders (mixed disorders) is seen almost exclusively in dogs and cats with DIC.

## CLINICOPATHOLOGIC EVALUATION OF THE BLEEDING PATIENT

Clinicopathologic evaluation of the hemostatic system is indicated primarily in two subsets of patients: in those with spontaneous or prolonged bleeding and before surgery in

those with disorders commonly associated with bleeding tendencies (e.g., splenic hemangiosarcoma [HSA] and DIC in dogs; liver disease and clotting factor deficiency) or with a suspected congenital coagulopathy (e.g., before ovariohysterectomy in a Doberman Pinscher suspected of having subclinical vWD).

When evaluating a cat or dog with a spontaneous bleeding disorder, one should keep in mind that the preliminary clinical diagnosis can usually be confirmed by performing a handful of simple cage-side tests. If these tests do not yield a definitive answer or if a more specific diagnosis is desirable (e.g., the identification of specific clotting factor deficiencies), a plasma sample can be submitted to a referral veterinary diagnostic laboratory or to a specialized coagulation laboratory (Dr. Marjorie Brooks, New York State Diagnostic Laboratory, Cornell University, Ithaca, N.Y.).

These simple cage-side tests include evaluation of a blood smear and determination of the ACT, fibrin degradation product (FDP) concentration, and bleeding time (Table 89-2). Examination of a good-quality, well-stained (e.g., Diff-Quik) *blood smear* provides important clues regarding platelet numbers and morphology. The first aspect of this examination should be to scan the smear at low power to identify platelet clumps; platelet clumping commonly results in pseudo-thrombocytopenia. Next, the oil immersion lens should be used to examine several representative monolayer fields (i.e., where approximately 50% of the red blood cells [RBCs] touch each other), and the number of platelets in five fields should be averaged. In dogs, 12 to 15 platelets should be present in each oil immersion field, whereas in normal cats, 10 to 12 platelets per field should be seen. As a general rule, each platelet in an oil immersion field represents 12,000 to 15,000 platelets/$\mu$l (i.e., number of platelets/oil immersion field $\times$ 15,000 = platelets/$\mu$l). Cats and dogs with platelet counts of more than 30,000/$\mu$l and normal platelet function do not bleed spontaneously. Therefore the cause of bleeding is usually not thrombocytopenia if more than two or three platelets are visualized in each oil immersion field. While evaluating platelet numbers, one should also evaluate the morphology of individual platelets, because abnormal platelet morphology may reflect impaired platelet function.

The second cage-side test of hemostatic ability is the ACT. In this test, 2 ml of whole fresh blood is added to a tube containing diatomaceous earth (Becton Dickenson; Franklin Lakes, N.J.); this activates the contact phase of coagulation, thus assessing the integrity of the intrinsic and common

TABLE 89-3

**Interpretation of Coagulation Screens**

| DISORDER | BT | ACT | OSPT* | APTT | PLATELETS | FIBRINOGEN | FDPs |
|---|---|---|---|---|---|---|---|
| Thrombocytopenia | ↑ | N | N | N | ↓ | N | N |
| Thrombocytopathia | ↑ | N | N | N | N | N | N |
| von Willebrand's disease | ↑ | N/↑? | N | N/↑? | N | N | N |
| Hemophilias | N | ↑ | N | ↑ | N | N | N |
| Rodenticide toxicity | N/↑? | ↑ | ↑ | ↑ | N/↓ | N/↓ | N/↑ |
| Disseminated intravascular coagulation | ↑ | ↑ | ↑ | ↑ | ↓ | N/↓ | ↑ |
| Liver disease | N/↑ | ↑ | N/↑ | ↑ | N/↓ | N/↓ | N |

*OSPT and APTT are considered prolonged if they are 25% or more than the concurrent controls.
*BT,* Bleeding time; *ACT,* activated coagulation test; *OSPT,* one-stage prothrombin time; *APTT,* activated partial thromboplastin time; *FDPs,* fibrin degradation products; ↑, high or prolonged; *N,* normal or negative; ↓, decreased or shortened; *?,* questionable.

pathways (i.e., factors XII, XI, IX, VIII, X, V, II, and I) (see Fig. 89-1). If the activity of individual clotting factors involved in these pathways has decreased by more than 70% to 75%, the ACT is prolonged (normal, 60 to 90 seconds). Common coagulopathies associated with prolongation of the ACT are listed in Table 89-3. A new cage-side instrument has recently become available in the veterinary market (SCA-2000, Synbiotics Corp., San Diego, Calif); this unit performs evaluation of the ACT, APTT, or one-stage prothrombin time (OSPT) using only a drop of blood for each test.

The third cage-side test that can be easily performed in practice is the determination of the *FDP concentration* (or titer) using the commercially available Thrombo Wellco Test, (Murex Diagnostics, Dartford, England). This latex agglutination test can detect circulating FDPs, which are generated during the cleavage of fibrin and fibrinogen (i.e., fibrinolysis). This test is commonly positive in dogs and cats with DIC. The FDP test is also positive in more than half of dogs with bleeding caused by rodenticide poisoning (e.g., warfarin). The mechanism of this is unknown, however, because these results cannot be reproduced by the intracavitary or intramuscular injection of anticoagulated blood in normal dogs. It is believed that vitamin K antagonists may activate fibrinolysis by inhibiting the production of plasminogen activator inhibitor.

A fourth cage-side test that can be performed primarily in dogs is the buccal mucosa *bleeding time* (BT) (Table 89-4), in which a template (Simplate-II; Organon Teknika Corp., Durham, N.C.) is used to make two incisions in the buccal mucosa and the time until bleeding completely ceases is determined. The BT is abnormal in cats and dogs with thrombocytopenia, platelet dysfunction and, possibly, vasculitis. In an animal with clinical signs of a primary bleeding disorder (i.e., petechiae, ecchymoses, mucosal bleeding) and a normal platelet count, a prolonged BT indicates an underlying platelet dysfunction (e.g., resulting from aspirin therapy or vWD) or, less likely, a vasculopathy.

By performing these simple tests after evaluating the clinical features of the bleeding disorder, the clinician should be able to narrow the number of differential diagnoses. For ex-

TABLE 89-4

**Procedure for Determining the Buccal Mucosa Bleeding Time in Dogs**

1. Position the animal in lateral recumbency, using manual restraint.
2. Place a 5 cm wide strip of gauze around the maxilla to fold up the upper lip, causing moderate engorgement of the mucosal surface.
3. Position the Simplate-II against the upper lip mucosa and push the trigger.
4. Start a stopwatch when the incisions are made.
5. Blot the blood with a gauze or blotting paper placed 1 to 3 mm ventral to the incision (without dislodging the clot).
6. Stop the stopwatch when the first of the two incisions ceases to bleed.
7. Both incisions usually cease bleeding almost simultaneously (if this does not occur, the last incision to cease bleeding has lacerated a vessel).
8. Normal times are 2 to 3 minutes.

ample, the blood smear evaluation reveals whether the patient is thrombocytopenic. If the patient is not thrombocytopenic but petechiae and ecchymoses are present, a prolonged BT supports the existence of a platelet function defect. A prolonged ACT indicates that there is an abnormality in the intrinsic or common pathways, and a positive test result for FDPs supports the presence of primary or secondary intravascular fibrinolysis.

If further confirmation of a presumptive diagnosis is required, plasma can be submitted to a referral laboratory or to a specialized coagulation laboratory (see p. 1187). Most commercial veterinary diagnostic laboratories evaluate hemostatic profiles routinely. Samples should be submitted in a purple-top (sodium ethylene diamine tetraacetic acid [EDTA]) tube for platelet count, a blue-top (sodium citrate)

## TABLE 89-5

### Specimens Required for Laboratory Evaluation of Hemostatis

| SAMPLE | TUBE TOP COLOR | TEST(S) |
|---|---|---|
| EDTA blood | Purple | Platelet count |
| Citrated blood | Blue | OSPT, APTT, fibrinogen, AT III |
| Thrombin | Blue | FDPs |

*EDTA,* Ethylenediamine tetraacetic acid; *OSPT,* one-stage prothrombin time; *APTT,* activated partial thromboplastin time; *AT III,* antithrombin III, *FDP,* fibrin degradation product.

## TABLE 89-6

### Congenital and Acquired Clotting Factor Defects

**Congenital Clotting Factor Defects**

Factor I or hypofibrinogenemia and dysfibrinogenemia (St. Bernards and Borzois)

Factor II or hypoprothrombinemia (Boxers, Otterhounds, English Cocker Spaniels)

Factor VII or hypoproconvertinemia (Beagles, Malamutes, Boxers, Bulldogs, Miniature Schnauzers)

Factor VIII or hemophilia A (many breeds but mainly German Shepherd Dogs)

Factor IX or hemophilia B (many breeds of dogs; domestic short-haired and British Shorthair cats)

Factor X or Stuart-Prower trait (Cocker Spaniels, Jack Russell Terriers)

Factor XI or hemophilia C (English Springer Spaniels, Great Pyrenees, Kerry Blue Terriers)

Factor XII or Hageman factor (Miniature and Standard Poodles, Sharpeis, German Shorthair Pointers; cats)

Prekallikrein (Fletcher factor) deficiency (various dog breeds)

**Acquired Clotting Factor Defects**

Liver disease
    Decreased production of factors
    Qualitative disorders?
Cholestasis
Vitamin K antagonists
Autoimmune disease (lupus anticoagulant)
Disseminated intravascular coagulation

---

tube for coagulation studies (OSPT, APTT, fibrinogen concentration), and a special blue-top tube (Thrombo Wellco Test) for FDP determination (the last tube is usually supplied by the diagnostic laboratory). It is important to submit the right samples in the appropriate anticoagulant. The guidelines for sample submission to commercial laboratories are summarized in Table 89-5.

A routine coagulation screen (or hemostatic profile) is usually composed of the OSPT, APTT, platelet count, fibrinogen concentration, and FDP concentration (or titer); in some laboratories, a D-dimer test and ATIII activity may also be included. The OSPT primarily evaluates the *extrinsic pathway*, whereas the APTT primarily evaluates the *intrinsic pathway*. Because the end product in these assays is always fibrin formation, both tests also evaluate the *common pathway* (see Fig. 89-1). The D-dimer assay, as does the FDP test, evaluates for systemic fibrinolysis. The interpretation of routine hemostasis profiles is summarized in Table 89-3.

As discussed previously, if an unusual coagulopathy or a specific clotting factor deficiency is suspected, blood should be submitted to a specialized veterinary coagulation laboratory (see p. 1187). Congenital and acquired clotting factor deficiencies that occur in cats and dogs are listed in Table 89-6.

Because thrombocytopenia can result from the decreased production or increased destruction/consumption/sequestration of platelets, a bone marrow aspiration to obtain material for cytologic evaluation is indicated in cats and dogs with thrombocytopenia of unknown cause. Other tests can also be performed in thrombocytopenic cats and dogs, including determinations of titers or PCR for tick-borne diseases, evaluation for retrovirus infection, radioactive platelet scanning, and antiplatelet antibody tests (see p. 1190).

## MANAGEMENT OF THE BLEEDING PATIENT

Several basic principles apply to the management of cats and dogs with spontaneous bleeding disorders. Specific principles are discussed in the following paragraphs. In general, a cat or dog with a spontaneous bleeding disorder should be managed aggressively (i.e., these disorders are potentially life-threatening), but iatrogenic bleeding should be minimized. As a general rule, trauma should be minimized and the patients must be kept quiet, preferably confined to a cage and leash-walked, if necessary. Exercise should be avoided or markedly restricted.

Venipunctures should be done with the smallest gauge needle possible, and pressure should be applied to the puncture site for a minimum of 5 minutes. A compressive bandage should also be applied to the area once pressure has been released. If repeated samples for packed cell volumes (PCVs) and plasma protein determinations are necessary, they should be obtained from a peripheral vein, with a 25-gauge needle used to fill a microhematocrit tube by capillarity. A bandage should be applied after each venipuncture.

Invasive procedures should be minimized. For example, urine samples should never be collected by cystocentesis because of the risk of intraabdominal, intravesical, or intramural bladder bleeding. Certain invasive procedures, however, can be performed quite safely. These include bone marrow aspiration from the iliac crest or wing of the ilium, fine-needle aspiration of lymph nodes or superficial masses, fine-needle aspiration of the spleen (the thick fibromuscular capsule of the carnivore spleen seals the needle hole as soon as the needle is removed), and intravenous catheter placement (although seepage from the catheter is common in thrombocytopenic patients).

Certain types of surgery can also be safely performed in some cats and dogs with coagulopathies. For example, pedicle surgery (e.g., splenectomy) can be performed with minimal bleeding (i.e., seepage from the abdominal wound) in dogs with marked thrombocytopenia (i.e., less than 25,000 platelets/μl).

A transfusion of blood or blood products is indicated in some dogs and cats with spontaneous bleeding disorders. Whole fresh blood (or a combination of packed red blood cells and fresh frozen plasma) should be used, when possible, if the animal is anemic and is lacking one or more clotting factors; plasma transfusions are of no benefit in thrombocytopenic animals. Fresh frozen plasma can be used to replenish clotting factors in a cat or dog with a normal or mildly decreased PCV (i.e., the animal is not symptomatic). Stored blood or frozen plasma is deficient in factors V and VIII. In general, whole fresh blood, platelet-rich plasma, and platelet transfusions rarely provide sufficient platelets to halt spontaneous bleeding in a cat or dog with thrombocytopenia, particularly if the bleeding is the result of platelet consumption. (Some guidelines for transfusion therapy are discussed on p. 1168.)

## PRIMARY HEMOSTATIC DEFECTS

Primary hemostatic defects are characterized by the presence of superficial and mucosal bleeding (e.g., petechiae, ecchymoses, hematuria, epistaxis) and are usually caused by thrombocytopenia. Platelet dysfunction is a rare cause of spontaneous bleeding. Primary hemostatic defects caused by vascular problems are extremely rare and thus are not discussed here. Primary hemostatic defects are the most common cause of spontaneous bleeding in dogs seen at our hospital.

### THROMBOCYTOPENIA

Thrombocytopenia represents the most common cause of spontaneous bleeding in dogs seen at our clinic. Decreased numbers of circulating platelets can be the result of one or more of the following abnormalities (Table 89-7):

- Decreased platelet production
- Increased platelet destruction
- Increased platelet consumption
- Increased platelet sequestration

Decreased platelet production appears to be the most common cause of thrombocytopenia in cats, resulting in particular from retrovirus-induced bone marrow disorders, but it is rare in dogs. Disorders that commonly result in the decreased production of platelets are listed in Table 89-7.

Increased platelet destruction represents the most common cause of thrombocytopenia in dogs in our clinic, but it is extremely rare in cats. Most commonly the peripheral destruction of platelets results from immune-mediated, drug-

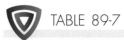

## TABLE 89-7

### Causes of Thrombocytopenia in Dogs and Cats

**Decreased Platelet Production**

Immune-mediated megakaryocytic hypoplasia
*Idiopathic bone marrow aplasia*
**Drug-induced megakaryocytic hypoplasia (estrogens, phenylbutazone, melphalan, lomustine β-lactams)**
**Myelophthisis**
Cyclic thrombocytopenia
*Retroviral infection*

**Increased Platelet Destruction/Sequestration/ Utilization**

**Immune-mediated thrombocytopenia**
*Live viral vaccine–induced thrombocytopenia*
**Drug-induced thrombocytopenia**
**Microangiopathy**
**Disseminated intravascular coagulation**
Hemolytic uremic syndrome/thrombotic thrombocytopenic purpura
Vasculitis
Splenomegaly
Splenic torsion
Endotoxemia
Acute hepatic necrosis
**Neoplasia** (immune mediated, microangiopathy)

**Common;** *relatively common;* rare.

related (including vaccination with modified-live viruses), and sepsis-related (see Table 89-7) mechanisms. Increased platelet consumption occurs most commonly in dogs and cats with DIC (see below), and sequestration is usually caused by splenomegaly or, rarely, hepatomegaly (see Table 89-7).

### Approach to the Patient with Thrombocytopenia

Once thrombocytopenia has been confirmed by a platelet count or by evaluation of a blood smear, its pathogenesis should be identified. The absolute platelet count may offer clues to its cause; for example, platelet counts of less than 25,000/μl are common in dogs with immune-mediated thrombocytopenia (IMT), whereas platelet counts of 50,000 to 75,000/μl are more common in dogs with ehrlichiosis, hypersplenism, lymphoma affecting the spleen, or rodenticide toxicity.

The patient's drug history should be obtained from the owner, and if the animal is receiving any medication, the thrombocytopenia should be considered drug-related until proven otherwise. The drug should be discontinued (if possible) and the platelet count reevaluated within 2 to 6 days. If the count returns to normal, a retrospective diagnosis of drug-associated thrombocytopenia is made. Drugs that have been associated with thrombocytopenia in cats and dogs can also cause anemia and neutropenia; these drugs are listed in Tables 85-2 and 87-1.

Because retroviral disorders commonly affect the bone marrow and result in thrombocytopenia in cats, bone marrow aspiration is indicated in a thrombocytopenic cat with no history of previous medication. The risk of bleeding during or after bone marrow aspiration in a thrombocytopenic animal is minimal. Feline leukemia virus (FeLV) and feline immunodeficiency virus tests should also be performed. If determined by the laboratory, a mean platelet volume is high in most cats with FeLV infection (i.e., macrothrombocytosis); however, macrothrombocytes are also seen in cats and dogs with peripheral platelet destruction/consumption/sequestration, in which they may be analogous to reticulocytes (i.e., young, immature, large platelets).

Bone marrow evaluation may also be indicated in dogs with thrombocytopenia. Given the high prevalence of IMT, at our clinic we usually elect to treat a dog with a presumed diagnosis of IMT. If the patient does not respond to immunosuppressive drugs within 2 to 3 days, a bone marrow aspiration is performed.

Hyperplasia of megakaryocytes occurs in response to peripheral destruction/consumption/sequestration of platelets. Occasionally in dogs and cats with IMT, there are decreased numbers of megakaryocytes and abundant free megakaryocyte nuclei in the bone marrow. This is thought to be mediated by antibodies directed against platelets that also destroy the megakaryocytes. Infiltrative or dysplastic bone marrow disorders causing thrombocytopenia are easy to identify on a bone marrow smear.

Because IMT is a diagnosis of exclusion, tick-borne diseases (i.e., canine ehrlichiosis, Rocky Mountain spotted fever, cyclic thrombocytopenia, babesiosis) should theoretically be ruled out by evaluating the appropriate titers or PCR and a blood smear. However, if the animal does not have clinical signs unrelated to the bleeding, it is unlikely that the thrombocytopenia is caused by sepsis or tick-borne diseases, although occasionally asymptomatic thrombocytopenic dogs have subclinical rickettsial diseases. If sepsis is suspected on the basis of clinical signs and clinicopathologic findings (e.g., fever, tachycardia, poor perfusion, degenerative left-shift in the leukogram, hypoglycemia, hyperbilirubinemia), urine and blood should be obtained for bacterial cultures (see p. 1110).

The presence of spherocytic hemolytic anemia or autoagglutination in a dog with thrombocytopenia is highly suggestive of Evans's syndrome (combination of IMT and immune hemolytic anemia [IHA]). A direct Coombs' test is usually positive in these cases. On rare occasions, a direct Coombs' test is positive in a dog with IMT and borderline anemia, further supporting a diagnosis of Evans's syndrome.

A hemostasis screen should always be performed to rule out DIC in a thrombocytopenic animal found to have RBC fragments in a blood smear or evidence of secondary bleeding (i.e., hematomas, bleeding into body cavities). The remainder of the hemostasis screen is usually normal in dogs and cats with selective thrombocytopenia.

Several tests are available to evaluate antiplatelet antibodies, including the platelet factor 3 release test, direct immunofluorescence of bone marrow megakaryocytes, and enzyme-linked immunosorbent assays for circulating or platelet-bound antibodies (also see Chapter 92). However, most of these are not clinically reliable, and a diagnosis of IMT can be made only after other causes of thrombocytopenia have been excluded (i.e., regardless of the results of the antiplatelet antibody tests).

Abdominal radiographs and ultrasonograms may reveal an enlarged spleen not evident during physical examination. Diffuse splenomegaly may be the cause of the thrombocytopenia (i.e., splenic sequestration of platelets), or it may reflect "work hypertrophy" (i.e., mononuclear phagocytic system hyperplasia) and extramedullary hematopoiesis in a dog with IMT.

Often a specific diagnosis of IMT is obtained only after a therapeutic trial with corticosteroids (see later discussion) results in resolution of the thrombocytopenia. If the clinician is in doubt as to whether the thrombocytopenia is caused by a rickettsial disease or IMT (in dogs), immunosuppressive doses of corticosteroids can be administered in conjunction with doxycycline (5 to 10 mg/kg PO q12-24h) until serologic or PCR test results become available. This combination of agents has no deleterious effects on dogs with rickettsial diseases.

Blood or blood products should be transfused as needed (see p. 1168). However, the transfusion of whole fresh blood, platelet-rich plasma, or platelets rarely, if ever, results in normalization of the platelet count or even in increases in the platelet count to "safe" levels.

## Immune-Mediated Thrombocytopenia

IMT is the most common cause of spontaneous bleeding in dogs but is extremely rare in cats. It affects primarily middle-aged, female dogs, and Cocker Spaniels and Old English Sheepdogs are overrepresented. The clinical signs are those of a primary hemostatic defect and include petechiae, ecchymoses, and mucosal bleeding. Acute collapse may occur if bleeding is pronounced; if the anemia is mild, most dogs are fairly asymptomatic. IMT is acute or peracute in onset in most dogs. During physical examination, signs of bleeding (e.g., petechiae, ecchymoses) with or without splenomegaly may be found.

The CBC in dogs with IMT is characterized by thrombocytopenia with or without anemia (depending on the degree of spontaneous bleeding and the presence or absence of concurrent IHA); leukocytosis with a left-shift may also be present. As a general rule, hematologic changes are limited to the thrombocytopenia. If IHA is associated with IMT (i.e., Evans's syndrome), a Coombs'-positive, regenerative anemia with spherocytosis or autoagglutination is usually present. Bone marrow cytologic studies typically reveal megakaryocytic hyperplasia, although megakaryocytic hypoplasia with free megakaryocyte nuclei is occasionally present. In addition to the thrombocytopenia, the bleeding time is the only other abnormal test result (i.e., ACT, APTT, OSPT, FDPs, and fibrinogen concentration are normal). There is usually an inverse linear correlation between the platelet count and the BT (i.e., a longer BT with lower platelet counts). Ideally, canine ehrlichiosis, drug-induced thrombocytopenia, and infectious thrombocytopenia *(Ehrlichia platys)* should be ruled out before one establishes a definitive diagnosis of IMT.

If the index of suspicion for IMT is high (i.e., a fairly asymptomatic dog with spontaneous primary hemostatic bleeding and thrombocytopenia as the sole hematologic abnormality), a therapeutic trial with immunosuppressive doses of corticosteroids (equivalent to 2 to 8 mg/kg/day of prednisone) should be instituted. Responses are usually seen within 24 to 96 hours. There is no clinical evidence that dexamethasone is more effective than prednisone in controlling IMT. Indeed, in my experience, acute gastrointestinal tract ulceration is considerably more prevalent in dogs receiving dexamethasone than in those receiving prednisone. Because an acute upper gastrointestinal tract bleed is usually catastrophic in a dog with thrombocytopenia, prednisone is my drug of choice. $H_2$-antihistamines, such as famotidine (0.5 mg/kg PO q24h), can be used in combination with the corticosteroids.

Fresh whole blood, stored blood, packed RBCs, or hemoglobin solutions should be administered as needed to maintain adequate oxygen-carrying capacity (see Transfusion Therapy in Chapter 85). In addition to immunosuppressive doses of corticosteroids, cyclophosphamide (Cytoxan; Mead Johnson, Evansville, Ind), given intravenously or orally in a single dose of 200 to 300 mg/m², is effective for inducing remission. However, it should not be used as a maintenance agent, because it usually causes sterile hemorrhagic cystitis when used on a long-term basis. Vincristine (Oncovin; Eli Lilly, Indianapolis, Ind), at a dose of 0.5 mg/m² given intravenously, traditionally has been recommended for dogs with IMT. This drug stimulates megakaryocyte endomitosis, resulting in early platelet release from the bone marrow. However, because vinca alkaloids bind to tubulin, the platelets released prematurely are not fully functional (i.e., tubulin is responsible for platelet aggregation), and the patients may experience further bleeding before the platelet count increases.

Failure to induce remission (i.e., to normalize the platelet count) is usually the result of insufficient drug (i.e., low doses or the need for a second agent), insufficient duration of therapy (the drugs have not yet had time to become effective), or a wrong diagnosis. In the event of one of these, the treatment protocol can easily be amended, with the thrombocytopenia usually resolving as a result.

Azathioprine (50 mg/m² PO q24-48h; Imuran; Burroughs Wellcome, Research Triangle Park, N.C.) is effective in maintaining remission but is not a good agent for inducing remission. In some dogs, azathioprine is better tolerated than long-term corticosteroid therapy, although close hematologic monitoring is recommended, given its myelosuppressive properties and potential for hepatotoxicity (see p. 1115). The androgenic steroid danazol (5 to 10 mg/kg PO q12h) may be beneficial in dogs with IMT, although its cost in large dogs is usually prohibitive. As discussed in Chapter 85, human IV immunoglobulin (0.5 to 1 g/kg, single dose) can also be used successfully in dogs with refractory IMT.

 TABLE 89-8

**Platelet Function Defects in Dogs and Cats**

**Hereditary**

von Willebrand disease (many breeds)
Canine thrombasthenic thrombopathia (Otterhounds)
Canine thrombopathia (Basset Hounds, Foxhounds)
Collagen-deficiency diseases or Ehlers-Danlos syndrome (many breeds)

**Acquired**

Drugs (prostaglandin inhibitors, antibiotics, phenothiazines, vaccines)
Secondary to diseases (myeloproliferative disorders, systemic lupus erythematosus, renal disease, liver disease, dysproteinemias)

The prognosis is good in most dogs with IMT, though they may require lifelong treatment. Dogs with refractory IMT can be successfully treated with vinca-loaded platelets, pulse-dose cyclophosphamide, human immunoglobulin (see p. 1163), or splenectomy. My limited experience in treating cats with IMT is that they are not nearly as responsive as dogs, even when corticosteroids are used in combination with other drugs such as chlorambucil or cyclophosphamide (see Chapter 93). However, as discussed previously, thrombocytopenic cats rarely bleed spontaneously.

## PLATELET DYSFUNCTION

The presence of primary hemostatic bleeding in a patient with a normal platelet count is highly suggestive of a platelet dysfunction syndrome, although vasculopathies and enhanced fibrinolysis should also be considered. Platelet dysfunction syndromes can be congenital or acquired (Table 89-8); however, they rarely result in spontaneous bleeding. More often, a prolonged BT is noted preoperatively in an otherwise healthy animal or there is a history of pronounced bleeding during a previous surgery. Congenital platelet dysfunction syndromes are rare, with the notable exception of vWD. Acquired platelet function disorders are more common; clinically they are mainly secondary to uremia, monoclonal gammopathies, ehrlichiosis, retroviral infections, or drug therapy. Because vWD is quite prevalent in dogs, it is used as an example of a platelet dysfunction syndrome (although vWD is actually a clotting factor deficiency).

### von Willebrand's Disease

vWD is the most common inherited bleeding disorder in humans and dogs but is rare in cats. It can be classified into three types (Table 89-9). Dogs with the disease typically have a decreased concentration or activity (type I vWD), or absence (type III vWF) of circulating vWF (also referred to as factor VIII–related antigen or F VIII:Ag), or low-to-normal concentrations of an abnormal vWF (type II vWF), which re-

## TABLE 89-9

**Classification of von Willebrand's Disease in Dogs**

| TYPE | DEFECT | BREEDS |
|------|--------|--------|
| I | Low concentration of normal von Willebrand factor (vWF) | Airedale Terrier, Akita, Corgi, Dachshund, Doberman Pinscher, German Shepherd Dog, Golden Retriever, Greyhound, Irish Wolfhound, Manchester Terrier, Poodle, Schnauzer, Shetland Sheepdog |
| II | Low concentration of abnormal vWF | German Shorthaired Pointer, German Wirehaired Pointer |
| III | Absence of vWF | *Familial:* Chesapeake Bay Retriever, Scottish Terrier, Shetland Sheepdog<br>*Sporadic:* Border Collie, Bull Terrier, Cocker Spaniel, Labrador Retriever, Pomeranian |

Modified from Brooks M: von Willebrand disease. In Feldman BF et al, editors: *Schalm's veterinary hematology,* ed 5, Philadelphia, 2000, Lippincott Williams & Wilkins, p 509.

sult in mild (if any) spontaneous bleeding or, more likely, in prolonged surgical bleeding. In dogs vWD can be inherited as an autosomal dominant trait with incomplete penetrance or, more rarely, as an autosomal recessive trait (see later discussion). This disorder has been reported to occur in more than 50 breeds of dogs but is more common in Doberman Pinschers, German Shepherd Dogs, Poodles, Golden Retrievers, and Shetland Sheepdogs. In these breeds the defect is inherited as an autosomal dominant trait with incomplete penetrance. In Scottish Terriers and Shetland Sheepdogs, it can be inherited as an autosomal recessive trait; homozygous dogs have no detectable vWF concentrations and are usually severely affected. Acquired vWD may purportedly occur in association with clinical hypothyroidism in dogs; however, most scientifically controlled studies have failed to prove an association between vWD and hypothyroidism.

vWF is produced by megakaryocytes and endothelial cells, circulates in plasma complexed to factor VIII coagulant (F VIII:C), and is one of the major adhesive proteins in the body. It is mainly responsible for causing platelets to adhere to the subendothelial structures (e.g., collagen) once endothelial cell damage has occurred, thus initiating the formation of the primary hemostatic plug (Fig. 89-2). As a consequence, vWD is usually characterized by primary hemostatic defects (i.e., petechiae, ecchymoses, mucosal bleeding). However, most dogs with vWD do not bleed spontaneously but rather bleed excessively during or after surgery; excessive bleeding during teething or estrus can also occur. Most dogs with vWD and spontaneous bleeding seen at our clinic are brought in for evaluation of diffuse oropharyngeal bleeding. People with vWD can also have low circulating concentrations of F VIII leading to spontaneous secondary hemostatic bleeding (i.e., the clinical findings of hemophilia A); however, this is extremely rare in dogs. Perinatal mortality or abortions/stillbirths are common in litters with vWD.

The hemostasis screens are normal in most dogs with vWD, with the possible exception of a mildly prolonged APTT in a patient that also has partial F VIII deficiency (al-

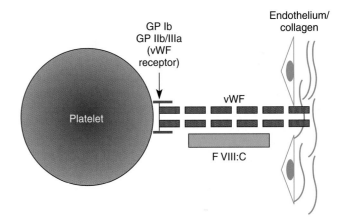

**FIG 89-2**

The interaction between vWF, platelet, and subendothelial surfaces. *GP,* Glycoprotein; *vWF,* von Willebrand factor, *FVIII:C,* factor VIII coagulant.

though this is rare). The platelet counts in dogs with vWD are also normal. However, the results of a buccal mucosal BT usually inversely correlate with the degree of vWF deficiency (i.e., the BT is prolonged if the vWF concentration or activity is low). Indeed, the BT is the most cost-effective method for screening dogs for vWD, although its results are not foolproof. It can be done before surgery in breeds at risk or if the owner or breeder is interested in determining whether the dog is likely to have this disorder. At our clinic the buccal mucosa BT is routinely evaluated before surgery in dogs at high risk for vWD so that appropriate therapy can be instituted before or during surgery (see following paragraph). However, a normal BT does not necessarily rule out vWD. Platelet retention in a glass bead column is also markedly decreased in affected dogs, indicating a severe platelet dysfunction; however, this test is not clinically reliable. A diagnosis of vWD can be confirmed by quantifying vWF in specialized veterinary coagulation laboratories.

Most dogs with type I vWD can be treated before surgery (or during a bleeding episode) with desmopressin acetate (DDAVP), which causes a massive release of vWF from the endothelial cells and results in shortening of the BT within 30 minutes of administration. A single 1μg/kg dose of DDAVP (intranasal preparation) given subcutaneously consistently lessens bleeding in dogs with type I vWD. DDAVP is not effective in dogs with types II or III vWD, because these dogs either lack or have an abnormal (i.e., nonfunctional) vWF. The administration of fresh frozen plasma, whole fresh blood, or cryoprecipitate causes the circulating vWF concentration to increase within minutes. DDAVP can also be administered to the blood donor dog 1 hour before blood is collected to maximize the yield of vWF. The use of topical hemostatic agents such as fibrin, collagen, or methacrylate is also indicated to control the local bleeding. As is the case in dogs with other inheritable disorders, dogs with congenital vWD should not be bred.

### Other Congenital Platelet Function Defects

Platelet function defects leading to spontaneous primary hemostatic bleeding have been reported to occur in at least three breeds of dogs (Otterhounds, Foxhounds, and Basset Hounds). The clinical signs and clinicopathologic abnormalities are similar to those seen in dogs with vWD, but the vWF concentrations are normal or high.

## SECONDARY HEMOSTATIC DEFECTS

Dogs with secondary hemostatic defects usually are evaluated because of collapse, exercise intolerance, dyspnea, abdominal distention, lameness, or masses. The collapse and exercise intolerance are usually caused by the anemia resulting from intracavitary bleeding; the dyspnea and abdominal distention also result from intracavitary bleeding; the lameness is usually caused by hemarthrosis; and the masses or lumps usually represent hematomas. Cats and dogs with secondary hemostatic disorders do not have petechiae or ecchymoses, and mucosal bleeding (e.g., melena, epistaxis) is rarely seen. In general the severity of the bleeding is directly related to the severity of the deficiency of the clotting factor or factors. Liver disease and rodenticide poisoning leading to vitamin K deficiency are the two most common causes of secondary hemostatic defects seen at our clinic. As noted previously, these disorders appear to be more common in dogs than in cats.

### CONGENITAL CLOTTING FACTOR DEFICIENCIES

Congenital clotting factor deficiencies, as well as the breeds affected, are listed in Table 89-6. Congenital factor deficiencies are relatively common in dogs but rare in cats. Hemophilia A and B are sex-linked traits; the modes of inheritance of other coagulopathies vary. In affected animals the severity of the bleeding is usually inversely proportional to the concentration of the individual clotting factor affected (i.e., bleeding is more severe in association with a very low factor activity). Clinical signs usually include spontaneous hematoma formation

(which the owners may describe as "lumps") and bleeding into body cavities, as well as signs compatible with "fading puppy syndrome" and protracted umbilical cord bleeding after birth; abortions or stillbirths in the litter are common. Petechiae and ecchymoses are not present in dogs with congenital clotting factor deficiencies. Cats with congenital clotting factor deficiency usually do not bleed spontaneously, but rather have intraoperative or delayed postoperative bleeding.

Carriers of the defect may be asymptomatic but usually have prolonged clotting times in vitro. Certain factor deficiencies (so called "contact factors"), including factors XII and XI, Fletcher factor (prekallikrein), and high-molecular-weight kininogen, are also found in otherwise asymptomatic animals (i.e., no excessive bleeding) with markedly prolonged APTTs. However, massive (and often life-threatening) postoperative bleeding (starting 24 to 36 hours after surgery) is common in dogs with factor XI deficiency.

Most dogs and cats with congenital coagulopathies are treated with supportive and transfusion therapies; no other treatments appear to be beneficial. As with animals with other congenital defects, dogs and cats with coagulopathies should not be bred.

## VITAMIN K DEFICIENCY

Vitamin K deficiency in small animals usually results from the ingestion of vitamin K antagonists (warfarin, diphacinone, or their derivatives, brodifacoum and bromadiolone), although it can also occur as a consequence of malabsorption in dogs and cats with obstructive cholestasis, infiltrative bowel disease, or liver disease. Four clotting factors are vitamin K-dependent: factors II, VII, IX, and X. Proteins C and S, two natural anticoagulants, are also vitamin K-dependent. Due to its clinical relevance, the following discussion focuses only on rodenticide poisoning.

Most dogs with rodenticide poisoning (this type of poisoning is extremely rare in cats) are evaluated because of acute collapse and a possible history of rodenticide ingestion; coughing, thoracic pain, and dyspnea are also common. These animals usually have clinical signs compatible with secondary bleeding, such as hematomas and bleeding into body cavities. The most common sites of bleeding in dogs evaluated at our clinic are intrathoracic and intrapulmonary; some dogs have superficial skin bruising in areas of friction, such as the axilla or the groin. Other abnormalities include pale mucous membranes, anemia (usually regenerative if sufficient time has elapsed since the acute bleeding episode), and hypoproteinemia. Sudden death may occur as a result of central nervous system or pericardial hemorrhage.

If the rodenticide has been ingested minutes to hours before presentation, induced vomiting and the administration of activated charcoal may eliminate or neutralize most of it. If the ingestion is questionable and there are no clinical signs of coagulopathy (e.g., hemothorax, hemoabdomen, bruising), determination of the OSPT is recommended. Because factor VII is the shortest-lived vitamin K–dependent protein (circulating half-life of 4 to 6 hours), the OSPT is usually prolonged before spontaneous bleeding becomes evident. Newer tests for proteins induced by vitamin K absence (PIVKA) may also aid in the early diagnosis of rodenticide toxicity, but they are not used in our clinic because they seem to lack clinical relevance.

The typical hemostasis screen in a dog with symptomatic vitamin K deficiency reveals marked prolongation of the OSPT and APTT. The FDP test is positive in more than half of affected dogs, and there is mild thrombocytopenia (70,000 to 125,000/μl), which is likely caused by an excessive consumption of platelets due to protracted bleeding.

These animals usually require immediate transfusions of whole fresh blood or fresh frozen plasma (or cryo-poor plasma) to replenish the coagulation factors (and packed RBCs if the animal is anemic). It may take 12 hours before vitamin K therapy appreciably shortens the OSPT (and subsequently decreases bleeding).

Vitamin K is available in several forms, but vitamin $K_1$ is the most effective. It is available for oral or parenteral use. Intravenous administration of vitamin K is not recommended because of the risk of anaphylactic reactions or Heinz body formation; intramuscular injections in a dog with a coagulopathy usually result in hematoma formation. Subcutaneous administration of vitamin $K_1$ using a 25-gauge needle (loading dose of 5 mg/kg, followed in 8 hours by 2.5 mg/kg SQ divided q8h) is preferred if the patient is properly hydrated. Administration of oral loading doses of vitamin $K_1$ has been advocated for the treatment of dogs with rodenticide poisoning (5 mg/kg with a fatty meal, then 2.5 mg/kg divided q8-12h); this is the treatment used in our clinic. Because vitamin K is lipid soluble, its absorption is enhanced if it is given with fatty meals. Animals with cholestatic or malabsorptive syndromes may require continued subcutaneous injections of vitamin K. In critical cases the OSPT should be monitored every 8 hours until it normalizes.

If the anticoagulant is known to be warfarin or another first-generation hydroxycoumarin, 1 week of oral vitamin $K_1$ is usually sufficient to reverse the coagulopathy. However, if it is indanedione or any of the second- or third-generation anticoagulants, oral vitamin $K_1$ therapy must be maintained for at least 3 weeks (and possibly as long as 6 weeks). Most currently available rodenticides contain second- and third-generation anticoagulants. If the rodenticide ingested is unknown, it is recommended that the animal be treated for 1 week, at which time vitamin K treatment is discontinued. An OSPT is then determined within 24 to 48 hours of the last dose. If the OSPT is prolonged, therapy should be reinstituted and maintained for 2 more weeks and the OSPT reevaluated at the end of this time.

# MIXED (COMBINED) HEMOSTATIC DEFECTS

## DISSEMINATED INTRAVASCULAR COAGULATION

DIC, previously called consumptive coagulopathy or defibrination syndrome, is a complex syndrome in which excessive intravascular coagulation leads to multiple-organ microthrombosis (multiple organ failure [MOF]) and paradoxical bleeding caused by the inactivation or excessive consumption of platelets and clotting factors secondary to enhanced fibrinolysis. DIC is not a specific disorder but rather a common pathway in a variety of disorders. Moreover, DIC constitutes a dynamic phenomenon in which the patient's status and the results of coagulation tests change markedly, rapidly, and repeatedly during treatment. This syndrome is relatively common in dogs and cats.

### Pathogenesis

Several general mechanisms can lead to activation of intravascular coagulation and therefore to the development of DIC. These include the following:

- Endothelial damage
- Platelet activation
- Release of tissue "procoagulants"

Endothelial damage commonly results from electrocution or heat stroke, although it may also play a role in sepsis-associated DIC. Platelets can be activated by a variety of stimuli, but mainly they are activated by viral infections (e.g., FIP in cats) or sepsis. Tissue procoagulants are released in several common clinical conditions, including trauma, hemolysis, pancreatitis, bacterial infections, acute hepatitis, and possibly some neoplasms (e.g., HSA).

The best way to understand the pathophysiology of DIC is to think of the entire vascular system as a single, giant blood vessel and the pathogenesis of the disorder as an exaggeration of the normal hemostatic mechanisms. Once the coagulation cascade has been activated in this "giant vessel" (i.e., it is widespread within the microvasculature in the body), several events take place. Although they are described sequentially, most of them actually occur simultaneously, and the intensity of each varies with time, thus making for an extremely dynamic process.

First, the primary and secondary hemostatic plugs are formed (see p. 1185); because this is happening in multiple small vessels simultaneously, multiple thrombi form in the microcirculation. If this process is left unchecked, eventually ischemia (resulting in MOF) develops. During this excessive intravascular coagulation, platelets are consumed in large quantities, leading to thrombocytopenia. Second, the fibrinolytic system is activated systemically, resulting in clot lysis and the inactivation (or lysis) of clotting factors and impaired platelet function. Third, AT III and possibly proteins C and S are consumed in an attempt to halt intravascular coagulation, leading to "exhaustion" of the normal anticoagulants. Fourth, the formation of fibrin within the microcirculation leads to the development of hemolytic anemia as the RBCs are sheared by these fibrin strands (i.e., fragmented RBCs or schistocytes).

When all these events are taken into consideration, it is easy to understand (1) why an animal with multiple organ thrombosis (caused by excessive intravascular coagulation and the depletion of natural anticoagulants) is bleeding spontaneously (as a result of thrombocytopenia, impaired platelet function, and inactivation of clotting factors), and (2) why one of the therapeutic approaches that appears to be beneficial in halting the bleeding in dogs and cats with DIC is to paradoxically administer heparin (i.e., if sufficient AT III is available, heparin halts intravascular coagulation, which in turn decreases activation of the fibrinolytic system, thus releasing its inhibitory effect on the clotting factors and platelet function).

In addition to the events just described, impaired tissue perfusion results in the development of secondary "enhancers" of DIC, including hypoxia; acidosis; and hepatic, renal, and pulmonary dysfunction; and the release of myocardial depressant factor. The function of the mononuclear-phagocytic system (MPS) also is impaired, so that FDPs and other byproducts, as well as bacteria absorbed from the intestine, cannot be cleared from the circulation. These factors also need to be dealt with therapeutically (see p. 1197).

A variety of disorders are commonly associated with DIC in dogs and cats (Table 89-10).

The prevalence of primary disorders associated with DIC in 50 dogs and 21 cats recently evaluated at the Ohio State University Veterinary Teaching Hospital (OSU-VTH) is depicted in Table 89-10. Neoplasia (primarily HSA), liver disease, and immune-mediated blood diseases are the most common disorders associated with DIC in dogs; liver disease (primarily hepatic lipidosis), neoplasia (mainly lymphoma), and feline infectious peritonitis are the disorders most frequently associated with DIC in cats.

At our clinic, symptomatic DIC in dogs (i.e., that associated with bleeding) is most commonly associated with HSA, followed by sepsis, pancreatitis, hemolytic anemia, gastric dilation-volvulus (GDV), liver disease, and others. Symptomatic DIC is extremely rare in cats, but hemostatic evidence of DIC is common, accounting for approximately two-thirds of the abnormal hemostatic profiles in this species. As discussed above, DIC is common in cats with liver disease, malignant neoplasms, or FIP. We have also observed symptomatic DIC in two cats receiving methimazole (Tapazole; Eli Lilly, Indianapolis, Ind). The pathogenesis of DIC in dogs with HSA appears to be complex and multifactorial; it was believed that the major mechanism triggering intravascular coagulation in dogs with this neoplasm was the abnormal irregular endothelium in the neoplasm (i.e., exposure to subendothelial collagen and the activation of coagulation). However, some canine HSAs appear to synthesize a procoagulant, because dogs with small HSAs can have severe DIC, whereas some dogs with widely disseminated HSA have normal hemostasis.

## Clinical Features

There are several clinical presentations in dogs with DIC; the two common forms are chronic, silent (subclinical) and acute (fulminant) DIC. In the chronic, silent form, the patient does not show evidence of spontaneous bleeding, but clinicopathologic evaluation of the hemostatic system reveals abnormalities compatible with this syndrome (see following paragraphs). This form of DIC appears to be common in dogs with malignancy or possibly other chronic disorders. The acute (fulminant) form may represent a true acute phenomenon (e.g., after heatstroke, electrocution, or acute pancreatitis), or more commonly, it represents acute decompensation of a chronic, silent process (e.g., HSA). Acute DIC is extremely rare in cats. Regardless of the pathogenesis, dogs with acute DIC often are brought in because

 TABLE 89-10

**Primary Disorders Associated with Disseminated Intravascular Coagulation in 50 Dogs and 21 Cats Evaluated at The Ohio State University Veterinary Teaching Hospital**

| DISEASE | DOGS (%) | CATS (%) |
|---|---|---|
| Neoplasia | 18 | 29 |
|   HSA | 8 | 5 |
|   Carcinoma | 4 | 10 |
|   LSA | 4 | 14 |
|   HA | 2 | 0 |
| Liver disease | 14 | 33 |
|   Cholangiohepatitis | 4 | 0 |
|   Lipidosis | 0 | 24 |
|   PSS | 4 | 0 |
|   Cirrhosis | 2 | 0 |
|   Unspecified | 4 | 10 |
| Pancreatitis | 4 | 0 |
| Immune-mediated diseases | 10 | 0 |
|   IHA | 4 | 0 |
|   IMT | 2 | 0 |
|   Evans's syndrome | 2 | 0 |
|   IMN | 2 | 0 |
| Infectious diseases | 10 | 19 |
|   FIP | 0 | 19 |
|   Sepsis | 8 | 0 |
|   Babesiosis | 2 | 2 |
| Rodenticide* | 8 | 0 |
| GDV | 6 | 0 |
| HBC | 4 | 0 |
| Miscellaneous | 18 | 19 |

From Couto CG: Disseminated intravascular coagulation in dogs and cats, *Vet Med* 94:547, 1999. This table originally appeared in the June 1999 issue of *Veterinary Medicine*. It is reprinted here by permission of Thomson Veterinary Healthcare Communications, 8033 Flint, Lenexa, KS 66214; (913) 492-4300; fax: (913) 492-4157; www.vetmedpub.com. All rights reserved.
*The results of hemostasis profiles in dogs with rodenticide toxicity mimic those seen in disseminated intravascular coagulation.
*HSA,* Hemangiosarcoma; *LSA,* lymphoma; *HA,* hemangioma; *PSS,* portosystemic shunt; *IHA,* immune-mediated hemolytic anemia; *IMT,* immune-mediated thrombocytopenia; *IMN,* immune-mediated neutropenia; *FIP,* feline infectious peritonitis; *GDV,* gastric dilation-volvulus.

of profuse spontaneous bleeding, plus constitutional signs secondary to anemia or to parenchymal organ thrombosis (i.e., MOF). The clinical signs of bleeding indicate both primary bleeding (i.e., petechiae, ecchymoses, mucosal bleeding) and secondary bleeding (i.e., blood in body cavities). There is also clinical and clinicopathologic evidence of organ dysfunction (see following paragraphs). Most cats with DIC seen at our clinic do not have evidence of spontaneous bleeding; clinical signs in these cats are those associated with the primary disease.

In a recent retrospective study of 50 dogs with DIC conducted in our clinic, only 26% had evidence of spontaneous bleeding; only 1 of 21 cats with DIC retrospectively evaluated in our clinic had evidence of spontaneous bleeding. Most patients were presented for evaluation of their primary problem and were not bleeding spontaneously; DIC was diagnosed as part of the routine clinical evaluation.

## Diagnosis

Because clinical DIC is uncommon in cats, the discussion on diagnosis and treatment focuses on dogs. Several hematologic findings help support a presumptive clinical diagnosis of DIC and include a regenerative hemolytic anemia (although occasionally, because the animal has a chronic disorder such as cancer, the anemia is nonregenerative), hemoglobinemia (caused by intravascular hemolysis), RBC fragments or schistocytes, thrombocytopenia, neutrophilia with a left-shift, and rarely neutropenia. Most of these features are evident with evaluation of a spun hematocrit and a blood smear.

Serum biochemical abnormalities in dogs with DIC include hyperbilirubinemia (secondary to hemolysis or hepatic thrombosis), azotemia and hyperphosphatemia (if severe renal microembolization has occurred), an increase in liver enzyme activities (caused by hypoxia or hepatic microembolization), a decreased total carbon dioxide content (caused by metabolic acidosis), and panhypoproteinemia, if the bleeding is severe enough. Another manifestation of MOF is the development of multifocal ventricular premature contractions (VPCs) detected in an EKG.

Urinalysis usually reveals hemoglobinuria and bilirubinuria, and occasionally proteinuria and cylindruria. Urine samples in dogs with acute DIC should not be obtained by cystocentesis, because severe intravesical or intramural bleeding may result.

Hemostatic abnormalities in dogs with DIC include thrombocytopenia, a prolongation of the OSPT or APTT (more than 25% of the concurrent control), normal or low fibrinogen concentration, a positive FDP or D-dimer test, and a decreased AT III concentration. If evaluated, fibrinolysis can also be documented to be enhanced in these animals (e.g., decreased plasminogen activity, enhanced clot lysis test). At our clinic, DIC is diagnosed if the patient has four or more of the hemostatic abnormalities just described, particularly if schistocytes are present.

The hemostatic abnormalities in 50 dogs and 21 cats with DIC evaluated in our clinic are listed in Table 89-11. In dogs, thrombocytopenia, prolongation of the APTT, anemia, and schistocytosis were common; in contrast with previous descriptions of the syndrome in dogs, regenerative anemia, prolongation of the OSPT, and hypofibrinogenemia were not. In cats, prolongation of the APTT and/or OSPT, schistocytosis, and thrombocytopenia were common, whereas the presence of FDPs and hypofibrinogenemia were rare.

## Treatment

Once a diagnosis of DIC has been established (or even if there is a high degree of suspicion that DIC is present), treatment should be instituted without delay. Unfortunately, there are no controlled clinical trials in veterinary medicine evaluating the effects of different treatments in dogs with DIC. Therefore the following discussion reflects my own beliefs in the management of dogs with the disorder (Table 89-12).

 TABLE 89-11

**Hemostatic Abnormalities in 50 Dogs and 21 Cats with Disseminated Intravascular Coagulation Evaluated at The Ohio State University Veterinary Teaching Hospital**

| ABNORMALITY | DOGS (%) | CATS (%) |
| --- | --- | --- |
| Thrombocytopenia | 90 | 57 |
| Prolonged APTT | 88 | 100 |
| Schistocytosis | 76 | 67 |
| Positive FDPs | 64 | 24 |
| Prolonged OSPT | 42 | 71 |
| Hypofibrinogenemia | 14 | 5 |

From Couto CG: Disseminated intravascular coagulation in dogs and cats, *Vet Med* 94:547, 1999.
*APTT,* Activated partial thromboplastin time; *FDPs,* fibrin degredation products; *OSPT,* one-stage prothrombin time.

 TABLE 89-12

**Treatment of Dogs and Cats with Disseminated Intravascular Coagulation**

1. Eliminate the precipitating cause
2. Halt intravascular coagulation:
   Heparin
      Mini dose: 5-10 IU/kg SQ q8h
      Low dose: 50-100 IU/kg SQ q8h
      Intermediate dose: 300-500 IU/kg SQ or IV q8h
      High dose: 750-1000 IU/kg SQ or IV q8h
   Blood or blood products (provide antithrombin III and clotting factors)
3. Maintain parenchymal organ perfusion:
   Aggressive fluid therapy
4. Prevent secondary complications:
   Oxygen
   Correct acid-base imbalance
   Antiarrhythmics
   Antibiotics

Unquestionably, removing or eliminating the precipitating cause constitutes the main therapeutic goal in patients with DIC. However, this is rarely possible. Those conditions in which the precipitating causes can be eliminated include a primary HSA (surgical excision), disseminated or metastatic HSA (chemotherapy; see p. 1142), sepsis (appropriate antimicrobial treatment), and immune hemolytic anemia in (immunosuppressive treatment). In most other situations (e.g., electrocution, heatstroke, pancreatitis), the cause can rarely be eliminated within a short time. Therefore the treatment of dogs with DIC is aimed at:

- Halting intravascular coagulation
- Maintaining good parenchymal organ perfusion
- Preventing secondary complications

It should be remembered that if blood and blood products were to be available in an unlimited supply (such as is the case in most human hospitals), dogs with DIC would not die of hypovolemic shock. Most dogs with DIC die of pulmonary or renal dysfunction. At our clinic, "DIC lungs" (i.e., intrapulmonary hemorrhages with alveolar septal microthrombi) appear to be a common cause of death in these patients.

**Halting intravascular coagulation.** At our clinic a dual approach is used to halt intravascular coagulation: the administration of heparin and the administration of blood or blood products. As mentioned previously, heparin is a cofactor for AT III and therefore is not effective in preventing the activation of coagulation unless there is sufficient AT III activity in the plasma. Because AT III activity in animals with DIC is usually low (as a result of consumption and possibly inactivation), the patient should be provided with sufficient quantities of this anticoagulant. The most cost-efficient way of achieving this is to administer whole fresh blood or fresh frozen plasma (or cryoprecipitate). The old adage that administering blood or blood products to a dog with DIC is analogous to "adding logs to a fire" has not been true in my experience. Therefore blood or blood products should never be withheld based solely on this belief.

Heparin has been used historically to treat DIC in humans and dogs. However, there is still controversy as to whether it is beneficial. At our clinic the survival rate in dogs with DIC has increased markedly since we routinely started using heparin and blood products. Although this can also be attributed to improvement in patient care, I believe that heparin is beneficial in such patients and indeed may be responsible for the increased survival rate.

Sodium heparin is given in a wide range of doses. Traditionally there are four dose ranges:

- Mini dose: 5 to 10 IU/kg SQ q8h
- Low dose: 50 to 100 IU/kg SQ q8h
- Intermediate dose: 300 to 500 IU/kg SQ or IV q8h
- High dose: 750 to 1000 IU/kg SQ or IV q8h

At our clinic we routinely use mini- or low-dose heparin in combination with the transfusion of blood or blood products. The rationale for this is that this dose of heparin does not prolong the ACT or APTT in normal dogs (a minimum of 150 to 250 IU/kg q8h is required to prolong the APTT in normal dogs), and it appears to be biologically active in these animals, given that some of the clinical signs and hemostatic abnormalities are reversed in animals receiving it. The fact that it does not prolong the APTT or ACT is extremely beneficial in dogs with DIC. For example, if a dog with DIC is receiving intermediate-dose heparin, it is then impossible to predict, on the basis of hemostatic parameters, whether a prolongation of the APTT is caused by excessive heparin administration or by progression of this syndrome. As laboratory heparin determinations become widely available, this may become a moot point. Until then, my clinical impression is that if an animal with DIC receiving mini- or low-dose heparin shows a prolonged ACT or APTT, the intravascular coagulation is deteriorating and a treatment change is necessary. The first dose of heparin is usually added to the blood or plasma to be transfused and allowed to sit at room temperature for approximately 30 minutes. This may allow for a better heparin–AT III interaction in vitro so that when the blood or plasma is administered, the heparin–AT III complex is already formed and active. The use of low-molecular weight heparin in dogs with DIC is currently being investigated.

If there is evidence of severe microthrombosis (e.g., marked azotemia with isosthenuria, increase in liver enzyme activity, VPCs), dyspnea, or hypoxemia, intermediate- or high-dose heparin can be used, with the goal of prolonging the ACT to 2 to 2.5 times the baseline value (or normal if the baseline time was already prolonged). If overheparinization occurs, protamine sulfate can be administered by slow intravenous infusion (1 mg for each 100 IU of the last dose of heparin; 50% of the calculated dose is given 1 hour after the heparin and 25% 2 hours after the heparin). The remainder of the dose can be administered if clinically indicated. Protamine sulfate should be administered with caution, because it can be associated with acute anaphylaxis in dogs. Once improvement in the clinical and clinicopathologic parameters has been achieved, the heparin dose should be tapered gradually (over 1 to 3 days) to prevent "rebound" hypercoagulability, a phenomenon commonly observed in people.

Aspirin can also be given to prevent platelet activation and thus halt intravascular coagulation. Doses of 5 to 10 mg/kg given orally every 12 hours in dogs and every third day in cats have been recommended, although in my experience aspirin is rarely of clinical benefit. If it is used, the patient should be closely watched for severe gastrointestinal tract bleeding, because this nonsteroidal antiinflammatory drug can cause gastroduodenal ulceration, which could be catastrophic in a dog with a severe coagulopathy such as DIC. New recombinant anticoagulants, such as hirudin, may also be of benefit in dogs and cats with DIC.

**Maintaining good parenchymal organ perfusion.** Good parenchymal organ perfusion is best achieved with aggressive fluid therapy consisting of crystalloids or plasma expanders such as dextran (see Table 89-11). The purpose of this therapy is to dilute out the clotting and fibrinolytic factors in the circulation, to flush out microthrombi from the microcirculation, and to maintain the precapillary arterioles patent, so that blood is shunted to areas in which oxygen exchange is efficient. However, care should be taken not to overhydrate an animal with compromised renal or pulmonary functions.

**Preventing secondary complications.** As discussed in previous paragraphs, numerous complications occur in dogs with DIC. Attention should be directed toward maintaining oxygenation (i.e., by oxygen mask, cage, or nasopharyngeal catheter), correcting acidosis, eliminating cardiac arrhythmias, and preventing secondary bacterial infections (i.e., the ischemic gastrointestinal mucosa no longer functions as an effective barrier to microorganisms, bacteria are absorbed and cannot be cleared by the hepatic MPS, and sepsis occurs).

**Prognosis.** The prognosis for dogs with DIC is still grave. Despite the numerous acronyms for DIC coined over the past few decades (i.e., Death Is Coming, Dead In Cage, Dog In Cooler), if the inciting cause can be controlled, most patients recover with appropriate treatment (see Fig. 89-2). In the retrospective study of DIC in dogs conducted at the OSU-VTH, the mortality rate was 54%; however, the mortality rate in dogs with minor changes in the hemostasis screen (i.e.; less than three abnormalities) was 37%, whereas that in the dogs with severe hemostatic abnormalities (i.e.; more than three hemostatic abnormalities) was 74%. In addition, marked prolongation of the APTT and marked thrombocytopenia were negative prognostic factors. The median APTT in dogs that survived was 46% over the controls, whereas in dogs that did not survive, it was 93% over the controls. Likewise, the median platelet count in dogs that survived was 110,000/$\mu$l, and in dogs that did not survive, it was 52,000/$\mu$l.

## THROMBOSIS

Thrombotic and thromboembolic disorders appear to be considerably less common in cats and dogs than in humans. The low prevalence of thrombotic disorders in cats and dogs appears to be real and not artificial (i.e., unrecognized).

Several situations can result in thrombosis or thromboembolism, including stasis of blood, activation of intravascular coagulation in an area of abnormal (or damaged) endothelium, decreased activity of natural anticoagulants, and decreased (or impaired) fibrinolysis. Thrombosis has been recognized clinically in association with cardiomyopathy, hyperadrenocorticism, protein-losing enteropathy and nephropathy, and IHA.

Stasis of blood (and possibly an irregular endothelial surface) appears to be the major cause in cats with aortic (iliac) thromboembolism secondary to hypertrophic cardiomyopathy (see p. 134). Decreased activity of the natural anticoagulant AT III is responsible for causing the thrombosis seen in dogs with protein-losing nephropathy or protein-losing enteropathy. This decreased activity stems from the fact that AT III is a relatively small molecule (approximately 60 kD) that is easily lost in the urine or gut contents in dogs with either of these two disorders. The thrombosis seen in dogs with hyperadrenocorticism is related to the inhibitory effect of corticosteroids on plasminogen activator synthesis by the macrophages (i.e., corticosteroids inhibit fibriuolysis). Recently an increased risk for thromboembolism has been recognized in dogs with IHA. Although the pathogenesis of these disorders is obscure, the release of "procoagulants" from the lysed RBCs has been postulated as a cause; sludging of autoagglutinated RBCs in the microcirculation is also likely to contribute to this procoagulant state.

Dogs and cats at high risk for thrombosis or thromboembolism should receive anticoagulants. The two drugs commonly used in cats and dogs at risk for this condition are aspirin and heparin. Coumarin derivatives are commonly used in humans, but in dogs and cats excessive bleeding has been documented in patients receiving these drugs. In recent re-

ports of humans with AT III deficiency, it has been suggested that certain anabolic steroids such as stanozolol (Winstrol V; Winthrop, New York, N.Y.) may also decrease the risk of thrombotic disorders as a result of their stimulatory effect on the fibrinolytic system. Dosages of heparin and aspirin are specified on pp. 134 and 1198. The recognition and management of pulmonary thromboembolism are discussed on p. 310.

### Suggested Readings

Bateman SW et al: Diagnosis of disseminated intravascular coagulation in dogs admitted to an intensive care unit, *J Am Vet Med Assoc* 215:805, 1999.

Bateman SW et al: Evaluation of point-of-care tests for diagnosis of disseminated intravascular coagulation in dogs admitted to an intensive care unit, *J Am Vet Med Assoc* 215:798, 1999.

Bick RL: Disseminated intravascular coagulation, *Hematol Oncol Clin North Am* 6:1259, 1992.

Brooks M: von Willebrand disease. In Feldman BF et al, editors: *Schalm's veterinary hematology*, ed 5, Philadelphia, 2000, Lippincott Williams & Wilkins, p 509.

Brooks M et al: Epidemiologic features of von Willebrand's disease in Doberman Pinschers, Scottish Terriers, and Shetland Sheepdogs, *J Am Vet Med Assoc* 200:1123, 1992.

Couto CG: Clinical approach to the bleeding patient, *Vet Med* 94:450, 1999.

Couto CG: Disseminated intravascular coagulation in dogs and cats, *Vet Med* 94:547, 1999.

Couto CG: Managing thrombocytopenia in the dog and cat, *Vet Med* 94:460, 1999.

Couto CG et al: Disorders of hemostasis. In Sherding RG, editor: *The cat: diseases and clinical management*, ed 2, New York, 1994, Churchill Livingstone.

Dodds WJ: Hereditary and acquired hemorrhagic disorders in animals, *Prog Hemost Thromb* 2:215, 1974.

Dodds WJ: Other hereditary coagulopathies. In Feldman BF et al, editors: *Schalm's veterinary hematology*, ed 5, Philadelphia, 2000, Lippincott Williams & Wilkins, p 1030.

Feldman BF: Coagulopathies in small animals, *J Am Vet Med Assoc* 179:559, 1981.

Feldman BF et al: Disseminated intravascular coagulation: antithrombin, plasminogen, and coagulation abnormalities in 41 dogs, *J Am Vet Med Assoc* 179:151, 1981.

Grindem CB et al: Epidemiologic survey of thrombocytopenia in dogs: a report on 987 cases, *Vet Clin Pathol* 20:38, 1991.

Kraus KH et al: Effect of desmopressin acetate on bleeding times and plasma von Willebrand factor in Doberman Pinscher dogs with von Willebrand's disease, *Vet Surg* 18:103, 1989.

Lewis DC et al: Canine idiopathic thrombocytopenic purpura, *J Vet Intern Med* 10:207, 1996.

Millis DL et al: Abnormal hemostatic profiles and gastric necrosis in canine gastric dilatation-volvulus, *Vet Surg* 22:93, 1993.

Panciera DL et al: Plasma von Willebrand factor antigen concentration in dogs with hypothyroidism, *J Am Vet Med Assoc* 205:1550, 1994.

Peterson JL et al: Hemostatic disorders in cats: a retrospective study and review of the literature, *J Vet Intern Med* 9:298, 1995.

Ramsey CC et al: Use of streptokinase in four dogs with thrombosis, *J Am Vet Med Assoc* 209:780, 1996.

Sheafor S et al: Clinical approach to the dog with anticoagulant rodenticide poisoning, *Vet Med* 94:466, 1999.

# CHAPTER 90

# Lymphadenopathy and Splenomegaly

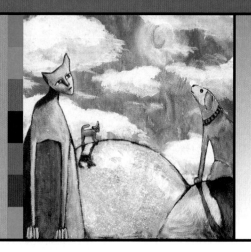

## CHAPTER OUTLINE

APPLIED ANATOMY AND HISTOLOGY, 1200
FUNCTION, 1200
LYMPHADENOPATHY, 1200
SPLENOMEGALY, 1204
APPROACH TO PATIENTS WITH LYMPHADENOPATHY
OR SPLENOMEGALY, 1206
MANAGEMENT OF PATIENTS WITH
LYMPHADENOPATHY OR SPLENOMEGALY, 1208

## APPLIED ANATOMY AND HISTOLOGY

The lymph nodes and spleen constitute the main source of immunologic and mononuclear-phagocytic (MP) cells in the body. Because these lymphoid structures are in a constant dynamic state, they continuously reshape and change in size in response to antigenic stimuli. In general the response of the cells within a lymph node to different stimuli is similar to that occurring in the spleen. However, the spleen responds primarily to blood-borne antigens (mainly nonopsonized organisms), whereas the lymph nodes respond to antigens arriving through the afferent lymphatics (i.e., local tissue response). The response of the lymph nodes and spleen to different stimuli is briefly reviewed in this chapter.

The canine and feline lymph nodes are reniform, encapsulated, well-developed structures responsible for filtering lymph and participating in immunologic reactions. Fig. 90-1 depicts the basic microscopic anatomy of a lymph node in a carnivore. It is composed of a capsule, subcapsular spaces, cortex, paracortex, and medulla. Each of these areas has specific functions. The capsule surrounds and supports all other structures within the node (stroma). The subcapsular spaces (or sinuses) contain mainly MP cells responsible for "filtering" particles arriving through the afferent lymphatics and presenting the antigens to the lymphoid cells. The cortex contains mainly B-cell areas in the germinal centers. The paracortex is composed primarily of T cells and is therefore involved in cell-mediated immunity. The medulla contains the medullary cords, where the committed B cells persist and

may expand to solid areas of plasma cells in response to antigenic stimulation. Between the medullary cords, the medullary sinuses form an endothelial sieve containing varying numbers of MP cells, which "screen" the efferent lymph. The lymph flows from the medulla to the efferent lymphatics in the hilus.

An understanding of the different histologic and functional characteristics of these anatomic areas aids in understanding the pathogenesis of lymphadenopathy. For example, a lymph node reacting to a bacterial infection has primarily B-cell hyperplasia, characterized by increased numbers of secondary follicles. This histologic/functional compartmentalization should be kept in mind when one interprets cytologic or histopathologic lymph node specimens.

## FUNCTION

The two main functions of the lymph nodes are to filter particulate material and to participate in immunologic processes. Particulate material is filtered as lymph flows through the areas rich in MP cells, while it moves from the afferent to the efferent lymphatics. During this transit, particulate material is taken up and processed by the MP cells and presented to the lymphoid cells to generate a humoral or cellular immune response.

The spleen has multiple functions, including hematopoiesis, filtration and phagocytosis, remodeling of red blood cells (RBCs), removal of intraerythrocytic inclusions, acting as a blood reservoir, metabolizing iron, and immunologic functions. Because of its nonsinusal nature, the feline spleen is be less efficient at removing intracellular inclusions than its canine counterpart.

## LYMPHADENOPATHY

### Etiology and Pathogenesis

In this chapter, lymphadenopathy is defined as lymph node enlargement. According to the distribution, the following terms are used to characterize lymphadenopathy. *Solitary*

**1200**

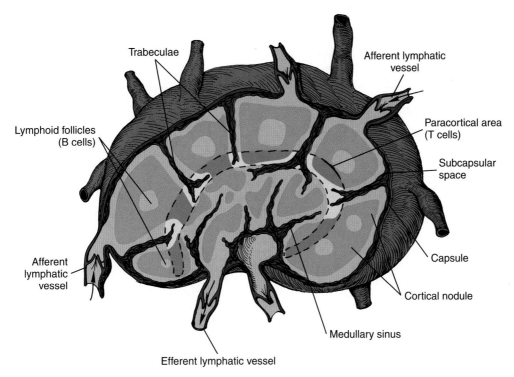

**FIG 90-1**
Microscopic anatomy of a typical lymph node in a carnivore. For a detailed discussion see text. (From Couto CG: Diseases of the lymph nodes and spleen. In Ettinger SJ, editor: *Textbook of veterinary internal medicine—diseases of the dog and cat,* ed 3, Philadelphia, 1989, WB Saunders.)

*lymphadenopathy* refers to the enlargement of a single lymph node. *Regional lymphadenopathy* is an enlargement of a chain of lymph nodes draining a specific anatomic area. *Generalized lymphadenopathy* is a multicentric lymph node enlargement affecting more than one anatomic area. Lymphadenopathies can also be classified as *superficial* or *deep* (or *visceral*), according to their anatomic location.

Lymph nodes enlarge as a consequence of the proliferation of normal cells or infiltration with normal or abnormal cells. Rarely, lymph nodes enlarge as a result of vascular changes (i.e., hyperemia, congestion, neovascularization, edema).

When normal cells proliferate within a lymph node in response to antigenic stimuli (e.g., vaccination, infection), the term *reactive lymphadenopathy* (or *lymph node hyperplasia*) is used to refer to the resultant lymphadenopathy. Lymphoid and MP cells proliferate in response to immunologic and infectious stimuli, although occasionally a clinician evaluates a dog or cat in which a cause for the reactive lymphadenopathy cannot be identified. Because these lymphoid structures are usually presented with many antigens simultaneously, the cell proliferation that occurs in reactive lymphadenopathies is polyclonal (i.e., a wide variety of morphologic types of lymphoid and MP cell types are present in a cytologic or histopathologic specimen).

When polymorphonuclear leukocytes or macrophages predominate in the cellular infiltrate, the term *lymphadenitis* is used. This is usually, but not always, secondary to infectious processes. Depending on the predominant cell type in the infiltrate, lymphadenitides are classified as *suppurative* (neutrophils predominate), *granulomatous* (macrophages predominate), *pyogranulomatous* (macrophages and neutrophils predominate), or *eosinophilic* (eosinophils predominate). A focal area of suppurative inflammation with marked liquefaction (i.e., pus) is referred to as a *lymph node abscess.* The etiologic agents that cause the different types of lymphadenitis are listed in Table 90-1.

*Infiltrative lymphadenopathies* usually result from the displacement of normal lymph node structures by neoplastic cells and, more rarely, from extramedullary hematopoiesis. Neoplasms affecting the lymph nodes can be either *primary* hematopoietic tumors or *secondary* (metastatic) neoplasms. Lymph node infiltration by hematopoietic malignancies (i.e., lymphoma) constitutes one of the most common causes of generalized lymphadenopathy in dogs.

## Clinical Features

From the clinical standpoint it is important to become familiar with the location and palpation characteristics of normal lymph nodes, which should always be evaluated during a routine physical examination. The following lymph nodes are palpable in normal dogs and cats: the mandibular, prescapular (or superficial cervical), axillary (in approximately one half of animals), superficial inguinal, and popliteal (Fig. 90-2). Lymph nodes that are palpable only when markedly enlarged include

TABLE 90-1

## Classification of Lymphadenopathies in Dogs and Cats

| TYPE | SPECIES | TYPE | SPECIES |
|---|---|---|---|
| **Proliferative and Inflammatory Lymphadenopathies** | | Viral | |
| *Infectious* | |     Canine viral enteritides | D |
| Bacterial | |     Feline immunodeficiency virus | C |
|     *Actinomyces* spp. | D, C |     Feline infectious peritonitis | C |
|     *Borrelia burgdorferi* | D |     Feline leukemia virus | C |
|     *Brucella canis* | D |     Infectious canine hepatitis | D |
|     *Corynebacterium* spp. | C | Unclassified | |
|     Mycobacteria | D, C |     *Pneumocystis carinii* | D |
|     *Nocardia* spp. | D, C | | |
|     Streptococci | D, C | *Noninfectious* | |
|         Contagious streptococcal | C | Dermatopathic lymphadenopathy | D, C |
|         lymphadenopathy | | Drug reactions | D, C |
|     *Yersinia pestis* | C | Idiopathic | D, C |
|     *Bartonella* spp. | D, C |     Distinctive peripheral lymph node hyperplasia | C |
|     Localized bacterial infection | D, C |     Plexiform vascularization of lymph nodes | C |
|     Septicemia | D, C | Immune-mediated disorders | |
| Rickettsial | |     Systemic lupus erythematosus | D, C |
|     Ehrlichiosis | D, C |     Rheumatoid arthritis | D |
|     Rocky Mountain spotted fever | D |     Immune-mediated polyarthritides | D, C |
|     Salmon poisoning | D |     Puppy strangles | D |
| Fungal | |     Other immune-mediated disorders | D, C |
|     Aspergillosis | D, C | Localized inflammation | D, C |
|     Blastomycosis | D, C | Postvaccinal | D, C |
|     Coccidioidomycosis | D | | |
|     Cryptococcosis | D, C | **Infiltrative Lymphadenopathies** | |
|     Histoplasmosis | D, C | *Neoplastic* | |
|     Phaeohyphomycosis | D, C | Primary hemolymphatic neoplasms | |
|     Phycomycosis | D, C |     Leukemias | D, C |
|     Sporotrichosis | D, C |     Lymphomas | D, C |
|     Other mycoses | D, C |     Lymphomatoid granulomatosis | D, C |
| Algal | |     Malignant histiocytosis | D, C |
|     Protothecosis | D, C |     Multiple myeloma | D, C |
| Parasitic | |     Systemic mast cell disease | D, C |
|     Babesiosis | D | Metastatic neoplasms | |
|     Cytauxzoonosis | C |     Carcinomas | D, C |
|     Demodicosis | D, C |     Malignant melanomas | D |
|     Hepatozoonosis | D |     Mast cell tumors | D, C |
|     Leishmaniasis | D |     Sarcomas | D, C |
|     *Neospora caninum* | D | | |
|     Toxoplasmosis | D, C | *Nonneoplastic* | |
|     Trypanosomiasis | D | Eosinophilic granuloma complex | C, D |
| | | Mast cell infiltration (nonneoplastic) | D, C |

Modified from Hammer AS et al: Lymphadenopathy. In Fenner NR: *Quick reference to veterinary medicine*, ed 2, Philadelphia, 1991, JB Lippincott.
*D*, Dogs; *C*, cats.

the facial, retropharyngeal, mesenteric, and iliac (sublumbar) lymph nodes.

When evaluating dogs and cats with lymphadenopathy or diffuse splenomegaly, the clinician can glean important information from the history. Certain diseases have a defined geographic or seasonal prevalence, including leishmaniasis (i.e., Mediterranean region of Europe), salmon poisoning (i.e., Pacific Northwest), and some systemic mycoses (e.g., histoplasmosis in the Ohio River Valley). Systemic (constitutional) clinical signs are usually present in dogs with systemic mycoses, salmon poisoning, Rocky Mountain spotted fever (RMSF), ehrlichiosis, leishmaniasis, and acute leukemia. Clin-

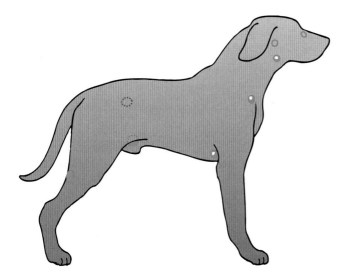

**FIG 90-2**
Anatomic distribution of clinically relevant lymph nodes in a dog. The nodes are in the same general location in cats. The lymph nodes depicted by the darkened circles include, from cranial to caudal, the mandibular, prescapular, axillary, superficial inguinal, and popliteal lymph nodes. The lymph nodes depicted by the open circles include, from cranial to caudal, the facial, retropharyngeal, and iliac or sublumbar lymph nodes. (From Couto CG: Diseases of the lymph nodes and spleen. In Ettinger SJ, editor: *Textbook of veterinary internal medicine—diseases of the dog and cat,* ed 3, Philadelphia, 1989, WB Saunders.)

 TABLE 90-2

Correlation Between Clinical Presentation and Etiology in Dogs and Cats with Lymphadenopathy in the Midwestern United States (in Relative Order of Importance)

| | SOLITARY/REGIONAL | |
| GENERALIZED | SUPERFICIAL | INTRACAVITARY |
| --- | --- | --- |
| Lymphoma | Abscess | Histoplasmosis (A, T) |
| Histoplasmosis | Periodontal disease | Blastomycosis (T) |
| Blastomycosis | Paronychia | Perianal gland aCA (A) |
| Postvaccinal | Deep pyoderma | Apocrine gland aCA (A) |
| Canine ehrlichiosis | Demodicosis | Primary lung tumors (T) |
| Leukemias | Mast cell tumor | Lymphoma (A, T) |
| Brucellosis | Malignant melanoma | Mast cell tumor (A, T) |
| Systemic mast cell disease | Eosinophilic granuloma complex | Prostatic aCA (A) |
| Multiple myeloma | Lymphoma | Malignant histiocytosis (A, T) |
| Malignant histiocytosis | | Lymphomatoid granulomatosis (T) |
| Systemic lupus erythematosus | | Tuberculosis (A, T) |
| Other | | |

*A, Abdomen; T, thorax; aCA, adenocarcinoma.*

ical signs are rare or absent in dogs and cats with chronic leukemias, most lymphomas, and reactive lymphadenopathies occurring after vaccination.

Clinical signs in dogs and cats with lymphadenopathy or splenomegaly are vague and nonspecific and are usually related to the primary disease; they include anorexia, weight loss, weakness, abdominal distention, vomiting, diarrhea, or polyuria-polydipsia (PU/PD) (the latter in dogs with lymphoma-associated hypercalcemia), or a combination of these. Occasionally, enlarged lymph nodes can result in obstructive or compressive signs (e.g., dysphagia resulting from enlarged retropharyngeal nodes, coughing resulting from enlarged tracheobronchial nodes, edema).

The distribution of the lymphadenopathy is also of diagnostic relevance. In patients with solitary or regional lymphadenopathy, the area drained by the lymph node or nodes should be examined meticulously, because generally the primary lesion is found there. Most cases of superficial solitary or regional lymphadenopathy in dogs and cats result from localized inflammatory (or infectious) processes or from metastatic neoplasia (less commonly), whereas most cases of deep (i.e., intraabdominal, intrathoracic) solitary or regional lymphadenopathy result from metastatic neoplasia or systemic infectious diseases (e.g., systemic mycoses). Most cases of generalized lymphadenopathy are caused by systemic fungal or rickettsial infections (in dogs), by nonspecific hyperplasia (mainly in cats), or by lymphoma (in dogs) (Table 90-2).

The characteristics of the lymph nodes on palpation are also important. In most dogs and cats with lymphadenopathy, regardless of the distribution, the lymph nodes are firm, irregular, and painless; their temperature is normal to the touch (i.e., cold lymphadenopathies); and they do not adhere to the surrounding structures. However, in patients with lymphadenitis the lymph nodes may be softer than usual and more tender and warmer than normal; they may also adhere to surrounding structures (i.e., fixed lymphadenopathy). Fixed lymphadenopathies may also be the presenting feature in dogs and cats with metastatic lesions or lymphomas with extracapsular invasion.

The size of the affected lymph nodes is also important. Massive lymphadenopathy (i.e., lymph node size five to ten times normal) occurs almost exclusively in dogs with lymphoma or lymphadenitis (i.e., lymph node abscess formation). In cats the syndrome of distinctive lymph node hyperplasia usually results in massive lymphadenopathy. Rarely, metastatic lymph nodes exhibit this degree of enlargement. Dogs with salmon poisoning may also have marked generalized lymphadenopathy as the presenting feature, preceded by or in conjunction with bloody diarrhea. Mild to moderate lymph node enlargement (i.e., two to four times the normal size) occurs mostly in a variety of reactive and inflammatory lymphadenopathies (e.g., ehrlichiosis, RMSF, systemic mycoses, leishmaniasis, immune-mediated diseases, skin diseases) and in leukemias.

As already discussed, the area draining the enlarged lymph node or nodes should always be thoroughly examined, paying particular attention to the skin, subcutis, and bone. In dogs and cats with generalized lymphadenopathy, it is also important to evaluate other hemolymphatic organs, including the spleen, liver, and bone marrow.

## SPLENOMEGALY

### Etiology and Pathogenesis

Splenomegaly is defined as a localized or diffuse splenic enlargement. The term *localized splenomegaly* (or *splenic mass*) refers to a localized, palpable enlargement of the spleen. Diffuse splenic enlargement occurs as a consequence of either the proliferation of normal cells or infiltration with normal or abnormal cells. Rarely, diffuse splenic enlargement can occur as a result of vascular changes (i.e., hyperemia, congestion). Focal splenomegaly is more common in dogs, and diffuse splenomegaly is more common in cats.

There are four major categories of *diffuse splenomegaly* in terms of its pathogenesis: lymphoreticular hyperplasia, inflammatory changes (i.e., splenitis), infiltration with abnormal cells (e.g., lymphoma) or substances (e.g., amyloidosis), and congestion (Table 90-3).

The spleen commonly reacts to blood-borne antigens and to RBC destruction with hyperplasia of the MP and lymphoid components. This hyperplasia has been referred to as *work hypertrophy*, because it usually results in varying degrees of splenic enlargement. Hyperplastic splenomegaly is relatively common in dogs with bacterial endocarditis, systemic lupus erythematosus, or chronic bacteremic disorders such as diskospondylitis and brucellosis.

It has been recognized for some time that RBC phagocytosis by the splenic MP system in humans leads to hyperpla-

sia of this cell population, resulting in splenomegaly. The same seems to occur in dogs and cats with certain hemolytic disorders, including immune hemolytic anemia, drug-induced hemolysis, pyruvate kinase deficiency anemia, phosphofructokinase deficiency anemia, familial nonspherocytic hemolysis in Poodles and Beagles, Heinz body hemolysis, and hemobartonellosis (see p. 1158).

As in the lymph nodes, if polymorphonuclear leukocytes or macrophages predominate in the cellular infiltrate, the term *splenitis* is used. The exudates are also classified according to the cell type as *suppurative, granulomatous, pyogranulomatous,* or *eosinophilic. Splenic abscesses* can also form, often in association with a perforation by a foreign body. *Necrotizing splenitis* caused by gas-forming anaerobes can occur in dogs in association with splenic torsion or neoplasia. *Lymphoplasmacytic splenitis* is also relatively common in dogs. The etiologic agents for different types of splenitis are listed in Table 90-3.

*Infiltrative splenomegalies* are also common in small animals. Marked splenomegaly is a common finding in dogs and cats with acute and chronic leukemias (although it appears to be more common in dogs), in dogs and cats with systemic mastocytosis, and in dogs with some forms of malignant histiocytosis. In addition, diffuse neoplastic infiltration of the spleen commonly occurs in dogs and cats with lymphoma and multiple myeloma (although the latter is not as common in cats). Metastatic splenic neoplasms usually result in focal splenomegaly, but are rare.

Nonneoplastic causes of infiltrative splenomegaly are uncommon, with the exception of *extramedullary hematopoiesis (EMH)*, which is more common in dogs than in cats. Because the spleen retains its fetal hematopoietic potential during adult life, a variety of stimuli, such as anemia, severe splenic or extrasplenic inflammation, neoplastic infiltration of the spleen, bone marrow hypoplasia, and splenic congestion, may cause the spleen to resume its fetal hematopoietic function and produce RBCs, white blood cells, and platelets. EMH has been detected in approximately one third of dogs with diffuse or focal splenomegaly evaluated at our hospital by means of percutaneous fine-needle aspiration (FNA) of the spleen. I have also observed splenic EMH in dogs with pyometra, immune-mediated hemolysis, immune-mediated thrombocytopenia, several infectious diseases, and a variety of malignant neoplasms, as well as in seemingly healthy dogs. Another disorder that commonly results in prominent infiltrative splenomegaly is the *hypereosinophilic syndrome* of cats, a disease characterized by peripheral blood eosinophilia, bone marrow hyperplasia of the eosinophil precursors, and multiple-organ infiltration by mature eosinophils (see p. 1177).

The canine and feline spleens have a great capacity to store blood, and under normal circumstances they store between 10% and 20% of the total blood volume. However, tranquilizers and barbiturates can cause splenic blood pooling to increase by relaxing the smooth muscle of the splenic capsule, leading to congestive splenomegaly. The blood that has pooled in an enlarged spleen can account for up to 30% of the total blood volume. Anesthetics such as halothane also

TABLE 90-3

## Pathogenetic Classification of Splenomegaly in Dogs and Cats

| TYPE | SPECIES | TYPE | SPECIES |
|---|---|---|---|
| **Inflammatory and Infectious Splenomegaly** | | | |
| *Suppurative splenitis* | | *Pyogranulomatous splenitis* | |
| Penetrating abdominal wounds | D, C | Blastomycosis | D, C |
| Migrating foreign bodies | D, C | Sporotrichosis | D |
| Bacterial endocarditis | D, C | Feline infectious peritonitis | C |
| Septicemia | D | Mycobacteriosis (i.e., tuberculosis) | D, C |
| Splenic torsion | D | | |
| Toxoplasmosis | D, C | **Hyperplastic Splenomegaly** | |
| Infectious canine hepatitis (acute) | D | Bacterial endocarditis | D |
| Mycobacteriosis (i.e., tuberculosis) | D, C | Brucellosis | D |
| | | Diskospondylitis | D |
| *Necrotizing splenitis* | | Systemic lupus erythematosus | D, C |
| Splenic torsion | D | Hemolytic disorders (see text) | D, C |
| Splenic neoplasia | D | | |
| Infectious canine hepatitis (acute) | D | **Congestive Splenomegaly** | |
| Salmonellosis | D, C | Pharmacologic (see text) | D, C |
| | | Portal hypertension | D, C |
| *Eosinophilic splenitis* | | Splenic torsion | D |
| Eosinophilic gastroenteritis | D, C | | |
| Hypereosinophilic syndrome | C, D | **Infiltrative Splenomegaly** | |
| | | *Neoplastic* | |
| *Lymphoplasmacytic splenitis* | | Acute and chronic leukemias | D, C |
| Infectious canine hepatitis (chronic) | D | Systemic mastocytosis | D, C |
| Ehrlichiosis (chronic) | D, C | Malignant histiocytosis | D, C |
| Pyometra | D, C | Lymphoma | D, C |
| Brucellosis | D | Multiple myeloma | D, C |
| Hemobartonellosis | D, C | Metastatic neoplasia | D, C (rare) |
| Bartonellosis | D, C | | |
| Leishmaniasis | D | *Nonneoplastic* | |
| | | Extramedullary hematopoiesis | D, C |
| *Granulomatous splenitis* | | Hypereosinophilic syndrome | C, D |
| Histoplasmosis | D, C | Amyloidosis | D |
| Mycobacteriosis (i.e., tuberculosis) | D, C | | |
| Leishmaniasis | D | | |

Modified from Couto CG: Diseases of the lymph nodes and the spleen. In Ettinger S, editor: *Textbook of veterinary internal medicine*, ed 3, Philadelphia, 1989, WB Saunders.
*D,* Dogs; *C,* cats.

may result in marked decreases in the packed cell volume and plasma protein concentrations in dogs (i.e., 10% to 20% decrease) as a result of the same mechanism.

Portal hypertension can lead to congestive splenomegaly; however, such splenic congestion does not appear to be as common in dogs and cats as it is in humans. Causes of portal hypertension that may lead to splenomegaly in small animals include right-sided congestive heart failure; obstruction of the caudal vena cava as a result of congenital malformations, neoplasia, or heartworm disease; and intrahepatic obstruction of the vena cava. Ultrasonographic evaluation in these patients may reveal markedly distended splenic, portal, or hepatic veins.

A relatively common cause of congestive splenomegaly in dogs is *splenic torsion*. Torsion of the spleen, either by itself or in association with the gastric dilatation-volvulus (GDV) syndrome, commonly results in marked splenomegaly caused by congestion. Splenic torsion can occur independently of the GDV syndrome. Most affected dogs are of large, deep-chested breeds, primarily Great Danes and German Shepherd Dogs. Clinical signs can be either acute or chronic. Dogs with acute splenic torsion are usually evaluated because of acute abdominal pain and distention, vomiting, depression, and anorexia. Dogs with chronic splenic torsion display a wide variety of clinical signs, including anorexia, weight loss, intermittent vomiting, abdominal distention, PU/PD, hemoglobinuria, and abdominal pain. Physical examination usually reveals marked splenomegaly, and radiographs typically reveal a C-shaped spleen. Ultrasonography of the abdomen in these patients may show greatly distended splenic veins.

Hematologic abnormalities usually include regenerative anemia, target cells, leukocytosis with a regenerative left shift, and leukoerythroblastosis. Disseminated intravascular coagulation appears to be a common complication in dogs with torsion of the spleen. A high percentage of dogs with splenic torsion have hemoglobinuria, possibly as a consequence of intravascular or intrasplenic hemolysis. Two dogs with splenic torsion and hemoglobinuria seen at our clinic had positive direct Coombs' tests. The treatment of choice for dogs with splenic torsion is splenectomy.

Splenic masses appear to be more common than diffuse splenomegaly in dogs, whereas the opposite is true for cats. Most splenectomies in dogs are done to remove splenic masses. Because there is a scarcity of information regarding splenic masses in cats, the following discussion pertains primarily to localized splenomegaly in dogs.

Splenic masses can be classified according to their histopathologic features and biologic behavior as either neoplastic or nonneoplastic. *Neoplastic splenic masses* can be benign or malignant and mainly include hemangiomas (HAs) and hemangiosarcomas (HSAs). Other neoplastic splenic masses that are occasionally found are leiomyosarcomas, fibrosarcomas, leiomyomas, myelolipomas, and occasionally lymphomas. *Nonneoplastic splenic masses* include primarily hematomas and abscesses, although splenic infarcts are occasionally described as splenic masses in dogs.

HAs and HSAs are vascular tumors of the spleen; they are extremely common in dogs, constituting the most common primary neoplasm in surgically collected splenic tissues (i.e., splenectomy). These neoplasms are extremely rare in cats. The clinicopathologic features of canine HSA are discussed on p. 1142.

## Clinical Features

The history-taking and physical examination in dogs with splenomegaly are similar to those in dogs with lymphadenopathy. The clinical signs in dogs with splenomegaly are vague and nonspecific and include anorexia, weight loss, weakness, abdominal distention, vomiting, diarrhea, or PU/PD, or a combination of these. PU/PD is relatively common in dogs with marked splenomegaly, particularly in those with splenic torsion. Although the pathogenesis of the PU/PD is unclear, psychogenic polydipsia provoked by abdominal pain and distention of the splenic stretch receptors may be a contributory mechanism. Splenectomy in these dogs usually results in prompt resolution of the signs. Other signs associated with splenomegaly are those resulting from the hematologic consequences of the splenic enlargement and include spontaneous bleeding caused by thrombocytopenia, pallor caused by anemia, and fever caused by neutropenia or the primary disorder.

During a routine physical examination in pups and cats, the normal spleen is easily palpated as a flat structure oriented dorsoventrally in the left anterior abdominal quadrant. In some deep-chested dogs (e.g., Irish Setters, German Shepherd Dogs), the normal spleen is also easily palpated during routine examination, either in the ventral midabdomen or in the left anterior quadrant. This is also the case in Miniature Schnauzers and in some Cocker Spaniels. The fullness of the stomach determines to what extent a normal spleen is palpable in other breeds of dogs. It is easily palpated postprandially, because its contour conforms to the greater curvature of the stomach, such that it lies parallel to the last rib. It should be kept in mind, however, that not all enlarged spleens are palpable, and not every palpable spleen is abnormal. The characteristics of the spleen on palpation vary. In dogs an enlarged spleen can be either smooth or irregular (i.e., "lumpy-bumpy"). In most cats with marked splenomegaly, the surface of the organ is smooth; a diffusely enlarged, "lumpy-bumpy" spleen in a cat suggests systemic mast cell disease. As discussed in preceding paragraphs, animals with hematologic abnormalities secondary to splenomegaly may also have pallor, petechiae, or ecchymoses.

# APPROACH TO PATIENTS WITH LYMPHADENOPATHY OR SPLENOMEGALY

## Clinicopathologic Features

It is important to obtain a complete blood count (CBC) and a serum biochemistry profile, particularly in dogs and cats with generalized or regional lymphadenopathies and in those with diffuse splenomegaly. Changes in the CBC may indicate a systemic inflammatory process (e.g., leukocytosis with neutrophilia, left shift, monocytosis) or hemolymphatic neoplasia (e.g., circulating blasts in acute leukemia or lymphoma, marked lymphocytosis suggestive of chronic lymphocytic leukemia or ehrlichiosis). Occasionally the etiologic agent may be identified during examination of a blood smear (i.e., histoplasmosis, hemobartonellosis, trypanosomiasis, babesiosis).

The spleen exerts a marked influence on the CBC, resulting in two patterns of hematologic changes in dogs and cats with splenomegaly: hypersplenism and hyposplenism (or asplenia). *Hypersplenism* results from increased MP activity, is rare, and is characterized by cytopenias in the presence of a hypercellular bone marrow; these changes resolve after splenectomy. *Hyposplenism* is more common and results in hematologic changes similar to those seen in splenectomized animals, such as thrombocytosis, schistocytosis, acanthocytosis, Howell-Jolly bodies, and increased numbers of reticulocytes and nucleated RBCs.

Anemia in dogs and cats with lymphadenopathy or splenomegaly can occur as a result of several mechanisms (see preceding paragraphs). Briefly, anemia of chronic disease can be seen in inflammatory, infectious, or neoplastic disorders; hemolytic anemia is usually present in patients with hemoparasitic lymphadenopathies or splenomegaly and in those with malignant histiocytosis. Severe nonregenerative anemia may be seen in dogs with chronic ehrlichiosis, in cats with feline leukemia virus–related disorders or feline immunodeficiency virus–related disorders, and in dogs and cats with primary bone marrow neoplasms (e.g., leukemias, multiple myeloma).

Thrombocytopenia is a common finding in patients with ehrlichiosis, RMSF, sepsis, lymphomas, leukemias, multiple myeloma, systemic mastocytosis, malignant histiocytosis, or some immune-mediated disorders. Pancytopenia is common in dogs with chronic ehrlichiosis or systemic immune-mediated disorders; in dogs and cats with lymphoma or leukemia; and in cats with disorders associated with retroviral infections.

Two major serum biochemical abnormalities are of diagnostic value in dogs and cats with lymphadenopathy: hypercalcemia and hyperglobulinemia. *Hypercalcemia* is a paraneoplastic syndrome that occurs in approximately 10% to 20% of dogs with lymphoma and multiple myeloma, although it may also occur in dogs with blastomycosis. It is extremely rare in cats with these diseases. Monoclonal *hyperglobulinemia* commonly occurs in dogs and cats with multiple myeloma and occasionally in dogs with lymphoma, ehrlichiosis, or leishmaniasis (see Chapter 91). Polyclonal hyperglobulinemia commonly occurs in dogs and cats with systemic mycoses; in cats with feline infectious peritonitis; and in dogs with ehrlichiosis or leishmaniasis (see Chapter 91).

Serologic and microbiologic studies should always be conducted in dogs and cats with suspected infectious lymphadenopathy-splenomegaly. Serologic tests or polymerase chain reaction (PCR) for canine ehrlichiosis, RMSF, brucellosis, and systemic mycoses may aid in the diagnosis of regional or systemic lymphadenopathies. Lymph node specimens for bacterial and fungal cultures should also be obtained if deemed necessary.

## Imaging

Radiographic abnormalities in dogs with lymphadenopathy can be related to the primary disorder, or they can reflect the location and degree of lymphadenopathy. In general, plain radiographs or computerized tomography (CT) are beneficial in dogs and cats with solitary lymphadenopathy (i.e., to search for primary bone inflammation or neoplasia), in those with generalized peripheral (superficial) lymphadenopathy (i.e., to detect intrathoracic or intraabdominal lymph node enlargement), and in those with deep regional lymphadenopathy involving the thoracic cavity (i.e., to determine the distribution and size of the affected nodes and the changes in the pulmonary parenchyma and pleura). Contrast studies (i.e., lymphangiograms) may be beneficial in evaluating lymph nodes draining highly metastatic primary neoplasms (e.g., apocrine gland adenocarcinoma). However, because of the technical difficulties involved in performing lymphangiography, this technique is rarely used in small animals.

The spleen is normally well visualized on plain abdominal radiographs, but there is a wide variation in its appearance. On dorsoventral or ventrodorsal views, the spleen is seen between the gastric fundus and the left kidney. The size and location of the spleen are more variable on lateral radiographs than on ventrodorsal or dorsoventral projections. On plain radiographs, large splenic masses usually appear in the caudal abdomen or the midabdomen. Tranquilization or anesthesia usually results in a diffuse congestive splenomegaly, making radiographic interpretation of splenic size

extremely difficult. CT is currently being evaluated in our clinic as a diagnostic tool in dogs with focal or diffuse splenomegaly.

Ultrasonography constitutes the noninvasive procedure of choice to evaluate intraabdominal lymphadenopathy and splenomegaly, because it can accurately image and show the size of both enlarged lymph nodes and the spleen, so that the patient's response to therapy can be monitored. In addition, ultrasound-guided FNA or biopsies can be performed with minimal complications. Abdominal ultrasonography can reveal diffuse splenomegaly, splenic masses, splenic congestion, hepatic nodules, or other changes; in addition, color-flow Doppler allows evaluation of the splenic blood supply. It should be pointed out, however, that the presence of hepatic nodules in a dog with a splenic mass does not constitute a valid reason for an owner to decline treatment or request euthanasia, because regenerative liver nodules are indistinguishable from metastatic lesions. Moreover, hypoechoic splenic nodules are frequently found in normal dogs.

Radionuclide imaging of the spleen (and less commonly of lymph nodes) using technetium-99m–labeled sulfur colloid has become an accepted method of splenic imaging in humans and small animals. However, this technique only evaluates the spleen's ability to clear particulate matter.

## Additional Diagnostics

Evaluation of bone marrow aspirates or core biopsy specimens may be beneficial in dogs and cats with generalized lymphadenopathy-splenomegaly caused by hemolymphatic neoplasia or systemic infectious diseases. For example, acute or chronic leukemia in dogs may be difficult to diagnose on the basis of lymph node cytologic findings alone, because the diagnosis is usually that of lymphoma (i.e., the presence of well-differentiated or poorly differentiated lymphoid cells). In those cases, the combination of hematologic and bone marrow findings is usually diagnostic. Bone marrow evaluation should always be done before splenectomy in patients with cytopenias, because the spleen may assume the primary hematopoietic function in dogs and cats with primary bone marrow disorders such as hypoplasia or aplasia. Splenectomy in these animals would remove the sole source of circulating blood cells, leading to death.

Cytologic evaluation of lymph node and splenic aspirates provides the clinician with a wealth of information and often constitutes the definitive diagnostic procedure in animals with lymphadenopathy or diffuse splenomegaly. In my experience, cytologic evaluation of appropriately collected specimens yields diagnostic findings in approximately 80% to 90% of dogs and 70% to 75% cats with lymphadenopathy and in approximately 70% of those with diffuse splenomegaly.

Although superficial lymph nodes can be aspirated with minimal difficulty, the successful aspiration of intrathoracic or intraabdominal lymph nodes or spleen requires some expertise and occasionally must be done under the guidance of imaging techniques (e.g., fluoroscopy, ultrasonography) (see Chapter 77). To obtain a fine-needle aspirate of a superficial node, the area does not have to be surgically prepared.

However, the aspiration of intrathoracic and intraabdominal structures (e.g., spleen) requires surgical preparation of the area and adequate restraint of the animal. Certain intraabdominal lymph nodes (e.g., markedly enlarged mesenteric or iliac nodes) are easily aspirated transabdominally using manual isolation of the mass. Iliac lymph nodes can also be aspirated transrectally using a 2- to 3-inch (5 to 7.5 cm) needle. Splenic aspirates are obtained with the animal in right lateral or dorsal recumbency, using manual restraint or mild sedation. Transabdominal splenic FNA in dogs or cats chemically restrained with phenothiazine tranquilizers or barbiturates usually yields blood-diluted specimens as a result of splenic congestion.

In a patient with generalized lymphadenopathy, the clinician must decide which lymph node to aspirate. Obviously, it is important to aspirate a node in which the tissue changes are representative of the ongoing disease. Therefore it is advisable not to obtain a specimen from the largest lymph node, because the central necrosis in such a node usually precludes a definitive diagnosis. Because clinical and subclinical gingivitis are common in older dogs and cats, mandibular lymph nodes should not be aspirated routinely, because they are usually reactive and findings may obscure the primary diagnosis. The techniques of FNA are described in Chapter 77.

Several reviews of the cytologic evaluation of lymphoid tissues have appeared in the veterinary literature (see Suggested Readings). Briefly, *normal lymph nodes* are composed primarily of small lymphocytes (80% to 90% of all cells); a low number of macrophages, medium or large lymphocytes, plasma cells, and mast cells can also be found. Normal spleens are similar, except that there is a high concentration of RBCs, given this organ's vascularity. *Reactive lymph nodes* and hyperplastic spleens are characterized by variable numbers of lymphoid cells in different stages of development (i.e., small, medium, and large lymphocytes; plasma cells). The cytologic features of *lymphadenitis-splenitis* vary with the etiologic agent and the type of reaction elicited (see preceding paragraphs). Etiologic agents can frequently be identified in cytologic specimens from nodes with lymphadenitis. *Metastatic neoplasms* have different cytologic features, depending on the degree of involvement and the cell type. Carcinomas, adenocarcinomas, melanomas, and mast cell tumors are easily diagnosed on the basis of cytologic findings. However, the cytologic diagnosis of sarcomas may be difficult, because the neoplastic cells that make up this tumor do not exfoliate easily. *Primary lymphoid neoplasms* (lymphomas) are characterized by a monomorphic population of lymphoid cells, which are usually immature (i.e., a fine chromatin pattern, one or more nucleoli, basophilic cytoplasm, vacuolation; Fig. 90-3). For a more detailed description of cytologic changes, see Chapter 77.

When the cytologic examination of an enlarged lymph node or spleen does not provide findings that can be used to make a definitive diagnosis, excision of the affected node or incisional (even excisional) splenic biopsy to obtain a specimen for histopathologic examination is indicated. It is preferable to excise the whole node, since core biopsy specimens are difficult to interpret because the lymph node architecture

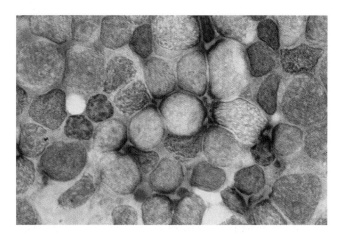

**FIG 90-3**
Cytologic characteristics of a lymph node aspirate from a dog with massive generalized lymphadenopathy (lymphoma). Note a monomorphic population of large, round cells with a lacy chromatin pattern (neoplastic cells), intermixed with small, darker, normal lymphocytes. (Wright-Giemsa stain, ×1000.)

is often poorly preserved. A wedge of tissue can be obtained during a splenic biopsy, or if the surgeon deems it necessary, a splenectomy can be performed. Care should be taken in handling the tissues during surgical manipulation, because trauma may induce considerable artifactual changes, which would preclude interpretation of the specimen. The popliteal lymph nodes are easily accessible and are the ones usually excised in dogs and cats with generalized lymphadenopathy.

Once a node is excised, it should be sectioned in half lengthwise, impression smears made for cytologic analysis, and the node fixed in 10% buffered formalin in a proportion of one part of tissue to nine parts of fixative. The specimen is then ready to be sent to a laboratory for evaluation. Samples can also be saved for cytochemical or immunohistochemical evaluation, ultrastructural studies, or microbiologic evaluation. The same guidelines apply to the preparation of splenic specimens.

## MANAGEMENT OF PATIENTS WITH LYMPHADENOPATHY OR SPLENOMEGALY

As discussed in previous paragraphs, there is no specific treatment for dogs or cats with local, regional, or generalized lymphadenopathy or with diffuse splenomegaly. Treatment should be directed at the cause or causes of the lymphadenopathy-splenomegaly rather than at the enlarged lymph nodes or spleen. Exploratory celiotomies provide considerable information regarding the gross morphology of an enlarged spleen and adjacent organs and tissues. However, direct visualization of these structures may be misleading, because it may be impossible to differentiate some benign splenic masses (i.e., hematoma, HA) from their malignant counterpart (i.e., HSA) on the basis of gross morphology alone. As discussed in the section on imaging, the surgeon may recommend to the owners that the animal be euthanized on the operating table because it has a splenic mass and nodules in the liver, only to find out that the hepatic nodules represent nodular hyperplasia or EMH and the primary mass was benign (e.g., HA or hematoma).

Splenectomy is indicated in the event of splenic torsion, splenic rupture, symptomatic splenomegaly, or splenic masses. The value of splenectomy is questionable in dogs with immune-mediated blood disorders, dogs and cats with splenomegaly caused by lymphoma in which chemotherapy has not induced splenic remission, and dogs and cats with leukemias. Splenectomy is contraindicated in patients with bone marrow hypoplasia in which the spleen is the main hematopoietic site.

Although rare, a syndrome of postsplenectomy sepsis has been documented in approximately 3% of dogs that undergo this surgical procedure in our clinic. The syndrome is similar to its human counterpart. Most dogs with postsplenectomy sepsis evaluated at our clinic were undergoing immunosuppressive therapy at the time of surgery or had undergone splenectomy for a neoplasm. This sepsis is usually rapid in onset (hours to days), so prophylactic bactericidal antibiotic therapy is recommended postoperatively. We routinely use cephalothin (20 mg/kg intravenously [IV] q8h) with or without amikacin (15 mg/kg IV q24h) for 2 to 3 days postoperatively. All dogs with clinically recognized postsplenectomy sepsis at our clinic have died within 12 hours of its onset, despite aggressive treatment.

Occasionally the clinician encounters a patient in which the enlarged lymph node mechanically compresses or occludes a viscus, airway, or vessel. This may result in marked clinical abnormalities, such as intractable coughing, caused by tracheobronchial lymphadenopathy; colonic obstruction, caused by iliac lymphadenopathy; or anterior vena cava syndrome, caused by cranial vena cava and thoracic duct obstruction. Several treatment options are available for these situations. If the lymph node is surgically resectable, excision (or drainage) should be attempted. If the node is not surgically resectable or if surgery or anesthesia poses a high risk for the animal, one or more of the following can be used:

1. Irradiation can shrink the lymph node and ameliorate the signs in animals with primary or metastatic neoplastic lesions. This can be accomplished using intraoperative irradiation or external-beam fractionated therapy.

2. Antiinflammatory doses of corticosteroids can be used (0.5 mg/kg orally q24h) in animals with fungal lesions such as *Histoplasma*-induced tracheobronchial lymphadenopathy.

3. Intralesional injections of corticosteroids (prednisolone, 50 to 60 mg/m²) can be successful in dogs and cats with solitary lymphomas or metastatic mast cell tumors, if irradiation is not feasible.

4. Systemic antibiotic therapy may be beneficial in animals with solitary suppurative lymphadenitis.

## Suggested Readings

Couto CG: A diagnostic approach to splenomegaly in cats and dogs, *Vet Med* 85:220, 1990.

Couto CG et al: Diseases of the lymph nodes and spleen. In Ettinger SJ et al, editors: *Textbook of veterinary internal medicine—diseases of the dog and cat*, ed 4, Philadelphia, 1995, WB Saunders.

Gamblin R et al: Lymphadenopathy and organomegaly. In Fenner WR: *Quick reference to veterinary medicine*, ed 3, Philadelphia, 2000, Lippincott Williams & Wilkins, p 91.

Gamblin RM et al: Nonneoplastic disorders of the spleen. In Ettinger SJ et al: *Textbook of veterinary internal medicine: diseases of the dog and cat*, ed 5, Philadelphia, 2000, WB Saunders, p 1857.

Hammer AS et al: Disorders of the lymph nodes and spleen. In Sherding RG, editor: *The cat: diseases and clinical management*, ed 2, New York, 1994, Churchill Livingstone.

Mills JN: Diagnosis from lymph node fine-aspiration cytology, *Aust Vet Pract* 14:14, 1984.

Mooney SC et al: Generalized lymphadenopathy resembling lymphoma in cats: six cases (1972-1976), *J Am Vet Med Assoc* 190:897, 1987.

Moore FM et al: Distinctive peripheral lymph node hyperplasia of young cats, *Vet Pathol* 23:386, 1986.

O'Keefe DA et al: Fine-needle aspiration of the spleen as an aid in the diagnosis of splenomegaly, *J Vet Intern Med* 1:102, 1987.

Spangler WL et al: Prevalence, type, and importance of splenic diseases in dogs: 1,480 cases (1985-1989), *J Am Vet Med Assoc* 200:829, 1992.

Spangler WL et al: Prevalence and type of splenic diseases in cats: 455 cases (1985-1991), *J Am Vet Med Assoc* 201:773, 1992.

Spangler WL et al: Pathologic factors affecting patient survival after splenectomy in dogs, *J Vet Intern Med* 11:166, 1997.

# CHAPTER 91

# Hyperproteinemia

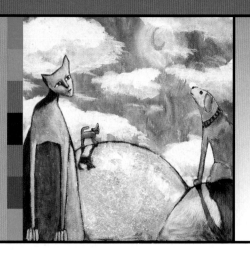

The plasma protein fraction is composed mainly of albumin, globulins, and fibrinogen; fibrinogen is absent in serum (i.e., as a result of clotting and conversion into fibrin). *Hyperproteinemia* is the term given to an absolute or relative increase in the serum or plasma protein concentration. Before further evaluating a cat or dog with hyperproteinemia, the clinician should make sure that the condition is not due to a laboratory artifact (i.e., interference of other substances in protein determination), which constitutes one of the most common causes of "hyperproteinemia." Lipemia and, to a lesser degree, hemolysis typically result in artifactual increases in the plasma or serum protein concentration.

Once it has been established that the hyperproteinemia is real, the clinician should determine whether it is *relative* or *absolute.* Relative hyperproteinemia is usually accompanied by erythrocytosis, and it is caused by hemoconcentration (i.e., dehydration). However, in an anemic cat or dog, relative hyperproteinemia may be present in association with a normal packed cell volume (PCV) (i.e., the PCV is low, but hemoconcentration results in an artifactual increase). The relative proportions (ratio) of albumin and globulin provide considerable information regarding the pathogenesis of hyperproteinemia. This information is usually contained in reports of serum biochemistry profiles from most referral diagnostic laboratories. Occasionally only the total serum protein and serum albumin concentrations are reported. In this event, the total globulin concentration can be determined by simply subtracting the albumin concentration from the total protein concentration.

In dogs and cats with *relative hyperproteinemia* (i.e., hemoconcentration), both the albumin and globulin concentrations are increased beyond reference values, whereas in those with *absolute hyperproteinemia,* only the globulin concentration is increased, usually in association with a mild or marked decrease in the albumin concentration. Hyperalbuminemia does not occur because the liver already is at its maximal synthetic capacity. The finding of "hyperalbuminemia" and hyperglobulinemia indicates either the presence of dehydration or a laboratory error. Rehydration causes relative hyperproteinemia to resolve.

When exposed to an electrical field (i.e., protein electrophoresis), the protein molecules migrate according to their shape, charge, and molecular weight. Staining of the electrophoresis gel after migration usually reveals six distinct protein bands: albumin (closer to the anode or negative electrode), α-1 globulin, α-2 globulin, β-1 globulin, β-2 globulin, and γ-globulin (closer to the cathode or positive electrode) (Fig. 91-1, *A*). The albumin fraction is responsible for conferring oncotic properties on body fluids. Acute phase reactants (APRs) migrate in the α-2 (and α-1) regions, whereas immunoglobulins (Igs) and complement usually migrate in the β and γ regions. Igs migrate in the following order (from anode to cathode and beginning in the α-2 region): IgA, IgM, and IgG. By evaluating a protein electrophoretogram, the clinician can gain insight into the pathogenesis of the hyperglobulinemia.

Increased production of globulins occurs in a variety of clinical settings but mainly in two groups of disorders: *inflammatory-infectious* and *neoplastic.* In inflammation (and infection), the hepatocytes elaborate a variety of globulins, collectively termed *APRs,* which result in increases in the α-2– and α-1–globulin fractions. Because the hepatocytes are "reprogrammed" to produce APRs, the albumin production is "switched off," resulting in hypoalbuminemia. In conjunction with these changes, the immune system produces a variety of immune proteins (mainly Igs), which result in increases in the α-2, β, or γ regions, or a combination of these.

Because the immune system reacts against an organism (e.g., a bacterium) by producing antibodies against each somatic antigen, several clones of lymphocytes–plasma cells are "instructed" to simultaneously produce specific antibody molecules (i.e., each clone is programmed to produce one specific antibody type against a specific antigen). As a consequence, immune stimulation leads to the appearance of a "polyclonal" band in the β or γ regions, or both. This polyclonal band is broad-based and irregular and contains most of the Igs (and complement) generated by the immune cells. A typical "inflammatory-infectious" electrophoretogram, therefore, consists of a normal to mildly decreased albumin concentration and hyperglobulinemia resulting from increased α-2– (i.e., APR) and β-γ–globulins (polyclonal gammopathy) (Fig. 91-1, *C*).

Typical inflammatory-infectious electrophoretograms are seen in several common disorders, including chronic pyo-

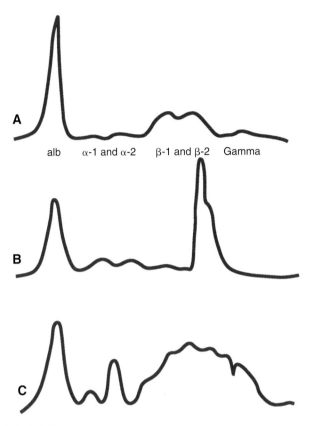

alb      α-1 and α-2      β-1 and β-2      Gamma

**FIG 91-1**

**A,** A normal canine or feline serum protein electrophoretogram. For a description, see text. **B,** Electrophoretogram from a dog with multiple myeloma and a monoclonal gammopathy in the β₂-γ region. Note the narrow spike approximately the same width as the albumin band. **C,** Electrophoretogram from a cat with feline infectious peritonitis and a typical polyclonal gammopathy. Note the α₂ spike (APRs) and the broad-based β-γ spikes.

derma, pyometra, and other chronic suppurative processes; feline infectious peritonitis; feline and canine hemobartonellosis (and other hemoparasite infections); canine ehrlichiosis and leishmaniasis; chronic autoimmune disorders (e.g., systemic lupus erythematosus, immune polyarthritis); and some neoplastic diseases (although they are rare) (Table 91-1). Polyclonal gammopathies are also common in otherwise healthy old cats.

Monoclonal gammopathies occur when one clone of immune cells produces the same type (and subtype) of Ig molecule. Because these molecules are identical, they migrate in a narrow band (monoclonal spike, or M-component) located typically in the β or γ regions (Fig. 91-1, *B*). Monoclonal gammopathies occur in dogs with chronic lymphocytic leukemia, multiple myeloma, and lymphoma; they are also present in dogs with ehrlichiosis and occasionally in dogs with leishmaniasis (Table 91-2). In most cats, monoclonal gammopathies occur in association with multiple myeloma or lymphoma, but they can occur in cats with feline infectious peritonitis. Occasionally an M-component is detected in an otherwise asymptomatic cat or dog but additional evaluation fails to reveal a

 TABLE 91-1

**Diseases Associated with Polyclonal Gammopathies in Dogs and Cats**

Infectious
  **Chronic pyoderma**
  **Pyometra**
  Chronic pneumonia
  **Feline infectious peritonitis**
  Hemobartonellosis
  Bartonellosis
  **Ehrlichiosis**
  **Leishmaniasis**
  Chagas' disease
  Babesiosis
  **Systemic mycoses**
Immune-mediated diseases
Neoplasia
  Lymphomas
  Mast cell tumors
  **Necrotic or draining tumors**

**Common;** uncommon.

 TABLE 91-2

**Diseases Associated with Monoclonal Gammopathies in Dogs and Cats**

Multiple myeloma
Chronic lymphocytic leukemia
Lymphoma
"Idiopathic" monoclonal gammopathy
Ehrlichiosis
Leishmaniasis
Feline infectious peritonitis

source for the monoclonal gammopathy. Although it is likely that this represents the counterpart of human "idiopathic monoclonal gammopathy," the patient should be reevaluated frequently for a clinically emerging malignancy.

The treatment of dogs and cats with monoclonal or polyclonal gammopathies is aimed at the primary disease. Please refer to specific sections throughout this book for discussion of these treatments.

## Suggested Readings

Breitschwerdt EB et al: Monoclonal gammopathy associated with naturally occurring canine ehrlichiosis, *J Vet Intern Med* 1:2, 1987.

Dorfman M et al: Paraproteinemias in small animal medicine, *Compend Contin Educ* 14:621, 1992.

Forrester SD et al: Serum hyperviscosity syndrome: its diagnosis and treatment, *Vet Med* 87:48, 1992.

Weiser MG et al: Granular lymphocytosis and hyperproteinemia in dogs with chronic ehrlichiosis, *J Am Anim Hosp Assoc* 27:84, 1991.

Williams DA: Gammopathies, *Compend Contin Educ* 3:815, 1981.

# CHAPTER 92

# Immune-Mediated Diseases: Overview and Diagnosis

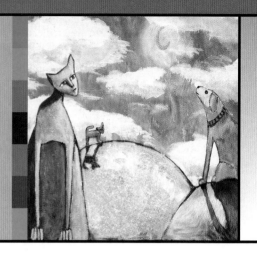

## CHAPTER OUTLINE

GENERAL CONSIDERATIONS, 1212
IMMUNOLOGY FOR THE CLINICIAN, 1212
DIAGNOSTIC TESTS, 1213
    Direct Coombs' test or direct antiglobulin test, 1213
    Antinuclear antibody test, 1214
    Direct immunofluorescence
       and immunohistochemistry, 1214
    Other tests, 1214

## GENERAL CONSIDERATIONS

Occasionally the immune system recognizes the host's tissues as foreign and directs a humoral or cellular immune response against specific target organs or tissues. This may result in clinically relevant organ or tissue damage. These disorders are collectively termed *immune-mediated disorders (IMDs)* but are referred to by some as *autoimmune disorders*. Because in most cases true autoantibodies (i.e., antibodies against the host's own antigens) are not produced, but rather antigen-antibody complexes (immune complexes [ICs]) are deposited in certain tissues or organs, the term *IMD* is preferred. Most IMDs that develop in dogs and cats are thought to be idiopathic or primary (i.e., no underlying cause can be found). However, IMDs occasionally develop during or after drug therapy (e.g., propylthiouracil in cats) or shortly after vaccination. IMDs are considerably more common in dogs than in cats. Thus the following discussion applies to dogs, unless otherwise stated. Most of these disorders are also more common in females than in males.

IMDs have a multitude of clinical manifestations. They can affect a solitary organ or tissue (e.g., immune hemolytic anemia [IHA], polyarthritis), or they can be multisystemic (systemic lupus erythematosus), and they are often associated with pyrexia or fever. Target organs and tissues commonly affected in dogs and cats with IMDs are listed in Table 92-1. Most IMDs have been discussed elsewhere in this book; this chapter focuses on the diagnostic approach to patients with suspected IMDs.

In addition to organ- or tissue-specific signs, such as proteinuria in dogs with glomerulonephritis or shifting-limb lameness in a dog with polyarthritis, dogs and cats with IMDs may be brought in for evaluation of fever of unknown origin (see Chapter 95) or persistent neutrophilic leukocytosis in association with nonspecific signs.

## IMMUNOLOGY FOR THE CLINICIAN

The immune system is composed of three main arms (Table 92-2): humoral, cellular, and phagocytic. The *humoral arm* is composed primarily of B-lymphocytes and their final product, the plasma cells. These cells secrete four types of immunoglobulins (Igs): G, A, M, and E. The first three recognize free or membrane-bound antigens and are involved in a variety of protective mechanisms but mainly agglutination, lysis (with or without complement), or phagocytosis of antigen. IgE is involved in type I (acute) hypersensitivity reactions (e.g., allergies) and is of no clinical relevance in IMDs. IgG or IgM or both are commonly the mediators of cell destruction in IHA and immune-mediated thrombocytopenia (IMT).

The *cellular arm* of the immune system includes mainly the T-lymphocytes, which are in charge of producing bioactive substances (lymphokines) and generating cytotoxic T cells. Most circulating lymphocytes in peripheral blood are T cells; they are classified as helper T cells (i.e., they stimulate immune reactivity) or suppressor T cells (i.e., they suppress immune reactivity). The natural killer cells, which are also part of the cellular arm, participate in direct cytotoxicity. The role of the cellular arm of the immune system in dogs with IMDs is largely unknown.

Finally, the *phagocytic arm* of the immune system is composed mainly of the mononuclear phagocytic cells (i.e., macrophages) and the neutrophils, although the eosinophils also participate in microphagocytic processes. Neutrophils are responsible for phagocytosing blood-borne and tissue particles, such as bacteria and fungi. Given their potent enzymatic arsenal, considerable tissue damage occurs when neutrophils release these enzymes in response to chemotactic stimuli such as IC deposition (e.g., in the synovium or the glomerular base-

## TABLE 92-1

Common Organ or Tissue Targets in Immune-Mediated Disorders

| ORGAN/ TISSUE AFFECTED | DISORDER |
|---|---|
| Red blood cells | Immune-mediated hemolytic anemia; pure red cell aplasia |
| Platelets | Immune-mediated thrombocytopenia |
| Neutrophils | Immune-mediated neutropenia |
| Synovium | Polyarthritis |
| Glomeruli/tubules | Glomerulonephritis |
| Skin | Dermatitis |
| Muscle/nerve/ end plate | Polymyositis, polyneuritis, myasthenia gravis |

## TABLE 92-2

Compartmentalization of the Immune System

| COMPARTMENT | FUNCTION |
|---|---|
| **Humoral Arm** | |
| B-lymphocytes and plasma cells | Produce immunoglobulins |
| **Cellular Arm** | |
| T-lymphocytes, natural killer cells | Cytotoxic lymphocytes Lymphokines ADCC |
| **Phagocytic Arm** | |
| Mononuclear phagocytic cells | Phagocytosis of particles and antigen presentation |
| Neutrophils, eosinophils | Phagocytosis of particles, ADCC |

*ADCC,* Antibody-dependent cell-mediated cytotoxicity.

ment membrane). Macrophages also phagocytose and kill particulate material and play a major role in the destruction of red blood cells (RBCs) and platelets in dogs with IHA or IMT. In addition, macrophages play a pivotal role in antigen presentation to immunocompetent cells. Neutrophils and macrophages are more active in phagocytosing target particles if these are coated with an antibody (opsonization).

The three arms of the immune system interact in a variety of ways. If they do not interact appropriately, either an IMD (i.e., hyperactive immune system) or immunosuppression (i.e., hypoactive immune system) develops in the host.

## *DIAGNOSTIC TESTS*

Unfortunately, with few exceptions, there is no diagnostic test that practicing clinicians can use to make a definitive diag-

## TABLE 92-3

Laboratory Diagnosis of Immune-Mediated Disease

| TEST | SPECIMEN | INTERPRETATION* |
|---|---|---|
| Direct Coombs' | Plasma† | IHA, RBC lysis in SLE |
| Antiplatelet antibodies | Serum | IMT |
| Antinuclear antibody | Serum | SLE, chronic antigenic stimulation |
| Rheumatoid factor | Serum | Rheumatoid arthritis |
| Direct immuno- fluorescence | Tissue | Antibody-complement deposition |

*IHA,* Immune hemolytic anemia; *RBC,* red blood cell; *SLE,* systemic lupus erythematosus; *IMT,* immune-mediated thrombocytopenia.
*For discussion, see text.
†Anticoagulated (EDTA) blood is commonly used as a source of RBCs.

nosis of IMD. Rather, a diagnosis of IMD is reached by a careful evaluation of the historical and clinicopathologic information in the patient in question.

Most laboratory tests included in "immune profiles" detect antibody molecules (Igs) on the surface of affected cells (e.g., direct Coombs' test), circulating autoantibodies (e.g., antinuclear antibody [ANA] test, rheumatoid factor [RF]), or antibodies-complement in the intercellular matrix or basement membrane (e.g., direct immunofluorescence [DIF]; Table 92-3). Most of these tests are species-specific, so the laboratory must know whether the specimen is from a dog or cat. With the possible exception of the direct Coombs' test, most tests for IMD are not very specific and have limited clinical application. A brief discussion of commonly used immune tests follows.

### DIRECT COOMBS' TEST OR DIRECT ANTIGLOBULIN TEST

The direct Coombs' test uses an antibody directed against canine (or feline) IgG, IgM, and complement and is fairly sensitive and specific. In dogs (and cats) with IHA, there is usually a considerable amount of Ig or complement on the surface of the RBCs (mainly IgG and complement). The Coombs' reagent (anticanine or antifeline Ig) binds to the IgG, IgM, or complement molecules already bound to the surface of the RBC, bridging them and causing agglutination. In humans the direct antiglobulin test (DAT) can detect more than 200 molecules of Ig on the surface of each RBC, but hemolysis can occur if there are only 30 to 40 molecules of Ig per cell. Therefore false-negative results can occur in animals with a small number of Ig molecules per RBC. False-negative results also occur in dogs receiving corticosteroids and stem from the elution of antibodies from the surface of the RBCs.

In humans the DAT is usually performed at 37° and 4° C; Coombs' tests performed at 4° C (cold agglutinins) are commonly positive if there is IgM on the surface of the RBCs.

However, cold agglutinins are rarely detected in canine specimens, so most laboratories perform this test at 37° C unless otherwise requested. The prevalence of IgM-mediated IHA in dogs is extremely low (<1%). Cold agglutinins can also be detected in some cats with hemobartonellosis.

At most veterinary laboratories, a DAT is considered positive if the titer is 1:32 or higher. However, a positive DAT only indicates that the animal has antibodies coating its RBCs, not that it has an "autoimmune disease." The RBCs may actually behave as innocent bystanders, in which antibodies directed against a different antigen bind to the RBC membrane. For example, the DAT may be positive in dogs with systemic mycoses, thus leading to the potential catastrophic use of immunosuppressive drugs in a patient with an infectious disease. A positive DAT should be interpreted with caution in patients with normal PCVs. In dogs with IHA, the titer does not correlate with either the severity of hemolysis or the response to treatment. The laboratory should always dilute the reagents for the Coombs' test, because occasionally the titer is negative in dogs with large amounts of Ig on the surface of their RBCs, the reason being that the antibody molecules are bridging with one another (i.e., forming a lattice), thus not leaving any empty binding sites for the Coombs' reagent (prozone effect).

## ANTINUCLEAR ANTIBODY TEST

The ANA test detects circulating antibodies against the host's DNA. This test is quite sensitive but not very specific; dogs with other chronic diseases such as inflammation and malignancy frequently have positive ANA tests. Dogs and cats receiving certain drugs such as propylthiouracil or procainamide may also have positive test results. This test involves the use of serum from the patient, which is evaluated against one of various substrates for the presence of antibodies against nuclear DNA. Most laboratories consider titers of more than 1:10 positive in dogs and of more than 1:40 positive in cats. Because chronic inflammatory and degenerative processes can result in enough cell damage to cause the release of single strands of deoxyribonucleic acid (DNA) (and therefore allow the immune system to generate antibodies against it), some laboratories now evaluate ANA directed against double-stranded DNA, which may be more representative of true autoimmune disease (i.e., antibody-mediated nuclear damage). ANA test results are commonly positive in dogs and cats with a variety of infectious diseases, and by itself (unless the titer is extremely high) it has little clinical relevance.

## DIRECT IMMUNOFLUORESCENCE OR IMMUNOHISTOCHEMISTRY

As discussed in previous paragraphs, in a variety of IMDs there is antibody directed against somatic antigens of the host or ICs deposited in certain tissues (e.g., glomerular basement membrane). These Igs (and complement) can be detected in specially fixed tissue samples by means of DIF or peroxidase-antiperoxidase (PAP) immunohistochemical stains. The sample (e.g., kidney or skin biopsy specimen) is fixed in a special fixative (provided by most diagnostic laboratories), and then it is processed and treated with an anticanine or antifeline Ig (or complement) reagent labeled with fluorescein or with a PAP system. After this the sample is washed and evaluated using fluorescence or light microscopy. Staining indicates antibody or complement deposition or both. In certain instances the pattern of antibody deposition indicates a specific pathologic process. For example, a positive band in the basement membrane of a skin biopsy specimen is suggestive of systemic lupus erythematosus (or discoid lupus), whereas the finding of intercellular epidermal staining is compatible with pemphigus vulgaris, pemphigus foliaceus, or pemphigus vegetans. Both staining patterns are usually seen in pemphigus erythematosus.

Samples fixed in Michelle's medium can be stored refrigerated for several weeks to months (even years). Therefore, if IMD is suspected in an animal, the clinician can submit a biopsy specimen for histopathologic studies and refrigerate a sample in Michelle's medium. If the histopathologic changes support IMD, the sample in the special fixative can then be submitted to a referral laboratory for DIF studies.

DIF is also used at some laboratories in the diagnosis of IMT. In these cases, a bone marrow smear is prepared as just described. Fluorescence of the megakaryocytes indicates the presence of antimegakaryocyte (or antiplatelet) antibodies. However, this technique is not specific, and samples from dogs with malignancy or chronic inflammatory disease and normal platelet counts are commonly positive.

## OTHER TESTS

Other tests commonly used in animals with suspected or confirmed IMD include the RF test and the test for antiplatelet-antimegakaryocyte or antineutrophil antibodies.

The RF test detects an IgM directed against canine Ig in the patient's serum and is typically present in dogs with rheumatoid arthritis; it is not very sensitive or specific, however. The substrate used for this test is variable (canine antibody–coated sheep RBCs [Rose-Waaler test] or latex particles coated with canine IgG). Most laboratories consider titers of more than 1:40 to be positive in dogs; this test has not been extensively evaluated in cats.

A variety of techniques, including enzyme-linked immunosorbent assays and radioimmunoassays, are currently being evaluated to detect circulating antiplatelet antibodies or platelet-bound Igs; their clinical value is still uncertain, since dogs with infectious or neoplastic causes of thrombocytopenia frequently have positive test results.

Several tests have been designed to detect antineutrophil antibodies, including leukoagglutination and immunofluorescence. However, their clinical value is still questionable.

### Suggested Readings

Bennett D et al: The laboratory identification of serum antinuclear antibody in the dog, *J Comp Pathol* 97:523, 1987.

Bennett D et al: The laboratory identification of serum rheumatoid factor in the dog, *J Comp Pathol* 97:541, 1987.

Day MJ: Immune-mediated hemolytic anemia. In Feldman BF et al: *Schalm's veterinary hematology,* ed 5, Philadelphia, 2000, Lippincott Williams & Wilkins, p 799.

Dunn JK et al: The diagnostic significance of a positive direct antiglobulin test in anemic cats, *Can J Comp Med* 48:349, 1984.

Jacobs RM et al: Use of a microtiter Coombs' test for study of age, gender, and breed distributions in immunohemolytic anemia in the dog, *J Am Vet Med Assoc* 185:66, 1984.

Slappendel RJ: The diagnostic significance of the direct antiglobulin test (DAT) in anemic dogs, *Vet Immunol Immunopathol* 1:49, 1979.

# CHAPTER 93

# Immunosuppressive Drugs

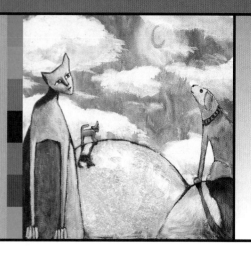

## CHAPTER OUTLINE

GENERAL CONSIDERATIONS, 1216
CORTICOSTEROIDS, 1216
CYCLOPHOSPHAMIDE, 1217
AZATHIOPRINE, 1217
CHLORAMBUCIL, 1218
GOLD SALTS, 1218
CYCLOSPORIN A, 1218
DANAZOL, 1218

## GENERAL CONSIDERATIONS

Immunosuppressive drugs are commonly used in small animal practice to induce or maintain remission in dogs and cats with immune-mediated (or "autoimmune") diseases (IMDs). These drugs usually act by a variety of mechanisms, but mainly they either suppress mononuclear-phagocytic activity or suppress antibody production by the humoral arm of the immune system (B-cells), or they do both; the effects of immunosuppressive drugs on cell-mediated immunity are largely unknown. Because the half-life of circulating immunoglobulin G in dogs is approximately 1 week, suppression of antibody production is a delayed effect. Most of the following observations are gleaned from my personal experience, mostly in dogs with immune-mediated blood disorders, because there are few published clinical trials of immunosuppressive drugs in veterinary medicine and the experimental studies conducted in dogs have been mostly short-term ones.

Similar to anticancer chemotherapy, the therapeutic approach used in dogs and cats with IMDs involves three (with a possible fourth) strategies or phases. These phases are (see p. 1126) (1) induction of remission, (2) intensification, (3) maintenance, and (4) reinduction of remission, or "rescue." The induction phase may not be necessary in patients with mild IMDs, and maintenance immunosuppressive treatment can be initiated at the time of diagnosis. As with chemotherapy, the induction phase is more aggressive and potentially associated with more adverse effects. The patient therefore must be more closely monitored during this phase than during the maintenance phase.

Drugs commonly used for induction of remission, intensification, maintenance, and rescue are listed in Table 93-1. A brief discussion of some pharmacologic principles that apply to commonly used immunosuppressive agents follows. General principles of treatment in dogs and cats with IMDs are discussed on p. 1162.

## CORTICOSTEROIDS

Corticosteroids are the most widely used immunosuppressants in dogs and cats. Two drugs are frequently used: prednisone (or prednisolone) and dexamethasone. Prednisone is used for both induction and maintenance, whereas dexamethasone is typically used in the induction phase, and only briefly. When dosing these agents, the clinician should bear in mind their relative potency: dexamethasone is seven to eight times more potent than prednisone.

Corticosteroids act by three major mechanisms: (1) they suppress mononuclear-phagocytic activity (immediate effect); (2) they cause elution of the antibody molecules from the surface of the target cells (immediate effect); and (3) they suppress the production of immunoglobulins (delayed effect). In addition, they appear to impair neutrophil bacterial killing ability and cell-mediated immunity.

During the induction phase of immunosuppression, prednisone (or equivalent doses of dexamethasone) is administered daily for 7 to 10 days in doses of approximately 2 to 4 mg/kg in dogs and 4 to 8 mg/kg in cats. After this, the dose is decreased and the interval between administration is lengthened to every other day to prevent interference with the hypothalamic-pituitary-adrenal axis. Once the disease is in remission, the doses of corticosteroids, as well as of other immunosuppressants, should be decreased gradually to prevent sudden relapses. Prednisone and prednisolone are considerably safer than dexamethasone for long-term treatment. Because in cats the liver is not effective at methylating, pred-

TABLE 93-1

Immunosuppressive Drugs Used for Induction,
Intensification, Maintenance, and Rescue in Dogs and Cats
with Immune-Mediated Diseases

**Induction of Remission**

Prednisone: 2-4 mg/kg PO q24h (dogs) or 4-8 mg/kg PO
  q24h (cats)
Dexamethasone sodium phosphate: 1-4 mg/kg IV **single
  dose** (dogs and cats)
Cyclophosphamide (Cytoxan): 200-300 mg/m² IV
  single dose (dogs) or 200-300 mg/m² PO single dose
  (cats)
Vincristine (Oncovin): 0.5 mg/m² IV single dose (dogs
  and cats)*
Human IV immunoglobulin: 0.5-1.5 g/kg IV single dose
  (dogs)

**Intensification**

Cyclophosphamide (Cytoxan): 200-300 mg/m² IV single
  dose (dogs) or 200-300 mg/m² PO single dose (cats)

**Maintenance**

Prednisone: 1-2 mg/kg PO q48h (dogs) or 2-4 mg/kg PO
  q48h (cats)
Azathioprine (Imuran): 50-75 mg/m² PO q24-48h (dogs)
Chlorambucil (Leukeran): 20 mg/m² PO every 2 weeks
  (dogs and cats)

**Rescue (Reinduction of Remission)**

Cyclophosphamide (Cytoxan): 200-300 mg/m² IV
  single dose (dogs) or 200-300 mg/m² PO single dose
  (cats)
Cyclophosphamide (Cytoxan): 50 mg/m² PO q48h, or
  q24h for 4 days and off for 3 days (alternating) (dogs);
  200-300 mg/ m² PO q3wk (cats)
Danazol (Danocrine): 5 mg/kg PO q12h (dogs)(cats?)
Human IV immunoglobulin: 0.5-1.5 g/kg IV, single dose
  (dogs)

*Of questionable efficacy in immune-mediated thrombocytopenia
(see p. 1191).

nisolone (methylated prednisone) may be a better choice than
prednisone.

Adverse effects of corticosteroid treatment include iatrogenic hyperadrenocorticism (see p. 778), gastrointestinal tract ulceration, recurrent urinary tract infections, and pancreatitis. In my clinical experience, acute gastrointestinal tract ulceration or pancreatitis is more common in dogs receiving dexamethasone than in those receiving prednisone. Indeed, we have observed gastroduodenal ulcers or severe acute pancreatitis in dogs within 24 to 48 hours of administering one dose of dexamethasone. There are minimal or no adverse effects in most cats, although diabetes mellitus (usually transient) may occur.

# CYCLOPHOSPHAMIDE

In my experience, cyclophosphamide (Cytoxan, Mead Johnson, Evansville, Ind) is a very effective immunosuppressive agent for inducing remission in dogs and possibly cats with IMDs. This drug is an alkylator anticancer agent, which appears to suppress cell-mediated and humoral immunity, as well as mononuclear-phagocytic function. It is activated and metabolized by the microsomal fraction of the liver and is available as 25 and 50 mg tablets and injectable vials of 100, 200, 500, and 1000 mg.

In my experience, cyclophosphamide has been effective in inducing or consolidating remission in dogs with immune-mediated hemolytic anemia (IHA) or immune-mediated thrombocytopenia (IMT). It is also effective in dogs with immune-mediated polyarthritis, dermatitis, or systemic lupus erythematosus (SLE). I commonly administer one dose of 200 to 300 mg/m² intravenously in dogs with steroid-nonresponsive or severe IHA or IMT. In cats the same dose is administered orally, because gastrointestinal adverse effects (e.g., vomiting, anorexia) appear to be more common after intravenous injections of this agent.

The oral form of cyclophosphamide can be given on a continuous basis either every other day or for 4 consecutive days followed by 3 days off, at a dose of 50 mg/m². However, one of the common adverse effects of long-term cyclophosphamide treatment in dogs is sterile hemorrhagic cystitis (see p. 1114), which frequently develops after 8 to 10 weeks of continuous treatment. Female dogs are at increased risk for this toxicity and should therefore undergo periodic urinalysis and physical examination while receiving the drug. The concurrent administration of prednisone appears to decrease the risk of cystitis in dogs receiving ongoing cyclophosphamide treatment. Cystitis caused by long-term cyclophosphamide treatment is extremely rare in cats.

Two other common adverse effects of cyclophosphamide include anorexia (mainly in cats) and myelosuppression (in both dogs and cats). Because of this agent's potential to cause myelosuppression, a complete blood count (CBC) should be performed every 2 to 4 weeks, and the dose adjusted accordingly (see Chapter 80). For a discussion of the diagnosis and management of these complications, see Chapter 80.

# AZATHIOPRINE

Azathioprine (Imuran; PrometheasLabs, San Diego, Calif) is an antimetabolite that is converted to 6-mercaptopurine in the liver. It is extremely effective as a maintenance drug, but because it appears to have a delayed action (2 to 4 weeks), it is not the drug of choice for induction of remission. It is usually given orally daily for 1 week and every other day thereafter in doses of 50 mg/m²; it is available in 50 mg tablets. In my experience, when azathioprine is used at doses of 2.2 mg/kg in dogs weighing over 30 kg, myelosuppression is extremely common (i.e., a dose of azathioprine for a 35-kg dog would be 50 mg when using 50 mg/m², and 75 mg when using 2.2 mg/kg). I use azathioprine routinely in dogs with IMDs that develop corticosteroid intolerance (e.g., polyuria, polydipsia, panting, psychosis) and in those in which corticosteroid therapy alone is not sufficient to induce or maintain remission.

Azathioprine is an excellent drug for the maintenance of remission in dogs with immune-mediated cytopenias, dermatopathies, polyarthritis, or SLE. The most common adverse effect is myelosuppression, particularly in larger dogs (see previous paragraph) and in cats. Given its severe myelosuppressive effect in cats, I do not use it in this species; chlorambucil is as effective and better tolerated (see following paragraphs). Because of azathioprine's potential to cause myelosuppression, a CBC should be performed every 2 to 4 weeks and the dose adjusted accordingly (see Chapter 80). A cholestatic hepatopathy can also develop in dogs receiving high doses of azathioprine.

## CHLORAMBUCIL

Chlorambucil (Leukeran; Burroughs Wellcome, Research Triangle Park, N.C.) is another alkylator anticancer agent with good immunosuppressive properties. It is effective in maintenance protocols because, like azathioprine, it appears to have a delayed onset of action (i.e., 2 to 4 weeks).

Chlorambucil is available as 2-mg tablets and is administered at doses of 20 mg/m² given orally every other week or 2 to 4 mg/m² given orally every other day. This drug is almost devoid of toxicity, although occasionally myelosuppression or anorexia occurs in both dogs and cats; we have also seen a cholestatic hepatopathy in a limited number of cats receiving chronic chlorambucil treatment. As discussed earlier, it is the drug of choice for the maintenance of remission in cats that do not tolerate or respond to corticosteroids; in this species it has been effective in lymphoplasmacytic gastroenteritis, stomatitis, and pododermatitis; in immune-mediated blood diseases; and in SLE.

## GOLD SALTS

Gold salts (chrysotherapy) are used for the management of steroid-refractory immune-mediated dermatopathies and polyarthritis, as well as for the treatment of other IMDs. These heavy metal derivatives are concentrated in the synovium, liver, kidneys, and mononuclear-phagocytic organs. Most of the administered drug is excreted by the kidneys. From an immunologic standpoint, gold salts apparently decrease phagocytosis, inhibit macrophage enzymes, and inhibit B- and T-lymphocyte–dependent blastogenesis.

Several gold salts are available for therapeutic use, including gold sodium thiomalate (Myochrysine; MSD, West Point, Pa), aurothioglucose (Solganal; Schering, Kenilworth, N.J.), and thiethylphosphine gold, or auranofin, (Ridaura; SKF, Philadelphia, Pa.). The first two are administered by intramuscular injection, whereas thiethylphosphine gold (auranofin) is an oral preparation. Adverse effects include cuta-

neous and mucosal reactions, cytopenias, and reversible renal tubular damage.

Auranofin is administered at a dose of 0.05 to 0.2 mg/kg given orally twice a day, up to a total of 9 mg/day. It is available in 3-mg capsules. Its major toxicity is reversible thrombocytopenia, and it has been effective in dogs with immune-mediated polyarthritis, pemphigus foliaceus, and pemphigus vulgaris.

## CYCLOSPORIN A

Cyclosporin A (CyA) (Sandimmune; Sandoz, East Hanover, N.J. or Neoral; Novartis, Summit, N.J. ) is a cyclic polypeptide metabolite of the fungus *Tolypocladium inflatum* that impairs cell-mediated immunity. It is extensively used in humans with IMDs and in organ transplant recipients. It has also been used extensively in dogs and cats undergoing bone marrow and kidney transplantation.

CyA is available in 25 and 100 mg gelatin capsules, an oral suspension (100 mg/ml), 50 mg ampules for intravenous injection, and an ophthalmic preparation (Optimune, Sandoz). The cost of using it in large dogs is usually prohibitive. The 50 mg ampule dose can cause anaphylaxis if it is administered intravenously in dogs. CyA has been dosed at 7 to 15 mg/kg/day, doses that result in therapeutic serum concentrations of 200 to 400 ng/ml; toxicity usually occurs if serum concentrations exceed 600 ng/ml.

Beneficial effects of CyA have been shown in dogs undergoing allogeneic bone marrow transplantation and in cats and dogs undergoing renal transplantation. No beneficial effects are apparent in dogs and cats with immune-mediated dermatitis, glomerulonephritis, or polyarthritis. However, topical CyA is beneficial in dogs with keratoconjunctivitis sicca and pannus. Some clinicians recommend that CyA be used for the treatment of dogs with refractory IHA or IMT, but my experience with this drug is limited. Adverse effects of CyA in dogs include gastrointestinal tract irritation, hirsutism, gingival hyperplasia, papillomatosis, and nephrotoxicosis.

## DANAZOL

Danazol (Danocrine; Winthrop, New York, N.Y.) is an androgenic steroid with minimal masculinizing properties. It has been used successfully in humans with steroid-refractory IMT and IHA and in those with azathioprine-resistant SLE. This steroid appears to exert its immunosuppressive effects mainly by decreasing expression of Fc receptors on the membrane of the mononuclear-phagocytes (i.e., antibody-coated cells are phagocytosed after adhering to the macrophage membrane via the Fc receptor). Danazol is available in 50, 100, and 200 mg capsules.

This agent has been used in dogs with steroid-resistant IMT or IHA, but beneficial responses have been noticed in a limited number of patients. We administer it at a dosage of 5 mg/kg given orally twice a day; at this dose, adverse effects are minimal. Danazol can be used in patients with IMD that have failed conventional immunosuppressive treatment; however, its cost may be prohibitive in large-breed dogs (i.e., $2 to $3 for a 100 mg tablet).

## Suggested Readings

Helton Rhodes K et al: Chlorambucil: effective therapeutic options for the treatment of feline immune-mediated dermatoses, *Fel Pract* 20:5, 1992.

Miller E, editor: Immunotherapy: augmentation and suppression, *Semin Vet Med Surg* 12(3), 1997 (the entire issue is devoted to immunomodulatory treatment).

Ogilvie GK et al: Short-term effects of cyclophosphamide and azathioprine on selected aspects of the canine blastogenic response, *Vet Immunol Immunopathol* 18:119, 1988.

Serra DA et al: Oral chrysotherapy with auranofin in dogs, *J Am Vet Med Assoc* 194:1327, 1989.

White JV: Cyclosporine: prototype of a T-cell selective immunosuppressant, *J Am Vet Med Assoc* 189:566, 1986.

White SD et al: Use of tetracycline and niacinamide for treatment of autoimmune skin disease in 31 dogs, *J Am Vet Med Assoc* 200:1497, 1992.

# CHAPTER 94

# Systemic Lupus Erythematosus

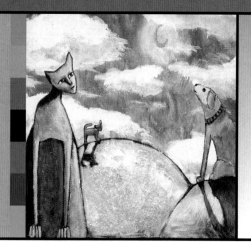

## CHAPTER OUTLINE

ETIOLOGY AND PATHOGENESIS, 1220
    Clinical features, 1220
    Diagnosis, 1220
    Treatment, 1221

## ETIOLOGY AND PATHOGENESIS

Systemic lupus erythematosus (SLE) is a chronic, multisystemic, immune-mediated disease in which immunity is directed against a variety of tissues or tissue components. In addition, circulating immune complexes cause type III hypersensitivity reactions (i.e., immune complex deposition–mediated tissue damage). Although the etiology of SLE is unknown, the occasional clustering of the disorder seen in colony dogs indicates that SLE may be genetically transmitted or infectious in nature. This disease is well characterized in both dogs and in cats.

### Clinical Features

Because several tissues and organs can be affected, SLE can mimic a variety of chronic inflammatory, infectious, and neoplastic disorders; thus it is frequently referred to as "the great imitator." Typical clinical findings in dogs with SLE include shifting-limb lameness caused by polyarthritis, bullous or erythematous skin lesions, petechiae and ecchymoses caused by thrombocytopenia or vasculitis, icteric mucous membranes resulting from immune-mediated hemolysis, and edema or ascites caused by hypoalbuminemia (i.e., secondary to immune complex glomerulonephritis). In addition, dogs with SLE usually have pyrexia, lymphadenopathy, splenomegaly, polyclonal gammopathies, or a combination of these. The clinical manifestations of SLE are listed in Table 94-1.

The complete blood count (CBC) usually reveals hemolytic anemia, thrombocytopenia, neutropenia, and/or hyperproteinemia; if severe glomerulonephritis is present, the protein-losing nephropathy may lead to hypoproteinemia. Changes in the serum biochemistry profile are variable and include hypoalbuminemia, hyperglobulinemia, hyperbiliru-

 TABLE 94-1

**Organs and Tissues Potentially Affected in Dogs with Systemic Lupus Erythematosus**

| ORGAN/TISSUE AFFECTED | DISORDER |
| --- | --- |
| Red blood cells | Immune-mediated hemolytic anemia/pure red cell aplasia |
| Platelets | Immune-mediated thrombocytopenia |
| Neutrophils | Immune-mediated neutropenia |
| Clotting factors | Coagulopathy |
| Synovium | Nonerosive polyarthritis |
| Glomeruli (tubules) | Glomerulonephritis |
| Blood vessels | Vasculitis |
| Epidermis | Dermatitis |
| Central nervous system | Seizures, focal signs |
| Skeletal muscle/ nerve end plate | Polymyositis, polyneuritis, myasthenia gravis |

binemia, azotemia, and high liver enzyme activities. The urinalysis may reveal proteinuria with or without bilirubinuria.

### Diagnosis

The diagnosis of SLE is reached after careful evaluation of the clinical, hematologic, and serum biochemical findings, as well as the results of immunologic tests (see Chapter 92). In humans, four of the following eleven criteria have to be fulfilled for SLE to be diagnosed: malar rash, diskoid rash, photosensitivity, oral ulceration, arthritis, serositis, renal disease, neurologic disorders, hematologic disorders (i.e., cytopenias), a positive antinuclear antibody (ANA) test, and positive LE cell preparation or false-positive results to serologic tests for syphilis.

If SLE is suspected in a dog, the following tests or procedures are indicated: joint radiography (to rule out erosive polyarthritis, as seen in rheumatoid arthritis); a joint tap for cytologic evaluation; a direct Coombs' test (if the dog has anemia); bone marrow aspiration (if the dog has nonregenerative anemia, neutropenia, or thrombocytopenia); a lymph node or splenic aspiration (if lymphadenopathy or splenomegaly is present); a skin biopsy for histopathologic and direct immunofluorescence or immunohistochemistry (if cutaneous lesions are present); and a renal biopsy for histopathologic and direct immunofluorescence or immunoperoxidase tests (if glomerulonephritis is suspected). A dog with two or more of the following findings should be considered to have SLE and treated accordingly: peripheral blood cytopenia, oligoarthritis or polyarthritis, glomerulonephritis, focal or multifocal central nervous system signs, dermatitis, polymyositis, myasthenia gravis, or vasculitis, together with a positive ANA test (i.e., more than 1:10).

Although SLE can mimic a variety of clinical entities, canine ehrlichiosis, multiple myeloma, and bacterial endocarditis are the most important differential diagnoses in affected dogs. Canine ehrlichiosis can be ruled out by performing serologic tests or polymerase chain reaction for *Ehrlichia canis* (see p. 1267); multiple myeloma by performing bone marrow aspiration, skeletal radiography, and serum protein electrophoresis (see p. 1210); and subacute bacterial endocarditis by auscultation for a murmur, echocardiography, and bacterial blood cultures (see p. 145).

## Treatment

The treatment of dogs with SLE is similar to that of dogs with other immune-mediated diseases and is discussed in Chapter 93 (see p. 1216).

## Suggested Readings

Day MJ: Systemic lupus erythematosus. In Feldman BF et al: *Schalm's veterinary hematology,* ed 5, Philadelphia, 2000, Lippincott Williams & Wilkins, p 818.

Grindem CB et al: Systemic lupus erythematosus: literature review and report of 42 cases, *J Am Anim Hosp Assoc* 19:481, 1983.

Hubert B et al: Spontaneous familial systemic lupus erythematosus in a canine breeding colony, *J Comp Pathol* 98:81, 1988.

Monier JC et al: Systemic lupus erythematosus in a colony of dogs, *Am J Vet Res* 49:46, 1988.

Shull RM et al: Investigation of the nature and specificity of antinuclear antibody in dogs, *Am J Vet Res* 44:2004, 1983.

White SD et al: Investigation of antibodies to extractable nuclear antigens in dogs, *Am J Vet Res* 53:1019, 1992.

# CHAPTER 95

# Fever of Undetermined Origin

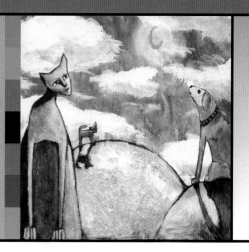

## CHAPTER OUTLINE

FEVER, 1222
FEVER OF UNDETERMINED ORIGIN, 1222
  Disorders associated with fever of undetermined
    origin, 1222
  Diagnostic approach to the patient with fever
    of undetermined origin, 1223
  Treatment, 1224

## FEVER

The term *fever* refers to a syndrome of malaise (or nonspecific systemic clinical signs) and pyrexia (or hyperthermia). In this chapter, however, the terms *fever* and *pyrexia* are used interchangeably. Fever constitutes a protective physiologic response to both infectious and noninfectious causes of inflammation that enhances the host's ability to eliminate a noxious agent.

A variety of stimuli, including bacteria, endotoxins, viruses, immune complexes, activated complement, and necrotic tissue, trigger the release of endogenous pyrogens by the phagocytic system (mainly the mononuclear cells, or macrophages). These endogenous pyrogens include interleukin-1, tumor necrosis factor, and interleukin-6, among others. They activate the preoptic nucleus of the hypothalamus, raising the set point of the thermostat by generating heat (through muscle contraction and shivering) and conserving heat (through vasoconstriction).

In humans, several patterns of fever have been associated with specific disorders; however, this does not appear to be the case in dogs and cats. In people with *continuous fever,* the pyrexia is maintained for several days or weeks; this type of fever is associated with bacterial endocarditis, central nervous system lesions, tuberculosis, and some malignancies. In people with *intermittent fever,* the body temperature decreases to normal but rises again for periods of 1 to 2 days; this is seen in brucellosis and some malignancies. In *remittent fever* the temperature varies markedly each day but is always above normal (i.e., 39.2° C); this type of fever is associated with bacterial infections. The term *relapsing fever* is used to refer to febrile periods that alternate with variable periods of normal body temperature, as seen in humans with malaria.

## FEVER OF UNDETERMINED ORIGIN

The term *fever of undetermined (or unknown) origin* (FUO) is used quite liberally in veterinary medicine to refer to a febrile syndrome for which a diagnosis is not evident. In human medicine, FUO refers to a febrile syndrome of more than 3 weeks' duration that remains undiagnosed after 1 week of thorough in-hospital evaluation. If the term FUO were to be used in the same way in animals as is recommended in people, very few dogs and cats would actually have it. Therefore in this chapter, the discussion focuses on the approach to a dog or cat with fever that does not respond to antibacterial antibiotic treatment and for which a diagnosis is not obvious after a minimum workup (i.e., complete blood count [CBC], serum biochemistry profile, urinalysis) has been performed.

As a general rule, the clinician typically presumes that a dog or cat with fever has an infection, until this is proved otherwise. This appears to be true in reality, as shown by the fact that a large proportion of dogs and cats with fever respond to nonspecific antibacterial treatment. No clinicopathologic evaluation is performed in most of these animals because the fever responds so promptly to treatment.

### DISORDERS ASSOCIATED WITH FEVER OF UNDETERMINED ORIGIN

In humans, certain infectious, neoplastic, and immune-mediated disorders are commonly associated with FUO. Approximately one third of patients have infectious diseases; one third have cancer (mainly hematologic malignancies, such as lymphoma and leukemia); and the remaining one third have immune-mediated, granulomatous, or miscellaneous disorders. In 10% to 15% of the patients with FUO, the underlying disorder remains undiagnosed despite intensive efforts to do so. However, most of the review articles describing dogs and cats with FUO that have appeared in the literature extrapolate data from human papers.

On the basis of observations made in dogs and cats evaluated at our clinic and case reports in the literature, the most common cause of FUO appears to be infectious diseases, followed by immune-mediated, neoplastic disorders, and miscellaneous (Table 95-1). However, it should be remembered that, despite aggressive evaluation, the cause of the fever

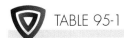 TABLE 95-1

Causes of Fever of Undetermined Origin in Dogs and Cats

| CAUSE | SPECIES AFFECTED | CAUSE | SPECIES AFFECTED |
|---|---|---|---|
| **Infectious** | | **Immune Mediated** | |
| Bacterial | | Polyarthritis | D, C |
|   Subacute bacterial endocarditis | D | Vasculitis | D |
|   Brucellosis | D | Meningitis | D |
|   Tuberculosis | D, C | Systemic lupus erythematosus | D, C |
|   Hemobartonellosis | D, C | Immune hemolytic anemia | D, C |
|   Plague | C | Steroid-responsive fever | D |
|   Lyme disease | D | Steroid-responsive neutropenia | D, C |
|   Bartonellosis | D, C | | |
|   Suppurative infection | D, C | **Neoplastic** | |
|     Abscesses (liver, pancreas, stump | | Acute leukemia | D, C |
|       pyometra) | | Chronic leukemia | D, C |
|     Prostatitis | | Lymphoma | D, C |
|     Diskospondylitis | | Malignant histiocytosis | D |
|     Pyelonephritis | | Multiple myeloma | D, C |
|     Peritonitis, pyothorax | | Necrotic solid tumors | D, C |
|     Septic arthritis | | **Miscellaneous** | |
| Rickettsial | | | |
|   Ehrlichiosis, Rocky Mountain spotted | D, C | Metabolic bone disorders | D |
|     fever, salmon poisoning | | Drug induced (tetracycline, | C, D |
| Mycotic | |   penicillins, sulfa) | |
|   Histoplasmosis | D, C | Tissue necrosis | D, C |
|   Blastomycosis | D, C | Hyperthyroidism | C, D |
|   Coccidioidomycosis | D | Idiopathic | D, C |
| Viral | | | |
|   Feline infectious peritonitis | C | | |
|   Feline leukemia virus infection | C | | |
|   Feline immunodeficiency virus | C | | |
|     infection | | | |
| Protozoal | | | |
|   Babesiosis | D | | |
|   Hepatozoonosis | D | | |
|   Cytauxzoonosis | C | | |
|   Chagas' disease | D | | |
|   Leishmaniasis | D | | |

*D*, Dog; *C*, cat; *?*, poorly documented.

cannot be determined in approximately 10% to 15% of small animals.

## DIAGNOSTIC APPROACH TO THE PATIENT WITH FEVER OF UNDETERMINED ORIGIN

A dog or cat with FUO should be evaluated in a systematic fashion. In general, a three-stage approach is used at our clinic (Table 95-2). The first stage consists of a thorough history-taking and physical examination, as well as a minimum database. The second stage consists of additional noninvasive and invasive diagnostic tests. The third stage consists of a therapeutic trial, which is instituted if no diagnosis can be obtained after completion of the second stage.

## History and Physical Examination

When a febrile patient fails to respond to antibacterial treatment, a course of action must be formulated. A thorough history should be obtained and a complete physical examination performed. The history rarely provides clues to the cause of the fever; however, a history of ticks may indicate a rickettsial or hemoparasitic disorder; previous administration of tetracycline (mainly to cats) may indicate a drug-induced fever; and travel to areas where systemic mycoses are endemic should prompt further investigation consisting of cytologic or serologic studies or fungal cultures.

During a physical examination it is important to evaluate the lymphoreticular organs, because numerous infectious and neoplastic diseases affecting these organs (e.g., ehrlichiosis,

## TABLE 95-2

**Diagnostic Evaluation of the Dog or Cat with Fever of Undetermined Origin**

### First Stage

CBC
Serum biochemistry profile and thyroxine concentration
Urinalysis
Urine bacterial culture and susceptibility
FNA of enlarged organs, masses, or swellings

### Second Stage

Thoracic and abdominal radiography
Abdominal ultrasonography
Echocardiography
Serial blood cultures
Immune tests (ANA, rheumatoid factor)
Serum protein electrophoresis
Serologic tests or PCR (see Table 95-1)
Arthrocentesis (cytologic studies and culture)
Biopsy of any lesion or enlarged organ
Bone marrow aspiration (for cytologic studies and
    bacterial/fungal culture)
Cerebrospinal fluid analysis
Leukocyte scanning
Exploratory celiotomy

### Third Stage

Therapeutic trial (antipyretics, antibiotics, corticosteroids)

*CBC,* Complete blood count; *FNA,* fine-needle aspiration; *ANA,* antinuclear antibody; *PCR,* polymerase chain reaction.

Rocky Mountain spotted fever, bartonellosis, leukemia, systemic mycoses) may cause fever. An enlarged lymph node or spleen should be evaluated cytologically using specimens obtained by fine-needle aspiration (FNA); an FNA sample can also be obtained for bacterial and fungal culture and susceptibility testing, should the cytologic studies reveal evidence of infection or inflammation. Any palpable mass or swelling should also be evaluated using specimens obtained by FNA to rule out granulomatous, pyogranulomatous, and suppurative inflammation, as well as neoplasia (for additional information, see Chapter 77).

The clinician should thoroughly inspect and palpate the oropharynx, searching for signs of pharyngitis, stomatitis, or tooth root abscesses. The bones should also be thoroughly palpated, particularly in young dogs, because metabolic bone disorders, such as hypertrophic osteodystrophy, can cause fever associated with bone pain. Palpation and passive motion of all joints is also indicated, in search of monoarthritis, oligoarthritis, or polyarthritis. A neurologic examination should be conducted to detect signs of meningitis or other central nervous system lesions (see p. 946). In older cats the ventral cervical region should be palpated to detect thyroid enlargement or nodules.

The thorax should be auscultated carefully in search of a murmur, which could indicate bacterial endocarditis. A thorough ocular examination may reveal changes suggestive of a specific cause (e.g., chorioretinitis in cats with feline infectious peritonitis [FIP] or in dogs with ehrlichiosis).

## Clinicopathologic Evaluation

A minimum database consisting of a CBC, serum biochemistry profile, urinalysis, and urine bacterial culture and susceptibility testing should always be carried out in dogs and cats with persistent fever. The CBC may provide important clues to the cause of the fever (Table 95-3). A serum biochemistry profile rarely yields diagnostic information in dogs and cats with FUO, although it can provide indirect information on parenchymal organ function. However, the finding of hyperglobulinemia and hypoalbuminemia may indicate an infectious, immune-mediated, or neoplastic disorder (see Chapter 91). The finding of pyuria or white blood cell casts in a urinalysis may indicate a urinary tract infection, which may be the cause of the FUO (i.e., pyelonephritis).

Other diagnostic tests that may be called for in patients with FUO are listed in Table 95-2. Echocardiography is indicated only if the patient has a heart murmur, because it rarely detects a valvular lesion in dogs without murmurs. Bacterial and fungal blood cultures are performed as described on p. 1229, and tests of immune function are performed as described on p. 1226. Some of the infectious diseases listed in Table 95-1 (i.e., systemic mycoses, rickettsial diseases, bartonellosis, FIP, feline immunodeficiency virus infection, feline leukemia virus infection, brucellosis, babesiosis, Lyme disease) can be diagnosed on the basis of serologic findings or polymerase chain reaction (PCR) testing (see appropriate sections for discussion).

Fluid from several joints should be aspirated for cytologic evaluation (and possibly bacterial culture), because polyarthritis may be the only manifestation of a widespread immune-mediated disorder. Thoracic radiography and abdominal ultrasonography should be performed to search for a silent septic focus. In dogs and cats with neurologic signs associated with fever, a cerebrospinal fluid tap should be performed; in dogs, immune-mediated vasculitis or meningitis can cause marked temperature elevations. If a diagnosis has still not been reached, bone marrow aspirates for cytologic studies and bacterial and fungal culture should also be obtained. A leukocyte scan may reveal a hidden septic focus. Finally, if a definitive diagnosis is ultimately not obtained, a therapeutic trial of specific antibacterial or antifungal agents or immunosuppressive doses of corticosteroids can be initiated.

## TREATMENT

If a definitive diagnosis is obtained, a specific treatment should be initiated (see appropriate sections for a discussion of the treatment of disorders that cause FUO).

The problem arises if the clinician cannot arrive at a definitive diagnosis. In these patients, changes in the CBC usually are the only clinicopathologic abnormality (see Table

TABLE 95-3

Hematologic Changes in Dogs and Cats with Fever of Undetermined Origin

| HEMATOLOGIC CHANGE | COMPATIBLE WITH |
| --- | --- |
| Regenerative anemia | Immune-mediated diseases, hemoparasites, drugs |
| Nonregenerative anemia | Infection, immune-mediated diseases, tissue necrosis, malignancy, endocarditis |
| Neutrophilia with left-shift | Infection, immune-mediated diseases, tissue necrosis, malignancy, endocarditis |
| Neutropenia | Leukemia, immune-mediated diseases, pyogenic infection, bone marrow infiltrative disease, drugs |
| Monocytosis | Infection, immune-mediated diseases, tissue necrosis, lymphoma, endocarditis, histiocytosis |
| Lymphocytosis | Ehrlichiosis, Chagas' disease, leishmaniasis, chronic lymphocytic leukemia |
| Eosinophilia | Hypereosinophilic syndrome, eosinophilic inflammation, lymphoma |
| Thrombocytopenia | Rickettsiae, leukemia, lymphoma, drugs, immune-mediated diseases |
| Thrombocytosis | Infections (chronic), immune-mediated diseases |

95-3). That is, results of bacterial and fungal cultures, serologic tests, PCR, imaging studies, and FNAs are negative or normal. If the patient has already been treated with a broad-spectrum bactericidal antibiotic, a therapeutic trial of immunosuppressive doses of corticosteroids is warranted (see p. 1216). However, before one institutes immunosuppressive treatment, the owners should be informed of the potential consequences of this approach, primarily that a dog or cat with an undiagnosed infectious disease may die as a result of systemic dissemination of the organism after the start of treatment. Dogs and cats undergoing a therapeutic trial of corticosteroids should be kept in the hospital and monitored frequently for worsening of clinical signs, in which case steroid therapy should be discontinued. In patients with immune-mediated (or steroid-responsive) FUO, the pyrexia and clinical signs usually resolve within 24 to 48 hours of the start of treatment. The animal is then treated as described on p. 1162.

If no response to corticosteroids is observed, two courses of action remain. In one, the patient can be released and given antipyretic drugs, such as aspirin (10 to 25 mg/kg PO q12h in dogs and 10 mg/kg PO q72h in cats), and then returned to the clinic for a complete reevaluation in 1 to 2 weeks. Antipyretics should be used with caution, however, because fever is a protective mechanism, and lowering the body temperature may be detrimental in an animal with an infectious disease. Moreover, drugs such as dipyrone and flunixin (Banamine) can result in marked hypothermia, which may have adverse effects. It should also be remembered that most nonsteroidal antiinflammatory drugs have ulcerogenic effects, can cause cytopenias, and may result in tubular nephropathy if the patient becomes dehydrated or receives other nephrotoxic drugs. The second course of action is to continue the trial of antibiotics using a combination of bactericidal drugs (e.g., ampicillin and enrofloxacin) for a minimum of 5 to 7 days.

## Suggested Readings

Feldman BF: Fever of undetermined origin, *Compend Contin Educ* 2:970, 1980.

Ward A: Fever of unknown origin in cats and dogs, *Vet Med* 81:40, 1985.

# CHAPTER 96

# Recurrent Infections

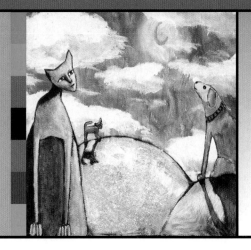

## CHAPTER OUTLINE

CLASSIFICATION AND CLINICAL FEATURES, 1226
Diagnosis, 1227
Management, 1227

Recurrent or persistent infections usually result from congenital or acquired abnormalities of the immune system. Although veterinary clinical immunology is not yet a well-developed specialty, great progress has been made over the past decade in elucidating the underlying immunologic abnormalities in dogs with recurrent infections. Most often these principles also apply to cats; however, with the exception of retrovirus-induced immunodeficiency syndromes (see Chapter 102) and Chédiak-Higashi syndrome, little is known about recurrent infections in this species.

## CLASSIFICATION AND CLINICAL FEATURES

*Congenital immunodeficiency syndromes* can affect the humoral, cellular, or phagocytic systems, either singly or in combination, and appear to be more common in dogs than in cats (Table 96-1). Humoral immunodeficiency syndromes usually result in recurrent upper and lower respiratory tract infections, dermatitis, and enteritis; some Beagles with a selective immunoglobulin A (IgA) deficiency also experience grand mal seizures of unknown pathogenesis and may be more susceptible to immune-mediated diseases. Cellular immunodeficiency syndromes are apparently less common; a T-cell abnormality has been documented in Weimaraners with pituitary dwarfism and in Bull Terriers with lethal acrodermatitis (see Table 96-1). The disease in Weimaraner pups is characterized by retarded growth and recurrent respiratory and gastrointestinal tract infections. Necropsy findings in affected dogs include hypoplastic thymuses with no thymic cortex. Related Bull Terriers with growth retardation, progressive acrodermatitis, chronic pyoderma and paronychia, pneumonia, and diarrhea have significantly decreased lym-

phocyte blastogenesis in response to phytohemagglutinin stimulation. Other diseases that involve inconsistent cell-mediated immunologic abnormalities include *Pneumocystis carinii* infection in Dachshunds and systemic aspergillosis, generalized demodicosis, and prototothecosis in other breeds. Bassett Hounds and Miniature Schnauzers have increased susceptibility to mycobacteriosis. Birman cats with congenital hypotrichosis and thymic atrophy resemble nude mice in that they are born hairless and have severe cell-mediated immune deficiency.

Abnormalities in the phagocytic system have been well documented in dogs and cats (see Table 96-1). They may occur as a consequence of decreased numbers of circulating phagocytes (e.g., in Grey Collies with cyclic hematopoiesis) or as a consequence of abnormal phagocytic function (e.g., defective neutrophil adhesion in Irish Setters with leukocyte adhesion deficiency, defective bactericidal capacity in Doberman Pinschers with recurrent respiratory tract infections). Occasionally the affected neutrophils are morphologically abnormal (e.g., Chédiak-Higashi syndrome in Persian cats). Setters with a deficiency of surface adhesion proteins have recurrent episodes of omphalophlebitis, gingivitis, lymphadenitis, pyoderma, respiratory tract infections, pyometra, and fulminant sepsis. Affected Dobermans exhibit recurrent episodes of rhinitis and pneumonia that respond transiently to antibiotic therapy.

Immunodeficiency syndromes affecting more than one arm of the immune system (X-linked severe combined immunodeficiency syndrome [SCIDS]) have been documented in Basset Hounds and Cardigan Welsh Corgis; they are associated with severe growth retardation and early death. Low serum IgG and IgA concentrations and abnormal lymphocyte blastogenesis in response to phytohemagglutinin are common in affected dogs; the defect is secondary to a mutation in the gene that encodes for the interleukin-2 receptor.

*Acquired immunodeficiency syndromes* include canine distemper virus, parvovirus, and ehrlichial infections, as well as generalized demodicosis in dogs and feline leukemia virus and feline immunodeficiency virus infections in cats. In addition, systemically administered anticancer agents may cause variable degrees of immunosuppression.

TABLE 96-1

Congenital Immunodeficiency Syndromes in Dogs and Cats

| ARM | DEFECT | BREED |
|---|---|---|
| Humoral | IgA deficiency | Beagle, Sharpei, German Shepherd Dog |
|  | IgM deficiency | Doberman Pinscher? |
|  | C3 deficiency | Brittany Spaniel |
|  | Transient hypogammaglobulinemia | Samoyed |
| Cellular | Hypotrichosis, thymic atrophy, acrodermatitis | Weimaraner, Bull Terrier, Dachshunds? Birman cats |
| Phagocytic | Cyclic hematopoiesis | Grey Collie |
|  | Abnormal granulation | Birman cat |
|  | Chédiak-Higashi syndrome | Persian cat |
|  | Mucopolysaccharidosis | Domestic short-haired cat, Siamese cat |
|  | Defective neutrophil adhesion | Irish Setter |
|  | Defective bactericidal capacity | Doberman Pinscher |
|  | Abnormal chemiluminescence | Weimaraner |
| Combined | Severe combined immunodeficiency | Basset Hound, Cardigan Welsh Corgi |

*IgA*, Immunoglobulin A; *IgM*, immunoglobulin M; *C3*, complement 3.

 TABLE 96-2

Laboratory Diagnosis of Immunodeficiency Syndromes in Dogs and Cats

| ARM | TESTS* |
|---|---|
| Humoral | Serum protein electrophoresis, immunoelectrophoresis, radial immunodiffusion for immunoglobulin concentrations, complement activity, immunophenotyping |
| Cellular | Lymphocyte blastogenesis in response to concanavalin A, pokeweed mitogen, and phytohemagglutinin; enumeration of circulating T cells; natural killer (NK) cell assays, immunophenotyping |
| Phagocytic | Nylon wool adhesion; migration under agarose; phagocytosis of bacteria, yeasts, or latex; phagocytosis of opsonized particles; chemiluminescence; nitroblue tetrazolium reduction test; bacterial killing assay; flow cytometry |

*Molecular genetic testing is available for some of the conditions discussed.

## Diagnosis

The type of infectious agent and the pattern of infection are usually determined by the nature of the defect. For example, defects in humoral immunity usually result in infections with pyogenic organisms affecting one or more sites; defects in T-cell function result in viral, fungal, or protozoal infections that are usually widespread; and abnormalities in the phagocytic system may result in skin, respiratory tract, meningeal, or systemic infections with pyogenic or enteric organisms. Therefore the type and pattern of the infection dictate which tests should be performed in these animals.

Several diagnostic tests can be used to evaluate dogs and cats with a suspected immunodeficiency syndrome. Some of these tests (i.e., neutrophil function tests, lymphocyte blastogenesis) require fresh blood samples (i.e., must be performed within 4 hours of sampling) and specialized laboratory equipment. They are therefore of limited use to general practitioners because such equipment is only available at teaching or research institutions. However, other tests can be performed on serum samples mailed to referral laboratories. Tests that can be used to evaluate animals with recurrent infections are listed in Table 96-2.

## Management

The clinical management of these animals includes appropriate antimicrobial drugs determined on the basis of the etiologic agent identified (i.e., bacterial or fungal culture and sensitivity testing). If an infectious agent cannot be isolated and the animal appears to have a bacterial infection, bactericidal antibiotics that attain high intraleukocyte concentrations (e.g., sulfa-trimethoprim, enrofloxacin) should be used. Dogs and cats with suspected or known immunodeficiencies should be current on their vaccinations. If a severe immunodeficiency is present, the use of modified-live vaccines should be avoided, because they may induce disease.

Nonspecific immunomodulators may be of benefit in dogs and cats with immunodeficiency. We have used levamisole (3 mg/kg orally [PO] two or three times per week) successfully in a limited number of dogs with recurrent infections; however, because of the potential for toxicity in cats, this drug should be used with caution in this species.

## Suggested Readings

Couto CG et al: Congenital and acquired neutrophil function abnormalities in the dog. In Kirk RW, editor: *Current veterinary therapy X*, Philadelphia, 1989, WB Saunders.

Degen MA et al: Canine and feline immunodeficiencies. I, *Compend Cont Ed* 8:313, 1986.

Degen MA et al: Canine and feline immunodeficiencies. II, *Compend Cont Ed* 8:379, 1986.

Giger U: Hereditary blood diseases. In Feldman BF et al: *Schalm's veterinary hematology*, ed 5, Philadephia, 2000, Lippincott Williams & Wilkins, p 955.

# CHAPTER 97

## Laboratory Diagnosis of Infectious Diseases

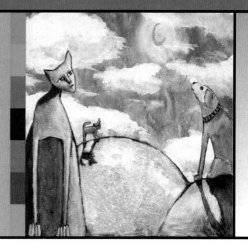

### CHAPTER OUTLINE

DEMONSTRATION OF THE ORGANISM, 1229
    Fecal examination, 1229
    Cytology, 1232
    Tissue techniques, 1235
    Culture techniques, 1235
    Immunologic techniques, 1236
    Polymerase chain reaction, 1236
    Animal inoculation, 1237
    Electron microscopy, 1237
ANTIBODY DETECTION, 1237
    Serum, 1237
    Body fluids, 1238

Clinical syndromes induced by infectious agents are common in small animal practice. The combination of signalment, history, and physical examination findings are used to develop a list of differential diagnoses ranking the most likely infectious agents involved. For example, young, unvaccinated cats with conjunctivitis generally are infected by herpesvirus type 1, *Chlamydophila felis,* or *Mycoplasma felis;* if a dendritic ulcer is present, herpesvirus type 1 is most likely. Results of complete blood count (CBC), serum biochemical panel, urinalysis, radiographs, or ultrasonography can also suggest infectious diseases. For example, a dog with polyuria, polydipsia, neutrophilic leukocytosis, azotemia, pyuria, and an irregularly marginated kidney on radiographic examination is likely to have pyelonephritis. After making a tentative diagnosis, the clinician then has to determine whether to "test or treat." Empiric treatment is often satisfactory in simple, first-time infections of dogs or cats without life-threatening disease (see Chapter 98). However, having a definitive diagnosis is usually preferred so that treatment, prevention, and zoonotic issues can be addressed optimally.

Demonstration of the infectious agent is the best way to make a definitive diagnosis. With some infectious agents, or-

ganism demonstration techniques have low sensitivity, are expensive, or are invasive. Antibody detection is commonly used to aid in the diagnosis of specific infectious diseases in these situations. Antibody detection is generally inferior to organism demonstration for three reasons: (1) antibodies can persist long after an infectious disease has resolved, (2) positive antibody test results do not confirm clinical disease induced by the infectious agent, and (3) in peracute infections, results of serum antibody tests can be negative if the humoral immune responses have not had time to develop. The following is a discussion of the common organism demonstration and antibody detection techniques used in small animal practice.

## DEMONSTRATION OF THE ORGANISM

### FECAL EXAMINATION

Examination of feces can be used to aid in the diagnosis of parasitic diseases of the gastrointestinal (Table 97-1; see Chapter 29) and respiratory tracts (Table 97-2; see Chapter 20). The techniques used most frequently include direct and saline smear, stained smear, fecal flotation, and Baermann technique; each procedure can easily be performed in small animal practice.

#### Direct Smear

Fresh, liquid feces or feces that contain large quantities of mucus should be microscopically examined immediately for the presence of protozoal trophozoites, including those of *Giardia* spp.(small bowel diarrhea) and *Tritrichomonas foetus* (large bowel diarrhea). A direct saline smear can be made to potentiate observation of these motile organisms. The amount of feces required to cover the head of a match is mixed thoroughly with one drop of 0.9% NaCl. The surface of the feces should be used. After application of a coverslip, the smear is evaluated for motile organism by examining it under 100× magnification.

TABLE 97-1

**Demonstration Techniques for Canine and Feline Gastrointestinal Parasites**

| ORGANISM | FORM IN STOOL | SPECIES INFESTED* | OPTIMAL FECAL EXAMINATION TECHNIQUE |
|---|---|---|---|
| **Cestodes** | | | |
| Dipylidium caninum | Egg | B | Identification of adult |
| Echinococcus granulosa | Egg | D | Identification of adult |
| Echinococcus multilocularis | Egg | B | Identification of adult |
| Taenia spp. | Egg | B | Identification of adult |
| **Protozoans** | | | |
| Balantidium coli | Trophozoite | B | Direct or saline smear |
| | Cyst | D | Zinc sulfate centrifugation; other flotations |
| Cryptosporidium parvum | Oocyst | B | Acid fast or monoclonal antibody stain |
| Cystoisospora spp. | Oocyst | B | Sugar or zinc sulfate centrifugation |
| Entamoeba histolytica | Trophozoite | B | Direct or saline smear |
| | Cyst | D | Zinc sulfate centrifugation; other flotations |
| Giardia spp. | Trophozoite | B | Direct or saline smear |
| | Cyst | B | Zinc sulfate centrifugation; other flotations |
| Toxoplasma gondii | Oocyst | B | Sugar or zinc sulfate centrifugation |
| Tritrichomonas foetus | Trophozoite | B | Direct or saline smear |
| | Cyst | D | Zinc sulfate centrifugation; other flotations |
| **Flukes** | | | |
| Eurytrema procyonis | Egg | C | Fecal sedimentation |
| Nanophyetus salmincola | Egg | D | Fecal sedimentation |
| Platynosomum fastosum | Egg | C | Fecal sedimentation |
| **Helminths** | | | |
| Ancylostoma spp. | Egg | B | Zinc sulfate centrifugation; other flotations |
| Ollulanus tricuspis | Egg | C | Zinc sulfate centrifugation; other flotations |
| Physaloptera spp. | Egg | B | Zinc sulfate centrifugation; other flotations |
| Spirocerca lupi | Egg | D | Zinc sulfate centrifugation; other flotations |
| Strongyloides stercoralis | Larvae | B | Baermann technique |
| Toxocara spp. | Egg | B | Zinc sulfate centrifugation; other flotations |
| Toxascaris spp. | Egg | B | Zinc sulfate centrifugation; other flotations |
| Trichuris vulpis | Egg | D | Zinc sulfate centrifugation; other flotations |
| Uncinaria stenocephala | Egg | B | Zinc sulfate centrifugation; other flotations |

*D, Dog; C, cat; B, dog and cat.

 TABLE 97-2

**Demonstration Techniques for Common Canine and Feline Respiratory Tract Parasites**

| ORGANISM | FORM IN STOOL | SPECIES INFECTED* | OPTIMAL FECAL EXAMINATION TECHNIQUE |
|---|---|---|---|
| Aelurostrongylus abstrusus (lungworm) | Larva | C | Baermann technique |
| Andersonstrongylus milksi (lungworm) | Larva | D | Baermann technique |
| Capillaria aerophila | Egg | D | Zinc sulfate or other flotation |
| Crenosoma vulpis (lungworm) | Egg | D | Zinc sulfate or other flotation |
| Eucoleus bohemi (nasal worm) | Egg | D | Zinc sulfate or other flotation |
| Filaroides hirthi (lungworm) | Larva | D | Baermann technique |
| Oslerus osleri (tracheal nodular worm) | Egg or larva | D | Zinc sulfate or other flotation and Baermann technique |
| Paragonimus kellicotti (lung fluke) | Egg | B | Fecal sedimentation |
| Pneumonyssoides caninum (nasal mite) | None | D | None; visualization of adults |

*D, Dog; C, cat; B, dog and cat.

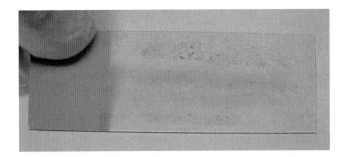

**FIG 97-1**
Diff-Quick stained fecal smear showing appropriate smear thickness.

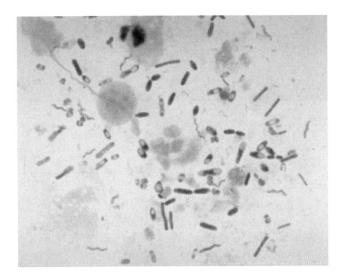

**FIG 97-2**
Wright's-stained, thin fecal smear. A neutrophil and spore-forming rods are present in the center of the field.

## Stained Smear

A thin smear of feces should be made from all dogs and cats with diarrhea. Material should be collected by rectal swab, if possible, to increase the chances of finding white blood cells (WBCs). A cotton swab is gently introduced 3 to 4 cm through the anus into the terminal rectum, directed to the wall of the rectum, and gently rotated several times. Placing a drop of 0.9% NaCl on the cotton swab will facilitate passage through the anus, but not adversely affect cell morphology. The cotton swab is rolled on a microscope slide gently multiple times to give areas with varying smear thickness (Fig. 97-1). After air drying, the slide can be stained. WBCs and bacteria morphologically consistent with *Campylobacter* spp. or *Clostridium perfringens* (Fig. 97-2) can be observed after staining with Diff-Quick or Wright's or Giemsa stains (see Cytology). *Histoplasma capsulatum* or *Prototheca* may be observed in the cytoplasm of mononuclear cells. Methylene blue in acetate buffer (pH 3.6) stains trophozoites of the enteric protozoans. Iodine stains and acid methyl green are also used for the demonstration of protozoans. Modified acid-fast staining of a thin fecal smear can be performed in dogs and cats with diarrhea to aid in the diagnosis of

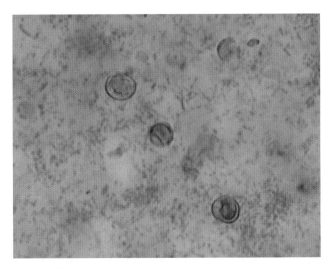

**FIG 97-3**
*Cryptosporidium parvum* oocysts stained with a modified acid-fast stain. The oocysts are approximately 4 × 6 μm.

  TABLE 97-3

**Zinc Sulfate Centrifugation Procedure**

1. Place 1 g fecal material in a 15 ml conical centrifuge tube.
2. Add 8 drops of Lugol iodine and mix well.
3. Add 7 to 8ml of $ZnSO_4$ (1.18 specific gravity)* and mix well.
4. Add $ZnSO_4$ until there is a slight positive meniscus.
5. Cover the top of the tube with a coverslip.
6. Centrifuge at 1500-2000 rpm for 5 minutes.
7. Remove the coverslip and place on a clean microscope slide for microscopic examination.
8. Examine the entire area under the coverslip for the presence of ova, oocysts, or larvae at 100×.

*Add 330 g $ZnSO_4$ to 670 ml of distilled water.

cryptosporidiosis. *Cryptosporidium* spp. are the only enteric organisms of approximately 4 to 6 μ in diameter that will stain pink to red with acid-fast stain (Fig. 97-3). Presence of neutrophils on rectal cytology can suggest inflammation induced by *Salmonella* spp., *Campylobacter* spp., or *Clostridium perfringens*; fecal culture is indicated in these cases.

## Fecal Flotation

Cysts, oocysts, and eggs in feces can be concentrated to increase the sensitivity of detection. Most eggs, oocysts, and cysts are easily identified after zinc sulfate centrifugal flotation (Table 97-3). This procedure is considered by many to be optimal for the demonstration of protozoan cysts (in particular, *Giardia* spp.; Fig. 97-4) and therefore is a good choice for a routine flotation technique in practice. Fecal sedimentation will recover most cysts and ova, but will also contain debris. This technique is superior to flotation procedures for the documentation of fluke eggs.

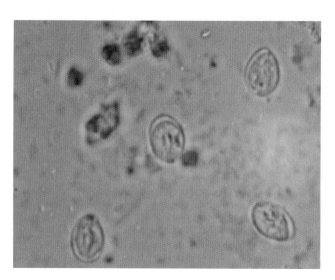

**FIG 97-4**
*Giardia* cysts after zinc sulfate flotation. The cysts are approximately 10 × 8 μm.

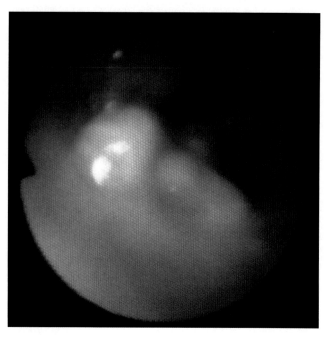

**FIG 97-5**
*Oslerus osleri* nodule in the lumen of the trachea of an infected dog as viewed by endoscopy.

## Baermann Technique

This technique is used to concentrate motile larva from feces. Some respiratory parasites are passed as larvated eggs but will release larvae shortly after being passed in feces. Eggs or larva from respiratory parasites can also be detected by cytologic evaluation of airway washings. Bronchoscopy is the procedure of choice for diagnosis of *Oslerus osleri* infection (Fig. 97-5).

## Preservation of Feces

Feces should be refrigerated, not frozen, until assayed. If a fecal sample is to be sent to a diagnostic laboratory for further analysis and will not be evaluated within 48 hours, it should be preserved. Polyvinyl alcohol, merthiolate-iodine-formalin, and 10% formalin preservation can be used. Ten percent formalin is commonly used because of its routine availability; the clinician should add 1 part feces to 9 parts formalin and mix well.

## CYTOLOGY

Cytologic evaluation of exudates, bone marrow aspiration, blood smears, synovial fluid, gastric brushings, duodenal secretions, urine, prostatic washings, airway washings, fecal smears, tissue imprints, and aspiration biopsies is an inexpensive and extremely valuable tool for the documentation of infectious agents (Table 97-4). Cytologic demonstration of some infectious agents constitutes a definitive diagnosis. Morphologic appearance and Gram stain of bacteria aids in the selection of empiric antibiotics while waiting for results of culture and antimicrobial susceptibility testing (see Chapter 98).

For demonstration of most infectious agents, thin smears are preferred. Blood can be prepared as follows: A drop of blood approximately the size of the head of a match is placed at one end of a clean microscope slide. The short edge of another slide (i.e., spreader slide) is placed against the slide at a 30-degree angle and pulled back until the blood and the spreader slide make contact. After the blood spreads across the width of spreader slide, the slide is smoothly and quickly pushed away from the blood, across the length of the slide (i.e., "push" smears). For materials other than blood, the spreader slide is laid gently on top of the material; the slides are then smoothly and rapidly pulled apart on parallel planes (i.e., "pull" smears). Alternately, the tip of a 22-gauge needle can be passed several times through the material, drawing it along the slide. Cells in airway washings, prostatic washings, urine, aqueous humor, and cerebrospinal fluid (CSF) should be pelleted by centrifugation at 2000 × g for 5 minutes before staining. For CSF, the clinician should add 1 drop of 22% albumin or normal canine serum before centrifugation to aid cell adherence to slides. Multiple slides should always be made, if possible. After being placed on the microscope slide, the material is air dried at room temperature, fixed if indicated by the procedure used, and stained. Slides that are not stained immediately should be fixed by dipping in 100% methanol and air dried.

Cytologic specimens can be stained with routine stains; immunocytochemical techniques for certain pathogens are available (see Immunologic Techniques, p. 1236). Stains routinely used for the diagnosis of infectious diseases in small animal practice include Wright's-Giemsa stain (CAMCO II, Baxter Scientific Products, McGraw Park, IL 60085-6787), Diff-Quik (various manufacturers), Gram stain (BBL Gram stain kit; Becton-Dickinson Microbiology Systems, Cock-

TABLE 97-4

**Characteristic Cytologic Morphology of Small Animal Bacterial and Rickettsial Agents**

| AGENT | MORPHOLOGIC CHARACTERISTICS |
|---|---|
| **Bacteria** | |
| *Actinomyces* spp. | Gram-positive, acid fast–negative filamentous rod within sulfur granules |
| Anaerobes | Usually occur in mixed morphologic groups |
| *Bacteroides fragilis* | Thin, filamentous, gram-negative rods |
| *Campylobacter* spp. | Seagull-shaped spirochete in feces |
| *Chlamydophila felis* | Large, cytoplasmic inclusions in conjunctival cells or neutrophils |
| *Clostridium* spp. | Large, gram-positive rods |
| *Clostridium perfringens* | Large, spore-forming rods in feces |
| *Haemobartonella felis** | Rod or ring-shaped on the surface of red blood cells (RBCs) |
| *Haemobartonella canis* | Rod or ring-shaped on the surface of RBCs |
| *Helicobacter* spp. | Tightly coiled spirochetes in gastric or duodenal brushings |
| *Mycobacterium* spp. | Intracytoplasmic acid-fast rods in macrophages or neutrophils |
| *Nocardia* spp. | Gram-positive, acid fast–positive filamentous rod within sulfur granules |
| *Leptospira* spp. | Spirochetes in urine; dark-field microscopy required |
| *Yersinia pestis* | Bipolar rods in cervical lymph nodes or airway fluids |
| **Rickettsia** | |
| *Ehrlichia canis* | Clusters of gram-negative bacteria (morulae) in mononuclear cells |
| *Ehrlichia ewingii* | Clusters of gram-negative bacteria (morulae) in neutrophils |
| *Ehrlichia equi†* | Clusters of gram-negative bacteria (morulae) in neutrophils and eosinophils |
| *Ehrlichia platys* | Clusters of gram-negative bacteria (morulae) in platelets |
| *Ehrlichia risticii* | Clusters of gram-negative bacteria (morulae) in mononuclear cells |

*Now *Mycoplasma hemofelis*.
†Renamed as *Anaplasma phagocytophila*.

eysville, MD 21030-0243), and acid-fast stain (TB Ziehl-Neelson stain kit; Baxter Scientific Products). Immunocytochemical techniques (e.g., fluorescent antibody staining of bone marrow cells for feline leukemia virus [FeLV]) are only performed in reference or research laboratories (see Immunologic Techniques, p. 1236). The laboratory should be contacted for specific specimen handling information.

## Bacterial Diseases

If bacterial disease is suspected, materials are collected aseptically and handled initially for culture (see Culture Techniques, p. 1235). After slides are prepared for cytologic evaluation, one is generally stained initially with Wright's-Giemsa or Diff-Quik stains. If bacteria are noted, Gram stain of another slide is performed to differentiate gram-positive and gram-negative agents. This information can be used to aid in the empiric selection of antibiotics (see Chapter 98). If filamentous, gram-positive rods are noted, acid-fast staining can help differentiate between *Actinomyces* (nonacid fast) and *Nocardia* (generally acid fast). If macrophages or neutrophils are detected, acid-fast staining is indicated to assess for *Mycobacterium* spp. within the cytoplasm. Bacteria can be present in small numbers, so failure to document organisms cytologically does not totally exclude the diagnosis. Bacterial culture of all samples with increased numbers of neutrophils or macrophages should always be considered. Some organisms

like *Mycoplasma* are rarely documented cytologically, whereas other organisms require special stains for optimal visualization. For example, *Helicobacter* spp. in cytologic specimens made from gastric brushings are easiest to see after staining with Warthin-Starry stain.

For some bacteria, culture has never been successful. For example *Haemobartonella felis* (previously classified as *Rickettsia;* now recognized as *Mycoplasma*) or *H. canis* can be detected on the surface of red blood cells (RBCs) but have never been successfully cultured. Until the advent of polymerase chain reaction (PCR; see p. 1236), documentation of infection was based on cytology; Wright's-Giemsa stain is the best stain to use in practice for these organisms. The duration of parasitemia is short-lived, and the organism commonly leaves the surface of the RBC if the blood is placed into ethylenediaminetetraacetic acid (EDTA), making it difficult to document the presence of the organism. Collection of blood from an ear margin vessel, making thin blood smears immediately with blood that has not been placed into anticoagulant, or collecting blood into a heparinized syringe may aid in finding *Haemobartonella* spp.

## Rickettsial Diseases

*Ehrlichia* spp. are occasionally found within the cytoplasm of cells in the peripheral blood, lymph node aspirates, bone marrow aspirates, or synovial fluid (see Chapter 101).

*Ehrlichia* spp. morulae are found in different cell types (see Table 97-4). Wright's-Giemsa stain is superior to Wright's or Diff-Quik stain for the demonstration of morulae. *Rickettsia rickettsii* in endothelial cells lining vessels can be documented by immunofluorescent antibody staining (see Immunologic Techniques, p. 1236).

## Fungal Diseases

Arthrospores and conidia of dermatophytes can be identified cytologically. Hairs plucked from the periphery of a lesion are covered with 10% to 20% potassium hydroxide on a microscope slide to clear debris. The slide is then heated but not boiled, and it is examined for dermatophytes. All cats with chronic, draining skin lesions should have imprints of the lesions made and stained with Wright's-Giemsa stain followed by microscopic examination for the characteristic round, oval, or cigar-shaped yeast phase of *Sporothrix schenckii* within the cytoplasm of mononuclear cells (see Chapter 103). Periodic acid-Schiff (PAS) stain is superior to Wright's-Giemsa stain for the demonstration of fungi. The cytologic appearance of the systemic fungi is presented in Table 103-1.

## Cutaneous Parasitic Diseases

*Cheyletiella* spp., *Demodex* spp., *Sarcoptes scabiei, Notoedres cati,* and *Otodectes cynotis* are the most common small animal cutaneous parasites. Definitive diagnosis is based on cytologic demonstration of the organisms. *Cheyletiella* is demonstrated by pressing a piece of transparent tape against areas with crusts, placing the tape on a microscope slide, and examining it microscopically. *Demodex* spp. are most commonly detected in deep skin scrapings and follicular exudates;

*Cheyletiella* spp., *Sarcoptes scabiei,* and *Notoedres cati* are detected in wide, more superficial scrapings. *Otodectes cynotis* or its eggs are detected in ceruminous exudates from the ear canals.

## Systemic Protozoal Diseases

The most common systemic protozoal diseases and the cytologic appearance and location of these agents are summarized in Table 97-5. Cytologic demonstration of these agents leads to a presumptive or definitive diagnosis of the disease. Wright's-Giemsa or Giemsa staining of thin blood films should be used to demonstrate *Leishmania* spp., *Trypanosoma cruzi, Babesia* spp., *Hepatozoon canis,* and *Cytauxzoon felis.* Collection of blood from an ear margin vessel may increase the chances of demonstrating the protozoans found in blood, particularly *Babesia* spp. and *Cytauxzoon felis. Toxoplasma gondii* and *Neospora caninum* cause similar syndromes in dogs, but their tachyzoites cannot be distinguished morphologically; serology or immunocytochemical staining is required to differentiate these agents. With the exception of *T. gondii* and *N. caninum,* systemic protozoans are rare and regionally defined in the United States. See Chapter 104 for further discussion of these agents.

## Viral Diseases

Viral inclusion bodies can be rarely detected cytologically after staining with Wright's-Giemsa. Distemper virus infection causes inclusions in circulating lymphocytes, neutrophils, and erythrocytes of some dogs. Rarely, feline infectious peritonitis virus results in intracytoplasmic inclusions in circulating neutrophils. Feline herpesvirus 1 (FHV-1) transiently results in intranuclear inclusion bodies in epithelial cells.

 TABLE 97-5

**Characteristic Cytologic Morphology of Small Animal Systemic Protozoal Agents**

| AGENT | MORPHOLOGIC CHARACTERISTICS |
|---|---|
| *Babesia canis* | Paired piroplasms (2.4 × 5.0 μm) in circulating red blood cells |
| *Babesia gibsoni* | Single piroplasms (1.0 × 3.2 μm) in circulating red blood cells |
| *Cytauxzoon felis* | Piroplasms (1.0 × 1.5 μm "signet ring" form; 1.0 × 2.0 μm oval form; 1.0 μm round form) in circulating red blood cells; macrophages or monocytes of lymph node aspirates, splenic aspirates, or bone marrow |
| *Hepatozoon canis* and *H. americanum* | Gamonts in circulating neutrophils and monocytes |
| *Leishmania* spp. | Ovoid to round amastigotes (2.5-5.0 μm × 1.5-2.0 μm) in macrophages found on imprints of exudative skin lesions, lymph node aspirates, or bone marrow aspirates |
| *Neospora caninum* | Free or intracellular (macrophages or monocytes) tachyzoites (5-7 μm × 1-5 μm) in CSF, airway washings, or imprints of cutaneous lesions |
| *Toxoplasma gondii* | Free or intracellular (macrophages or monocytes) tachyzoites (6 × 2 μm) in pleural effusions, peritoneal effusions, or airway washings |
| *Trypanosoma cruzi* | Flagellated trypomastigotes (one flagellum; 15-20 μm long) free in whole blood, lymph node aspirates, and peritoneal fluid |

*CSF,* Cerebrospinal fluid.

## TISSUE TECHNIQUES

Tissues collected from animals with suspected infectious diseases can be evaluated by several different techniques. Tissue samples should be aseptically placed in appropriate transport media for culture procedures or inoculated into laboratory animals, if indicated, before further handling.

Gently blotting the cut edge of the tissue on a paper towel to remove excess blood and then lightly touching the tissue multiple times to a microscope slide make tissue impressions for cytologic examination. Tissue specimens can then be frozen, placed into 10% buffered formalin solution, or placed into glutaraldehyde-containing solutions. Frozen specimens are generally superior for immunohistochemical staining and PCR. Routine histopathologic evaluation is performed on formalin-fixed tissues. Special stains can be used to maximize the identification of some infectious agents. The clinician should alert the histopathology laboratory to the infectious agents most suspected to allow for appropriate stain selection. Glutaraldehyde-containing fixatives are superior to other fixatives for electron microscopic examination of tissues; this technique can be more sensitive than other procedures for demonstration of viral particles.

## CULTURE TECHNIQUES

Bacteria, fungi, viruses, and some protozoans can be cultured. In general, a positive culture can be used to establish a definitive diagnosis. Bacterial culture can be combined with antimicrobial susceptibility testing to determine optimal drug therapy. Successful culture is dependent on collecting the optimal materials without contamination, transporting the materials to the laboratory as quickly as possible in the most appropriate medium to minimize organism death or overgrowth of nonpathogens, and by using the most appropriate culture materials.

Culture results of body systems with normal bacterial and fungal flora, including the skin, ears, mouth, nasal cavity, trachea, feces, and vagina are the most difficult to interpret. Finding positive culture results and inflammatory cells cytologically suggests the organism is inducing disease. Culture of a single agent, particularly if the organism is relatively resistant to antimicrobials, is more consistent with a disease-inducing infection than if multiple, antibiotic-susceptible bacteria are cultured. Materials for routine aerobic bacterial culture can be placed on sterile swabs if the swabs remain moist and are placed on appropriate culture media within 3 hours of collection. If a delay of greater than 3 hours is expected, swabs containing transport medium (Culturette; American Scientific Products, McGraw Park, Ill) should be used. These swabs should be refrigerated or frozen to inhibit bacterial growth if cultures are not to be started within 4 hours; some bacteria will grow more rapidly than others, potentially masking fastidious organisms. Most aerobes will survive at 4° C (routine refrigeration temperature) in tissue or on media-containing swabs for 48 hours. Solid phase transport media (BBL CultureSwab Plus; Becton Dickinson Microbiology Systems, Sparkes, Md) is also routinely available. This material will sup-

port the growth of most aerobes, anaerobes, *Mycoplasma* spp., and fungi for several days if refrigerated. Routine aerobic culture is generally successful on fluid samples (e.g., urine, airway washings) stored at 20° C for 1 to 2 hours, 4° C for 24 hours, or 4° C for 72 hours if placed in transport medium.

Anaerobes can be successfully cultured from fluid collected aseptically into a syringe and the needle covered with a rubber stopper if the material is to be placed on culture media within 10 minutes of collection. Because of time limitations, transport media (BBL CultureSwab Plus; Becton Dickinson Microbiology Systems, Sparkes, Md) is generally required for samples from animals with suspected anaerobic infections. These media will support the growth of most anaerobes for 48 hours if stored at 4° C.

Samples for blood culture should be collected aseptically from a large vein after surgical preparation of the surface. In general, three 5 ml samples are collected over a 24-hour period in stable patients or a 1- to 3-hour period in septic patients. Unclotted whole blood is placed directly into transport media (BBL Septi-Chec; Becton Dickinson) that will support the growth of aerobic and anaerobic bacteria, and it is incubated at 20° C for 24 hours. Culture for *Bartonella henselae* from the blood of cats is generally performed on a 1.5 ml whole blood sample collected aseptically and placed into an EDTA-containing tube.

Culture of feces for *Salmonella* spp., *Campylobacter* spp., and *Clostridium perfringens* is occasionally indicated in small animal practice. Approximately 2 to 3 g of fresh feces should be submitted to the laboratory immediately for optimal results; however, *Salmonella* and *Campylobacter* are usually viable in refrigerated fecal specimens for 3 to 7 days. To increase the likelihood of achieving positive culture results, a transport medium should be used if a delay is expected (Cary-Blair selective media; Becton-Dickinson). The laboratory should be notified of the suspected pathogen so that appropriate culture media can be used.

*Mycoplasma* and *Ureaplasma* cultures are most commonly performed on airway washings, synovial fluid, exudates from chronic draining tracts in cats, urine from animals with chronic urinary tract disease, and the vagina of animals with genital tract disease. Samples should be transported to the laboratory in Amies medium or modified Stuart bacterial transport medium (Becton-Dickinson). *Mycoplasma* spp. culture should be specifically requested.

*Mycobacterium* spp. grow very slowly, and culture is often limited by overgrowth of other bacteria. Special medium is required; therefore the laboratory should be specifically instructed to culture for *Mycobacterium* spp. Tissue samples or exudates from animals with suspected *Mycobacterium* spp. infection should be refrigerated immediately after collection and transported to the laboratory as soon as possible. Exudates should be placed in transport media (BBL Culture Swap Plus; Becton-Dickinson Microbiology Systems).

Cutaneous fungal agents can be cultured in the small animal office using routine available culture media (Dermatophyte test media, Pittman Moore, Mundelein, Ill; Derm duet,

Bacti Lab, Mountain View, Calif). Materials from dogs or cats with suspected systemic fungal infection can be transported to the laboratory as described for bacteria, and the laboratory can be told specifically that fungal culture is needed. The yeast phase of the systemic fungi occurs in vivo and are not zoonotic; the mycelial phase of *Blastomyces, Coccidioides,* and *Histoplasma* grows in culture and will infect humans. Thus, in-house culture for these agents is not recommended.

Viral agents can be isolated from tissues or secretions at some laboratories. Contact the laboratory before submitting samples. Samples should be collected aseptically as for bacteria, placed in transport media (i.e., Culturette), and immediately stored under refrigeration to inhibit bacterial growth. The samples should be transported to the laboratory on cold packs but not frozen.

## IMMUNOLOGIC TECHNIQUES

Infectious agents or their antigens can be detected in body fluids, feces, cells, or tissues using immunologic techniques. In general, polyclonal or monoclonal antibodies against the agent in question are used in a variety of different test methodologies, including direct fluorescent antibody assay with cells or tissue, agglutination assays, and enzyme-linked immunosorbent assay. Sensitivities and specificities vary among tests but are generally high for most assays. Positive results with these tests generally prove infection; this is in contrast to antibody detection procedures, which only document exposure to an infectious agent. Contact the laboratory for details concerning specimen transport before collection.

Commercially available assays for the detection of antigens in serum or plasma are routinely available for *Dirofilaria immitis, Cryptococcus neoformans,* and FeLV. The *Cryptococcus neoformans* latex agglutination procedure can also be performed on aqueous humor, vitreous humor, and CSF.

Parvovirus, *Cryptosporidium parvum,* and *Giardia* spp. antigen detection procedures are available for use with feces. The parvovirus assay detects both canine and feline parvovirus antigen. Little sensitivity and specificity data exists for the currently available *C. parvum* and *Giardia* spp. assays when used with feces from naturally infected small animals. The assays were designed for use with human feces containing human isolates of the organisms. Whether currently available assays detect dog- or cat- specific species of *C. parvum* and *Giardia* is unknown. Therefore if used, results of these assays should be interpreted in conjunction with results from fecal examination techniques.

Immunocytochemistry and immunohistochemistry techniques are widely available for the documentation of a variety of infectious diseases. These procedures are particularly valuable for the detection of viral diseases, detection of agents present in small numbers, and for differentiating among agents with similar morphologic features. In general, these techniques are more sensitive and specific than histopathologic techniques, and are comparable to culture. For example, focal feline infectious peritonitis granulomatous disease can be documented by immunohistochemical staining (see Chapter 102).

## POLYMERASE CHAIN REACTION

PCR amplifies small quantities of DNA to detectable levels (Fig. 97-6). By use of a reverse transcriptase step, RNA is converted to DNA; therefore the technique can also be used to detected RNA (RT-PCR). In general, PCR is much more sensitive than cytologic or histopathologic techniques and is comparable to culture and laboratory animal inoculation. PCR assays are of great benefit for documentation of infections, particularly if the organism in question is difficult to culture (e.g., *Ehrlichia* spp.) or cannot be cultured (e.g., *Haemobartonella* spp.). Specificity can be very high, depending on the primers used in the reaction. For example, primers can be designed to detect one bacterial genus but no others. Primers can also be designed to identify only one species. For example a PCR assay can be developed to detect all *Ehrlichia* spp. or just one species such as *E. canis.*

Because of the inherent sensitivity of the reaction, PCR can give false-positive results if sample contamination occurs

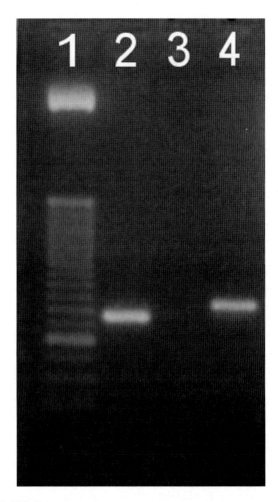

**FIG 97-6**
Photograph of a PCR assay for *Haemobartonella felis* showing the 2 different band sizes that differentiate the two species, *Mycoplasma haemofelis (Lane 2)* and *M. haemominutum (Lane 4)*. Lane 1 is a base pair ladder and Lane 3 is a negative sample.

during collection or at the laboratory performing the procedure. False-negative results can occur if the sample is handled inappropriately; this is of particular importance for detection of RNA viruses by RT-PCR. Results may also be affected by treatment. Another potential problem is that no standardization exists among commercial assays offering PCR assays; in addition, no external quality control exists.

Although PCR assays can be one of the most sensitive for documentation of infections, positive test results do not always prove that the infection is resulting in clinical illness. For example, because the technique detects DNA of both live and dead organisms, positive test results may be achieved even if the infection has been controlled. When the organism being tested for commonly infects the background population of healthy pets, interpretation of results for a single animal can be difficult. For example, FHV-1 commonly infects cats and is commonly carried by healthy cats. Thus although PCR is the most sensitive way to document infection by FHV-1, the positive predictive value for disease of a FHV-1 PCR result is actually very low. In one study, more positive FHV-1 PCR results were detected in the healthy control group than the group with conjunctivitis (Burgesser and colleagues, 1999). Based on these findings, it is very important that small animal practitioners carefully assess the predictive values of currently available PCR. New PCR assays are being developed almost daily. To date in small animal practice, diagnostic utility of PCR assays for canine and feline *Ehrlichia* spp. (blood), canine and feline *Bartonella* spp. (blood, aqueous humor), feline *Haemobartonella* spp. (blood), *Toxoplasma gondii* (aqueous humor, CSF), feline coronavirus (tissues and body fluids), FHV-1 (conjunctival swabs, aqueous humor), feline calicivirus (conjunctival swabs), *Mycoplasma felis* (conjunctival swabs, joint fluid), and *Chlamydophila felis* (conjunctival swabs) have been assessed the most. See specific chapters for a discussion of the use of PCR for the detection of the agents.

## ANIMAL INOCULATION

Animal inoculation can be used to identify some infectious diseases. For example, oocysts of *Toxoplasma gondii* cannot be distinguished morphologically from those of *Hammondia hammondi* or *Besnoitia darlingi;* only *T. gondii* is infectious for human beings. *Toxoplasma gondii* can be differentiated from the other coccidians by inoculation of sporulated oocysts into mice and monitoring for *T. gondii*-specific antibody production. However, because live animals are required, animal inoculation is rarely used in small animal practice.

## ELECTRON MICROSCOPY

Electron microscopy is a very sensitive procedure for organism identification in body fluids and tissues. Glutaraldehyde-containing fixatives are used most commonly. One of the most clinically relevant uses of electron microscopy is for the detection of viral particles in feces of animals with gastrointestinal signs of diseases. Approximately 1 to 3 g of feces without fixative should be transported to the laboratory (Diagnostic Laboratory, Colorado State University, College of Veterinary Medicine and Biomedical Sciences, Fort Collins, Colo) by overnight mail on cold packs.

## ANTIBODY DETECTION

### SERUM

A variety of different methods exist for detecting serum antibodies against infectious agents; complement fixation, hemagglutination inhibition, serum neutralization, agglutination assays, agar gel immunodiffusion, indirect fluorescent antibody assay (IFA), enzyme-linked immunosorbent assays (ELISA), and western blot immunoassay are commonly used methodologies. Complement fixation, hemagglutination inhibition, serum neutralization, and agglutination assays generally detect all antibody classes in a serum sample. Western blot immunoassay, IFA, and ELISA can be adapted to detect specific IgM, IgG, or IgA responses.

Comparison of IgM, IgA, and IgG antibody responses against an infectious agent can be used to attempt to prove recent or active infection. In general, immunoglobulin M (IgM) is the first antibody produced after antigenic exposure (Fig. 97-7). Antibody class shift to IgG occurs in days to weeks. Serum and mucosal IgA immune responses have also been studied for some infectious agents, including *T. gondii,* feline coronaviruses, and *Helicobacter felis.*

Timing of antibody testing is important. In general, serum antibody tests in puppies and kittens cannot be interpreted as specific responses until at least 8 to 12 weeks of age because of the presence of antibodies from the dam passed to the puppy or kitten in colostrum. Most infectious agents can induce disease within 3 to 10 days after initial exposure; using many assays, serum IgG antibodies are usually not detected until 2 to 3 weeks after initial exposure. Based on these facts, falsely negative serum antibody tests during acute disease are probably common in small animal practice. If specific serum antibody testing is negative initially in an animal with acute disease, repeat antibody testing should be performed in 2 to 3 weeks to assess for seroconversion. Documentation of increasing antibody titers is consistent with recent or active infection. It is preferable to assess both the acute and convalescent sera in the same assay on the same day to avoid interassay variation.

Sensitivity is the ability of an assay to detect a positive sample; specificity is the ability of an assay to detect a negative sample. Sensitivity and specificity vary with each assay. Positive predictive value is the ability of a test result to predict presence of disease; negative predictive value is the ability of a test result to predict absence of disease. Many of the infectious agents encountered in small animal practice infect a large percentage of the population, resulting in serum antibody production. However, they only induce disease in a small number of animals in the infected group. Examples include coronaviruses, canine distemper virus, *Toxoplasma gondii,* and *Borrelia burgdorferi.* For these examples, even though assays with good sensitivity and specificity for the

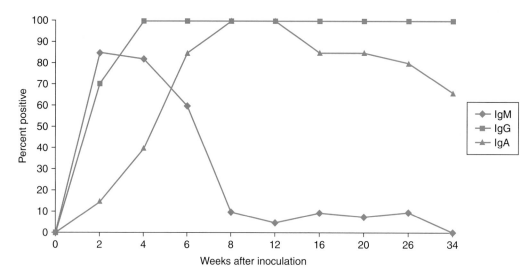

**FIG 97-7**

Serum *Toxoplasma gondii* IgM, IgG, and IgA immune responses after experimental inoculation in cats.

detection of serum antibodies are available, the predictive value of a positive test for presence of disease is extremely low. This is because antibodies are commonly detected in nondiseased animals. Diagnostic utility of some serologic tests are also limited because of the presence of antibodies induced by vaccination. Examples include feline coronaviruses, some *Borrelia burgdorferi* assays, FHV-1, parvoviruses, calicivirus, and canine distemper virus.

The clinician should interpret positive results in serum antibody tests only as evidence of present or prior infection by the agent in question. Recent or active infection is suggested by the presence of IgM, an increasing antibody titer over 2 to 3 weeks, or seroconversion (negative antibody result on the first test and positive antibody result on convalescent testing). However, detection of recent infection based on antibody testing does not always prove disease because of the agent in question. Conversely, failure to document recent or active infection based on serologic testing does not exclude a diagnosis of clinical disease. For example, many cats with toxoplasmosis develop clinical signs of disease after serum antibody titers have reached their plateau. The magnitude of antibody titer does not always correlate with active or clinical disease. For example, many cats with clinical toxoplasmosis have IgM and IgG titers that are at the low end of the titer scale; conversely, many healthy cats have IgG titers greater than 1:16,384 years after infection with *T. gondii*. The clinical diagnosis of an infectious disease usually includes the combination of the following:

- Clinical signs referable to the agent
- Serologic evidence of exposure to the agent
- Exclusion of other causes of the clinical syndrome
- Demonstration of the agent or response to treatment

## BODY FLUIDS

Some infectious agents induce disease of the eyes and central nervous system (CNS). Documentation of agent-specific antibodies in aqueous humor, vitreous humor, or CSF can be used to support the diagnosis of infection of these tissues. Quantification of ocular and CSF antibodies is difficult to interpret if serum antibodies and inflammatory disease are present; serum antibodies leak into ocular fluids and CSF in the face of inflammation. Detection of local production of antibodies within the eye or CNS has been used to aid in the diagnosis of canine distemper virus infection and feline toxoplasmosis (see Chapters 102 and 104). The following is a method to prove local antibody production by the eye or CNS:

$$\frac{\text{Aqueous humor or CSF specific antibody}}{\text{Serum specific antibody}} \times \frac{\text{Serum total antibody}}{\text{Aqueous humor or CSF total antibody}}$$

If this ratio is greater than 1, it suggests that the antibody in the aqueous humor or CSF was produced locally. This formula has been used extensively in the evaluation of cats with uveitis. Approximately 60% of cats with uveitis in the United States have *T. gondii*-specific IgM, IgA, or IgG C values over 1 (see Chapter 104). The technique was also used to help prove that FHV-1 and *Bartonella henselae* are causes of uveitis in cats.

### Suggested Readings

Burgesser KM et al: Comparison of PCR, virus isolation, and indirect fluorescent antibody staining in the detection of naturally occurring feline herpesvirus infections, *J Vet Diagn Invest* 11:122, 1999.

Jensen WA et al: Prevalence of *Haemobartonella felis* infection in cats, *Am J Vet Res* 62:604, 2001.

Lappin MR et al: Enzyme-linked immunosorbent assays for the detection of *Toxoplasma gondii*–specific antibodies and antigens in the aqueous humor of cats, *J Am Vet Med Assoc* 201:1010, 1992.

Lappin MR et al: Polymerase chain reaction for the detection of *Toxoplasma gondii* in aqueous humor of cats, *Am J Vet Res* 57:1589, 1996.

Lappin MR et al: Laboratory diagnosis of protozoal infections. In Greene CE, editor: *Infectious diseases of the dog and cat,* ed 2, Philadelphia, 1998, WB Saunders Co, p 437.

Lappin MR: Microbiology and infectious disease. In Willard MD et al, editors: *Small animal clinical diagnosis by laboratory methods,* ed 3, Philadelphia, 1999, WB Saunders Co, p 288.

Lappin MR et al: *Bartonella* spp. antibodies and DNA in aqueous humor of cats, *Fel Med Surg* 2:61, 2000.

Lappin MR et al: Use of serologic tests to predict resistance to feline herpesvirus 1, feline calicivirus, and feline parvovirus infection in cats, *J Am Vet Med Assoc* 220:38, 2002.

# CHAPTER 98

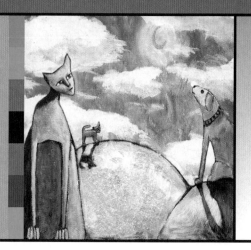

# Practical Antimicrobial Chemotherapy

## CHAPTER OUTLINE

ANAEROBIC INFECTIONS, 1240
BACTEREMIA AND BACTERIAL ENDOCARDITIS, 1244
SKIN AND SOFT TISSUE INFECTIONS, 1245
GASTROINTESTINAL TRACT AND HEPATIC
INFECTIONS, 1245
MUSCULOSKELETAL INFECTIONS, 1246
CENTRAL NERVOUS SYSTEM INFECTIONS, 1247
RESPIRATORY TRACT INFECTIONS, 1247
UROGENITAL TRACT INFECTIONS, 1248

In small animal practice, decisions to institute antimicrobial chemotherapy are almost always made without the benefit of results of culture and antimicrobial susceptibility testing. In simple, first-time infections, culture and antimicrobial susceptibility testing is often not performed. In life-threatening infections, decisions on the choice of antimicrobials must be made prior to obtaining the culture results; patient survival may depend on the selection of optimal treatment regimens.

Recognition of the most common infectious agents (gram-positive, gram-negative, aerobic, or anaerobic) associated with infection of different organ systems is imperative in the empirical selection of antimicrobials. Cytologic findings and the results of Gram's staining can be used to identify microbes and aid in choosing appropriate antimicrobials. The antimicrobial selected must have an appropriate mechanism of action against the suspected pathogen and must achieve an adequate concentration in infected tissues. Bacteriostatic agents may be less effective for treatment of infections in immunosuppressed animals because normal immune responses are required for the drugs to have maximal effect (Table 98-1).

The owner must be willing to administer the drug using the appropriate interval, and the drug must be affordable. Whether the antimicrobial has potential for toxicity is also an important consideration (Table 98-2). In animals with simple, first-time infections or when drugs with the potential for toxicity are used, the low end of the antimicrobial dose and the longest dosage interval should be used. Intracellular

pathogens, anaerobic infections, and life-threatening infections, including bacteremia and central nervous system infections should be treated with the high end of the dose and the shortest dosage interval. In all animals with life-threatening infections, antibiotics should be administered parenterally for at least the first 3 to 5 days. Parenteral antibiotic administration is also indicated in animals with vomiting or regurgitation. Oral administration of antibiotics can be initiated when vomiting, regurgitation, or the life-threatening condition have resolved.

Most simple, first-time infections in immunocompetent animals respond adequately to 10 to 14 days of antibiotic therapy. Chronic infections, bone infections, infections in immunosuppressed animals, infections resulting in granulomatous reactions, and those caused by intracellular pathogens are generally treated for a minimum of 1 to 2 weeks beyond resolution of clinical or radiographic signs of disease; the duration of therapy commonly exceeds 4 to 6 weeks.

When the results of antimicrobial susceptibility tests become available, the antibiotic choice is changed, if indicated. If there is poor therapeutic response to an antibiotic in 72 hours and if an antibiotic-responsive infectious disease is likely, an alternative treatment should be considered. Conditions resulting in devitalized, granulomatous, or consolidated tissues, such as aspiration pneumonia, may not show radiographic signs of improvement before 7 days. Devitalized tissues should be debrided, if possible, to aid in the resolution of infection.

The following is a brief discussion of the empirical antimicrobial choices for treatment of infections of various body systems or types of infections. The reader is referred to individual chapters for further information concerning adjunct treatments.

## ANAEROBIC INFECTIONS

The anaerobic bacteria of clinical significance in dog and cats are *Bacteroides* spp., *Fusobacterium* spp., *Peptostreptococcus* spp., *Peptococcus* spp., *Clostridium* spp., *Actinomyces* spp., *Propionibacterium* spp., and *Eubacterium* spp. *Actinomyces* is a

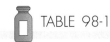

## TABLE 98-1

**Antibiotics and General Dosing Guidelines\* for the Treatment of Bacterial Infections in Dogs and Cats**

| DRUG | MECHANISM | BACTERIOSTATIC OR BACTERIOCIDAL | SPECIES | DOSAGE | ROUTE OF ADMINISTRATION |
|---|---|---|---|---|---|
| **Aminoglycosides†** | Protein synthesis inhibition | Bacteriocidal | | | |
| Amikacin | | | B | 15-20 mg/kg q24h | IV, IM, SC |
| Gentamicin | | | B | 6 mg/kg q24h | IV, IM, SC |
| Neomycin | | | B | 2.5-10 mg/kg q8-12h | PO |
| Tobramycin | | | B | 2 mg/kg q8h | IV, IM, SC |
| **Carbapenems** | Cell wall synthesis inhibition | Bacteriocidal | | | |
| Imipenem | | | B | 2-10 mg/kg q6-8h | IV, SC, IM |
| **Cephalosporins** | Cell wall synthesis inhibition | Bacteriocidal | | | |
| Cefadroxil (first generation) | | | D | 22 mg/kg q12h | PO |
| | | | C | 22 mg/kg q24h | PO |
| Cephalexin (first generation) | | | B | 20-60 mg/kg q8-12h | PO |
| Cefazolin (first generation) | | | B | 20-33 mg/kg q8-12h | SC, IM, IV |
| Cefoxitin (second generation) | | | B | 15-30 mg/kg q8h | SC, IM, IV |
| Cefixime (third generation) | | | D | 5-12.5 mg/kg q12-24h | PO |
| Cefotaxime (third generation) | | | B | 20-80 mg/kg q8h | SC, IM, IV |
| **Chloramphenicol** | Protein synthesis inhibition | Bacteriostatic | D | 25-50 mg/kg q8h | PO, SC, IV, IM |
| | | | C | 15-25 mg/kg q12h | PO, SC, IV, IM |
| **Macrolides/ Lincosamides** | Protein synthesis inhibition | Bacteriostatic | | | |
| Azithromycin‡ | | | D | 5-10 mg/kg q12-24h | PO |
| | | | C | 7-15 mg/kg q24h | PO |
| Clarithromycin | | | B | 5-10 mg/kg q12h | PO |
| Clindamycin | | | D | 5-20 mg/kg q12h | PO, SC, IM, IV |
| | | | C | 5-25 mg/kg q12-24h | PO, SC, IM, IV |
| Erythromycin | | | B | 10-25 mg/kg q8-12h | PO |
| Lincomycin | | | B | 11-22 mg/kg q12h | PO, IM, IV, SC |
| Tylosin | | | B | 10-40 mg/kg q12-24h | PO |
| **Metronidazole§** | Protein synthesis inhibition | Bacteriocidal | D | 10-30 mg/kg q8-24h | PO |
| | | | C | 10-30 mg/kg q12-24h | PO |
| **Penicillins** | Cell wall synthesis inhibition | Bacteriocidal | | | |
| Amoxicillin | | | B | 10-22 mg/kg q8-12h | PO, SC |
| Amoxicillin and clavulanate | | | D | 12.5-25 mg/kg q8-12h | PO |
| | | | C | 62.5 mg q8-12h | PO |
| Ampicillin sodium | | | B | 22 mg/kg q8h | SC, IM, IV |
| Oxacillin | | | B | 22-40 mg/kg q8h | PO, SC, IM, IV |
| Penicillin G | | | B | 22,000 U/kg q6-8h | PO, IM, IV |
| Ticarcillin and clavulanate | | | B | 15-50 mg/kg q6-8h | IM, IV, SC |

\*The dose ranges and intervals in this table are general. Please see the appropriate sections to determine the optimal dose for specific syndromes or infections.
†For parenterally administered aminoglycosides, giving the total daily dose at one time may lessen the potential for renal toxicity.
‡For simple infections, azithromycin can be given daily for 3 days and then every third day.
§The maximal total daily dose should be 50 mg/kg.

*Continued*

TABLE 98-1

Antibiotics and General Dosing Guidelines for the Treatment of Bacterial Infections in Dogs and Cats—cont'd

| DRUG | MECHANISM | BACTERIOSTATIC OR BACTERIOCIDAL | SPECIES | DOSAGE | ROUTE OF ADMINISTRATION |
|------|-----------|--------------------------------|---------|--------|------------------------|
| **Quinolones** | Nucleic acid inhibition | Bacteriocidal | | | |
| Ciprofloxacin | | | B | 5-15 mg/kg q24h | PO |
| Difloxacin | | | D | 5-10 mg/kg q24h | PO |
| Enrofloxacin | | | B | 2.5-10 mg/kg q24h | PO, IM, SC, IV |
| Marbofloxacin | | | B | 2.75-5.5 mg/kg q24h | PO |
| Orbifloxacin | | | B | 2.5-7.5 mg/kg q24h | PO |
| **Potentiated Sulfas** | Intermediary metabolism inhibition | Bacteriocidal | | | |
| Ormetoprim-sulfadimethoxine | | | B | 27.5 mg/kg q24h | PO |
| Trimethoprim-sulfonamide | | | B | 15-30 mg/kg q12h | PO |
| **Tetracyclines** | Protein synthesis inhibition | Bacteriostatic | | | |
| Doxycycline‖ | | | B | 5-10 mg/kg q12h | PO, IV |
| Minocycline | | | B | 5-12.5 mg/kg q12h | PO, IV |
| | | | B | 22 mg/kg q8-12h | PO |

‖The drug can be given once daily to cats for the treatment of simple infections and to dogs and cats with ehrlichiosis.

 TABLE 98-2

Common Antibiotic Toxicities

| ANTIBIOTICS | TOXICITY |
|-------------|----------|
| Aminoglycosides | Renal tubular disease |
| | Neuromuscular blockade |
| | Ototoxicity |
| Cephalosporins | Immune-mediated diseases |
| Chloramphenicol | Bone marrow—aplastic anemia (predominantly cats) |
| | Inhibition of drug metabolism |
| Doxycycline | Esophagitis/strictures in cats given generic tablets |
| Macrolides/lincosamides | Vomiting or diarrhea |
| | Cholestasis |
| Metronidazole | Neutropenia |
| | Central nervous system toxicity |
| Penicillins | Immune-mediated cytopenias |
| Quinolones | Failure of cartilage development in young, growing animals |
| | Retinal dysfunction in some cats |
| | Potentiation of seizures |
| Sulfonamides | Hepatic—cholestasis or acute hepatic necrosis (rare) |
| | Macrocytic anemia (long-term administration in cats) |
| | Thrombocytopenia |
| | Suppurative, nonseptic polyarthritis (Doberman Pinschers predominantly) |
| | Keratoconjunctivitis sicca |
| | Renal crystalluria (rare) |
| Tetracyclines | Renal tubular disease |
| | Cholestasis |
| | Fever (particularly in cats) |
| | Inhibition of drug metabolism |

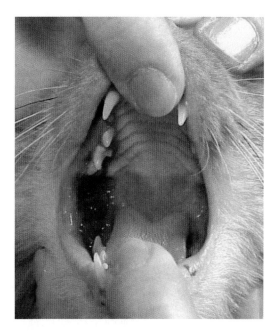

**FIG 98-1**
Severe stomatitis in a cat. Anaerobic bacteria are often
involved as secondary invaders.

 TABLE 98-3

**Clinical Findings Consistent with Anaerobic Infections
in Dogs and Cats**

**Signalment**

All ages and breeds, both genders

**History**

Fighting
Foreign body
Vomiting or regurgitation with aspiration
Recent surgery, open wound or fracture, or dentistry
History of immunosuppressive drugs or diseases
Infection resistant to sulfonamides or aminoglycosides
Neutrophilic inflammation with cytologically evident
    bacteria but negative aerobic culture results

**Physical Examination**

Flaccid paralysis *(Clostridium botulinum)*
Rigid paralysis and trismus *(Clostridium tetani)*
Subcutaneous gas production
Putrid odor from lesion
Serosanguineous discharge from a painful lesion
Necrotic tissue
Open wound or fracture
High fever
"Sulphur" granules
Abscesses
Blackish exudate

**Cytologic Findings**

Degenerate and nondegenerate neutrophils with mixed
    population of bacteria
Large gram-positive rods with minimal neutrophils
"Sulphur" granules
Branching filamentous rods *(Actinomyces* or *Nocardia)*

facultative anaerobe; the other organisms are obligate
anaerobes, which cannot utilize oxygen metabolically and
die in its presence. Anaerobic bacteria are part of the normal flora in areas with low oxygen tension and low oxygen-
reduction potential, such as the mucous membranes of the
oral cavity and vagina. The origin of most anaerobic infections is the animal's own flora. Anaerobic infections are
potentiated by poor blood supply, tissue necrosis, prior infection, or immunosuppression. Anaerobic bacteria produce a number of enzymes and factors that induce tissue
injury and promote colonization. Most infections involving anaerobes usually have coexisting aerobic bacterial infection, which should be considered when selecting an antimicrobial agent or agents.

Anaerobic infections are commonly associated with infections of the oropharynx, the central nervous system (CNS), the
subcutaneous space, the musculoskeletal system, the gastrointestinal tract, the liver, and the female genital tract, and they
are relatively common in animals with aspiration pneumonia
or consolidated lung lobes. Dogs and cats with gingivitis/
stomatitis (Fig. 98-1), rhinitis, retrobulbar abscesses, retropharyngeal abscesses, aspiration pneumonia, pyothorax, otitis media or interna, CNS infection, bite wounds, open wounds, open
fractures, osteomyelitis, peritonitis, bacterial hepatitis, pyometra, vaginitis, bacteremia, and valvular endocarditis should be
suspected to be infected with anaerobes (Table 98-3). The
reader is referred to Chapter 97 for a discussion of the cytologic and cultural characteristics of anaerobic infections.

Improving the blood supply and oxygenation of the infected area is the primary goal for treatment of anaerobic infections. Antibiotic therapy should be used concurrently with

drainage or debridement. Parenteral antibiotics should be administered for several days in dogs or cats with pyothorax,
pneumonia, peritonitis, and clinical signs consistent with bacteremia. Penicillin derivatives, clindamycin, metronidazole,
cephalosporins (first and second generation), and chloramphenicol are used commonly for the treatment of anaerobic
infections (Table 98-4). With the exception of *Bacteroides
fragilis,* penicillin derivatives have excellent activity against
anaerobes. If gram-negative coccobacilli are detected cytologically in a neutrophilic exudate, particularly if associated
with the oral cavity, metronidazole, a first-generation
cephalosporin, or clindamycin should be administered instead of a penicillin derivative. Because concurrent anaerobic and aerobic infections occur frequently, combination antimicrobial treatment is often indicated, particularly if
life-threatening signs of bacteremia exist (see Bacteremia and
Bacterial Endocarditis, below, for a discussion of antibiotic
combinations).

TABLE 98-4

Empirical Antibiotic Choices for Dogs and Cats
with Cutaneous or Soft Tissue Infections

| INFECTIOUS AGENT | ANTIBIOTIC CHOICES |
|---|---|
| Staphylococcal pyoderma | 1. First-generation cephalosporins<br>2. Amoxicillin-clavulanate or cloxacillin or oxacillin<br>3. Clindamycin or lincomycin or erythromycin<br>4. Trimethoprim-sulfadiazine or ormetoprim-sulfadimethoxine (superficial pyoderma) |
| Gram-negative pyoderma | 1. Quinolones |
| Abscesses (anaerobes) | 1. Penicillin derivatives<br>2. First- or second-generation cephalosporins<br>3. Clindamycin<br>4. Metronidazole<br>5. Chloramphenicol |
| L-form bacteria | 1. Doxycycline<br>2. Quinolones<br>3. Chloramphenicol |
| Atypical Mycobacteria | 1. Doxycycline or minocycline<br>2. Chloramphenicol<br>3. Quinolones<br>4. Trimethoprim-sulfadiazine<br>5. Aminoglycosides<br>6. Clarithromycin |
| Nocardia | 1. Penicillins (high dose)<br>2. Penicillins combined with trimethoprim-sulfadiazine for penicillin-resistant *Nocardia* infections<br>3. Minocycline<br>4. Erythromycin<br>5. Amikacin<br>6. Imipenem |
| Actinomyces | 1. Penicillins<br>2. Clindamycin<br>3. Erythromycin<br>4. Chloramphenicol<br>5. Minocycline |

 TABLE 98-5

Empirical Antibiotic Choices for Dogs and Cats
with Cardiopulmonary Infections

| ORGAN SYSTEM OR INFECTIOUS AGENT | ANTIBIOTIC CHOICES |
|---|---|
| Sepsis, bacteremia, and bacterial endocarditis | 1. Enrofloxacin and penicillin (or ampicillin or amoxicillin or clindamycin or first-generation cephalosporin)<br>2. Aminoglycoside and penicillin (or ampicillin or amoxicillin or clindamycin or first-generation cephalosporin)<br>3. Second- or third-generation cephalosporin<br>4. Imipenem<br>5. Ticarcillin and clavulanate |
| Upper respiratory | 1. Amoxicillin or amoxicillin-clavulanate<br>2. First-generation cephalosporin<br>3. Potentiated sulfas<br>4. Clindamycin<br>5. Doxycycline*<br>6. Chloramphenicol*<br>7. Enrofloxacin |
| Bacterial pneumonia with bacteremia† | 1. Enrofloxacin and penicillin (or ampicillin or amoxicillin or clindamycin or metronidazole or first-generation cephalosporin)<br>2. Imipenem |
| Bacterial pneumonia | 1. Amoxicillin-clavulanate<br>2. Potentiated sulfas<br>3. First-generation cephalosporin<br>4. Chloramphenicol |
| Pyothorax† | 1. Penicillin derivatives<br>2. Clindamycin<br>3. Metronidazole<br>4. Chloramphenicol<br>5. First-generation cephalosporin |
| Toxoplasmosis/ neosporosis | 1. Clindamycin<br>2. Potentiated sulfas |

*This drug should be used if *Bordetella, Mycoplasma,* or *Chlamydophila* infection is suspected.
†These are generally mixed infections, often with gram-negative, gram-positive, aerobic, and anaerobic combinations. If signs of bacteremia or sepsis are present, a four-quadrant antibiotic is administered parenterally as discussed for sepsis until culture and antimicrobial susceptibility results are available.

## BACTEREMIA AND BACTERIAL ENDOCARDITIS

Bacteremia can be transient, intermittent, or continuous. Routine dentistry is a common cause of transient bacteremia. Immunosuppressed or critically ill animals commonly develop intermittent bacteremia; the source of infection is commonly the urinary or gastrointestinal systems. Continuous bacteremia occurs most frequently in association with bacterial endocarditis. Bacteremic animals have intermittent fever, depres-

sion, and clinical signs associated with the primary organ system infected. Sepsis is the systemic response to infection and is manifested by peripheral circulatory failure (septic shock).

*Staphylococcus, Streptococcus, Klebsiella, Enterobacter, Pseudomonas, Clostridium,* and *Bacteroides* organisms, as well as *Escherichia coli,* are commonly isolated from the blood of bacteremic animals. Bacterial endocarditis is usually due to *Staphylococcus aureus, E. coli,* or β-hemolytic *Streptococcus* infection. If the source of bacteremia or bacterial endocarditis is from an area with mixed flora, such as the gastrointestinal tract, or if the animal has life-threatening clinical signs of disease, an antibiotic or combination of antibiotics that is effective against gram-positive, gram-negative, aerobic, and anaerobic organisms (four-quadrant approach) should be used. An aminoglycoside or quinolone for gram-negative organisms combined with ampicillin, a first-generation cephalosporin, or clindamycin for gram-positive and anaerobic organisms is a commonly prescribed combination treatment (Table 98-5). Second- and third-generation cephalosporins, ticarcillin combined with clavulanate, and imipenem are some of the agents with a four-quadrant spectrum. After parenteral treatment with these drugs for 5 to 7 days, oral treatment is selected on the basis of culture and antimicrobial susceptibility results. Oral treatment is continued for at least 4 to 6 weeks, particularly in dogs or cats with bacterial endocarditis. The blood culture should be rechecked 1 and 4 weeks after discontinuation of therapy to confirm control of the infection. The prognosis in dogs and cats with bacterial endocarditis is guarded to poor, owing to damage of the infected heart valves.

## SKIN AND SOFT TISSUE INFECTIONS

*Staphylococcus intermedius* is the most common cause of pyoderma in dogs and cats. Deep pyoderma can be induced by any organism, including the gram-negative types. Most soft tissue infections, including open wounds and abscesses, are infected with a mixed population of bacteria; the aerobic and anaerobic flora from the mouth are often involved. Recommended empirical antibiotic choices for routine cases of pyoderma and soft tissue infections are listed in Table 98-4. Antibiotics with a broad spectrum, such as first-generation cephalosporins and amoxicillin-clavulanate, are often first choices. Other β-lactamase–resistant penicillins, such as oxacillin and cloxacillin, also can be used. Potentiated sulfas can be used to treat dogs and cats with superficial pyoderma but should be avoided if long-term treatment is needed because bacterial resistance occurs quickly. Cutaneous and soft tissue infections that do not respond to these antibiotics may be caused by gram-negative bacteria, L-form bacteria, *Mycoplasma* organisms, atypical *Mycobacterium* spp., systemic fungi, or *Sporothrix schenckii*. Quinolones are the antibiotic class of choice for the treatment of gram-negative infections. Animals that fail to respond to empirical antibiotic treatment should undergo further diagnostic testing or should be treated with antibiotics known to have an effect against the less common pathogens (see Table 98-4). If not previously done, microscopic examination of tissue or pustule aspirates should be performed for the presence of *Sporothrix* organisms and bacteria morphologically similar to *Mycobacterium* spp. After surgical preparation of the skin, deep tissues should be obtained for aerobic, anaerobic, *Mycoplasma,* fungal, and atypical *Mycobacterium* spp. culture (see Chapter 97).

 TABLE 98-6

**Empirical Antibiotic Choices for Dogs and Cats with Hepatic and Gastrointestinal Infections**

| INFECTIOUS AGENT | ANTIBIOTIC CHOICES |
| --- | --- |
| Bacterial cholangiohepatitis | 1. Amoxicillin<br>2. First-generation cephalosporin<br>3. Chloramphenicol<br>4. Metronidazole<br>5. Quinolones |
| Bacterial overgrowth | 1. Penicillin derivative<br>2. Tetracycline derivative<br>3. Tylosin<br>4. Metronidazole |
| *Campylobacter* spp. | 1. Erythromycin<br>2. Quinolones<br>3. Tetracycline derivative<br>4. Chloramphenicol |
| *Clostridium perfringens* | 1. Penicillin derivative<br>2. Tylosin<br>3. Metronidazole<br>4. Tetracycline derivative |
| Hepatic encephalopathy | 1. Neomycin<br>2. Ampicillin<br>3. Metronidazole |
| *Salmonella* spp. | 1. Quinolones<br>2. Trimethoprim-sulfadiazine<br>3. Amoxicillin<br>4. Aminoglycosides<br>5. Chloramphenicol |

## GASTROINTESTINAL TRACT AND HEPATIC INFECTIONS

Oral administration of antibiotics is indicated for the treatment of small intestinal bacterial overgrowth, hepatic encephalopathy, cholangiohepatitis, hepatic abscessation, and infection by *Helicobacter felis, Campylobacter* spp., *Clostridium perfringens, Giardia* spp., *Cryptosporidium* spp., *Balantidium coli, Entamoeba histolytica, Tritrichomonas foetus, Toxoplasma gondii,* and *Cystoisospora* spp. (Table 98-6). Administration of parenteral antibiotics is indicated in dogs and cats with bacteremia from translocation of enteric flora or *Salmonella* infection.

Clinical signs associated with infection by *Entamoeba, Giardia, Balantidium,* and *Tritrichomonas* organisms generally respond to metronidazole, 25 mg/kg given orally twice a day for 8 days. This is the maximum dose of metronidazole that should be used; progressively lower doses should be used in larger dogs to lessen the potential for toxicity. Albendazole, fenbendazole, and the combination of febantel/praziquantel/pyrantel are also effective for the treatment of giardiasis; fenbendazole and febantel/praziquantel/pyrantel are preferred because they are less toxic (see Chapter 30). Administration

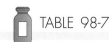

## TABLE 98-7

Empirical Antibiotic Choices for Dogs and Cats with Central Nervous System and Musculoskeletal Infections

| ORGAN SYSTEM OR INFECTIOUS AGENT | ANTIBIOTIC CHOICES |
|---|---|
| **Central Nervous System** | |
| Encephalitis | 1. Chloramphenicol<br>2. Amoxicillin<br>3. Trimethoprim-sulfa<br>4. Quinolone |
| Otitis media/ interna | 1. Amoxicillin *or* amoxicillin-clavulanate<br>2. Chloramphenicol<br>3. Clindamycin<br>4. First-generation cephalosporin<br>5. Quinolone |
| Toxoplasmosis/ neosporosis | 1. Clindamycin<br>2. Trimethoprim-sulfadiazine<br>3. Pyrimethamine |
| **Musculoskeletal System** | |
| Diskospondylitis | 1. First-generation cephalosporin<br>2. Amoxicillin-clavulanate<br>3. Clindamycin<br>4. Chloramphenicol<br>5. Quinolone |
| Hepatozoonosis | 1. *Acute:* Clindamycin, trimethoprim-sulfa, and pyrimethamine<br>2. *Chronic:* Decoquinate |
| Osteomyelitis | 1. Amoxicillin-clavulanate<br>2. Clindamycin<br>3. First-generation cephalosporin<br>4. Chloramphenicol<br>5. Quinolone |
| Toxoplasmosis/ neosporosis | 1. Clindamycin<br>2. Trimethoprim-sulfadiazine<br>3. Pyrimethamine |
| **Polyarthritis** | |
| Bacterial | 1. First-generation cephalosporin<br>2. Quinolone |
| *Borrelia burgdorferi* | 1. Doxycycline<br>2. Amoxicillin |
| *Ehrlichia* spp. | 1. Doxycycline<br>2. Chloramphenicol<br>3. Imidocarb |
| L-form bacteria or *Mycoplasma* | 1. Doxycycline<br>2. Quinolone<br>3. Chloramphenicol |
| Rocky Mountain spotted fever | 1. Doxycycline<br>2. Enrofloxacin<br>3. Chloramphenicol |

of tylosin at 10 to 15 mg/kg given orally twice a day lessens clinical signs of cryptosporidiosis in some infected dogs and cats. Paromomycin (Parke-Davis, Morris Plains, N.J.) is the drug of choice for the treatment of cryptosporidiosis in humans, and when administered at a dosage of 150 mg/kg given orally once or twice daily for 5 days, it lessened the clinical signs of cryptosporidiosis in experimentally infected cats (Lappin MR, unpublished data). This drug should be avoided if hemorrhagic diarrhea is present because it can be absorbed systemically in this situation and has been associated with acute renal failure and hearing deficits. The *T. gondii* oocyst shedding period can be shortened by administration of clindamycin at 12 mg/kg given orally twice a day for 10 days. *Cystoisospora* spp. generally are responsive to the administration of sulfadimethoxine at 25 mg/kg given orally once a day for 7 days, with the treatment regimen repeated again 7 days later.

*C. perfringens* and bacterial overgrowth generally respond to treatment with tylosin, ampicillin, amoxicillin, tetracyclines, or metronidazole. Campylobacteriosis usually responds clinically to the oral administration of quinolones, erythromycin, chloramphenicol, or tetracyclines. Appropriate empirical antibiotics for the treatment of bacteremia from salmonellosis include quinolones, sulfonamide combinations, and penicillins. *Helicobacter* infection is usually treated with the combination of metronidazole and tetracycline derivatives, or amoxicillin and metronidazole. Macrolide antibiotics, such as azithromycin and clarithromycin, may also be effective for helicobacteriosis.

Hepatic infections generally respond to first-generation cephalosporins, amoxicillin, or chloramphenicol. Decreasing numbers of enteric flora by oral administration of penicillins, metronidazole, or neomycin can lessen the clinical signs of hepatic encephalopathy. Animals with apparent bacteremia due to enteric bacteria should be treated with parenteral antibiotics that have a spectrum against anaerobic and gram-negative organisms, as discussed previously. Bacterial overgrowth is secondary to many diseases of the gastrointestinal tract and may be induced by oral administration of broad-spectrum antimicrobial agents. This condition may be managed by resolution of the primary etiology and administration of tylosin or tetracycline derivatives.

## MUSCULOSKELETAL INFECTIONS

Osteomyelitis and diskospondylitis are commonly associated with infections by *Staphylococcus, Streptococcus, Proteus,* and *Pseudomonas* spp., *E. coli,* and anaerobes. First-generation cephalosporins, amoxicillin-clavulanate, and clindamycin are logical antibiotics for empirical therapy of these conditions, owing to their spectrum of activity against the gram-positive organisms and anaerobic bacteria and their ability to achieve high concentrations in bone (Table 98-7). Quinolones should be used if gram-negative organisms are suspected. Antibiotic treatment should be continued for a minimum of 2 weeks beyond resolution of radiographic changes.

Dogs and cats with septic polyarthritis should be treated in the same way as those with osteomyelitis. The source of infection should be removed if possible. *Ehrlichia* spp., *Rickettsia rickettsii*, *Borrelia burgdorferi*, *Mycoplasma* organisms, and L-form bacteria can induce nonseptic, suppurative polyarthritis. Occasionally, morulae of *Ehrlichia* spp. are identified cytologically in the joint fluid. In general, the cytologic findings in joint fluid that are induced by these agents are similar to those of immune-mediated polyarthritis. For this reason, doxycycline is a logical empirical antibiotic choice for dogs with nonseptic, suppurative polyarthritis pending the results of further diagnostic tests. Amoxicillin is an alternative drug for the treatment of *B. burgdorferi* infection. Enrofloxacin can also be used for *R. rickettsii*, *Mycoplasma*, and L-form bacteria infections.

Muscle disease from *T. gondii* infection often resolves during treatment with clindamycin hydrochloride. Although many dogs with neosporosis die, some have survived after treatment with trimethoprim-sulfadiazine combined with pyrimethamine; sequential treatment with clindamycin hydrochloride, trimethoprim-sulfadiazine, and pyrimethamine; or clindamycin alone. For treatment of acute *Hepatozoon americanum* infection, the combination of trimethoprim-sulfadiazine, pyrimethamine, and clindamycin for 14 days is very successful; use of decoquinate at 10 to 20 mg/kg given every12 hours with food lessens the likelihood of recurrence of clinical disease and prolongs survival time.

## CENTRAL NERVOUS SYSTEM INFECTIONS

Chloramphenicol, the sulfonamides, trimethoprim, metronidazole, and the quinolones penetrate the CNS and should be chosen for empirical treatment of suspected bacterial infections of this system (see Table 98-7). Anaerobic bacterial infection and rickettsial infections (*Ehrlichia* spp. and *R. rickettsii*) of the CNS occur in some cases, making chloramphenicol a logical first choice. Doxycycline and erythromycin may cross into the cerebrospinal fluid when inflammation exists. Clindamycin achieves adequate brain tissue concentrations in normal cats for the treatment of toxoplasmosis. Potentiated sulfas are alternate anti-*Toxoplasma* drugs.

## RESPIRATORY TRACT INFECTIONS

Most bacterial upper respiratory infections are secondary to other primary diseases, including foreign bodies, viral infections, tooth root abscesses, neoplasms, trauma, and fungal infections. After the epithelium of the nose and sinuses is inflamed, normal bacterial flora can colonize and perpetuate inflammation; deep infection can result in chondritis and osteomyelitis. Since the upper respiratory passageways have a normal flora, it is difficult to assess the results of culture and antimicrobial susceptibility testing in these tissues. The source of the primary insult should always be removed if possible.

Broad-spectrum antibiotics with an anaerobic spectrum including amoxicillin, amoxicillin-clavulanate, potentiated sulfas, and first generation cephalosporins are commonly prescribed empirically to treat upper respiratory infections secondary to normal flora overgrowth (see Table 98-5). Treatment duration is generally 1 to 2 weeks for acute, first-time infections. Dogs and cats with chronic rhinitis suspected to have osteochondritis that respond to antibiotics should be treated for a minimum of 4-6 weeks or until clinical signs have been resolved for 2 weeks. Chronic rhinitis often responds to treatment with clindamycin because of the excellent anaerobic and gram-positive spectrum, and its ability to penetrate cartilage and bone well. *Bordetella bronchiseptica*, *Mycoplasma* spp., and *Chlamydophila felis* infection of cats are primary bacterial pathogens that infect the upper respiratory tissues. If the animal responds poorly to broad spectrum antibiotics, doxycycline, azithromycin, chloramphenicol, or quinolones can be administered; *Chlamydophila*, *Bordetella*, and *Mycoplasma* organisms generally respond to these drugs. Chloramphenicol is an excellent first choice for the treatment of upper respiratory infection in immunocompetent animals owing to its broad spectrum, efficacy against primary pathogens, and tissue penetration.

Canine kennel cough syndrome caused by *Bordetella* or *Mycoplasma* spp. is usually effectively treated with doxycycline, chloramphenicol, quinolones, or amoxicillin-clavulanate. Bacterial bronchitis in cats generally responds to administration of doxycycline or chloramphenicol. In dogs and cats with chronic bronchitis, doxycycline, chloramphenicol, uinolones, or amoxicillin-clavulanate are rational empirical antibiotic choices.

Common bacteria associated with pneumonia in dogs include *E. coli*; *Klebsiella*, *Pasteurella*, and *Pseudomonas* spp.; *B. bronchiseptica*; and *Streptococcus*, *Staphylococcus*, and *Mycoplasma* spp. In cats, *Bordetella*, *Pasteurella*, and *Mycoplasma* organisms are commonly isolated. Aspiration of gastrointestinal contents is a common cause of bacterial pneumonia with a mixed population of bacteria. Multiple species of bacteria are typically cultured from dogs and cats with bronchopneumonia. *B. bronchiseptica* is the most important primary pathogen in dogs and cats; most other bacteria colonize after airways have been previously inflamed. If consolidated lung lobes are detected radiographically, an anaerobic infection should be assumed. It is unknown whether species of *Mycoplasma* infecting dogs and cats are capable of being primary respiratory pathogens. *Chlamydophila* infection in cats is not a common cause of lower respiratory tract infection. *Yersinia pestis* causes pneumonia in cats in the western states (see Chapter 105); aminoglycosides, tetracycline derivatives, and quinolones are antibiotics that can be used successfully for treatment.

In dogs and cats with bacterial pneumonia, culture and antimicrobial susceptibility testing should be performed on secretions collected by transtracheal wash or bronchoalveolar lavage. If the animal is showing signs of bacteremia or if radiographic evidence of consolidated lung lobes is present, parenteral administration of a four-quadrant antibiotic choice as discussed for bacteremia should be used initially. Quinolones combined with clindamycin or azithromycin, or chloramphenicol alone, are good choices for animals with consolidated lung lobes due to their broad spectrum, excellent tissue penetration, and efficacy against *B. bronchiseptica* (see Table 98-5). In animals with pneumonia but without clinical signs of bacteremia or consolidated lung lobes, broad-spectrum antibiotics, including amoxicillin, amoxicillin-clavulanate, potentiated sulfas, and first-generation cephalosporins, may be effective. Surface-dwelling organisms such *as B. bronchiseptica* and *Mycoplasma* may respond to nebulization of gentamicin diluted in sterile saline (25 to 50 mg in 3 to 5 ml saline/nebulization). Treatment for bacterial pneumonia should be continued for at least 4 weeks or 1 to 2 weeks beyond resolution of clinical and radiographic signs of disease.

*T. gondii* and *Neospora caninum* occasionally causes pneumonia in neonatally infected, transplacentally infected, and immunosuppressed cats (see Chapter 104). Clindamycin or potentiated sulfas should be used if toxoplasmosis is suspected.

If pyothorax is due to penetration of foreign material from an airway or esophagus into the pleural space, thoracotomy is usually required for removal of devitalized tissue and the foreign body (see Chapter 23). Occasionally, pyothorax is from hematogenous spread of bacteria to the pleural space; this may be common in cats. Pleural lavage through chest tubes is the most effective treatment for patients with pyothorax and no obvious foreign material. Most dogs and cats with pyothorax have mixed aerobic and anaerobic bacterial infections. Animals with pyothorax and clinical signs of bacteremia should initially receive parenteral four-quadrant antibiotics, as discussed for bacteremia.

## UROGENITAL TRACT INFECTIONS

Microscopic examination and Gram's staining of a urine sediment aids in the empirical choice of an antibiotic in dogs and cats with signs of urinary tract infection. Culture and antimicrobial susceptibility testing should always be performed, if possible. Approximately 75% of urinary tract infections in dogs are caused by gram-negative organisms; *E. coli, Proteus, Klebsiella, Pseudomonas,* and *Enterobacter* infections are common. In cats that have been previously catheterized, *E. coli* is most common; *Staphylococcus* and *Streptococcus* organisms are common after urethrostomy (see Chapter 45).

In bitches with simple, first-time urinary tract infections, amoxicillin or amoxicillin-clavulanate should be used if cocci are observed; potentiated sulfas or first-generation cephalosporins should be used if rods are observed. Quinolones should be reserved for life-threatening or resistant infections. Many antibiotics do not penetrate the prostate unless it is markedly inflamed. Because the prostate can be a source of recurrent urinary tract infection, it should be assumed that all male dogs with urinary tract infection have prostatitis, and antibiotics that penetrate the prostate should be chosen

(Table 98-8). The majority of urinary tract infections in cats respond to amoxicillin. Administration of antibiotics for 10 to 14 days is generally sufficient for simple urinary tract infections. Urinalysis, culture, and antimicrobial susceptibility testing should be performed 7 days after finishing treatment, if possible.

*Mycoplasma* and *Ureaplasma* infections have been documented in dogs with clinical signs of urinary tract infections. If poor response to penicillin derivatives, cephalosporins, or potentiated sulfas is observed, further diagnostics should be performed. If empirical therapy is deemed necessary, chloramphenicol, doxycycline, or quinolone treatment can be administered and may be more effective for *Mycoplasma* and *Ureaplasma* organisms.

All dogs and cats with urinary tract infection and azotemia should be assumed to have pyelonephritis and should be treated accordingly, even if further diagnostic procedures are not performed. Treatment for pyelonephritis should be based on susceptibility results, if possible; potentiated sulfa combinations or quinolones are good empirical choices. If renal insufficiency exists, the tetracyclines (except doxycycline) and

 **TABLE 98-8**

**Empirical Antibiotic Choices for Dogs and Cats with Urogenital Infections**

| ORGAN SYSTEM OR INFECTIOUS AGENT | ANTIBIOTIC CHOICES |
| --- | --- |
| Aerobic urinary tract infection | 1. Amoxicillin or amoxicillin-clavulanate<br>2. First-generation cephalosporin<br>3. Sulfonamide combinations<br>4. Quinolone |
| *Brucella canis* | 1. Minocycline or doxycycline cycled with a quinolone |
| *Leptospira* spp. | 1. Penicillin G or ampicillin given IV during acute phase; amoxicillin given PO during chronic phase<br>2. Doxycycline to eliminate renal carriers |
| Mastitis | 1. First-generation cephalosporin<br>2. Amoxicillin or amoxicillin-clavulanate |
| *Mycoplasma/ Ureaplasma* | 1. Doxycycline<br>2. Chloramphenicol<br>3. Quinolone |
| Prostatitis | 1. Potentiated sulfas<br>2. Quinolone<br>3. Chloramphenicol<br>4. Erythromycin<br>5. Clindamycin |
| Pyometra | 1. Quinolone and amoxicillin<br>2. Chloramphenicol<br>3. Potentiated sulfas<br>4. Amoxicillin-clavulanate |

aminoglycosides should be avoided, and the dosage or dosing interval of quinolones and cephalosporins should be reduced according to the diminution in renal function. The new dosage can be calculated by multiplying the current dosage by the result obtained when the mean normal creatinine concentration is divided by the patient's creatinine concentration. The new dosing interval can be calculated by multiplying the current dosing interval by the result obtained when the patient's creatinine concentration is divided by the mean normal creatinine concentration. Treatment for pyelonephritis and other chronic, complicated urinary tract infections should be continued for at least 6 weeks. Urinalysis, culture, and antimicrobial susceptibility testing should be performed 7 and 28 days after treatment. Some infections cannot be eliminated and require administration of pulse antibiotic therapy.

Most bacterial prostatic infections involve gram-negative bacteria. During acute prostatitis almost all antibiotics penetrate the prostate well due to inflammation. After reestablishment of the blood-prostate barrier in dogs with chronic prostatitis, the acidic prostatic fluid allows only the basic antibiotics (pKa <7) to penetrate well (see Table 98-8). Chloramphenicol, because of its high lipid solubility, also penetrates prostatic tissue well. In acute prostatitis, administration of acidic antibiotics, including penicillins and first-generation cephalosporins, may initially penetrate well, lessening clinical signs of disease but not eliminating the infection; this predisposes to chronic bacterial prostatitis and prostatic abscessation. For this reason, the use of penicillins and first-generation cephalosporins is contraindicated for the treatment of urinary tract infections in male dogs. In dogs with chronic prostatitis, antimicrobial therapy should be continued for at least 6 weeks. Urine and prostatic fluid should be cultured 7 days and 28 days after therapy.

*Brucella canis* causes a number of clinical syndromes in dogs, including epididymitis, orchitis, endometritis, stillbirths, abortion, diskospondylitis, and uveitis (see Chapter 63 for a complete discussion of the clinical manifestations and diagnostic procedures). Ovariohysterectomy or neutering lessens contamination of the human environment (see Chapter 105 for a discussion of the zoonotic potential). Long-term antibiotic administration usually does not lead to a complete cure. Some dogs become antibody-negative, but the organism can still be cultured from tissues (see Chapter 63). Several antibiotic protocols have been suggested for dogs with brucellosis (see Table 98-8 and p. 936), but overall, treatment should be discouraged because of human health risks.

Vaginitis generally results from overgrowth of normal flora secondary to primary diseases, including herpesvirus infection, urinary tract infection, foreign bodies, vulvar or vaginal anomalies, vaginal or vulvar masses, or urinary incontinence. In dogs and cats with bacterial vaginitis from overgrowth of flora and resolution of the primary insult, broad-spectrum antibiotics, including amoxicillin, potentiated sulfas, first-generation cephalosporins, tetracycline derivatives, and chloramphenicol, are commonly successful (see Chapter 63). Because *Mycoplasma* and *Ureaplasma* organisms are part of the normal vaginal flora, it is virtually impossible to provide a clinical disease association; positive cultures do not confirm disease due to the organism (see Chapter 100). Hence a positive vaginal culture from an asymptomatic dog (excluding *B. canis*) is meaningless.

In all dogs and cats with pyometra, ovariohysterectomy or medically induced drainage of the uterus is imperative. Antibiotic treatment is for the bacteremia that commonly occurs concurrently (i.e., *E. coli* and anaerobes). Animals with clinical signs of bacteremia or sepsis should be treated with a four-quadrant antibiotic choice (see Table 98-5). Broad-spectrum antibiotics with efficacy against *E. coli,* such as potentiated sulfas or amoxicillin-clavulanate, are appropriate empirical choices pending the results of culture and antimicrobial susceptibility testing. Potentiated sulfas and the quinolones commonly are effective for *E. coli* but are not as effective as other drugs for the treatment of anaerobic infections in vivo.

Ampicillin, amoxicillin, and first-generation cephalosporins achieve good concentrations in milk and are relatively safe for the neonate, therefore they can be used in the empirical treatment of mastitis. Chloramphenicol, quinolones, and tetracycline derivatives should be avoided due to potential adverse effects on the neonate.

## Suggested Readings

Brady CA et al: Severe sepsis in cats: 29 cases (1986-1998), *J Am Vet Med Assoc* 217:531, 2000.

Calvert CA: Cardiovascular infections. In Greene CE, editor: *Infectious diseases of the dog and cat,* Philadelphia, 1998, WB Saunders, p 567.

Chandler JC et al: Mycoplasmal respiratory infections in small animals: 17 cases (1988-1999), *J Am Anim Hosp Assoc* 38:111, 2002.

Dow SW: Diagnosis of bacteremia in critically ill dogs and cats. In Bonagura JD, editor: *Kirk's current veterinary therapy XII,* Philadelphia, 1995, WB Saunders, p 137.

Ferguson DC et al: Antimicrobial therapy. In Lorenz LMD et al, editors: *Small animal medical therapeutics,* Philadelphia, 1992, JB Lippincott, p 457.

Hardie EM: Life-threatening bacterial infection, *Comp Contin Educ Pract Vet* 17:763, 1995.

Jameson PH et al: Comparison of clinical signs, diagnostic findings, organisms isolated, and clinical outcome in dogs with bacterial pneumonia: 93 cases (1986-1991), *J Am Vet Med Assoc* 206:206, 1995.

Jang SS et al: *Mycoplasma* as a cause of canine urinary tract infection, *J Am Vet Med Assoc* 185:45, 1984.

Jang SS et al: Organisms isolated from dogs and cats with anaerobic infections and susceptibility to selected antimicrobial agents, *J Am Vet Med Assoc* 210:1610, 1997.

Johnson CA et al: Clinical signs and diagnosis of *Brucella canis* infection, *Comp Contin Educ Pract Vet* 14:763, 1992.

Kirby R: Septic shock. In Bonagura JD, editor: *Kirk's current veterinary therapy XII,* Philadelphia, 1995, WB Saunders, p 139.

Walker AL et al: Bacteria associated with pyothorax of dogs and cats: 98 cases (1989-1998), *J Am Vet Med Assoc* 216:359, 2000.

# CHAPTER 99

## Prevention of Infectious Diseases

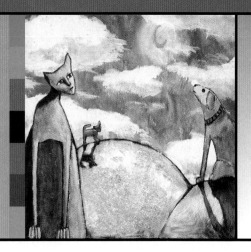

### CHAPTER OUTLINE

BIOSECURITY PROCEDURES FOR SMALL ANIMAL
HOSPITALS, 1250
    General biosecurity guidelines, 1250
    Patient evaluation, 1251
    Hospitalized patients, 1251
    Basic disinfection protocols, 1252
BIOSECURITY PROCEDURES FOR CLIENTS, 1252
VACCINATION PROTOCOLS, 1252
    Vaccine types, 1252
    Vaccine selection, 1253
    Vaccination protocols for cats, 1254
    Vaccination protocols for dogs, 1256

It is always preferred to prevent rather than treat infections. Consequently, avoiding exposure is the most effective way to prevent infections. Most infectious agents of dogs and cats are transmitted in fecal material, respiratory secretions, reproductive tract secretions, or urine; by bites or scratches; or by contact with vectors or reservoirs. Some infectious agents can be transmitted by direct contact with clinically normal, infected animals. Many infectious agents are environmentally resistant and can be transmitted by contact with a contaminated environment (fomites). It is extremely important to avoid zoonotic transfer of infectious agents, because some zoonotic diseases, such as plague and rabies, are life-threatening (see Chapter 105). Recognition of risk factors associated with infectious agents is the initial step in prevention of infectious diseases. Veterinarians should strive to understand the biology of each infectious agent so that they can counsel clients and staff on the best strategies for prevention. Vaccines available for some infectious agents can prevent infection or lessen clinical illness when infection occurs. However, vaccines are not uniformly effective, are not available for all pathogens, and sometimes induce serious adverse effects; thus it is paramount to develop sound biosecurity procedures to avoid exposure to infectious agents when developing a preventive medicine program.

## BIOSECURITY PROCEDURES FOR SMALL ANIMAL HOSPITALS

Most hospital-borne infections (nosocomial) can be prevented by following simple biosecurity guidelines (Table 99-1). The following is a suggested format for control of infectious diseases in small animal hospitals that is adapted from those used at Colorado State University (http://www.vth.colostate.edu/biosecurity/biosecurity.html).

### GENERAL BIOSECURITY GUIDELINES

Contaminated hands are the most common source of infectious disease transmission in the hospital environment. Fingernails of personnel having patient contact should be cut short. Hands should be washed before and after attending to each individual animal as follows: collect clean paper towels and use to turn on water faucets, wash hands for 30 seconds with antiseptic soap being sure to clean under fingernails, rinse hands thoroughly, use the paper towel to dry hands, and use the paper towel to turn off the water faucets. Use of antiseptic lotion should be encouraged. Personnel should not touch patients, clients, food, doorknobs, drawer or cabinet handles or contents, equipment, or medical records with soiled hands or gloves.

All employees should wear an outer garment, such as a smock or scrub suit, when attending to patients. Footwear should be protective, clean, and cleanable. A minimum of two sets of outer garments should always be available, and they should be changed immediately after contamination with feces, secretions, or exudates. Equipment such as stethoscopes, pen lights, thermometers, bandage scissors, lead ropes, percussion hammers, and clipper blades can be fomites and should be cleaned and disinfected after each use with animals likely to have a transmissible infectious disease. Disposable thermometer covers or thermometers should be used.

To avoid zoonotic transfer of infectious diseases, food or drink should not be consumed in areas where animal care is provided. All areas where animals are examined or treated should be cleaned and disinfected immediately after use, irrespective of infectious disease status of the individual animal.

TABLE 99-1

**General Hospital Biosecurity Guidelines**

Wash hands before and after each patient contact.

Wear gloves when handling patients when zoonotic diseases are on the list of differential diagnoses.

Minimize contact with hospital materials (instruments, records, door handles, etc.) while hands or gloves are contaminated.

Always wear an outer garment, such as a smock or scrub shirt, when handling patients.

Change outer garments when soiled by feces, secretions, or exudates.

Clean and disinfect equipment (stethoscopes, thermometers, bandage scissors, etc.) after each use with animals likely to have an infectious disease.

Do not consume fluid or drink in areas where patient care is provided.

Examination tables, cages, and runs should be cleaned and disinfected after each use.

Litter boxes and dishes should be cleaned and disinfected after each use.

Place animals with suspected infectious diseases immediately into an examination room or an isolation area on admission into the hospital.

Treat animals with suspected infectious diseases as outpatients, if possible.

Procedures using general hospital facilities, such as surgery and radiology, should be postponed until the end of the day, if possible.

## PATIENT EVALUATION

Prevention of infectious diseases starts with the front desk personnel. Staff should be trained to recognize the owner presenting complaints for the infectious agents in the geographic area of the hospital. Animals with gastrointestinal or respiratory diseases are the most likely to be contagious. Infectious gastrointestinal disease should be suspected in all dogs and cats with small or large bowel diarrhea, whether the syndrome is acute or chronic. Infectious respiratory disease should be suspected in all dogs and cats with sneezing (especially those with purulent oculonasal discharge) or coughing (especially if productive). The index of suspicion for infectious diseases is increased for dogs or cats with acute disease and fever, particularly if the animal is from a crowded environment, such as a breeding facility, boarding facility, or humane society.

Front desk personnel should indicate clearly on the hospital record that gastrointestinal or respiratory disease is occurring. If the presenting complaint is known before admission into the hospital, it would be optimal to meet the client in the parking area to determine the infectious disease risk before entering the hospital. If infectious gastrointestinal or respiratory disease is suspected, the animal should be transported (i.e., not allowed to walk on the premises) to an ex-

amination room or the isolation facility. If a patient with acute gastrointestinal or respiratory disease is presented directly to the reception desk, the receptionist should contact the receiving clinician or technician immediately and coordinate placement of the animal in an examination room to minimize hospital contamination. Animals with suspected infectious diseases should be treated as outpatients if possible. If hospitalization is required, the animal should be transported to the appropriate housing area by the shortest route possible, preferably using a gurney to lessen hospital contamination. The gurney and any hospital material contacted by potentially contaminated employees (including examination tables and doorknobs) should be immediately cleaned and disinfected (see Basic Disinfection Protocols).

## HOSPITALIZED PATIENTS

If possible, all animals with suspected infectious diseases, such as *Salmonella* spp., *Campylobacter* spp., parvoviral infection, kennel cough syndrome, feline upper respiratory disease syndrome, rabies, or plague, should be housed in an isolated area of the hospital (see Chapter 15 for a discussion of the control of respiratory infections). The number of staff members entering the isolation area should be kept to a minimum. On entry into the isolation area, outerwear should be left outside and surgical booties or other disposable shoe covers should be placed over the shoes. Alternatively, a foot bath filled with disinfectant should be placed by the exit and used when leaving the area. The room should be entered and a disposable gown (or smock designated for the patient) and latex gloves should be put on. A surgical mask should be worn when attending cats with plague. Separate equipment and disinfectant supplies should be used in the isolation area.

All biologic materials submitted to clinical pathology laboratories or diagnostic laboratories from animals with suspected or proven infectious diseases should be clearly marked as such. Fecal material should be placed in a plastic, screw-capped cup using a tongue depressor or while wearing gloves. Place the cup in a clean area, and place the lid on with a clean, gloved hand. Remove the used gloves, and place the cup in a second bag clearly marked with the name of the infectious disease suspected. The outer surface of the bag should be disinfected before leaving the isolation area.

Disposable materials should be placed in plastic bags in the isolation area. The external surfaces of the bags should be sprayed with a disinfectant before being removed from the isolation area. After attending to the patient, contaminated equipment and surfaces should be cleaned and disinfected, and contaminated outer garments and shoe covers should be removed. Hands should be washed after discarding the contaminated outerwear. Dishes and litter pans should be cleansed thoroughly with detergent before you return them to the central supply area. Optimally, materials such as outerwear and equipment to be returned to the central supply area should be placed in plastic bags and sprayed with a disinfectant before transport. Procedures requiring general hospital facilities such as surgery and radiology should be postponed to the end of the day, if possible, and the contaminated areas disinfected before use with other animals. Animals should be discharged using the shortest path to the parking lot possible.

Some animals with infectious diseases can be maintained in the general hospital boarding or treatment areas with special management techniques. For example, feline leukemia virus–positive cats or feline immunodeficiency virus–positive cats should not be placed in the isolation area, if possible, to avoid exposing them to other infectious diseases. Since neither of these two viruses is transmitted by aerosolization, cats with these infectious diseases can be housed in close proximity to other cats. The cages should be labeled appropriately, and the infected cats should not be caged next to or above seronegative cats. In addition, there should not be direct contact between infected and naïve cats and there should be no sharing of litter boxes or food bowls.

## BASIC DISINFECTION PROTOCOLS

To lessen spread of potential contagions, hospitalized animals should never be moved from cage to cage. The key to effective disinfection is cleanliness. Cage papers and litter boxes soiled by feces, urine, blood, exudates, or respiratory secretions should be removed and placed in trash receptacles. Bulk fecal material should also be placed in trash receptacles.

The Veterinary Teaching Hospital at Colorado State University uses A464N disinfectant (Airkem Professional Products, Ecolab Center, St. Paul, MN 55102) as its primary disinfectant. This quaternary ammonium compound has been shown to inactivate most viruses, including parvoviruses, as well as bacteria such as *Salmonella,* when used at a concentration of 1:64 (2 oz/1 gallon of water). Many agents are resistant to disinfectants or require prolonged contact time to be inactivated (Greene, 1998a). Contaminated surfaces, including the cage or run floor, walls, ceiling, door, and door latch, should be wetted thoroughly with a disinfectant that is then blotted with clean paper towels or mops. Surfaces should be in contact with the disinfectant for 10 to 15 minutes if possible, particularly if known infectious agents are present. Soiled paper towels should be placed in trash receptacles. If infectious diseases are suspected, the trash bags should be sealed, the surface of the bag sprayed with a disinfectant, and the trash bags discarded.

Contaminated surfaces in examination rooms should be cleaned to remove hair, blood, feces, and exudates. Examination tables, countertops, floors, canister lids, and water taps should be saturated with disinfectant for 10 minutes. Surfaces should be blotted with paper towels until dry, and the soiled towels should be placed in a trash receptacle. Urine or feces on the floor should be contained with paper towels, blotted, and placed in trash receptacles. The soiled area of the floor should be mopped with disinfectant.

Disinfectants are relatively effective for viral and bacterial agents but require high concentrations and long contact times to kill parasite eggs, cysts, and oocysts. Cleanliness is the key to lessening hospital-borne infection with these agents; detergent or steam cleaning inactivates most of these agents. Litter pans and dishes should be thoroughly cleaned with detergent and scalding water.

## BIOSECURITY PROCEDURES FOR CLIENTS

Housing animals indoors in a human environment to prevent exposure to other animals, fomites, or vectors is the optimal way to prevent infectious diseases. Some infectious agents can be carried into the home environment with the owners, by vectors, or by paratenic or transfer hosts. Although most infections will occur in both immunocompromised and immunocompetent animals, clinical disease is often more severe in immunocompromised animals. Puppies, kittens, old animals, debilitated animals, animals with immunosuppressive diseases (e.g., hyperadrenocorticism, diabetes mellitus), animals with concurrent infections, and animals treated with glucocorticoids or cytotoxic agents are examples of immunocompromised patients. In this group, it is of particular importance to avoid exposure to infectious agents because of the increased susceptibility to disease. These animals are also less likely to have appropriate responses to immunization. Kennels, veterinary hospitals, dog and cat shows, and humane societies have an increased likelihood for infectious agent contact because of the concentration of potentially infected animals and should be avoided when possible. Areas such as parks are common sources of infectious agents that survive for long periods in the environment; parvoviruses are classic examples. Owners should avoid bringing new animals with unknown histories into the home environment that has other pets until the new animal is evaluated by a veterinarian for infectious disease risk. If people are in contact with animals outside the home environment, hands should be washed before being in contact with their own pet. The owner should consult the veterinarian concerning vaccination protocols and other preventive medical procedures (e.g., routine deworming) most indicated for each individual patient.

## VACCINATION PROTOCOLS

### VACCINE TYPES

Vaccines are available for some infectious diseases of dogs and cats and can be administered to prevent infection or limit disease. Vaccination stimulates humoral, mucosal, or cell-mediated immune responses. Humoral immune responses are characterized by the production of immunoglobulin M (IgM), IgG, IgA, and IgE class antibodies, which are produced by B-lymphocytes and plasma cells after being presented antigen by macrophages. Binding of antibodies to an infectious agent or its toxins helps prevent infection or disease by facilitating agglutination (viruses), improving phagocytosis (opsonization), neutralizing toxins, blocking attachment to cell surfaces, initiating the complement cascade, and antibody-dependent cell-mediated cytotoxicity. Antibody responses are most effective in controlling infectious agents during extracellular replication or toxin production. Cell-mediated immune responses are mediated principally by T-lymphocytes. Antigen-specific T-lymphocytes either destroy the infectious agent or mediate destruction of the agent by producing cytokines that stimulate other white blood cells, including macrophages, neutrophils, and natural killer cells. Cell-mediated immunity is required for the control of most cell-associated infections.

Attenuated (modified-live), noninfectious, and vector vaccines are the types of vaccines currently available commercially for dogs and cats. Attenuated vaccines generally have low antigen mass and so almost never induce local vaccine reactions; they can be given locally (e.g., modified-live *Bordetella bronchiseptica* intranasal vaccine) or parenterally (e.g., modified-live canine distemper vaccine). However, these are living vaccines that must replicate in the host to effectively stimulate an immune response (Table 99-2).

Noninfectious vaccines include killed virus, killed bacteria (bacterins), and subunit vaccines. In general, noninfectious vaccines require higher antigen mass than modified-live vaccines to stimulate immune responses since they do not replicate in the host. Noninfectious vaccines stimulate immune responses of lesser magnitude and shorter duration than attenuated vaccines unless adjuvants are added. Adjuvants improve immune responses by stimulating uptake of antigens by macrophages that present the antigens to lymphocytes. Adjuvants can cause or potentiate adverse vaccine reactions; induction of vaccine-associated (or injection site) sarcomas in cats may be one example. Most vaccines with added adjuvants studied in cats have led to pyogranulomatous reactions that could undergo malignant transformation to soft tissue sarcomas (see Chapter 84). Subunit vaccines can be superior to killed vaccines that use the entire organism since only the immunogenic parts of the organism are used. This decreases the potential for vaccine reactions.

Deoxyribonucleic acid (DNA) of infectious agents has been incorporated into some vector vaccines, which combines the advantages of attenuated and subunit vaccines. The DNA that codes for the immunogenic components of the infectious agent is inserted into the genome of a nonpathogenic organism (vector) that will replicate in the species being vaccinated. As the vector replicates in the host, it expresses the immunogenic components of the infectious agent, resulting in the induction of specific immune responses. Because the vector vaccine is live and replicates in the host, adjuvants and high-antigen mass are not required. Since only DNA from the infectious agent is incorporated into the vaccine there is no risk of reverting to the virulent parent strain, as occasionally occurs with attenuated vaccines. Only vectors that do not induce disease in the animal being vaccinated are used. Native DNA vaccines are also being evaluated for a number of infectious diseases.

## VACCINE SELECTION

Selection of optimal vaccines for use in dogs and cats is complicated. Multiple products for most infectious agents are available, but efficacy studies allowing for direct comparison of different products are generally lacking. Not all vaccines for a given infectious disease are comparable. For example, some high-antigen mass parvovirus vaccines for dogs break through maternal immunity by 12 weeks of age whereas other parvovirus vaccines fail to induce protective titers in normal animals. Long-term duration of immunity studies and studies evaluating a vaccine's ability to block infection by multiple field strains are not available for most individual products. The practitioner should request information concerning efficacy challenge studies, duration of immunity studies, adverse reactions, and cross-protection capability when evaluating a new vaccine. Vaccine issues are commonly debated in veterinary journals and continuing education meetings; these are excellent sources of current information.

 TABLE 99-2

Potential Advantages and Disadvantages of Vaccines

|  | ADVANTAGES | DISADVANTAGES |
| --- | --- | --- |
| **Attenuated** | Rapid protection<br>Long-lasting immunity<br>May require only one dose<br>Adjuvants not required<br>Inexpensive to produce<br>Induce good cell-mediated responses<br>Potentially induce immunoglobulin A (IgA) responses<br>May stimulate interferon production | Potential reversion to virulence<br>Potential virulence in immune suppressed<br>Potentially immunosuppressive<br>Adverse fetal effects |
| **Noninfectious** | Cannot revert to virulence<br>Infrequent contamination<br>Rarely immunosuppressive<br>Relatively safe in pregnancy | Hypersensitivity reactions<br>Require two or more doses<br>Short duration of immunity<br>Adjuvants usually required<br>Poor cell-mediated immune stimulation<br>Poor stimulation of secretory IgA |

Modified from Larson RL et al: Immunologic principles and immunization strategy, *Comp Contin Educ Pract Vet* 18:963, 1996.

Not all dogs and cats need all available vaccines. Vaccines are not innocuous and should only be given if indicated. The type of vaccine and route of administration for the disease in question should also be considered. A benefit, risk, and cost assessment should be discussed with the owner of each individual animal before determining the optimal vaccination protocol. For example, feline leukemia virus only lives outside the host for minutes, and so it is very unlikely that an owner would bring the virus into the household; thus cats housed indoors are not likely to come in contact with the virus. Feline leukemia virus vaccines are not 100% efficacious, and products containing adjuvant may induce soft tissue sarcomas in up to 1 in 1000 vaccinated cats. In this situation, the cat is significantly more likely to have a vaccine reaction than develop feline leukemia virus infection, and so vaccination is of questionable benefit.

Before administering vaccines, the animal should be evaluated for factors that may influence ability to respond to the vaccine (Table 99-3) or that may affect whether vaccination could be detrimental. Hypothermic animals have poor T-lymphocyte and macrophage function and are unlikely to respond appropriately to vaccination. Dogs with body temperature above 39.7° C respond poorly to canine distemper virus vaccines; this may be true for other vaccines as well. Immunosuppressed animals, including those with feline leukemia virus infection, feline immunodeficiency virus infection, canine parvovirus infection, *Ehrlichia canis* infection, and debilitating diseases, may not respond appropriately to vaccination; modified-live vaccines occasionally induce the disease in these animals. If high levels of specific antibodies are present, vaccine efficacy is diminished. This is a particularly important consideration when vaccinating puppies or kittens from well-vaccinated dams. Disease may also develop in vaccinated puppies and kittens because infection had already occurred and was incubating when the animal was vaccinated. Vaccines can be rendered ineffective from mishandling (Table 99-4). Vaccines should not be administered while the animal is under anesthesia because efficacy can be diminished and if a vaccine reaction occurs, it may be masked by the anesthesia.

Adverse reactions can potentially occur with any vaccine. Administration of any vaccine to animals with proven immune-mediated diseases, such as immune-mediated polyarthritis, immune-mediated hemolytic anemia, immune-mediated thrombocytopenia, glomerulonephritis, or polyradiculoneuritis, is questionable because immune stimulation may exacerbate these conditions. Modified-live vaccines can induce transient thrombocytopenia; therefore routine surgical procedures should be delayed for 4 weeks after immunization. Modified-live products may cause disease. For example, modified-live canine distemper virus vaccines occasionally induce clinical signs of central nervous system canine distemper virus infection when administered to dogs with concurrent parvovirus infection (see Chapter 6, p. 102). Bacterins are commonly associated with anaphylactoid or anaphylactic reactions. Vaccination has been associated with soft tissue sarcomas in some cats. Intranasal products can result in transient sneezing and coughing. Feline vaccines for which the viruses were grown on Crandall Reese feline kidney cell cultures induce antibodies that cross-react with feline renal tissues (Lappin and colleagues, 2002a). Whether this results in renal disease is currently unknown.

## VACCINATION PROTOCOLS FOR CATS

A physical examination, fecal parasite screen, and vaccine risk assessment should be performed yearly for all cats. The American Association of Feline Practitioners and Academy of Feline Medicine recently published vaccination guidelines for cats that have been endorsed by the American Animal Hospital Association and the American College of Veterinary Internal Medicine. The following recommendations were adapted from those guidelines.

 TABLE 99-3

**Potential Causes of Vaccine Failure**

Protective immune responses were not stimulated by the antigens in the vaccine (humoral versus cell-mediated).
The animal was exposed to a field strain of the organism the vaccine fails to protect against.
The vaccine-induced immune response waned by the time of exposure.
The vaccine-induced immune response was overwhelmed by the degree of exposure.
The vaccine was handled or administered improperly.
The animal was incubating the disease when vaccinated.
The animal was unable to respond to the vaccine because of immunosuppression.
The animal was unable to respond to the vaccine because of hypothermia or fever.
The animal had maternal antibodies that lessened the response to vaccination.
The modified-live product induced disease.

 TABLE 99-4

**Proper Vaccine Handling**

Maintain at the manufacturer's recommended temperature until administered.
Protect from contact with ultraviolet light.
Reconstitute immediately before use.
Do not mix vaccines in the same syringe.
Do not use chemically sterilized syringes with modified-live products.
If multiuse vials are used, mix well before withdrawing a dose.
Discard expired vaccines.

Modified from Larson RL et al: Immunologic principles and immunization strategy, *Comp Contin Educ Pract Vet* 18:963, 1996.

All healthy kittens and adult cats without a known vaccination history should be routinely vaccinated subcutaneously (SC) or intramuscularly (IM) for panleukopenia, rhinotracheitis, and calicivirus (FVRCP); intranasal products can also be used. Most vaccine-associated soft tissue sarcomas have been associated with feline leukemia virus and rabies virus vaccines with adjuvants added. However, tumors at injection sites have also been documented after both killed and modified-live FVRCP vaccines. Thus, intranasal FVRCP vaccines may be safer than injectable FVRCP vaccines.

Modified-live products should not be administered to clinically ill, debilitated, or pregnant animals but are preferred over killed products in healthy cats, since cell-mediated immune responses are superior. Kittens presented at 6 to 12 weeks of age should receive a modified-live or killed FVRCP with boosters given every 3 to 4 weeks until 12 weeks of age. Kittens presented past 12 weeks of age and adult cats with unknown vaccination history should receive two killed or two modified-live FVRCP doses 3 to 4 weeks apart.

All cats should be vaccinated against rabies. Rabies vaccine should be administered SC or IM in the lower right rear limb at 12 or 16 weeks of age depending on local ordinances. A new canarypox vector rabies vaccine (Merial, Duluth, Ga) that has minimal tissue irritation is available and so may be less likely than vaccines with adjuvants to be associated with soft tissue sarcomas.

At 1 year of age or 1 year after the last vaccination, booster FVRCP and rabies virus vaccines should be administered. After 1 year of age, risk of infection by herpesvirus 1, calicivirus, and panleukopenia should be assessed yearly. Based on several challenge studies, it has been recommended that FVRCP vaccines be given no more frequently than every third year; it is possible the duration of immunity is much longer. Colorado State University has recommended a 3-year FVRCP interval for over 4 years and has detected no significant problems. If a rabies product with known duration of immunity of 3 years is used, it should then be administered every 3 years; more frequent vaccination is not required for immunity and only increases the risk for vaccine reactions. The canarypox vector rabies vaccine is only approved for intervals of 1 year.

Serology can be used in lieu of arbitrary vaccination with FVRCP. In a study of 72 vaccinated and control cats that assessed three different vaccines, the positive predictive value of antibody titers against panleukopenia, calicivirus, and herpesvirus 1 were 100%, 100%, and 90%, respectively (Lappin and colleagues, 2002b). Both cats for which susceptibility to herpesvirus 1 infection was predicted incorrectly had only been vaccinated once. Results were similar using virus neutralization (New York State Veterinary Diagnostic Laboratory, Ithaca, N.Y.) or ELISA (Heska Corporation, Fort Collins, Colo). In the same study, 70.7%, 92.4%, and 68.5% of randomly screened, client-owned cats had titers predictive of protection against herpesvirus 1, calicivirus, and panleukopenia virus, respectively. These results suggest that use of an arbitrary vaccine interval leads to unneeded vaccination of the majority of cats.

Optional vaccines currently available for use in cats include *Chlamydophila felis* (previously *Chlamydia*), *Bordetella bronchiseptica*, feline leukemia virus, feline immunodeficiency virus, feline infectious peritonitis virus, *Giardia*, and ringworm. These vaccines should only be considered for use under special circumstances.

*Chlamydophila felis* infection in cats generally only results in mild conjunctivitis, and so whether vaccination is ever required is controversial. The use of this vaccine should be reserved for cats with a high risk of exposure to other cats and in catteries with endemic disease. Duration of immunity for *Chlamydophila* vaccines may be short-lived, so high-risk cats should be immunized before a potential exposure.

Many cats have antibodies against *Bordetella bronchiseptica*, the organism is commonly cultured from cats of crowded environments, and there are sporadic reports of severe lower respiratory disease caused by bordetellosis in kittens and cats of crowded environments or other stressful situations. However, the significance of infection in otherwise healthy pet cats appears to be minimal. For example, in client-owned cats in north central Colorado, the organism was rarely cultured from cats with rhinitis or lower respiratory disease. *Bordetella* vaccination should be considered primarily for use in cats at high risk for exposure and disease, such as those with a history of respiratory problems and living in humane shelters. Since the disease is apparently not life-threatening in adult cats, is uncommon in pet cats, and responds to a variety of antibiotics, routine use of this vaccine in client-owned cats seems unnecessary.

Several feline leukemia virus vaccines are currently available. Because of difficulties in assessment of efficacy studies it is unclear which vaccine is optimal. Feline leukemia virus vaccines are potentially indicated in cats allowed to go outdoors or that have other exposure to cats of unknown FeLV status. The vaccines are likely to be most helpful in kittens because as cats age, there is an acquired resistance to FeLV infection that limits usefulness of vaccination. Vaccinated cats should receive two vaccinations initially. Products with adjuvants should be administered SC or IM in the distal left rear thigh because of the risk for development of soft tissue sarcomas. A product without adjuvant is available and induces less inflammation than products with adjuvants (Merial, Athens, Ga). Maximal duration of immunity is unknown, so annual or biannual boosters are currently recommended. The vaccine is not effective in persistently viremic cats and so is not indicated. However, administration of the vaccine to viremic or latently infected cats does not pose an increased risk of vaccine reaction. FeLV testing should be performed before vaccination because the retrovirus serologic status of all cats should be known so appropriate husbandry can be maintained.

A killed vaccine containing immunogens from two FIV isolates was recently licensed for use in the United States (Fel-O-Vax FIV; Fort Dodge Animal Health, Overland Park, Kan). In prelicensing studies, 689 cats received 2051 doses of vaccine with side effects detected in less than 1%. In a challenge study performed 375 days after inoculation with three doses (3 weeks apart), 84% of the vaccinated cats did not become

FIV-infected and 90% of the controls became FIV-infected, giving a preventable fraction of 82%. However, the efficacy and safety of the vaccine have not been assessed under field conditions in large numbers of cats with multiple FIV strains (see Chapter 102). Whether the vaccine will induce vaccine sarcomas is currently unknown. The primary problem with FIV vaccination at this time is that the vaccine induces antibodies detectable by the currently available antibody test. Thus, after vaccination, the practitioner will be unable to determine whether the cat is infected by FIV. Polymerase chain reaction (PCR) for detection of FIV provirus is available in some laboratories, but as discussed in Chapter 97, standardization and external quality control for laboratories providing PCR testing are not currently performed.

A relatively safe, intranasal coronavirus vaccine that may protect some cats from developing feline infectious peritonitis is currently available. In pet cats, the seroprevalence of coronavirus infection is approximately 20% to 70%, but the incidence of disease caused by feline infectious peritonitis virus infection is only 1 in 5000 single-cat households. Because the incidence of disease is low, cats are commonly exposed to coronaviruses before vaccination, the duration of immunity is short, and the efficacy is less than 100%, coronavirus vaccination is currently considered optional for pet cats. The vaccine is indicated for seronegative cats entering a known feline infectious peritonitis–infected household or cattery. The efficacy of this vaccine has not been proven in cats with positive coronavirus serology. Many cats that are to be exposed to coronaviruses have done so by 16 weeks of age, and so if used, the vaccine may be more effective at 8 and 12 weeks of age.

A *Giardia* spp. vaccine has been introduced for use in cats. When given twice, the vaccine lessened numbers of cysts shed and lessened clinical disease after challenge with one heterologous strain. Although the company reported no significant adverse effects in preliminary studies, the vaccine is adjuvanted and given SC and so may ultimately be proven to be associated with fibrosarcomas. Because giardiasis is usually not life-threatening and usually responds to therapy, routine use in client-owned cats seems unnecessary. In addition, it is now known that there are multiple *Giardia* spp., including a feline-specific strain. It is unknown whether the vaccine is protective against strains other than the one used in challenge studies. Based on one study in dogs, it was proposed that the vaccine has utility as an immunotherapeutic agent. However, in one study of experimentally infected cats, the vaccine was ineffective for the treatment of giardiasis.

A killed ringworm vaccine is available for use in cats. This vaccine is indicated for treatment of disease in some situations but not as a preventative. Since the product contains adjuvants, granuloma formation occurs in some cats.

## VACCINATION PROTOCOLS FOR DOGS

The American Animal Hospital Association and the American College of Veterinary Internal Medicine formed a committee to develop canine vaccination guidelines. The following recommendations were adapted in part from those guidelines.

Routine vaccines include canine distemper virus, parainfluenza, adenovirus 2, and parvovirus (DA2PP). As in cats, modified-live products should not be administered to clinically ill, debilitated, or pregnant animals. Puppies born to vaccinated bitches and presented at 6 to 12 weeks of age should be vaccinated every 3 to 4 weeks until 14 to 16 weeks of age. Puppies presented between 12 and 16 weeks of age and adult dogs with unknown vaccination history should be given two vaccines, 3 to 4 weeks apart. Puppies between 6 and 8 weeks of age should receive a distemper-measles vaccine at that time and then receive routine vaccines at 10, 13, and 16 weeks of age. High-antigen mass, low-passage parvovirus vaccines are not needed after 16 weeks of age and are likely to be effective in most puppies that are vaccinated to 12 weeks of age.

Rabies vaccine is administered at 12 or 16 weeks of age depending on local ordinances. In areas in which rabies is endemic and exposure may occur before 16 weeks of age, vaccination at 8, 10, or 12 weeks of age may be indicated.

At 1 year of age or 1 year later the dog should return for a DA2PP and rabies booster vaccinations. If a rabies product with known duration of immunity of 3 years is used, it should then be administered every 3 years; more frequent vaccination is not required for immunity and only increases the risk for local and systemic vaccine reaction.

Dogs should be evaluated at least yearly for risk of infection by canine distemper virus, parainfluenza, adenovirus 2, and parvovirus while performing a physical examination and checking for enteric parasites. In one study of client-owned dogs, canine distemper virus titers and canine parvovirus titers suggestive of protection were detected in 97.6% and 95.1% of the dogs tested, respectively. Canine parvovirus vaccines may provide life-long immunity, and distemper virus titers are detected for up to 10 years in many dogs. Thus, in low-risk dogs, DA2PP vaccines should be administered no more often than every third year. Colorado State University has recommended a 3-year DA2PP vaccination interval for dogs after 1 year of age for more than 6 years. Canine parvovirus or canine distemper virus infection has not been detected in any dog. Positive serologic tests for canine distemper virus and canine parvovirus are predictive of resistance (New York State Veterinary Diagnostic Laboratory, Ithaca, N.Y.) and are used in lieu of arbitrary vaccination interval by some veterinarians.

Optional vaccines for use in dogs with high risk for developing the disease include *Bordetella bronchiseptica, Borrelia burgdorferi, Leptospira* spp., coronavirus, and *Giardia* spp.

*Bordetella bronchiseptica* vaccines are considered optional since the agent rarely causes life-threatening disease in otherwise healthy animals and is not the only cause of kennel cough syndrome. In addition, genetic information suggests that field strains of the bacterium vary considerably from vaccine strains. Thus it is unknown which field strains are protected against by currently available vaccines. In one study, concurrent use of an intranasal and parenteral product gave optimal protection in previously naïve dogs. In another study based on serum antibody anamnestic responses, administration of a parenteral product was superior to an intranasal product in previously vaccinated dogs. Serum antibody titers persist for months, so most dogs only need only one or two immunizations yearly. Optimally, booster vaccines should be administered 5 days before potential exposure.

*Borrelia burgdorferi* and *Leptospira* spp. vaccines can be administered to dogs residing in endemic areas but are generally not indicated for dogs in nonendemic areas. Efficacy of the vaccines is still in question. Vaccine reactions are common with bacterins. For *Leptospira,* products containing the most serovars are indicated. However, there are serovars in the environment that are not in any vaccines and there is minimal cross-protection between serovars. Thus it is important that clients realize that even though their dog has been given a *Leptospira* vaccine, 100% protection cannot be guaranteed. A product containing serovars *canicola, icterohemorrhagiae, grippotyphosa,* and *pomona* is now available (Fort Dodge Animal Health) and provides the greatest spectrum of protection (see Chapter 105). Dogs in endemic areas should receive three vaccinations 2 to 3 weeks apart. Duration of immunity is more than 1 year in dogs receiving three vaccinations.

For *Borrelia burgdorferi,* even in endemic areas the potential for vaccine reaction approximates the potential for developing Lyme disease. Thus, in endemic areas, vaccination may hurt as many dogs as it helps. In nonendemic areas, vaccination will hurt many more dogs than it helps. Dogs previously naturally infected with *B. burgdorferi* likely do not benefit from vaccination. Maintaining tick control is an important part of prevention of this disease.

Coronavirus infection in dogs results in mild gastrointestinal disease unless concurrent infection with parvovirus occurs. The virus rarely causes disease in dogs after 6 weeks of age. In one study of healthy dogs and dogs with diarrhea, coronavirus was only detected in one healthy dog. Based on these findings, vaccination against coronarvirus is not indicated in adult dogs.

A *Giardia* spp. vaccine has been introduced for use in dogs. The vaccine is given to dogs older than 8 weeks of age SC, twice, 2 to 4 weeks apart. In a clinical study of 755 dogs, adverse reactions were not reported. In a challenge study performed 12 months after the second inoculation, only 9 of 20 vaccinated dogs shed cysts, whereas all 10 placebo-inoculated dogs shed cysts. Vaccinated dogs shed cysts for an average of 7 days versus 37 days for placebo dogs. Average number of cysts shed per gram of feces per day was 0.8 and 670, for the vaccinated dogs and placebo dogs, respectively. It is now apparent that there are dog-specific *Giardia* strains; vaccine efficacy against these strains is unknown. Since the disease is usually not life-threatening and has a response to therapy of at least 90%, routine use in client-owned dogs as a preventive seems unnecessary. Immunotherapy with the *Giardia* vaccine has aided in the elimination of cyst shedding and diarrhea in some infected dogs. In one study of 17 dogs with resistant giardiasis, cyst shedding and diarrhea resolved in all dogs after administration of 2 doses of *Giardia* vaccine (Olson and colleagues, 2001).

## Suggested Readings

Appel MJ: Forty years of canine vaccination, *Adv Vet Med* 41:309, 1999.

Carmichael LE: Canine viral vaccines at a turning point—a personal perspective, *Adv Vet Med* 41:289, 1999.

Chalmers WSK et al: A comparison of canine distemper vaccine and measles vaccine for the prevention of canine distemper in young puppies, *Vet Rec* 135:349, 1994.

Dodds WJ: Vaccination protocols for dogs predisposed to vaccine reactions, *J Am Anim Hosp Assoc* 37:211, 2001.

Duval D et al: Vaccine-associated immune mediated hemolytic anemia in the dog, *J Vet Intern Med* 10:290, 1996.

Ellis JA et al: Effect of vaccination on experimental infection with *Bordetella bronchiseptica* in dogs, *J Am Vet Med Assoc* 218:367, 2001.

Greene CE: Environmental factors in infectious disease. In Greene CE, editor: *Infectious diseases of the dog and cat,* ed 2, Philadelphia, 1998a, WB Saunders, p 673.

Greene CE: Vaccine induced complications versus overvaccination. In *Proceedings of the sixty-fifth annual AAHA meeting,* Chicago, 1998b, p 368.

Greene CE et al: Canine vaccination, *Vet Clin North Am Small Anim Pract* 31:473, 2001.

Hoskins JD et al: Challenge trial of an intranasal feline infectious peritonitis vaccine, *Fel Pract* 22:9, 1994.

Kass PH et al: Epidemiologic evidence for a causal relationship between vaccination and fibrosarcoma tumorigenesis in cats, *J Am Vet Med Assoc* 203:396, 1993.

Keil DJ et al: Evaluation of canine *Bordetella bronchiseptica* isolates using randomly amplified polymorphic DNA fingerprinting and ribotyping, *Vet Microbiol* 66:41, 1999.

Lappin MR et al: Parenteral administration of FVRCP vaccines induces antibodies against feline renal tissues, *J Vet Intern Med* 16:351, 2002a.

Lappin MR et al: Use of serologic tests to predict resistance to feline herpesvirus 1, feline calicivirus, and feline parvovirus infection in cats, *J Am Vet Med Assoc* 220:38, 2002b.

Larson RL et al: Immunologic principles and immunization strategy, *Comp Contin Educ Pract Vet* 18:963, 1996.

McCaw DL et al: Serum distemper virus and parvovirus antibody titers among dogs brought to a veterinary hospital for revaccination, *J Am Vet Med Assoc* 213:72, 1998.

Macy DW: Vaccination against feline retroviruses. In August JR, editor: *Consultations in feline internal medicine,* ed 2, Philadelphia, 1994, WB Saunders, p 33.

Macy DW: Are we vaccinating too much? *J Am Vet Med Assoc* 207:421, 1995.

Olson P et al: Duration of immunity elicited by canine distemper virus vaccinations in dogs, *Vet Rec* 141:654, 1997.

Olson ME et al: The use of a *Giardia* vaccine as an immunotherapeutic agent in dogs, *Can Vet J* 42:865, 2001.

Postorino Reeves NC et al: Long-term follow-up study of cats vaccinated with a temperature-sensitive feline infectious peritonitis vaccine, *Cornell Vet* 82:117, 1992.

Roth JA: The principles of vaccination: the factors behind vaccine efficacy and failure, *Vet Med* 86:406, 1991.

Roth JA: Characterization of protective antigens and the protective immune response, *Vet Microbiol* 37:193, 1993.

Schultz RD: Current and future canine and feline vaccination programs, *Vet Med* 3:233, 1998.

Scott FW et al: Duration of immunity in cats vaccinated with an inactivated feline panleukopenia, herpesvirus, and calicivirus vaccine, *Fel Pract* 25:12, 1997.

Scott FW et al: Long term immunity in cats vaccinated with an inactivated trivalent vaccine, *Am J Vet Res* 60:652, 1999.

Smith CA: Current concepts: are we vaccinating too much? *J Am Vet Med Assoc* 207:421, 1995.

Tizard I: Risks associated with the use of live vaccines, *J Am Vet Med Assoc* 196:1851, 1990.

Twark L et al: Clinical use of serum parvovirus and distemper virus antibody titers for determining revaccination strategies in healthy dogs, *J Am Vet Med Assoc* 217:1021, 2000.

Van Kampen KR: Recombinant vaccine technology in veterinary medicine, *Vet Clin North Am Small Anim Pract* 31:535, 2001.

# CHAPTER 100

# Polysystemic Bacterial Diseases

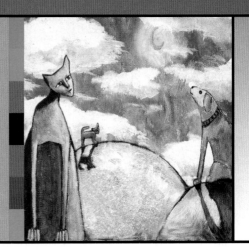

## CHAPTER OUTLINE

FELINE PLAGUE, 1259
LEPTOSPIROSIS, 1260
*MYCOPLASMA* AND *UREAPLASMA*, 1262

## FELINE PLAGUE

### Etiology and Epidemiology

*Yersinia pestis* is the facultatively anaerobic gram-negative coccobacillus that causes plague. The organism is maintained in a sylvan life cycle between rodent fleas and infected rodents, including rock squirrels, ground squirrels, and prairie dogs. Cats are susceptible to infection and can die after natural or experimental infection; dogs are very resistant to infection. Clinical disease is recognized most frequently from spring through early fall, when rodents and rodent fleas are most active. Most of the cases in humans and cats have been documented in New Mexico, Arizona, and California. Of the cases of human plague diagnosed from 1977 to 1998, 23 (7.7%) resulted from contact with infected cats (Gage and colleagues, 2000).

Cats are infected after being bitten by infected rodent fleas, after ingestion of bacteremic rodents, or after inhalation of the organism. After ingestion, the organism replicates in the tonsils and pharyngeal lymph nodes, disseminates in the blood, and results in a neutrophilic inflammatory response and abscess formation in infected tissues. The incubation period is 2 to 6 days after a flea bite, and 1 to 3 days after ingestion or inhalation of the organism. Outcomes in experimentally infected cats include death (6 of 16 cats; 38%), transient febrile illness with lymphadenopathy (7 of 16 cats; 44%), or inapparent infection (3 of 16 cats; 18%) (Gasper and colleagues, 1993).

### Clinical Features

Bubonic, septicemic, and pneumonic plague develop in infected humans and cats (Table 100-1); clinical disease is extremely rare in dogs. Bubonic plague is the most common form of the disease in cats, but individual cats can show clin-ical signs of all three syndromes. Most infected cats are housed outdoors and have a history of hunting. Anorexia, depression, cervical swelling, dyspnea, and cough are common presenting complaints; fever is detected in most infected cats. Unilateral or bilateral enlarged tonsils, mandibular lymph nodes, and anterior cervical lymph nodes are detected in approximately 50% of infected cats. Cats with pneumonic plague commonly have respiratory difficulty and may cough.

### Diagnosis

Hematologic and serum biochemical abnormalities reflect bacteremia and are not specific for *Y. pestis* infection. Neutrophilic leukocytosis, left shift and lymphopenia, hypoalbuminemia, hyperglobulinemia, hyperglycemia, azotemia, hypokalemia, hypochloremia, hyperbilirubinemia, and increased activities of alkaline phosphatase and alanine transaminase are common. Pneumonic plague causes increased alveolar and diffuse interstitial densities on thoracic radiographs. Cytologic examination of lymph node aspirates reveals lymphoid hyperplasia, neutrophilic infiltrates, and bipolar rods (Fig. 100-1).

Cytologic demonstration of bipolar rods on examination of lymph node aspirates, exudates from draining abscesses, or airway washings combined with a history of potential exposure, the presence of rodent fleas, and appropriate clinical signs lead to a presumptive diagnosis of feline plague. Since some cats survive infection and antibodies can be detected in serum for at least 300 days, detection of antibodies alone may indicate only exposure, not clinical infection. However, demonstration of a fourfold increase in antibody titer is consistent with recent infection. Definitive diagnosis is made by culture or fluorescent antibody demonstration of *Y. pestis* in smears of the tonsillar region, lymph node aspirates, exudates from draining abscesses, airway washings, or blood.

### Treatment

Supportive care should be administered as indicated for any bacteremic animal (see Chapter 98). Cervical lymph node abscesses should be drained and flushed while wearing gloves, a mask, and a gown. Parenteral antibiotics should be administered until anorexia and fever resolve. Streptomycin

TABLE 100-1

Clinical Findings in Cats with *Yersinia Pestis* Infection (Plague)

**Signalment**

All ages, breeds, and gender

**History and Physical Examination**

Outdoor cats
Male cats
Hunting of rodents or exposure to rodent fleas
Depression
Cervical swellings, draining tracts, lymphadenopathy
Dyspnea or cough

**Clinicopathologic and Radiographic Evaluation**

Neutrophilia with or without a left shift
Lymphopenia
Neutrophilic lymphadenitis or pneumonitis
Homogenous population of bipolar rods cytologically
   (lymph node aspirate or airway washings)
Serum antibody titers, either negative (peracute) or
   positive
Interstitial and alveolar lung disease

**Diagnosis**

Culture of blood, exudates, tonsillar region, respiratory
   secretions
Fluorescent antibody identification of organism in exudates
Fourfold increase in antibody titer and appropriate clinical
   signs

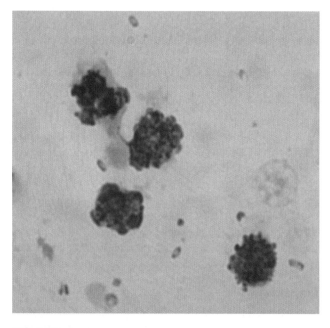

**FIG 100-1**
Lymph node aspirate from a cat with bubonic plague stained with Wright's stain. Bipolar rods are scattered throughout the field.

administered intramuscularly at 5 mg/kg every 12 hours, gentamicin administered intramuscularly or intravenously at 2 to 4 mg/kg every 12 to 24 hours, or enrofloxacin administered intramuscularly or intravenously at 5.0 mg/kg every 12 hours should be used initially. Although controlled studies on the efficacy of enrofloxacin for the treatment of feline plague are not available, I have successfully treated three cats with the combination of enrofloxacin and doxycycline. Chloramphenicol administered orally or intravenously at 15 mg/kg every 12 hours can be used in animals with central nervous system signs. Antibiotics should be administered orally for 21 days after the animal has survived the bacteremic phase; tetracycline at 20 mg/kg every 8 hours or doxycycline at 5 mg/kg every 12 hours are appropriate choices. In one study, 90.9% of cats treated with antibiotics survived, while only 23.8% of untreated cats survived (Eidson and colleagues, 1991). The prognosis is poor for cats with pneumonic or septicemic plague.

## Zoonotic Aspects and Prevention

Cats should be housed indoors and not allowed to hunt. Flea control should be used, and rodents should be controlled, if possible. Tetracycline or doxycycline at the doses listed for therapy should be administered for 7 days to animals with potential exposure. Human infection occurs following contact with infected fleas; contact with the tissues or exudates from infected animals, including cats; and from bites and scratches from infected cats. Even though fomite transmission is unlikely, since the organism is sensitive to drying, it can survive for weeks to months in infected carcasses and for up to 1 year in infected fleas. Cats from endemic areas with clinical signs of bacteremia, respiratory tract disease, or cervical draining areas or masses in the spring, summer, and early fall months should immediately be treated for fleas and handled while wearing gloves, a mask, and a gown until the diagnosis is made or denied. While hospitalized, infected cats should be handled by as few personnel as possible while in isolation. Exposed people should see their physician to discuss prophylactic antibiotic therapy. Cats are not infectious to humans after 3 days of antibiotic therapy. Areas where infected cats are handled should be thoroughly cleaned with routine disinfectants (see Chapter 99).

## *LEPTOSPIROSIS*

### Etiology and Epidemiology

Leptospires are 0.1 to 0.2 μm wide by 6 to 12 μm long, motile, filamentous spirochetes that infect animals and humans. Leptospirosis can be caused by many different serovars of *Leptospira interrogans* (Table 100-2). Dogs are infected by *L. australis, L. autumnalis, L. ballum, L. bratislava, L. bataviae, L. canicola, L. grippotyphosa, L. harjo, L. icterohaemorrhagiae, L. pomona,* and *L. tarassovi.* Cats are infected by *L. bratislava, L. canicola, L. grippotyphosa,* and *L. pomona* but appear to be resistant to clinical disease.

Prevalence and risk factors for cases of canine leptospirosis diagnosed at Veterinary Teaching Hospitals in North

TABLE 100-2

Reservoirs for *Leptospira interrogans* Serovars Known to Infect Dogs

| SEROVAR | PRIMARY RESERVOIR |
| --- | --- |
| *L. bataviae* | Dog, rat, mouse |
| *L. bratislava* | Pig, horse, dog (?) |
| *L. canicola* | Dog |
| *L. grippotyphosa* | Vole, raccoon, skunk, opossum |
| *L. harjo* | Cow |
| *L. icterohaemorrhagiae* | Rat |
| *L. pomona* | Pig, skunk, opossum |
| *L. tarassovi* | Cow, pig |

America between 1970 and 1998 were recently reviewed; the hospital prevalence was 37 cases per 100,000 dogs examined (Ward and colleagues, 2002). The numbers of cases diagnosed has increased since 1983. Infection by leptospires occurs in both rural and suburban environments in semitropical areas of the world with alkaline soil conditions. Clinical cases are most commonly diagnosed in the summer and early fall, and numbers of cases often increase in years with heavy rainfall. Infection by host-adapted species results in subclinical infection, and the host acts as a reservoir, shedding the organism intermittently. Infection by non–host-adapted species results in clinical illness. Leptospires are passed in urine and enter the body through abraded skin or intact mucous membranes. Transmission also occurs through bite wounds; by venereal contact; transplacentally; and by ingestion of contaminated tissues, soil, water, bedding, food, and other fomites. Hosts with preexisting antibody titers usually eliminate the organism quickly and remain subclinically infected. Leptospires replicate in multiple tissues of nonimmune hosts or hosts infected by a non–host-adapted species; in the dog the liver and kidneys develop the highest levels of infection. Inflammation induced by organism replication and by production of toxins leads to renal or hepatic disease. Clinical signs develop approximately 7 days after exposure; animals that are treated or develop appropriate immune responses usually survive. Some animals will clear the infection 2 to 3 weeks after exposure without treatment but develop chronic active hepatitis or chronic renal disease. Cats are generally subclinically affected but may shed the organism into the environment for variable periods of time after exposure.

## Clinical Findings

Dogs of any age, breed, or gender can develop leptospirosis if not previously immune. Male, middle-aged, herding dogs; hounds; working dogs; and mixed breeds are at greater risk than companion dogs younger than 1 year of age (Ward and colleagues, 2002). Most dogs have subclinical infection. Dogs with peracute clinical disease are usually presented for evaluation of anorexia, depression, generalized muscle hyperes-

 TABLE 100-3

Clinical Findings in Dogs with Leptospirosis

**Signalment**

All ages, breeds, and gender
Greatest risk in young adult, male, working dogs

**History**

Exposure to appropriate reservoir host or contaminated environment
Anorexia, depression, lethargy

**Physical Examination**

Fever
Anterior uveitis
Hemorrhagic tendencies, including melena, epistaxis, petechiae, and ecchymoses
Vomiting, diarrhea
Muscle or meningeal pain
Renomegaly with or without renal pain
Hepatomegaly
Polyuria/polydipsia
Icterus
Coughing or respiratory distress

**Clinicopathologic and Radiographic Evaluation**

Thrombocytopenia
Leukopenia (acute)
Leukocytosis (subacute)
Azotemia
Suboptimal urine-concentrating ability
Pyuria and hematuria without obvious bacteriuria
Hyperbilirubinemia and bilirubinuria
Increased activities of ALT, AST, ALP, and CK
Interstitial to alveolar lung disease
Hepatomegaly or renomegaly

**Diagnosis**

Culture of urine, blood, or tissues
Demonstration of the organism in urine by darkfield or phase-contrast microscopy
Demonstration of organismal DNA in urine, blood, or tissues by PCR
Combination of increasing antibody titer with clinical signs and response to therapy

thesia, tachypnea, and vomiting (Table 100-3). Fever, pale mucous membranes, and tachycardia are usually present. Petechiae, ecchymoses, melena, and epistaxis occur frequently from thrombocytopenia and disseminated intravascular coagulation. Peracute infections may rapidly progress to death before marked renal or hepatic disease is recognized.

Fever, depression, and clinical signs or physical examination findings consistent with hemorrhagic syndromes, hepatic disease, renal disease, or a combination of hepatic and renal disease are common in subacutely infected dogs. Conjunctivitis, rhinitis, tonsillitis, cough, and dyspnea occur occasionally. Oliguric or anuric renal failure can develop during the subacute phase.

Some dogs that survive peracute or subacute infection develop chronic interstitial nephritis or chronic active hepatitis. Polyuria, polydipsia, weight loss, ascites, and signs of hepatic encephalopathy due to hepatic insufficiency are the most common manifestations of chronic leptospirosis.

## Diagnosis

Multiple nonspecific clinicopathologic and radiographic abnormalities occur in dogs with leptospirosis and vary depending on the host, the serovar, and whether the disease was peracute, subacute, or chronic. Leukopenia (peracute leptospiremic phase), leukocytosis with or without a left shift, thrombocytopenia, regenerative anemia (from blood loss), or nonregenerative anemia (from chronic renal or hepatic disease) are common hematologic abnormalities. Hyponatremia; hypokalemia; hyperphosphatemia; hypoalbuminemia; hypocalcemia; azotemia; hyperbilirubinemia; decreased total carbon dioxide concentrations; and increased activities of alanine transaminase (ALT), alkaline phosphatase (ALP), and aspartate transaminase (AST) are common serum biochemical abnormalities that develop from renal disease, hepatic disease, gastrointestinal losses, or acidosis. Hyperglobulinemia is detected in some dogs with chronic leptospirosis. Dogs with myositis may have increased creatine kinase (CK) activity. Urinalysis abnormalities include bilirubinuria, suboptimal urine specific gravity in the face of azotemia, granular casts, and increased numbers of granulocytes and erythrocytes. The organism is not seen in the urine sediment by light microscopy. Renomegaly, hepatomegaly, and interstitial or alveolar pulmonary infiltrates are common radiographic abnormalities. Mineralization of the renal pelves and cortices can occur with chronic leptospirosis.

Detection of anti-*Leptospira* antibodies is commonly done by a microscopic agglutination test (MAT). Because of the wide range of leptospires infecting dogs, as many serovars as possible should be used for screening. *L. bratislava, L. canicola, L. grippotyphosa, L. harjo, L. icterohaemorrhagiae,* and *L. pomona* are commonly used. Positive titers can result from active infection, previous infection, or vaccination. Antibody titers can be negative in animals with peracute disease; seronegative dogs with classical clinical disease should be retested in 2 to 4 weeks.

Documentation of seroconversion (negative result becoming positive over time), a single MAT titer greater than 1:3200, or a fourfold increase in antibody titers combined with appropriate clinicopathologic abnormalities and clinical findings are suggestive of clinical leptospirosis. Definitive diagnosis is made by demonstrating the organism in urine, blood, or tissues. The organism can be seen in urine using darkfield or phase-contrast microscopy, but owing to intermittent shedding of small numbers of organisms, these procedures can be falsely negative. The organism can be cultured from urine collected by cystocentesis, blood, or renal or hepatic tissue. Materials for culture should be collected before administration of antibiotics, placed in transport media im-

mediately after collection, and transported to the laboratory as quickly as possible. Leptospiremia can be of short duration, and urine shedding of the organism can be intermittent, giving false-negative results. Polymerase chain reaction (PCR) can be used to demonstrate the organism in urine, blood, or tissues, but PCR is not widely available at this time.

## Treatment

Fluid therapy is required for most dogs; intense diuresis for renal involvement may be required (see Chapter 44). Hemodialysis may increase the probability of survival in dogs with oliguric or anuric renal failure. Dogs should be treated during the initial treatment period with ampicillin administered intravenously at 22 mg/kg every 8 hours or penicillin G administered intramuscularly or intravenously at 25,000 to 40,000 units/kg every 12 hours. Some quinolones have effect against leptospires and can be used in combination with penicillins during the acute phase of infection. Ampicillin and enrofloxacin were used concurrently in one study; 83% of infected dogs survived (Adin and colleagues, 2000). Penicillins should be administered for 2 weeks. Doxycycline administered orally at 2.5 to 5.0 mg/kg every 12 hours for 2 weeks following penicillin therapy should be used to eliminate the renal carrier phase.

## Zoonotic Aspects and Prevention

All mammalian serovars should be considered zoonotic to humans. Infected urine, contaminated water, and reservoir hosts should be avoided. Infected dogs should be handled while wearing gloves. Contaminated surfaces should be cleaned with detergents and disinfected (see Chapter 99).

Vaccines are available for some serovars, and they reduce severity of disease but not the chronic carrier state. Vaccination against serovars *L. canicola* and *L. icterohemorrhagiae* do not always cross-protect against other serovars. A product containing serovars *L. canicola, L. icterohemorrhagiae, L. grippotyphosa,* and *L. pomona* is now available (Fort Dodge Animal Health, Overland Park, Kan) and provides the greatest spectrum of protection (see Chapter 99). Dogs in endemic areas should receive three vaccinations 2 to 3 weeks apart. The duration of immunity is greater than 1 year in dogs receiving three vaccinations.

## MYCOPLASMA *AND* UREAPLASMA

### Etiology and Epidemiology

*Mycoplasma* spp. and *Ureaplasma* spp. are small, free-living microorganisms that lack a rigid, protective cell wall and depend on the environment for nourishment. Some *Mycoplasma* spp. and *Ureaplasma* spp. are considered normal flora of mucous membranes. For example, *Mycoplasma* spp. have been isolated from the vagina of 75% of healthy dogs (Doig and colleagues, 1981), the pharynx of 100% of healthy dogs (Randolph and colleagues, 1993a), and the pharynx of 35% of healthy cats (Randolph and colleagues, 1993b). Recently, *Haemobartonella felis* was shown to be a *Mycoplasma* with two species. Both *M. haemofelis* and *M. haemominutum* are associated with red blood cells and may result in development of anemia. These organisms are discussed in Chapter 85.

*M. cynos, M. spumans,* and *M. canis* are the species most commonly associated with disease in dogs. *M. felis* and *M. gateae* are the species most commonly associated with disease in cats. *Ureaplasma* spp. have been cultured from the vagina (40%) and prepuce (10%) of healthy dogs (Doig and colleagues, 1981).

The pathogenic potential for most *Mycoplasma* spp. or *Ureaplasma* spp. is difficult to determine because the organisms can be cultured from both healthy and sick animals. In many cases, *Mycoplasma* spp. or *Ureaplasma* spp. may be colonizing diseased tissues as opportunists secondary to inflammation induced by other etiologies. Other bacteria are usually isolated concurrently with *Mycoplasma* spp. or *Ureaplasma* spp., making it difficult to determine which agent is inducing disease.

*M. felis* conjunctivitis in cats, *M. felis* upper respiratory tract infection in cats, *M. gateae* polyarthritis in cats, and *M. cynos* (one strain) pneumonia in dogs have been induced experimentally. *Mycoplasma* spp. were isolated in pure culture from 20 of 2900 dogs with clinical signs of urinary tract inflammation (Jang and colleagues, 1984). *Mycoplasma* spp. were the only organism cultured from 7 of 93 dogs (Jameson and colleagues, 1995), 5 of 38 dogs (Randolph and colleagues, 1993a), 4 of 28 cats (Randolph and colleagues, 1993b), and 17 of 17 dogs or cats (Chandler and colleagues, 2002) with lower respiratory tract disease. These findings suggest that some species may be primary pathogens.

## Clinical Findings

*Mycoplasma* spp. or *Ureaplasma* spp. infection should be considered a potential differential diagnosis for cats presented for evaluation of conjunctivitis, sneezing and mucopurulent nasal discharge, coughing, dyspnea, fever, lameness with or without swollen painful joints, subcutaneous abscessation, or abortion (Table 100-4). In cats, *Mycoplasma* spp. or *Ureaplasma* spp. are not involved with lower urinary tract inflammation. *Mycoplasma* spp. or *Ureaplasma* spp. infection should be considered a potential differential diagnosis for dogs presented for evaluation of coughing, dyspnea, fever, pollakiuria,

hematuria, lameness with or without swollen painful joints, mucopurulent vaginal discharge, or infertility (see Table 100-4). *Mycoplasma* spp. and *Ureaplasma* spp. are generally not recognized cytologically and do not grow on aerobic media; infection should be suspected in animals with neutrophilic inflammation without visible bacteria or negative aerobic culture. The index of suspicion for *Mycoplasma* spp. or *Ureaplasma* spp. infection is higher if the animal has neutrophilic inflammation and has been poorly responsive to cell wall–inhibiting antibiotics such as penicillins or cephalosporins.

## Diagnosis

The clinical laboratory and radiographic abnormalities associated with *Mycoplasma* spp. or *Ureaplasma* spp. infections are similar to those induced by other bacterial infections. Neutrophilia and monocytosis are common in dogs with pneumonia; pyuria and proteinuria occur in dogs with urinary tract disease.

Preputial discharges, vaginal discharges, chronic draining wounds, airway washings, and synovial fluid from animals with *Mycoplasma* spp. or *Ureaplasma* spp. infections have nondegenerate neutrophils as the most common cell type. Dogs with lower respiratory tract disease and pure *Mycoplasma* cultures have alveolar lung patterns that cannot be differentiated from those in dogs with mixed bacterial and *Mycoplasma* cultures. In some dogs and cats with small airway disease evident radiographically, *Mycoplasma* spp. are isolated from the airways in pure culture (Chandler and colleagues, 2002). Joint radiographs of animals with *Mycoplasma*-associated polyarthritis reveal nonerosive changes.

Specimens for *Mycoplasma* spp. or *Ureaplasma* spp. culture should be plated immediately or transported to the laboratory in Hayflicks broth medium, Amies medium without charcoal, or modified Stuart bacterial transport medium. Specimens should be shipped on ice packs if the transport time is expected to be less than 24 hours and on dry ice if the transport time is expected to be longer than 24 hours. Since the organisms are part of the normal flora, culture of the mucous membranes of healthy animals is never indicated. Since *Mycoplasma* spp. or *Ureaplasma* spp. can be cultured from healthy animals, interpretation of positive culture results in sick animals is difficult. The disease association is strong if *Mycoplasma* spp. or *Ureaplasma* spp. are isolated in pure culture from tissues from which isolation is unusual (lower airway, uterus, joints). Response to treatment with drugs with known activity against *Mycoplasma* spp. or *Ureaplasma* spp. may help support the diagnosis of disease induced by these agents. Polymerase chain reaction assays are now available for detection of mycoplasmal DNA in several diagnostic laboratories (Veterinary Diagnostic Laboratory, Colorado State University, Fort Collins, Colo) but has the same diagnostic limitations as culture.

## Treatment

Tylosin, erythromycin, clindamycin, lincomycin, tetracyclines, chloramphenicol, aminoglycosides, and enrofloxacin are effective for treatment of *Mycoplasma* spp. or *Ureaplasma*

TABLE 100-4

Clinical Findings in Dogs and Cats with *Mycoplasma* spp. or *Ureaplasma* spp. Infections

| CATS | DOGS |
|---|---|
| Conjunctivitis | Pneumonia |
| Pneumonia | Nephritis, cystitis |
| Reproductive diseases or infertility | Reproductive diseases or infertility |
| Polyarthritis | Polyarthritis |
| Abscesses | |

spp. infections (see Chapter 98). Doxycycline administered orally at 5 mg/kg every 12 hours is generally effective in animals with a competent immune system or without life-threatening disease and is proposed to have the added benefit of being antiinflammatory. In animals with mixed infections or life-threatening disease, enrofloxacin administered orally at 2.5 to 5.0 mg/kg every 12 hours is a good treatment choice. In one cat with mycoplasmal polyarthritis, enrofloxacin therapy, but not doxycycline therapy, eliminated infection. Treatment for 4 to 6 weeks is usually required for lower airway, subcutaneous, or joint infections. Erythromycin administered orally at 20 mg/kg every 8 to 12 hours or lincomycin administered orally at 22 mg/kg every 12 hours should be used in pregnant animals.

## Zoonotic Aspects and Prevention

Although risk of zoonotic transfer is likely minimal, bite wound transmission of *Mycoplasma* spp. from an infected cat to the hand of a human has been reported (McCabe and colleagues, 1987). Most *Mycoplasma* spp. or *Ureaplasma* spp. infections in dogs and cats are opportunistic and associated with other causes of inflammation; thus they are not likely to be directly contagious from animal to animal. However, *M. felis* may be transmitted from cat to cat by conjunctival discharges. *Mycoplasma* spp. have been associated with respiratory tract disease in dogs and cats as primary pathogens and may be spread from animal to animal like *M. pneumoniae* in humans. Animals with conjunctivitis or respiratory tract disease should be isolated from other animals until clinical signs of disease have resolved (see Chapter 99). *Mycoplasma* spp. and *Ureaplasma* spp. are susceptible to routine disinfectants and rapidly die outside the host.

## Suggested Readings

FELINE PLAGUE

Eidson M et al: Feline plague in New Mexico: risk factors and transmission to humans, *Am J Publ Health* 78:1333, 1988.

Eidson M et al: Clinical, clinicopathologic, and pathologic features of plague in cats: 119 cases (1977-1988), *J Am Vet Med Assoc* 199:1191, 1991.

Gage KL et al: Cases of cat-associated human plague in the Western US, 1977-1998, *Clin Infect Dis* 30:893, 2000.

Gasper PW et al: Plague *(Yersinia pestis)* in cats: description of experimentally induced disease, *J Med Entomol* 30:20, 1993.

Kirkpatrick C: Plague. In Greene CE, editor: *Infectious diseases of the dog and cat,* ed 2, Philadelphia, 1998, WB Saunders, p 806.

Orloski KA et al: *Yersinia pestis* infection in three dogs, *J Am Vet Med Assoc* 207:316, 1995.

LEPTOSPIROSIS

Adin CA et al: Treatment and outcome of dogs with leptospirosis: 36 cases (1990-1998), *J Am Vet Med Assoc* 216:371, 2000.

Batza HJ et al: Occurrence of *Leptospira* antibodies in cat serum samples, *Kleintierpraxis* 32:171, 1987.

Birnbaum N et al: Naturally acquired leptospirosis in 36 dogs: serological and clinicopathological features, *J Small Anim Pract* 39:231, 1998.

Brown CA et al: *Leptospira interrogans* serovar *grippotyphosa* infection in dogs, *J Am Vet Med Assoc* 209:1265, 1996.

Greene CE: Leptospirosis. In Greene CE, editor: *Infectious diseases of the dog and cat,* ed 2, Philadelphia, 1998, WB Saunders, p 588.

Heath SE et al: Leptospirosis, *J Am Vet Med Assoc* 205:1518, 1994.

Rentko VT et al: Canine leptospirosis, *J Vet Intern Med* 6:235, 1992.

Ward MP et al: Prevalence of and risk factors for leptospirosis among dogs in the United States and Canada: 677 cases (1970-1998), *J Am Vet Med Assoc* 220:53, 2002.

Watson ADJ: *Leptospira interrogans* serovar *bratislava* infection, *J Am Vet Med Assoc* 199:1239, 1991.

Wohl JS: Canine leptospirosis, *Compend Contin Educ Pract Vet* 18:1215, 1996.

MYCOPLASMA AND UREAPLASMA

Chandler JC et al: Mycoplasmal respiratory infections in small animals: 17 cases (1988-1999), *J Am Anim Hosp Assoc* 38:111, 2002.

Doig PA et al: The genital mycoplasma and ureaplasma flora of healthy and diseased dogs, *Can J Comp Med* 45:233, 1981.

Foster SF et al: Pneumonia associated with *Mycoplasma* spp. in three cats, *Aust Vet J* 76:460, 1998.

Hooper PT et al: *Mycoplasma* polyarthritis in a cat with probable severe immune deficiency, *Aust Vet J* 62:352, 1985.

Jameson PH et al: Comparison of clinical signs, diagnostic findings, organisms isolated, and clinical outcome in dogs with bacterial pneumonia: 93 cases (1986-1991), *J Am Vet Med Assoc* 206:206, 1995.

Jang SS et al: *Mycoplasma* as a cause of canine urinary tract infection, *J Am Vet Med Assoc* 185:45, 1984.

Kirchner BK et al: Spontaneous bronchopneumonia in laboratory dogs with untyped *Mycoplasma* sp., *Lab Anim Sci* 40:625, 1990.

McCabe SJ et al: *Mycoplasma* infection of the hand acquired from a cat, *J Hand Surg* 12:1085, 1987.

Moise NS et al: *Mycoplasma gateae* arthritis and tenosynovitis in cats: case report and experimental reproduction of the disease, *Am J Vet Res* 44:16, 1983.

Moise NS et al: Clinical, radiographic, and bronchial cytologic features of cats with bronchial disease: 65 cases (1980-1986), *J Am Vet Med Assoc* 194:1467, 1989.

Randolph JF et al: Prevalence of mycoplasmal and ureaplasmal recovery from tracheobronchial lavages and prevalence of mycoplasmal recovery from pharyngeal swab specimens in dogs with or without pulmonary disease, *Am J Vet Res* 54:387, 1993a.

Randolph JF et al: Prevalence of mycoplasmal and ureaplasmal recovery from tracheobronchial lavages and of mycoplasmal recovery from pharyngeal swab specimens in cats with or without pulmonary disease, *Am J Vet Res* 54:897, 1993b.

Rosendal S: *Mycoplasma* infections. In Greene CE, editor: *Infectious diseases of the dog and cat,* ed 2, Philadelphia, 1998, WB Saunders, p 446.

Senior DF et al: The role of *Mycoplasma* species and *Ureaplasma* species in feline lower urinary tract disease, *Vet Clin North Am Small Anim Pract* 26:305, 1996.

Slavik MF et al: *Mycoplasma* infections of cats, *Fel Pract* 20:12, 1992.

## CHAPTER 101

# Polysystemic Rickettsial Diseases

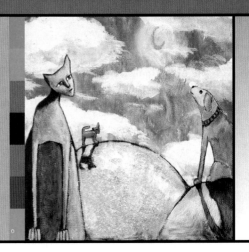

## CHAPTER OUTLINE

ROCKY MOUNTAIN SPOTTED FEVER, 1265
CANINE EHRLICHIOSIS, 1267
FELINE EHRLICHIOSIS, 1271
OTHER RICKETTSIAL INFECTIONS, 1271

## ROCKY MOUNTAIN SPOTTED FEVER

**Etiology and epidemiology.** Rocky Mountain spotted fever (RMSF) is caused by *Rickettsia rickettsii*. Other members of the genus also infect dogs in the United States; however, they are not associated with clinical disease but result in the production of antibodies that cross-react with *R. rickettsii* (see Diagnosis). For example, 17 of 22 canine sera submitted for *R. akari* (rickettsialpox in humans) indirect fluorescent antibody (IFA) testing serologically cross-reacted with *R. rickettsii* (Comer and colleagues, 2001). In another study of dogs coinfected with several tick-borne pathogens, infection with an uncharacterized rickettsial agent commonly induced cross-reacting antibodies to *R. rickettsii* (Kordick and colleagues, 1999). Canine RMSF is recognized predominantly in the southeastern states from April through September when the tick vectors are most active; cats are resistant to clinical infection. From 1993 to 1996, 52% of human cases of RMSF were reported from the south Atlantic region (Treadwell and colleagues, 2000). *Dermacentor andersoni* (i.e., American wood tick), *Dermacentor variabilis* (i.e., American dog tick), and *Amblyomma americanum* (i.e., Lone Star tick) are the principal vectors, host, and reservoir of *R. rickettsii*. The organism is maintained in nature in a cycle between ticks and small mammals like voles, ground squirrels, and chipmunks, and it is transmitted transovarially in ticks, so nymphs and larvae can be infected without feeding. *R. rickettsii* replicates in endothelial tissues (causing vasculitis) and so can lead to diverse and sometimes severe clinical manifestations of disease as soon as 2 to 3 days after exposure. Antiplatelet antibodies can be detected in many infected dogs, suggesting an immune-mediated component to the thrombocytopenia that is frequently present.

**Clinical features.** Any dog not previously exposed to *R. rickettsii* can develop RMSF. Frequently, the tick has fed and left the dog before the development of clinical signs. In one study, only 5 of 30 owners knew their dogs had been infested by ticks (Gasser and colleagues, 2001). After infection, the majority of dogs are subclinical; some develop acute disease with a clinical course of approximately 14 days. No age or sex predilection exists.

Fever and depression are the most common clinical signs (Table 101-1). Interstitial pulmonary disease, dyspnea, and cough occur in some dogs and gastrointestinal signs occur in some acutely infected dogs. Because the disease is generally acute, lymphadenopathy and splenomegaly are not as common as in dogs with ehrlichiosis. Petechiae, epistaxis, subconjunctival hemorrhage, hyphema, anterior uveitis, iris hemorrhage, retinal petechiae, and retinal edema occur frequently. Cutaneous manifestations can include hyperemia, petechiae, edema, and dermal necrosis. Hemorrhage results from vasculitis, thrombocytopenia from consumption of platelets at sites of vasculitis, thrombocytopenia from immune destruction, and in some dogs, disseminated intravascular coagulation. Central nervous system (CNS) signs include vestibular lesions (nystagmus, ataxia, head tilt), seizures, and hyperesthesia. Fatal RMSF is generally secondary to cardiac arrhythmias and shock, pulmonary disease, acute renal failure, or severe CNS disease.

**Diagnosis.** Clinicopathologic and radiographic abnormalities are common but do not definitively document RMSF. Neutrophilic leukocytosis, with or without a left shift and toxic cells, is found in most clinically affected dogs. Platelet counts are variable, but in one study, 14 of 30 dogs had less than 75,000 platelets/µl without evidence of disseminated intravascular coagulation (Gasser, 2001). In other dogs, coagulation abnormalities consistent with disseminated intravascular coagulation occur. Anemia occurs in some dogs, primarily from blood loss. Increased activities of alanine aminotransferase, aspartate aminotransferase, and alkaline phosphatase, as well as hypoalbuminemia from blood loss or third spacing of albumin in tissues secondary to vasculitis occur frequently. Because *R. rickettsii* does not result in chronic intracellular infection like ehrlichiosis, hyperglobulinemia is

## TABLE 101-1

### Clinical Abnormalities in Human Beings and Dogs with Rocky Mountain Spotted Fever

| CLINICAL ABNORMALITY | HUMAN BEINGS (N = 262) N (%) | DOGS (N = 79) N (%) |
|---|---|---|
| Low fever | 99 (37.8) (>37.8° C) | 67 (84.8) (>39.2° C) |
| High fever | 90 (34.4) (>38.9° C) | 54 (68.4) (>40° C) |
| Headache | 91 (34.7) | NR |
| Rash/petechiae | 88 (33.6) | 19 (24.1) |
| Myalgia/arthralgia | 83 (31.7) | 49 (62.0) |
| Anorexia | NR | 51 (64.6) |
| Known tick exposure | 67 (25.6) | 52 (65.8) |
| Nausea/vomiting | 60 (22.9) | 18 (22.8) |
| Diarrhea | 19 (7.3) | 16 (20.3) |
| Abdominal pain | 52 (19.8) | 30 (38.0) |
| Conjunctivitis/scleral congestion | 30 (11.5) | 34 (43.0) |
| Lymphadenopathy | 27 (10.3) | 43 (54.4) |
| Hepatomegaly | 12 (4.6) | 3 (3.8) |
| Splenomegaly | 16 (6.1) | 3 (3.8) |
| Depression/altered mental status | 26 (9.9) | 65 (83.0) |
| Vestibular deficits | 18 (6.9) | 41 (51.9) |
| Coma/unconsciousness | 9 (3.4) | 4 (5.1) |
| Seizures | 8 (3.1) | 10 (12.7) |
| Edema of face/ extremities | 18 (6.9) | 25 (31.6) |
| Polyuria/polydipsia | NR | 5 (6.3) |
| Pneumonitis/dyspnea/ cough | 12 (4.6) | 39 (49.4) |
| Icterus | 9 (3.4) | 4 (5.1) |
| Cardiac arrhythmias | 7 (2.7) | 8 (10.1) |
| Death | 4 (1.5) | 3 (3.8) |

Modified from Greene CE et al: Rocky Mountain spotted fever and Q fever. In Greene CE, editor: *Infectious diseases of the dog and cat,* ed 2, Philadelphia, 1998, WB Saunders, p 155 and Helmick CG et al: Rocky Mountain spotted fever: clinical, laboratory, and epidemiologic features of 262 cases, *J Infect Dis* 150:480, 1984. *NR,* Not reported.

rare. Renal insufficiency in some dogs causes azotemia and metabolic acidosis. Serum sodium, chloride, and potassium concentrations decrease in many dogs with gastrointestinal tract signs or renal insufficiency. In contrast to dogs with chronic ehrlichiosis, chronic proteinuria from glomerulonephritis is rare. Positive direct Coombs' test results occur in some dogs.

Nonseptic, suppurative polyarthritis occurs in some dogs. CNS inflammation usually causes increased protein concentrations and neutrophilic pleocytosis in CSF; some dogs may have mononuclear cell pleocytosis or mixed inflammation. No pathognomonic radiographic abnormalities are associated with RMSF, but both experimentally- and naturally-infected dogs commonly develop unstructured pulmonary interstitial patterns.

A presumptive diagnosis of canine RMSF can be based on the combination of appropriate clinical, historical, and clinicopathologic evidence of disease, serologic test results, exclusion of other causes of the clinical abnormalities, and response to antirickettsial drugs. Documentation of seroconversion or an increasing titer 2 to 3 weeks after initial serologic testing suggests recent infection. Diagnostic criteria used in one recent study included a fourfold rise in antibody titer or a single titer of greater than 1:1024 if the initial titer was submitted 1 week or more after initial onset of clinical abnormalities (Gasser and colleagues, 2001). Positive serum antibody test results alone do not prove RMSF because subclinical infection is common. In addition, positive serum antibody tests do not document infection by *R. rickettsii* because infection with nonpathogenic spotted fever group agents induce cross-reacting antibodies. Demonstration of *R. rickettsii* by inoculating affected tissues or blood into susceptible laboratory animals or by documenting the organism in endothelial cells using direct fluorescent antibody staining leads to a definitive diagnosis of RMSF but are not clinically practical. Polymerase chain reaction (PCR) can be used to document the presence of rickettsial agents in blood, other fluids, or tissues and will likely be clinically useful in the future.

**Treatment.** Supportive care for gastrointestinal tract fluid and electrolyte losses, renal disease, disseminated intravascular coagulation, and anemia should be provided as indicated. Overzealous fluid therapy may worsen respiratory or CNS manifestations of disease if vasculitis is severe.

Tetracycline derivatives, chloramphenicol, and enrofloxacin are the antirickettsial drugs used most frequently. Trovafloxacin and to a lesser extent, azithromycin, were beneficial for treatment of RMSF in experimentally inoculated dogs (Breitschwerdt and colleagues, 1999). Tetracycline (22 mg/kg PO q8h for 14 to 21 days) was commonly used historically. Doxycycline (5 to 10 mg/kg PO q12h for 14 to 21 days) is an alternative to tetracyclines; GI absorption and CNS penetration are superior to tetracycline, owing to increased lipid solubility. Chloramphenicol (22 to 25 mg/kg PO q8h for 14 days) can be used in puppies less than 5 months of age to avoid dental staining associated with tetracyclines. Enrofloxacin (3 mg/kg PO q12h for 7 days) is as effective as tetracycline or chloramphenicol. In one study of 30 dogs with RMSF, all dogs survived and there were no apparent differences in response rate between tetracycline, doxycycline, chloramphenicol, or enrofloxacin (Gasser and colleagues, 2001). Fever, depression, and thrombocytopenia often begin to resolve within 24 to 48 hours after starting therapy. Administration of prednisolone at antiinflammatory or immunosuppressive doses in combination with doxycycline did not potentiate RMSF in experimentally infected dogs. The prognosis for canine RMSF is fair; death occurs in less than 5% of affected dogs.

**Zoonotic aspects and prevention.** Because RMSF has not been reported twice in the same dog, permanent immunity is likely. Infection can be prevented by providing strict tick control. It is unlikely that people acquire *R. rickettsii* from contact with dogs, but dogs may increase human exposure to RMSF by bringing ticks into the human environment. People can also be infected when removing ticks with activated *R. rickettsii* from the dog by hand. As in dogs, RMSF in people is almost exclusively recognized from April to September when the tick vectors are most active. Untreated RMSF is fatal in approximately 20% of infected people.

## CANINE EHRLICHIOSIS

**Etiology and epidemiology.** *Ehrlichia* spp. are tick-borne *Rickettsia* that form intracellular clusters called morulae (Fig. 101-1). Clinical ehrlichiosis in dogs can be caused by infection with a variety of ehrlichial agents. Species from naturally-infected dogs include *Ehrlichia canis, E. risticii* var *atypicalis, E. platys, E. ewingii, E. chaffeensis,* and *Anaplasma phagocytophila.* The latter organism was previously known in different reports as *E. equi, E. phagocytophila,* and human granulocytic ehrlichia (HGE) but has now been designated a single species based on genetic sequencing (Dumler and colleagues, 2001). Vectors and primary clinical syndromes for the *Ehrlichia* species infecting dogs are summarized in Table 101-2. An individual dog can be infected by more than one ehrlichial agent.

*Ehrlichia canis* is the most common and causes the most severe clinical disease; it is maintained in the environment from passage from ticks to dogs, and *Rhipicephalus sanguineus* (i.e., brown dog tick) is the vector. The organism is not passed transovarially in the tick, so unexposed ticks must feed on a rickettsemic dog in the acute phase to become infected and perpetuate the disease. *Ehrlichia* spp. can be transmitted by blood transfusions, so blood donors should be serologically screened for evidence of infection. Dogs seropositive for *E. canis* have been identified in many regions of the world and most of the United States, but the majority of cases occur in areas with high concentrations of *R. sanguineus* such as the Southwest and Gulf Coast. *E. risticii* var *atypicalis* has been detected only in the United States to date. *E. platys* is most common in the southeastern United States, southern Europe, and South America. *E. ewingii* is most common in the southern parts of the mideastern states. *E. chaffeensis* infections are detected primarily in the southeastern United States. The distribution of *A. phagocytophila* is defined by the range of *Ixodes* ticks and so is most common in California, Wisconsin, Minnesota, and the northeastern states. This agent is also found in Europe, Asia, and Africa.

*Ehrlichia canis* infection causes acute, subclinical, and chronic phases of disease. Infected mononuclear cells marginate in small vessels or migrate into endothelial tissues, inducing vasculitis during the acute phase. The acute phase begins 1 to 3 weeks after infection and lasts 2 to 4 weeks; most immunocompetent dogs survive. The subclinical phase lasts months to

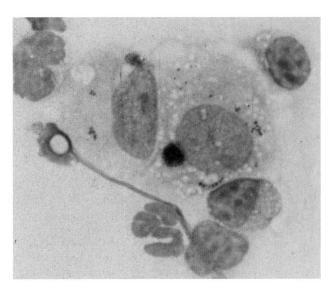

**FIG 101-1**
A morula consistent with *Ehrlichia* spp. is present in a mononuclear cell from a cat with clinical ehrlichiosis.

years in naturally infected dogs. Although some dogs clear the organism during the subclinical phase, the organism persists intracellularly in some, leading to the chronic phase of infection. Many of the clinical and clinicopathologic abnormalities developing during the chronic phase are from immune reactions against the intracellular organism. The variable duration of the subclinical phase of disease explains why *E. canis* infection does not have a distinct seasonal incidence like RMSF. However, acute phase disease is recognized most frequently in the spring and summer when the tick vector is most active.

**Clinical features.** Clinical disease from ehrlichial infection can occur in any dog, but its severity varies depending on the organism, host factors, and presence of coinfections. Virulence is thought to vary with different field strains of *E. canis.* Dogs with depressed cell-mediated immunity develop severe disease.

Clinical findings in dogs with *E. canis* infections vary with the timing of infection (Table 101-3). The clinical manifestations of acute phase disease are very similar to those of RMSF, owing to the development of vasculitis. Ticks are most commonly noted or reported on dogs during the acute phase of infection. Fever can occur in both clinical phases of infection but is more common in dogs with acute ehrlichiosis. Petechiae or other evidence of bleeding noted during the acute phase are generally caused by a combination of mild thrombocytopenia (consumption or immune-mediated destruction) and vasculitis; thrombocytopenia (consumption, immune-mediated destruction, sequestration, decreased production), vasculitis, and platelet function abnormalities occur in the chronic phase. The thrombocytopenia in the acute phase is generally not severe enough to result in spontaneous bleeding and so bleeding may be primarily from vasculitis and decreased platelet function.

TABLE 101-2

*Ehrlichia* spp. that Infect Dogs

| SPECIES | VECTOR | PRIMARY CLINICAL SYNDROMES |
|---------|--------|----------------------------|
| *Ehrlichia canis* | *Rhipicephalus sanguineus* | See text and Tables 101-3 and 101-4 |
| *Ehrlichia chaffeensis* | *Amblyomma americanum* *Dermacentor variabilis* | Subclinical; unclear in natural infections |
| *Ehrlichia ewingii* | *Amblyomma americanum* *Otobius megnini* *Ixodes?* | Polyarthritis, fever, meningitis |
| *Ehrlichia platys* | *Rhipicephalus sanguineus?* | Fever, thrombocytopenia, uveitis |
| *Ehrlichia risticii* | Unknown in dogs* | Unclear in natural infections, but similar to *E. canis* |
| *Anaplasma phagocytophila†* | *Ixodes* spp. | Fever, polyarthritis |

*Horses are infected by ingestion of *E. risticii*–infected metacercariae of trematodes found in intermediate host such as aquatic insects or snails.
†Previously *E. equi, E. phagocytophila,* and the human granulocytic ehrlichia (HGE) agent.

 TABLE 101-3

Clinical Abnormalities Associated with *Ehrlichia canis* Infection in Dogs

| STAGE OF INFECTION | ABNORMALITIES |
|--------------------|---------------|
| Acute | Fever |
| | Serous or purulent oculonasal discharge |
| | Anorexia |
| | Weight loss |
| | Dyspnea |
| | Lymphadenopathy |
| | Tick infestation often evident |
| Subclinical | No clinical abnormalities |
| | Ticks often not present |
| Chronic | Ticks often not present |
| | Depression |
| | Weight loss |
| | Pale mucous membranes |
| | Abdominal pain |
| | Evidence of hemorrhage; epistaxis, retinal hemorrhage, etc. |
| | Lymphadenopathy |
| | Splenomegaly |
| | Dyspnea, increased lung sounds, interstitial or alveolar lung infiltrates |
| | Ocular; perivascular retinitis, hyphema, retinal detachments, anterior uveitis, corneal edema |
| | CNS; meningeal pain, paresis, cranial nerve deficits, seizures |
| | Hepatomegaly |
| | Arrhythmias and pulse deficits |
| | Polyuria and polydipsia |
| | Stiffness and swollen, painful joints |

Pale mucous membranes usually only occur in the chronic phase during the development of pancytopenia. Hepatomegaly, splenomegaly, and lymphadenopathy are from chronic immune stimulation (i.e. lymphoreticular hyperplasia) and are detected most frequently in dogs in the chronic phase. Interstitial or alveolar edema secondary to vasculitis, pulmonary parenchymal hemorrhage secondary to vasculitis or thrombocytopenia, or secondary infections from neutropenia are mechanisms resulting in dyspnea or cough in some dogs with ehrlichiosis. Polyuria, polydipsia, and proteinuria are reported in some dogs that develop renal insufficiency.

Stiffness, exercise intolerance, and swollen painful joints occur in some dogs with suppurative nonspecific polyarthritis. Most dogs with polyarthritis from which the organism has been demonstrated have been infected with *E. ewingii* or *A. phagocytophila.* Ophthalmic manifestations of disease are

## TABLE 101-4

Clinicopathologic Abnormalities Associated with *Ehrlichia canis* Infection in Dogs

| STAGE | ABNORMALITIES |
| --- | --- |
| Acute | Thrombocytopenia |
| | Leukopenia followed by neutrophilic leukocytosis and monocytosis |
| | Morulae |
| | Low-grade, nonregenerative anemia unless hemorrhage has occurred |
| | Variable *Ehrlichia* titer |
| | PCR positive |
| Subclinical | Hyperglobulinemia |
| | Thrombocytopenia |
| | Neutropenia |
| | Lymphocytosis |
| | Monocytosis |
| | Positive *Ehrlichia* titer |
| | PCR positive |
| Chronic | Monocytosis |
| | Lymphocytosis |
| | Thrombocytopenia |
| | Nonregenerative anemia |
| | Hyperglobulinemia |
| | Hypocellular bone marrow |
| | Bone marrow/spleen plasmacytosis |
| | Hypoalbuminemia |
| | Proteinuria |
| | Polyclonal or IgG monoclonal gammopathy |
| | CSF mononuclear cell pleocytosis |
| | Nonseptic, suppurative polyarthritis |
| | Rare azotemia |
| | Increased ALT and ALP activities |
| | Positive *Ehrlichia* titer |
| | PCR positive |

common; tortuous retinal vessels, perivascular retinal infiltrates, retinal hemorrhage, anterior uveitis, and exudative retinal detachment occur. CNS signs can include depression, pain, ataxia, paresis, nystagmus, and seizures.

**Diagnosis.** Clinicopathologic abnormalities and radiographic abnormalities consistent with *E. canis* infection are summarized in Table 101-4. Neutropenia is common during acute phase vasculitis and after bone marrow suppression in the chronic phase. Chronic immune stimulation causes monocytosis and lymphocytosis; lymphocytes often have cytoplasmic azurophilic granules (i.e., large granular lymphocytes). Regenerative anemia is from blood loss (acute and chronic phases); normocytic, normochromic nonregenerative anemia is from bone marrow suppression or anemia of chronic disease (chronic phase). Thrombocytopenia can occur with either acute or chronic ehrlichiosis, but is generally more severe with chronic phase disease. Thrombocytopathies from hyperglobulinemia potentiate bleeding in some dogs with chronic ehrlichiosis. Chronic ehrlichiosis is classically

associated with pancytopenia, but any combination of neutropenia, thrombocytopenia, and anemia can occur. Changes in bone marrow cell lines associated with ehrlichiosis vary from hypercellular (acute phase) to hypocellular (chronic phase). Bone marrow plasmacytosis is common in dogs with subclinical and chronic ehrlichiosis and the disease can be confused with multiple myeloma, particularly in those dogs with monoclonal gammopathies.

Hypoalbuminemia in the acute phase is probably caused by third spacing of albumin in tissues because of vasculitis, whereas in chronic phase disease it is due to glomerular loss from immune complex deposition or chronic immunostimulation (i.e., monoclonal or polyclonal gammopathy). Prerenal azotemia can occur with acute or chronic disease; renal azotemia develops in some dogs with severe glomerulonephritis from chronic ehrlichiosis. The combination of hyperglobulinemia and hypoalbuminemia is consistent with subclinical or chronic ehrlichiosis. Polyclonal gammopathies are most common, but monoclonal (e.g., IgG) gammopathies can also occur.

Aspirates of enlarged lymph nodes and spleen reveal reactive lymphoreticular and plasma cell hyperplasia. Nondegenerate neutrophils are the primary cells in synovial fluid from dogs with polyarthritis caused by any *Ehrlichia* spp.; *E. ewingii* and *A. phagocytophila* morulae can be identified in synovial neutrophils from some dogs. Bone marrow aspirates in dogs with chronic ehrlichiosis typically reveal myeloid, erythroid, and megakaryocytic hypoplasia in association with lymphoid and plasma cell hyperplasia. Morulae from *E. canis* are rarely detected in the cytoplasm of mononuclear cells. Ehrlichiosis generally causes mononuclear pleocytosis and increased protein concentrations in CSF. Antiplatelet antibodies, antinuclear antibodies (ANA), antierythrocyte antibodies (by direct Coombs' test), and rheumatoid factors are detected in some dogs with ehrlichiosis, leading to an inappropriate diagnosis of primary immune-mediated disease.

No pathognomonic radiographic signs appear in dogs with ehrlichiosis. The polyarthritis is nonerosive, and dogs with respiratory signs most commonly have increased pulmonary interstitial markings, but alveolar patterns can occur.

Most commercial laboratories (using IFAs) and one point-of-care diagnostic test (IDEXX Laboratories, Portland, Me) use reagents that detect antibodies against *E. canis* in serum. These tests are generally used as the first screening procedures in dogs suspected to have ehrlichiosis. The American College of Veterinary Internal Medicine (ACVIM) Infectious Disease Study Group suggests that *E. canis* IFA antibody titers between 1:10 and 1:80 be rechecked in 2 to 3 weeks because of the potential for false-positive results at these titer levels (Neer and colleagues, 2002). If serum antibodies against *E. canis* are detected in a dog with clinical signs consistent with ehrlichiosis, a presumptive diagnosis of canine ehrlichiosis infection should be made and appropriate treatment begun. However, detection of antibodies alone is not diagnostic of ehrlichiosis (because of the existence of cross-reactive antibodies between *E. canis, Neorickettsia helminthoeca,* and *Cowdria ruminantium*). Additionally, negative test results do not totally exclude ehrlichiosis from the differential list, because clinical disease can be detected before seroconversion and the *E. canis* assays do not reliably detect antibodies against the other ehrlichial agents. IFA using *E. platys, A. phagocytophila,* and *E. risticii* are available commercially and may be indicated for the evaluation of dogs that are *E. canis* seronegative but still suspected to have ehrlichiosis.

Identification of morulae in cells documents *Ehrlichia* infection, but it is uncommon (with the exception of granulocytic strains). Examination of buffy coat smears or blood smears made from blood collected from an ear margin vessel may increase the chances of finding morulae. Some ehrlichia can be cultured, but the procedure is low-yield and expensive and so is not clinically useful.

PCR is now available commercially and can be used to detect organism-specific DNA in peripheral blood. It can be performed on joint fluid, aqueous humor, cerebrospinal fluid, and tissues. Blood PCR results can be positive before seroconversion in some experimentally inoculated dogs, and positive results document infection, whereas positive serologic tests only document exposure. However, as for serology, no standardization between laboratories currently exists, and insufficient quality control can lead to both false-positive and false-negative results. Until more information is available, the ACVIM Infectious Disease Study Group suggests using PCR with serology, not in lieu of it. Because antibiotic treatment rapidly induces negative blood PCR results, the clinician should draw the blood sample for testing and place it in an EDTA tube before treatment.

**Treatment.** Supportive care should be provided as indicated. Several different tetracycline, doxycycline, chloramphenicol, and imidocarb diproprionate protocols have been used. The ACVIM Infectious Disease Study Group currently recommends doxycycline (10 mg/kg PO q24h for 28 days). Clinical signs and thrombocytopenia should rapidly resolve. If clinical abnormalities are not resolving within 7 days, other differential diagnoses should be considered. Imidocarb diproprionate (5 to 7 mg/kg IM or SQ repeated in 14 days) has been used to successfully treat canine ehrlichiosis. Some patients develop pain at the injection site, salivation, oculonasal discharge, diarrhea, tremors, and dyspnea after administration of this drug. Quinolones are not effective for the treatment of ehrlichiosis.

Positive antibody titers have been detected for up to 31 months after therapy in some naturally infected dogs. Dogs with low (<1:1024) antibody titers generally revert to negative within 1 year after therapy. Dogs with antibody titers greater than 1:1024 often maintain positive antibody titers after therapy. It is undetermined whether these dogs are persistent carriers of the organism. Based on these findings, antibody titers are considered to be ineffective for monitoring response to therapy. The ACVIM Infectious Disease Study Group recommends monitoring resolution of thrombocytopenia and of hyperglobulinemia as markers of therapeutic elimination of the organism.

It is currently unknown whether ehrlichial infections are cleared by treatment. If PCR is to be used to monitor treatment, the ACVIM Infectious Disease Study Group recommends the following steps be taken: The PCR test should be repeated 2 weeks after stopping treatment. If still positive, treatment should be reinstituted for 4 weeks and retesting performed. If PCR results are still positive after 2 treatment cycles, an alternate antiehrlichia drug should be used. If PCR results are negative, the test should be repeated in 8 weeks, and if still negative it can be assumed therapeutic elimination is likely.

Whether to treat seropositive, healthy dogs is controversial. Arguments for and against testing or treating healthy dogs were reviewed by the ACVIM Infectious Disease Study Group (Neer and colleagues, 2002). The primary reason to treat a seropositive, healthy dog is to try to eliminate infection before development of chronic phase disease. However, treatment of healthy dogs is controversial for six reasons: (1) it is unknown whether treatment halts progression to the chronic phase; (2) not all seropositive dogs are infected; (3) not all seropositive dogs progress to the chronic phase; (4) it is unknown whether treatment eliminates infection; (5) even if infection is eliminated, reinfection can occur; and (6) treatment of healthy carriers may result in antimicrobial resistance.

Because further data are needed to make definitive recommendations, owners should be given the pros and cons and asked to make treatment decisions.

The prognosis is good for dogs with acute ehrlichiosis, and it is variable to guarded for those with chronic ehrlichiosis. Fever, petechiation, vomiting, diarrhea, epistaxis, and thrombocytopenia often resolve within days after initiation of therapy in acute cases. Bone marrow suppression from chronic phase ehrlichiosis may not respond for weeks to months, if at all. Anabolic steroids and other bone marrow stimulants can be administered but are unlikely to be effective because precursor cells are often lacking. Immune-mediated events resulting in the destruction of red blood cells or thrombocytes are likely to occur with ehrlichiosis, leading to the recommendation to administer antiinflammatory or immunosuppressive doses of glucocorticoids to acutely affected animals. Prednisone (2.2 mg/kg PO divided q12h during the first 3 to 4 days after diagnosis) may be beneficial in some cases.

**Zoonotic aspects and prevention.** Dogs and people are both infected by *Ehrlichia canis, E. chaffeensis,* and *A. phagocytophila.* Although people cannot acquire ehrlichiosis from handling an infected dog, dogs may be reservoirs for these agents and may play a role in the human disease by bringing vectors into the human environment. Ticks should be removed and handled with care.

Tick control should be maintained at all times. Because *Ehrlichia canis* is not passed transovarially in the tick, it can be eliminated in the environment by tick control or by treating all dogs through a generation of ticks. *Rhipicephalus* can only transmit *E. canis* for approximately 155 days; if tick control is not feasible, tetracycline can be administered (6.6 mg/kg PO daily for 200 days). During this time, infected dogs will not infect new ticks and previously infected ticks will lose the ability to transmit the organism. Blood donors should be screened serologically yearly.

# FELINE EHRLICHIOSIS

**Etiology and epidemiology.** *Ehrlichia canis* DNA (United States and Canada) and *Anaplasma phagocytophila* (previously *E. equi, E. phagocytophila,* and HGE) DNA (United States, Sweden, United Kingdom, Denmark) have been amplified from naturally exposed cats in several countries. *Ehrlichia*-like morula have been detected in mononuclear cells or neutrophils of naturally-exposed cats in the United States, Kenya, Brazil, France, Sweden, and Thailand. Cats experimentally infected with *E. risticii* develop morulae in mononuclear cells and occasionally develop clinical signs of disease, including fever, depression, lymphadenopathy, anorexia, and diarrhea. Cats experimentally infected with *A. phagocytophila* developed morulae in neutrophils and eosinophils, not mononuclear cells.

A presumptive diagnosis of ehrlichiosis has been based on detection of morulae or DNA in clinically ill cats or by the combination of positive serology, clinical or laboratory findings consistent with ehrlichial infection, exclusion of other causes, and response to an antirickettsial drug. Currently over 50 cases of suspected or proven cases of feline ehrlichiosis appear in the literature. It is unknown how the clinically ill, naturally exposed cats described in the literature were infected. Exposure to arthropods has been reported in about 30% of the cases. *Ixodes* spp. ticks have been associated with several cases of *A. phagocytophila* infection. Pathogenesis of disease associated with ehrlichiosis in cats is unknown.

**Clinical features.** All ages of cats have been infected; most cats were domestic short haired, and both males and females have been affected. Anorexia, fever, inappetence, lethargy, weight loss, hyperesthesia or joint pain, pale mucous membranes, splenomegaly, dyspnea, and lymphadenomegaly were the most common historical and physical examination abnormalities. Concurrent diseases are rarely reported but have included *Haemobartonella felis* (i.e., *Mycoplasma*) infection and lymphoma.

**Diagnosis.** Anemia is common and is usually nonregenerative. Leukopenia; leukocytosis characterized by neutrophilia, lymphocytosis, monocytosis; and intermittent thrombocytopenia were reported for some cats. Hyperglobulinemia was reported for multiple cats; protein electrophoresis documented polyclonal gammopathy in the cat assayed. An epidemiologic link has been made between the presence of *Ehrlichia* spp. antibodies in serum and monoclonal gammopathy (Stubbs and colleagues, 2000).

Some cats with suspected clinical ehrlichiosis seroreacted to *E. canis, E. risticii,* or *A. phagocytophila* morulae. Antibodies that seroreact to more than one ehrlichia are sometimes detected. Some cats infected with *E. canis* are seronegative. In contrast, most *A phagocytophila* infected cats have strongly positive antibody test results. Western blot immunoassay has been used to confirm some *E. risticii* positive results. Positive serologic test results occur in both healthy and clinically ill cats, and so a diagnosis of clinical ehrlichiosis should not be based on serologic test results alone. A tentative diagnosis of feline clinical ehrlichiosis can be based on the combination of positive serologic test results, clinical signs of disease consistent with *Ehrlichia* infection, exclusion of other causes of the disease syndrome, and response to antirickettsial drugs. *Ehrlichia* spp. has been cultured from some cats on monocyte cell cultures. PCR and gene sequencing can also be used to confirm infection and should be considered the tests of choice at this time. However, as for dogs no standardization exists among laboratories providing *Ehrlichia* PCR.

**Treatment.** Clinical improvement after therapy with tetracycline, doxycycline, or imidocarb dipropionate was reported for most cats. However, for some cats a positive response to therapy was a criterion for the diagnosis of ehrlichiosis. The current recommendation of the ACVIM Infectious Disease Study Group is to give doxycycline (10 mg/kg PO q24h for 28 days). For cats with treatment failure or those intolerant of doxycycline, imidocarb diproprionate can be given safely (5 mg/kg IM or SQ twice, 14 days apart) (Lappin and colleagues, 2002). Salivation and pain at the injection site are the common side effects.

**Zoonotic aspects and prevention.** Cats are known to be infected by *E. canis* and *A. phagocytophila,* agents that also infect people. However, direct transmission of *Ehrlichia* does not occur. Care should be taken when removing ticks, and arthropod control should be maintained at all time for cats, particularly if allowed outdoors.

# OTHER RICKETTSIAL INFECTIONS

*Neorickettsia helminthoeca* (i.e., salmon poisoning) causes enteric signs of disease in dogs from the Pacific Northwest. *Coxiella burnetii* infection is associated with parturient or aborting cats and is primarily a zoonotic disease (see Chapter 105). *Haemobartonella felis* has been reclassified as a *Mycoplasma* (see Chapter 85).

## Suggested Readings

ROCKY MOUNTAIN SPOTTED FEVER

Breitschwerdt EB et al: Efficacy of chloramphenicol, enrofloxacin, and tetracycline for treatment of experimental Rocky Mountain spotted fever in dogs, *Antimicrob Agents Chemother* 35:2375, 1991.

Breitschwerdt EB et al: Prednisolone at anti-inflammatory or immunosuppressive dosages in conjunction with doxycycline does not potentiate the severity of *Rickettsia rickettsii* infection in dogs, *Antimicrob Agents Chemother* 41:141, 1997.

Breitschwerdt EB et al: Efficacy of doxycycline, azithromycin, or trovafloxacin for treatment of experimental Rocky Mountain spotted fever in dogs, *Antimicrob Agents Chemother* 43:813, 1999.

Comer JA et al: Serologic evidence of *Rickettsia akari* infection among dogs in a metropolitan city, *J Am Vet Med Assoc* 218:1780, 2001.

Davidson MG et al: Identification of *Rickettsiae* in cutaneous biopsy specimens from dogs with experimental Rocky Mountain spotted fever, *J Vet Int Med* 3:8, 1989.

Davidson MG et al: Ocular manifestations of Rocky Mountain spotted fever in dogs, *J Am Vet Med Assoc* 194:777, 1989.

Drost WT et al: Thoracic radiographic findings in dogs infected with *Rickettsia rickettsii, Vet Radiol Ultrasound* 38:260, 1997.

Gasser AM et al: Canine Rocky Mountain spotted fever: a retrospective study of 30 cases, *J Am Anim Hosp Assoc* 37:41, 2001.

Greene CE et al: Rocky Mountain spotted fever and Q fever. In Greene CE, editor: *Infectious diseases of the dog and cat,* ed 2, Philadelphia, 1998, WB Saunders, p 155.

Grindem CB et al: Platelet-associated immunoglobulin (antiplatelet antibody) in canine Rocky Mountain spotted fever and ehrlichiosis, *J Am Anim Hosp Assoc* 35:56, 1999.

Helmick CG et al: Rocky Mountain spotted fever: clinical, laboratory, and epidemiological features of 262 cases, *J Infect Dis* 150:480, 1984.

Kordick SK et al: Coinfection with multiple tick-borne pathogens in a Walker Hound kennel in North Carolina, *J Clin Microbiol* 37:2631, 1999.

Suksawat J et al: Serologic and molecular evidence of coinfection with multiple vector-borne pathogens in dogs from Thailand, *J Vet Intern Med* 15:453, 2001.

Weiser IB et al: Dermal necrosis associated with Rocky Mountain spotted fever in four dogs, *J Am Vet Med Assoc* 195:1756, 1989.

CANINE EHRLICHIOSIS

Anderson BE et al: *Ehrlichia chaffeensis,* a new species associated with human ehrlichiosis, *J Clin Microbiol* 29:2838, 1991.

Anderson BE et al: *Ehrlichia ewingii* sp. nov., the etiologic agent of canine granulocytic ehrlichiosis, *Int J System Bacteriol* 42:299, 1992.

Bartsch RC et al: Post-therapy antibody titers in dogs with ehrlichiosis: follow-up study on 68 patients treated primarily with tetracycline and/or doxycycline, *J Vet Int Med* 10:271, 1996.

Breischtwerdt E et al: Monoclonal gammopathy associated with naturally occurring canine ehrlichiosis, *J Vet Intern* 1:2, 1987.

Chen SM et al: Identification of a granulocytic *Ehrlichia* species as the etiologic agent of human disease, *J Clin Microbiol* 32:589, 1994.

Dawson JE et al: Polymerase chain reaction evidence of *Ehrlichia chaffeensis,* an etiologic agent of human ehrlichiosis, in dogs from southeast Virginia, *Am J Vet Res* 57:1175, 1996.

Dumler JS et al: Reorganization of genera in the families Rickettsiaceae and Anaplasmataceae in the order Rickettsiales: unification of some species of *Ehrlichia* with *Anaplasma, Cowdria* with *Ehrlichia* and *Ehrlichia* with *Neorickettsia,* descriptions of six new species combinations and designation of *Ehrlichia equi* and "HGE agent" as subjective synonyms of *Ehrlichia phagocytophila, Int J Syst Evol Microbiol* 51:2145, 2001.

Iqbal Z et al: Comparison of PCR with other tests for early diagnosis of canine ehrlichiosis, *J Clin Microbiol* 32:1658, 1994.

Iqbal Z et al: Reisolation of *Ehrlichia canis* from blood and tissues of dogs after doxycycline treatment, *J Clin Microbiol* 32:1644, 1994.

Kakoma I et al: Serologically atypical canine ehrlichiosis associated with *Ehrlichia risticii* "infection," *J Am Vet Med Assoc* 199:1120, 1991.

Lewis GE et al: Experimentally induced infection of dogs, cats, and nonhuman primates with *Ehrlichia equi,* etiologic agent of equine ehrlichiosis, *J Am Vet Med Assoc* 36:85, 1975.

Neer TM et al: Consensus statement on ehrlichial disease of small animals from the Infectious Disease Study Group of the ACVIM, *J Vet Int Med,* 2002 (in press).

Ristic M et al: Susceptibility of dogs to infection with *Ehrlichia risticii,* causative agent of equine monocytic ehrlichiosis (Potomac horse fever), *Am J Vet Res* 49:1497, 1988.

Stockham SL et al: Evaluation of granulocytic ehrlichiosis in dogs of Missouri, including serologic status to *Ehrlichia canis, Ehrlichia equi,* and *Borrelia burgdorferi, Am J Vet Res* 53:63, 1992.

Weiser MG et al: Granular lymphocytosis and hyperproteinemia in dogs with chronic ehrlichiosis, *J Am Anim Hosp Assoc* 27:84, 1991.

FELINE EHRLICHIOSIS

Artursson K et al: Diagnosis of borreliosis and granulocytic ehrlichiosis of horses, dogs, and cats in Sweden, *Svensk Veterinartidning* 45:331, 1994.

Beaufils JP: Ehrlichiosis: clinical aspects in dogs and cats, *Compend Contin Educ* 19(suppl):57, 1997.

Beaufils JP et al: *Ehrlichia* infection in cats: a review of three cases, *Pratique Medicale Chirurgicate de l'Animale de Compagnie* 30:397, 1995.

Bjoersdorff A et al: Feline granulocytic ehrlichiosis—a report of a new clinical entity and characterization of the new infectious agent, *J Sm Anim Pract* 40:20, 1999.

Bouloy RP et al: Clinical ehrlichiosis in a cat, *J Am Vet Med Assoc* 204:1475, 1994.

Breitschwerdt E et al: Molecular evidence of *Ehrlichia canis* infection in cats from North America. Proceedings of the ACVIM Forum, Denver Colo, May 2001.

Buoro IBJ et al: Feline anaemia associated with *Ehrlichia*-like bodies in three domestic short-haired cats, *Vet Rec* 125:434, 1989.

Charpentier F et al: Probable case of ehrlichiosis in a cat, *Bull Acad Vet Fr* 59:287, 1986.

Dawson JE et al: Susceptibility of cats to infection with *E. risticii,* causative agent of equine monocytic ehrlichiosis, *Am J Vet Res* 49:2096, 1988.

Jittapalapong S et al: Preliminary survey on blood parasites of cats in Bangkhen District Area, *Kasetsart J Nat Sci* 27:330, 1993.

Lappin MR et al: *Ehrlichia equi* infection of 2 cats from Massachusetts, *American Society of Rickettsiology,* August 2001 (abstract).

Lappin MR et al: Effects of imidocarb diprorionate in cats with chronic haemobartonellosis, *Vet Ther* 3:144, 2002.

Lewis GE et al: Experimentally induced infection of dogs, cats, and nonhuman primates with *Ehrlichia equi,* etiologic agent of equine ehrlichiosis, *J Am Vet Med Assoc* 36:85, 1975.

Maeda K et al: Human infection with *Ehrlichia canis,* a leukocytic rickettsia, *N Engl J Med* 316:853, 1987.

Matthewman LA et al: Antibodies in cat sera from southern Africa react with antigens of *Ehrlichia canis, Vet Rec* 138:364, 1996.

Peavy GM et al: Suspected ehrlichial infection in five cats from a household, *J Am Vet Med Assoc* 210:231, 1997.

Stubbs CJ et al: Feline ehrlichiosis; literature review and serologic survey, *Compend Contin Educ* 22:307, 2000.

# C H A P T E R 102

# Polysystemic Viral Diseases

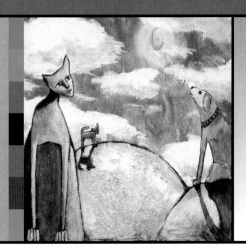

## CHAPTER OUTLINE

CANINE DISTEMPER VIRUS, 1273
FELINE CORONAVIRUS, 1275
FELINE IMMUNODEFICIENCY VIRUS, 1278
FELINE LEUKEMIA VIRUS, 1281

There are multiple viral infections of dogs and cats. Several, including canine distemper virus (CDV), some feline coronaviruses, feline leukemia virus (FeLV), and feline immunodeficiency virus (FIV), can cause systemic signs of disease. Please see other chapters for a discussion of viral diseases more specific to one organ system.

## CANINE DISTEMPER VIRUS

### Etiology and Epidemiology

Canine distemper virus induces disease predominantly in terrestrial carnivores, but other species, including seals, ferrets, porpoises, exotic Felidae, and a nonhuman primate have been infected by either CDV or a related virus. The virus replicates in lymphoid, nervous, and epithelial tissues and is shed in respiratory exudates, feces, saliva, urine, and conjunctival exudates for up to 60 to 90 days after natural infection. After inhalation, the virus is engulfed by macrophages and within 24 hours is carried by lymphatics to tonsillar, pharyngeal, and bronchial lymph nodes, where replication occurs. Central nervous system (CNS) and epithelial tissues are infected approximately 8 to 14 days after infection.

The degree of clinical illness and the tissues involved vary depending on the strain of the virus and the immune status of the host (Greene and colleagues, 1990). Nonimmune dogs of any age are susceptible, but disease is most common in puppies between 3 and 6 months of age. Massive replication of the virus in the epithelial cells of the respiratory tract, gastrointestinal system, and genitourinary system occurs in dogs with poor immune responses by days 9 to 14 after infection; these dogs usually die due to polysystemic disease. In those dogs with moderate immune responses by day 9 to 14 after infection, the virus replicates in epithelial tissues and may have resultant clinical signs of disease. Dogs with good cell-mediated responses and virus-neutralizing antibody titers by day 14 after infection clear the virus from most tissues and may not be clinically affected. Most infected dogs develop CNS infection, but clinical signs of CNS disease occur only in dogs with low or no antibody response. Acute demyelination results from restrictive infection of oligodendrogliocytes and subsequent necrosis; chronic demyelination is due to immune-mediated mechanisms, including antimyelin antibodies and CDV immune complex formation and removal.

### Clinical Features

Many clinically affected dogs are unvaccinated, failed to receive colostrum from an immune bitch, were inappropriately vaccinated, or are immunosuppressed, and also have a history of exposure to infected animals. Owners generally present affected dogs for evaluation of depression, malaise, oculonasal discharge, cough, vomiting, diarrhea, or CNS signs. Dogs with poor immune responses generally have the most severe signs and progress rapidly to life-threatening disease. Some partially immune dogs have only mild respiratory disease, presumptively diagnosed as kennel cough syndrome. Tonsillar enlargement, fever, and mucopurulent ocular discharge are common physical examination findings. Increased bronchial sounds, crackles, and wheezes are usually ausculted in dogs with bronchopneumonia.

Hyperesthesia, seizures, cerebellar or vestibular disease, paresis, and chorea myoclonus are common CNS signs that generally develop within 21 days of recovery from systemic disease (Table 102-1; also see Chapter 71). CNS disease is generally progressive and carries a poor prognosis. Systemic signs of disease are not recognized in approximately 30% of dogs with CNS signs of disease. Old-dog encephalitis is a chronic progressive panencephalitis in older dogs (>6 years of age) thought to be due to CDV infection in which microglial proliferation and neuronal degeneration in the cerebral cortex result in depression, circling, head-pressing, and visual deficits (see Chapter 71 of the neurology section for further discussion of CNS distemper).

TABLE 102-1

**Clinical Manifestations of Canine Distemper Virus Infection**

| | |
|---|---|
| *In utero* infection | Stillbirth |
| | Abortion |
| | Fading puppy syndrome in the neonatal period |
| | Central nervous system signs at birth |
| Gastrointestinal tract disease | Vomiting |
| | Small bowel diarrhea |
| Respiratory tract disease | Mucoid to mucopurulent nasal discharge |
| | Sneezing |
| | Coughing with increased bronchovesicular sounds or crackles on auscultation |
| | Dyspnea |
| Ocular disease | Retinochoroiditis, medallion lesions (see Fig. 102-1), optic neuritis |
| | Keratoconjunctivitis sicca |
| | Mucopurulent ocular discharge |
| Neurologic disease | |
|   Spinal cord disease | Paresis and ataxia |
|   Central vestibular disease | Head tilt, nystagmus, other cranial nerve and conscious proprioception deficits |
|   Cerebellar disease | Ataxia, head bobbing, hypermetria |
|   Cerebral disease | Generalized or partial seizures ("chewing gum fits"), depression, unilateral or bilateral blindness |
|   Chorea myoclonus | Rhythmic jerking of single muscles or muscle groups |
| Miscellaneous | Fever |
| | Anorexia |
| | Tonsillar enlargement |
| | Dehydration |
| | Pustular dermatosis |
| | Hyperkeratosis of the nose and footpads |
| | Enamel hypoplasia in surviving puppies |

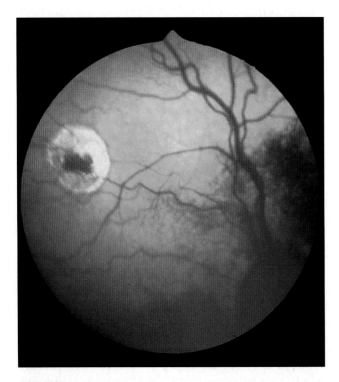

**FIG 102-1**
Medallion lesions resulting from canine distemper virus infection. (Courtesy Dr. Cynthia Powell, Colorado State University, Fort Collins, Colo.)

Ocular abnormalities associated with CDV infection include anterior uveitis, optic neuritis with resultant blindness and dilated pupils, and retinochoroiditis. The combination of retinochoroiditis and encephalitis are detected in approximately 40% of affected dogs. Keratoconjunctivitis sicca and hyperreflective retinal scars called *medallion lesions* occur in some dogs with chronic infection (Fig. 102-1).

A number of other, less common syndromes have been attributed to CDV infection. Dogs infected prior to the development of permanent dentition usually have enamel hypoplasia. Hyperkeratosis of the nose and footpads and pustular dermatosis are the most common dermatologic abnormalities. Puppies infected transplacentally can be stillborn, aborted, or born with CNS disease.

## Diagnosis

The combination of clinical findings and routine clinicopathologic and radiographic evaluation usually leads to a presumptive diagnosis of CDV infection. Lymphopenia and mild thrombocytopenia are consistent hematologic abnormalities. Interstitial and alveolar pulmonary infiltrates are common radiographic findings in dogs with respiratory disease. Although some dogs with CNS infection have normal cerebrospinal fluid (CSF) analyses, most have mononuclear cell pleocytosis and increased protein concentrations. The ratio of serum-to-CSF IgG and albumin is commonly high in dogs with encephalitis but only documents inflammation of the CNS, not CDV infection.

Measurement of serum or CSF antibodies can aid in the diagnosis of CDV infection. Documentation of a fourfold increase in the serum IgG titer over a 2- to 3-week period or detection of IgM antibodies in serum is consistent with recent infection or recent vaccination but does not prove clinical disease. CSF antibodies to CDV are increased in some dogs with encephalitis. False-positive results can occur in CSF samples contaminated with blood; if CSF antibody titers are greater than those in serum, the antibody in CSF had to be produced locally and is consistent with CNS distemper virus infection. If increased CSF protein concentrations, lymphocytic pleocytosis, and antibodies against CDV are detected in a CSF sample not contaminated with peripheral blood, a presumptive diagnosis of CDV encephalitis can be made.

Definitive diagnosis of CDV infection requires demonstration of viral inclusions by cytologic examination, direct fluorescent antibody staining of cytologic or histopathologic specimens, histopathologic evaluation, or polymerase chain reaction documentation of CDV DNA in peripheral blood, CSF, or conjunctival scrapings (Colorado State University Veterinary Diagnostic Laboratories, Fort Collins, Colo). Viral inclusions can rarely be found in erythrocytes, leukocytes, and leukocyte precursors of infected dogs. Inclusions are generally present for only 2 to 9 days following infection and therefore often are not present when clinical signs occur. Inclusions may be easier to find in smears made from buffy coats or bone marrow aspirates than in those made from peripheral blood. Viral particles can be detected by immunofluorescence in cells from the tonsils, respiratory tree, urinary tract, conjunctival scrapings, and CSF for 5 to 21 days following infection.

### Treatment

Therapy for CDV infection is nonspecific and supportive. Secondary bacterial infections of the gastrointestinal tract and respiratory system are common and, if indicated, should be treated with appropriate antibiotics (see Chapter 98). Anticonvulsants are administered as needed to control seizures (see Chapter 69), but there is no known effective treatment for chorea myoclonus. Glucocorticoid administration may be beneficial in some dogs with CNS disease from chronic CDV infection, but it is contraindicated in acutely infected dogs. The prognosis for dogs with CNS distemper is poor.

### Prevention and Zoonotic Aspects

The CDV survives in exudates only for approximately 20 minutes and is susceptible to most routine hospital disinfectants. Dogs with gastrointestinal or respiratory signs of disease should be housed in isolation to avoid aerosolization to susceptible populations. Care should be taken to avoid transmission by contaminated fomites (see Chapter 99). Dogs with only CNS signs of infection are not generally shedding the virus into the environment.

Puppies should be vaccinated with a modified-live vaccine at 6 to 8 weeks of age and should receive boosters every 3 weeks until at least 14 weeks of age (see Chapter 99). Ma-

ternal antibodies can block CDV vaccines; therefore, in high-risk puppies, measles virus vaccines can be administered to induce heterologous antibodies that will protect puppies against CDV as maternal antibodies wane. Measles vaccine can be given concurrently with modified-live distemper vaccine but should not be given before 6 weeks of age or after 12 weeks of age. At least two distemper boosters should be given after the initial measles vaccine. Vaccination is not as effective if the body temperature is 39.9° C or higher or if other systemic diseases are detected (see Chapter 99). Vaccines should be boosted at 1 year of age. Recent data suggest that after the 1-year booster, repeat boosters are not needed again for a minimum of 3 years (see Chapter 99).

Disease from CDV infection has occurred in some vaccinated dogs and rarely is attributed to modified-live virus vaccination. Clinical disease in vaccinated dogs develops if the host was immunocompromised, infected with the virus prior to vaccination, had vaccine-suppressive levels of maternal antibodies, or was incompletely vaccinated (see Chapter 99). Alternately, the vaccine may have been inactivated by improper handling or may not have protected against all field strains of CDV. Distemper virus encephalitis develops after modified-live vaccination of some dogs coinfected with canine parvovirus; administration of modified-live CDV vaccines should be delayed in dogs with clinical signs of disease consistent with parvovirus infection. Mild, transient, thrombocytopenia can be induced by modified CDV vaccination but has not been associated with spontaneous bleeding. There is no proven public health risk associated with CDV.

## FELINE CORONAVIRUS

### Etiology and Epidemiology

Coronaviruses causing disease in cats include feline infectious peritonitis virus (FIPV) and feline enteric coronavirus (FECV). Enteric infection generally results in mild gastrointestinal signs; systemic infection can induce a clinical syndrome with diverse manifestations commonly referred to as *feline infectious peritonitis* (FIP). There are multiple field strains of FECV and FIPV with varying degrees of virulence. Mutations or recombinant strains of endemic FECV capable of inducing FIP develop in the gastrointestinal tract of some infected cats.

Enteric coronaviruses are commonly shed in feces and rarely in saliva (Addie and colleagues, 2001) and are very contagious. Although the prevalence of transplacental transmission is unknown, one epidemiologic study suggested that it is unlikely (Addie and colleagues, 1993). By use of reverse transcriptase polymerase chain reaction (RT-PCR) testing, coronaviruses can be detected in feces as early as 3 days after infection. In studies of FECV-infected, closed cat colonies, almost every cat becomes infected. In one study of 155 pet cats with naturally occurring FECV infection, viral RNA was shed continuously (n = 18) or intermittently (n = 44) in the feces of some cats (Addie and colleague, 2001). Others were initially shedding viral RNA and then ceased shedding (n = 56), and some were resistant to infection (n = 4). The cats that stopped viral shedding were susceptible to reinfection. Viral RNA was detected in the ileum, colon, and rectum of cats with persistent shedding.

Coronaviruses with the ability to infect monocytes can cause viremia and disseminate throughout the body, potentially resulting in FIP. Between 1986 and 1995, one of every 200 feline accessions at veterinary teaching hospitals in North America were given a clinical diagnosis of FIP (Rohrbach and colleagues, 2001). Most cases of FIP develop in multicat households or catteries. The effusive form of disease develops in cats with poor cell-mediated immune responses; the noneffusive form develops in cats with partial cell-mediated immunity. The effusive form of disease is an immune-complex vasculitis characterized by leakage of protein-rich fluid into the pleural space, the peritoneal cavity, the pericardial space, and the subcapsular space of the kidneys. In the noneffusive form, pyogranulomatous or granulomatous lesions develop in multiple tissues, in particular the eyes, brain, kidneys, omentum, and liver. Some cats have characteristics of both forms of FIP.

Clinical disease associated with FIPV may be influenced by a number of factors, including the virulence of the strain, the dose of the virus, the route of infection, the immune status of the host, genetically determined host factors, the presence of other concurrent infections, and whether or not the cat had been previously exposed to a coronavirus. Inheritance of susceptibility appears to be polygenic. Feline leukemia virus infection and respiratory tract infection results in a higher incidence of FIP, suggesting that the immune status of the host is important in determining the development of clinical disease. Cats concurrently infected with FIV shed 10 to 100 times more FECV in stool than FIV-naive cats. Experimentally infected, seropositive kittens develop accelerated FIP compared to seronegative kittens when exposed to FIPV. This antibody-dependent enhancement of virus infectivity occurs because macrophages are more effectively infected by virus complexed with antibody than by virus alone. This phenomenon appears to be rare in naturally infected cats.

## Clinical Features

Enteric replication of coronaviruses commonly results in fever, vomiting, and mucoid diarrhea. With FECV infection, clinical signs are self-limiting and generally respond within days to supportive care. Fulminant FIP can occur in cats of any age but is generally recognized in cats under 5 years; most cases are under 1 year of age. Intact males are overrepresented in some studies. In cattery outbreaks, usually only one or two kittens in a litter are clinically affected. Anorexia, weight loss, and general malaise are common presenting complaints (Table 102-2). Icterus, ocular inflammation, abdominal distension, dyspnea, or CNS abnormalities are occasionally noted by the owner.

Fever and weight loss are common with both the effusive and noneffusive forms of the disease. Pale mucous membranes or petechiation are noted in some cats. FIP is one of the most common causes of icterus in cats under 2 years of age; liver size

## TABLE 102-2

**Clinical Findings Suggestive of Feline Infectious Peritonitis in Cats**

### Signalment and History

Cats <5 years of age or >10 years of age
Purebred cat
Cat purchased from a cattery or multicat household
Previous history of a mild, self-limiting gastrointestinal or respiratory disease
Serologic evidence of infection by feline leukemia virus
Nonspecific signs of anorexia, weight loss, or depression
Seizures, nystagmus, or ataxia
Acute, fulminant course in cats with effusive disease
Chronic, intermittent course in cats with noneffusive disease

### Physical Examination

Fever
Weight loss
Pale mucous membranes with or without petechiae
Dyspnea with a restrictive breathing pattern
Muffled heart or lung sounds
Abdominal distension with a fluid wave, with or without scrotal swelling
Abdominal mass from focal intestinal granuloma or lymphadenopathy
Icterus with or without hepatomegaly
Chorioretinitis or iridocyclitis
Multifocal neurologic abnormalities
Irregularly marginated kidneys with or without renomegaly
Splenomegaly

### Clinicopathologic Abnormalities

Nonregenerative anemia
Neutrophilic leukocytosis with or without a left shift
Lymphopenia
Hyperglobulinemia characterized as a polyclonal gammopathy; rare monoclonal gammopathies
Nonseptic, pyogranulomatous exudate in pleural space, peritoneal cavity, or pericardial space
Increased protein concentrations, neutrophilic pleocytosis, and coronavirus antibodies in cerebrospinal fluid
Positive coronavirus antibody titer in the majority (especially noneffusive)
Pyogranulomatous or granulomatous inflammation in perivascular location on histologic examination of tissues
Positive results of immunofluorescence or reverse transcriptase polymerase chain reaction (RT-PCR) testing performed on pleural or peritoneal exudate

can be normal or enlarged, and the margination is generally irregular. Abdominal distension is common, a fluid wave can often be balloted, and occasionally masses (pyogranulomas or lymphadenopathy) can be palpated in the omentum, mesentery, and intestines. A solitary ileocecocolic or colonic mass, resulting in obstruction leading to vomiting and diarrhea, occurs in some cats. Kidneys can be small (chronic disease) or large (acute disease or subcapsular effusion); renal margins are usually irregular. Pleural effusion can result in dyspnea and a restrictive breathing pattern (shallow and rapid) as well as muffled heart and lung sounds. Male cats sometimes have scrotal enlargement due to fluid accumulation.

Anterior uveitis and chorioretinitis occur most frequently with the noneffusive form of the disease and can be its only manifestation. Pyogranulomatous disease can develop anywhere in the CNS, leading to a variety of neurologic signs that include seizures, posterior paresis, and nystagmus.

Feline coronaviruses have been suggested as a cause of failure to conceive, abortion, stillbirth, and congenital defects, as well as the fading kitten syndrome (kitten mortality complex). However, one epidemiologic study failed to link feline coronavirus with reproductive failure or neonatal kitten mortality (Addie and colleagues, 1993).

## Diagnosis

Multiple hematologic, serum biochemical, urinalysis, diagnostic imaging, and CSF abnormalities develop in cats with FIP, but none are pathognomonic. Normocytic, normochromic, nonregenerative anemia; neutrophilic leukocytosis; and lymphopenia are common. Disseminated intravascular coagulation resulting in thrombocytopenia occurs in some cats. Hyperproteinemia with or without hypoalbuminemia can occur. Polyclonal gammopathies due to increases in $\alpha_2$- and $\gamma$-globulin concentrations are most commonly detected; monoclonal gammopathies are rare. Most findings are consistent with chronic inflammation and do not prove FIP.

Hyperbilirubinemia with variable increases in alanine aminotransferase and alkaline phosphatase activities occur in some cats with hepatic disease. Increases in lipase and amylase activities in serum or peritoneal effusions can be detected in cats with pancreatic involvement. Prerenal azotemia, renal azotemia, and proteinuria are the most common renal abnormalities. Radiographs can reveal pleural, pericardial, or peritoneal effusions; hepatomegaly; or renomegaly. Mesenteric lymphadenopathy may result in mass lesions in some cats. Ultrasonography can be used to confirm the presence of abdominal fluid in cats with minimal fluid volumes and to evaluate the pancreas, liver, lymph nodes, and kidneys. Magnetic resonance imaging showed periventricular contrast enhancement, ventricular dilation, and hydrocephalus in one group of cats with neurologic FIP (Foley and colleagues, 1998). Protein concentrations ($>30$ mg/dl) and nucleated cell counts (40 to 1600 cells/$\mu$l; neutrophils predominate in most cases) are commonly increased in CSF from cats with CNS involvement. High coronavirus antibody titers are common in the CSF of cats with neurologic FIP.

Effusions from cats with FIP are sterile, colorless to straw colored, may contain fibrin strands, and may clot when exposed to air. The protein concentration on fluid analysis commonly ranges from 3.5 g/dl to 12 g/dl and is generally higher than that associated with other diseases. Mixed inflammatory cell populations of lymphocytes, macrophages, and neutrophils occur most commonly; neutrophils predominate in most cases, but in some cats, macrophages are the primary cell type seen. In some cats the coronavirus antibody titers are greater in the effusion than in serum. Measurement of protein concentrations in effusions can aid in the diagnosis of effusive FIP. If the albumin-to-globulin ratio of the effusion is greater than 0.81 or the albumin component is greater than 48% of the total protein concentration, FIP is unlikely. If the $\gamma$-globulin concentration is greater than 32% of the total protein concentration, FIP is likely. If the total protein concentration is greater than 3.5 g/dl and the globulin component is greater than 50% of the total protein concentration, FIP is likely. Coronavirus antigens are commonly detected by direct immunofluorescence in the effusions of cats with FIP but not in the effusions of cats with other diseases. Additionally, viral RNA can be detected by RT-PCR in effusions. Based on limited numbers of cases, the sensitivity and specificity of RT-PCR used with effusions is approximately 90%.

Detection of serum antibodies is of limited benefit in the evaluation of cats for FIP. Infection of cats by any coronavirus can cause cross-reacting antibodies, therefore a positive antibody titer does not diagnose FIP, protect against disease, or predict when a cat may develop clinical FIP. Because coronavirus antibody tests are not standardized, results from different laboratories commonly do not correlate. The presence of coronavirus antibodies in the CNS can aid in the diagnosis of neurologic FIP. Cats with FIP are occasionally serologically negative because of rapidly progressive disease with a delayed rise in titer, disappearance of antibody in terminal stages of the disease, or immune complex formation. Maternal antibodies decline to undetectable concentrations by 4 to 6 weeks of age; kittens infected in the postnatal period become seropositive at 8 to 14 weeks of age. Thus serologic testing of kittens can be used to prevent the spread of coronaviruses (see Prevention and Zoonotic Aspects, below).

A presumptive diagnosis of FIP is usually based on the combination of clinical and clinicopathologic findings. The effusive form of the disease can be diagnosed using assessment of effusions as discussed. The positive and negative predictive values of individual tests and combinations of tests for the diagnosis of FIP were reported (Sparkes and colleagues, 1991 and 1994). The combination of hyperglobulinemia, a serum antibody titer greater than 160, and lymphopenia had a positive predictive value of 88%.

Definitive diagnosis of FIP is based on detection of characteristic histopathologic findings, virus isolation, demonstration of the virus in effusions or tissue by use of immunocytochemical or immunhistochemical staining, or on demonstration of viral RNA in effusions or tissues by RT-PCR. Because virus isolation is not practical clinically, RT-PCR is used most frequently to detect coronaviruses in feces. Based on currently available RT-PCR technology, detection of coronavirus RNA in whole blood does not always correlate with the development of FIP.

## Treatment

Because an antemortem diagnosis of FIP is difficult to make, assessment of studies reporting successful treatment is virtually impossible. A small percentage of cats have spontaneous remission, adding to the confusion concerning therapeutic response. Supportive care, including correction of electrolyte and fluid balance abnormalities, should be provided to cats with FIP as needed.

Optimal treatment of cats with FIP would combine virus elimination with suppression of B-lymphocyte function and stimulation of T-lymphocyte function. In vitro inhibition of FIPV replication has been demonstrated with a number of drugs, including ribavirin, human interferon-α, feline fibroblastic interferon-β, adenine arabinoside, and amphotericin B. However, to date there has been no uniformly successful antiviral treatment.

Because disease due to FIP is secondary to immune-mediated reactions against the virus, modulation of the inflammatory reaction is the principal form of palliative therapy. Low-dose prednisolone (1 to 2 mg/kg PO q24h) may lessen clinical manifestations of noneffusive FIP. However, the use of immune-suppressive drugs is controversial, because cats with FIP have impaired immune responses (Knotek, 2000). Antibiotics do not have primary antiviral effects but may be indicated for the treatment of secondary bacterial infection. Other supportive care treatments, such as anabolic steroids (stanozolol, 1 mg PO q12h), aspirin (10 mg/kg PO q48-72h), and ascorbic acid (125 mg PO q12h) have also been recommended for the treatment of FIP. Most cats with systemic clinical signs of FIP die or require euthanasia within days to months of diagnosis. The effusive form of disease carries a grave prognosis. Depending on the organ system involved and the severity of polysystemic clinical signs, cats with noneffusive disease have variable survival times. Cats with only ocular FIP may respond to antiinflammatory treatment or enucleation of the affected eye(s) and have a better prognosis than cats with systemic FIP.

## Prevention and Zoonotic Aspects

Prevention of coronavirus infections is best accomplished by avoiding exposure to the virus. Although viral particles of FIPV can survive in dried secretions for up to 7 weeks, routine disinfectants inactivate the virus. Epidemiologic studies suggest the following:

- Some healthy, coronavirus-seropositive cats shed the virus.
- Seronegative cats do not usually shed the virus.
- Kittens are usually not infected by coronaviruses transplacentally.
- Maternally derived coronavirus antibodies wane by 4 to 6 weeks of age.
- Kittens are most likely to become infected by contact with cats other than their queens after maternal antibodies wane.
- Coronavirus antibodies due to natural infection develop by 8 to 14 weeks of age.

These findings have lead to recommendations that kittens born in a breeding situation with coronavirus-seropositive cats should be housed only with the queen and littermates until sold, should be tested for coronavirus antibodies at 14-16 weeks of age, and should be sold only if seronegative. It would be optimal to maintain a coronavirus-seronegative household and not allow cats to have contact with other cats. Cats can eliminate coronavirus infections; a previously infected cat should be shown to be negative for viral RNA in feces for 5 months and should be seronegative in order to be considered coronavirus naïve (Addie and colleagues, 2001).

An intranasally administered, mutant strain of coronavirus that induces mucosal immune response but minimal systemic immune response is available (Primucell FIP, Pfizer Animal Health, Exton, Pa). This strain does not induce FIP; the majority of cats with adverse effects have exhibited only mild signs associated with placement of liquid in the nares; and the vaccine does not appear to potentiate antibody-dependent enhancement of virus infectivity when administered to previously seropositive cats (see Chapter 99). The vaccine appears to be effective in at least some cats, but whether the vaccine protects against all field strains, mutations, or recombinants is unknown. It is unlikely the vaccine is effective in cats that have previously been infected by a coronavirus. Vaccination induces serum antibody titers, making the interpretation of serologic test results difficult in vaccinated cats showing clinical signs of FIP. The only indication for the vaccine is for seronegative cats with risk of exposure to coronaviruses (see Chapter 99). There is no known zoonotic transfer of FIP coronavirus or enteric coronavirus to humans.

## FELINE IMMUNODEFICIENCY VIRUS

### Etiology and Epidemiology

Feline immunodeficiency virus is an exogenous, single-strand RNA virus in the family Retroviridae, subfamily Lentivirinae. The virus is morphologically similar to the human immunodeficiency virus, but it is antigenically distinct. Like FeLV, FIV produces reverse transcriptase to catalyze the insertion of viral RNA into the host genome. There are multiple subtypes of the virus, and some isolates have differing biologic behavior. For example, immune deficiency is induced much more quickly by some isolates, and clinical diseases, such as uveitis, are induced by some but not all isolates.

Aggressive biting behavior is thought to be the primary route of transmission of FIV; older, male, outdoor cats are most commonly infected. FIV is present in semen and can be transmitted by artificial insemination. Transplacental and perinatal transmission occurs from infected queens to kittens. Arthropod transmission appears to be unlikely. Transmission by routes other than biting is less common because high levels of viremia are of short duration. FIV infection of cats has worldwide distribution, and prevalence rates vary greatly by region and the lifestyle of the cats tested. Outdoor, fighting males are most commonly at risk.

FIV replicates in T-lymphocytes (CD4+ and CD8+), B-lymphocytes, macrophages, and astrocytes. Monocytotropic characteristics may be related to virulence. The primary phase of infection occurs as the virus disseminates throughout the body, initially leading to low-grade fever, neutropenia, and generalized reactive lymphadenopathy. A subclinical, latent period of variable length then develops; the length of this period is related in part to the strain of virus and the age of the cat when infected. The median age of healthy, naturally infected cats and clinically ill naturally infected cats is approximately 3 years and 10 years, respectively, suggesting a latent period of years for most strains of FIV. Chronic experimental and naturally occurring infection results in a slow decline in circulating CD4+ lymphocyte numbers, response to mitogens, and decreased production of cytokines involved with cell-mediated immunity, such as IL-2 and IL-10; neutrophil function and natural killer cell function are also affected. Humoral immune responses are often intact, and a polyclonal gammopathy develops from nonspecific B-lymphocyte activation. Within months to years, an immune deficiency stage similar to acquired immunodeficiency syndrome (AIDS) in humans develops. Coinfection with FeLV potentiates the primary and immune deficiency phases of FIV. Coinfection with *Haemobartonella felis (Mycoplasma hemofelis), Toxoplasma gondii,* feline herpesvirus, and feline calicivirus, as well as immunization, failed to potentiate FIV-associated immunodeficiency.

## Clinical Features

Clinical signs of infection with FIV can arise from direct viral effects or from secondary infections that ensue following the development of immunodeficiency (Table 102-3). Most of the clinical syndromes diagnosed in FIV-seropositive cats also occur in FIV-naive cats, which makes proving disease causation difficult during the subclinical stage of infection. A positive FIV antibody test does not prove immunodeficiency or disease due to FIV and does not necessarily indicate a poor prognosis. The only way to accurately determine whether an FIV-seropositive cat with a concurrent infectious disease has a poor prognosis is to treat the concurrent infection.

Primary (acute) FIV is characterized by fever and generalized lymphadenopathy. Owners commonly present FIV-infected cats in the immunodeficiency stage for evaluation of nonspecific signs such as anorexia, weight loss, and depression or for evaluation of abnormalities associated with specific organ systems. When a clinical syndrome is diagnosed in a cat seropositive for FIV, the workup should include diagnostic tests for other potential causes (see Table 102-3).

Clinical syndromes reportedly due to primary viral effects include chronic small bowel diarrhea, nonregenerative anemia, thrombocytopenia, neutropenia, lymphadenopathy, pars planitis (inflammation in the anterior vitreous humor), anterior uveitis, glomerulonephritis, renal insufficiency, and hyperglobulinemia. There was no link between FIV infection and lower urinary tract disease in one study (Barsanti and colleagues, 1996). Behavioral abnormalities, with dementia, hiding, rage, inappropriate elimination, and roaming are the most common neurologic manifestations of FIV infection. Occasionally, seizures, nystagmus, ataxia, and peripheral nerve abnormalities may be due to primary viral effects. Lymphoid malignancies, myeloproliferative diseases, and several carcinomas and sarcomas have been detected in FIV-infected,

TABLE 102-3

**Clinical Syndromes Associated with FIV Infection and Possible Opportunistic Agents**

| CLINICAL SYNDROME | PRIMARY VIRAL EFFECT | OPPORTUNISTIC AGENTS |
|---|---|---|
| Dermatologic/otitis externa | None | Bacterial; atypical *Mycobacterium* spp.; *Otodectes cynotis; Demodex cati; Notoedres cati;* dermatophytosis; *Cryptococcus neoformans;* cowpox |
| Gastrointestinal | Yes; small bowel diarrhea | *Cryptosporidium, Cystoisospora, Giardia,* and *Salmonella* spp.; *Campylobacter jejuni;* others |
| Glomerulonephritis | Yes | Bacterial; FeLV, FIP, SLE |
| Hematologic | Yes; nonregenerative anemia, neutropenia, thrombocytopenia | *Haemobartonella felis;* FeLV; *Bartonella henselae?* |
| Neoplasia | Yes; myeloproliferative disorders, lymphoma | FeLV |
| Neurologic | Yes; behavioral abnormalities | *Toxoplasma gondii; C. neoformans;* FIP; FeLV; *B. henselae?* |
| Ocular | Yes; pars planitis, anterior uveitis | *T. gondii;* FIP; *C. neoformans;* FHV-1; *B. henselae* |
| Pneumonia/pneumonitis | None | Bacterial; *T. gondii; C. neoformans* |
| Pyothorax | None | Bacterial |
| Renal failure | Yes | Bacterial; FIP; FeLV |
| Stomatitis | None | Calicivirus; overgrowth of bacterial flora; candidiasis; *B. henselae?* |
| Upper respiratory tract | None | FHV-1; calicivirus; overgrowth of bacterial flora; *C. neoformans* |
| Urinary tract infection | None | Bacterial |

*FeLV,* Feline leukemia virus; *FIP,* feline infectious peritonitis; *SLE,* systemic lupus erythematosus; *FHV-1,* feline herpesvirus-1.

FeLV-naive cats, suggesting a potential association between FIV and malignancy; FIV-infected cats are at higher risk for the development of lymphoma.

## Diagnosis

Neutropenia, thrombocytopenia, and nonregenerative anemia are the most common hematologic abnormalities associated with FIV infection. Monocytosis and lymphocytosis occur in some cats and may be due to the virus or chronic infection with opportunistic pathogens. Cytologic examination of bone marrow aspirates may reveal maturation arrest (i.e., myelodysplasia), lymphoma, or leukemia. A progressive decline in CD4+ lymphocytes, a plateau or progressive increase in CD8+ lymphocytes, and an inversion of the CD4+/CD8+ ratio occurs in experimentally infected cats over time. A multitude of serum biochemical abnormalities are possible, depending on what FIV-associated syndrome is occurring. Renal azotemia and polyclonal gammopathy are the changes most likely to be due to direct viral effects. There are no pathognomonic radiographic abnormalities associated with FIV infection.

Antibodies against FIV are detected in serum in clinical practice most frequently by enzyme-linked immunosorbent assay (ELISA). Clinical signs can occur before seroconversion in some cats, and some infected cats never seroconvert; thus false-negative reactions can occur. Results of virus isolation or PCR on blood are positive in some antibody-negative cats. False-positive reactions are common using ELISA; hence, positive ELISA results in healthy or low-risk cats should be confirmed using Western blot immunoassay or PCR. Kittens can have detectable, colostrum-derived antibodies for several months. Kittens less than 6 months of age that are FIV seropositive should be tested every 60 days until the result is negative. If antibodies persist at 6 months of age, the kitten is likely infected. Virus isolation or PCR on blood can also be performed to confirm infection. A vaccine against FIV has been licensed in the United States (see Chapter 99). This vaccine induces antibodies that cannot be distinguished from those induced by naturally occurring disease using currently available tests.

Detection of antibodies against FIV in the serum of cats that have not been vaccinated against FIV documents exposure and correlates well with persistent infection but does not correlate to disease induced by the virus. Because many of the clinical syndromes associated with FIV can be due to opportunistic infections, further diagnostic procedures may determine treatable etiologies (see Table 102-3). For example, some FIV-seropositive cats with uveitis are coinfected by *T. gondii* and often respond to the administration of anti-*Toxoplasma* drugs (see Chapter 104).

## Treatment

Because FIV-seropositive cats are not necessarily immunosuppressed or diseased due to FIV, the cat should be evaluated and treated for other potential causes of the clinical syndrome. Some FIV-seropositive cats are immunodeficient; if infectious diseases are identified, bacteriocidal drugs administered at the upper end of the dosage should be chosen. Long-term antibiotic therapy or multiple treatment periods may be required. The only way to determine if an FIV-seropositive cat with a concurrent infection has a poor prognosis is to treat the concurrent infection.

A variety of antiviral drugs and immune stimulation therapies have been administered to cats with FIV or FeLV infections (Table 102-4). Administration of antiviral agents such as the reverse transcriptase inhibitor azidothymidine (AZT) have had mixed success in the treatment of FIV. Use of AZT at a dosage of 5 mg/kg given orally or subcutaneously every 12 hours improved overall quality of life and stomatitis in FIV-infected cats and is thought to aid in the treatment of neurologic signs (Hartmann and colleagues, 1995a and 1995b). Cats treated with AZT should be monitored for the development of anemia. Administration of bovine lactoferrin by mouth was beneficial in the treatment of intractable stomatitis in FIV-seropositive cats. Removal of all premolar and molar teeth has also been effective for treatment of in-

 TABLE 102-4

**Drug Treatment Regimens for Viremic, Clinically Ill Cats with FIV Or FeLV Infections***

| THERAPEUTIC AGENT† | ADMINISTRATION |
| --- | --- |
| Acemannan | 2 mg/kg IP once weekly for 6 weeks |
| Azidothymidine (AZT) | 5 mg/kg PO or SQ q12h; monitor for development of anemia |
| Bovine lactoferrin | 175 mg PO in milk or VAL syrup q12-24h; for treatment of stomatitis |
| Diethylcarbamazine | 3-12 mg/kg PO q24h; to lessen risk of FeLV-associated lymphoma |
| Erythropoietin | 100 U/kg SQ three times weekly and then titrate to effect |
| Interferon-α | 30 U in 1 ml saline PO q24h as long as effective *or* 100,000-1 million U SQ q24h for 6-12 weeks |
| *Staphylococcus* protein A | 10 µg/kg IP twice weekly for 10 weeks and then monthly |
| *Propionibacterium acnes* | 0.5 ml IV once or twice weekly to effect |

*Limited information from controlled studies is available for any of these protocols. See the text for discussion of specific studies.
†These are general guidelines; controlled studies are lacking for the most part.

tractable stomatitis in some FIV-seropositive cats (see Chapter 31). Immunomodulators have not been shown to have reproducible clinical effect, but the owners sometimes report positive responses. Human recombinant erythropoietin administration increased red blood cell and white blood cell counts in FIV-infected cats when compared to placebo, did not increase viral load, and had no measurable adverse clinical effects (Arai and colleagues, 2000). In contrast, although administration of human recombinant granulocyte-monocyte colony-stimulating factor (GM-CSF) to FIV-infected cats increased white blood cell counts in some treated cats, it also induced fever, anti GM-CSF antibodies, and increased viral load. GM-CSF therefore appears to be contraindicated for the treatment of FIV in cats.

## Prevention and Zoonotic Aspects

Housing cats indoors to avoid fighting and testing new cats before introduction to a FIV-seronegative, multiple-cat household will prevent most cases of FIV. Transmission by fomites is unusual because the virus is not easily transmitted by casual contact, is susceptible to most routine disinfectants, and dies when out of the host for minutes to hours, especially when dried. Cleaning litter boxes and dishes shared between cats using scalding water and detergent inactivates the virus. Cats with potential exposure from fighting should be retested 60 days after the potential exposure. Cats that are FIV infected should be housed indoors at all times to avoid exposing FIV-naive cats in the environment to the virus and to lessen the affected animal's chance of acquiring an opportunistic infection. Kittens queened by FIV-infected cats should not be allowed to nurse to avoid transmission by ingestion of milk. Kittens queened by FIV-infected cats should be shown to be serologically negative at 6 months of age to document failure of lactogenic or transplacental transmission prior to being sold. A killed vaccine containing immunogens from two FIV isolates was recently licensed for use in the United States (Fel-O-Vax FIV, Fort Dodge Animal Health, Overland Park, Kan). However, the efficacy and safety of the vaccine has not been assessed under field conditions in large numbers of cats (see Chapter 99). Additionally, the vaccine induces antibodies that cannot be distinguished from those induced by natural exposure by use of currently available tests.

The human immunodeficiency virus and FIV are morphologically similar but antigenically distinct. Antibodies against FIV have not been documented in the serum of human beings, even after accidental exposure to virus-containing material. Cats with FIV infection resulting in immunodeficiency may be more likely to spread other zoonotic agents into the human environment (see Chapter 105).

## *FELINE LEUKEMIA VIRUS*

### Etiology and Epidemiology

Feline leukemia virus is a single-strand RNA virus in the family Retroviridae, subfamily Oncovirinae. The virus produces reverse transcriptase, which catalyzes the reaction, resulting in the formation of a DNA copy (provirus) of FeLV viral RNA in the cytoplasm of infected cells; provirus is inserted into the host cell genome. On subsequent host cell divisions, provirus serves as a template for new virus particles formed in the cytoplasm and is released across the cell membrane by budding. FeLV is made up of several core and envelope proteins. Envelope protein p15e is associated with the development of immunosuppression. Core protein p27 is present in the cytoplasm of infected cells, peripheral blood, saliva, and tears of infected cats; detection of p27 is the basis of most FeLV tests. The envelope glycoprotein 70 (gp70) contains the subgroup antigens A, B, or C, which are associated with the infectivity, virulence, and disease caused by individual strains of the virus. Neutralizing antibodies are produced by some cats after exposure to gp70. Antibodies against feline oncornavirus-associated cell membrane antigen (FOCMA) are formed by some cats.

The principal route of infection by FeLV is prolonged contact with infected cat saliva and nasal secretions; grooming or sharing of common water or food sources effectively results in infection. Because the organism does not survive in the environment, feces, or urine, fomite and aerosol transmissions are unlikely. Transplacental, lactational, and venereal transmission are less important than casual contact. FeLV infection has worldwide distribution; the seroprevalence of infection varies geographically and by the population of cats tested. Infection is most common in outdoor male cats between 1 and 6 years of age.

The virus replicates first in the oropharynx, followed by dissemination through the body to the bone marrow (Table 102-5). If persistent bone marrow infection occurs, infected white blood cells and platelets leave the bone marrow with ultimate infection of epithelial structures, including salivary and lacrimal glands. Whether or not infection occurs following natural exposure to FeLV is determined by the virus subtype or strain, the virus dose, the age of the cat when exposed, and the cat's immune responses. Approximately 30% of exposed cats become persistently viremic; self-limiting infection occurs in the remaining cats. Cats with persistent viremia usually die of an FeLV-related illness within 2 to 3 years. Approximately 30% of exposed cats are transiently viremic, develop neutralizing antibodies, and clear the infection within 4 to 6 weeks. Latent or sequestered infections occur in the remainder of the cats. Latent infections occur when provirus is inserted into the cat's genome but the cat is not viremic. In sequestered infections, the organism can be found in the bone marrow, spleen, lymph node, and small intestine but not in the blood. Latent and sequestered infections can be activated by the administration of glucocorticoids or other immunosuppressive drugs.

The pathogenesis of various syndromes induced by FeLV is complex but includes induction of lymphoma from activation of oncogenes by the virus or insertion of provirus into the genome of lymphoid precursors; subgroup C induction of aplastic anemia from increased secretion of tumor necrosis factor-$\alpha$; immunodeficiency secondary to T-lymphocyte depletion (both CD4+ and CD8+ lymphocytes) or dysfunction;

TABLE 102-5

Stages of Feline Leukemia Virus Infection with Corresponding Test Results

| STAGE | ORGANISM LOCALIZATION | TIMING | PERIPHERAL BLOOD RESULT | | |
|---|---|---|---|---|---|
| | | | IFA | ELISA | PCR |
| I | Replication in local lymphoid tissues (tonsillar and pharyngeal tissues with oronasal exposure) | 2-4 days | neg | neg | neg |
| II | Dissemination in circulating lymphocytes and monocytes | 1-14 days | neg | pos | pos |
| III | Replication in the spleen, distant lymph nodes, and gut-associated lymphoid tissue | 3-12 days | neg | pos | pos |
| IV | Replication in bone marrow cells and intestinal epithelial crypts | 7-21 days | neg* | pos | pos |
| V | Peripheral viremia; dissemination via infected bone marrow–derived neutrophils and platelets | 14-28 days | pos | pos | pos |
| VI | Disseminated epithelial cell infection with virus secretion in saliva and tears | Day 28 | pos | pos† | pos |

Modified from Rojko JL et al: Pathogenesis of infection by the feline leukemia virus, *J Am Vet Med Assoc* 199:1305, 1991; and Wolf AM: Feline leukemia virus. In Bonagura J, editor: *Kirk's current veterinary therapy XIII*, Philadelphia, 2000, WB Saunders, p 280.
*IFA result may be positive on bone marrow.
†Saliva and tears may test positive.
*IFA,* Immunofluorescent antibody testing; *ELISA,* enzyme-linked immunosorbent assay; *PCR,* polymerase chain reaction; *neg,* negative; *pos,* positive.

neutropenia; neutrophil function disorders; malignant transformation; and viral induction of bone marrow growth, promoting substances leading to myeloproliferative diseases.

## Clinical Features

Owners generally present FeLV-infected cats for evaluation of nonspecific signs such as anorexia, weight loss, and depression or for evaluation of abnormalities associated with specific organ systems. Of the FeLV-infected cats evaluated at necropsy, 23% had evidence of neoplasia (96% lymphoma/leukemia), and the remainder died due to numerous other nonneoplastic diseases (Reinacher, 1989). Specific clinical syndromes can result from specific effects of the virus or from opportunistic infections secondary to immunosuppression. A positive FeLV test result does not prove disease induced by FeLV. When a clinical syndrome is diagnosed in an FeLV-seropositive cat, the workup should include diagnostic tests for other potential causes. The opportunistic agents discussed for FIV also are common in FeLV-infected cats (see Table 102-3).

Bacterial or calicivirus-induced stomatitis occurs in some FeLV-infected cats due to immunosuppression. FeLV infection can result in vomiting or diarrhea from a form of enteritis clinically and histopathologically resembling panleukopenia, from alimentary lymphoma, or from secondary infections due to immunosuppression. Icterus in FeLV-infected cats can be prehepatic from immune-mediated destruction of red blood cells induced by FeLV or secondary infection by *H. felis* (*Mycoplasma haemofelis* and *Mycoplasma haemominutum*); hepatic from hepatic lymphoma, hepatic lipidosis, or focal liver necrosis; or posthepatic from alimentary lymphoma. Some FeLV-infected cats with icterus may be concurrently infected by feline infectious peritonitis virus or *T. gondii.*

Clinical signs of rhinitis or pneumonia occur in some FeLV-infected cats from secondary infections. Dyspnea from mediastinal lymphoma occurs in some cats. These cats are generally less than 3 years of age and may have decreased cranial chest compliance on palpation, as well as muffled heart and lung sounds if pleural effusion is present.

Mediastinal, multicentric, and alimentary lymphoma are the most common neoplasms associated with FeLV; lymphoid hyperplasia also occurs. Alimentary lymphoma most commonly involves the small intestines, mesenteric lymph nodes, kidneys, and liver of older cats. Renal lymphoma can involve one or both kidneys, which are usually enlarged and irregularly marginated on physical examination. Fibrosarcomas occasionally develop in young cats coinfected with FeLV and feline sarcoma virus. Lymphocytic, myelogenous, erythroid, and megakaryocytic leukemia all are reported secondary to FeLV infection; erythroleukemia and myelomonocytic leukemia are the most common. The history and physical examination findings are nonspecific.

Renal failure occurs in some FeLV-infected cats from renal lymphoma or glomerulonephritis. Affected cats are presented for evaluation of polyuria, polydipsia, weight loss, and inappetence during the last stages of disease. Urinary incontinence due to either sphincter incompetence or detrusor hyperactivity occurs in some cats; small bladder, nocturnal incontinence is reported most frequently.

Some FeLV-infected cats are presented for miosis, blepharospasm, or cloudy eyes from ocular lymphoma. Aqueous flare, mass lesions, keratic precipitates, lens luxations, and glaucoma are often found on ocular examination. It is unlikely FeLV induces uveitis without lymphoma. Neurologic abnormalities associated with FeLV infection include anisocoria, ataxia, weakness, tetraparesis, paraparesis, behavioral changes, and urinary incontinence. Nervous system disease is likely to develop due to polyneuropathy or lymphoma. Intraocular and nervous system disease in FeLV-infected cats can occur from infection with other agents including FIPV, *Cryptococcus neoformans,* or *T. gondii.*

Abortion, stillbirth, or infertility occurs in some FeLV-infected queens. Kittens infected in utero that survive to parturition generally develop accelerated FeLV syndromes or die as part of the kitten mortality complex.

Some FeLV-seropositive cats present for lameness or weakness due to neutrophilic polyarthritis attributed to immune complex deposition. Multiple cartilaginous exostoses occurs in some cats and may be FeLV-related.

## Diagnosis

A variety of nonspecific hematologic, biochemical, urinalysis, and radiographic abnormalities occur in FeLV-infected cats. Nonregenerative anemia alone or in combination with decreases in lymphocyte, neutrophil, and platelet counts are common in FeLV-infected cats. The presence of increased numbers of circulating nucleated red blood cells or macrocytosis without appropriate reticulocytosis occurs frequently; examination of bone marrow often documents a maturation arrest in the erythroid line (erythrodysplasia). Immune-mediated destruction of erythrocytes can be induced by FeLV and occurs in cats coinfected with *H. felis;* regenerative anemia, microagglutination or macroagglutination of erythrocytes, and a positive result on the direct Coombs' test are common in these cats. Neutropenia and thrombocytopenia occur from bone marrow suppression or immune-mediated destruction. FeLV-infected cats with the panleukopenia-like syndrome have gastrointestinal tract signs and neutropenia and are difficult to differentiate from cats with panleukopenia virus infection or salmonellosis. Cats with FeLV-induced panleukopenia-like syndrome usually have anemia and thrombocytopenia, abnormalities rarely associated with panleukopenia virus infection. Azotemia, hyperbilirubinemia, bilirubinuria, and increased activity of liver enzymes are common biochemical abnormalities. Proteinuria occurs in some FeLV-infected cats with glomerulonephritis. Cats with lymphoma have mass lesions radiographically, depending on the organ system affected. Mediastinal lymphoma can result in pleural effusion; alimentary lymphoma can cause obstructive intestinal patterns.

Lymphoma can be diagnosed by cytologic or histopathologic evaluation of affected tissues (see Chapters 77 and 82). Because lymphoma can be diagnosed cytologically and treated with chemotherapy, cats with mediastinal masses, lymphadenopathy, renomegaly, hepatomegaly, splenomegaly, or intestinal masses should be evaluated cytologically prior to surgical intervention. Malignant lymphocytes are also occasionally identified in peripheral blood smears, in effusions, and in CSF.

Most cats with suspected FeLV infection are screened for FeLV antigens in neutrophils and platelets by immunofluorescent antibody (IFA) testing or, in whole blood, plasma, serum, saliva, or tears, by ELISA. IFA results are not positive until the bone marrow has been infected (see Table 102-5). The results of IFA testing are accurate more than 95% of the time. False-negative reactions may occur when leukopenia or thrombocytopenia prevents evaluation of an adequate number of cells. False-positive reactions can occur if the blood smears submitted for evaluation are too thick. A positive IFA result indicates that the cat is viremic and contagious; approximately 90% of cats with positive IFA results are viremic for life. The rare combination of IFA-positive and ELISA-negative results suggests technique-related artifact. Negative ELISA results correlate well with negative IFA results and an inability to isolate FeLV.

The virus can be detected in serum by ELISA prior to infection of bone marrow and so can be positive in some cats during early stages of infection or during self-limiting infection, even though IFA results are negative. Other possibilities for discordant results (ELISA positive, IFA negative) are false-positive ELISA results or false-negative IFA results. Cats with positive ELISA results and negative IFA results are probably not contagious at that time but should be isolated until retested 4 to 6 weeks later, because progression to persistent viremia and epithelial cell infection may be occurring.

ELISA-positive cats that revert to negative have developed neutralizing antibodies, latent infection, or sequestered infection. Virus isolation, IFA performed on bone marrow cells, immunohistochemical staining of tissues for FeLV antigen, and PCR can be used to confirm latent or sequestered infection in some cats. Cats with latent or sequestered infection are not likely contagious to other cats, but infected queens may pass the virus to kittens during gestation, parturition, or by milk. Cats with localized or latent infection can be immunodeficient and may become viremic (IFA and ELISA positive) after receiving corticosteroids or following extreme stress.

There is generally a delay of 1 to 2 weeks after the onset of viremia before ELISA tear and saliva test results become positive, therefore these tests can be negative even when results using serum are positive. Antibody titers to FeLV envelope antigens (neutralizing antibody) and against virus-transformed tumor cells (FOCMA antibody) are available in some research laboratories, but the diagnostic and prognostic significance of results from these tests is unknown.

## Treatment

A number of antiviral agents have been proposed for the treatment of FeLV; the reverse transcriptase inhibitor, 3'-azido-3'-deoxythymidine (AZT) has been studied the most (see Table 102-4). Unfortunately, administration of AZT to persistently viremic cats does not appear to clear viremia in most cats, and it had minimal benefits for clinically ill cats in a recent study. Immunotherapy with drugs such as α-interferon, *Staphylococcus* protein A, *Propionibacterium acnes,* or acemannan (see Table 102-4) improves clinical signs of disease in some cats.

Chemotherapy should be administered to cats with FeLV-associated neoplasia (see Chapters 79 and 82). Opportunistic agents should be managed as indicated; the upper dose range and duration of antibiotic therapy are generally required. Administration of supportive therapies such as hematinic agents, vitamin $B_{12}$, folic acid, anabolic steroids, and erythropoietin generally has been unsuccessful in the management of the nonregenerative anemia. Blood transfusion is required in many cases. Cats with autoagglutinating hemolytic anemia require immunosuppressive therapy, but this may activate virus replication. The prognosis for persistently viremic cats is guarded; the majority die within 2 to 3 years.

## Prevention and Zoonotic Aspects

Avoiding contact with FeLV by housing cats indoors is the best form of prevention. Potential fomites such as water bowls and litter pans should not be shared between seropositive and seronegative cats. Testing and removal of seropositive cats can result in virus-free catteries and multiple-cat households.

Due to variation in challenge study methodology and the difficulty of assessing the preventable fraction of a disease with a relatively low infection rate, long subclinical phase, and multiple field strains, the efficacy of individual vaccines continues to be in question (see Chapter 99). Vaccination of cats not previously exposed to FeLV should be considered in cats at high risk (i.e., contact with other cats), but owners should be warned of the potential efficacy of less than 100%. Cats with persistent FeLV viremia do not benefit from vaccination. Vaccination is related to the development of fibrosarcoma in some cats, particularly if adjuvanted products are used.

FeLV-infected cats should be housed indoors to avoid infecting other cats and to avoid exposure to opportunistic agents. Flea control should be maintained to avoid exposure to *H. felis* and *Bartonella henselae*. FeLV-infected cats should not be allowed to hunt or be fed undercooked meats to avoid infection by *T. gondii*, *Cryptosporidium parvum*, *Giardia* spp., and other infectious agents carried by transport hosts.

Antigens of FeLV have never been documented in the serum of human beings, suggesting that the zoonotic risk is minimal. However, FeLV-infected cats may be more likely than FeLV-naive cats to pass other zoonotic agents, such as *C. parvum* and *Salmonella* spp., into the human environment.

## Suggested Readings

CANINE DISTEMPER VIRUS

Greene CE et al: Canine distemper. In Greene CE, editor: *Infectious diseases of the dog and cat,* ed 2, Philadelphia, 1990, WB Saunders, p 226.

Krakowka S et al: Experimental and naturally occurring transplacental transmission of canine distemper virus, *Am J Vet Res* 38:919, 1977.

Krakowka S et al: Canine parvoviruses potentiate canine distemper encephalitis attributable to modified live-virus vaccine, *J Am Vet Med Assoc* 180:137, 1982.

McCandlish IAP et al: Distemper encephalitis in pups after vaccination of the dam, *Vet Rec* 130:27, 1992.

Raw ME et al: Canine distemper infection associated with acute nervous signs in dogs, *Vet Rec* 130:291, 1992.

Shell LG: Canine distemper, *Comp Contin Educ Pract Vet* 12:173, 1990.

Sorjonen DC et al: Electrophoretic determination of albumin and gamma globulin concentrations in the cerebrospinal fluid of dogs with encephalomyelitis attributable to canine distemper virus infection: 13 cases (1980-1987), *J Am Vet Med Assoc* 195:977, 1989.

Thomas WB et al: A retrospective evaluation of 38 cases of canine distemper encephalomyelitis, *J Am Anim Hosp Assoc* 29:129, 1993.

Tipold A et al: Neurological manifestations of canine distemper virus infection, *J Small Anim Pract* 33:466, 1992.

Tipold A et al: Determination of the IgG index for the detection of intrathecal immunoglobulin synthesis in dogs using an ELISA, *Res Vet Sci* 54:40, 1993.

Tizard I: Risks associated with use of live vaccines, *J Am Vet Med Assoc* 196:1851, 1990.

Zurbriggen A et al: The pathogenesis of nervous distemper, *Prog Vet Neurol* 5:109, 1994.

FELINE INFECTIOUS PERITONITIS VIRUS

Addie DD et al: Control of feline coronavirus infection in kittens, *Vet Rec* 126:164, 1990.

Addie DD et al: A study of naturally occurring feline coronavirus infections in kittens, *Vet Rec* 130:133, 1992.

Addie DD et al: Feline coronavirus is not a major cause of neonatal kitten mortality, *Fel Pract* 21:13, 1993.

Addie DD et al: Use of a reverse-transcriptase polymerase chain reaction for monitoring the shedding of feline coronavirus by healthy cats, *Vet Rec* 148:649, 2001.

Foley JE et al: The inheritance of susceptibility to feline infectious peritonitis in purebred catteries, *Fel Pract* 24:14, 1996.

Foley JE et al: Risk factors for feline infectious peritonitis among cats in multiple-cat environments with endemic feline enteric coronavirus, *J Am Vet Med Assoc* 210:1313, 1997.

Foley JE et al: Diagnostic features of clinical neurologic feline infectious peritonitis, *J Vet Intern Med* 12:415, 1998.

Gunn-Moore DA et al: Detection of feline coronaviruses by culture and reverse transcriptase-polymerase chain reaction of blood samples from healthy cats and cats with clinical feline infectious peritonitis, *Vet Microbiol* 62:193, 1998.

Harvey CJ et al: An uncommon intestinal manifestation of feline infectious peritonitis: 26 cases (1986-1993), *J Am Vet Med Assoc* 209:1117, 1996.

Heil-Franke G et al: The importance of the polymerase chain reaction (PCR) for the diagnosis of feline infectious peritonitis (FIP) *Kleintierpraxis,* 46:629, 2001.

Herrewegh AA et al: Persistence and evolution of feline coronavirus in a closed cat-breeding colony, *Virology* 234:349, 1997.

Kennedy MA et al: Correlation of genomic detection of feline coronavirus with various diagnostic assays for feline infectious peritonitis, *J Vet Diagn Invest* 10:93, 1998.

Knotek Z et al: Clinical and immunological characteristics of cats affected with feline infectious peritonitis, *Acta Veterinaria Brno* 69:51, 2000.

Paltrinieri S et al: Some aspects of humoral and cellular immunity in naturally occurring feline infectious peritonitis, *Vet Immunol Immunopathol* 65:205, 1998.

Paltrinieri S et al: In vivo diagnosis of feline infectious peritonitis by comparison of protein content, cytology, and direct immunofluorescence test on peritoneal and pleural effusions, *J Vet Diagn Invest* 11:358, 1999.

Paltrinieri S et al: Laboratory profiles in cats with different pathological and immunohistochemical findings due to feline infectious peritonitis (FIP), *J Fel Med Surg* 3:149, 2001.

Poland AM et al: Two related strains of feline infectious peritonitis virus isolated from immunocompromised cats infected with a feline enteric coronavirus, *J Clin Microbiol* 34:3180, 1996.

Rohrbach BW et al: Epidemiology of feline infectious peritonitis among cats examined at veterinary medical teaching hospitals, *J Am Vet Med Assoc* 218:1111, 2001.

Shelly SM et al: Protein electrophoresis in effusions from cats as a diagnostic test for feline infectious peritonitis, *J Am Anim Hosp Assoc* 24:495, 1998.

Sparkes AH et al: Feline infectious peritonitis: a review of clinicopathological changes in 65 cases and a critical assessment of their diagnostic value, *Vet Rec* 129:209, 1991.

Sparkes AH et al: An appraisal of the value of laboratory tests in the diagnosis of feline infectious peritonitis, *J Am Anim Hosp Assoc* 30:345, 1994.

Telford D et al: PCR-based diagnosis of feline infectious peritonitis, *Vet Rec* 140:379, 1997.

Vennema H et al: Feline infectious peritonitis viruses arise by mutation from endemic feline enteric coronaviruses, *Virology* 243:150, 1998.

## FELINE IMMUNODEFICIENCY VIRUS

Arai M et al: The use of human hematopoietic growth factors (rhGM-CSF and rhEPO) as a supportive therapy for FIV-infected cats, *Vet Immunol Immunopathol* 77:71, 2000.

Barlough JE et al: Acquired immune dysfunction in cats with experimentally induced feline immunodeficiency virus infection: comparison of short-term and long-term infections, *J Acquir Immune Defic Syndr* 4:219, 1991.

Barsanti JA et al: Relationship of lower urinary tract signs to seropositivity for feline immunodeficiency virus in cats, *J Vet Intern Med* 10:34, 1996.

Butera ST et al: Survey of veterinary conference attendees for evidence of zoonotic infection by feline retroviruses, *J Am Vet Med Assoc* 217:1475, 2000.

Celer V Jr et al: Detection of feline immunodeficiency provirus by seminested polymerase chain reaction, *Folia Microbiol* 45:161, 200.

Dow SW et al: In vivo monocyte tropism of pathogenic feline immunodeficiency viruses, *J Virol* 73:6852, 1999.

English R et al: Preliminary report of the ocular manifestations of feline immunodeficiency virus infections, *J Am Vet Med Assoc* 196:1116, 1990.

English RV et al: In vivo lymphocyte tropism of feline immunodeficiency virus, *J Virol* 67:5175, 1993.

Hartmann K et al: AZT in the treatment of feline immunodeficiency virus infection. I, *Fel Pract* 23:16, 1995a.

Hartmann K et al: AZT in the treatment of feline immunodeficiency virus infection. II, *Fel Pract* 23:16, 1995b.

Jordan HL et al: Transmission of feline immunodeficiency virus in domestic cats via artificial insemination, *J Virol* 70:8224, 1996.

Jordan HL et al: Shedding of feline immunodeficiency virus in semen of domestic cats during acute infection, *Am J Vet Res* 60:211, 1999.

Kohmoto M et al: Eight-year observation and comparative study of specific pathogen-free cats experimentally infected with feline immunodeficiency virus (FIV) subtypes A and B: terminal acquired immunodeficiency syndrome in a cat infected with FIV petaluma strain, *J Vet Med Sci* 60:315, 1998.

Lappin MR et al: Primary and secondary *Toxoplasma gondii* infection in normal and feline immunodeficiency virus–infected cats, *J Parasitol* 82:733, 1996.

Leutenegger CM et al: Rapid feline immunodeficiency virus provirus quantitation by polymerase chain reaction using the TaqMan R fluorogenic real-time detection system, *J Virol Methods* 78:105, 1999.

Obert LA et al: Relationship of lymphoid lesions to disease course in mucosal feline immunodeficiency virus type C infection, *Vet Pathol* 37:386, 2000.

O'Neil LL et al: Frequent perinatal transmission of feline immunodeficiency virus by chronically infected cats, *J Virol* 70:2894, 1996.

Papasouliotis K et al: Assessment of intestinal function in cats with chronic diarrhea after infection with feline immunodeficiency virus, *Am J Vet Res* 59:569, 1998.

Pedersen NC et al: Isolation of a T-lymphotrophic virus from domestic cats with an immunodeficiency-like syndrome, *Science* 235:790, 1987.

Pedersen NC et al: Feline leukemia virus infection as a potentiating cofactor for the primary and secondary stages of experimentally induced feline immunodeficiency virus infection, *J Virol* 64:598, 1990.

Poli A et al: Renal involvement in feline immunodeficiency virus infection: a clinicopathological study, *Nephron* 64:282, 1993.

Reubel GH et al: Effects of incidental infections and immune activation on disease progression in experimentally feline immunodeficiency virus–infected cats, *J AIDS* 7:1003, 1994.

Sato R et al: Oral administration of bovine lactoferrin for treatment of intractable stomatitis in feline immunodeficiency virus (FIV)–positive and FIV-negative cats, *Am J Vet Res* 57:1443, 1996.

Shelton GH et al: Prospective hematologic and clinicopathologic study of asymptomatic cats with naturally acquired feline immunodeficiency virus infection, *J Vet Intern Med* 9:133, 1995.

Steigerwald ES et al: Effects of feline immunodeficiency virus on cognition and behavioral function in cats, *J Acquir Immune Defic Syndr Hum Retrovirol* 20:411, 1999.

## FELINE LEUKEMIA VIRUS

Addie DD et al: Long-term impact on a closed household of pet cats of natural infection with feline coronavirus, feline leukaemia virus and feline immunodeficiency virus, *Vet Rec* 146:419, 2000.

Hartmann K et al: Treatment of feline leukemia virus infection with 3'-azido-2,3-dideoxythymidine and human alpha-interferon, *J Vet Intern Med* 16:345, 2002.

Hayes KA et al: Incidence of localized feline leukemia virus infection in cats, *Am J Vet Res* 53:604, 1992.

Herring ES et al: Detection of feline leukaemia virus in blood and bone marrow of cats with varying suspicion of latent infection, *J Fel Med Surg* 3:133, 2001.

Hoover EA et al: Feline leukemia virus infection and diseases, *J Am Vet Med Assoc* 199:1287, 1991.

Jackson ML et al: Feline leukemia virus detection by ELISA and PCR in peripheral blood from 68 cats with high, moderate, or low suspicion of having FeLV-related disease, *J Vet Diagn Invest* 8:25, 1996.

Kass PH et al: Epidemiologic evidence for a causal relationship between vaccination and fibrosarcoma tumorigenesis in cats, *J Am Vet Med Assoc* 203:396, 1993.

Lafrado LJ et al: Immunodeficiency in latent feline leukemia virus infections, *Vet Immunol Immunopathol* 21:39, 1989.

Lubkin SR et al: Evaluation of feline leukemia virus control measures, *J Theor Biol* 178:53, 1996.

Macy DW: Vaccination against feline retroviruses. In August JR, editor: *Consultations in feline internal medicine,* ed 2, Philadelphia, 1994, WB Saunders, p 33.

McCaw DL et al: Immunomodulation therapy for feline leukemia virus infection, *J Am Anim Hosp Assoc* 37:356, 2001.

O'Connor TP et al: Report of the national FeLV/FIV awareness project, *J Vet Med Assoc* 199:1348, 1991.

Reinacher M: Feline leukemia virus–associated enteritis: a condition with features of feline panleukopenia, *Vet Pathol* 24:1, 1987.

Reinacher M: Diseases associated with spontaneous feline leukemia virus (FeLV) infection in cats, *Vet Immunol Immunopathol* 21:85, 1989.

Rojko JL et al: Pathogenesis of infection by the feline leukemia virus, *J Am Vet Med Assoc* 199:1305, 1991.

Sellon R et al: Therapeutic effects of diethylcarbamazine and 3'-azido-3'-deoxythymidine on feline leukemia virus lymphoma formation, *Vet Immunol Immunopathol* 46:181, 1995.

Wolf AM: Feline leukemia virus. In Bonagura J, editor: *Kirk's current veterinary therapy XIII,* Philadelphia, 2000, WB Saunders, p 280.

# CHAPTER 103

# Polysystemic Mycotic Infections

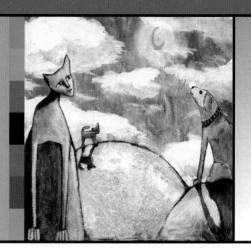

## CHAPTER OUTLINE

CRYPTOCOCCOSIS, 1287
BLASTOMYCOSIS, 1290
HISTOPLASMOSIS, 1291
COCCIDIOIDOMYCOSIS, 1293

## CRYPTOCOCCOSIS

**Etiology and epidemiology.** *Cryptococcus neoformans* is a 3.5 to 7.0 μm yeastlike organism with worldwide distribution. It has a thick polysaccharide capsule and reproduces by narrow-based budding (Table 103-1). Many human and animal infections are reported in southern California and the eastern coast of Australia. Environmental associations include bird excrement (i.e., *C. neoformans* var. *neoformans*) and *Eucalyptus* trees (i.e., *C. neoformans* var. *gatti*). Birds rarely develop clinical cryptococcosis because their high body temperature inhibits fungal replication.

The route of transmission for *C. neoformans* is thought to be inhalation. Nasal and pulmonary disease manifestations are common; however, based on culture and serologic studies of healthy animals, an inapparent carrier state also occurs (Malik and colleagues, 1997a; Malik and colleagues, 1999b). The organism probably spreads to extrapulmonary sites hematogenously; the central nervous system (CNS) may also be infected by direct extension across the cribriform plate from the nasal cavity. Immunity is cell-mediated; individuals with incomplete responses fail to completely remove the organism, thus resulting in granulomatous lesions. The polysaccharide capsule of the organism inhibits plasma cell function, phagocytosis, leukocyte migration, and opsonization, potentiating infection.

Preexisting immunosuppressive conditions are documented in approximately 50% of people with cryptococcosis and have been documented in some infected cats and dogs. Serologic evidence of coinfection with feline immunodeficiency virus or feline leukemia virus (FeLV) occurs in some cats with cryptococcosis. Potentially immunosuppressive conditions such as corticosteroid administration, ehrlichiosis, heartworm disease, and neoplasia are identified in less than 10% of dogs with cryptococcosis.

**Clinical features.** Cryptococcosis is the most common systemic fungal infection of cats and should be considered a differential diagnosis for cats with respiratory tract disease, subcutaneous (SC) nodules, lymphadenopathy, intraocular inflammation, fever, or CNS disease. All ages of cats have been infected, and male cats are overrepresented in most studies. Infection of the nasal cavity resulting in sneezing and nasal discharge (Fig. 103-1) is reported most frequently. The nasal discharge can be unilateral or bilateral, ranges from serous to mucopurulent, and often contains blood. Granulomatous lesions extruding from the external nares, facial deformity over the bridge of the nose, and ulcerative lesions on the nasal planum are common. Mandibular lymphadenopathy is detected in most cats with rhinitis. The nasopharynx is the primary site of involvement in some infected cats and dogs, resulting in snoring and stertor as the predominant clinical signs.

Single or multiple, small (<1 cm), cutaneous or SC masses also have been reported commonly in cats infected with *C. neoformans*. The masses can be either firm or fluctuant and have a serous discharge if ulcerated. Anterior uveitis, chorioretinitis, or optic neuritis occur in association with ocular infection; lens luxations and glaucoma are common sequelae. Chorioretinitis lesions can be punctate or large; suppurative retinal detachment occurs in some infected cats. CNS signs of disease result from diffuse or focal meningoencephalitis or focal granuloma formation.

Manifestations include depression, behavioral changes, seizures, blindness, circling, ataxia, loss of sense of smell, and paresis, depending on the location of the lesion; peripheral vestibular disease can also occur. Nonspecific signs of anorexia, weight loss, and fever occur in some infected cats.

Clinical findings in dogs with cryptococcosis are dependent on the organ systems involved and are similar to those that occur in the cat. Cryptococcosis is diagnosed most commonly in young purebred dogs; Doberman Pinschers and Great Danes were overrepresented in one study (Malik and colleagues, 1995). Clinical manifestations include respiratory tract infection, disseminated disease including intraabdominal masses, CNS disease, disease of the orbit or eye, skin lesions, nasal cavity disease, and lymph node involvement. Seizures, ataxia, central vestibular syndrome, cranial nerve deficits, and clinical signs of cerebellar disease are the most common CNS manifestations in dogs.

TABLE 103-1

Morphologic Appearance of Systemic Canine and Feline Fungal Agents

| AGENT | CYTOLOGIC APPEARANCE |
|---|---|
| *Blastomyces dermatitidis* | Extracellular yeast, 5 to 20 μm in diameter, thick, refractile double-contoured wall, broad-based bud, routine stains are adequate |
| *Cryptococcus neoformans* | Extracellular yeast, 3.5 to 7.0 μm in diameter, thick unstained capsule, thin-based bud, violet color with light red capsule with Gram stain, unstained capsule with India ink |
| *Coccidiodes immitis* | Extracellular spherules (20 to 200 μm in diameter) containing endospores, deep red to purple double outer wall with bright red endospores with PAS stain |
| *Histoplasma capsulatum* | Intracellular yeast in mononuclear phagocytes, 2 to 4 μm in diameter, basophilic center with lighter body with Wright's stain |
| *Sporothrix schenckii* | Round, oval, or cigar-shaped intracellular yeast that is 2 to 3 μm × 3 to 6 μm |

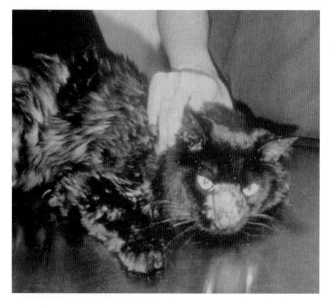

**FIG 103-1**
Severe nasal cryptococcosis in a cat. (Courtesy Dr. Faith Flower, Albuquerque, N.M.)

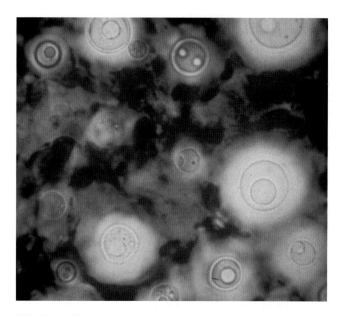

**FIG 103-2**
Cytologic appearance of *Cryptococcus neoformans*. The organism is 3.5 to 7.0 μm in diameter and has a thick polysaccharide capsule. (Courtesy Dr. Dennis Macy, College of Veterinary Medicine and Biomedical Sciences, Colorado State University.)

**Diagnosis.** Nonregenerative anemia and monocytosis are the most common hematologic abnormalities; neutrophil counts and biochemical panels are generally normal. In dogs with CNS involvement, cerebrospinal fluid (CSF) protein concentrations vary from normal to 500 mg/dl, and cell counts vary from normal to 4,500/μl; neutrophils and mononuclear cells predominate, but eosinophils are present in some cases. Radiographic changes consistent with cryptococcosis include increased soft tissue density in the nasal cavity caused by fungal granuloma formation, as well as nasal bone deformity and lysis. Hilar lymphadenopathy and diffuse to miliary pulmonary interstitial patterns are common thoracic radiographic abnormalities.

Because circulating *C. neoformans* antibodies can be detected in both healthy and diseased animals, their presence does not document clinical disease. Additionally, in one study,

all infected cats were seronegative (Flatland and colleagues, 1996). Cryptococcal antigen can be detected in serum, aqueous humor, or CSF using latex agglutination (LA); serum antigen tests are positive in most cats and dogs with cryptococcosis. Animals with acute disease, chronic low-grade infections, drug-induced remission, or in nondisseminated disease can be LA-negative. The LA performed on CSF is positive in almost all animals with CNS cryptococcosis.

A definitive diagnosis of cryptococcosis is based on cytologic, histopathologic, or culture demonstration of the organism (Fig. 103-2). The organism is found during cytologic evaluation of nasal lesions, cutaneous lesions, lymph node aspirates, CSF, and bronchoalveolar lavage fluid in most af-

## TABLE 103-2

Antifungal Drugs Used in the Management of the Systemic Canine and Feline Fungal Diseases

| DRUG | SPECIES* | DOSE | ORGANISM† |
|---|---|---|---|
| Amphotericin B (regular) | D | 0.25 mg/kg IV as test dose, then 0.5 mg/kg IV, up to 3 times weekly‡<br>0.5-0.8 mg/kg SC 2-3 times weekly§ | B,H,Cr,Co |
| | C | 0.25 mg/kg IV, up to 3 times weekly‖<br>0.5-0.8 mg/kg SC 2-3 times weekly§ | B,H,Cr,Co |
| Amphotericin B (liposomal) | B | 0.5 mg/kg IV as test dose, then 1.0 mg/kg, IV, 3-5 times weekly¶ | B,H,Cr,Co |
| Fluconazole | C | 50 mg/cat PO q12h | Cr |
| Flucytosine¶ | B | 50 mg/kg PO q6h | Cr |
| Ketoconazole | B | 10 mg/kg PO q24h | B,H,Cr,Co,Sp |
| Itraconazole | D | 5 mg/kg PO q12h for 4 days, then 5 mg/kg PO q24h | B,Cr,H,Co,Sp |
| | C | 50-100 mg/cat PO q24h | B,Cr,H,Co,Sp |

*D, dog; C, cat; B, dog and cat.
†B, *Blastomyces*; H, *Histoplasma*; Cr, *Cryptococcus*; Co, *Coccidioides*; Sp, *Sporothrix*.
‡In dogs with normal renal function, dilute in 60-120 ml 5% dextrose and administer IV over 15 min; in dogs with renal insufficiency but BUN <50 mg/dl, dilute in 500 ml-1 L 5% dextrose and administer IV over 3-6 hours. Cumulative dose of at least 12 mg/kg if used alone or 6 mg/kg if combined with another antifungal drug.
§Mix in 400 ml (cats) or 500 ml (dogs) of 0.45% saline and 2.5% dextrose solution and administer SQ.
‖In cats with normal renal function, dilute in 50-100 ml 5% dextrose and administer IV over 3-6 hours. Dilute the contents of a vial with 5% dextrose to a final concentration of 1.0 mg/ml and shake for 30 seconds. Draw up needed volume and filter through 18 gauge Monoject filter into 100 ml of 5% dextrose. Infuse IV over 15 minutes (Abelcet; Liposome Co., Princeton, N.J.).
¶Should be used in combination with amphotericin B.

fected animals; it can also be cultured from CSF in animals with neurologic involvement. Because the organism can be cultured from the nasal cavity of some asymptomatic animals, positive results do not always correlate to disease in this region of the body.

**Treatment.** Dogs and cats with cryptococcosis have been treated with amphotericin B, ketoconazole, itraconazole, fluconazole, and 5-flucytosine alone and in varying combinations (Table 103-2). Amphotericin B is usually not indicated unless life-threatening disseminated disease requiring rapid response to therapy is required (see Blastomycosis). If amphotericin B is deemed necessary, the animal should be well hydrated with 0.9% NaCL before treatment, and treatment should be discontinued if the blood urea nitrogen (BUN) exceeds 50 mg/dl. Intravenous (IV) administration of lipid or liposomal encapsulated amphotericin is likely optimal in this situation. However, for clients that cannot afford this therapy, a less expensive SC protocol for administration of regular amphotericin B has been used successfully for the treatment of cryptococcosis in dogs and cats and is likely effective for other systemic fungi (Malik and colleagues, 1996a; Table 103-2).

Ketoconazole, itraconazole, or fluconazole are used as singe agents in dogs or cats without life-threatening disease. In cats with cryptococcosis, there have been variations in reported success rates for fluconazole (96.6%; Malik and colleagues, 1992), itraconazole (57.1%; Medleau and colleagues, 1995), and ketoconazole (34.6%; Flatland and colleagues, 1996). Ketoconazole commonly leads to inappetence, vomit-

ing, diarrhea, weight loss, and increases in liver enzyme activities in some dogs and cats. In dogs, chronic use of ketoconazole can suppresses testosterone and cortisol production and has been associated with cataracts. Because of these problems, ketoconazole is used less frequently.

Itraconazole administration to cats at 100 mg/day can induce anorexia, depression, and increase activity of alamine aminotrausferase (ALT); only one thirteenth of cats receiving 50 mg/day developed toxicity (Medleau and colleagues, 1995). Itraconazole and 5-flucytosine can induce drug eruptions in some dogs. If toxicity develops, drug therapy should be stopped and then reinstituted at 50% of the original dose after signs of toxicity abate. Inappetence in a few cats was the only adverse effect attributed to fluconazole. Itraconazole and fluconazole have less adverse effects than ketoconazole; therefore the author prescribes them more frequently.

Flucytosine crosses the blood-brain barrier better than ketoconazole or amphotericin B, so it has been used primarily for the treatment of CNS cryptococcosis. It has to be used in combination with other antifungal drugs and has many adverse effects including vomiting, diarrhea, hepatotoxicity, cutaneous reactions, and bone marrow suppression. Fluconazole and itraconazole are very lipid soluble; therefore they are also effective for the treatment of CNS disease.

Nasal and cutaneous cryptococcosis generally resolve with treatment, but cats with CNS or ocular disease are less likely to respond. Treatment should continue for at least 1 to 2 months past resolution of clinical disease. Serum and CSF LA antigen titers can diminish with therapy and have been used to monitor response. Antigen titers fail to decrease in some animals without clinical evidence of disease, suggesting persistence of the organism in tissues or false-positive results. It has been recommended that clinically ill animals be treated until clinically normal and the LA titer is less than 1 or the titer has decreased thirty-twofold or more (Malik and colleagues, 1996a).

**Zoonotic aspects and prevention.** People and animals can have the same environmental exposure to *C. neoformans,* but zoonotic transfer from contact with infected animals is unlikely. Prevention is achieved by decreasing potential for exposure; avoiding areas with high concentrations of pigeon droppings is indicated. Application of hydrated lime solution (40 g/L water) at 1.36 L/m² can reduce numbers of organism in contaminated areas.

## BLASTOMYCOSIS

**Etiology and epidemiology.** *Blastomyces dermatitidis* is a saprophytic yeast found primarily in the Mississippi, Missouri, and Ohio River valleys; the mid-Atlantic states; and southern Canada. Recently, two humans acquired blastomycosis in Colorado. An extracellular yeast form (5 to 20 μm in diameter) with broad-based budding develops in the vertebrate host (see Table 103-1). The infectious mycelial phase occurs in the soil and in culture.

Most clinical cases occur from "point source" exposure; multiple cases are diagnosed in an area. Blastomycosis develops most frequently in areas exposed to high humidity, fog, excavation sites, and sandy, acid soils near bodies of water. Most cases in dogs are diagnosed in the autumn. Potential for disease varies with the virulence of the field strain, the inoculum dose, and the immune status of the host.

Transmission is from inhalation or contamination of open wounds with spores from the environment. The organism probably replicates in the lungs initially and then spreads hematogenously to other tissues including the skin and subcutaneous tissues, eyes, bones, lymph nodes, external nares, brain, testes, nasal passages, prostate, liver, mammary glands, vulva, and heart. The organism can be swallowed and passed in feces. Incomplete clearance of the organism by individuals with poor cell-mediated immune responses results in pyogranulomatous inflammation in affected organs, which can cause clinical signs of disease. Subclinical infection is uncommon in dogs.

**Clinical features.** Large-breed, young male, sporting dogs are infected most commonly by *B. dermatitidis* because of an increased chance for exposure to the organism. Anorexia, cough, dyspnea, exercise intolerance, weight loss, ocular disease, skin disease, depression, or lameness are the most common presenting complaints.

Fever occurs in approximately 40% of affected dogs. Interstitial lung disease and hilar lymphadenopathy result in cough, dry harsh lung sounds, and dyspnea; hypertrophic osteopathy occurs in some dogs. Dyspnea from chylothorax

caused by cranial vena cava syndrome has been described. Lymphadenopathy and cutaneous or subcutaneous nodules, abscesses, plaques, or ulcers occur in 20% to 40% of infected dogs. Splenomegaly is common. Lameness from fungal osteomyelitis of the spine or appendicular skeleton occurs in approximately 30% of dogs with blastomycosis. Infection of the testes, prostate, urinary bladder, and kidneys occurs rarely.

Ocular manifestations are recognized in approximately 30% of dogs with blastomycosis; anterior uveitis, endophthalmitis, posterior segment disease, and optic neuritis occur. Depression and seizures from diffuse or multifocal CNS involvement occur in some dogs.

Blastomycosis can occur in any cat, but is most common in young males. Infected cats develop respiratory tract disease, CNS disease, regional lymphadenopathy, dermatologic disease, ocular disease, gastrointestinal tract disease, and urinary tract disease. Pleural or peritoneal effusion resulting in dyspnea or abdominal distension occurs in some cats. Ocular disease usually involves the posterior segment.

**Diagnosis.** Hematologic abnormalities commonly identified in dogs or cats with blastomycosis are normocytic normochromic nonregenerative anemia, lymphopenia, and neutrophilic leukocytosis with or without a left shift. Hypoalbuminemia and hyperglobulinemia (i.e., polyclonal gammopathy) caused by chronic inflammation are common serum biochemical abnormalities; hypercalcemia occurs rarely. Most infected dogs and cats with respiratory disease have diffuse, miliary, or nodular interstitial lung patterns and intrathoracic lymphadenopathy on thoracic radiographs (Fig. 103-3); single masses and pleural effusion from chylothorax sometimes occur. Bone lesions induced by blastomycosis are lytic with a secondary periosteal reaction and soft tissue swelling.

Serum antibodies develop in some infected animals; an antigen test is not available. Many cats with blastomycosis are negative for serum antibodies by agar gel immunodiffusion

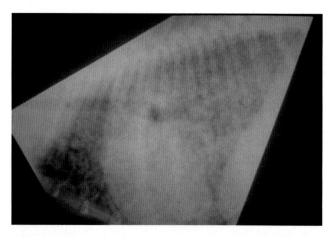

**FIG 103-3**
Miliary interstitial lung pattern consistent with blastomycosis in a dog. (Courtesy Dr. Lynelle Johnson, College of Veterinary Medicine, University of California, Davis.)

(AGID). False-negative results can occur in animals with peracute infection, immunosuppression, or advanced infection that overwhelms the immune system. Antibody titers do not always revert to negative after successful treatment. Because blastomycosis rarely causes subclinical infection, positive serologic results combined with appropriate clinical signs and radiographic abnormalities allow presumptive diagnosis if the organism cannot be demonstrated.

Definitive diagnosis of blastomycosis is based on cytologic, histopathologic, or culture demonstration of the organism (Fig. 103-4). Impression smears from skin lesions and aspirates from enlarged lymph nodes and focal lung lesions usually reveal pyogranulomatous inflammation and organisms that can usually be seen at low power; recovery of organisms from urine is less consistent. Bronchoalveolar lavage is more sensitive than transtracheal wash for organism demonstration. Growth in culture requires 10 to 14 days and is of lower yield than cytology or biopsy.

**Treatment.** Amphotericin B, ketoconazole, amphotericin B and ketoconazole, and itraconazole alone are used most frequently for the treatment of blastomycosis in dogs (see Table 103-2). Amphotericin B is generally used in animals with life-threatening disease; the liposomal encapsulated product is less likely to cause toxicity. If amphotericin B is used, the animal should be well hydrated with 0.9% NaCL before treatment, and treatment should be discontinued if the BUN exceeds 50 mg/dl. Because itraconazole is as effective as amphotericin B and ketoconazole alone or in combination, and has fewer adverse effects (see Therapy for Cryptococcosis) it is the drug of choice for the treatment of blastomycosis (see Table 103-2). Dogs treated with 5 mg/kg/day (53.6%) had a similar success rate as dogs treated with 10 mg/kg/day

(54.3%; Legendre and colleagues, 1996). Treatment should be continued for 60 to 90 days or for 2 to 4 weeks beyond resolution of measurable disease (i.e., thoracic radiographic abnormalities or skin lesions).

Relapses occur in 20% to 25% of treated dogs. When they occur, a complete course of therapy should be reinstituted. Posterior segment ocular disease responds well to itraconazol, but anterior uveitis and endophthalmitis often require enucleation of the affected eye. In one study of 23 cats with blastomycosis, successful results were reported for 2 cats treated with amphotericin B and ketoconazole, 1 cat treated with amputation, and 1 cat treated with potassium iodide (Miller and colleagues, 1990).

**Zoonotic aspects and prevention.** Direct zoonotic transmission from infected animals is unlikely because the yeast phase is not as infectious as the mycelial phase. One veterinarian was infected after material from a pulmonary aspirate from an infected dog was injected intramuscularly (IM), and another developed disease after being bitten by an infected dog. The mycelial phase develops at temperatures lower than body temperature; positive cultures and contaminated bandages are infectious. There have been multiple reports of canine and human blastomycosis that developed from the same environment exposure. Decreasing potential for exposure by avoiding lakes and creeks in endemic areas is the only way to prevent the disease.

## HISTOPLASMOSIS

**Etiology and epidemiology.** *Histoplasma capsulatum* is a saprophytic dimorphic fungus found in the soil in all regions with tropic and subtropic climates; histoplasmosis is diagnosed most frequently in the Mississippi, Missouri, and Ohio River valleys and in the mid-Atlantic states. The organism has been associated with disease in a dog in Australia and a dog in Japan. The microconidia (2 to 4 μm) and macroconidia (5 to 18 μm) of the mycelial phase are found in the environment. In the vertebrate host, the 2 to 4 μm yeast phase is found in the cytoplasm of mononuclear phagocytes (Fig. 103-5; see Table 103-1).

*H. capsulatum* is concentrated most heavily in soil contaminated with bird or bat excrement. Point sources for infection are found within endemic areas; 2 dogs and 20 people developed pulmonary histoplasmosis after removing a tree that had served as a bird roost (Ward and colleagues, 1979). Subclinical infections are common in dogs. Dogs in endemic areas are commonly exposed, but the incidence of disease is low. Immunosuppression may predispose to clinical infection in dogs and cats.

Infection is by ingestion or inhalation of microconidia from the environment. The organism is engulfed by mononuclear phagocytes, transformed to the yeast phase, and transported throughout the body in the blood and lymph. Granulomatous inflammation results in persistently infected organs and clinical signs of disease. Disseminated disease is common in cats.

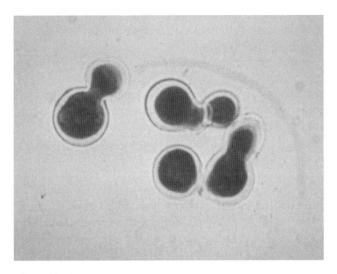

**FIG 103-4**
Cytologic appearance of the budding yeast, *Blastomyces dermatitidis*. The organism is 5 to 20 μm in diameter with a thick, refractile double-contoured wall. (Courtesy Dr. Dennis Macy, College of Veterinary Medicine and Biomedical Sciences, Colorado State University.)

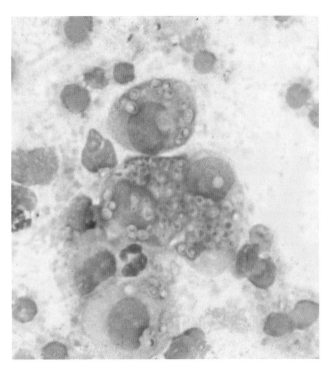

**FIG 103-5**
*Histoplasma capsulatum* (2 to 4 μm in diameter) in a mononuclear cell. (Courtesy Dr. Dennis Macy, College of Veterinary Medicine and Biomedical Sciences, Colorado State University.)

**Clinical features.** Most dogs with histoplasmosis are outdoor sporting breeds less than 7 years of age. Subclinical infection, pulmonary infection, and disseminated infection are recognized most frequently. Most affected dogs are presented for evaluation of anorexia, fever, depression, weight loss, cough, dyspnea, or diarrhea. Large bowel diarrhea is most common, but small bowel diarrhea, mixed bowel diarrhea, and protein-losing enteropathy occurs in some.

Physical examination abnormalities often include depression, increased lung sounds, respiratory wheezes, fever, evidence of diarrhea, pale mucous membranes, hepatomegaly, splenomegaly, icterus, ascites, and intraabdominal lymph node enlargement. Airway obstruction from massive hilar lymphadenopathy occurs in some dogs (Schulman and colleagues, 1999). Lameness from bone infection or polyarthritis, peripheral lymphadenopathy, chorioretinitis, CNS disease, and skin disease occur occasionally. Subcutaneous nodules rarely drain or ulcerate and are less common than in dogs with cryptococcosis or blastomycosis.

Infected cats are either normal or develop disseminated disease. Most clinically affected cats are less than 4 years of age, and some are coinfected with FeLV. Depression, weight loss, anorexia, lameness, or dyspnea are common presenting complaints. Weight loss can be severe and develop in as little as 2 weeks. Fever (103.5° to 105° F), pale mucous membranes, abnormal lung sounds, oral erosions or ulcers, peripheral or visceral lymphadenopathy, icterus, soft tissue swelling around osseous lesions, hepatomegaly, skin nodules, and, rarely,

splenomegaly are physical examination abnormalities potentially consistent with histoplasmosis. Disseminated disease has a grave prognosis in cats. Osseous histoplasmosis is most common in bones of the appendicular skeleton distal to the stifle or elbow joints, and one or more limbs can be involved. Feline ocular histoplasmosis manifests with conjunctivitis, chorioretinitis, retinal detachment, or optic neuritis and may induce glaucoma and blindness. Other than depression, CNS signs are uncommon.

**Diagnosis.** A variety of nonspecific clinicopathologic and radiographic abnormalities are associated with histoplasmosis. Normocytic, normochromic, nonregenerative anemia is the most common hematologic abnormality in both dogs and cats. Neutrophil counts can be normal, increased, or decreased. Unlike the other systemic fungi, *H. capsulatum* is occasionally seen in circulating cells, particularly on examination of a buffy coat smear; mononuclear cell infection is most common, followed by eosinophils. Thrombocytopenia from disseminated intravascular coagulation of microangiopathic destruction occurs in approximately 50% of dogs and some cats. Some affected cats develop pancytopenia from bone marrow infection. Hypoproteinemia and increased activities of alkaline phosphatase and ALT occur in some infected animals.

Lysis predominates in animals with bone infection; periosteal and endosteal new bone production occurs in some cases. In dogs with pulmonary infection, radiographic abnormalities include diffuse interstitial, miliary-to-nodular interstitial disease; hilar lymphadenopathy; pleural effusion; and calcified pulmonary parenchyma caused by chronic disease. In some dogs, massive hilar lymphadenopathy is the only radiographic finding. Alveolar lung disease, tracheobronchial lymphadenopathy, and calcified lymph nodes are uncommon in cats. Colonoscopic findings in dogs with gastrointestinal infection include increased mucosal granularity, friability, ulceration, and thickness.

Several tests have been evaluated for the detection of circulating antibodies against *H. capsulatum* in the serum of dogs and cats, but the sensitivity and specificity are poor for all. Serologic diagnosis is unreliable and should be used only to establish a presumptive diagnosis when the organism cannot be demonstrated by cytology, histopathology, or culture and the clinical signs are suggestive of the disease.

Definitive diagnosis requires demonstration of the organism by cytology, biopsy, or culture (see Fig. 103-5). The organism is found most frequently in rectal scrapings or biopsies from dogs with large bowel diarrhea, in bone marrow or buffy coat cells from cats with disseminated disease, and in other locations (e.g., lymph nodes, lung, spleen, liver, skin nodules). The organism has also been identified in pleural and peritoneal effusions and in CSF.

**Treatment.** Because of its effectiveness and minimal toxicity, itraconazole is the initial drug of choice for dogs and cats with histoplasmosis (see Table 103-2). Animals should be treated for 60 to 90 days or until clinical evidence of disease has been resolved for at least 1 month. Amphotericin B can be used in animals with life-threatening disease or in those unable to absorb oral medications because of intestinal disease. Ketoconazole and fluconazole are also effective in some animals. The overall success rate for the treatment of histoplasmosis in cats was 33% in one study (Clinkenbeard and colleagues, 1989b). In another study, all 8 cats treated with itraconazole (5 mg/kg q12h) were eventually cured (Hodges and colleagues, 1994). Pulmonary disease in dogs has a fair-to-good prognosis, whereas disseminated disease has a poor prognosis.

Administration of glucocorticoids with or without antifungal drugs lessened clinical signs associated with chronic hilar lymphadenopathy much more quickly than administration of antifungal drugs alone and did not result in disseminated histoplasmosis (Schulman and colleagues, 1999). However, if the infection is active, administration of glucocorticoids may exacerbate clinical disease.

**Zoonotic aspects and prevention.** Like blastomycosis, direct zoonotic transmission from infected animals is unlikely because the yeast phase is not as infectious as the mycelial phase. Care should be taken when culturing the organism. Prevention is by avoiding potentially contaminated soil. Organism numbers in contaminated areas can be decreased by application of 3% formalin.

# COCCIDIOIDOMYCOSIS

**Etiology and epidemiology.** *Coccidioides immitis* is a dimorphic fungus found deep in sandy alkaline soils in regions with low elevation, low rainfall, and high environmental temperatures, including the southwestern United States, California, Mexico, Central America, and South America. In the United States, coccidioidomycosis is diagnosed most frequently in California, Arizona, New Mexico, Utah, Nevada, and southwest Texas. The environmental mycelial phase produces arthrospores (2 to 4μm wide, 3 to 10 μm long) that enter the vertebrate host by inhalation or wound contamination. Large numbers of arthrospores return to the surface after periods of rainfall and are dispersed by the wind; the prevalence of coccidioidomycosis increase in years after high rainfall. Most cases (67%) of feline coccidioidomycosis are diagnosed between December and May.

Inhaled arthrospores induce neutrophilic inflammation followed by infiltrates of histiocytes, lymphocytes, and plasma cells. Infection is cleared if cell-mediated immune responses are normal; most people, dogs, and cats exposed to the organism are subclinically affected. The organism disseminates to mediastinal and tracheobronchial lymph nodes, bones and joints, visceral organs (i.e., liver, spleen, kidneys), heart and pericardium, testicles, eyes, brain, and spinal cord of some individuals. Spherules (20 to 200 μm in diameter) containing endospores (see Table 103-1) form in tissues of infected hosts. Endospores are released by cleavage and produce new spherules. Respiratory signs and signs of disseminated disease occur 1 to 3 weeks and 4 months after exposure, respectively.

**Clinical features.** Clinical disease in dogs is most common in young males. Approximately 90% of clinically af-

fected dogs have lameness with swollen, painful bones or joints. Cough, dyspnea, anorexia, weakness, weight loss, lymphadenopathy, lameness, clinical signs of ocular inflammation, and diarrhea are other presenting complaints. Crackles, wheezes, or muffled lung sounds from pleural effusion are common. If subcutaneous abscesses, nodules, ulcers, and draining tracts occur, they are usually associated with infected bones. Myocarditis, icterus, renomegaly, splenomegaly, hepatomegaly, orchitis, epididymitis, keratitis, iritis, granulomatous uveitis, and glaucoma are detected in some dogs. Depression, seizures, ataxia, central vestibular disease, cranial nerve deficits, and behavioral changes are the most common signs of CNS infection.

The median age of cats with coccidioidomycosis is 5 years; no obvious sex or breed predilection exists. The most common clinical manifestations include skin disease (56%), respiratory disease (25%), musculoskeletal disease (19%), and either ophthalmic or neurologic disease (19%) (Greene and colleagues, 1995).

**Diagnosis.** Normocytic, normochromic nonregenerative anemia; leukocytosis; leukopenia; and monocytosis are the most common hematologic abnormalities. Hyperglobulinemia (i.e., polyclonal gammopathy), hypoalbuminemia, renal azotemia, and proteinuria occur in some infected animals.

Diffuse interstitial lung patterns are more common than bronchial, miliary interstitial, nodular interstitial, or alveolar patterns radiographically in dogs and cats with respiratory coccidioidomycosis. Pleural effusion secondary to pleuritis, right-sided heart failure, or constrictive pericarditis can occur. Hilar lymphadenopathy is common in dogs and cats; however, sternal lymphadenopathy or calcification of lymph nodes is not. Bone lesions usually involve the distal diaphysis, epiphysis, and metaphysis of one or more long bones, and they are more proliferative than lytic.

Serum antibodies are detected by complement fixation (CF), AGID, and tube precipitin (TP) tests; TP detects IgM antibodies; CF and AGID detect IgG antibodies. False-negative results can occur in dogs and cats with early infections (<2 weeks), chronic infection, rapidly progressive acute infection, and primary cutaneous coccidioidomycosis. False-positive results in the CF test can occur as a result of anticomplementary serum, which may be caused by bacterial contaminants or immune complexes. The assays can cross-react with antibodies against *Histoplasma capsulatum* and *Blastomyces dermatitidis*. The combination of positive serologic tests and radiographic signs of interstitial lung disease, dermatologic disease, or osteomyelitis in animals from endemic areas can be used to make a presumptive diagnosis if the organism cannot be demonstrated. Titers may persist for months to years after resolution of clinical disease.

Definitive diagnosis requires demonstration of the organism by cytology, biopsy, or culture. The organism is often difficult to demonstrate by cytology; transtracheal aspiration or bronchoalveolar lavage is commonly negative. Extracellular spherules (Fig. 103-6) are most commonly found in lymph node aspirates, draining masses, and pericardial fluid; wet mount examination of unstained smears or Periodic

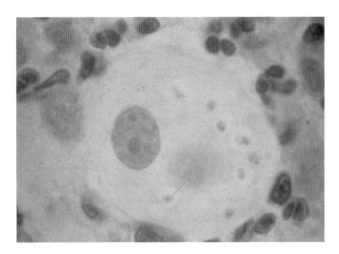

**FIG 103-6**
*Coccidiodes immitis* spherule (20 to 200 μm in diameter) in muscle tissue.

Acid-Schiff (PAS)-stained smears are more suitable than are dry mounts.

**Treatment.** Ketoconazole is the drug of choice for treatment of coccidioidomycosis in dogs (see Table 103-1), but it commonly leads to inappetence, vomiting, diarrhea, weight loss, and increases in liver enzyme activities in some dogs and cats. In dogs, chronic use of ketoconazole can suppress testosterone and cortisol production and has been associated with cataracts. Amphotericin B should be used if life-threatening disease is present or if response to ketoconazole is poor. Itraconazole can be used in animals with toxicity from ketoconazole.

Fluconazole should be used for animals with meningoencephalitis. Cats and dogs should be treated for 60 to 90 days or until clinical illness has been resolved for at least 1 month. Bone infections are often incurable; therefore repeated treatments are often required. When treated with ketoconazole, itraconazole, or fluconazole, 32 of 44 cats with coccidioidomycosis were asymptomatic during or after treatment (Greene and colleagues, 1995). Relapse occurred in 11 cats during or after treatment.

**Zoonotic aspects and prevention.** People exposed to *C. immitis* develop asymptomatic infection or mild, transient respiratory signs. The organism is not transmitted from infected animals to people. However, the mycelial phase occurs outside the vertebrate host and so fomites, such as bandage material and cultures, should be handled carefully. Avoiding endemic areas is the only way to prevent the disease.

## Suggested Readings

CRYPTOCOCCOSIS

Beatty JA et al: Peripheral vestibular disease associated with cryptococcosis in three cats, *J Feline Med Surg* 2:29, 2000.

Berthelin CF et al: Cryptococcosis of the nervous system in dogs. I. Epidemiologic, clinical, and neuropathological features, *Prog Vet Neurol* 5:88, 1994.

Berthelin CF et al: Cryptococcosis of the nervous system in dogs. II. Diagnosis, treatment, monitoring, and prognosis, *Prog Vet Neurol* 5:136, 1994.

Como JA et al: Oral azole drugs as systemic antifungal therapy, *N Engl J Med* 330:263, 1994.

da Costa PD et al: Cataracts in dogs after long-term ketoconazole therapy, *Vet Comp Ophthalmol* 6:176, 1996.

Flatland B et al: Clinical and serologic evaluation of cats with cryptococcosis, *J Am Vet Med Assoc* 209:1110, 1996.

Jacobs GJ et al: Cryptococcal infection in cats: factors influencing treatment outcome and results of sequential serum antigen titers in 35 cats, *J Vet Intern Med* 11:1, 1997.

Kano R et al: PCR detection of the *Cryptococcus neoformans* CAPS9 gene from a biopsy specimen from a case of feline cryptococcosis, *J Vet Diagn Invest* 13:439, 2001.

Legendre AM: Antimycotic drug therapy. In Bonagura JD et al, editors: *Kirk's current veterinary therapy XII,* Philadelphia, 1995, WB Saunders Co, p 327.

Malik R et al: Cryptococcosis in cats: clinical and mycological assessment of 29 cases and evaluation of treatment using orally administered fluconazole, *J Med Vet Mycol* 30:133, 1992.

Malik R et al: Cryptococcosis in dogs: a retrospective study of 20 consecutive cases, *J Med Vet Mycol* 33:291, 1995.

Malik R et al: Combination chemotherapy of canine and feline cryptococcosis using subcutaneously administered amphotericin B, *Aust Vet J* 73:124, 1996a.

Malik R et al: A latex cryptococcal antigen agglutination test for diagnosis and monitoring of therapy for cryptococcosis, *Aust Vet J* 74:358, 1996b.

Malik R et al: Suspected drug eruption in seven dogs during administration of flucytosine, *Aust Vet J* 74:285, 1996c.

Malk R et al: Asymptomatic carriage of *Cryptococcus neoformans* in the nasal cavity of dogs and cats, *J Med Vet Mycol* 35:27, 1997a.

Malik R et al: Nasopharyngeal cryptococcosis, *Aust Vet J* 75:483, 1997b.

Malik R et al: Intra-abdominal cryptococcosis in two dogs, *J Small Amim Pract* 40:387, 1999a.

Malik R et al: Serum antibody response to *Cryptococcus neoformans* in cats, dogs and koalas with and without active infection, *Med Mycol* 37:43, 1999b.

Mancianti F et al: Mycological findings in feline immunodeficiency virus-infected cats, *J Med Vet Mycol* 30:257, 1992.

Medleau L et al: Itraconazole for the treatment of cryptococcosis in cats, *J Vet Intern Med* 9:39, 1995.

BLASTOMYCOSIS

Anonymous: Blastomycosis acquired occupationally during prairie dog relocation—Colorado, 1998, *Morb Mortal Wkly Rep* 48:98, 1999.

Arceneaux KA et al: Blastomycosis in dogs: 115 cases (1980-1995), *J Am Vet Med Assoc* 213:658, 1998.

Baumgardner DJ et al: An outbreak of human and canine blastomycosis, *Rev Infect Dis* 13:898, 1991.

Baumgardner DJ et al: Blastomycosis in dogs: a fifteen-year survey in a very highly endemic area near Eagle River, Wisconsin, USA, *Wilderness Environ Med* 7:1, 1996.

Baumgardner DJ et al: Identification of *Blastomyces dermatitidis* in the stool of a dog with acute pulmonary blastomycosis, *J Med Vet Mycol* 35:419, 1997.

Bloom JD et al: Ocular blastomycosis in dogs: 73 cases, 108 eyes (1985-1993), *J Am Vet Med Assoc* 209:1271, 1996.

Breider MA et al: Blastomycosis in cats: five cases (1979-1986), *J Am Vet Med Assoc* 193:570, 1988.

Brooks DE et al: The treatment of canine ocular blastomycosis with systemically administered itraconazole, *Prog Vet Comp Ophthalmol* 1:263, 1991.

Côté E et al: Possible transmission of *Blastomycosis dermatitidis* via culture specimen., *J Am Vet Med Assoc* 210:479, 1997.

Dow SW et al: Hypercalcemia associated with blastomycosis in dogs, *J Am Vet Med Assoc* 188:606, 1986.

Gnann JW et al: Human blastomycosis after a dog bite, *Ann Intern Med* 98:48, 1983.

Hawkins EC et al: Cytologic analysis of tracheal wash specimens and bronchoalveolar lavage fluid in the diagnosis of mycotic infections in dogs, *J Am Vet Med Assoc* 197:79, 1990.

Howard J et al: Blastomycosis granuloma involving the cranial vena cava associated with chylothorax and cranial vena caval syndrome in a dog, *J Am Anim Hosp Assoc* 36:159, 2000.

Krawieck DR et al: Use of an amphotericin B lipid complex for treatment of blastomycosis in dogs, *J Am Vet Med Assoc* 209:2073, 1996.

Legendre AM et al: Treatment of blastomycosis with itraconazole in 112 dogs, *J Vet Intern Med* 10:365, 1996.

McCune MB: A blastomycosis field investigation: canine outbreak suggests risk to human health, *J Environ Health* 51:22, 1988.

Miller PE et al: Feline blastomycosis: a report of three cases and literature review (1961 to 1988), *J Am Anim Hosp Assoc* 26:417, 1990.

Ramsey DT: Blastomycosis in a veterinarian, *J Am Vet Med Assoc* 205:968, 1994.

Rudmann DG et al: Evaluation of risks factors for blastomycosis in dogs: 857 cases (1980-1990), *J Am Vet Med Assoc* 201:1754, 1992.

Wood EF et al: Ultrasound-guided fine-needle aspiration of focal parenchymal lesions of the lung in dogs and cats, *J Vet Intern Med* 12:338, 1998.

HISTOPLASMOSIS

Clinkenbeard KD et al: Identification of Histoplasma organisms in circulating eosinophils of a dog, *J Am Vet Med Assoc* 192:217, 1988.

Clinkenbeard KD et al: Thrombocytopenia associated with disseminated histoplasmosis in dogs, *Comp Cont Ed Pract Vet* 11:301, 1989.

Clinkenbeard KD et al: Canine disseminated histoplasmosis, *Comp Cont Ed Pract Vet* 11:1347, 1989a.

Clinkenbeard KD et al: Feline disseminated histoplasmosis, *Comp Cont Ed Pract Vet* 11:1223, 1989b.

Davies C et al: Deep mycotic infections in cats, *J Am Anim Hosp Assoc* 32:380, 1996.

Davies SF et al: Concurrent human and canine histoplasmosis from cutting decayed wood, *Ann Intern Med* 113:252, 1990.

Hodges RD et al: Itraconazole for the treatment of histoplasmosis in cats, *J Vet Intern Med* 8:409, 1994.

Kagawa Y et al: Histoplasmosis in the skin and gingiva in a dog, *J Vet Med Sci* 60:863, 1998.

Mackie JT et al: Confirmed histoplasmosis in an Australian dog, *Aust Vet J* 75:362, 1997.

Schulman RL et al: Use of corticosteroids for treating dogs with airway obstruction secondary to hilar lymphadenopathy caused by chronic histoplasmosis: 16 cases (1979-1997), *J Am Vet Med Assoc* 214:1345, 1999.

Ward JI et al: Acute histoplasmosis: clinical, epidemiologic and serologic finding of an outbreak associated with exposure to a fallen tree, *Am J Med* 66:587, 1979.

Wolf AM: *Histoplasma capsulatum* in the cat, *J Vet Intern Med* 1:158, 1987.

Wolf AM: Successful treatment of disseminated histoplasmosis with osseous involvement in two cats, *J Am Anim Hosp Assoc* 24:511, 1988.

Wolf AM: Histoplasmosis. In Greene CE, editor: *Infectious diseases of the dog and cat*, ed 2, Philadelphia, 1990, WB Saunders Co, p 679.

Wolf AM et al: The radiographic appearance of pulmonary histoplasmosis in the cat, *Vet Radiol* 28:34, 1987.

COCCIDIOIDOMYCOSIS

Angell JA et al: Ocular lesions associated with coccidioidomycosis in dogs: 35 cases (1980-1985), *J Am Vet Med Assoc* 190:1319, 1987.

Armstrong PJ et al: Canine coccidioidomycosis: a literature review and report of 8 cases, *J Am Anim Hosp Assoc* 19:937, 1983.

Barsanti JA et al: Coccidioidomycosis. In Greene CE, editor: *Infectious diseases of the dog and cat*, ed 2, Philadelphia, 1990, WB Saunders Co, p 696.

Burtch M: Granulomatous meningitis caused by in a dog, *J Am Vet Med Assoc* 212:827, 1998.

Coccidioidomycosis—United States, 1991-1992, *Morb Mortal Wkly Rep* 42:21, 1993.

Greene RT et al: Coccidioidomycosis in 48 cats: a retrospective study (1984-1993), *J Vet Intern Med* 9:86, 1995.

Hinsch BG: Ketoconazole treatment of disseminated coccidioidomycosis in a dog, *Mod Vet Pract* 69:161, 1988.

Jackson JA et al: Treatment of canine coccidioidomycosis with ketoconazole: serological aspects of a case study, *J Am Anim Hosp Assoc* 21:572, 1985.

Millman TM et al: Coccidioidomycosis in the dog; its radiographic diagnosis, *J Am Vet Rad Soc* 20:50, 1979.

Pappagianis D: Evaluation of the protective efficacy of the killed *Coccidioides immitis* spherule vaccine in humans, *Am Rev Respir Dis* 148:656, 1993.

Shubitz LF et al: Constrictive pericarditis secondary to *Coccidioides* infection in a dog, *J Am Vet Med Assoc* 218:537, 2001.

## CHAPTER 104

# Polysystemic Protozoal Infections

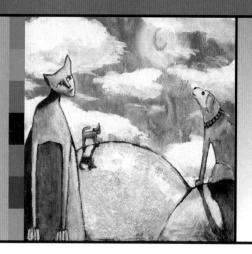

## CHAPTER OUTLINE

FELINE TOXOPLASMOSIS, 1296
CANINE TOXOPLASMOSIS, 1299
NEOSPOROSIS, 1299
BABESIOSIS, 1300
CYTAUXZOONOSIS, 1301
HEPATOZOONOSIS, 1302
LEISHMANIASIS, 1303
AMERICAN TRYPANOSOMIASIS, 1304

## FELINE TOXOPLASMOSIS

**Etiology and epidemiology.** *Toxoplasma gondii* is one of the most prevalent parasites infecting warm-blooded vertebrates. Only cats complete the coccidian life cycle and pass environmentally resistant oocysts in feces. Sporozoites develop in oocysts after 1 to 5 days of exposure to oxygen and appropriate environmental temperature and humidity. Tachyzoites disseminate in blood or lymph during active infection and replicate rapidly intracellularly until the cell is destroyed. Bradyzoites are the slowly dividing, persistent tissue stage that form in the extraintestinal tissues of infected hosts as immune responses attenuate tachyzoite replication. Tissue cysts form readily in the central nervous system (CNS), muscles, and visceral organs.

Infection of warm-blooded vertebrates occurs following ingestion of any of the three life stages of the organism or transplacentally. Most cats are not coprophagic and so are infected most commonly by ingesting *T. gondii* bradyzoites during carnivorous feeding; oocysts are shed in feces from 3 to 21 days. Sporulated oocysts can survive in the environment for months to years and are resistant to most disinfectants (Fig. 104-1). Bradyzoites may persist in tissues for the life of the host. Approximately 30% to 40% of cats and people in the United States are seropositive and so presumed to be infected.

**Clinical features.** Approximately 10% to 20% of experimentally inoculated cats develop self-limiting, small bowel diarrhea for 1 to 2 weeks following primary oral inoculation with *T. gondii* tissue cysts; this is presumed to be due to enteroepithelial replication of the organism. However, detection of *T. gondii* oocysts in feces is rarely reported in studies of naturally exposed cats with diarrhea. *T. gondii* enteroepithelial stages were found in intestinal tissues from two cats with inflammatory bowel disease. Positive response to anti-*Toxoplasma* drugs in these two cats suggests that toxoplasmosis may occasionally induce inflammatory bowel disease.

Fatal extraintestinal toxoplasmosis can develop from overwhelming intracellular replication of tachyzoites following primary infection; hepatic, pulmonary, CNS, and pancreatic tissues are commonly involved. Transplacentally or lactationally infected kittens develop the most severe signs of extraintestinal toxoplasmosis and generally die of pulmonary or hepatic disease. Common clinical findings in cats with disseminated toxoplasmosis include depression, anorexia, and fever followed by hypothermia, peritoneal effusion, icterus, and dyspnea. If a host with chronic toxoplasmosis is immunosuppressed, bradyzoites in tissue cysts can replicate rapidly and disseminate again as tachyzoites; this is common in people with acquired immunodeficiency syndrome (AIDS). Disseminated toxoplasmosis has been documented in cats concurrently infected with feline leukemia, feline immunodeficiency, or feline infectious peritonitis viruses, as well as following renal transplantation.

Sublethal, chronic toxoplasmosis occurs in some cats. *T. gondii* infection should be on the differential diagnoses list for cats with anterior or posterior uveitis, fever, muscle hyperesthesia, weight loss, anorexia, seizures, ataxia, icterus, diarrhea, or pancreatitis (Fig. 104-2). Based on results of *T. gondii*–specific aqueous humor antibody and polymerase chain reaction (PCR) studies, toxoplasmosis appears to be a common infectious cause of uveitis in cats. Kittens infected transplacentally or lactationally commonly develop ocular disease. Immune complex formation and deposition in tissues and delayed hypersensitivity reactions may be involved in chronic, sublethal clinical toxoplasmosis. Since none of the anti-*Toxoplasma* drugs totally clear the body of the organism, recurrence of disease is common.

**Diagnosis.** Cats with clinical toxoplasmosis can have a variety of clinicopathologic and radiographic abnormalities, but none document the disease. Nonregenerative anemia,

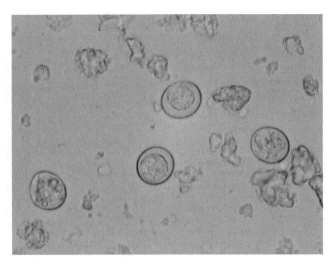

**FIG 104-1**
Unstained *Toxoplasma gondii* unsporulated oocysts. The oocysts are 10 × 12 μm.

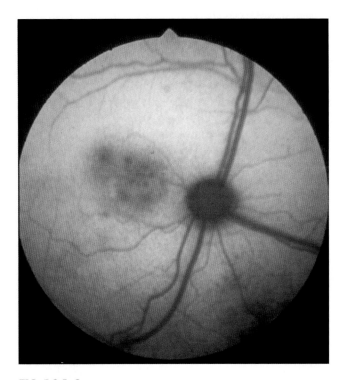

**FIG 104-2**
Punctate chorioretinitis caused by *Toxoplasma gondii* in an experimentally inoculated cat.

neutrophilic leukocytosis, lymphocytosis, monocytosis, neutropenia, eosinophilia, proteinuria, bilirubinuria, as well as increases in serum protein and bilirubin concentrations, and creatinine kinase, alanine aminotransferase, alkaline phosphatase, and lipase activities occur in some cats. Pulmonary toxoplasmosis most commonly causes diffuse interstitial to alveolar patterns or pleural effusion. Cerebrospinal fluid (CSF) protein concentrations and cell counts are often higher

than normal. The predominant white blood cells in CSF are small mononuclear cells, but neutrophils also are commonly found.

The antemortem definitive diagnosis of feline toxoplasmosis can be made if the organism is demonstrated; however, this is uncommon, particularly if sublethal disease is occurring. Bradyzoites or tachyzoites are rarely detected in tissues, effusions, bronchoalveolar lavage fluids, aqueous humor, or CSF. Detection of 10 × 12 μm oocysts in feces in cats with diarrhea suggests toxoplasmosis but is not definitive, since *Besnoitia* and *Hammondia* infections of cats produce morphologically similar oocysts.

*T. gondii*–specific antibodies (immunoglobulin [Ig]: IgM, IgG, IgA), antigens, and immune complexes can be detected in the serum of normal cats, as well as in those with clinical signs of disease, so it is impossible to make an antemortem diagnosis of clinical toxoplasmosis based on these tests alone. Of the serum tests, IgM correlates the best with clinical feline toxoplasmosis since this antibody class is rarely detected in serum of healthy cats. The antemortem diagnosis of clinical toxoplasmosis can be tentatively based on the combination of the following:

- Demonstration of antibodies in serum, which documents exposure to *T. gondii*
- Demonstration of an IgM titer above 1:64 or a fourfold or greater increase in IgG titer, which suggests recent or active infection
- Clinical signs of disease referable to toxoplasmosis
- Exclusion of other common causes for the clinical syndrome
- Positive response to appropriate treatment

Some cats with clinical toxoplasmosis will have reached their maximal IgG titer or will have undergone antibody class shift from IgM to IgG by the time they are serologically evaluated, so the failure to document an increasing IgG titer or a positive IgM titer does not exclude the diagnosis of clinical toxoplasmosis. Since some healthy cats have extremely high serum antibody titers and some clinically ill cats have low serum antibody titers, the magnitude of titer is relatively unimportant in the clinical diagnosis of toxoplasmosis. Because the organism cannot be cleared from the body, most cats will be antibody-positive for life, so there is little reason to repeat serum antibody titers after the clinical disease has resolved.

The combination of aqueous humor or CSF *T. gondii*–specific antibody detection and organism deoxyribonucleic acid (DNA) detection by PCR is the most accurate way to diagnose ocular or CNS toxoplasmosis (Diagnostic Laboratory, College of Veterinary Medicine and Biomedical Sciences, Colorado State University, Fort Collins, CO 80523). Whereas *T. gondii*–specific IgA, IgG, and organism DNA can be detected in aqueous humor and CSF of both normal and clinically ill cats, *T. gondii*–specific IgM has only been detected in the aqueous humor or CSF of clinically ill cats and so may be the best indicator of clinical disease. Since *T. gondii* DNA can be detected in blood of healthy cats, positive PCR results do not correlate to clinical disease.

**Treatment.** Supportive care should be instituted as needed. Clindamycin hydrochloride (Antirobe; Pharmacia Animal Health, Kalamazoo, Mich) administered (10 to 12 mg/kg, PO, q12h) for 4 weeks or a trimethoprim-sulfonamide combination administered (15 mg/kg, PO, q12h) for 4 weeks has been used most frequently by the author for the treatment of clinical feline toxoplasmosis. Azithromycin administered (7.5 mg/kg, PO, q12h) has been used successfully in a limited number of cats, but the optimal duration of therapy is unknown. Pyrimethamine combined with sulfa drugs is effective for the treatment of human toxoplasmosis but commonly results in toxicity in cats. Cats with systemic clinical signs of toxoplasmosis, such as fever or muscle pain combined with uveitis, should be treated with anti-*Toxoplasma* drugs in combination with topical, oral, or parenteral corticosteroids to avoid secondary lens luxations and glaucoma. *T. gondii*–seropositive cats with uveitis that are otherwise normal can be treated with topical glucocorticoids alone unless the uveitis is recurrent or persistent. In these situations, administration of a drug with anti–*T. gondii* activity may be beneficial.

Clinical signs not involving the eyes or the CNS usually resolve within the first 2 to 3 days of clindamycin or trimethoprim-sulfonamide administration; ocular and CNS toxoplasmosis responds more slowly to therapy. If fever or muscle hyperesthesia is not decreasing after 3 days of treatment, other causes should be considered. Recurrence of clinical signs may be more common in cats treated for less than 4 weeks. There is no evidence to suggest that any drug can totally clear the body of the organism, so recurrences are common and infected cats will always be seropositive. The prognosis is poor for cats with hepatic or pulmonary disease caused by organism replication, particularly in those that are immunocompromised.

**Zoonotic aspects and prevention.** *T. gondii* is a major zoonosis. Primary infection of mothers during gestation can lead to clinical toxoplasmosis in the fetus; stillbirth, CNS disease, and ocular disease are common clinical manifestations. Primary infection in immunocompetent individuals results in self-limiting fever, malaise, and lymphadenopathy. As T-helper cell counts decline, approximately 10% of people with AIDS develop toxoplasmic encephalitis from activation of bradyzoites in tissue cysts.

People most commonly acquire toxoplasmosis by ingesting sporulated oocysts or tissue cysts, or transplacentally. To prevent toxoplasmosis, avoid eating undercooked meats or ingesting sporulated oocysts (Table 104-1). Although owning a pet cat was epidemiologically associated with acquiring toxoplasmosis in one study of pregnant women, touching individual cats is probably not a common way to acquire toxoplasmosis for the following reasons:

- Cats generally only shed oocysts for days to several weeks after primary inoculation.
- Repeat oocyst shedding is rare, even in cats receiving glucocorticoids or in those infected with feline immunodeficiency virus or feline leukemia virus.

 TABLE 104-1

**Prevention of Human Toxoplasmosis**

**Prevention of Oocyst Ingestion**

Avoid feeding cats undercooked meats.
Do not allow cats to hunt.
Clean the litter box daily, and incinerate or flush the feces.
Clean the litter box daily with scalding water, or use a litter box liner.
Wear gloves when working with soil.
Wash hands thoroughly with soap and hot water following gardening.
Wash fresh vegetables well before ingestion.
Keep children's sandboxes covered.
Boil water for drinking that has been obtained from the general environment.
Control potential transport hosts.
Treat oocyst shedding cats with anti-*Toxoplasma* drugs.

**Prevention of Tissue Cyst Ingestion**

Cook all meat products to 66° C.
Wear gloves when handling meats.
Wash hands thoroughly with soap and hot water after handling meats.
Freeze all meat for a minimum of 3 days before cooking.

- Cats with toxoplasmosis inoculated with tissue cysts 16 months after primary inoculation did not shed oocysts.
- Cats are very fastidious and usually do not allow feces to remain on their skin for time periods long enough to lead to oocyst sporulation; the organism was not isolated from the fur of cats shedding millions of oocysts 7 days previously.
- Increased risk of acquired toxoplasmosis was not associated with cat ownership in people with AIDS or in veterinary health care providers.

However, since some cats will repeat oocyst shedding when exposed a second time, feces should always be handled carefully. If a fecal sample from a cat is shown to contain oocysts measuring $10 \times 12$ μm it should be assumed that the organism is *T. gondii*. The feces should be collected daily until the oocyst shedding period is complete; administration of clindamycin (25 to 50 mg/kg, divided q12h, PO) or sulfonamides (100 mg/kg, divided q12h, PO) can reduce levels of oocyst shedding.

Since humans are not commonly infected with *T. gondii* from contact with individual cats, testing healthy cats for toxoplasmosis is not recommended. Fecal examination is an adequate procedure to determine when cats are actively shedding oocysts but cannot predict when a cat has shed oocysts in the past. There is no serologic assay that accurately predicts when a cat shed *T. gondii* oocysts in the past, and most cats that are shedding oocysts are seronegative. Most seropositive cats have completed the oocyst shedding period and are unlikely to repeat shedding; most seronegative cats would shed the organism if infected. If owners are concerned that they may have toxoplasmosis, they should see their physician for testing.

## CANINE TOXOPLASMOSIS

**Etiology and epidemiology.** Dogs do not produce *T. gondii* oocysts like cats, but they can mechanically transmit oocysts after ingesting feline feces. The tissue phases of *T. gondii* infection occur in dogs and can induce clinical disease. Approximately 20% of dogs in the United States are seropositive for *T. gondii* antibodies. Before 1988, many dogs diagnosed with toxoplasmosis based on histologic evaluation were truly infected with *Neospora caninum* (see Neosporosis section).

**Clinical features.** Respiratory, gastrointestinal, or neuromuscular infection resulting in fever, vomiting, diarrhea, dyspnea, and icterus occurs most commonly in dogs with generalized toxoplasmosis. Generalized toxoplasmosis is most common in immunosuppressed dogs, such as those with canine distemper virus infection or those receiving cyclosporine to prevent rejection of a transplanted kidney. Neurologic signs depend on the location of the primary lesions and include ataxia, seizures, tremors, cranial nerve deficits, paresis, and paralysis. Dogs with myositis present with weakness, stiff gait, or muscle wasting. Rapid progression to tetraparesis and paralysis with lower motor neuron dysfunction can occur. Some dogs with suspected neuromuscular toxoplasmosis probably had neosporosis. Myocardial infection resulting in ventricular arrhythmias occurs in some infected dogs. Dyspnea, vomiting, or diarrhea occurs in dogs with polysystemic disease. Retinitis, anterior uveitis, iridocyclitis, and optic neuritis occur in some dogs with toxoplasmosis, but they are less common than in cats.

**Diagnosis.** As in cats, hematologic, biochemical, urinalysis, and radiographic abnormalities are not specific. Increased protein concentrations and mixed inflammatory cell infiltrates occur in dogs with CNS toxoplasmosis.

Demonstration of the organism associated with inflammation in tissues or exudates can lead to a definitive diagnosis. More commonly, an antemortem diagnosis is based on the combination of appropriate clinical signs, exclusion of other likely etiologies, positive serum antibody tests, exclusion of *Neospora caninum* infection by serologic testing, and response to an anti-*Toxoplasma* drug. Interpretation of serum, aqueous humor, and CSF antibody and PCR test results is as discussed for toxoplasmosis in cats.

**Therapy.** Clindamycin hydrochloride (10-12 mg/kg, PO, q12h) has been used most frequently for treatment of canine toxoplasmosis by the author. Trimethoprim-sulfa (15 mg/kg, PO, q12h) is an alternative protocol. Treatment should be continued for a minimum of 4 weeks. If uveitis occurs, topical glucocorticoid treatment should also be used.

**Zoonotic aspects and prevention.** Dogs do not complete the enteroepithelial phase of *T. gondii* but can mechanically transmit oocysts after ingesting feline feces. Like all other warm-blooded vertebrates, dogs are infected by the ingestion of sporulated oocysts or tissue cysts. Toxoplasmosis in dogs can be prevented by not allowing dogs to be coprophagic and to feed only cooked meat and meat byproducts.

## NEOSPOROSIS

**Etiology and epidemiology.** *Neospora caninum* is a coccidian previously confused with *T. gondii* because of similar morphology. The sexual cycle is completed in the gastrointestinal tract of dogs and results in the passage of oocysts in feces. Sporozoites develop in oocysts within 24 hours of passage. Tachyzoites (rapidly dividing stage) and tissue cysts containing hundreds of bradyzoites (slowly dividing stage) are the other two life stages. Dogs are infected by ingestion of bradyzoites but not tachyzoites. Infection has been documented after ingestion of infected bovine placental tissue. Transplacental infection has been well documented; dams that give birth to infected offspring can repeat transplacental infection during subsequent pregnancies. Pathogenesis of disease is primarily related to the intracellular replication of tachyzoites. Although organism replication occurs in many tissues including the lungs, in dogs clinical illness is primarily neuromuscular. Encephalomyelitis and myositis develop in experimentally infected kittens, but clinical disease in naturally infected cats has not been reported.

Canine neosporosis has been reported in many countries around the world. Seroprevalence of infection has varied from 0% to 29%. Whether other intermediate hosts play a role in maintenance of infection is unknown, but white-tailed deer are commonly seropositive. Thus free-roaming dogs may be at increased risk of infection. Since repeated transplacental infections occur, there is increased risk for puppies from a bitch previously birthing infected puppies. Administration of glucocorticoids may activate bradyzoites in tissue cysts resulting in clinical illness.

**Clinical features.** Ascending paralysis with hyperextension of the hindlimbs in congenitally infected puppies is the most common clinical manifestation of the disease. Muscle atrophy occurs in many cases. Polymyositis and multifocal CNS disease can occur alone or in combination. Clinical signs can be evident soon after birth or may be delayed for several weeks. Neonatal death is common. Although disease tends to be most severe in congenitally infected puppies, dogs as old as 15 years have been clinically affected. In one dog presented primarily for respiratory disease, cough was the principal sign. Myocarditis, dysphagia, ulcerative dermatitis, pneumonia, and hepatitis occur in some dogs. It is unknown whether clinical disease in older dogs is due to acute, primary infection or exacerbation of chronic infection. Administration of glucocorticoids may activate bradyzoites in tissue cysts resulting in clinical illness. Disease is due to intracellular replication of *Neospora caninum* tachyzoites. Infection of CNS structures causes mononuclear cell infiltrates, which suggests an immune-mediated component to the pathogenesis of disease. Intact tissue cysts in neural structures are generally not associated with inflammation, but ruptured tissue cysts induce inflammation. The untreated disease generally results in death.

**Diagnosis.** Hematologic and biochemical findings are nonspecific. Myositis commonly results in increased creatine kinase (CK) and aspartase aminotransferase (AST) activities. CSF abnormalities include increased protein concentration (20 to 50 mg/dl) and a mild, mixed inflammatory cell pleocytosis (10 to 50 cells/μl) consisting of monocytes, lymphocytes, neutrophils, and rarely, eosinophils. Interstitial and alveolar patterns can be noted on thoracic radiographs.

Definitive diagnosis is based on demonstration of the organism in CSF or tissues. Tachyzoites are rarely identified on cytologic examination of CSF, imprints of dermatologic lesions, and bronchoalveolar lavage. Mixed inflammation with neutrophils, lymphocytes, eosinophils, plasma cells, macrophages, and tachyzoites was noted on transthoracic aspirate of one dog with lung disease. *Neospora caninum* tissue cysts have a wall thicker than 1 μm; *T. gondii* tissue cysts have a wall thinner than 1 μm (Fig. 104-3). Oocysts can be detected in feces by microscopic examination after flotation or by PCR. The organism can be differentiated from *T. gondii* by electron microscopy, immunohistochemistry, and PCR.

A presumptive diagnosis of neosporosis can be made by combining appropriate clinical signs of disease and positive serology or presence of antibodies in CSF with the exclusion of other etiologies inducing similar clinical syndromes, in particular, *T. gondii*. IgG antibody titers of at least 1:200 have been detected in most dogs with clinical neosporosis; there is minimal serologic cross-reactivity with *T. gondii* at titers of 1:50 or higher.

**Treatment.** Although many dogs with neosporosis die, some have survived after treatment with trimethoprim-sulfadiazine combined with pyrimethamine; sequential treatment with clindamycin hydrochloride, trimethoprim-

sulfadiazine, and pyrimethamine; or clindamycin alone. Administration of trimethoprim-sulfadiazine (15 mg/kg, PO, q12h) with pyrimethamine (1 mg/kg, PO, q24h) for 4 weeks or clindamycin (10 mg/kg, PO, q8h) for 4 weeks is currently recommended for the treatment of canine neosporosis. Treatment of clinically affected dogs should be initiated before the development of extensor rigidity, if possible. The prognosis for dogs presented with severe neurologic involvement is grave.

**Zoonotic aspects and prevention.** *Neospora caninum* antibodies have been detected in people, but in one study, there was no link to repeated abortion. There has been an epidemiologic link between dogs and cattle, and so efforts should be made to lessen dog fecal contamination of livestock feed, and dogs should not be allowed to ingest bovine placentas. White-tailed deer are commonly seropositive, so it is possible that intermediate hosts play a role in canine infection. Bitches that whelp clinically affected puppies should not be bred. Glucocorticoids should not be administered to seropositive animals, if possible, since a potential exists for activation of infection.

## BABESIOSIS

**Etiology and epidemiology.** Babesiosis in dogs is most commonly associated with *Babesia canis* and *B. gibsoni*, protozoans that parasitize red blood cells, leading to progressive anemia. *B. canis* has worldwide distribution including Africa, Asia, Australia, Europe, Central America, South America, Japan, and the United States. There are three subspecies of *B. canis* that have been proposed to be separate species. *B. canis rossi* is transmitted by *Haemaphysalis leachi* and is the most pathogenic; *B. canis canis* is transmitted by *Dermacentor reticulatus* and is moderately pathogenic; *B. canis vogeli* is the least pathogenic and is transmitted by *Rhipicephalus sanguineus* (brown dog tick). *B. gibsoni* infects dogs in the United States, Japan, India, Sri Lanka, Korea, Malaysia, and Egypt. North American and Asian isolates of *B. gibsoni* vary genetically enough to be proposed as different species. In countries other than the United States, *H. bispinosa* and *H. longicornis* are known vectors for *B. gibsoni*. *R. sanguineus* is proposed but not proven to be a vector in the United States. *B. gibsoni* has been detected in at least 16 of the United States. A *Babesia* spp. that genetically varies considerably from other *B. canis* or *B. gibsoni* isolates was described in Oklahoma. None of the *Babesia* spp. that infect cats (*B. cati* [India], *B. felis* [South Africa, Sudan], *B. herpailuri* [South America, Africa], *B. pantherae* [Kenya]) have been recognized in the United States. *Babesia* spp. can also be transmitted by blood transfusions.

Following infection with *B. canis*, the incubation period varies from 10 to 21 days. Parasitemia can be detected transiently from day 1; recurrent parasitemia is detected by day 14, with peak organism levels occurring on day 20. The organism replicates intracellularly in red blood cells, resulting in intravascular hemolytic anemia. Immune-mediated reactions against the parasite or altered self-antigens worsen the he-

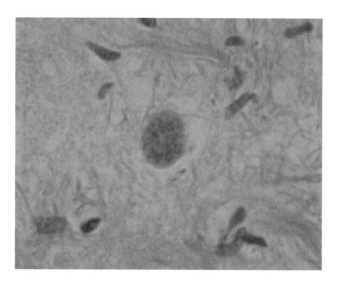

**FIG 104-3**
*Neospora caninum* cyst filled with bradyzoites in canine central nervous system (CNS) tissue.

molytic anemia and commonly result in a positive direct Coombs' test. Stimulation of macrophages leads to fever and hepatosplenomegaly. Severe hypoxia occurs because of rapid breakdown of red blood cells. Disseminated intravascular coagulation occurs in some infected dogs during acute infection. Severity of disease depends on the species and strain of *Babesia* and the host's immune status; chronic, subclinical infection can be common with some. Administration of glucocorticoids or splenectomy may activate chronic disease.

**Clinical features.** Peracute or acute *Babesia* infections result in anemia and fever, leading to pale mucous membranes, tachycardia, tachypnea, depression, anorexia, and weakness. Icterus, petechiae, and hepatosplenomegaly are present in some dogs depending on the stage of infection and the presence of disseminated intravascular coagulation. Severe anemia, disseminated intravascular coagulation, metabolic acidosis, and renal disease are most common during acute infection. The main differential diagnosis for acute babesiosis is primary immune-mediated hemolytic anemia. Chronically infected dogs commonly have weight loss and anorexia. Ascites, gastrointestinal signs, CNS disease, edema, and clinical evidence of cardiopulmonary disease occur in some dogs with atypical infection. Subclinical infection occurs as well.

**Diagnosis.** Regenerative anemia, hyperbilirubinemia, bilirubinuria, hemoglobinuria, thrombocytopenia, metabolic acidosis, azotemia, polyclonal gammopathy, and renal casts are common in dogs with babesiosis. A presumptive diagnosis can be based on historical findings, physical examination findings, test results, and positive serology. Indirect fluorescent antibody tests for *B. canis* and *B. gibsoni* are available commercially. However, there is serologic cross-reactivity between *B. canis* and *B. gibsoni,* and so antibody test results cannot be used to definitively determine the infective species. Demonstration of increasing titers over 2 to 3 weeks is consistent with recent or active infection. There is currently no standardization between laboratories, and so suggested positive cutoff titers vary. False-negative serologic test results can occur in peracute cases or in dogs with concurrent immunosuppression. A titer above 1:320 was suggested as diagnostic for *B. gibsoni,* but not all infected dogs achieve this titer magnitude (Birkenheuer and colleagues, 1999). Many dogs are seropositive but clinically normal, so serology alone cannot be used to make a definitive diagnosis. Definitive diagnosis is based on organism demonstration in red blood cells using Wright's or Giemsa stains on thin blood smears (see Chapter 97). *B. canis* is typically found as paired, piriform bodies measuring 2.4 × 5.0 μm. *B. gibsoni* is typically found as single, annular bodies measuring 1.0 × 3.2 μm. PCR is now available commercially and can be used to document organism presence, but positive results do not always correlate with clinical illness.

**Treatment.** Supportive care, including blood transfusion, sodium bicarbonate therapy for acidosis, and fluid therapy, should be administered as indicated. There are no drugs available known to eliminate infection, and so it is unknown whether it is beneficial to treat healthy, seropositive dogs.

Phenamidine isethionate reportedly is effective for lessening clinical disease associated with *Babesia* spp. infections when administered at 15 mg/kg of a 5% solution subcutaneously (SC) once daily for 2 days, but it is not available in the United States. Imidocarb diproprionate may be effective for the treatment of babesiosis when administered (5 to 6.6 mg/kg SC or intramuscularly [IM]) twice, 14 days apart or (7.5 mg/kg, SC or IM) once. Adverse effects include transient salivation, diarrhea, dyspnea, lacrimation, and depression. Metronidazole administered (25 mg/kg, PO, q8-12h) for 2 to 3 weeks or clindamycin hydrochloride administered (12.5 mg/kg, PO, q12h) for 2 to 3 weeks may lessen clinical disease if other drugs are not available. Diminazene aceturate, pentamidine isethionate, parvaquone, and niridazone have also been used.

**Zoonotic aspects and prevention.** There is currently no evidence to suggest that *Babesia* spp. infecting dogs and cats can cause human disease. Ticks should be controlled if possible. Administration of immunosuppressive drugs and splenectomy should be avoided in previously infected dogs. Dogs used as blood donors should be assessed for infection by PCR or serologic screening.

## CYTAUXZOONOSIS

**Etiology and epidemiology.** *Cytauxzoon felis* is a protozoal disease of cats in the southeastern and south central United States. Bobcats are usually subclinically affected and so may be the natural host of the organism. The organism can be passed experimentally from infected bobcats to domestic cats by *Dermacentor variabilis* (American dog tick); clinical illness occurs after an incubation period of 5 to 20 days. Following infection, schizonts and macroschizonts form in mononuclear phagocytes. The infected macrophages line the lumen of veins throughout the body. Merozoites released from the infected macrophages infect erythrocytes. Clinical disease results from obstruction of blood flow through tissues by the mononuclear infiltrates and from hemolytic anemia. Recently, sublethal cytauxzoonosis was described in cats in Oklahoma and Arkansas. Results suggest that variants that are less virulent to cats also exist.

**Clinical features.** Most cases of cytauxzoonosis are in cats allowed to go outdoors. Fever, anorexia, dyspnea, depression, icterus, pale mucous membranes, and death are the most common clinical findings. A primary differential diagnosis is haemobartonellosis. Ticks are generally not identified on affected cats.

**Diagnosis.** Regenerative anemia and neutrophilic leukocytosis are the most common hematologic findings; thrombocytopenia occurs in some cats. Hemoglobinemia, hemoglobinuria, hyperbilirubinemia, and bilirubinuria are uncommon. Antemortem diagnosis is based on demonstration of the erythrocytic phase on thin blood smears (Fig. 104-4) stained with Wright's or Giemsa stains (see Chapter 97). Infected macrophages can be detected cytologically in bone marrow, spleen, liver, or lymph node aspirates. The organism is easily identified on histopathologic evaluation of most organs. Serologic

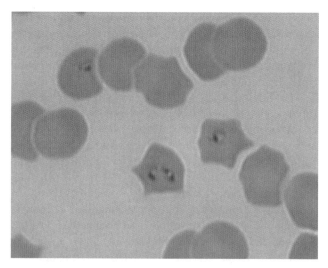

**FIG 104-4**
*Cytauxzoon felis* in the red blood cells of a cat. (Courtesy Dr. Terry M. Curtis, Gainesville, Fla.)

testing is not commercially available. PCR can be used to amplify organism DNA from blood.

**Treatment.** Supportive care including fluid therapy and blood transfusion should be administered as indicated. Treatment with diminazene (five cats) or imidocarb (one cat) (2 mg/kg, IM) twice 14 days apart was used in cats that survived infection (Greene and colleagues, 1999). Historically, parvaquone administered (10 to 30 mg/kg, IM or SC, q24h) for 2 to 3 days, buparvaquone administered (10 mg/kg, IM or SC, q24h) for 2 to 3 days, or thiacetarsamide administered (0.1 mg/kg, IV, q12h) for 2 days have been attempted. Parvaquone and buparvaquone are not routinely available; thiacetarsamide is toxic for cats (see Chapter 10) and should not be used in this species.

**Zoonotic aspects and prevention.** *Cytauxzoon felis* is not known to be zoonotic. The disease can only be prevented by avoiding exposure. Ticks should be controlled, and cats in endemic areas should be housed during periods of peak tick activity.

## HEPATOZOONOSIS

**Etiology and epidemiology.** Hepatozoonosis in dogs is caused by the protozoal agents *Hepatozoon canis* and *H. americanum*. In North America, *H. americanum* predominates, is transmitted by *Amblyomma maculatum* (Gulf Coast tick), and is most common in the Texas Gulf Coast, Mississippi, Alabama, Georgia, Florida, Louisiana, and Oklahoma. In Africa, southern Europe, and Asia, *H. canis* predominates and is transmitted by *Rhipicephalus sanguineus* (brown dog tick). A *Hepatozoon* species is occasionally found in the blood of cats in Europe. Clinical disease associations are currently unclear, but the cats are commonly coinfected with feline leukemia virus or feline immunodeficiency virus. Vertebrate hosts develop macrogametes and microgametes in neu-

trophils and monocytes. The tick ingests the organism during a blood meal, and oocysts develop. After a dog ingests an infected tick, sporozoites are released and infect mononuclear phagocytes and endothelial cells of the spleen, liver, muscle, lungs, and bone marrow and ultimately form cysts containing macromeronts and micromeronts. Micromeronts develop into micromerozoites, which infect leukocytes and develop into gamonts. Tissue phases induce pyogranulomatous inflammation resulting in clinical disease. Glomerulonephritis or amyloidosis may occur secondary to chronic inflammation and immune complex disease.

**Clinical features.** *H. americanum* can be a primary pathogen, resulting in clinical illness without concurrent immune deficiency. Clinically affected dogs have been in all age-groups, but disease is most commonly recognized in puppies. Fever, weight loss, and severe hyperesthesia over the paraspinal regions are common findings. Anorexia, pale mucous membranes from anemia, depression, oculonasal discharge, and bloody diarrhea occur in some dogs. Clinical signs can be intermittent and recurrent.

**Diagnosis.** Neutrophilic leukocytosis (20,000 to 200,000 cells/μl) with a left shift is the most common hematologic finding. Thrombocytopenia is unusual unless co-infection by *Ehrlichia canis* occurs. Normocytic, normochromic nonregenerative anemia is common and is likely from chronic inflammation. Increased activity of alkaline phosphatase but not creatine kinase occurs in *H. americanum*–infected dogs. Hypoalbuminemia, hypoglycemia, and rarely, polyclonal gammopathy occur in some dogs. Periosteal reactions from the inflammatory reaction directed at tissue phases in muscle can occur in any bone except the skull, are most common in young dogs, do not occur in every case, and are not pathognomonic for hepatozoonosis. Definitive diagnosis is based on identification of gamonts in neutrophils or monocytes in Giemsa or Leishman's stained blood smears or by demonstration of the organism in muscle biopsy sections. An indirect enzyme-linked immunosorbent assay (ELISA) for detection of serum antibodies against *H. americanum* was developed and compared with tissue biopsy; the sensitivity and specificity were 93% and 96%, respectively (Mathew and colleagues, 1998).

**Treatment.** No therapeutic regimen has been shown to eliminate *H. canis* or *H. americanum* infection from tissues. However, clinical disease resolves rapidly with several drug protocols. For treatment of *H. americanum*, the combination of trimethoprim-sulfadiazine (15 mg/kg PO q12h), pyrimethamine (0.25 mg/kg PO q24h), and clindamycin (10 mg/kg PO q8h) for 14 days is very successful in the acute stage (Macintire and colleagues, 2001). Use of decoquinate (10 to 20 mg/kg q12h) with food lessens the likelihood of recurrence of clinical disease and prolongs survival time. Imidocarb dipropionate administered (5 to 6 mg/kg, IM or SC) once or twice 14 days apart is the drug of choice for treatment of *H. canis* and may also be effective for *H. americanum*. Administration of nonsteroidal antiinflammatory agents may lessen discomfort for some dogs.

**Zoonotic aspects and prevention.** There is no evidence for zoonotic transfer of *H. americanum* or *H. canis* from infected dogs to people. Tick control is the best form of prevention. Glucocorticoid administration should be avoided since it may exacerbate clinical disease.

## LEISHMANIASIS

**Etiology and epidemiology.** *Leishmania* spp. are flagellates that cause cutaneous, mucocutaneous, and visceral diseases in dogs, humans, and other mammals. Rodents and dogs are primary reservoirs of *Leishmania* spp., people and cats are probably incidental hosts, and sandflies are the vectors. Leishmaniasis was considered unimportant in the United States until recently with cases only reported occasionally. In 2000, *L. donovani* infection was confirmed in multiple dogs in a Foxhound kennel in New York state (Breitschwerdt, 2001). Further investigation documented *L. donovani* or *Leishmania* spp. infection in 30 other Foxhound kennels in 20 states and Ontario, Canada, suggesting a competent vector exists in North America. A clinically affected cat in Texas was infected by *L. mexicana mexicana* (Craig and colleagues, 1986). Flagellated promastigotes develop in the sandfly and are injected into the vertebrate host when the sandfly feeds. Promastigotes are engulfed by macrophages and disseminate through the body. After an incubation period of 1 month to 7 years, amastigotes (nonflagellate) form and cutaneous lesions develop; sandflies are infected during feeding. The intracellular organism induces extreme immune responses: polyclonal gammopathies (and occasionally monoclonal); proliferation of macrophages, histiocytes, and lymphocytes in lymphoreticular organs; and immune complex formation resulting in glomerulonephritis and polyarthritis are common.

**Clinical features.** Dogs generally develop visceral leishmaniasis. A subclinical phase of infection may persist for months or years. Weight loss in the face of a normal to increased appetite, polyuria, polydipsia, muscle wasting, depression, vomiting, diarrhea, cough, epistaxis, sneezing, and melena are common presenting complaints. Splenomegaly, lymphadenopathy, facial alopecia, fever, rhinitis, dermatitis, increased lung sounds, icterus, swollen painful joints, uveitis, and conjunctivitis are commonly identified on physical examination. Cutaneous lesions are characterized by hyperkeratosis, scaling, thickening, mucocutaneous ulcers, and intradermal nodules on the muzzle, pinnae, ears, and foot pads. Bone lesions are detected in some dogs (Turrel and colleagues, 1982). Cats are usually subclinically infected; one cat had cutaneous nodules on the ear pinna.

**Diagnosis.** The principal clinicopathologic abnormalities include hyperglobulinemia, hypoalbuminemia, proteinuria, increased liver enzyme activities, thrombocytopenia, azotemia, lymphopenia, and leukocytosis with left shift. The hyperglobulinemia is usually polyclonal, but an IgG monoclonal gammopathy was reported in a dog (Font and colleagues, 1994). Neutrophilic polyarthritis occurs in some dogs as a manifestation of a type III hypersensitivity reaction. Demonstration of amastigotes (2.5 to 5.0 μm × 1.5 to 2.0 μm) in lymph node aspirates, bone marrow aspirates, or skin

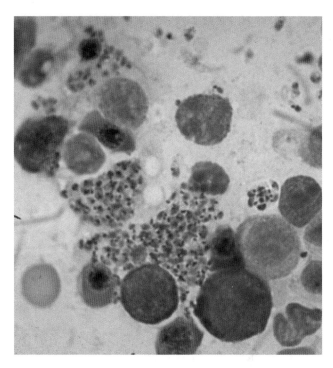

**FIG 104-5**
Impression smear of a lymph node of a *Leishmania* spp.–infected dog showing intracellular amastigotes. (Courtesy Dr. Arturo Font, Barcelona, Spain.)

imprints stained with Wright's or Giemsa stain gives a definitive diagnosis (Fig. 104-5). The organism can also be identified by histopathologic or immunoperoxidase evaluation of skin or organ biopsy, culture, inoculation of hamsters, or PCR. Antibodies against *Leishmania* can be detected in serum; IgG titers develop 14 to 28 days after infection and decline 45 to 80 days after treatment. Serological cross-reactivity occurs between *Trypanosoma cruzi* and *Leishmania*. Since dogs are unlikely to eliminate infection spontaneously, a true-positive antibody test indicates infection. PCR can be performed on EDTA-anticoagulated blood, bone marrow, or lymph node aspirates.

**Treatment.** No drug or drug combination has been used to successfully clear *Leishmania* from the body. One study showed that the combination of antimony and allopurinol (15 mg/kg PO q12h) was superior to treatment with either drug alone (Denerolle and colleagues, 1999). Antimony drugs are not available in the United States. Liposomal amphotericin B administered (3.0 to 3.3 mg/kg IV q48h) for three to five treatments has been prescribed. The prognosis is variable; most cases are recurrent. Dogs with renal insufficiency have a poor prognosis.

**Zoonotic aspects and prevention.** The primary zoonotic risk for canine leishmaniasis is from dogs acting as a reservoir host for the organism. Direct contact with amastigotes in draining lesions is unlikely to result in human infection. Avoidance of infected sandflies is the only means of prevention. If in endemic areas, house animals during night hours, and control breeding places of sandflies.

## AMERICAN TRYPANOSOMIASIS

**Etiology and epidemiology.** *Trypanosoma cruzi* is a flagellate that infects many mammals and causes American trypanosomiasis. The disease is diagnosed primarily in South America, but several cases have been detected in dogs of North America. Infected reservoir mammals (dogs, cats, raccoons, opossums, armadillos) and vectors (reduviid [kissing] bugs) are found in the United States, but infection in dogs or people is rare; this may relate to differences in vector behavior and sanitation standards in the United States. In one study in Texas, the number of serologically positive dogs increased between 1987 and 1996 (Meurs and colleagues, 1998). The organism has three life stages: trypomastigotes (flagellated stage found free in blood), amastigotes (nonflagellated intracellular form), and epimastigotes (flagellated form found in the vector). When infected kissing bugs defecate during feeding, epimastigotes enter the vertebrate host, infect macrophages and myocytes, and transform into amastigotes. Amastigotes divide by binary fission until the host cell ruptures, releasing trypomastigotes into the circulation. The vector is then infected by ingesting trypomastigotes during a blood meal. Transmission can also occur by ingesting the vector, by blood transfusions, by ingestion of infected tissues or milk, or transplacentally. Peak parasitemia occurs 2 to 3 weeks after infection causing acute disease. Disease in dogs is primarily a cardiomyopathy that develops from parasite-induced damage to myocardial cells or immune-mediated reactions.

**Clinical features.** Exercise intolerance and weakness are nonspecific presenting complaints that relate to myocarditis or heart failure during acute infection. Generalized lymphadenopathy, pale mucous membranes, tachycardia, pulse deficits, hepatomegaly, and abdominal distension can be detected on physical examination. Anorexia, diarrhea, and neurologic signs occasionally occur. Dogs that survive acute infection can present for evaluation of chronic dilative cardiomyopathy. In one study of 11 dogs with chronic infection, right-sided cardiac disease, conduction disturbances, ventricular arrhythmias, and supraventricular arrhythmias were most common (Meurs and colleagues, 1998).

**Diagnosis.** Common clinicopathologic abnormalities include lymphocytosis and increased activities of liver enzymes and CK. Thoracic radiographic, abdominal radiographic, and echocardiographic findings are consistent with cardiac disease and failure but are not specific for trypanosomiasis. The primary electrocardiogram (ECG) findings are ventricular premature contractions, heart block, and T-wave inversion. Definitive diagnosis is based on organism demonstration. Trypomastigotes (one flagellum, 15 to 20 μm long) can be identified during acute disease on thick blood film (see Chapter 97) or buffy coat smears stained with Giemsa or Wright's stain. The organism is sometimes detected in lymph node aspirates or in abdominal effusions. Histopathologic evaluation of cardiac tissue may reveal amastigotes (1.5 to 4.0 μm). Trypomastigotes can also be cultured from blood or grown by bioassay in mice. In North American cases, positive serologic test results correlate with infection. PCR can also be used to detect infection.

**Treatment.** Nifurtimox administered (2 to 7 mg/kg, PO, q6h) for 3 to 5 months has been prescribed most frequently, but it is not routinely available. Glucocorticoid therapy may improve survival of infected dogs. Therapy for arrhythmias or heart failure should be instituted as needed. Most dogs that survive acute infection will develop dilative cardiomyopathy. Survival time in 11 dogs ranged from 0 to 60 months (Meurs and colleagues, 1998).

**Zoonotic aspects and prevention.** Infected dogs can serve as a reservoir of *T. cruzi* for vectors, and blood from infected dogs can be infectious to humans. Vector control is the primary means of prevention. Dogs should be kept from other reservoir hosts, such as opossums, and should not be fed raw meat. Potential blood donors from endemic areas should be serologically screened.

## Suggested Readings

TOXOPLASMOSIS

Angulo FJ et al: Caring for pets of immunocompromised persons, *J Am Vet Med Assoc* 205:1711, 1994.

Baril L et al: Risk factors for *Toxoplasma* infection in pregnancy: a case-control study in France, *Scand J Infect Dis* 31:305, 1999.

Bernstein L et al: Acute toxoplasmosis following renal transplantation in three cats and a dog, *J Am Vet Med Assoc* 215:1123, 1999.

Brownlee L et al: Diagnosis of naturally occurring toxplasmosis by bronchoalveoloar lavage in a cat, *J Am Anim Hosp Assoc* 37:251, 2001.

Burney DP et al: Detection of *Toxoplasma gondii* parasitemia in experimentally inoculated cats, *J Parasitol* 5:947, 1999.

Davidson MG: Toxoplasmosis, *Vet Clin North Am Small Anim Pract* 30:1051, 2000.

Davidson MG et al: Feline immunodeficiency virus predisposes cats to acute generalized toxoplasmosis, *Am J Pathol* 143:1486, 1993.

Dubey JP: Duration of immunity to shedding *Toxoplasma gondii* oocysts by cats, *J Parasitol* 81:410, 1995.

Dubey JP et al: Fatal neonatal toxoplasmosis in cats, *J Am Anim Hosp Assoc* 18:461, 1982.

Dubey JP et al: *Toxoplasmosis of animals and man*, Boca Raton, Fla, 1988, CRC Press, p 1.

Dubey JP et al: Fatal toxoplasmosis in dogs, *J Am Anim Hosp Assoc* 25:659, 1989.

Dubey JP et al: Histologically confirmed clinical toxoplasmosis in cats: 100 cases (1952-1990), *J Am Vet Med Assoc* 203:1556, 1993.

Dubey JP et al: Neonatal toxoplasmosis in littermate cats, *J Am Vet Med Assoc* 203:1546, 1993.

Dubey JP et al: Toxoplasmosis and neosporosis. In Greene CE, editor: *Infectious diseases of the dog and cat*, ed 2, Philadelphia, 1998, WB Saunders, p 493.

Hass JA et al: Neurological manifestations of toxoplasmosis: a literature review and case summary, *J Am Anim Hosp Assoc* 25:253, 1989.

Hawkins EC et al: Cytologic identification of *Toxoplasma gondii* in bronchoalveolar lavage fluid of experimentally infected cats, *J Am Vet Med Assoc* 210:648, 1997.

Lappin MR: Feline toxoplasmosis: interpretation of diagnostic test results, *Semin Vet Med Surg* 11:154, 1996.

Lappin MR et al: Clinical feline toxoplasmosis: serologic diagnosis and therapeutic management of 15 cases, *J Vet Intern Med* 3:139, 1989.

Lappin MR et al: The effect of glucocorticoid administration on oocyst shedding, serology, and cell-mediated immune responses of cats with recent or chronic toxoplasmosis, *J Am Anim Hosp Assoc* 27:625, 1992.

Lappin MR et al: Polymerase chain reaction for the detection of *Toxoplasma gondii* in aqueous humor of cats, *Am J Vet Res* 57:1589, 1996.

Lappin MR et al: Primary and secondary *Toxoplasma gondii* infection in normal and feline immunodeficiency virus-infected cats, *J Parasitol* 82:733, 1996.

Lindsay DS et al: Mechanical transmission of *Toxoplasma gondii* oocysts by dogs, *Vet Parasitol* 73:27, 1997.

Powell CC, Lappin MR: Clinical ocular toxoplasmosis in neonatal kittens, *Vet Ophthalmol* 4:87, 2001.

Wallace MR et al: Cats and toxoplasmosis risk in HIV-infected adults, *JAMA* 269:76, 1993.

NEOSPORIOSIS

Barber TS et al: Clinical aspects of 27 cases of neosporosis in dogs, *Vet Rec* 139:439, 1996.

Basso W et al: First isolation of *Neospora caninum* from the feces of a naturally infected dog, *J Parasitol* 87:612, 2001.

Cuddon P et al: *Neospora caninum* infection in English Springer spaniel littermates: diagnostic evaluation and organism isolation, *J Vet Intern Med* 6:325, 1992.

Dijkstra T et al: Dogs shed *Neospora caninum* oocysts after ingestion of naturally infected bovine placenta but not after ingestion of colostrum spiked with *Neospora caninum* tachyzoites, *Int J Parasitol* 31:747, 2001.

Dubey JP: *Neospora caninum*: a look at a new *Toxoplasma*-like parasite of dogs and other animals, *Comp Contin Educ Pract Vet* 12:653, 1990.

Dubey JP et al: Neonatal *Neospora caninum* infection in dogs: isolation of the causative agent and experimental transmission, *J Am Vet Med Assoc* 193:1259, 1988.

Dubey JP et al: Newly recognized fatal protozoan disease of dogs, *J Am Vet Med Assoc* 192:1269, 1988.

Dubey JP et al: Neosporosis in cats, *Vet Pathol* 27:335, 1990.

Dubey JP et al: Repeated transplacental transmission of *Neospora caninum* in dogs, *J Am Vet Med Assoc* 197:857, 1990.

Dubey JP et al: High prevalence of antibodies to *Neospora caninum* in white-tailed deer (*Odocoileus virginianus*), *Int J Parasitol* 29:1709, 1999.

Greig B et al: *Neospora caninum* pneumonia in an adult dog, *J Am Vet Med Assoc* 206:1000, 1995.

Hill DE et al: Specific detection of *Neospora caninum* oocysts in fecal samples from experimentally-infected dogs using the polymerase chain reaction, *J Parasitol* 87:395, 2001.

Lindsay DS et al: Evaluation of anti-coccidial drug inhibition of *Neospora caninum* development in cell cultures, *J Parasitol* 175:990, 1989.

Lindsay DS et al: *Neospora caninum* and the potential for parasite transmission, *Comp Contin Educ Pract Vet* 21:317, 1999.

Lindsay DS et al: Canine neosporosis, *J Vet Parasitol* 14:1, 2000.

McAllister MM et al: Dogs are definitive hosts of *Neospora caninum*, *Int J Parasitol* 28:1473, 1998.

Petersen E et al: *Neospora caninum* infection and repeated abortions in humans, *Emerg Infect Dis* 5:278, 1999.

Ruehlmann D et al: Canine neosporosis: a case report and literature review, *J Am Anim Hosp Assoc* 31:174, 1995.

Tranas J et al: Serological evidence of human infection with the protozoan *Neospora caninum*, *Clin Diagn Lab Immunol* 6:765, 1999.

Wouda W et al: Seroepidemiological evidence for a relationship between *Neospora caninum* in dogs and cattle, *Int J Parasitol* 29:1677, 1999.

BABESIOSIS

Ano H et al: Detection of *Babesia* species from infected dog blood by polymerase chain reaction, *J Vet Med Sci* 63:111, 2001.

Birkenheuer AJ et al: *Babesia gibsoni* infections in dogs from North Carolina, *J Am Anim Hosp Assoc* 35:125, 1999.

Breitschwerdt EB et al: Babesiosis in the greyhound, *J Am Vet Med Assoc* 182:978, 1983.

Carret C et al: *Babesia canis canis, Babesia canis vogeli, Babesia canis rossi*: differentiation of the three subspecies by a restriction fragment length polymorphism analysis on amplified small subunit ribosomal RNA genes, *J Eukaryot Microbiol* 46:298, 1999.

Conrad P et al: Hemolytic anemia caused by *Babesia gibsoni* infection in dogs, *J Am Vet Med Assoc* 199:601, 1991.

Futter GJ et al: Studies on feline babesiosis. 4. Chemical pathology; macroscopic and microscopic postmortem findings, *J S Afr Vet Assoc* 52:5, 1981.

Geulfi JF: Use of imidocarb dipropionate to treat babesiosis in dogs: chemoprophylaxis trial, *Rev Med Vet* 133:617, 1982.

Kocan AA et al: A genotypically unique *Babesia gibsoni*-like parasite recovered from a dog in Oklahoma, *J Parasitol* 87:437, 2001.

Kordick SK et al: Coinfection with multiple tick-borne pathogens in a Walker Hound kennel in North Carolina, *J Clin Microbiol* 37:2631, 1999.

Lobetti RG et al: Renal involvement in dogs with babesiosis, *J S Afr Vet Assoc* 72:23, 2001.

Schetters TP et al: Different *Babesia canis* isolates, different diseases, *Parasitology* 115:485, 1997.

Wlosniewski A et al: Asymptomatic carriers of *Babesia canis* in an enzootic area, *Comp Immunol Microbiol Infect Dis* 20:75, 1997.

Wozniak EJ et al: Clinical, anatomic, and immunopathologic characterization of *Babesia gibsoni* infection in the domestic dog (*Canis familiaris*), *J Parasitol* 83:692, 1997.

Zahler M et al: Characteristic genotypes discriminate between *Babesia canis* isolates of differing vector specificity and pathogenicity to dogs, *Parasitol Res* 84:544, 1998.

Zahler M et al: "*Babesia gibsoni*" of dogs from North America and Asia belong to different species, *Parasitology* 120:365, 2000.

Zahler M et al: Detection of a new pathogenic *Babesia microti*-like species in dogs, *Vet Parasitol* 89:241, 2000.

CYTAUXZOONOSIS

Greene CE et al: Administration of diminazene aceturate or imidocarb dipropionate for treatment of cytauxzoonosis in cats, *J Am Vet Med Assoc* 215:497, 1999.

Hoover JP et al: Cytauxzoonosis in cats: eight cases (1985-1992), *J Am Vet Med Assoc* 205:455, 1994.

Kier AB et al: Experimental transmission of *Cytauxzoon felis* from bobcats (*Lynx rufus*) to domestic cats (*Felis domesticus*), *Am J Vet Res* 43:97, 1982.

Meier HT et al: Feline cytauxzoonosis: a case report and literature review, *J Am Anim Hosp Assoc* 36:493, 2000.

Meinkoth J et al: Cats surviving natural infection with *Cytauxzoon felis*: 18 cases (1997-1998), *J Vet Intern Med* 14:521, 2000.

Walker DB et al: Survival of a domestic cat with naturally acquired cytauxzoonosis, *J Am Vet Med Assoc* 206:1363, 1995.

HEPATOZOONOSIS

Baneth G et al: *Hepatozoon* spp. parasitemia in a domestic cat, *Fel Pract* 23:10, 1995.

Baneth G et al: Antibody response to *Hepatozoon canis* in experimentally infected dogs, *Vet Parasitol* 74:299, 1998.

Baneth G et al: *Hepatozoon* species infection in domestic cats: a retrospective study, *Vet Parasitol* 79:123, 1998.

Baneth G et al: Genetic and antigenic evidence supports the separation of *Hepatozoon canis* and *Hepatozoon americanum* at the species level, *J Clin Microbiol* 38:1298, 2000.

Ewing GO: Granulomatous cholangiohepatitis in a cat due to a protozoan resembling *Hepatozoon canis, Fel Pract* 7:37, 1977.

Macintire DK et al: Treatment of dogs infected with *Hepatozoon americanum:* 53 cases (1989-1998), *J Am Vet Med Assoc* 218:77, 2001.

Mathew JS et al: Experimental transmission of *Hepatozoon americanum* to dogs by the Gulf Coast tick, *Amblyomma maculatum, Vet Parasitol* 80:1, 1998.

Panciera RJ et al: Skeletal lesions of canine hepatozoonosis caused by *Hepatozoon americanum, Vet Pathol* 37:225, 2000.

Vincent-Johnson N et al: Canine hepatozoonosis: pathophysiology, diagnosis, and treatment, *Comp Contin Educ Pract Vet* 19:51, 1997.

Vincent-Johnson NA et al: A new *Hepatozoon* species from dogs: description of the causative agent of canine hepatozoonosis in North America, *J Parasitol* 83:1165, 1997.

### Leishmaniasis

Ashford DA et al: Comparison of the polymerase chain reaction and serology for the detection of canine visceral leishmaniasis, *Am J Trop Med Hyg* 53:251, 1995.

Bravo L et al: Canine leishmaniasis in the United States, *Comp Contin Educ Pract Vet* 15:699, 1993.

Breitschwerdt EB: Visceral leishmaniasis in North America. In *Proceedings of the Nineteenth Annual Forum, American College of Veterinary Internal Medicine,* Denver, 2001, p 756.

Cavaliero T et al: Clinical, serologic, and parasitologic follow-up after long-term allopurinol therapy of dogs naturally infected with *Leishmania infantum, J Vet Intern Med* 13:330, 1999.

Craig TM et al: Dermal leishmaniasis in a Texas cat, *Am J Trop Med Hyg* 35:1100, 1986.

Denerolle P et al: Combination allopurinol and antimony treatment versus antimony alone and allopurinol alone in the treatment of canine leishmaniasis (96 cases), *J Vet Intern Med* 13:413, 1999.

Eddlestone SM: Visceral leishmaniasis in a dog from Maryland, *J Am Vet Med Assoc* 217:1686, 2000.

Ferrer L et al: Serological diagnosis and treatment of canine leishmaniasis, *Vet Rec* 136:514, 1995.

Font A et al: Monoclonal gammopathy in a dog with visceral leishmaniasis, *J Vet Intern Med* 8:233, 1994.

Kirkpatrick CE et al: *Leishmania chagasi* and *L. donovani:* experimental infections in domestic cats, *Exp Parasitol* 58:125, 1984.

Kontos UJ et al: Old World canine leishmaniasis, *Comp Contin Educ Pract* 15:949, 1993.

Oliva G et al: Activity of liposomal amphotericin B (AmBisone) in dogs naturally infected with *Leishmania infantum, J Antimicrob Chemother* 36:1013, 1995.

Pena MT et al: Ocular and periocular manifestations of leishmaniasis in dogs: 105 cases (1993-1998), *Vet Ophthalmol* 3:35, 2000.

Reale S et al: Detection of *Leishmania infantum* in dogs by PCR with lymph node aspirates and blood, *J Clin Microbiol* 37:2931, 1999.

Slappendel RJ: Canine leishmaniasis: a review based on 95 cases in the Netherlands, *Vet Q* 10:1, 1988.

Turrel JM et al: Bone lesions in four dogs with visceral leishmaniasis, *Vet Radiol* 23:243, 1982.

### American Trypanosomiasis

Baer S et al: Trypanosomiasis and laryngeal paralysis in a dog, *J Am Vet Med Assoc* 188:1307, 1986.

Barr SC et al: Chronic dilatative myocarditis caused by *Trypanosoma cruzi* in two dogs, *J Am Vet Med Assoc* 195:1237, 1989.

Barr SC et al: *Trypanosoma cruzi* infection in Walker Hounds from Virginia, *Am J Vet Res* 56:1037, 1995.

Berger SL et al: Neurologic manifestations of trypanosomiasis in a dog, *J Am Vet Med Assoc* 198:132, 1991.

Bradley KK et al: Prevalence of American trypanosomiasis (Chagas disease) among dogs in Oklahoma, *J Am Vet Med Assoc* 217:1853, 2000.

Fox JC et al: *Trypanosoma cruzi* infection in a dog from Oklahoma, *J Am Vet Med Assoc* 189:1583, 1986.

Meurs KM et al: Chronic *Trypanosoma cruzi* infection in dogs: 11 cases (1987-1996), *J Am Vet Med Assoc* 213:497, 1998.

Snider TG: Myocarditis caused by *Trypanosoma cruzi* in a native Louisiana dog, *J Am Vet Med Assoc* 177:247, 1980.

# CHAPTER 105

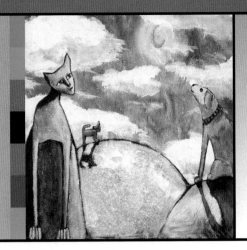

# Zoonoses

## CHAPTER OUTLINE

ENTERIC ZOONOSES, 1307
    Nematodes, 1307
    Cestodes, 1310
    Coccidians, 1310
    Flagellates, amoeba, and ciliates, 1311
    Bacteria, 1312
BITE, SCRATCH, OR EXUDATE EXPOSURE
ZOONOSES, 1312
    Bacteria, 1312
    Fungi, 1314
    Viruses, 1315
RESPIRATORY TRACT AND OCULAR
ZOONOSES, 1315
GENITAL AND URINARY TRACT ZOONOSES, 1316

Zoonotic diseases are defined as being common to, shared by, or naturally transmitted between humans and other vertebrate animals. Most of the agents discussed in this chapter can infect and cause disease in immunocompetent people, but disease is generally more prevalent or more severe in immunodeficient people. Immunosuppression is common in humans. People with acquired immunodeficiency syndrome (AIDS) are discussed most frequently, but there are many other immunodeficient individuals, including the very old, the very young, and those receiving chemotherapy for immune-mediated diseases, organ transplantation, or neoplasia. Immunosuppressed people are commonly advised to give up their pets. However, it appears that humans are unlikely to contract zoonotic diseases from contact with their pets, so in most cases they do not need to relinquish their animals. The Centers for Disease Control and Prevention online publication, *Preventing Infections from Pets: A Guide for People with HIV Infection,* states, "You do *not* have to give up your pet."* The author believes that all human and

*http://www.cdc.gov/hiv/pubs/brochure/oi_pets.htm.

other animal health care providers should provide accurate information to pet owners concerning the risks and benefits of pet ownership so that an informed decision about acquiring and keeping pets can be made.

For some zoonoses, including *Rickettsia rickettsii, Ehrlichia* spp., and *Borrelia burgdorferi,* the pet brings the vector of the organism into the environment, resulting in exposure of the human. With other zoonoses, including *Dirofilaria immitis, Histoplasma capsulatum, Coccidioides immitis, Blastomyces dermatitidis, Cryptococcus neoformans, Trypanosoma cruzi,* and *Leishmania* spp., the owner and pet are infected by shared environmental exposure to the agent or its vector. Many infectious agents can infect humans by direct contact with pets, their exudates, or their excrement. These agents are the most important to veterinary health care providers and to dog and cat owners.

The following is a brief description of the more common canine and feline zoonoses that are encountered in small animal practice. General guidelines for the avoidance of zoonotic transfer of disease for veterinarians and pet owners are listed in Tables 105-1 and 105-2, respectively.

## ENTERIC ZOONOSES

There are multiple infectious agents of the gastrointestinal tract that can be shared between animals and humans. Prevalences recently reported in two studies in cats and one in dogs are listed in Table 105-3. These findings emphasize that diagnostic workups for enteric infections are indicated because of potential human health risks. The minimum diagnostic plan to assess for enteric zoonoses includes a fecal flotation, *Cryptosporidum* spp. screening procedure, fecal wet mount, and rectal cytology. Fecal culture should be considered if infection with *Salmonella* spp. or *Campylobacter* spp. is on the list of differential diagnoses.

### NEMATODES

Visceral larva migrans can be induced by infection of humans with *Toxocara cati, Toxocara canis,* or *Baylisascaris procyonsis* (Table 105-4). In the United States, infection of humans is

TABLE 105-1

### General Guidelines for Veterinarians to Avoid Zoonotic Transfer of Disease

- Veterinarians and their staff should familiarize themselves with zoonotic issues and take an active role in discussing the health risks and benefits of pet ownership with clients so that logical decisions concerning ownership and management of individual animals can be made.
- The veterinary clinic should make it clear that the staff understands conditions associated with immune deficiency, is discreet, and is willing to help; use of signs or posters can be effective for this purpose.
- Pet owners should be provided information concerning veterinary or public health aspects of zoonoses, but veterinarians should not diagnose diseases in humans or discuss specific treatments.
- Clinically ill pet owners should always be referred to a physician for additional information and treatment.
- Veterinarians and physicians have different experiences concerning zoonoses; veterinarians should volunteer to speak to the pet owner's physician to clarify zoonotic issues when indicated.
- When public health–related advice is offered, it should be documented in the medical record.
- When reportable zoonotic diseases are diagnosed, appropriate public health officials should be contacted.
- Diagnostic plans to assess for the presence of organisms with zoonotic potential should be offered, particularly to owners with clinically ill pets.
- All dogs and cats should be vaccinated for rabies.
- Dogs and cats should be routinely dewormed with a drug that kills hookworms and roundworms.
- Flea and tick control should be maintained at all times.

 TABLE 105-2

### General Guidelines for Pet Owners to Avoid Zoonotic Transfer of Disease

- If a new pet is to be adopted, the dog or cat least likely to be a zoonotic risk is a clinically normal, arthropod-free, adult animal from a private family.
- Once the animal to be adopted is identified, it should be quarantined from any immunocompromised persons until a thorough physical examination and zoonotic risk assessment is performed by a veterinarian.
- Seek veterinary care for all clinically ill pets.
- Physical examination and fecal examination should be performed at least once or twice yearly.
- Fecal material produced in the home environment should be removed daily, preferably by someone other than an immunocompromised individual.
- Use litterbox liners and periodically clean the litterbox with scalding water and detergent.
- Do not allow dogs or cats to drink from the toilet.
- Wear gloves when gardening and wash hands thoroughly when finished.
- Filter or boil water from sources in the environment.
- Wash hands after handling animals.
- Do not handle animals that you are unfamiliar with.
- Clinically ill animals should not be handled by immunocompromised people, if possible.
- Maintain pets within the home environment to lessen exposure to other animals that may carry zoonotic agents, exposure to excrement of other animals, and exposure to fleas and ticks.
- Feed pets only commercially processed food.
- People should not share food utensils with pets.
- Avoid being licked by animals.
- Claws of cats should be clipped frequently to lessen the risk of skin penetration.
- To lessen the risk of bites and scratches, do not tease or physically restrain dogs or cats.
- If bitten or scratched by a dog or cat, seek medical attention.
- Control potential transport hosts such as flies and cockroaches, which may bring zoonotic agents into the home.
- Cook meat for human consumption to 80° C for 15 minutes minimum (medium-well).
- Wear gloves when handling meat and wash hands thoroughly with soap and water when finished.

still common; the seroprevalence of antibodies against *Toxocara* is 2.8% in the general human population and from 4.6% to 7.3% in children 1 to 11 years of age. These common roundworms are passed as eggs in feces. The eggs larvate and become infectious after 1 to 3 weeks and can survive in the environment for months. Humans are infected after ingesting larvated eggs. Dogs are considered more of a significant problem than cats for the spread of eggs. However, areas such as children's sandboxes may be contaminated with *T. cati* because of the defecation habits of cats. It is extremely unlikely that human infection will develop following direct contact with dogs or cats, since the eggs are not immediately infectious.

Dogs and cats can be subclinically affected or may develop poor haircoats, poor weight gain, and gastrointestinal signs. Following ingestion of infectious eggs, larvae penetrate the intestinal wall and migrate through the tissues. Eosinophilic granulomatous reactions involving the skin, lungs, central nervous system (CNS), or eyes then occur, potentially leading to clinical signs of disease. Clinical signs and physical examination abnormalities in affected humans include skin rash, fever, failure to thrive, CNS signs, cough, pulmonary infiltrates, and

hepatosplenomegaly. Peripheral eosinophilia is common. Ocular larva migrans most commonly involves the retina and can cause reduced vision; uveitis and endophthalmitis can also occur. Visceral larva migrans is most common in children between 1 and 4 years of age, whereas ocular larva migrans is most common in older children. Diagnosis in humans is confirmed by biopsy or can be presumed in cases with classic clinical manifestations, eosinophilia, and positive serology.

*Ancylostoma caninum, Ancylostoma braziliense, Ancylostoma tubaeforme, Uncinaria stenocephala,* and *Strongyloides*

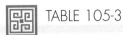

TABLE 105-3

Prevalence of Enteric Zoonoses in Dogs and Cats of the United States

|  | ADULT DOGS* (n = 130) | ADULT CATS† (n = 206) | CATS <1 YR‡ (n = 263) |
|---|---|---|---|
| Ancylostoma spp. | 0.8% | 0.0% | 0.0% |
| Campylobacter spp. | 0.8% | 1.0% | 0.8% |
| Cryptosporidium spp. | 3.8% | 5.4% | 3.8% |
| Giardia spp. | 5.4% | 2.4% | 7.2% |
| Salmonella spp. | 2.3% | 1.0% | 0.8% |
| Toxocara canis | 3.1% | 0.0% | 0.0% |
| Toxocara cati | 0.0% | 3.9% | 32.7% |
| Toxoplasma gondii | 0.0% | 0.0% | 1.1% |
| Any zoonotic agent | 14.6% | 13.1% | 40.7% |

*Colorado dogs (Hackett T et al: Prevalence of enteric pathogens in dogs, *Proceedings of the 2000 American College of Veterinary Internal Medicine Forum*, Fort Collins, Colo, May 2000).
†Colorado cats (Hill and colleagues, 2000).
‡New York State cats (Spain and colleagues, 2001).

TABLE 105-4

Characteristics of Common Enteric Zoonoses

| ORGANISM | SPECIES* | INCUBATION |
|---|---|---|
| **Bacterial** | | |
| Campylobacter jejuni | B | Immediately infectious |
| Eschericia coli | B | Immediately infectious |
| Helicobacter spp.† | B | Immediately infectious |
| Salmonella spp. | B | Immediately infectious |
| Yersinia enterocolitica | B | Immediately infectious |
| **Parasitic—Amoeba‡** | | |
| Entamoeba histolytica | D | Cysts are immediately infectious |
| **Parasitic—Cestodes** | | |
| Echinococcus multilocularis | C | Ova are immediately infectious |
| Echinococcus granulosa | D | Ova are immediately infectious |
| Multiceps multiceps | D | Ova are immediately infectious |
| **Parasitic—Coccidians** | | |
| Cryptosporidium spp. | B | Oocysts are immediately infectious |
| Toxoplasma gondii | C | Oocysts are infectious after 1- to 5-day incubation-exposure from environment |
| **Parasitic—Flagellates** | | |
| Giardia spp. | B | Cysts are immediately infectious |
| **Parasitic—Helminths** | | |
| Ancylostoma spp. | B | Larvae are infectious after >3-day incubation-exposure from environment Skin penetration from larvae in environment |
| Baylisascaris procyonis | D | Larvated ova are infectious after 1- to 3-week incubation-exposure from environment |
| Strongyloides stercoralis | B | Larvae are immediately infectious |
| Toxocara canis | D | Larvated ova are infectious after 1- to 3-week incubation-exposure from environment |
| Toxocara cati | C | As for T. canis |
| Uncinaria stenocephala | B | As for Ancylostoma |

*D, Dog; C, cat; B, dog and cat.
†Zoonotic potential is undetermined.
‡Dogs occasionally are infected by the ciliate *Balantidium coli*.

*stercoralis* have been associated with cutaneous larva migrans in the United States. Following the passage of hookworm eggs into the environment in feces, infectious larvae are released after incubating for 1 to 3 days; humans are infected by skin penetration. Eosinophilic enteritis in humans was reported following ingestion of larvated *A. caninum* eggs.

Animals are either subclinically ill or have nonspecific signs such as poor haircoats, failure to gain weight, vomiting, or diarrhea. Heavily infested puppies and kittens may have pale mucous membranes from blood loss anemia. In humans the larvae cannot penetrate the dermoepidermal junction and usually die in the epidermis. Clinical signs are related to migration of the larvae, which results in an erythematous, pruritic cutaneous tunnel. Cutaneous signs usually resolve within several weeks. Abdominal pain was the most common clinical sign in humans with *A. caninum* intestinal infection.

Prevention of hookworm and roundworm infestation is achieved by control of animal excrement in human environments. All puppies and kittens should have a fecal flotation performed and should be routinely treated with an anthelmintic such as pyrantel pamoate twice, 21 days apart, during their initial vaccination period. Roundworm and hookworm infestation are occasionally occult, so all puppies or kittens should receive an anthelmintic whether or not eggs are detected on microscopic examination of feces. In puppies with high worm burdens, deworming with pyrantel pamoate can be initiated at 1 to 2 weeks of age and repeated at 2-week intervals. In heavily infested kittens, deworming with pyrantel should be done at 6, 8, and 10 weeks of age. Heartworm preventatives that also control hookworms and roundworms are indicated in areas with a high prevalence. Fenbendazole administered orally at 50 mg/kg for 5 days is an effective treatment for *S. stercoralis* infection.

## CESTODES

*Dipylidium caninum, Echinococcus granulosa,* and *Echinococcus multilocularis* are cestodes that can infest humans. Wild carnivores are more common definitive hosts of *Echinococcus* spp. and shed infestive eggs into the environment. *E. granulosa* eggs can be transmitted in feces of dogs following ingestion of infected sheep tissues; *E. multilocularis* can be transmitted in feces of dogs or cats after ingestion of an infected vole. Transmission to humans occurs following ingestion of the intermediate host (flea, *Dipylidium*) or by ingestion of eggs (*Echinococcus* spp.).

Infestation of dogs and cats with cestodes is generally subclinical. *Dipylidium* infestation is most common in children and can lead to diarrhea and pruritis ani. In humans following ingestion of eggs, which are immediately infectious, *Echinococcus* enters the portal circulation and spreads throughout the liver and other tissues. *E. multilocularis* is most common in the northern and central parts of North America but seems to be spreading with the fox population (most common definitive host). Prevention or control of cestodes is based on sanitation procedures and use of taeniacides. Praziquantel has been shown to be effective for the treatment of *Echinococcus* spp. and *Dipylidium caninum* in-

festation in dogs and cats. Dogs and cats should not be allowed to hunt and should be fed only commercial foods.

## COCCIDIANS

*Cryptosporidium parvum* inhabits the respiratory and intestinal epithelium of many vertebrates, including birds, mammals, reptiles, and fish. Once thought to be a commensal, *C. parvum* is now known to cause gastrointestinal tract disease in a number of mammalian species, including rodents, dogs, cats, calves, and humans. *C. parvum* has an enteric life cycle similar to that of other coccidians; it culminates in the production of thin-walled, autoinfective oocysts and thick-walled, environmentally resistant oocysts that are passed in feces (Fig. 105-1). Oocysts (4 to 6 μm in diameter) are passed sporulated and are immediately infectious to other hosts. It is now apparent that there are multiple species of *Cryptosporidium* spp., including *C. felis* and *C. canis*. Although some isolates infect multiple species, others have a limited host range. However, strains that infect both pets and people cannot be differentiated by light microscopy from those that infect only pets, so all *Cryptosporidium* spp. should be considered potentially zoonotic.

The prevalence of *Cryptosporidium* spp. oocysts in dog and cat feces approximates that of *Giardia* (see Table 105-3), leading to the recommendation that all dogs or cats with diarrhea in the homes of immunosuppressed people be assessed for this infection. In the United States, the seroprevalence of immunoglobulin G (IgG) antibodies in serum is 8.6% in cats and up to 58% in humans, suggesting that exposure is very common. Person-to-person contact with oocysts by fecal-oral contamination and ingestion of contaminated water are the most likely routes of exposure. *C. parvum* infection of humans following exposure to infected calves has been recog-

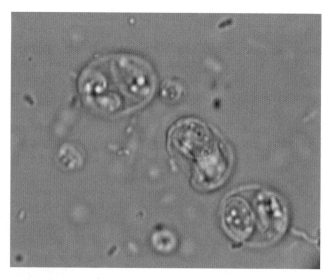

**FIG 105-1**
*Cryptosporidium parvum* and *Toxoplasma gondii* oocysts on a fecal flotation. The *C. parvum* oocysts are approximately 4 × 5 μm, and the *T. gondii* oocysts are approximately 10 × 12 μm.

nized for years. Human infection associated with contact with infected dogs and cats has been reported but is thought to be unusual. In one study, cat or dog ownership was not statistically associated with cryptosporidiosis in human immunodeficiency virus (HIV)–infected people (Glaser and colleagues, 1999).

Infection of dogs and cats by *Cryptosporidium* spp. is usually subclinical, but small bowel diarrhea occurs in some cases. Immunosuppression may potentiate disease; several dogs and cats had concurrent feline leukemia virus infection, canine distemper virus infection, or intestinal lymphoma. Clinical cryptosporidiosis is characterized by small bowel diarrhea and is generally self-limiting in immunocompetent humans, but fatal infection is common in humans with AIDS. Ten to 20% of humans with AIDS will be infected by *C. parvum* during the course of their illness.

The small size (approximately 4 to 6 μm in diameter) of *C. parvum* oocysts leads to difficulty in diagnosis. Routine salt solution flotation and microscopic examination at ×100 magnification will commonly lead to false-negative results. The combination of concentration techniques with fluorescent antibody staining or acid-fast staining appears to be more sensitive. Enzyme-linked immunosorbent assays for the detection of *C. parvum* antigen in feces is commercially available, but it is unknown whether they detect *C. felis* or *C. canis*. Polymerase chain reaction (PCR) is the most sensitive test to date, but assays are not routinely available and are not standardized among laboratories. No drug has been shown to eliminate *Cryptosporidium* spp. from the gastrointestinal tract. However, clinical signs usually resolve when paromomycin (Parke-Davis, Morris Plains, N.J.) administered orally at 150 mg/kg daily for 5 days or tylosin administered orally at 10 to 15 mg/kg three times a day for 14 to 21 days is given. Avoiding exposure is the most effective prevention. Routine disinfectants require extremely long contact with the organism to be effective. Drying, freeze-thawing, and steam-cleaning can inactivate the organism. Surface water collected in the field for drinking should be boiled or filtered.

*Toxoplasma gondii* is an ubiquitous coccidian with worldwide distribution. Most seroprevalence studies performed in the United States suggest that at least 30% of cats and humans have previously been exposed. Cats are the only known definitive host of the organism, and they complete the enteroepithelial cycle (sexual phase) that results in the passage of environmentally resistant unsporulated oocysts in feces. Oocyst sporulation occurs in 1 to 5 days in the presence of oxygen; sporulated oocysts are infectious to most warm-blooded vertebrates (see Fig. 105-1). Following infection by *T. gondii,* an extraintestinal phase that ultimately leads to the formation of tissue cysts containing the organism develops. Infection by *T. gondii* occurs after ingestion of sporulated oocysts, after ingestion of tissue cysts, or transplacentally. Transplacental infection of humans and cats usually occurs only if the mother is infected for the first time during gestation.

In dogs and cats, clinical disease from *T. gondii* infection occurs occasionally and is manifested most commonly by fever, uveitis, pulmonary disease, hepatic disease, and CNS

disease (see Chapter 104). Infected immunocompetent humans are generally asymptomatic; self-limiting fever, lymphadenopathy, and malaise occur occasionally. Transplacental infection of humans results in clinical manifestations, including stillbirth, hydrocephalus, hepatosplenomegaly, and retinochoroiditis. Chronic tissue infection in humans can be reactivated by immunosuppression leading to dissemination and severe clinical illness; this has been commonly associated with drug-induced immunosuppression, as well as AIDS. Approximately 10% of humans with AIDS will develop toxoplasmic encephalitis. Oocysts are most effectively demonstrated in cat feces following sugar solution centrifugation. Clinical toxoplasmosis is difficult to diagnose in humans, dogs, and cats but usually involves the combination of clinical signs, serologic test results, organism demonstration techniques, and response to anti-*Toxoplasma* drugs (see Chapter 104).

Although *T. gondii* is recognized as one of the most common zoonoses, humans are usually not infected by direct contact with cats. The oocyst shedding period usually lasts several days to several weeks (approximately 7 to 10 days if the cat was infected by tissue cyst ingestion). Since oocysts have to sporulate in order to be infectious, contact with fresh feces cannot cause infection. Cats are very fastidious and usually do not allow feces to remain on their skin for time periods long enough to lead to oocyst sporulation; oocysts were not isolated from the fur of cats 7 days after completion of the oocyst shedding period. There was no association between cat ownership and *T. gondii* seroprevalence in a group of HIV-infected humans. Veterinary health care providers do not have an increased incidence of toxoplasmosis when compared with the general population. Thus cats do not need to be removed from households with immunodeficient people or pregnant women because of the risk for acquiring toxoplasmosis. Prevention of *T. gondii* infection is summarized in Table 104-1, p. 1298.

## FLAGELLATES, AMOEBA, AND CILIATES

*Giardia* spp. (flagellate), *Entamoeba histolytica* (amoeba), and *Balantidium coli* (ciliate) are enteric protozoans that can be transmitted to humans by contact with feces; the cysts do not require an incubation period to become infectious. *E. histolytica* infection is extremely rare in dogs and cats; *B. coli* infection is rare in dogs and has never been reported in cats.

*Giardia* spp. infection of dogs and cats is common and can be detected in feces of normal dogs and cats and in those with small bowel diarrhea (and occasionally mixed bowel diarrhea in cats). Clinical signs of disease are generally more severe in immunodeficient individuals. Because the organism is immediately infectious when passed as cysts in stool, there is a potential for direct zoonotic transfer. Although it is known that some *Giardia* spp. will infect humans, dogs, and cats, that may not be the case with all species. In one study, cats were relatively resistant to infection by a *Giardia* sp. isolated from humans. On the basis of genetic studies, it is now known that there are multiple *Giardia* spp. Assemblage A has been found in infected humans and many other mammals, including dogs and cats. Assemblage B has been found in infected humans and dogs, but not cats. It also appears that there is a specific genotype of *Giardia* that infects cats but not humans, and one that infects dogs but not humans. However, as is the case with *Cryptosporidium*, since it is impossible to determine zoonotic strains of *Giardia* spp. by microscopic examination, it seems prudent to assume that feces from all dogs and cats infected with *Giardia* spp. are a potential human health risk.

Fecal examination should be performed on all dogs and cats at least yearly, and treatment with drugs with anti-*Giardia* activity, such as fenbendazole, metronidazole, or febantel/praziquantel/pyrantel, should be administered if indicated (see Chapter 30). Zinc sulfate centrifugation is considered by most parasitologists to be the optimal fecal flotation technique to demonstrate cysts (see Fig. 97-3, p. 1231). If fresh stool is available from dogs or cats with diarrhea, examination of a wet mount to detect the motile trophozoites may improve sensitivity. Monoclonal antibody–based immunofluorescent antibody tests and fecal antigen tests are available but have not been validated for detection of dog and cat strains. Thus these techniques should be used in addition to, not in lieu of, fecal flotation, which can also reveal other parasites.

*Giardia* vaccines for subcutaneous administration are now available for both dogs and cats (see Chapter 99). The feline *Giardia* vaccine is not currently recommended for routine prophylactic use in cats, but vaccination against *Giardia* could be considered in cats or dogs with recurrent infection and is being evaluated as a therapeutic agent. Prevention of zoonotic giardiasis includes boiling or filtering surface water for drinking and washing hands that have handled fecally contaminated material, even if gloves were worn. It is unknown whether treated dogs and cats are cured, and it is likely that if a treated dog or cat is exposed again, it will be reinfected.

## BACTERIA

*Salmonella* spp., *Campylobacter* spp., *Escherichia coli*, *Yersinia enterocolitica*, and *Helicobacter* spp. each infect dogs and cats and can cause disease in humans. Transmission from animals to humans is by fecal-oral contact. Dogs can be subclinical carriers of *Shigella* spp., but humans are the natural hosts. Although *Helicobacter pylori* was isolated from a colony of cats, it is unclear whether dogs and cats are a common source of *Helicobacter* infection in humans. However, on the basis of epidemiologic studies, it is unlikely. In three recent prevalence studies of enteric zoonoses, *Salmonella* spp. and *Campylobacter* spp. infections were uncommon in pet dogs and cats (see Table 105-3). The prevalence of *Salmonella* and *Campylobacter* infections is greater in young animals housed in unsanitary or crowded environments.

Gastroenteritis can occur in dogs or cats following infection by *Salmonella* spp., *Campylobacter* spp., or *E. coli*; *Y. enterocolitica* is probably a commensal agent in animals but causes fever, abdominal pain, polyarthritis, and bacteremia in humans. *Helicobacter* infections cause gastritis, which is commonly manifested as vomiting, belching, and pica. *Salmonella* spp. infection in dogs and cats is often subclinical. Approximately 50% of clinically affected cats have gastroenteritis;

many are presented with signs of bacteremia. Salmonellosis of cats and humans has been associated with songbirds (songbird fever). Abortion, stillbirth, and neonatal death can result from *in utero* infection. Diagnosis of *Salmonella* spp., *Campylobacter jejuni*, *E. coli*, and *Y. enterocolitica* is based on culture of feces (see Chapter 97). A single negative culture may not rule out infection. Rectal cytology (see Chapter 97) should be performed on all animals with diarrhea. If neutrophils are noted, culture for enteric bacteria is indicated, particularly if the animal is owned by an immunodeficient individual.

Antibiotic therapy can control clinical signs of disease from infection by *Salmonella* spp. or *Campylobacter* spp. (see Chapter 30) but should not be administered orally to animals that are subclinical carriers of *Salmonella* because of the risk for antibiotic resistance. Strains of *Salmonella* that were resistant to most antibiotics have been detected in several cats. Prevention of enteric bacterial zoonoses is based on sanitation and control of exposure to feces. Immunodeficient people should avoid young animals and animals from crowded or unsanitary housing, particularly if clinical signs of gastrointestinal tract disease are occurring.

## BITE, SCRATCH, OR EXUDATE EXPOSURE ZOONOSES

### BACTERIA

*Bartonella henselae* is the most common cause of cat scratch disease, as well as bacillary angiomatosis and bacillary peliosis—common disorders in humans with AIDS (Table 105-5). Cats can also be infected with *Bartonella clarridgeiae*, *Bartonella koehlerae*, and *Bartonella weissii*. *B. henselae* has been isolated from the blood of subclinically ill, seropositive cats and also from some cats with a variety of clinical manifestations such as fever, lethargy, lymphadenopathy, uveitis, gingivitis, and neurologic diseases. Seroprevalence in cats varies by region, but as many as 55% to 81% of cats in some geographic areas of the United States are *Bartonella* spp. seropositive. The organism is transmitted between cats by fleas, so the prevalence is greatest in cats from states where fleas are common. Transmission to humans commonly occurs after cat bites or scratches; the disease appears to be transmitted most commonly from kittens.

Humans with cat scratch disease develop a variety of clinical signs such as lymphadenopathy, fever, malaise, weight loss, myalgia, headache, conjunctivitis, skin eruptions, and arthralgia. Bacillary angiomatosis is a diffuse disease resulting in vascular cutaneous eruptions. Bacillary peliosis is a diffuse systemic vasculitis of parenchymal organs, particularly the liver. The incubation period for cat scratch disease is approximately 3 weeks. Most cases of cat scratch disease are self-limiting but may take several months to completely resolve. Blood culture, blood PCR, and serologic testing can be used to determine the risk of individual cats.

Cats that are culture-negative or PCR-negative and antibody-negative, and cats that are culture-negative or PCR-

TABLE 105-5

Select Canine or Feline Zoonoses Associated with Bites, Scratches, or Contact with Exudates

| ORGANISM | SPECIES* | CLINICAL DISEASE |
|---|---|---|
| **Bacterial** | | |
| *Bartonella* spp. | C | Cat—subclinical, fever, uveitis, gingivitis, lymphadenopathy, neurologic disease<br>Human—fever, malaise, lymphadenopathy, bacillary angiomatosis, bacillary peliosis |
| *Capnocytophaga canimorsus* | B | Dog and cat—subclinical oral carriage<br>Human—bacteremia |
| *Francisella tularensis* | C | Cat—septicemia, pneumonia<br>Human—ulceroglandular, oculoglandular, glandular, pneumonic, or typhoidal depending on route of infection) |
| L-form bacteria | C | Cat—chronic draining tracts<br>Humans—chronic draining tracts |
| *Yersinia pestis* | C | Cat—bubonic, bacteremic, or pneumonic<br>Human—bubonic, bacteremic, or pneumonic |
| **Fungal** | | |
| Dermatophytes | B | Dog, cat, and human—superficial dermatologic disease |
| *Sporothrix schenkii* | C | Cat—chronic draining cutaneous tracts<br>Human—chronic draining cutaneous tracts |
| **Viral** | | |
| Rabies | B | Dog and cat—progressive CNS disease<br>Human—progressive CNS disease |

*C, Cat; B, dog and cat.

negative and antibody positive are probably not shedding *Bartonella* into the human environment. However, bacteremia can be intermittent, and false-negative culture or PCR results may occur. With PCR, false-positive results can occur, and positive results do not necessarily indicate that the organism is alive. Although serologic testing can be used to determine whether an individual cat has been exposed, both seropositive and seronegative cats can be bacteremic, limiting the diagnostic utility of serologic testing. Thus testing healthy cats for *Bartonella* spp. infection is not currently recommended (Lappin and colleagues, 2002). Testing should be reserved for cats with suspected clinical bartonellosis.

Administration of doxycycline, tetracycline, erythromycin, amoxicillin-clavulanate, or enrofloxacin can limit bacteremia but does not cure infection in all cats and has not been shown to lessen the risk of cat scratch disease. Thus antibiotic treatment of healthy bacteremic cats is controversial. Treatment should be reserved for cats with suspected clinical bartonellosis. Strict flea control should be maintained. Kittens should be avoided by immunodeficient people. Cat claws should be kept clipped, and cats should never be teased. Cat-induced wounds should immediately be cleansed, and medical advice sought.

Feline plague is caused by *Yersinia pestis,* a gram-negative coccobacillus found most commonly in midwestern and far-western states, particularly New Mexico and Colorado. Rodents are the natural hosts for this bacterium; cats are most commonly infected by ingestion of bacteremic rodents or lagomorphs or by being bitten by *Yersinia*-infected rodent fleas. Dogs are more resistant to infection and have not been associated with zoonotic transfer. Humans are most commonly infected by rodent flea bites, but there have been many documented cases of transmission by exposure to wild animals and infected domestic cats. From 1977 to 1998, 23 cases of human plague (7.7% of the total cases) resulted from contact with infected cats. Infection can be induced by inhalation of respiratory secretions of cats with pneumonic plague, through bite wounds, or by contamination of mucous membranes or abraded skin with secretions or exudates.

Bubonic, septicemic, and pneumonic plague can develop in cats and humans; each form has accompanying fever, headache, weakness, and malaise. Since cats are most commonly infected by ingestion of bacteremic rodents, suppurative lymphadenitis (buboes) of the cervical and submandibular lymph nodes is the most common clinical manifestation. Exudates from cats with lymphadenopathy should be examined cytologically for the presence of large numbers of the characteristic bipolar rods (see Fig. 100-1, p. 1260). The diagnosis is confirmed by fluorescent antibody staining of exudates; culture of exudates, the tonsillar area, and saliva; and documentation of increasing antibody titers. People who are exposed to infected cats should be urgently referred to physicians for antimicrobial therapy, and public health officials alerted. Doxycycline, enrofloxacin, chloramphenicol, or aminoglycosides can be used successfully for the treatment of plague. Parenteral antibiotics should be used during the bacteremic phase. Drainage of lymph nodes may be required. Cats with suppurative lymphadenitis should be considered plague suspects, and extreme caution should be exercised when handling exudates or treating draining wounds. Suspect animals should be treated for fleas and housed in isolation. Cats are not infectious to humans after 4 days of antibiotic treatment.

*Francisella tularensis* is the gram-negative bacillus found throughout the continental United States that causes tularemia. *Dermacentor variabilis* (American dog tick), *Dermacentor andersoni* (American wood tick), and *Amblyomma americanum* (Lone Star tick) are known vectors. Human tularemia occurs most commonly following exposure to ticks and less commonly from contact with infected animals. There have been at least 51 cases of human tularemia resulting from contact with infected cats. Dogs are not considered a source of human tularemia but may facilitate human exposure by bringing infected ticks into the environment. Cats are infected most frequently by tick bites or ingestion of infected rabbits or rodents. Most cases of feline tularemia have been documented in the midwestern states, particularly Oklahoma.

Infected cats exhibit generalized lymphadenopathy and abscess formation in organs such as the liver and spleen, which leads to fever, anorexia, icterus, and death. Ulceroglandular, oculoglandular, glandular, oropharyngeal, pneumonic, and typhoidal forms have been described in humans and develop depending on the route of exposure. Unlike the situation with plague, the organism is not often recognized in exudates or lymph node aspirates from infected cats. Cultures and documentation of increasing antibody titers can be used to confirm the diagnosis in cats and humans. Most cases of tularemia in cats have been diagnosed at necropsy, so optimal treatment is unknown. Streptomycin and gentamicin are the drugs used most commonly to treat humans. Tetracycline or chloramphenicol can be used in cases not requiring hospitalization but may be associated with relapses. The disease is prevented by avoiding exposure to lagomorphs, ticks, and infected cats. All cats dying with bacteremia should be handled carefully.

Approximately 300,000 emergency room visits per year are made by people bitten by animals in the United States. Most of the aerobic and anaerobic bacteria associated with bite or scratch wounds cause only local infection in immunocompetent individuals. However, 28% to 80% of cat bites become infected, and severe sequelae, including meningitis, endocarditis, septic arthritis, osteoarthritis, and septic shock, can occur. The majority of the aerobic and anaerobic bacteria associated with dog or cat bite or scratch wounds lead only to local infection in immunocompetent individuals. Immunodeficient humans or humans exposed to *Pasteurella* spp., *Capnocytophaga canimorsus* (DF-2), or *Capnocytophaga cyn-*

*odegmi* more consistently develop systemic clinical illness. Splenectomized humans are at increased risk for developing bacteremia. *Pasteurella multocida* from a cat was cultured from the lungs of a man with AIDS who had only passive contact with the cat.

Dogs and cats are subclinical carriers of multiple bacteria in the oral cavity. After a human is bitten or scratched, local cellulitis is noted initially, followed by evidence of deeper tissue infection. Bacteremia and the associated clinical signs of fever, malaise, and weakness are common, and death can occur within hours following infection with *Capnocytophaga* spp. in immunodeficient humans. Diagnosis is confirmed by culture. Treatment of carrier animals is not needed. Treatment of clinically affected humans includes local wound management and parenteral antibiotic therapy. Penicillin derivatives are very effective against most *Pasteurella* infections; penicillins and cephalosporins are effective against *Capnocytophaga* spp. *in vitro*.

*Mycoplasma* spp. infections of humans secondary to cat bites, one with cellulitis and one with septic arthritis, have been reported. L-form bacteria are cell wall–deficient organisms associated with chronic draining skin wounds in cats that are commonly resistant to cell wall–inhibiting antibiotics, such as penicillins and cephalosporins. Infection of a human after a cat bite has been documented. Diagnosis can be confirmed only by histologic examination of tissue. Doxycycline has been used to successfully treat cats and people. Gloves should be worn when attending cats with draining tracts, and hands should be cleansed thoroughly.

## FUNGI

Of the many fungal agents that infect both humans and animals, only *Sporothrix schenckii* and the dermatophytes have been shown to infect humans on direct exposure. *Histoplasma*, *Blastomyces*, *Coccidioides*, *Aspergillus*, and *Cryptococcus* infections of humans and animals can occur in the same household but generally result from a common environmental exposure (see Chapter 103).

*Sporothrix* is cosmopolitan in distribution, and the soil is thought to be the natural reservoir. Infection of cats and humans usually occurs after the organism contaminates broken skin. Cats are thought to be infected by scratches from contaminated claws of other cats; infection is most common in outdoor males. Humans can be infected by contamination of cutaneous wounds with exudates from infected cats. *Sporothrix* infection in cats can be cutaneolymphatic, cutaneous, or disseminated. Chronic draining cutaneous tracts are common. Cats commonly produce large numbers of the organism in feces, tissues, and exudates; thus veterinary care personnel are at high risk when treating infected cats (Fig. 105-2). The clinical disease in humans is similar to that in cats. Dogs generally do not produce large numbers of *Sporothrix* in exudates, so they are less of a zoonotic risk. The organism can be demonstrated by cytologic examination of exudates or culture. Fluconazole, itraconazole, or ketoconazole are effective treatments. Gloves should be worn when attending cats with draining tracts, and hands should be cleansed thoroughly.

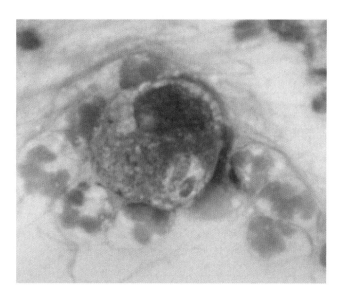

**FIG 105-2**
*Sporothrix schenckii* in a macrophage from an infected cat. There are two rod-shaped organisms in the cytoplasm.

## VIRUSES

Rabies is still the only significant small animal viral zoonosis in the United States. See Chapter 71 for a discussion of this agent.

Pseudorabies is a herpesvirus that infects pigs; dogs and humans can develop self-limiting pruritic skin disease following exposure. Dogs occasionally develop CNS disease characterized by depression and seizures. Diagnosis is suspected on the basis of the exposure history, and prevention is by avoiding exposure.

Some authorities have been concerned as to whether the retroviruses of cats—feline leukemia virus (FeLV), feline immunodeficiency virus (FIV), and feline foamy virus (FeFV)—can infect humans, because FeLV subtypes B and C can replicate in human cell lines. However, to date, humans have not been shown to be infected with any of the feline retroviruses. In the most recent study, 204 veterinarians and others potentially exposed to feline retroviruses were assessed for antibodies against FIV and FeFV, FeLV p27 antigen, and FeLV provirus; test results on all were negative (Butera and colleagues, 2000). Since both FeLV and FIV can induce immune deficiency, infected cats should be considered more likely than retrovirus-naive cats to be carrying other potential zoonotic agents, particularly if gastrointestinal tract signs are occurring.

## *RESPIRATORY TRACT AND OCULAR ZOONOSES*

*Bordetella bronchiseptica* is a bacterium that induces respiratory tract infections in dogs and cats (see Chapter 21). The classic clinical manifestation is tracheobronchitis, but the or-

ganism can also cause pneumonia, sneezing, and nasal discharge. Humans rarely develop clinical disease caused by *B. bronchiseptica* unless they are immunologically compromised. Only 39 cases of *B. bronchiseptica* infection in humans had been reported by 1998; most of these people were immunodeficient. Association with a cat has only been reported once, in a person coinfected with HIV and *B. bronchiseptica*. Amoxicillin-clavulanate, chloramphenicol, enrofloxacin, and tetracycline derivatives are all effective treatments. Animals with upper or lower respiratory tract inflammatory disease should be kept away from immunodeficient people until the animals are clinically normal. However, treated animals can still shed the organism.

*Chlamydophila felis* (formerly *Chlamydia psittaci*) causes mild conjunctival disease and rhinitis in cats (Table 105-6). In Japan the prevalence rates of antibodies against an isolate of *C. felis* were 51.1% in stray cats, 15.0% in pet cats, 3.1% in the general human population, and 5.0% in small animal clinic veterinarians, suggesting that transfer between cats and humans may occur (Yan and colleagues, 2000). Conjunctivitis in humans following direct contact with ocular discharges from cats has been described. A human isolate of *Chlamydia* spp. was inoculated into cats, resulting in conjunctivitis and persistent infection, suggesting that the isolate was a feline strain. Occasionally the organism is associated with systemic disease; atypical pneumonia was diagnosed in an apparently immunocompetent 48-year-old man, malaise and cough were diagnosed in an immunosuppressed woman, and endocarditis and glomerulonephritis were diagnosed in a 40-year-old woman. Diagnosis is based on organism demonstration by culture, cytologic documentation of characteristic inclusion bodies, or fluorescent antibody staining of conjunctival scrapings. Tetracycline or chloramphenicol-containing eye ointments generally are effective in the treatment of infection. Care should be taken to avoid direct conjunctival contact with discharges from the respiratory or ocular secretions of cats, especially by immunosuppressed persons (see Table 105-2). Employees should be directed to wear gloves or wash hands carefully when attending cats with conjunctivitis.

Humans are the principal natural hosts for *Streptococcus* group A bacteria, *Streptococcus pyogenes,* and *Streptococcus pneumoniae,* which cause "strep throat" in humans. Dogs and cats in close contact with infected humans can develop transient, subclinical colonization of pharyngeal tissues and can transmit the infection to other humans. However, this is poorly documented and thought to be unusual. The organism can be cultured from the tonsillar crypts. Culture-positive animals should be treated with penicillin derivatives. If animals are to be treated in a household with chronic, recurrent "strep throat," all humans should also be treated, since they also could be chronic subclinical carriers.

*Yersinia pestis* and *Francisella tularensis* can be transmitted from cats to humans in respiratory secretions (see Bite, Scratch, or Exudate Exposure Zoonoses). In endemic areas, cats with clinical signs or radiographic abnormalities consistent with pneumonia should be handled as plague or tularemia suspects.

TABLE 105-6

**Select Canine or Feline Zoonoses Associated with Contact with Respiratory or Ocular Secretions of Dogs or Cats**

| ORGANISM | SPECIES* | CLINICAL SIGNS |
| --- | --- | --- |
| *Bordetella bronchiseptica*† | B | Dog and cat—upper respiratory; rarely, pneumonia<br>Immunosuppressed humans—pneumonia |
| *Chlamydophila felis*† | C | Cat—conjunctivitis, mild upper respiratory<br>Human—conjunctivitis |
| *Francisella tularensis* | C | Cat—septicemia, pneumonia<br>Human—ulceroglandular, oculoglandular, glandular, pneumonic, or<br>typhoidal (depending on route of infection) |
| *Streptococcus* group A‡ | B | Dog and cat—subclinical, transient carrier<br>Human—"strep throat," septicemia |
| *Yersinia pestis* | C | Cat—bubonic, bacteremic, or pneumonic<br>Human—bubonic, bacteremic, or pneumonic |

*C, Cat; B, dog and cat.
†Zoonotic potential is largely unknown.
‡Minimal zoonotic potential.

 TABLE 105-7

**Select Canine and Feline Zoonoses Associated with Contact with Urine or Genital Secretions**

| ORGANISM | SPECIES* | CLINICAL DISEASE |
| --- | --- | --- |
| **Bacterial** | | |
| *Brucella canis* | D | Dog—orchitis, epididymitis, abortion, stillbirth, vaginal discharge, uveitis, diskospondylitis,<br>fever, malaise<br>Human—fever, malaise |
| *Leptospira* spp. | B† | Dog—fever, malaise, inflammatory urinary tract or hepatic disease, uveitis, CNS disease<br>Human—Fever, malaise, inflammatory urinary tract or hepatic disease, uveitis, CNS disease |
| **Rickettsial** | | |
| *Coxiella burnetii* | C | Cat—subclinical, abortion, or stillbirth<br>Human—fever, pneumonitis, lymphadenopathy, myalgia, arthritis |

*D, Dog; C, cat; B, dog and cat.
†Cats are of minimal significance.

Gloves, mask, gown, and eye protection should be worn while performing transoral airway washings in suspect cats.

## GENITAL AND URINARY TRACT ZOONOSES

*Coxiella burnetii* is a rickettsial agent found throughout the world, including North America (Table 105-7). Many ticks, including *Rhipicephalus sanguineus,* are naturally infected with *C. burnetii.* Cattle, sheep, and goats are commonly subclinically infected and pass the organism into the environment in urine, feces, milk, and parturient discharges. Seropositive dogs have been detected, but zoonotic transfer to humans from dogs has not been documented. Infection of cats most commonly occurs following tick exposure, ingestion of contaminated carcasses, or aerosolization from a con-

taminated environment. Fever, anorexia, and lethargy develop in some experimentally infected cats. Infection has been associated with abortion in cats, but the organism can also be isolated from normal parturient cats. Infection of cats appears to be common; 20% of cats from a humane society in southern California and 20% of cats in Maritime Canada were seropositive, and the organism was grown from the vagina of healthy cats in Japan (Nagaoka and colleagues, 1998).

Human illness associated with direct contact with infected cats occurs after aerosol exposure to the organism passed by parturient or aborting cats; clinical signs develop 4 to 30 days after contact. Humans commonly develop acute clinical signs similar to those associated with other rickettsial diseases, including fever, malaise, headache, pneumonitis, myalgia, and arthralgia. After primary infection, chronic Q fever develops in approximately 1% and can manifest as hepatic inflammation or valvular endocarditis. Tetracyclines, chloramphenicol, and quinolones are usually effective therapeutic agents in humans. Gloves and masks should be worn when attending to parturient or aborting cats. People who develop fever or respiratory tract disease after exposure to parturient or aborting cats should seek medical attention.

*Leptospira* spp. can be transmitted in urine from infected dogs and cats to humans, resulting in clinical disease. Host-adapted species cause subclinical infection; infection by non–host-adapted species commonly results in clinical illness. The organisms enter the body through abraded skin or intact mucous membranes. (See Chapter 100 for a detailed discussion of the clinical manifestations of this disease and its treatment in dogs and cats.) Human clinical syndromes vary with the serovar but are similar to those that occur in the dog. Animals with suspected leptospirosis should be handled while wearing gloves. Contaminated surfaces should be cleaned with detergents and disinfected with iodine-containing products.

*Brucella canis* is a bacterium that preferentially infects the testicles, prostate, uterus, and vagina of dogs (see Chapter 63). The infection is maintained in dogs primarily by venereal transmission. Humans can be infected by direct contact with vaginal and preputial discharges from dogs. Clinical syndromes in dogs are diverse but commonly include abortion, stillbirth, failure to conceive, orchitis, epididymitis, vaginal discharge, uveitis, diskospondylitis, and bacteremia. Intermittent fever, depression, and malaise are common in infected people. Diagnosis is based on serologic testing or demonstration of the organism by culture. Dogs with clinical signs of brucellosis should be evaluated serologically for *Brucella* infection using the 2-mercaptoethanol rapid slide agglutination card test. Seronegative dogs are unlikely to be harboring *Brucella* unless the clinical syndrome was peracute. Seropositive dogs should have results confirmed by tube agglutination or agar gel immunodiffusion. Long-term antibiotic treatment (tetracyclines, aminoglycosides, quinolones) usually does not clear the infection. Ovariohysterectomy or castration will lessen contamination of the environment. Genital tract secretions should be avoided.

## Suggested Readings

Angulo FJ et al: Caring for pets of immunocompromised persons, *J Am Vet Med Assoc* 205:1711, 1994.

Blagburn BL et al: Strategic control of intestinal parasites: diminishing the risk of zoonotic disease, *Compend Contin Educ Pract Vet* 19(suppl):4, 1997.

Breitschwerdt EB et al: *Bartonella* infection in animals: carriership, reservoir potential, pathogenicity, and zoonotic potential for human infection, *Clin Microbiol Rev* 13:428, 2000.

Burton B: Pets and PWAs: Claims of health risk exaggerated, *AIDS Patient Care*, p 34, Feb 1989.

Butera ST et al: Survey of veterinary conference attendees for evidence of zoonotic infection by feline retroviruses, *J Am Vet Med Assoc* 217:1475, 2000.

Capellan J et al: Tularemia from a cat bite: case report and review of feline-associated tularemia, *Clin Infect Dis* 16:472, 1993.

Carmack B: The role of companion animals for persons with AIDS/HIV, *Holist Nurs Pract* 5:24, 1991.

Chomel BB et al: Experimental transmission of *Bartonella henselae* by the cat flea, *J Clin Microbiol* 34:1952, 1996.

Croese J et al: Occult enteric infection by *Ancylostoma caninum*: a previously unrecognized zoonosis, *Gastroenterology* 106:3, 1994.

Drabick JJ et al: *Pasteurella multocida* pneumonia in a man with AIDS and nontraumatic feline exposure, *Chest* 103:7, 1993.

Dworkin MS et al: *Bordetella bronchiseptica* infection in human immunodeficiency virus–infected patients, *Clin Infect Dis* 28:1095, 1999.

Dubey JP: Duration of immunity to shedding *Toxoplasma gondii* oocysts by cats, *J Parasitol* 81:410, 1995.

Dubey JP et al: Toxoplasmosis and neosporosis. In Greene CE, editor: *Infectious diseases of the dog and cat,* ed 2, Philadelphia, 1998, WB Saunders, p 493.

Dunston RW et al: Feline sporotrichosis: a report of five cases with transmission to humans, *J Am Acad Dermatol* 15:37, 1986.

Eidson M et al: Clinical, clinicopathologic and pathologic features of plague in cats: 119 cases (1977-1988), *J Am Vet Med Assoc* 199:1191, 1991.

Foley JE et al: Seroprevalence of *Bartonella henselae* in cattery cats: association with cattery hygiene and flea infestation, *Vet Q* 20:1, 1998.

Fox JG: *Campylobacter* infections. In Greene CE, editor: *Infectious diseases of the dog and cat,* ed 2, Philadelphia, 1998, WB Saunders, p 226.

Gage KL et al: Cases of cat-associated human plague in the Western US, 1977-1998, *Clin Infect Dis* 30:893, 2000.

Glaser CA et al: Animal associated opportunistic infections among persons infected with the human immunodeficiency virus, *Clin Infect Dis* 18:14, 1994.

Grant S et al: Preventing zoonotic diseases in immunocompromised persons: the role of physicians and veterinarians, *Emerg Infect Dis* 5:159, 1999.

Greene CE: Immunocompromised people and pets. In Greene CE, editor: *Infectious diseases of the dog and cat,* ed 2, Philadelphia, 1998, WB Saunders, p 710.

Greene CE et al: *Bartonella henselae* infection in cats: evaluation during primary infection, treatment, and rechallenge infection, *J Clin Microbiol* 34:1682, 1996.

Greene CE et al: Streptococcal and other gram-positive bacterial infections. In Greene CE, editor: *Infectious diseases of the dog and cat,* ed 2, Philadelphia, 1998, WB Saunders, p 205.

Hill S et al: Prevalence of enteric zoonotic agents in cats, *J Am Vet Med Assoc* 216:687, 2000.

Jensen WA et al: Rapid identification and differentiation of *Bartonella* species using a single-step PCR assay, *J Clin Microbiol* 38:1717, 2000.

Juranek DD: Cryptosporidiosis: sources of infection and guidelines for prevention, *Clin Infect Dis* 21(suppl):57, 1995.

Kirkpatrick CE et al: Susceptibility of domestic cats to infections with *Giardia lamblia* cysts and trophozoites from human sources, *J Clin Microbiol* 21:678, 1985.

Kordick DL et al: Efficacy of enrofloxacin or doxycycline for treatment of *Bartonella henselae* or *Bartonella clarridgeiae* infection in cats, *Antimicrob Agents Chemother* 41:2448, 1997.

Lappin MR: Feline toxoplasmosis: interpretation of diagnostic test results, *Semin Vet Med Surg* 11:154, 1996.

Lappin MR et al: Cryptosporidiosis and inflammatory bowel disease in a cat, *Fel Pract* 3:10, 1997.

Lappin MR et al: Enzyme-linked immunosorbent assay for the detection of *Cryptosporidium* spp. IgG in the serum of cats, *J Parasitol* 83:957, 1997.

Lappin MR et al: *Bartonella* spp. antibodies and DNA in aqueous humor of cats, *J Fel Med Surg* 2:61, 2000.

Low JC et al: Multiresistant *Salmonella typhimurium* DT104 in cats, *Lancet* 348:1391, 1996.

MacKenzie WR et al: A massive outbreak in Milwaukee of cryptosporidium infection transmitted through the public water supply, *N Engl J Med* 331:161, 1994.

Macy DW: Plague. In Greene CE, editor: *Infectious diseases of the dog and cat,* ed 2, Philadelphia, 1998, WB Saunders, p 295.

Marcus LC: Medical aspects of visceral and cutaneous larva migrans and hydatid disease in humans, *Compend Contin Educ Pract Vet* 23(suppl):11, 2001.

Marrie TJ: *Coxiella burnetii* (Q fever) pneumonia, *Clin Infect Dis* 21(suppl):S253, 1995.

McReynolds C et al: Regional seroprevalence of *Cryptosporidium parvum* IgG specific antibodies of cats in the United States, *Vet Parasitol* 80:187, 1998.

Meloni BP et al: Isoenzyme electrophoresis of 30 isolates of *Giardia* from humans and felines, *Am J Trop Med Hyg* 38:65, 1988.

Morgan UM et al: Differentiation between human and animal isolates of *Cryptosporidium parvum* using rDNA sequencing and direct PCR analysis, *J Parasitol* 83:825, 1997.

Morgan U et al: Which genotypes/species of *Cryptosporidium* are humans susceptible to? *J Eukaryot Microbiol* 46(suppl):42, 1999.

Morgan U et al: Molecular characterization of *Cryptosporidium* isolates obtained from human immunodeficiency virus–infected individuals living in Switzerland, Kenya, and the United States, *J Clin Microbiol* 38:1180, 2000.

Nagaoka H et al: Isolation of *Coxiella burnetii* from the vagina of feline clients at veterinary clinics, *J Vet Med Sci* 60:251, 1998.

Neiger R et al: *Helicobacter* infection in dogs and cats: facts and fiction, *J Vet Intern Med* 14:125, 2000.

Olson ME et al: *Giardia* vaccination, *Parasitol Today* 16:213, 2000.

Pieniazek NJ et al: New *Cryptosporidium* genotypes in HIV-infected persons, *Emerg Infect Dis* 5:444, 1999.

Pinsky RL et al: An outbreak of cat-associated Q fever in the United States, *J Infect Dis* 164:202, 1991.

Pretorius AM et al: An update on human bartonelloses, *Cent Afr J Med* 46:194, 2000.

Prociv R et al: Human enteric infection with *Ancylostoma caninum:* hookworms reappraised in the light of a "new" zoonosis, *Acta Trop* 62:23, 1996.

Regnery RL et al: Characterization of a novel *Rochalimaea* species, *R. henselae* sp. nov., isolated from blood of a febrile, human immunodeficiency virus–positive patient, *J Clin Microbiol* 30:265, 1992.

Sargent KD et al: Morphological and genetic characterisation of *Cryptosporidium* oocysts from domestic cats, *Vet Parasitol* 77:221, 1998.

Simpson K et al: The relationship of *Helicobacter* spp. infection to gastric disease in dogs and cats, *J Vet Intern Med* 14:223, 2000.

Spain CV et al: Prevalence of enteric zoonotic agents in cats less than 1 year old in central New York State, *J Vet Intern Med* 15:33, 2001.

Spencer L: Study explores health risks and the human animal bond, *J Am Vet Med Assoc* 201:1669, 1992.

Sykes JE: Feline upper respiratory tract pathogens: *Chlamydophila felis, Compend Contin Educ Pract Vet* 23:231, 2001.

Talan DA et al: Bacteriologic analysis of infected dog and cat bites, *N Engl J Med* 340:84, 1999.

Tauni MA et al: Outbreak of *Salmonella typhimurium* in cats and humans associated with infection in wild birds, *J Small Anim Pract* 41:339, 2000.

Thompson RCA et al: Nomenclature and genetic groupings of *Giardia* infecting mammals, *Parasitol Today* 16:210, 2000.

Valtonen M et al: *Capnocytophaga canimorsus* septicemia: fifth report of a cat-associated infection and five other cases, *Eur J Clin Microbiol Infect Dis* 14:520, 1995.

Wallace M et al: Cats and toxoplasmosis risk in HIV-infected adults, *J Am Med Assoc* 269:76, 1993.

Yan C et al: Seroepidemiological investigation of feline chlamydiosis in cats and humans in Japan, *Microbiol Immunol* 44:155, 2000.

## Drugs Used to Treat Infectious Diseases of Dogs and Cats and General Dosing Guidelines*

| DRUG | TRADE NAME | CANINE DOSAGE | FELINE DOSAGE |
|---|---|---|---|
| **Antibiotics** | | | |
| ***Aminoglycosides*** | | | |
| Amikacin | Amiglyde-V | 15-20 mg/kg, q24h, IV, IM, SC | 15-20 mg/kg, q24h, IV, IM, SC |
| Gentamicin | | 6 mg/kg, q24h, IV, IM, SC | 6 mg/kg, q24h, IV, IM, SC |
| Neomycin | | 22 mg/kg, q8-12h, PO | 22 mg/kg, q8-12h, PO |
| Tobramycin | Nebcin | 2 mg/kg, q8h, IV, IM, SC | 2 mg/kg, q8h, IV, IM, SC |
| ***Carbapenems*** | | | |
| Imipenem | Primaxin | 2-10 mg/kg, q6-8h, IV, IM | 2-10 mg/kg, q6-8h, IV, IM |
| ***Cephalosporins*** | | | |
| Cefadroxil (first generation) | Cefa-Tabs | 22 mg/kg, q12h, PO | 22 mg/kg, q24h, PO |
| Cephalexin (first generation) | | 20-60 mg/kg, q8-12h, PO | 20-60 mg/kg, q8-12h, PO |

*IM,* Intramuscular; *IV,* intravenous; *SC,* subcutaneous; *PO,* oral.

*The dose ranges and intervals in this table are general. Please see appropriate sections to determine the optimal dose and duration of therapy for specific syndromes or infections.

## Drugs Used to Treat Infectious Diseases of Dogs and Cats and General Dosing Guidelines—cont'd

| DRUG | TRADE NAME | CANINE DOSAGE | FELINE DOSAGE |
|---|---|---|---|
| **Antibiotics—cont'd** | | | |
| ***Cephalosporins—cont'd*** | | | |
| Cefazolin (first generation) | | 20-33 mg/kg, q8-12h, SC, IM, IV | 20-33 mg/kg, q8-12h, SC, IM, IV |
| Cefoxitin (second generation) | Mefoxin | 15-30 mg/kg, q8h, SC, IM, IV | 15-30 mg/kg, q8h, SC, IM, IV |
| Cefixime (third generation) | Suprax | 5-12.5 mg/kg, q12-24h, PO | 5-12.5 mg/kg, q12-24h, PO |
| Cefotaxime (third generation) | | 20-80 mg/kg, q8h, SC, IM, IV | 20-80 mg/kg, q8h, SC, IM, IV |
| Ceftiofur | Naxcel | 2.2 mg/kg, q24h, SC | 2.2 mg/kg, q24h, SC |
| ***Chloramphenicol*** | | 25-50 mg/kg, q8h, PO, SC, IV, IM | 15-25 mg/kg, q12h, PO, SC, IV, IM |
| ***Macrolides/lincosamides*** | | | |
| Azithromycin† | Zithromax | 5-10 mg/kg, q12-24h, PO | 7-15 mg/kg, q24h, PO |
| Clindamycin | Antirobe | 5-20 mg/kg, q12-24h, PO, SC, IM, IV | 5-25 mg/kg, q12-24h, PO, SC, IM, IV |
| Erythromycin | | 10-25 mg/kg, q8-12h, PO | 10-25 mg/kg, q8-12h, PO |
| Lincomycin | | 11-22 mg/kg, q12h, PO, IM, IV, SC | 11-22 mg/kg, q12h, PO, IM, IV, SC |
| Tylosin | | 10-40 mg/kg, q12-24h, PO | 10-40 mg/kg, q12-24h, PO |
| ***Metronidazole‡*** | Flagyl | 10-30 mg/kg, q8-24h, PO | 10-30 mg/kg, q12-24h, PO |
| ***Penicillins*** | | | |
| Amoxicillin | | 10-22 mg/kg, q8-12h, PO, SC | 10-22 mg/kg, q8-12h, PO, SC |
| Amoxicillin clavulanate | Clavamox | 12.5-25 mg/kg, q8-12h, PO | 62.5 mg, q8-12h, PO |
| Ampicillin sodium | | 22 mg/kg, q8h, SC, IM, IV | 22 mg/kg, q8h, SC, IM, IV |
| Carbenicillin | Geocillin | 22-33 mg/kg, q8h, PO | 22-33 mg/kg, q8h, PO |
| Oxacillin | Prostaphlin | 22-40 mg/kg, q8h, PO, SC, IM, IV | 22-40 mg/kg, q8h, PO, SC, IM, IV |
| Penicillin G | | 22,000 U/kg, q6-8h, PO, IM, IV | 22,000 U/kg, q6-8h, PO, IM, IV |
| ***Quinolones*** | | | |
| Ciprofloxacin | Cipro | 5-15 mg/kg, q24h, PO | 5-15 mg/kg, q24h, PO |
| Difloxacin | Dicural | 5-10 mg/kg, q24h, PO | |
| Enrofloxacin | Baytril | 5-20 mg/kg, q12-24h, PO, IM, SC, IV | 5 mg/kg, q24h, PO, IM, SC, IV |
| Marbofloxacin | Zeniquin | 2.75-5.5 mg/kg, q24h, PO | 2.0 mg/kg, q24h, PO |
| Orbafloxacin | Orbax | 2.5-7.5 mg/kg, q24h, PO | 2.5-7.5 mg/kg, q24h, PO |
| ***Potentiated sulfas*** | | | |
| Ormetoprim-sulfadimethoxine | Primor | 27.5 mg/kg, q24h, PO | |
| Trimethoprim-Sulfonamide | Tribrissen (sulfadiazine) | 15-30 mg/kg, q12h, PO | 15-30 mg/kg, q12h, PO |
| ***Tetracyclines*** | | | |
| Doxycycline§ | | 5-20 mg/kg, q12-24h, PO, IV | 5-20 mg/kg, q12-24h, PO, IV |
| Minocycline | Minocin | 5-12.5 mg/kg, q12h, PO, IV | |
| Tetracycline | | 22 mg/kg, q8-12h, PO | 22 mg/kg, q8-12h, PO |
| **Antiviral** | | | |
| Acyclovir | Zovirax | | 25 mg/kg, q12h, PO |
| Alpha interferon (routine infections) | Intron A | | 30 IU, q24h, PO |

†For simple infections, azithromycin can be given daily for 3 days and then every third day.
‡The maximum daily dose should be 50 mg/kg.
§The drug can be given once daily to cats for the treatment of simple infections and animals with ehrlichiosis.

*Continued*

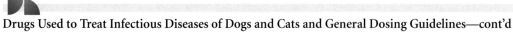

## Drugs Used to Treat Infectious Diseases of Dogs and Cats and General Dosing Guidelines—cont'd

| DRUG | TRADE NAME | CANINE DOSAGE | FELINE DOSAGE |
|---|---|---|---|
| **Antiviral—cont'd** | | | |
| Alpha interferon (life-threatening viral infection) | Intron A | 10,000-20,000 IU/kg, SC | 10,000-20,000 IU/kg, SC |
| AZT | Retrovir | | 5-10 mg/kg, q8-12h, PO |
| **Antiprotozoal** | | | |
| *Babesia* spp. | | | |
| Clindamycin hydrochloride | Antirobe | 12.5 mg/kg, q12h, PO | |
| Imidocarb diproprionate | Imizol | 5-6.6 mg/kg, q14d, SC or IM | |
| Metronidazole | Flagyl | 25 mg/kg, q8-12h, PO | |
| *Cryptosporidium* spp. | | | |
| Azithromycin | Zithromax | 10 mg/kg, q12-24h, PO | 10 mg/kg, q12-24h, PO |
| Paromomycin | | 150 mg/kg, q12-24h, PO × 5 days | 150 mg/kg, q12-24h, PO × 5 days |
| Tylosin | | 15 mg/kg, q12h, PO | 15 mg/kg, q12h, PO |
| *Cytauxzoon felis* | | | |
| Diminazene | | | 2 mg/kg, q14d, IM |
| Imidocarb | | | 2 mg/kg, q14d, IM |
| Parvaquone | | | 10-30 mg/kg, q24h, IM or SC |
| Buparvaquone | | | 10 mg/kg, q24h, IM or SC |
| *Giardia* spp. | | | |
| Febantel/pyrantel/praziquantel | Drontal Plus | Label dose, PO, daily × 3 days | |
| Fenbendazole | | 50 mg/kg, PO, q24h × 3-5 days | 50 mg/kg, PO, q24h × 3-5 days |
| Metronidazole | | 15-25 mg/kg, PO, q24h × 7 days | 25 mg/kg, PO, q24h × 7 days |
| *Hepatozoon canis*‖ | | | |
| Trimethoprim-sulfadiazine | | 15 mg/kg, q12h, PO | |
| Pyrimethamine | | 0.25 mg/kg, q24h, PO | |
| Clindamycin | Antirobe | 10 mg/kg, q8h, PO | |
| Decoquinate | Deccox | 10 to 20 mg/kg, q12h, PO | |

‖Clindamycin, pyrimethamine, and trimethoprim-sulfa are generally used together for acute disease, and decoquinate is used for long-term maintenance therapy.

**Drugs Used to Treat Infectious Diseases of Dogs and Cats and General Dosing Guidelines—cont'd**

| DRUG | TRADE NAME | CANINE DOSAGE | FELINE DOSAGE |
|---|---|---|---|
| **Antiprotozoal—cont'd** | | | |
| Imidocarb dipropionate | | 5-6 mg/kg, q14d, IM or SQ | |
| *Neospora caninum* | | | |
| Trimethoprim-sulfadiazine | | 15 mg/kg, q12h, PO | |
| Pyrimethamine | | 1 mg/kg, q24h, PO | |
| Clindamycin | | 10 mg/kg, q8h, PO | |
| *Toxoplasma gondii* | | | |
| Azithromycin | | 10 mg/kg, q12-24h, PO | 10 mg/kg, q12-24h, PO |
| Clindamycin | | 12.5 mg/kg, q12h, PO | 12.5 mg/kg, q12h, PO |
| Trimethoprim-sulfadiazine | | 15 mg/kg, q12h, PO | 15 mg/kg, q12h, PO |
| **Antifungal** | | | |
| Amphotericin B (regular) | | 0.25 mg/kg, IV as test dose, then 0.5 mg/kg, IV, up to 3 times weekly | 0.25 mg/kg, IV, up to 3 times weekly |
| Amphotericin B (regular) | | 0.5-0.8 mg/kg, SQ, 2-3 times weekly | 0.5-0.8 mg/kg, SQ, 2-3 times weekly |
| Amphotericin B (liposomal) | Abelcet | 0.5 mg/kg, IV as test dose, then 1.0 mg/kg, IV, 3-5 times weekly | 0.5 mg/kg, IV as test dose, then 1.0 mg/kg, IV, 3-5 times weekly |
| Fluconazole | Diflucan | 2.5-5.0 mg/kg, q12-24h, PO | 50-100 mg/cat, q12-24h, PO |
| Flucytosine¶ | Ancobon | 25-50 mg/kg, q6h, PO | 25-50 mg/kg, q6h, PO |
| Itraconazole | Sporonox | 5 mg/kg, q12h, PO for 4 days, then 5 mg/kg, q24h, PO | 50-100 mg/cat, PO, daily |
| Ketoconazole | Nizofal | 10 mg/kg, q24h, PO | 10 mg/kg, q24h, PO |
| Anti-rickettsial | | | |
| *Ehrlichia* spp. | | | |
| Doxycycline | | 10 mg/kg, q24h, PO | 10 mg/kg, q24h, PO |
| Chloramphenical | | 25-50 mg/kg, q8h, PO, SC, IV, IM | |
| Imidocarb | | 5.0-6.6 mg/kg, q14d, IM, SC | 5.0 mg/kg, q14d, IM, SC |
| *Rickettsia rickettsii* | | | |
| Doxycycline | | 10 mg/kg, q24h, PO | |
| Chloramphenicol | | 25-50 mg/kg, q8h, PO, SC, IV, IM | |
| Enrofloxacin | | 5 mg/kg, q24h, PO, SC, IM, IV | |

¶This drug is generally used in combination with other antifungal drugs.

# A

Abdomen
  acute, 361-362, 361t, 362f
  distention of, in digestive disorders, 363-364, 364t
  effusions in, 360-361, 474-476, 475f, 476f
  enlargement of
    from abdominal muscular hypotonia, 476
    in digestive disorders, 363-364, 364t
    in hepatobiliary disease, 472-476, 473f, 473t, 474t, 475f, 476f
  fluid in, accumulation of, mechanisms of, 475f
  muscles of, hypotonia of, 476, 476f
  pain in, in digestive disorders, 362-363, 363t
  radiography of, without contrast media, 371-374, 372f, 374f
Abdominal carcinomatosis, 469
Abdominal hemangiosarcoma, 468
Abdominocentesis
  in acute pancreatitis, 557
  for ascites, 550
  in hepatobiliary disorders, 491, 491t
  in septic peritonitis diagnosis, 466
Abelcet. See Amphotericin B
Abiotrophy, cerebellar neuronal, 978, 978t
Abortifacients, 898-900, 898t
Abortion
  Brucella canis infection and, 936
  herpesvirus infection and, 934
  spontaneous, 900-901
Abscess(es)
  antibiotics for, 1244t
  hepatic, 541-542, 541f
  laryngoscopy/pharyngoscopy of, 244-245
  lymph node, 1201
  pancreatic, in acute pancreatitis, 555t
  prostatic, 930-931
  pulmonary, interstitial pattern in, 258, 260t
  splenic, 1204
  tooth root, radiographic signs of, 220t
AC protocol
  for carcinomas, 1155t
  for hemangiosarcoma, 1143, 1144
  for lymphoma, 1127t
  for soft-tissue sarcomas, 1154t
Acanthocytes, in hepatobiliary disorders, 485f, 486
Acanthocytosis, disorders associated with, 1159t
Acanthomatous epulis, 406t
Acarbose
  in diabetes management, 736-737, 755t, 757
  for endocrine disorders, 813t
Accelerated ventricular rhythm, 22
ACEIs. See Angiotensin-converting enzyme inhibitors (ACEIs)
Acemannan
  for feline immunodeficiency virus, 1280t
  for infectious diseases, 1319t

Acepromazine
  for detrusor atony in urethral obstruction, 648
  dosages of, 206t, 341t
  for hypertension, 202t, 203
  for respiratory distress, 334t
  for tetanus, 981
Acetaminophen hepatotoxicity, 522t
  treatment for, 523t
Acetylcholine receptors
  antibodies to, in alimentary tract disease, 379
  deficiency of, in myasthenia gravis, 1059, 1060
Acetylpromazine, for neurologic disorders, 1069t
Acetylsalicylic acid
  for degenerative joint disease, 1080, 1080t
  for disseminated intravascular coagulation, 1198
  for fever of undetermined origin, 1225
  hepatotoxicity of, 522t
  for joint disease, 1092t
  low-dose, for glomerulonephritis, 605-606
  for neurologic disorders, 1069t
  for pulmonary thromboembolism, 311
  for urinary tract disorders, 658t
Achalasia, cricopharyngeal, 409
Acid-base status, 285
Acidification, urinary, for urinary tract infections, 629-630
Acidophil cells, 529
Acidosis, minimization of, in cardiopulmonary resuscitation, 104
Aclarubicin, for myelodysplastic syndromes, 1140
Acoustic enhancement, in echocardiography, 36
Acoustic shadow, in echocardiography, 36
Acromegaly, feline, 673-677. See also Feline acromegaly
ACT. See Activated coagulation time (ACT)
ACTH. See Adrenocorticotropic hormone (ACTH)
Actinomyces
  antibiotics for, 1244t
  lymphadenopathy associated with, 1202t
  morphologic characteristics of, 1233t
Actinomycin D
  gastrointestinal complications of, 1111
  for lymphoma, 1127t, 1129, 1153t
Activated coagulation time (ACT), in bleeding patient evaluation, 1187-1188, 1187t
Actos. See Pioglitazone
Acute respiratory distress syndrome (ARDS), 312, 313
Acute tumor lysis syndrome (ATLS), complicating chemotherapy, 1115-1116, 1116f
Addisonian crisis, acute, therapy for, 807-808
Addison's disease, electrocardiography in, 26, 28f

Adenocarcinoma(s)
  anal sac, 461-462
  esophageal, endoscopic view of, 380f
  intestinal, 457-458
  large intestinal, 459
  mammary, 884-885
  metastatic behavior of, 1118t
  pancreatic, 564
  prostatic, 932-933
  pulmonary, 260f
  thyroid, 725f, 726f, 1119t
    hyperthyroidism from, 712, 715f
  uterine, 877
Adenoma
  of pars distalis, hyperadrenocorticism from, 778
  of pars intermedia, hyperadrenocorticism from, 778
  pituitary
    hyperparathyroidism from, 681, 682f
    ultrasound image of, 684f
Adenosine
  for arrhythmias, 96
  commercial preparations of, 88t
  dosages of, 80t
  metabolism of, 640f
Adenovirus, canine, canine infectious tracheobronchitis from, 287
Adenovirus 2, vaccination for, 1256
Adequan. See Polysulfated glycosaminoglycan
ADH. See Antidiuretic hormone (ADH)
ADIC protocol
  for lymphoma, 1127t, 1129, 1153t
  for soft- tissue sarcomas, 1154t
Adrenal-dependent sex hormone imbalance, endocrine alopecia differentiated from, 669-670
Adrenal gland
  disorders of, 778-813
    hyperadrenocorticism as, 778-804 (See also Hyperadrenocorticism)
    hypoadrenocorticism as, 804-809 (See also Hypoadrenocorticism)
    incidental adrenal mass as, 812-813
    pheochromocytoma as, 809-812 (See also Pheochromocytoma)
  tumors of, 811t
Adrenal insufficiency
  primary, maintenance therapy for, 808-809
  secondary, therapy for, 809
Adrenalectomy
  for adrenal mass, 812
  for hyperadrenocorticism, in cats, 803
  indications for, 812-813
  medical, using mitotane, 795
  for pituitary-dependent hyperadrenocorticism, 796-797
Adrenaline chloride. See Epinephrine
Adrenocortical insufficiency, 804-809. See also Hypoadrenocorticism
Adrenocortical tumors (ATs)
  deoxycorticosterone-secreting, 812
  hyperadrenocorticism from, 778-779, 779f
  low-dose dexamethasone suppression in, 790, 791f
  progesterone-secreting, 804f, 812
  ultrasonographic appearance of, 783, 785f, 786f

Adrenocorticotropic hormone (ACTH)
  endogenous, tests of
    in hyperadrenocorticism diagnosis
      in cats, 801t, 802
      in dogs, 787f, 792
    in hypoadrenocorticism diagnosis, 807, 807t
  pituitary tumor secreting, hyperadrenocorticism from, 778
Adrenocorticotropic hormone (ACTH) stimulation test
  dexamethasone suppression combined with, in hyperadrenocorticism diagnosis, 787t, 790-791
  in hyperadrenocorticism diagnosis, 787t, 789-790, 789f
  in hypoglycemia diagnosis, 731
Adrenocorticotropic hormone (ACTH) suppression test
  in hyperadrenocorticism diagnosis in cats, 801t, 802
  in hypoadrenocorticism diagnosis, 806-807, 807t
Adrenomegaly
  bilateral, 785, 786f
  in pheochromocytoma, 810
Adriamycin. See Doxorubicin
Adulticide therapy
  in cats, 182
  in dogs, 174-176, 175t
Aelurostrongylus abstrusus, fecal examination for, 1230t
Aelurostrongylus obstrusus
  characteristics of eggs or larvae of, 263t
  larva of, 263f
  lung disease from, 302, 303
Aeromonas hydrophila, enterocolitis from, 439
Afghan hound, hereditary myelopathy in, 1044t
Aflatoxin, hepatotoxicity of, 522t
Afrin. See Oxymetazoline
Agalactia, 895-896
Agar gel immunodiffusion (AGID) tests, for Brucella canis infection, 937
Age
  advanced, acute renal failure and, 612
  litter size and, 888
  male sexual function and, 906
AGID tests. See Agar gel immunodiffusion (AGID) tests
Aglipristone, as abortifacient, 899-900
Airway(s)
  in cardiopulmonary resuscitation, 99, 100f
  hydration of, for bacterial pneumonia, 300t, 301
  large, disease of, 333-335, 334t, 335f
  obstruction of, feline, factors contributing to, 291t
  upper, obstruction of, 334-335, 334t, 335f
Alaskan Husky, laryngeal paralysis in, 1046t
Alaskan Malamutes, hereditary polyneuropathy of, 1045t
Albendazole
  dosages of, 402t, 469t
  for giardiasis, 445
  for infectious diseases, 1320t
  use of, 402t

Page numbers followed by "f" indicate figures; page numbers followed by "t" indicate tables.

Albon. *See* Sulfadimethoxine

Albumin concentration
in digestive disorders, 366
in hepatobiliary system assessment, 487, 492t

Albuterol, for feline bronchitis, 294

Aldactone. *See* Spironolactone

Aleukemic, 1133

Algal infections, lymphadenopathy associated with, 1202t

Alimentary lymphoma, 1123
treatment of, 1131

Alimentary tract, 343-471. *See also* Digestive system

Alkaline phosphatase (AP)
activity of, in hepatobiliary disorders, 486-487, 492t
seminal, 909-910

Alkaloids, plant, 1107

Alkeran. *See* Melphalan

Alkylating agents, 1106
for digestive disorders, 401

Allantoin, decreased production of, urate urolithiasis and, 634

Allergic bronchitis, 295
bronchial pattern in, 258f

Allergic reactions to insulin, 747

Allergic rhinitis, 239-240
radiographic signs of, 220t

Allopurinol
for infectious diseases, 1320t
for leishmaniasis, 1303
for urate uroliths, 639-640
for urinary tract disorders, 657t

Alopecia
from chemotherapy drugs, 1113, 1113f
endocrine, 667-670, 667f (*See also* Endocrine alopecia)
in hypothyroidism
in cats, 709
in dogs, 693, 695f
in pituitary dwarfism, 678

Alpha-adrenergic blockade, before pheochromocytoma surgery, 811

Alpha-amylase, 553t

Alpha-blockers, for hypertension, 202t, 203

Alpha-interferon, for infectious diseases, 1319t

Alpha-mannosidosis, cerebellar dysfunction in, 979t

Aluminum carbonate
for hyperphosphatemia in chronic renal failure, 619, 621
for urinary tract disorders, 657t

Aluminum hydroxide
as antacid, 397
for chronic renal failure, 618t
dosages of, 469t
for hypercalcemia, 839
for hyperphosphatemia in chronic renal failure, 619, 621
for urinary tract disorders, 657t

Alveolar-arterial oxygen gradient (A-*a* gradient), 284, 284t, 285t

Alveolar pattern in lung radiography, 258, 259f, 259t

*Amanita phalloides,* hepatotoxicity of, 522f

*Amblyomma americanum,* as vector for Rocky Mountain spotted fever, 1265

Ambulatory electrocardiography, 29, 31f

American trypanosomiasis, 1304

Amicar. *See* Aminocaproic acid (EACA)

Amiglyde. *See* Amikacin

Amikacin
for abdominal sepsis, 401
for bacterial pneumonia, 301
for cutaneous and soft tissue infections, 1244t
dosages of, 341t, 469t, 1241t
for hepatobiliary and pancreatic disorders, 566t

Amikacin—cont'd
for infection in chemotherapy patient, 1110
for infectious diseases, 1318t
for inflammatory hepatobiliary disease, 516
for liver abscesses, 542
for parvoviral enteritis, 434, 435t
for postsplenectomy sepsis, 1209
for sepsis in liver failure, 551

Amino acids
aromatic, 480
branched chain, 480

Aminocaproic acid (EACA)
for degenerative myelopathy, 1037-1038
for neurologic disorders, 1069t

Aminoglutethimide
for endocrine disorders, 813t
for hyperadrenocorticism in cats, 803

Aminoglycosides
for aspiration pneumonia, 306
for bacterial pneumonia, 301
for cardiopulmonary infections, 1244t
for cutaneous and soft tissue infections, 1244t
for digestive disorders, indications for, 401
for hepatic and gastrointestinal infections, 1245t
for infectious diseases, 1318t
for infective endocarditis, 149
for inflammatory hepatobiliary disease, 516
ototoxicity of, 1008
for septic peritonitis, 468
toxicities of, 1242t

Aminopentamide
as antiemetic, 396t
dosages of, 469t

Aminophylline
for dilated cardiomyopathy, 111t, 112-113
dosages of, 292t, 341t
for fulminant congestive heart failure, 59, 59t

Amiodarone
for arrhythmias, 93-94
commercial preparations of, 87t
dosages of, 79t, 207t
for ventricular tachyarrhythmias, 82

Amitriptyline, for urinary tract disorders, 657t

Amlodipine besylate
for chronic renal failure, 618t
for congestive heart failure, 71
for dilated cardiomyopathy, 111t, 112
dosages of, 62t, 206t
for hypertension, 202t, 203
preparations of, 63t
for urinary tract disorders, 658t

Ammonia concentrations
hepatic encephalopathy and, 479, 480f
in hepatobiliary system assessment, 489-490, 490t, 492t

Ammoniagenesis, in chronic renal failure, 618-619

Ammonium biurate crystals
in hepatobiliary disorders, 490, 490f
in urine sediment, 571f, 571t

Ammonium chloride
for urinary tract disorders, 658t
for urinary tract infections, 629-630

Ammopathy(ies)
monoclonal, 1211, 1211t
polyclonal, 1210-1211, 1211t

Amoeba, zoonotic, 1309t, 1311-1312

Amoxi-drop. *See* Amoxicillin

Amoxi-tab. *See* Amoxicillin

Amoxicillin
for antibiotic responsive enteropathy, 450
for bacterial meningitis/myelitis, 1015
for cardiopulmonary infections, 1244t
for chronic hepatic encephalopathy, 547

Amoxicillin—cont'd
with clavulanate
for bacterial pneumonia, 300
for canine infectious tracheobronchitis, 288
for cardiopulmonary infections, 1244t
for cutaneous and soft tissue infections, 1244t
for diskospondylitis, 1033
dosages of, 341t, 1241t
for facial nerve paralysis, 1053
for infectious diseases, 1319t
for Lyme disease, 1084
for pyothorax, 327
for urogenital infections, 1248t
with clavulanic acid, for septic arthritis, 1082
for clostridial disease, 438
dosages of, 341t, 469t, 1241t
for esophagitis, 412
for feline upper respiratory infections, 229, 230
for *Helicobacter*-associated disease, 420
for *Helicobacter* gastritis, 401
for hepatobiliary and pancreatic disorders, 566t
for hepatic and gastrointestinal infections, 1245t
for hepatobiliary inflammation, 540
for infectious diseases, 1319t
for inflammatory hepatobiliary disease, 516
for joint disease, 1092t
for Lyme disease, 1084
for urinary tract infections, 627
for urogenital infections, 1248t

*Amphimerus pseudofelieus,* extrahepatic bile duct obstruction from, 518

Amphojel. *See* Aluminum hydroxide

Amphotericin B
for blastomycosis, 1291
for cryptococcosis, 1289, 1289t
dosages of, 469-470t
for histoplasmosis, 440, 1291-1292
for infectious diseases, 1320t
for leishmaniasis, 1303
liposomal, for pythiosis, 429
for prototheosis, 440

Ampicillin
for abdominal sepsis, 401
for bacterial meningitis/myelitis, 1015
for cardiopulmonary infections, 1244t
for diskospondylitis, 1033
dosages of, 341t, 470t, 1241t
for feline upper respiratory infections, 229
for hepatobiliary and pancreatic disorders, 566t
for hepatic and gastrointestinal infections, 1245t
for hepatobiliary inflammation, 540
for infection in chemotherapy patient, 1110
for infectious diseases, 1319t
for joint disease, 1092t
for leptospirosis, 1262
for Lyme disease, 1084
for neurologic disorders, 1069t
for parvoviral enteritis, 434, 435t
for septic peritonitis, 468
with sulbactam
for aspiration pneumonia, 306
for bacterial pneumonia, 301
dosages of, 341t
for pyothorax, 327
for urogenital infections, 1248t

Amprolium
for coccidiosis, 444
dosages of, 470t

Amputation, for osteosarcoma, 1145

Amrinone
for congestive heart failure, 70
for dilated cardiomyopathy, 111t, 112

Amrinone—cont'd
dosages of, 67t, 206t
for fulminant congestive heart failure, 59, 59t
preparations of, 67t

Amylase activity, serum, in acute pancreatitis, 556

Amyloidosis
glomerular, 602-603, 603f
treatment of, 606
islet, in diabetes mellitus in cats, 749-750, 749f

ANA test. *See* Antinuclear antibody (ANA) test

Anabolic steroids
for feline infectious peritonitis, 1278
for nonregenerative anemia in chronic renal failure, 622

Anaerobes
culture techniques for, 1235
morphologic characteristics of, 1233t

Anaerobic infections
antibiotics for, 1240, 1243, 1243f, 1243t, 1244t
clinical findings in, 1243t

Anafen. *See* Ketoprofen

Anal sac
adenocarcinoma of, 461-462
inflammation of, 461

Anal sacculitis, 461

Analgesics, for severe pancreatitis, 559

Anaphylactic reactions, to chemotherapy drugs, 1112

Ancef. *See* Cefazolin

Ancobon. *See* Flucytosine

*Ancylostoma,* 443
as enteric zoonosis, 1309t
fecal examination for, 1230t

*Andersonstrongylus milksi,* fecal examination for, 1230t

Andro-Cyp. *See* Testosterone cypionate

Androgen-binding protein, 906

Androgens
for estrus suppression, 867
for false pregnancy, 887
for short interestrous intervals, 862

Anechoic tissues, 36

Anemia(s), 1156-1169
blood loss, 1160
of chronic disease, 1165, 1165t
clinical evaluation of, 1156-1158
clinical manifestations of, 1157t
clinicopathologic evaluation of, 1156-1158
in cytauxzoonosis, 1301
definition of, 1156
disorders associated with, 1158t
drugs associated with, 1157t
in ehrlichiosis, 1271
grading of, 1157
in hemangiosarcoma, 1142
hemolytic, 1160-1164 (*See also* Hemolytic anemia[s])
in hepatobiliary disorders, 485-486
iron deficiency, 1167-1168
distinguishing features of, 1165, 1165t
in gastric tumor, 429
in lymphadenopathy, 1206
management principles for, 1160
nonregenerative, 1164-1167
causes of, 1164t
in chronic renal failure, management of, 622
classification of, 1164t
pathogenetic classification of, 1159t
regenerative, 1160-1164
of renal disease, 1166-1167
semiregenerative, 1167-1168
in splenomegaly, 1206
toxins associated with, 1157t
transfusions for, 1168-1169

Anesthesia
for laryngoscopy, 243, 244
for pharyngoscopy, 243

Anesthesia—cont'd
for radiography, of oral cavity, 369
for rhinoscopy, 221
Anestrus, 860-862
canine, 848f, 850-851
vaginoscopy in, 853-854
Angiocardiography, 47
Angiography
in feline dilated cardiomyopathy, 131f, 132
in lower respiratory tract disorders, 262
in pulmonary thromboembolism, 311
Angiosarcomas, 1142-1144
*Angiostrongylus vasorum* infection, myocarditis in, 117
Angiotensin, glomerulonephritis and, 600, 602
Angiotensin-converting enzyme inhibitors (ACEIs)
for congestive heart failure, 57, 64-65
in AV valve degeneration, 144-145
for dilated cardiomyopathy, 111t, 112
dosages of, 62t, 206t
for feline hypertrophic cardiomyopathy, 128-129
for glomerulonephropathies, 606-607
for hypertension, 202t, 203
Angiotensin II, in congestive heart failure, 53, 53f
Animal inoculation, in infectious disease detection, 1237
Aninoglycosides, dosages of, 1241t
Anisocoria, 986-987
Anorexia
in chronic renal failure, management of, 621-622
complicating chemotherapy, 1111
in digestive disorders, 360, 360f, 361t
in gastrinomas, 775
in hypoadrenocorticism, 805
Antacids, 397, 397t
for gastroesophageal reflux, 411
for *Helicobacter* gastritis, 401
Anthelmintic drugs
for digestive disorders, 401-402, 402t
for hookworms, 443
for roundworms, 443
Antiacetylcholine receptor antibody, in neuromuscular disorders, 973
Antiarrhythmic drugs, 86-96
anticholinergic, 95-96
commercial preparations of, 88t
class I, 87-88t, 87-91
commercial preparations of, 87t
dosages of, 79t
class II, 91-93
commercial preparations of, 87t
dosages of, 79t
class III, 93-94
commercial preparations of, 87t
dosages of, 79t
class IV, 94-95
commercial preparations of, 88t
dosages of, 79t
classes and effects of, 78t
dosages of, 79-80t
proarrhythmic effects of, 78
sympathomimetic, 96
commercial preparations of, 88t
therapy with, goals of, 73-74
Antibacterial drugs, for digestive disorders, 401
Antibiotic(s)
for acute enteritis, 433
for anaerobic infections, 1240, 1243, 1243f, 1243t, 1244t
for anal sacculitis, 461
for antibiotic responsive enteropathy, 450
antitumor, 1107
for aspiration pneumonia, 306
for bacteremia, 1244-1245
for bacterial endocarditis, 1244-1245

Antibiotic(s)—cont'd
for bacterial infections, dosing guidelines or, 1241-1242t
for bacterial meningitis/myelitis, 1015
for bacterial pneumonia, 300-301, 300t
for canine chronic bronchitis, 297
for canine infectious tracheobronchitis, 288
for canine lymphocytic-plasmacytic enteritis, 447
for chronic hepatic encephalopathy, 547
for clostridial disease, 438
for CNS infections, 1246t, 1247
for cutaneous infections, 1244t, 1245
for cystic endometrial hyperplasia-pyometra complex, 879
for digestive disorders, 401
for digestive infections, 1245-1246, 1245t
for diskospondylitis, 1032-1033
for ehrlichiosis, 1270
for esophagitis, 412
for exocrine pancreatic insufficiency, 564
for facial nerve paralysis, 1053
for feline infectious peritonitis, 1278
for feline plague, 1259-1260
for feline upper respiratory infections, 229, 230
for gastric dilation/volvulus, 425
for gingivitis, 408
for *Helicobacter*-associated disease, 420
for hepatobiliary inflammation, 540
for hepatic infections, 1245-1246, 1245t
for immunodeficiency syndromes, 1227
for infectious diseases, 1318-1319t
for infective endocarditis, 149
for leptospirosis, 1262
for liver abscesses, 542
for Lyme disease, 1018
for mastitis, 882
for metritis, 897
for musculoskeletal infections, 1246-1247, 1246t
for *Mycoplasma* genital infections, 936
for *Mycoplasma* infections, 1263-1264
for neonates, 897, 897t
for parvoviral enteritis, 434, 435t
for perianal fistulae, 461
for periodontitis, 408
for postsplenectomy sepsis, 1209
in practical antimicrobial chemotherapy, 1240-1249
for pyothorax, 327-328
for respiratory distress in lung disease, 336
for respiratory tract infections, 1247-1248
for salmonellosis, 438
for sclerosing, encapsulating peritonitis, 468
for sepsis in liver failure, 551
for septic arthritis, 1082
for septic peritonitis, 468
for soft tissue infections, 1244t, 1245
for stomatitis, 408
toxicities of, 1242t
for *Ureaplasma* genital infections, 936
for *Ureaplasma* infections, 1263-1264
for urinary tract infections, 627-629, 629t
urine concentration of, 588t
for urogenital tract infections, 1248-1249, 1248t
for vaginitis, 875
Antibiotic-responsive enteropathy (ARE), 450
serum concentrations of vitamins in evaluation of, 378-379

Antibody(ies)
to acetylcholine receptors, in alimentary tract disease, 379
anti-LH, in population control, 866
detection of, in infectious disease detection, 1237-1238, 1238f
insulin-binding, circulating
in cats, 762
in dogs, 746-747
to 2M muscle fibers, in alimentary tract disease, 379
Antibody tests, for pulmonary pathogens, 264
Anticancer drugs
mechanism of action of, 1106
toxicity of, 1109t
types of, 1106-1107
Anticholinergic drugs
as antiemetics, 396t
for arrhythmias, 95-96
for diarrhea, 399t
dosages of, 80t, 208t
for irritable bowel syndrome, 452
for nonischemic priapism, 919
Anticoagulants
for glomerulonephropathies, 607
for pulmonary thromboembolism, 311
Anticonvulsants, 1001-1004, 1001t
alkaline phosphatase activity and, 486
chronic hepatitis from, 529
clonazepam as, 1003-1004
clorazepate as, 1003-1004
diazepam as, 1003
felbamate as, 1004
phenobarbital as, 1001-1002
potassium bromide as, 1002-1003
valproic acid as, 1004
Antidiarrheals, for acute enteritis, 432
Antidiuretic hormone (ADH)
exogenous, response to, in urinary disorder evaluation, 587-588
release of, in congestive heart failure, 53-54
Antiemetics, 396-397, 396t
for acute enteritis, 432
for gastrointestinal complications of chemotherapy, 1111
for parvoviral enteritis, 434, 435t
for severe pancreatitis, 558-559
Antifibrotic agents, for chronic hepatitis, 537
Antifungal drugs, 1320t
for cryptococcosis, 1289, 1289t
Antigen, heartworm, 170, 170t
Antigen tests, heartworm
in cats, 181
in dogs, 170, 170t
Antiglobulin test (AT), direct, for immune-mediated disorders, 1213-1214
Antihelmintics, for parvoviral enteritis, 435t
Antihistamines
for allergic rhinitis, 239
as antiemetics, 396t, 397
for hypersensitivity reactions to chemotherapy drugs, 1112
for nonischemic priapism, 919
Antiinflammatory drugs, for digestive disorders, 399-401
Antimetabolites, 1106-1107
Antimony, for leishmaniasis, 1303
Antinuclear antibody (ANA) test
for immune-mediated disorders, 1214
for systemic lupus erythematosus, 1073, 1077, 1086
Antioxidants
for chronic hepatitis, 537
in congestive heart failure, 62
for hepatobiliary and pancreatic disorders, 566t
Antiprotozoals, for infectious diseases, 1319-1320t
Antirobe. *See* Clindamycin

Antisecretory drugs, for digestive disorders, 399-401
Antispasmodics, for detrusor hyperreflexia, 656
Antithyroid drugs, 721-722, 721t
for thyroid neoplasia, 727
Antitumor antibiotics, 1107
Antiviral agents
for feline immunodeficiency virus, 1280-1281, 1280t
for feline leukemia virus infection, 1283
for infectious diseases, 1319t
Antral mucosal hypertrophy, gastric, 421, 423, 423f
Aortic root, diameter of, M-mode scan in evaluation of, 42
AP. *See* Alkaline phosphatase (AP)
Apocrine gland adenocarcinoma, 461-462
Apomorphine
dosages of, 470t
for neurologic disorders, 1069t
Appetite
in congestive heart failure, stimulating, 60
ravenous, in exocrine pancreatic insufficiency, 561
stimulants of, 391
for hepatobiliary and pancreatic disorders, 566t
for hepatic lipidosis, 508
Apresoline. *See* Hydralazine
Aquamethyton. *See* Vitamin K$_1$
Arava. *See* Leflunomide
ARDS. *See* Acute respiratory distress syndrome (ARDS)
ARE. *See* Antibiotic responsive enteropathy (ARE)
Arginine vasopressin (AVP), disorders of, in diabetes insipidus, 661
ARMD. *See* Autosomal recessive muscular dystrophy (ARMD)
Aromatic amino acids, 480
Arrhythmia(s)
in acute pancreatitis, 555t
bradyarrhythmias as, 84-86, 85f
cardiogenic shock from, 119t
catecholamine-induced, 103
common, 74-86
complicating atrioventricular valve disease, 140, 140t
differential diagnoses for, 74t
drugs for, 86-96, 207t (*See also* Antiarrhythmic drugs)
factors predisposing to, 76t
in feline hypertrophic cardiomyopathy, 124
in hyperkalemia, 833, 833t
irregular tachyarrhythmias as, 75-83
rapid, regular, 83-84
sinus, 16, 18f, 18t
ECG in, 18f
syncope or intermittent weakness from, 2t, 3
Arrhythmogenic right ventricular cardiomyopathy
in cat, 133
in dog, 116
Arsenicals, inorganic, hepatotoxicity of, 522t
treatment of, 523t
Arterial blood pressure measurement, 200
Arterial carbon dioxide tension
indications for, 281
results of, interpretation of, 282-285, 282t, 283f, 283t, 284t, 285t
techniques for, 281-282, 281f, 282f
Arterial pulses
in cardiovascular examination, 6, 6t
hyperkinetic, in patent ductus arteriosus, 153
Arterial thromboembolism, in cat, 134-137. *See also* Thromboembolism, arterial, in cat

Arteriolar vasodilators, in congestive heart failure management, 65-66

Arteriosclerosis, dilated cardiomyopathy and, 107

Arteriovenous shunts, extracardiac, 153-155

Artery(ies), pulmonary
echocardiographic view of, 37f
enlarged, differential diagnosis of, 257, 257t
evaluation of, 35
in heartworm disease, 169-170
small, differential diagnosis of, 257, 257t

Arthritis. *See also* Polyarthritis
bacterial L form-associated, 1083
fungal, 1084-1085
immunologically mediated, 1072
rheumatoid, 1089-1091, 1089f, 1090f
(*See also* Rheumatoid arthritis [RA])
septic, 1081-1083, 1081t, 1082f, 1083f
viral, 1085, 1085f

Arthrocentesis, for synovial fluid collection, 1073-1074, 1074f, 1075-1076f

Artifacts, electrocardiographic, 29, 30f

Artificial insemination (AI), 940-944
advantages of, 940
principles of, 940-941
semen for
cat, 943-944
chilled extended, 943
fresh, 942
frozen, 942-943
handling of, 940-941
technique of, 941-942
timing of, 940

Ascites, 474
complicating hepatic failure, 549-550

Ascorbic acid
for feline infectious peritonitis, 1278
for hepatibiliary and pancreatic disorders, 567t

ASD. *See* Atrial septal defect (ASD)

Aspergillosis
lymphadenopathy associated with, 1202t
nasal, 211, 212f, 220f, 220t
rhinoscopic view of, 223f

*Aspergillus*, nasal infection from, 235-237

Aspiration
complicating nasal biopsy, 226
fine-needle, 1093-1094 (*See also* Fine-needle aspiration [FNA])
in solitary mass evaluation, 1117
lung, transthoracic, 274-276, 276f

Aspiration pneumonia, 304-307, 306t

Aspirin. *See* Acetylsalicylic acid

Asthma, feline, 291-295. *See also* Feline bronchitis

AT. *See* Antiglobulin test (AT)

Ataxia, 974, 975t, 975t, 976f
hereditary
in Jack Russell terriers, 1044t
in smooth-coated Fox Terriers, 1044t

Atelectasis, interstitial patterns in, 260

Atenolol
for arrhythmias, 92
characteristics of, 91t
commercial preparations of, 87t
dosages of, 79t, 207t
for feline hypertrophic cardiomyopathy, 127, 128, 128t
for hypertension, 202t, 203

Atlantoaxial instability and luxation, in young animals, 1046-1047, 1047f

ATLS. *See* Acute tumor lysis syndrome (ATLS)

Atrial arrhythmias, factors predisposing to, 76t

Atrial fibrillation, 21, 22f, 82-83, 83f
M-mode echocardiogram in, 75f

Atrial flutter, 21

Atrial gallop, 9

Atrial septal defect (ASD), 151, 162
breed dispositions for, 152t
murmurs in, 152f, 162
pulmonary hypertension in, 164-166
radiographic findings in, 154t

Atrial standstill, 23, 86

Atrioventricular (AV) block, 23-24, 24f

Atrioventricular (AV) node, conduction disturbances within, 23-24, 24f

Atrioventricular (AV) valve
disease of, degenerative
with asymptomatic regurgitation, treatment of, 144
clinical signs of, 141
complications of, 140-141, 140t
with congestive heart failure, treatment of, 144-145
echocardiography in, 142-143, 142f, 143f
electrocardiography in, 142
epidemiology of, 141
etiology of, 139
pathology of, 139
pathophysiology of, 139-140
patient monitoring in, 145
prognosis in, 143-145
reevaluation in, 145
treatment of, 143-145
malformations of, 162-163, 163f
mitral dysplasia as, 162
tricuspid dysplasia as, 162-163, 163f

Atrium
left
diameter of, M-mode scan in evaluation of, 42-43
enlargement of
in feline hypertrophic cardiomyopathy, 127, 127f
radiography in, 33t, 34, 34f
right, enlargement of, radiography in, 33t, 34, 34f

Atromid-S. *See* Clofibrate

Atrophic gastritis, 419-420

Atrophic myositis, 409

Atropine
for arrhythmias, 95-96
in cardiopulmonary resuscitation, dosages of, 99t
commercial preparations of, 88t
dosage of, 208t, 209t
dosages of, 80t, 341t, 470t
for neurologic disorders, 1069t

ATs. *See also* Adrenocortical tumors (ATs)

Auranofin
immune-mediated disorders, 1218
for joint disease, 1092t
for rheumatoid arthritis, 1090

Aurothioglucose
for immune-mediated disorders, 1218
for joint disease, 1092t
for rheumatoid arthritis, 1090

Auscultation, thoracic, in lower respiratory tract disease diagnosis, 252-253

Autoagglutination, disorders associated with, 1159t

Autoimmune disorders, 1212-1214. *See also* Immune-mediated disorders (IMDs)

Autonomic bladder, treatment of, 655

Autonomic innervation, of bladder, 650-651, 651f

Autosomal recessive muscular dystrophy (ARMD), 1067

Avandia. *See* Rosiglitazone

AVP. *See* Arginine vasopressin (AVP)

Axid. *See* Nizatidine

Axillary nerve, trauma to, 1050t

Axis
lead, 12
mean electrical, 13, 14f, 15

Axonal neuropathy, giant, in German Shepherds, 1045t

Axonopathy
central, in Scottish Terriers, 1044t
Labrador Retriever, 1044t
progressive, of Boxers, 1045t

Azathioprine
for canine lymphocytic-plasmacytic enteritis, 447
for chronic hepatitis, 537
chronic hepatitis from, 529
for digestive disorders, 400
dosages of, 470t
for idiopathic, immune-mediated polyarthritis, 1088
for immune hemolytic anemia, 1163
for immune-mediated thrombocytopenia, 1192
for immunoproliferative enteropathy in Basenjis, 450
as immunosuppressant, 1217-1218
indication and dosage of, 565t
for joint disease, 1092t
for masticatory muscle myositis, 409
for masticatory myositis, 1063
for meningeal vasculitis, 1012
for myasthenia gravis, 1061
for neurologic disorders, 1069t
for perianal fistulae, 461
for rheumatoid arthritis, 1090
for steroid-responsive suppurative meningitis, 1011
for urinary tract disorders, 658t

Azidothymidine (AZT)
for feline immunodeficiency virus, 1280, 1280t
for feline leukemia virus infection, 1283
for infectious diseases, 1319t

Azithromycin
for bacterial pneumonia, 301
dosages of, 1241t
for feline bronchitis, 292
for feline upper respiratory infections, 229
for *Helicobacter*-associated disease, 420
for *Helicobacter* gastritis, 401
for infectious diseases, 1319t
for toxoplasmosis, 1298

Azium. *See* Dexamethasone

Azoospermia, 915-916

Azotemia, 581-583
in acute renal failure, 611
in arterial thromboembolism, 134
definition of, 608
prerenal
acute renal failure differentiated from, 582t
in dilated cardiomyopathy, 109
renal, definition of, 608

AZT. *See* Azidothymidine (AZT)

Azulfidine. *See* Sulfasalazine

**B**

*Babesia*, drugs for, 1319t

*Babesia canis*
infection with, 1300-1301
morphologic characteristics of, 1234t
myocarditis from, 117

*Babesia gibsoni*
infection with, 1300-1301
morphologic characteristics of, 1234t

Babesiosis, 1300-1301
lymphadenopathy associated with, 1202t

Bacteremia
antibiotics for, 124t, 1244-1245
infective endocarditis from, 145-146

Bacteria
cultures for
in feces, 367-368
in semen, 911-912, 911f
cytologic examination for, 1233, 1233f
fetal death from, 900
L-form, antibiotics for, 1244t, 1246t
overgrowth of, antibiotics for, 1245t

Bacteria—cont'd
polysystemic diseases from, 1259-1264
feline plague as, 1259-1260, 1260f, 1260t
leptospirosis as, 1260-1262, 1261t
*Mycoplasma*, 1262-1264, 1263t
*Ureaplasma*, 1262-1264, 1263t
urinary tract infections from, 624, 625t
in urine, significant numbers of, by collection method, 569t
virulence of, factors affecting, 624, 625t
zoonotic, 1312-1314, 1309t

Bacterial antibiotic sensitivity testing
in urinary tract disorders, 588-589, 588t
in urinary tract infections, 627

Bacterial arthritis, 1081-1083, 1081t, 1082f, 1083f

Bacterial endocarditis, antibiotics for, 1244-1245, 1244t

Bacterial infections, halitosis in, 344t

Bacterial L form-associated arthritis, 1083

Bacterial meningitis, 1014-1015, 1014f
CSF analysis in, 964t

Bacterial myelitis, 1014-1015, 1014f

Bacterial myocarditis
canine, 116
feline, 133-134

Bacterial pneumonia, 299-302, 300t, 301f
antibiotics for, 1244t

Bacterial prostatitis, 930-931
chronic, 931-932

*Bacteroides fragilis*, morphologic characteristics of, 1233t

BAER. *See* Brainstem auditory evoked response (BAER)

Baermann technique
for *Aelurostrongylus abstrusus* diagnosis, 303
for concentration of larvae, 264t
for fecal examination, 1232, 1232f

BAL. *See* Bronchoalveolar lavage (BAL)

BAL in oil. *See* Dimercaprol

Balanoposthitis, 920

*Balantidium coli*, fecal examination for, 1230t

Balloon valvuloplasty, for pulmonic stenosis, 160

Banamine. *See* Flunixin meglumine

Barbiturates
ECG changes from, 27t
in head trauma management, 984

Barium sulfate
in contrast-enhanced esophagraphy, 371, 372f
in contrast-enhanced gastrography, 374-376
in contrast-enhanced studies of small intestine, 376
enemas using, 376-377, 378f
as intestinal protectant, 398
in radiography, of esophagus, 369

*Bartonella*, lymphadenopathy associated with, 1202t

*Bartonella henselae*, cat scratch disease from, 1312-1314, 1313t

*Bartonella vinsonii*, myocarditis from, 116

Basal gel. *See* Aluminum carbonate

Basenjis, immunoproliferative enteropathy in, 449-450

Basopenia, 1178

Basophilia, 1178, 1178t

*Baylisascaris procyonis*, as enteric zoonosis, 1309t

Baytril. *See* Enrofloxacin

Bedlington Terriers, familial chronic hepatitis in, 526-527, 527f

Behavior, hypothyroidism and, 695

Benadryl. *See* Diphenhydramine

Benazepril
for chronic renal failure, 618t
in congestive heart failure management, 65
dosages of, 62t, 206t

Benazepril—cont'd
preparations of, 63t
for urinary tract disorders, 658t
Benign prostatic hyperplasia (BPH), 928-930, 929f
Bentylol. *See* Dicyclomine
Benztropine, for nonischemic priapism, 919
Beta-blockers
for arrhythmias, 91-93
atenolol as, 92
for atrial fibrillation, 83, 83f
characteristics of, 91t
for dilated cardiomyopathy, 113
for feline hypertrophic cardiomyopathy, 127-128, 128t
for hypertension, 202t, 203
for hypertrophic cardiomyopathy, 116
for paroxysmal AV reciprocating tachycardia, 77
propranolol as, 92
for pulmonic stenosis, 160
for respiratory distress in lung disease, 336
for restrictive cardiomyopathy, 130
for subaortic stenosis, 158
for supraventricular premature contractions, 76-77, 77f
for supraventricular tachycardias, 77, 77f
for tetralogy of Fallot, 164
for ventricular tachyarrhythmias, 80, 81, 81f, 82
for ventricular tachycardia, 84
Beta cell tumors, insulin-secreting, 769-775. *See also* Insulin-secreting β-cell neoplasia
Beta-lactam antibiotics, for septic peritonitis, 468
Betapace. *See* Sotalol
Bethanechol
for detrusor atony in urethral obstruction, 648
in detrusor hypocontractility diagnosis, 654
for diarrhea, 399
dosages of, 470t
for dysautonomia, 413
for neurologic disorders, 1069t
for urinary tract disorders, 658t
Biaxin. *See* Clarithromycin
Bicarbonate
for acute addisonian crisis, 807t, 808
for acute renal failure, 614
for cardiogenic shock, 119
for cardiopulmonary resuscitation, dosages of, 99t
for chronic renal failure, 618t
for diabetic ketoacidosis, 765t, 767
dosage of, 208t
for hyperkalemia, 834, 834t, 846t
Bicytopenia, 1181
causes of, 1182t
Biguanides, 755t, 757
Bile
extravasation of, from biliary tract rupture, 475-476
"white," 479
in lymphocytic cholangitis, 516, 516f
Bile acid, serum concentrations of
in congenital portosystemic shunt, 521
in hepatobiliary system assessment, 488-489, 492t
Bile acid sequestrates for hypercholesterolemia, 827
Bile duct
common, anatomic relationship of, with pancreas and duodenum in cat, 513f
obstruction of, 477
extrahepatic, 518-520, 519f, 519t
(*See* Extrahepatic bile duct obstruction)
Bile peritonitis, 539

Bile pigment, absence of, acholic feces from, 479, 479f
Biliary tract
disorders of, in dogs, 538-540
ruptured, bile extravasation from, 475-476
ultrasonographic findings in, 497t
Bilious vomiting syndrome, 427
Bilirubin
concentrations of, total, 477
excretion of, disorders impeding, 478
hepatobiliary disease and, 476-479, 477f, 478f
serum concentration of, in hepatobiliary system assessment, 487-488, 492t
Bilirubinuria, 476-479
Biliverdin, 477
Biochemical markers, of myocardial injury, 48
Biochemistry profile
in acute pancreatitis, 554, 556
in diabetes mellitus, 733t
in neuromuscular disorders, 961
Biologic response modifiers, for hemangiosarcoma, 1144
Biopsy(ies)
in antral mucosal hypertrophy diagnosis, 423
in canine lymphocytic-plasmacytic colitis diagnosis, 448
colonoscopic, 384, 384f
in digestive disorder evaluation, 343-344
endomyocardial, 48
gastric, in gastritis diagnosis, 419
gastroduodenoscopy and, in alimentary tract disease, 380-381, 382-383f
gastrointestinal
endoscopic, 384-385
fine-needle aspiration, 384
full-thickness, 385
intestinal
in canine eosinophilic gastroenterocolitis diagnosis, 448-449
for enteropathy in Shar-Peis diagnosis, 450
in feline eosinophilic enteritis/hypereosinophilic syndrome diagnosis, 449
liver, 499-504, 499t, 500f, 501f, 502-503f, 504f, 505f (*See* Liver, biopsy of)
lung
in lower respiratory tract specimen collection, 265t
open-chest, 281
transbronchial, 278, 281
transthoracic, 274-276, 276f
in metastatic lung lesion, 1118
muscle
in canine idiopathic polymyositis diagnosis, 1064
for neuromuscular disorders, 972-973
nasal, 224-226, 225f, 226f
in aspergillosis, 235
in tumor diagnosis, 234
nerve, for neuromuscular disorders, 973
renal, 598
in acute renal failure, 610-611
in solitary mass evaluation, 1117
synovial membrane, 1077
testicular, in functional assessment, 912
transthoracic, in mediastinal masses, 319
in vomiting, 349
Biosecurity guidelines
for clients, 1252
for small animal hospitals, 1250-1252, 1251t
Biosol. *See* Neomycin sulfate

Bisacodyl dosages, 403t, 470t
Bismuth subsalicylate
for acute enteritis, 432
as antiemetic, 396t
for diarrhea, 399, 399t
dosages of, 470t
for gastrointestinal complications of chemotherapy, 1111
Bisphosphonates, for hypercalcemia, 839, 839t
Bitch
estrous cycle in, 847-851, 848f (*See also* Estrous cycle, canine)
estrus induction in, 868-869
false pregnancy in, 886-887
infertility in, diagnostic approach to, 861f
mature, vaginitis in, treatment of, 875
ovulation induction in, 869
pregnant, alterations in, 890-891
prepubertal, vaginitis in, treatment of, 874-875
Bite zoonoses, 1312-1315, 1313t
Bladder
autonomic, treatment of, 655
autonomic innervation of, 650-651, 651f
distended
micturition disorders associated with, 651-652, 652t
urinary incontinence with, 576
expression of, for lower motor neuron disorders, 655
function of, diagnostic tests of, 588
innervation of, 650-651, 651f
small or normal-sized
micturition disorders associated with, 652-653, 652t
urinary incontinence with, 576-577
transitional cell carcinoma of, 570, 593f, 597f
ultrasonography of, 589t, 596, 596f, 597f
Bland diet, 389, 389t
for acute colitis/proctitis, 458
for acute gastritis, 418
for dietary-induced diarrhea, 433
for parvoviral enteritis, 434
Blastocysts, 887-888
*Blastomyces dermatitidis*
cytologic appearance of, 1288t
infection from, 1290-1291, 1290f, 1291f
in tracheal wash specimen, 268f
Blastomycosis, 1290-1291, 1290f, 1291f
lymphadenopathy associated with, 1202t
pulmonary, interstitial pattern in, 260f, 260t
Bleeding
complicating chemotherapy, 1110
spontaneous, in hemangiosarcoma, 1142
Bleeding disorders, spontaneous, clinical manifestations of, 1186-1187, 1186t
Bleeding patient, management of, 1189-1190
Bleeding time (BT), buccal mucosal
in bleeding patient evaluation, 1187t, 1188, 1188t
in von Willebrand's disease, 1193
Blindness, 984-990. *See also* Vision, loss of
in diabetes mellitus, in dogs, 732, 732f, 748
Blood
administration of, 1168-1169
clotting of (*See* Hemostasis)
crossmatching of, 1168, 1169t
culture of, in infectious disease diagnosis, 1235
fecal
fresh, 355-356, 356t
occult, 367

Blood—cont'd
flow of, patterns of, Doppler echocardiography detecting, 44-47, 45f, 46f, 47f
groups of, 1168
loss of
acute and peracute, anemia from, 1167
hemolytic anemias differentiated from, 1160
transfusion of
for bleeding patient, 1190
complications of, 1169
crossmatching for, 1168, 1169t
for immune hemolytic anemia, 1164
principles of, 1168-1169
transfusions of, for cytauxzoonosis, 1302
Blood culture
in diskospondylitis, 1032
in infective endocarditis diagnosis, 147-148
Blood gases
abnormalities of, clinical correlations of, 283t
analysis of, 281-285
in aspiration pneumonia, 305-306
indications for, 281
results of, interpretation of, 282-285, 282t, 283f, 283t, 284t, 285t
techniques of, 281-282, 281f, 282f
arterial, measurements of, relationships of, 284t
Blood glucose curve, serial, in diabetes management, 739-741, 740f, 741f, 742f, 743f
Blood glucose-monitoring device, in diabetes diagnosis, 732
Blood pressure
elevated (*See* Hypertension)
measurement of, 200-201
Blood smear
in anemia, 1158
platelet estimation in, in bleeding patient evaluation, 1187, 1187t
Blood vessels
disorders of, seizures from, 999
hepatobiliary, ultrasonographic findings in, 498t
intrathoracic, radiography of, 34-35
pulmonary, thoracic radiography of, 256-257, 257f, 257t
systemic lupus erythematosus and, 1220t
Body condition scoring system, 818, 818t
Body fluids, antibody detection in, 1238
Bone marrow
aspirates from, in ehrlichiosis, 1269
disorders of, anemia in, 1165-1166, 1166t
evaluation of
in leukoerythroblastosis, 1184
in lymphadenopathy-splenomegaly, 1207
hypercellular, pancytopenia in, diagnostic algorithm for, 1183f
hypocellular, pancytopenia in, diagnostic algorithm for, 1183f
Bone marrow aplasia-hypoplasia
anemia in, 1165-1166, 1166t
cytopenias in, 1184
Bone neoplasms, 1144-1146, 1144f, 1145f, 1145t
*Bordetella bronchiseptica*
canine infectious tracheobronchitis from, 287-289, 288f
pulmonary infection from, 299
respiratory zoonoses associated with, 1315
vaccination against, 1255, 1256-1257
*Bordetella* vaccines, 230
Boron neutron capture therapy (BNCT), for brain tumors, 999

*Borrelia burgdorferi*
  antibiotics for, 1246t
  lymphadenopathy associated with, 1202t
  vaccination against, 1257
Botulism, 1058
Bouvier des Flandres, laryngeal paralysis of, 1045t
Bovine lactoferrin, for stomatitis, 408
Boxers
  cardiomyopathy in, 113-114
  central-peripheral neuropathy in, 1044t
  progressive axonopathy of, 1045t
  sudden death predisposition in, 73
BPH. *See* Benign prostatic hyperplasia (BPH)
Brachial plexus avulsion, 1050t
Brachycephalic airway syndrome, 248-249, 248f
Bradyarrhythmia(s), 84-86, 85f
  atrial standstill as, 86
  definition of, 16
  second-degree AV blocks as, 86
  sick sinus syndrome as, 85-86, 85f
  sinus bradycardia as, 84, 85f
  syncope or intermittent weakness from, 2t
  third-degree AV blocks as, 86
Bradycardia, sinus, 84
  causes of, 18t
  ECG in, 18f
Brain
  infarction in, CSF analysis in, 964t
  injury to, from cardiac arrest and resuscitation, 105
  neurologic abnormality in, localization of, 957, 959t
  trauma to, complicating nasal biopsy, 225
  tumors of
    clinical signs of, 996
    CSF analysis in, 997-998
    diagnostic imaging in, 997
    neurologic deficits from, 996-997
    seizures and, 996-999
    treatment of, 998-999
Brainstem auditory evoked response (BAER), in neuromuscular disorders, 971
Bran, wheat, dosage of, 403t
Branched chain amino acids, 480
Branchial cysts, as mediastinal masses, 1119t
Breathing
  in cardiopulmonary resuscitation, 99-100, 100f
  patterns of, in laryngeal disease, 241
Breeding, canine, management of, 849-850
Breeding behavior, male, 907
  age-related effects on, 906
Brethine. *See* Terbutaline
Bretylium
  for arrhythmias, 94
  in cardiopulmonary resuscitation, dosages of, 99t
  commercial preparations of, 87t
  dosages of, 79t, 207t
Bretylol. *See* Bretylium
Brevibloc. *See* Esmolol
Bricanyl. *See* Terbutaline
Brittany Spaniels, spinal muscular atrophy of, 1045t
Bromocriptine
  as abortifacient, 899
  for false pregnancy, 887
  for reproductive disorders, 944t
Bronchial disorders, differential diagnosis of, 251f
Bronchial patterns
  in feline bronchitis, 292
  in lung radiography, 257-258, 258f, 258f, 259f

Bronchiectasis, in canine chronic bronchitis, 295, 295f, 296
Bronchitis
  allergic, 295
    bronchial pattern in, 258f
  bacterial, 299
  canine, chronic, 295-297, 295f
  feline, 291-295 (*See also* Feline bronchitis)
Bronchoalveolar lavage (BAL)
  bronchoscopic, 277-278
  in lower respiratory tract specimen collection, 265t
  nonbronchoscopic, 270-274, 271f, 272f, 273f, 274f, 274t
  in pulmonary neoplasia, 308f
Bronchodilators, 292t
  for aspiration pneumonia, 306
  for bacterial pneumonia, 300t, 301
  for canine chronic bronchitis, 296-297
  for dilated cardiomyopathy, 112-113
  for feline bronchitis, 293-294
  for respiratory distress in lung disease, 336
Bronchopneumonia, bacterial, 299
Bronchopneumopathy, eosinophilic, 303
Bronchoscopy, 276-281, 278-279f, 280t
  in aspiration pneumonia, 305
  bronchoalveolar lavage by, 277-278
  in canine chronic bronchitis, 296
  indications for, 276
  technique of, 276-277, 278-279f
Bronchus(i)
  abnormalities of, 280t
  bronchoscopic view of, 279f
  disorders of, 291-298
    feline, classification of, 291t
  nomenclature of, 280t
  *Oslerus osleri* in, 297-298
*Brucella canis*
  antibiotics for, 1248t, 1249
  genital infections from, 936-938
  genitourinary zoonoses from, 1317
  lymphadenopathy associated with, 1202t
Bubonic plague, feline, 1259-1260
Buccal mucosal bleeding time
  in bleeding patient evaluation, 1187t, 1188, 1188t
  in von Willebrand's disease, 1193
Budesonide
  for digestive disorders, 400
  for feline lymphocytic-plasmacytic enteritis, 448
Bulk laxatives, 403, 403t
Bull Mastiffs, spongiform degeneration of gray matter in, 1044t
Bundle branch blocks (BBBs), 15, 15t, 16f, 16t
  left, 25
  right, 24-25
Bupaparavaquone, for infectious diseases, 1320t
Buparvaquone, for cytauxzoonosis, 1302
Buprenorphine, in respiratory distress, 334t
Butazolidin. *See* phenylbutazone
Butorphanol
  for acute intervertebral disk disease, 1026
  for arterial thromboembolism, 135
  for cough in dogs, 288, 288f
  dosages of, 341t, 565t
  for gastrointestinal complications of chemotherapy, 1111
  indications for, 565t
  in respiratory distress, 334t
  for severe pancreatitis, 559

**C**

Cabergoline
  as abortifacient, 899
  in estrus induction in bitch, 868-869
  for false pregnancy, 887
Cachexia, cardiac, 60

Caesarian section, in dystocia management, 895
Cage confinement, in acute intervertebral disk disease management, 1026
Cairn Terriers, neuronal chromatolysis of, 1045t
Calan. *See* Verapamil
Calcimar. *See* Calcitonin
Calcitonin
  actions of, on calcium and phosphorus metabolism, 682t
  for hypercalcemia, 839, 845t
Calcitriol
  for chronic renal failure, 621
  for urinary tract disorders, 658t
Calcium
  deficiency of (*See* Hypocalcemia)
  for endocrine disorders, 814t
  excess of (*See* Hypercalcemia)
  for hypocalcemia, 686
  metabolism of, hormones affecting, biologic actions of, 682t
  plasma concentrations of, interactions of, with phosphorus, parathyroid hormone and vitamin D concentrations, 620f
    in chronic renal failure, 621f
  preparations of, for hypocalcemia, 845t
  serum concentration of
    depressed, 840-841
    elevated, 836-839, 838f, 839t (*See also* Hypercalcemia)
  supplemental
    during lactation, 896
    for primary hypoparathyroidism, 688-689, 688t
Calcium chloride
  for cardiac arrest, 103-104
  in cardiopulmonary resuscitation, dosages of, 99t
  dosage of, 208t
Calcium EDTA, for neurologic disorders, 1069t
Calcium entry blockers
  for arrhythmias, 94-95
  for congestive heart failure, 71
  for hypertension, 202t, 203
  verapamil as, 95
Calcium gluconate
  in cardiopulmonary resuscitation, dosages of, 99t
  dosage of, 208t
  for dystocia, 895
  for hyperkalemia, 845t
    in acute renal failure, 614-615
  for hypocalcemia, 840
  for neurologic disorders, 1069t
  for puerperal hypocalcemia, 896
  for reproductive disorders, 944t
Calcium oxalate crystals in urine sediment, 570f, 571t
Calcium oxalate uroliths
  canine
    etiology and pathogenesis of, 633-634, 634f
    factors predicting composition of, 632t
    treatment of, 639
  feline, 644
    in feline lower urinary tract inflammation, 644
Calculi, renal, 590f
Calicivirus, feline, 228
  vaccination for, 230, 1255
*Campylobacter*
  antibiotics for, 1245t
  culture techniques for, 1235
  cytologic evaluation of feces for, 368, 437
  as enteric zoonosis, 1309t
  infection by, 437
  morphologic characteristics of, 1233t

*Campylobacter jejuni*, as enteric zoonosis, 1309t
Campylobacteriosis, 437
Cancer. *See also* Oncology
  humoral hypercalcemia of malignancy in, 837-839, 838
*Candida*, fecal culture for, 368
Canine adenovirus
  type 1 (CAV1), chronic hepatitis from, 529
  type 2 (CAV2), canine infectious tracheobronchitis from, 287
Canine chronic bronchitis, 295-297, 295f
Canine coronaviral enteritis, 436
Canine distemper, 1015-1016, 1273-1275, 1274t. *See also* Distemper, canine
Canine ehrlichiosis, 1267-1270
Canine eosinophilic gastroenterocolitis, 448-449
Canine estrous cycle, 847-851, 848f
Canine granulomatous enteritis/gastritis, 449
Canine idiopathic polymyositis, 1063-1064
Canine infectious hepatitis, lymphadenopathy associated with, 1202t
Canine infectious tracheobronchitis, 287-289, 288f
Canine lymphocytic-plasmacytic colitis, 448
Canine lymphocytic-plasmacytic enteritis, 447-448
Canine parvoviral enteritis, 433-435t
Canine transmissible venereal tumor, 938-939
Canine urolithiasis, 631-641
  calcium oxalate, 633-634, 634f
  clinical features of, 636, 636f
  cystine, 635-636, 635f
  diagnosis of, 636, 637f
  etiology of, 631-636
  pathogenesis of, 631-636
  prevention of, 638-639, 638t
  reevaluation of patient with, 641
  silicate, 635, 635f
  struvite, 633, 633f
  treatment of, 636-641, 637t, 638t
  urate, 634-635, 634f
  urohydropropulsion for, 637, 638t
Canine viral enteritides, lymphadenopathy associated with, 1202t
Canine wobbler syndrome, 1040-1043, 1041-1042f, 1043f
Caparsolate. *See* Thiacetarsamide
*Capillaria aerophila*
  characteristics of eggs or larvae of, 263t
  fecal examination for, 1230t
  lung disease from, 302, 303
*Capillaria boehmi*, nasal, rhinoscopic view of, 223f
*Capillaria* sp., ova or, 263t
Capillariasis, nasal, 238-239
Capillary refill time (CRT), in cardiovascular examination, 4
*Capnocytophaga canimorsus*, zoonoses associated with, 1313t
Capoten. *See* Captopril
Captopril
  for congestive heart failure, 65
  dosages of, 62t, 206t
  for hypertension, 202t
  preparations of, 63t
Capture beat, 22
Carafate. *See* Sucralfate
Carbamates, neurologic dysfunction from, 995t
Carbapenems, for infectious diseases, 1318t
Carbergoline, for reproductive disorders, 944t
Carbimazole
  for endocrine disorders, 814t
  for hyperthyroidism, 722

Carbohydrates, dietary, restriction of, for diabetes in cats, 753, 753t, 754t
Carbopenems, dosages of, 1241t
Carboplatin
  for carcinomas, 1155t
  for injection site sarcomas, 1152
  for oropharyngeal masses, 1151
  for osteosarcoma, 1145-1146, 1155t
  for soft-tissue sarcomas, 1155t
Carcinoma(s)
  chemotherapy protocols for, 1155t
  cholangiocellular, 517
  in cytologic specimen interpretation, 1095, 1096f
  hepatocellular, 517
    radiography of, 494f
  intraabdominal, abdominal effusion from, 475
  metastatic, lymphadenopathy associated with, 1202t
  nasal cavity, 219f
  pulmonary, 307-309
  squamous cell
    metastatic behavior of, 1118b
    oropharyngeal, 1150
  thyroid, 725f, 726f
    hyperthyroidism from, 712, 715f
  transitional cell
    of bladder, 570, 593f, 597f
    metastatic behavior of, 1118t
Carcinomatosis, abdominal, 469
Cardiac arrest, recurrence of, 104-105
Cardiac cachexia, 60
Cardiac catheterization, 47-48
Cardiac cycle, 8f
Cardiac output
  decreased, in dilated cardiomyopathy, 108
  forward, impaired, syncope or intermittent weakness from, 2t
Cardiac rhythm(s)
  disturbances of, 73-96 (See also Arrhythmia[s])
  in ECG interpretation, 28
  gallop, 8-9
  sinus, electrocardiography in, 15-16, 17t, 18f, 18t
  stabilization of, in cardiopulmonary resuscitation, 104
  ventricular, accelerated, 22
Cardiac tamponade
  in pericardial effusion, 186
  syncope or intermittent weakness from, 2t
Cardiac ultrasonography, 35-47. See also Echocardiography
Cardiogenic edema, acute, management of, 60
Cardiogenic shock
  canine, 118-120
  in dilated cardiomyopathy, 110, 111
Cardiology, nuclear, 48-49
Cardiomegaly
  in dilated cardiomyopathy, 109
  in feline dilated cardiomyopathy, 132
  precordial impulses in, 6
  radiographic signs of, 32, 33t
  in tetralogy of Fallot, 164
Cardiomyopathy
  arrhythmogenic right ventricular
    in cat, 133
    in dog, 116
  in Boxers, 113-114
  dilated (See Dilated cardiomyopathy [DCM])
  in Doberman Pinschers, 110f, 114-115
  hypertrophic (See Hypertrophic cardiomyopathy [HCM])
  restrictive, in cat, 129-130
  thyrotoxic, 714, 716
Cardioplasty, dynamic, for dilated cardiomyopathy, 113
Cardiopulmonary arrest, impending, signs of, 98-99

Cardiopulmonary disease, episodic weakness in, 976-977
Cardiopulmonary infections, antibiotics for, 1244t
Cardiopulmonary resuscitation (CPR), 98-105
  airway in, 99, 100f
  approach to, 99-105
  breathing in, 99-100, 100f
  circulation in, 100-102, 100f
  defibrillation in, 102
  drugs in, 100-101f, 102-104, 208-209t
    dosages of, 99f
  electrocardiogram in, 104
  follow-up of, 104-105
Cardioquin, Se Quinidine
Cardiotoxicity
  of chemotherapy drugs, 1114
  doxorubicin-induced, 106-107, 1114
Cardiovascular system
  anomalies of, 166-167
  diagnostic tests for, 12-50
    angiocardiography as, 47
    biochemical markers of myocardial injury as, 48
    cardiac catheterization as, 47-48
    central venous pressure measurement as, 48
    echocardiography as, 35-47 (See also Echocardiography)
    electrocardiography as, 12-31 (See also Electrocardiography [ECG])
    endomyocardial biopsy as, 48
    nuclear cardiology as, 48-49
    pneumopericardiography as, 49
    thoracic radiography as, 32-35
  examination of, 1-11
    clinical signs in, 1, 2t, 3-4
    physical examination of, 4-11
      arterial pulses in, 6, 6t
      cardiac murmurs in, 9-11, 9f, 9t, 10f
      fluid accumulation evaluation in, 6
      jugular veins in, 5-6, 5f, 5t
      mucous membranes in, 4-5, 5t
      precordium in, 6
      thoracic auscultation in, 6-7, 7f
      transient heart sounds in, 7-9, 8f
Cardizem. See Diltiazem
Cardoxin. See Digoxin
Carina
  bronchoscopic abnormalities of, 280t
  bronchoscopic view of, 279f
  *Olserus osleri* in, 297-298, 298f
Carnitine
  deficiency of, dilated cardiomyopathy and, 107
  for dilated cardiomyopathy, 111t, 113
  supplemental, for weight loss, 821
Carprofen
  for degenerative joint disease, 1080, 1080t
  hepatotoxicity of, 522t
  for joint disease, 1092t
Carvedilol
  for arrhythmias, 93
  characteristics of, 91t
  for dilated cardiomyopathy, 113
Castration
  for squamous metaplasia of prostate, 930
  for testicular tumors, 926
Cat(s). See under Feline or specific disorder, organ, or system
  diuretic dosages for, 62t
  echocardiographic measurement guidelines for, 44t
  electrocardiographic reference ranges for, 17t
  myocardial diseases in, 122-137
  upper respiratory infections in, 228-232 (See also Feline upper respiratory infection)
  vasodilator dosages for, 62t
Cat scratch disease, 1312-1314

Cataracts, in diabetes mellitus in dogs, 732, 732f, 748
Catecholamines
  in congestive heart failure management, 69-70
  secretion of, excessive, in pheochromocytoma, 810
Cathartics, 403, 403t
  in emergency treatment of intoxications, 997t
Catheter(s)
  nasal, for oxygen supplementation, 338-339, 338t, 339f
  transtracheal, for oxygen supplementation, 338t, 339
Catheterization
  cardiac, 47-48
  urethral
    in feline lower urinary tract inflammation management, 647
    for lower motor neuron disorders, 655
    urinary tract infections and, 626
Cauda equina syndrome, 1038-1039, 1038f, 1039f, 1040f
Caudal agenesis, of Manx cats, 1047
Caudal vena cava (CaVC), 35
CAV2. See Canine adenovirus 2 (CAV2)
Caval syndrome, in heartworm disease, 169
  treatment of, 177-178
CaVC. See Caudal vena cava (CaVC)
Cavitary lung disease, interstitial patterns in, 260-261, 262f
Cavitation, in pulmonary neoplasia, 307
CCNU. See Lomustine
Cecocolic intussusception, 456f, 458
Ceenu. See Lomustine
Cefa-Tabs. See Cefadroxil
Cefadroxil
  dosages of, 1241t
  for infectious diseases, 1318t
  for neurologic disorders, 1069t
Cefazolin
  for diskospondylitis, 1033
  dosages of, 341t, 470t, 1241t
  for gastric dilation/volvulus, 425
  for infectious diseases, 1318t
Cefixime, dosages of, 1241t
Cefotaxime
  for bacterial meningitis/myelitis, 1015
  dosages of, 1241t
  for hepatobiliary and pancreatic disorders, 566t
  for infectious diseases, 1318t
  for severe pancreatitis, 559
Cefoxitin
  for abdominal sepsis, 401
  dosages of, 470t, 1241t
  for infectious diseases, 1318t
  for septic peritonitis, 468
Ceftiofur, for infectious diseases, 1318t
Ceftriazone sodium, for joint disease, 1092t
CEH. See Cystic endometrial hyperplasia (CEH)
Celiotomy, in estrous cycle disorders, 858-859
Cellular debris in vulvar discharge, 872
Cellular immunodeficiency syndromes, 1226, 1227t
Central nervous system (CNS)
  feline leukemia virus infection and, 1282-1283
  infections of, antibiotics for, 1246t, 1247
  inflammation of, 1010-1019
    ancillary diagnostics for, 1011t
    bacterial meningitis as, 1014-1015, 1014f
    bacterial myelitis as, 1014-1015, 1014f
    in canine distemper, 1015-1016
    clinical features of, 1010, 1011f, 1011t

Central nervous system (CNS)—cont'd
  inflammation of—cont'd
    feline immunodeficiency virus encephalopathy as, 1014
    in feline infectious peritonitis, 1016-1017
    feline polioencephalomyelitis as, 1013-1014
    granulomatous meningoencephalitis as, 1012-1013, 1012f
    in Lyme disease, 1018
    meningeal vasculitis as, 1011f, 1012
    in mycotic infections, 1018
    in neosporosis, 1017-1018
    parasitic, 1018-1019
    Pug meningoencephalitis as, 1013
    in rabies, 1016, 1273, 1274t
    in rickettsial diseases, 1018
    steroid-responsive suppurative meningitis as, 1010-1011
    in toxoplasmosis, 1017
  lymphoma of
    CSF analysis in, 964t
    true, 1124
  neoplasia of, CSF analysis in, 964t
  parasite migration to, CSF analysis in, 964t
  systemic lupus erythematosus and, 1220t
  toxicity for, lidocaine, 88
Central venous pressure (CVP), measurement of, 48
Centrine. See Aminopentamide
Cephalexin
  for bacterial pneumonia, 300
  for diskospondylitis, 1033
  dosages of, 341t, 1241t
  for facial nerve paralysis, 1053
  for hepatobiliary and pancreatic disorders, 566t
  for infectious diseases, 1318t
  for joint disease, 1092t
  for Lyme disease, 1084
  for neurologic disorders, 1069t
  for septic arthritis, 1082
Cephalosporin(s)
  for abdominal sepsis, 401
  for bacterial meningitis/myelitis, 1015
  for cardiopulmonary infections, 1244t
  for cutaneous and soft tissue infections, 1244t
  for diskospondylitis, 1033
  dosages of, 1241t
  for facial nerve paralysis, 1053
  for hepatic and gastrointestinal infections, 1245t
  for hepatobiliary inflammation, 540
  for infectious diseases, 1318t
  for infective endocarditis, 149
  for parvoviral enteritis, 434
  for septic arthritis, 1082
  toxicities of, 1242t
  for urinary tract infections, 627
  for urogenital infections, 1248t
Cephalothin
  for infection in chemotherapy patient, 1110
  for neurologic disorders, 1069t
  for postsplenectomy sepsis, 1209
Cephazolin
  for hepatobiliary and pancreatic disorders, 566t
  for inflammatory hepatobiliary disease, 516
  for sepsis in liver failure, 551
Cephulac. See Lactulose
Cerebellar disorders
  locomotion disorders from, 977-980 (See also Dysmetria; Hypermetria)
  signs of, disorders resulting in, 978t
Cerebellar neuronal abiotrophy, 978, 978t
Cerebellar syndromes, inherited and congenital, 978t

Cerebrospinal fluid (CSF) analysis, 962-965
  in acute intervertebral disk disease, 1026
  in bacterial meningitis/myelitis diagnosis, 1014-1015
  in canine distemper, 1016-1017
  contraindications for, 962
  indications for, 962
  in intracranial neoplasia, 997-998
  procedure for, 963, 964f, 965
  in spinal neoplasia, 1035, 1036f
  technique for, 962-963, 962f, 963f
  in toxoplasmosis, 1017
  in various neurologic diseases, 964t
Ceroid lipofuscinosis, cerebellar dysfunction in, 979t
Cervical disk disease, 1025, 1029, 1029t
Cervical vertebral instability/malformation, 1040-1043, 1041-1042f, 1043f
Cervical vertebral malformation malarticulation syndrome, 1025
Cestex. *See* Episprantel
Cestodes
  fecal examination for, 1230t
  zoonotic, 1309t, 1310
Chagas' disease, myocarditis in, 117
Charcoal, activated, for neurologic disorders, 1069t
Chédiak-Higashi syndrome, 1174
Chemical defibrillation, 102
Chemical intoxication, mentation abnormalities from, 983
Chemicals, ototoxic, 1008
Chemodectomas, 195
  treatment of, 190-191
Chemotherapy, 1103-1116
  for abdominal carcinomatosis, 469
  for alimentary lymphoma, 457
  antimicrobial, practical, 1240-1249
    (*See also* Antibiotic[s])
  basic principles of, 1103, 1105
  for brain tumors, 998
  for cardiac tumors, 196
  cell kinetics and, 1103, 1104f
  chronic hepatitis from, 529
  complications of, 1108-1116
    acute tumor lysis syndrome as, 1115-1116, 1116f
    cardiotoxicity as, 1114
    dermatologic toxicity as, 1112-1113
    gastrointestinal toxicity as, 1111
    hematologic toxicity as, 1108-1111
    hepatotoxicity as, 1115
    hypersensitivity reactions as, 1112
    neurotoxicity as, 1115
    pancreatitis as, 1113-1114
    pulmonary toxicity as, 1115
    urotoxicity as, 1114-1115
  drugs in
    mechanism of action of, 1106
    types of, 1106-1107
  for feline leukemia virus infection, 1283
  for hemangiosarcoma, 1143-1144
  indications and contraindications of, 1105-1106
  for injection site sarcomas, 1152
  for leukemias
    acute, 1137t
    chronic, 1138t
  for lymphoma, 1126-1131, 1127t
    alimentary, 1131
    central nervous system, 1130-1131
    cutaneous, 1131
    for induction of remission, 1127t, 1128
    for intensification, 1127t, 1129
    in "low-budget" protocols, 1127t, 1131
    for maintenance, 1127t, 1128-1129
    ocular, 1131
    for reinduction of remission, 1127t, 1129

Chemotherapy—cont'd
  for lymphoma—cont'd
    for rescue, 1127t, 1129
    solitary/extranodal, 1130
  for mammary neoplasia, 885
  for mast cell tumors, 1148-1149, 1148t
  for mediastinal masses, 1120
  for nasal tumors, 234
  for oropharyngeal masses, 1151
  for osteosarcoma, 1145-1146, 1145t
  for pulmonary neoplasia, 308
  for spinal neoplasia, 1036
  for thyroid neoplasia, 727
  for transmissible venereal tumor, 938-939
  tumor kinetics and, 1103, 1104f
Cheque. *See* Mibolerone
Chest tubes, 323-326, 324-325f
  complications of, 323
  indications for, 323
  placement of, 323-326, 324-325f
  for pyothorax, 328-329
*Chlamydophila felis*
  morphologic characteristics of, 1233t
  ocular zoonoses associated with, 1315
  vaccination against, 1255
*Chlamydophila* vaccines, 230
Chlorambucil
  for digestive disorders, 400, 401
  dosages of, 470t
  for feline chronic progressive polyarthritis, 1091
  for feline eosinophilic granuloma, 407
  for feline lymphocytic-plasmacytic enteritis, 448
  for feline lymphocytic-plasmacytic gingivitis/pharyngitis, 408
  for immune hemolytic anemia, 1163-1164
  as immunosuppressant, 1218
  for leukemias, chronic, 1138t, 1154t
  for lymphoma, 1127t, 1128, 1153t
  for mast cell tumors, 1149
Chloramphenicol
  for bacterial L form-associated arthritis, 1083
  for bacterial meningitis/myelitis, 1015
  for bacterial pneumonia, 300
  for canine infectious tracheobronchitis, 288
  for cardiopulmonary infections, 1244t
  for cutaneous and soft tissue infections, 1244t
  dosages of, 341t, 470t, 1241t
  for feline bronchitis, 292, 293
  for feline plague, 1260
  for feline upper respiratory infections, 229, 230
  for hepatic and gastrointestinal infections, 1245t
  for infectious diseases, 1319t
  for joint disease, 1092t
  for *Mycoplasma* polyarthritis, 1083
  for neurologic disorders, 1069t
  for rickettsial diseases, 1018
  for rickettsial polyarthritis, 1084
  for Rocky Mountain spotted fever, 1266
  for salmonellosis, 438
  toxicities of, 1242t
  for urogenital infections, 1248t
Chlorazepate dipotassium, for neurologic disorders, 1069t
Chlorhexidine digluconate, injection of, into epididymis, 866
Chloride, in commercial reduced-sodium diets, 61t
Chlorinated hydrocarbons, neurologic dysfunction from, 995t
Chlorothiazide
  in congestive heart failure management, 64
  dosages of, 62t, 206t
  for endocrine disorders, 814t
  preparations of, 63t

Chlorpheniramine
  for allergic rhinitis, 239-240
  dosages of, 341t
Chlorpromazine
  as antiemetic, 396t
  for chronic renal failure, 618t
  dosages of, 470t, 565t
  indications for, 565t
  for neurologic disorders, 1069t
  for severe pancreatitis, 558-559
  for tetanus, 981
  for urinary tract disorders, 658t
  for vomiting in chronic renal failure, 621
Chlorpropamide, for diabetes insipidus, 666, 666t
Cholangiocellular carcinoma, 517
Cholangiohepatitis
  bacterial, antibiotics for, 1245t
  in inflammatory hepatobiliary disease, 513-514, 514f
Cholangitis, 513, 538
  lymphocytic, 514-515, 515f
  sclerosing, 515, 515f
Cholecystitis, 538
Choledyl. *See* Oxtriphylline; Oxtriphylline elixir
Choleliths
  in cats, extrahepatic bile duct obstruction from, 518, 519f
  in dogs, 540
Cholestasis, sepsis and, 543
Cholesterol, serum concentration of, in hepatobiliary system assessment, 488, 492t
Cholestyramine
  for digitalis toxicity, 69
  for hypercholesterolemia, 827, 845t
Chondroitin sulfate
  for degenerative joint disease, 1081
  for rheumatoid arthritis, 1090
Chondroprotective agents
  for degenerative joint disease, 1080-1081
  for rheumatoid arthritis, 1090
CHOP protocol
  for lymphoma, 1153t
  for thymomas, 1120
Chordae tendineae
  echocardiographic view of, 37f
  ruptured
    in atrioventricular valve disease, 140
    in AV valve degeneration, 143, 143f
Chorioretinitis, punctate, in toxoplasmosis, 1296, 1297f
Chromium, in diabetes management, 757
Chylomicron test, 824
Chylomicrons, 822
Chylothorax, 330-332, 331t
Chymotrypsinogen, 553t
Chyrsotherapy, for immune-mediated disorders, 1218
Cicatrix
  endoscopic view of, 380, 381f
  esophageal, 414-415, 415f
Ciliary dyskinesia, in canine chronic bronchitis, 296
Ciliates, zoonotic, 1309t, 1311-1312
Cimetidine
  as antacid, 397, 397t
  for chronic renal failure, 618t
  dosages of, 470t
  for hepatobiliary and pancreatic disorders, 567t
  for neurologic disorders, 1069t
  for urinary tract disorders, 658t
Cipro. *See* Ciprofloxacin
Ciprofloxacin
  dosages of, 1242t
  for infectious diseases, 1319t
Circulation
  in cardiopulmonary resuscitation, 100-102, 100f
  support of, in CPR, 103-104

Cisapride
  for congenital esophageal weakness, 410
  for diarrhea, 399
  dosages of, 470t
  for esophagitis, 412
  for gastroesophageal reflux, 411
  for hepatic lipidosis, 508
  for hepatobiliary and pancreatic disorders, 567t
  for idiopathic gastric motility, 427
  for idiopathic megaesophagus, 411
Cisplatin
  for abdominal carcinomatosis, 469
  for carcinomas, 1155t
  gastrointestinal complications of, 1111
  for oropharyngeal masses, 1151
  for osteosarcoma, 1145-1146, 1145t, 1155t
Cisternal myelography, 965
Claforan. *See* Cefotazime
Clarithromycin
  for cutaneous and soft tissue infections, 1244t
  dosages of, 1241t
  for infectious diseases, 1319t
Clavamox. *See* Amoxocillin with clavulanate
Clavulanate
  amoxicillin with
    for bacterial pneumonia, 300
    for canine infectious tracheobronchitis, 288
    for cardiopulmonary infections, 1244t
    for cutaneous and soft tissue infections, 1244t
    for diskospondylitis, 1033
    dosages of, 341t, 1241t
    for facial nerve paralysis, 1053
    for infectious diseases, 1319t
    for pyothorax, 327
    for urogenital infections, 1248t
  ticarcillin with
    for cardiopulmonary infections, 1244t
    dosages of, 1241t
    for infectious diseases, 1319t
Cleansing enema administration, 402-403
Cleocin. *See* Clindamycin
Clindamycin
  for abdominal sepsis, 401
  for babesiosis, 1301
  for bacterial pneumonia, 301
  for cardiopulmonary infections, 1244t
  for cutaneous and soft tissue infections, 1244t
  dosages of, 341t, 470t, 1241t
  for esophagitis, 412
  for feline idiopathic polymyositis, 1064
  for hepatobiliary and pancreatic disorders, 566t
  for hepatozoonosis, 1302
  for infectious diseases, 1319t, 1320t
  for liver abscesses, 542
  for neosporosis, 1017-1018, 1300
  for neurologic disorders, 1069t
  for oropharyngeal masses, 1150
  for protozoal myositis, 1065
  for *Toxoplasma* meningoencephalomyelitis, 1017
  for toxoplasmosis, 1298, 1299
  for urogenital infections, 1248t
Clitoral hypertrophy, 873, 874f
Clofibrate, for hypertriglyceridemia, 845t
Clonapin. *See* Clonazepam
Clonazepam
  as anticonvulsant, 1003-1004
  for neurologic disorders, 1069t
Clonidine-stimulation test, for growth hormone-responsive dermatosis in adult dog, 671
CLOP protocol
  for acute lymphoid leukemia, 1153t
  for lymphoma, 1153t

Cloprostenol
  as abortifacient, 899
  for reproductive disorders, 944t
Clor-Trimeton. *See* Chlorpheniramine
Clorazepate, as anticonvulsant, 1003-
  1004
Clostridial infections
  fecal culture for, 367
  gastrointestinal, 438-439
*Clostridium*
  culture techniques for, 1235
  morphologic characteristics of, 1233t
*Clostridium botulinum,* LMN paralysis
  from, 1058
*Clostridium perfringens,* antibiotics for,
  1245t
Clotrimazole, for nasal aspergillosis, 236-
  237, 236f, 237f
Clotting. *See* Hemostasis
Clotting factors
  congenital deficiencies in, 1194
  defects in, congenital and acquired,
    1189t
  systemic lupus erythematosus and,
    1220t
Cloxacillin
  for cutaneous and soft tissue infec-
    tions, 1244t
  for neurologic disorders, 1069t
CMF protocol, for carcinomas, 1155t
CNS. *See* Central nervous system (CNS)
Coagulation. *See also* Hemostasis
  disseminated intravascular, 1195-1199
    (*See also* Disseminated in-
    travascular coagulation
    [DIC])
  pathways of, 1185-1186, 1186f
Coagulation proteins, synthesized by
  liver, 481t
Coagulation tests
  in hepatobiliary disease, 492, 492t
  before liver biopsy, 500-501
Coagulopathy(ies), 481-482, 481t
  complicating liver failure, 550-551
COAP protocol
  for acute lymphoid leukemia, 1153t
  for lymphoma, 1127t, 1128-1131,
    1153t
  for thymomas, 1120
Cobalamin
  for feline lymphocytic-plasmacytic en-
    teritis, 448
  serum concentrations of, in digestive
    disorders, 378-379
Cobalt irradiation, for thyroid neoplasia,
  727
Cobalt teletherapy, for feline acromegaly,
  676
Coccidians, zoonotic, 1309t, 1310-1311,
  1310f
*Coccidioides immitis*
  cytologic appearance of, 1288t, 1293f
  infection with, 1293-1294
Coccidioidomycosis, 1292-1293, 1293f
  lymphadenopathy associated with,
    1202t
Coccidiosis, 444
Cocker Spaniels, multisystem neuronal
  degeneration in, 1044t
Colace. *See* Dioctyl sodium sulfosuccinate
Colchicine
  for amyloidosis, 606
  for chronic hepatitis, 537
  indication and dosage of, 565t
Colitis
  acute, 458
  lymphocytic-plasmacytic, 448
Collapse, episodic, in pheochromocytoma, 810
Colloidal solutions, 832t
Colloids, for shock, 388
Colonoscopy, 381, 383-384, 383-384f
  in constipation, 357
Color, mucous membrane, in cardiovas-
  cular examination, 4-5, 5t

Color flow mapping, 46, 46f, 47f
Coma, characteristics of, 948t
Compazine. *See* Prochlorperazine
Complete blood count (CBC)
  in acute pancreatitis, 554
  in anemia, 1158
  in chylothorax, 331t
  in diabetes mellitus, 733t
  in digestive disorders, 365-366
  in gastrinomas, 775
  in hematuria evaluation, 574-575
  in hepatobiliary disorders, 485-486
  in lower respiratory tract disease, 253
  in nasal discharge, 213
Computed tomography (CT)
  in acute intervertebral disk disease,
    1026
  in fibrocartilaginous embolism, 1030
  in hyperadrenocorticism
    in cats, 802-803
    in dogs, 785-786
  in intracranial neoplasia, 997
  in lower respiratory tract disorders,
    262
  nasal, 221
  in nasal discharge evaluation, 214, 215f
  in nasal tumor diagnosis, 234
  in neuromuscular disorders, 970, 971f
  in solitary mass evaluation, 1117
  in thyroid neoplasia, 726
Conduction system, cardiac, 13f
  disturbances of, 23-25
Congenital adrenal hyperplasia-like syndrome, 670
Congenital anomalies
  cardiac, 151-167 (*See also* Heart, con-
    genital anomalies of)
  penile, 919-920, 920f
  seizures from, 994-995
  vaginal, 872-873
  vulvar, 872-873
Congenital cerebellar hypoplasia, 978, 978t
Congenital immunodeficiency syndromes, 1226, 1227t
Congenital infertility, 916
Congenital nystagmus, 1009
Congestive heart failure
  in AV valve degeneration, treatment of,
    144-145
  causes of, general, 55, 55t
  fulminant, treatment of, 58-60, 59t
  in infective endocarditis, 146
  management of, 51-72, 55-58
    calcium entry blockers in, 71
    dietary, 60-62, 61t
    diuretics in, 62-64, 62t, 63t
    goals of, by pathophysiologic group,
      56t
    patient monitoring in, 58
    phosphodiesterase inhibitors in, 70-
      71
    positive inotropic drugs in, 66-69
    principles of, basic, 56
    sympathomimetic agents in, 69-70
    vasodilators in, 64-66
  in patent ductus arteriosus, 155
  pathophysiology of, 51-55
    cardiac responses in, 54
    neurohormonal mechanisms in, 52-
      54, 52f, 53f
    renal effects in, 54
  right-sided
    fluid accumulation in, 6
    in heartworm disease, treatment of,
      177
  severity of, classification systems for,
    57t
  signs of, 1, 2t, 3-4, 3f
  in subaortic stenosis, 157
  in ventricular septal defect, 161
Conray 400. *See* Iothalamate sodium
Consciousness, disorders of, 948, 948t
Consolidation
  alveolar, 258
  lung lobe, 260

Constant-rate infusion, formulas to cal-
  culate, 89t
Constipation, 357, 462-463
  causes of, 358t
  fiber-enriched diet for, 390
Constrictive pericardial disease, 194
Continuous wave (CW) Doppler
  echocardiography, 45-46, 46f
Contralac. *See* Meterfoline
Contrast echocardiography, 43-44
Contrast media, for myelography, 965
Contusion, pulmonary, 309-310
Convulsions, 991-1004. *See also* Seizures
Coombs' test, direct
  for hemolytic anemia, 1162
  for immune-mediated disorders, 1213-
    1214
Coonhound paralysis, 1056-1057, 1057f
COP protocol
  for acute lymphoid leukemia, 1153t
  for lymphoma, 1153t
  for thymomas, 1120
Copper
  chelation of, for copper hepatotoxico-
    sis, 536
  dietary reduction of, for copper hepa-
    totoxicosis, 535-536, 535t
  intestinal absorption of, reduced, for
    copper hepatotoxicosis, 536
Copper hepatotoxicosis
  copper chelation for, 536
  dietary copper reduction for, 535-536,
    535t
  familial chronic hepatitis and, 526-528,
    526t, 527f, 528f
  reducing intestinal copper absorption
    for, 536
Cor pulmonale, from heartworm disease,
  169
Cor triatriatum, 166-167
Cordarone. *See* Amiodarone
Core biopsy, nasal, 225, 226f
Corgard. *See* Nadolol
Cornification, 848
Coronavirus
  enteritis from, 436
  feline, 1275-1278, 1276t
    clinical features of, 1276-1277, 1276t
    diagnosis of, 1277
    epidemiology of, 1275-1276
    etiology of, 1275-1276
    prevention of, 1278
    treatment of, 1277-1278
    zoonotic aspects of, 1278
  vaccination against, 1256, 1257
Corpora luteal function, 888
Corticosteroid-responsive neutropenia,
  1175, 1175t
Corticosteroids
  for acute spinal injury, 1023
  alkaline phosphatase activity and, 486-
    487
  for anal sacculitis, 461
  for brain tumors, 999
  for canine eosinophilic gastroentero-
    colitis, 449
  for canine lymphocytic-plasmacytic
    colitis, 448
  for canine lymphocytic-plasmacytic
    enteritis, 447
  for digestive disorders, 400
  for esophagitis, 412
  for feline eosinophilic enteritis/
    hypereosinophilic syndrome,
    449
  for feline eosinophilic granuloma, 407
  for feline idiopathic polymyositis, 1064
  for feline lymphocytic-plasmacytic en-
    teritis, 448
  for feline lymphocytic-plasmacytic
    gingivitis/pharyngitis, 408
  for fever of undetermined origin, 1225
  for fibrocartilaginous embolism, 1031
  gamma-glutamyltransferase activity
    and, 487

Corticosteroids—cont'd
  for granulomatous meningoencephali-
    tis, 1013
  for heat trauma, 984
  for hemolytic anemia, 1162
  for hypercalcemia, 839, 839t
  for idiopathic, immune-mediated
    polyarthritis, 1088
  for immune hemolytic anemia, 1162-
    1163
  for immunoproliferative enteropathy
    in Basenjis, 450
  as immunosuppressants, 1216-1217
  for inflammatory hepatobiliary dis-
    ease, 516, 517
  for lymphocytic-plasmacytic gastritis,
    419
  for masticatory muscle myositis, 409
  for masticatory myositis, 1063
  for meningeal vasculitis, 1012
  for myasthenia gravis, 1061
  for neurologic signs of hydrocephalus,
    994
  for optic neuritis, 986
  for pulmonary arterial disease in heart-
    worm disease, 177
  for sclerosing, encapsulating peritoni-
    tis, 468
  for spinal neoplasia, 1036
  for steroid-responsive suppurative
    meningitis, 1011
  for toxoplasmosis, 1298
  for type II intervertebral disk disease,
    1037
  for wobbler syndrome, 1042-1043
Cortisol, serum concentrations of, signaling parturition, 891
Cortisol/creatinine ratios, urine, in
  hyperadrenocorticism
  diagnosis
    in cats, 801, 801t
    in dogs, 788f, 789
*Corynebacterium*
  infective endocarditis from, 146
  lymphadenopathy associated with,
    1202t
Cosequin
  for degenerative joint disease, 1081
  for rheumatoid arthritis, 1090
Cosmogen. *See* Actinomycin D
Cough
  in degenerative AV valve disease, 141
  in heart disease/failure, 3-4
  "kennel," 287-289, 288f
    antibiotics for, 1247
  in laryngeal paralysis, 246
  in lower respiratory tract disorders,
    250-251
  productive, differential diagnoses for,
    251f
  in tracheal collapse, 289
"Cough-drop," 3
Cough suppressants, for dogs, 288t
Cough syncope, 3
Coumadin. *See* Warfarin
*Coxiella burnetii,* genitourinary zoonoses
  from, 1316-1317
CPR. *See* Cardiopulmonary resuscitation
  (CPR)
Crackles, 252
  in respiratory distress in lung disease,
    336
Cranial nerves
  functional assessment of, 958t
  in neurologic examination, 957, 958t
Craniotomy, in head trauma manage-
  ment, 984
Creatinine clearance, endogenous, calcu-
  lation of, 585t
*Crenosoma vulpis*
  characteristics of eggs or larvae of, 263t
  fecal examination for, 1230t
Cretinism, in hypothyroidism, 695-696,
  696f, 696t
Cricopharyngeal achalasia/dysfunction,
  409

CRT. *See* Capillary refill time (CRT)
Cryopreservation, of semen, 942-943
Cryptococcosis, 1287-1290
  ancillary diagnostics for, 1011t
  clinical features of, 1287, 1288f
  CSF analysis in, 964t
  diagnosis of, 1288-1289
  epidemiology of, 1287
  etiology of, 1287
  lymphadenopathy associated with, 1202t
  nasal, 235
  prevention of, 1290
  radiographic signs of, 220t
  treatment of, 1289-1290
  zoonotic aspects of, 1290
*Cryptococcus*, nasal, 211, 212f
  fundic findings in, 211, 213f
*Cryptococcus neoformans*
  cytologic appearance of, 1288t
  immunologic techniques for, 1236
  infection by, 1287-1290 (*See also* Cryptococcosis)
  meningoencephalitis from, 1018
Cryptorchidism, 922-923, 924f
Cryptosporidiosis, 444-445
  fecal evaluation for, 366
*Cryptosporidium*
  drugs for, 1320t
  as enteric zoonosis, 1309t, 1310-1311
*Cryptosporidium parvum*, 444-445
  as enteric zoonosis, 1310-1311
  fecal examination for, 1230t
  immunologic techniques for, 1236
  oocysts of, 1231f
Crystallization inhibitor theory, of urolith pathogenesis, 631, 633
Crystalluria, urolithiasis and, 570, 570f, 571f, 571t, 631
Crystodigin. *See* Digitoxin
CSF. *See* Cerebrospinal fluid (CSF)
Culture(s)
  bacterial
    fecal, 367-368
    seminal, 911-912, 911f
      in infertility evaluation, 916
    vaginal, 854, 854t
  blood
    in diskospondylitis, 1032
    in infective endocarditis diagnosis, 147-148
    in infectious disease diagnosis, 1235-1236
    in *Mycoplasma* detection, 1263
    nasal, 226-227
    synovial fluid, 1076-1077
    in *Ureaplasma* detection, 1263
Cuprimine. *See* D-Penicillamine
Cutaneous lymphoma, 1123
  treatment of, 1131
*Cuterebra* fly larvae, brain migration of, seizures from, 999
CVP. *See* Central venous pressure (CVP)
CVP protocol, for mast cell tumors, 1148, 1149, 1154t
CW Doppler echocardiography. *See* Continuous wave (CW) Doppler echocardiography
CyA. *See* Cyclosporin A
Cyanosis
  cardiac anomalies causing, 163-166
  in lower respiratory tract disorders, 251
  mucous membrane, 5t
  oxygen partial pressure and, 282
  in pulmonary hypertension with shunt reversal, 165
  in tetralogy of Fallot, 164
Cyanotic heart disease, syncope or intermittent weakness from, 2t
Cyclophosphamide
  for carcinomas, 1155t
  dosages of, 341t
  for eosinophilic lung disease, 304
  for feline chronic progressive polyarthritis, 1091

Cyclophosphamide—cont'd
  gastrointestinal complications of, 1111
  for granulomatous meningoencephalitis, 1013
  for hemangiosarcoma, 1143-1144
  hemorrhagic cystitis from, 1114-1115
  for immune hemolytic anemia, 1163
  as immunosuppressant, 1217
  for injection site sarcomas, 1152
  for joint disease, 1092t
  for leukemias
    acute, 1137t
    chronic, 1138t, 1154t
  for lymphoma, 1127t, 1128-1131, 1153t
  for mast cell tumors, 1148, 1149, 1154t
  for oropharyngeal masses, 1151
  for soft-tissue sarcomas, 1154-1155t
  for thymomas, 1120
  for urinary tract disorders, 658t
Cyclosporin A (CyA), as immunosuppressant, 1218
Cyclosporine
  for immune hemolytic anemia, 1163
  for perianal fistulae, 461
  for urinary tract disorders, 658t
Cyproheptadine
  as appetite stimulant, 391
  dosages of, 341t, 470t
  for feline bronchitis, 294
  for hepatic lipidosis, 508
  for hepatobiliary and pancreatic disorders, 566t
Cyst(s)
  branchial, as mediastinal masses, 1119t
  follicular, prolonged estrus from, 863-864, 863f
  *Giardia*, after zinc sulfate flotation, 1232f
  intraspinal articular, 1036
  *Neospora caninum*, 1299-1300, 1300f
  paraprostatic, 932, 932f
  pericardial, 192
  pulmonary, interstitial patterns in, 260-261, 262f
Cysteine, structure of, 640f
Cysteine-penicillamine disulfide, structure of, 640f
Cystic endometrial hyperplasia (CEH)-pyometra complex, 877-880
  clinical features of, 878
  diagnosis of, 878-879, 878f
  etiology of, 877-878
  treatment of, 879-880, 880t
Cystine, structure of, 640f
Cystine crystals in urine sediment, 571f, 571t
Cystine uroliths
  factors predicting composition of, 632t
  treatment of, 640-641
Cystitis
  bacterial, struvite-induced inflammation and, 643-644
  clinical signs of, 645t
  hemorrhagic, from cyclophosphamide, 1114-1115
Cystocentesis
  for urine collection in UTI diagnosis, 627
  urine sample from, 574
Cystography, contrast-enhanced, 589t, 595, 595f
*Cystoisospora*, fecal examination for, 1230t
Cystorelin. *See* Gonadotropin-releasing hormone (GnRH)
Cystoscopy, 596, 598
  in feline lower urinary tract inflammation, 645
Cystouroliths, radiography of, 594f
Cytadren. *See* Aminoglutethimide
*Cytauxzoon felis*, 1301-1302, 1302f
  drugs for, 1320t
  morphologic characteristics of, 1234t

Cytauxzoonosis, 1301-1302, 1302f
  lymphadenopathy associated with, 1202t
Cytology
  in anal sac adenocarcinoma diagnosis, 461
  in bacterial diseases, 1233, 1233t
  in blastomycosis, 1291, 1291f
  in canine distemper, 1275
  in cardiac tumors, 196
  in chylothorax, 331t
  in coccidioidomycosis, 1293-1294, 1294f
  in cryptococcosis, 1288-1289, 1288f, 1288t
  in cutaneous parasitic diseases, 1234
  in fecal evaluation, 368
  in feline plague, 1259, 1260f
  in feline upper respiratory infections, 228
  in fever of undetermined origin, 1224
  fine-needle aspiration for, 1093-1094
  in fungal diseases, 1234
  in hemangiosarcoma, 1143, 1143f
  in hepatic lipidosis, 507, 507f
  in histoplasmosis, 439-440, 440f, 1292, 1292f
  impression smears in, 1094
  in infectious diseases, 1232-1234, 1233t, 1234t
  in inflammatory hepatobiliary disease, 514f, 515f, 516
  in lymphadenopathy-splenomegaly, 1207-1208
  in lymphoma diagnosis, 11
  in mammary neoplasia, 884
  in mast cell tumors, 1147
  in metastatic lesion, 1117
  in nasal aspergillosis, 235, 235f
  in nasal discharge evaluation, 213
  in oncology, 1093-1099
  in osteosarcoma, 1145, 1145f
  in pleural effusion, 315-316
  in prostate gland disorders, 927-928
  in pyothorax, 327
  in rickettsial diseases, 1233-1234, 1233t
  in semen evaluation, 909
  in septic arthritis, 1081
  in septic peritonitis diagnosis, 466, 467f
  in solitary mass evaluation, 1117
  specimens in
    interpretation of, 1094-1099
    staining of, 1094
  in synovial fluid analysis, 1074, 1076, 1076f, 1076t, 1077f
  in systemic protozoal diseases, 1234, 1234t
  in transmissible venereal tumor diagnosis, 938
  vaginal
    in breeding management, 849
    in cystic endometrial hyperplasia-pyometra complex, 879
    diagnostic uses of, 853
    in estrus, 849
    in proestrus, 848-849
    in vulvar discharge assessment, 870, 871f, 872t
  in viral diseases, 1234
Cytopenias, combined, 1181-1184
  causes of, 1182t
  clinicopathologic features of, 1181-1182, 1184
  diagnostic algorithms for, 1183f
Cytosar. *See* Cytosine arabinoside
Cytosar-U. *See* Cytosine arabinoside
Cytosine arabinoside
  for granulomatous meningoencephalitis, 1013
  for leukemias, acute, 1137t, 1139, 1154t
  for lymphoma, 1127t, 1128-1131, 1153t
  for myelodysplastic syndromes, 1140
  for thymomas, 1120

Cytotec. *See* Misoprostol
Cytoxan. *See* Cyclophosphamide

**D**

D-MAC protocol, for lymphoma, 1127t, 1129, 1153t
D-Penicillamine
  for copper chelation, 536
  for cystine uroliths, 640-641
  for hepatobiliary and pancreatic disorders, 566t
  structure of, 640f
  for urinary tract disorders, 659t
Dacarbazine
  gastrointestinal complications of, 1111
  for lymphoma, 1127t, 1129
  for oropharyngeal masses, 1151
  for soft-tissue sarcomas, 1154t
Dachshund, long-haired, sensory neuropathy in, 1046t
Dalmatians
  chronic hepatitis in, 528
  laryngeal paralysis in, 1045t
  leukodystrophy of, 1044t
  polyneuropathy in, 1045t
Dam, neonatal morbidity/mortality and, 902
Danazol
  for immune hemolytic anemia, 1163
  for immune-mediated thrombocytopenia, 1192
  as immunosuppressant, 1218-1219
Danocrine. *See* Danazol
Daraprim. *See* Pyrimethamine
DAT. *See* Direct antiglobulin test (DAT)
DCM. *See* Dilated cardiomyopathy (DCM)
DDAVP. *See* Desmopressin
DEC. *See* Diethylcarbamazine
Deca-Durabolin. *See* Nandrolone decanoate
Decapeptyl. *See* Gonadotropin-releasing hormone (GnRH) analog
Decerebrate rigidity, 980-981
Decompression, gastric, for gastric dilation/volvulus, 424-425
Decoquinate, for hepatozoonosis, 1302
Defecation, painful or difficult, 356-357, 357t
Defibrillation, in CPR, 102
Degenerative disorders, of nervous system, 1044-1046t
  seizures in, 995-996
Degenerative joint disease (DJD), 1079-1081, 1080f, 1080t
Degenerative myelopathy, 1037-1038, 1044t
  CSF analysis in, 964t
Dehydration
  acute renal failure and, 612
  fluid therapy for, 388-389
Delirium, characteristics of, 948t
Delivery, difficult, 892-895. *See also* Dystocia
Demodicosis, lymphadenopathy associated with, 1202t
Denosyl SD4. *See* S-adenosylmethionine
Deoxycorticosterone-secreting adrenocortical carcinoma, 812
Deoxyribonucleic acid (DNA), of infectious agents in vector vaccines, 1253
Depakene. *See* Valproic acid
Depo-Medrol. *See* Methylprednisolone acetate
Depoprovera. *See* Medroxyprogesterone
Depression, characteristics of, 948t
*Dermacentor andersoni*
  tick paralysis from, 1057-1058
  as vector for Rocky Mountain spotted fever, 1265
*Dermacentor variabilis*
  tick paralysis from, 1057-1058
  as vector for Rocky Mountain spotted fever, 1265

Dermatologic toxicity, of chemotherapy drugs, 1112-1113
Dermatomyositis, 1064-1065
Dermatopathic lymphadenopathy, 1202t
Dermatophytes, zoonoses associated with, 1313t
Dermatosis, growth hormone-responsive in adult dog, 670-671, 672-673f, 673, 673t
    endocrine alopecia differentiated from, 668
Desmopressin
    for diabetes insipidus, 666, 666t
    for endocrine disorders, 814t
    for hepatobiliary and pancreatic disorders, 567t
    response to, in diabetes insipidus diagnosis, 664-665
Desoxycorticosterone pivalate
    for acute addisonian crisis, 808
    after adrenalectomy in cats, 803
    for endocrine disorders, 814t
Detrusor atony, in obstructed feline lower urinary tract inflammation, management of, 648
Detrusor hyperreflexia, 576-577
    incontinence from, 653
    treatment of, 656
Detrusor-urethral dyssynergia, 576, 652
Dexamethasone
    as abortifacient, 899
    in brain tumor management, 999
    in cardiopulmonary resuscitation, dosages of, 99t
    for cystic endometrial hyperplasia-pyometra complex, 879
    dosages of, 341t, 470t
    for feline bronchitis, 294
    for feline ischemic encephalopathy, 999
    in head trauma management, 984
    in hydrocephalus management, 994
    for hypersensitivity reactions to chemotherapy drugs, 1112
    for immune hemolytic anemia, 164, 1162, 1163
    for lymphoma, 1127t, 1129, 1153t
    for neurologic disorders, 1069t
Dexamethasone sodium phosphate, for endocrine disorders, 814t
Dexamethasone SP, dosage of, 209t
Dexamethasone suppression test
    combined with ACTH stimulation test, in hyperadrenocorticism diagnosis, 787t, 790-791
    high-dose, in hyperadrenocorticism diagnosis, 787t, 791-792
    in hyperadrenocorticism diagnosis in cats, 801-802, 801t, 802f
    low-dose, in hyperadrenocorticism diagnosis, 787t, 790, 791f
Dexate. *See* Dexamethasone
Dexrazoxane, for doxorubicin-induced cardiomyopathy, 1114
Dextran, 832t
Dextromethorphan
    for cough in dogs, 288, 288t
    dosages of, 341t
Dextrose
    for hyperkalemia in ARF, 614
    for hypoglycemia, 731
    for neurologic disorders, 1069t
    solutions of, 832t
        for hyperkalemia, 834, 834t
Diaβeta. *See* Glyburide
Diabetes insipidus, 661-667
    central, 662
        therapies for, 666t
    clinical features of, 662-663
    diagnosis of, 663-666
        desmopressin response in, 664-665
        plasma osmolality in, random, 665, 665f
        water deprivation test in, modified, 663-664, 664f, 664t
    etiology of, 661-662, 662t

Diabetes insipidus—cont'd
    nephrogenic, 662
        therapies for, 666t
    prognosis for, 667
    treatment of, 666, 666t
Diabetes mellitus, 729-776
    in acute pancreatitis, 555t
    in cats, 749-762
        clinical features of, 751, 751f
        complications of, chronic, 762
        diagnosis of, 752
        etiology of, 749-750, 749f, 751f
        prognosis or, 762
        treatment of, 752-762
            concurrent problems identification/control in, 753
            insulin in, 752-753, 758-762 (*See also* Insulin in diabetes management for cats)
            oral hypoglycemic drugs in, 753, 755-757, 756t, 757t
        clinical signs of, recurrence of, complicating insulin therapy, 744-748, 745f, 746f, 747f, 748f
    complications of, 734t
        chronic, 748-749
    concurrent with pituitary-dependent hyperadrenocorticism, management of, 793-794
    in dogs, 731-749
        after surgery for insulin-secreting β-cell neoplasia, 773
        clinical features of, 732, 732f
        diagnosis of, 732-733, 733t
        etiology of, 731-732
        prognosis for, 749
        treatment of, 733-737
            acarbose in, 736-737
            concurrent problem identification/control in, 737
            dietary, 734-736, 735f, 735t, 736t
            exercise in, 736
            insulin in, 733-734, 734t (*See also* Insulin in diabetes management for dogs)
    hypercholesterolemia and, 824
    ketoacidosis in, 762-769 (*See also* Diabetic ketoacidosis [DKA])
    polyneuropathy in, 1055, 1056f
    uncomplicated, clinicopathologic abnormalities found in, 733t
Diabetic ketoacidosis (DKA), 762-769
    bicarbonate therapy for, 765t, 767
    clinical features of, 763
    clinicopathologic abnormalities in, 765t
    etiology of, 762-763
    fluid therapy for, 764, 765t
    insulin therapy for, 765t, 767-768
    magnesium supplementation for, 767
    phosphate supplementation for, 765t, 766-767, 766f
    potassium supplementation for, 764, 765t, 766, 766f
    prognosis for, 769
    treatment of
        complications of, 769
        in "healthy" animals, 764
        in sick animals, 764-769
Diabetic neuropathy, in cats, 762
Diabinese. *See* Chlorpropamide
Dialume. *See* Aluminum hydroxide
Dialysis, peritoneal, for acute renal failure, 613, 615
Diaphragmatic hernia
    peritoneopericardial, 192, 193f
    pleural effusions and, 316-317
Diarrhea, 432-440
    in acute enteritis, 432-433
    in campylobasteriosis, 437
    in canine lymphocytic-plasmacytic colitis, 448
    in clostridial diseases, 438-439
    dietary-induced, 433
    in digestive disorders, 352-355, 352t, 353t, 354f, 355t

Diarrhea—cont'd
    in enteropathy in Shar-Peis, 450
    in exocrine pancreatic insufficiency, 446
    feline immunodeficiency virus-associated, 436-437
    fiber-enriched diet for, 390
    in gastrinomas, 775
    hemorrhagic, in canine coronaviral enteritis, 436
    in histoplasmosis, 439-440, 440f
    in hypertriglyceridemia, 824
    infectious, 433-440
    large intestinal, 354-355
        chronic, causes of, 355t
        small intestinal diarrheas differentiated from, 353t
    motility modifiers for, 398-399, 399t
    in parvoviral enteritis
        canine, 433-435, 435t
        feline, 435-436
    in prothecosis, 440
    in salmon poisoning, 437
    in salmonellosis, 437-438
    small intestinal, 352-354, 354f
        large intestinal diarrheas differentiated from, 353t
Diastolic murmurs, 9f, 10-11
Diazepam
    as anticonvulsant, 1003
    as appetite stimulant, 391
    dosages of, 341t, 470t
    in head trauma management, 984
    for hepatic lipidosis, 508
    for hepatobiliary and pancreatic disorders, 566t
    hepatotoxicity of, 522, 522t
    for neurologic disorders, 1069t
    for status epilepticus, 996t
    for tetanus, 981
    for urinary tract disorders, 658t
Diazoxide
    for endocrine disorders, 814t
    for hypoglycemia in insulin-secreting β-cell neoplasia, 772t, 774
Dibenzyline. *See* Phenoxybenzamine
DIC. *See* Disseminated intravascular coagulation (DIC)
Dicyclomine
    dosages of, 470t
    for irritable bowel syndrome, 452
    for urinary tract disorders, 658t
Didronel. *See* Etidronate
Diestrus
    canine, 848f, 850
    vaginoscopy in, 853
Diet(s)
    for acute enteritis, 432-433
    for acute renal failure, 615
    bland, 389, 389t (*See also* Bland diet)
    for calcium oxalate uroliths, 639
    carbohydrate-restricted, for diabetes in cats, 753, 753t, 754t
    for chronic gastritis, 419
    for chronic hepatic encephalopathy, 546-547
    commercial, for weight loss, nutrients in, 820t, 821t
    for congenital esophageal weakness, 410-411
    constipation and, 463
    for cystine uroliths, 640
    for diabetes
        for cats, 753, 753t
        for dogs, 734-736, 735f, 735t, 736t
        diarrhea induced by, 352t, 433
    for digestive disorders, 389-396
    elemental, 390
        for canine lymphocytic-plasmacytic enteritis, 447
        for immunoproliferative enteropathy in Basenjis, 449-450
    elimination, 389-390
        for canine eosinophilic gastroenterocolitis, 449
        for canine lymphocytic-plasmacytic enteritis, 447

Diet(s)—cont'd
    elimination—cont'd
        for feline lymphocytic-plasmacytic enteritis, 448
        for immunoproliferative enteropathy in Basenjis, 449-450
    enteral, 392t, 395-396
        for exocrine pancreatic insufficiency, 564
        for feline lower urinary tract inflammation, 647, 648
        for feline lymphocytic-plasmacytic colitis, 448
    fiber-supplemented, 390
        for diabetes
            in cats, 753, 753t, 754f, 754t
            in dogs, 734-736, 735f, 735t
        for idiopathic megacolon, 463
        for irritable bowel syndrome, 452
        for weight loss, 821
    for glomerulonephropathies, 606
    for hyperlipidemia, 825-827, 825t, 826t
    hypoallergenic, 389, 390t
        for canine eosinophilic gastroenterocolitis, 449
    litter size and, 888
    low phosphorus, for hyperphosphatemia in chronic renal failure, 619, 621
    low protein
        for chronic renal failure, 619
        homemade recipes for, 620t
    low sodium, 60
        for ascites, 549
        commercial, 61t
        for mild pancreatitis, 558
        modifications of, for chronic hepatitis, 537
    partially hydrolyzed, 390
    for relapsing and chronic pancreatitis, 560
    for severe pancreatitis, 559
    for silicate uroliths, 640
    for struvite uroliths, 639
    ultra-low-fat, 390
        for intestinal lymphangiectasia, 451
    for urate uroliths, 639-640
Dietary therapy, for insulin-secreting β-cell neoplasia, 772, 772t, 773-774
Diethylcarbamazine
    dosage of, 209t
    for feline immunodeficiency virus, 1280t
    in heartworm prevention, 179-180
Diethylcarbamazine-oxibendazole
    chronic hepatitis from, 529
    hepatotoxicity of, 522t
Diethylstilbestrol (DES)
    as abortifacient, 898
    for endocrine disorders, 814t
    for estrus induction in bitch, 868
    for incontinence with decreased sphincter tone, 656
    for urinary tract disorders, 658t
DIF. *See* Direct immunofluorescence (DIF)
Diffusion abnormalities, in hypoxemia, 282-283
Difloxacin, dosages of, 1242t
Diflucan. *See* Fluconazole
Digestion, fecal tests of, 366-367
Digestive enzyme supplementation, 398
Digestive system. *See also* Oral cavity; Stomach; *specific segment, e.g. Esophagus*
    biopsy techniques for, 384-385
    diagnostic tests for, 365-385
    disorders of
        abdominal distention or enlargement in, 363-364, 364t
        abdominal effusion in, 360-361
        abdominal pain in, 362-363, 363t

Digestive system—cont'd
　disorders of—cont'd
　　acute abdomen in, 361-362, 361t, 362f
　　anorexia in, 360, 360f, 361t
　　antacids for, 397, 397t
　　anthelmintic drugs for, 401-402, 402t
　　antibacterial drugs for, 401
　　antibodies to acetylcholine receptors in, 379
　　antibodies to 2M muscle fibers in, 379
　　antiemetics for, 396-397, 396t
　　antiinflammatory and antisecretory drugs for, 399-401
　　cathartics for, 403, 403t
　　clinical manifestations of, 343-364
　　complete blood count in, 365-366
　　constipation in, 357, 358t
　　diarrhea in, 352-355, 352t, 353t, 354f, 355t
　　dietary management of, 389-396 (See also Diet[s])
　　digestive enzme supplementation for, 398
　　dysphagia in, 343-345, 344t
　　enemas for, 402-403
　　fecal digestion tests in, 366-367
　　fecal incontinence in, 358
　　fecal parasitic evaluation in, 366
　　fluid therapy in, 387-389
　　hematemesis in, 350f, 351-352, 351t
　　hematochezia in, 355-356, 356t
　　in hyperthyroidism, 716
　　intestinal permeability testing in, 379
　　intestinal protectants for, 398, 398t
　　laxatives for, 403, 403t
　　melena in, 356, 356t
　　motility modifiers for, 398-399, 399t
　　peritoneal fluid analysis in, 377
　　physical examination in, 365
　　polyphagia with weight loss and, 816
　　regurgitation in, 346-347, 346f, 347t
　　serum concentrations of vitamins in, 378-379
　　serum gastrin concentrations in, 379
　　serum trypsin-like immunoreactivity in, 378
　　tenesmus in, 356-357, 357t
　　urase activity in gastric mucosa in, 379
　　vomiting in, 347-349, 348t, 349f
　　weight loss in, 358-360, 359t, 360f
　endoscopy of, 38f, 379-384, 381-383f, 384f
　hemorrhage in, complicating liver failure, 550-551
　infections of, antibiotics for, 1245-1246, 1245t
　lymphoma of, 1123
　　treatment of, 1131
　obstruction in, vomiting from, 348t
　parasites of, demonstration techniques for, 1230t
　radiography of, 368
　toxicity for
　　of chemotherapy drugs, 1111
　　of digitalis, 69
　ultrasonography of, 368
Digitalis, toxicity of, 68-69
Digitalis glycosides, in congestive heart failure management, 66-69
Digitoxin
　in congestive heart failure management, 68
　dosages of, 67t, 206t
　preparations of, 67t
Digoxin
　for atrial fibrillation, 82-83, 83f
　commercial preparations of, 88t
　for congestive heart failure, 57, 66-68
　　in AV valve degeneration, 144, 145
　for dilated cardiomyopathy
　　in cat, 132
　　in dog, 109, 111, 112

Digoxin—cont'd
　dosages of, 67t, 80t, 206t
　ECG changes from, 27t
　for paroxysmal atrial tachycardia, 76
　preparations of, 67t
　for supraventricular premature contractions, 76
　for supraventricular tachycardias, 77
　for ventricular tachyarrhythmias, 80
Digoxin-immune Fab, 69
Dihydrate calcium oxalate crystals in urine sediment, 570f, 571t
Dihydrostreptomycin, for *Brucella canis* infection, 937
1,25-Dihydroxycholecalciferol, for urinary tract disorders, 658t
Dilacor XR. *See* Diltiazem
Dilantin. *See* Phenytoin
Dilated cardiomyopathy (DCM)
　canine, 106-115, 110f, 111f, 111t
　　clinical features of, 108
　　clinical findings in, 108-109
　　clinical pathology in, 109
　　in Doberman Pinschers, 110f, 114-115
　　echocardiography in, 109, 111f
　　electrocardiography in, 109
　　etiology of, 106-108
　　pathology of, 108
　　pathophysiology of, 108
　　prognosis of, 113
　　radiography in, 109, 110f
　　secondary myocardial diseases in, 106-108
　　treatment of, 109-113, 111t
　feline, 130-133
　　clinical features of, 132
　　diagnosis of, 132
　　etiology of, 130-131
　　pathophysiology of, 131-132
　　prognosis for, 132-133
　　treatment of, 132-133
　M-mode echocardiogram in, 75f
Diltiazem
　for arrhythmias, 94-95
　for atrial fibrillation, 83, 83f
　commercial preparations of, 88t
　for congestive heart failure, 71
　　in AV valve degeneration, 144
　for dilated cardiomyopathy, 111
　dosages of, 79t, 207t
　for feline hypertrophic cardiomyopathy, 127, 128, 128t
　for fulminant congestive heart failure, 60
　for hypertrophic cardiomyopathy, 116
　for paroxysmal atrial tachycardia, 76
　for supraventricular premature contractions, 76
　for supraventricular tachyarrhythmias, 77
　for sustained supraventricular tachycardia, 84
Dimercaprol, indication and dosage of, 565t
Dimethyl sulfoxide, for neurologic disorders, 1069t
Dimethylsulfoxide (DMSO), for amyloidosis, 606
Diminazene, for cytauxzoonosis, 1302
Diminazene aceturate, for infectious diseases, 1319t
Dioctyl sodium sulfosuccinate
　dosage of, 403t
　dosages of, 470t
Dipentum. *See* Olsalazine
*Dipetalonema reconditum*, *Dirofilaria immitis* differentiated from, 171t
Diphallia, 920
Diphenhydramine
　as antiemetic, 396t
　dosages of, 341t, 470t
　for feline ischemic encephalopathy, 999
　for hypersensitivity reactions to chemotherapy drugs, 1112
　for neurologic disorders, 1069t

Diphenoxylate
　for diarrhea, 399, 399t
　dosages of, 470t
Diphenylthiocarbozone, indication and dosage of, 565t
Dipstick test, for proteinuria, 580
*Dipylidium caninum*, 443
　as enteric zoonosis, 1310
　fecal examination for, 1230t
Direct antiglobulin test (DAT), for immune-mediated disorders, 1213-1214
Direct immunofluorescence (DIF), for immune-mediated disorders, 1214
*Dirofilaria immitis*, 169-183
　*Dipetalonema reconditum* differentiated from, 171t
　immunologic techniques for, 1236
　lung disease from, 302
Disinfection protocols, 1252
Disk, intervertebral
　disease of (*See* Intervertebral disk disease)
　prolapse of, CSF analysis in, 964t
Diskospondylitis, 1031-1034, 1032f, 1033f
　antibiotics for, 1246, 1246t
　clinical features of, 1032
　diagnosis of, 1032, 1032f, 1033f
　treatment of, 1032-1034
Disofenin, indication and dosage of, 565t
Disopyramide, for arrhythmias, 91
Disseminated intravascular coagulation (DIC), 1195-1199
　in acute pancreatitis, 555t
　clinical features of, 1196-1197
　diagnosis of, 1197
　hemangiosarcoma and, 1142
　hemostatic abnormalities in, 1197t
　pathogenesis of, 1195-1196
　primary disorders associated with, 1196t
　prognosis for, 1198-1199
　treatment of, 1197-1198, 1197t
Distemper
　canine, 1015-1016
　　acute, ancillary diagnostics for, 1011t
　　clinical features of, 1273-1274, 1274t
　　CSF analysis in, 964t
　　diagnosis of, 1274-1275
　　epidemiology of, 1273
　　etiology of, 1273
　　immunologic and serologic tests for, 973
　　prevention of, 1275
　　treatment of, 1275
　　vaccination for, 1256
　　zoonotic aspects of, 1275
　feline, 435-436
　myoclonus related to, 982
Ditropan. *See* Oxybutynin
Diuresis
　for acute renal failure, 613-614
　for emergency treatment of intoxications, 997t
　forced, for chemotherapy urotoxicity, 1114-1115
　rapid, for fulminant congestive heart failure, 59, 59t
Diuretics, 566t
　for ascites, 549-550
　for congestive heart failure, 57
　for dilated cardiomyopathy, 112
　dosage of, 206t
　dosages of, 62t
　for hypertension, 202t
　preparations of, 63t
　for pulmonary edema, 313
　for respiratory distress in lung disease, 336
　syncope or intermittent weakness from, 2t, 3
Diuril. *See* Chlorothiazide
Diverticuli, vesicourachal, feline lower urinary tract inflammation and, 644-645

DJD. *See* Degenerative joint disease (DJD)
DKA. *See* Diabetic ketoacidosis (DKA)
DMSO. *See* Dimethylsulfoxide (DMSO)
DNA. *See* Deoxyribonucleic acid (DNA)
Doberman Pinschers
　cardiomyopathy in, 110f, 114-115
　distal polyneuropathy of, 1045t
　familial chronic hepatitis in, 527-528, 528f
　sudden death predisposition in, 73
Dobutamine
　for congestive heart failure, 70
　for dilated cardiomyopathy
　　in cat, 132
　　in dog, 111
　dosages of, 67t, 206t
　for fulminant congestive heart failure, 59, 59t
　preparations of, 67t
Dobutrex. *See* Dobutamine
DOCP. *See* Desoxycorticosterone pivalate
Dofetilide, for arrhythmias, 94
Dog(s). *See also under* Canine *or specific disorder, organ, or system*
　cardiomyopathy in, dilated, 106-115, 110f, 111f, 111t
　diuretic dosages for, 62t
　echocardiographic measurements for, 43t
　electrocardiographic reference ranges for, 17t
　myocardial diseases in, 106-120
　vasodilator dosages for, 62t
Dopamine
　for cardiogenic shock, 119
　for cardiopulmonary resuscitation, dosages of, 99t
　for chronic renal failure, 618t
　for circulatory support, 103
　for congestive heart failure, 69-70
　for dilated cardiomyopathy
　　in cat, 132
　　in dog, 111
　dosages of, 67t, 206t, 208t
　preparations of, 67t
　for urinary tract disorders, 658t
Dopamine agonists
　for estrus induction in bitch, 868
　for false pregnancy, 887
Doppler echocardiography, 44-47, 45f, 46f, 47f
　in atrial septal defect, 162
　in patent ductus arteriosus, 154, 156f
　in subaortic stenosis, 157-158, 157f
　in ventricular septal defect, 161, 161f
Doppler ultrasound method of blood pressure measurement, 201
Dostinex. *See* Cabergoline
Doxorubicin
　for carcinomas, 1155t
　cardiotoxicity of, 106-107, 1114
　for endocrine disorders, 814t
　gastrointestinal complications of, 1111
　for hemangiosarcoma, 1143-1144
　hypersensitivity reactions to, 1112
　for injection site sarcomas, 1152
　for leukemias, acute, 1137t
　for lymphoma, 1127t, 1128, 1129, 1153t
　for oropharyngeal masses, 1151
　for osteosarcoma, 1145-1146, 1155t
　for soft-tissue sarcomas, 1154t
　for thymomas, 1120
　urotoxicity of, 1114
Doxycycline
　for bacterial L form-associated arthritis, 1083
　for bacterial pneumonia, 300-301
　for canine infectious tracheobronchitis, 288
　for cardiopulmonary infections, 1244t
　for cutaneous and soft tissue infections, 1244t
　dosages of, 341t, 470t, 1242t

Doxycycline—cont'd
for ehrlichiosis, 1270, 1271
for feline bronchitis, 292
for feline plague, 1260
for feline upper respiratory infections, 229, 230
for hemolytic anemia, 1162
for infectious diseases, 1319t
for joint disease, 1092t
for leptospirosis, 1262
for Lyme disease, 1084
for *Mycoplasma* infections, 1264
for *Mycoplasma* polyarthritis, 1083
for neurologic disorders, 1069t
for rickettsial diseases, 1018
for rickettsial polyarthritis, 1084
for Rocky Mountain spotted fever, 1266
toxicities of, 1242t
for *Ureaplasma* infections, 1264
for urogenital infections, 1248t
Drainage
of septic exudate, in pyothorax, 328-329
for septic peritonitis, 467
Droncit. *See* Praziquantel
Drooling
causes of, 344t
in digestive disorders, 343, 345
Drug(s)
in acute pancreatitis development, 553t
affecting male reproduction, 914t
alkaline phosphatase activity and, 486-487
anthelmintic, for digestive disorders, 401-402, 402t
antiacid, 397, 397t
antiarrhythmic, 207t
antibacterial, for digestive disorders, 401
anticancer
mechanism of action of, 1106
toxicity of, 1109t
types of, 1106-1107
antiemetic, 396-397, 396t
antithyroid, 721-722, 721t
in cardiopulmonary resuscitation, 100-101f, 102-104
dosages of, 99t
cardiovascular, syncope or intermittent weakness from, 2t, 3
causing chronic hepatitis, 526t, 528-529
for chronic renal failure, 618t
to decrease stress in respiratory distress, 334t
for electrolyte imbalances, 845-846t
emetogenic, 348t
for endocrine disorders, 813-815t
for feline hypertrophic cardiomyopathy, 128t
for gastrointestinal disorders, 469-471t
for hepatobiliary disorders, 565-567t
in hyperlipidemia management, 826-827
for hypertension, 202-203, 202t
hypoglycemic, for diabetes management in cats, 753, 755-757, 755t, 756f, 757t
immunosuppressive, 1216-1219 (*See also* Immunosuppressive drugs)
for infectious diseases, 1318-1320t
intoxication with, mentation abnormalities from, 983
for joint disease, 1092t
for metabolic disorders, 845-846t
for neurolgic disorders, 1069-1070t
overdose of, cardiogenic shock from, 119t
for pancreatic disorders, 565-567t
pregnancy risk from, 900, 900t
reactions to, lymphadenopathy associated with, 1202t
for reproductive disorders, 944-945t

Drug(s)—cont'd
for respiratory disorders, 341-342t
toxicities of, electrocardiography in, 25-26, 27t
for urinary tract disorders, 657-659t
Dry-cleaning fluid, hepatotoxicity of, 522t
DTIC. *See* Dacarbazine
Dulcolax. *See* Bisacodyl
Duodenal reflux, in acute pancreatitis development, 553t
Duodenum
anatomic relationship of, with pancreas and common bile duct in cat, 513f
obstruction of, in acute pancreatitis, 555t
Dwarfism
in hypothyroidism, in cats, 709, 710f
pituitary, 677-680 (*See also* Pituitary dwarfism)
Dyrenium. *See* Triamterene
Dysautonomia, 412-413, 1059
pupil dilatation in, 987
Dyschezia, 356-357, 357t
Dyskinesias, 980
Dysmetria, 977-980
diagnostic approach to, 979-980
etiology of, 978, 978t, 979t
Dysphagia
causes of, 344t
cricopharyngeal, 409
in digestive disorders, 343-345
of muscular origin, 345
neurogenic, 345
pharyngeal, 409-410
regurgitation and, 346
Dysphagias, 409
Dyspnea. *See also* Respiratory distress
in acute pancreatitis, 555t
in congestive heart failure, 3, 4f
in heart disease/failure, 3, 4f
in pulmonary thromboembolism, 310
Dyssynergia
detrusor-urethral, 576
reflex, 576, 652
treatment of, 655
Dystocia, 892-895
causes of, 892
diagnosis of, 893-894
history of, 892-893
indicators of, 893t
treatment of, 894-895
Dysuria, in micturition disorders, 653
Dysuria-stranguria, 568, 569f

**E**

Ear, middle, inflammation of. *See* Otitis media-interna
EBDO. *See* Extrahepatic bile duct obstruction (EBDO)
Ecchinocytosis, disorders associated with, 1159t
ECG. *See* Electrocardiography (ECG)
*Echinococcus granulosa*
as enteric zoonosis, 1309t, 1310
fecal examination for, 1230t
*Echinococcus multilocularis*
as enteric zoonosis, 1309t, 1310
fecal examination for, 1230t
Echocardiography, 35-47
in arterial thromboembolism, 134
in atrial septal defect, 162
basic principles of, 36
benefits of, 35
in cardiac tumors, 196
contrast, 43-44
in degenerative AV valve disease, 142-143, 142f, 143f
in dilated cardiomyopathy, 109, 111f
Doppler, 44-47, 45f, 46f, 47f
in feline dilated cardiomyopathy, 132
in feline hypertrophic cardiomyopathy, 124, 126-127f, 127
in heartworm diagnosis in cats, 181

Echocardiography—cont'd
in heartworm disease in dogs, 173, 173f
in hypertrophic cardiomyopathy, in dogs, 115
in infective endocarditis diagnosis, 148, 149f
limitations of, 35-36
M-mode, 38-43
in atrial fibrillation, 75f
diastolic measurements with, 39
in dilated cardiomyopathy, 75f
indices of myocardial function and, 39-40, 42f
measurements with, 39-40, 42-43, 42f
for cats, guidelines for, 44t
for dogs, approximate, 43t
views with, 39, 41f
in patent ductus arteriosus, 154, 155f
in pericardial effusion, 188, 189f
in pulmonary edema, 312
in pulmonary hypertension with shunt reversal, 166
in pulmonary thromboembolism, 310
in pulmonic stenosis, 159-160, 160f
in subaortic stenosis, 157-158, 157f
in tetralogy of Fallot, 164
transesophageal, 47
in tricuspid dysplasia, 163, 163f
two-dimensional, 36-38, 37f, 38f, 39f, 40f
in ventricular septal defect, 161, 161f
Eclampsia, 896
Ectopic impulses, 16, 19-23
accelerated ventricular rhythm as, 22
atrial fibrillation as, 21, 22f
atrial flutter as, 21
escape complexes as, 20-21f, 23
supraventricular premature complexes as, 19, 19f, 23
supraventricular tachycardia as, 21
ventricular fibrillation as, 22-23, 23f
ventricular premature complexes as, 20-21f, 21-22
ventricular tachycardia as, 20-21f, 22
Edema
cardiogenic, acute, management of, 60
pulmonary, 312-313
alveolar pattern in, 258
radiographic signs of, 35
Edrophonium chloride, for neurologic disorders, 1069t
Effusion(s)
abdominal, 360-361, 474-476, 475f, 476f
in hepatobiliary disease, characteristics of, 491t
pericardial, 185-192 (*See also* Pericardial effusion)
pleural (*See* Pleural effusion)
EGE. *See* Eosinophilic gastroenterocolitis (EGE)
Eggs, parasitic
characteristics of, 263t
concentration of, sedimentation of feces for, 264t
*Ehrlichia canis,* infection with, 1267-1270. *See also* Ehrlichiosis, canine
Ehrlichiosis, 1267-1271
ancillary diagnostics for, 1011t
antibiotics for, 1246t
canine, 1267-1270
clinical features of, 1267-1269, 1268t
diagnosis of, 1269-1270, 1269t
epidemiology of, 1267
etiology of, 1267, 1267f
prevention of, 1270
treatment of, 1270
zoonotic aspects of, 1270
CNS involvement in, 1018
CSF analysis in, 964t
feline, 1271
lymphadenopathy associated with, 1202t
morphologic characteristics of, 1233t

Ehrlichiosis—cont'd
neutropenia in, 1175t
polyarthritis in, 1084
serologic tests for, 973
Eisenmenger's physiology, 165
Ejaculation disorders, oligospermia from, 915
Ejection murmur, 9, 9f
Elavil. *See* Amitriptyline
Eldepryl. *See* L-Deprenyl
Electrical defibrillation, 102
Electrocardiography (ECG), 12-31
ambulatory, 29, 31f
artifacts in, 29, 30f
assessment of, heart rate variability in, 29, 31
benefits of, 12
in bundle branch block, 15, 15t, 16f
in cardiopulmonary resuscitation, 104
in chamber enlargement, 15, 15t, 16f, 16t
conduction disturbances in, 23-25
in degenerative AV valve disease, 142
in dilated cardiomyopathy, 109
in drug toxicities, 25-26, 27t
ectopic impulses in, 16, 19-23 (*See also* Ectopic impulses)
in electrolyte imbalances, 25-26, 27f, 27t, 28f
in feline hypertrophic cardiomyopathy, 124
in heartworm diagnosis
in cats, 181-182
in dogs, 173
in hypoadrenocorticism, 806
in infective endocarditis diagnosis, 148-149
interpretation guide for, 74t
interpretation of, approach to, 26, 28-29
lead systems for, 12-13, 14f, 14t
limitations of, 12
mean electrical axis in, 13, 14f, 15
in pericardial effusion, 188, 188f
in pulmonic stenosis, 159
in sick sinus syndrome, 85, 85f
signal-averaged, 31
in sinus rhythms, 15-16, 17t, 18f, 18t
ST-T abnormalities in, 25, 26t
in tricuspid dysplasia, 163
waveforms on, normal, 12, 13f, 13t
Electrodiagnostic testing
for neuromuscular disorders, 970-972
in traumatic neuropathies, 1049
Electroencephalography, in neuromuscular disorders, 971-972
Electrofulguration, for perianal fistulae, 461
Electrolyte imbalances, 828-845
drugs for, 845-846t
hypercalcemia as, 836-839, 838f, 839t (*See also* Hypercalcemia)
hyperkalemia as, 832-834, 833t, 834t
hypermagnesemia as, 843
hypernatremia as, 828-830, 829t
hyperphosphatemia as, 841-842, 841t
hypocalcemia as, 840-841
hypokalemia as, 833t, 834-836, 835t
hypomagnesemia as, 843-845, 844t
hyponatremia as, 830-832, 830t, 831t
hypophosphatemia as, 842-843, 842t
Electrolyte(s)
imbalances of, electrocardiography in, 25-26, 27f, 27t, 28f
serum concentrations of, in hepatobiliary system assessment, 488
Electromechanical dissociation (EMD), 98
Electromyography (EMG)
in cauda equina syndrome, 1039
in masticatory myositis, 1062-1063
in myasthenia gravis, 1060
in neuromuscular disorders, 970-971
Electron microscopy
in fecal analysis, 367
in infectious disease detection, 1237

Electrophoresis
  lipoprotein, 824-825
  protein, 1210-1211, 1211f
  urine and serum protein, in protein-
    uria identification, 586
Electroretinography (ERG), in neuro-
    muscular disorders, 971
Elemental diet(s), 390
  for canine lymphocytic-plasmacytic
    enteritis, 447
  for hepatobiliary and pancreatic disor-
    ders, 567t
  for immunoproliferative enteropathy
    in Basenjis, 449-450
Elimination diet(s), 389-390
  for canine eosinophilic gastroentero-
    colitis, 449
  for canine lymphocytic-plasmacytic
    enteritis, 447
  for feline lymphocytic-plasmacytic en-
    teritis, 448
  for immunoproliferative enteropathy
    in Basenjis, 449-450
ELISA. See Enzyme-linked immunosor-
    bent assay (ELISA)
Elliptocytosis, disorders associated with,
    1159t
Elspar. See L-Asparaginase
Embolism, fibrocartilaginous, 1030-1031,
    1031f
Embolization, in infective endocarditis,
    146
EMD. See Electromechanical dissociation
    (EMD)
Emergency management
  of respiratory distress, 333-336
  of status epilepticus, 1004
Emesis, induction of
  for acute renal failure, 613
  for intoxications, 997t
EMG. See Electromyography (EMG)
EMH. See Extramedullary hematopoiesis
    (EMH)
Emphysema, feline, features of, 291t
Enacard. See Enalapril
Enalapril
  for chronic renal failure, 618t
  for congestive heart failure, 65
    in AV valve degeneration, 144, 145
  dosages of, 62t, 206t
  for feline hypertrophic cardiomyop-
    athy, 128-129
  for glomerulonephropathies, 606
  for hypertension, 202t
  preparations of, 63t
  for restrictive cardiomyopathy, 130
  for urinary tract disorders, 658t
Encephalitis
  antibiotics for, 1246t
  parasitic, 1018-1019
  seizures in, 999
Encephalomyelitis, rabies, 1017
Encephalopathy
  feline immunodeficiency virus, 1014
  hepatic, 479-481, 480f, 480t
    antibiotics for, 1245t
    complicating liver failure
      acute, treatment of, 547-548
      chronic, treatment of, 546-547
  ischemic, feline, seizures from, 999
Encephalotoxins, in pathogenesis of he-
    patic encephalopathy, 480t
Endocardial fibroelastosis, 167
Endocarditis
  bacterial, antibiotics for, 1244-1245,
    1244t
  infective, 145-150 (See also Infective
    endocarditis)
Endocrine alopecia, 667-670, 667f
  disorders causing, 668t
  in hyperadrenocorticism, 779f, 780,
    780t, 781f
  in hypothyroidism, 693, 695f
  sex hormone-responsive, 669-670
    treatment of, 670

Endocrine disorders, 660-815
  diabetes insipidus as, 661-667 (See also
    Diabetes insipidus)
  endocrine alopecia as, 667-670 (See
    also Endocrine alopecia)
  feline acromegaly as, 673-677 (See also
    Feline acromegaly)
  growth hormone-responsive dermato-
    sis in adult dog as, 670-673
    (See also Growth hormone-
    responsive dermatosis in
    adult dog)
  pituitary dwarfism as, 677-680 (See
    also Pituitary dwarfism)
  polydipsia as, 660-661, 661t
    primary, 667
  polyuria as, 660-661, 661t
Endocrine pancreas, 729-776. See also
    Pancreas, endocrine
Endocrinology, reproductive, in male,
    905-906
Endometrium
  cystic hyperplasia of, with pyometra,
    877-880 (See also Cystic en-
    dometrial hyperplasia
    [CEH]-pyometra complex)
  inflammation of, Mycoplasma canis
    causing, 935
Endomyocardial biopsy, 48
Endoscope, for rhinoscopy, 221f
Endoscopy
  in alimentary tract disease, 379-384,
    380f, 381f, 382-383f, 384f
  in foreign body removal, from esopha-
    gus, 414
  in gastric foreign body removal, 424
  in gastrostomy tube placement, 508,
    510-511f
  in hematemesis, 351
  in vomiting, 349
Endotoxic shock, hypertonic saline solu-
    tion for, 387-388
Endotracheal tubes, for oxygen supple-
    mentation, 338t, 339
Enema(s)
  in acute hepatic encephalopathy man-
    agement, 547-548
  barium contrast, 376-377, 378f
  cleansing
    administration of, 402-403
    for constipation from dietary
      indiscretion, 463
  hypertonic, administration of, 403
  retention
    administration of, 402
    for constipation from dietary
      indiscretion, 463
    for digestive disorders, 400
English Pointers
  progressive neurogenic muscular atro-
    phy in, 1045t
  sensory neuropathy in, 1046t
Enilconazole, for nasal aspergillosis, 236
Enrofloxacin
  for cardiopulmonary infections, 1244t
  dosages of, 341t, 470t, 1242t
  for feline plague, 1260
  for hepatobiliary and pancreatic disor-
    ders, 566t
  for infection in chemotherapy patient,
    1110
  for infectious diseases, 1319t
  for leptospirosis, 1262
  for liver abscesses, 542
  for Mycoplasma infections, 1264
  for neurologic disorders, 1006t
  for parvoviral enteritis, 434
  for rickettsial diseases, 1018
  for Rocky Mountain spotted fever,
    1266
  for septic peritonitis, 468
  for severe pancreatitis, 559
  for Ureaplasma infections, 1264
  for urinary tract infections, 627

Entamoeba histolytica
  as enteric zoonosis, 1309t
  fecal examination for, 1230t
Enteral diets, 392t, 395-396
Enteric zoonoses, 1307-1312, 1308t,
    1309t, 1310f
Enteritis
  acute, diarrhea in, 432-433
  coronaviral, 436
  eosinophilic, in hypereosinophilic syn-
    drome, 449
  granulomatous, with gastritis, 449
  intussusception in, 455-456
  lymphocytic-plasmacytic
    canine, 447-448
    feline, 448
  parvoviral
    canine, 433-435, 435t
    feline, 435-436
Enterobacter
  antimicrobial agents for, 627, 629t
  urinary tract infections from, 624, 625t
Enterococcus
  antimicrobial agents for, 627, 629t
  urinary tract infections from, 624, 625t
Enteropathy
  antibiotic-responsive, 450
    serum concentrations of vitamins in
      evaluation of, 378-379
  immunoproliferative, in Basenjis, 449-
    450
  protein-losing, 451
    causes of, 355t
    diarrhea in, 353
    in Shar-Peis, 450
Enterostomy tubes, 395
  uses of, 395-396
Environment, neonatal morbidity/
    mortality and, 901-902
Enzyme(s)
  pancreatic
    dosages of, 471t
    for exocrine pancreatic insufficiency,
      447
    for hepatobiliary and pancreatic
      disorders, 567t
    supplemental
      for exocrine pancreatic
        insufficiency, 563-564
      for relapsing and chronic
        pancreatitis, 560
  serum
    activities of, in hepatobiliary
      disorders, 486-487, 492t
    in extrahepatic bile duct obstruction
      diagnosis, 518
Enzyme-linked immunosorbent assay
    (ELISA)
  antigen capture, for microalbuminuria,
    586
  in canine parvovirus detection, 434
  in fecal analysis, 367
  in feline immunodeficiency virus diag-
    nosis, 1280
  in feline leukemia virus detection, 1283
  in progesterone measurement, 855
Eosinopenia, 1177, 1177t
Eosinophil(s), pulmonary infiltrates with,
    303
  differential diagnosis of, 251t
Eosinophilia, 1177-1178, 1177t
Eosinophilic enteritis/hypereosinophilic
    syndrome, feline, 449
Eosinophilic gastritis, 419-420
Eosinophilic gastroenterocolitis (EGE),
    canine, 448-449
Eosinophilic granuloma
  feline, 407
  lymphadenopathy associated with,
    1202t
Eosinophilic granulomatosis, pulmonary,
    in heartworm disease, treat-
    ment of, 176-177
Eosinophilic lung disease, 303-304

Ephedrine, for urinary tract disorders, 658t
EPI. See Exocrine pancreatic insufficiency
    (EPI)
Epicardium, 185
Epidermis, systemic lupus erythematosus
    and, 1220t
Epididymis, sclerosing agent injection
    into, 866
Epididymitis, 921-922, 922f
  Mycoplasma canis causing, 935
Epidural lymphoma, 1124
Epidurography, in neuromuscular disor-
    ders, 967-968, 969f
Epilepsy, 1000-1001
  idiopathic, 1000-1001
  trauma/scar-related, 1000
Epinephrine
  in cardiopulmonary resuscitation,
    dosages of, 99t
  in circulatory support, 103
  in congestive heart failure manage-
    ment, 70
  dosage of, 208t
  for hypersensitivity reactions to che-
    motherapy drugs, 1112
Episodic weakness, 976-977, 977t
Episprantel
  dosages of, 402t, 470t
  for tapeworms, 443
  uses of, 402t
Epistaxis, 211, 211t
Epoetin alfa, for urinary tract disorders,
    658t
Epogen. See Erythropoietin
Epulides, oropharyngeal, 1150
ERG. See Electroretinography (ERG)
Erosion, turbinate, differential diagnosis
    of, 223t
Erysipelothrix rhusiopathiae, infective en-
    docarditis from, 146
Erythrocytes, morphology of, in hepato-
    biliary disorders, 485-486,
    485f
Erythrocytosis, 1170-1172
Erythromycin
  for campylobacteriosis, 437
  for cutaneous and soft tissue infec-
    tions, 1244t
  for diarrhea, 399
  dosages of, 470t, 1241t
  for Helicobacter gastritis, 401
  for hepatic and gastrointestinal infec-
    tions, 1245t
  for idiopathic gastric motility, 427
  for infectious diseases, 1319t
  for joint disease, 1092t
  for Mycoplasma infections, 1264
  for perianal fistulae, 461
  for Ureaplasma infections, 1264
  for urogenital infections, 1248t
Erythropoietin
  for chronic renal failure, 618t
  for feline immunodeficiency virus,
    1280t, 1281
  for urinary tract disorders, 658t
Escape complexes, 19f, 20-21f, 23
Escherichia coli
  antimicrobial agents for, 627, 629t
  as enteric zoonosis, 1309t
  infective endocarditis from, 146
  pulmonary infection from, 299
  urinary tract infections from, 624, 625t
Esmolol
  characteristics of, 91t
  commercial preparations of, 87t
  dosages of, 79t, 207t
  for hypertension, 202t
Esophagitis, 412
  endoscopic view of, 381f
  secondary to parvoviral enteritis, treat-
    ment of, 435t
Esophagoscopy
  in alimentary tract disease, 380, 380f,
    381f, 382f
  in esophageal neoplasm detection, 415
  in regurgitation evaluation, 347

Esophagostomy tube(s), 392
  placement of, 508, 509f
  uses of, 395
Esophagraphy
  contrast-enhanced, 371, 372f
  of esophageal neoplasms, 416f
  in hiatal hernia, 413f
Esophagus
  cicatrix of, 414-415, 415f
  disorders of, 410-416
  foreign objects in, 414
  imaging of, 369-371, 370-371f, 372f
  in myasthenia gravis, 1059-1060
  neoplasms of, 415-416, 416f
  obstruction of, 413-416, 414f, 415f, 416f
    causes of, 347t
    regurgitation from, 346
  vascular ring anomalies of, 413-414, 414f
  weakness of
    acquired, 411-412
    causes of, 347t
    congenital, 410-411
    regurgitation from, 346-347
Estradiol, assessment of, 856
Estrogens
  as abortifacients, 898, 898t
  in estrus induction in bitch, 868
  neutropenia from, 1175t
  in ovulation induction in bitch, 868
  in proestrus, 848
Estrous cycle
  canine, 847-851, 848f
    anestrus in, 848f, 850-851
    in breeding management, 849-850
    diestrus in, 848f, 850
    estrus in, 848f, 849
    proestrus in, 847-849, 848f
  disorders of
    celiotomy and, 858-859
    estrus induction in, 868-869
    estrus suppression in, 865-867
    in female infertility, 859-865, 860t
      (See also Infertility, female)
    karyotyping and, 858
    laparoscopy and, 858-859
    ovarian remnant syndrome as, 867-868
    ovulation induction in, 869
    population control and, 865-867
    radiology and, 858
    reproductive hormone assessment in, 855-858
    ultrasonography and, 858, 859f
  feline, 851-852, 851f, 852f, 853f
Estrumate. *See* Cloprostenol
Estrus
  abnormal, 863
  canine, 848f, 849
  feline, 851, 853f
  induction of, 862, 868-869
  prolonged, 863-864, 863f
  resolution of vaginitis and, in prepubertal bitch, 874-875
  short, 864
  suppression of, population control and, 865-867
  vaginoscopy in, 853
Ethanol
  injection of, for parathyroid disorders, 683
  myocardial depression from, 107
Ethyl alcohol. *See* Ethanol
Ethylene glycol
  ingested, ultrasonographic appearance of kidney with, 611f
  neurologic dysfunction from, 995t
Etidronate, for hypercalcemia, 839, 839t, 845t
Etodolac, for degenerative joint disease, 1080t
Etogesic. *See* Etodolac
Etoposide, hypersensitivity reactions to, 1112

*Eucoleus bohemi,* fecal examination for, 1230t
Eurovet BV. *See* Bromocriptine
*Eurytrema procyonis,* fecal examination for, 1230t
Euthyroid sick syndrome, 702, 705f
Evan's syndrome, 1191
Event recording, cardiac, 29
Excretory urography, 589t
Exercise(s)
  capacity for, reduced, in heart failure, 55
  in congestive heart failure management, 58
  for degenerative myelopathy, 1037
  in diabetes management, 736
  in dystocia management, 894
Exercise intolerance, in lower respiratory tract disorders, 251-252
Exocrine pancreas. *See also* Pancreas, exocrine
Exocrine pancreatic insufficiency (EPI), 446-447, 560-564
  clinical features of, 561, 561f
  diagnosis of, 561-563, 562f, 562t
  diarrhea from, 352-353
  pancreatic enzyme supplementation for, 398
  pathogenesis of, 560-561
  prognosis for, 563-564
  serum TLI for, 378
  treatment of, 563-564, 563f
Extracardiac arteriovenous shunts, 153-155
Extracardiac obstruction, cardiogenic shock from, 119t
Extrahepatic bile duct obstruction (EBDO), 518-520, 519f, 519t
  in acute pancreatitis, 555t
  causes of, 516t
  clinical features of, 518
  diagnosis of, 518-519
  etiology of, 518
  pathogenesis of, 518
  treatment of, 519-520
  ultrasonographic appearance of, 496f
Extramedullary hematopoiesis (EMH), infiltrative splenomegaly from, 1204
Extranodal lymphoma, 1123, 1123t
Extrathoracic airway obstruction, 334-335, 334f, 335f
Exudate exposure zoonoses, 1312-1315, 1313t
Exudates
  in abdominal effusions in hepatobiliary disease, 491t
  pericardial effusion from, 186
  in pleural effusion, 316t, 317
  septic
    in pleural cavity, 327-329
    in pyothorax, drainage of, 328-329
Eye(s)
  in blastomycosis, 1290
  color of, in congenital portosystemic shunt, 520, 520f
  in distemper, 1274, 1274f
  feline leukemia virus infection and, 1282
  fluids of, antibody detection in, 1238
  hypertension and, 201
  lymphoma of, 1124
    treatment of, 1131
  sympathetic innervation of, 988f
  zoonoses of, 1315-1316
Eyelid, third, protrusion of, 989-990

**F**

FAC protocol, for carcinomas, 1155t
Face, deformity of, 216, 216f
Facial nerve paralysis, 1051-1053, 1052f, 1053f
Fading puppy syndrome, 1194
Familial reflex myoclonus, 982
Famotidine
  for acute spinal injury, 1023
  as antacid, 397, 397t

Famotidine—cont'd
  from chronic renal failure, 618t
  dosages of, 470t
  for gastrointestinal hemorrhage in liver failure, 550
  for *Helicobacter*-associated disease, 420
  for *Helicobacter* gastritis, 401
  for hepatobiliary and pancreatic disorders, 567t
  for mast cell tumors, 1148
  for urinary tract disorders, 659t
Fascicular block, left anterior, 25
Fast Fourier transformation, in heart rate variability analysis, 31
Fat(s)
  in commercial reduced-sodium diets, 61t
  fecal, quantitated analysis of, 367
Fat absorption testing, 378
FCE. *See* Fibrocartilaginous embolism (FCE)
FCV. *See* Feline calicivirus (FCV)
Febantel, dosages of, 470t
Fecal flotation, in digestive disorders, 366
Fecal incontinence, 358
Fecal sedimentation, 366
Feces
  acholic, 479, 479f
  assays for bacterial toxins in, 367
  bacterial culture of, 367-368
  coal tar black, 356, 356t
  color of, changes in, 477-479, 479f
  culture of, in infectious disease diagnosis, 1235
  cytologic evaluation of, 368
  digestion tests on, 366-367
  electron microscopy of, for viral particles, 367
  evaluation of, in hepatobiliary disorders, 491
  examination of
    Baermann technique in, 1232, 1232f
    direct smear in, 1229
    fecal flotation in, 1231, 1231t, 1232f
    in infectious diseases, 1229-1232, 1230t, 1231f, 1231t, 1232f
    preservation of feces for, 1232
    stained smear in, 1231, 1231f
  fat analysis in, quantitated, 367
  fresh blood in, 355-356, 356t
  impacted, removal of, for idiopathic megacolon, 463
  occult blood in, 367
  sedimentation of, for concentration of eggs, 264t
  smears of, in clostridial disease diagnosis, 438, 438f
Feeding tube(s), 391-392, 393-394f, 395
  enterostomy, 395
    uses of, 395-396
  esophagostomy, 392
    placement of, 508, 509f
    uses of, 395
  gastrostomy, 392, 393-394f, 395
    for acquired megaesophagus, 411
    in congenital esophageal weakness management, 411
    in esophagitis management, 412
    uses of, 395
  nasoesophageal, 391-392
    uses of, 395
  orogastric
    for decompression in gastric dilation/volvulus, 425
    intermittent, 391
  pharyngostomy, 392
    uses of, 395
  placement of
    endoscopic, 508, 510-511f
    nonendoscopic, devices for, 508, 511f
    percutaneous, 508, 509f
Felbamate, as anticonvulsant, 1004
Felbatol. *See* Felbamate
Feldene. *See* Piroxicam

Feline acromegaly, 673-677
  clinical features of, 674-676, 675f, 675t
  clinical pathology of, 676
  diagnosis of, 676, 676f
  etiology of, 671-672
  prognosis for, 677
  treatment of, 676-677
Feline acute pancreatitis, 560
Feline bronchitis, 291-295
  classification of, 291t
  clinical features of, 291
  diagnosis of, 292
  differential diagnosis of, 292t
  etiology of, 291, 291t
  prognosis in, 295
  treatment of, 94f, 292-295, 292t, 295t
Feline calicivirus (FCV), 228
  vaccine for, 230, 1255
Feline chronic progressive polyarthritis, 1091
Feline coronavirus, 1275-1278, 1276t. *See also* Coronavirus, feline
Feline distemper, 435-436
Feline ehrlichiosis, 1271
Feline endocrine alopecia, 667-668
Feline eosinophilic enteritis/hypereosinophilic syndrome, 449
Feline eosinophilic granuloma, 407
Feline granulomatous enteritis/gastritis, 449
Feline herpesvirus (FHV), vaccine for, 230
Feline idiopathic polymyositis, 1064
Feline idiopathic vestibular syndrome, 1008
Feline immunodeficiency virus (FIV), 1278-1281, 1279t, 1280t
  clinical features of, 1279-1280, 1279t
  diagnosis of, 1280
  diarrhea associated with, 436-437
  encephalopathy from, 1014
  epidemiology of, 1278-1279
  etiology of, 1278-1279
  lymphadenopathy associated with, 1202t
  in nasal discharge, 213
  prevention of, 1281
  treatment of, 1280-1281, 1280t
  vaccines for, 1255-1256
  zoonotic aspects of, 1281
Feline infectious peritonitis (FIP), 469, 1017-1018, 1275-1278, 1276t
  ancillary diagnostics for, 1011t
  CSF analysis in, 964t
  lymphadenopathy associated with, 1202t
  vaccination for, 1278
Feline ischemic encephalopathy (FIE), seizures from, 999
Feline leukemia virus (FeLV), 1281-1284, 1282t
  acute leukemia and, 1138
  clinical features of, 1282-1283
  diagnosis of, 1283
  epidemiology of, 1281-1282
  etiology of, 1281-1282
  lymphadenopathy associated with, 1202t
  in nasal discharge, 213
  panleukopenia associated with, 436
  prevention of, 1284
  stages of, 1282t
  treatment of, 1283-1284
  vaccine for, 1255
  zoonotic aspects of, 1284
Feline lower urinary tract inflammation (FLUTI), 571-572, 573f, 642-649
  clinical features of, 645, 645t
  diagnosis of, 645
  etiology of, 642-645
  management of, 645, 646f, 646t, 647-649
    in obstructed cats, 647-649
    in unobstructed cats, 645, 646f, 646t, 647
  pathogenesis of, 642-645

Feline lymphocytic-plasmacytic colitis, 448
Feline lymphocytic-plasmacytic enteritis, 448
Feline lymphocytic-plasmacytic gingivitis/pharyngitis, 408-409
Feline mammary hyperplasia and hypertrophy, 883-884, 883f
Feline panleukopenia, 435-436
Feline parvoviral enteritis, 435-436
Feline plague, 1259-1260, 1260f, 1260t, 1313-1314
Feline polioencephalomyelitis, 1013-1014
Feline polyarthritis, diagnosis of, 1073
Feline semen, 943-944
Feline upper respiratory infection, 228-232
    clinical features of, 228
    diagnosis of, 228-229
    etiology of, 228
    prevention of, 230-232, 231t
    prognosis for, 230
    treatment
        with acute signs, 229
        with chronic signs, 229-230, 229t
Feline urologic syndrome, 642
FeLV. See Feline leukemia virus (FeLV)
Femoral arterial pulses, 6
Femoral nerve, damage to, 1050t
Fenbendazole
    for *Aelurostrongylus abstrusus,* 303
    for *Capillaria,* 303
    dosages of, 341t, 402t, 470t
    for giardiasis, 445
    for hookworms, 443
    for infectious diseases, 1320t
    for nasal capillariasis, 239
    for paragonimiasis, 303
    for roundworms, 443
    for strongyloidiasis, 444
    uses of, 402t
    for whipworms, 441
Fentanyl patch, for arterial thromboembolism, 135
Fertile period, in canine, 849
Fertilization, 887-888
Fetal resorption-abortion-stillbirth complex, 900-901
Fetus
    death of, radiographic signs of, 894t
    nonviable, 889, 890f
Fever, 1222
    complicating chemotherapy, 1110
    of undetermined origin (FUO), 1222-1225
        diagnostic approach to, 1223-1224, 1224t
        disorders associated with, 1222-1223, 1223t
        hematologic changes in, 1225t
        treatment of, 1224-1225
FHV. See Feline herpesvirus (FHV)
Fiber
    diet high in, for weight loss, 821
    dietary, 403
        in diabetes management
            for cats, 753, 754f, 754t
            for dogs, 734-736, 735f, 735t
        supplemental
            in digestive disorders, 390
            for idiopathic megacolon, 463
            for irritable bowel syndrome, 452
Fibrillation
    atrial, 21, 22f (*See also* Atrial fibrillation)
    ventricular, 22-23, 23f
Fibrin degradation products (FDP), concentration of, in bleeding patient evaluation, 1187t, 1188
Fibrocartilaginous embolism (FCE), 1030-1031, 1031f
Fibroelastosis, endocardial, 167
Fibromatous epulis, 406t
Fibrosarcoma (FSA)
    oral, 406t
    oropharyngeal, 1150

Fibrosis
    hepatic, idiopathic, 530-531
    hepatoportal, 534
FIE. See Feline ischemic encephalopathy (FIE)
Filaribits. See Diethylcarbamazine
*Filaroides hirthi,* fecal examination for, 1230t
Finasteride
    for benign prostatic hyperplasia, 930
    for reproductive disorders, 944t
Fine-needle aspiration (FNA), 1093-1094
    in lymphadenopathy-splenomegaly, 1208
    in mast cell tumor diagnosis, 1147
    in mediastinal masses, 1120
    in metastatic lung lesion, 1118
    in solitary mass evaluation, 1117
FIP. See Feline infectious peritonitis (FIP)
Fistula, perianal, 461
FIV. See Feline immunodeficiency virus (FIV)
Flagellates, zoonotic, 1309t, 1311-1312
Flagging, 849
Flagyl. See Metronidazole
Flavoxate, for urinary tract disorders, 659t
Flecainide, for arrhythmias, 91
Florinef. See Fludrocortisone acetate
Flotation, fecal, 1231, 1231t, 1232f
Flovent. See Fluticasone propionate
Floxacin, for abdominal sepsis, 401
Fluconazole
    for coccidioidomycosis, 1294
    for cryptococcosis, 1289, 1289t
    for histoplasmosis, 1292
    for infectious diseases, 1320t
Flucytosine
    for cryptococcosis, 1289, 1289t
    for infectious diseases, 1320t
Fludrocortisone acetate
    for acute addisonian crisis, 808
    after adrenalectomy in cats, 803
    for endocrine disorders, 814t
Fluid(s)
    abdominal
        accumulation of, mechanisms of, 475f
        analysis of, in hepatobiliary disorders, 491, 491t
    accumulation of, evaluation for, in cardiovascular examination, 6
    dry-cleaning, hepatotoxicity of, 522t
    parenteral, administration of, 387
Fluid therapy
    for acute addisonian crisis, 807t, 808
    for acute enteritis, 432
    for acute renal failure, 614-615, 614t
    for canine coronaviral enteritis, 436
    for canine urolithiasis, 636
    for chylothorax, 331
    for cytauxzoonosis, 1302
    for diabetic ketoacidosis, 764, 765t
    for digestive disorders, 387-389
    for digitalis toxicity, 69
    for dilated cardiomyopathy, 112
    for feline lower urinary tract inflammation, 648
    for gastrointestinal complications of chemotherapy, 1111
    for hemorrhagic gastroenteritis, 419
    for hypernatremia, 829-830
    for hyponatremia, 831-832, 832t
    for leptospirosis, 1262
    for mastitis, 883
    for metritis, 897
    parenteral, for acute gastritis, 418
    for parvoviral enteritis, 434, 435t
    for severe pancreatitis, 558
Fluke(s)
    fecal examination for, 1230t
    liver, extrahepatic bile duct obstruction from, 518, 519f
    lung, fecal examination for, 1230t

Flumazenil
    for acute hepatic encephalopathy, 548
    for hepatobiliary and pancreatic disorders, 567t
Flunixin meglumine
    dosages of, 470t
    for endotoxemia from gastric dilation/volvulus, 425
    gastrointestinal ulceration/erosion from, 427-428
    for parvoviral enteritis, 435t
Fluorescent antibody tests, for feline upper respiratory infections, 228
Fluoroquinolone(s)
    for aspiration pneumonia, 306
    for bacterial pneumonia, 300-301
    for chronic feline upper respiratory infections, 230
    for feline bronchitis, 293
    for inflammatory hepatobiliary disease, 516
Fluoroscopy, in degenerative AV valve disease, 141
5-Fluorouracil
    for abdominal carcinomatosis, 469
    for carcinomas, 1155t
    gastrointestinal complications of, 1111
Flush, nasal, 224
Fluticasone propionate, for feline bronchitis, 293
FNA. See Fine-needle aspiration (FNA)
Folate, serum concentrations of, in digestive disorders, 378, 379
Folinic acid, for neurologic disorders, 1069t
Follicle-stimulating hormone (FSH)
    in anestrus, 850
    assessment of, 856-857, 857t
    in estrus, 849
    in estrus induction in queen, 868
    evaluation of, in male reproductive function assessment, 913
    in male sexual development, 905, 906
    in proestrus, 847-848
Foreign body(ies)
    esophageal, 370-371f, 371, 414
        endoscopic view of, 380f, 381f
    gastric, 423-424
    gastrointestinal, endoscopic view of, 383f
    intestinal, radiography of, 372
    intestinal obstruction by, 454-455, 454f
    nasal
        radiographic signs of, 220t
        sneezing from, *215*
Fosinopril
    in congestive heart failure management, 65
    dosages of, 62t, 206t
    preparations of, 63t
Fox Terriers, smooth-coated, hereditary ataxia in, 1044f
Fractional clearance (FC), of solutes, 585-586
Fractional shortening, 40, 42f
Fracture(s)
    of canine os penis, 918
    pelvic, 1023
        old, malaligned healing of, pelvic canal obstruction from, constipation from, 462
    sacral, 1023
    spinal, radiographic evaluation of, three-compartment model for, 1021, 1022f, 1023
*Francisella tularensis*
    respiratory zoonoses associated with, 1315-1316
    zoonoses associated with, 1313t, 1314
Frank-Starling mechanism, in heart failure, 54
Frenulum, penile, persistent, 919, 920f
Frequency-domain analysis, of heart rate variability, 31

Frontal sinus
    ablation of, for feline upper respiratory infection, 230
    radiography of, 217, 218f
Fructosamine, serum, in stress-induced hyperglycemia
    in cats, 758
    in dogs, 741-742
FSA. See Fibrosarcoma (FSA)
FSH. See Follicle-stimulating hormone (FSH)
Fucosidosis, cerebellar dysfunction in, 979t
Fulminant congestive heart failure, treatment of, 58-60, 59t
Fundus, examination of, in nasal discharge evaluation, 211, 213, 213f
Fungal arthritis, 1084-1085
Fungal pneumonia, 302
Fungizone. See Amphotericin B
Fungus(i)
    cutaneous, culture techniques for, 1235-1236
    cytologic examination for, 1234
    fecal examination for, 368
    lymphadenopathy associated with, 1202t
    myocarditis from, 117
    nasal plaques from, differential diagnosis of, 223t
    zoonotic, 1314, 1315f
FUO. See Fever of undetermined origin (FUO)
Furazolidone
    dosages of, 402t, 470t
    for giardiasis, 445
    uses of, 402t
Furosemide
    for ascites, 550
    for chronic renal failure, 618t
    for congestive heart failure, 57, 62-63
        in AV valve degeneration, 144, 145
        in patent ductus arteriosus, 155
    for cyclophosphamide-induced hemorrhagic cystitis, 1115
    for dilated cardiomyopathy
        in cat, 132
        in dog, 109, 110, 111t, 112
    dosage of, 206t
    dosages of, 62t, 341t
    for electrolyte disorders, 845t
    gentamicin-induced nephrotoxicity and, 612
    for head trauma, 984
    for hepatobiliary and pancreatic disorders, 566t
    for hydrocephalus, 994
    for hypercalcemia, 839, 839t
    for hypertension, 202t
    for massive hepatic necrosis, 548
    for neurologic disorders, 1069t
    preparations of, 63t
    for pulmonary edema, 313
    for pulmonary edema in cats, 128, 128t
    for respiratory distress in lung disease, 336
    for restrictive cardiomyopathy, 130
    for urinary tract disorders, 659t
Furoxone. See Furazolidone

**G**

GABA. See Gamma-aminobutyric acid (GABA)
Gagging, in laryngeal paralysis, 246
Gait
    abnormal
        diagnostic approach to, 976f
        in joint disorders, 1071
    in neurologic examination, 948, 949f
    in wobbler syndrome, 1041
Galactorrhea, 883
Galactostasis, 882-883
Galastop. See Cabergoline

Gallbladder
  dilated, ultrasonographic appearance
    of, 495, 496f
  mucocele in, 539, 539f
  ultrasonographic findings in, 497t
Gallop sounds, 8-9
Gamma-aminobutyric acid (GABA), in
    hepatic encephalopathy
    pathogenesis, 481
Gamma-glutamyl transpeptidase (GGT),
    in urine, monitoring of, in
    patients at risk for ARF, 613
Gamma-glutamyltransferase (GGT), ac-
    tivity of, in hepatobiliary dis-
    orders, 486-487, 492t
Gammopathy(ies)
  monoclonal, 1211, 1211t
    in chronic leukemias in dogs, 1139
  polyclonal, 1211, 1211t
Gangliosidosis, cerebellar dysfunction in,
    979t
Gastric dilation/volvulus (GVD), 424-
    426, 425f
Gastric lavage, in emergency treatment of
    intoxications, 997t
Gastric outflow obstruction, 421-427
  from benign muscular pyloric hyper-
    trophy, 421, 422f
  from gastric antral mucosal hypertro-
    phy, 421, 423, 423f
  from gastric dilation/volvulus, 424-
    426, 425f
  from gastric foreign objects, 423-424
  radiography of, 372, 373f
Gastric stasis, 421-427
Gastrin, serum concentrations of, in ali-
    mentary tract disease, 379
Gastrinoma, 775-776, 775t
Gastritis
  acute, 418-419
  atrophic, 419-420
  chronic, 419-420
  endoscopic view of, 382f
  eosinophilic, 419-420
  granulomatous, 419-420
  granulomatous enteritis with, 449
  *Helicobacter*, 420, 420f
    drug therapy for, 401
  lymphocytic-plasmacytic, 419-420
  *Ollulanus tricuspis*, 421
  *Physaloptera*, 419, 420-421
Gastroduodenal ulceration and erosion,
    hematemesis in, 351
Gastroduodenoscopy
  biopsy and, in alimentary tract disease,
    380-381, 382-383f
  in gastrinomas, 775-776
Gastroenteritis, hemorrhagic, 419
Gastroenterocolitis
  complicating chemotherapy, 1111
  eosinophilic, canine, 448-449
Gastrography, contrast-enhanced, 374-376
Gastrointestinal adsorbents, in emer-
    gency treatment of intoxica-
    tions, 997t
Gastrointestinal tract, 343-471. *See also*
    Digestive system
Gastrointestinal ulceration/erosion
    (GUE), 427-428, 428f
Gastropexy, for gastric dilation/volvulus,
    425
Gastrostomy tube(s), 392, 393-394f, 395
  for acquired megaesophagus, 411
  in congenital esophageal weakness
    management, 411
  in esophagitis management, 412
  placement of, 508, 510-511f
  uses of, 395
Gaucher's disease, cerebellar dysfunction
    in, 979t
GDV. *See* Gastric dilation/volvulus
    (GVD)
Gemfibrozil
  in hyperlipidemia management, 826
  for hypertriglyceridemia, 845t

Genital infections, 934-938
  *Brucella canis*, 936-938
  herpesvirus, 934-935
  *Mycoplasma*, 935-936
  *Ureaplasma*, 935-936
  zoonotic, 1316-1317
Gentamicin
  dosages of, 1241t
  for feline plague, 1260
  for infectious diseases, 1318t
  nephrotoxicity induced by, furosemide
    and, 612
Geriatric canine vestibular disease, 1007-
    1008, 1007f
Geriatric incontinence, 577, 653
German Shepherds
  giant axonal neuropathy in, 1045t
  spinal muscle atrophy in, 1045t
  sudden death predisposition in, 73
Gestation length, 891
GGT. *See* Gamma-glutamyltransferase
    (GGT)
GH. *See* Growth hormone (GH)
Giant axonal neuropathy, in German
    Shepherds, 1045t
*Giardia*, 366
  drugs for, 1320t
  as enteric zoonosis, 1309t, 1311-1312
  fecal examination, 366, 1230t
  immunologic techniques for, 1236
  infection with, 445-446, 445f
  trophozoites of, *Trichomonas* tropho-
    zoites compared with, 446f
  vaccination against
    in cats, 1256
    in dogs, 1257
*Giardia* cysts, after zinc sulfate flotation,
    1232f
Giardiasis, 445-446, 445f
Gingiva
  inflammation of, 407-408
    feline lymphocytic-plasmacytic,
    408-409
  squamous cell carcinoma of, 406t
Gland(s)
  adrenal, disorders of, 778-813 (*See also*
    Adrenal gland, disorders of)
  apocrine, adenocarcinoma of, 461-462
  parathyroid, disorders of, 681-689
    hyperparathyroidism as, 681-686
    (*See also*
    Hyperparathyroidism)
    hypoparathyroidism as, 686-689
    (*See also*
    Hypoparathyroidism)
  perianal, tumors of, 462
  pituitary, disorders of, 660-680 (*See
    also* Pituitary disorders)
  prostate, disorders of, 927-933 (*See also*
    Prostate gland)
  salivary, necrosis of, 405-406
  thyroid, disorders of, 691-728 (*See also*
    Thyroid disorders)
Glipizide, 755, 755t, 756f, 757t
  for endocrine disorders, 814t
Globoid cell leukodystrophy, cerebellar
    dysfunction in, 979t
Glomerular amyloidosis, 602-603, 603f
  treatment of, 606
Glomerular filtration, acute renal failure
    and, 609-610
Glomerular filtration rate (GFR), 584-585
Glomerulonephropathies, 600-607
  clinical features of, 603-605, 604t
  diagnosis of, 605
  diseases associated with, 601t
  etiology of, 600-603, 601f
  immune complexes and, 600, 601f
  membranoproliferative, 602, 602f
  pathogenesis of, 604f
  pathophysiology of, 600-603, 601f,
    602f, 603f, 604f
  prognosis of, 607
  treatment of, 605-607, 605t

Glomerulus, systemic lupus erythemato-
    sus and, 1220t
Glucagon, for endocrine disorders, 814t
Glucocerebrosidosis, cerebellar dysfunc-
    tion in, 979t
Glucocorticoids
  for acute addisonian crisis, 807t, 808
  for allergic rhinitis, 240
  for American trypanosomiasis, 1304
  for aspiration pneumonia, 306
  for brachycephalic airway syndrome,
    248
  for canine chronic bronchitis, 297
  for canine distemper, 1017
  for chronic hepatitis, 536-537
  chronic hepatitis from, 529
  for cystic endometrial hyperplasia-
    pyometra complex, 879
  for eosinophilic lung disease, 304
  excess of
    endocrine alopecia from, 667-668,
    668t
    myopathy associated with, 1065
  for feline bronchitis, 293-294
  for feline upper respiratory infection,
    230
  hepatotoxicity of, 522t
  for histoplasmosis, 1292
  for hypocortisolism from mitotane ex-
    cess, 794
  for hypoglycemia in insulin-secreting
    β-cell neoplasia, 772t, 774
  for idiopathic, immune-mediated
    polyarthritis, 1088
  for laryngeal paralysis, 247
  for obstructive laryngitis, 249
  for pericardial effusion, 190
  for respiratory distress in lung disease,
    336
  for rickettsial polyarthritis, 1084
  for status epilepticus, 996t
Glucophage. *See* Metformin
Glucosamine
  for degenerative joint disease, 1081
  for rheumatoid arthritis, 1090
Glucose
  blood concentrations of
    decreased, 729-731
    elevated, 729
    measurement of, in diabetes
    diagnosis, 732
    serial measurement of, curve of, in
    diabetes management
    in cats, 758, 759f
    in dogs, 739-741, 740f, 741f, 742f,
    743f
  counterregulation of, in insulin ther-
    apy, 744-745, 745f
  for hypoglycemia, 731
  serum concentration of, in hepatobil-
    iary system assessment, 488,
    492t
Glucotrol. *See* Glipizide
Glutamine, in enteral diets, 392
Glyburide, 755, 755t, 757
  for endocrine disorders, 814t
Glycogenosis IV, cerebellar dysfunction
    in, 979t
Glycoproteinosis, neuronal, cerebellar
    dysfunction in, 979t
Glycopyrrolate
  for arrhythmias, 95-96
  commercial preparations of, 88t
  dosages of, 80t, 208t, 341t
Glycosaminoglycans
  decreased concentration of, in urine,
    urate urolithiasis and, 634-
    635
  polysulfated, for joint disease, 1092t
Glycosuria
  monitoring for, in diabetes manage-
    ment, 739
  testing for, in diabetes diagnosis, 732,
    733

GME. *See* Granulomatous meningoen-
    cephalitis (GME)
Gold salts, as immunosuppressants, 1218
Gold sodium thiomalate, for immune-
    mediated disorders, 1218
Golden Retrievers
  hypomyelinating polyneuropathy of,
    1045t
  muscular dystrophy of, 1066
Gonadal-dependent sex hormone imbal-
    ance, endocrine alopecia dif-
    ferentiated from, 668-669
Gonadotropin-releasing hormone
    (GnRH)
  antagonists of, in reproductive func-
    tion suppression, 867
  assessment of, 857-858, 857t
  in ovulation induction, 869
  for reproductive disorders, 944t
Gonadotropin-releasing hormone
    (GnRH) analog, in estrus in-
    duction, 868
Gonadotropins
  assessment of, 856-857, 857t
  in male sexual development, 905, 906
Gram-negative pyoderma, antibiotics for,
    1244t
Granulocyte colony-stimulating factor,
    for myelosuppression in che-
    motherapy patient, 1111
Granulocyte-macrophage colony-
    stimulating factor, for myelo-
    suppression in chemother-
    apy patient, 1111
Granuloma(s)
  eosinophilic
    feline, 407
    lymphadenopathy associated with,
    1202t
  laryngoscopy/pharyngoscopy of, 244-
    245
Granulomatosis
  eosinophilic, pulmonary, in heartworm
    disease, treatment of, 176-
    177
  lymphomatoid, 309
    lymphadenopathy associated with,
    1202t
  pulmonary, eosinophilic, 303-304
Granulomatous enteritis, 449
Granulomatous gastritis, 419-420, 449
Granulomatous meningoencephalitis
    (GME), 1012-1013, 1012f
  CSF analysis in, 964t
Gray matter, spongiform degeneration of,
    in Bull Mastiffs, 1044t
Greyhounds, erosive polyarthritis of,
    1091
Griseofulvin
  hepatotoxicity of, 522t
  neutropenia from, 1175t
Growth hormone (GH)
  excessive secretion of, feline
    acromegaly from, 673-674
  for pituitary dwarfism, 679
  porcine
    for endocrine disorders, 814t
    for growth hormone-responsive
    dermatosis in adult dog, 671,
    673f
Growth hormone-responsive dermatosis
    in adult dog, 670-671, 672-673f, 673,
    673t
  clinical features of, 671, 672f
  clinical pathology of, 671
  clinical signs of, 671, 672f
  dermatohistopathology of, 671
  diagnosis of, 671, 673t
  etiology of, 670-671
  prognosis for, 673
  treatment of, 671, 673, 673f
  endocrine alopecia differentiated from,
    668
GUE. *See* Gastrointestinal ulceration/
    erosion (GUE)

**H**

*Haemobartonella canis,* morphologic characteristics of, 1233t

*Haemobartonella felis,* morphologic characteristics of, 1233t

Hair growth, delayed, from chemotherapy drugs, 1113

Haircoat
in diabetes mellitus, in dogs, 732
in hypothyroidism, 692-693, 695f

Halitosis
causes of, 344t
in digestive disorders, 343, 345
from oropharyngeal mass, 1150

Halothane
ECG changes from, 27t
hepatotoxicity of, 522t

Haw syndrome, 989-990

HCM. *See* Hypertrophic cardiomyopathy (HCM)

HE. *See* Hepatic encephalopathy (HE)

Head tilt, 1005-1009
in central vestibular disease, 1009
in congenital nystagmus, 1009
disorders causing, 1006t
lesion localization in, 1005-1006
in peripheral vestibular disease, 1006-1009, 1007f
bilateral, 1009

Head trauma, neuromuscular disorders from, 983-984, 984t

Heart
base of, tumors of, 195, 1119t
treatment of, 190-191
catheterization of, 47-48
chambers of, enlargement of
electrocardiography in, 15, 15t, 16f, 16t
radiography in, 32, 33t, 34, 34f
conduction system of, 13f
congenital anomalies of, 151-167
atrial septal defect as, 151, 162
atrioventricular valve malformations as, 162-163, 163f
breed dispositions for, 152t
causing cyanosis, 163-166
intracardiac shunts as, 160-162
mitral dysplasia as, 162
patent ductus arteriosus as, 152, 153-155
pulmonary hypertension with shunt reversal as, 164-166
pulmonic stenosis as, 151, 158-160, 159f, 160f
subaortic stenosis as, 152, 156-158, 157f
tetralogy of Fallot as, 164
tricuspid dysplasia as, 162-163, 163f
ventricular outflow obstructions as, 155-160
ventricular septal defect as, 151, 161-162, 161f
disease of
cyanotic, syncope or intermittent weakness from, 2t
history in, 1, 2t
signs of, 1, 2t, 3-4
failure of
congestive, 51-72 (*See also* Congestive heart failure)
signs of, 1, 2t, 3-4
in hyperkalemia, 833, 833t
hypertrophy of, in heart failure, 54
in hypokalemia, 835
massage of
external, in CPR, 100-101, 100f
internal, in CPR, 101-102
murmurs in, 9-11, 9f, 9t, 10f
remodeling of, in heart failure, 54
responses of, to congestive heart failure, 54
rhythms of (*See* Cardiac rhythm[s])
tumors of, 194-196
dog breed incidence of, 195t

Heart rate
in ECG interpretation, 28
normal, ranges for, 17t

Heart rate variability (HRV), in ECG assessment, 29, 31

Heart sounds
thoracic auscultation of, 6-11
transient, in cardiovascular examination, 7-9, 8f

Heartgard. *See* Ivermectin

Heartworm antibody tests
for cats, 171
in chylothorax, 331t

Heartworm disease, 169-183
in cats, 180-183
clinical features of, 180-181
diagnosis of, 181-182
microfilaricide therapy for, 183
prevention of, 183
treatment of, 182-183
diagnostic testing for, 170-171, 170t
in dogs, 171-180
adulticide therapy for, 174-176, 175t
pulmonary thromboembolic complications of, 176
classification of, 174, 175t
clinical features of, 172
complicated, treatment of, 176-178
diagnosis of, 172-173, 172f, 173f
microfilaricide therapy for, 178
pretreatment evaluation of, 173-174
prevention of, 178-180
drugs for, 209t
heartworm life cycle and, 169
microfilariae detection in, 171
pathophysiology of, 169-170
prevention of, drugs for, 209t
chronic hepatitis from, 529
pulmonary artery dilation in, 257f
serologic tests for, 170-171, 170t

Heat, 847
split, 862
standing, 849

Heat ablation, of parathyroid masses, 685, 685f

Heinz bodies, disorders associated with, 1159t

*Helicobacter*
as enteric zoonosis, 1309t
gastritis from, 419, 420, 420f
drug therapy for, 401
morphologic characteristics of, 1233t

Helminths, fecal examination for, 1230t

Hemangioendotheliomas, 1142-1144

Hemangiosarcoma (HSA), 195
abdominal, 468
in dogs, 1142-1144
hemorrhagic pericardial effusion from, 185
metastatic behavior of, 1118t
ultrasonographic appearance of, 495, 496f

Hematemesis, 350f, 351-352, 351t

Hematochezia, 355-356, 356t
in feline lymphocytic-plasmacytic colitis, 448

Hematologic toxicity, of cancer chemotherapy, 1108-1111

Hematology
anemia in, 1156-1169 (*See also* Anemia[s])
in blastomycosis diagnosis, 1290
combined cytopenias in, 1181-1184
erythrocytosis in, 1170-1172
fever of undetermined origin and, 1225t
hemostatic disorders in, 1185-1199 (*See also* Hemostasis)
leukocytosis in, 1173-1179
leukoerythroblastosis in, 1181-1184
leukopenia in, 1173-1179
in neuromuscular disorder diagnosis, 91

Hematomas, thymic, as mediastinal masses, 1119t

Hematopoiesis, extramedullary, infiltrative splenomegaly from, 1204

Hematuria, 572-575, 573t, 574f
causes of, 573t

Hemoabdomen, 468

Hemoculture, in *Brucella canis* infection diagnosis, 936

Hemoglobin, bovine, for immune hemolytic anemia, 1164

Hemolysis, acute and peracute, anemia from, 1167

Hemolytic anemia(s)
acquired, 1161
blood loss differentiated from, 1160
causes of, 1161t
congenital, 1161
evaluation of, 1161-1162
extravascular, 1160
immune, 1162-1164
intravascular, 1160-1161

Hemophilia, 1194

Hemoptysis, 250, 251t

Hemorrhage
in alveoli, alveolar patterns in, 258, 259t
complicating heparin therapy, 311
complicating nasal biopsy, 225
gastrointestinal, complicating liver failure, 550-551
pericardial effusion from, 185-186
into spinal canal, 1024

Hemorrhagic cystitis, from cyclophosphamide, 1114-1115

Hemorrhagic effusions, 316t, 317-318

Hemorrhagic gastroenteritis, 419

Hemorrhagic nasal discharge, 211, 211t

Hemorrhagic vulvar discharge, 870-872

Hemostasis, 1185-1199
defects in
classification of, cage-side tests for, 1187-1188, 1187t
clinical manifestations of, 1186-1187, 1186t
in disseminated intravascular coagulation, 1197t
mixed (combined), 1195-1199
disseminated intravascular coagulation as, 1195-1199 (*See also* Disseminated intravascular coagulation [DIC])
primary, 1190-1194
platelet dysfunction as, 1192-1194, 1192t, 1193f, 1193t
thrombocytopenia as, 1190-1192, 1190t
secondary, 1194-1195
thrombosis as, 1199
laboratory evaluation of, specimens for, 1188-1189, 1189t
normal, 1185-1186, 1186f

Hemostatic plugs, formation of, 118

Heparin
for arterial thromboembolism, 135-136
for coagulopathy in liver failure, 550-551
for disseminated intravascular coagulation, 1198
dosages of, 341t
for hepatobiliary and pancreatic disorders, 567t
for immune hemolytic anemia, 1163
for pulmonary thromboembolism, 311
for severe pancreatitis, 559

Hepatic encephalopathy (HE), 479-481, 480f, 480t
antibiotics for, 1245t
complicating liver failure
acute, treatment of, 547-548
chronic, treatment of, 546-547
conditions accentuating or precipitating, 548t

Hepatic fibrosis, idiopathic, 530-531

Hepatic lipidosis, in cat, 506-513
clinical features of, 506-507
diagnosis of, 507, 507f
etiology of, 506
pathogenesis of, 506
treatment of, 507-508, 508f, 509-512f, 512-513

Hepatitis
chronic, 525-530
acquired canine hepatic disease known as, 526t
in Bedlington Terriers, 526-527, 527f
in Dalmatians, 528
in Doberman Pinschers, 527-528, 528f
drugs causing, 526t, 528-529
familial, 526-528
glucocorticoids for, 536-537
idiopathic, 530
infectious agents causing, 529-530
in Skye Terriers, 528
treatment of, 535-537, 535t
in West Highland White Terriers, 528
infectious, canine, lymphadenopathy associated with, 1202t
lobular dissecting, 530
portal, lymphocytic, 515-516

Hepatobiliary system
clinical manifestations of, 472-482, 473t
diagnostic tests for, 483-505
disorders of, 472-551
abdominal effusion in, 474-476, 475f, 476f
abdominal enlargement in, 472-476, 473f, 473t, 474t, 475f, 476f
abdominal muscular hypotonia as, 476
abdominocentesis/fluid analysis in, 491, 491t
biliary tract, 538-540
bilirubinuria in, 476-479, 477f
in cat, 506-524
acute toxic hepatopathy as, 521-523, 522t, 523t
congenital portosystemic shunt as, 520-521, 520f, 521f
hepatic lipidosis as, 506-513 (*See also* Hepatic lipidosis in cat)
inflammatory, 513-517, 513f, 514f, 515f, 516f, 516t
neoplastic, 517-518
secondary hepatobiliary disease as, 523-524
clinically relevant, 484t
coagulation tests in, 492, 492f
coagulopathies as, 481-482, 481t
complete blood count in, 485-486
diagnostic approach to, 483-484
diagnostic imaging in, 492-499, 493f, 494f, 495-496f, 497-498f, 498f
in dog, 525-543
acute toxic hepatopathy as, 537-538
arterioportal fistula as, 535
chronic hepatitis as, 525-530
congenital portosystemic shunt as, 531-533, 531f, 531t, 532f
focal hepatic lesions as, 541-542, 541f
hepatoportal fibrosis as, 534
idiopathic hepatic fibrosis as, 530-531
idiopathic noncirrhotic portal hypertension as, 534-535
of liver, treatment of, 535-537, 535t
neoplastic, 542
primary portal vein hypoplasia as, 534
drugs for, 565-567t
fecal evaluation in, 491

Hepatobiliary system—cont'd
  disorders of—cont'd
    hepatic encephalopathy as, 479-481, 480f, 480t
    jaundice in, 476-479, 477f, 478f
    microvascular dysplasia as, 533
    polydipsia as, 482, 482t
    polyuria as, 482, 482t
    radiography in, 492-494, 493f, 494f, 495f
    scintigraphy of, 498f, 499
    ultrasonography in, 494-499, 495f, 496f, 497-498t
    urinalysis in, 490-491, 490f
  function of, assessment of, 487-490
    plasma ammonia concentration in, 489-490, 490t, 492t
    serum albumin concentration in, 487, 492t
    serum bile acid concentrations in, 488-489, 492t
    serum bilirubin concentration in, 487-488, 492t
    serum cholesterol concentration in, 488, 492t
    serum electrolyte concentrations in, 488
    serum enzyme activities in, 486-487
    serum glucose concentration in, 488, 492t
    serum urea nitrogen concentration in, 487, 492t
    status of, tests to assess, 486-487
Hepatocellular carcinoma, 517
  radiography of, 494f
Hepatocellular dysfunction, mechanisms of polyuria and polydipsia in, 482, 482t
Hepatomegaly, 472
  differential diagnosis of, 474t, 476f
  in hepatic lipidosis, 507
  radiography of, 493, 493f
Hepatopathy, toxic, acute, 521-523, 522t, 523t, 537-538
Hepatoportal fibrosis, 534
Hepatosplenomegaly, 472
  differential diagnosis of, 476f
*Hepatozoon americanum*, morphologic characteristics of, 1234t
*Hepatozoon canis*
  drugs for, 1320t
  morphologic characteristics of, 1234t
  myocarditis from, 117
Hepatozoonosis, 1302-1303
  antibiotics for, 1246t
  lymphadenopathy associated with, 1202t
Heptolite. See Disofenin
Hereditary Afghan myelopathy, 1044t
Hereditary ataxia
  in Jack Russell terriers, 1044t
  in smooth-coated Fox Terriers, 1044t
Hereditary factors, in cryptorchidism, 923
Hereditary polyneuropathy, of Alaskan Malamutes, 1045t
Hernia(s)
  diaphragmatic
    peritoneopericardial, 192, 193
    pleural effusions and, 316-317
  hiatal, 412, 413f
  perineal, 460-461
Herpesvirus
  canine
    genital infections from, 934-935
    reproductive problems from, 854-855
  feline
    genital infections from, 934-935
    reproductive problems from, 854-855
    upper respiratory infection from, 228
HES. See Hypereosinophilic syndrome (HES)

Hetastarch, 832t
  for shock, 388
Hiatal hernia, 412, 413f
Histamine₂-receptor antagonists
  for acute spinal injury, 1023
  as antacids, 397, 397t
  for gastrointestinal ulceration/erosion, 428
  for vomiting, in chronic renal failure, 621
Histiocytosis, malignant, lymphadenopathy associated with, 1202t
*Histoplasma capsulatum*
  cytologic appearance of, 1288t
  infection from, 1291-1293, 1292f
  in tracheal wash specimen, 268f
Histoplasmosis, 1291-1293, 1292f
  gastrointestinal, 439
  lymphadenopathy associated with, 1202t
History, failure of, history in, 1, 2t
HMG-CoA reductase inhibitors, for hypercholesterolemia, 827
Holter monitoring, 29, 31f
Hoods, oxygen, 337, 338f
Hookworms, 442f, 443
Hormonal therapy, adjunct, for mammary neoplasia, 885
Hormone(s)
  anticancer, 1107
  antidiuretic
    exogenous, response to, in urinary disorder evaluation, 587-588
    release of, in congestive heart failure, 53-54
  diabetogenic
    increased levels of, in diabetic ketoacidosis, 763
    secretion of, in insulin therapy, 745
  follicle-stimulating, 847-852 (See also Follicle-stimulating hormone [FSH])
  luteinizing, 847-852 (See also Luteinizing hormone [LH])
  parathyroid, plasma concentrations of, interactions of, with calcium, phosphorus and vitamin D concentrations, 620f
    in chronic renal failure, 621f
  reproductive, assessment of, 855-858, 857t
  sex
    evaluation of, in male reproductive function assessment, 912-913
    imbalance of
      adrenal-dependent, endocrine alopecia differentiated from, 669-670
      gonadal-dependent, endocrine alopecia differentiated from, 668-669
    thyroid, tests of, 697-700, 697f, 698f, 699f, 699t
    thyroid-stimulating, endogenous concentration of, baseline, 700, 701f
Hormone replacement therapy
  for incontinence with decreased sphincter tone, 656
  in micturition disorder diagnosis, 654-655
Horner's syndrome, 987-989, 987f, 987t, 988f, 989f
  anisocoria in, 986
  from spinal neoplasia, 1034
  third eyelid protrusion in, 989
Host defense mechanisms, urinary tract infections and, 625-626, 625t
Host response, in antibiotic responsive enteropathy, 450
Howell-Jolly bodies, disorders associated with, 1159t
HRV. See Heart rate variability (HRV)
HSA. See Hemangiosarcoma (HSA)

Human chorionic gonadotropin (hCG)
  in ovulation induction, 869
  for reproductive disorders, 945t
Humidification, for bacterial pneumonia, 301
Humoral hypercalcemia of malignancy, 836-837, 838
Humoral immunodeficiency syndromes, 1226, 1227t
Husky
  Alaskan, laryngeal paralysis in, 1046t
  Siberian, laryngeal paralysis in, 1046t
Hycodan. See Hydrocodone bitartrate
Hydralazine
  for chronic renal failure, 618t
  for congestive heart failure, 65-66
    in AV valve degeneration, 144, 145
  for dilated cardiomyopathy, 111t, 112
  dosages of, 62t, 206t
  for fulminant congestive heart failure, 59, 59t
  for hypertension, 202t, 203
  preparations of, 63t
  for urinary tract disorders, 659t
Hydration, airway, for bacterial pneumonia, 300t, 301
Hydrocarbons, chlorinated, neurologic dysfunction from, 995t
Hydrocephalus
  CSF analysis in, 964t
  seizures in, 994, 998f
Hydrochlorothiazide
  for calcium oxalate uroliths, 639
  dosages of, 62t, 206t
  for hypertension, 202t
  preparations of, 63t
Hydrocodone bitartrate
  for cough in dogs, 288, 288t
  dosages of, 341t
Hydrocortisone hemisuccinate, for acute addisonian crisis, 808
Hydrocortisone phosphate, for acute addisonian crisis, 808
Hydrocortisone sodium succinate, for endocrine disorders, 814t
Hydrodiuril. See Hydrochlorothiazide
Hydromorphone
  dosages of, 341t, 565t
  indications for, 565t
  in respiratory distress, 334t
  for severe pancreatitis, 559
Hydromyelia, 1048
Hydroxyurea
  for leukemias, chronic, 1138t, 1154t
  for polycythemia rubra vera, 1172
  for pulmonary hypertension with shunt reversal, 166
Hyperactivity, in hyperthyroidism, 713
Hyperadrenocorticism
  adrenal-dependent sex hormone imbalance associated with, 669
  in cats, 798-804
    clinical features of, 798, 799f, 799t, 800-801, 800f
    diagnosis of, 803
      imaging in, 802-803
    etiology of, 798
    prognosis for, 803-804
    treatment of, 803
  in dogs, 778-798
    clinical features of, 779f, 780-782, 780t, 781f, 782f
    clinical pathology of, 782-783, 782t
    diagnosis of, 782-792
      imaging in, 783-786, 783t, 784-785f, 786f
      pituitary-adrenocortical axis tests in, 786, 787t, 788-792
    etiology of, 778-780, 779f
    iatrogenic, 779-780
    medical complications of, 780-782, 782t
    pituitary-dependent, 778, 779f
      treatment of, 792-797
        adrenalectomy in, 796-797
        ketoconazole in, 795-796

Hyperadrenocorticism—cont'd
  in dogs—cont'd
    pituitary-dependent—cont'd
      treatment of—cont'd
        L-Deprenyl in, 796
        mitotane in, 792-795 (See also Mitotane for pituitary-dependent hyperadrenocorticism)
        radiation therapy in, 797, 798f
        trilostane in, 796
      prognosis for, 797-798
  hypertriglyceridemia and, 824
Hyperammonemia, postchallenge, in congenital portosystemic shunt, 521
Hyperbilirubinemia, 476
  in feline coronavirus, 1277
Hypercalcemia, 836-839, 838f, 839t
  in anal sac adenocarcinoma, 461-462
  clinical features of, 837
  diagnosis of, 837-839, 838f
  ECG changes in, 27t
  etiology of, 836-837
  identification of, 836
  in lymphadenopathy, 1207
  in lymphoma, 1124
  of malignancy, 836-837, 838
  treatment of, 839, 839t
Hypercalciuria, in calcium oxalate urolithiasis, 633
Hypercholesterolemia, 822
  clinical signs of, 824t
  management of, 826-827
  in nephrotic syndrome, 603-604
Hyperchylomicronemia, 823
  peripheral nerve disorders in, 1054
Hypercoagulability, in nephrotic syndrome, 605
Hyperechoic tissues, 36
Hypereosinophilic syndrome (HES), 1177, 1204
  feline eosinophilic enteritis in, 449
Hyperglobulinemia, in lymphadenopathy, 1207
Hyperglycemia, 729, 730t
  in acute pancreatitis, 554
  persistent, in diabetes diagnosis, 733
  stress-induced
    in cats
      complicating insulin therapy, 759-760, 760f
      serum fructosamine in, 758
    in dogs, serum fructosamine in, 741-742
Hyperhomocysteinemia, in thromboembolism, 137
Hyperinsulinemia, in diabetes mellitus, 731
Hyperkalemia, 832-834, 833t, 834t
  in acute renal failure, management of, 614-615
  atrial function and, 23
  electrocardiography in, 26, 27f, 27t, 637t
  in hypoadrenocorticism, 805-806, 806t
  treatment recommendations for, 637t
Hyperkinetic arterial pulses, 6
  in patent ductus arteriosus, 153
Hyperlipidemia, 822-827
  causes of, 823t
  classification of, 823-824
  clinical features of, 824, 824t, 825t
  diagnosis of, 824-825
  management of, 825-827, 825t, 826t
  pathophysiology of, 822-823
Hyperlipoproteinemia, in acute pancreatitis development, 553t
Hypermagnesemia, 843
Hypermetria, 977-980
  diagnostic approach to, 979-980
  etiology of, 978, 978t, 979t
Hypernatremia, 828-830, 829t

Hyperparathyroidism, 681-686
  classification of, 681
  primary, 681-686
    clinical features of, 682-683, 683t
    diagnosis of, 683, 684f, 684t, 685f
    etiology of, 681-682, 682f, 682t, 684t
Hyperpathia, in neurologic examination, 955-957, 956f, 957t
Hyperphosphatemia, 841-842, 841t
  in chronic renal failure, management of, 619, 621
  in hypoparathyroidism, 687
Hyperplasia, in cytologic specimen interpretation, 1094
Hyperplastic lymphadenopathy, cytologic evaluation of, 1098-1099
Hyperpnea, 333
Hyperproteinemia, 1210-1211, 1211f, 1211t
  in lymphoma, 1125
Hyperreflexia, detrusor, 576-577
  incontinence from, 653
Hypersensitivity reactions, to chemotherapy drugs, 1112
Hypersplenism, 1206
Hypertension, 198-204
  in chronic renal failure, management of, 618
  clinical features of, 201
  complications of, 199t
  diagnosis of, 201
  drugs for, 202-203, 202t
  etiology of, 198-199, 199t
  in hyperthyroidism, 716
  pathology of, 199-200
  pathophysiology of, 199
  portal
    congestive splenomegaly from, 1205
    noncirrhotic, idiopathic, 534-535
    portal venous, intrahepatic, ascites in, 474
  pulmonary
    from heartworm disease, 169
    with shunt reversal, 164-166
  therapy of, 201-203, 202t, 204t
Hypertensive crisis, drugs for, 202t, 203
Hyperthermia, malignant, 1068
Hyperthyroidism
  in cats, 712-724
    clinical features of, 712-713, 715t
    clinical pathology of, 713-714
    diagnosis of, 716-720, 717f, 717t, 718-719f
      baseline serum free $T_4$ concentration in, 717, 718f
      baseline serum $T_4$ concentration in, 716, 717f, 718f
      radionuclide thyroid scanning in, 713f, 714f, 715f, 720
      $T_3$ suppression test in, 717-718, 719f, 720
      TRH stimulation test in, 720
    etiology of, 712, 713f, 714f, 715f
    feline hypertrophic cardiomyopathy and, 122-123
    problems concurrent with, 714, 716
    prognosis for, 724
    treatment of, 720-724, 721t, 722f, 723t
      antithyroid drugs in, 721-722, 721t
      radioactive iodine in, 723-724
      surgery in, 722-723, 723t
  digitalis toxicity and, 69
  hepatobiliary disease secondary to, 523
Hypertonic enemas, administration of, 403
Hypertonic saline
  for hyponatremia, 832
  for shock, 387-388
Hypertriglyceridemia, 822, 823
  clinical signs of, 824t
  management of, 825-826, 825t

Hypertrophic cardiomyopathy (HCM)
  in dogs, 115-116
  feline, 122-129
    clinical features of, 124
    echocardiography in, 124, 126-127f, 127
    electrocardiography in, 124
    etiology of, 122
    radiography in, 124, 125f
    treatment of, 127-129, 128t
  pathology of, 123-124
  pathophysiology of, 123
Hyperventilation, in head trauma management, 984
Hypoadrenocorticism, 804-809
  clinical features of, 805-806, 805t
  clinicopathologic abnormalities in, 805-806, 806t
  diagnosis of, 806-807, 807t
  etiology of, 804-805
  prognosis for, 809
  treatment of, 807-809, 807t
Hypoalbuminemia
  in acute pancreatitis, 554
  in digestive disorders, 366
  in ehrlichiosis, 1269
  pleural effusions secondary to, 316
Hypoaldosteronism, from mitotane excess, 795
Hypoallergenic diet, 389, 390t
  for canine eosinophilic gastroenterocolitis, 449
Hypocalcemia, 840-841
  in acute pancreatitis, 554
  after parathyroid surgery, management of, 686
  causes of, 688t
  complicating thyroidectomy, 723, 723t
  ECG changes in, 27t
  in hypoparathyroidism, 687
  puerperal, 896
Hypochloremia, in hypoadrenocorticism, 805-806, 806t
Hypochromia, disorders associated with, 1159t
Hypoechoic tissues, 36
Hypoglycemia, 729-731, 730t
  chronic, in insulin-secreting β-cell neoplasia, medical treatment of, 772t, 773-774
  complicating insulin therapy
    in cats, 760-761
    in dogs, 744
  episodic weakness from, 977
  in insulin-secreting β-cell neoplasia, 770-771
  neonatal mortality from, 903
  polyneuropathy in, 1055
Hypoglycemic drugs, oral, for diabetes management in cats, 753, 755-757, 755t, 756f, 757t
Hypogonadism, in pituitary dwarfism, 677
Hypokalemia, 833t, 834-836, 835t
  acute renal failure and, 612
  electrocardiography in, 26, 27t
  myocardial toxicity of digitalis and, 69
Hypokalemic polymyopathy, 1065-1066
Hypokinetic arterial pulses, 6
Hypomagnesemia, 843-845, 844t
Hypomotility, gastric, idiopathic, 427
Hypomyelinating polyneuropathy, of Golden Retrievers, 1045t
Hyponatremia, 830t, 831t, 832-838
  in hypoadrenocorticism, 805-806, 806t
Hypoparathyroidism
  complicating thyroidectomy, 723
  primary, 686-689
    clinical features of, 687, 687t
    diagnosis of, 687-688, 688t
    etiology of, 686-687, 688t
    prognosis of, 689
    treatment of, 688-689, 689t
Hypophosphatemia, 842-843, 842t

Hypophysectomy, transsphenoidal, microsurgical, for feline acromegaly, 677
Hypoproteinemia, fluid therapy in, 389
Hyposplenism, 1206
Hypospadia, 919-920
Hypotension, from phenoxybenzamine, 655
Hypothalamic disorders, 660-680
  in cats, clinical pathology of, 800-801
  diabetes insipidus as, 661-667 (See also Diabetes insipidus)
  endocrine alopecia as, 667-670 (See also Endocrine alopecia)
  feline acromegaly as, 673-677 (See also Feline acromegaly)
  growth hormone-responsive dermatosis in adult dog as, 670-673 (See also Growth hormone-responsive dermatosis in adult dog)
  pituitary dwarfism as, 677-680 (See also Pituitary dwarfism)
  polydipsia as, 660-661, 661t
  primary, 667
  polyuria as, 660-661, 661t
Hypothalamic-pituitary-gonadal axis disorders of, anestrus from, 862
  feline, 851, 852f, 856-857
Hypothalamic-pituitary-thyroid gland complex, 691, 692f
Hypothermia, neonatal mortality from, 902-903
Hypothyroidism, 691-712
  in cats, 709-712
    clinical signs of, 709-710, 709t
    diagnosis of, 711-712
    etiology of, 709
    prognosis for, 712
    treatment of, 712
  complicating thyroidectomy, 723
  digitalis toxicity and, 69
  in dogs, 691-709
    clinical features of, 691-697, 694t, 695f, 696f, 696t
    clinical pathology of, 697
    cretinism in, 695-696, 696f, 696t
    dermatohistopathologic findings in, 697
    dermatologic signs in, 692-693, 694t, 695f
    diagnosis of, 703-705
    etiology of, 691, 692f, 692t, 693f
    immunoendocrinopathy syndromes in, 696-697
    neuromuscular signs in, 693-694
    primary, 691
    prognosis for, 709
    reproductive signs in, 694, 694t
    secondary, 691
    tertiary, 691
    thyroid gland function tests in, 697-702
    treatment of, 706-709, 707t, 708f
  endocrine alopecia from, 667-668, 668t
  false pregnancy and, 887
  hypercholesterolemia and, 823
  infertility and, 862
  myopathy in, 1065
  peripheral vestibular disease in, 1008
  polyneuropathy in, 1055, 1056f
Hypotonia, abdominal muscular, 476, 476f
Hypoventilation
  in hypoxemia, 282
  ventilation/perfusion abnormalities differentiated from, 284
Hypovolemic shock, hypertonic saline solution for, 387-388
Hypoxemia
  diagnosis of, 282
  mechanisms of, 282-284
  in pulmonary thromboembolism, 310

**I**

IBD. See Inflammatory bowel disease (IBD)
IBS. See Irritable bowel syndrome (IBS)
Ibuprofen, gastrointestinal ulceration/erosion from, 427-428
Ibutilide fumarate, for arrhythmias, 94
Icteric mucous membranes, 5t
Icterus, 476-479, 477f, 478f. See also Jaundice
IDA. See Iron deficiency anemia (IDA)
Idioventricular tachycardia, 22
IFA test. See Indirect fluorescent antibody (IFA) test
Ig. See Immunoglobulin (Ig)
Ileocolic intussusception, 455, 456f
  ultrasonography of, 375f
Ileocolic valve, endoscopic view of, 384f
Ileus, radiography of, 372, 373f
IMDs. See Immune-mediated disorders (IMDs)
Imidocarb dipropionate
  for babesiosis, 1301
  for cytauxzoonosis, 1302
  for ehrlichiosis, 1270, 1271
  for hepatozoonosis, 1302
  for infectious diseases, 1319t
Imipenem
  for aspiration pneumonia, 306
  for bacterial pneumonia, 301
  for cardiopulmonary infections, 1244t
  for cutaneous and soft tissue infections, 1244t
  dosages of, 1241t
  for infectious diseases, 1318t
Imipenem-cilastin, dosages of, 341t
Imipramine, for urinary tract disorders, 659t
Immiticide. See Melarsomine
Immune complexes, glomerular response to, 600, 601f
Immune hemolytic anemia, 1162-1164
Immune-mediated disorders (IMDs), 1212-1214
  diagnostic tests for, 1213-1214, 1213t
  fever of undetermined origin in, 1223t
  immunosuppressive drugs for, 1216-1219, 1217t (See also Immunosuppressive drugs)
  organ or tissue targets in, 1213t
  systemic lupus erythematosus as, 1220-1221 (See also Systemic lupus erythematosus [SLE])
Immune-mediated lymphadenopathies, 1202t
Immune-mediated neutropenia, 1175t
Immune-mediated polyarthritides, lymphadenopathy associated with, 1202t
Immune-mediated thrombocytopenia (IMT), 1191-1192
Immune modulators, for infectious diseases, 1319t
Immune system
  cellular arm of, 1212
  compartmentalization of, 1212-1213, 1213t
  humoral arm of, 1212
  phagocytic arm of, 1212-1213
Immunocytochemistry techniques, in infectious disease detection, 1236
Immunodeficiency syndromes, 1226-1228, 1227t
Immunodeficiency virus, feline, 1278-1281. See also Feline immunodeficiency virus (FIV)
Immunoendocrinopathy syndromes, in hypothyroidism, 696-697
Immunofluorescence, direct, for immune-mediated disorders, 1214
Immunofluorescent techniques, in canine distemper virus detection, 1015

Immunoglobulin (Ig)
  for immune hemolytic anemia, 1163
  for immune-mediated thrombocy-
    topenia, 1192
Immunohistochemistry techniques
  for immune-mediated disorders, 1214
  in infectious disease detection, 1236
Immunologic tests
  for infectious diseases, 1236
  for joint disorders, 1077-1078
  for neuromuscular disorders, 973
Immunology
  for clinician, 1212-1213
  immune-mediated diseases in, 1212-
    1214
  leukocytosis in, 1173-1179
  leukopenia in, 1173-1179
  lymphadenopathy in, 1200-1204 (*See
    also* Lymphadenopathy)
  splenomegaly in, 1204-1209 (*See also*
    Splenomegaly)
Immunoproliferative enteropathy, in
    Basenjis, 449-450
Immunoreglan. *See Propionibacterium
    acnes*
Immunosuppressive drugs, 1216-1219
  azathioprine as, 1217-1218
  chlorambucil as, 1218
  corticosteroids as, 1216-1217
  cyclophosphamide as, 1217
  cyclosporin A as, 1218
  danazol as, 1218-1219
  for digestive disorders, 400
  gold salts as, 1218
  for localized myasthenia gravis, 411
  for perianal fistulae, 461
Immunotherapy, for feline leukemia virus
    infection, 1283
Imodium. *See* Loperamide
Implantation, 887-888
IMT. *See* Immune-mediated thrombocy-
    topenia (IMT)
Imuran. *See* Azathioprine
Incarcerated intestinal obstruction, 452-
    453, 453f
Incontinence
  fecal, 358
  urinary, 575-577
    with decreased sphincter tone,
      treatment of, 656
    with distended bladder, 651-652,
      652t
    geriatric, 653
    paradoxic, 652
    with small or normal-sized bladder,
      652-653, 652t
Incoordination, 974, 975f, 975t, 976f
Inderal. *See* Propranolol
Indirect fluorescent antibody (IFA) tests
  for babesiosis, 1301
  for rickettsial infections, 1077
Indomethacin, gastrointestinal
    ulceration/erosion from,
    427-428
Infarction
  brain, CSF analysis in, 964t
  spinal cord, 1024
    CSF analysis in, 964t
Infection(s)
  anaerobic
    antibiotics for, 1240, 1243, 1243f,
      1243t, 1244t
    clinical findings in, 1243t
  in aspiration pneumonia, 305
  cardiopulmonary, antibiotics for, 1244t
  chronic hepatitis from, 529-530
  CNS, antibiotics for, 1246t, 1247
  complicating chemotherapy, 1110
  cutaneous, antibiotics for, 1244t, 1245
  diarrhea from, 352t
  genital, 934-938 (*See also* Genital
    infections)
  hepatobiliary disease secondary to,
    523-524
  musculoskeletal, antibiotics for, 1246-
    1247, 1246t

Infection(s)—cont'd
  mycotic, CNS involvement in, 1018
  neonatal mortality from, 903, 903t
  parvovirus, neutropenia in, 1175t
  *Physaloptera*, of stomach, endoscopic
    view of, 383f
  recurrent, 1226-1228
  respiratory tract, 1247-1248
  soft-tissue, antibiotics for, 1244t, 1245
  upper respiratory tract, feline, 228-232
    (*See also* Feline upper respi-
      ratory infection)
  urinary tract, 568-569, 569t, 624-630
    (*See also* Urinary tract, infec-
      tions of)
  urogenital tract, antibiotics for, 1248-
    1249, 1248t
  uterine, postpartum, 896-897
Infectious diarrhea, 433-440
Infectious diseases, 1229-1320
  bacterial, polysystemic, 1259-1264 (*See
    also* Bacteria, polysystemic
    diseases from)
  cytologic morphology of, 1232-1234,
    1233t, 1234t
  drugs for, 1318-1320t
  fever of undetermined origin in, 1223t
  laboratory diagnosis of, 1229-1238
    animal inoculation in, 1237
    culture techniques in, 1235-1236
    cytology in, 1232-1234, 1232f, 1233t,
      1234t
    demonstration of organism in,
      1229-1237
    electron microscopy in, 1237
    fecal examination in, 1229-1232,
      1230t, 1231f, 1231t, 1232f
    immunologic techniques in, 1236
    polymerase chain reaction in, 1236-
      1237, 1236f
    tissue techniques in, 1235
  mycotic, polysystemic, 1287-1294 (*See
    also* Mycotic infections,
    polysystemic)
  neutropenia in, 1175t
  prevention of, 1250-1257
    biosecurity procedures for
      for clients, 1252
      for small animal hospitals, 1250-
        1252, 1251t
    disinfection protocols in, 1252
    in hospitalized patients, 1251-1252
    patient evaluation in, 1251
    vaccination protocols in, 1252-1257
      (*See also* Vaccination
        protocols)
  protozoal, polysystemic, 1296-1304
    (*See also* Protozoa, polysys-
      temic infections from)
  rickettsial, polysystemic, 1265-1271
    (*See also* Rickettsiae, polysys-
      temic diseases from)
  viral, polysystemic, 1273-1284 (*See also*
    Virus(es), polysystemic dis-
    eases from)
  zoonotic, 1307-1317 (*See also*
    Zoonoses)
Infectious hepatitis, canine, lymphade-
    nopathy associated with,
    1202t
Infectious inflammatory disease, spinal
    cord dysfunction in, 1031
Infectious pericarditis, treatment of, 191
Infectious peritonitis, feline, 469, 1016-
    1017, 1275-1278. *See also* Fe-
    line infectious peritonitis
    (FIP)
Infectious tracheobronchitis, canine, 287-
    289, 288f
Infective endocarditis, 145-150
  clinical features of, 146-147
  diagnosis of, 147-149, 148t, 149f
  etiology of, 145-146
  pathophysiology of, 146
  prognosis of, 149-150

Infective endocarditis—cont'd
  sequelae of, 147t
  treatment of, 149-150
Infective myocarditis, canine, 116-118
Infertility
  female, 859-865, 860t
    abnormal proestrus and estrus in,
      863
    diagnostic approach to, 861f
    failure to cycle in, 860-862
    with normal cycles, 864-865
    normal cycles in, 864-865
    prolonged estrus in, 863-864, 863f
    prolonged interestrous interval in,
      862
    short estrus in, 864
    short interestrous interval in, 862-
      863
  herpesvirus infection and, 934
  male, 905-917
    acquired, 916-918
    azoospermia and, 915-916
    in *Brucella canis* infection, 936
    congenital, 916
    diagnostic approach to, 910f, 913-
      915
    historical information for, 913t
    oligospermia and, 915-916
Infiltrative gastric diseases, 428-429
Infiltrative lymphadenopathies, 1201,
    1202t
Infiltrative splenomegaly, 1204
Inflammation
  central nervous system, 1010-1019 (*See
    also* Central nervous system
    [CNS], inflammation of)
  in cytologic specimen interpretation,
    1094-1095
  epididymal, 921-922, 922f
  esophageal, 412
  gastrointestinal, vomiting from, 348t
  glomerular, 600-602, 601f, 601t, 602f
  hyperproteinemia in, 1210-1211
  large intestinal, 458
  liver (*See* Hepatitis)
  localized, lymphadenopathy associated
    with, 1202t
  lower urinary tract, feline, 571-572,
    573f, 642-649 (*See also* Feline
    lower urinary tract inflam-
    mation [FLUTI])
  mammary gland, 882
  myocardial
    canine, 116-118
    feline, 133-134
  nasal, differential diagnosis of, 223t
  optic nerve, 985-986, 986t
  pancreatic, 552-560 (*See also*
    Pancreatitis)
  peritoneal, 466-468, 467f (*See also*
    Peritonitis)
  prostatic, bacterial, 930-931
    chronic, 931-932
  stomach, 418-421 (*See also* Gastritis)
  testicular, 921-922
    infertility from, 916-917
  thyroid, lymphocytic, tests for, 700-702
  tracheal wash and, 269-270
  vaginal, 874-875
Inflammatory bowel disease (IBD), 447-
    450. *See also* Malabsorptive
    diseases
  endoscopic view of, 383f
  in hyperthyroidism, 716
  metronidazole for, 401
Inflammatory disease(s)
  infectious, spinal cord dysfunction in,
    1031
  noninfectious, spinal cord dysfunction
    in, 1031
  seizures from, 999
Inflammatory hepatobiliary disease, 513-
    517, 513f, 514f, 515f, 516f,
    516t
  clinical features of, 513-516, 514f, 515f
  diagnosis of, 516

Inflammatory hepatobiliary disease—
    cont'd
  etiology of, 513
  pathogenesis of, 513
  prognosis of, 517
  treatment of, 516-517
Inflammatory nodules, pulmonary inter-
    stitial, 258
Infusion, constant-rate, formulas to cal-
    culate, 89t
Inherited myopathies, 1066-1068
Injection site sarcomas (ISSs), in cats,
    1151-1152
Inocor. *See* Amrinone
Inotropic drugs
  for dilated cardiomyopathy, 111-112
  positive
    in congestive heart failure
      management, 66-69
    dosages of, 67t, 206t
    preparations of, 67t
Inotropic therapy, positive, for fulminant
    congestive heart failure, 59-
    60, 59t
Insemination, artificial, 940-944. *See also*
    Artificial insemination (AI)
Insulin
  blood concentration of, in hypo-
    glycemia in insulin-secreting
    β-cell neoplasia, 770-771
  deficiency of, in diabetic ketoacidosis,
    762-763
  in diabetes management
    for cats
      circulating insulin-binding
        antibodies in, 762
      complications of, 758-762, 760f
        hypoglycemia as, 760-761
        recurrence of clinical signs as,
          761-762
        stress hyperglycemia as, 759-
          760, 760f
      concurrent disorders causing
        insulin resistance in, 762
      glucose counterregulation in, 761
      inadequate insulin absorption in,
        762
      initial adjustments in, 758
      initial therapy with, 752-753
      insulin underdosing in, 761
      monitoring techniques for, 758,
        759f
      overdosing in, 761
      prolonged duration of insulin
        effect in, 762
      short duration of insulin effect in,
        761
      Somogyi phenomenon in, 761
      during surgery, 758
    for dogs, 733-734, 734t
      allergic reactions to, 747
      circulating insulin-binding
        antibodies in, 746-747
      complications of, 744-748
        hypoglycemia as, 744
        recurrence of clinical signs as,
          744-748, 745f, 746f, 747f,
          747t, 748t
      concurrent disorders causing
        insulin resistance in, 747-
        748, 747t
      diluted insulin in, 744
      inadequate insulin absorption in,
        746
      initial adjustments in, 737
      monitoring of, 737-748
        history in, 738
        physical examination in, 738
        serial blood glucose curve in,
          739-742, 740f, 741f, 742f,
          743f
        serum fructosamine concen-
          tration in, 738-739, 738t
      during surgery, 742, 744
      urine glucose monitoring in,
        739

Insulin—cont'd
in diabetes management—cont'd
for dogs—cont'd
overdosing in, 744-745, 745f
prolonged duration of insulin
effect in, 746, 747f
short duration of insulin effect in,
746, 746f, 747f
during surgery, 742, 744
underdosing in, 744
for diabetic ketoacidosis, 765t, 767-768
for endocrine disorders, 814t
for hyperkalemia, 845t
for hyperkalemia in ARF, 614
recombinant human, properties of,
734t
for relapsing and chronic pancreatitis,
560
resistance to
in cats, concurrent disorders
causing, 762
in dogs, evaluation of, 748t
Insulin-secreting β-cell neoplasia, 769-
775
clinical features of, 769-770, 769t
diagnosis of, 770-772, 771f
etiology of, 769
prognosis for, 774
treatment of, 772-774
Interceptor. *See* Milbemycin
Interferon-α
for feline immunodeficiency virus,
1280t
for feline leukemia virus infection,
1283
Interstitial cell tumors, 925
Interstitial pattern in lung radiography,
258-260, 260f, 260t, 261f,
261t
Intervertebral disk, prolapse of, CSF
analysis in, 964t
Intervertebral disk disease
acute, 1024-1030
cervical, 1029, 1029t
clinical features of, 1024-1026, 1025f
diagnosis of, 1026, 1026f, 1027-
1028f
postoperative care in, 1030, 1030f
thoracolumbar, 1028-1029
treatment of, 1026, 1028
classification of, 1024, 1025f
type II, 1025f, 1036-1037
Intestinal lymphangiectasia, 451
Intestinal protectants, 398
Intestine. *See also* Digestive system
adenocarcinoma of, 457-458
biopsy of
in canine eosinophilic
gastroenterocolitis diagnosis,
448-449
in feline eosinophilic
enteritis/hypereosinophilic
syndrome diagnosis, 449
disorders of, 431-463
constipation as, 462-463
diarrhea as, 432-440 (*See also*
Diarrhea)
foreign objects in, linear, 454-455, 454f
functional diseases of, 452
inflammatory disease of, 447-450 (*See
also* Malabsorptive diseases)
endoscopic view of, 383f
in hyperthyroidism, 716
metronidazole for, 401
intussusception of, 455-456, 456f
irritable bowel syndrome in, 452
large
diseases of, diarrhea in,
differentiated from small
intestinal diarrheas, 353t
inflammation of, 458
inflammatory disease of,
metronidazole for, 401
intussusception/prolapse of, 458-459
neoplasms of, 459, 459f
pythiosis of, 460, 460f

Intestine—cont'd
leiomyoma/leiomyosarcoma of, 458
malabsorptive diseases of, 447-450
maldigestive disease of, 446-447
obstruction of, 452-455
in acute pancreatitis, 555t
incarcerated, 452-453, 453f
by linear foreign objects, 454-455,
454f
parasites in, 440-446
permeability testing for, 379
preparation of, for colonoscopy and
proctoscopy, 383
protein-losing enteropathy and, 451
short bowel syndrome in, 456-457
small
contrast-enhanced studies of, 376,
377f
diseases of, diarrhea in,
differentiated from large
intestinal diarrheas, 353t
neoplasms of, 457-458
obstruction of, radiography of, 372,
373f, 374f
radiography of, without contrast
media, 371-374, 373f, 374f
Intoxication
chemical/drug, mentation abnormalities from, 983
emergency treatment of, 997t
Intracardiac obstruction, cardiogenic
shock from, 119t
Intracardiac shunts, 160-162
Intracranial injury, 983-984, 984t
Intracranial pressure, control of
in head trauma management, 984-985
in hydrocephalus, 994
Intrahepatic portal venous hypertension,
ascites in, 474
Intraspinal articular cysts, 1036
Intraventricular conduction disturbances,
24-25
Intron A. *See* Alpha-interferon
Intropin. *See* Dopamine
Intussusception
cecocolic, 456f, 458
ileocolic, 455, 456f
ultrasonography of, 375f
jejunojejunal, 455-456
Iodine, radioactive
for hyperthyroidism, 723-724
for thyroid neoplasia, 727
Iohexol, for myelography, 965
Iopamidol, for myelography, 965
Iothalamate sodium, indication and
dosage of, 565t
Ipecac syrup, for neurologic disorders,
1069t
Iron deficiency anemia (IDA), 1167-1168
distinguishing features of, 1165, 1165t
in gastric tumor, 429
Irritable bowel syndrome (IBS), 452
Irritative laxatives, 403, 403t
Ischemia, in acute pancreatitis development, 553
Islet cells, vacuolar degeneration of, in diabetes mellitus in cats, 749,
749f
Isopropanol, hepatotoxicity of, 522t
Isoproterenol
for arrhythmias, 96
commercial preparations of, 88t
in congestive heart failure management, 70
dosage of, 208t
dosages of, 80t
Isoptin. *See* Verapamil
Isordil Titradone. *See* Isosorbide dinitrate
Isosorbide dinitrate
in congestive heart failure management, 66
dosages of, 62t, 206t
preparations of, 63t
*Isospora*, 444
Isovue. *See* Iopamidol

ISSs. *See* Injection site sarcomas (ISSs)
Isuprel. *See* Isoproterenol
Itraconazole
for blastomycosis, 1291
for coccidioidomycosis, 1294
for cryptococcosis, 1289, 1289t
dosages of, 341t, 470t
for histoplasmosis, 440, 1291
for infectious diseases, 1320t
for nasal aspergillosis, 236
for pythiosis, 429
Ivermectin
for *Aelurostrongylus abstrusus*, 303
dosages of, 209t, 341t, 402t, 470t
for feline ischemic encephalopathy, 999
in heartworm prevention, 179
in cats, 183
in microfilaricide therapy, 178
for nasal capillariasis, 239
for nasal mites, 238
for parasitic CNS disease, 1019
for *Physaloptera* gastritis, 421
for strongyloidiasis, 444
uses of, 402t
Ivomec. *See* Ivermectin

**J**

Jack Russell Terrier, hereditary ataxia in,
1044t
Jaundice, 476-479, 477f, 478f
in biliary tract disorders, 539
evaluation of, preliminary, 478f
medical and surgical causes of, differentiation of, 540
Jejunojejunal intussusception, 455-456
Joint(s)
disorders of, 1071-1092
arthritis as, 1072-1073 (*See also*
Arthritis; Polyarthritis)
classification of, 1072t
clinical manifestations of, 1071-1073
degenerative, 1079-1081, 1080f,
1080t
diagnostic tests for, 1073-1078
immunologic, 1077-1078
radiography as, 1073
serologic, 1077-1078
synovial fluid analysis as, 1074,
1076, 1076f, 1076t, 1077f
synovial fluid collection for, 1073-
1074, 1074f, 1075-1076f
synovial fluid culture as, 1076-
1077
synovial membrane biopsy as,
1077
drugs for, 1092t
inflammatory
diagnosis of, 1072
infectious, 1081-1085
noninfectious
erosive, 1089-1091
nonerosive, 1085-1089
noninflammatory, 1079-1081, 1080f,
1080t
pain in, diagnostic algorithm for, 1087f
swelling of, in joint disorders, 1071
Jugular veins, in cardiovascular examination, 5-6, 5f, 5t

**K**

Kaon Elixir. *See* Potassium gluconate
Kaopectate
as antiemetic, 396t
dosages of, 470t
as intestinal protectant, 398
Karyotyping, 858
KBr. *See* Potassium bromide (KBr)
Keflex. *See* Cephalexin
Keflin. *See* Cephalothin
Kennel cough, 287-289, 288f
antibiotics for, 1247
Ketamine, dosages of, 341t, 470t
Ketaset. *See* Ketamine
Ketoacidosis, diabetic, 762-769. *See also*
Diabetic ketoacidosis (DKA)

Ketoconazole
for blastomycosis, 1291
for coccidioidomycosis, 1294
for cryptococcosis, 1289, 1289t
dosages of, 470t
for endocrine disorders, 814t
hepatotoxicity of, 522t
for histoplasmosis, 1292
for infectious diseases, 1320t
for perianal fistulae, 461
for pituitary-dependent hyperadrenocorticism, 795-796
Ketonuria
in diabetes, diagnosis of, 763-764
in diagnosis of diabetic ketoacidosis,
763
monitoring for, in diabetes management, 739
Ketoprofen, for joint disease, 1092t
Key-Gaskell syndrome, pupil dilatation
in, 987
Kidney(s)
biopsy of, 598
in acute renal failure, 610-611
disease of
anemia of, 1166-1167
preexisting, acute renal failure and,
612
enlargement of, 583
excretory function of, tests of, 584-586
failure of, 608-622
acute, 608-615
in acute pancreatitis, 555t
chronic renal failure differentiated
form, 582t
clinical features of, 611, 611f
diagnosis of, 611
etiology of, 608-611, 609t, 610t
monitoring patients at risk for,
613
pathogenesis of, 608-611
phases of, 610
prerenal azotemia differentiated
from, 582t
risk factors for, 611-613, 612t
treatment of, 613-615, 614t
chronic, 615-622
acute renal failure differentiated
from, 582t
drugs used in, 618t
etiology of, 615-616, 616t
pathogenesis of, 615-616
treatment of, 617-622, 617t, 618t,
620f, 620t, 621f
definition of, 608
from feline leukemia virus infection,
1282
gastrointestinal ulceration/erosion
from, 427-428
hypercalcemia in, 837
function of, stages of, 609f
in heart failure, 54
hydronephrotic, 592f
in hyperthyroidism, 716
lymphoma of, 591f, 1124
toxicity of chemotherapy drugs for,
1114
ultrasonography of, 590, 591-592f
*Klebsiella*
pulmonary infection from, 299
urinary tract infections from, 624, 625t
*Klebsiella pneumoniae*, antimicrobial
agents for, 627, 629t
Klonopin. *See* Clonazepam
Krabbe's disease, cerebellar dysfunction
in, 979t
Kussmaul's respirations, in diabetic ketoacidosis, 763

**L**

L-Asparaginase
hypersensitivity reactions to, 1112
for leukemias, acute, 1137t
for lymphoma, 1127t, 1129, 1153t
pancreatitis from, 1113-1114

L-Deprenyl
for endocrine disorders, 815t
for pituitary-dependent hyperadrenocorticism, 796
L-form bacteria
antibiotics for, 1244t, 1246t
zoonoses associated with, 1313t
Labetalol, characteristics of, 91t
Labor
predicting, 891
stages of, 891-892
Laboratory evaluation, in digestive disorders, 365-366
Labrador Retrievers
axonopathy in, 1044t
hereditary myopathy in, 1067, 1067f
spongy degeneration of white matter
in, 1044t
Lactafal. See Bromocriptine
Lactated Ringer's solution, 832t
for hyperkalemia, 834
for hyponatremia, 832
Lactescence, 824
Lactitol, for hepatobiliary and pancreatic
disorders, 567t
Lactoferrin, bovine
for feline immunodeficiency virus,
1280t
for stomatitis, 408
Lactulose, 403, 403t
in chronic hepatic encephalopathy
management, 547
dosages of, 403t, 470t
for hepatobiliary and pancreatic disorders, 567t
for idiopathic megacolon, 463
rectal administration of, for acute hepatic encephalopathy, 547-
548
Lacty. See Lactitol
Laminectomy, for thoracolumbar disk
disease, 1029
Lanoxin. See Digoxin
Lansoprazole, as antacid, 397
Laparoscopic liver biopsy, 504, 504f
Laparoscopy, in estrous cycle disorders,
858-859
Laplace's law, 54
Lapland Dogs, Swedish, spinal muscular
atrophy in, 1046t
Larva migrans, visceral, 1307-1308, 1310
Larvae, parasitic
characteristics of, 263t
concentration of, Baermann technique
for, 264t
Larvae, *Cuterebra* fly, brain migration of,
seizures from, 999
Laryngitis, obstructive, 249
Laryngoplasty, for laryngeal paralysis, 247
Laryngoscopy, 243-245, 244f
in laryngeal paralysis diagnosis, 246
Larynx
brachycephalic airway syndrome and,
248-249, 248f
collapse of, 245
diseases of
clinical signs of, 241
differential diagnoses for, 242,
242t
diagnostic tests for, 243-245
neoplasia of, 249
paralysis of, 246-247, 247t
in Bouvier des Flandres, 1045t
in Dalmatians, 1045t
in Siberian and Alaskan Huskies,
1046t
Lasix. See Furosemide
Latex agglutination capsular antigen test
(LCAT), in nasal discharge
evaluation, 213
Laxatives, 403, 403t
osmotic, for idiopathic megacolon, 463
LCAT. See Latex agglutination capsular
antigen test (LCAT)
LE cell test. See Lupus erythematosus
(LE) cell test

Lead, neurologic dysfunction from, 995t
Lead arsenate, hepatotoxicity of, 522t
Lead axis, 12
Lead systems, ECG, 12-13, 14f, 14t
Leflunomide
for granulomatous meningoencephalitis, 1013
for rheumatoid arthritis, 1090
Leiomyoma, 877
endoscopic view of, 380, 381f
hemorrhagic discharge from, 871
Leiomyoma/leiomyosarcoma, intestinal,
458
Leiomyosarcoma, endoscopic view of,
382f
*Leishmania*
drugs for, 1320t
infection with, 1303
morphologic characteristics of, 1234t
Leishmaniasis, 1303
lymphadenopathy associated with,
1202t
Lens-induced uveitis, complicating diabetes mellitus, in dogs, 748-
749
*Leptospira*
antibiotics for, 1248t
genitourinary zoonoses from, 1317
morphologic characteristics of, 1233t
reservoirs of, 1261t
vaccination against, 1257, 1262
Leptospirosis, 1260-1262, 1261t
chronic hepatitis and, 530
LER. See Leukoerythroblastic reaction
(LER)
Lesion localization, in neurologic examination, 957
Lethargy, in hypoadrenocorticism, 805
Leukemia(s), 1133-1140
in cats, 1138-1140
vaccination against, 1255
chemotherapy protocols for, 1153-
1154t
classification of, 1133, 1134t
definition of, 1133
in dogs, 1133-1138
acute, 1134-1136, 1134t, 1135f,
1136t
chronic, 1136-1138, 1138t
lymphadenopathy associated with, 1202t
Leukemoid reaction, 1176
Leukeran. See Chlorambucil
Leukocyte(s)
changes in, in disease, 1174-1179
morphology of, normal, 1173-1174
physiology of, normal, 1173-1174
Leukocytosis, 1173-1179
in chronic leukemias in dogs, 1137
neutrophilic
in cytauxzoonosis, 1301
in hepatozoonosis, 1302
Leukodystrophy
of Dalmatians, 1044t
globoid cell, cerebellar dysfunction in,
979t
Leukoencephalomyelopathy, in Rottweilers, 1044t
Leukoerythroblastic reaction (LER), 1181
causes of, 1182t
clinicopathologic features of, 1181-
1182, 1184
Leukoerythroblastosis, 1181-1184
Leukogram, 1173
Leukopenia, 1173-1179
disorders associated with, 1159t
Leukotriene inhibitors, for feline bronchitis, 294
Levamisole
for *Capillaria*, 303
for immunodeficiency syndromes,
1227-1228
Levophed. See Norepinephrine
Levothyroxine, sodium, for hypothyroidism, 706-707, 707t
Leydig cells, in male sexual development,
905

LH. See Luteinizing hormone (LH)
Lidocaine
for arrhythmias, 87-89
in cardiopulmonary resuscitation,
dosages of, 99t
commercial preparations of, 87t
for digitalis toxicity, 69
dosages of, 79t, 207t, 209t
ECG changes from, 27t
for sustained ventricular tachycardia,
84
toxic effects of, 88
for ventricular tachyarrhythmias, 80,
81f, 82
Ligation, tubal, 866
Light, in estrus induction in queen, 868
Limb reflexes, 952, 952t, 953f
Lincomycin
for cutaneous and soft tissue infections, 1244t
dosages of, 1241t
for infectious diseases, 1319t
for *Mycoplasma* infections, 1264
for *Ureaplasma* infections, 1264
Lincosamides
dosages of, 1241t
for infectious diseases, 1319t
toxicities of, 1242t
Lipase, 553t
activity of, serum, in acute pancreatitis,
556
Lipidosis, hepatic, in cat, 506-513. See also
Hepatic lipidosis in cat
Lipofuscinosis, ceroid, cerebellar dysfunction in, 979t
Lipoma, as mediastinal mass, 1119t
Lipoprotein electrophoresis, 824-825
Lipoproteins, classes of, 822
Liposomal amphotericin B, for pythiosis,
429
Lisinopril
for chronic renal failure, 618t
in congestive heart failure management, 65
dosages of, 62t, 206t
preparations of, 63t
for urinary tract disorders, 659t
Lissencephaly
CSF analysis in, 964t
seizures in, 994-995
Lithium carbonate, for myelosuppression
in chemotherapy patient,
1111
Litter size, 888
Liver
abscesses of, 541-542, 541f
asymmetrical, differential diagnosis of,
474t
biopsy of, 499-504, 499t, 500f, 501f,
502-503f, 504f, 505f
patient and operator considerations
for, 499t
specimens from, comparison of, 504,
505f
techniques for, 501-504
laparoscopic, 504, 504f
operative, 504, 504f
percutaneous, 501, 501f, 502-503f,
503
visualized percutaneous needle,
503, 503f
coagulation proteins and inhibitors
synthesized by, 481t
disease of, 483-484
secondary, 542-543
disorders of, chronic, treatment of,
535-537, 535t
enlargement of, 472, 474t
differential diagnosis of, 474t
radiography of, 493, 493f
failure of, 484
ascites complicating, treatment of,
549-550
coagulopathy complicating,
treatment of, 550-551

Liver—cont'd
failure of—cont'd
complications of, treatment of, 546-
551
fulminant, 548
gastrointestinal hemorrhage
complicating, treatment of,
550-551
gastrointestinal ulceration/erosion
from, 427-428
hepatic encephalopathy
complicating, treatment of,
546-548
massive hepatic necrosis
complicating, treatment of,
548, 549f
sepsis complicating, treatment of,
551
fibrosis of, idiopathic, 530-531
functional lobule of, Rappaport
scheme of, 477f
infections of, antibiotics for, 1245-
1246, 1245t
inflammation of (See Hepatitis)
injury to, toxic, 521-523, 522t, 523t
lesions of, focal, 541-542, 541f
necrosis of, massive, 548, 549f
nodular hyperplasia of, 542
portal vascular path to, scintigraphy of,
498f
position of, 473f
reduced size of, differential diagnosis
of, 474t
toxicity of chemotherapy drugs for,
1115
Liver fluke, extrahepatic bile duct obstruction from, 518, 519t
Liver function test, in hypoglycemia diagnosis, 731
LMP protocol, for lymphoma, 1127t,
1128-1130, 1153t
Lobular dissecting hepatitis, 530
Locomotion disorders, 974-982
ataxia as, 974, 975f, 975t, 976f
dysmetria as, 977-980 (See also
Dysmetria)
episodic weakness as, 976-977, 977t
generalized lower motor neuron paresis and paralysis ad, 976
hypermetria as, 977-980 (See also
Hypermetria)
from involuntary alterations in muscle
tone, 980-982, 981f
paralysis as, 974-975
paresis as, 974-975, 975t
spinal cord lesion localization in, 975-
976
Lomotil. See Diphenoxylate
Lomustine
for lymphoma, 1127t, 1128, 1131
for mast cell tumors, 1148-1149, 1154t
Long-haired Dachshund, sensory neuropathy in, 1046t
Loop diuretics, in congestive heart failure
management, 62-63
Loperamide
for diarrhea, 399, 399t
dosages of, 471t
Lopid. See Gemfibrozil
Lopressor. See Metroprolol
Lotensin. See Benazepril
Lovastatin, for hypercholesterolemia, 827,
845t
Lower motor neuron (LMN)
disorders of
paralysis from (See Paralysis, LMN)
paresis and paralysis from,
generalized, 976
functional anatomy of, 946, 947f
ischemic damage to, pelvic limb paralysis from, 1054, 1054f
lesions of
bladder distention from, 651
treatment of, 655
signs from, 952t

LPC. *See* Lymphocytic-plasmacytic colitis (LPC)
LPE. *See* Lymphocytic-plasmacytic enteritis (LPE)
Lumbar myelography, 965, 966f
Lung(s)
    aspiration of, in lower respiratory tract specimen collection, 265t
    auscultation of, 252-253
    biopsy of
        in lower respiratory tract specimen collection, 265t
        open-chest, 281
        transbronchial, 278, 281
    blood vessels of, evaluation of, 35
    cavitary lesions of, interstitial patterns in, 260-261, 262f
    complications of heartworm disease involving, treatment of, 176-177
    contusion of, 309-310
    disorders of, 299-313
        eosinophilic, 303-304
        pneumonia as, 299-302, 304-307 (*See also* Pneumonia)
        pulmonary parasites as, 302-303
        toxoplasmosis as, 302
    inflammatory infiltrates of, alveolar patterns in, 258, 259t
    lobe of, torsion of, radiography of, 261
    metastatic lesion of, approach to, 1118
    neoplasia of, 307-309
    parenchyma, disorders of, differential diagnosis of, 251t
    pathogens of, serologic tests for, 264
    thoracic radiography of, 256-261, 257f, 257t, 258f, 258t, 259f, 259t, 260f, 260t, 261f, 261t, 262f
    vascular pattern in, 256-257, 257f, 257t
    toxicity of chemotherapy drugs for, 1115
Lung fluke, fecal examination for, 1230t
Lungworm, fecal examination for, 1230t
Lupus erythematosus (LE) cell test, for systemic lupus erythematosus, 1077, 1086
Luteinizing hormone (LH)
    in anestrus, 850-851
    antibodies against, in population control, 866
    assessment of, 856-857, 857t
    in breeding management, 849-850
    in diestrus, 850
    in estrus, 849
        in queen, 851, 852f, 853f
    evaluation of, in male reproductive function assessment, 913
    in male sexual development, 905
    in proestrus, 847-848
Lyme carditis, 117
Lyme disease, 1018
    joint disorders in, 1084
    titers for, 1077
Lymph nodes
    abscess of, 1201
    anatomic distribution of, in dogs, 1203f
    anatomy of, 1200, 1201f
    aspirates from
        in bubonic plague, 1260f
        in ehrlichiosis, 1269
    cytologic evaluation of, 1098-1099, 1098f
    enlargement of, 1200-1204 (*See also* Lymphadenopathy)
    function of, 1200
    histology of, 1200
    peripheral, hyperplasia of, 1202t
    plexiform vascularization of, 1202t
    reactive, 1208
Lymphadenitis, 1201
    cytologic evaluation of, 1099
Lymphadenitis-splenitis, 1208

Lymphadenopathy, 1200-1204
    approach to, 1206-1208
    classification of, 1201, 1202t
    clinical features of, 1201-1204
    clinicopathologic features of, 1206-1207
    correlation between clinical presentation and etiology in, 1203t
    cytologic evaluation of, 1098-1099, 1098f
    dermatopathic, 1202t
    diagnosis of, 1207-1208
    etiology of, 1200-1201
    imaging in, 1207
    immune-mediated, 1202t
    infiltrative, 1201, 1202t
    management of, 1208-1209
    pathogenesis of, 1200-1201
    reactive, 1201
    regional, 1201
    solitary, 1200-1201
Lymphangiectasia, intestinal, 451
Lymphangiography, in chylothorax, 331t
Lymphocytic cholangitis, 514-515, 515f
Lymphocytic-plasmacytic colitis (LPC), 448
Lymphocytic-plasmacytic enteritis (LPE)
    canine, 447-448
    feline, 448
Lymphocytic-plasmacytic gastritis, 419-420
Lymphocytic-plasmacytic gingivitis/pharyngitis, feline, 408-409
Lymphocytic portal hepatitis, 515-516
Lymphocytic thyroiditis, tests for, 700-702
Lymphocytosis, 1179t, 1197
    in chronic leukemias in dogs, 1137
Lymphoma(s), 1122-1131
    alimentary, 457, 1123
        treatment of, 1131
        ultrasonography of, 375f
    brain, treatment of, 998
    in cats, 195
    chemotherapy protocols for, 1153t
    clinical features of, 1122-1125, 1123t
    CNS
        CSF analysis in, 964t
        treatment of, 1130-1131
    cutaneous, 1123
        treatment of, 1131
    diagnosis of, 1125-1126
    epidemiology of, 1122, 1123t
    epidural, 1124
    etiology of, 1122
    extranodal, 1123, 1123t
    feline leukemia virus infection and, 1282, 1283
    gastric, 428-429
    hematologic features of, 1124-1125
    hypercalcemia induced by, 836-837, 838
    imaging in, 1125
    lymphadenopathy associated with, 1202t
    mediastinal, 1119, 1123
        neoplastic effusions from, 332
    multicentric, 1122-1123
    nasopharyngeal, 1124
    neural, 1124
    neuropil, 1124
        treatment of, 1130-1131
    ocular, 1124
        treatment of, 1131
    peripheral nerve, 1124
    renal, 591f, 1124
    serum biochemical features of, 1124-1125
    staging of, 1125-1126, 1125t
    treatment of, 1126-1131, 1127f
    true CNS, 1124
        treatment of, 1130
Lymphomatoid granulomatosis, 309
    lymphadenopathy associated with, 1202t

Lymphopenia, 1179, 1179t
Lymphoplasmacytic rhinitis, 239
    radiographic signs of, 220t
Lymphoplasmacytic splenitis, 1204
Lymphoplasmacytic synovitis, 1088-1089
Lymphoproliferative disorders, neutropenia in, 1175t
Lysine
    dosages of, 341t
    for herpesvirus infections in cats, 230
Lysodren. *See* Mitotane

**M**

M-mode echocardiogram
    in atrial fibrillation, 75f
    in dilated cardiomyopathy, 75f
Macrocytosis
    disorders associated with, 1159t
    in hepatobiliary disorders, 485, 485f
Macrolides
    dosages of, 1241t
    for *Helicobacter*-associated disease, 420
    for *Helicobacter* gastritis, 401
    for infectious diseases, 1319t
    toxicities of, 1242t
Magnesium
    in commercial reduced-sodium diets, 61t
    depletion of, hypoparathyroidism from, 687
    dietary, struvite crystal/urolith formation and, 642-643
    for digitalis toxicity, 69
    for hypomagnesemia, 845t
    serum concentration of
        depressed, 843-845, 844t
        elevated, 843
    supplemental, for diabetic ketoacidosis, 767
Magnesium ammonium phosphate uroliths
    etiology and pathogenesis of, 633
    factors predicting composition of, 632t
Magnesium chloride, for hypomagnesemia, 844
Magnesium hydroxide
    as antacid, 397
    dosages of, 471t
Magnesium sulfate
    for hypomagnesemia, 844
    for ventricular tachyarrhythmias, 81, 81f
Magnetic resonance imaging (MRI)
    in acute intervertebral disk disease, 1026, 1028f
    in cauda equina syndrome, 1039, 1040f
    in fibrocartilaginous embolism, 1030-1031
    in hyperadrenocorticism
        in cats, 802-803
        in dogs, 785-786
    in intracranial neoplasia, 997
    in intraparenchymal spinal cord abnormalities, 1048
    in lower respiratory tract disorders, 262
    in neuromuscular disorders, 970, 972f
    in thyroid neoplasia, 726, 726f
Maine Coon Cats, spinal muscular atrophy in, 1045t
Malabsorptive diseases, 353, 447-450
    canine eosinophilic gastroenterocolitis as, 448-449
    causes of, 355t
    lymphocytic-plasmacytic colitis as, 448
    lymphocytic-plasmacytic enteritis as
        canine, 447-448
        feline, 448
Maldigestive disease, 352, 446-447
Malignancy(ies)
    in cytologic specimen interpretation, 1095, 1095t, 1096-1097f, 1097-1098, 1098f
    hepatobiliary, abdominal effusion from, 475

Malignant histiocytosis, lymphadenopathy associated with, 1202t
Malignant hyperthermia, 1068
Malignant melanoma (MM)
    lymphadenopathy associated with, 1202t
    metastatic behavior of, 1118t
    oral, 406t
    oropharyngeal, 1150
Mammary gland disorders, 882-885
    feline mammary hyperplasia and hypertrophy as, 883-884, 883f
    galactorrhea as, 883
    galactostasis as, 882-883
    mastitis as, 882
    neoplastic, 884-885
Mannitol
    for chronic renal failure, 618t
    for head trauma, 984
    for hepatobiliary and pancreatic disorders, 566t
    for hydrocephalus, 994
    for massive hepatic necrosis, 548
    for neurologic disorders, 1070t
    for status epilepticus, 996t
    for urinary tract disorders, 659t
Manx cats, caudal agenesis of, 1047
Marbofloxacin
    dosages of, 341t, 1242t
    for hepatobiliary and pancreatic disorders, 566t
    for inflammatory hepatobiliary disease, 516
Marine-life oil supplements, 845t
Masks, oxygen, 337, 338t
Mass(es)
    mediastinal, approach to, 1119-1120, 1119f, 1119t
    solitary, approach to, 1117-1118
    splenic, 1206
Massage, cardiac
    external, in CPR, 100-101, 100f
    internal, in CPR, 101-102
Massive hepatic necrosis, 548, 549f
Mast cell infiltration, lymphadenopathy associated with, 1202t
Mast cell tumors (MCTs), 1146-1149
    in cats, 1149
    chemotherapy protocols for, 1154t
    in dogs, 1146-1149
        biologic behavior of, 1147
        clinical features of, 1146
        clinical staging of, 1148t
        diagnosis of, 1147-1148
        epidemiology of, 1146
        etiology of, 1146
        pathologic features of, 1146-1147
        prognosis for, 1148-1149
        treatment of, 1148-1149, 1148t
    lymphadenopathy associated with, 1202t
    metastatic behavior of, 1118t
Mastectomy, for mammary neoplasia, 884
Masticatory muscles, myositis of, 409
Masticatory myositis, 1062-1063, 1063f
Mastiffs, Tibetan, inherited hypertrophic neuropathy in, 1046t
Mastitis, antibiotics for, 1248t, 1249
Mastocytoma, 1146
MAT. *See* Microscopic agglutination test (MAT)
Matrix nucleation theory of urolith pathogenesis, 631
MCT oil. *See* Medium-chain triglycerides for hepatobiliary and pancreatic disorders, 566t
MCTs. *See* Mast cell tumors (MCTs)
MD. *See* Muscular dystrophy (MD)
MDS. *See* Myelodysplastic syndrome (MDS)
MEA. *See* Mean electrical axis (MEA)
Mean electrical axis (MEA), 13, 14f, 15
    normal, ranges for, 17t
Mebendazole, hepatotoxicity of, 522t

MED technique. *See* Modified equilibrium dialysis (MED) technique
Medallion lesions, in distemper, 1274, 1274f
Median nerve, trauma to, 1050t
Mediastinum
lymphoma of, neoplastic effusions from, 332
mass(es) in, 318-319, 319f
approach to, 1119-1120, 1119f, 1119t
radiography of, 320-322, 322f
Medium-chain triglycerides, dosages of, 471t
Medroxyprogesterone, for reproductive disorders, 945t
Medroxyprogesterone acetate (MPA), for benign prostatic hyperplasia, 930
Mefoxin. *See* Cefoxitin
Megacolon, idiopathic, constipation from, 463
Megaesophagus
aspiration pneumonia and, 305
endoscopic view of, 382f
in myasthenia gravis, 1059-1060
Megestrol acetate
as appetite stimulant, 391
dosages of, 471t
for endocrine disorders, 815t
for estrus control, 866-867
for false pregnancy, 887
for feline eosinophilic granuloma, 407
hepatotoxicity of, 522t
for reproductive disorders, 945t
Meglumine antimonate, for infectious diseases, 1320t
Melanoma, malignant
lymphadenopathy associated with, 1202t
metastatic behavior of, 1118t
oral, 406t
oropharyngeal, 1150
Melarsomine
dosage of, 209t
for heartworm disease in dogs, 174-175, 175t
Melatonin, for endocrine disorders, 815t
Melena, 356, 356t
Meloxicam, for degenerative joint disease, 1080t
Melphalan
for lymphoma, 1127t, 1129
for multiple myeloma, 1154t
Membranes, mucous, in cardiovascular examination, 4-5, 5t
Membranoproliferative glomerulonephritis, 602, 602f
Meningeal vasculitis, 1011f, 1012
CSF analysis in, 964t
Meningioma(s)
cerebral, treatment of, 998
CSF analysis in, 964t
Meningitis
bacterial, 1014-1015, 1014f
CSF analysis in, 964t
parasitic, 1018-1019
steroid-responsive
CSF analysis in, 964t
suppurative, 1010-1011
Meningoencephalitis
*Cryptococcus neoformans*, 1018
distemper, 1015-1016
granulomatous, 1012-1013, 1012f
CSF analysis in, 964t
parasitic, 1018-1019
Pug Dog, 1013
CSF analysis in, 964t
Meningoencephalomyelitis, *Toxoplasma*, 1017
Mental state, in neurologic examination, 948, 948t
Mentation abnormalities, 983

Mephentermine
in cardiopulmonary resuscitation, dosages of, 99t
dosage of, 208t
Mephyton. *See* Vitamin K₁
*N*-(2-mercaptopropionyl)-glycine, for urinary tract disorders, 659t
Mesalamine
for canine lymphocytic-plasmacytic colitis, 448
for digestive disorders, 400
dosages of, 471t
Mesenteric torsion/volvulus, 453
Mesenteric volvulus, radiography of, 372, 374f
Mesoesophagus
acquired, 411-412
congenital, 410-411
Mestinon. *See* Pyridostigmine
Metabolic disorders, 816-827
affecting male reproduction, 914t
drugs for, 845-846t
hyperlipidemia as, 822-827 (*See also* Hyperlipidemia)
obesity as, 817-822 (*See also* Obesity)
polyphagia with weight loss as, 816, 817t
seizures in, 994
Metabolic myopathies, 1065-1066
Metabolic storage diseases
cerebellar dysfunction in, 979t
seizures in, 995-996
spinal dysfunction in, 1043, 1046
Metacam. *See* Meloxicam
Metaldehyde, neurologic dysfunction from, 995t
*Metametorchis intermedius,* extrahepatic bile duct obstruction, 540
Metamucil. *See* Psyllium hydrochloride
Metaraminol
in cardiopulmonary resuscitation, dosages of, 99t
dosage of, 208t
Metarubricytosis, disorders associated with, 1159t
Metastatic lesion, approach to, 1118-1119
Metastatic neoplasms, lymphadenopathy associated with, 1202t
Metered dose inhaler (MDI), for drug administration in feline bronchitis, 293-294, 294f
Metergoline, for reproductive disorders, 945t
Metformin, 755t, 757
for endocrine disorders, 815t
Methenamine mandelate, for urinary tract infections, 630
Methimazole
for endocrine disorders, 815t
for hyperthyroidism, 721-722, 721t
for thyroid neoplasia, 727
Methio-Form. *See* Racemethionine
Methocarbamol, for neurologic disorders, 1070t
Methotrexate
gastrointestinal complications of, 1111
for inflammatory hepatobiliary disease, 517
for lymphoma, 1127t, 1128-1130
for rheumatoid arthritis, 1090
urotoxicity of, 1114
Methoxamine
in cardiopulmonary resuscitation, dosages of, 99t
dosage of, 208t
Methoxyflurane, ECG changes from, 27t
Methscopolamine
for diarrhea, 399t
dosages of, 471t
Methylprednisolone acetate
dosages of, 341t, 471t
for feline bronchitis, 293
for feline eosinophilic granuloma, 407
Methylprednisolone sodium, in brain tumor management, 999

Methylprednisolone sodium succinate
in head trauma management, 984
for neurologic disorders, 1070t
Methyltestosterone
for endocrine disorders, 815t
for short interestrous intervals, 862
Methylxanthine, for sick sinus syndrome, 86
Methylxanthines
dosages of, 292t
for feline bronchitis, 293
Methyoxyflurane, hepatotoxicity of, 522t
Metoclopramide
for acute enteritis, 432
as antiemetic, 396t, 397
for chronic renal failure, 618t
for diarrhea, 399
dosages of, 471t
for esophagitis, 412
for gastrointestinal complications of chemotherapy, 1111
for hepatic lipidosis, 508
for hepatobiliary and pancreatic disorders, 567t
for idiopathic gastric hypomotility, 427
for parvoviral enteritis, 434, 435t
for urinary tract disorders, 659t
for vomiting, in chronic renal failure, 621
Metopirone. *See* Metyrapone
Metoprolol
characteristics of, 91t
for dilated cardiomyopathy, 113
dosages of, 79t, 207t
Metoprolol tartrate, commercial preparations of, 87t
Metritis, 896-897
Metronidazole
for abdominal sepsis, 401
for babesiosis, 1301
for bacterial meningitis/myelitis, 1015
for canine lymphocytic-plasmacytic colitis, 448
for canine lymphocytic-plasmacytic enteritis, 447
for cardiopulmonary infections, 1244t
for chronic hepatic encephalopathy, 547
for cutaneous and soft tissue infections, 1244t
for digestive disorders, 401
dosages of, 341t, 402t, 1241t
for exocrine pancreatic insufficiency, 564
for feline lymphocytic-plasmacytic colitis, 448
for feline lymphocytic-plasmacytic enteritis, 448
for giardiasis, 445
for *Helicobacter*-associated disease, 420
for hepatic and gastrointestinal infections, 1245t
for hepatobiliary and pancreatic disorders, 566t
for hepatobiliary inflammation, 540
for immunoproliferative enteropathy in Basenjis, 450
for infectious diseases, 1319t, 1320t
for inflammatory bowel disease, 401
for inflammatory hepatobiliary disease, 517
for liver abscesses, 542
for neurologic disorders, 1070t
for oropharyngeal masses, 1150
for perianal fistulae, 461
for septic peritonitis, 468
toxicity of, 1009, 1242t
uses of, 402t
Metyrapone
for endocrine disorders, 815t
for hyperadrenocorticism in cats, 803
Mevacor. *See* Lovastatin
Mexiletine
for arrhythmias, 90
commercial preparations of, 87t

Mexiletine—cont'd
dosages of, 79t, 207t
for ventricular tachyarrhythmias, 82
Mexitil. *See* Mexiletine
MG. *See* Myasthenia gravis (MG)
Mibolerone
for estrus suppression, 867
hepatotoxicity of, 522t
MiC protocol
for carcinomas, 1155t
for lymphoma, 1127t
for soft-tissue sarcomas, 1154t
MiCA protocol, for lymphoma, 1127t
MiCO protocol, for soft-tissue sarcomas, 1155t
Microalbuminuria, 586
Microbubbles, in contrast echocardiography, 43-44
Microcytosis, disorders associated with, 1159t
Microfilariae, detection of, in heartworm screening, 171
Microfilaricide therapy
in cats, 183
in dogs, 178
drugs for, 209t
Microhepatia
differential diagnosis of, 474t
radiography of, 493, 493f
Micronase. *See* Glyburide
Microscopic agglutination test (MAT), in *Leptospira* detection, 1262
Microscopy, electron, in infectious disease detection, 1237
Microsurgical transsphenoidal hypophysectomy for feline acromegaly, 677
Microvascular dysplasia, 533
Micturition
abnormal, urinary tract infections and, 626
disorders of, 650-657
clinical features of, 651-653
diagnosis of, 653-655
pharmacologic testing in, 654-655
etiology of, 651-653, 652t
initial evaluation of, 654
prognosis of, 656-657
treatment of, 655-656
physiology of, 650-651
Mifepristone, as abortifacient, 899
Milbemycin
dosages of, 341t, 402t, 471t
uses of, 402t
Milbemycin oxime
dosage of, 209t
in heartworm prevention, 179
in cats, 183
in microfilaricide therapy, 178
for nasal mites, 238
Milk of Magnesia. *See* Magnesium hydroxide
Milrinone
in congestive heart failure management, 70
dosages of, 67t, 206t
in fulminant congestive heart failure therapy, 59
preparations of, 67t
Mineralocorticoids, for acute addisonian crisis, 807t, 808
Minipress. *See* Prazosin
Minocin. *See* Minocycline
Minocycline
for *Brucella canis* infection, 937
for cutaneous and soft tissue infections, 1244t
dosages of, 1242t
for hemangiosarcoma, 1144
for infectious diseases, 1319t
for joint disease, 1092t
for urogenital infections, 1248t
Minute virus of canines, 433-435
Mismating management, 898-900, 898t

Misoprostol
for acute spinal injury, 1023
for degenerative joint disease, 1080
dosages of, 471t
in gastrointestinal ulceration/erosion
prevention, 428
as intestinal protectant, 398
Mites, nasal, 238
fecal examination for, 1230t
Mitochondrial myopathies, 1068
Mitotane
for endocrine disorders, 815t
for pituitary-dependent hyperadrenocorticism, 792-795
adverse reactions to, 794-795, 795t
diabetes concurrent with,
management of, 793-794
induction of therapy with,
monitoring of, 793
induction phase of therapy with, 792
maintenance therapy with, 794
medical adrenalectomy using, 795
Mitoxantrone
for carcinomas, 1155t
for injection site sarcomas, 1152
for leukemias, acute, 1137t, 1153t
for lymphoma, 1127t, 1129, 1153t
for oropharyngeal masses, 1151
for soft-tissue sarcomas, 1154-1155t
Mitral dysplasia
breed dispositions for, 152t
radiographic findings in, 154t
Mitral valve
degenerative disease of, 139-145
clinical signs of, 141
complicating factors in, 140-141,
140t
echocardiography in, 142-143, 142f,
143f
electrocardiography in, 142
epidemiology of, 141
etiology of, 139
pathology of, 139
pathophysiology of, 139-140
patient monitoring in, 145
prognosis in, 143-145
radiography in, 141-142, 142t
reevaluation in, 145
treatment of, 143-145
dysplasia of, 162
echocardiographic view of, 37f
motion of, M-mode scan in evaluation
of, 40, 41f, 42, 42f
MM. *See* Malignant melanoma (MM)
Mobitz type I AV block, 23, 24f
Mobitz type II AV block, 23-24, 24f
Modified equilibrium dialysis (MED)
technique of serum free thyroxine measurement, 698-
699
Modrenal. *See* Trilostane
Monoclonal gammopathies, 1211, 1211t
in chronic leukemias in dogs, 1139
Monocytopenia, 1178
Monocytosis, 1178-1179, 1178t
Monohydrate calcium oxalate crystals in
urine sediment, 570f, 571t
Monopril. *See* Fosinopril
Morphine
dosages of, 341t
in respiratory distress, 334t
Morulae, *Ehrlichia,* 1267, 1267f, 1269-
1270, 1271
Mosquito, in heartworm life cycle, 169
Motor neurons. *See also* Lower motor
neuron (LMN); Upper mo-
tor neuron (UMN)
diseases of, in cats, 1045t
functional anatomy of, 946, 947f
signs from, 952t
Mouth. *See* Oral cavity
Moxidectin
dosage of, 209t
in heartworm prevention, 179

MPA. *See* Medroxyprogesterone acetate
(MPA)
MTP. *See* Muramyl tripeptide (MTP)
Mucocele, gallbladder, 539, 539f
Mucoid vulvar discharge, 872
Mucomyst. *See* *N*-acetylcysteine
Mucopolysaccharidosis, cerebellar dys-
function in, 979t
Mucopurulent nasal discharge, 210, 211t
Mucosa
gastric, urease activity in, testing for,
379
nasal, rhinoscopic view of, 222, 223f
Mucous membranes, in cardiovascular
examination, 4-5, 5t
Multicentric lymphoma, 1122-1123
*Multiceps multiceps,* as enteric zoonosis,
1309t
Multiple myeloma
chemotherapy protocols for, 1154t
lymphadenopathy associated with,
1202t
Muramyl tripeptide (MTP), liposomal,
for hemangiosarcoma, 1144
Murmur(s), cardiac, 9-11, 9f, 9t, 10f
in atrial septal defect, 152f, 162
in cardiac tumors, 195
continuous, 11
in degenerative AV valve disease, 141
diastolic, 9f, 10-11
differentiating, flow chart for, 152f
ejection, 9, 9f
in feline hypertrophic cardiomyopathy,
124
grading of, 9t
in hypertension, 201
location of, 10f
in pulmonary hypertension with shunt
reversal, 165
in pulmonic stenosis, 152f, 158-159
shapes and descriptions of, 9f
in subaortic stenosis, 152f, 157
systolic, 9-10, 9f
in tetralogy of Fallot, 152f, 164
thoracic auscultation of, 7
to-and-fro, 11
Muscle(s)
abdominal, hypotonia of, 476, 476f
in arterial thromboembolism, 134
atrophy of, neurogenic, progressive, in
English Pointers, 1045t
biopsy of
in canine idiopathic polymyositis
diagnosis, 1064
for neuromuscular disorders, 972-
973
cricopharyngeus, achalasia/dysfunction
of, 409
disorders of, 1062-1068 (*See also*
Myopathy[ies])
masticatory, myositis of, 409, 1062-
1063, 1063f
pain in, in neurologic examination,
956-957
papillary, echocardiographic view of,
37f
skeletal, systemic lupus erythematosus
and, 1220t
spinal, atrophy of
in German Shepherds, 1045t
in Maine Coon Cats, 1045t
in Rottweilers, 1046t
in Swedish Lapland Dogs, 1046t
tone of
involuntary alterations in, 980-982,
981f
in neurologic examination, 949f, 950
Muscle fibers, 2M, antibodies to, in alimentary tract disease, 379
Muscular dystrophy (MD), 1066-1067
autosomal recessive, 1067
dilated cardiomyopathy and, 107-108
Musculocutaneous nerve, trauma to,
1050t

Musculoskeletal infections, antibiotics
for, 1246-1247, 1246t
Myasthenia gravis (MG), 1059-1061,
1060t, 1061f
localized, esophageal weakness in, 411
Mycobacteria
atypical, antibiotics for, 1244t
lymphadenopathy associated with,
1202t
*Mycobacterium*
culture techniques for, 1235
morphologic characteristics of, 1233t
*Mycoplasma*
antibiotics for, 1246t, 1248t
culture techniques for, 1235
genital infections from, 935-936
infections from, secondary to cat bites,
1314
pneumonia and, 299
polysystemic disease from, 1262-1264,
1263t
urinary tract infections from, 624-625
*Mycoplasma* polyarthritis, 1083
Mycotic infections
CNS involvement in, 1018
interstitial pattern in, 258, 260f, 260t
nasal, 235-237
polysystemic, 1287-1294
blastomycosis as, 1290-1291, 1290f,
1291f
coccidioidomycosis as, 1293-1294,
1294f
cryptococcosis as, 1287-1290, 1288f,
1288t, 1289t (*See also*
Cryptococcosis)
histoplasmosis as, 1291-1293, 1292f
Mydriasis, unilateral, 986
Myelitis
bacterial, 1014-1015, 1014f
parasitic, 1018-1019
Myelodysplastic syndrome (MDS), 1133,
1140
Myelofibrosis, 1184
Myelography
in acute intervertebral disk disease,
1026
in fibrocartilaginous embolism, 1030
in neuromuscular disorders, 066f, 965-
967, 967f, 968f
in spinal neoplasia, 1035-1036
in wobbler syndrome, 1041-1042,
1042f, 1043f
Myeloma, multiple
chemotherapy protocols for, 1154t
lymphadenopathy associated with,
1202t
Myelopathy
degenerative, 1037-1038, 1044t
CSF analysis in, 964t
hereditary Afghan, 1044t
Myelophthisis, 1182t, 1184
Myeloproliferative disease, 1133
Myelosuppression, complicating chemotherapy, 1111
Myocardial ischemia, in feline hypertrophic cardiomyopathy, 123
Myocarditis
canine, 116-118
feline, 133-134
Myocardium
contractility of
in atrioventricular valve disease,
140
poor, in dilated cardiomyopathy,
131-132, 131f
diseases of
in cat, 122-137
in dog, 106-120
failure of
chronic heart failure from, 55t
therapeutic goals for, 56t
hypertrophy of, secondary, 122-129
(*See also* Hypertrophic cardiomyopathy [HCM], feline)

Myocardium—cont'd
inflammation of
canine, 116-118
feline, 133-134
injury to, biochemical markers of, 48
toxicity of digitalis glycosides for, 68-69
Myochrysine. *See* Gold sodium thiomalate; Sodium aurothiomalate
Myoclonus, 981-982
Myofibers, type IIM, antibody against, in
neuromuscular disorders,
973
Myopathic cardiogenic shock, 119t
Myopathy(ies), 1062-1068
hereditary, Labrador Retriever, 1067,
1067f
inflammatory, 1062-1065
canine idiopathic polymyositis as,
1063-1064
dermatomyositis as, 1064-1065
feline idiopathic polymyositis as,
1064
masticatory myositis as, 1062-1063,
1063f
protozoal myositis as, 1065
inherited, 1066-1068
metabolic, 1065-1066
mitochondrial, 1068
Myositis
atrophic, 409
masticatory, 1062-1063, 1063f
masticatory muscle, 409
in neosporosis, 1299-1300
protozoal, 1065
Myotomy, cricopharyngeal, 409
Myotonia, 1067-1068
Myringotomy, in facial nerve paralysis,
1053
Myxedema, in hypothyroidism
in cats, 709
in dogs, 693

**N**

*N*-(2-mercaptopropionyl)-glycine
(MPG), for cystine uroliths,
641
*N*-acetyl glucosaminidase (NAG), in
urine, monitoring of, in patients at risk for ARF, 613
*N*-acetylcysteine, indication and dosage
of, 565t
Nadolol
characteristics of, 91t
dosages of, 79t, 207t
NAG. *See* *N*-acetyl glucosaminidase
(NAG)
Nandrolone decanoate
for chronic renal failure, 618t
for urinary tract disorders, 659t
*Nanophyetus salmincola*
fecal examination for, 1230t
fecal flotation for, 366
Naproxen
gastrointestinal ulceration/erosion
from, 427-428
hepatotoxicity of, 522t
Narcon. *See* Norfloxacin
Narcotic analgesics, for acute interverte-
bral disk disease, 1026
Narcotics, as antiemetics, 396t, 397
Nares, rhinoscopic views of, 222f
Nasal catheters, for oxygen supplementa-
tion, 338-339, 338t, 339f
Nasal cavity. *See* Nose
Nasal flush, 224
Nasal mite, fecal examination for, 1230t
Nasal swab, 224
Nasal worm, fecal examination for, 1230t
Nasoesophageal tubes, 391-392
uses of, 395
Nasopharynx
lymphoma of, 1124
polyps of, 219f, 232-233, 233f
clinical features of, 232
diagnosis of, 233

Nasopharynx—cont'd
  polyps of—cont'd
    prognosis for, 233
    radiographic signs of, 220t
    treatment of, 233
Natriuretic peptides, in heart failure, 54
Nausea, complicating chemotherapy, 1111
Naxcel. *See* Ceftiofur
NB-BAL. *See* Nonbronchoscopic bronchoalveolar lavage (NB-BAL)
Nebcin. *See* Tobramycin
Nebulization, for bacterial pneumonia, 300t, 301
Neck pain, in neurologic examination, 955, 956f, 957t
Necrotizing splenitis, 1204
Needles, biopsy, 502f
Nemacide. *See* Diethylcarbamazine
Nematodes, zoonotic, 1307-1308, 1309t, 1310
Nembutal. *See* Pentobarbital
Nemex. *See* Pyrantel pamoate
Neo-Mercazole. *See* Carbimazole
Neo-Synephrine. *See* Phenylephrine
Neomycin
  for campylobacteriosis, 437
  for chronic hepatic encephalopathy, 547
  dosages of, 471t, 1241t
  for hepatic and gastrointestinal infections, 1245t
  for hepatobiliary and pancreatic disorders, 567t
  for infectious diseases, 1318t
Neonate(s)
  antimicrobial therapy for, 897t
  herpesvirus infection in, 934
  illness in, clinical features of, 902
  morbidity and mortality of, 901-903, 903t
Neoplasia. *See* Tumor(s)
Neoplasms. *See* Tumor(s)
Neoral. *See* Cyclosporine
*Neorickettsia helminthoeca*, salmon poisoning from, 437
Neosar. *See* Cyclophosphamide
*Neospora caninum*, 1299-1300, 1300f
  lymphadenopathy associated with, 1202t
  morphologic characteristics of, 1234t
  polyradiculoneuritis from, 1058
  serologic tests for, 973
Neosporosis, 1017-1018, 1299-1300, 1300f
  ancillary diagnostics for, 1011t
  antibiotics for, 124, 1244t, 1246t
  CSF analysis in, 964t
*Neosporum caninum*, myocarditis from, 117
Neostigmine
  for myasthenia gravis, 1061
  for neurologic disorders, 1070t
Nephrogenic diabetes insipidus, 662
  therapies for, 666t
Nephrotic syndrome, 603-605
Nephrotoxicants, 609, 610t
Nephrotoxicity, of chemotherapy drugs, 1114
Nerve(s)
  axillary, trauma to, 1050t
  biopsy of, for neuromuscular disorders, 973
  cranial
    functional assessment of, 958t
    in neurologic examination, 957, 958t
  facial, paralysis of, 1051-1053, 1052f, 1053f
  femoral, damage to, 1050t
  median, trauma to, 1050t
  musculocutaneous, trauma to, 1050t
  peripheral, disorders of, 1049-1061
    (*See also* Peripheral nerves, disorders of)

Nerve(s)—cont'd
  radial
    peripheral, damage to, 1050t
    trauma to, 1050t
  sciatic, damage to, 1050t
  suprascapular, trauma to, 1050t
  trigeminal, paralysis of, 1053-1054, 1054f
  ulnar, trauma to, 1050t
Nerve conduction velocities, in neuromuscular disorders, 971
Nervous system
  central (*See* Central nervous system [CNS])
  degenerative disorders of, 1044-1046t
  deterioration of, after myelography, 966-967
  functional anatomy of, 946-947, 947f, 947t
  lymphoma of, 1124
  toxicity of chemotherapy drugs for, 1115
Neural lymphoma, 1124
Neuritis, optic, 985-986, 986t
Neuroaxonal dystrophy, in Rottweilers, 1044t
Neurogenic dysphagia, 345
Neurogenic muscular atrophy, progressive, in English Pointers, 1045t
Neurohormonal mechanisms, in congestive heart failure, 52-54, 52f, 53f
Neurologic disorders, drugs in, 1069-1070t
Neurologic examination, 946-959
  in fibrocartilaginous embolism, 1030
  functional anatomy in, 946-947, 947f, 947t
  screening, 948-959
    animal history in, 957-958
    cranial nerves in, 957, 958t
    diagnostic approach and, 957, 959t
    disease onset and progression in, 958-959, 959t
    gait in, 948, 949f
    hyperpathia in, 955-957, 956f, 957t
    lesion localization in, 957
    localization within brain in, 957, 959t
    mental state in, 948, 948t
    muscle tone in, 949f, 950
    pain in, 955-957, 956f, 957t
    postural reactions in, 948, 950, 950f
    posture in, 948, 949-950f
    sensation in, 953, 955, 955f
    spinal reflexes in, 950-953, 952t, 953f, 954f, 954t
    urinary tract function in, 957
  in spinal cord trauma, 1021
Neurologic signs
  of distemper, 1273
  of feline leukemia virus infection, 1282-1283
  of hypernatremia, 828
  of hyponatremia, 831
  of pituitary macrotumor syndrome, 780, 780t
Neuromuscular disorders, 946-1070
  biopsy for, 972-973
  CNS inflammation and, 1010-1019
  computerized tomography in, 970, 971f
  diagnostic tests for, 961-973
    cerebrospinal fluid analysis as, 962-965, 962f, 963f, 964f, 964t
    electrodiagnostic, 970-972
    hematologic, 961
    immunologic, 973
    serologic, 973
    serum biochemistry profile as, 961
    urinalysis as, 961
  dysphagia in, 34t
  epidurography of, 967-968, 969f
  focal, 1049-1054

Neuromuscular disorders—cont'd
  head tilt as, 1005-1009 (*See also* Head tilt)
  head trauma and, 983-984, 984t
  of locomotion, 974-982 (*See also* Locomotion disorders)
  magnetic resonance imaging in, 970, 972f
  mentation abnormalities in, 983
  muscular, 1062-1068 (*See also* Myopathy[ies])
  myelography in, 965-967, 966f, 967f, 968f
  neurologic examination in, 946-959 (*See also* Neurologic examination)
  pneumoventriculography of, 968, 969-970f, 970
  pupillary abnormalities and, 984-990
  radiography of, 961-962
    contrast-enhanced, 965-970
  seizures as, 991-1004 (*See also* Seizures)
  spinal cord, 1020-1048 (*See also* Spinal cord, dysfunction of)
  vision loss and, 984-990
Neuromuscular junction, disorders of, botulism as, 1058
Neuromuscular signs
  of hypoparathyroidism, 687
  in hypothyroidism, 693-694, 694t
Neuron(s)
  degeneration of, 1043
    multisystem, in Cocker Spaniels, 1044t
  motor
    functional anatomy of, 946, 947f
    signs from, 952t
Neuronal abiotrophy(ies), 1043
  cerebellar, 978, 978t
Neuronal chromatolysis, of Cairn Terriers, 1045t
Neuronal glycoproteinosis, cerebellar dysfunction in, 979t
Neuropathy(ies)
  axonal, giant, in German Shepherds, 1045t
  central-peripheral, in Boxer, 1044t
  diabetic, in cats, 762
  focal, 1049-1054
  hypertrophic, inherited, in Tibetan Mastiffs, 1046t
  sensory
    in English Pointers, 1046t
    in long-haired Dachshund, 1046t
  traumatic, 1049, 1050t, 1051f
Neuropil lymphoma, 1124
Neutering, 865-866
Neutropenia, 1174-1176, 1175f, 1175t
  from chemotherapy, 1109-1110
Neutrophil pools, 1174
Neutrophilia, 1176-1177
  in cystic endometrial hyperplasia-pyometra complex, 878
Neutrophils
  morphologic abnormalities in, 1173-1174
  systemic lupus erythematosus and, 1220t
Niacin
  for hyperlipidemia, 826
  for hypertriglyceridemia, 846t
Niemann-Pick disease, cerebellar dysfunction in, 979t
Nifurtimox, for American trypanosomiasis, 1304
Nitrobid. *See* Nitroglycerine ointment
Nitroglycerine
  in congestive heart failure management, 66
  preparations of, 63t
Nitroglycerine ointment, dosages of, 62t, 206t
Nitrol. *See* Nitroglycerine ointment
Nitropress. *See* Sodium nitroprusside

Nitroprusside, for hypertension, 202t
Nizatidine
  as antacid, 397
  for diarrhea, 399
  dosages of, 471t
Nizoral. *See* Ketoconazole
*Nocardia*
  antibiotics for, 1244t
  lymphadenopathy associated with, 1202t
  morphologic characteristics of, 1233t
Nodular hyperplasia, hepatic, 542
Nodular panniculitis, in acute pancreatitis, 555t
Nonbronchoscopic bronchoalveolar lavage (NB-BAL), 270-274, 271f, 272f, 273f, 274f, 274t
  complications of, 270
  diagnostic yield of, 274
  indications for, 270, 271f
  recovery following, 273
  results of, interpretation of, 273-274, 274f, 274t
  specimen handling from, 273
  technique for
    in cats, 270, 271f, 272, 272f
    in dogs, 272-273, 272f, 273f
Noninfective myocarditis, 118
Nonsteroidal antiinflammatory drugs (NSAIDs)
  for acute intervertebral disk disease, 1026
  acute renal failure and, 612
  for degenerative joint disease, 1080, 1080t
  gastrointestinal ulceration/erosion from, 427-428
Norepinephrine
  in cardiopulmonary resuscitation, dosages of, 99t
  dosage of, 208t
Norfloxacin, dosages of, 471t
Normosol, 832t
Norvasc. *See* Amlodipine besylate
Nose
  biopsy of, 224-226, 225f, 226f
  computed tomography of, 221
  cultures from, 226-227
  discharge from, 210-214
    classification of, 210-211
    diagnostic approach to, 211-214, 212-213f, 214f
    differential diagnosis of, 211t
    etiology of, 210-211
    mucopurulent, 210, 211t
    persistent pure hemorrhagic, 211, 211t
    serous, 210, 211t
  disorders of, 228-240
    allergic rhinitis as, 239-240
    bacterial rhinitis as, 238
    feline upper respiratory infection as, 228-232 (*See also* Feline upper respiratory infection)
    lymphoplasmacytic rhinitis as, 239
    nasal mycoses as, 235-237, 236f, 237f
    nasal parasites as, 238-239
    nasal tumors as, 233-235
    nasopharyngeal polyps as, 232-233, 233f
  facial deformity involving, 216, 216f
  foreign bodies of, radiographic signs of, 220t
  radiography of, 217-221, 218-220f, 220t
  rhinoscopy of, 221-222f, 221-224, 223f, 223t
  sneezing and, 215-216
  stretor and, 216
  tumors of, 219f, 233-235
    radiographic signs of, 220t
Novantrone. *See* Mitoxantrone
Noxious substance ingestion, halitosis from, 344t
NSAIDs. *See* Nonsteroidal antiinflammatory drugs (NSAIDs)

Nuclear cardiology, 48-49
Nuclear imaging, in lower respiratory tract disorders, 262
Nutrition, parenteral, 396
    total (*See* Total parenteral nutrition)
Nutritional factors, in acute pancreatitis development, 553t
Nutritional needs, calculation of, 390-391, 391t
Nutritional therapy
    for hepatic lipidosis, 507-512
    for inflammatory hepatobiliary disease, 517
    in parvoviral enteritis, 435t
Nyquist limit, 45, 46f
Nystagmus, 1005
    congenital, 1009

**O**

Obesity, 817-822
    adverse effects of, 817t
    causes of, 817-818, 818t
    in diabetes in cats, 753
    diagnosis of, 818-819, 818t, 819f
    heart failure and, 61
    management of, 819-822, 820t, 821t
    prevention of, 822
Obstipation, 357
Obstructive laryngitis, 249
Occipital cortex lesions, 986
Octreotide. *See* Somatostatin
Ocular lymphoma, 1124
    treatment of, 1131
Oil, marine-life, supplemental, 845t
Oligospermia, 915-916
*Ollulanus tricuspis*
    fecal examination for, 1230t
    gastritis from, 421
    granulomatous gastritis from, 419-420
Olsalazine
    for canine lymphocytic-plasmacytic colitis, 448
    for digestive disorders, 400
    dosages of, 471t
Omeprazole
    in acute spinal injury management, 1023
    as antacid, 397, 397t
    dosages of, 471t
    for esophagitis, 412
    for gastroesophageal reflux, 411
    for gastrointestinal hemorrhage in liver failure, 550
    for *Helicobacter*-associated disease, 420
    for *Helicobacter* gastritis, 401
    for hepatobiliary and pancreatic disorders, 567t
Omnipaque. *See* Iohexol
Omnizole. *See* Thiabendazole
Oncology, 1093-1155
    chemotherapy in, 1103-1116 (*See also* Chemotherapy)
    cytology in, 1093-1099
    mass and, 1117-1120 (*See also* Mass)
    treatment principles in, 1100-1102
        owner-related factors in, 1100-1101
        patient-related factors in, 1100, 1101t
        treatment-related factors in, 1101-1102, 1102t
Oncovin. *See* Vincristine
Ondansetron
    for acute enteritis, 432
    as antiemetic, 396t, 397
    dosages of, 471t
    for gastrointestinal complications of chemotherapy, 1111
    for parvoviral enteritis, 434, 435t
Oocysts, *Cryptosporidium parvum*, 1231f
o,p'-DDD. *See* Mitotane
Open-chest lung biopsy, 281
Opiates, for diarrhea, 399, 399t
Opisthotonos, 980-981
Optic chiasm lesions, 986, 987f
Optic neuritis, 985-986, 986t

Oral cavity
    disorders of, 405-409
    imaging of, 368-369
    masses in, 405
    neoplasms of, 406-407, 406t
Orbax. *See* Orbifloxacin
Orbifloxacin
    dosages of, 1242t
    for infectious diseases, 1319t
Orchitis, 921-922
    infertility from, 916-917
    *Mycoplasma canis* causing, 935
Organomegaly, 472, 473f, 474f
Organophosphates, neurologic dysfunction from, 995t
Ormetoprim-sulfadimethoxine
    for cutaneous and soft tissue infections, 1244t
    dosages of, 1242t
    for infectious diseases, 1319t
Orogastric tube
    for decompression in gastric dilation/volvulus, 425
    feeding by, intermittent, 391
Oropharyngeal neoplasms, 1149-1151
OSA. *See* Osteosarcoma (OSA)
Oscillometric method of blood pressure measurement, 200-201
*Oslerus osleri*, 297-298, 298f, 302
    characteristics of eggs or larvae of, 263t
    endoscopic view of, 1232f
    fecal examination for, 1230t
    parasitologic evaluation for, 262, 264
Osmitrol. *See* Mannitol
Osmolality
    plasma
        measurement of, in urinary disorder evaluation, 587
        random, in diabetes insipidus diagnosis, 665, 665f
    urine, measurement of, in urinary disorder evaluation, 587
Osmotic laxatives, 403
    for idiopathic megacolon, 463
Osteomyelitis, antibiotics for, 1246, 1246t
Osteopetrosis, 1184
Osteosarcoma (OSA), 1144-1146, 1144f, 1145f, 1145t
    chemotherapy protocols for, 1155t
    metastatic behavior of, 1118t
Osteosclerosis, 1184
Osteotomy, ventral bulla, in facial nerve paralysis management, 1053
Ostium secundum, 162
Otitis media-interna
    antibiotics for, 1246t
    facial nerve paralysis from, 1051
    vestibular extension of, 1006-1007, 1007f
Ototoxicity
    aminoglycoside, 1008
    chemical, 1008
Ovaban. *See* Megestrol acetate
Ovarian remnant syndrome, 867-868
Ovaries, cystic, prolonged estrus from, 863-864, 863f
Ovariohysterectomy, 865
    diabetes mellitus after, in dogs, 731-732
    mastectomy with, 884
    for pyometra, 879
    for uterine neoplasia, 877
    for vaginal hyperplasia and prolapse, 876
Overhydration, signs of, 388-389
Ovulation
    in bitch, timing of, 850
    for artificial insemination, 940
    induction of, 869
    in queen, 851
Oxacillin
    for cutaneous and soft tissue infections, 1244t
    dosages of, 1241t
    for infectious diseases, 1319t

Oxazepam
    as appetite stimulant, 391
    dosages of, 471t
    for hepatic lipidosis, 508
    for hepatobiliary and pancreatic disorders, 566t
Oxfendazole, for *Ollulanus tricuspis* infection, 421
Oximetry, pulse, 285-286, 286f
Oxtriphylline, dosages of, 341t
Oxtriphylline elixir, dosages of, 292t
Oxybutynin, for urinary tract disorders, 659t
Oxygen
    concentrations of, maximum achievable, by supplemental methods, 338t
    supplemental, 337-340
        for aspiration pneumonia, 306
        endotracheal tubes for, 338t, 339
        for fulminant congestive heart failure, 58-59, 59t
        for head trauma, 984
        nasal catheters for, 338-339, 338t, 339f
        oxygen cages for, 338t, 340
        oxygen hoods for, 337, 338f
        oxygen masks for, 337, 338t
        tracheal tubes for, 338t, 339-340
        transtracheal catheters for, 338t, 339
Oxygen cages, for oxygen supplementation, 338t, 340
Oxygen content of arterial blood, 284-285
Oxygen-hemoglobin dissociation curve, 282, 283f
    pulse oximetry and, 286
Oxygen hoods, 337, 338f
Oxygen masks, 337, 338t
Oxygen partial pressure
    indications for, 281
    results of, interpretation of, 282-285, 282t, 283f, 284t, 285t
    techniques for, 281-282, 281f, 282f
Oxygen therapy, for respiratory distress in lung disease, 336
Oxymetazoline, dosages of, 341t
Oxymorphone, for acute intervertebral disk disease, 1026
Oxytetracycline
    dosages of, 471t
    for joint disease, 1092t
Oxytocin
    in dystocia management, 895
    in metritis management, 897
    for milk letdown stimulation, 895-896
    for uterine evacuation following abortion, 901

**P**

P wave, normal, ranges for, 17t
P' wave, 19
Pacemaker, wandering, 16
PaCO₂. *See* Arterial carbon dioxide tension
Pain
    abdominal, in digestive disorders, 362-363, 363t
    in cauda equina syndrome, 1038-1039, 1039f
    in intervertebral disk disease, 1025, 1025f
    joint, diagnostic algorithm for, 1087f
    in joint disorders, 1071
    in neurologic examination, 955-957, 956f, 957t
    oral, dysphagia in, 344t
Palpation
    abdominal, in pregnancy confirmation, 888
    of intussusceptions, 455, 456
Pamine. *See* Methscopolamine
Panacur. *See* Fenbendazole
Pancreas
    abscess of, in acute pancreatitis, 555t
    anatomic relationship of, with common bile duct and duodenum in cat, 513f

Pancreas—cont'd
    endocrine, disorders of, 729-776
        diabetes mellitus as, 731-762 (*See also* Diabetes mellitus)
        diabetic ketoacidosis as, 762-769 (*See also* Diabetic ketoacidosis [DKA])
        gastrinoma as, 775-776, 775t
        hyperglycemia as, 729, 730t
        hypoglycemia as, 729-731, 730t
        insulin-secreting β-cell neoplasia as, 769-775 (*See also* Insulin-secreting β-cell neoplasia)
    exocrine, 552-564
        diseases of, 553t
        disorders of, drugs for, 565-567t
        inflammation of, 552-560 (*See also* Pancreatitis)
        insufficiency of (*See* Exocrine pancreatic insufficiency [EPI])
        neoplasia of, 564
        substances secreted by, 553t
        pseudocyst of, in acute pancreatitis, 555t
Pancreatic enzyme powder
    for exocrine pancreatic insufficiency, 398, 563-564
    for hepatobiliary and pancreatic disorders, 567t
Pancreatic enzymes
    dosages of, 471t
    for exocrine pancreatic insufficiency, 447
    for hepatobiliary and pancreatic disorders, 567t
    supplemental, 398
        for exocrine pancreatic insufficiency, 563-564
        for relapsing and chronic pancreatitis, 560
Pancreatic lipase immunoreactivity (PLI), in acute pancreatitis, 557-558
Pancreatitis
    acute, 552-560
        clinical features of, 552, 554, 554f, 555t
        clinical signs and findings in, 555t
        development, factors involved in, 553t
        diagnosis of, 554-558, 555t, 556f, 557f
        feline, 560
        mild, treatment of, 558, 558t
        pathogenesis of, 552, 553t
        prognosis for, 558-560
        severe
            complications of, 555t
            treatment of, 558-560, 558t
    chronic, 560
        in diabetes mellitus in cats, 749, 749f, 750, 751f
    complicating chemotherapy, 1113-1114
    hepatic lipidosis with, nutritional support for, 512
    liver disease secondary to, 543
    relapsing, 560
Pancreazyme. *See* Pancreatic enzymes; Pancreatic enzymes, supplemental
    for exocrine pancreatic insufficiency, 398
Pancytopenia, 1181
    causes of, 1182t
    diagnostic algorithm for, 1183f
    disorders associated with, 1159t
Panleukopenia
    feline, 435-436
    vaccination for, 1255
Panniculitis, nodular, in acute pancreatitis, 555t
Panniculus reflex, 952-953, 954f
Panting, in hyperadrenocorticism, 780, 780t, 781f

PaO₂. See Oxygen partial pressure

Papillary muscle, echocardiographic view of, 37f

Papillomatosis, oral, 406t

Paradoxic incontinence, 652

Paradoxical incontinence, 576

*Paragonimus kellicotti*
  characteristics of eggs or larvae of, 263t
  fecal examination for, 1230t
  lung disease from, 302, 303
  ova of, 263f

Parainfluenza virus (PIV)
  canine infectious tracheobronchitis from, 287
  vaccination for, 1256

Paralysis, 974-975
  Coonhound, 1056-1057, 1057f
  facial nerve, 1051-1053, 1052f, 1053f
  laryngeal, 246-247, 247t
    in Bouvier des Flandres, 1045t
    in Dalmatians, 1045t
    in Siberian and Alaskan Huskies, 1046t
  LMN
    in botulism, 1058
    in protozoal polyradiculoneuritis, 1058
  lower motor neuron, generalized, 976
  in neosporosis, 1299
  pelvic limb, LMN, 1054, 1054f
  sciatic nerve, 1050t
  tick, 1057-1058
  trigeminal nerve, 1053-1054, 1054f

Paraneoplastic syndromes, thymomas and, 1119

Paraphimosis, 920-921, 921f

Paraplegic cart, 1030, 1030f

Paraprostatic cysts, 932, 932f

Parasites
  alimentary tract, 440-446
    demonstration techniques for, 1230t
  CNS migration of, CSF analysis in, 964t
  cutaneous, cytologic examination for, 1234
  diarrhea from, 352t
  fecal, evaluation for, 366-367
  lower respiratory tract, evaluation for, 262-264, 263f, 263t, 264t
  nasal, 238-239
    differential diagnosis of, 223t
  pulmonary, 302-303
    interstitial pattern in, 258, 260t
  respiratory tract, demonstration techniques for, 1230t

Parasitic encephalitis, 1018-1019

Parasitic infections, lymphadenopathy associated with, 1202t

Parasitic meningitis, 1018-1019

Parasitic myelitis, 1018-1019

Parathyroid gland disorders
  hyperparathyroidism as, 681-686 (*See also* Hyperparathyroidism)
  hypoparathyroidism as, 686-689 (*See also* Hypoparathyroidism)

Parathyroid hormone (PTH)
  actions of, on calcium and phosphorus metabolism, 682t
  decreased secretion of, in hypoparathyroidism, 686-689
  increased secretion of, in hyperparathyroidism, 681
  plasma concentrations of, interactions of, with calcium, phosphorus and vitamin D concentrations, 620f
  in chronic renal failure, 621f

Paregoric
  for diarrhea, 399t
  dosages of, 471t

Parenteral fluids
  administration of, 387
  solutions of, 832t
  therapy with, for acute gastritis, 418

Parenteral nutrition, 396
  total (*See* Total parenteral nutrition)

Parenteral solutions, formulation of, 391t

Paresis, 974-975, 975t
  lower motor neuron, generalized, 976
  in neurologic examination, 948
  peripheral nerve and neuromuscular junction disorders causing, 1055t

Parlodel. *See* Bromocriptine

Paromomycin, for infectious diseases, 1320t

Paroxysmal AV reciprocating tachycardia, treatment of, 77

Paroxysmal tachycardias, 75-82, 77f

Pars distalis, adenoma of, hyperadrenocorticism from, 778

Pars intermedia, adenoma of, hyperadrenocorticism from, 778

Partially hydrolyzed diet, 390

Parturition, 891

Parvaquone
  for cytauxzoonosis, 1302
  for infectious diseases, 1320t

Parvoviral enteritis
  canine, 433-435, 435t
  feline, 435-436

Parvoviral myocarditis, 116

Parvovirus
  enzyme-linked immunosorbent assays for, 367
  immunologic techniques for, 1236
  infection with, neutropenia in, 1175t
  vaccination for, 1256

*Pasteurella*
  infective endocarditis from, 146
  pulmonary infection from, 299

Patent ductus arteriosus (PDA), 34-35, 152, 153-155, 153f, 155f, 156f
  breed dispositions for, 152t
  murmurs in, 152f
  pulmonary hypertension in, 164-166
  radiographic findings in, 154t

PB. *See* Phenobarbital (PB)

PCR. *See* Polymerase chain reaction (PCR)

PCWP. *See* Pulmonary capillary wedge pressure (PCWP)

PDA. *See* Patent ductus arteriosus (PDA)

PDH. *See* Pituitary-dependent hyperadrenocorticism (PDH)

Pelger-Huët anomaly, 1174

Pelvic canal obstruction, from malaligned healing of old pelvic fractures, constipation from, 462

Pelvic fracture, 1023

Penicillin(s)
  for bacterial meningitis/myelitis, 1015
  for cardiopulmonary infections, 1244t
  for cutaneous and soft tissue infections, 1244t
  derivatives of
    for cutaneous and soft tissue infections, 1244t
    for hepatic and gastrointestinal infections, 1245t
  for diskospondylitis, 1033
  dosages of, 1241t
  for infectious diseases, 1319t
  for infective endocarditis, 149
  toxicities of, 1242t

Penicillin G
  dosages of, 1241t
  for infectious diseases, 1319t
  for joint disease, 1092t
  for leptospirosis, 1262
  for neurologic disorders, 1070t
  for urogenital infections, 1248t

Penile frenulum, persistent, 919, 920f

Penis
  congenital disorders of, 919-920, 920f
  trauma to, 918

Pentasa. *See* Mesalamine

Pentobarbital
  for neurologic disorders, 1070t
  for status epilepticus, 996t
  for tetanus, 981

Pepcid. *See* Famotidine

Peptides, natriuretic, in heart failure, 54

Pepto-Bismol. *See* Bismuth subsalicylate

Percorten-V. *See* Desoxycorticosterone pivalate

Percutaneous liver biopsy, 501, 501f, 502-503f, 503

Perfusion, and ventilation, mismatched, in hypoxemia, 283

Periactin. *See* Cyproheptadine

Perianal fistulae, 461

Perianal gland tumors, 462

Perianal neoplasms, 461-462

Pericardial effusion, 185-192
  clinical features of, 186-187, 187f
  clinical pathology in, 188, 190
  complications of, 191
  diagnosis of, 187-188, 187f, 188f, 189f
  etiology of, 185-186
  pathophysiology of, 186
  prognosis of, 190-191
  treatment of, 190-191

Pericardiectomy
  subtotal, surgical, for pericardial effusion, 190
  surgical, for constrictive pericardial disease, 194

Pericardiocentesis
  for cardiac tamponade, 191-192
  for cardiogenic shock, 119
  complications of, 192
  in pericardial effusion, 190

Pericarditis
  constrictive, syncope or intermittent weakness from, 2t
  infectious, treatment of, 191

Pericardium
  constrictive disease of, 194
  cysts of, 192
  disorders of, congenital, 192, 193f
  visceral, 185

Perineal hernia, 460-451

Perineal urethrostomy, for urethral obstruction, 648

Periodontitis, 407-408

Peripheral nerves
  disorders of
    acute polyradiculoneuritis as, 1056-1057, 1057f
    botulism as, 1058
    dysautonomia as, 1059
    facial nerve paralysis as, 1051-1053, 1052f, 1053f
    focal neuropathies as, 1049-1054
    in hyperchylomicronemia, 1054
    ischemic neuromyopathy as, 1054, 1054f
    myasthenia gravis as, 1059-1061, 1060t, 1061f
    neoplastic, 1049-1051, 1051f
    polyneuropathy as, 1055-1056, 1055t, 1056f
    protozoal polyradiculoneuritis as, 1058
    tick paralysis as, 1057-1058
    traumatic, 1049, 1050t, 1051f
    trigeminal nerve paralysis as, 1053-1054, 1054f
  lymphoma of, 1124
  trauma to, 1050t
  tumors of, 1049-1051, 1051f

Peritoneal dialysis, for acute renal failure, 613, 615

Peritoneopericardial diaphragmatic hernia (PPDH), 192, 193f

Peritoneum
  disorders of, 466-469
    abdominal carcinomatosis as, 469
    hemoabdomen as, 468
    fluid in, analysis of, 377
    inflammation of, 466-468, 467f (*See also* Peritonitis)

Peritonitis
  bile, 539
  infectious, feline, 469, 1016-1017, 1275-1278 (*See also* Feline infectious peritonitis [FIP])

Peritonitis—cont'd
  sclerosing, encapsulating, 468
  septic, 466-468, 467f

Peroneal branch, damage to, 1050t

Pertechnetate, indication and dosage of, 565t

pH, seminal, 909

Phaeohyphomycosis, lymphadenopathy associated with, 1202t

Phagocytic immunodeficiency syndromes, 1226, 1227t

Pharmacologic testing, in Horner's syndrome, 989, 990t

Pharyngeal dysphagia, 409-410

Pharyngitis, feline lymphocytic-plasmacytic, 408-409

Pharyngoscopy, 243-245

Pharyngostomy tubes, 392
  uses of, 395

Pharynx
  diseases of
    clinical signs of, 241-242
      differential diagnoses for, 242, 242t
    diagnostic tests for, 243-245
  disorders of, 409-410

Phenamidine isethionate
  for babesiosis, 1301
  for infectious diseases, 1320t

Phenazopyridine, hepatotoxicity of, 522t

Phenobarbital (PB)
  alkaline phosphatase activity and, 486
  as anticonvulsant, 1001-1002
  chronic hepatitis from, 529
  hepatotoxicity of, 522t
  for neurologic disorders, 1070t
  for seizures, from brain tumors, 999
  for tetanus, 981

Phenols, hepatotoxicity of, 522t

Phenothiazine derivatives, an antiemetics, 396-397, 396t

Phenoxybenzamine
  for detrusor atony in urethral obstruction, 648
  dosage of, 206t
  for endocrine disorders, 815t
  for hypertension, 202t, 203
  for neurologic disorders, 1070t
  before pheochromocytoma surgery, 811
  for reflex dyssynergia, 655
  for urinary tract disorders, 659t

Phentolamine
  dosage of, 206t
  for hypertension, 202t, 203

Phenylbutazone
  hepatotoxicity of, 522t
  for joint disease, 1092t
  for neurologic disorders, 1070t
  neutropenia from, 1175t

Phenylephrine
  in cardiopulmonary resuscitation, dosages of, 99t
  dosages of, 208t, 341t

Phenylpropanolamine
  for incontinence with decreased sphincter tone, 656
  for micturition disorder diagnosis, 654-655
  for urinary tract disorders, 659t

Phenytoin
  alkaline phosphatase activity and, 486
  for arrhythmias, 90-91
  commercial preparations of, 87t
  for digitalis toxicity, 69
  dosages of, 79t, 207t
  hepatotoxicity of, 522t

Pheochromocytoma, 809-812
  clinical features of, 810, 810t
  diagnosis of, 810-811, 811t
  etiology of, 809-810
  prognosis for, 811-812
  surgical complications in, 811
  treatment of, 811

Phimosis, 920

Phlebotomy(ies)
  periodic
    for pulmonary hypertension with
      shunt reversal, 166
    for tetralogy of Fallot, 164
  therapeutic
    for erythrocytosis, 1171
    for polycythemia rubra vera, 1172
Phosphate, supplemental
  for diabetic ketoacidosis, 765t, 766-
    767, 766f
  for hypophosphatemia, 842-843
Phosphodiesterase inhibitors
  in congestive heart failure manage-
    ment, 70-71
  for dilated cardiomyopathy, 111-112
Phosphorus
  binders of, for hypercalcemia, 839, 839t
  in commercial reduced-sodium diets,
    61t
  diet low in, for hyperphosphatemia in
    chronic renal failure, 619,
    621
  metabolism of, hormone affecting, bio-
    logic actions of, 682t
  plasma concentrations of, interactions
    of, with calcium, parathyroid
    hormone and vitamin D
    concentrations, 620f
  in chronic renal failure, 621f
  serum concentration of
    depressed, 842-843, 842t
    elevated, 841-842, 841t
  white, hepatotoxicity of, 522t
Photodynamic therapy, for esophageal
    neoplasms, 415
Photomicrography, in clostridial disease
    diagnosis, 438f
Phycomycosis, lymphadenopathy associ-
    ated with, 1202t
*Physaloptera*, fecal examination for, 1230t
*Physaloptera rara*
  gastritis from, 419
  in stomach, 420-421
    endoscopic view of, 383f
Physical examination, in digestive disor-
    ders, 365
Physiologic nystagmus, 1005
Physiologic saline
  for hyperkalemia, 834, 834t
  for hyponatremia, 832
Physiotherapy, for bacterial pneumonia,
    300t, 301
Pimobendan
  in congestive heart failure manage-
    ment, 70-71
  for dilated cardiomyopathy, 113
Pinch biopsy, nasal, 224, 225f
Pindolol, characteristics of, 91t
Pine oil, hepatotoxicity of, 522t
Pioglitazone, 755t, 757
Piperazine, dosages of, 471t
Piroxicam
  for degenerative joint disease, 1080t
  for nasal tumors, 234
Pituitary-adrenocortical axis tests
  in cats, 801-802, 801t, 802f
  in dogs, 786, 787t, 788-792
Pituitary-dependent hyperadrenocorti-
    cism (PDH)
  in cats, 798
  in dogs, 778
  ultrasonographic appearance of, 783,
    784f, 786f
Pituitary dwarfism, 677-680
  clinical features of, 677-678, 677t, 678f
  clinical pathology of, 678
  diagnosis of, 678-679, 679f
  etiology of, 677, 678t
  prognosis for, 680
  treatment of, 679-680
Pituitary gland
  adenoma of
    hyperparathyroidism from, 681,
      682f
    ultrasound image of, 684f

Pituitary gland—cont'd
  disorders of, 660-680
    diabetes insipidus as, 661-667 (*See
      also* Diabetes insipidus)
    endocrine alopecia as, 667-670 (*See
      also* Endocrine alopecia)
    feline acromegaly as, 673-677 (*See
      also* Feline acromegaly)
    growth hormone-responsive
      dermatosis in adult dog as,
      670-673 (*See also* Growth
      hormone-responsive
      dermatosis in adult dog)
    pituitary dwarfism as, 677-680 (*See
      also* Pituitary dwarfism)
    polydipsia as, 660-661, 661t
      primary, 667
    polyuria as, 660-661, 661t
  hyperadrenocorticism dependent on,
    in dogs, 778
Pituitary macrotumor syndrome, 779f,
    780
PIV. *See* Parainfluenza virus (PIV)
Placenta, delivery of, 891-892
Placental sites, subinvolution of, 871-872,
    897-898
Plague, feline, 1259-1260, 1260f, 1260t,
    1313-1314
Plant alkaloids, 1107
Plantigrade stance, in polyneuropathy,
    1055, 1056f
Plasma, concentration of substances in,
    increasing, 616t
Plasma osmolality
  estimation of, in hyponatremia, 831f,
    8308-831
  measurement of, in urinary disorder
    evaluation, 587
  random, in diabetes insipidus diagno-
    sis, 665, 665f
Platelet(s)
  adhesion of, in hemostasis, 1185
  dysfunction of, 1192-1194, 1192t,
    1193f, 1193t
  estimation of, in blood smear in bleed-
    ing patient evaluation, 1187,
    1187f
  systemic lupus erythematosus and,
    1220t
Platelet count, in digestive disorders, 366
*Platynosomum concinnum*, extrahepatic
    bile duct obstruction from,
    518, 519f
*Platynosomum fastosum*, fecal examina-
    tion for, 1230t
PLE. *See* Protein-losing enteropathy
    (PLE)
*Plesiomonas shigelloides*, enterocolitis
    from, 439
Pleural cavity
  disorders of, 327-332
    chylothorax as, 330-332, 331f
    neoplastic effusion as, 332
    pyothorax as, 327-329, 328f, 329f,
      330f
    respiratory distress in, 336
    spontaneous pneumothorax as, 332
  effusions in, 315-318 (*See also* Pleural
    effusion[s])
  radiography of, 320, 321f
  septic exudates in, 327-329
Pleural effusion(s), 315-318
  chylous, 316t, 317
  diagnostic approach to, 315-318
  due to neoplasia, 318
  exudative, 316t, 317
  in feline dilated cardiomyopathy, 132
  in feline hypertrophic cardiomyopathy,
    123
    treatment of, 128, 129
  fluid classification in, 315-318
  hemorrhagic, 316t, 317-318
  neoplastic, 332
  in pulmonary thromboembolism, 310
  radiography of, 320, 321f
  respiratory distress in, 336

Pleural effusion(s)—cont'd
  thoracocentesis in, 322
  transudative, 316-317, 316t
Pleural fissure lines, 320
Pleural thickening, 320
Plexiform vascularization of lymph
    nodes, 1202t
PLI. *See* Pancreatic lipase immunoreac-
    tivity (PLI)
PLR. *See* Pupillary light reflex (PLR)
PMNs. *See* Polymorphonuclear cell
    (PMNs)
*Pneumocystis carinii*, lymphadenopathy
    associated with, 1202t
Pneumomediastinum, 319, 321, 321f
Pneumonia
  aspiration, 304-307, 306t
  bacterial, 299-302, 300t, 301f
    antibiotics for, 1244t, 1247-1248
  fungal, 302
  viral, 299
Pneumonic plague, feline, 1259-1260
Pneumonitis, immune-mediated, in
    heartworm disease, treat-
    ment of, 176
*Pneumonyssoides caninum*, 238
  fecal examination for, 1230t
  nasal, rhinoscopic view of, 223f
  sneezing from, 215
Pneumopericardiography, 49
Pneumoperitoneum, radiography of, 374
Pneumothorax, 318, 321f
  chest tubes for, 323
  radiography of, 320, 321f
  respiratory distress in, 336
  spontaneous, 332
Pneumoventriculography, in neuromus-
    cular disorders, 968, 969-
    970f, 970
Poikilocytosis
  disorders associated with, 1159t
  in hepatobiliary disorders, 485f, 486
Pointers, English
  progressive neurogenic muscular atro-
    phy in, 1045t
  sensory neuropathy in, 1046t
Poisoning
  rodenticide, vitamin K deficiency from,
    1194-1195
  salmon, 437, 1271
    lymphadenopathy associated with,
      1202t
Polioencephalomyelitis, feline, 1013-1014
Pollakiuria, 568, 569f
Polyarthritis. *See also* Arthritis
  antibiotics for, 1246t, 1247
  breed-specific, 1088
  chronic progressive, feline, 1091
  classification of, 1081t
  erosive, of Greyhounds, 1091
  feline, diagnosis of, 1073
  immune-mediated
    diagnosis of, 1072-1073
    idiopathic nonerosive, 1086-1088
    lymphadenopathy associated with,
      1202t
  Lyme disease, 1084
  *Mycoplasma*, 1083
  reactive, 1086, 1086f
  rickettsial, 1084
  systemic lupus erythematosus-
    induced, 1085-1086
    diagnosis of, 1073
Polychromasia, disorders associated with,
    1159t
Polyclonal gammopathies, 1211, 1211t
Polycythemia rubra vera (PRV), 1170
  treatment of, 1172
Polydipsia, 482, 482t, 577-579, 660-661,
    661t
  causes of, 577t
  in diabetes insipidus, 662-663
  in diabetes mellitus
    in cats, 751
    in dogs, 732

Polydipsia—cont'd
  diagnostic approach to, 578f
  endocrine disorders causing, 661t
  evaluation of, diagnostic tests in, 579t
  in hyperadrenocorticism, 780, 780t
    in cats, 798, 799t
  in hypertension, 201
  primary, 667
  psychogenic, 667
  urinalysis results in, 661t
Polymerase chain reaction (PCR)
  in ehrlichiosis, 1270
  in infectious disease diagnosis, 1236-
    1237, 1236f
  serologic studies for, in combined cy-
    topenias, 1182
  in toxoplasmosis diagnosis, 1297
Polymorphonuclear cells (PMNs), in pu-
    rulent vulvar discharge, 872
Polymyopathy, hypokalemic, 1065-1066
Polymyositis, idiopathic
  canine, 1063-1064
  feline, 1064
Polyneuropathy
  in Dalmatians, 1045t
  distal
    in Doberman Pinschers, 1045t
    sensorimotor, in Rottweilers, 1045t
  hereditary, of Alaskan Malamutes,
    1045t
  hypomyelinating, of Golden Retrievers,
    1045t
Polyp(s)
  bladder, benign, 596f
  gastric, ultrasonography of, 375f
  nasopharyngeal, 219f, 232-233, 233f
    (*See also* Nasopharyngeal
    polyps)
    radiographic signs of, 220t
  rectal, 459
Polyphagia
  in diabetes mellitus, in cats, 751
  in hyperadrenocorticism, in cats, 798,
    799t
  in hyperthyroidism, 713
  with weight loss, 816, 817t
Polyradiculoneuritis
  acute, 1056-1057, 1057f
  CSF analysis in, 964t
  protozoal, 1058
Polysulfated glycosaminoglycan
  for degenerative joint disease, 1080-
    1081
  for joint disease, 1092t
Polyuria, 482, 482t, 577-579, 660-661,
    661t
  causes of, 577t
  in chronic renal failure, management
    of, 617-618
  in diabetes insipidus, 662-663
  in diabetes mellitus
    in cats, 751
    in dogs, 732
  diagnostic approach to, 578f
  endocrine disorders causing, 661t
  evaluation of, diagnostic tests in, 579t
  in hyperadrenocorticism, 780, 780t
    in cats, 798, 799t
  in hypertension, 201
  urinalysis results in, 661t
Population control, estrus suppression
    and, 865-867
Portacaval shunt
  portal venography in, 495f
  ultrasonographic appearance of, 496f
Portal hepatitis, lymphocytic, 515-516
Portal hypertension
  congestive splenomegaly from, 1205
  noncirrhotic, idiopathic, 534-535
Portal vein hypoplasia, primary, 534
Portal venous hypertension, intrahepatic,
    ascites in, 474
Portal venous occlusion, prehepatic, ab-
    dominal effusion in, 474

Portosystemic shunt (PSS)
 congenital
  in cats, 520-521, 520f, 521f
  in dogs, 531-533, 531f, 532f
 hepatic encephalopathy and, 479, 480f
Portovascular disorders, congenital
 with high portal pressure, 533-535, 534f
 with normal portal pressure, 531-533, 531f, 531t, 532f
Positional nystagmus, 1005
Postcoital lock, 907
Postpartum disorders, 895-898
 agalactia as, 895-896
 metritis as, 896-897
 puerperal hypocalcemia as, 896
 subinvolution of placental sites as, 897-898
Postural reactions, in neurologic examination, 948, 950-951f
Posture, in neurologic examination, 948, 949f
Potassium
 abnormalities of, electrocardiography in, 26, 27f, 27t
 in commercial reduced-sodium diets, 61t
 deficiency of (See Hypokalemia)
 for digitalis toxicity, 69
 excess of (See Hyperkalemia)
 serum concentration of
  depressed, 833t, 834-836, 835t (See also Hypokalemia)
  elevated, 832-834, 833t, 834t (See also Hyperkalemia)
 supplemental
  for acute renal failure, guidelines for, 615t
  for diabetic ketoacidosis, 764, 765t, 766, 766f
  for hepatic lipidosis, 508
  for hypernatremia, 829t
  for hypokalemia, 835-836
  in IV fluids, 388, 388t
Potassium bromide (KBr)
 as anticonvulsant, 1002-1003
 for neurologic disorders, 1070t
Potassium chloride
 for hypokalemia, 836
 for hypokalemic polymyopathy, 1066
Potassium citrate
 for calcium oxalate uroliths, 639
 for chronic renal failure, 618t
 for cystine uroliths, 640
Potassium gluconate
 for hypokalemia, 835, 846t
 for hypokalemic polymyopathy, 1066
 for neurologic disorders, 1070t
Potassium phosphate
 for hepatic lipidosis, 508
 for hypokalemia, 836
Potassium-sparing diuretics, in congestive heart failure management, 64
PPDH. See Peritoneopericardial diaphragmatic hernia (PPDH)
PR interval, normal, ranges for, 17t
Pralidoxime chloride, for neurologic disorders, 1070t
Praziquantel
 dosages of, 341t, 402t, 471t
 for hepatobiliary and pancreatic disorders, 566t
 for liver flukes in cat, 520
 for tapeworms, 443
 uses of, 402t
Prazosin
 dosages of, 62t, 206t
 for hypertension, 202t, 203
 preparations of, 63t
 for urinary tract disorders, 659t
Precipitation-crystallization theory of urolith pathogenesis, 631
Precordial thrill, in cardiovascular examination, 6

Precordium, in cardiovascular examination, 6
Precose. See Acarbose
Prednisolone
 for canine lymphocytic-plasmacytic enteritis, 447
 for digestive disorders, 400
 dosages of, 471t
 for esophagitis, 412
 for feline eosinophilic enteritis/hypereosinophilic syndrome, 449
 for feline eosinophilic granuloma, 407
 for feline infectious peritonitis, 1278
 for feline lymphocytic-plasmacytic colitis, 448
 for feline lymphocytic-plasmacytic gingivitis/pharyngitis, 408
 for lymphocytic-plasmacytic gastritis, 419
 for masticatory muscle myositis, 409
Prednisolone sodium succinate
 for acute addisonian crisis, 808
 for cystic endometrial hyperplasia-pyometra complex, 879
 dosages of, 342t
 for endocrine disorders, 815t
 for feline bronchitis, 292
 for respiratory distress in lung disease, 336
Prednisone
 for allergic rhinitis, 240
 for aspiration pneumonia, 306
 for brachycephalic airway syndrome, 248
 for brain tumors, 999
 for canine chronic bronchitis, 297
 for canine idiopathic polymyositis, 1064
 for chronic hepatitis, 536-537
 chronic hepatitis from, 529
 for cyclophosphamide-induced hemorrhagic cystitis, 1115
 dosages of, 342t, 565t
 for ehrlichiosis, 1270
 for endocrine disorders, 815t
 for eosinophilic lung disease, 304
 for feline bronchitis, 293, 294
 for feline chronic progressive polyarthritis, 1091
 for feline idiopathic polymyositis, 1064
 for granulomatous meningoencephalitis, 1013
 for hypercalcemia, 839, 839t, 846t
 for hypocortisolism from mitotane excess, 794
 for idiopathic, immune-mediated polyarthritis, 1088
 for immune hemolytic anemia, 1162, 1163
 indications for, 565t
 for inflammatory hepatobiliary disease, 517
 for joint disease, 1092t
 for laryngeal paralysis, 247
 for leukemias
  acute, 1137t
  chronic, 1138t, 1154t
 for lymphoma, 1127t, 1128-1131, 1153t
 for lymphoplasmacytic rhinitis, 239
 for mast cell tumors, 1148, 1148t, 1149, 1154t
 for meningeal vasculitis, 1012
 for multiple myeloma, 1154t
 for myasthenia gravis, 1061
 for neurologic disorders, 1070t
 for neurologic signs of hydrocephalus, 994
 for obstructive laryngitis, 249
 for parasitic CNS disease, 1019
 for pulmonary arterial disease in heartworm disease, 177
 for rheumatoid arthritis, 1090
 for rickettsial polyarthritis, 1084

Prednisone—cont'd
 for steroid-responsive suppurative meningitis, 1011
 for thymomas, 1120
 for type II intervertebral disk disease, 1037
 for wobbler syndrome, 1043
Preeclampsia, 896
Preexcitation, ventricular, 25, 25f
Preganglionic cell bodies, trauma to, Horner's syndrome from, 987t, 988
Pregnancy
 alterations in bitch and queen during, 890-891
 confirmation of, 888-890, 889-890f
 disorders of, 886-895
 drugs risking, 900, 900t
 false, 886-887
 fetal resorption-abortion-stillbirth complex in, 900-901
 gestation length and, 891
 normal events in, 887-981
Prehensile disorder, dysphagia in, 345
Preleukemic syndrome, 1133
Premature contractions, 75-82, 77f
 supraventricular, treatment of, 7f, 76-77, 78t, 79-80t
Premature ventricular complexes (PVCs), 19f, 20-21f, 21-22
Preputial disorders, 920-921, 920f, 921f
Pressure gradients, across stenotic/regurgitant valves, Doppler estimation of, 46
Pressure overload
 chronic heart failure from, 55t
 therapeutic goals for, 56t
Presystolic gallop, 9
Prevacid. See Lansoprazole
Priapism, 918-919
Prilosec. See Omeprazole
Primacor. See Milrinone
Primaquine phosphate, for infectious diseases, 1320t
Primaxin. See Imipenem-cilastin
Primidone
 alkaline phosphatase activity and, 486
 hepatotoxicity of, 522t
 for neurologic disorders, 1070t
Primor. See Ormetoprim-sulfadimethoxine
Prinivil. See Lisinopril
Pro-Banthine. See Propantheline
Proarrhythmic effects, 78
Probucol, for hypercholesterolemia, 827
Procainamide
 for arrhythmias, 89
 commercial preparations of, 87t
 dosages of, 79t, 207t
 ECG changes from, 27t
 for paroxysmal AV reciprocating tachycardia, 77
 for sustained supraventricular tachycardia, 84
 for ventricular tachyarrhythmias, 80, 82
Procan SR. See Procainamide
Procarboxypeptidases A and B, 553t
Prochlorperazine
 for acute enteritis, 432
 as antiemetic, 396-397, 396t
 dosages of, 471t, 565t
 for gastrointestinal complications of chemotherapy, 1111
 indications for, 565t
 for parvoviral enteritis, 434, 435t
 for severe pancreatitis, 558-559
Procolipase, 553t
Proctitis, acute, 458
Proctoscopy, 381, 383-384, 383-384f
Proelastase, 553t
Proestrus
 abnormal, 863
 canine, 847-849, 848f

Proestrus—cont'd
 feline, 851
 vaginoscopy in, 853
Progesterones
 assessment of, 855-856
 cystic endometrial hyperplasia and, 877-878
 feline mammary hyperplasia and hypertrophy and, 883-884
 serum concentrations of, in corpora luteal function assessment, 888
Progestins
 for benign prostatic hyperplasia, 930
 for false pregnancy, 887
Proglycem. See Diazoxide
ProHeart. See Moxidectin
Prolactin
 antagonists of, in estrus induction in bitch, 868
 false pregnancy and, 886
Prolapse, rectal, 458-459
Pronestyl. See Procainamide
Propagest. See Phenylpropanolamine
Propantheline
 as antiemetic, 396t
 commercial preparations of, 88t
 for diarrhea, 399t
 dosages of, 80t, 208t, 471t
 for irritable bowel syndrome, 452
 for urinary tract disorders, 659t
Prophospholipase A, 553t
Propicia. See Finasteride
*Propionibacterium acnes*
 for feline immunodeficiency virus, 1280t
 for infectious diseases, 1319t
Propofol, for status epilepticus, 996t
Propranolol
 for arrhythmias, 92
 characteristics of, 91t
 commercial preparations of, 87t
 dosages of, 79t, 207t
 for feline hypertrophic cardiomyopathy, 127-128, 128t
 for hypertension, 202t, 203
Proprioceptive deficits, gait abnormalities from, 948
Propulsid. See Cisapride
Propylthiouracil (PTU), for endocrine disorders, 815t
Proscar. See Finasteride
Prostaglandins
 as abortifacients, 899
 for cystic endometrial hyperplasia-pyometra complex, 879-880, 880f
 for metritis, 897
 for reproductive disorders, 945t
 serum concentrations of, signaling parturition, 891
Prostaphlin. See Oxacillin
Prostate gland
 abscess of, 930-931
 bacterial infection of, 930-931
 disorders of, 927-933
  benign prostatic hyperplasia as, 928-930, 929f
  clinical features of, 927, 928t
  diagnosis of, 927-928
  inflammatory, 930-932
  neoplastic, 932-933
 hyperplasia of, benign, 928-930, 929f
 neoplasia of, 932-933
 squamous metaplasia of, 930
Prostatitis
 antibiotics for, 1248t, 1249
 bacterial, 930-931
 chronic, 931-932
Prostigmin. See Neostigmine
Protein(s)
 androgen-binding, 906
 coagulation, synthesized by liver, 481t
 in commercial reduced-sodium diets, 61t

Protein(s)—cont'd
dietary
acute renal failure and, 612-613
reduced
in chronic hepatic encephalopathy management, 546-547
for chronic renal failure, 619
homemade recipes for, 620t
plasma, molecular weights of, 579t
serum/plasma concentrations of, increased, 1210-1211, 1211f, 1211t
Protein-losing enteropathy (PLE), 451
causes of, 355t, 451
diarrhea in, 353
intestinal lymphangiectasia and, 451
in Soft-Coated Wheaten Terriers, 451
Proteinuria, 579-581
classification of, 580t
in glomerulonephropathies, 603-604, 604t
quantification of, 586
Proteolytic activity, fecal analysis for, 367
*Proteus*
antimicrobial agents for, 627, 629t
urinary tract infections from, 624, 625t
Proton pump inhibitors
in acute spinal injury management, 1023
as antacids, 397, 397t
Protopam. *See* Pralidoxime chloride
Prototothecosis, 440, 441f
lymphadenopathy associated with, 1202t
Protozoa
fecal examination for, 1230t
polysystemic infections from, 1296-1304
American trypanosomiasis as, 1304
babesiosis as, 1300-1301
cytauxzoonosis as, 1301-1302, 1302f
hepatozoonosis as, 1302-1303
leishmaniasis as, 1303, 1303f
neosporosis as, 1299-1300, 1300f
toxoplasmosis as, 1296-1299 (*See also* Toxoplasmosis)
systemic, cytologic examination for, 1234, 1234t
Protozoal myocarditis, 117
Protozoal myositis, 1065
Protozoal polyradiculoneuritis, 1058
PRV. *See* Polycythemia rubra vera (PRV)
PS. *See* Pulmonic stenosis (PS)
Pseudocyesis, 886
Pseudocyst, pancreatic, in acute pancreatitis, 555t
Pseudohyperkalemia, 833, 833t
Pseudohypokalemia, 834, 835t
Pseudohyponatremia, 830
*Pseudomonas*
antimicrobial agents for, 627, 629t
pulmonary infection from, 299
urinary tract infections from, 624, 625t
*Pseudomonas aeruginosa*, infective endocarditis from, 146
Pseudopregnancy, 886
Pseudoptyalism, drooling in, 344t
PSS. *See* Portosystemic shunt (PSS)
Psychogenic polydipsia, 667
Psychomotor seizures, 991
Psyllium hydrocolloid, dosages of, 403t, 471t
PTE. *See* Pulmonary thromboembolism (PTE)
PTH. *See* Parathyroid hormone (PTH)
PTU. *See* Propylthiouracil (PTU)
Ptyalism, drooling in, 344t
Puberty
in female, 847
in male, 905
Pug meningoencephalitis, 1013
Pulmonary artery(ies)
echocardiographic view of, 37f
in heartworm disease, 169-170, 172-173, 172f

Pulmonary capillary wedge pressure (PCWP), monitoring of, 48
Pulmonary edema, 312-313
in feline hypertrophic cardiomyopathy, treatment of, 128, 128t
radiographic signs of, 35
Pulmonary hypertension
from heartworm disease, 169
with shunt reversal, 164-166
Pulmonary infiltrates, with eosinophils, 303-304
differential diagnosis of, 251t
Pulmonary thromboembolism (PTE), 310-312, 310t
in hyperadrenocorticism, 780-782, 782t
Pulmonary vessels, radiographic assessment of, 34-35
Pulmonic stenosis (PS), 151, 158-160
breed dispositions for, 152t
murmurs in, 152f, 158
radiographic findings in, 154t
Pulse(s), arterial
in cardiovascular examination, 6, 6t
hyperkinetic, in patent ductus arteriosus, 153
Pulse oximetry, 285-286, 286f
Pulsed wave (PW) Doppler echocardiography, 45, 45f
Pulsus paradoxus, 6
in pericardial effusion, 186
Pulsus parvus et tardus, 6, 157
Pumpkin pie filling for dietary fiber, 390, 403t
Punctate chorioretinitis, in toxoplasmosis, 1296, 1297f
Pupil(s)
abnormalities of, 984-990
asymmetrical, 986-987
Pupillary light reflex (PLR)
absence of, in head trauma, 983
in visual pathway lesion localization, 984, 985t
Puppies, diagnosis of hypothyroidism in, 705
Puppy strangles, lymphadenopathy associated with, 1202t
Purulent vulvar discharge, 872
Pyelography, intravenous, 593-594f
Pyelonephritis, bacterial, clinicopathologic findings associated with, 627t
Pyloric hypertrophy, benign muscular, 421, 422f
Pyloric stenosis, 421, 422f
Pyloroplasty, for benign muscular pyloric hypertrophy, 421
Pyoderma
antibiotics for, 1245
gram-negative, antibiotics for, 1244t
in hypothyroidism, 693
staphylococcal, antibiotics for, 1244t
Pyometra
antibiotics for, 1248t, 1249
cystic endometrial hyperplasia and, 877-880 (*See also* Cystic endometrial hyperplasia [CEH]-pyometra complex)
Pyothorax, 327-329, 328t, 329f, 330f
antibiotics for, 1244t, 1248
chest tubes for, 323
Pyrantel pamoate
dosages of, 402, 471t
for *Physaloptera* gastritis, 421
for roundworms, 443
use of, 402t
Pyrexia, 1222
Pyridostigmine
for diarrhea, 399
dosages of, 471t
for myasthenia gravis, 1060
for neurologic disorders, 1070t
Pyrimethamine
for hepatozoonosis, 1302
for infectious diseases, 1320t
for neosporosis, 1300

Pyrimethamine—cont'd
for neurologic disorders, 1070t
for toxoplasmosis, 1298
Pythiosis, 429, 460, 460f

**Q**

QRS complex(es)
in dilated cardiomyopathy, 109
normal, ranges for, 17t
QT interval
abnormalities in, 25, 26t
duration of, normal, ranges for, 17t
Qualitative fecal analysis, in exocrine pancreatic insufficiency, 562, 562t
Queen
estrous cycle in, 851-852, 851f, 852f, 853f
estrus induction in, 868
infertility in, diagnostic approach to, 861f
ovulation induction in, 869
pregnancy, alterations in, 890-891
Questran. *See* Cholestyramine
Quinacrine, for giardiasis, 445
Quinaglute Dura-Tabs. *See* Quinidine
Quinidex Extentabs. *See* Quinidine
Quinidine
for arrhythmias, 89-90
dosages of, 79t, 207t
ECG changes from, 27t
for ventricular tachyarrhythmias, 80
Quinidine gluconate, commercial preparations of, 87t
Quinidine polygalacturonate, commercial preparations of, 87t
Quinidine sulfate, commercial preparations of, 87t
Quinolones
for bacterial meningitis/myelitis, 1015
for cutaneous and soft tissue infections, 1244t
for diskospondylitis, 1033
dosages of, 1242t
for hepatic and gastrointestinal infections, 1245t
for infectious diseases, 1319t
for leptospirosis, 1262
for salmonellosis, 438
for septic arthritis, 1082
toxicities of, 1242t
for urogenital infections, 1248t

**R**

R factor resistance, to antimicrobials, 624
R-HuEPO. *See* Erythropoietin
R wave, height of, normal, ranges for, 17t
Rabies, 1017
CSF analysis in, 964t
vaccination for
in cats, 1255
in dogs, 1256
zoonoses associated with, 1313t, 1315
Racemethionine, for urinary tract disorders, 659t
Radial nerve
peripheral, damage to, 1050t
trauma to, 1050t
Radiation therapy. *See* Radiotherapy
Radiography
in abdominal hemangiosarcoma diagnosis, 468
in acute abdomen, 361-362
in acute intervertebral disk disease, 1026, 1026f, 1027f, 1028f
in acute pancreatitis, 556-557, 556f
in adrenal mass detection, 812
of alimentary tract, 368
in aspiration pneumonia, 305
in atlantoaxial instability and luxation, 1047, 1047f
in atrial septal defect, 162

Radiography—cont'd
in atrioventricular valve disease, 141-142, 142f
in canine urolithiasis, 636f, 637f
in cardiac chamber enlargement, 32, 33t, 34, 34f
in cardiac tumors, 195-196
in cardiomegaly, 32, 33t
in cauda equina syndrome, 1039, 1040f
in chylothorax, 331t
in congenital heart defects, 154t
contrast-enhanced, of small intestine, 376, 377f
in cystic endometrial hyperplasia-pyometra complex, 878, 879
in dilated cardiomyopathy, 109, 110f
in diskospondylitis, 1032, 1032f, 1033f
in dysphagia, 344
in esophageal neoplasms, 416f
of esophagus, 369-371, 370-371f
in estrous cycle disorders, 858
in facial nerve paralysis, 1052, 1053f
in feline hypertrophic cardiomyopathy, 124, 125f
in feline lower urinary tract inflammation, 645
in foreign body detection, in intestine, 454-455, 454f
in gastric dilation/volvulus, 424, 425f
in gastric volvulus, 426f
in gastrinomas, 775
in gastrointestinal ulceration/erosion, 428, 428f
in heartworm disease
in cats, 181
in dogs, 172-173, 172f
in hepatic lipidosis, 507
in hepatobiliary disorders, 492-494, 493f, 494f, 495f
in hiatal hernia, 413f
in hyperadrenocorticism, 783, 784f
in hypertension, 201
in intracranial neoplasia, 997
in intrathoracic blood vessel assessment, 34-35
in intussusceptions, 455, 456, 456f
in joint disorders, 1071-1072, 1073
of larynx, 243
in liver abscesses, 541-542, 541f
in lower respiratory tract disease, 253
in lymphadenopathy, 1207
in lymphoma, 1125
in male reproductive function assessment, 912
in mediastinal masses, 318-319, 319f, 1119-1120
of mediastinum, 320-322, 322f
in mesenteric torsion/volvulus, 453
in metastatic hemangiosarcoma, 1143
in myasthenia gravis, 1060
nasal, 217-221, 220t, 228-220f
in nasal aspergillosis, 235
in nasal discharge evaluation, 213
in nasal tumor diagnosis, 234
in neuromuscular disorders, 961-962
contrast-enhanced, 965-970
in osteosarcoma, 1144-1145, 1144f
in paraprostatic cysts, 932
in pericardial effusion, 187-188, 187f
in peritoneopericardial diaphragmatic hernia, 192, 193f
of pharynx, 243
of pleural cavity, 320, 321f
in pleural effusion, 315, 320, 321f
in pneumothorax, 320, 321f
in pregnancy confirmation, 889-890
in prostate gland disorders, 927
in pulmonary edema, 35, 312
in pulmonary hypertension with shunt reversal, 166
in pulmonic stenosis, 159, 159f
in pyloric stenosis, 421, 422f
in pyothorax, 327
in septic arthritis, 1082f, 1083f
in solitary mass evaluation, 1117

Radiography—cont'd
  in spinal cord trauma, three-compartment model for, 1021, 1022f, 1023
  in spinal neoplasia, 1035, 1035f, 1036f
  in splenomegaly, 1207
  in subaortic stenosis, 157
  in tetralogy of Fallot, 164
  thoracic, 32-35, 255-261
    general principles of, 255-261
    lungs in, 256-261, 257f, 257t, 258f, 258t, 259f, 259t, 260f, 260t, 261f, 261t, 262f
    trachea in, 256, 256f
  in tricuspid dysplasia, 163
  in type II intervertebral disk disease, 1037
  in urinary disorders, 589-590, 590f, 593f, 594f
    findings in, 589t
  in ventricular septal defect, 161
  in wobbler syndrome, 1041, 1041f
Radioimmunoassay (RIA)
  in gonadotropin measurement, 856
  in progesterone measurement, 855-856
  in serum thyroxine measurement, 698
Radionuclide imaging, of spleen, 1207
Radionuclide thyroid scanning, 713f, 714f, 715f, 720
Radiotherapy
  for brain tumors, 998-999
  for CNS lymphoma, 1130
  cobalt, for thyroid neoplasia, 727
  for feline acromegaly, 676
  for mast cell tumors, 1148
  for mediastinal masses, 1120
  for nasal tumors, 234
  for oropharyngeal masses, 1150, 1151
  for pituitary-dependent hyperadrenocorticism, 797, 798f
  for spinal neoplasia, 1036
Ranitidine
  for acute spinal injury, 1023
  as antacid, 397, 397t
  for chronic renal failure, 618t
  for diarrhea, 399
  dosages of, 471t
  for gastrointestinal hemorrhage in liver failure, 550
  for hepatobiliary and pancreatic disorders, 567t
  for urinary tract disorders, 659t
  for vomiting, in chronic renal failure, 621
Rapid immunomigration (RIM) test, in relaxin detection, 858
Rapid slide agglutination test (RSAT), for *Brucella canis* infection, 937
Rappaport scheme, of hepatic functional lobule, 477f
RBCs. See Red blood cells (RBCs)
Reactive lymphadenopathy, cytologic evaluation of, 1098-1099, 1098f
Reactive polyarthritis, 1086, 1086f
Rectum
  polyps of, 459
  prolapse of, 458-459
  stricture of, benign, constipation from, 462
Red blood cells (RBCs)
  decrease in, 1156 (See also Anemia)
  increase in, 1170-1172
  morphologic abnormalities of, interpretation of, 1159t
  systemic lupus erythematosus and, 1220t
  in vulvar discharge, 870-871
Reflex(es)
  limb, 952, 952t, 953f
  panniculus, 952-953, 954f
  pupillary light
    absence of, in head trauma, 983
    in visual pathway lesion localization, 984, 985t

Reflex(es)—cont'd
  spinal, in neurologic examination, 950-953, 952t, 953f, 954f, 954t
  vasodepressor, syncope or intermittent weakness from, 2t
Reflex dyssynergia, 576, 652
  treatment of, 655
Reflux esophagitis, endoscopic view of, 381f
Regenerative anemias, 1160-1164
Regitine. See Phentolamine
Reglan. See Metoclopramide
Regurgitation
  aspiration pneumonia and, 305
  definition of, 345
  distinguishing vomiting from, 345, 345t
  in esophageal cicatrix, 415
Rehydration, for acute renal failure, 614-615
Rehydration therapy, 389
Relaxin, assessment of, 858
Renal azotemia, definition of, 608
Renal insufficiency, 608
  in hyperthyroidism, 716
Renal lymphoma, 1124
Renal reserve, 608
Renin-angiotensin system, in heart failure, 53, 53f
Renomegaly, 583
Reproductive function, male
  age-related effects on, 906
  diagnostic assessment of, 907-913
    hormonal evaluation in, 912-913
    radiography in, 912
    semen collection and evaluation in, 907-911 (See also Semen, collection and evaluation of)
    testicular aspiration and biopsy in, 912
    ultrasonography in, 912
  drugs affecting, 914t
  metabolic disorders affecting, 914t
  normal sexual development and behavior and, 905-907
Reproductive signs, in hypothyroidism, 694, 694t
Reproductive system
  artificial insemination and, 940-944 (See also Artificial insemination [AI])
  disorders of, 847-945
    canine transmissible venereal tumor as, 938-939
    drugs for, 944-945t
    estrous cycle disorders as, 847-869 (See also Estrous cycle, disorders of)
    genital infections as, 934-938 (See also Genital infections)
    infertility as
      female, 859-865 (See also Infertility, female)
      male, 905-917 (See also Infertility, male)
    mammary gland, 882-885 (See also Mammary gland disorders)
    penile, 918-920, 920f
    pregnancy-related, 886-895 (See also under Pregnancy)
    preputial, 920-921, 920f, 921f
    prostatic, 927-933
    testicular, 921-926, 922f, 924f, 925f, 925t
    uterine, 877-880
    vaginal, 870-877 (See also under Vagina)
  estrous cycle and, 847-852
    canine, 847-851, 848f
    estrous cycle in, feline, 851-852, 851f, 852f, 853f
    female, diagnostic tests for, 853-859
Respiratory arrest, 98
Respiratory distress
  in aspiration pneumonia, 305
  emergency management of, 333-336

Respiratory distress—cont'd
  in extrathoracic airway obstruction, 334-335, 334t, 335f
  in intrathoracic large airway obstruction, 335
  in large airway disease, 333-335, 334t, 335f
  in laryngeal disease, 241
  in laryngeal paralysis, 246
  in lower respiratory tract disorders, 251-252
  in pleural space disease, 336
  in pulmonary parenchymal disease, 335-336
Respiratory tract
  disorders of, 210-342
    localization of, by physical examination findings, 334t
    nasal, 210-240 (See also Nose)
    oxygen supplementation for, 337-340, 338f, 338t, 339f (See also Oxygen, supplemental)
    ventilatory support for, 340
  infections of, antibiotics for, 1247-1248
  lower
    disorders of, 250-314
      angiography in, 262
      bronchoscopy in, 276-281, 278-279f, 280t (See also Bronchoscopy)
      clinical signs of, 250-252
      computed tomography in, 262
      diagnostic approach to, 252-254, 253f
      diagnostic tests for, 255-286
      differential diagnoses for, 251t
      magnetic resonance imaging in, 262
      nonbronchoscopic bronchoalveolar lavage in, 270-274, 271f, 272f, 273f, 274f, 274t
      nuclear imaging in, 262
      open-chest lung biopsy in, 281
      parasitologic evaluation in, 262-264, 263t, 264t
      pulse oximetry in, 285-286
      radiography in, 255-261, 262f
      serologic tests for, 264
      thoracoscopy in, 281
      tracheal wash for, 264-270 (See also Tracheal wash)
      transthoracic lung aspiration and biopsy in, 274-276, 276f
      ultrasonography in, 262
    specimen collection from, comparison of techniques for, 265t
  parasites of, demonstration techniques for, 1230t
  upper, infection of, feline, 228-232 (See also Feline upper respiratory infection)
  zoonoses of, 1315-1316
Restlessness, in hyperthyroidism, 713
Restrictive cardiomyopathy, in cat, 129-130
Retention enemas, administration of, 402
Reticular interstitial pattern, 260, 261f, 261t
Reticulocyte count, in anemia, 1158
Reticulocyte index (RI), calculation of, in dogs, 1159t
Retrievers
  Golden
    hypomyelinating polyneuropathy of, 1045t
    muscular dystrophy of, 1066
  Labrador
    axonopathy in, 1044t
    hereditary myopathy in, 1067, 1067f
    spongy degeneration of white matter in, 1044t
Retrovir. See Azidothymidine (AZT)
Revolution. See Selamectin

Rheumatoid arthritis (RA), 1089-1091, 1089f, 1090f
  clinical features of, 1089, 1089f, 1090f
  diagnosis of, 1073, 1089-1090
  etiology of, 1089
  lymphadenopathy associated with, 1202t
  treatment of, 1090-1091
Rheumatoid factor, laboratory test for, 1078, 1089-1090
Rhinitis
  allergic, 239-240
    radiographic signs of, 220t
  bacterial, 238
  lymphoplasmacytic, 239
    radiographic signs of, 220t
  viral, radiographic signs of, 220t
Rhinoscopy, 221-222f, 221-224, 223f, 223t
  in aspergillosis, 235
Rhinotomy, exploratory, in nasal discharge evaluation, 224
Rhinotracheitis, vaccination for, 1255
Rhinotracheitis virus, feline, 228
*Rhipicephalus sanguineus,* as vector for ehrlichiosis, 1267
Rhythms. See Cardiac rhythm(s)
RIA. See Radioimmunoassay (RIA)
*Rickettsia rickettsii,* Rocky Mountain spotted fever from, 1265-1267. See also Rocky Mountain spotted fever (RMSF)
Rickettsiae
  cytologic examination for, 1233-1234, 1233t
  diseases from, CNS involvement in, 1018
  lymphadenopathy associated with, 1202t
  myocarditis from, 117
  polyarthritis from, 1084
  polysystemic diseases from, 1265-1271
    ehrlichiosis as, 1267-1271 (See also Ehrlichiosis)
    Rocky Mountain spotted fever as, 1265-1267, 1266t
  titers of, 1077
Ridaura. See Auranofin
Right aortic arch, persistent, breed dispositions for, 152t
Right ventricular cardiomyopathy, arrhythmogenic
  in cat, 133
  in dog, 116
Rigidity, decerebrate, 980-981
RIM test. See Rapid immunomigration (RIM) test
Rimadyl. See Carprofen
Ringer's solution, 832t
Ringworm vaccine, killed, 1256
Rintal. See Febantel
Risus sardonicus, in tetanus, 981, 981f
RMSF. See Rocky Mountain spotted fever (RMSF)
Robaxin. See Methocarbamol
Robinul. See Glycopyrrolate
Rocaltrol. See 1,25-Dihydroxycholecalciferol
Rocky Mountain spotted fever (RMSF), 1265-1267
  ancillary diagnostics for, 1011t
  antibiotics for, 1246t
  clinical features of, 1265, 1266t
  CNS involvement in, 1018
  CSF analysis in, 964t
  diagnosis of, 1265-1266
  epidemiology of, 1265
  etiology of, 1265
  lymphadenopathy associated with, 1202t
  myocarditis in, 117
  polyarthritis in, 1084
  prevention of, 1267
  serologic tests for, 973
  treatment of, 1266
  zoonotic aspects of, 1267

Rodenticide poisoning, vitamin K deficiency from, 1194-1195
Romazicon. *See* Flumazenil
Rompun. *See* Xylazine
Root signature, in intervertebral disk disease, 1025, 1025f
Rosiglitazone, 755t, 757
Rottweilers
 distal sensorimotor polyneuropathy in, 1045t
 leukoencephalomyelopathy in, 1044t
 neuroaxonal dystrophy in, 1044t
 spinal muscular atrophy in, 1046t
Round cell tumors, in cytologic specimen interpretation, 1097-1098, 1097-1098f
Roundworms, 441, 443
RSAT. *See* Rapid slide agglutination test (RSAT)
Rutin, for chylothorax, 331

**S**

S-adenosylmethionine
 for chronic hepatitis, 537
 for hepatobiliary and pancreatic disorders, 566t
Sacculitis, anal, 461
Sacral fracture, 1023
Saddle thrombus, 134
SAECG. *See* Signal-averaged electrocardiography (SAECG)
Salicylazosulfapyridine, for digestive disorders, 399-400
Saline, hypertonic, solution of, for shock, 387-388
Saline solution
 hypertonic, for hyponatremia, 832
 physiologic
  for hyperkalemia, 834, 834t
  for hyponatremia, 832
Salivary gland necrosis, 405-406
Salmon poisoning, 437, 1271
 lymphadenopathy associated with, 1202t
*Salmonella*
 antibiotics for, 1245t
 culture techniques for, 1235
 digestive disease caused by, 437-438
 as enteric zoonosis, 1309t
 fecal culture for, 367-368
Salmonellosis, 437-438
Salt, dietary, restricted, in congestive heart failure management, 60
Sandimmune. *See* Cyclosporine
Sandostatin. *See* Somatostatin
Sandoz. *See* Bromocriptine
Sarcoma(s)
 in cytologic specimen interpretation, 1095, 1096f, 1097, 1097f
 esophageal, 415
 injection site, in cats, 1151-1152
 lymphadenopathy associated with, 1202t
 mast cell, 1146
 soft-tissue
  chemotherapy protocols for, 1154-1155t
  vaccine-associated, 1255
SAS. *See* Subaortic stenosis (SAS)
Saw palmetto berry extract, for benign prostatic hyperplasia, 930
Scar, cerebral, epilepsy related to, 1000
SCC. *See* Squamous cell carcinoma (SCC)
Schistocytosis, disorders associated with, 1159t
Sciatic nerve, paralysis of, 1050t
Scintigraphy
 in hepatobiliary disorders, 498f, 499
 renal, in glomerular filtration rate evaluation, 585
Sclerosing, encapsulating peritonitis, 468
Sclerosing agents, injection of, into epididymis, 866
Sclerosing cholangitis, 515, 515f

Scottish Terriers, central axonopathy in, 1044t
Scratch zoonoses, 1312-1315, 1313t
Season, 847
Seborrhea, in hypothyroidism, 693
Sedimentation, fecal, 366
Seizures, 991-1004
 alternative therapies for, 1004
 anticonvulsants for, 1001-1004, 1001t
 classification of, 991, 992t
 clonazepam for, 1003-1004
 clorazepate for, 1003-1004
 complicating myelography, 965-966
 in degenerative diseases, 995-996
 diagnostic approach to, 991-993, 993f
 diazepam for, 1003
 disorders resulting in, 991-992, 992t, 994-1001
  congenital, 994-995
  metabolic, 994
 in epilepsy, 1000-1001
 felbamate for, 1004
 in feline ischemic encephalopathy, 999
 focal partial motor, 991, 992t
 generalized motor, complicating portosystemic shunt repair, 532-533
 generalized tonic-clonic, 991, 992t
 in hydrocephalus, 994, 998f
 in hypocalcemia, 840
 in hypoglycemia, 730
 inflammatory diseases causing, 999
 from insulin-secreting β-cell neoplasia, medical therapy for, 773, 774t
 in lissencephaly, 994-995
 neoplasia and, 996-999 (*See also* Brain, tumors of)
 phenobarbital for, 1001-1002
 potassium bromide for, 1002-1003
 psychomotor, 991
 valproic acid for, 1004
 vascular diseases causing, 999
Selamectin
 dosage of, 209t, 402t
 dosages of, 471t
 in heartworm prevention, 179
  in cats, 183
 uses of, 402t
Semen
 for artificial insemination
  cat, 943-944
  chilled extended, 943
  fresh, 942
  frozen, 942-943
  handling of, 940-941
 bacterial culture of, 911-912, 911f
 collection and evaluation of, 907-911
  color in, 908
  cytology in, 909
  indications for, 907
  interpretation of, 910-911
  seminal alkaline phosphatase in, 909-910
  seminal pH in, 909
  sperm morphology in, 909
  sperm motility in, 908-909
  spermatozoa concentration in, 908
  technique for, 907-908
  volume in, 908
 evaluation of
  interpretation of, 910-911
  in male infertility diagnosis, 914-915
Sensation, in neurologic examination, 953, 955, 955f
Sensory neuropathy
 in English Pointers, 1046t
 in long-haired Dachshund, 1046t
Sensory pathways, functional anatomy of, 946-947, 947f
Sepsis
 abdominal, of alimentary tract origin, 401
 in acute pancreatitis, 555t
 complicating liver failure, 551

Sepsis—cont'd
 liver disease secondary to, 543
 systemic, of alimentary tract origin, 401
Septic arthritis, 1081-1083, 1081t, 1082f, 1083f
Septic exudates
 in pleural cavity, 327-329
 in pleural effusion, 316t, 317
 in pyothorax, drainage of, 328-329
Septic peritonitis, 466-468, 467f
Septic vulvar discharge, 872
Septra. *See* Trimethoprim-sulfamethoxazole
Serax. *See* Oxazepam
*Serenoa repens* berry extract, for benign prostatic hyperplasia, 930
Serologic tests
 for *Brucella canis* infection, 936-937
 for joint disorders, 1077-1078
 for neuromuscular disorders, 973
 for polymerase chain reaction in combined cytopenias, 1182
 for pulmonary pathogens, 264
Serous nasal discharge, 210, 211t
Sertoli cells
 in male sexual development, 906
 tumors of, 924-925
  estrogen-secreting, squamous metaplasia of prostate from, 930
Serum antibody tests
 in infectious disease detection, 1237-1238, 1238f
 in nasal aspergillosis diagnosis, 235-236
 for toxoplasmosis, 1297
Serum biochemistry profile
 in digestive disorders, 366
 in hepatobiliary disease evaluation, 483
Serum enzymes, activities of, in hepatobiliary disorders, 486-487, 492t
Sex hormone imbalance
 adrenal-dependent, endocrine alopecia differentiated from, 669-670
 gonadal-dependent, endocrine alopecia differentiated from, 668-669
Sexual development, male, normal, 905-907
Sexual function, male, age-related effects on, 906
Shar-Peis, enteropathy in, 450
Shepherds, German
 giant axonal neuropathy in, 1045t
 spinal muscle atrophy in, 1045t
Shock
 in acute abdomen, 361
 cardiogenic
  canine, 118-120
  in dilated cardiomyopathy, 110, 111
 fluid therapy for, 387-389
Short bowel syndrome, 456-457
Shunt(s)
 arteriovenous, extracardiac, 153-155
 intracardiac, 160-162
 portacaval
  portal venography in, 495f
  ultrasonographic appearance of, 406f
 portosystemic, congenital
  in cats, 520-521, 520f, 521f
  in dogs, 531-533, 531f, 532f
  reversal of, pulmonary hypertension with, 164-166
Shunting
 in patent ductus arteriosus, 153
 portosystemic, hepatic encephalopathy and, 479, 480f
Sialoadenitis, 405-406
Sialoadenosis, 405-406
Sialocele, 405
Siberian Husky, laryngeal paralysis in, 1046t

Sick sinus syndrome, 85-86, 85f
Signal-averaged electrocardiography (SAECG), 31
Silicate uroliths
 factors predicting composition of, 632t
 treatment of, 640
Sinoatrial block, 23
Sinus(es), frontal
 ablation of, for feline upper respiratory infection, 230
 radiography of, 217, 218f
Sinus arrest, 16
Sinus arrhythmia(s), 16, 18f, 18t
 ECG in, 18f
Sinus bradycardia, 84
 causes of, 18t
 ECG in, 18f
Sinus rhythms, electrocardiography in, 15-16, 17t, 18f, 18t
Sinus tachycardia, 83
 causes of, 18t
Skeletal muscle, systemic lupus erythematosus and, 1220t
Skin
 in hypothyroidism, 692-693, 695f
 infections of, antibiotics for, 1244t, 1245
 lymphoma of, 1123
  treatment of, 1131
 tumors of, mast cell, 1146-1149 (*See also* Mast cell tumors [MCTs])
Skye Terriers, chronic hepatitis in, 528
SLE. *See* Systemic lupus erythematosus (SLE)
Smears
 blood
  in anemia, 1158
  platelet estimation in, in bleeding patient evaluation, 1187, 1187t
 fecal
  direct, 1229
  stained, 1231, 1231f
 impression, 1094
Sneezing, 215-216
 reverse, 215-216
Sodium
 balance of, maintaining, in chronic renal failure, 618
 in commercial reduced-sodium diets, 61t
 dietary
  reduced, for hypertension, 202
  restricted
   for ascites, 549
   for congestive heart failure, 60
 fractional excretion of, in hyponatremia, 831, 831f
 serum concentration of
  depressed, 830-832, 830t, 831f
  elevated, 828-830, 829t
Sodium arsenate, hepatotoxicity of, 522t
Sodium aurothiomalate, for joint disease, 1092t
Sodium bicarbonate. *See* Bicarbonate; Bicarbonate therapy
Sodium levothyroxine
 for endocrine disorders, 815t
 for hypothyroidism, 706-707, 707t
Sodium nitroprusside
 dosages of, 62t, 206t
 in fulminant congestive heart failure therapy, 59
 preparations of, 63t
Sodium pentobarbital, for status epilepticus, 996t
Sodium stibogluconate, for infectious diseases, 1320t
Sodium sulfate, for neurologic disorders, 1070t
Soft-Coated Wheaten Terriers, protein-losing enteropathy in, 451

Soft tissues
  infections of, antibiotics for, 1244t,
      1245
  sarcomas of
    chemotherapy protocols for, 1154-
        1155t
    vaccine-associated, 1255
Solganol. *See* Aurothioglucose
Solu-Cortef. *See* Hydrocortisone sodium
    succinate
Solu-Delta-Cortef. *See* Prednisolone
    sodium succinate
SoluMedrol. *See* Methylprednisolone
    sodium succinate
Somatostatin
  for digestive disorders, 399
  for endocrine disorders, 815t
  for feline acromegaly, 676-677
  for hypoglycemia in insulin-secreting
      β-cell neoplasia, 772t, 774
Somogyi phenomenon
  in cats, 761
  in dogs, 744-745, 745f
Sonolucent tissues, 36
Sotalol
  for arrhythmias, 93
  characteristics of, 91t
  commercial preparations of, 87t
  dosages of, 79t, 207t
  for ventricular tachyarrhythmias, 82
Spaniels, Brittany, spinal muscular atro-
    phy of, 1045t
Spaying, 865-866
  false pregnancy and, 887
Specimens
  cytologic
    interpretation of, 1094-1099
    staining of, 1094
  synovial fluid
    analysis of, 1074, 1076, 1076f, 1076t,
        1077f
    collection of, 1073-1074, 1074f,
        1075-1076f
    culture of, 1076-1077
Spermatogenesis, 906, 906f
Spermatozoa, 906, 906f
  concentration of, in semen evaluation,
      908
  morphology of, 909
  motility of, assessment of, 908
Spherocytosis, disorders associated with,
    1159t
Sphingomyelinosis, cerebellar dysfunc-
    tion in, 979t
Spina bifida, 1047
Spinal cord
  cystic accumulation of fluid in, 1048
  dysfunction of, 1020-1048
    acute, 1021-1031
      in acute intervertebral disk
          disease, 1024-1030 (*See also*
          Intervertebral disk disease)
      from fibrocartilaginous
          embolism, 1030-1031, 1031f
      hemorrhagic, 1024
      infarction causing, 1024
      traumatic, 1021-1024, 1022f,
          1023f
    causes of, 1021t
    clinical signs of, 1020
    congenital, 1047-1048
    diagnosis of, 1020
    general considerations on, 1020
    progressive
      chronic, 1034-1043
        in cauda equina syndrome,
            1038-1039, 1038f, 1039f,
            1040f
        in cervical vertebral
            instability/malformation,
            1040-1043, 1041-1042f,
            1043f
        from degenerative myelopathy,
            1037-1038
        from intraspinal articular cysts,
            1036

Spinal cord—cont'd
  dysfunction of—cont'd
    progressive—cont'd
      chronic—cont'd
        neoplastic, 1034-1036, 1034f,
            1035f, 1036f
        in type II intervertebral disk
            disease, 1036-1037
      subacute, 1031-1034
      in young animals, 1043, 1044t-
          1046t, 1046f, 1046-1047
    infarction in, CSF analysis in, 964t
    lesions of
      causing locomotion disorder,
          localization of, 975-976
      neurologic findings in, 976t
    masses of, myelographic appearance
        of, 967, 967f
    neoplasia of, 1034-1036, 1034f, 1035f,
        1036f
    radiography of, in neuromuscular dis-
        orders, 961-962
    segments of, 947f
      localization of, within vertebral
          bodies in dog, 1021t
      position of, 1022f
    trauma to, 1021-1024
      clinical features of, 1021
      diagnosis of, 1021, 1022f, 1023
      prognosis for, 1024
      treatment of, 1023-1024
Spinal dysraphism, 1047-1048
Spinal muscular atrophy
  in Brittany Spaniels, 1045t
  in German Shepherds, 1045t
  in Maine Coon Cats, 1045t
  in Rottweilers, 1046t
  in Swedish Lapland Dogs, 1046t
Spinal reflexes, in neurologic examina-
    tion, 950-953, 952t, 953f,
    954f, 954t
*Spirocerca lupi*
  esophageal sarcomas from, 415
  fecal examination for, 1230t
Spironolactone
  for ascites, 549-550
  for congestive heart failure, 57, 64
    in AV valve degeneration, 145
  for dilated cardiomyopathy, 112
  dosages of, 62t, 206t
  for hepatobiliary and pancreatic disor-
      ders, 566t
  preparations of, 63t
Spleen
  abscess of, 1204
  anatomy of, 1200
  enlargement of, 472, 1204-1209 (*See
      also* Splenomegaly)
  function of, 1200
  histology of, 1200
  masses in, 1206
  position of, 473f
  torsion of, 1205-1206
  work hypertrophy of, 1204
Splenectomy, 1209
Splenitis
  lymphoplasmacytic, 1204
  necrotizing, 1204
Splenomegaly, 1204-1209
  approach to, 1206-1208
  clinical features of, 1206
  clinicopathologic features of, 1206-
      1207
  diagnosis of, 1207-1208
  diffuse, 1204
  etiology of, 1204-1206
  imaging in, 1207
  infiltrative, 1204
  localized, 1204
  management of, 1208-1209
  pathogenesis of, 1204-1206, 1205t
Spongiform degeneration, of gray matter
    in Bull Mastiffs, 1044t
Spongy degeneration, of white matter in
    Labrador Retrievers, 1044t

Spontaneous nystagmus, 1005
Spontaneous pneumothorax, 332
Sporanox. *See* Itraconazole
*Sporothrix schenckii*
  cytologic appearance of, 1288t
  zoonoses associated with, 1313t, 1314,
      1315f
Sporotrichosis, lymphadenopathy associ-
    ated with, 1202t
Springomyelia, 1048
Squamous cell carcinoma (SCC)
  metastatic behavior of, 1118t
  oral, 406-407, 406f
  oropharyngeal, 1150
Squamous metaplasia, of prostate, 930-
    931
ST segment, normal, ranges for, 17t
ST-T interval, abnormalities in, 25, 26t
Staging, of lymphomas, 1125t
Standing heat, 849
Stanozolol
  for feline infectious peritonitis, 1278
  hepatotoxicity of, 522, 522t
Staphylococcal pyoderma, antibiotics for,
    1244t
*Staphylococcus*
  antimicrobial agents for, 627, 629t
  infective endocarditis from, 146
  pulmonary infection from, 299
  urinary tract infections from, 624, 625t
*Staphylococcus A,* for infectious diseases,
    1319t
*Staphylococcus intermedius,* pyoderma
    from, antibiotics for, 1245
*Staphylococcus* protein A, for feline im-
    munodeficiency virus, 1280t
Statins, in hyperlipidemia management,
    826
Status epilepticus
  emergency therapy for, 1004
  treatment of, 996t
Sterilization, 865-866
Steroid-responsive meningitis, CSF analy-
    sis in, 964t
Steroid-responsive neutropenia, 1175,
    1175t
Steroids
  anabolic
    for feline infectious peritonitis, 1278
    for nonregenerative anemia in
        chronic renal failure, 622
    suppurative meningitis responsive to,
        1010-1011
Stertor, 216
Stethoscope, 7, 7f
Stiglyn. *See* Neostigmine
Stillbirths, 900-901
  herpesvirus infection and, 934
Stomach
  biopsy of, in gastritis diagnosis, 419
  decompression of, for gastric
      dilation/volvulus, 424-425
  dilation of, with volvulus, 424-426,
      425f
  disorders of, 418-429
  foreign objects in, 423-424
  hypomotility of, idiopathic, 427
  infiltrative diseases of, 428-429
  inflammation of, 418-421 (*See also*
      Gastritis)
  lymphoma of, 428-429
  mucosa of, urease activity in, testing
      for, 379
  neoplasms of, 428-429
  outflow obstruction in, 421-427 (*See
      also* Gastric outflow
      obstruction)
    radiography of, 372, 373f
  polyps of, ultrasonography of, 375f
  pythiosis involving, 429
  radiography of, without contrast me-
      dia, 371-374, 373f, 374f
  ulcer of, endoscopic view of, 380, 382f
  volvulus of
    gastric dilation with, 424-426, 425f
    partial or intermittent, 426-427, 426f

Stomatitis, 408, 408t
Stranguria, in micturition disorders, 653
*Streptococcus*
  antimicrobial agents for, 627, 629t
  infective endocarditis from, 146
  lymphadenopathy associated with,
      1202t
  pulmonary infection from, 299
  respiratory zoonoses associated with,
      1315
  urinary tract infections from, 624, 625t
Streptokinase, for arterial thromboem-
    bolism, 136
Streptomycin, for feline plague, 1259-
    1260
Streptozotocin
  for endocrine disorders, 815t
  for hypoglycemia in insulin-secreting
      β-cell neoplasia, 772t, 774
Stress
  avoidance of, in chronic renal failure,
      622
  hyperglycemia induced by
    in cats
      complicating insulin therapy, 759-
          760, 760f
      serum fructosamine in, 758
    in dogs, serum fructosamine in, 741-
        742
Stress ulceration, gastrointestinal, 427-
    428
Stridor
  in laryngeal disease, 241
  in laryngeal paralysis, 246
*Strongyloides stercoralis*, 444
  as enteric zoonosis, 1309t
  fecal examination for, 1230t
Strongyloidiasis, 444
Struvite, feline lower urinary tract in-
    flammation related to, 642-
    644, 643f
Struvite crystals in urine sediment, 570f,
    571f
Struvite uroliths
  canine
    etiology and pathogenesis of, 633,
        633f
    factors predicting composition of,
        632t
    treatment of, 639
  feline, in feline lower urinary tract in-
      flammation, 642-644, 643f
Strychnine, neurologic dysfunction from,
    995t
Stupor
  characteristics of, 948t
  in pituitary-dependent hyperadreno-
      corticism, 780
Subaortic stenosis (SAS), 152, 156-158
  breed dispositions for, 152t
  murmurs in, 152f, 157
  radiographic findings in, 154t
Subinvolution of placental sites, 871-872,
    897-898
Subleukemia, 1133
Sucralfate
  dosages of, 471t
  for esophagitis, 412
  for gastrointestinal hemorrhage in liver
      failure, 550
  for gastrointestinal ulceration/erosion
      prevention, 428
  for hepatobiliary and pancreatic disor-
      ders, 567t
  as intestinal protectant, 398
  for mast cell tumors, 1148
Sulbactam, ampicillin with
  for aspiration pneumonia, 306
  for bacterial pneumonia, 301
  dosages of, 341t
  for pyothorax, 327
Sulfa drugs
  for salmonellosis, 438
  for toxoplasmosis, 1298

Sulfa-trimethoprim
for carcinomas, 1155t
for lymphoma, 1153t
for soft-tissue sarcomas, 1154t
Sulfadiazine-trimethoprim, for infection in chemotherapy patient, 1110
Sulfadimethoxine
for coccidiosis, 444
dosages of, 402t, 471t
uses of, 402t
Sulfas, potentiated
for cardiopulmonary infections, 1244t
dosages of, 1242t
for urogenital infections, 1248t
Sulfasalazine
for canine lymphocytic-plasmacytic colitis, 448
for digestive disorders, 399-400
dosages of, 471t
Sulfonamides
for infectious diseases, 1319t
toxicities of, 1242t
for urogenital infections, 1248t
Sulfonylureas, 755-757, 755t, 756f, 757t
Sulfosalicylic acid test, for proteinuria, 580-581
Summation gallop, 8
Suppurative meningitis, steroid-responsive, 1010-1011
Suprascapular nerve, trauma to, 1050t
Supraventricular ectopic complexes, 19, 19f, 20-21f, 21
Supraventricular premature complexes, 19, 19f, 20-21f, 21
Supraventricular premature contractions, 75-82, 77f
treatment of, 76-77, 77f, 78t, 79-80t
Supraventricular tachycardia (SVT), sustained, 84
Surface area, conversion of, to body weight
in cats, 1106t
in dogs, 1105t
Surgery
for abdominal hemangiosarcoma, 468
for acute spinal injury, 1023
for antral mucosal hypertrophy, 423
for atrial septal defect, 162
for benign muscular pyloric hypertrophy, 421
for bile peritonitis, 540
for brachycephalic airway syndrome, 248
for brain tumors, 998
for cardiac tumors, 196
for cauda equina syndrome, 1039
for caval syndrome in heartworm disease, 177-178
for cervical disk disease, 1029
for chylothorax, 331
for congenital portosystemic shunt, 521
for diskospondylitis, 1033
for esophageal neoplasms, 415
for esophageal vascular ring anomalies, 414
for extrahepatic bile duct obstruction, 540
for gallbladder mucocele, 540
for gastric dilation/volvulus, 425
for gastrinomas, 776
for heartworm disease, in cats, 182
for hemangiosarcoma, 1143
for hepatic neoplasia, 542
for hepatobiliary neoplasia in cats, 518
for hiatal hernia, 412
for hyperthyroidism, 722-723, 723t
for injection site sarcomas, 1152
for insulin-secreting β_cell neoplasia, 772-773, 773f
insulin therapy during, 742, 744
for intestinal foreign object, 455
for intestinal obstruction, 452, 453
for intussusception, 455

Surgery—cont'd
for large intestinal tumors, 459
for laryngeal paralysis, 247
for lymphadenopathy, 1208-1209
for mast cell tumors, 1148, 1148t
for mesenteric torsion/volvulus, 453
for nasal tumors, 234
for oral neoplasms, 407
for oropharyngeal masses, 1150, 1151
for pancreatic mass complicating pancreatitis, 559-560
for paraprostatic cysts, 932
for parathyroid disorders, 683, 685-686
for patent ductus arteriosus, 154
for perianal fistulae, 461
for pericardial effusion, 190
for peritoneopericardial diaphragmatic hernia, 192
for pheochromocytoma, 811
for portosystemic shunt, 532
for pythiosis, 429
for septic peritonitis, 466-468
for spinal neoplasia, 1036
for splenomegaly, 1208-1209
for spontaneous pneumothorax, 332
for subaortic stenosis, 158
for tetralogy of Fallot, 164
for thoracolumbar disk disease, 1029
for thyroid neoplasia, 727
for vaginal hyperplasia and prolapse, 876-877
for vascular ring anomalies, 166
for ventricular septal defect, 161-162
for wobbler syndrome, 1043
SVT. *See* Supraventricular tachycardia (SVT)
Swab, nasal, 224
Swedish Lapland Dogs, spinal muscular atrophy in, 1046t
Sympathetic innervation, of bladder, 650-651
Sympathetic nervous system, stimulation of, in congestive heart failure, 53
Sympathomimetic drugs
for arrhythmias, 96
for congestive heart failure, 69-70
dosages of, 80t, 208t, 292t
for feline bronchitis, 293
Syncope
causes of, 2t, 3
in degenerative AV valve disease, 141
in heart disease/failure, 1, 2t, 3, 3f
Synovial fluid
analysis of
gross appearance in, 1074, 1076f
microscopic appearance in, 1074, 1076, 1076f, 1076t, 1077f
collection of, in joint disorder diagnosis, 1073-1074, 1074f, 1075-1076f
culture of, 1076-1077
Synovial membrane, biopsy of, 1077
Synovium
inflammation of, lymphoplasmacytic, 1088-1089
systemic lupus erythematosus and, 1220t
Syprine. *See* Trientine
Systemic lupus erythematosus (SLE), 1220-1221
clinical features of, 1220
diagnosis of, 1220-1221
tests in, 1077
etiology of, 1220
lymphadenopathy associated with, 1202t
organs and tissues affected by, 1220t
pathogenesis of, 12204
polyarthritis induced by, 1085-1086
diagnosis of, 1073
polyneuropathy in, 1056
treatment of, 1221
Systolic clicks, 9

Systolic dysfunction, in dilated cardiomyopathy, 108
Systolic murmurs, 9-10, 9f

**T**

T3. *See* 3,5,3'-Triiodothyronine (T3)
T4. *See* Thyroxine (T4)
T wave, normal, ranges for, 17t
Tachyarrhythmia(s)
definition of, 16
syncope or intermittent weakness from, 2t
ventricular, chronic oral therapy of, 81-82
Tachycardia(s)
idioventricular, 22
paroxysmal, 75-82, 77f
AV reciprocating, treatment of, 77
sinus, 83
causes of, 18t
supraventricular, 19, 19f, 21
sustained, 84
ventricular
acute treatment of, 78, 80-81
sustained, 84
Tachypnea, in congestive heart failure, 3
Tacrolimus, for perianal fistulae, 461
*Taenia*, fecal examination for, 1230t
Tagamet. *See* Cimetidine
Tamoxifen, for mammary neoplasia, 885
Tapazole. *See* Methimazole
Tapeworms, 443
fecal evaluation for, 366
TAT. *See* Tube agglutination test (TAT)
Taurine
deficiency of
in cats, 61-62
dilated cardiomyopathy and
in cat, 130-131
in dog, 107
for dilated cardiomyopathy
in cat, 132-133
in dog, 111t, 113
TCC. *See* Transitional cell carcinoma (TCC)
Teasing, 849
Tegopen. *See* Cloxacillin
Teletherapy, cobalt
for feline acromegaly, 676
for thyroid neoplasia, 727
Temperature, body, in predicting labor, 891
Tenesmus, 356-357, 357t
Tenormin. *See* Atenolol
Tensilon. *See* Edrophonium chloride
Tensilon test, for myasthenia gravis, 1060, 1060t
Teratospermia, 909
Terbutaline
commercial preparations of, 88t
dosages of, 80t, 208t, 292t, 342t
for feline bronchitis, 292, 293
for respiratory distress in lung disease, 336
for sick sinus syndrome, 86
Terriers
Bedlington, familial chronic hepatitis in, 526-527, 527f
Cairn, neuronal chromatolysis of, 1045t
Fox, smooth-coated, hereditary ataxia in, 1044t
Jack Russell, hereditary ataxia in, 1044t
Scottish, central axonopathy in, 1044t
Skye, chronic hepatitis in, 528
Soft-Coated Wheaten, protein-losing enteropathy in, 451
West Highland White, chronic hepatitis in, 528
Testis(es)
aspiration of, in functional assessment, 912
biopsy of, in functional assessment, 912

Testis(es)—cont'd
cryptorchid, 922-923, 924f
descent of, 905
disorders of, 921-926
functional compartments of, 905
inflammation of, 921-922
infertility from, 916-917
neoplasia of, 924-926, 924f, 925f, 925t
torsion of, 923
Testosterone
evaluation of, in male reproductive function assessment, 912-913
for incontinence with decreased sphincter tone, 656
in male sexual development, 905-906
Testosterone cypionate, for urinary tract disorders, 659t
Tetanus, 980-981, 981f
Tetany
hypocalcemic, 840
puerperal, 896
Tetracycline(s)
for antibiotic responsive enteropathy, 450
for *Brucella canis* infection, 937
for campylobacteriosis, 437
derivatives of, for hepatic and gastrointestinal infections, 1245t
for digestive disorders, 401
dosages of, 342t, 471t, 1242t
for exocrine pancreatic insufficiency, 564
for feline plague, 1260
hepatotoxicity of, 522, 522t
for infectious diseases, 1319t
for joint disease, 1092t
for *Mycoplasma* polyarthritis, 1083
for neurologic disorders, 1070t
for rickettsial diseases, 1018
for Rocky Mountain spotted fever, 1266
toxicities of, 1242t
for urinary tract infections, 627
Tetralogy of Fallot, 164
breed dispositions for, 152t
radiographic findings in, 154t
2,3,2, -tetramine, for copper chelation, 536
Tg. *See* Thyroglobulin (Tg)
Thallium, hepatotoxicity of, 522t
treatment of, 523t
Theophylline(s)
for canine chronic bronchitis, 296-297
dosages of, 292t, 342t
for feline bronchitis, 293
for respiratory distress in lung disease, 336
Thiabendazole
dosages of, 471t
for strongyloidiasis, 444
Thiacetarsamide
for cytauxzoonosis, 1302
dosage of, 209t
for heartworm disease in cats, 182
for heartworm disease in dogs, 175
hepatotoxicity of, 522t
Thiamine
deficiency of, seizures from, 1000
for neurologic disorders, 1070t
for status epilepticus, 996t
Thiazide diuretics
for calcium oxalate uroliths, 639
for congestive heart failure, 64
for diabetes insipidus, 666, 666t
Thiazolidinediones, 755t, 757
Thiethylphosphine gold, for immune-mediated disorders, 1218
Thiobarbiturates, ECG changes from, 27t
6-Thioguanine, for leukemias, acute, 1137t, 1154t
Thirst, increased, 482, 482t
Thoracocentesis, 322-323
for chylothorax, 331
for mediastinal masses, 319

Thoracocentesis—cont'd
for paragonimiasis, 303
for pleural effusion in cat
in feline dilated cardiomyopathy, 132
in hypertrophic cardiomyopathy, 128, 129
for spontaneous pneumothorax, 332
Thoracolumbar disk disease, 1028-1029
Thoracoscopy, 281, 326
Thoracotomy, 326
in foreign body removal from esophagus, 414
in lower respiratory tract specimen collection, 265t
in pyothorax, 329, 329f
in thymomas, 1120
Thorax
auscultation of, in cardiovascular examination, 6-7, 7f
radiography of, 32-35, 255-261 (*See also* Radiography, thoracic)
Thorazine. *See* Chlorpromazine
Thrombocytopenia, 1190-1192, 1190t
approach to, 1190-1191
causes of, 1190t
from chemotherapy, 1109
disorders associated with, 1159t
immune-mediated, 1191-1192
Thromboembolism
arterial, in cat, 134-137
clinical features of, 134, 134f, 135t
complicating hypertrophic cardiomyopathy, 129
diagnosis of, 134
prevention of, 136-137
prognosis of, 134-136
treatment of, 134-136
in nephrotic syndrome, 605
pulmonary, 310-312, 310t
complicating adulticide heartworm therapy, 176
in hyperadrenocorticism, 780-782, 782t
in restrictive cardiomyopathy, 130
Thrombolytic therapy, for arterial thromboembolism, 136
Thrombosis, 1199
Thromboxane synthetase inhibitors, for glomerulonephritis, 606
Thymic hematomas, as mediastinal masses, 1119t
Thymoma, 1119, 1119f, 1119t
Thyroglobulin (Tg) autoantibodies, in lymphocytic thyroiditis, 700
Thyroid gland
adenocarcinoma of, 1119t
atrophy of, idiopathic, 691
carcinoma of, hyperthyroidism from, 712, 715f
disorders of, 691-728
hyperthyroidism as, 712-724 (*See also* Hyperthyroidism)
hypothyroidism as, 691-712 (*See also* Hypothyroidism)
neoplastic, 724-728
function tests on, 697-702
baseline endogenous canine TSH concentration as, 700, 701f
baseline serum free thyroxine concentrations as, 698-699, 699t
baseline serum thyroxine concentration as, 698, 699t
factors affecting, 702, 703t, 704f, 705f
for lymphocytic thyroiditis, 700-702
TSH and TRH stimulation tests as, 700
neoplasia of, canine, 724-728
clinical features of, 724-726, 725f, 725t, 726f
diagnosis of, 726
diagnostic imaging in, 725-726, 726f

Thyroid gland—cont'd
neoplasia of, canine—cont'd
etiology of, 724
prognosis for, 727-728
treatment of, 726-727
radionuclide scanning of, 713f, 714f, 715f, 720
Thyroid hormone autoantibodies, breeds with increased prevalence of, 692t
Thyroid hormones
serum concentrations of, in thyroid neoplasia, 725
tests of, 697-700, 697f, 698f, 699f, 699t
Thyroid-stimulating hormone (TSH)
endogenous concentration of, baseline, 700, 701f
stimulation test using, 700
Thyroidectomy, 722-723, 723t
Thyroiditis, lymphocytic, tests for, 700-702
Thyrotoxic cardiomyopathy, 714, 716
Thyrotoxicosis, 707, 709
Thyrotropin-releasing hormone (TRH) stimulation test for hypothyroidism
in cats, 711
in dogs, 700, 702f
Thyroxine (T$_4$)
synthetic, for endocrine disorders, 815t
Thyroxine (T$_4$)
autoantibodies to, in lymphocytic thyroiditis, 701-702
free, serum concentrations of baseline
in cats, 717, 718f
in dogs, 698-699, 699t
in cats, 710-711, 711f
serum concentration of baseline
in cats, 716, 717f, 718f
in dogs, 698, 699t
in cats, 710-711f, 711
synthetic, for hypothyroidism, 706-707, 707t
Tibetan Mastiffs, inherited hypertrophic neuropathy in, 1046f
Tibial branch, damage to, 1050t
Ticarcillin, with clavulanate
for cardiopulmonary infections, 1244t
dosages of, 1241t
for infectious diseases, 1319t
Tick paralysis, 1057-1058
Ticks, as vectors
for ehrlichiosis, 1267
for Rocky Mountain spotted fever, 1265
Tie, 907
Tigan. *See* Trimethobenzamide
Timentin. *See* Ticarcillin with clavulanate
Timolol, characteristics of, 91t
Tissue factor, in hemostasis, 1185-1186
Tissue necrosis, local, from chemotherapy drug extravasation, 1112-1113, 1112t
Tissue plasminogen activator (TPA), for arterial thromboembolism, 136
TLI. *See* Trypsin-like immunoreactivity (TLI); Trypsinlike immunoreactivity (TLI)
Tobramycin
dosages of, 1241t
for infectious diseases, 1318t
Tocainide
for arrhythmias, 90
commercial preparations of, 87t
dosages of, 79t, 207t
for ventricular tachyarrhythmias, 82
Tofranil. *See* Imipramine
Toltrazuril
for coccidiosis, 444
for infectious diseases, 1320t
Toluene, hepatotoxicity of, 522t

Tongue, squamous cell carcinoma of, 406t
Tonocard. *See* Tocainide
Tonsil, squamous cell carcinoma of, 406t
Tooth root abscess, radiographic signs of, 220t
Torbugesic. *See* Butorphanol
Torbutrol. *See* Butorphanol
Torsades de pointes, 81, 93
Torsion
mesenteric, 453
splenic, 1205-1206
testicular, 923
uterine, 877
Total parenteral nutrition, for parvoviral enteritis, 434, 435t
*Toxacara canis,* 441, 442f, 443
*Toxascaris,* fecal examination for, 1230t
*Toxascaris leonina,* 441, 443
Toxic hepatopathy, acute, 521-523, 522t, 523t, 537-538
Toxicants, renal, 609, 610t
Toxicity
antibiotic, 1242t
chemotherapy drug
cardiovascular, 1114
dermatologic, 1112-1113
gastrointestinal, 1111
hematologic, 1108-1111
hepatic, 1115
neurologic, 1115
pancreatic, 1113-1114
pulmonary, 1115
urologic, 1114-1115
digitalis, 68-69
lidocaine, 88-89
procainamide, 89
quinidine, 90
Toxins
polyneuropathy from, 1056
seizures from, 994, 995t
*Toxocara,* fecal examination for, 1230t
*Toxocara canis*
as enteric zoonosis, 1309t
lung disease from, 302
*Toxocara cati,* 441, 443
as enteric zoonosis, 1309t
*Toxoplasma gondii*
drugs for, 1320t
as enteric zoonosis, 1309t, 1311
fecal examination for, 1230t
infection with, 1296-1299 (*See also* Toxoplasmosis)
morphologic characteristics of, 1234t
myocarditis from, 117
polyradiculoneuritis from, 1058
*Toxoplasma gondii* tachyzoites, in tracheal wash specimen, 269f
Toxoplasmosis, 302, 1017
ancillary diagnostics for, 1011t
antibiotics for, 1244t, 1246t
canine, 1299
CSF analysis in, 964t
feline, 1296-1299
clinical features of, 1296, 1297f
diagnosis of, 1296-1297
epidemiology of, 1296
etiology of, 1296
prevention of, 1298-1299
treatment of, 1298
zoonotic aspects of, 1298-1299
immunologic and serologic tests for, 973
lymphadenopathy associated with, 1202t
Trachea
bronchoscopic abnormalities of, 280t
bronchoscopic view of, 278f
collapsing, 289-291
bronchoscopic view of, 278f
radiography of, 289f, 290f
disorders of, 287-291
differential diagnoses for, 251t
hypoplastic, 256, 256f
thoracic radiography of, 256, 256f

Tracheal nodular worm, fecal examination for, 1230t
Tracheal tubes, for oxygen supplementation, 338t, 339-340
Tracheal wash, 264-270
for aspiration pneumonia, 306-307
in aspiration pneumonia diagnosis, 305
in canine chronic bronchitis, 296
complications of, 264-265, 265t
endotracheal technique of, 268
indications for, 264-265, 265t
in lower respiratory tract specimen collection, 265t
problems with, overcoming, 267t
results of, interpretation of, 268-270, 269f
specimen handling from, 268-269f
techniques of, 266-268, 266f
transtracheal technique of, 266-268, 266f
Tracheobronchitis, canine infectious, 287-289, 288f
Tranquilizers, in fulminant congestive heart failure management, 59, 59t
Transbronchial lung biopsy, 278, 281
Transesophageal echocardiography, 47
Transfusion, blood/blood product
for bleeding patient, 1190
complications of, 1169
crossmatching for, 1168, 1169t
for immune hemolytic anemia, 1164
principles of, 1168-1169
Transfusions, blood/blood product
for cytauxzoonosis, 1302
Transitional cell carcinoma (TCC)
of bladder, 570, 593f, 597f
metastatic behavior of, 1118t
Transmissible venereal tumor (TVT), canine, 938-939
Transsphenoidal hypophysectomy, microsurgical, for feline acromegaly, 677
Transthoracic lung aspiration and biopsy, 274-276, 276f
Transtracheal catheters, for oxygen supplementation, 338t, 339
Transudates
in abdominal effusions in hepatobiliary disease, 491t
pericardial effusion from, 186
in pleural effusion, 316-317, 316t
Trauma
brain, complicating nasal biopsy, 225
epilepsy related to, 1000
head, neuromuscular disorders from, 983-984, 984t
neonatal mortality from, 903
oral, dysphagia in, 344t
spinal cord, 1021-1024, 1022f, 1023f
stomatitis from, 408t
Traumatic myocarditis, 118
Traumatic neuropathies, 1049, 1050t, 1051f
Traxene. *See* Clorazepate
Tremors, 980
TRH. *See* Thyrotropin-releasing hormone (TRH)
Triamterene
dosages of, 62t, 206t
preparations of, 63t
Tribrissen. *See* Trimethoprim-sulfadiazine
Trichlorethane, hepatotoxicity of, 522t
*Trichomonas*
fecal evaluation for, 366
trophozoites of, *Giardia* trophozoites compared with, 446f
*Trichomonas foetus,* fecal examination for, 1230t
Trichomoniasis, 446, 446f
*Trichuris vulpis,* 440-441, 442f
fecal examination for, 1230t

Tricuspid dysplasia
  breed dispositions for, 152t
  radiographic findings in, 154t
Tricuspid valve
  degenerative disease of, 138-145
    clinical signs of, 141
    complicating factors in, 140-141, 140t
    echocardiography in, 142-143, 142f, 143f
    electrocardiography in, 142
    epidemiology of, 141
    etiology of, 139
    pathology of, 139
    pathophysiology of, 139-140
    patient monitoring in, 145
    prognosis in, 143-145
    radiography in, 141-142, 142f
    reevaluation in, 145
    treatment of, 143-145
  dysplasia of, 162-163, 163f
Trientine
  for copper chelation, 536
  for hepatobiliary and pancreatic disorders, 566t
Trigeminal nerve paralysis, 1053-1054, 1054f
Triglyceride challenge test, in exocrine pancreatic insufficiency, 561-562, 562f, 562t
Triglycerides, 822-823
  medium-chain, dosages of, 471t
3,5,3'-Triiodothyronine (T$_3$)
  serum concentration of, baseline, 698, 698f
  synthetic, for endocrine disorders, 815t
3,5,3'-Triiodothyronine (T$_3$) suppression test in hyperthyroidism diagnosis, 717-718, 719f, 720
Trilostane
  for endocrine disorders, 815t
  for pituitary-dependent hyperadrenocorticism, 796
Trimethobenzamide
  as antiemetic, 396t, 397
  for chronic renal failure, 618t
  dosages of, 471t
  for urinary tract disorders, 659t
  for vomiting, in chronic renal failure, 621
Trimethoprim-sulfa
  for coccidiosis, 444
  hepatotoxicity of, 522t
  for urinary tract infections, 627
Trimethoprim-sulfadiazine
  for cutaneous and soft tissue infections, 1244t
  dosages of, 342t, 402t, 471t
  for feline upper respiratory infections, 230
  for hepatic and gastrointestinal infections, 1245t
  for hepatozoonosis, 1302
  for infectious diseases, 1320t
  for neosporosis, 1300
  for neurologic disorders, 1070t
  for *Toxoplasma* meningoencephalomyelitis, 1017
  uses of, 402t
Trimethoprim-sulfamethoxasole
  for hepatobiliary and pancreatic disorders, 566t
Trimethoprim-sulfamethoxazole
  for severe pancreatitis, 559
Trimethoprim-sulfonamide
  dosages of, 1242t
  for infectious diseases, 1319t
  for toxoplasmosis, 1298, 1299
Troponins, cardiac, as myocardial injury markers, 48
*Trypanosoma cruzi*, 1304
  morphologic characteristics of, 1234t
  myocarditis from, 117

Trypanosomiasis
  American, 1304
  lymphadenopathy associated with, 1202t
Trypsin-like immunoreactivity (TLI)
  in exocrine pancreatic insufficiency, 562-563
  serum, 378
Trypsinlike immunoreactivity (TLI), serum, in acute pancreatitis, 557
Trypsinogen, 553t
Tubal ligation, 866
Tube(s)
  chest, 323-326, 324-325f
    complications of, 323
    indications for, 323
    placement of, 323-326, 324-325f
    for pyothorax, 328-329
  endotracheal, for oxygen supplementation, 338t, 339
  feeding, 391-392, 393-394f, 395 (*See also* Feeding tube[s])
  tracheal, for oxygen supplementation, 338t, 339-340
Tube agglutination test (TAT), for *Brucella canis* infection, 937
Tumil-K. *See* Potassium gluconate
Tumor(s)
  adrenal, 811t
  adrenocortical, 778-792 (*See also* Adrenocortical tumors [ATs])
  beta-cell, insulin-secreting, 769-775 (*See also* Insulin-secreting β-cell neoplasia)
  bone, 1144-1146, 1144f, 1145f, 1145t
  brain (*See also* Brain, tumors of)
    seizures and, 996-999
  canine transmissible venereal, 938-939
  cardiac, 194-196
    dog breed incidence of, 195t
  CNS, CSF analysis in, 964t
  effusions due to, 318
  esophageal, 415-416, 416f
  extrahepatic bile duct obstruction from, 518
  fever of undetermined origin in, 1223t
  gastric, 428-429
  heart base, 195, 1119t
    treatment of, 190-191
  hepatic, 542
  hepatobiliary, in cat, 517-518
  interstitial cell, 925
  large intestinal, 459, 459f
  laryngeal, 249
  laryngoscopy/pharyngoscopy of, 244-245
  lung, interstitial pattern in, 259-260, 260f
  lymph node, cytologic evaluation of, 1099
  lymphoid, metastatic, 1208
  malignant, cytologic characteristics of, 1095t
  mammary, 884-885
  mast cell
    gastrointestinal ulceration/erosion from, 427-428
    lymphadenopathy associated with, 1202t
    metastatic behavior of, 1118t
  mediastinal, 318
  metastatic, lymphadenopathy associated with, 1202t
  metastatic behavior of, 1118t
  nasal, 219f, 233-235
    radiographic signs of, 220t
  oral, 406-407, 406t
    dysphagia in, 344t
  oropharyngeal, 1149-1151
  pancreatic, 564
    gastrin-secreting, 775-776, 775f
    in severe pancreatitis, management of, 559-560

Tumor(s)—cont'd
  perianal, 461-462
  perianal gland, 462
  peripheral nerve, 1049-1051, 1051f
  prostatic, 932-933
  pulmonary, 307-309
  round cell, in cytologic specimen interpretation, 1097-1098, 1097-1098f
  Sertoli cell, 924-925
  small intestinal, 457-458
  spinal cord, 1034-1036, 1034f, 1035f, 1036f
  testicular, 924-926, 924f, 925f, 925t
  thyroid, canine, 724-728 (*See also* Thyroid gland, neoplasia of, canine)
  uterine, 877
  vestibular, 1008
Tums. *See* Calcium gluconate
Turbinates, erosion of, differential diagnosis of, 223t
Turbinectomy, 225
  exploratory, 214
  for feline upper respiratory infection, 230
TVT. *See* Transmissible venereal tumor (TVT)
Tylan. *See* Tylosin
Tylosin
  for antibiotic responsive enteropathy, 450
  for clostridial disease, 438
  dosages of, 471t, 1241t
  for exocrine pancreatic insufficiency, 564
  for hepatic and gastrointestinal infections, 1245t
  for hepatobiliary and pancreatic disorders, 566t
  for infectious diseases, 1319t, 1320t
  for joint disease, 1092t
  for *Mycoplasma* polyarthritis, 1083
Tympanic bullae, in nasal radiography, 217, 219f
Typhlectomy, for cecocolic intussusception, 458

**U**

Ulcers
  gastric, endoscopic view of, 380, 382f
  gastroduodenal, erosion and, hematemesis in, 351
Ulnar nerve trauma, 1050t
Ultra-low-fat diet, 390
Ultrasonography (US)
  in abdominal hemangiosarcoma diagnosis, 468
  in acute abdomen, 361
  in acute pancreatitis, 557, 557f
  in adrenal mass detection, 812
  of alimentary tract, 368
  in biliary tract disorders, 539f, 540
  of bladder, 589t, 596, 596f, 597f
  cardiac, 35-47 (*See also* Echocardiography)
  in chylothorax, 331
  in cystic endometrial hyperplasia-pyometra complex, 878, 878f, 879
  in dystocia assessment, 893
  in estrous cycle disorders, 858, 859f
  in feline lower urinary tract inflammation, 645
  in hemangiosarcoma, 1143, 1143f
  in hepatic lipidosis, 507
  in hepatobiliary disorders, 494-499, 495f, 496f, 497-498f
  in hyperadrenocorticism
    in cats, 802
    in dogs, 783, 784-785f, 785, 786f
  in hypoadrenocorticism, 806
  in insulin-secreting β-cell neoplasia diagnosis, 770, 771f
  of larynx, 243

Ultrasonography (US)—cont'd
  in lower respiratory tract disorders, 262
  in lymphadenopathy, 1207
  in lymphoma, 1125
  in male reproductive function assessment, 912
  in mediastinal masses, 1119
  of mediastinal masses, 319
  of mediastinum, 322
  of pharynx, 243
  in pheochromocytoma diagnosis, 810
  of pleural cavity, 322
  in pleural effusion, 315
  in pregnancy confirmation, 889-890f
  in prostate gland disorders, 927, 928f
  renal, 590, 591-592f
    findings in, 589t
  in septic peritonitis, 466
  of small intestine, 374, 375f
  in splenomegaly, 1207
  of stomach, 374
  in thyroid neoplasia, 725-726, 726f
Unasyn. *See* Ampicillin with sulbactam
*Uncinaria*, 443
*Uncinaria stenocephala*, as enteric zoonosis, 1309t
Upper airway obstruction syndrome, 248-249, 248f
Upper motor neuron (UMN)
  functional anatomy of, 946, 947f
  injury to, Horner's syndrome from, 987-988, 987t
  lesions of
    bladder distention from, 651-652
    treatment of, 655
  signs from, 952t
Upper respiratory tract, infection of, feline, 228-232. *See also* Feline upper respiratory infection
Urate uroliths
  factors predicting composition of, 632t
  treatment of, 639-640
*Urcinaria stenocephala*, fecal examination for, 1230t
Urea nitrogen, serum concentration of, in hepatobiliary system assessment, 487, 492t
*Ureaplasma*
  antibiotics for, 1248t
  culture techniques for, 1235
  genital infections from, 935-936
  polysystemic disease from, 1262-1264, 1263t
Urease activity, in gastric mucosa, testing for, 379
Urecholine. *See* Bethanechol
Uremia, definition of, 608
Uremic syndrome, definition of, 608
Ureter, unilateral ectopic, 594f
Urethra
  catheterization of
    in feline lower urinary tract inflammation management, 647
    for lower motor neuron disorders, 655
    urinary tract infections and, 626
  function of, diagnostic tests of, 588
  inflammation of, clinical signs of, 645t
  obstruction of, 568
    anatomic, treatment of, 656
    clinical signs of, 645t
    functional, treatment of, 655-656
Urethral sphincter mechanism incompetence, treatment of, 656
Urethritis, clinical signs of, 645t
Urethrography, 596, 597f, 598f
  contrast-enhanced, 589t
Urethrostomy, perineal, for urethral obstruction, 648
Urinalysis
  in acute pancreatitis, 556
  in diabetes mellitus, 733t
  in digestive disorders, 366

Urinalysis—cont'd
  in feline lower urinary tract inflamma-
      tion management, 648-649
  findings of, in urinary tract infection,
      626-627
  in hematuria evaluation, 574
  in hepatobiliary disorders, 490-491,
      490f
  in neuromuscular disorders, 961
  in polydipsia, results of, 661t
  in polyuria, results of, 661t
Urinary incontinence, 575-577
  causes of, 575t
  with distended bladder, 576
  evaluation in, initial, 575
  geriatric, 577
  paradoxical, 576
  pharmacologic testing in, 576
  with small or normal-sized bladder,
      576-577
  treatment of, 576
Urinary tract
  diagnostic tests for, 584-598
      bacterial antibiotic sensitivity testing
          as, 588-589, 588t
      for bladder function, 588
      diagnostic imaging as, 589-596,
          589t, 590f, 591-595f, 592t,
          596f
      fractional clearance as, 585-586
      glomerular filtration rate as, 584-585
      plasma osmolality measurement as,
          587
      proteinuria quantification as, 586
      response to exogenous antidiuretic
          hormone as, 587-588
      urine osmolality measurement as,
          587
      water deprivation test as, 587
  disorders of, 568-659
      azotemia in, 581-583
      clinical manifestations of, 568-583
      drugs used in, 657-659t
      dysuria-stranguria in, 568, 569f
      feline lower urinary tract
          inflammation as, 571-572,
          573f
      glomerulonephropathies as, 600-607
          (See also
          Glomerulonephropathies)
      hematuria in, 572-575, 573t, 574f
      pollakiuria in, 568, 569f
      polydipsia as, 577-579
      polyuria as, 577-579
      proteinuria in, 579-581
      renal failure as, 608-622 (See also
          Kidney[s], failure of)
      renomegaly in, 583
      transitional cell carcinoma as, 570
      urethral obstruction in, 568
      urinary incontinence in, 575-577
      urinary tract infection as, 568-569,
          569f
      urolithiasis as, 570-571, 570f, 571f,
          571t
  function of, in neurologic examina-
      tion, 957
  infections of, 568-569, 569t, 624-630
      antibiotics for, 1248-1249, 1248t
      clinical features of, 626-627
      complicated *versus* uncomplicated,
          626
      etiology of, 624-625, 625t
      host defense mechanisms in, 625-
          626, 625t
      prognosis for, 629-630
      relapses of, *versus* reinfections, 626
      treatment of, 627-630, 628f, 629t
      zoonotic, 1316-1317
  lower, inflammation of, feline, 642-649
      (See also Feline lower urinary
      tract inflammation [FLUTI])
  toxicity of chemotherapy drugs for,
      1114-1115

Urination
  increased frequency of, 568, 569f
  increased volume of, 482, 482t
  straining at, 568, 569f
      ineffectual or painful, 356-357, 357t
Urine
  glucose in, monitoring of, in diabetes
      management, 739
  osmolality of, measurement of, in uri-
      nary disorder evaluation, 587
  production of, monitoring of, in pa-
      tients at risk for ARF, 613
  protein in, 579-581
  specific gravity of, in hypernatremia,
      828-829
Urine reagent test strips, in diabetes diag-
      nosis, 732
Urispas. See Flavoxate
Uroeze. See Racemethionine
Urogenital tract infections, antibiotics
      for, 1248-1249, 1248t
Urography
  excretory, 589t
  intravenous, 590
      technique for, 592t
Urohydropulsion, 637, 638t
Urolith(s)
  calcium oxalate
      canine, 632t, 633-634, 639
      feline, 644
  composition of, factors predicting,
      632t
  cystine
      factors predicting composition of,
          632t
      treatment of, 640-641
  intraluminal, 597f
  silicate
      factors predicting composition of,
          632t
      treatment of, 640
  struvite
      canine, 632t, 633, 639
      feline, in feline lower urinary tract
          inflammation, 642-644, 643f
  urate
      factors predicting composition of,
          632t
      treatment of, 639-640
Urolithiasis, 570-571, 570f, 571f, 571t
  canine, 631-641 (See also Canine
      urolithiasis)
Urologic syndrome, feline, 642
Uropathy, obstructive, 598f
Urotoxicity, of chemotherapy drugs,
      1114-1115
Ursodeoxycholic acid
  for chronic cholestatic hepatopathies,
      517
  indication and dosage of, 565t
Ursodiol. See Ursodeoxycholic acid
  for chronic hepatitis, 537
US. See Ultrasonography (US)
Uteroverdin, 872
Uterus
  disorders of, 877-880
  infection of, postpartum, 896-897
  torsion of, 877
Uveitis, lens-induced, complicating dia-
      betes mellitus in dogs, 748-
      749

**V**

VAC protocol
  for carcinomas, 1155t
  for hemangiosarcoma, 1143-1144
  for soft-tissue sarcomas, 1154t
Vaccination
  for feline infectious peritonitis, 1278
  for feline leukemia virus, 1284
  for parvovirus, canine, 434-435
  rabies, 1017
Vaccination protocols, 1252-1257
  for cats, 1254-1256
  for dogs, 1256-1257

Vaccination protocols—cont'd
  vaccine selection for, 1253-1254
  vaccine types for, 1252-1253, 1253t
Vaccines
  advantages and disadvantages of, 1253t
  for canine infectious tracheobronchi-
      tis, 288-289
  during chemotherapy, 1109-1110
  failure of, causes of, 1254t
  handling of, proper, 1254t
  lymphadenopathy associated with,
      1202t
  selection of, 1253-1254
  types of, 1252-1253, 1253t
Vaccine(s)
  *Bordetella*, 230
  *Chlamydophila*, 230
  feline calcivirus, 230
  feline herpesvirus, 230
VAF protocol, for carcinomas, 1155t
Vagal maneuver, for sustained supraven-
      tricular tachycardia, 84
Vagina
  bacterial cultures in, 854, 854t
  congenital anomalies of, 872-873
  disorders of, 870-877
  epithelial cells of, cytologic changes in,
      848-849, 848f
  hyperplasia of, 875-877, 876f
  inflammation of, 874-875
  prolapse of, 875-877, 876f
Vaginitis
  antibiotics for, 1249
  diagnosis of, 874
  etiology of, 874
  treatment of, 874-875
Vaginography, in congenital anomalies,
      873
Vaginoscopy, 853-854
  in congenital anomalies, 873
Vagolytic drugs, for arrhythmias, 96
Valbazen. See Albendazole
Valium. See Diazepam
Valproic acid
  as anticonvulsant, 1004
  for neurologic disorders, 1070t
Valve(s), cardiac
  disease of, complications of, 140t
  locations of, on chest wall, 8f
  mitral (See Mitral valve)
  tricuspid (See Tricuspid valve)
Valvular cardiogenic shock, 119t
Valvuloplasty, balloon, for pulmonic
      stenosis, 160
Vanadium, 757
Vascular. See also Blood vessels
Vascular ring anomalies, 166
  esophageal, 413-414, 414f
Vasculature. See Blood vessels
Vasculitis, meningeal, 1011f, 1012
  CSF analysis in, 964t
Vasectomy, 866
Vasodepressor reflexes, syncope or inter-
      mittent weakness from, 2t
Vasodilators
  for dilated cardiomyopathy, 112
  dosages of, 62t, 206t
  for fulminant congestive heart failure,
      59, 59t
  preparations of, 63t
  syncope or intermittent weakness
      from, 2t, 3
Vasopressin
  arginine (See Arginine vasopressin
      [AVP])
  release of, in congestive heart failure,
      53-54
Vasotec. See Enalapril
Vasoxyl. See Methoxamine
Vein(s)
  congestion of, abdominal effusion
      from, 474
  jugular, in cardiovascular examination,
      5-6, 5f, 5t

Vein(s)—cont'd
  portal, hypoplasia of, primary, 534
  pulmonary
      enlarged, differential diagnosis of,
          257, 257t
      evaluation of, 35
      small, differential diagnosis of, 257,
          257t
Vena cava, caudal, 35
  radiographic assessment of, 35
Venodilators, in congestive heart failure
      management, 66
Venography, in portosystemic shunt, 532,
      532f
Ventilation, and perfusion, mismatched,
      in hypoxemia, 283
Ventilatory support, 340
Ventral bulla osteotomy, in facial nerve
      paralysis management, 1053
Ventricle(s)
  contractility of, decreased, in dilated
      cardiomyopathy, 108
  filling of, restricted
      chronic heart failure from, 55t
      therapeutic goals for, 56t
  left, enlargement of
      electrocardiography in, 15, 15t, 16f,
          16t
      in feline hypertrophic
          cardiomyopathy, 123, 124,
          125f, 126f
      radiography in, 33t, 34, 34f
  remodeling of, 51-52
  right, enlargement of
      electrocardiography in, 15, 15t, 16f,
          16t
      in pulmonic stenosis, 159, 159f
      radiography in, 33t, 34, 34f
Ventricular arrhythmias, factors predis-
      posing to, 76t
Ventricular fibrillation, 22-23, 23f
  in cardiopulmonary arrest, 98
  defibrillation for, 102
Ventricular gallop, 8
Ventricular outflow obstructions, 155-160
  pulmonic stenosis as, 158-160, 159f,
      160f
  subaortic stenosis as, 156-158, 157f
  syncope or intermittent weakness
      from, 2t
Ventricular preexcitation, 25, 25f
Ventricular premature complexes, 19f,
      20-21f, 21-22
Ventricular premature contractions
      (VPCs), 76
  acute treatment of, 78, 80-81
Ventricular rhythm, accelerated, 22
Ventricular septal defect (VSD), 151, 161-
      162, 161f
  breed dispositions for, 152t
  murmurs in, 152f
  pulmonary hypertension in, 164-166
  radiographic findings in, 154f
Ventricular tachyarrhythmias, chronic
      oral therapy of, 81-82
Ventricular tachycardia, 20-21f, 22
  acute treatment of, 78, 80-81
  sustained, 84
Ventricular tap, in hydrocephalus man-
      agement, 994
Verapamil
  for arrhythmias, 95
  commercial preparations of, 88t
  dosages of, 79t, 207t
  for supraventricular tachycardias, 77
  for sustained supraventricular tachy-
      cardia, 84
Versenate. See Calcium EDTA
Vertebrae
  cartilaginous exostosis of, myelogram
      of, 968f
  cervical, instability/malformation of,
      1040-1043, 1041-1042f,
      1043f
  localization of spinal cord segments in,
      1021t

Vertebral heart score (VHS), 32, 33f
Vesicourachal diverticuli, feline lower urinary tract inflammation and, 644-645
Vestibular syndromes, 1008
Vestibular system
disease of, 1006t
central, 1009
geriatric canine, 1007-1008, 1007f
peripheral, 1006-1009, 1006t, 1007f
bilateral, 1009
diagnosis of, 1008-1009
etiology of, 1006-1008, 1007f
lesion of, head tilt from, 1005-1009 (See also Head tilt)
neoplasia of, 1008
Vetalar. See Ketamine
VHS. See Vertebral heart score (VHS)
Vibramycin. See Doxycycline
Vinblastine, for mast cell tumors, 1148, 1149, 1154t
Vincristine
for carcinomas, 1155t
for hemangiosarcoma, 1143-1144
for leukemias
acute, 1137t
chronic, 1138t
for lymphoma, 1127t, 1128-1131, 1153t
for soft-tissue sarcomas, 1154-1155t
for thymomas, 1120
for transmissible venereal tumor, 938-939
Viokase-V. See Pancreatic enzyme powder; Pancreatic enzymes
Viral arthritis, 1085, 1085f
Viral myocarditis, canine, 116
Viral pneumonia, 299
Virology, 854-855
Virus(es)
canine distemper, 1015-1016
canine parvovirus-1, 433-435
canine parvovirus-2, 433-435
chronic hepatitis from, 529
coronaviral, enteritis from, 436
culture techniques for, 1236
cytologic examination for, 1234
diarrhea from, 352t
feline immunodeficiency (See Feline immunodeficiency virus [FIV])
feline leukemia (See Feline leukemia virus [FeLV])
in feline lower urinary tract inflammation, 644
fetal death from, 900
immunodeficiency, feline, encephalopathy from, 1014
infections with, lymphadenopathy associated with, 1202t
isolation tests for, in feline upper respiratory infections, 228
polysystemic diseases from, 1273-1284
canine distemper as, 1273-1275, 1274f, 1274t (See also Distemper, canine)
feline coronavirus infection as, 1275-1278, 1276t

Virus(es)—cont'd
polysystemic diseases from—cont'd
feline immunodeficiency virus infection as, 1278-1281, 1279t, 1280t
feline leukemia virus infection as, 1281-1284, 1282t
rabies, 1017
zoonotic, 1315
Visceral larva migrans, 1307-1308, 1310
Visceral pericardium, 185
Vision loss, 984-990
in anisocoria, 986-987
in occipital cortex lesions, 986
in optic chiasm lesions, 986, 987f
in optic neuritis, 985-986, 986t
Vitamin(s)
serum concentrations of, in digestive disorders, 378-379
supplemental, for degenerative myelopathy, 1037
Vitamin B$_1$. See Thiamine
Vitamin B$_{12}$, for hepatobiliary and pancreatic disorders, 567t
Vitamin D
actions of, on calcium and phosphorus metabolism, 682t
for endocrine disorders, 815t
for hypocalcemia, 686, 841, 846t
plasma concentrations of, interactions of, with calcium, phosphorus and parathyroid hormone concentrations, 620f
for primary hypoparathyroidism, 688-689, 689f
Vitamin E
for chronic hepatitis, 537
for hepatobiliary and pancreatic disorders, 566t
Vitamin K$_1$
dosages of, 342t
in hepatic lipidosis management, 512
for hepatobiliary and pancreatic disorders, 567t
Vitamin K deficiency, 1194-1195
Voiding. See Micturition
Volume-flow overload
chronic heart failure from, 55t
therapeutic goals for, 56t
Volvulus
gastric, partial or intermittent, 426-427, 426f
gastric dilation with, 424-426, 425f
mesenteric, 453
radiography of, 372, 374f
Vomiting
in bilious vomiting syndrome, 427
in chronic renal failure, management of, 621-622
complicating chemotherapy, 1111
definition of, 345
in digestive disorders, 347-349, 348t, 349f
distinguishing regurgitation from, 345, 345t
in gastric foreign object, 424
in gastrinomas, 775
in hypoadrenocorticism, 805
in parvoviral enteritis, 434
in *Physaloptera* gastritis, 420-421
waxing-and-waning, in hypertriglyceridemia, 824

Von Willebrand's disease (vWD), 1192-1194, 1193f, 1193t
VPCs. See Ventricular premature contractions (PVCs)
VSD. See Ventricular septal defect (VSD)
Vulva
congenital anomalies of, 872-873
discharge from
cellular debris in, 872
in cystic endometrial hyperplasia-pyometra complex, 878
diagnostic approach to, 870, 871f, 871t
hemorrhagic, 870-872
mucoid, 872
purulent, 872
septic, 872
uteroverdin in, 872
vWD. See von Willebrand's disease (vWD)

**W**

Wandering pacemaker, 16
Warfarin
dosages of, 342t
for glomerulonephropathies, 607
for pulmonary thromboembolism, 311
for thromboembolism prevention, 136-137
Water deprivation test
in diabetes insipidus diagnosis, 663-664, 664f, 664t
in urinary disorder evaluation, 587
Waveforms
ECG, normal, 12, 13f, 13t
in ECG interpretation, 28-29
Weakness
in degenerative AV valve disease, 141
episodic, 976-977, 977t
in heart disease/failure, 1, 2t, 3
in hyperkalemia, 833
in hypokalemia, 835
intermittent, causes of, 2t
in myasthenia gravis, 1059-1060
in pheochromocytoma, 810
Weight
body, conversion of, to surface area
in cats, 1106t
in dogs, 1105t
loss of
in diabetes mellitus, in cats, 751
in digestive disorders, 358-360, 359t, 360f
in exocrine pancreatic insufficiency, 561, 561f
in gastrinomas, 775
in hyperthyroidism, 713
in hypoadrenocorticism, 805
polyphagia with, 816, 817t
Wenckebach block, 23, 24f
West Highland White Terriers, chronic hepatitis in, 528
Wheat bran, dosage of, 403t
Wheaten Terriers, Soft-Coated, protein-losing enteropathy in, 451
Wheezes, 252
Whipworms, 440-441, 442f
White bile syndrome, 479
White matter, spongy degeneration of, in Labrador Retrievers, 1044t
Wobbler syndrome, 1025
canine, 1040-1043, 1041-1042f, 1043f

Wolf-Parkinson-White syndrome, tricuspid dysplasia and, 162
Wolf-Parkinson-White (WPW) preexcitation, 25, 25f
Worms, respiratory tract, fecal examination for, 1230t
WPW preexcitation. See Wolff-Parkinson-White (WPW) preexcitation

**X**

Xylazine
dosages of, 471t
ECG changes from, 27t
for neurologic disorders, 1070t
Xylocaine. See Lidocaine

**Y**

*Yersinia enterocolitica*
as enteric zoonosis, 1309t
enterocolitis from, 439
*Yersinia pestis*
feline plague from, 1259-1260
lymphadenopathy associated with, 1202t
morphologic characteristics of, 1233t
zoonoses associated with, 1313-1314, 1313t

**Z**

*Zamia floridana,* hepatotoxicity of, 522t
Zantac. See Ranitidine
Zeniquin. See Marbofloxacin
Zestril. See Lisinopril
Zidovudine, for feline immunodeficiency virus encephalopathy, 1014
Zinacard. See Dexrazoxane
Zinc, hepatotoxicity of, 522t
Zinc acetate, for hepatobiliary and pancreatic disorders, 566t
Zinc phosphide, hepatotoxicity of, 522t
Zinc salts, in copper hepatotoxicosis management, 536
Zinc sulfate, for hepatobiliary and pancreatic disorders, 566t
Zinc sulfate centrifugal flotation, in fecal examination, 1231, 1231t, 1232f
Zithromax. See Azithromycin
Zofran. See Ondansetron
Zollinger-Ellison syndrome, 775-776, 775t
Zoonoses, 1307-1317
amoeba as, 1309t, 1311-1312
bite, 1312-1315, 1313t
cestodes as, 1309t, 1310
ciliates as, 1309t, 1311-1312
coccidians as, 1309t, 1310-1311, 1310f
disease transfer in, avoidance of, 1308t
enteric, 1307-1312, 1308t, 1309t, 1310f
characteristics of, 1309t
prevalence of, 1309t
exudate exposure, 1312-1315, 1313t
flagellates as, 1309t, 1311-1312
genitourinary, 1316-1317
nematodes as, 1307-1308, 1309t, 1310
ocular, 1315-1316
respiratory tract, 1315-1316
scratch, 1312-1315, 1313t
Zyloprim. See Allopurinol